Pediatric Anesthesia

Pediatric Anesthesia

Fourth Edition

George A. Gregory, M.D.

Professor
Departments of Anesthesia and Pediatrics
University of California, San Francisco
School of Medicine
San Francisco, California

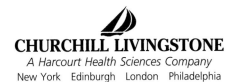

CHURCHILL LIVINGSTONE
A Harcourt Health Sciences Company
New York   Edinburgh   London   Philadelphia

CHURCHILL LIVINGSTONE
A Harcourt Health Sciences Company

The Curtis Center
Independence Square West
Philadelphia, Pennsylvania 19106

Library of Congress Cataloging-in-Publication Data

Pediatric anesthesia / [edited by] George A. Gregory.—4th ed.
     p. ;   cm.
   Includes bibliographical references and index.
   ISBN 0–443–06561–6
     1. Pediatric anesthesia.   I. Gregory, George A.
   [DNLM: 1. Anesthesia—Child.   2. Anesthesia—Infant. WO 440 P371 2002]
   RD139 .P4 2002
   617.9′6798—dc21
                                                              00-065825

PEDIATRIC ANESTHESIA   ISBN 0–443–06561–6

Printed in the United States of America.

Last digit is the print number: 9   8   7   6   5   4   3   2   1

◆

This book is dedicated to my wife Ann
who continues to make my career possible
and my life enjoyable.
It also is dedicated to
all of the anesthesia and pediatric residents
and to all of the patients
who have taught me so much and
continue to do so every day.

◆

Contributors

◆   ◆   ◆

Charles B. Berde, M.D., Ph.D.
Professor of Anaesthesia and Pediatrics, Harvard
Medical School; Senior Associate in Anesthesia, and
Director, Pain Treatment Service, Children's Hospital,
Boston, Massachusetts
*Pediatric Regional Anesthesia; Pediatric Pain
Management*

Frederic A. Berry, M.D.
Professor, Departments of Anesthesiology and
Pediatrics, University of Virginia Health System,
Charlottesville, Virginia
Anesthesia for Genitourinary Surgery

Bruno Bissonnette, M.D.
Professor, Department of Anaesthesia, University of
Toronto; Director, Neurosurgical Anaesthesia,
Department of Anesthesia, The Hospital for Sick
Children, Toronto, Ontario, Canada
Anesthesia for Neurosurgical Procedures

Claire M. Brett, M.D.
Professor of Anesthesia and Pediatrics, University of
California, San Francisco, School of Medicine, San
Francisco, California
Eyes, Ears, Nose, Throat, and Dental Surgery

Barbara A. Castro, M.D.
Assistant Professor of Anesthesiology and Pediatrics,
University of Virginia Health System, Charlottesville,
Virginia
Anesthesia for Genitourinary Surgery

Charles B. Cauldwell, M.D., Ph.D.
Clinical Professor of Anesthesia, Department of
Anesthesia and Perioperative Services, University of
California, San Francisco; Chief, Division of Pediatric
Anesthesia, University of California, San Francisco,
Medical Center, San Francisco, California
*Induction, Maintenance, and Emergence;
Anesthesia for Transplantation*

Dennis M. Fisher, M.D.
Medical Director, DURECT Corporation, Cupertino,
California
Anesthesia Equipment for Pediatrics

Jeremy M. Geiduschek, M.D.
Associate Professor, Department of Anesthesiology,
University of Washington School of Medicine; Attending
Physician, Department of Anesthesiology, Children's
Hospital and Regional Medical Center, Seattle,
Washington
Anesthesia for Thoracic Surgery

Christine D. Greco, M.D.
Instructor of Anaesthesia, Harvard Medical School;
Associate Director, Pain Treatment Service, and
Assistant in Anesthesia, Children's Hospital, Boston,
Massachusetts
Pediatric Pain Management

George A. Gregory, M.D.
Professor, Departments of Anesthesia and Pediatrics,
University of California, San Francisco, School of
Medicine, San Francisco, California
*Ethical Considerations; Pharmacology; Monitoring
During Surgery; Anesthesia for Premature Infants;
Anesthesia for Transplantation*

Alvin Hackel, M.D.
Emeritus Active Professor of Anesthesia and Pediatrics,
Stanford School of Medicine; Attending
Anesthesiologist, Stanford University Hospital, Lucile
Salter Packard Children's Hospital at Stanford, Stanford,
California
Training and Practice of Pediatric Anesthesia

Steven C. Hall, M.D.
Professor of Anesthesiology, Northwestern University
Medical School; Arthur C. King Professor of Pediatric
Anesthesia, and Anesthesiologist-in-Chief, Department of
Pediatric Anesthesia, Children's Memorial Hospital,
Chicago, Illinois
Anesthesia Outside the Operating Room

Raafat S. Hannallah, M.D.
Professor, Departments of Anesthesiology and
Pediatrics, George Washington University Medical
Center; Chairman, Department of Anesthesiology,
Children's National Medical Center, Washington, D.C.
Outpatient Anesthesia

John W. Holl, M.D.
Attending Physician, Children's Hospital and Health
Center, San Diego, California
Anesthesia for Abdominal Surgery

Constance S. Houck, M.D.
Assistant Professor, Department of Anaesthesia, Harvard
Medical School; Associate in Anesthesia, Children's
Hospital, Boston, Massachusetts
Pediatric Pain Management

Arthur J. Klowden, M.D.
Clinical Assistant Professor, Department of
Anesthesiology, University of Illinois College of
Medicine; Attending Anesthesiologist, Department of
Anesthesiology, Illinois Masonic Medical Center;
Attending Anesthesiologist, Shriner's Hospital for
Children, Chicago Unit, Chicago, Illinois
Anesthesia for Orthopedic Surgery

Peter C. Laussen, M.B.B.S.
Associate Professor, Harvard Medical School; Clinical
Director, Cardiac Anesthesia, and Associate Director,
Cardiac Intensive Care Unit, Children's Hospital, Boston,
Massachusetts
Anesthesia for Congenital Heart Disease

Jerrold Lerman, M.D.
Professor, Department of Anaesthesia, University of
Toronto; Siemens Chair in Paediatric Anaesthesia,
Department of Anaesthesia, The Hospital for Sick
Children, Toronto, Ontario, Canada
*Special Techniques: Acute Normovolemic
Hemodilution, Controlled Hypotension and
Hypothermia and ECMO*

Jeffrey P. Morray, M.D.
Professor, Department of Anesthesiology, University of
Washington School of Medicine; Director, Department
of Anesthesiology, Children's Hospital and Regional
Medical Center, Seattle, Washington
Anesthesia for Thoracic Surgery

Barbara W. Palmisano, M.D.
Associate Professor of Anesthesiology and Pediatrics,
Medical College of Wisconsin; Attending Physician,
Children's Hospital of Wisconsin, Milwaukee, Wisconsin
Anesthesia for Plastic Surgery

Robert C. Pascucci, M.D.
Instructor in Anaesthesia (Pediatrics), Department of
Anaesthesia, Harvard Medical School; Associate
Director, Multidisciplinary Intensive Care Unit,
Children's Hospital, Boston, Massachusetts
Pediatric Intensive Care

Lynne M. Reynolds, M.D.
Associate Professor of Anesthesiology, University of
California, San Francisco, School of Medicine, San
Francisco, California
*Appendix A: Useful Drugs in the Perioperative
Period; Appendix B: Normal Laboratory Values*

Mark C. Rogers, M.D.
Clinical Professor, Department of Anesthesiology and
Critical Care Medicine, Johns Hopkins University School
of Medicine; Former Professor and Chairman,
Department of Anesthesiology and Critical Care
Medicine, Johns Hopkins Hospital, Baltimore, Maryland
Cardiopulmonary Resuscitation

Lynn M. Rusy, M.D.
Associate Professor of Anesthesiology, Medical College
of Wisconsin; Attending Anesthesiologist, and Associate
Director, Jane B. Pettit Comprehensive Pediatric Pain
Clinic, Children's Hospital of Wisconsin, Milwaukee,
Wisconsin
Anesthesia for Plastic Surgery

Parvine Sadeghi, M.D.
Clinical Fellow, Department of Anaesthesia, The
Hospital for Sick Children, Toronto, Ontario, Canada
Anesthesia for Neurosurgical Procedures

M. Ramez Salem, M.D.
Chair, Department of Anesthesiology, and Advocate,
Illinois Masonic Medical Center; Clinical Professor,
Department of Anesthesiology, University of Illinois
College of Medicine, Chicago, Illinois
Anesthesia for Orthopedic Surgery

Charles L. Schleien, M.D.
Professor, Departments of Pediatrics and
Anesthesiology, Columbia University College of
Physicians and Surgeons; Medical Director, Division of
Pediatric Critical Care Medicine, Children's Hospital of
New York
Cardiopulmonary Resuscitation

Daniel I. Sessler, M.D.
Assistant Vice-President for Health Affairs, Associate
Dean for Research, Director, Outcomes Research
Institute, and Weakley Professor and Acting Chair in
Anesthesiology, University of Louisville, Louisville,
Kentucky
Temperature Disturbances

Navil F. Sethna, M.B., Ch.B.
Associate Professor, Department of Anaesthesia,
Harvard Medical School; Senior Associate, Department
of Anesthesia, and Associate Director, Pain Treatment
Service, Children's Hospital, Boston, Massachusetts
Pediatric Regional Anesthesia

Donald H. Shaffner, M.D.
Associate Professor, Department of Anesthesiology and
Critical Care Medicine, Johns Hopkins University School
of Medicine; Assistant Director, Division of Pediatric
Intensive Care, Johns Hopkins Hospital, Baltimore,
Maryland
Cardiopulmonary Resuscitation

Laura Siedman, M.D.
Assistant Clinical Professor of Anesthesiology, University
of California, San Francisco, San Francisco, California
Anesthesia for the Expremature Infant

Daniel Siker, M.D.
Associate Professor, Departments of Anesthesiology and
Pediatrics, Medical College of Wisconsin; Staff
Physician, Children's Hospital of Wisconsin, Milwaukee,
Wisconsin
Pediatric Fluids, Electrolytes, and Nutrition

Linda Stehling, M.D.
Former Professor, Departments of Anesthesiology and
Pediatrics, State University of New York Health Science
Center at Syracuse College of Medicine, Syracuse,
New York
Blood Transfusion and Component Therapy

David J. Steward, M.B.B.S.
Professor, Department of Anesthesiology, University of
Southern California School of Medicine; Senior
Anesthesiologist, Children's Hospital of Los Angeles, Los
Angeles, California
*Preoperative Evaluation and Preparation for
Surgery*

Theodore W. Striker, M.D.
Professor, Departments of Anesthesia and Pediatrics,
University of Cincinnati College of Medicine;
Anesthesiologist-in-Chief, and Director, Department of
Anesthesia, Children's Hospital Medical Center,
Cincinnati, Ohio
Anesthesia for Trauma in the Pediatric Patient

George Ulma, M.D.
Clinical Pediatric Anesthesiologist, University of
California, San Diego; Children's Hospital and Health
Center, San Diego, California
Anesthesia for Thoracic Surgery

David L. Wessel, M.D.
Associate Professor of Pediatrics (Anaesthesia),
Department of Pediatrics, Harvard Medical School;
Director, Cardiac Intensive Care Unit, Children's
Hospital, Boston, Massachusetts
Anesthesia for Congenital Heart Disease

A. Andrew Zimmerman, M.D.
Clinical Staff Pediatric Anesthesiologist, University of
California, San Diego; Staff Pediatric Anesthesiologist,
Children's Hospital and Health Center, San Diego,
California
   Anesthesia for Thoracic Surgery

Maurice S. Zwass, M.D.
Professor, Departments of Anesthesia and Pediatrics,
University of California, San Francisco, School of
Medicine; Associate Director, Pediatric Critical Care
Medicine, University of California, San Francisco,
Medical Center, San Francisco, California
   Eyes, Ears, Nose, Throat, and Dental Surgery

Preface

◆　◆　◆

This, the fourth edition of *Pediatric Anesthesia,* has been expanded and updated. I am truly grateful to many people for the production of this book, especially the authors of the chapters who have worked so hard. I believe they have achieved their goals of providing the latest information available and of doing so in a readable and interesting manner. The chapters have been revised significantly. New information and references have been added. Several new chapters have been included to reflect the change in our specialty, especially the interesting subject of how to educate anesthesiologists who provide anesthesia for infants and children. This subject is dear to all anesthesiologists, especially those interested in the care of pediatric patients.

It is my belief that anyone who anesthetizes infants and children must understand the differences in physiology and pharmacology that exist between children and adults. The anesthesiologist who fails to understand these differences will have a hard time responding appropriately to unexpected events. The results can be disastrous for the patient. For these reasons, we have tried to include as much physiology and pharmacology as possible in each chapter and to integrate this information with practical care of patients.

I thank Eduardo Mabolo for his secretarial help and good humor throughout the production of this new edition of *Pediatric Anesthesia.* He efficiently and effectively saw to many of the details and kept me on track. I thank Allan Ross of Harcourt Health Sciences for his encouragement and willingness to do whatever needed to be done to complete this edition, and for his strong support of this project. He kept me on the straight and narrow.

Finally, I thank all of the residents I have had the privilege to teach over the past 33 years. I have learned as much from them as they learned from me. Their constant questioning has kept me interested and excited about academic medicine. I also thank the thousands of patients I have had the privilege of caring for in the operating rooms and the intensive care units for these many years. They have taught me the most. I continue to learn from them everyday. They are great teachers.

George A. Gregory, M.D.

Preface to the First Edition

◆　　◆　　◆

For years pediatric patients have been cared for without a clear understanding of whether the care being provided was appropriate or not. There was inadequate information available on which to decide. This was due in part to the misguided feeling that research should not be done in children. Recently, things have changed. As a result, there has been an explosion of such information, much of which has come from neonatal and pediatric intensive care units. Because of this information it has been recognized that infants and children really are not small adults (some of us believe that adults are large children) and that we cannot apply adult standards to the care of pediatric patients. Unfortunately, this knowledge is widely dispersed throughout the medical literature. As a consequence, the busy practitioner and house officer, as well as the academician, may not have time to find the information he or she needs, especially in the middle of the night. Therefore, the task of writing and editing this book was undertaken. My goal was to produce a book that provided a physiologic and pharmacologic approach to anesthesia for the pediatric patient, as well as the clinical information needed to care for these patients. To reach this goal, I have gently coerced a combination of pediatricians and anesthesiologists to contribute their talents and clinical experience to the writing of this book. My dictum to them was to produce chapters that stressed physiology, embryology, pharmacology, and anatomy wherever possible. This, I believe, has been done.

The first volume of the book provides the basic information needed to understand the differences between children and adults and to understand the abnormal states described in the second volume of the book. Both volumes are designed to complement one another.

I sincerely thank Ms. Jenna Haynes for her invaluable secretarial assistance, for correcting my spelling, and for maintaining her good humor throughout the production of this book. In addition I thank Lewis Reines, president of Churchill Livingstone, for his unflagging encouragement, and William Schmitt, for his patience with the process and with my constant questions. I thank Ann Ruzycka for her excellent editorial work. Without her help, the book would never have been completed. Finally, but certainly not least, I thank the families of the authors who may have been confronted by spouses and parents disgruntled because they had received another phone call from me urging them to get their chapter in. I apologize for this, but I wanted the book to be as up-to-date as possible when published. I believe that this goal has been accomplished. It is our sincere hope that this book will be of aid to you in your care of patients. Like any such venture, it can be improved. Therefore, I would be grateful for any comments you have on how this can be accomplished.

George A. Gregory, M.D.

Contents

◆ ◆ ◆

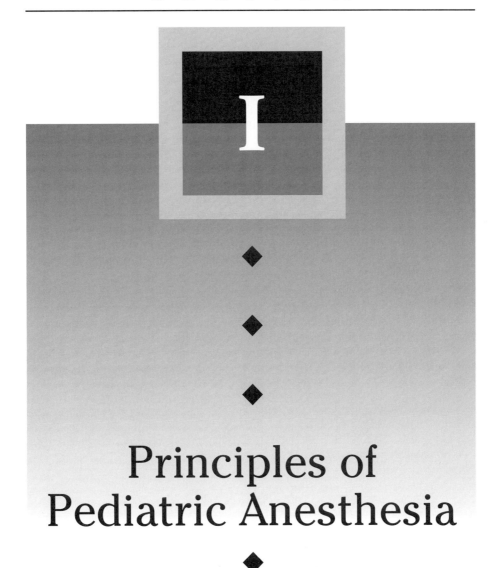

SECTION

I

Principles of
Pediatric Anesthesia

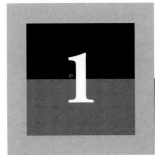

Ethical Considerations

GEORGE A. GREGORY

◆ ◆ ◆

Discussions and disputations about medical ethics have increased during the past 20 years. Everyone, from Congresspersons to our neighbors, seems to have the answers to how medicine should be practiced and who should make decisions about how patient care should be provided. The positive side of this debate is that it has led physicians to rethink what they do and why they do it. In some cases, this discussion has had a profound effect on patient care (e.g., providing anesthesia for premature infants).

Ethics is defined in Webster's Dictionary[1] as (1) the discipline dealing with what is good and bad and with moral duty and obligation and (2) (a) a set of moral principles and values, (b) a theory or system of moral values, (c) the principles of conduct governing an individual or a group (profession). What is "correct" depends on what the majority of people in a society believe at a given time. Even so, very respected ethicists have views that are entirely opposite. Neither can be proven to be right or wrong.

Perceptions of what is right (ethical) or wrong (unethical) can change, as exemplified by occurrences in Germany during this century. In the 1930s, it was thought ethical by the leaders of Germany to perform medical research on people without their consent and without benefit to those on whom the research was conducted. Today, medical research in Germany is governed by the rules of the Nuremberg Convention and is performed only with consent of the subject and under strict protocols. The latter is now the ethical standard.

CONSENT

Children present special problems when consent for procedures must be obtained, because they frequently do not understand the nature of the procedure. Consequently, consent for medical care, surgery, and permission to be a research subject must be given by surrogates, such as parents, legal guardians, and courts. The person giving consent usually does so with the patient's best interests in mind. However, factors rooted in their own mores (moral attitudes), past experience, and ability to accept a situation may prevent caregivers from giving consent. If parents or guardians believe that "everything must be done" no matter what, they will allow or insist on many forms of therapy that may not be beneficial and, in fact, may be futile and harmful, may delay dying, and may increase the child's suffering. On the other hand, if they feel the child has suffered too much, they may want all treatment stopped, even when there is no legal or medical reason to do so. The beliefs of parents or guardians or their inability to make a decision often prevents them from permitting extraordinary support to be withdrawn and allowing the patient to die, even though it is appropriate to do so. The person who obtains informed consent for procedures must be aware that outside factors may affect whether the parent or guardian agrees to a form of therapy.

Whether the parents or guardians give consent for a procedure depends on how information about the procedure is presented. If the person obtaining the consent tells them that there will be no problems and that everything

3

will be wonderful after the procedure, the parent or guardian will consent willingly. Unfortunately, many physicians are reluctant to give parents "bad news,"[2] and fail to tell them that the patient's long-term condition may not be changed by the procedure or that it could be worse. This is not informed consent.

Informed consent fully discloses the benefits, the therapeutic or nontherapeutic alternatives, and the potential complications of the procedure. Consent obtained for research is more likely to be informed because it is required by law to list in writing the benefits and potential problems associated with the study. This is seldom true of surgical or medical consents.

Informed consent for medical treatment must provide enough information in language the parent or guardian can understand so that a rational decision can be made about whether the procedure should be performed.[3] In our multicultural society, it is important that the information be conveyed in a language the parents understand. For example, if the consent is obtained in English, and the parents only speak Spanish, consent for the procedure is not informed. Nor is consent informed if it is obtained in "broken" Spanish that the parents do not understand. Whenever possible, consent should be obtained with the help of a translator who is fluent in both English and the parent's or guardian's primary language. The translator should be someone who understands medical terms and their translation.

Anesthesiologists have an obligation to inform the parent or guardian about the types of anesthesia available. The information should be presented in a way that enables the parent(s) to understand the options, potential benefits, and complications of the various anesthetic techniques. Only pertinent information should be presented. Too much information is confusing and clouds the issues. There is no reason to discuss forms of anesthesia that are inappropriate or to provide information about complications that are very unlikely to occur. Whereas it is appropriate to discuss the possibility that death may occur during anesthesia and surgery in a child who has sepsis and a necrotic bowel, it is not necessary to do so if the patient is having a digital block to incise and drain a small abscess. There is no requirement that all possible complications be discussed. Only complications that have a reasonable possibility of occurring should be presented and discussed (see below). The goal is to inform, not to frighten.

Obtaining informed consent is often complicated by whether the parents want to hear what is being said. Parents or guardians who either are unwilling to hear "bad news" or cannot accept it often block out the information and, at a later time, believe that they were never told of the potential problems or alternatives for one form of anesthesia or the other. Consequently, the anesthesiologist should document clearly and concisely in the chart what the parents were told and should state that they were given the opportunity to ask questions and to have them answered. This is the only effective defense in case of subsequent litigation. If the plan of anesthesia must be changed after informed consent is obtained, the parents should be told as soon as possible. At times, surgery must proceed before the anesthesiologist can talk with the parents. If so, it should be documented in the chart that the anesthesiologist tried to talk with the parents or guardians, either in person or by telephone, and was unable to do so. The anesthesiologist should never believe that because the plan in mind is "standard practice" there is no need to discuss it with the parents or guardians.

Papadatos[4] suggested that there is "widespread ignorance and misunderstanding and misstatements regarding consent and [that the consents] are usually meaningless unless one knows how fully the patient was informed of the risks." He feels that "Consent is obtained but is seldom informed" and that many physicians believe the reason for obtaining consent is to protect the physician and the institution, not to inform the parents, guardians, or subject of potential risks. How much all concerned parties should be told depends on their age, their ability to understand, and their desire to know. Some parents or guardians who give consent for a surgical procedure do not want to know of the potential complications; this should be noted in the chart.[5]

Assent

There is a move to have pediatric patients who are able to give their assent for surgery and/or research before the procedure occurs. This is based on the belief that no one can give consent for another person for surgery or to be a research subject.[6] The American Academy of Pediatrics (AAP) now suggests that the physician seek *permission* (not consent) from the parents and that the physician seek *assent* from the child whenever possible. This is done because the AAP is encouraging the development of healthy, involved, fully decisional adults through helpful encounters with their pediatricians (and others). It is suggested that there are four elements that are pertinent when obtaining assent from a child.[6]

1. Discussions between the child and parents to ensure that the child understands the present illness and what is to be done, especially when it comes to surgery. However, this is often tricky for physicians because some parents fail to tell their child that he or she is having surgery or what that entails. When the anesthesiologist arrives to discuss anesthesia with the family and child, there is confusion. Discussion of surgery and anesthesia often leads to conflicts between the anesthesiologist and the family, and between the child and parents or guardians, at a time when anesthesia and surgery are about to begin. Failure to properly inform the child that he or she is having surgery and what that entails may have serious postoperative consequences. Many postoperative problems can be allayed by a preoperative evaluation that includes play therapy and a video that describes what will occur.

2. Telling the child what he or she should expect during the induction of anesthesia and after awakening from anesthesia. A discussion of pain and its treatment or prevention is important, if the child is able to understand these concepts.

3. Determining the child's understanding of his or her illness. Depending on the parents, the child may have little or no understanding of the problem, or may be

very well informed. If the physician begins to discuss the illness with the child, and they have told her or him nothing about the surgery, the parents may become angry and feel that their authority is being impugned. Other parents will be pleased that someone can and will discuss the child's illness with their child.

4. Solicitation of the child's assent to anesthesia can lead to problems. If the child withholds assent, he or she will usually have the surgery anyway. This can lead to serious behavioral problems during the induction of anesthesia. When this occurs, anesthesia should be induced as quickly and safely as possible.

Children can feel betrayed in this situation. They were asked their opinion, they stated it, and others did whatever they wanted to anyway. This can lead to relational problems with the parents and the anesthesiologist. It is better to have discussions about surgery and anesthesia before the child arrives in the operating room area. Ideally, these discussions should be initiated by the family pediatrician and should be reinforced by the parents. These discussions should be continued during the preanesthesia visit.

It is unclear at what age assent should be attained from the child. Certainly, it is appropriate for teenagers. Some believe that assent should be sought as early as 7 or 8 years of age. This is a developing area that requires much more work.

Consent to Be a Research Subject

Some people believe that research should never be performed in infants and children unless the patient will benefit directly from the experiment; they believe this because children cannot consent to the procedure.[7] Most clinicians believe, however, that research should be done in infants and children because failure to perform appropriate studies in children may subject them to unproven, dangerous therapies, as has occurred in the past.

Mitchell[8] suggested that research can be conducted in infants and children under one of the following conditions:

1. The experimental treatment attempts to cure the disease.
2. The experiment will give new information about the child's condition and the disease that causes it.
3. The child is well or suffers from another disease and information obtained will provide information about a particular disease.
4. The experiment will give information from a healthy child about children in general.

The United States Congress[9] has affirmed that research in infants and children is appropriate if (1) the studies have been approved by a multidisciplinary ethics advisory committee, (2) the parents consent to the experiment, and (3) the risk/benefit ratio is determined. The British Pediatric Association,[10] on the other hand, feels that studies should not be performed in children if the same information can be obtained in adults. However, children often respond differently than adults to a disease or drug. For instance, if adult minimum anesthetic concentration values were used for young infants, infants would receive too little anesthesia to meet their needs. On the other hand, if a premature infant receives the same dose of inhaled anesthetic as a 30-year-old adult, the anesthetic dose of the premature infant will be too great, and the infant might become hypotensive.

The United States National Commission for the Protection of Human Subjects of Biomedical Research[9] stated that:

1. Research in infants and children is important and may be done if (a) the research is scientifically sound; (b) prior research has been done in animals and adults; (c) the risk is minimized as much as possible; and (d) the privacy and confidentiality of the child and parents is maintained as much as possible.
2. Research that involves more than minimal risk may be conducted if there is an anticipated benefit to the subject and if informed consent is obtained from the parent or guardian and from the child when possible.
3. Research that is without benefit to the patient may be conducted if the risk is minor and consent is obtained.
4. Research that does not fall under the previous categories can be done if there is a possibility that the information gained will alleviate serious problems affecting the health of children.
5. Research can be done only after consent is obtained from the parent or guardian and from the child when possible. If the child refuses to permit the research, the study cannot be done unless there is direct benefit to the child from the study.
6. Parental consent is necessary unless it is not required to protect the patient.
7. Institutionalized children may be included as subjects if all other conditions are met.

The United States Department of Public Health added that (1) a child's objection to being a research subject is not binding but parental consent is, and (2) there is no specific age at which consent by the child is mandatory. In most institutions, children between 7 and 14 years of age are asked to participate in the study. Failure to give their consent is usually sufficient to prevent the study from being done. If a child over 14 years of age refuses to participate in the study, it should not be done.[11]

The risk/benefit ratio of doing each study must be determined. If there is little or no risk, as occurs for most anesthesia studies, the study can be done. If there is a significant risk of a complication (e.g., hypotension or hypoxia), research committees usually will not allow studies to be performed in children unless they have been previously performed in adults and there is a compelling reason to perform them in children. Risk can never be eliminated totally. Because there were no complications in the first 50 subjects does not mean that one will not occur in the next 10 subjects. If complications are rare, thousands of subjects may have to be studied before a complication is detected.

Since most anesthesia studies entail minimal risk, it is important to provide a frame of reference of what "minimal risk" means so that the parents can make an informed decision about allowing their child to participate in a study.[11] Risk rates are usually derived from the literature and are, for the most part, educated guesses. It is helpful for the parents if the risks are described in terms of real-life events (e.g., a comparison with the risk of injury or death from riding in an automobile for 100 miles).

The United States Department of Health, Education, and Welfare listed the important elements of informed consent for research:

1. An explanation of the procedures and the reasons for doing the study.
2. A description of the risks and discomforts (including pain) that can be reasonably expected. The consent does not, however, have to cover every possible problem that could occur, only those that have some likelihood of occurring.
3. A description of possible benefits (if there are none, this should be stated).
4. A description of the alternatives to participation in the research, including a statement that the subject's medical care (if any) will not be affected by refusal to participate in the study.
5. A statement that the subject is free to withdraw from the study at any time without jeopardizing ongoing medical care.
6. The parents and the subject must have the opportunity to ask questions about the study and must receive answers in language they can understand.

Koren[12, 13] identified the reasons why approximately 5 percent of the studies submitted to the Committee on Research were rejected. Three fourths of them were drug studies; they were rejected because there were major scientific flaws in the study design or because the studies would not answer the questions asked. For nine physically invasive studies, the committee felt that the studies were without direct benefit to the subject. In three cases, the committee indicated that patients with serious medical conditions might be randomized to receive a placebo when there is already a drug with proven efficacy for their condition. All committees must determine whether the proposed studies are "me too" studies or whether they will actually add new information.

Jehovah's Witnesses

One of the most difficult ethical problems anesthesiologists face is that of obtaining informed consent for children of Jehovah's Witnesses. Because of their religious beliefs, Jehovah's Witnesses are prohibited from receiving or allowing blood and blood components to be administered to their children, even if it means that a child will die from anemia. This is a very difficult situation for the family because they, like all parents or guardians, want the child to survive and do well. It is the anesthesiologist's responsibility to help them as much as possible with this moral dilemma, not to "punish" them. Rather than being ignorant, uncaring, or "bad" people, the parents happen to have a set of beliefs that differ from those of the majority of society. The anesthesiologist should understand this and should respect these religious convictions as much as possible, without compromising either the safety of the child or the ethical position of the anesthesiologist. Although all parties involved should understand the risks they are taking, it should be clear what the risks really are. Since the problem is transfusion, the reason(s) a child will need a transfusion should be clear in the surgeon's and anesthesiologist's minds before there is any discussion with the family. Clearly, patients without cardiorespiratory disease, and even those with renal failure, can tolerate hemoglobin concentrations of 7 g/dl or less without serious effects. Consequently, transfusion of patients with hemoglobin concentrations above this level is seldom necessary.

Blood transfusion should become an issue with the parent or guardian only when there is a significant likelihood that it will be necessary for the patient's well-being. If there is no likelihood that the child will need a blood transfusion (e.g., incision and drainage of an abscess of the toe), the parents or guardians should be told this and other matters discussed. If there is a high likelihood that the patient will need a blood transfusion to prevent serious harm or death and the parent or guardian refuses to allow a transfusion, there are several steps to follow.

First, and most importantly, the true potential for requiring transfusion must be determined and discussed with the surgeon and the family *before* the need for transfusion is imminent. The goal is not to have the parents or guardians change their minds and agree to a blood transfusion, but rather to be certain that everyone understands what will happen if a transfusion is required. The point at which blood is required to save the patient's life is not the time to discover that the surgeon has promised the parents or guardians that no blood will be given, even if this means that the patient would die. An anesthesiologist who knows before surgery that such an agreement was made between the family and the surgeon can either accept and go along with it or find another anesthesiologist who will do so. This cannot be done during a life-threatening situation.

It is unclear how a given court will respond if a physician agrees not to transfuse an unemancipated minor and the patient dies. There have been no judgments against a physician for this to date, but the court has taken the view that it (the court) has jurisdiction over this matter and has never prevented a transfusion from taking place if it was in the best interest of the child. The court has said that "parents may be free to make martyrs of themselves, but they are not free to make martyrs of their children before they have reached the age when they can make that choice for themselves" (*Prince v Massachusetts*, 1944). Therefore, agreement to withhold a life-saving blood transfusion from an unemancipated minor might be viewed as thwarting the will of the court if someone decided to pursue this matter in court. Physicians who withhold treatment from incompetent patients may be held liable unless they take reasonable steps to authorize treatment.[14]

Courts in the United States will make a child a ward of the court for the perioperative period if the parents or guardians refuse to allow a blood transfusion and there is a reasonable likelihood that blood administration will be required to prevent death or serious harm to the child. The court order should be obtained before surgery, not at the last minute. If the surgeon and anesthesiologist have promised that they will not transfuse the child, a court order should not be obtained later if the patient is dying from blood loss. In many instances, obtaining a court order for blood transfusion is important for the family. This relieves them of the enormous responsibility for preventing a needed transfusion, and it affords their child the opportunity to survive without the parents having to compromise their religious beliefs. It should not be assumed, however, that this is always the case.

The parents should be told that a court order is going to be obtained, and they should be given the opportunity to contact the court to present their side of the question. The hospital should help the family by giving them the telephone number of the court and by providing transportation to meet with the judge if this becomes necessary. This has been very helpful in a number of such cases because, after making their own petition to the court (and failing), the parents were relieved. They had done all that they could to prevent the transfusion.

Before surgery, the anesthesiologist should discuss with the parent or guardian in clear, concise terms what will happen if the child requires a blood transfusion. Preferably, this discussion should take place with the surgeon and the family in the same room. If the family or guardian wish to have someone from the Jehovah's Witnesses church present at the time transfusion is discussed, they should be allowed to do so. Members of the church are told to have a "teacher" present when these discussions take place. The teacher will put enormous pressure on the family members not to allow the transfusion, which is usually very disturbing to the physicians and nurses involved, but the teacher is there at the parents' request. Arguing with the teacher will solve nothing, nor will it change anyone's mind. Physicians should only present the facts and should do so as unemotionally as possible.

The parents should be told the following:

1. Everything will be done to avoid transfusing their child. The steps that will be taken to accomplish this goal should be outlined. It should be made clear that no one wishes to violate the religious beliefs of the family and transfuse the child against their wishes unless the child's life is in danger or unless there is a high likelihood that not transfusing the child would cause the child serious harm.
2. The criteria for which transfusion will be necessary (e.g., metabolic acidosis, decreased cardiac output, severe anemia). This information gives the parent or guardian concrete criteria for transfusion and demonstrates that the anesthesiologist is attempting to work with them. The parent or guardian should understand that although the child may tolerate severe, acute anemia while anesthetized, because of reduced oxygen consumption, serious problems may occur when the child awakens.[15]
3. The ways to decrease the risk of transfusion: (1) not having surgery; (2) delaying surgery and giving iron therapy and/or erythropoietin for several weeks to increase the hematocrit; (3) hypervolemic hemodilu-

tion[16] or hemodilution with possible hypothermia, and controlled hypotension[17–19] (see Chapter 13); and (4) staging the surgery (i.e., performing only part of the surgery, allowing the patient to recover for several weeks while the hemoglobin concentration returns to normal, and finishing the operation at a later time).
4. A court order will be obtained to allow a blood transfusion during surgery if this becomes necessary. The parent or guardian should always be told the truth. They should never be told that the child will not be transfused, only to discover later that the child was given blood or blood products.

DO NOT RESUSCITATE

Cardiopulmonary resuscitation (CPR) is performed reflexively and with great skill by many physicians. Despite this, there has been no improvement in the outcome of CPR since it was first described in the late 1950s.[20] Approximately 15 percent of in-hospital cardiac arrest in adults can be "successfully" resuscitated, and about 10 percent leave the hospital alive.[21] Of the latter, many do not recover their former lifestyle. The outcome of resuscitation in infants and children is usually worse (see Chapter 7) because the cause of arrest is hypoxia rather than coronary artery disease. The heart often can be revived, but the brain cannot. When this happens, long-term care of the patient devastates families and is very expensive for society. The dying process is prolonged[22, 23] and the patient often survives with "multiple invasive, painful, and dehumanizing procedures."[24]

DECISIONS ABOUT THE APPROPRIATENESS OF SURGERY

Those who care for infants and children often make decisions that have far-reaching implications for the child's survival. Technology has made it possible for patients to survive for long periods in a persistent vegetative state. The challenge is to apply the technology appropriately and to know when enough is enough. Many physicians have difficulty doing this because they are taught to do everything they can to preserve life. They often feel they have failed if a patient dies.

In the past there was only one definition of death: absence of pulses and respiration. Because it is now possible to maintain patients on cardiopulmonary life-support (e.g., extracorporeal membrane oxygenation) for months at great expense to the family, the child, and society, and because there was a need to obtain organs for transplantation, the concept of brain death came into use. Brain death occurs when there is a lack of function of the entire brain, including the brain stem. However, the American Medical Association's Council on Ethical and Judicial Affairs indicated that if death is imminent or there is irreversible coma, "with the concurrence of those who have responsibility for the care of the patient, it is ethical to discontinue all means of life-prolonging medical treatment."[25] This is different from declaring the patient brain dead and is not sufficient to obtain organs for transplantation. If those caring for a patient have differing opinions about whether to continue life support, the hospital ethics committee can be very helpful in resolving these conflicts, or at least in clarifying the issues. Rarely should the courts have to intervene. An overriding principle should be that if life support is not expected to lead to the patient's recovery, support may be withdrawn. Physicians must be the patient's advocate, which on occasion includes withdrawing support and allowing the patient to die. "The concept of a 'good death' does not mean simply the withholding of technological treatments that serve only to prolong the act of dying. It also requires the art of deliberately creating a medical environment that allows a peaceful death."[26]

Serious conflicts arise when the medical staff "knows" that further treatment is futile, and the family is unable to accept this. "Such conflict can be emotionally draining, ethically unsettling, and legally troublesome to physicians involved in the patient's care. The ideal resolution to this conflict is to reach an ethically defensible agreement: either the parents convince the physicians to continue treating the child or the physicians convince the parents to forego further treatment."[27] Often this matter cannot be resolved, despite serious efforts on the part of both parties, because outside forces (e.g., family, religion, or society) prevent its resolution. Many clinicians believe that physicians must always continue care if the family insists on doing so, but this is not always true. A physician can refuse to treat a child if the treatment is contrary to the best interests of the child (i.e., if it is futile, harmful, or disproportionately burdensome to the patient[27] and the treatment is not in the best interests of the child). This satisfies the "first principle" of Hippocrates: "Above all be useful, or at least do no harm." Physicians should intervene if parents or guardian make decisions that are contrary to a child's best interests, but these interventions should not be made in a vacuum. They should be made in conjunction with others and should be based on as many facts as possible. Since care usually is withdrawn because further treatment is believed to be futile, physicians should be clear about what "futile" means. Nelson and Nelson[27] suggest that "futile" should be used when the therapy is without any benefit to the patient and that "disproportionate burden" be used when the burden of continued treatment outweighs the expected benefits. Futility is a reason to withhold treatment.[23, 28, 29] When an impasse is reached between physicians and the family, it is time to seek help from the ethics committee and the family's religious counselor, if there is one. Nelson and Nelson clearly and concisely discuss the steps to take in resolving conflicts of this type.[27]

One problem faced in the practice of modern medicine is that of continuing or discontinuing life support once it is started. From the moment life support is instituted, physicians should question whether continuing therapy is in the best interests of the patient. If it is not, strong consideration should be given to withdrawing therapy.

"Do Not Resuscitate" Orders

A major reason why physicians are forced to decide whether to continue or discontinue treatment is that CPR is sometimes initiated in emergency rooms or on the hospital ward, often without sufficient information to determine if doing so is appropriate. This occurs because physicians are reluctant to write do not resuscitate (DNR) orders, even when they know that CPR is useless. This stems in part from fear of being sued and from lack of clear policies or guidelines for writing DNR orders in many hospitals. CPR can reasonably be withheld when there is virtually no likelihood of restoring cardiopulmonary function for more than a short time. Examples of this are resuscitation of anencephalic infants or of children with anomalies incompatible with life. When some clinicians are faced with resuscitating a patient who is unknown to them, they reasonably resuscitate the patient with the intent of withdrawing support if it becomes clear that the therapy is futile. This gives the parents or guardian the opportunity to see the child while still "alive," but does not commit the patient to long-term care.

Many problems associated with discontinuing CPR can be avoided if DNR orders are written in the charts of patients who will not benefit from CPR or for whom CPR may be harmful. However, all DNR orders are not the same. Physicians should be clear about and should document what actually is meant by DNR in any given patient. In most instances, DNR means that the trachea should not be intubated and that mechanical ventilation and cardioversion should be withheld. Intravenous fluids, antibiotics, and narcotics are usually given. DNR orders should never be verbal, but should be written in the chart. Each member of the medical team should be aware of the DNR order and any restrictions placed on it, so that inappropriate care will not be provided.

There have been recent ongoing discussions about whether to continue DNR orders when patients require surgery, usually to insert a gastrostomy or a central venous line or to palliate a lesion and provide comfort for the patient. DNR orders are initiated to prevent patients from becoming dependent on cardiopulmonary life support and from prolonging the dying process.[30] "The general assumption is that the DNR order is intended to apply specifically to situations where the dying process cannot be reversed and respiratory and/or cardiac arrest is simply a manifestation of death."[31] Consequently, endotracheal intubation, mechanical ventilation, defibrillation, and use of vasopressors for arterial blood pressure support are prohibited.[32] However, fluids and vasopressors are used to treat hypotension, tracheal intubation and mechanical ventilation are used to treat apnea and hypoventilation, and oxygen is used to treat hypoxia during anesthesia. Brief periods of chest compression are occasionally required because of an overdose of anesthetic. It is often difficult to determine where anesthesia ends and resuscitation begins. If a DNR order is intended to avoid therapy for an untreatable cause of death, there is no reason to believe that the same order applies when treatable and easily reversible problems (e.g., hypotension, acidosis, apnea) occur during anesthesia. Therefore, DNR orders written to cover nonsurgical events are usually not applicable during surgery unless the family has specifically stated that they should continue in effect.[33] If they have done so, the anesthesiologist who chooses to ignore their wishes may be subject to the law because "resuscitating a patient with a DNR order may be viewed as disregard for patient autonomy and as [grounds for] potential accusations of battery."[33] Truog[34] points out that many seriously ill patients choose DNR status because resuscitation outside the operating room often increases suffering and has a poor outcome (see Chapter 7). Resuscitation in the operating room, on the other hand, is much more effective and is not associated with pain.[35] Each institution should have a policy regarding whether to suspend DNR orders during surgery, and that policy should be understood by all members of the surgery and anesthesia team. This matter should be discussed with the family before surgery. If a child requires emergency surgery, and the parents or guardian are unavailable, the DNR order should probably be suspended. Every anesthesiologist should read and be familiar with the guidelines promulgated by the American Society of Anesthesiology.[36]

Recently, goal-directed orders have been promulgated for the perioperative period in relationship to DNR orders.[37] This allows patients "to guide therapy by prioritizing outcomes rather than procedures."[38] Clinicians are allowed to use clinical judgment to achieve the patient's stated outcome goals. These goals are usually defined by the patient in terms of what he or she is willing to accept (i.e., a reasonable chance of leaving the hospital without undue pain or suffering). Waisel[38] lists four possibilities that could occur.

1. *Full resuscitation.* The patient wants all means of resuscitation for problems that are related to the surgery and anesthesia
2. *Limited resuscitation: Procedure-directed.* This means that the patient or his or her surrogate refuses certain resuscitative efforts (i.e., he or she refuses tracheal intubation but will accept vasopressors and alkali, etc.)
3. *Limited resuscitation: Goal-directed #1.* The patient desires resuscitative measures during and after anesthesia only if the adverse advents are both reversible and temporary in the judgment of the anesthesiologist and surgeon.
4. *Limited resuscitation: Goal-directed #2.* The patient desires resuscitation efforts to take place only if they support the specified goals and values of the patient. A statement of the patient's desires must be provided.

Whatever occurs, it is important for the anesthesiologist to define the benefits and the possible burdens that accrue to the patient as a result of the anesthesiologist's actions. The benefits might include improved quality of life. The burden might include increased pain. These should be discussed with the child if he or she is old enough to understand, and with the parents or guardians.

How long endotracheal intubation, mechanical ventilation, and administration of pressor drugs started in the operating room should be continued postoperatively, and the circumstances under which they are to be discontinued, should be addressed before surgery. Some patients who were not dependent on life support preoperatively will require life support postoperatively, not because of their primary disease process but because of the surgery and anesthesia. For example, patients with upper abdominal incisions may not breathe adequately for several days and may require oxygen and mechanical ventilation during that time. If the reason for the delay in weaning from mechanical ventilation and tracheal extubation is surgical, therapy should be continued in most cases. If it is clearly because of the basic disease process for which the DNR order was originally written, therapy should be stopped and nature allowed to take its course.[34] It seems reasonable, as Troug[34] has suggested, to continue mechanical ventilation as long as the patient's pulmonary status is improving. If it reaches a plateau or begins to worsen, withdrawing support should be considered. Life-support measures that will not reverse the patient's condition should be discontinued. Before surgery, the family should be informed about the conditions under which support will be continued or discontinued, and this should be documented in the chart. Once the life-support measures engendered by surgery and anesthesia can be withdrawn, the original DNR order should be reinstituted.

When life-support measures instituted in the operating room cannot be withdrawn, appropriate consultation should be obtained to determine if there are other reasons why the patient cannot be weaned. Some clinicians have dealt with this problem by limiting the duration of support (e.g., 7 days). Although this is tempting, it fails to take into account the differences in the recovery rates among sick patients after anesthesia and surgery.

Some anesthesiologists feel themselves unable to honor a DNR order, no matter what the circumstances. In one study, 34 percent of anesthesiologists reported that they would resuscitate a patient who had a cardiac arrest caused by intrinsic disease, and 68 percent would do so if the arrest was due to another cause.[31] This is difficult to defend if the parent or guardian truly wishes the DNR order to be in effect at all times. Resuscitating patients against their will violates their rights and may leave the anesthesiologist open to prosecution for assault and battery, or worse.[34] An anesthesiologist who cannot honor an appropriately executed DNR order should withdraw from care of that patient after finding someone who can honor the order.

Futility

Futile is defined as "serving no useful purpose, completely ineffective." When futility is applied to medical care, it means that the care would serve no useful purpose for the patient. Truog et al.[39] suggest that a better term is "physiologic futility" (i.e., the treatment "offers no physiological benefit to the patient").[39] In this case, the physician has no obligation to provide the therapy. This was reinforced by the Baby Doe rules, which specifically exempted physicians from having to provide treatment that is "virtually futile."[40]

Examples of futile therapy would be performing CPR on a baby with anencephaly, on a patient who has been declared brain dead, or on a patient in whom it is impossible to do so effectively (aortic or pulmonic atresia). The problem is, can we really know that therapy is futile? Physicians have difficulty estimating the likelihood of success of a therapeutic intervention because frequently there are no data on which to base conclusions except their own experience, which may be limited or tainted by the memory of one or two exceptional cases. To the extent possible, decisions to provide or not provide therapy should be based on data that indicate how effective the therapy is. When these data are available it is useful to record them in the patient's chart. Physicians should constantly keep in mind that what was futile in the past may not be futile today. Fifteen years ago, therapy for hypoplastic left hearts was usually futile. Today, a significant number of infants with this anomaly undergo surgery to palliate this lesion, and they survive.

Each institution should provide for the staff guidelines that delineate the conditions under which therapy should be considered futile. This helps the staff make more appropriate decisions and reduces the likelihood that decisions will be made without consultation. If one of the recommendations is to consult the ethics committee, the committee's help will be sought earlier rather than later or not at all. Decisions about futility should never be made on the basis of cost alone, because hidden, unconscious agendas may deny care to one patient and not to another.

"Providers are obligated to make an effort to clarify precisely what the patient/parents/guardians intends to achieve with continued treatment. If the goals appear to reflect unrealistic expectations about the probable course of the underlying illness or the probable effects of medical interventions, providers should attempt to correct those impressions."[39] Frank, honest discussions with the family will resolve most of these conflicts.[29, 41] If this fails, involving members of the ethics committee, and the family's clergy may be very helpful.

Omission or Cessation of Therapy

Because physicians are taught that they must always *do something*, it is difficult for them to do nothing, even when doing so is appropriate. When therapy does not improve or stabilize the patient's condition, or when the patient is harmed by the therapy, the therapy should not be instituted or, if it has been started, it should be discontinued. It is often difficult for physicians to realize that "In some circumstances, the death of a child is not merely to be condoned but is morally required."[42]

Whether to continue or to omit treatment should not be based on judgments concerning the quality of life. The Child Abuse Act specifies that withdrawal of treatment can only be done when (1) the infant is chronically or irreversibly comatose, (2) the provision of treatment would only prolong dying and not effectively correct or ameliorate the infant's life-threatening conditions, and (3) the provision of such treatment would be virtually futile in terms of survival of the infant and the treatment itself under such circumstances would be inhumane.[43]

Parental Requests

Our society demands perfection and, in some instances, has devalued life in the search for perfection. Physicians are at times requested by parents to discontinue care of an infant when there is no clear reason to do so except that the infant is "not perfect" at birth. I have received such requests from several parents of normal term infants

who had infections or mild hyaline membrane disease. These highly educated parents were unable to differentiate between illnesses that are easily treated and severe congenital anomalies that will persist for life. The physician is faced with a difficult problem because there is no guarantee that the infant will be "perfect," although the likelihood of abnormalities is very low. Furthermore, there is no legal criterion under which care can be discontinued. Physicians should discuss the problem with the parents and determine why they believe that this child is "imperfect" and what that means to them. In most instances, these discussions solve the problem. However, in a small number of cases this question cannot be resolved. The ethics committee should be contacted and asked to review the circumstances of the case and make recommendations. Members of the committee may wish to meet with the family. It is often helpful to have someone in whom the parents have faith present during these discussions. This can be a family member or their religious advisor, if they have one. The last resort is to involve the court, which will usually make the child a ward of the court until the crisis is over. If the child requires surgery, the parents are often very hostile because the need for surgery is a further sign that their child is not "perfect."

The parents of such infants require close follow-up. When the baby has recovered, the parents are often angry and frustrated because they now have a child that in their mind may still be "imperfect," and they have to care for the child.

Rights of the Anesthesiologist

Anesthesiologists are often placed in a position in which they must make ethical decisions about the care of infants and children in the operating room and the intensive care unit. Since the anesthesiologist is usually not the primary physician (except in some intensive care units), decisions often have been made and confirmed with the parents or guardian by other physicians, without input from the anesthesiologist. However, it is often the anesthesiologist who must then live with the decision or find someone else to provide care for the patient. An anesthesiologist who cannot agree with the majority opinion should withdraw from the case, after first ensuring that the required care will be provided by another physician. The fact that the anesthesiologist has withdrawn should be documented in the patient's chart, and the name of the physician to whom the anesthesia care was transferred also should be noted.

CONCLUSION

This chapter has addressed some ethical questions that confront anesthesiologists who anesthetize infants and children. The underlying theme is communication with the parents or guardian, surgeons, and others involved in the child's care. The solution to most ethical conflicts is full discussion with the parents or guardian and listening to what they have to say. The latter allows the anesthesiologist to determine why the parents or guardian hold the opinion(s) they do. When it is understood why these opinions are held, the conflict(s) between parents or guardians and the medical team can be addressed logically. Although this does not always resolve the conflict, it does in most cases.

It is seldom productive to argue with the parents or guardians about conflicts, because this usually hardens the positions of both sides and prevents conflict resolution. It take enormous restraint on the part of anesthesiologists and family not to argue with each other, because each side holds strong beliefs and each side is sure that it is "right." If an argument begins, joining in the argument is counterproductive. Presenting facts in a kind, gentle, and reassuring way without patronizing the family is much more successful. Communication is the solution to conflicts. Failure to communicate effectively makes the conflict worse and often leads to intervention by the courts.

REFERENCES

1. Webster's Ninth New Collegiate Dictionary. Springfield, MA, Mirriam-Webster,1983.
2. Miyaji NT: The power of compassion: truth-telling among American doctors in the care of dying patients. Soc Sci Med 36:249, 1993.
3. Lipson JG, Meleis AI: Methodological issues in research with immigrants. Med Anthropol 12:103, 1989.
4. Papadatos CJ: Guidelines for medical research in children. Infection 17:411, 1989.
5. Singer PA, Choudhry S, Armstrong J: Public opinion regarding consent to treatment. J Am Geriatr Soc 41:112, 1993.
6. Morganweck CS, Nelson RM: Pediatric assent: can children understand, assess or communicate their wishes? Am Soc Anesthesiol Newslett 63:11, 1999.
7. Ramsey P: The Patient as a Person. New Haven, CT, Yale University Press, 1970.
8. Mitchell RG: The child and experimental medicine. BMJ 4:721, 1964.
9. National Commission for the Protection of Human Subjects of Biomedical and Behavioral Research: Research involving children. Report and recommendations. 77-0004 Appendix 770005. Washington, DC, Department of Health, Education and Welfare, 1977.
10. British Paediatric Association: Guidelines to aid ethical committees considering research involving children. Arch Dis Child 55:75, 1980.
11. Nicholson HR: Medical Research with Children, Ethics, Law and Practice. Oxford, Oxford University Press, 1986.
12. Koren G: Ethical boundaries of medical research in infants and children in the 80s: analysis of rejected protocols and a new solution for drug studies. Dev Pharmacol Ther 15:130, 1990.
13. Koren G: Medical research in infants and children in the eighties: analysis of rejected protocols. Pediatr Res 27:432, 1990.
14. Roth LH, Meisel A, Lidz CW: Tests of competency to consent to treatment. Am J Psychiatry 134:279, 1977.
15. Wong DH, Jenkins LC: Surgery in Jehovah's Witnesses. Can J Anaesth 36:578, 1989.
16. Trouwborst A, Hagenouw RR, Jeekel J, Ong GL: Hypervolaemic haemodilution in an anaemic Jehovah's Witness. Br J Anaesth 64:646, 1990.
17. Brodsky JW, Dickson JH, Erwin WD, Rossi CD: Hypotensive anesthesia for scoliosis surgery in Jehovah's Witnesses. Spine 16:304, 1991.
18. Schaller RJ, Schaller J, Morgan A, Furman EB: Hemodilution anesthesia: a valuable aid to major cancer surgery in children. Am J Surg 146:79, 1983.
19. Wong KC, Webster LR, Coleman SS, Dunn HK: Hemodilution and induced hypotension for insertion of a Harrington rod in a Jehovah's Witness patient. Clin Orthop 152:237, 1980.
20. Schneider AW, Nelson DJ, Brown DJ: In-hospital cardiopulmonary resuscitation: a 30-year review. J Am Board Fam Pract 6:91, 1993.
21. Beuret P, Feihl F, Vogt P, et al: Cardiac arrest: prognostic factors and outcome at one year. Resuscitation 25:171, 1993.
22. Baskett PJF: The ethics of resuscitation. BMJ 283:189, 1986.
23. Blackhall LJ: Must we always use CPR? N Engl J Med 317:1281, 1987.
24. Davies JM, Reynolds BM: The ethics of cardiopulmonary resuscitation. I. Background to decision making. Arch Dis Child 67:1498, 1992.
25. American Medical Association Council on Judicial and Ethical Affairs: Withholding or withdrawing life-prolonging medical treatment. JAMA 256:471, 1986.
26. Wanzer SH, Federman DD, Adelstein SJ, et al: The physician's responsibility towards hopelessly ill patients: a second look. N Engl J Med 320:844, 1989.
27. Nelson LJ, Nelson RM: Ethics and the provision of futile, harmful, or burdensome treatment to children. Crit Care Med 20:427, 1992.
28. Schneiderman LJ, Jecker NS, Jonsen AR: Medical futility: its meaning and ethical implications. Ann Intern Med 112:949, 1990.
29. Murphy DJ: Do not resuscitate orders: time for reappraisal in long-term care institutions. JAMA 260:2098, 1988.
30. Rabkin MT, Gillerman G, Rice NR: Orders not to resuscitate. N Engl J Med 295:364, 1976.
31. Franklin CM, Rothenberg DM: Do-not-resuscitate orders in the presurgical patient. J Clin Anesth 4:181, 1992.
32. Franklin CM: Do not resuscitate policies. Acute Care 11:208, 1985.
33. Swartz M: The patient who refuses medical treatment. A dilemma for hospitals and physicians. Am J Law Med 11:147, 1985.
34. Truog RD: "Do-not-resuscitate" orders during anesthesia and surgery. Anesthesiology 74:606, 1991.
35. Peatfield RC, Sillett RW, Taylor D, McNicol MW: Survival after cardiac arrest in hospital. Lancet 1:1223, 1977.
36. American Society of Anesthesiologists ethical guidelines for the anesthesia care of patients with do-not-resuscitate orders or other directives that limit care. American Society of Anesthesiologist 1999 Directory of Members. Park Ridge, IL, American Society of Anesthesiologists, 1998, p 470.
37. Truog RD, Waisel DB, Burns JP: DNR in the OR: A goal-directed approach. Anesthesiology 90:289, 1999.
38. Waisel DB: Preoperative DNR orders: new options, greater flexibility. Am Soc Anesthesiol Newslett 63:9, 1999.
39. Truog RD, Brett AS, Frader J: The problem with futility. N Engl J Med 326:1560, 1992.
40. 1984 Amendments to the Child Abuse Prevention and Treatment Act: Public Law 98–457, 1984.
41. Younger JS: Who defines futility? JAMA 260:2094, 1988.
42. Goldworth A: Human rights and the omission or cessation of treatment for infants. J Perinatol 19:79, 1989.
43. Federal Regulations: Vol. 50, No. 72, p 14878, 1985.

2

Training and Practice of Pediatric Anesthesia

ALVIN HACKEL

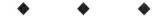

HISTORY

This chapter reviews the history of the development of the practice and training of pediatric anesthesia. It also discusses the current status of recent initiatives and clarifies issues pertaining to them. Much of the information in this chapter is the result of work of local and national anesthesiology organizations that has focused on problems of teaching and defining pediatric anesthesia over the past 10 years. The ultimate goal of these organizations and of all anesthesiologists is to provide optimal care of all infants and children requiring anesthesia care.

Pediatric anesthesia has evolved over the past 150 years. Very early on, it became clear that pediatric patients had anatomic and physiologic differences that made the administration of anesthesia to them different and more dangerous than administering anesthesia to adults. This led early pioneers such as Dr. Charles H. Robson at the Hospital for Sick Children in Toronto to become the first anesthesiologist to specialize in anesthesia for infants and children.[1] Others followed in his footsteps, including Digby Leigh at the Children's Hospital in Montreal, Robert Cope at the Hospital for Sick Children in London, Robert Smith at the Children's Hospital in Boston, Ernest Salanitre and Herbert Rackow at the Babies Hospital in New York, Alan Conn and David Steward at the Hospital for Sick Children in Toronto, Jack Downes at the Children's Hospital in Philadelphia, and George Gregory at the University of California in San Francisco. They created an environment in which major contributions have been made to the perioperative care of infants and children.

Improved anesthesia and surgery spawned the need for neonatal and pediatric intensive care units. Technological and pharmaceutical advances made the practice of anesthesia safer and more complicated. The application of these advances to the pediatric patient has led to the need for additional training and repetitive experience in the care of pediatric patients. Expensive technology and the applicability of this technology to a relatively small portion of the pediatric anesthesia population has led many politicians and bureaucrats to consider regionalization of pediatric care.

Because of extensive developments in the field of pediatric anesthesiology, it has become customary for anesthesiologists who wish to focus on the care of infants and children to take additional clinical training in an academic pediatric anesthesia environment. Consequently, pediatric anesthesia fellowship programs have developed across the United States and Canada. Anesthesiology groups and hospitals that wish to provide anesthesia for pediatric surgery recruit individuals with additional training in pediatric anesthesia to oversee the care of these patients. Thus, an environment has developed in the United States in which an individual with additional training and experience in pediatric anesthesiology has skills with professional value.

13

Development of an environment in which the teaching of pediatric anesthesia flourished has led anesthesiologists with a particular interest in the care of pediatric patients to take additional training, usually 1 year in length, at these pediatric anesthesia centers of excellence. Graduates of these centers have gone on to establish their own pediatric anesthesia training programs, which in turn created more fellowship training centers in pediatric anesthesia. Today there are more than 50 such centers offering excellent training in pediatric anesthesia.[2]

Other factors also have stimulated the development of pediatric anesthesia. An increase in the American population, the requirement for a third year of anesthesiology residency training by the American Board of Anesthesiology, and the movement of American medicine to managed care accelerated the process of adding anesthesiologists with special training in pediatric anesthesia to anesthesia practices. The third year of anesthesiology residency provided the opportunity for residents to take up to 6 months in a subspecialty area. Because pediatric anesthesia is interesting, challenging, and something many residents are fearful of, pediatric anesthesia electives became popular. Graduates of anesthesiology residencies who took 6 months of elective time on a pediatric anesthesia service were hired into anesthesiology practice groups as "pediatric anesthesiologists." As a result of this practice, questions arose regarding whether 6 months was long enough to qualify someone as a pediatric anesthesiologist. Most experts felt that the curriculum and clinical experience required that would allow someone to be considered a pediatric anesthesiologist could not be provided in this amount of time. This became even clearer when data on outcome of pediatric anesthesia became available.

QUALITY ASSURANCE AND PEDIATRIC ANESTHESIA

Studies comparing the perioperative anesthesia-related morbidity and mortality of pediatric and adult patients have demonstrated that both the morbidity and the mortality are increased for pediatric patients.[3-5] The publications of Cohen[4] and Morray[5] have been particularly important in this regard. Cohen demonstrated increases in airway and cardiovascular morbidity in pediatric patients compared to adult patients. Morray found a higher percentage of adverse outcomes in the pediatric age group in a closed claim study co-sponsored by the American Society of Anesthesiologists (ASA) and the American Academy of Pediatrics (AAP). In England, Campling demonstrated similar adverse outcomes for the pediatric age group.[6] In an allied study, Keenan showed an increase in the frequency of cardiac arrests in infants cared for by nonpediatric anesthesiologists compared with children cared for by pediatric anesthesiologists.[7]

This information suggests that the practice of pediatric anesthesia is different from the practice of anesthesia for adults and that people providing anesthesia care for children require knowledge, training, and repetitive experience that are different as well. Anesthesiologists who wish to provide anesthesia for infants and children need special training and experience if they are to care for this unique

group of patients safely. British anesthesiologists recommended, as a result of their work, "that surgeons and anesthetists should not undertake 'occasional pediatric practice', as outcome was found to be related to the experience of the clinicians involved."[8-10] They recommended the development of a minimum requirement for the number of pediatric cases that anesthesiologists and surgeons must perform annually and the development of a regional system for pediatric anesthesia with the transfer of patients with more complex medical problems to special centers for pediatric anesthesia. This recommendation is supported by data from the United States that compare the outcome of patients undergoing repair of congenital cardiac defects who are cared for in centers with small volumes of pediatric patients versus those cared for in centers with large surgical volumes.[11, 12] Clearly, patients cared for in larger centers do better.

WHAT IS THE PRACTICE OF PEDIATRIC ANESTHESIA?

Pediatric anesthesia is defined as the provision of anesthesia care for infants and children. The clear anatomic, physiologic, and psychological differences between pediatric and adult patients, and the pathophysiologic differences that affect the types and severity of illnesses found in the two groups of patients, are the basis for this textbook. The "cutoff age" between adult and pediatric anesthesia is difficult to determine. There is a continuum that varies depending on the above-noted differences and the psychological development of the child. The younger the patient, the clearer the differentiation is.

WHERE AND BY WHOM IS PEDIATRIC ANESTHESIA PRACTICED?

A central question in the development of appropriate training for pediatric anesthesia is, "Where and by whom is pediatric anesthesia practiced?" Unfortunately, there are few data with which to answer this question. The practice of pediatric anesthesia is distributed widely among inpatient and outpatient facilities with and without special expertise in the care of infants and children. Macario et al. studied the distribution of the inpatient pediatric anesthesia population among hospitals in northern California.[13] Their data indicated 162 of the 205 hospitals in the region had at least one surgical procedure per year that required anesthesia in patients less than 6 years of age. This accounted for a total of 14,435 surgeries on 13,188 patients. Seventy-two percent of the hospitals had less than 50 cases per year. The 10 hospitals performing more than 100 cases per year performed 61 percent of all the anesthesia cases. Thus, most pediatric anesthesia was done in hospitals with large pediatric anesthesia practices, but most hospitals in the region performed at least a small number of cases. The findings of this study are supported by data obtained for the Study Group on Pediatric Anesthesia by Hoffman, Kain and Viney.[14-16] The question is, who should anesthetize children in those hospitals where only a few cases are performed each year? It is likely that many anesthesiologists may perform only one case every few years.

WHO SHOULD PROVIDE PEDIATRIC ANESTHESIA?

Despite what is said, all pediatric patients requiring anesthesia cannot and do not have to be cared for by anesthesiologists with training in pediatric anesthesia beyond their anesthesiology residency. It is more important that the anesthesiologists have demonstrated continuing experience and competency in providing anesthesia care for this population of patients.

To try and clarify the differences in training and competency required by anesthesiologists who care for infants and children, the Study Group on Pediatric Anesthesia was formed.*

The first project of the Study Group was to clarify differences in the level of competency required and the training required of general and pediatric anesthesiologists who will provide pediatric anesthesia. The Study Group divided the patients into infants and children and into less severe and more severe conditions for which anesthesia was required.

This resulted in the following statement.[17]:

"Clinical Competency Objectives for Training of the General Anesthesiologist and the Pediatric Anesthesiologist in Pediatric Anesthesiology."

1. The general anesthesiologist by the end of the CA3 year shall be competent to:
   a. Provide safe anesthesia and postanesthesia care for infants and children undergoing routine surgical, diagnostic and therapeutic procedures; and
   b. To recognize when the clinical condition of the patient or the proposed procedure requires skills, facilities, or support beyond the capability of the anesthesiologist or institution; and
   c. Resuscitate neonates, infants, and children.
2. The specialist in pediatric anesthesiology after at least one year of subspecialty training shall be proficient in providing:
   a. Anesthesia care for neonates, infants and children undergoing all types of surgical, diagnostic, and therapeutic procedures; and
   b. Resuscitation, pain management, and routine and critical perioperative care for neonates, infants and children.

Thus, pediatric patients with an ASA status of 1 or 2 who require anesthesia for routine surgical, diagnostic, or therapeutic procedures that do not require special anesthesia techniques or intensive care during the perioperative period can be cared for by anesthesiologists whose training

---

* This study group consisted of an ad-hoc group of pediatric anesthesiologists whose membership included the leadership of the various committees and societies representing pediatric anesthesiology in formal anesthesiology organizations, the directors of pediatric anesthesia training programs, and the directors of pediatric anesthesia services in children's and university hospitals.

in pediatric anesthesia occurred during their anesthesiology residency.

Anesthesiologists with at least 1 year additional training in pediatric anesthesiology beyond their anesthesiology residency would have the competency and proficiency to care for pediatric patients with any degree of illness who require anesthesia.

HOW SHOULD ANESTHESIOLOGISTS BE TRAINED IN PEDIATRIC ANESTHESIA?

Training of the General Anesthesiologist in Pediatric Anesthesia

Requirements of the American Council on Graduate Medical Education (ACGME) for clinical competency of graduates of accredited anesthesiology residencies are the basis for the training of anesthesiologists in pediatric anesthesia. The *general aspects* of residency training in pediatric anesthesia are not different from those of all other areas of anesthesiology. Anesthesiologists in training must learn all aspects of perioperative anesthesia care through both didactic and clinical teaching. Graduates of accredited anesthesiology residencies are expected to be competent in the provision of anesthesia care for routine pediatric anesthesia cases, as noted in the Study Group definition of clinical competency for the general anesthesiologist. There is, however, a specific requirement for the minimum number of pediatric cases to be performed during the residency, as there is for other subspecialties. The ACGME anesthesiology residency program requirements state, "A minimum clinical experience in anesthesia for one hundred (100) children under the age of twelve, with the inclusion of anesthesia for fifteen (15) infants less than forty-five weeks post-conceptual age, is required."[18] Required clinical experience in other aspects of the practice of anesthesia during the residency (e.g., neuroanesthesia, cardiac anesthesia, and regional anesthesia) provides valuable experience that can be applied to pediatric anesthesia training.

Training of the Specialist in Pediatric Anesthesiology: The Fellowship Year

Fellowship training in pediatric anesthesiology provides the opportunity to achieve "proficiency" in anesthesia care of infants and children by focusing for 12 months or more on the care of pediatric patients with complicated medical problems. Thus, the focus is on patients with major birth defects and other medical problems that cause airway deformities (with their attendant metabolic and electrolyte abnormalities) that require surgical intervention. These patients often require pre- and/or postoperative intensive care.

As part of its work, The Study Group on Pediatric Anesthesia formed by the Society for Pediatric Anesthesia surveyed pediatric anesthesiology fellowship training programs with regard to the composition of their training programs. The concern of both groups was the absence of an agreed upon definition of the training and experience required to call oneself a pediatric anesthesiologist and the desire of both groups to come up with satisfactory definitions. The findings of this investigation indicated that there was no commonality concerning the length of the training program, the curriculum, the numbers and types of cases performed by a fellow, or the number or caliber of the faculty of the programs. As an example, some fellowship programs focused on the performance of the anesthesia management of infants with congenital heart disease. Other training programs focused on other types of surgical patients to the exclusion of the cardiac cases. Some fellowships were 3 months in length during the third year of an anesthesiology residency. Others were 2 years in length and began after completion of the anesthesiology residency. Although most fellowship programs took place in large pediatric environments, there were some that did not. Some training programs were based in free-standing children's hospitals that were not affiliated with an anesthesiology residency training program, but they were accredited by the American Council on Graduate Medical Education. The unaffiliated fellowship training programs were in danger of losing their accreditation by the ACGME even though they were recognized as outstanding teaching centers in pediatric anesthesia.

As a result of this information, the Society for Pediatric Anesthesia, the Section on Anesthesiology of the American Academy of Pediatrics, and the Study Group on Pediatric Anesthesia (with the support of the Committee on Pediatric Anesthesia of the American Society of Anesthesiology) jointly requested formal accreditation of fellowship training programs in pediatric anesthesiology. This application was approved in 1998. The ACGME indicated that

Accreditation of a subspecialty program in pediatric anesthesiology will be granted only when the program is associated with a core residency program in anesthesiology that is accredited by the ACGME. Therefore, subspecialty training in pediatric anesthesiology can occur only in an institution in which there is an ACGME-accredited residency program in anesthesiology or in an institution related to a core program by a formal agreement. The director of the core anesthesiology residency program is responsible for the appointment of the director of the pediatric anesthesiology subspecialty program and determines the activities of the appointee and the duration of the appointment.

Accredited fellowship training programs must provide a minimum of 1 year of clinical training. An established curriculum is required. The range of clinical cases must be broad, inclusive of all types of cases anticipated in practice, and have a case volume acceptable to the ACGME. Its faculty must be composed of pediatric anesthesiologists.[19]

WHERE SHOULD PEDIATRIC ANESTHESIA BE PRACTICED?

Until recently, little attention was paid to the perioperative environment in which surgery and anesthesia care for infants and children are provided. Standards exist for the care of pediatric patients receiving intensive care, but standards do not exist for the perioperative period. The lack of standards puts the anesthesiologist in an awkward position. No matter how extensive his or her training and experience is, he or she may be faced with the need to provide anesthesia care for a pediatric patient in circumstances that are not optimal. Work on this matter began in the San Francisco Bay Area Pediatric Anesthesia Consortium (BAYPAC). The results of their deliberations were carried forward by the Committee on Quality Assurance of the Section on Anesthesiology of the American Academy of Pediatrics with continual cooperation, comments, and endorsement by the Study Group on Pediatric Anesthesia and the Society for Pediatric Anesthesia. Comments were also received from the Committee on Pediatric Anesthesia of the American Society of Anesthesiologists. A document entitled "Guidelines for the Pediatric Perioperative Anesthesia Environment" was prepared and has been endorsed and published by the American Academy of Pediatrics.[20] This document also has been recognized by the Accreditation Association for Ambulatory Health Care (AAAHC) as an important resource document.[21]

The goal of the work of these committees is to ensure that anesthesiologists have the appropriate facilities and support to provide optimal care for pediatric patients during the perioperative period. The document clearly recognizes the importance of the entire patient care team and of the facilities in the provision of high-quality anesthesia care. It establishes minimum requirements for patient care facilities if pediatric anesthesia care is to be provided, and it provides recommendations for a hospital policy that considers case selection on the basis of the facilities available, the ability of the anesthesiologist, and the anesthesia risk. The document's recommendations for the patient care facility and medical staff are presented in Table 2–1. There are other recommendations for the patient care units; including the preoperative evaluation units, the operating room suite, health care providers (other than the anesthesiologist), clinical laboratory and radiology services, and pediatric anesthesia equipment and drugs.

THE EFFECT OF THE RECENT CHANGES IN THE PRACTICE AND TRAINING OF PEDIATRIC ANESTHESIA

What effect will this activity have on the practice of pediatric anesthesiology? We believe it will be beneficial. The differences between the general anesthesiologist and the pediatric anesthesiologist have been defined, and the cases each group is asked to perform are more clearly differentiated. This makes it easier for anesthesiologists who feel uncomfortable anesthetizing a sick infant in a given hospital or outpatient care facility to point out to the hospital administration what the guidelines are. It also makes it easier for hospital and outpatient care facility administrators to know what is required if they want pediatric surgery to be performed in their institution. Does it mean that a pediatric anesthesiologist will be required for every pediatric case? Definitely not! Pediatric patients constitutes approximately 25 percent of the total number

TABLE 2-1
PATIENT CARE FACILITY AND MEDICAL STAFF POLICIES—DESIGNATION OF OPERATIVE PROCEDURES/CATEGORIZATION OF PEDIATRIC PATIENTS UNDERGOING ANESTHESIA: THE ANNUAL MINIMUM CASE VOLUME TO MAINTAIN CLINICAL COMPETENCE

There should be a written policy designating and categorizing the types of pediatric operative, diagnostic, and therapeutic procedures requiring anesthesia on an elective and emergent basis, and indicating the minimum number of cases required in each category for the facility to maintain its clinical competence in their performance. This policy should be based on the capability of the patient care facility and its medical staff to care for pediatric patients requiring anesthesia. The categories should identify patients at increased anesthesia risk. They will be used to determine facility capability and whether or not anesthesiologists providing or directly supervising the anesthesia care for patients in a specific category will require special clinical privileges. The categories should include patient age, procedures for which postoperative intensive care is anticipated, and patients with special anesthesia risks based on coexisting medical conditions. Information available on anesthesia adverse outcomes suggests neonates are at higher risk than older infants, and, in turn, older infants are at greater risk than pediatric patients more than 2 years of age. The following age categories are recommended: 0 to 1 month, 1 to 6 months, 6 months to 2 years, and older than 2 years. Because of the anatomic, physiologic, and psychological differences between children and adults, further differentiation of pediatric age groups for patients older than 2 years is recommended.

Anesthesia care for pediatric patients should be provided or supervised by anesthesiologists with clinical privileges as noted below. The annual minimum case volume required to maintain clinical competence in each patient care category should be determined by the facility's department of anesthesia.

Clinical Privileges of Anesthesiologists
I. Regular Clinical Privileges
Anesthesiologists providing clinical care to pediatric patients should be graduates of an anesthesiology residency training program accredited by the Accreditation Council for Graduate Medical Education (ACGME) or its equivalent.

II. Special Clinical Privileges
In addition to the above requirement, anesthesiologists providing or directly supervising the anesthesia care of patients in the categories designated by the facility's department of anesthesia as being at increased anesthesia risk should be graduates of an ACGME pediatric anesthesiology fellowship training program or its equivalent, or have documented demonstrated historical and continuous competence in the care of such patients.

From Hackel A, Badgwell JM, Binding RR, et al: Guidelines for the pediatric perioperative anesthesia environment. American Academy of Pediatrics. Section on Anesthesiology. Pediatrics 103:512, 1999.)

of anesthesia cases performed in the United States each year. There are not enough pediatric anesthesiologists available to perform all of these cases, even if they wanted to. Does it mean that a pediatric anesthesiologist should be on the staff of every hospital or outpatient care facility in which anesthesia is performed for a pediatric patient? That really depends on the types of cases to be performed in an individual patient care facility, the capabilities of the facility, and the policy adopted by its department of anesthesia concerning anesthesiologist competence and capability. Clearly, there cannot be a pediatric anesthesiologist on the staff of every patient care facility that performs one pediatric anesthesia case or less a week. Nor can a small rural patient care facility have a full-time pediatric anesthesiologist on staff. The latter may perform only one or less cases involving anesthesia for pediatric patients each year. And what will be the result if a patient with a serious problem arrives at a hospital and the patient cannot be transferred because the condition of the patient is life threatening? How will care be provided and by whom? If there is no pediatric anesthesiologist on staff, what will be done? How does the average anesthesiologist maintain a modicum of ability to care for sick pediatric patients when they have little or no experience doing these cases anymore. These are real and serious problems for the future delivery of anesthesia care to sick infants and children. Each patient care facility and its department of anesthesia have to address these problems. State and national organizations have to address them as well. State government agencies in Florida and California are developing policies to address these issues and more will follow.

The answers have to be based on the provision of the best quality of anesthesia to infants and children within the confines of the many aspects of modern-day life. The present residency requirements in anesthesiology prepare the general anesthesiologist to provide pediatric anesthesia under emergency circumstances. As noted above, the residency training, the number of cases performed annually in a given age group or on specific types of cases, such as those requiring perioperative intensive care, may not be deemed adequate preparation for the performance of such cases on a regular basis. These factors will influence the policy determination of the patient care facility and its department of anesthesia on the provision of pediatric anesthesia care.

The regional, state, and national policies of referral for regional care in place for neonatal and pediatric intensive care can be models for perioperative pediatric anesthesia and surgical care. Initially, all infants and children requiring intensive care were transferred to a small defined group of regional centers. With time, as the concepts of intensive care spread and the delivery of neonatal and pediatric intensive care became more simplified, the number of regional intensive care centers increased. Their requirements changed. Neonatal and pediatric intensive care has become stratified, with a stepwise incremental increase in the patient care facility requirements. Now, "deregionalization" of neonatal and pediatric intensive care is occurring. With time, the same can occur with perioperative pediatric anesthesia care.

Demographic concepts used in the development of many aspects of modern life, such as the centralization of business and shopping centers, have to be incorporated into our thinking. Is it reasonable for every hospital, outpatient care facility, and even dental and surgical offices to have the capabilities required for the provision of perioperative pediatric anesthesia care? No matter how many cases are performed, and no matter what the perioperative environment is, is that what we want for our community and ourselves? Can we afford it? What value does our culture place on the delivery of the best patient care as compared to traveling an extra 30 minutes or 1 hour to obtain it?

The answers to the question of where and by whom anesthesia will be provided for pediatric patients will come at several levels. First, they will be based on the information and the logic available to us at the present time. That is the basis for the new policies that have been and are being developed. In time, the results of our present actions will be determined by measuring their outcome.

REFERENCES

1. Downes JJ: What is a paediatric anaesthesiologist? The American perspective. Paediatr Anaesth 5:277, 1995.
2. Directory of Fellowship Programs in Pediatric Anesthesia: Society for Pediatric Anesthesia, Richmond, Virginia, 1998.
3. Rackow H, Salanitre E, Green L: Frequency of cardiac arrest associated with anesthesia in infants and children. Pediatrics 28:697, 1961.
4. Cohen MM, Cameron CB, Duncan PG: Pediatric anesthesia morbidity and mortality in the perioperative period. Anesth Analg 70:160, 1990.
5. Morray JP, Geiduschek JM, Caplan RA, et al: A comparison of pediatric and adult anesthesia closed malpractice claims. Anesthesiology 78:461, 1993.
6. Campling EA, Devlin HB, Lunn JN: The Report of the National Confidential Enquiry into Perioperative Deaths 1989 (NCEPOD). London, UK, The Royal College of Surgeons of England, 1990.
7. Keenan RL, Shapiro JH, Dawson K: Frequency of anesthetic cardiac arrests in infants: effect of pediatric anesthesiologists. J Clin Anesth 3:433, 1991.
8. Lunn JN: Implications of the National Confidential Inquiry into Perioperative Deaths for paediatric anaesthesia. Paediatr Anaesth 2:69, 1992.
9. Audit Commission: Children First—A Study of Hospital Services. London, UK, HMSO, 1993.
10. The Report of the Joint Working Group: The Transfer of Infants and Children for Surgery. London, UK, British Paediatric Association, 1993.
11. Hannan EL, Racz M, Kavey RE, et al: Pediatric cardiac surgery: the effect of hospital and surgeon volume on in-hospital mortality. Pediatrics 101:963, 1998.
12. Jenkins KJ, Newburger JW, Lock JE, et al: In-hospital mortality for surgical repair of congenital heart defects: preliminary observations of variation by hospital caseload. Pediatrics 95:323, 1995.
13. Macario A, Hackel A, Gregory GA, Forseth D: Demographics of inpatient pediatric anesthesia: implications for performance-based credentialing. J Clin Anesthesiology 7:507, 1995.
14. Hoffman GM: Personal correspondence. A survey of the distribution of pediatric anesthesia cases among community and tertiary care patient care facilities in the State of Wisconsin. May 23, 1999.
15. Kain Z: Personal correspondence. An analysis of the distribution of pediatric anesthesia cases in a random survey of members of the American Society of Anesthesiologists participating in a survey on premedication of infants and children. May 23, 1999.
16. Viney J: Personal correspondence. A survey of the distribution of pediatric anesthesia cases among community and tertiary care patient care facilities in the State of Utah. May 23, 1999.
17. Minutes, Study Group on Pediatric Anesthesiology, October 16, 1994.
18. Program requirements for residency education in anesthesiology: Accreditation Council for Graduate Medical Education, Chicago, Illinois, 1995.
19. Program requirements for residency education in Pediatric Anesthesiology: Accreditation Council for Graduate Medical Education, Chicago, Illinois, 1997.
20. Hackel A, Badgwell JM, Binding RR, et al: Guidelines for the pediatric perioperative anesthesia environment. American Academy of Pediatrics. Section on Anesthesiology. Pediatrics 103:512, 1999.
21. 2000 Accreditation Handbook for Ambulatory Health Care: American Association for Ambulatory Health Care, Inc., Wilmette, Illinois, 2000.

3

Pharmacology

GEORGE A. GREGORY

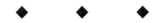

Inadequate knowledge of pediatric pharmacology has led to disasters such as the "gray baby" syndrome,[1] which occurred because physicians were unaware that low levels of glucuranyl transferase in neonates reduced their ability to remove chloramphenicol. Development of powerful analytic methods has enabled us to determine drug concentrations in small volumes of blood, to determine the appropriate dose of drug for each patient, and to reduce the potential for disasters.

Adverse drug reactions are common in neonates, especially in those who are premature.[2, 3] In one study, at least 30 percent of neonates had one or more acute drug reactions, and in 8 percent at least one of these reactions was life threatening. The incidence of these adverse reactions does not seem to be decreasing.

Aranda et al.[4] found that 27 percent of 1,200 patients admitted to the neonatal intensive care unit (ICU) had at least one acute drug reaction. These patients were less mature and were hospitalized longer; those born at less than 28 weeks' gestation had the most reactions. Neonates with respiratory distress syndrome, intraventricular hemorrhage, necrotizing enterocolitis, and neonatal apnea had more drug reactions than those without these problems, probably because they were in the hospital longer, and they required more drugs.

Premature neonates receive three to four times more drugs than older patients,[5] which probably accounts for many of these reactions, but the immaturity of their kidneys, livers, and immune systems also may be important factors.

This chapter discusses some of the differences between infants, children, and adults, and the ways in which these differences affect their responses to drugs. For the purposes of this chapter, a *neonate* is any newborn, premature or full-term, between birth and 1 month of age; an *infant* is between 1 and 12 months of age; and a *child* is between 1 year of age and puberty.

PHARMACOLOGY

Most drugs exert their effects by binding reversibly to receptors. The availability of the drug to the receptor depends on the concentration of drug in the fluid surrounding the receptor, which in turn depends on the plasma concentration of the drug. To reach its receptor, a drug must actively or passively cross several phospholipid membranes. Active movement requires energy; passive movement does not. The latter occurs when a concentration or an electrochemical gradient is established across the cell membrane. The rapidity with which these gradients develop depends on several factors. Lipid-soluble (lipophilic) drugs cross membranes more rapidly than lipophobic drugs. Small molecules cross more rapidly than large ones. Only nonionized lipid-soluble drugs cross lipid membranes by passive diffusion in significant quantities. Ionized molecules do so poorly, if at all. The degree of drug ionization depends on the dissociation constant (pKa) of the drug and on the local pH. Changes in pH most often affect drugs whose nonionized fraction can be reduced or increased at physiologic pH. At equilibrium, the nonionized fraction is identical on both sides of the membrane. Equilibrium is delayed or prevented when a drug diffuses from a small space to a large one or when the drug is rapidly removed from the inside of the membrane by rapid metabolism.

Drugs follow *first-order kinetics* when the rate of drug transfer is proportional to the amount of drug remaining in the plasma. A semilogarithmic plot of concentration versus time gives a straight line. *Zero-order kinetics* occurs when drug transfer across membranes is constant and is unrelated to concentration. *Facilitated diffusion* occurs when drugs that are normally too large to cross membranes can do so after combining with a carrier substance. No energy is required for facilitated diffusion. *Active transport* enables drugs to move across cell membranes against a concentration gradient, a process requiring metabolic energy. Changes in metabolism or temperature alter the rate of active transport. It is unknown whether the cell membranes of neonates differ from those of adults. Certainly, some drugs (e.g., barbiturates and narcotics) enter the central nervous system (CNS) of neonates more rapidly than in adults, possibly because the neonatal blood–brain barrier is more "porous." Increased entry of these drugs is not due to active transport.

ROUTES OF ADMINISTRATION

Oral Administration

The efficacy of orally administered drugs depends on the rate and extent of absorption from the gastrointestinal tract, on how well the drug dissolves in physiologic solutions, and on the physicochemical nature of the drug. It also depends on the composition of the membranes through which the drug must pass, the nature of the gastrointestinal juices, the rate of gastric emptying, the degree of gastrointestinal motility, and the amount of gut blood flow. Several of these factors are altered in young patients. At birth the gastric pH is usually 6 to 8, but it decreases to 1 to 2 within 24 hours.[6] This decrease in gastric pH is independent of age.[7] There is wide variability in the gastric pH over the first few months of life.[8] Some neonates are achlorhydric and others are not. By 6 weeks of age, all have a gastric pH of less than 4. Adult pH levels are present in all patients by 6 months to 3 years of age. Serum gastrin concentrations are elevated in term neonates for several days after birth,[9] but gastric acid secretion is less than expected.[10] Pentagastrin stimulation has minimal effects on gastric acid secretion for at least the first 2 days of life.[11] Achlorhydria develops after the first 24 hours of extrauterine life, and the gastric pH rises, gradually decreasing to adult levels by 3 years of age. Preterm infants secrete less gastric acid during the perinatal period than term infants, but stimulation with pentagastrin almost doubles gastric acid production after 1 week of age.[12] Basal acid concentration reaches that of term infants after 4 weeks, regardless of gestational age. The volume of bile acids may be reduced in neonates[13, 14] and may therefore reduce the rate and degree of absorption of lipid-soluble drugs. Liver disease may interfere with bile acid secretion and further reduce absorption of fat-soluble drugs.

Most drugs given orally are absorbed in the small intestine, and delayed gastric emptying delays drug absorption. The rate of gastric emptying varies during the neonatal period. The amount of 5 percent glucose and water retained in the stomach is inversely related to age.[15] Gastric emptying is slowed by increasing caloric density but not by osmolarity[16] in premature neonates. Long-chain fatty acids (as found in some neonatal formulas) delay gastric emptying; short-chain fatty acids do not. This should be considered when premature neonates are designated NPO (nothing by mouth).

Some drugs used to premedicate infants affect the pH and volume of gastric juice in children.[17] Neither premedication with morphine sulfate or pentobarbital nor the inclusion of atropine or scopolamine with these drugs alters the volume of gastric fluid.[18] Glycopyrrolate (Robinul) reduced the gastric fluid volume by one third and increased the pH of 68 percent of gastric samples to above 2.5; atropine increased the pH of the gastric fluid in 32 percent of patients. Sixty percent of the bile-stained samples had a pH below 2.5. Therefore, we cannot assume that the pH of gastric fluid is "safe" if the fluid is bile stained. Because these studies were done by inserting a nasogastric tube and collecting gastric fluid, the volumes of gastric fluid were probably greater than those measured by dilution of a marker substance.

Only weakly acidic or alkaline lipid-soluble drugs that are nonionized at physiologic pH are absorbed in the stomach and small bowel. Highly ionized strong acids are poorly absorbed; moderately strong acids (e.g., aspirin) are well absorbed. Drugs are usually better absorbed from the upper gastrointestinal tract, owing to its larger surface area.

Intramuscular and Subcutaneous Drug Administration

Drug administration by the intramuscular (IM) or subcutaneous (SC) route ensures that the patient receives the prescribed amount of drug. However, drug availability to the receptor still depends on drug uptake from the administration site and delivery to the receptor. Drugs given by either route are rapidly absorbed if the drugs are stable in aqueous solution and are lipophilic. Absorption of poorly soluble acids or bases may be delayed, and drugs with a high or low pH may precipitate at normal tissue pH levels. Drugs with high pH levels often cause pain (midazolam, pentobarbital), tissue necrosis, and sterile abscesses when injected intramuscularly.

Capillary perfusion alters the absorption of drugs given IM or SC. Peripheral vasoconstriction (e.g., associated with shock, hypothermia, or acidosis) delays drug uptake. Arterial blood pressure and tissue perfusion are low at birth and increase during the first 2 weeks of life, which increase the rapidity of drug uptake from deposition sites.[19] The rate and the amount of drug absorption also depend on the surface area of absorptive tissue available, which is reduced in neonates, infants, and small children. The site of injection also is important. Drugs injected in the lower extremity are absorbed more slowly than those injected into an upper extremity.[20] Drugs injected into the tongue are absorbed most rapidly of all.[21]

Percutaneous Drug Absorption

Percutaneous absorption of drugs is inversely related to the thickness of the stratum corneum and is directly related to skin hydration.[22] Neonates have a larger ratio of surface area to body weight. Therefore, if the same amount of drug is applied to the skin, a neonate will absorb about 2.7 times more drug per kilogram of body weight.[23] More drug is absorbed in patients with dehydrated skin.[24] The advent of transdermal drugs has increased the potential for drug overdoses in neonates. The use of transdermal drugs has made possible the use of lidocaine 2.5 percent and prilocaine 2.5 percent (EMLA) to prevent pain with needlesticks or starting an intravenous line.[25] However, the drug mixture (lidocaine 2.5 percent and prilocaine 2.5 percent) must be applied for approximately 1 hour before the painful procedure is done to ensure that needlesticks will be painless. Transdermal drugs, such as clonidine and fentanyl, are also being used to treat acute and chronic pain.[26]

INTRAVENOUS DRUG ADMINISTRATION

Intravenous (IV) drug administration avoids the problems of uptake and is the preferred route of administration for most drugs given in the operating room, postanesthesia care unit, and ICU. Intravenous drugs usually should be infused slowly, and the patient's vital signs should be monitored carefully for adverse effects (e.g., hypotension, cardiorespiratory arrest, anaphylactic reactions).

Some drugs injected into the IV tubing or bottles may be lost because the drug is adsorbed to the glass or plastic infusion system or to the filtration system.[27] Furthermore, drug may be lost when the tubing is changed. When the flow rate of fluid is slow, large amounts of drug may adhere to the tubing. Even when drug is not lost, its effect may be delayed by several hours if the IV rate is very slow. This may lead to incorrect conclusions about the patient's need for more or less drug and may lead to the administration of a drug overdose in infants. Drugs must be injected in a standard way to ensure that peak and trough levels are obtained at the appropriate times.[28]

Rectal Drug Administration

Drugs are often administered to pediatric patients per rectum to avoid IM or SC injection. However, care should be taken to avoid this route of administration in patients on chemotherapy or patients who have immune defficiency. Problems of residual drug in the stomach (as occurs with barbiturates and diazepam) and aspiration of gastric contents during the induction of anesthesia are reduced by rectal administration of drugs. Drugs can be administered per rectum to patients who have nausea and vomiting or diseases of the upper gastrointestinal tract. Most drugs readily cross the rectal mucosa, but because the surface area of the rectal mucosa is small, absorption of rectally administered drugs is often slow and erratic.

The rectum is usually an empty, flat organ lined with predominantly columnar or cuboidal epithelium. Its main blood supply is derived from the inferior rectal arteries, which originate from the pudendal and middle rectal arteries. The inferior rectal vein drains the anal canal below the anorectal line, including the hemorrhoidal plexus. The rectal columns drain into the middle and inferior rectal veins, and the inferior and middle rectal veins drain into the inferior vena cava, bypassing the liver and avoiding first-pass metabolism of the drug. The superior rectal veins drain into the portal vein, and drugs absorbed by these veins are subject to first-pass metabolism. There are, however, significant anastomoses among these veins. The variable uptake of drugs from the rectum may be related in part to the amount of drug absorbed by each portion of the rectal venous system. The blood supply and other factors affecting drug absorption from the rectum have been reviewed elsewhere.[29]

Some drugs are well absorbed from the rectum and sigmoid colon, but their absorption can be erratic. The onset of sleep varies from 4 to 22 minutes in patients premedicated for surgery with rectal barbiturates, owing in part to the location at which the drug is deposited in the bowel. Drugs deposited below the dentate line have no first-pass effect because they enter the iliac veins and are circulated to the brain and heart before they reach the liver. Drugs deposited above the dentate line enter the hepatic circulation before they reach the central circulation. Therefore, some of the drug is metabolized, which delays the onset of sedation.

Uptake of drugs from the rectum is also affected by whether the drugs are given in the form of suppositories, rectal capsules, or enemas. Metabolism of drugs by the gut wall and by microorganisms in the rectal lumen also can reduce drug uptake from the rectum.[30]

Several drugs used for premedication are commonly given per rectum to infants and children, including thiopentone (Pentothal), methohexitone (methohexital [Brevital], diazepam [Valium]), and atropine. Rectal methohexital 18 to 25 mg/kg is used to induce sleep before infants and children are taken to the operating room.[31, 32] Goresky and Steward[33] recommended giving 22 to 31 mg/kg. Liu et al.[34] reported that 93 percent of unpremedicated children fell asleep with 30 mg/kg of rectal methohexitone. Evidence suggests that a more dilute 1 or 2 percent solution of 25 mg/kg methohexital is superior to the same dose in higher concentrations.[35] Loss of consciousness after rectal methohexital administration is correlated with the plasma concentration of the drug.[36, 37] In healthy patients, there are no significant effects of methohexital on cardiovascular variables[38] or oxygen saturation.[39]

Rectal methohexital does not delay discharge from the recovery room after surgery.[33] High concentrations of rectal methohexital are associated with proctitis.[40] Methohexital has been associated with apnea in patients with meningomyelocele.[41]

Rectal thiopentone has been used successfully as an aqueous suspension.[42] Its onset of action is rapid, but recovery from anesthesia is delayed. Consequently, methohexital is usually used for premedication.

Diazepam 0.75 mg/kg (maximum 20 mg) also has been given rectally to sedate children preoperatively.[43] Although most children were awake and calm during anesthesia induction, two thirds were agitated (crying) during awakening from anesthesia. This agitation was significantly reduced by giving 0.25 ml/kg of a lytic cocktail (28 mg meperidine, 7 mg chlorpromazine, and 7 mg promethazine per milliliter of cocktail) either as premedication (30 minutes before administering the diazepam) or after induction of anesthesia. Adding morphine 0.15 mg/kg and hyoscine 0.01 mg/kg to the rectal diazepam[44] also reduced agitation on awakening.

Atropine can be given rectally to premedicate children for surgery,[45] but larger doses are usually required to achieve the same effects seen in adults.[46] When given rectally, the maximal concentration of atropine in the blood is less in patients weighing less than 15 kg than it is in larger patients,[47] and the plasma concentration of atropine decreases much more rapidly in smaller patients. The plasma atropine concentration was about 0.1 ng/ml compared with about 0.5 ng/ml in larger patients 240 minutes after the drug was administered. Whether this difference is caused by differences in kinetics or by a first-pass effect is unclear. The maximal depression of salivation occurs later than the maximal effect on heart rate and later than the maximal plasma concentrations of atropine.

Acetaminophen has been used rectally to treat the postoperative pain of infants and children,[48] primarily to avoid administering narcotics to premature infants and to children who are to be discharged home shortly after surgery. Progressively larger doses of rectally administered acetaminophen have been used over the years. The average dose today is about 40 mg/kg. In children, the absorption half-life is about 35 minutes and the clearance is 13.5 L/h.[49] This compares with an absorption half-life of 4.5 minutes from the stomach. The relative bioavailability by the rectal route was 0.54 compared to the oral route. A blood concentration of 10 mg/L was required to give a pain score of 3.6 out of 10. When acetaminophen is given to children after a tonsillectomy, 60 mg/kg/day orally or 90 mg/kg/day rectally, 22 to 73 percent of children rated their pain as severe.[48] Clearly this dose of drug was insufficient. The pharmocokinetics of rectal acetaminophen have been studied in infants and children.[49, 50]

UPTAKE AND DISTRIBUTION

Distribution

Before drugs can exert their effect, they must be removed from the site of administration and distributed to the effector site. Both removal and distribution depend on cardiac output, tissue perfusion, and the blood–tissue partition coefficient of the drug.[51] At equilibrium, drugs are distributed into their *apparent volume of distribution*. V_d is the volume of fluid and tissue into which a drug appears to distribute with concentrations equal to those in plasma. V_d assumes that the body is a single compartment with respect to the drug. This is not an anatomic compartment or space and is often much larger (0.5 to 500 L) than true body water spaces. (V_d is often larger in neonates due to increased total body water). V_d is the product of a drug's tissue plasma partition coefficient and the tissue volume. Highly protein-bound and extremely water-soluble drugs (e.g., salicylates, penicillin) usually have low V_d values. The V_d of bases is usually large.

Protein Binding

Drugs bind to proteins to various degrees, which reduces their effect, diminishes their penetration into cells, and delays their clearance from plasma. Only unbound drug diffuses through membranes, is available for binding to receptors, and exerts a pharmacologic action.

The protein-bound fraction is a reservoir that helps maintain the concentration of free drug in plasma and tissues. Caffeine and digoxin[52] are highly protein bound and their concentration in tissues, such as the heart, is greater than in plasma. Barbiturates,[53] lidocaine (Xylocaine),[54] and theophylline[55] are less highly bound. Diazepam is poorly bound.[56] When all plasma protein-binding sites are occupied, addition of more drug increases the unbound fraction (salicylates), making more drug available to the tissues. The latter can be a problem when the serum albumin concentration is low, as it is in neonates and sick young patients, or when other compounds occupy the binding sites (e.g., bilirubin, sulfa).[57]

Protein binding is usually determined in vitro, but in vitro studies may give a false picture of how drugs distribute in the body. For example, the V_d in the test tube is limited, but it may be very large in vivo. Binding can also be affected by cerebral blood flow. Decreasing cerebral blood flow increases the extraction of some drugs (e.g., phenytoin [Dilantin], phenobarbital) from plasma because more time is available for drugs to dissociate from protein when the blood flow is slower.[58] This could account for some of the increased drug accumulation in the neonatal brain (see below).

Several factors affect protein binding in neonates. First, they have low serum albumin concentrations, which increase to adult levels by 5 months of age (Table 3–1).[59] Second, their albumin has a lower binding capacity and affinity for drugs.[60, 61] Third, several substances commonly found in the plasma of neonates reduce protein binding of drugs (free fatty acids, bilirubin, maternal steroids, and drugs such as sulfonamides).

α_1-Acid glycoprotein is present in plasma in much smaller concentrations than albumin and binds basic drugs, including many of interest to anesthesiologists.[62] *d*-Tubocurarine, metocurine, propranolol, and lidocaine are all less highly bound to α_1-acid glycoprotein in children than in adults; diazepam is more highly bound in children than in pregnant women and less highly bound than in nonpregnant women or in men. There is a strong correlation between the amount of unbound drug and the plasma concentration of α_1-acid glycoprotein. Infants have very low concentrations of this protein. Because albumin accounts for only a small fraction of drug binding,[63] reduced

T A B L E   3 – 1
PROTEIN BINDING IN NEONATES AND ADULTS

Drug	% Bound Neonate	% Bound Adult
Ampicillin	9–11	15–29
Digoxin	14–26	23–40
Diazepam	84	94–98
Phenytoin	75–84	89–92
Phenobarbitone	28–36	46–48
Pentobarbitone	37–40	39–45

From Morselli PL: Clinical pharmacokinetics in neonates. Clin Pharmacokinet 1:81, 1976, with permission.

amounts of α_1-acid glycoprotein are probably responsible for a significant proportion of unbound drug.

Many drugs have reduced plasma binding, increased concentration of free drug, and increased V_d. Among these are salicylates,[64] ampicillin, nafcillin (Nafcil), pentobarbital, bupivacaine, lidocaine,[54] diazepam,[56] and phenobarbital.[53] Reduced plasma protein binding increases the apparent V_d and the amount of free (active) drug in the tissues of neonates. For example, twice as much morphine and barbiturate accumulate in the CNS of neonates compared with adults because binding of these drugs to plasma proteins is reduced in neonates and because the neonatal blood–brain barrier less effectively prevents substances from reaching the brain. Although both drugs are highly lipid soluble, less meperidine than morphine accumulates in the CNS of neonates, even though the lipid solubility of meperidine exceeds that of morphine. The combination of reduced CNS uptake and reduced CNS sensitivity to meperidine produces one tenth the respiratory depression and considerably less sedation than occurs with morphine in neonates.[65] Meperidine's activity also may be less because the opioid receptors of the brain are more primitive and do not recognize structural analogues.

METABOLISM

Enzymes that oxidize, reduce, and hydrolyze drugs (phase I reactions) are present in the endoplasmic reticulum of the liver, kidney, and gastrointestinal cells and in the plasma early in fetal life, but these enzymes are relatively inactive.[66] They convert drugs to water-soluble, nonpolar, excretable compounds. Parent compounds may also be converted into active substances (e.g., theophylline to caffeine). Conjugation (phase II reactions) is accomplished with acetate, glycine, sulfate, and glucuronic acids. Some of these pathways are less active in neonates (glucuronidation), and others are active (sulfonation).

Drug clearance is expressed as blood flow times the difference in the amount of drug entering and leaving the liver:

$$Q\ (Ca–Cv)$$

where Q is liver blood flow and Ca and Cv are the arterial and venous drug concentrations, respectively. Only unbound drug is cleared. Drugs with high extraction ratios are almost completely removed before blood leaves the liver, and their metabolism is limited by hepatic blood flow. Drugs with low extraction ratios are unaffected by liver blood flow or diffusion of the compound to the site of metabolism. Drugs with very low extraction ratios have little hepatic clearance. When all enzyme sites are occupied, the rate of drug metabolism becomes maximal, constant (zero order), and independent of drug dose.

The microsomal endoplasmic reticulum of the liver catalyzes many drug reactions, usually by oxidation (cytochrome P-450) but also by reduction and conjugation. Both phase I (cytochrome P-450–dependent, mixed-function oxidases) and phase II (conjugation) reactions are decreased in the neonate but can be induced by barbiturates. Some reactions, such as glucuronidation,

may be reduced in neonates but compensated for by others, such as sulfonation. Neonates can demethylate diazepam[67] and mepivacaine (Carbocaine),[68] but they hydroxylate these agents poorly, which prolongs the elimination half-lives of these drugs. The ability of neonates to conjugate salicylic acid with glucuronide is reduced, but their ability to conjugate salicylic acid with glycine is equal to that of adults.[69] Development of these enzyme systems and the ability to metabolize drugs is a function of postnatal rather than gestational age. Development also may depend on the mother's exposure to drugs during pregnancy. Fetal exposure to drugs may increase metabolism of some drugs and may account for some of the variability in drug metabolism in the neonatal period.

These differences in metabolism alter the way in which neonates and infants reduce the plasma concentration of drugs. For example, neonates hydroxylate and N-demethylate diazepam less well than adults or children do, which prolongs the elimination half-life of diazepam (75 ± 38 hours in preterm infants, 31 ± 2 hours in term neonates, and 18 ± 3 hours in children) and prolongs its effect.[67] If the hydroxylating enzymes of neonates are induced with phenobarbital, the half-life of diazepam is reduced to that of children.

Theophylline is demethylated. The activity of this phase I pathway is also reduced during the neonatal period, which prolongs the elimination half-life of theophylline in neonates (30 hours in preterm neonates, 17 hours in term neonates, 3 hours in children, and 5 hours in adults).[70] Phase I enzymes function at adult levels by 6 months of age.

Some phase II pathways are mature at birth (sulfonation), and some are not (acetylation, glycination, glucuronidation). All are mature by 1 year of age.[71]

Salicylate, although seldom given to children nowadays, is an example of a drug that is metabolized differently by neonates, but its elimination half-life is less prolonged than might be expected because of functioning parallel metabolic pathways. The glucuronide pathway accounts for 34 percent of this drug's metabolism in adults, but this pathway accounts for less than 10 percent of salicylate metabolism in neonates. However, the glycine pathway accounts for 74 percent of salicylate metabolism in neonates and only 49 percent in adults. The gentisic acid pathway accounts for 12 percent of the drug's metabolism in neonates and 4 percent in adults. Because of these parallel pathways, the elimination half-life of salicylate is only slightly longer in neonates than in adults (4 to 11 hours vs. 2 to 3 hours).[69]

Acetaminophen is conjugated with both glucuronic acid and sulfate.[72] The former pathway is reduced in neonates; the latter is not. Consequently, the elimination half-life of the drug is similar in neonates and adults (3.5 hours).

EXCRETION

The adult kidney receives 20 to 25 percent of the total cardiac output, whereas the kidney of the neonate receives only 5 to 6 percent (see Chapter 21). Only 2 to 3 percent of renal blood flow is filtered by the glomeruli. Less than 1 percent of the filtrate appears in the urine.

The neonate's glomerular filtration rate is lower than that of the adult.[73] Infants born before 34 weeks' gestation have reduced glomerular filtration rates and decreased tubular resorption of water, bicarbonate, glucose, and salt.[74] After 34 weeks' gestation, the neonate's renal function is more mature, although less mature than that of adults.[75] Immature renal function impedes the ability of infants to remove drugs that depend on renal excretion. In addition, renal drug clearance is affected by the *renal extraction ratio* (the amount of drug removed from the renal capillaries per unit time) and by glomerular pore size. Pore size increases with age. When the extraction ratio is low (0 to 0.2), clearance is sensitive to changes in protein binding. When it is high (0.9 to 1.0), clearance is affected by renal flow but not by protein binding or partitioning of drug into blood cells. In most instances, the *extraction rate* is directly related to the drug's plasma concentration (extraction rate = renal clearance × plasma concentration). Clearance can be greater than, less than, or equal to the glomerular filtration rate. When the clearance of a drug is constant, its excretion rate is directly proportional to its plasma concentration. The solute load and pH of the filtrate are the same as those of plasma, and the protein content is lower. Drugs also are cleared by renal tubular secretion.

Despite adequate glomerular and tubular secretion, renal clearance of many drugs is low because of resorption by the renal tubules. The amount of resorption depends on the lipid solubility of the drug and on its concentration in the tubular fluid. As water is absorbed from the tubule, the drug concentration in tubular fluid increases and establishes a concentration gradient that favors drug resorption. The pH of blood and renal fluid affects renal clearance of a drug to the extent that its clearance is pKa dependent. Drugs that are strong acids (pKa < 2) exist in urine primarily in their ionized form and are poorly resorbed, regardless of their concentration in tubular fluid or of blood pH. Renal clearance is high. Weak acids (of pKa > 7 [e.g., barbital]) are sufficiently nonionized over the entire physiologic pH range and are almost entirely resorbed by the renal tubules. Resorption of drugs with a pKa between 3.0 and 7.5 is sensitive to changes in pH, and their renal clearance is greatly affected by pH. The same is true of weak bases (pKa < 6). They are resorbed at all tubular fluid pHs; those with a pKa of 6 to 12 are sensitive to changes in pH, and those with a pKa above 17 are little affected by the pH of tubular fluid. Renal insufficiency or immaturity alters the renal clearance of drugs and may necessitate a reduction in the drug dose, a longer interval between doses, or both.

The glomerular filtration rate (GFR) of term infants is approximately 40 percent that of adults and is proportional to gestational age.[75-77] That of preterm neonates is only 20 to 30 percent that of adults (per 1.73 m^2). GFR increases significantly during the first week of life as arterial blood pressure and renal perfusion increase, but tubular secretion reaches adult levels at approximately 1 year of age.

GFR, tubular secretion, and tubular resorption of compounds mature at different rates. Term neonates have a full complement of glomeruli; preterm neonates do not. The renal blood flow of both groups is low at birth, increases over the first week of life, and increases further during the first year of life. The slightly acidic urine at birth (pH 6.0 to 6.5) decreases the elimination of weak acids (see above).

If the kidney is the primary route of a drug's elimination, the neonate's reduced renal function delays the drug's elimination (e.g., natural and synthetic penicillins).[77] Aminoglycosides are removed more slowly after birth because their elimination depends on glomerular filtration. The aminoglycoside dose must be adjusted as GFR increases over the first week of life.

PHARMACOKINETICS

Drugs administered IV are simultaneously diluted by blood and taken up by tissues. Initial drug uptake occurs primarily in well-perfused tissues (e.g., heart, brain, liver, and kidney) and later in less well-perfused tissues. For example, thiopental, a highly lipid-soluble compound, rapidly equilibrates with the brain and produces sleep. However, despite thiopental's slow metabolism, adults awaken within 10 to 20 minutes after receiving the drug because it is redistributed from the brain to less well-perfused tissues. Little drug is redistributed to fat, despite thiopental's high liposolubility, because blood flow to fat is low. Less thiopental is apportioned to fat and muscle in neonates owing to their low body fat and muscle content. Consequently, the concentration of drugs in the CNS may remain high for a longer time and delay awakening.

The initial drug distribution phase is followed by an elimination phase ($t_{1/2\beta}$), during which the plasma and total body drug concentrations decline exponentially. Kinetics are usually first order during this phase. If the drug dose at time zero and the *elimination rate constant* (K_d) are known, the amount of drug present in the body at any given time can be calculated. K_d is determined from the slope of a semilogarithmic plot of the declining plasma concentration of drug. K_d also is used to determine the *plasma half-life* of drugs ($t_{1/2} = 0.693\ K_d$) (Table 3–2). In asphyxiated neonates, the volume of distribution of thiopental was 66 ml/h/kg and the clearance was 36 (29 to 70) hours. Eight of 10 infants required vasopressors to maintain their arterial blood pressures in a normal range.[78]

T A B L E　3 – 2
PLASMA HALF-LIVES OF DRUGS DEPENDENT ON OXIDATION FOR ELIMINATION

Drug	Half-life (h)	
	Newborn	Adult
Amylbarbitone	17–60	12–27
Bupivacaine	25	1.3
Caffeine	95	4
Diazepam	25–100	15–25
Indomethacin	14–20	2–11
Mepivacaine	8.7	3.2
Meperidine	22	3–4
Phenytoin	21	11–29
Theophylline	24–36	3–9

From Rane A: Basic principles of drug disposition and action in infants and children. *In* Yaffee SJ (ed): Pediatric Pharmacology: Therapeutic Principles in Practice. New York, Grune & Stratton, 1980, p 15, with permission.

Drug clearance is defined as the volume of drug removed by metabolism or excretion per unit of time. The *rate of elimination* (Cl) is equal to the product of the elimination rate constant and the plasma concentration of drug:

$$Cl = K_d \times V_d$$

or

$$Cl = 0.693 \, V_d/t_{1/2}$$

V_d can be calculated if clearance and $t_{1/2}$ are known. Maximal clearance usually is related to the sum of the blood flows to both the liver and kidneys. Clearance also can be determined by dividing the bolus dose of a drug by the total area under its plasma concentration curve (AUC) between zero time and the time no drug remains in the body

$$Cl = dose/AUC$$

where AUC is the area under the curve (Fig. 3–1).

Some drugs (e.g., isoproterenol, dopamine, aminophylline, fentanyl) are best infused continuously to avoid the peaks and troughs of drug concentration seen after bolus drug injections. Constant infusion of a drug increases its plasma concentration until the concentration reaches a plateau (i.e., when the rate of drug infusion equals its rate of elimination). Because clearance is constant under these conditions, doubling the drug infusion rate doubles its plasma level. In three half-lives (*half-life* is the time required for a 63 percent change in drug concentration), the plasma concentration of a constantly infused drug reaches 88 percent of its plateau level. In four half-lives it reaches 94 percent of the level.

When a given plasma concentration of drug must be attained quickly, a bolus of drug is administered and the drug is infused continuously. The bolus size is usually based on the average therapeutic dose of the drug and the infusion rate is determined by the formula

$$K_d \times D_o \ (D_o = 0.63/t_{1/2})$$

where D_o is the dose. This formula enables one to rapidly reach and maintain constant blood levels of aminophylline, antibiotics, and muscle relaxants in infants and children.

Drug dosages must be altered for patients with renal or liver disease because V_d often is increased. When V_d is increased, the initial dose of drug (loading dose) must be larger to obtain the desired effect. Giving a larger dose increases the store of drug in the body and prolongs the drug's half-life. The only way to determine that appropriate plasma levels of drug are present in these patients is to measure the levels. Curare, for example, has a prolonged half-life in neonates because they have increased extracellular fluid volume and decreased renal function (see below).

The desired plasma concentration of a drug at steady state (Cp_{ss}) can be calculated for patients with renal disease by the formula

$$Cp_{ss} = F \times dose/Cl \times T$$

where F is the fraction of drug absorbed (F = 1 for drugs given IV), Cl is the clearance of the drug (as determined from several blood levels of drug obtained several hours apart), and T is the interval between doses. Renal impairment reduces clearance. By rearranging the equation, the time between doses can be calculated.

INHALED DRUGS

The uptake of inhaled drugs is affected by inspired anesthetic concentration (F_I), alveolar ventilation, blood/gas

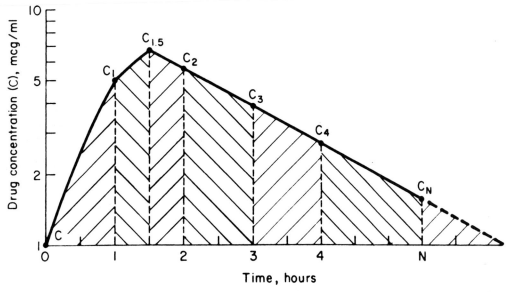

FIGURE 3–1. Typical serum concentration data needed for area under the curve. (From Rane A: Basic principles of drug disposition and action in infants and children. *In* Yaffee SJ [ed]: Pediatric Pharmacology: Therapeutic Principles in Practice. New York, Grune & Stratton, 1980, p 15, with permission.)

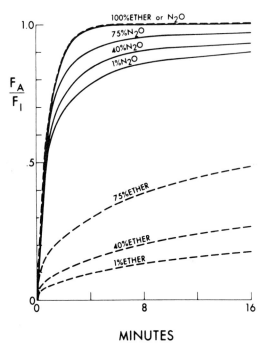

FIGURE 3–2. Relation between anesthetic concentration and anesthetic solubility or the ratio of the rate of rise of the alveolar concentration (F_A) to the inspired anesthetic concentration (F_I). (From Eger EI II: Anesthetic Uptake and Action. Baltimore, Williams & Wilkins, 1974.)

partition coefficient (λ), and cardiac output and its distribution. All affect the rate at which end-tidal anesthetic concentration (F_E) rises towards inspired concentration (F_E/F_I).[79, 80] F_E/F_I is a measure of how rapidly gas equilibrates between lung and blood. Drugs that are poorly soluble in blood and tissue (nitrous oxide, cyclopropane, desflurane [Suprane]), sevoflurane [Ultane]) rapidly equilibrate. Those that are more soluble (halothane [Fluothane], isoflurane [Forane], enflurane [Ethrane]) equilibrate more slowly (Fig. 3–2). When the tissues are fully saturated with drug (which takes several days in adults), end-tidal and inspired anesthetic concentrations are equal.

The body can be divided into several compartments on the basis of blood flow. The vessel-rich group (VRG) is composed of the brain, heart, and viscera; the muscle group (MG) is composed of all striated muscle except the heart; the fat group (FG) includes all adipose tissues; and the vessel-poor group (VPG) is made up of bone, tendons, and other poorly perfused tissues. Table 3–3 shows the

TABLE 3 – 3
TISSUE VOLUMES

Age Group	% of Total Body Volume		
	Vessel-Rich Group	Muscle Group	Fat Group
Newborn	22.0	38.7	13.2
1 Year	17.3	38.7	25.4
4 Years	16.6	40.7	23.4
8 Years	13.2	44.8	21.4
Adult	10.2	50.0	22.4

From Eger EI II, Bahlman SH, Munson ES: The effect of age on the rate of increase of alveolar anesthetic concentration. Anesthesiology 35:365, 1971, with permission.

distribution of these tissues in the body. Proportionately, the VRG is larger and the MG and FG are smaller in neonates than in adults.

The inspired anesthetic concentration affects the rate at which F_E/F_I rises (Fig. 3–3). The higher the inspired concentration, the more quickly F_E rises towards F_I (concentration effect), because more drug is removed from the lung. This decreases lung volume and increases the alveolar gas concentration. Less anesthetic is removed when the anesthetic concentration is low. Furthermore, removal of large volumes of gas from the lung causes more gas to be "drawn" into the lung to offset the "negative pressure" created by the uptake of gas. The gas "drawn" in has a high anesthetic concentration. The magnitude of the concentration effect is greater with more soluble gases.

Changes in ventilation alter the rate at which F_E rises toward F_I (Fig. 3–3). The greater the minute ventilation, the more rapidly the rise occurs (assuming a constant cardiac output). The more soluble the gas, the greater its effect of ventilation. The ratio of F_E/F_I also is affected by tidal volume and functional residual capacity (FRC). The smaller the FRC, the faster F_E/F_I increases (cardiac output constant). The FRC of infants is smaller than that of adults, but their tidal volume per kilogram body weight is the same as that of adults.[81] Figure 3–4 shows the rapidity with which an insoluble gas (helium) is washed into the lungs of a neonate.

Right-to-left shunting of blood through the lung increases F_E/F_I because each breath removes less gas than occurs when the circulation is normal. Induction of anesthesia is slowed because the blood concentration of the anesthetic rises more slowly. Neonates, infants, and chil-

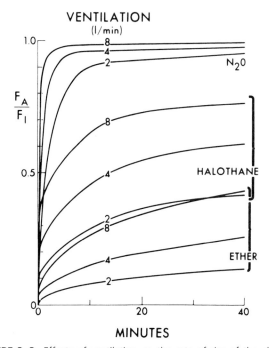

FIGURE 3–3. Effects of ventilation on the rate of rise of the alveolar concentration (F_A) relative to the inspired anesthetic concentration (F_I). (From Eger EI II: Anesthetic Uptake and Action. Baltimore, Williams & Wilkins, 1974.)

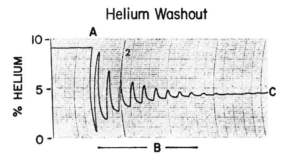

Helium Washout

FIGURE 3–4. Washout of helium in a term infant. Note that equilibrium occurs within 10 breaths.

dren often have right-to-left shunting of blood (see Chapter 18).

Anesthetic solubility in blood also affects the rate at which F_E/F_I rises. The F_E/F_I of an insoluble gas, such as nitrous oxide, increases rapidly. That of more soluble gases, such as halothane, increases more slowly. The blood/gas partition coefficients of halothane, enflurane, and isoflurane are 18 percent lower (12 percent for methoxyflurane) in neonates than in young adults (20 to 40 years); in children (1 to 7 years) the coefficients are 12 percent lower than in young adults.[82-84] This difference is due in part to lower blood albumin concentrations, which accounts for the more rapid rise of F_E/F_I in neonates. However, this also reduces the rate of rise of anesthetic in tissue.

Anesthetic solubility in brain, heart, and liver increases by approximately 50 percent between the newborn period and middle age.[85] This change is probably due to a decrease in water content and an increase in lipid content with increasing age.[86]

The solubility of inhaled anesthetics in muscles increases linearly with age, probably due to an increase in the protein concentration of muscle during the first 5 decades of life and an increase in fat content during subsequent decades.[87]

The rate of increase in the partial pressure of anesthetics in tissue is approximately 30 percent more rapid in neonates than in adults, which partially explains the more rapid rise of F_E/F_I in neonates. Because the blood flow per unit tissue mass is greater in neonates, tissue, blood, and alveolar anesthetic partial pressure increase more rapidly in neonates, and the onset of anesthesia is rapid. During anesthesia, the blood/gas partition coefficient decreases by approximately 10 percent due to hemodilution with crystalloid and reduction in hematocrit.[87]

Despite its lower solubility in the blood of infants, the concentration of halothane in the blood of neonates and adults is similar (17.1 vs. 18.5 mg/dl) at minimum anesthetic concentration (MAC). Therefore, neonates require higher end-tidal halothane concentrations to attain the same blood halothane concentration as adults. Cook and co-workers[88] found lower concentrations of halothane in the brains of 15-day-old rats compared with older animals, even though younger animals had a higher median effective dose for halothane (ED_{50}). This difference disappeared when they corrected for the higher brain water content of younger animals. They concluded that younger animals require the same concentration of halothane per gram of dry brain tissue to produce anesthesia and that a higher

partial pressure of drug is needed to reach this concentration. Increased cardiac output reduces the rate of rise of the alveolar concentration of anesthetic because more anesthetic is removed from the alveolus per unit of time. The cardiac output of neonates per kilogram is normally twice that of adults (see Chapter 18).[89] Distribution of blood among tissues affects the rate at which F_E rises towards F_I. Directing more blood to the VRG and less to other tissues (as occurs in young pediatric patients) saturates the VRG with anesthetic sooner, and less drug is extracted from the blood. The anesthetic concentration of pulmonary arterial blood is higher, which reduces the anesthetic gradient between blood and alveoli and increases the alveolar anesthetic concentration more quickly. Because much of the infant's cardiac output is directed to the VRG, F_E/F_I rises more rapidly.

Congenital heart disease also affects the uptake of inhaled anesthetics. When there is a right-to-left shunt (Fig. 3–5), the anesthetic concentration of blood rises more slowly and induction of anesthesia is delayed. The larger the shunt, the slower the induction of anesthesia. Whether a left-to-right shunt affects F_E/F_I depends on the size of the shunt. If the shunt is large (> 80 percent), recirculating blood has the same anesthetic concentration as blood leaving the systemic ventricle. Consequently, the anesthetic concentration of blood perfusing the alveolar capillaries is high and F_E/F_I rises rapidly. If the shunt is equal to half or less of the cardiac output, the effect on F_E/F_I is small because blood that mixes outside the lung has the same anesthetic concentration as that of patients with normal circulations.

The alveolar concentrations of halothane,[90] nitrous oxide,[91] and cyclopropane[92] rise more rapidly in pediatric

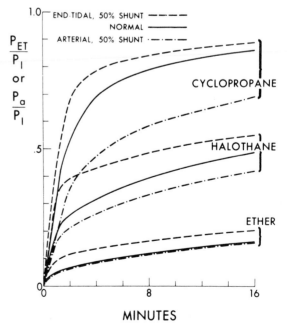

FIGURE 3–5. Effects of a 50 percent right-to-left shunt of blood on the ratio of the rate of rise of the end-tidal (P_{ET}) to the inspired (P_I) anesthetic concentration or on the ratio of the pulmonary arterial blood (P_a) to the inspired anesthetic concentration. (From Eger El II: Anesthetic Uptake and Action. Baltimore, Williams & Wilkins, 1974.)

patients than in adults, shortening the time for induction of anesthesia. This occurs because the minute ventilation of pediatric patients is larger, the FRC is smaller, and anesthetics are less soluble in the blood of pediatric patients. Deming[93] found higher concentrations of cyclopropane in the blood of neonates than in adults at comparable depths of anesthesia. The anesthetic requirement (MAC) for halothane is age dependent (0.55 ± 0.02 percent in infants of 33 weeks' or less gestation, 0.87 ± 0.03 percent in 0- to 1-month-old neonates, and 1.20 ± 0.06 percent at 1 to 6 months of age.)[94] Similar changes occur with isoflurane.[95, 96] After 6 months of age, MAC progressively decreases.[97, 98] Similar changes are reported for sevoflurane and desflurane.[99–101]

Neonates also require larger doses of ketamine per kilogram to produce anesthesia.[102] It is unclear why this is so. It may be related to a high metabolic rate, the greater number of neurons per unit mass of brain, greater cerebral oxygen consumption and cerebral blood flow, or all of these factors. It may also be that these concentrations of drugs in the brain are not different from those of adults (see above).[88] A higher percentage of the neonate's cardiac output is distributed to the VRG because it constitutes a larger fraction of the body (Table 3–3). As a result, the VRG is more rapidly saturated with anesthetic, reducing induction time. Drugs can penetrate the CNS of neonates more easily than they can in adults, either because the neonatal blood–brain barrier is more permeable[103] or because cerebral blood flow is slower and the drugs have longer to dissociate from plasma proteins.[57] The blood–brain barrier of neonates also is more easily disrupted by hypoxia and acidosis than it is in adults.

Anesthetics are apparently metabolized by pediatric patients to a lesser degree than by adults. Fewer methoxyflurane breakdown products are present in the urine of pediatric patients than in adults.[104] Carbon tetrachloride and chloroform are less hepatotoxic to young animals.[105] Further evidence for the lack of or a reduced rate of anesthetic metabolism by patients below the age of puberty is the low incidence of halothane-induced hepatitis in this age group, despite repeated use of halothane for such procedures as dressing changes and radiation therapy. This may in part be due to the fact that halothane reduces the hepatic blood flow of prepubescent children rather than increases it as it does in adults.[106] Consequently, less drug reaches the liver and fewer potentially toxic metabolites are produced. Infants metabolize halothane less (produce less bromine) than adults, and peak levels of metabolites occur earlier (12 to 24 hours) than in adults (48 hours).[107] These data suggest that infants can biotransform halothane but do so to a lesser extent than adults and that infants clear inhaled anesthetics more quickly.

Respiratory Effects of Inhaled Anesthetics

As in adults, inhaled anesthetics depress the respiration of infants and children in a dose-dependent manner.[108] A mixture of 1.5 percent inspired halothane and 70 percent nitrous oxide decreases minute ventilation by about 25 percent, tidal volume by about 35 percent, mean inspiratory flow by about 20 percent, and the duty cycle (inspiratory time/total respiratory time) by less than 5 percent. Expired CO_2 and respiratory frequency increase by 15 and 10 percent, respectively. The net effect is a decrease in alveolar ventilation and a rise in CO_2, which is probably a central effect of halothane but may, as with enflurane, have some peripheral component as well.[109] Sevoflurane reduces minute ventilation and respiratory frequency significantly more than halothane.[110] There was less thoracoabdominal asynchrony during sevoflurane. The increase in P_{ETCO_2} was modest in both groups.

In newborn lambs, 0.75 MAC halothane in oxygen decreases tidal volume (20 percent), minute ventilation (34 percent), work of breathing (20 percent), and functional residual capacity (32 percent).[111] Lung and airway resistance increased by 59 percent, whereas lung compliance was unchanged. $Paco_2$ increased by 50 percent and (A–a)Do_2 increased by 26 percent. The rise in CO_2 was the result of decreased ventilation, increased airway resistance, and unchanged work of breathing.

Low concentrations of added CO_2 increase minute ventilation during halothane/nitrous oxide anesthesia. However, increasing concentrations of halothane shift the CO_2 response curve to the right and flatten it, decreasing tidal volume and minute ventilation. This indicates decreased sensitivity to CO_2 with increasing doses of halothane. At 1.1 MAC, the mean slope of the CO_2 response was 38 percent of control; at 2 MAC, it was only 17 percent of the control value. This difference is due to a direct central effect of halothane on regulatory and integratory mechanisms.[112]

Adding increased respiratory loads to the airways of children during 0.5 percent halothane anesthesia initially decreased tidal volume,[113] but it returned to normal within 5 minutes. Respiratory rate and duration of inspiration were unchanged, suggesting that the decrease in tidal volume was not due to a lung or airway stretch receptor-mediated on–off, switch–reflex mechanism. The respiratory compensation that occurred within 5 minutes was due to chemoreceptor stimulation or to reflexes from joint receptors or respiratory muscle spindles.

All of these data suggest that anesthesia depresses the ventilation of infants and young children and that it is appropriate to control their ventilation during anesthesia.

Cardiovascular Effects of Inhaled Anesthetics

All inhaled anesthetics depress the myocardium in vitro in a dose-dependent relationship. Similar effects occur in vivo.

In lambs, 0.5 MAC halothane decreases oxygen consumption by 25 percent; 1 MAC decreases it by 43 percent.[114] Similarly, 1 MAC halothane decreases cardiac output by 48 percent from control levels without causing metabolic acidosis, suggesting that tissue oxygen requirements were satisfied. It therefore appears that the decrease in cardiac output was the result of decreased oxygen demand. Organ blood flow was similar during control and 0.5 MAC halothane. It was, however, significantly reduced by 1 MAC halothane. One MAC halothane also reduced plasma epinephrine and norepinephrine concentrations significantly, suggesting that halothane anesthesia alleviates rather than produces stress. Similar responses have been shown for fentanyl[115] and halothane.[116]

At 0.5 and 1.0 MAC halothane, hypoxia reduced oxygen consumption even more than occurred in normoxic animals[114]; no increase in metabolic acidosis occurred. Cardiac output was unchanged between hypoxia and normoxia. Blood flow was redistributed from the periphery to the brain and heart, as it was in awake, hypoxic animals. Consequently, oxygen delivery to the brain and heart was normal. One MAC halothane also significantly decreased plasma catecholamine concentrations in hypoxic animals. We conclude that hypoxia does not inhibit redistribution of blood flow from the periphery to the heart and brain during halothane anesthesia, leaving this protective mechanism intact.

Anesthesia reduces the arterial blood pressure of neonates more than that of adults[117–120] without altering the heart rate. This indicates that inhaled anesthetics depress the baroreceptor reflexes, which has been confirmed in preterm neonates[121] and animals.[122, 123] Ebert et al.[124] showed in adults that both the cardiopulmonary reflexes and the arterial baroreflexes are reduced by halothane. Krane and Su[125] showed that halothane caused more depression of the peak tension developed by right ventricular muscle strips from neonatal hearts than occurred in muscle strips from adults. This was probably due to different cellular composition of neonatal cardiac myocytes.[126] Wolf et al.[118] showed that halothane depressed the myocardium of 2- to 7-year-old children more than isoflurane. Both anesthetics had similar effects on heart rate and arterial blood pressure. Neither anesthetic altered the left ventricular end-diastolic dimension or preload. The decrease in myocardial function with halothane was, therefore, due to a decrease in myocardial contractility. It is unclear if isoflurane causes myocardial depression. If so, it is less than with halothane. Similar changes have been seen in adult rabbit papillary muscles.[127] In infants, both 1 MAC halothane and 1 MAC isoflurane reduced cardiac output by approximately 25 percent and stroke volume by approximately 20 percent. Ejection fraction was reduced by 25 percent.[128]

Nitrous oxide also has cardiovascular effects in neonates. It depresses the baroreflex of neonatal rabbits[123] and increases the pulmonary vascular resistance of normoxic and hypoxic lambs[129] and of children.[130]

Sevoflurane

Sevoflurane (Ultane) is a relatively new halogenated anesthetic that has a low blood/gas partition coefficient (low solubility in blood). Consequently, the induction of anesthesia is about 1 minute faster when done with 8 percent inspired sevoflurane than with and 5 percent halothane. Interestingly, when sevoflurane was tested against halothane, only 56 percent of anesthesiologists could correctly identify which anesthetic was being administered for the induction of anesthesia.[131] Anesthesia is induced more rapidly when 8 percent sevoflurane is used compared to starting with 1 percent sevoflurane and increasing the concentration every two to three breaths.[132] To most people, the smell of sevoflurane is slightly less pungent than

that of halothane. The MAC that allows smooth tracheal extubation is 1.87 percent end-tidal sevoflurane.[133]

The passage of sevoflurane through the soda lime of a carbon dioxide absorber produces compound-A, which is potentially toxic. The production of compound-A is related to body size and habitus, as well as the temperature of the soda lime. At least two studies have shown that the administration of sevoflurane to children results in low concentrations of compound-A[134] and that the concentration of this compound has decreased by two thirds 24 hours later.[135] The maximum inspiratory concentration of compound-A was 5.5 ± 4.4 ppm and the corresponding expired concentration was 3.7 ± 2.7 ppm. The maximum concentration of compound-A in any patient was 15 ppm. The concentration of compound-A remained relatively constant during the anesthetic. Peak inorganic fluoride concentrations were higher in patients anesthetized with sevoflurane than with halothane.[135] The fluoride concentrations decreased by two thirds over 24 hours. Neither the fluoride nor the compound-A concentrations were high enough to pose a danger to the children. There was no evidence of renal or hepatic injury in any of the children. Both sevoflurane and isoflurane have been associated with a marked increase in creatinine phosphatase following administration of succinylcholine.[136] The significance of this finding is unclear.

One proposed advantage of sevoflurane is more rapid induction of anesthesia and intubation of the trachea. However, several studies have shown that the time to tracheal intubation occurs more quickly and with less coughing with halothane than with sevoflurane.[137, 138] Another proposed advantage of the use of sevoflurane is the rapid awakening from anesthesia. This advantage exists if no narcotics are administered in the operating room. If they are, the awakening times for sevoflurane and halothane are similar. The incidence of postoperative delirium was greater with sevoflurane than with halothane, probably due to the more rapid awakening from anesthesia.[139, 140] More patients given sevoflurane required postoperative narcotics. Therefore, the time to discharge from the recovery room was no different than that of patients who were anesthetized with halothane (approximately 2 hours).[141]

There is a greater reduction in ventilation with sevoflurane compared with halthane.[110] In fact, it is common for infants and children to become apneic during the administration of high concentrations of sevoflurane. Minute ventilation (4.5 vs. 5.4 L/m²) and respiratory rate (37.5 vs. 47.6 bpm) were significantly lower with sevoflurane than with halothane. There was, however, no difference in respiratory drive, but there was a difference in the flow waveform with the two agents. Peak expiratory flow occurred sooner with sevoflurane. There was significantly less thoracoabdominal asynchrony during sevoflurane anesthesia.

There are in general few differences in the cardiovascular effects of sevoflurane and halothane. Sevoflurane is associated in one study with a 20 percent increase in heart rate and arterial blood pressure compared with halothane.[142] However, most studies show no difference in heart rate or arterial blood pressure with sevoflurane or halothane.[143] In one study, both halothane and sevoflurane decreased arterial blood pressure and increased cerebral blood-flow velocity as measured by transcranial Doppler.[144] There is no difference in the SpO2 with either agent.

Although there are no differences in blood flow velocity, some children who receive sevoflurane develop twitching and abnormal muscle movements during anesthesia. In at least one patient, a seizure has been documented in an otherwise normal child.[145]

There has been no evidence of renal or hepatic damage associated with sevoflurane administration. There have been a few patients who have developed malignant hyperthermia with the administration of this drug.

INTRAVENOUS AGENTS

Muscle Relaxants

Nondepolarizing Muscle Relaxants

For years there was controversy about whether neonates and infants are more sensitive to nondepolarizing muscle relaxants than adults. Several investigators said that they were[146–151]; others said that they were not.[152, 153] One study suggested that infants are more resistant to d-tubocurarine (curare). In great part, this controversy is due to methodologic differences and failure to measure anesthetic concentrations. Claims that neonates are more sensitive to nondepolarizing muscle relaxants are based on data that demonstrate a greater reduction of ventilation in neonates with the same or smaller doses of muscle relaxant. This difference may be due to differences in the shape of the infant's diaphragm or to earlier fatigue and stress than occurs in the diaphragm of adults.[154] The composition of the muscle of the infant diaphragm also differs from that of adults.[155] The neonatal diaphragm is paralyzed at the same time as the peripheral muscles, not later as in adults.

When the sensitivity to nondepolarizing muscle relaxants is studied by stimulating a peripheral nerve and observing the response of muscles innervated by the nerve (twitch), the neonate's response is similar to that of adults. However, these studies were done without regard to anesthetic concentration, which significantly affects the results.[156] When adults and neonates are anesthetized with the same inspired anesthetic concentration, neonates and infants are less deeply anesthetized than adults, and the twitch response of older patients is depressed more than that of neonates.

Fisher et al.[157] resolved the question by using a pharmacodynamic–pharmacokinetic model that enabled them to determine both the drug effect (depression of twitch height) and the sensitivity of the neuromuscular junction. These authors concluded that neonates are indeed more sensitive to curare but that they require the same dose of curare per square meter of surface area as adults because neonates have a larger volume of distribution. Neonates also eliminated curare more slowly because of the larger volume of distribution and reduced glomerular filtration. Curare is mostly (40 percent) excreted unchanged in the urine of adults[158]; about 12 percent is excreted in bile. Whether the same is true in pediatric patients is unknown.

Kroenigsberger et al.[159] demonstrated posttetanic exhaustion in preterm infants after nerve stimulation at 20 Hz and in term infants after 60 Hz stimulation. Exhaustion did not occur at either stimulation rate in adults. Nitrous oxide and methohexital (Brevital) also caused exhaustion of neuromuscular transmission in neonates.[160] These two studies and that of Fisher et al.[157] support the idea that neonates and infants are more sensitive to curare than adults and that the myoneural junction of neonates and infants not only is different from that of adults but is also more sensitive to anesthetics. Therefore, any study of the effects of muscle relaxants in neonates and infants should include a measurement of anesthetic depth.

The onset of action of curare is more rapid in neonates (1.56 ± 0.34 minutes) than in 3- to 10-year-olds (5.20 ± 1.16 minutes).[161] The time to recovery from paralysis is prolonged. Administering pancuronium 0.07 mg/kg 3 minutes before giving curare speeded the onset of paralysis in all age groups. Recovery from paralysis was delayed in infants given pancuronium plus curare but not in older patients. Aminoglycosides potentiate the block caused by curare and other nondepolarizing muscle relaxants because aminoglycosides inhibit release of acetylcholine from the prejunctional membrane and stabilize the postjunctional membrane.

Cameron et al.[162] found that d-tubocurarine and pancuronium (Pavulon) had no effect on the oxygen consumption of normoxic lambs. Both drugs reduced the oxygen consumption of hypoxic lambs by about 35 percent. Hypoxia increased the plasma lactic acid concentration whether or not the animals were paralyzed. Cardiac output was unaffected by muscle paralysis. The surprising finding was that both drugs increased the right ventricular rate–pressure product, pulmonary vascular resistance, and mean pulmonary artery pressure. The mechanism of this increase is not known, but it is probably not due to histamine because pancuronium does not release histamine. Furthermore, histamine dilates the pulmonary arteries of neonates. It is possible that muscle relaxants potentiate the effects of hypoxia-induced angiotensin and catecholamine release. Burned patients require more nondepolarizing muscle relaxants to produce the same amount of paralysis as unburned patients. This seems to be due to circulating inhibitors of muscle relaxants.[163]

Pancuronium

Pancuronium bromide is a bisquaternary compound that produces a competitive block. It is 5 to 10 times more potent than curare, although the onset of action of both drugs is similar (1.5 ± 0.2 minutes with a range of 0.5 to 3.0 minutes). A dose of 0.06 mg/kg of pancuronium reduces the muscle twitch height by 95 percent with ulnar nerve stimulation when patients are anesthetized with halothane/nitrous oxide.[164] Recovery of twitch height occurred at 54.7 ± 11.1 minutes, similar to that of adults. Meretoja and Luosto[165] found that infants required less pancuronium than children and that all age groups recovered from paralysis at the same rate. In unanesthetized infants, recovery from pancuronium-induced muscle paralysis may be prolonged if the patient is premature, has renal disease, or has anasarca. Goudsouzian et al.[166] found that the muscle paralysis of infants could be successfully reversed after days of paralysis if 3 or more hours had elapsed since the last dose of drug was given. The more premature the infant, the more difficult it was to reverse the paralysis. They attributed this finding to the fact that premature infants have fewer type I (slow-twitch, high-oxidation) fibers in their peripheral muscles.[167]

Muscle relaxants that depend primarily on renal excretion for clearance may behave similarly to or differently from drugs cleared by other methods, depending on the maturity of the metabolic pathways and other routes of excretion.[168] About 30 to 40 percent of a pancuronium dose is excreted unchanged in the bile.[169] Another 45 percent is metabolized, primarily by hydroxylation. One third of this metabolite is active and is approximately one half as potent as the parent drug. The hydroxylation pathway is less effective at birth, but other pathways may compensate for this lack of effectiveness. Therefore, it is difficult to predict if the kinetics of neonatal pancuronium metabolism differ between pediatric patients and adults. If alternate metabolic pathways are not functional, the drug may be cleared more slowly. If these pathways are functional, metabolism may proceed normally. On the basis of clinical experience, this effect is probably small.

Pancuronium causes mild to severe tachycardia in some pediatric patients whether they are anesthetized[170] or not.[171] At times, the tachycardia is severe enough to cause congestive heart failure. Both curare and pancuronium inhibit the increase in cardiac output normally seen with hypoxemia, and both drugs markedly increase myocardial blood flow. They do not prevent redistribution of blood flow from the periphery to the heart and brain of hypoxic animals.[162]

The arterial blood pressure of premature infants increases with pancuronium, and this, combined with the increase in circulating epinephrine and norepinephrine caused by pancuronium, may account for the increased incidence of intracranial hemorrhage in neonates paralyzed with pancuronium.[172] Pancuronium has little effect on arterial blood pressure when the patient is adequately anesthetized. Paralysis with pancuronium has no effect on the plasma volume of premature neonates.[173] However, it reduces variability in cerebral blood flow,[174] which has been associated with less intracranial hemorrhage in these patients.[175-177]

The cerebral oxygen consumption of anesthetized dogs is unchanged by paralysis with pancuronium.[178] The total body oxygen consumption of sedated infants decreased after paralysis with pancuronium if the infants were moving about before they were paralyzed. If they were quiet, oxygen consumption did not change.[179]

Atracurium

Atracurium (Tracrium) is a quaternary ammonium, half of which is eliminated by Hofmann elimination and ester hydrolysis and the remainder by poorly defined tissue-based mechanisms.[180] Atracurium is stable in normal saline but spontaneously degrades to a small extent (about 6 percent over 5 hours) in lactated Ringer's solution, which may be of some importance if the drug is to be infused continuously.[181] The onset of block with atracurium occurs within 3.8 ± 0.09 minutes in children,[182] which is similar to that in adults. The ED_{50} of atracurium varies with age,

being least in neonates,[183] next lowest in children,[184-186] and highest in adolescents. These data suggest that neonates are more sensitive to the effects of atracurium than older patients. As with other muscle relaxants, the ED_{50} of atracurium is affected by anesthetics, being 170 $\mu g/kg$ with thiopental/fentanyl, 130 $\mu g/kg$ with halothane and 120 $\mu g/kg$ with isoflurane. Recovery from the effects of atracurium averages 20 to 30 minutes in all age groups and does not differ among groups, probably because of the unique method by which this drug is eliminated. In neonates, the effect of this drug is influenced by time and temperature.[187]

Neonates less than 48 hours old require less atracurium to induce almost complete paralysis than neonates more than 48 hours old (300 vs. 500 $\mu g/kg$).[187] Recovery from the effects of atracurium takes longer in patients less than 48 hours old than it does in those over 48 hours of age (32.4 ± 7 vs. 23.1 ± 3.4 minutes). Neonates with body temperatures below 36°C have a longer duration of paralysis (47.5 ± 11.8 minutes). Therefore, if it is desirable for neonates to breathe spontaneously at the end of surgery, their body temperature should be normal at that time.

The atracurium block lasts about 32 minutes. Recovery of twitch height from 25 to 95 percent of control occurs within about 10 minutes, which differs from pancuronium and vecuronium and is probably due to atracurium's unique metabolism.

Atracurium releases histamine in adults, but this action does not appear to cause significant problems in neonates, infants, and children, because there are no significant changes in heart rate or arterial pressure, even when twice the ED_{95} of atracurium was given. It is unknown if laudanosine, a major breakdown product of atracurium and a potential cause of seizures, crosses the blood–brain barrier of neonates more easily than in adults. However, no seizures have been reported in infants treated with this drug. The "immature" kidney of neonates should have little effect on the kinetics of atracurium because its pharmacokinetics and pharmacodynamics are similar in adults with renal failure and those with normal renal function.[188]

Vecuronium

Vecuronium (Norcuron) is a monoquaternary compound that is approximately 10 times more potent than pancuronium and has a shorter duration of action,[189] which makes it useful for short surgical procedures. The onset of paralysis occurs sooner (1.5 ± 0.6 minutes) in infants than in children and adults (2.4 ± 1.4 and 2.9 ± 0.2 minutes) who are anesthetized with equipotent doses of halothane/nitrous oxide, which makes it a useful drug when rapid tracheal intubation must be accomplished. However, one must give 0.4 mg/kg to attain the same conditions for tracheal intubation as occur with succinylcholine.[190] The ED_{50} of vecuronium is 0.16 mg/kg in neonates, 0.19 mg/kg in infants, and 0.15 mg/kg in children, indicating that the sensitivity of infants, neonates, and older children to vecuronium is about the same. Meretoja et al.[191] found significantly longer ED_{50} values in infants and children than did Fisher et al., probably because Meretoja et al. used the cumulative-dose technique and Fisher et al. used the single-bolus technique.[191, 192] The duration of block also varied with the age of the patient.[193, 194] It was almost twice as long in the neonates (73 ± 23 minutes) as in adults and about 30 percent longer in neonates than in children, probably because of a larger volume of distribution in neonates at steady state. The recovery time was longer in neonates (20 ± 8 minutes) than in children (9 ± 3 minutes) or adults (13 ± 7 minutes), which is due to a larger volume of distribution rather than to reduced clearance of the drug. The elimination half-life of vecuronium was longer in infants than in children and adults, but clearance was not different. However, recovery from paralysis was 55 minutes in neonates and 20 to 24 minutes in 3- to 15-year-old patients.[195] The V_d of vecuronium was much larger and its blood concentration significantly smaller at 50 percent twitch depression. These findings are similar to those for curare and probably have the same meaning. There is no change in heart rate or arterial blood pressure after vecuronium administration. Vecuronium is apparently safe for use in patients who are susceptible to malignant hypothermia.[196]

Mivacurium

Mivacurium is a bis-benzylisoquinolinium nondepolarizing muscle relaxant that has been studied in children.[197] In patients anesthetized with halothane/nitrous oxide and with nitrous oxide/narcotic, the ED_{95} was similar (0.051 and 0.059 mg/kg, respectively). Ninety-five percent recovery of the block occurred in approximately 10 minutes in both groups. The neuromuscular block was satisfactorily reversed with 0.03 mg/kg of atropine and 0.3 mg/kg of edrophonium. There was no clinically significant change in heart rate or arterial blood pressure. Similar results were obtained in another study.[198] There was no difference in the time to maximum block or the time to 90 percent recovery with 66 percent nitrous oxide and 1.5 MAC sevoflurane or isoflurane or propofol.[199] In burned patients, 0.2 mg/kg of mivacurium caused good muscle relaxation in the expected time.[200] There was decreased metablolism of mivacurium due to the decreased concentrations of plasma cholinesterase activity caused by the burns. These data make mivacurium a useful arternative to succinylcholine (which is contraindicated in burn patients). Markakis et al.[201] demonstrated a positive relationship between pseudocholinesterase activity and rocuronium infusion rates. The severity of liver disease did not affect the duration of block with mivacurium.[202] In patients with liver disease, the intubating conditions 2 minutes after the administration of mivacurium was the same as 1 minute after succinylcholine. Recovery from muscle paralysis was inversely related to the plasma cholinesterase activity.

Rocuronium

The search for a drug to replace succinylcholine continues. To this end, rocuronium, an aminosteroidal neuromuscular blocking agent, was developed. Several studies demonstrate that 1.0 to 1.2 mg/kg of rocuronium gives similar intubating conditions as succinylcholine in approximately 60 seconds after the drug is given intravenously.[203, 204] Recovery from intravenous rocuronium takes approximately eight times longer than recovery from succinylcholine.[204, 205] Reynolds et al.[206] found good intubating conditions in infants following 1 mg/kg and in children following 1.8 mg/kg of rocuronium given into the deltoid muscle. Good to excellent intubating conditions were present 3.0 and 2.5 minutes, respectively, in infants and children. Recovery times to first twitch were 70 ± 23 minutes in children and 57 ± 13 minutes in infants following intramuscular injection of the drug. Approximately 80 percent of the drug is bioavailable when administered by this route.[206]

The pharmacokinetics of rocuronium have been studied in both infants and children. Infants differed from children in plasma clearance (4.2 ± 0.4 vs. 6.7 ± 1.1 ml/kg/min) and in volume of distribution at steady state (V_{dss}) (231 ± 32 vs. 165 ± 44 ml/kg), and the slope of the concentration–effect relationship was 5.7 ± 1.3 versus 3.9 ± 0.5, respectively.[207–209] Clearance of the drug is not significantly influenced by dysfunction of the liver and kidneys.[210] The potency of rocuronium is greatest in infants and least in children (251 ± 73 vs. 409 ± 71 μg/kg) for an ED_{95}.[211]

Rocuronium increased the heart rate a mean of 6 bpm and mean arterial pressure decreased slightly.[212] The mean arterial pressure was significantly greater in rocuronium-treated than in vecuronium-treated infants. However, if the anesthetic depth is light, there may be a significant increase in heart rate and arterial blood pressure. Muscle paralysis induced by rocuronium is easily reversed with neostigmine.[213] Twenty micrograms of neostigmine produces a greater than 80 percent train-of-four ratio after 10 minutes in infants but at least 50 μg/kg are required to reverse a 90 percent block in adults. The time course for recovery from an approximately 94 percent block was 6.6 minutes in infants, children, and adults.[211]

Rapacuronium

Rapacuronium is a new drug that also was developed to replace succinylcholine. It is another of the steroid nondepolarizing muscle relaxants. It has been administered both intramuscularly and intravenously. When given intravenously with halothane,[214] satisfactory conditions for tracheal intubation occurred after 1.5 mg/kg of the drug was administered in neonates and 2.0 mg/kg in children. Recovery of the third twitch of a train-of-four occurred in less than 10 minutes in both age groups. With balanced anesthesia, there was no difference in the onset or the maximum block among neonates, infants, or toddlers whether 1 or 2 mg/kg of drug was given.[215] Maximum neuromuscular blockade occurred in the same amount of time (1 ± 0.5 minute) following drug injection. The degree of block was similar in both groups 60 seconds after the drug was injected. Recovery of a train-of-four (T4/T1) occurred in 10 to 11 minutes. Compared with succinylcholine, 1 to 1.5 mg/kg of rapacuronium induces 98 to 100 percent depression of the muscle twitch in 60 seconds. Recovery of the train-of-four was shorter, 5.7 minutes with succinylcholine compared with rapacuronium (8 minutes). Meakin et al. reported several complications with injecting rapacuronium intravenously, including bronchospasm, tachycardia, and increased salavation.[214] Apparently none of these complications was serious.

Reynolds et al. studied the pharmacokinetics of rapacuronium following intravenous and intramuscular injection of rapacuronium in infants and children during light halothane anesthesia.[216] In this study, clearance of rapacuronium was more rapid in infants than in children and both were slower than in adults. Plasma clearance was approximately 5 mg/kg/min and the drug was 56 percent bioavailable. Plasma concentrations peaked in 4 to 5 minutes following intramuscular injection of the drug. Rapacuronium has a metabolite that has significant muscle paralyzing activity. However, because the parent compound decreases rapidly, the metabolite does not seem to be a problem. It might be a problem if repeated doses of rapacuronium are administered or if the drug is administered for long periods of time in an intensive care unit.

Reversal of rapacuronium's effects are possible with either edrophonium 1 mg/kg or neostigmine 0.05 mg/kg,[217] although no studies have been reported in infants and children. Following repeated doses of rapacuronium (0.5 mg/kg each), reversal of the muscle block took longer.

Reversal of Nondepolarizing Muscle Relaxants

Until the studies of Fisher et al.[218] there were no studies in pediatric patients that defined the dose of drugs required for reversal of muscle paralysis. These authors showed that the ED_{50} of neostigmine (Prostigmin) was 13.1 μg/kg for children, 15.5 μg/kg for infants, and 22.0 μg/kg for adults. The time to 70 percent antagonism of the block was similar in all three groups (5 to 8 minutes). The only difference in the kinetic data was the $t_{1/2\beta}$, which was shorter in infants and children than in adults. Clearance of the drug was longer in infants and children than in adults. On the basis of these data, infants and children require one half to two thirds as much neostigmine as adults to antagonize muscle paralysis with curare.

A similar study with edrophonium (Tensilon) showed that its ED_{50} is larger in infants and children than in adults (145, 233, and 128 μg/kg, respectively).[219] The mean time to 100 percent antagonism of the block was about twice as long (2.5 vs. 1.5 minutes) in infants as in adults. The duration of antagonism was similar in all age groups. When patients were given atropine 10 to 20 μg/kg 30 seconds before administration of edrophonium, edrophonium had no effect on heart rate or arterial blood pressure. When the two drugs were given simultaneously, both heart rate and systolic blood pressure decreased. Giving atropine 20 μg/kg 30 seconds before administering edrophonium increased the heart rate and arterial blood pressure for 5 minutes or more in all patients. Because the patients' response to edrophonium varied widely, the authors recommended giving edrophonium 1 mg/kg to infants and children 30 seconds after giving atropine 10 to 20 μg/kg.

The onset of edrophonium's action is significantly shorter (< 1 minute) in infants and children than that of neostigmine (7 to 8 minutes). This difference may make edrophonium more useful than neostigmine for reversing drug-induced muscle paralysis.

Paralysis caused by nondepolarizing muscle relaxants should be reversed at the end of each operation (unless postoperative mechanical ventilation is planned) because

Rackow and Salanitre[220] found that 20 percent of neonates had respiratory failure postoperatively and required assisted ventilation when they had been paralyzed with curare and the block was not reversed. Thirty percent of patients less than 8 days old had respiratory failure after paralysis with curare. Forty-eight percent required assisted ventilation if their body temperature fell below 35.5°C versus 12 percent of normothermic patients. Respiratory support was required more often after long surgical procedures. More expremature neonates required mechanical ventilation postoperatively when they had received muscle relaxants.[221] The likelihood of prolonged muscle paralysis is reduced or eliminated if the degree of neuromuscular block is monitored with a nerve stimulator and only enough drug is administered to achieve the desired degree of block.

Depolarizing Muscle Relaxants

Succinylcholine (Anectine) is the only depolarizing muscle relaxant commonly used today. When given IV (2 mg/kg at < 1 year of age, 1 mg/kg in those > 1 year) or IM (2 to 4 mg/kg), succinylcholine depolarizes the postjunctional membrane for 3 to 10 minutes. Its effects are not reversible with neostigmine. Neonates and infants are apparently less sensitive to succinylcholine when sensitivity is tested by either respiration or twitch height.[222, 223] Their response to an equivalent dose of drug is approximately 50 percent less than that of adults. When this drug is given IV, paralysis occurs within 20 to 30 seconds. When it is given IM, paralysis occurs within 40 to 60 seconds if peripheral blood flow is normal.

Ninety percent of an IV dose of succinylcholine is rapidly hydrolyzed in the plasma by pseudocholinesterase. Only 10 percent is delivered to the active site in muscle. Pseudocholinesterase deficiency (e.g., caused by liver disease or a genetic defect) hastens the onset of muscle paralysis and prolongs its effects by delaying hydrolysis of succinylcholine. The plasma pseudocholinesterase concentration in term neonates is about 50 percent that of adults,[224, 225] and the pseudocholinesterase activity of premature neonates is similar to that of term neonates.[226] However, a larger percentage of premature neonates have abnormally low values, although not low enough to affect the hydrolysis of succinylcholine significantly or to prolong its effects. By 2 weeks of age, all neonates have plasma pseudocholinesterase concentrations similar to those of adults.

The duration of neuromuscular blockade following succinylcholine administration may be prolonged if the patient has an abnormal variant of pseudocholinesterase. Dibucaine inhibits the activity of normal pseudocholinesterase much more than it does that of the abnormal enzyme (80 percent vs. 20 percent).[227, 228] This difference is used to test for the presence of abnormal pseudocholinesterase.

Patients can have normal pseudocholinesterase levels and low dibucaine numbers and still have a prolonged response to succinylcholine if the enzyme is atypical. Alternatively, a patient may have a low level of pseudocholinesterase, a normal dibucaine number, and a normal or only slightly prolonged response to succinylcholine (e.g., premature infants, patients with severe liver disease).[229] This pattern indicates that all of the pseudocholinesterase formed is normal but that the quantity is reduced. Thus, the dibucaine number reflects the enzyme's ability to hydrolyze succinylcholine, not the amount of pseudocholinesterase present.

Viby-Mogensen[230] demonstrated that 75 percent of patients with at least one abnormal gene for pseudocholinesterase have muscle fasciculations when given succinylcholine 1 mg/kg. The presence of one normal and one abnormal gene only slightly prolongs the duration of apnea beyond that of patients who are homozygous for the normal gene. If both genes are abnormal, recovery from paralysis is prolonged approximately fivefold. The train-of-four is the same as that of patients with a phase II block if both genes are abnormal.

In Viby-Mogensen's study,[230] 46 percent of patients with one normal and one abnormal gene required 15 to 20 minutes for twitch height to return to control levels. In 11 percent of patients this took more than 20 minutes. This increase in the duration of neuromuscular blockade is seldom significant. However, if the pseudocholinesterase activity is low (e.g., in neonates and those with liver disease) and the patient has an abnormal gene, the block may be markedly prolonged. If patients with abnormal genes are allowed to recover some amount of muscle function (respiration, movement) before the dose of succinylcholine is repeated, there is little likelihood of a prolonged block occurring.

The duration of muscle paralysis with succinylcholine is considerably shorter in neonates and children than in adults, probably owing to differences in extracellular space.

On a per-kilogram basis, neonates are more resistant than older patients to succinylcholine. On the basis of surface area (which corrects for extracellular water), their response is similar to that of adults. Cook and Fischer[231] found that succinylcholine 0.5 mg/kg produced less neuromuscular blockade in infants and neonates than in adults, probably because of differences in extracellular fluid volume. Infants also recovered from this dose of succinylcholine more rapidly, in part because the drug is more rapidly redistributed away from the effector site by the relatively greater cardiac output of neonates.

Neonates developed tachyphylaxis after succinylcholine 3.0 ± 0.4 mg/kg.[232] Thereafter, more drug is required to maintain adequate paralysis, which led to a phase II block in 21 of 22 1- to 15-year-old patients. Seventy-five percent of control twitch height was recovered within 41 minutes. However, recovery from a continuous infusion of succinylcholine is variable (3 to 81 minutes) and occurs in two phases. The first phase is relatively rapid and is probably due to metabolism of succinylcholine by plasma cholinesterase. The second phase is slower and is probably due to binding of the drug to myoneural junctions or to "inherent alteration of the receptor." All children eventually recover spontaneously from a phase II block. Because of the variability in the duration of paralysis, only that dose of succinylcholine should be given that allows the return of some twitch when the infusion is interrupted for 60 to 90 seconds. Use of a nerve stimulator allows early detection of phase II block and adjustment of the amount

of drug being infused. A phase II block occurs sooner and with a significantly lower dose of succinylcholine during isoflurane anesthesia than during nitrous oxide/fentanyl anesthesia.[233] Neonates and infants are more likely than adults to develop a phase II block following the administration of depolarizing muscle relaxants, although this was not the case in one study.[232]

The muscles of neonates and infants seldom fasciculate after succinylcholine 1 to 2 mg/kg IV, probably because of dilution of succinylcholine by the large extracellular fluid volume of neonates and infants and their small muscle mass. Fasciculations occur, and the increase in intragastric pressure caused by succinylcholine administration can be inhibited by alfentanil 50 μg/kg.[234]

There are several potential side effects of succinylcholine administration to pediatric patients. Ryan et al.[235] reported that 60 percent of prepubescent children had an increase in plasma myoglobin following 1 to 2 mg/kg of succinylcholine IV, despite the absence of obvious muscle fasciculation. This increase is probably the result of a small increase in baseline muscle tension, as occurs with halothane and succinylcholine in vitro. The serum myoglobin concentration does not increase with puberty.

Approximately 75 percent of patients given succinylcholine have a non–age-related increase in plasma creatinine phosphokinase, an indicator of muscle injury. Forty-six percent develop muscle pain even though muscle fasciculation is absent. Muscle fasciculation seldom occurs in children after IM or continuous infusion of succinylcholine. An IV bolus of succinylcholine may give rise to bradycardia, and repeated doses of succinylcholine increase the incidence of this complication. Bradycardia is more common with halothane than with isoflurane. Atropine 0.03 mg/kg prevents bradycardia.[236]

In normal patients, serum potassium increases 0.5 mEq/L after IV succinylcholine.[237] It increases considerably more in burned patients, enough to occasionally cause cardiac arrest.[238] It also increases when succinylcholine is given to patients with muscle trauma, tetanus, or upper and lower motor neuron lesions.[239] Increased sensitivity to succinylcholine usually appears 5 to 15 days after the injury occurs, and persists for 2 to 3 months in burned and traumatized patients and for 3 to 6 months in patients with neuromotor diseases. It is usually safer to paralyze such patients with a nondepolarizing muscle relaxant. Administering a small dose of nondepolarizing muscle relaxant before administering a dose of succinylcholine does not necessarily prevent the rise in potassium.

Administering succinylcholine to patients with abnormal musculature (e.g., Duchenne's muscular dystrophy) may lead to cardiac arrest[240] owing to massive contracture of the abnormal muscles. In one study, the concentration of creatinine phosphokinase (CPK) rose to 17,850 U/L after succinylcholine. Patients with these diseases may have elevated CPK levels when they are well. Lavach et al. also found that young male children who appear to be normal may develop cardiac arrest following succinylcholine administration if they have occult muscle disease.[241]

Succinylcholine administration causes masseter muscle spasm (resistance to mouth opening) and is said to be associated with an increased incidence of malignant hyperthermia.[242, 243] More recent evidence suggests that this is not the case. Van Der Spek et al.[244] showed that succinylcholine decreased jaw opening and increased jaw tone but found no association between this and malignant hyperthermia. Similarly, Carroll[245] showed an increased incidence of masseter spasm with halothane and succinylcholine, but found no evidence of malignant hyperthermia in 1,468 children. Masseter spasm occurred in 2.8 percent of children with strabismus and 1.02 percent of all others. The blood CPK concentration also increased without associated malignant hyperthermia occurring.

The findings of Van Der Spek et al.[244] differed from those of Rosenberg and Fletcher.[246] Fifty percent of patients with masseter spasm had caffeine contracture tests suggestive of malignant hyperthermia. CPK was measured in 52 patients and all values were above normal. Only 6 of 30 patients diagnosed as being susceptible to malignant hyperthermia had elevated plasma CPK concentrations. All of the patients studied were referred for evaluation of possible malignant hyperthermia, which may account for the correlation of masseter spasm and malignant hyperthermia. It seems safe to conclude that masseter spasm may be present in patients with malignant hyperthermia, but its occurrence seldom is a sign of malignant hyperthermia. Recently, Meaken et al.[247] demonstrated that much higher doses of succinylcholine were required in infants to obtain a rapid onset of paralysis. They suggested that the high incidence of masseter spasm is related to inadequate doses of succinylcholine and that infants and young children require 3 mg/kg of succinylcholine rather than 2 mg/kg as previously believed.

Succinylcholine increases the incidence of dreaming during anesthesia in children.[248] Giving curare 80 μg/kg 1 minute before induction of anesthesia with thiopentone significantly reduces the incidence of dreaming (2.8 percent treated vs. 16.8 percent nontreated).

Barbiturates

Barbiturates are commonly administered to pediatric patients for premedication, induction of anesthesia, and treatment of seizures. Absorption is rapid and complete for most members of this family of drugs. Renal elimination of barbiturates is relatively unimportant, at least for nonmetabolized (parent) drug. Younger children require larger doses of barbiturates than adults. The recommended dosage of IV thiopental in pediatric patients has been 1 to 2 mg/kg, a figure that has been revised upward by Cote et al.,[249] who found that all the children studied had normal eyelid reflexes and that none would accept an anesthesia mask without fussing if they were given a 2 mg/kg dose of thiopental. Six milligrams per kilogram of thiopental abated the eyelid reflex of 5- to 15-year-old children, but the corneal reflexes were blocked in only 62.5 percent of the patients. Five milligrams per kilogram of thiopental were required before 100 percent of the patients accepted an anesthesia mask without responding. Brett and Fisher[250] found similar responses in 1-month to 5-year-old patients. The doses of thiopental needed to abate the responses of younger children were similar to those for adults.[251]

The elimination half-life of thiopental in children is about half that of adults (6 ± 3 vs. 12 ± 6 hours), whereas clearance of thiopental from plasma is about twice as great (6.6 ± 2.2 vs. 3.1 ± 0.5 ml/kg/min).[252] There is, however, no difference between groups in V_{dss} or in volume of the central compartment. In both age groups, 13 percent of the drug is unbound.

Children with burns over greater than 9 percent of their body required more thiopental to induce anesthesia than unburned children of the same age.[249] This was attributed to the development of resistance to the drug. Even 1 year later, 6- to 16-year-old burned patients required much higher doses of thiopental to abate lid and corneal reflexes. Only 50 percent of previously burned children tolerated placing a mask on their faces without response after thiopental 8 mg/kg, whereas no nonburned children responded after 6 mg/kg. Even with these "large" doses of thiopental, there were no significant effects on the heart rate and arterial blood pressures of burned patients. There is no good explanation for this difference in drug requirement between burned and nonburned children, but it is possible that thiopental inhibitors are present in the serum of burned patients.

Thiopental 10.3 ± 0.9 mg/kg did not alter cardiac function or cardiac output.[253] There was no change in arterial pressure or heart rate. In neonates undergoing tracheal intubation in the neonatal ICU, heart rate increased without a change in arterial blood pressure following the administration of 6 mg/kg of pentothal.[254] In fact, the heart rate and arterial blood pressures were nearer to baseline than occurred when these neonates were intubated without sedation.

Barbiturates have greater depressant effects in very young animals compared with the effects in older animals.[255] Pentobarbital 35 mg/kg produces anesthesia for approximately 1 hour in adult rabbits but kills 80 percent of newborn rabbits. The sleep times of young animals are much longer than those of adults following a dose of barbiturate (Table 3–4). These data contrast with data in human neonates that show rapid awakening from a dose of thiopental given to their mothers.[256]

Domek et al.[257] found more pentobarbital in the brains of newborn kittens than in those of adult cats. Penetration of drug into the brain was inversely related to the degree of nerve myelination. The plasma half-life of amobarbital is approximately 2.5 times longer in neonates than in adults, probably because neonates have less ability to metabolize and conjugate the drug. Enzymes that metabolize and conjugate amobarbital are reduced at birth but increase 10- to 30-fold over the first month of life[258] and can be

	T A B L E 3 – 4			
SLEEP TIMES AFTER HEXOBARBITONE IN MICE OF VARIOUS AGES				
Dose (mg/kg)	1 Day Old	7 Days Old	21 Days Old	Adult
10	>360	107 ± 26	27 ± 11	<5
50	Died	243 ± 30	64 ± 17	17 ± 5
100	Died	>360	94 ± 27	47 ± 11

From Jandorf WR, Maickel RP, Brodie BB: Inability of newborn mice and guinea pigs to metabolize drugs. Biochem Pharmacol 1:352, 1958, with permission.

induced with phenobarbital or benzopyrene. Microsomal enzyme activity and the hepatic metabolism of pentobarbital are low in neonatal rats and increase to adult levels by 1 month of age.[259] Dose–response curves for barbiturates are parallel in neonates and adults but are shifted to the left in neonates, indicating greater sensitivity to these drugs. The barbiturate concentration required for sleep, awakening, ataxia, and death is much lower in neonates than in adults. Hepatic metabolism of phenobarbital by neonates is 10 percent that of adults. Differences in sleep times and the quantity of drug present in neonatal brain are probably related to the greater water content of neonatal brain (89 vs. 78 percent) and differences in the ratio of glial cells to neurons (1:1 in neonates and 2:1 in older animals). If one assumes that the drug is equally divided between the two cell types, less drug will be found in the neurons of older animals.

Onishi et al.[260] determined the concentration of phenobarbital in the serum and organs of premature and full-term neonates and of children at necropsy. The serum/brain ratio was 0.82 to 0.95, whereas that of the liver, kidney, spleen, and lung exceeded 1.0.

Gal et al.[261] demonstrated that infants with Apgar scores of 3 or lower 1 or 5 minutes after birth, those with cardiopulmonary arrest or apnea lasting more than 1 minute who required ventilatory support, or those with a PaO_2 of 30 mm Hg or less (FIO_2 1.0) had significant differences in the pharmacokinetics of phenobarbital. Although no difference existed in the V_d of the drug in the two populations, it varied from 0.66 to 1.22 L/kg. Almost 60 percent less phenobarbital was cleared in nonasphyxiated neonates (4.1 ± 1.0 vs. 8.7 ± 3.9 mg/kg/min). During hypothermia, the V_d was 30 to 40 percent greater in hypothermic than in normothermic infants.[212] Elimination half-life was prolonged, metabolite excretion was altered, and about twice as much drug was excreted unchanged. The concentrations of phenobarbital metabolites (hydroxyphenobarbital, conjugated hydroxyphenobarbital, and phenobarbital N-glucoside) were about half of those found at normal body temperature. On return to normothermia, the maximum serum concentration of phenobarbital increased. The excretion rate for phenobarbital was decreased during hypothermia, partly owing to concomitant furosemide (Lasix) administration.

Propofol (Diprivan)

Propofol is a 2,6-diisopropylphenol which, because it is only slightly soluble in water, is dissolved in a solution of soybean oil, lecithin, and glycerol. Its pH is 7.0 to 8.5. Because it is an incomplete anesthetic under most circumstances, it must be administered in conjunction with another injectable agent or with an inhaled agent. Propofol best fits a three-compartment model.[263] Phase I, the rapid distribution phase, is 2 to 3 minutes; phase II, the high-clearance phase, lasts 34 to 56 minutes; and phase III, the clearance phase from poorly perfused tissues, lasts 184 to 480 minutes. More than 70 percent of the drug is cleared in phases I and II, mostly by the liver, where the drug is conjugated by glucuronidation and by sulfonation. Glucuronidation of the drug may be decreased in neonates, but this will probably be compensated for by sulfonation.

The dose of propofol required for induction of anesthesia is increased in young children, probably because their volume of distribution is increased. The V_{dss} is 0.0394 L/kg/min, and the serum concentration on awakening is 2.3 µg/ml.[264]

Anesthesia can be induced with more than 2.4 mg/kg of propofol in 95 percent of patients. With increasing age, as little as 1.5 mg/kg may effectively induce sleep. Apnea occurs more frequently in older patients and in patients given larger doses of propofol. Propofol reduces minute ventilation compared with halothane.[265] There is a decrease in thoracic volume without a change in abdominal volume, which may account for the reduction in functional residual volume.[266] The maintenance dose of propofol is often 50 to 200 µg/kg/min or more, especially in younger patients. Recovery from anesthesia is faster in children in whom anesthesia is induced with propofol 3 mg/kg than in those given thiopental 5 mg/kg.[267] The reduction of arterial blood pressure occurring with propofol is similar to that seen with other anesthetics.[268] The arterial blood pressure is reduced by approximately 30 percent 5 minutes after the drug is administered and the heart rate (HR) is decreased by approximately 20 percent. In piglets, HR and left ventricular end-diastolic pressures are unchanged from control values. Both dp/dt max and min were slightly decreased. Indices of right ventricular function were unchanged from control. Vomiting during the first 24 hours after surgery was significantly reduced by propofol anesthesia compared with inhaled anesthetics.[269] There was no difference in the time to tracheal extubation, recovery scores, time in the postanesthesia recovery unit, or pain scores between the two groups.

Continuous infusion of propofol has been used to sedate patients in intensive care units. However, unexplained metabolic acidosis and cardiac failure occurred in some patients, and some of these patients died.[270] This may be due to agglutination of the lipid vehicle of propofol and lipid microemboli production. There also are potential neurologic sequelae after prolonged administration of propofol.[271] Fewer patient shiver following propofol anesthesia than with other anesthetics.[272]

Narcotics

Morphine and Meperidine

Narcotics are frequently used to provide pain relief, sedation, and anesthesia in pediatric patients, and to sedate children to facilitate mechanical ventilation in ICUs. Neonates and infants respond to these drugs differently than adults. Two to four times more morphine accumulated in the CNS of young animals than in the CNS of adults, even though their plasma concentrations were similar.[273] This is probably due to a "defect" in the blood–brain barrier of neonates.

Morphine is more rapidly absorbed from SC injection sites of unweaned rats than of adults. Meperidine appears in the blood of fetal lambs approximately 2 minutes after it is given IV to the mother[274] and appears in the fetal brain shortly thereafter. Equilibrium of the drug between mother and fetus occurs 20 to 25 minutes after its injection into the mother.

More meperidine than normeperidine is excreted by human neonates during the first 2 days of life.[275] By 3 days of age the reverse is true, indicating that neonates are able to N-demethylate meperidine but can do this less efficiently than adults. The kinetics of morphine in 0- to 15-year-old patients undergoing surgery were not age related.[276] However, the youngest patient studied was 1 month of age and patients of all ages were lumped together, which may have masked differences. These authors reported a $t_{1/2\beta}$ of 133 minutes and a clearance rate of 6.2 to 6.7 ml/min/kg. Pain occurred when the plasma concentration of morphine fell below 65 ng/ml.

Koren et al.[277] demonstrated significant differences in some pharmacologic variables between neonates and older patients when morphine sulfate 6.2 to 40 μg/kg/h was infused continuously. The plasma concentration of morphine was three times higher in neonates than in older children. Some patients given 18.2 to 24 μg/kg/h of morphine developed seizures. The elimination half-life of morphine was significantly longer in neonates (13.9 $\pm$ 6.4 hours) than in older children and adults (2 hours). In several patients, the plasma concentration of morphine increased after the drug was discontinued, suggesting the presence of enterohepatic circulation of morphine. Significant amounts of β-glucuronidase activity in the gut of neonates would allow hydrolyzation of morphine glucuronide and reabsorption of morphine. Reabsorption of morphine from the gut and the presence of high serum morphine concentrations suggest that care must be taken when morphine is infused continuously to spontaneously breathing infants.

The terminal half-life of morphine in the serum of 2- to 15-year-old children[278] was considerably shorter than in neonates.[277] Greater clearance of the drug in young patients is probably responsible for this difference and probably can be attributed to their relatively large livers, their increased hepatic microsomia (P-450) activity,[279] or both.

Morphine and meperidine depress the CO_2 response curves of neonates more than those of adults. These drugs alter both the set-point and the slope of the CO_2 response. As a result, the resting $Paco_2$ rises and the ventilatory response to the added CO_2 decreases. Differences in the responses of morphine and meperidine are in part related to the different solubilities of the drugs in the CNS. Morphine is more soluble and more drug accumulates in the brain, which may account for its lower LD_{50} in young animals. In older children, morphine depresses the CO_2 response of the respiratory system to the same degree as general anesthesia. However, the depression is more protracted with morphine.

Morphine is often used to sedate infants who require mechanical ventilation. This does not appear to have any adverse effect on the intelligence, motor function, or behavior of those children when tested at 5 to 6 years of age.[280]

Buprenorphine

Buprenorphine (Buprenex), a potent long-acting analgesic, can be given orally or sublingually for postoperative pain relief.[281] Its duration of action is about twice that of morphine. However, the incidence of nausea and vomiting is also almost twice that of morphine (28 percent vs. 16 percent).

Methadone

Methadone, a long-acting narcotic, has been used to treat drug addiction. Recently, it has been used to prevent postoperative pain.[282] A dose of 0.2 mg/kg given during surgery provided 6 to 9 hours of postoperative pain relief, and patients receiving methadone required fewer doses of narcotics postoperatively than did patients receiving the same dose of morphine. Patients given methadone 0.08 mg/kg plus trimeprazine 1 mg/kg and droperidol 0.15 mg/kg were sleepy at the induction of anesthesia and required less pentothal for induction of anesthesia.[283] Methadone has been used successfully in the treatment of patients with chronic pain.[284] Importantly, its use has decreased the total amount of narcotic needed and provided better pain relief. When used in doses of 0.1 mg/kg, methadone administration had a higher incidence of mild hypercarbia and mild oxygen desaturation following ophthalmologic surgery.[285] Berde et al. found no significant complications with administering 0.2 mg/kg of methadone to 3- to 7-year-old children to relieve postoperative pain.[286]

Fentanyl

Fentanyl (Innovar, Sublimaze) is a potent synthetic narcotic used extensively for anesthesia in infants and children. The effective dose (MAC) of adult rats is 52 $\pm$ 7 μg/kg.[287] Pretreatment with phenobarbital increases MAC about 50 percent. Fentanyl is not a complete anesthetic unless given in high concentrations,[288] but when given with nitrous oxide it abolishes heart rate changes and increases arterial blood pressure during surgery. It is cleared primarily by N-dealkylation and hydroxylation in the liver. Only 6 percent of the drug is cleared by the kidney.

Infants have lower serum concentrations of fentanyl than children and adults, despite being given larger doses.[289] Secondary peaks of fentanyl occur in about one-half of infants. Koehntop et al.[290] reported similar pharmacokinetics for fentanyl in preterm and term neonates. However, the data varied greatly. Mean elimination half-life, total body clearance, V_d, and V_{dss} were larger in all pediatric age groups than in adults. The lower initial and steady-state plasma fentanyl concentrations were due to larger initial values for V_d and V_{dss}. The latter prolongs the elimination half-life of fentanyl in neonates. The elimination half-lives were 1.5 to 3.0 times longer in patients with increased abdominal pressures than in those patients with lower intra-abdominal pressures, probably because liver blood flow was altered, cardiac output was decreased, or a compartment (e.g., abdominal viscera, lower extremities) was poorly perfused.[291, 292]

The effects of fentanyl have been studied in acyanotic[293] and cyanotic[294] infants and children. In cyanotic infants, fentanyl 75 μg/kg plus diazepam 0.4 mg/kg caused a slight decrease in heart rate and had no effect on plasma catecholamine concentrations. No increase in arterial or central venous pressure occurred with tracheal intubation or skin incision. Isoflurane, on the other hand, was associated with a significant increase in heart rate and epinephrine concentrations and no change in arterial or central venous pressure. The combination of fentanyl and diazepam produced better cardiovascular stability than either fentanyl 50 to 75 μg/kg[295] or fentanyl 30 μg/kg plus 50 percent nitrous oxide.[296]

The kinetics of fentanyl in infants and children with cyanotic congenital heart disease differ from those of acyanotic patients. The V_d of patients with tetralogy of Fallot increased with increasing age.[294] Clearance of the drug was highest in infants and decreased with increasing age. Pao_2 increased inversely with V_{dss}. The increased elimination half-life of fentanyl in neonates was the result of a two- to threefold smaller V_{dss}. Neonates with tetralogy of Fallot cleared fentanyl better than older patients. V_d at steady state, clearance, and elimination half-life were greater in older patients with tetralogy of Fallot than in adults. Fentanyl infusion blocks the increase in pulmonary vascular resistance and pulmonary arterial pressure that occur with stress in normoxic neonates.[297]

Preterm neonates have a prolonged elimination half-life (6 to 32 hours; mean, 17.7 $\pm$ 0.3 hours)[297] compared with that in older children (4 to 7 hours). Chest wall rigidity has been reported in a preterm infant and following administration of fentanyl to mothers.

Fentanyl significantly affects both the pressor and depressor baroreceptor responses in neonates[298] without affecting resting heart rate and blood pressure. The slopes of both curves were decreased and shifted to the left, suggesting that fentanyl affects the CNS without altering the ratio of parasympathetic tone to sympathetic tone. Fentanyl significantly reduced the total compliance of the lung and chest wall in children,[299] but this effect can be prevented by muscle relaxants.

Fentanyl has been used frequently as a continuous infusion in patients in intensive care units. Tolerance to the drug develops rapidly and escalating doses of fentanyl are required to achieve the same amount of sedation/pain relief.[300] Furthermore, abstinence syndrome occurs with prolonged use of fentanyl.[301]

Oral transmucosal fentanyl citrate (OTFC) has been used to provide preoperative sedation in children.[302] Patients given 10 to 15 or 15 to 20 μg/kg had greater sedation in 40 minutes and 20 minutes, respectively, than control patients. There was no difference in awakening from anesthesia, but patients receiving fentanyl had more vomiting and pruritus and were delayed in taking fluids postoperatively. Other studies have reported similar findings.[303] In addition, they found a decreased respiratory rate and decreased oxygen saturation in the preoperative period. Of special concern is the high incidence of pre- and postoperative vomiting (30 to 85 percent) that occurs with this form of drug administration.

Fentanyl also can be deliverd transdermally. When given by this method, fentanyl takes 18 to 66 hours to reach peak plasma concentrations.[304] The mean clearance and volume of distribution of fentanyl administered transdermally are similar to those of adults. One problem with this form of drug administration is the high incidence of vomiting (85 percent) that occurs.[305] Furthermore, oxygen desaturation and somnolence are also common. There-

fore, it is necessary to monitor infants and children closely if this form of fentanyl administration is used.

Sufentanil

Sufentanil (Sufenta) is a synthetic narcotic that is 5 to 10 times more potent than fentanyl and is used for anesthesia alone or with other drugs. In 2- to 8-year-old children, the elimination half-life is 97 $\pm$ 30 minutes and the V_{dss} is 1.5 times that of adults as a function of body weight, but it is similar to that of adults on the basis of surface area. Clearance of the drug is twice that of adults.[307] In neonates, the clearance, the V_{dss}, and the $t_{1/2\beta}$ are longer than in adults and children.[306] There is great variation in the data, probably due to the differences in extracellular fluid volume. The Clearance and V_{dss} increase and the $t_{1/2\beta}$ decreases with increasing age. Greeley et al. suggested that neonates were less sensitive to sufentanil because they had to supplement the ansthesia at higher serum levels of the drug.[307]

Anxiety is effectively reduced in infants and children when sufentanil is given intranasally as premedication.[308] Most often it is used for cardiovascular surgery.[309, 310] When 10 or 20 μg/kg of sufentanil was used as the sole induction agent for anesthesia, systolic and diastolic arterial blood pressures increased significantly with tracheal intubation and surgical incision.[309] Heart rate increased in patients receiving 5 or 10 μg/kg but decreased in patients receiving 20 μg/kg. Sufentanil 20 μg/kg prolonged the pre-ejection period and pre-ejection period/left ventricle ejection time ratio, suggesting that higher doses of sufentanil have a mild negative inotropic effect. Children receiving sufentanil 20 μg/kg had lower serum epinephrine concentrations than children receiving 5 or 10 μg/kg.

Infants given sufentanil 5 or 10 μg/kg for cardiac surgery had small decreases in heart rate and arterial blood pressure with the induction of anesthesia and a return to baseline with tracheal intubation.[310] A small rise in arterial pressure occurred with sternotomy. This finding differs from that seen with fentanyl 50 or 75 μg/kg, in which sternotomy increased systolic blood pressure by about 20 percent. The difference may be due to sufentanil's short elimination half-life (53 $\pm$ 15 and 55 $\pm$ 10 minutes in infants and children, respectively) and a V_d that is about half as large in infants as in older patients. Both would shorten the duration of anesthesia. Deep hypothermia had no effect on the pharmacokinetics of sufentanil in neonates.

Sufentanil 0.5, 1.0, and 1.5 μg/kg were used to supplement halothane/nitrous oxide for orthopedic surgery.[311] All three doses prevented the increases in heart rate and arterial blood pressure with tracheal intubation and provided good postoperative pain relief. However, 1.0 and 1.5 μg/kg were associated with bradycardia and hypotension during induction of anesthesia and with increased vomiting after surgery.

Intranasal sufentanil 1.5, 3.0, and 4.5 μg/kg has been administered to infants and children as premedication.[312] Treated patients were more likely to separate from their parents without fuss and were less likely to cough during tracheal intubation. However, 25 percent of those receiving 4.5 μg/kg had decreased pulmonary compliance and vomited more often during the first 24 hours after surgery.

Epidural sufentanil 0.75 μg/kg provided pain relief in children within 3.0 $\pm$ 0.3 minutes.[310] In 33 percent of patients, nausea and vomiting occurred 60 to 120 minutes after sufentanil was injected. Sufentanil did, however, decrease the slope of the CO_2 response curve and the minute ventilation beyond that caused by the isoflurane/nitrous oxide given for anesthesia. The slope of the CO_2 response returned to control levels after 120 minutes. The delay in return of the CO_2 response curve and minute ventilation to preanesthesia levels may be due to rostral spread of the drug in the cerebrospinal fluid and premedullary vascular channels.[313]

Alfentanil

Alfentanil (Alfenta) is a potent synthetic narcotic that is about one third as potent as fentanyl. Alfentanil has a rapid onset of action, and there is a rapid recovery from its effects.[314] Because of its relatively small V_d (1.03 $\pm$ 0.71 L/kg) and more rapid clearance from plasma, its elimination half-life is about 30 percent shorter in neonates and infants than in adults.[315] The V_d of alfentanil does not differ between adults and children. Because of its short duration of action, alfentanil is useful for short surgical procedures and lends itself to a continuous infusion technique.[316] The free fraction of drug is similar in adults and children (0.82 $\pm$ 0.30 vs. 1.03 $\pm$ 0.71 L/kg), but there are no data on the effects of continuous infusion of this drug in neonates. On the basis of data with fentanyl and sufentanil, one would predict that the plasma concentration would be higher and that clearance would be faster. In premature infants, the apparent volume of distribution is 1.0 versus the 0.48 L/kg in infants and children. Clearance of the drug was less, 2.2 versus 5.6 ml/kg/min. The elimination half-life was 525 versus 60 minutes. Similar data were found in mechanically ventilated premature infants.[317] A 20 μg/kg bolus of alfentanil was associated with about 20 percent decrease in arterial blood pressure and a significant decrease in heart rate.[318] If the drug was administered over 30 minutes, there was no change in either heart rate or arterial blood pressure.[319] Sixty-five percent of neonates given 9 to 15 μg/kg of alfentanil over 1 minute developed muscle rigidity.[318] Four of the infants had convulsive activity that impaired ventilation and oxygenation.[320]

Remifentanil

Remifentanil is a synthetic narcotic with very rapid onset and offset of action. It has not been widely studied in neonates, infants, and children. Because of its rapid offset, plans must be made to control postoperative pain before the patient awakens. Postoperative pain can be controlled with conduction anesthesia and still allow rapid awakening from anesthesia.[321] Doses of 0.25 μg/kg of remifentanil plus halothane or sevoflurane provided adequate anesthesia for tonsillectomy. The trachea could be extubated sooner, but the children had significant pain postoperatively. Therefore, discharge from the recovery room was not shortened. In one study, 10 percent of patients required ephedrine to restore arterial blood pressure to normal.[322]

Benzodiazepines

Benzodiazepines all exert qualitatively similar effects. These include sedation, hypnosis, decreased anxiety, anticonvulsive activity, and antegrade amnesia. Benzodiazepines potentiate neural inhibition mediated by γ-aminobutyric acid (GABA). There are two types of benzodiazepine receptors, type I and type II. The relative distribution of these receptors varies with development. Type II receptors predominate in the 27-week fetus and type I in the term fetus. Both receptor types are equally present in adults in the eye.

Diazepam

Diazepam (Valium) is commonly used to premedicate patients for surgical and diagnostic procedures and to treat seizures. It is metabolized by hydroxylation and demethylation, both of which are reduced in the neonate,[66] which prolongs the half-life of diazepam. Induction of these metabolic pathways with phenobarbital reduces the half-life of diazepam in neonates (31 $\pm$ 2 hours) to that of children (18 $\pm$ 3 hours). The prolonged half-life of diazepam in neonates may contribute to the level of anesthesia, even when the diazepam is given hours before induction.

The plasma and brain diazepam concentrations of 6- and 18-month-old rats were the same.[323] However, in older animals the $t_{1/2\beta}$ of diazepam was shorter and clearance was increased.

Midazolam

Midazolam (Versed) is a short-acting benzodiazepine that is used for premedication and for induction and maintenance of anesthesia. It also is anxiolytic, hypnotic, and anticonvulsant, like other benzodiazepines. It is three to four times more potent than diazepam and produces anterograde amnesia. Because it is an aqueous solution, midazolam causes little or no local irritation after IM or IV injection. It can be mixed in the same syringe with morphine, meperidine, atropine, or scopolamine. Because it is highly lipid soluble at physiologic pH levels, midazolam readily crosses the blood–brain barrier and has a rapid onset of action. Midazolam is rapidly metabolized by the liver, mainly by microsomal oxidation.[324] About 97 percent of the drug is plasma protein bound, the degree of binding being independent of the dose administered.[325]

Midazolam 0.15 mg/kg and diazepam 0.3 mg/kg have similar effects on the arterial blood pressure of children when used as induction agents for anesthesia.[326] Most studies found no change in heart rate, arterial blood pressure, or respiratory rate when midazolam was used for preoperative sedation.[327]

A study of midazolam found that the pharmacokinetics were dose related in children,[330] making it different from other benzodiazepines. Increasing doses of midazolam increased both drug clearance and AUC. There was no correlation between its pharmacokinetics and the patient's age and weight. The elimination half-life (1.24 to 1.72 hours) is, on average, less than that of adults (1.7 to 4.0 hours). After intranasal administration of 1 mg/kg of midazolam, the plasma concentration of midazolam rose quickly and reached a maximum of 72 ng/ml.[331] Ten minutes after administration, the plasma concentration was 57 percent of that after injection of the same dose IV.

Midazolam has been used to premedicate infants and children. Its effects are dose related. In one study,[328] all children who received intramuscular midazolam became drowsy or sleepy, but those who received less than 0.06 mg/kg were awake and crying within 15 minutes. All children who received 0.1 mg/kg were sleepy or drowsy. However, if anesthesia was delayed 45 to 60 minutes, the patients awoke. Patients (0 to 10 years of age) who received midazolam 0.06 to 0.09 mg/kg were euphoric, not sleepy or drowsy; older children were not euphoric. Patients who received midazolam 0.08 mg/kg had smooth inductions of anesthesia. In another study, midazolam 0.8 mg/kg was required to ensure adequate preoperative sedation. The drug more effectively produced relief of anxiety in 0- to 5-year-olds than in older patients or in those given morphine alone. Both midazolam and morphine produced similar degrees of sedation in older patients. In addition, induction of anesthesia was smoother with midazolam than with morphine premedication, especially in 1- to 5-year-old children.

Taylor et al.[329] found no difference between the effects of intramuscular midazolam 0.2 mg/kg with atropine 0.02 mg/kg and papaveretum 0.4 mg/kg with hyoscine 0.008 mg/kg when these drugs were given 30 to 60 minutes before surgery. The amount of anxiety and the state of awakeness before induction of anesthesia were similar between the two groups. About 75 percent of patients were awake and calm. Induction of anesthesia was satisfactory in 78 percent of midazolam-treated and 89 percent of papaveretum-treated children. Fewer midazolam-treated than papaveretum-treated patients had postoperative nausea and vomiting. Anterograde memory loss was greater in the midazolam-treated patients 2 hours after surgery.

Midazolam has been given rectally for premedication and provides good sedation and memory loss when given by this route.[332, 333] There is no difference in the arterial blood pressure or heart rate with 0.25 and 0.45 mg/kg of rectal midazolam for premedication, but the oxygen saturations of patients given 0.45 mg/kg were lower than those given the smaller dose.[334] The 0.45 mg/kg dose was associated with disinhibition in 25 percent of patients.[335] When more than 1 mg/kg of midazolam was given rectally, all patients were well sedated; discharge from the recovery room was delayed.[336]

Midazolam also has been administered nasally for premedication, with good results. Sixty-three percent of children did not respond to placement of an ear oximeter, 33 percent reacted negatively, and 4 percent could be reassured.[337] The investigators waited only 10 minutes after the drug was administered before they tested the patients' responses. Clinical experience suggests that a delay of 15 to 30 minutes may be more appropriate.

Oral midazolam is used widely to sedate patients for surgery. In doses of 0.5 to 0.75 mg/kg, there is significant sedation in some patients,[338] but more often they become silly. Most of the children will separate from their parents without problems. Children given 0.5 to 0.75 mg/kg of midazolam orally (PO) had no change in heart rate, arterial blood pressure, or oxygen saturation after administration of the drug.[339] However, significant numbers of patients given 0.75 or 1.0 mg/kg of midazolam lost their balance and head control and/or had blurred vision and dysphoria. Between 80 and 90 percent of the patients had good anxiolysis. A major problem with oral administration of midazolam is its bitter taste, which can be partially hidden by juices, chocolate syrup, or other things, but nothing completely masks the taste of this drug. The new oral formulation of the drug has significantly improved the acceptance of midazolam by children. Most of them take it willingly.

Cole[326] reported that all patients lost consciousness with midazolam 0.15 to 0.30 mg/kg IV if they were premedicated with papaveretum and hyoscine. Their vital signs were stable, and breathing was little affected. Therefore, this author suggested that midazolam could be used to induce anesthesia under these circumstances. The combination of ketamine 3 mg/kg and midazolam 0.5 mg/kg was associated with better premedication than with either drug alone.[340]

Ketamine

Ketamine (Ketalar, Ketaject) is a cyclohexylamine anesthetic with a rapid onset and short duration of action. It has the fewest side effects of all such compounds tested.[341] The solution is slightly acidic and contains a mixture of both the *d* and *l* forms of the drug. It has two major metabolites.[342] Metabolite I is formed by demethylation and metabolite II by dehydration. Both metabolites are formed by the hepatic P-450 microsomal system. Because the P-450 enzyme system is less active in the neonate and because infants are less able to conjugate drugs, infants take longer to recover from ketamine anesthesia.

Ketamine has many of the same properties as morphine.[343] Both bind to μ receptors. Ketamine, however, does not bind to other opioid receptors. Binding of ketamine to the receptor occurs at a concentration about one order of magnitude greater than morphine.

Waterman and Livingston[344] demonstrated that the onset of anesthesia was more rapid and its duration prolonged in rats anesthetized with ketamine during the first week of life. Over the next 6 weeks, the induction time was prolonged and the duration of anesthesia decreased. Similar changes have been reported in children.[345, 346] The sleep times of female rats were longer than those of male rats of the same age, which was probably related to differences in the formation of the metabolites.[344] Differences in oxidation are probably responsible for these findings. Similar sex differences for the metabolism of hexobarbital also have been reported.[347]

The kinetics of PO and IM ketamine have been determined.[348] After IM injection, its bioavailability is 93 percent and its peak concentration is about 240 ng/ml. The peak concentration of ketamine occurred 22 minutes after injection. The mean terminal half-life of IM ketamine is 155 ± 12 minutes, not different from that after IV injection.[349] Plasma concentrations of norketamine are 90 ± 10 ng/ml 77 ± 14 minutes after injection.

After PO administration of ketamine, peak plasma ketamine concentrations reach 45 ± 10 ng/ml within 30 ± 5 minutes. The mean bioavailability is 16.5 percent. The mean peak norketamine concentration is 20 ± 44 ng/ml after 63 ± 13 minutes, indicating a significant first-pass effect. This is the reason that the incidence of postoperative psychiatric problems are fewer than would be expected from the dose of oral keatamine usually administered. Part of the decreased sensitivity to pain with ketamine is thought to be due to norketamine. Oral ketamine (6 mg/kg) produces good preoperative sedation in children[350] and in adults.[348, 349]

Intravenous ketamine causes a loss of consciousness within approximately 30 seconds that lasts about 10 minutes.[351] Anesthesia is produced in older children with 2 to 3 mg/kg of drug. Higher concentrations of drug are required to produce the same level of anesthesia in younger children, probably because their V_d is larger.[352]

The route of administration of ketamine affects sleep time. Patients recover from an IV dose in 131 minutes but require 201 minutes to recover when the drug is given IM. By comparison, the average recovery time is 51 minutes for patients anesthetized with halothane.[353] Approximately one half the original dose of ketamine is needed to maintain anesthesia, but the time between doses varies greatly; it increases with increasing doses of drug.[333]

After injection of ketamine, patients blink, stare, and exhibit nystagmus, and they lose their eyelid reflexes. They fall into a dissociative, cataleptic state with their eyes wide open. The brain cannot interpret afferent impulses in this state because normal connections between the sensory cortex and the association areas are disrupted.[354] Depression of evoked activity of the lamina V layer of dorsal horn cells may be responsible for the analgesic effects of ketamine. Analgesia may persist for some time after the last dose of anesthetic,[355] which decreases the need for postoperative analgesia.[352–355]

Gag and cough reflexes are better maintained with ketamine than with other anesthetics, but not well enough to prevent aspiration of gastric contents during anesthesia.[356] Some patients anesthetized with ketamine have died after aspiration of gastric contents.

The cardiovascular effects of ketamine are dose related. In adults, 0.5 mg/kg increases both the systolic and diastolic arterial pressures and the heart rate.[341] Maximal changes occur with 1.5 mg/kg. In children, there is either a small increase or no change in arterial blood pressure and a large increase in heart rate. Similar cardiovascular changes occur after 1 or 2 mg/kg of ketamine IV.[357] Smaller increases in arterial blood pressure occur after IM ketamine. Hypotension is uncommon after ketamine administration unless the blood volume is diminished or the patient's ability to produce and release catecholamines is diminished. Plasma norepinephrine levels are significantly increased after injection of ketamine, probably on a central basis.[358] Although ketamine is a direct myocardial depressant, this effect is short-lived and is usually masked by the catecholamine and sympathetic stimulation. The increased myocardial work (tachycardia) and increased peripheral vascular resistance increase myocardial oxygen demand, as indicated by increased rate–pressure products. Therefore, ketamine is relatively contraindicated in patients with increased myocardial oxygen demands.[359] Baroreflexes are preserved in healthy adult volunteers. Right and left atrial, pulmonary arterial, and left ventricular pressures are unchanged when ketamine is given to children with heart disease. Heart rate and arterial pressure increase significantly. Low-dose ketamine (1 to 2 mg/kg IV) has no effect on left atrial, mean pulmonary arterial, and mean arterial pressures, nor does it affect the pulmonary or systemic vascular resistances or cardiac output of lambs.[357]

Both respiratory rate and tidal volume are significantly decreased by modest doses of ketamine 2 mg/kg IV, and these changes are associated with hypoxemia in both adult and pediatric patients.[359] The Pa_{CO_2} rises for up to 10 minutes after the drug is injected and then returns towards normal. Surgical stimulation hastens the return of the Pa_{CO_2} to normal. These adverse effects of ketamine on gas exchange may occur more quickly and may be more severe in young infants, because their functional residual capacity is relatively smaller than that of adults and because their cardiac output and oxygen consumption are larger. Brief periods of apnea can lead to severe hypoxemia. Consequently, patients should be preoxygenated before they are given IM or IV ketamine. Ketamine caused apnea in some patients,[353, 360] especially those who were premature[361] or those who had preexisting respiratory disease. Apnea is more common after large doses of ketamine. However, ketamine 6 mg/kg IM did not cause hypoxemia in children with cyanotic congenital heart disease.[362] In fact, their oxygen saturation increased from 72 percent to 89 percent with either ketamine or halothane. No change in arterial blood pressure occurred with ketamine; it decreased 25 percent with halothane. The authors concluded that both ketamine and halothane safely and effectively induced anesthesia in infants and children.

Corssen et al.[360] suggested that ketamine dilates the bronchi of adults, and Betts and Pankin[363] reported similar results in children. Cabanas et al.[364] found that ketamine relaxed bronchial smooth muscle and prevented histamine release in guinea pigs. However, inhalation of ketamine did not prevent bronchospasm.[365] A dose of 6 mg/kg produced good sedation in 20 to 25 minutes without changes in ventilation or oxygen saturation. An IV could be started in approximately 60 percent of the patients without response to the needlestick. There was no incidence of laryngospasm or prolonged recovery from anesthesia.

Ketamine 0.3 mg/kg also has been administered rectally to provide preoperative sedation.[366] Thirty minutes after administration, ketamine caused good anxiolysis, good sedation, and good cooperation in children. There was no significant change in vital signs.

Coughing occurs with ketamine administration,[346, 353] and at times it can be severe enough to require muscle relaxants or use of another anesthetic. Ketamine increases muscle tone and occasionally causes myoclonic movements. The latter may become so annoying that they require treatment.[346, 353, 367, 368] Nonpurposeful movements are common. Frank seizures are uncommon but electrical seizures are not.[367, 369] Despite its effects on muscle, the drug has been used successfully to anesthetize patients who have primary muscle disease[370] or malignant hyperthermia.[371, 372]

Plasma cortisol,[373] blood sugar, and free fatty acid[374] levels are increased by ketamine. These substances displace bilirubin from albumin, which may increase the likelihood of kernicterus in infants with hyperbilirubinemia.

Ketamine has no known effect on liver function. The transaminase (SGOT, SGPT) and alkaline phosphatase activities and the bilirubin concentration of blood are normal in healthy adult volunteers despite repeated doses of ketamine.[375] There have been no reports of acute or chronic renal failure.

Dreams and hallucinations are a major complication of ketamine administration. They occur in as many as 30 to 50 percent of adults[372–378] and 5 to 10 percent of prepubescent children.[352, 355, 379–382] In older children, the incidence of dreams and hallucinations is similar to that of adults. The adverse CNS effects of ketamine are manifested as picking at the air, increased agitation, personality changes, and enuresis. They can usually be prevented by premedicating the patient with barbiturates or diazepam.[383–386] When such problems occur, they can usually be aborted with IV barbiturates or diazepam. At times, these mental aberrations can be long-lasting and may pose a serious problem not only to the patient but also to the parents and other family members.[379]

Local Anesthetics

Local anesthetics are administered to neonates, infants, and children for conduction anesthesia and for pain relief (see Chapters 12 and 25). They are also administered to pregnant women for relief of pain during labor, and some of the drug crosses the placenta.

Lidocaine Hydrochloride

Peak levels of lidocaine (Xylocaine) are higher in lambs than in adult sheep, and clearance of the drug takes 25 percent longer in lambs.[387] V_d is 50 percent larger in lambs than in adult sheep. Twenty percent more drug is cleared by lambs, but the amount cleared by metabolism is equal in the two age groups. Renal clearance of the drug is increased in neonates, possibly because protein binding of lidocaine is 50 percent less than in adults and because the blood pH is lower and the urine pH higher in lambs. A change of 0.04 pH units doubles renal clearance of lidocaine. Despite increased clearance, the half-life of lidocaine is longer in neonates because of the large V_d.

Asphyxia increases uptake of lidocaine by fetal lambs.[388] About 50 percent more drug is present in the umbilical vein and artery than in maternal vessels. Cerebral lidocaine delivery is approximately doubled in lambs and uptake of lidocaine by the brain is quadrupled. This may account for the occasional toxic effects of lidocaine in asphyxiated neonates after maternal pudendal, spinal, or epidural anesthesia. The increased uptake of lidocaine is probably due to disruption of the blood–brain barrier and to decreased blood concentrations of α_1-acid glycoprotein.[389] Children with severe liver disease have decreased concentrations of this protein and increased serum concentrations of lidocaine.[390] Children with cyanotic congenital heart disease do not have altered lidocaine kinetics, but their free fraction of lidocaine is related to the concentration of α_1-acid glycoprotein in their blood.[391]

In infants and children (0.5 to 3 years of age), the elimination half-life, V_d, and clearance of IV lidocaine are similar to those of adults.[392] After caudal lidocaine, 3- to 9-year-old children have a larger V_d.[393] Neonates also have a larger V_d and prolonged elimination of lidocaine.[394, 395] None of the last three studies compared their findings to simultaneously studied adults. Finholt et al.[392] measured lidocaine kinetics in both adults and neonates.

Mepivacaine Hydrochloride

Mepivacaine (Carbocaine) is an anilide anesthetic that is primarily eliminated by oxidation, hydrolysis, and conjugation in the liver.[396] All three of these pathways are reduced in the neonate. Therefore, hepatic clearance of mepivacaine is reduced to one third that of the adult (16 vs. 48 ml/min/kg). The blood/plasma ratio of mepivacaine is higher in neonates than in older patients because more drug is bound to red blood cells. Total clearance of mepivacaine is higher in neonates due to lower plasma protein binding of the drug and higher urine pHs. The latter prevents resorption of mepivacaine by the renal tubules. Table 3–5 compares the kinetics of mepivacaine and lidocaine.

Etidocaine Hydrochloride

The blood/plasma ratio of etidocaine (Duranest) is greater in neonates than in adults, due in part to the fact that neonates have higher hematocrits and lower protein binding of the drug.[397] The reduced protein binding is the reason more drug is excreted as unchanged parent compound and N-demethylated metabolite by the kidneys than one would predict. The N-demethylated metabolite may be decreased in neonates.

T A B L E   3 – 5
COMPARISON OF PHARMACOKINETICS OF MEPIVACAINE AND LIDOCAINE IN NEONATES

Parameter	Mepivacaine	Lidocaine
Volume of distribution		
Liters	3.72	5.3
L/kg	1.75	2.75
t½ (h)	8.69	3.61
Hepatic clearance		
ml/min	2.57	15.70
ml/min/kg	1.37	8.00
% Dose excreted unchanged in urine	43.3	19.7
Renal plasma clearance		
ml/min	1.48	2.08
ml/min/kg	0.76	1.37

From Moore RG, Thomas J, Triggs DB, et al: The pharmacokinetics and metabolism of anilide anesthetics in neonates. III. Mepivacaine. Eur J Clin Pharmacol 14:203, 1978. Copyright 1978 Springer-Verlag, with permission.

Bupivacaine Hydrochloride

Bupivacaine (Marcaine) is frequently used to provide caudal, epidural, and local anesthesia in infants and children because of its relatively long duration of action. After caudal anesthesia in 7.25- ± 0.75-year-old children, the maximal plasma concentration of bupivacaine occurred within 29.1 ± 3.1 minutes.[398] Serum concentrations were 1.25 ± 0.09 μg/ml and the elimination half-life was 277 ± 34 minutes. The volume of distribution at steady state was 2.7 ± 0.2 L/kg and the clearance 10.0 ± 0.7 ml/kg/min. Therefore, bupivacaine is rapidly absorbed from the caudal space. The maximal bupivacaine concentration is slightly higher than that reported in adults.[399] The clearance of bupivacaine is the same as in adults.[400] The V_d of bupivacaine is about three times larger in neonates than in adults, and the terminal half-life of bupivacaine in children is longer than in adults. Midazolam has no effect on the kinetics of bupivacaine.[401, 402]

Cholinergic Drugs

Neonates, infants, and children have a greater response to vagal stimulation than adults. Bradycardia with succinylcholine, halothane, enflurane, laryngoscopy, and traction on the lateral and medial rectus muscles is more intense in infants and young children than in adults.[403] The usual dose of atropine required in neonates (0.03 to 0.04 mg/kg) is about 5- to 10-fold greater than that required by adults.

Atropine

Atropine competitively blocks the effects of acetylcholine on tissues innervated by postganglionic nerves. It is partly metabolized (39 ± 17 percent) and partly excreted unchanged in the kidney (57 percent).[404] Little of the drug is excreted in stool. The V_d (3.2 ± 1.5 L/kg) and the elimination half-life (6.9 ± 3.3 hours) are more than twice as large as those of adults.[405] The prolonged elimination half-life of atropine is probably due to the increased V_d of this drug.

Oral atropine (0.02 to 0.04 mg/kg) given to infants (5.6 ± 3.0 months of age) 30 to 90 minutes before induction of anesthesia increased heart rate and maintained higher heart rates during surgery better than a placebo.[406] There was no significant difference in arterial blood pressure among the three groups. Atropine did, however, increase the time to the lowest arterial blood pressure. Atropine did not prevent hypotension. Atropine given intravenously increased heart rate and cardiac output, and these increases were not age dependent.[407]

Intravenous atropine rapidly decreases lower esophageal sphincter pressure in infants and children.[408] Therefore, appropriate precautions should be taken when this drug is administered to patients with reduced gastroesophageal sphincter tone. Atropine given orally enhances the risk for gastric aspiration because it is associated with a greater number of children with a gastric pH of less than 2.5 and a gastric volume of more than 0.04 ml/kg. Glycopyrrolate given IV was associated with a low pH and significant gastric volume in about half as many patients.

The sight of atropine injection is important. When the drug was injected intralingually, the onset time of heart rate acceleration was 3 ± 1.1 minutes. When injected into the deltoid muscle it was 4.4 ± 1.1 minutes, and when it was injected into the vastus lateralis it was 6.4 ± 2.4 minutes.[21]

Glycopyrrolate

Glycopyrrolate (Robinul) is a quaternary amine that penetrates the CNS poorly.[409] It is rapidly absorbed after IM injection and has prolonged antisialogogue activity. It is excreted unchanged in both bile and urine.[409] The only difference in pharmacokinetic parameters between infants and children is that 1- to 3-year-olds exhibit a shorter elimination half-life.[410]

In children, IV glycopyrrolate 10 μg/kg dried the mouth significantly more effectively than IV atropine 20 μg/kg or PO atropine 30 μg/kg.[411] IV atropine and glycopyrrolate more effectively increased heart rate than did PO atropine, although the latter increased the heart rate significantly. Neither drug nor route of drug administration changed the axillary temperature. Forty-one percent of patients receiving atropine PO had arrhythmias with the induction of anesthesia. Only 19 percent of the other two groups had arrhythmias. Only 3.3 to 13.3 percent of glycopyrrolate given orally is bioavailable.[412] There are only small differences in the pharmacokinetics of glycopyrrolate in infants and children, and these are minor and not of clinical importance.[410]

REFERENCES

1. Weiss CF, Glazko AJ, Weston JK: Chloramphenicol in the newborn; a physiologic explanation of its toxicity when given in excessive doses. N Engl J Med 262:787, 1960.
2. Aranda JV, Portuguez-Malavasi A, Collinge JM, et al: Epidemiology of adverse drug reactions in the newborn. Dev Pharmacol Ther 5:173, 1982.
3. Turner S, Nunn AJ, Fielding K, Choonara I: Adverse drug reactions to unlicensed and off-label drugs on paediatric wards: a prospective study. Acta Paediatr 88:965, 1999.
4. Aranda JV, Cohen S, Neims AH: Epidomology of drug utilization in the newborn period. J Pediatr 89:315, 1976.
5. Aranda JV: Factors associated with adverse drug reactions in the newborn. Pediatr Pharmacol 3:245, 1983.
6. Weber WW, Cohen SN: Aging effects and drugs in man. In Gillette JR, Mitchell JR (eds): Concepts in Biochemical Pharmacology. Vol 28, Part 3. New York, Springer-Verlag, 1975, p 213.
7. Ames MD: Gastric acidity in the first ten days of life in the prematurely born baby. Am J Dis Child 100:123, 1960.
8. Hyman PE, Feldman EJ, Ament ME, et al: Effect of enteral feeding on the maintenance of gastric acid secretory function. Gastroenterology 84:341, 1983.
9. Rogers BM, Dix PM, Tolbert JL, McGuigan JE: Fasting and postprandial serum gastrin in normal human neonates. J Pediatr Surg 13:13, 1978.
10. Rooney PJ, Dow TG, Brooks PM, et al: Immunoreactive gastrin and gestation. Am J Obstet Gynecol 122:834, 1975.
11. Euler AR, Byrne WJ, Meis PJ, et al: Basal and pentagastrin stimulated acid secretion in newborn human infants. Pediatr Res 13:36, 1979.
12. Hyman PE, Clarke DD, Everett SL, et al: Gastric acid secretory function in preterm infants. J Pediatr 106:467, 1985.
13. Watkins JB, Ingall D, Szczepanik P, et al: Bile salt metabolism in the newborn: measurement of pool size and synthesis by stable isotope technique. N Engl J Med 288:431, 1973.
14. Murphy GM, Singer E: Bile acid metabolism in infants and children. Gut 15:151, 1974.
15. Gumpta M, Brans YW: Gastric retention in neonates. Pediatrics 62:26, 1978.

16. Siegel M, Lebentahl E, Krantz B: Effect of caloric density on gastric emptying in premature infants. J Pediatr 104:118, 1984.
17. Salem MR, Wong AU, Mani M, et al: Premedicant drugs and gastric juice pH and volume in pediatric patients. Anesthesiology 44:216, 1976.
18. Ong BY, Palahniuk RJ, Cumming M: Gastric volume and pH in outpatients. Anesthesiology 44:216, 1976.
19. Morselli PL: Pediatric clinical pharmacology—routine monitoring for clinical trials. In International Symposium on Clinical Pharmacology. Amsterdam, Excerpta Medica, 1976.
20. Reynolds LM, Lau M, Brown R, et al: Intramuscular rocuronium in infants and children. Anesthesiology 85:231, 1996.
21. Sullivan KJ, Berman LS, Koska J, et al: Intramuscular atropine sulfate in children: comparison of injection sites. Anesth Analg 84:54, 1997.
22. Morselli PL, Franco-Morselli R, Bossi L: Clinical pharmacokinetics in newborns and infants: age related differences and therapeutic implications. Clin Pharmacokinet 5:485, 1980.
23. Lester RS: Topical formulary for the pediatrician. Pediatr Clin North Am 30:749, 1983.
24. Nachman RL, Esterly NB: Increased skin permeability in preterm infants. J Pediatr 79:628, 1971.
25. Taddio A, Ohlsson A, Einarson TR, et al: A sysematic review of lidocaine-pricolaine cream (EMLA) in the treatement of acute pain in neonates. Pediatrics 101:E1, 1998.
26. Golianu B, Krane EJ, Galloway KS, Yaster M: Pediatric acute pain management. Pediatr Clin North Am 47:559, 2000.
27. Petty C, Cunningham NL: Insulin adsorption by glass bottles, polyvinylchloride infusion containers, and intravenous tubing. Anesthesiology 40:400, 1974.
28. Roberts RJ: Intravenous administration of medication in pediatric patients: problems and solutions. Pediatr Clin North Am 28:23, 1981.
29. De Boer AG, Moolenaar F, de Leede LGJ, Briemer DD: Rectal drug administration: clinical pharmacokinetic considerations. Clin Pharmacokinet 7:285, 1982.
30. Boxenbaum HG, Bekersky L, Jack ML, Kaplan SA: Influence of gut microflora on bioavailability. Drug Metab Rev 9:259, 1979.
31. Quaynor H, Corbey M, Bjorkman S: Rectal induction of anaesthesia in children with methohexitone. Br J Anaesth 57:573, 1985.
32. Bjorkman S, Gabrielsson H, Quaynor H, Corbey M: Pharmacokinetics of I.V. and rectal methohexitone in children. Br J Anaesth 59:1541, 1987.
33. Goresky GV, Steward DJ: Rectal methohexitane for induction of anaesthesia in children. Can Anaesth Soc J 26:213, 1979.
34. Liu LMP, Goudsouzian NG, Liu PC: Rectal methohexital premedication in children, a dose comparison study. Anesthesiology 53:343, 1980.
35. Forbes RB, Murray DJ, Dull DL, Mahoney LT: Haemodynamic effects of rectal methohexitone for induction of anaesthesia in children. Can J Anaesth 36:526, 1989.
36. Liu LMP, Gandreault P, Friedman PA, Goudsouzian NG: Methohexital plasma concentrations in children following rectal administration. Anesthesiology 62:567, 1985.
37. Forbes RB, Murray DJ, Dillman JB, Dull DL: Pharmacokinetics of two percent rectal methohexitone in children. Can J Anaesth 36:160, 1989.
38. Audenaert SM, Lock RL, Johnson GL, Pedigo NJ: Cardiovascular effects of rectal methohexital in children. J Clin Anesth 4:116, 1992.
39. Daniels AL, Cote CJ, Polaner DM: Continuous oxygen saturation monitoring following rectal methohexitone induction in paediatric patients. Can J Anaesth 39:27, 1992.
40. Hinkle AJ, Winlander CM: Rectal mucosal injury after rectal premedication with methohexital. Anesthesiology 61:A436, 1984.
41. Yemen TA, Pullerits J, Stillman R, Hershey M: Rectal methohexital causing apnea in two patients with meningomyeloceles. Anesthesiology 74:1139, 1991.
42. Burkart GJ, White TJ, Siegle RL, et al: Rectal thiopental versus IM cocktail for sedating children before computerized tomography. Am J Hosp Pharm 37:222, 1980.
43. Ahn NC, Andersen GW, Thomsen A, Valentin N: Preanesthetic medication with rectal diazepam in children. Acta Anaesthesiol Scand 25:158, 1981.
44. Haagensen RE: Rectal premedication in children: comparison of diazepam with a mixture of morphine, scopolamine and diazepam. Anaesthesia 40:956, 1985.
45. Lindahl S, Olsson AK, Thompson D: Rectal premedication in children. Anesthesia 36:376, 1981.
46. Kanto J: New aspects in the use of atropine. Int J Clin Pharmacol Ther Toxicol 21:92, 1983.
47. Bejersten A, Olsson GL, Palmer L: The influence of body weight on plasma concentration of atropine after rectal administration in children. Acta Anaesthesiol Scand 29:782, 1985.
48. Romsing J, Hertel S, Harder A, Rasmussen M: Examination of acetaminophen for outpatient management of postoperative pain in children. Paediatr Anaesth 8:235, 1998.
49. Anderson BJ, Holford NH, Woollard GA, et al: Perioperative pharmacodynamics of acetaminophen analgesia in children. Anesthesiology 90:411, 1999.
50. van Lingen RA, Deinum HT, Quak CM, et al: Multiple-dose pharmacokinetics of rectally administered acetaminophen in term infants. Clin Pharmacol Ther 66:509, 1999.
51. Oie S: Drug distribution and binding. J Clin Pharmacol 26:583, 1986.
52. Berman W Jr, Musselman J: The relationship of age to the metabolism and protein binding of digoxin in sheep. J Pharmacol Exp Ther 208:263, 1979.
53. Boreus LO, Jalling B, Kalberg N: Clinical pharmacology of phenobarbital in the neonatal period. In Morselli PL, Garattini S, Sereni F (eds): Basic and Therapeutic Aspects of the Perinatal Pharmacology. New York, Raven Press, 1975, p 331.
54. Tucker GT, Boyes RN, Bridenbaugh PO: Binding of analide-type local anesthetics in human plasma. II. Implications in vivo, with special reference to trans-placental distribution. Anesthesiology 33:304, 1970.
55. Aranda JV, Sitar DS, Parsons WD, et al: Pharmacokinetic aspects of theophylline in premature newborns. N Engl J Med 295:413, 1976.
56. Kanto J, Erkkola R, Sellman R: Prenatal metabolism of diazepam. BMJ 1:641, 1974.
57. Morselli PL: Clinical pharmacokinetics in neonates. Clin Pharmacokinet 1:81, 1976.
58. Cornford EM, Pardridge WM, Braun LD, Oldendorf WH: Increased blood-brain barrier transport of protein-bound anticonvulsant drugs in the newborn. J Cereb Blood Flow Metab 3:280, 1983.
59. Hyvarinen M, Zeltzer P, Oh W, et al: Influences of gestational age on serum levels of α-1 feto-protein, IgG globulin and albumin in newborn infants. J Pediatr 82:430, 1973.
60. Odell GB: Studies in kernicterus. I. The protein binding of bilirubin. J Clin Invest 38:823, 1959.
61. Odell GB: Influence of binding on the toxicity of bilirubin. Ann N Y Acad Sci 226:225, 1973.
62. Wood M, Wood AJJ: Changes in plasma drug binding and α-acid glycoprotein in mother and newborn infant. Clin Pharmacol Ther 29:522, 1981.
63. Sager G, Nilsen OG, Jacobsen S: Variable binding of propranolol in human serum. Biochem Pharmacol 28:905, 1979.
64. Windorfer A Jr, Kuenzer W, Urbanek R: The influence of age on the activity of acetylsalicylic acid esterase and protein binding. Eur J Clin Pharmacol 7:227, 1974.
65. Way WL, Costley EC, Way EL: Respiratory sensitivity of newborn infants to meperidine and morphine. Clin Pharmacol Ther 6:454, 1965.
66. Gladtke E, Heimann G: The rate of development of elimination functions of kidney and liver of young infants. In Morselli PL, Garattini S, Sereni F (eds): Basic and Therapeutic Aspects of Perinatal Pharmacology. New York, Raven Press, 1975, p 393.
67. Morselli PL, Principi N, Togoni G, et al: Diazepam elimination in premature and full term infants and children. J Perinat Med 1:167, 1973.
68. Meffin P, Long GL, Thomas J: Clearance and metabolism of mepivacaine in the human neonate. Clin Pharmacol Ther 14:218, 1973.
69. Alan SN, Roberts RJ, Fischer LJ: Age related differences in salicylamide and acetaminophen conjugation in man. J Pediatr 1:30, 1977.
70. Jenne JW, Nagasawa HT, Thompson RD: Relationship of urinary metabolites of theophylline to serum theophylline levels. Clin Pharmacol Ther 19:453, 1968.
71. Sereni F, Principi N: Developmental pharmacology. Annu Rev Pharmacol 8:453, 1968.
72. Levy G, Khanna NN, Soda DM, et al: Pharmacokinetics of acetaminophen in the human neonate: formation of acetaminophen glucuronide and sulfate in relation to plasma bilirubin concentrations and D-glucuronic acid excretion. Pediatrics 55:1461, 1966.

73. van den Anker JN: Pharmacokinetics and renal function in preterm infants. Acta Paediatr 85:1393, 1996.
74. Arant BS: Developmental patterns of renal functional maturation compared in the human neonate. Pediatrics 92:705, 1978.
75. Haycock GB: Development of glomerular filtration and tubular sodium reabsorption in the human fetus and newborn. Br J Urol 81(Suppl 2):33, 1998.
76. Leake RD, Trygstad CW: Glomerular filtration rate during the period of adaptation to extrauterine life. Pediatr Res 11:959, 1977.
77. Tognoni G: Antibiotics. In Morselli PL (ed): Drug Disposition During Development. New York, Spectrum, 1976, p 123.
78. Garg DC, Goldberg RN, Woo MR, Weidler DJ: Pharmacokinetics of thiopental in the asphyxiated neonate. Dev Pharmacol Ther 11:213, 1988.
79. Eger EI II: Anesthetic Uptake and Action. Baltimore, Williams & Wilkins, 1974.
80. Eger EI II: Effect of inspired anesthetic concentration on the rate of rise of alveolar concentration. Anesthesiology 24:153, 1963.
81. Avery ME, Fletcher BD: The Lung and its Disorders in the Newborn Infant. Philadelphia, WB Saunders Company, 1974.
82. Gibbs CP, Munson ES, Tham MK: Anesthetic solubility coefficients for maternal and fetal blood. Anesthesiology 43:100, 1975.
83. Lerman J, Gregory GA, Willis MM, Eger EI II: Age and solubility of volatile anesthetics in blood. Anesthesiology 61:139, 1984.
84. Lerman J, Schmitt-Bantel BI, Gregory GA, et al: Effect of age on the solubility of volatile anesthetics in human tissues. Anesthesiology 65:307, 1986.
85. Dobbing J, Sands J: Quantitative growth and development of human brain. Arch Dis Child 48:757, 1973.
86. Widdowson EM: Changes in body composition during growth. In Davis JA, Dobbing J (eds): Scientific Foundations of Pediatrics. 2nd ed. London, William Heinmann Medical Books, 1981, p 337.
87. Lerman J, Gregory GA, Eger EI II: Effects of anaesthesia and surgery on the solubility of volatile anaesthetics in blood. Can J Anaesth 34:14, 1987.
88. Cook DR, Brandom BW, Shiu G, Wolfson B: The inspired median effective dose, brain concentration at anesthesia, and cardiovascular index for halothane in young rats. Anesth Analg 60:182, 1981.
89. Rudolph AM: Congenital Diseases of the Heart. Chicago, Year Book Medical Publishers, 1974.
90. Salanitre E, Rackow H: The pulmonary exchange of nitrous oxide and halothane in infants and children. Anesthesiology 30:338, 1969.
91. Steward DI, Creighton RE: The uptake of nitrous oxide in the newborn. Can Anaesth Soc J 25:215, 1978.
92. Rackow H, Salanitre E: The pulmonary equilibration of cyclopropane in infants and children. Br J Anaesth 46:35, 1974.
93. Deming MV: Agents and techniques for induction of anesthesia in infants and young children. Anesth Analg 31:113, 1952.
94. Lerman J, Robinson S, Willis MM, Gregory GA: Anesthetic requirements for halothane in young children 0-1 month and 1-6 months of age. Anesthesiology 59:421, 1983.
95. LeDez KM, Lerman J: The minimum alveolar concentration (MAC) of isoflurane in preterm neonates. Anesthesiology 67:301, 1987.
96. Cameron CB, Robinson S, Gregory GA: The minimum anesthetic concentration of isoflurane in children. Anesth Analg 63:418, 1984.
97. Gregory GA, Eger EI, Munson ES: The relationship between age and halothane requirement in man. Anesthesiology 30:488, 1969.
98. Nicodemus NF, Nassiri-Rhimi C, Bachman L: Median effective doses (ED$_{50}$) of halothane in adults and children. Anesthesiology 31:344, 1969.
99. Katoh T, Ikeda K: Minimum alveolar concentration of sevoflurane in children. Br J Anaesth 68:139, 1992.
100. Fisher DM, Zwass M: MAC of desflurane in 60% nitrous oxide in infants and children. Anesthesiology 76:354, 1992.
101. Taylor RH, Lerman J: Minimum alveolar concentration of desflurane and hemodynamic response in neonates, infants, and children. Anesthesiology 75:975, 1991.
102. Lockhart CH, Nelson WL: The relationship of ketamine requirement to age in pediatric patients. Anesthesiology 40:507, 1974.
103. Wenzel D, Felgenhauer K: The development of the blood-CSF barrier after birth. Neuropadiatrie 7:175, 1976.
104. Stolting RK, Peterson C: Methoxyflurane anesthesia in pediatric patients: evaluation of anesthetic metabolism and renal function. Anesthesiology 42:26, 1975.
105. Uehleke H, Werner T: Postnatal development of halothane and other haloalkane metabolism and covalent bonding in rat liver microsomes. In Morselli PL, Garattini S, Sereni F (eds): Basic and Therapeutic Aspects of Perinatal Pharmacology. New York, Raven Press, 1975, p 277.
106. Mortensson W, Nilsson J: Effect of halothane on arterial hepatic blood flow as reflected at coeliac angiography. Pediatr Radiol 5:183, 1977.
107. Resurreccion MA, Castely P, Pimentel C, et al: Serum bromide posthalothane in infants and young children. Anesthesiology 54:A327, 1981.
108. Murat I, Delleur MM, MacGee K, Saint-Maurice C: Changes in ventilatory pattern during halothane anaesthesia in children. Br J Anaesth 57:569, 1985.
109. Wahba WM: Analysis of ventilatory depression by enflurane during clinical anesthesia. Anesth Analg 59:103, 1980.
110. Brown K, Aun C, Stocks J, et al: A comparsion of the respiratory effects of sevoflurane and halothane in infants and young children. Anesthesiology 89:86, 1998.
111. Robinson SL, Richardson CA, Willis MM, Gregory GA: Halothane anesthesia reduces pulmonary function in the newborn lamb. Anesthesiology 62:578, 1985.
112. Nagi SH, Katz RL, Farhie SE: Respiratory effects of trichlorethylene, halothane, and methoxyflurane in the cat. J Pharmacol Exp Ther 148:123, 1965.
113. Lindahl SGE, Charlton AJ, Hatch DJ, Phythyon JM: Ventilatory response to inspiratory mechanical loads in spontaneously breathing children during halothane anesthesia. Acta Anaesthesiol Scand 30:122, 1986.
114. Cameron CB, Gregory GA, Rudolph AM, Heymann M: The cardiovascular and metabolic effects of halothane in normoxic and hypoxic newborn lambs. Anesthesiology 62:732, 1985.
115. Anand JK, Sippell WG, Aynsley GA: Randomised trial of fentanyl anaesthesia in preterm babies undergoing surgery: effects on the stress response. Lancet 1:62, 1987.
116. Anand KJ: Neonatal stress responses to anesthesia and surgery. Clin Perinatol 17:207, 1990.
117. Crane L, Gootman N, Gootman PM: Age dependent cardiovascular effects of halothane anesthesia in neonatal pigs. Arch Int Pharmacodyn Ther 214:180, 1975.
118. Wolf WJ, Neal MB, Peterson MD: The hemodynamic and cardiovascular effects of isoflurane and halothane anesthesia in children. Anesthesiology 64:328, 1986.
119. Friesen RH, Lichtor JL: Cardiovascular depression during halothane anesthesia in infants: a study of three induction techniques. Anesth Analg 61:42, 1982.
120. Friesen RH, Lichtor JL: Cardiovascular effects of inhalation induction with isoflurane in infants. Anesth Analg 62:411, 1983.
121. Gregory GA: The baroresponses of preterm infants during halothane anaesthesia. Can Anaesth Soc J 29:105, 1981.
122. Ware R, Robinson S, Gregory GA: The effect of halothane on the baroresponse of adult and baby rabbits. Anesthesiology 56:188, 1982.
123. Duncan PG, Gregory GA, Wade JG: The effect of nitrous oxide on baroreceptor function in newborn and adult rabbits. Can Anaesth Soc J 28:339, 1981.
124. Ebert TJ, Kotrly KJ, Vucins EJ, et al: Halothane anesthesia attenuates cardiopulmonary baroreflex control of peripheral resistance in humans. Anesthesiology 63:668, 1985.
125. Krane EJ, Su JY: Comparison of the effects of halothane on newborn and adult rabbit myocardium. Anesth Analg 66:1240, 1987.
126. Friedman WF: The intrinsic physiologic properties of the developing heart. Prog Cardiovasc Dis 15:87, 1972.
127. Komai H, Rusy BF: Negative inotropic effects of isoflurane and halothane in rabbit papillary muscles. Anesth Analg 66:29, 1987.
128. Murray DJ, Forbes RB, Mahoney LT: Comparative hemodynamic depression of halothane versus isoflurane in neonates and infants: an echocardiographic study. Anesth Analg 74:329, 1992.
129. Eisele JH Jr, Milstein JM, Goetzman BW: Pulmonary vascular responses to nitrous oxide in newborn lambs. Anesth Analg 65:62, 1986.
130. Landry LD, Emerson CW, Philbin SM, et al: The effect of nitrous oxide on pulmonary vascular resistance in children. Anesth Analg 59:548, 1980.

131. Bacher A, Burton AW, Uchida T, Zornow MH: Sevoflurane or halothane anesthesia: can we tell the difference? Anesth Analg 85:1203, 1997.
132. Epstein RH, Stein AL, Marr AT, Lessin JB: High concentration versus incremental induction of anesthesia with sevoflurane in children: a comparison of induction times, vital signs, and complications. J Clin Anesth 10:41, 1998.
133. Inomata S, Suwa T, Toyooka H, Suto Y: End-tidal sevoflurane for tracheal extubation and skin incision in children. Anesth Analg 87:1263, 1998.
134. Frink EJ Jr, Green WB Jr, Brown EA, et al: Compound A concentrations during sevoflurane anesthesia in children. Anesthesiology 84:566, 1996.
135. Levine MF, Sarner J, Lerman J, et al: Plasma inorganic fluoride concentrations after sevoflurane anesthesia in children. Anesthesiology 84:348, 1996.
136. Kudoh A, Sakai T, Ishihara H, Matsuki A: Increase in serum creatine phosphokinase concentrations after suxamethonine during sevoflurane or isoflurane anaesthesia in children. Br J Anaesth 78:372, 1997.
137. O'Brien K, Kumar R, Morton NS: Sevoflurane compared with halothane for tracheal intubation in children. Br J Anaesth 80:452, 1998.
138. O'Brien K, Robinson DN, Morton NS: Induction and emergence in infants less than 60 weeks post-conceptual age: comparison of thiopental, halothane, sevoflurane and desflurane. Br J Anaesth 80:456, 1998.
139. Aono J, Ueda W, Mamiya K, et al: Greater incidence of delirium during recovery from sevoflurane anesthesia in preschool boys. Anesthesiology 87:1298, 1997.
140. Sury MR, Black A, Hemington L, et al: A comparison of the recovery characteristics of sevoflurane and halothane in children. Anaesthesia 51:543, 1996.
141. Welborn LG, Hannallah RS, Norden JM, et al: Comparison of emergence and recovery characteristics of sevoflurane, desflurane, and halothane in pediatric ambulatory patients. Anesth Analg 83:917, 1996.
142. Kern C, Erb T, Frei FJ: Haemodynamic responses to sevoflurane compared with halothane during inhalational induction in children. Paediatr Anaesth 7:439, 1997.
143. Lerman J: Sevoflurane in pediatric anesthesia. Anesth Analg 81(Suppl):S4, 1995.
144. Berkowitz RA, Hoffman WE, Cunningham F, McDonald T: Changes in cerebral blood flow velocity in children during sevoflurane and halothane anesthesia. J Neurosurg Anesthesiol 8:194, 1996.
145. Woodforth IJ, Hicks RG, Crawford MR, et al: Electroencephalographic evidence of seizure activity under deep sevoflurane anesthesia in nonepileptic patient. Anesthesiology 87:1579, 1997.
146. Stead AL: The response of the newborn infant to muscle relaxants. Br J Anesth 27:124, 1955.
147. Bush GH, Stead AL: The use of d-tubocurarine in neonatal anesthesia. Br J Anaesth 34:721, 1962.
148. Walts LF, Dillon JB: The response of newborns to succinylcholine and d-tubocurarine. Anesthesiology 31:35, 1969.
149. Lim HS, Davenport HT, Robson JG: The response of infants and children to muscle relaxants. Anesthesiology 25:161, 1964.
150. Churchill-Davidson HC, Wise RP: The response of the newborn infant to muscle relaxants. Can Anaesth Soc J 11:1, 1964.
151. Goudsouzian N, Donlon JV, Savarese JJ, Ryan JF: Re-evaluation of dosage and duration of d-tubocurarine in the pediatric age group. Anesthesiology 43:416, 1975.
152. Matteo RS, Lieberman IG, Salanitre E, et al: Distribution, elimination, and action of d-tubocurarine in neonates, infants, children and adults. Anesth Analg 63:799, 1984.
153. Long G, Bachman L: Neuromuscular blockage by d-tubocurarine in children. Anesthesiology 28:723, 1967.
154. Bryan AC, Bryan MH: Control of respiration in the newborn. In Thibeault DW, Gregory GA (eds): Neonatal Pulmonary Care. Menlo Park, CA, Addison-Wesley Publishing, 1979, p 2.
155. Keens TG, Bryan AC, Levison H, Zanuzzo CD: Developmental pattern of muscle fiber types in human ventilatory muscles. J Appl Physiol 144:909, 1978.
156. Miller RD, Way WL, Dolan WM, et al: The dependence of pancuronium and d-tubocurarine induced neuromuscular blockades on alveolar concentrations of halothane. Anesthesiology 37:573, 1972.
157. Fisher DM, O'Keeffe C, Stanski DR, et al: Pharmacokinetics and pharmacodynamics of d-tubocurarine in infants, children and adults. Anesthesiology 55:203, 1982.
158. Miller RD, Matteo R, Benet L, et al: Influence of renal failure on the pharmacokinetics of d-tubocurarine in man. J Pharmacol Exp Ther 202:1, 1977.
159. Kroenigsberger MR, Patten B, Lovelace RE: Studies of neuromuscular function in the newborn. I. A comparison of myoneural function in the full term and the premature infant. Neuropaediatrie 4:351, 1973.
160. Crumrine RS, Yodlowski EH: Assessment of neuromuscular function in infants. Anesthesiology 54:29, 1981.
161. Smith CE, Baxter M, Bevan JC, et al: Accelerated onset and delay of recovery of d tubocurarine blockade with pancuronium in infants and children. Can Anaesth Soc J 34:555, 1978.
162. Cameron CB, Gregory GA, Rudolph AM, Heymann MA: Cardiovascular effects of d tubocurarine and pancuronium in newborn lambs during normoxia and hypoxia. Pediatr Res 20:246, 1986.
163. Storella RJ, Martyn JA, Bierkamper GG: Anti-curare effect of plasma from patients with thermal injury. Life Sci 43:35, 1988.
164. Goudsouzian NG, Ryan JF, Savarese JJ: The neuromuscular effects of pancuronium in infants and children. Anesthesiology 41:9, 1974.
165. Meretoja OA, Luosto T: Dose-response characteristics of pancuronium in neonates, infants and children. Anaesth Intensive Care 18:455, 1990.
166. Goudsouzian NG, Crone RD, Todres ID: Recovery from pancuronium blockade in the neonatal intensive care unit. Br J Anaesth 53:1303, 1981.
167. Curless RG: Developmental pattern of peripheral nerve, myoneural junction and muscle: a review. Prog Neurobiol 9:197, 1977.
168. Agoston S, Crul JF, Kersten UW, et al: The fate of pancuronium in man. Acta Anaesthesiol Scand 17:267, 1973.
169. Somogyi AA: Pancuronium clearance with age. Br J Anaesth 52:360, 1980.
170. Bennett EJ, Daugherty MJ, Bowyer DE, et al: Pancuronium bromide: experience in 100 pediatric patients. Anesth Analg 50:798, 1971.
171. Runkle B, Bancalari E: Acute cardiopulmonary effects of pancuronium bromide in mechanically ventilated newborn infants. J Pediatr 104:614, 1984.
172. Cabal LA, Siassi B, Artal R, et al: Cardiovascular and catecholamine changes after administration of pancuronium in distressed neonates. Pediatrics 75:284, 1985.
173. Buckner PS, Todd DA, Lui K, John E: Effect of short-term muscle relaxation on neonatal plasma volume. Crit Care Med 19:1357, 1991.
174. Colditz PB, Williams GL, Berry AB, Symonds PJ: Variability of Doppler flow velocity and cerebral perfusion pressure is reduced in the neonate by sedation and neuromuscular blockade. Aust Paediatr J 25:171, 1989.
175. Goldstein DM, Davis PJ, Kretchman E, et al: Double-blind comparison of oral transmucosal fentanyl citrate with oral meperidine, diazepam, and atropine as preanesthetic medication in children with congenital heart disease. Anesthesiology 74:28, 1991.
176. Miall-Allen VM, de Vries LS, Dubowitz LM, Whitelaw AG: Blood pressure fluctuation and intraventricular hemorrhage in the preterm infant of less than 31 weeks' gestation. Pediatrics 83:657, 1989.
177. Perlman JM, Volpe JJ: Fluctuating blood pressure and intraventricular hemorrhage. Pediatrics 85:620, 1990.
178. Lanier WL, Milde JH, Michenfelder JD: The cerebral effects of pancuronium and atracurium in halothane-anesthetized dogs. Anesthesiology 63:589, 1985.
179. Palmisano BW, Fisher DM, Willis MM, et al: The effect of paralysis on oxygen consumption in normoxic children after cardiac surgery. Anesthesiology 61:518, 1984.
180. Fisher DM, Canfell PC, Fahey MR, et al: Elimination of atracurium in humans: contribution of the Hofmann elimination and ester hydrolysis versus organ-based elimination. Anesthesiology 65:6, 1986.
181. Fisher DM, Canfell C, Miller RD: Stability of atracurium administered by infusion. Anesthesiology 61:347, 1984.
182. Goudsouzian N, Martyn J, Rudd D, et al: Continuous infusion of atracunium in children. Anesthesiology 64:171, 1986.
183. Brandom BW, Woelfel SK, Cook DR, et al: Clinical pharmacology of atracurium in infants. Anesth Analg 63:309, 1984.
184. Brandom BW, Rudd GD, Cook DR: Clinical pharmacology of atracurium in paediatric patients. Br J Anaesth 55:117S, 1983.

185. Brandom BW, Cook DR, Woelfel SK, et al: Atracurium infusion requirements in children during halothane, isoflurane, and narcotic anesthesia. Anesth Analg 64:471, 1981.
186. Meakin G, Shaw EA, Baker RD, Morris P: Comparison of atracurium-induced neuromuscular blockade in neonates, infants and children. Br J Anaesth 60:171, 1988.
187. Nightingale DA: Use of atracurium in neonatal anaesthesia. Br J Anaesth 55(Suppl 1):1155, 1983.
188. Fahey MR, Rupp SM, Fisher DM, et al: The pharmacokinetics and pharmacodynamics of atracurium in patients with and without renal failure. Anesthesiology 61:699, 1984.
189. Fisher DM, Miller RD: Neuromuscular effects of vecuronium (ORG NC45) in infants and children during N₂O, halothane anesthesia. Anesthesiology 58:519, 1983.
190. Sloan MH, Lerman J, Bissonnette B: Pharmacodynamics of high-dose vecuronium in children during balanced anesthesia. Anesthesiology 74:656, 1991.
191. Meretoja OA, Wirtavuori K, Neuvonen PJ: Age-dependence of the dose-response curve of vecuronium in pediatric patients during balanced anesthesia. Anesth Analg 67:21, 1988.
192. Fisher DM, Fahey MR, Cronnelly R, Miller RD: Potency determination for vecuronium (ORG NC45): comparison of cumulative and single-dose techniques. Anesthesiology 57:309, 1982.
193. Fisher DM, Castagnoli K, Miller RD: Vecuronium kinetics and dynamics in anesthetized infants and children. Clin Pharmacol Ther 37:402, 1985.
194. Meretoja OA: Is vecuronium a long-acting neuromuscular blocking agent in neonates and infants? Br J Anaesth 62:184, 1989.
195. Kalli I, Meretoja OA: Duration of action of vecuronium in infants and children anaesthetized without potent inhalation agents. Acta Anaesthesiol Scand 33:29, 1989.
196. Ording H, Fonsmark L: Use of vecuronium and doxapram in patients susceptible to malignant hyperthermia. Br J Anaesth 60:445, 1988.
197. Goudsouzian NG, Alifimoff JK, Eberly C, et al: Neuromuscular and cardiovascular effects of mivacurium in children. Anesthesiology 70:237, 1989.
198. Sarner JB, Brandom BW, Woelfel SK, et al: Clinical pharmacology of mivacurium chloride (BW B1090U) in children during nitrous oxide-halothane and nitrous oxide-narcotic anesthesia. Anesth Analg 68:116, 1989.
199. Jalkanen L, Meretoja OA: The influence of the duration of isoflurane anaesthesia on neuromuscular effects of mivacurium. Acta Anaesthesiol Scand 41:248, 1997.
200. Martyn JA, Goudsouzian NG, Chang Y, et al: Neuromuscular effects of mivacurium in 2- to 12-yr-old children with burn injury. Anesthesiology 92:31, 2000.
201. Markakis DA, Hart PS, Lau M, et al: Does age or pseudocholinesterase activity predict mivacurium infusion rate in children? Anesth Analg 82:39, 1996.
202. Green DW, Fisher M, Sockalingham I: Mivacurium compared with succinylcholine in children with liver disease. Br J Anaesth 81:463, 1998.
203. McCourt KC, Salmela L, Mirakhur RK, et al: Comparison of rocuronium and suxamethonium for use during rapid sequence induction of anaesthesia. Anaesthesia 53:867, 1998.
204. Mazurek AJ, Rae B, Hann S, et al: Rocuronium versus succinylcholine: are they equally effective during rapid-sequence induction of anesthesia? Anesth Analg 87:1259, 1998.
205. Woolf RL, Crawford MW, Choo SM: Dose-response of rocuronium bromide in children anesthetized with propofol: a comparison with succinycholine. Anesthesiology 87:1368, 1997.
206. Reynolds LM, Lau M, Brown R, et al: Bioavailabilty of intramuscular rocuronium in infants and children. Anesthesiology 87:1096, 1997.
207. Wierda JM, Meretoja OA, Taivainen T, Proost JH: Pharmacokinetics and pharmacokinetic-dynamic modeling of rocuronium in infants and children. Br J Anaesth 78:690, 1997.
208. Vuksanaj D, Fisher DM: Pharmacokinetics of rocuronium in children aged 4-11 years. Anesthesiology 82:1104, 1995.
209. O'Kelly B, Fiset P, Meistelman C, Ecoffey C: Pharmacokinetics of rocuronium bromide in paediatric patients. Eur J Anaesthesiol Suppl 9:57, 1994.
210. Khuenl-Brady KS, Sparr H: Clinical pharmacokinetics of rocuronium bromide. Clin Pharmacol 31:174, 1996.
211. Meretoja OA, Taivainen T, Erkola O, et al: Dose-response and time-course of effect of rocuronium bromide in paediatric patients. Eur J Anaesthesiol Suppl 11:19, 1995.
212. Wierda JM, Schuringa M, van den Broek L: Cardiovascular effects of an intubating dose of rocuronium 0.6 mg kg-1 in anaesthetized patients, paralysed with vecuronium. Br J Anaesth 78:586, 1997.
213. Abdulatif M, Mowafi H, al-Ghamdi A, el-Sanabary M: Dose-response relationships for neostigmine antagonism of rocuronium-induced neuromuscular block in children and adults. Br J Anaesth 77:710, 1996.
214. Meakin GH, Meretoja OA, Motsch J, et al: A dose-ranging study of rapacuronium in pediatric patients. Anesthesiology 92:1002, 2000.
215. Brandon BW, Margolis JO, Bikhazi GB, et al: Neuromuscular effects of rapacuronium in pediatric patients during nitrous oxide-halothane anesthesia: comparison with mivacuronium. Can J Anaesth 47:143, 2000.
216. Reynolds LM, Infosino A, Brown R, et al: Pharmacokinetics of rapacuronium in infants and children with intravenous and intramuscular administration. Anesthesiology 92:376, 2000.
217. Mills KG, Wright PM, Pollard BJ, et al: Antagonism of rapacuronium using edrophonium or neostigmine: pharmacodynamics and pharmacokinetics. Br J Anaesth 83:727, 1999.
218. Fisher DM, Cronnelly R, Miller RD, Sharma M: The neuromuscular pharmacology of neostigmine in infants and children. Anesthesiology 59:220, 1983.
219. Fisher DM, Cronnelly R, Sharma M, Miller RD: Clinical pharmacology of edrophonium in infants and children. Anesthesiology 61:428, 1984.
220. Rackow H, Salanitre E: Modern concepts in pediatric anesthesiology. Anesthesiology 30:208, 1969.
221. Liu LMP, Cote CJ, Goudsouzian NG, et al: Life-threatening apnea in infants recovering from anesthesia. Anesthesiology 59:506, 1983.
222. Cook DR, Fisher BH: Neuromuscular blocking effects of succinylcholine in infants and children. Anesthesiology 42:662, 1975.
223. Goudsouzian NG, Liu LMP: The neuromuscular response of infants to continuous infusion of succinylcholine. Anesthesiology 60:97, 1984.
224. Escobichon DJ, Stephens DS: Perinatal development of human esterases. Clin Pharmacol Ther 14:41, 1973.
225. Mirakhur RK, Elliott P, Lavery TD: Plasma cholinesterase activity and the duration of suxamethonium apnoae in children. Ann R Coll Surg 66:43, 1984.
226. Strauss AA, Modanlou HD: Transient plasma cholinesterase deficiency in preterm infants. Dev Pharamcol Ther 9:82, 1986.
227. Kalow W, Benst K: A method for the detection of atypical forms of human serum cholinesterase; determination of dibucaine numbers. Can J Biochem Phys 35:339, 1957.
228. Pantuck EJ, Pantuck CB: Cholinesterases and anticholinesterases. In Katz RL (ed): Muscle Relaxants. Amsterdam, Excerpta Medica, 1975, p 143.
229. Viby-Mogensen J: Correlation of succinylcholine duration of action with plasma cholinesterase activity in subjects with a genotypically normal enzyme. Anesthesiology 53:517, 1980.
230. Viby-Mogensen J: Succinylcholine neuromuscular blockade in subjects heterozygous for abnormal plasma cholinesterase. Anesthesiology 55:231, 1981.
231. Cook R, Fischer CG: Characteristics of succinylcholine in infants and children. Anesthesiology 42:662, 1975.
232. DeCook TH, Goudsouzian NG: Tachyphylaxis and phase II block development during infusion of succinylcholine in children. Anesth Analg 59:639, 1980.
233. Donati F, Bevan DR: Potentiation of succinylcholine phase II block with isoflurane. Anesthesiology 58:552, 1983.
234. Lindgren L, Saarnivaara L: Increase in intragastric pressure during suxamethonium induced muscle fasciculations in children: inhibition by alfentanil. Br J Anaesth 60:176, 1988.
235. Ryan JF, Kagen LJ, Hyman AL: Myoglobinemia after a single dose of succinylcholine. N Engl J Med 285:824, 1971.
236. Lerman J, Robinson S, Willis MM, et al: Succinylcholine-induced heart rate changes in children during isoflurane and halothane. Anesthesiology 59:A443, 1983.
237. Gronert GA, Theye RL: Pathophysiology of hyperkalemia induced by succinylcholine. Anesthesiology 43:89, 1975.
238. Schaner PJ, Brown RL, Kirsey TD, et al: Succinylcholine induced hyperkalemia in burned patients. Anesth Analg 48:764, 1969.
239. Delphin E, Jackson D, Rothstein P: Use of succinylcholine during elective pediatric anesthesia should be reevaluated. Anesth Analg 66:1190, 1987.

240. Kepes ER, Martinez LR, Andrews IC, et al: Anesthetic problems in hereditary muscular abnormalities. N Y State J Med 72:1051, 1972.

241. Larach MG, Rosenberg H, Gronert GA, Allen GC: Hyperkalemic cardiac arrest during anesthesia in infants and children with occult myopathies. Clin Pediatr 36:9, 1997.

242. Danlon JV, Newfield P, Sreter F, Ryan JF: Implications of masseter spasm after succinylcholine. Anesthesiology 49:298, 1978.

243. Flewellen EH, Nelson TE: Halothane-succinylcholine induced masseter spasm: indicative of malignant hyperthermia susceptibility? Anesth Analg 63:393, 1984.

244. Van Der Spek AFL, Fang WB, Ashton-Miller JA, et al: The effects of succinylcholine on mouth opening. Anesthesiology 67:459, 1987.

245. Carroll JB: Increased incidence of masseter spasm in children with strabismus anesthetized with halothane-succinylcholine. Anesthesiology 67:559, 1987.

246. Rosenberg H, Fletcher JE: Masseter muscle rigidity and malignant hyperthermia susceptibility. Anesth Analg 65:161, 1986.

247. Meakin G, Walker RW, Dearlove OR: Myotonic and neuromuscular blocking effects of increased doses of suxamethonium in infants and children. Br J Anaesth 65:816, 1990.

248. O'Sullivan EP, Childs D, Bush GH: Perioperative dreaming in paediatric patients who receive suxamethonium. Anaesthesia 43:104, 1988.

249. Cote CJ, Petkau AJ: Thiopental requirements may be increased in children reanesthetized at least one year after recovery from extensive thermal injury. Anesth Analg 64:1156, 1985.

250. Brett CM, Fisher DM: Thiopental dose-response relations in unpremedicated infants, children, and adults. Anesth Analg 66:1024, 1987.

251. Sorbo S, Hudson RJ, Loomis JC: The pharmacokinetics of thiopental in pediatric surgical patients. Anesthesiology 61:666, 1984.

252. Cote DJ, Goudsouzian NG, Liu LMP, et al: The dose response of intravenous thiopental for the induction of general anesthesia in unpremedicated children. Anesthesiology 55:703, 1981.

253. Wodey E, Chonow L, Beneux X, et al: Haemodynamic effects of propofol vs thiopental in infants: an echocardiographic study. Br J Anaesth 82:516, 1999.

254. Bhutada A, Sahni R, Rastogi S, Wung JT: Randomised controlled trial of thiopental for intubation in neonates. Arch Dis Child Fetal Neonatal Ed 82:F34, 2000.

255. Carmichael EB: The median lethal dose (LD_{50}) of pentothal sodium for both young and old guinea pigs and rats. Anesthesiology 8:589, 1947.

256. Koska Y, Takahashi E, Mark LC: Intravenous thiobarbiturate anesthesia for cesarean section. Anesthesiology 31:489, 1959.

257. Domek NS, Barlow CF, Roth LJ: An octogenetic study of phenobarbital C-14 in cat brain. J Pharmacol Exp Ther 130:285, 1960.

258. Brown AK, Zwelzin WW, Burnett HH: Studies on the neonatal development of the glucuronide conjugation system. J Clin Invest 37:332, 1958.

259. Kalser SC, Forbes E, Kunig R: Relation of brain sensitivity of hepatic metabolism of hexobarbitone to dose-response relations in infant and young rats. J Pharmacol 21:109, 1969.

260. Onishi S, Ohki Y, Nishimura Y, et al: Distribution of pentobarbital in serum, brain, and other organs from pediatric patients. Dev Pharmacol Ther 7:153, 1984.

261. Gal P, Toback J, Erkan NV, Boer HR: The influence of asphyxia on phenobarbital dosing requirments in neonates. Dev Pharmacol Ther 7:145, 1984.

262. Kadar D, Tang BK, Conn AW: The fate of pentobarbitone in children in hypothermia and at normal body temperature. Can Anaesth Soc J 29:16, 1982.

263. Kanto J, Gepts E: Pharmacokinetic implications for the clinical use of propofol. Clin Pharmacokinet 17:308, 1989.

264. Vandermeersch E, Van JH, Byttebier G, Van AH: Pharmacokinetics of propofol during continuous infusion for pediatric anesthesia. Acta Anaesthiol Belg 40:161, 1989.

265. Kulkarni P, Brown KA: Ventilatory parameters in children during propofol anaesthesia: a comparison with halothane. Can J Anaesth 43:653, 1996.

266. Spens HJ, Drummond GB, Wraith PK: Changes in chest wall compartment volumes on induction of anaesthesia with eltanolone, propofol and thiopentone. Br J Anaesth 76:369, 1996.

267. Runcie CJ, Mackenzie SJ, Arthur DS, Morton NS: Comparison of recovery from anaesthesia induced in children with either propofol or thiopenton. Br J Anaesth 70:192, 1993.

268. Short SM, Aun CS: Haemodynamic effects of propofol in children. Anaesthesia 46:783, 1991.

269. Martin TM, Nicolson SC, Bargas MS: Propofol anesthesia reduces emesis and airway obstruction in pediatric outpatients. Anesth Analg 76:144, 1993.

270. Parke TJ, Stevens JE, Rice AS, et al: Metabolic acidosis and fatal myocardial failure after propofol infusion in children: five case reports. BMJ 305:613, 1992.

271. Trotter C, Serpell MG: Neurological sequelae in children after prolonged propofol infusion. Anaesthesia 47:340, 1992.

272. Cheong KF, Low TC: Propofol and postanaesthetic shivering. Anaesthesia 50:550, 1995.

273. Kupferberg HG, Way EL: Pharmacologic basis for the increased sensitivity of the newborn rat to morphine. Pharmacol Exp Ther 151:105, 1963.

274. Szeto HH, Clapp JF, Abrams R, et al: Brain uptake of meperidine in the fetal lamb. Am J Obstet Gynecol 138:528, 1980.

275. Kuhnert BR, Kuhnert PM, Prochaska AL, et al: Meperidine disposition in mother, neonate and non-pregnant females. Clin Pharmacol Ther 27:486, 1980.

276. Dahlstrom B, Blome P, Feychting H, et al: Morphine kinetics in children. Clin Pharmacol Ther 26:354, 1979.

277. Koren G, Butt W, Chinyanga H, et al: Postoperative morphine infusion in newborn infants: assessment of disposition characteristics and safety. J Pediatr 107:963, 1985.

278. Attia J, Ecoffey C, Sandouk P, et al: Epidural morphine in children: pharmacokinetics and CO_2 sensitivity. Anesthesiology 65:590, 1986.

279. Udkow G: Pediatric clinical pharmacology. Am J Dis Child 132:1025, 1978.

280. MacGregor R, Evans D, Sugden D, et al: Outcome at 5-6 years of prematurely born children who received morphine as neonates. Arch Dis Child Fetal Neonatal Ed 79:F40, 1998.

281. Maunuksela E-L, Korpela R, Olkkola KT: Comparison of buprenorphine with morphine in the treatment of postoperative pain in children. Anesth Analg 67:233, 1988.

282. Berde CB, Beyer JE, Bournaki MC, et al: Comparison of morphine and methadone for prevention of postoperative pain in 3- to 7-year-old children. J Pediatr 119:136, 1991.

283. Phillips GH, Mian T, Becker U, et al: Oral premedication in children. A comparison of trimeprazine with a trimeprazine, droperidol and methadone mixture. Anaesthesia 45:870, 1990.

284. Crews JC, Sweeney NJ, Denson DD: Clinical efficacy of methadone in patients refractory to other mu-opioid receptor agonist analgesics for management of terminal cancer pain. Case presentations and discussion of incomplete cross-tolerance among opioid agonist analgesics. Cancer 72:2266, 1993.

285. Hamunen K: Ventilatory effects of morphine, pethidine and methadone in children. Br J Anaesth 70:414, 1993.

286. Berde CB, Beyer JE, Bournaki MC, et al: Comparison of morphine and methadone for prevention of postoperative pain in 3- to 7-year-old children. J Pediatr 119:136, 1991.

287. Shingu K, Eger EI II, Johnson BH, et al: MAC values of thiopental and fentanyl in rats. Anesth Analg 62:151, 1983.

288. Crean P, Koren G, Goresky G, et al: Fentanyl-oxygen versus fentanyl-N_2O/oxygen anaesthesia in children undergoing cardiac surgery. Can Anaesth Soc J 33:36, 1986.

289. Singleton MA, Rosen JI, Fisher DM: Plasma concentrations of fentanyl in infants, children and adults. Can J Anaesth 34:152, 1987.

290. Koehntop DE, Rodman JH, Brundage DM, et al: Pharmacokinetics of fentanyl in neonates. Anesth Analg 65:227, 1986.

291. Bragg P, Zwass MS, Lau M, Fisher DM: Opioid pharmacodynamics in neonatal dogs: differences between morphine and fentanyl. J Appl Physiol 79:1519, 1995.

292. Luks AM, Zwass MS, Brown RC, et al: Opioid-induced analgesia in neonatal dogs: pharmacodynamic differences between morphine and fentanyl. J Pharmacol Exp Ther 284:136, 1998.

293. Morgan P, Lynn AM, Parrot C, Morray JP: Hemodynamic and metabolic effects of two anesthetic techniques in children undergoing surgical repair of acyanotic congenital heart disease. Anesth Analg 66:1028, 1987.

294. Koren G, Goresky G, Crean P, et al: Unexpected alterations in fentanyl pharmacokinetics in children undergoing cardiac surgery: age related or disease related? Dev Pharmacol Ther 9:183, 1986.

295. Hickey PR, Hansen DD: Fentanyl- and sufentanil-oxygen-pancuronium anesthesia for cardiac surgery in infants. Anesth Analg 63:117, 1984.

296. Hickey PR, Hansen DD, Wessel DL, et al: Blunting of stress responses in the pulmonary circulation of infants by fentanyl. Anesth Analg 64:1137, 1985.

297. Collins C, Koren G, Crean P, et al: Fentanyl pharmacokinetics and hemodynamic effects in preterm infants during ligation of patent ductus arteriosus. Anesth Analg 64:1078, 1985.

298. Murat I, Levron J-C, Berg A, Saint-Maurice C: Effects of fentanyl on baroreceptor reflex control of heart rate in newborn infants. Anesthesiology 68:717, 1988.

299. Marty J, Desmonts JM: Effects of fentanyl on respiratory pressure-volume curves in supine children. Acta Anaesthesiol Scand 25:293, 1991.

300. Arnold JH, Truog RD, Orav EJ, et al: Tolerance and dependence in neonates sedated with fentanyl during extracorporeal membrane oxygenation. Anesthesiology 73:1136, 1990.

301. Franck LS, Vilardi J, Durand D, Powers R: Opioid withdrawal in neonates after continuous infusions of morphine or fentanyl during extracorporeal membrane oxygenation. Am J Crit Care 37:857, 1990.

302. Ashburn MA, Streisand JB, Tarver SD, et al: Oral transmucosal fentanyl citrate for premedication in paediatric outpatients. Can J Anaesth 37:857, 1990.

303. Friesen RH, Lockhart CH: Oral transmucosal fentanyl citrate for preanesthetic medication of pediatric day surgery patients with and without droperidol as a prophylactic anti-emetic. Anesthesiology 76:46, 1992.

304. Collins JJ, Dunkel IJ, Gupta SK, et al: Transdermal fentanyl in children with cancer pain: feasibility, tolerability, and pharmacokinetic correlates. J Pediatr 134:319, 1999.

305. Yee LY, Lopez JR: Transdermal fentanyl. Ann Pharmacother 26:1393, 1992.

306. Guay J, Gaudreault P, Tang A, et al: Pharmacokinetics of sufentanil in normal children. Can J Anaesth 39:14, 1992.

307. Greeley WJ, de Bruijn NP: Changes in sufentanil pharmacokinetics within the neonatal period. Anesth Analg 67:86, 1988.

308. Henderson JM, Brodsky DA, Fisher DM, et al: Pre-induction of anesthesia in pediatric patients with nasally administered sufentanil. Anesthesiology 68:671, 1988.

309. Moore RA, Yang SS, McNicholas KW, et al: Hemodynamic and anesthetic effects of sufentanil as the sole anesthetic for pediatric cardiovascular surgery. Anesthesiology 62:725, 1985.

310. David PJ, Cook DR, Stiller RL, Davin-Robinson KA: Pharmacodynamics and pharmacokinetics of high-dose sufentanil in infants and children undergoing cardiac surgery. Anesth Analg 66:203, 1987.

311. Glenski JA, Friesen RH, Lane GA, et al: Low-dose sufentanil as a supplement to halothane/N$_2$O anaesthesia in infants and children. Can J Anaesth 35:379, 1988.

312. Henneberg S, Nilsson A, Hok B, Persson MP: Anesthesia and monitoring during whole body radiation in children. J Clin Anesth 2:76, 1990.

313. Benlabed M, Ecoffey C, Levron J-C, et al: Analgesia and ventilatory response to CO$_2$ following epidural sufentanil in children. Anesthesiology 67:948, 1987.

314. Mulroy JJ, Davis PJ, Rymer DB, et al: Safety and efficacy of alfentanil and halothane in paediatric surgical patients. Can J Anaesth 38:445, 1991.

315. Roure P, Jean N, Leclerc A-C, et al: Pharmacokinetics of alfentanil in children undergoing surgery. Br J Anaesth 59:1437, 1987.

316. White PF, Coe V, Shafer V, Sung M-L: Comparison of altfentanil with fentanyl for outpatient anesthesia. Anesthesiology 64:99, 1986.

317. Marlow N, Weindling AM, Van PA, Heykants J: Alfentanil pharmacokinetics in preterm infants. Arch Dis Child 349, 1990.

318. Hiller A, Klemola UM, Saarnivaara L: Tracheal intubation after induction of anaesthesia with propofol, alfentanil and lidocane without neuromuscular blocking drugs in children. Acta Anaesthesiol Scand 37:725, 1993.

319. Hiller A: Comparison of cardiovascular changes during anaesthesia and recovery from propofol-alfentanil-nitrous oxide and thiopentone-halothane-nitrous oxide anaesthesia in children undergoing otolaryngological surgery. Acta Anaesthesiol Scand 37:737, 1993.

320. Pokela ML, Ryhanen PT, Koivisto ME, et al: Alfentanil-induced rigidity in newborn infants. Anesth Analg 75:252, 1992.

321. Wee LH, Moriarty A, Cranston A, Bagshaw O: Remifentanil infusion for major abdominal surgery in small infants. Paediatr Anaesth 9:415, 1991.

322. Woods A, Grant S, Davidson A: Duration of apnoea with two different intubating doses of remifentanil. Eur J Anaesthesiol 16:634, 1999.

323. Klotz U: Effect of age on levels of diazepam in plasma and brain of rats. Arch Pharmacol 307:167, 1979.

324. Reves JG, Fragen RJ, Vinik R, Greenbalt DJ: Midazolam: pharmacology and uses. Anesthesiology 62:310, 1985.

325. Moschitto LJ, Greenbalt DJ: Concentration-independent plasma protein binding of benzodiazepines. J Pharm Pharmacol 35:179, 1983.

326. Cole WJH: Midazolam in pediatric anaesthesia. Anesth Intensive Care 10:36, 1982.

327. Rita L, Seleny FL, Goodarzi M, et al: Dose-finding study of intramuscular midazolam in children. Anesthesiol Rev 7:40, 1985.

328. Rita L, Seleny FL, Mazurek A, Rabins SY: Intramuscular midazolam for pediatric preanesthetic sedation: a double-blind controlled study with morphine. Anesthesiology 63:528, 1985.

329. Taylor MB, Vine PR, Hatch DJ: Intramuscular midazolam premedication in small children: a comparison with papaveretum and hyoscine. Anaesthesia 41:21, 1986.

330. Salonen M, Kanto J, Iisalo E, Himberg JJ: Midazolam as an induction agent in children: a pharmacokinetic and clinical study. Anesth Analg 66:625, 1987.

331. Walbergh EJ, Wills RJ, Eckhert J: Plasma concentrations of midazolam in children following intranasal administration. Anesthesiology 74:233, 1991.

332. De Jong PC, Verburg MP: Comparison of rectal to intramuscular administration of midazolam and atropine for premedication of children. Acta Anaesthesiol Scand 32:485, 1988.

333. Holm KR, Clausen TG, Eno D: Rectal administration of midazolam versus diazepam for preanesthetic sedation in children. Anesth Prog 37:29, 1990.

334. Roelofse JA, de V Joubert JJ: Arterial oxygen saturation in children receiving rectal midazolam as premedication for oral surgical procedures. Anesth Prog 37:286, 1990.

335. Roelofse JA, van der Bijl P, Stegman DH, Hartshorne JE: Preanesthetic medication with rectal midazolam in children undergoing dental extractions. J Oral Maxillofac Surg 48:791, 1990.

336. Spear RM, Yaster M, Berkowitz ID, et al: Preinduction of anesthesia in children with rectally administered midazolam. Anesthesiology 74:670, 1991.

337. Karl HW, Keifer AT, Rosenberger JL, et al: Comparison of the safety and efficacy of intranasal midazolam or sufentanil for preinduction of anesthesia in pediatric patients. Anesthesiology 76:209, 1992.

338. Felt LH, Negus JB, White PF: Oral midazolam preanesthetic medication in pediatric outpatients. Anesthesiology 73:831, 1990.

339. McMillan CO, Spahr SI, Sikich N, et al: Premedication of children with oral midazolam. Can J Anaesth 39:545, 1992.

340. Funk W, Jakob W, Riedl T, Taeger K: Oral preanaesthetic medication for children: double-blind randomized study of a combination of midazolam and ketamine vs midazolam or ketamine alone. Br J Anaesth 84:335, 2000.

341. Domino E, Chodoff P, Corssen G: Pharmacologic effects of Cl-581, a new dissociative anesthetic in man. Clin Pharmacol Ther 6:279, 1965.

342. Lau SS, Domino EF: Gas chromatography mass spectrometry assay for ketamine and its metabolites in plasma. Biomed Mass Spectrum 4:317, 1977.

343. Smith DJ, Bouchal RL, deSanctis CA, et al: Properties of the interaction between ketamine and opiate binding sites in vivo and in vitro. Neuropharmacology 26:1253, 1987.

344. Waterman AE, Livingston A: Effects of age and sex on ketamine anaesthesia in the rat. Br J Anaesth 50:885, 1978.

345. Mayhew JF, Lanier RJ: Ketamine: its use in the pediatric patient for radiotherapy. AANA J 45:178, 1977.

346. Wyant GM: Intramuscular ketalar (Cl 581) in pediatric anaesthesia. Anaesth Soc J 18:72, 1971.

347. Streicher E, Garbus J: The effect of age and sex on the duration of hexobarbital anesthesia in rats. J Gerontol 10:441, 1955.

348. Grant IS, Nimmo WS, Clements JA: Pharmacokinetics and analgesic effects of IM and oral ketamine. Br J Anaesth 53:805, 1981.

349. Clements JA, Nimmo WS: The pharmacokinetics and analgesic effect of ketamine in man. Br J Anaesth 53:27, 1981.

350. Gutstein HB, Johnson KL, Heard MB, Gregory GA: Oral ketamine preanesthetic medication in children. Anesthesiology 76:28, 1992.

351. Idvall J, Ahlgren I, Aronsen KF, et al: Hemodynamic and respiratory effects of ketamine in relation to its plasma levels. Excerpta Med Int Congr Ser 452:443, 1978.

352. Hollister GR, Burn JMB: Side effects of ketamine in pediatric anesthesia. Anesth Analg 53:264, 1974.

353. Roper AL, Kramer RJ: Ketamine anesthesia in minor otologic procedures. Laryngoscope 9:1423, 1971.

354. Kitahata LM, Taub A, Kosaka Y: Lamina specific suppression of dorsal-horn unit activity by ketamine hydrochloride. Anesthesiology 38:4, 1973.

355. Roberts FW: A new intramuscular anaesthetic for small children. Anaesthesia 22:23, 1967.

356. Carson IW, Moore J, Balmer JP, et al: Laryngeal competence with ketamine and other drugs. Anesthesiology 38:128, 1973.

357. Burrows FA, Norton JB, Fewel J: Cardiovascular and respiratory effects of ketamine in the neonatal lamb. Can Anaesth Soc J 33:10, 1986.

358. Zsigmond EK, Kelsch RC: Elevated plasma norepinephrine concentration during ketamine anesthesia. Clin Pharmacol Ther 14:149, 1973.

359. Zsigmond EK, Matsuki A, Kothary SP, et al: Arterial hypoxemia caused by intravenous ketamine. Anesth Analg 55:311, 1976.

360. Corssen G, Gutierrez J, Reves JG, et al: Ketamine in the anesthetic management of asthmatic patients. Anesth Analg 51:588, 1972.

361. Welborne LG, Rice LJ, Hannallah RS, et al: Postoperative apnea in former preterm infants: prospective comparison of spinal and general anesthesia. Anesthesiology 72:838, 1990.

362. Greeley WJ, Bushman GA, Davis DP, Reves JG: Comparative effects of halothane and ketamine on systemic arterial oxygen saturation in children with cyanotic heart disease. Anesthesiology 65:666, 1986.

363. Betts EK, Pankin CE: Use of ketamine in an asthmatic child: a case report. Anesth Analg 50:420, 1971.

364. Cabanas A, Souhrada JF, Aldrete JA: Effects of ketamine in normal and asthmatic airway smooth muscle of guinea pigs. In International Anesthesiology Research Society, Cleveland, Scientific Program Abstracts, 1979, p 86.

365. Rock MJ, Reyes de la Rocha S, Lerner M, et al: Effect on airway resistance of ketamine by aerosol in guinea pigs. Anesth Analg 68:506, 1989.

366. van der Bijl P, Roelofse JA, Stander IA: Rectal ketamine and midazolam for premedication in pediatric dentistry. J Oral Maxillofac Surg 49:1050, 1991.

367. Radnay PA, Badola RP: Generalized extensive spasm in infants following ketamine anesthesia. Anesthesiology 39:459, 1973.

368. Pandit UA, Sotyanaroyana CV, Paul BN, et al: Dissociative anaesthesia in pediatric surgery. J Indian Med Assoc 62:104, 1974.

369. Corssen G, Domino EF, Bree RL: Electroencephalographic effects of ketamine anesthesia in children. Anesth Analg 48:141, 1969.

370. Lees D, Emma P, Hittner K, et al: The safety of ketamine in pediatric neuromuscular disorders: a study of 100 patients. In International Anesthesiology Research Society. Cleveland, Scientific Program Abstracts, 1979, p 75.

371. Zsigmond EK: Comment on case history—case #65: malignant hyperthermia with subsequent uneventful general anesthesia. Anesth Analg 50:1111, 1971.

372. Wadhwa RK, Tantisira B: Parotidectomy in a patient with a family history of malignant hyperthermia. Anesthesiology 40:191, 1974.

373. Oyama T, Matsumoto F, Kudo T: Effects of ketamine on adrenocortical function in man. Anesth Analg 49:697, 1970.

374. Kanairis P, Lekakis D, Kykoniatis M, et al: Serum free fatty acids and blood sugar levels in children under halothane, thiopentone and ketamine anesthesia. Can Anaesth Soc J 22:509, 1975.

375. Zsigmond EK, Domino EF: Ketamine: clinical pharmacology, pharmacokinetics and current clinical uses. Anesthesiol Rev 4:13, 1980.

376. Coppel DL, Bovill JG, Dundee JW: The taming of ketamine. Anesthesia 28:293, 1972.

377. Hefer A, Monyi G: Neuropsychiatric manifestations of ketamine. Isr Ann Psychiatry Relat Discipl 10:180, 1972.

378. Dundee JW, Knox JWD, Black CW, et al: Ketamine as an induction agent in anaesthetics. Lancet 1:B70, 1970.

379. Meyers EF, Charles P: Prolonged adverse reactions to ketamine in children. Anesthesiology 49:39, 1978.

380. Wilson RD, Nichols RJ, McCoy NR: Dissociative anesthesia with CI-581 in burned children. Anesth Analg 46:719, 1967.

381. Spoerel WC, Kandel PF: CI-581 in anesthesia for tonsillectomies in children. Can Anaesth Soc J 17:172, 1970.

382. Page P, Morgan M, Loh L: Ketamine anesthesia in paediatric practice. Acta Anaesthiol Scand 16:155, 1972.

383. Becsey L, Malamed S, Radnay P, et al: Reduction of the psychotometric and circulatory side-effects of ketamine by droperidol. Anesthesiology 37:536, 1972.

384. Sadove MS, Hatano S, Redlin T, et al: Clinical study of droperidol in the prevention of side-effects of ketamine anesthesia. Anesth Analg 50:526, 1971.

385. DeCastro J: The use of ketamine and RO 5-4200 in 1/100 ratio in I.V. subvigile anesthesia. Ars Med 8:1287, 1972.

386. Kothary SP, Zsigmond EK: Prevention of ketamine induced psychic sequelae by diazepam. Clin Pharmacol Ther 17:238, 1975.

387. Morishima HO, Finster M, Pedersen H, et al: Pharmacokinetics of lidocaine in fetal and neonatal lambs and adult sheep. Anesthesiology 50:431, 1979.

388. O'Brien WF, Cefalo RC, Grissom MP, et al: The influence of asphyxia on fetal lidocaine toxicity. Am J Obstet Gynecol 142:205, 1982.

389. Lerman J, Strong HA, LeDez KM, et al: Effects of age on the serum concentration of alpha 1-acid glycoprotein and the binding of lidocaine in pediatric patients. Clin Pharmacol Ther 46:219, 1989.

390. Barry M, Keeling PW, Weir D, Feely J: Severity of cirrhosis and the relationship of alpha 1-acid glycoprotein concentration to plasma protein binding of lidocaine. Clin Pharmacol Ther 47:366, 1990.

391. Burrows FA, Lerman J, LeDez KM, Strong HA: Pharmacokinetics of lidocaine in children with congenital heart disease. Can J Anaesth 38:196, 1991.

392. Finholt DA, Stirt JA, DiFazio CA, Moscicki JC: Lidocaine pharmacokinetics in children during general anesthesia. Anesth Analg 65:279, 1986.

393. Ecoffey C, Desparmet J, Berdeaux A, et al: Pharmacokinetics of lignocaine in children following caudal anesthesia. Br J Anaesth 56:1399, 1984.

394. Mihaly GW, Moore RG, Thomas J, et al: The pharmacokinetics and metabolism of anilide local anesthetics in neonates. K. Lignocaine. Eur J Clin Pharmacol 13:143, 1978.

395. Brown WV, Bell GC, Lurie AO, et al: Newborn blood levels of lidocaine and mepivacaine in the first postnatal day following maternal epidural anesthesia. Anesthesiology 42:698, 1975.

396. Moore RG, Thomas J, Triggs DB, et al: The pharmacokinetics and metabolism of anilide anesthetics in neonates. III. Mepivacaine. Eur J Clin Pharmacol 14:203, 1978.

397. Morgan D, McQuillan D, Thomas J: Pharmacokinetics and metabolism of the anilide local anesthetics in neonates. II. Etidacaine. Eur J Clin Pharmacol 13:365, 1981.

398. Ecoffey C, Desparmet J, Maury M, et al: Bupivacaine in children: pharmacokinetics following caudal anesthesia. Anesthesiology 63:447, 1985.

399. Freund P, Bowdle TA, Slattery JT, Bell LE: Caudal anesthesia with lidocaine or bupivicaine: plasma local anesthetic concentration and extent of sensory spread in old and young patients. Anesth Analg 63:1017, 1984.

400. Mather LE, Tucker GT: Pharmacokinetics and biotransformation of local anesthetics. Int Anesthesiol Clin 16:23, 1978.

401. Giaufre E, Bruguerolle B, Morrison LG, Rousset RB: The influence of midazolam on the plasma concentrations of bupivacaine and lidocaine after caudal injection of a mixture of the local anesthetics in children. Acta Anaesthesiol Scand 34:44, 1990.

402. Bruguerolle B, Giaufre E, Morisson LG, et al: Bupivacaine free plasma levels in children after caudal anaesthesia: influence of pretreatment with diazepam? Fundam Clin Pharmacol 4:159, 1990.

403. Kanto J, Klotz U: Pharmacokinetic implications for the clinical use of atropine, scopolamine, and glycopyrrolate. Acta Anaesthesiol Scand 2:69, 1988.

404. Hinderling PH, Gundert-Remy U, Schmidlin O: Integrated pharmacokinetics and pharmacodynamics of atropine in healthy humans. J Pharm Sci 74:703, 1985.

405. Virtanen R, Kanto J, Iisalo E, et al: Pharmacokinetic studies on atropine with special reference to age. Acta Anaesthesiol Scand 26:297, 1982.

406. Miller BR, Friesen RH: Oral atropine premedication in infants attenuates cardiovascular depression during halothane anesthesia. Anes Analg 67:180, 1988.

407. McAuliffe G, Bissonnette B, Cavalle-Garrido T, Boutin C: Heart rate and cardiac output after atropine in anaesthetised infants and children. Can J Anaesth 44:154, 1997.
408. Opie JC, Chaye H, Steward DJ: Intravenous atropine rapidly reduces lower esophageal sphincter pressure in infants and children. Anesthesiology 67:989, 1987.
409. Katiala E, Penttila A, Vapaatalo H, Larmi T: The fate of intravenous (3H) glycopyrrolate in man. J Pharm Pharmacol 26:352, 1974.
410. Rautakorpi P, Ali-Melkkila T, Kaila T, et al: Pharmacokinteics of glycopyrrolate in children. J Clin Anesth 6:217, 1994.
411. Rautakorpi P, Manner T, Ali-Melkkila T, et al: Pharmacokinetics and oral bioavailabilty of glycopyrrolate in children. Pharmacol Toxicol 83:132, 1998.
412. Warran P, Radford P, Manford MLM: Glycopyrrolate in children. Br J Anaesth 53:1273, 1981.

Temperature Disturbances

DANIEL I. SESSLER

◆　　◆　　◆

Core body temperature is among the most jealously guarded of the physiologic parameters. Core body temperature varies slightly during the course of each day (circadian rhythm), monthly in women, and seasonally in some animals. Nonetheless, at any given time, body temperature is usually within a few tenths of a degree of the expected value. Anesthesia and surgery dramatically impair this delicate control; core body temperatures of 1° to 3°C below normal are common in postoperative patients. Although much less common than hypothermia, hyperthermia is a significant clinical problem when it occurs. This chapter first discusses the malignant hyperthermia syndrome, then it describes how anesthesia and surgery impair thermoregulation and body heat balance.

MALIGNANT HYPERTHERMIA

Malignant hyperthermia (MH) is an acute hypermetabolic syndrome triggered by succinylcholine and volatile anesthetics. Onset of malignant hyperthermia may be fulminant and its course may be rapid. Its symptoms include skeletal muscle rigidity, hypercarbia, and fever, and these symptoms can progress within 30 minutes to a premorbid state in which the arterial pH is as low as 6.6 units. Until recently, malignant hyperthermia was among the leading causes of anesthetic death, with a mortality exceeding 65 percent.[1]

Denborough and Lovell first reported the syndrome in 1960 in a letter to the editor of Lancet.[2] They described a young man with a broken leg who was justifiably concerned about his anesthetic risk because 10 of his 24 relatives had died during general anesthesia. The patient also developed the syndrome during general anesthesia with halothane; he survived. As early as 1953, a similar syndrome had been noted in swine (porcine stress syndrome),[3] but it was not until 1966 that the similarities between species were recognized by Nelson et al.[4] The syndrome has since been recognized in the dog, cat, horse, goat, deer, elk, and giraffe. It was the development of the porcine model that permitted significant research on this rare disease to begin.

Another factor that helped reduce mortality was the in vitro caffeine/halothane contracture test which determines if muscle from a patient suspected of having MH responds abnormally to caffeine. This test was first described in 1970 by Kalow et al.[5] and is the only proven test that reliably diagnoses the syndrome. Initially, the pathophysiology of MH was a mystery, although a defect of intracellular calcium regulation in skeletal muscle was suspected.[6] We have now acquired a reasonable understanding of the biochemical abnormalities involved and of the epidemiology and genetics of the syndrome. Nontriggering anesthetic drugs have been identified, and patients known to be susceptible can have safe anesthesia and surgery.

A final breakthrough was the recognition by Harrison in 1975 that dantrolene sodium inhibited triggering of the syndrome and provided effective treatment.[7] Initially available only in oral form, the use of dantrolene was limited to pretreatment of susceptible individuals. Since 1979, however, an intravenous formulation of the drug has been marketed, permitting rapid treatment of acute crises.

Increased knowledge, a sensitive diagnostic test, timely recognition, and appropriate treatment of MH have reduced the current mortality from MH to less than 1 percent. Malignant hyperthermia and its treatments have been described in over 1,500 articles, including a number of reviews published since 1986.[8-11]

Pathophysiology

Although most research on malignant hyperthermia has been done in swine, the major findings have been confirmed in humans. The syndrome is common in Landrace and Pietrain pigs, and is presumed to result from breeding for lean, heavily muscled animals. The porcine model of MH closely resembles the human syndrome, but malignant hyperthermia is more easily triggered and even more fulminant in pigs than in humans.

Affected Tissues

The biochemical changes of malignant hyperthermia are limited to skeletal muscle and hematologic tissues. In normal muscle, a nerve impulse depolarizes the sarcolemma. This impulse travels down the transverse tubules, where the signal is transferred to the sarcoplasmic reticulum by excitation-contraction coupling. The sarcolemma calcium concentration then increases 1,000-fold, binding troponin, which allows actin and myosin to interact. Susceptible skeletal muscle is similar to normal muscle in its histologic and tissue culture characteristics.[12, 13] It has a normal protein electrophoretic pattern,[14, 15] its calcium and magnesium contents are normal,[16-18] and the neuromuscular junction functions normally.[19] The actin, myosin, and troponin of susceptible muscle are normal,[20, 21] as are adenylate cyclase activity[22] and monoamine oxidase activity.[23]

The only other tissues that are primarily affected by the malignant hyperthermia syndrome are those of the hematopoietic system. Erythrocyte fragility is increased,[24] but the reason for this increase remains unknown, and erythrocyte fragility is not enhanced by exposure to the potent inhalation anesthetics.[25] Abnormal adenosine triphosphate (ATP) metabolism of halothane-exposed platelets was observed by one group, but other laboratories were unable to confirm this observation.[26] However, the ultrastructural morphology of platelets from susceptible patients is abnormal, suggesting that these cells are in some way affected by the syndrome.[27, 28] Mononuclear cytoplasmic calcium concentration is normal, but the concentration of calcium in susceptible cells is significantly increased by exposure to halothane.[29, 30]

Triggering

Triggering of susceptible muscle takes place during excitation-contraction coupling.[31] Initial evidence suggested that type I muscle is more sensitive than type II,[32] but this has been disputed.[33] Although the mean sarcoplasmic reticulum membrane potential in susceptible muscle is normal,[34] contraction occurs at -86 mV, whereas normal muscle is depolarized to -54 mV.[35] This is significant because halothane depolarizes susceptible (but not normal) muscle by 5 to 15 mV, which is sufficient to cause a contraction.[34] Presumably, the other potent inhalation anesthetics have similar effects. Succinylcholine depolarizes both normal and susceptible muscle but triggers MH only in susceptible muscle. It is not known under what circumstances depolarization and contraction in susceptible muscle progresses to contracture and clinical symptoms. A two-site excitation-contraction coupling mechanism has been proposed with succinylcholine, halothane, and dantrolene acting at the first site and caffeine acting at the second.[31]

Contraction

Once triggering has occurred in muscle that is susceptible to malignant hyperthermia, a contraction is propagated and maintained by a complex series of biochemical changes. The primary defect may be an increase in the phospholipase A_2 activity, which causes an increase in mitochondrial free fatty acid content that stimulates calcium release.[36] (More recent evidence suggests that the affected enzyme actually may be hormone-sensitive lipase.[37]) In turn, the abnormal mitochondria cause changes in the sarcoplasmic reticulum that result in contraction.

This mechanism was demonstrated in elegant experiments in which exogenous phospholipase A_2 caused a prolonged contraction when normal muscle was exposed to succinylcholine and halothane. The effect was blocked by the phospholipase A_2 inhibitors[38, 39] indomethacin and spermine. Similarly, exogenous free fatty acid was shown to decrease calcium uptake and to increase calcium release by normal sarcoplasmic reticulum.[40] In both humans and animals, halothane-stimulated contraction is attenuated by inhibitors of phospholipase A_2.[41, 42] The common link between abnormal activation-contraction coupling and increased phospholipase A_2 activity is probably an abnormality of the ryanodine (calcium-control) receptor in the sarcoplasmic reticulum.[43, 44]

In the presence of free fatty acid, the release of sarcoplasmic reticulum calcium is increased and reuptake of calcium is inhibited.[18, 45, 46] Both calcium-induced and halothane-induced calcium release are increased in susceptible sarcoplasmic reticulum.[47, 48] The resulting high sarcoplasmic calcium concentration allows actin and myosin fibers to interact. As in normal muscle, contraction in malignant hyperthermia–prone muscle is energy dependent. Aerobic metabolism, however, is insufficient, possibly because increased free fatty acid concentrations inhibit citrate synthase, which is the pacemaker step of the Krebs cycle.[45] (Even prior to triggering, susceptible muscle ATPase activity is increased,[49] and phosphocreatine, creatine, and ATP concentrations are diminished.[50-52]) As a result, energy needs are largely supplied by glycolysis.[46, 53] In late stages, when the muscle temperature rises above 43.5°C, actin-myosin binding is no longer calcium dependent, and the muscle contraction is irreversible (Fig. 4–1).[21, 54]

The clinical signs and laboratory findings of malignant hyperthermia result from the sustained contraction and

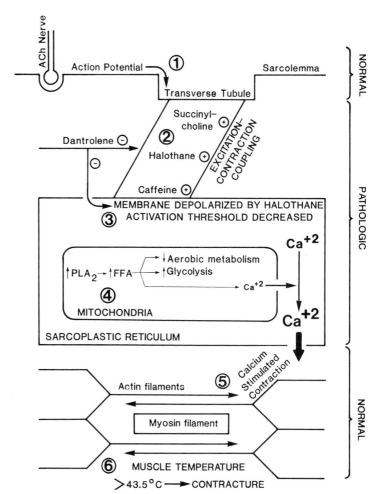

FIGURE 4–1. (*1*) Action potential from neuromuscular junction is propagated into transverse tubule. (*2*) Signal is transferred to sarcoplasmic reticulum by excitation-contraction coupling. Process is enhanced by succinylcholine, halothane, and caffeine, but inhibited by dantrolene. (*3*) Sarcoplasmic reticulum activation threshold is lowered sufficiently in susceptible patients such that small depolarization caused by halothane stimulates calcium release. Both effects are alleviated by dantrolene. (*4*) Elevated phospholipase A₂ (PLA₂) activity increases concentration of free fatty acid (FFA). This results in decreased aerobic metabolism, compensatory increase in glycolysis, and release of mitochondrial calcium. (*5*) Increased myoplasmic calcium concentration binds troponin. Actin and myosin then interact, causing contraction. (*6*) At muscle temperature greater than 43.5°C, calcium is no longer required for actin–myosin interaction, and contraction becomes an irreversible contracture. (From Sessler DI: Malignant hyperthermia. J Pediatr 109:9, 1986, with permission.)

increased glycolysis necessary to sustain ATP production with uncoupled aerobic metabolism. The increase in temperature, lactate concentration, and Pco₂ all result from this muscle pathology; most other organs react passively to these changes.[46]

Epidemiology

The reported incidence of malignant hyperthermia crises is approximately 1 per 14,000 anesthetics in children and 1 per 40,000 in adults. This approximation is based on the number of crises diagnosed at the Hospital for Sick Children in Toronto, Canada, divided by the number of anesthetics administered during this time.[55] Until recently, however, the syndrome was not well known and, as a result, the diagnosis was probably missed in some patients whose temperatures were not monitored or whose symptoms were mild. In addition, even patients known to be susceptible to malignant hyperthermia typically undergo anesthesia several times before a clinical episode occurs.[56] Thus, the actual population at risk may be considerably greater than previously believed.

Because malignant hyperthermia is a lifelong disease, the higher incidence in children is an anomaly. The syndrome does, however, appear more difficult to trigger in adults. Apparent resistance may result because anesthesia in adults is frequently induced with sodium thiopental and a nondepolarizing muscle relaxant, both of which

inhibit triggering.[57-59] In contrast, anesthesia in children is frequently induced using halothane followed by succinylcholine, a combination that is a particularly effective trigger. An additional factor is that triggering and severity of the syndrome are markedly reduced by just a couple of degrees Celsius core hypothermia.[60, 61] Since adults frequently become hypothermic during surgery and infants and children are kept warm, a greater incidence of malignant hyperthermia in pediatric patients may result in part from their higher core temperatures.

Malignant hyperthermia is rarely diagnosed in the extremes of age, possibly because muscle mass is diminished in both populations. However, it has been reported at birth (after cesarean section with general anesthesia)[62] and in infants as young as 5 and 6 months of age.[63-66] It has not been reported in patients over the age of 78 years.[67] Sex distribution until puberty is equal; after that, it is more common in men.[55] The sex-related change in the incidence of malignant hyperthermia may be because of the greater muscle mass in men, which would make the diagnosis more apparent during mild presentations. The syndrome has been reported several times during pregnancy without apparent adverse fetal effects.[68, 69]

Malignant hyperthermia is a familial disease, but its genetics remain unclear. Identifying genetic patterns has been complicated because (1) triggering drugs may not have been administered to many family members, (2) the response of a susceptible individual to anesthetic drugs may be poorly documented, (3) susceptibility varies with age, and (4) susceptible patients frequently do not develop clinical symptoms, even when exposed to known triggering agents.

The syndrome was initially thought to be autosomal dominant, on the basis of two extensive pedigrees.[70, 71] Further evaluation suggested that the inheritance in most families was multigenetic, with variable expressivity and incomplete penetrance. Studies of other populations indicated that susceptible patients do not share a common human leukocyte antigen (HLA) pattern and demonstrated no strict pattern of inheritance.[72] Instead, a familial tendency was apparent; first-degree relatives of a proband had a markedly increased susceptibility to malignant hyperthermia, whereas second-degree relatives had a lower risk (which was still higher than that of the normal population).

An isolated defect in the gene coding for the ryanodine receptor (sarcoplasmic reticulum calcium channel) has been identified in swine.[73] A similar defect initially was reported in humans, but subsequent analysis indicated that the human syndrome is genetically heterogeneous.[74] At least 10 genes contribute to malignant hyperthermia susceptibility.

Association with Myopathies

Since malignant hyperthermia is a disease of skeletal muscle, it is not surprising to find myopathies reported in susceptible patients. In one study, the incidence of mild myopathies (muscle cramping, ptosis, squint, and increased muscle volume) was 66 percent in susceptible patients, 36 percent in first-degree relatives, and 7 percent in controls.[55] However, these myopathies are common in the population at large, and most people in whom they occur are not susceptible to malignant hyperthermia.

Noonan's phenotype (also called King syndrome) presents with short stature, undescended testes, and scoliosis. King and Denborough described four such cases among the 19 patients in Australia and New Zealand who were known at the time to be susceptible to malignant hyperthermia.[75, 76] The syndrome has also been reported in a number of other patients with Noonan phenotype.[77–79] However, the correlation King and Denborough identified may not apply to other populations. A study of 27 patients with the Noonan phenotype failed to reveal evidence of malignant hyperthermia susceptibility. Although these patients did not undergo biopsy, 14 underwent 25 anesthetics without a hyperthermic crisis. One patient in the series had an elevated creatinine kinase (CK) concentration, yet underwent four halothane anesthetics without mishap. The authors concluded that no large subgroup equivalent to those found by King and Denborough existed among patients having the Noonan phenotype.[80] More recent series also have failed to identify patients with the Noonan phenotype among susceptible populations. The best relation is probably to central core disease, a mild myopathy that has been observed in association with malignant hyperthermia.[81–83] There is good genetic evidence linking central core disease with malignant hyperthermia.[84]

Although congenital myopathies have been associated with malignant hyperthermia, the evidence supporting a causal relationship is, in many cases, poor.[85] Evans syndrome (proximal muscle wasting, short stature, and scoliosis) has been demonstrated in a susceptible patient. Myotonia congenita has been reported in several susceptible subjects,[75, 86, 87] although it has not been possible to induce malignant hyperthermia in animals suffering from this myopathy.[88] Duchenne muscular dystrophy also has been described in a number of apparently susceptible patients,[89–92] but most have not been tested for malignant hyperthermia, making any correlation conjectural. One possible episode of malignant hyperthermia has been reported in a patient with Schwartz-Jampel syndrome.

When evaluating such reports, it is helpful to remember that well over 10,000 people have experienced documented malignant hyperthermia crises. It is therefore not surprising that some patients have coexisting diseases. Because some of these diseases increase the need for surgery, they increase the chances of diagnosing a patient's susceptibility to malignant hyperthermia.

Triggering Agents

The only well-documented triggering agents for malignant hyperthermia in humans are succinylcholine and the volatile anesthetics (Table 4–1). Halothane triggers the syndrome more easily than the other volatile anesthetics, but all can trigger the syndrome. Exercise and coffee frequently cause cramps in susceptible patients, but are not considered disease triggers in humans. Malignant hyperthermia reactions have been reported in patients receiving drugs such as iopanoic acid (Telepaque), phencyclidine, and cocaine. Reports of malignant hyperthermia reactions in patients using these drugs are exceedingly rare, and may represent stress-induced malignant hyperthermia, allergic reactions, or drug fever. They should not be considered triggering drugs.

Porcine malignant hyperthermia is triggered by α- (but not β-) adrenergic agonists. Phenylephrine and norepinephrine (with or without concurrent administration of propranolol) will cause triggering. However, isoproterenol does not cause triggering,[93] and reserpine and phentolamine actually prevent triggering by succinylcholine.[94] Triggering by dopamine and dobutamine have not been evaluated. Thus, if drugs are required to support the arterial blood pressure of patients susceptible to malignant hyperthermia, isoproterenol might be the best choice (although there is no evidence that any vasopressors trigger the syndrome in susceptible humans). Total epidural anesthesia reportedly blocked triggering in susceptible swine,[95] but total spinal anesthesia did not,[96] suggesting that the epidural report was erroneous. Malignant hyperthermia is

TABLE 4 – 1	
KNOWN TRIGGERS OF MALIGNANT HYPERTHERMIA	
In Humans	**In Swine**
Succinylcholine	Succinylcholine
Volatile anesthetics	Potent inhalation anesthetics
Stress (very rarely)	Stress
	α-Adrenergic agonists
	Exercise

not triggered by hypercarbia, hypercalcemia, or digoxin administration.[97]

Porcine malignant hyperthermia also is triggered by exercise and stress.[97] Neither is an important factor in the human disease, although there have been occasional reports of malignant hyperthermia induced by stress alone.[1] One particularly well-documented case involved a biopsy-positive, 42-year-old with stress-induced fevers that were relieved by dantrolene administration.[98] Other reports include a susceptible family in whom there were frequent, unexplained, sudden deaths,[99] and five subjects with "stress syndrome."[100] It is possible that stress is responsible for the rare crises observed during anesthesia with nontriggering drugs.[101–103]

Hypermetabolic fever after use of psychotropic drugs, such as phenothiazines, tricyclic antidepressants, and monoamine oxidase inhibitors, is known as neuroleptic malignant syndrome.[104, 105] Although clinically similar, this syndrome's relationship to malignant hyperthermia has yet to be determined. Several patients with neuroleptic malignant syndrome have had positive caffeine-contracture muscle biopsies, suggesting similar pathophysiology.[106, 107] A number of patients with neuroleptic malignant syndrome have been treated successfully with dantrolene.[108, 109]

Symptoms and Signs

The symptoms and signs of malignant hyperthermia all result from skeletal muscle hypermetabolism and injury. Thus, although the pulmonary, cardiovascular, and hepatic systems are involved during a crisis, their participation is secondary and results from the compensatory responses necessary to support generalized, prolonged muscular contracture. Renal involvement also is secondary and results from the release of myoglobin by injured muscle.

Malignant hyperthermia usually presents during the first 2 hours of anesthesia,[67] although the syndrome has appeared after prolonged anesthesia,[110] during recovery from anesthesia[102, 111, 112] and, very rarely, many hours after anesthesia and surgery when the patient has returned to the ward.[113]

Masseter Muscle Rigidity

Triggering of the syndrome is especially rapid when succinylcholine has been administered,[53, 114] with masseter spasm often being the first symptom in these patients. Masseter spasm or rigidity is a powerful trismus of the jaw observed within minutes of succinylcholine administration. It is not simply inadequate relaxation or "stiffness."

Jaw stiffness occurs in up to 1 percent of children in whom inhaled halothane is followed by intravenous succinylcholine[115] and 2.8 percent of children given the same anesthetic for strabismus surgery.[116] It is likely that most of this stiffness is not masseter rigidity. Supporting this frequency of stiffness are studies showing that succinylcholine initially *increases* jaw tone before providing relaxation.[117, 118] Masseter rigidity likely represents extreme tone in occasional children. Masseter rigidity is rare in adults, even when they are given succinylcholine.

Initially, masseter spasm occurring during the induction of anesthesia was reported to correlate perfectly with malignant hyperthermia.[115] However, the test of susceptibility used to make this determination was subsequently shown not to correlate with clinical crises or with the standard, in vitro caffeine-contracture test.[119] The best current estimate is that 50 percent of children who display masseter spasm upon induction of anesthesia are susceptible to malignant hyperthermia.[120, 121]

Acute Malignant Hyperthermia

The first symptoms of a crisis presenting during anesthesia are sinus tachycardia, hypertension, and tachypnea. These common signs are usually misinterpreted as inadequate anesthetic depth and "treated" by administering a higher concentration of inhaled anesthetic. The skin then becomes mottled with cyanotic areas and patches of bright red flushing. Generalized, rigor mortis-like skeletal muscle rigidity occurs in approximately 70 percent of such crises,[55] and is usually associated with a more fulminant course. Swollen and tender muscles are common after crises. However, rigidity and dystonic reactions to succinylcholine also may occur in patients with various myopathies who are not susceptible to malignant hyperthermia.[122, 123]

Central thermoregulation presumably remains intact during malignant hyperthermia. Temperature increases because continuous muscle contracture generates more heat than the body can dissipate to the environment. Although hyperthermia is a relatively late finding, the temperature can increase at a rate of 1°C every 5 minutes; the body temperature can rise above 46°C. Hyperthermia may be minimal in indolent cases or in crises so fulminant that the patient progresses in as few as 20 minutes to severe acidosis, shock, and ventricular fibrillation.

One retrospective study evaluated presenting symptoms and signs (e.g., generalized rigidity, masseter spasm, tachycardia, and fever) to determine which of these signs and symptoms are useful predictors of malignant hyperthermia susceptibility.[120] The authors found that generalized muscle rigidity was the only single symptom predicting a positive in vitro contracture test. Although masseter spasm after succinylcholine administration was not predictive, 50 percent of patients who experienced masseter spasm tested positive for malignant hyperthermia. All patients whose tests were ultimately positive had at least two symptoms, suggesting that assessment of the entire clinical situation is more useful than reliance on a single factor.

Cardiac muscle abnormalities have been suggested, but there is little evidence to support a primary myocardial defect. Although subtle histopathologic changes have been observed in heart muscle of patients who died of malignant hyperthermia, these findings probably reflect the stress of the lethal crises.[12, 22, 124] An increased incidence of cardiac arrhythmias has been suggested, but the only reports are anecdotal or from uncontrolled studies.[124–126]

Laboratory Findings

Because hyperthermia is secondary to skeletal muscle hypermetabolism,[46] most abnormal laboratory values can be detected before the temperature increases (Table 4–2).[127] The most notable finding is a severe metabolic and respiratory acidemia (both abnormalities are more pronounced in venous than in arterial blood). Otherwise unexplained hypercarbia is the first distinct physiologic evidence of malignant hyperthermia[52] and can be easily detected by monitoring end-tidal P_{CO_2}.[128, 129]

Oxygen consumption increases by less than a factor of five, which is considerably less than the maximum increase possible during vigorous exercise.[127] Skeletal muscle alone is the source of increased lactate,[130] and only half the temperature increase can be explained by increased oxygen consumption, indicating significant anerobic metabolism or an uneven distribution of heat within the body.[46, 53] Arterial oxygenation remains adequate despite pronounced cyanosis; however, mixed venous P_{O_2} decreases and P_{CO_2} increases, reflecting a sixfold increase in oxygen extraction by skeletal muscle. These responses are qualitatively similar to those observed during severe exercise.

Circulating norepinephrine concentrations are 20 times normal and cause vasoconstriction. The vasoconstriction prevents adequate peripheral blood flow and inhibits heat dissipation. Early in the course, serum potassium values rise to between 6 and 14 mEq/L.[131, 132] After several hours, hypokalemia may develop as a result of potassium redistribution and diuretic administration. In the liver, some lactate is metabolized. Glucose and potassium are released, presumably from the breakdown of glycogen.[133] Cardiac output and cardiac oxygen extraction increase substantially, apparently as a result of increased concentrations of circulating catecholamines.[134] Metabolic changes in the brain apparently are passive reflections of systemic changes, and normal cerebral blood flow is maintained.[135]

Severe crises are associated with microscopic areas of muscle necrosis, which releases myoglobin. Large amounts of circulating myoglobin cause disseminated intravascular coagulation and myoglobinurea, both of which may be associated with oliguria. Relapses used to be common for up to 3 days following untreated malignant hyperthermia crises, even without reexposure to triggering agents; however, such recrudescence is unusual in patients adequately treated with dantrolene.

Several early reports describe cardiomyopathy and ventricular arrhythmias in awake, susceptible patients who were not exposed to triggering agents.[125, 136] One investigator found that one third of susceptible subjects had abnormal electrocardiograms, most commonly atrioventricular conduction defects and ischemic changes.[126] However, that study was retrospective and the observed changes

were not compared to those in a control group. Moreover, susceptible cardiac muscle histology is normal.[137, 138] Malignant hyperthermia also has been proposed to be one cause of sudden infant death syndrome,[139, 140] but there currently is little evidence to suggest an important link between the two syndromes.

Prognosis and Treatment

Prior to the introduction of dantrolene, mortality from malignant hyperthermia crises was approximately 65 percent.[55] Treatment consisted of terminating anesthetic administration, hyperventilation with oxygen, and administration of sodium bicarbonate and drugs of questionable efficacy, such as procainamide, procaine, haloperidol, steroids, and ketanserin (a serotonin receptor blocker) (Table 4–3). Patients were aggressively cooled by submersion in iced water; lavage of the gastric, rectal, peritoneal, and pleural cavities with iced saline solution; and intravenous administration of refrigerated fluids. One patient with fulminant malignant hyperthermia (pH 6.85, P_{CO_2} 179 mm Hg) was successfully treated using partial cardiopulmonary bypass.[141]

Then, as now, early recognition of a crisis was critical. There are few reports of mortality in patients given anesthesia for fewer than 10 minutes. Conversely, nearly all patients in whom treatment of a severe crisis is delayed more than 2 hours die.[142] Rapid recognition and appropriate treatment, including intravenous administration of dantrolene, have reduced mortality to less than 1 percent of acute episodes. Aggressive follow-up of first- and second-degree relatives has resulted in increased awareness among both physicians and patients and, consequently, fewer crises.

Treatment and Monitoring

Current recommendations for treating acute malignant hyperthermia include discontinuing triggering drugs, hyperventilating with 100 percent oxygen, and administering dantrolene 2.5 mg/kg intravenously as quickly as possible. Within 45 minutes of the initial dantrolene dose, all symptoms (rigidity, acidosis, tachycardia) should disappear. If not, an additional 2.5 mg/kg dose should be administered intravenously every 30 minutes (to a maximum of 10 mg/kg) until the symptoms resolve. Sodium bicarbonate (1 or 2 mEq/kg intravenously) also is commonly administered.

T A B L E   4 – 3
RECOMMENDED TREATMENT OF A MALIGNANT HYPERTHERMIA CRISIS

Treatment	Monitor
Discontinue succinylcholine	Arterial and venous blood gases
Discontinue potent inhaled anesthetics	Serum creatine phosphokinase
Administer 100% oxygen	Serum potassium
Dantrolene 2.5 mg/kg IV	Twitch depression
Increase ventilation (per blood gases)	Urine myoglobin content
Administer bicarbonate	Urine output

T A B L E   4 – 2
TYPICAL LABORATORY ABNORMALITIES DURING A MALIGNANT HYPERTHERMIA CRISIS

Acute	Late
Hypercarbia	Hypokalemia
Lactic acidosis	Myoglobinuria
Decreased mixed venous P_{O_2}	Disseminated intravascular coagulation
Hyperkalemia	
Increased plasma catecholamines	Oliguria

Because the carbon dioxide that is released by the reaction of bicarbonate with metabolic acids can aggravate respiratory acidosis, bicarbonate should not be administered unless ventilation is adequate and arterial P_{CO_2} is near normal. Supplemental potassium should be avoided, if possible, because there may be rebound hyperkalemia 6 to 12 hours after the crises has ended. Immediate consultation with an expert is available 24 hours per day through the Malignant Hyperthermia Association of the United States. They can be reached at 800-MH-HYPER.

Frequent arterial blood gas, electrolyte, and serum creatine phosphokinase (CPK) measurements will assist management. At least one postoperative urine sample should be obtained because myoglobinuria, followed by acute tubular necrosis, may occur even when other symptoms are minimal. If the clinical and laboratory findings return to normal following dantrolene therapy, cooling measures are not needed. Intravenous dantrolene probably should be continued at 2.5 mg/kg every 6 hours for approximately 24 hours after the symptoms resolve. (Magnetic resonance spectroscopy studies indicate that muscle metabolism remains abnormal many hours after the clinical symptoms resolve.[143]) Before dantrolene was available, relapses were common in the first few days after crises and were manifested by anxiety, muscle rigidity, hyperkalemia, and anuria.[113] Such relapses in patients given dantrolene are rare. Nonetheless, it is prudent to observe patients in the hospital for at least 24 hours after the laboratory values return to normal and the symptoms resolve.

Masseter Muscle Rigidity

The first clinical symptom of malignant hyperthermia is frequently masseter spasm, but masseter spasm also occurs in patients who are not susceptible.[120, 121] The anesthesiologist presented with masseter spasm must decide whether to cancel surgery (often causing considerable inconvenience and expense) or to continue and risk a malignant hyperthermia crisis.

Some authorities believe it prudent to discontinue anesthesia when masseter spasm is detected, citing the risk of developing an MH crisis.[144] Others point out that masseter rigidity is relatively common compared with acute malignant hyperthermia. They recommend changing to nontriggering anesthetics and evaluating the patient for signs of crisis. If a blood gas is normal and there are no signs of hyperthermia, they suggest continuing surgery.[145]

In virtually every case so far evaluated, masseter rigidity plus a plasma CPK concentration exceeding 20,000 IU has indicated malignant hyperthermia susceptibility or another myopathy.[121] Consequently, any patient experiencing masseter rigidity should have blood sampled for CPK analysis 6, 12, and 24 hours afterwards. Patients having masseter spasm should also be tested for the presence of myoglobin in the urine, as myoglobinuria may be an isolated sign of muscle injury. However, it is not routinely necessary to keep such patients in the hospital.[146]

Anesthesiologists may wish to minimize the incidence of masseter spasm by avoiding the use of succinylcholine in patients in whom anesthesia is induced with potent inhaled anesthetics, because the combination of succinylcholine and volatile anesthetics is a particularly effective method of inducing masseter spasm. Occasionally, the administration of succinylcholine to young children (usually boys) provokes immediate cardiac arrest, which is usually caused by hyperkalemia associated with unrecognized muscular dystrophies.[147] Immediate treatment should be undertaken in this circumstance to reduce the plasma potassium concentration and should include administration of bicarbonate and glucose/insulin.

Dantrolene

Oral dantrolene (a drug related to diphenylhydantoin) was developed in 1967 for the treatment of muscle spasms in cerebral palsy and similar diseases. First reported effective in porcine malignant hyperthermia in 1975,[7] it was proven in 1977 to be more effective in humans than procainamide and other drugs in use at that time.[148, 149] However, attempts to dissolve oral capsules were hindered by the drug's poor solubility, which limited the use of dantrolene to oral prophylaxis in patients known to be susceptible to malignant hyperthermia. A U.S. Food and Drug Administration (FDA)-approved, lyophilized preparation for intravenous use finally became available in November 1979.

Administered intravenously, 3.5 mg/kg of dantrolene depresses muscle twitch in swine by 95 percent.[150] Both this dose and 5 mg/kg appear to be effective in inhibiting triggering of malignant hyperthermia in swine.[131] Malignant hyperthermia in swine (which is more fulminant than in humans) can be treated effectively with 7.5 mg/kg. Twitch depression in humans is approximately 73 percent inhibited by 2.5 mg/kg of the drug.[151, 152] This same dose was shown to be effective treatment of MH in a multicenter trial.[153] Originally, 1 mg/kg of dantrolene administered intravenously was recommended for both prophalaxis and initial treatment, but the current concensus is that the initial treatment dose should be at least 2.5 mg/kg.

The elimination half-life of dantrolene during anesthesia is approximately 9 hours and is not significantly influenced by pregnancy or preoperative medication with diazepam or phenobarbital.[68, 154] In contrast to earlier reports, dantrolene administered orally is well absorbed and reliably produces adequate blood concentrations.[155] The drug is metabolized in the liver primarily to 5-hydroxydantrolene, which is excreted in the urine. 5-Hydroxydantrolene pharmacologically has roughly half the activity of the parent compound and has a half-life of approximately 15 hours.[154] The pharmacokinetics are similar in pediatric patients.[156] The drug cannot be removed to any appreciable extent by dialysis.

Although dantrolene inhibits excitation-contraction coupling,[157, 158] its major, direct action appears to be on the sarcoplasmic reticulum. It increases the contraction activation threshold voltage in susceptible[35] and normal muscle,[159] and prevents the depolarization of susceptible muscle by halothane.[34] Dantrolene also decreases intracellular calcium concentrations, resulting in minimal concentrations at doses above 2 mg/kg.[152, 160] It also slows calcium release by the sarcoplasmic reticulum and decreases the total amount released.[161] Although this decreases twitch tension, dantrolene alone cannot completely abolish it. The effects of this drug on twitch tension height are similar in normal and susceptible muscle.[151] Dantrolene has no central effect, no effect on the neuromuscular junction,[158] and no direct effect on actin/myosin binding.[21]

Dantrolene also has primary antiarrhythmic effects, including increased atrial and ventricular refractory periods.[162] Cardiac contractility decreases and the duration of the action potential increases.[163] Systemic vascular resistance increases and cardiac index decreases. Mean arterial pressure does not change.[164] These effects are, to some extent, reversed by calcium, although they do not resemble the changes apparent with calcium channel blockers. Nevertheless, the toxicities of diltiazem and dantrolene appear to be synergistic, causing hyperkalemia and cardiac arrest when they are combined.[165] The potential toxicity of combined verapamil/dantrolene remains unclear.[166, 167] In contrast, the combination of nifedipine and dantrolene appears to be safe.[165]

No adverse effects have been observed in infants or fetuses exposed to dantrolene. Although uterine atony following dantrolene pretreatment was once reported, there is probably no contraindication to its use during pregnancy. Fetal blood levels are approximately half those of the mother.[68, 69] Hepatotoxicity can occur with prolonged oral use (3 to 6 months),[168] and acute changes in liver biochemistry have been detected.[169–171] However, clinical hepatotoxicity has never been reported during the treatment of hyperthermic crises. Chronic eosinophilic pleuropericardial effusion (apparently a hypersensitivity to the drug) may occur during prolonged treatment, but has not presented during acute treatment.[172] Dantrolene also decreases the LD_{50} of bupivacaine[173] and may cause drowsiness, dizziness, headache, and nausea. Occasionally, dantrolene administration causes profound muscle weakness and the need for mechanical ventilation.[174]

Because intravenous dantrolene treatment so effectively reduces mortality, this drug should be available wherever volatile anesthetics or succinylcholine are administered. (It is difficult to defend lawsuits in which malignant hyperthermia causes complications and dantrolene was not available.) Stocking intravenous dantrolene is expensive: a case of 36 vials (containing a total of 720 mg) costs hospitals approximately $1,000. Because, the shelf-life is short, keeping dantrolene available is a continuing expense. The oral preparation is about 30 times less expensive than the intravenous formulation.[175] A water-soluble analogue of dantrolene (azumolene) has been developed, but it is not commercially available.[176]

Elective Anesthesia in Susceptible Patients

Elective surgery is not contraindicated for patients who are known to be susceptible to malignant hyperthermia. Both regional and general anesthesia can be safely administered, although care should be taken with either technique to avoid unnecessary stress. Any type of conduction anesthesia, using any type of local anesthetic, is acceptable. Interestingly, when the first patient in whom the syndrome was described[2] required another operation 1 year after his near-lethal exposure to halothane, Denborough et al. administered spinal anesthesia using cinchocaine without complication.[71]

Lidocaine and other amide local anesthetics were avoided for many years because they were thought to increase intracellular calcium concentrations. However, administration of amide anesthetics does not trigger malignant hyperthermia in susceptible pigs,[177, 178] and there is only one reported case of malignant hyperthermia in humans following (but not necessarily caused by) administration of lidocaine. Consequently, these drugs can be used safely in patients who are susceptible to malignant hyperthermia.[179]

General anesthesia can be safely administered using a balanced anesthesia technique by combining nitrous oxide, narcotics, and nondepolarizing muscle relaxants.[46, 47, 180] Other safe drugs include benzodiazipines, ketamine, althesin, propofol, and etomidate.[181, 182] Barbiturates are known to inhibit triggering of MH,[57] as are the nondepolarizing muscle relaxants.[58, 59] Droperidol is probably safe, although it can theoretically trigger the neuroleptic malignant syndrome, which is clinically similar to MH.[104, 105] Anticholinergic drugs do not trigger the syndrome but may increase fever during a malignant hyperthermia crisis because these drugs inhibit heat dissipation to the environment by preventing sweating. Although a few reports of MH crisis during "nontriggering" anesthesia exist,[112, 183–185] it is now apparent that balanced anesthetic techniques can be used safely in susceptible patients. Nonetheless, there is a small incidence of mild malignant hyperthermia reactions (i.e., 0.5 percent) in patients given nontriggering drugs.[186] All episodes occurred immediately after anesthesia and were easily treated.

Anesthetic washout from anesthesia machines is rapid, even if all rubber and plastic components are left in place. When these components are removed (a new or disposable circuit is used) residual anesthetic concentrations are approximately 1/1,000 MAC (<10 parts per million) within 5 minutes of washout (Fig. 4–2). It is unlikely that this concentration of inhaled anesthetic will trigger the syndrome, even in patients at greatest risk for malignant hyperthermia. Thus, an anesthesia machine can probably be prepared for safe use in susceptible patients simply by removing the vaporizers (which may leak) and replacing easily accessible rubber and plastic components; it is not necessary to change the soda-lime CO_2 absorber.

Dantrolene Prophylaxis

It is unclear whether dantrolene prophylaxis prior to surgery is beneficial: some physicians use preoperative oral or intravenous dantrolene, while others believe it unnecessary. The historical context is important: prophylaxis of susceptible patients became standard after the efficacy of dantrolene was established in 1975 but before an intravenous preparation became available in 1979. Any treatment that might prevent triggering of malignant hyperthermia was prudent at the time because no existing treatment was effective once a crisis began, and mortality from the syndrome was high.

Intravenous dantrolene, 2.5 mg/kg, will yield therapeutic concentrations of the drug when the drug is administered 30 minutes prior to anesthesia.[151] Alternatively, the drug can be administered orally over the course of several days. However, pretreatment with an adequate dose of

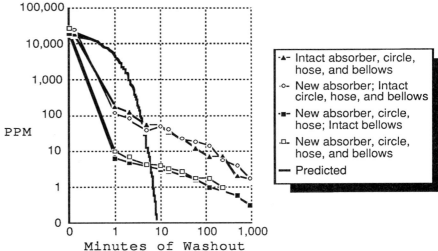

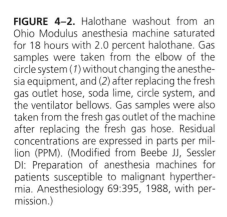

FIGURE 4–2. Halothane washout from an Ohio Modulus anesthesia machine saturated for 18 hours with 2.0 percent halothane. Gas samples were taken from the elbow of the circle system (1) without changing the anesthesia equipment, and (2) after replacing the fresh gas outlet hose, soda lime, circle system, and the ventilator bellows. Gas samples were also taken from the fresh gas outlet of the machine after replacing the fresh gas hose. Residual concentrations are expressed in parts per million (PPM). (Modified from Beebe JJ, Sessler DI: Preparation of anesthesia machines for patients susceptible to malignant hyperthermia. Anesthesiology 69:395, 1988, with permission.)

intravenous dantrolene can cause significant muscle weakness and depress respiration; several patients have required unexpected and prolonged ventilatory support after dantrolene administration.[174] Moreover, the cost of administering 2.5 mg/kg of dantrolene to a 70-kg patient is about $350.

Consequently, most investigators and clinicians now believe that dantrolene pretreatment is unnecessary because (1) crises are rare when nontriggering anesthetics are administered, (2) severe crises may be easily reversed with intravenous dantrolene in most cases, and (3) pretreatment may cause complications.[102] Large series of patients who did not receive pretreatment (because they were undergoing muscle biopsy) demonstrate that malignant hyperthermia crises during nontriggering anesthetics are extremely rare.[102, 180]

Diagnostic Tests

In general, malignant hyperthermia is suspected only after a crisis or when a patient is a relative of a proband.

Caffeine/Halothane Contracture

The in vitro caffeine/halothane contraction test developed by Kalow in 1970 is the only widely accepted test for malignant hyperthermia.[5] The diagnosis is established by evaluating a fresh, intact muscle segment to determine if muscle contraction occurs in response to halothane and caffeine. Both drugs have little effect on normal muscle. This test is difficult both to perform and to interpret. Consequently, it is not a routine procedure and is available only at approximately 10 medical centers in the United States.

The in vitro contracture test requires an intact muscle segment that is attached to a strain gauge and suspended in physiologic buffer (Fig. 4–3). Graded concentrations of halothane are bubbled through the buffer and changes in the muscle tension are measured. The caffeine concentration also is incrementally increased to 8 mM and the change in muscle tension again measured. Generally, a sustained contraction (e.g., ≥0.2 g) at a low caffeine concentration indicates that the muscle is malignant hyperthermia susceptible. Since 1989, there has been an agree-

ment among North American centers to standardize testing protocols.[187] The European countries also have a standardized (but slightly different) protocol.[188]

Some laboratories also identify an intermediate (phenotype K) response in which a contracture develops during halothane exposure only when the muscle is previously

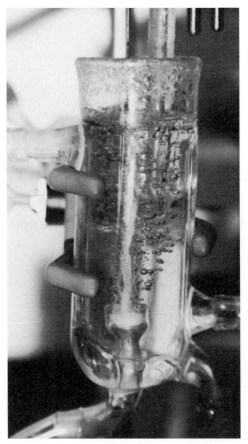

FIGURE 4–3. Muscle biopsy sample attached to a strain gauge and suspended in physiologic buffer. The in vitro contracture test is performed by adding caffeine and halothane to the buffer and measuring tension generated by the muscle. Sustained tension indicates that the muscle is susceptible to malignant hyperthermia. (Photograph by Imad Rasool, MD, PhD, University of California, Irvine, CA.)

exposed to succinylcholine.[189] This response correlates with patients who develop masseter muscle spasm but are not diagnosed as malignant hyperthermia susceptible using the conventional biopsy technique.[190] Phenotype K patients are not susceptible to malignant hyperthermia.[191] There does not appear to be a simple correlation between biopsy results and rigid versus nonrigid malignant hyperthermia.

Fresh tissue is required for the in vitro contracture test. Consequently, patients must travel to testing centers to undergo muscle biopsy and muscle contracture testing. Approximately 1 g of tissue is needed and it is usually taken from the quadriceps muscle. Because a relatively large piece of muscle is required, biopsy is usually postponed until a child is a few years old, unless biopsy is indicated because another myopathy is suspected. Anesthesia for biopsy often consists of femoral and lateral femoral cutaneous nerve blockade.[192] General anesthesia with nontriggering drugs also is acceptable. Field blocks are usually avoided because local anesthetic in the biopsy specimen may cause false-negative results. Patients undergoing biopsy must *not* be pretreated with dantrolene because dantrolene also interferes with performing the test.

The sensitivity of the test appears to be high: few false-negative results have been documented. However, triggering anesthetics have only been administered to a small number of patients who tested negative by caffeine/halothane contracture testing.[193] In contrast, the specificity of this test is relatively poor; the false-positive rate approaches 50 percent.

A modification of the in vitro contracture test uses skinned muscle fibers.[194] An advantage of this modification of the test is that it permits use of frozen muscle and does not require patients to travel to testing centers. It also allows a much smaller muscle segment to be used, which is beneficial in infants. Although the test correlates well with the conventional in vitro test, it is difficult to perform and, consequently, is not routinely available.[195] A recently proposed variant of the contracture test that uses 4-Chlorom-cresol instead of caffeine may improve its sensitivity.[196]

Creatine Phosphokinase and Microscopy

Measurement of preoperative CPK activity has been used to assist in diagnosing malignant hyperthermia–susceptible patients. The average CPK value is 152 IU in susceptible patients, 93 IU in first-degree relatives, and only 43 IU in normal subjects. The CPK value in normal subjects does not change with age. However, in susceptible subjects, the CPK concentration has a strong positive correlation with age in patients who are 10 and 50 years old.[55] This distribution obviously limits its use as a screening test in pediatric and geriatric patients. Neither the CPK activity nor the combination of this activity, myopathy, and family history is sufficient to confirm or exclude the diagnosis of malignant hyperthermia in any population.[13] An exception to this rule is that CPK activity greater than 20,000 IU after masseter spasm is highly correlated with positive caffeine-contracture tests (see above).[120, 121]

Conventional and electron microscopic analysis have been considered and rejected as reliable tests of susceptibility to malignant hyperthermia. Both analyses are usually normal in young children, nonspecific in adults (internal nuclei, single-fiber atrophy, fiber necrosis and regeneration, moth-eaten fibers, and core-targetoid fibers). The neuromuscular junction appears normal and there is no evidence of denervation. These changes are similar to those observed after many kinds of muscle injury, suggesting that they result from a crisis rather than indicate susceptibility.

Calcium Uptake

A test using calcium uptake in thin, frozen muscle slices was proposed in 1978 and subsequently used in about 2,000 patients.[197] One advantage of the test was that a small muscle specimen could be frozen and mailed to a central laboratory for processing. The developers reported that 1 percent of 1,460 children (whose induction of anesthesia included halothane plus succinylcholine) developed masseter spasm. They also found a nearly perfect correlation between masseter spasm and malignant hyperthermia susceptibility.[115] These findings concerned many other investigators because a 1 percent incidence of masseter spasm implied a 1 percent incidence of malignant hyperthermia susceptibility, which is far greater than previously estimated.

Because the calcium uptake test detected so many apparently susceptible patients, there have been several efforts to validate the test by comparing its results to those from the in vitro contracture test. None of these studies demonstrated a correlation between the two tests. Similarly, no correlation between positive calcium uptake tests and clinical crises was demonstrated.[119, 121] As a result, this test no longer is used. Patients identified as susceptible by this test should obviously be reevaluated using the in vitro caffeine contracture test.

Other Proposed Tests

Many diagnostic techniques less invasive than the in vitro contracture test have been proposed. A test based on platelet and muscle ATP depletion was suggested in 1980, but later was found not to predict susceptibility to malignant hyperthermia. Despite the similarities between the dense tubular system of platelets and skeletal muscle, platelet aggregation in response to halothane was normal in susceptible patients. Although osmotic fragility of red cells is slightly increased in swine and dogs susceptible to malignant hyperthermia, it does not appear to be increased in humans. Even in swine, overlap between normal and susceptible blood is so great that the difference cannot be used for diagnosis; moreover, red cell fragility is not enhanced by exposure to halothane.

Electrophoresis of muscle protein from patients who were susceptible to malignant hyperthermia initially revealed two abnormal bands. Subsequently, both bands were shown to represent contamination of the muscle by blood. Tests based on muscle stress, including measurement of plasma cyclic adenosine monophosphate (cAMP) activity following exercise and measurement of twitch strength of tourniqueted muscle, also do not predict susceptibility to malignant hyperthermia. Skeletal muscle adenylate cyclase activity initially was reported to be increased in MH-susceptible patients but has been shown to be normal. ATP depletion in susceptible muscle was proposed as a diagnostic test, but this test was subsequently determined to be inadequate. Other tests, such as electromyographic counts of motor neurons in various muscle groups, muscle phosphoralase, mitochondrial calcium efflux, chemiluminescence in susceptible erythrocytes, and total body calcium content determined by neutron activation also are not reliable methods of determining susceptibility to malignant hyperthermia.

Several recently observed differences between normal and susceptible tissues may provide a basis for minimally invasive tests. These include electron spin resonance of sarcoplasmic reticulum exposed to halothane,[198] cytoplasmic ionized calcium concentrations in lymphocytes exposed to halothane,[29, 30] electron microscopic morphology of platelets following exposure to halothane,[27, 28] and magnetic resonance evaluation of muscle.[199, 200] Use of these diagnostic techniques requires further evaluation of their sensitivity and specificity before they can be used clinically.

Counseling

Patients who have had a typical hyperthermic crisis and their first-degree relatives must be considered susceptible to malignant hyperthermia until a muscle biopsy proves otherwise. Second-degree relatives with either a myopathy or increased CPK activity should also be considered susceptible. These patients should be told about malignant hyperthermia and must inform their anesthesiologists that they may be susceptible. It is helpful to give patients a letter describing the basis for believing they may be susceptible (e.g., triggering anesthetic and occurrence of masseter spasm, fever, CPK activity, urine myoglobin, family history, and muscle biopsy results). They should wear a Med-Alert bracelet that reads "Malig. hyperthermia—no volatile anesth. or succinylcholine." They may also be referred to the Malignant Hyperthermia Association of the United States* to receive additional information and a monthly bulletin from the organization. The association maintains a 24-hour/day physician referral service to assist with both crisis and elective management in malignant hyperthermia susceptible individuals.

During the 1960s and 1970s, intraoperative temperature monitoring was rare, end-tidal CO_2 monitoring was unknown, and many anesthesiologists were unaware of malignant hyperthermia. Consequently, the syndrome was not usually appreciated until a crisis was advanced. Even when a crisis was recognized early, no effective treatment was available and symptoms frequently progressed further. Although this situation was unfortunate for victims of the syndrome, it at least made retrospective diagnosis and counseling straightforward.

Now that awareness of malignant hyperthermia is the rule and intraoperative temperature and end-tidal P_{CO_2} monitoring standard, crises are rarely allowed to progress to the point of being unequivocal. Most anesthesiologists

respond to even slight fever, tachycardia, and hypercapnea by changing to a nontriggering anesthetic technique; frequently, dantrolene also is administered. Increased awareness and early treatment have decreased the number of severe crises and have substantially reduced mortality. They also have introduced a diagnostic dilemma: although these patients may be susceptible, they are more likely to have experienced only a febrile reaction from excessive heating, tissue trauma, pyrogen release, drug administration, or blood incompatibility.

Counseling patients with clinically equivocal or aborted crises is difficult because the only generally accepted diagnostic test is both expensive and invasive. Options include discounting the episode, telling patients they may be susceptible, and referring them for muscle biopsy. Mild fever and tachycardia that resolve without treatment and are not accompanied by muscle rigidity, acidemia, or myoglobinuria reasonably can be attributed to causes other than malignant hyperthermia. Patients whose symptoms are more convincing must be told that they may be malignant hyperthermia susceptible, but that a muscle biopsy is required to establish the diagnosis. A biopsy is by no means mandatory because malignant hyperthermia has few, if any, manifestations except during anesthesia. Since nontriggering anesthetics are safe, susceptible patients can still undergo elective surgery and otherwise lead normal lives. The decision to perform a biopsy should be made jointly by the anesthesiologist and the patient, and must take into account the expense and inconvenience of the in vitro contracture test and the probability that minimally invasive tests will soon be available.

Perhaps the most common diagnostic and therapeutic problem posed by malignant hyperthermia is the patient whose only symptom is masseter spasm during the induction of anesthesia. Other symptoms may not have occurred because (1) 50 percent of masseter spasm occurs in patients who are not malignant hyperthermia susceptible[120, 121]; (2) anesthesia was discontinued (with or without dantrolene treatment), allowing little opportunity for other symptoms to develop; or, (3) the patient is susceptible but malignant hyperthermia was not triggered (susceptible patients typically have been exposed to triggering anesthetics without complication several times prior to diagnosis[56]). These patients should be told that their risk of susceptibility is about 50 percent, and that a muscle biopsy is necessary to determine the diagnosis. As in other equivocal cases, the decision to perform a biopsy should be made by both the anesthesiologist and the patient.

THERMOREGULATION AND HEAT BALANCE

Thermal disturbances in the perioperative period are common, even in adults. Virtually all pediatric surgical patients become hypothermic unless their temperatures are actively maintained. Hypothermia results partially from environmental exposure, but results mostly from anesthetic-induced failure of thermoregulatory control. Hypothermia is beneficial occasionally, but more commonly, is an unnecessary risk. Understanding anesthetic effects on thermoregulation and the consequent changes in heat bal-

*Malignant Hyperthermia Association of the United States, 39 East State Street, PO Box 1069, Sherburne, NY 13460-1069. Telephone: 800-MH-HYPER.

ance will facilitate optimal thermal management of pediatric surgical patients.

First the relevant aspects of normal thermoregulatory control are reviewed. Then the responses during general and epidural anesthesia are presented separately because these situations are physiologically distinct. During general anesthesia, central control is impaired, but peripheral responses remain available. In contrast, central regulation is intact during epidural anesthesia but afferent thermal input and peripheral effector mechanisms are inhibited directly by blocked nerves. Finally, perianesthetic fever and hyperthermia are reviewed.

Temperature Monitoring

Fever has long been recognized as a useful clinical sign and was correlated with disease in the oldest medical text: the *Edwin Smith Surgical Papyrus* (~1,700 years B.C.).[201] By the time of Hippocrates, fever patterns of some diseases (e.g., those of malaria) were accurately described.[202] Such descriptions are remarkable when one considers that thermometers were not invented for an additional 23 centuries! Furthermore, initial thermometers provided only relative indications of temperature using arbitrary units; it was not until 1714 that Gabriel Fahrenheit provided a reliable clinical thermometer reading in absolute units.[202]

During subsequent years, temperature monitoring was increasingly incorporated into medical practice, eventually becoming one of the critical "vital signs." However, it was not until the 1970s that concerns about the malignant hyperthermia syndrome prompted routine temperature monitoring in the perianesthetic period. Current American Society of Anesthesiologists guidelines require that a method for measuring body temperature be available during anesthesia; however, the Society has yet to adapt more rigorous standards. Once temperature monitoring was done routinely, it became apparent that nearly all patients became significantly hypothermic during anesthesia and surgery, and that the hypothermia sometimes triggered substantial physiologic responses.

Thermometers

Traditionally, medicine has used mercury-in-glass thermometers for measuring body temperature. Recently, glass thermometers have been supplanted by electronic thermometers, which are faster, safer to use, provide continuous readings, and are more accurate. Consequently, there is now little indication for the clinical use of glass thermometers.

Thermocouples and thermisters are the most common electronic temperature sensors. Both are so accurate and sufficiently inexpensive that they can be discarded after a single use. Although thermocouples and thermisters can be used to measure skin temperature, two methods are available specifically for this purpose: liquid crystal temperature sensors and infrared thermography. Infrared systems have a far broader detection range, are faster, and are considerably more accurate than liquid crystals.

Forehead skin-surface temperatures estimate core temperature better than might be expected.[203] Skin temperatures may not reliably confirm the clinical signs of malignant hyperthermia (tachycardia and hypercarbia), and they are not suitable for use during triggering anesthetics (Fig. 4–4).[204] Infrared aural canal temperatures have been shown to be insufficiently accurate and precise for clinical use.[205–207] More esoteric measures of temperature (including magnetic resonance spectroscopy) remain intriguing research tools, but are not currently clinically useful.

Temperature Monitoring Sites

Far more difficult than determining the type of thermometer to use is choosing an appropriate temperature monitoring site. Body temperature is far from uniform: a core of well-perfused tissues tends to be at the same (and relatively high) temperature. This is considered "core" temperature and is, in most cases, the best single indicator of body temperature. In contrast, "peripheral" tissues (representing up to half the body mass) may have considerably lower temperatures.[208] Furthermore, peripheral temperatures are far from uniform and can vary many degrees over short distances.

Both core and peripheral tissue temperatures contribute to thermoregulatory responses (see section "Afferent Input," below), but core temperature is usually the most important thermoregulatory controller by far, and is therefore of primary clinical interest. Common core temperature monitoring sites include the distal esophagus, the tympanic membrane, the pulmonary artery, and the nasopharynx. Even during rapid temperature change (e.g., cardiopulmonary bypass), these temperature-monitoring sites remain reliable.[209, 210] When core temperature is changing slowly, rectal and bladder temperatures reflect core temperature well.[211, 212] Core temperature also may be assessed orally or in the axilla, but the accuracy and precision of measurements in these sites tends to be low.[211] From a practical point of view, distal esophageal temperatures are the easiest, most reliable site for core temperature-monitoring during general anesthesia. The validity of these temperature-monitoring sites is comparable in adults and pediatric patients.[213]

Peripheral temperatures are useful to assess cutaneous input to the thermoregulatory system,[214, 215] to evaluate body heat content (e.g., during rapid rewarming on cardiopulmonary bypass), and to assess thermoregulatory vasoconstriction.[216] Cutaneous input to the thermoregulatory system is conventionally calculated from four area-weighted sites using the formula of Ramanathan: $0.3(T_{chest} + T_{arm}) + 0.2(T_{thigh} + T_{calf})$.[217] Although greater accuracy will be obtained using formulae that use temperatures from more sites,[218] the additional measurements are not usually necessary.

Similarly, mean skin temperature can be combined with core temperature to estimate average body temperature; from this value and the specific heat of humans (~0.83 kcal $\cdot$ kg^{-1} $\cdot$ °C$^{-1,219}$), body heat content can be calculated. A variety of formulae have been proposed for calculating mean body temperature from average skin temperature and core temperature. Among the best are those of Colin et al: $0.66 \cdot T_{core} + 0.34 \cdot T_{skin}$ in a neutral environment and $0.79 \cdot T_{core} + 0.21 \cdot T_{skin}$ in a warm environment.[208]

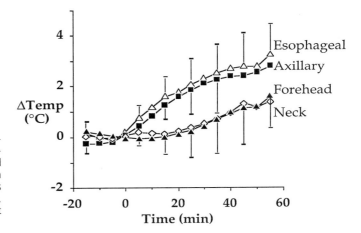

FIGURE 4–4. Acute malignant hyperthermia was induced in susceptible baby pigs at elapsed time zero. Esophageal (core) and axillary temperatures correlated well, but forehead and neck skin temperatures did not. An additional problem with using skin-surface temperatures as a substitute for valid core measurement sites is that skin temperatures do not reliably indicate absolute core temperature. (From Iaizzo PA, Kehler CH, Zink RS, et al: Thermal response in acute porcine malignant hyperthermia. Anesth Analg 82:803, 1996.)

It is important to realize that these formulae have been validated only in young healthy volunteers and in a limited number of steady-state circumstances. The extent to which they are valid in the perianesthetic period is unclear. For example, should one use the "warm" or "neutral" coefficients in an unanesthetized, hypothermic patient who is in a cold environment, yet vasodilated? Pending further validation, these formulae should be applied with caution to perianesthetic situations, especially those involving rapid thermal changes (e.g., rapid rewarming during recovery from general anesthesia).

When Intraoperative Temperature Monitoring Is Required

There are two major reasons for monitoring body temperature in the perianesthetic period: to evaluate body heat content and to confirm the other clinical signs of malignant hyperthermia.

The drugs used during monitored anesthesia care or regional anesthesia do not trigger malignant hyperthermia.[178, 220] However, core hypothermia does occur during conduction anesthesia, especially when surgery involves major body cavities,[221] and often is manifested as shivering.[222, 223] Core temperature should be measured during spinal or epidural anesthesia if the patient is likely to become hypothermic.

Core temperature monitoring is appropriate during most general anesthetics, both to facilitate detection of malignant hyperthermia and to quantify hyperthermia and hypothermia. Malignant hyperthermia is best detected by tachycardia and an increase in end-tidal P_{CO_2} out of proportion to minute ventilation.[129] Nonetheless, increasing core temperature helps confirm the diagnosis and is recommended by the Malignant Hyperthermia Association of the United States.

Normal core temperature is between 36.5° and 37.5°C, with the average being very nearly 37.0°C. Core temperature usually decreases 0.5° to 1.5°C in the first 30 minutes after the induction of anesthesia. Hypothermia results from internal redistribution of heat and from a variety of other factors whose importance in individual patients is hard to predict.[224] As a result, core temperature perturbations during the first 30 minutes of anesthesia are difficult to interpret. Significant subsequent decreases in core temperature are most likely in patients undergoing major surgery, but malignant hyperthermia remains a risk in all patients. Consequently, body temperature should be monitored in most patients undergoing general anesthesia that exceeds 30 minutes in duration and in all patients whose surgery lasts longer than 1 hour. Temperature changes tend to be particularly rapid in infants; consequently, temperature measurements should start as soon after induction of anesthesia as is practical in these patients.

Normal Thermoregulation

There are three major components to the thermoregulatory system: afferent input, central control, and efferent responses. Full control of body temperature in extreme environments requires effective function of each component. Almost certainly, the thermoregulatory system did not develop de novo. Instead, evolution progressively coopted preexisting regulatory systems and subsequently modified them into efficient regulators. Consequently, Satinoff has proposed a caudal–rostral hierarchy of regulatory control.[225] Lower centers exhibit modest degrees of control, but generally are supplanted by more precise regulatory centers higher in the neuroaxis.

Afferent Input

Temperature is sensed by Aδ fibers (most cold signals) and C-fibers (most warm signals).[226, 227] These sensors are distributed throughout the body, and it is likely that most tissues contribute at least somewhat to thermoregulatory control. Even after decades of research, the precise thermal contributions of various tissues remains unclear. However, the thermal core (neuraxis and deep abdominal and thoracic tissues) certainly contributes most.[228–230] The skin quantitatively contributes less than core temperature; but because the skin provides the major contact with the environment, its importance remains substantial.[214, 215] Specifically, the skin contributes 20 percent to control of autonomic responses[231, 232] and 50 percent to control of behavioral responses (thermal comfort).[233] The importance of cutaneous input is such that, in most cases, core temperature perturbations are trivial in a wide range of environments.

It is well established that the rate of change of skin temperature alters its apparent importance: rapid changes contribute about five times as much to the central regulatory system as comparable changes made slowly.[234] At least within the rates experienced by patients not undergoing cardiopulmonary bypass, the rate of change of core temperature does not appear to substantially influence the magnitude of provoked regulatory responses.

In mammals, the hypothalamus, other portions of the brain, the spinal cord, and deep abdominal and thoracic tissues each contribute roughly 20 percent to central thermoregulatory control. The precise values are not known in humans, and certainly have not been established in pediatric patients. In birds, the spinal cord is the major thermal detector, contributing far more than the hypothalamus. The extent to which the relatively high surface core ratio in infants and in children augments cutaneous thermal input is unknown.

Central Control

Satinoff has proposed that thermoregulatory control is hierarchical. The phylogenetically oldest, and least precise, control is likely to be at the level of the spinal cord. Responses at this level are modified by "newer" rostral centers that are more precise. The most precise control, in most cases, appears to emanate from the preoptic area of the hypothalamus. While this model was a huge advance over those proposing exclusive cutaneous or hypothalamic control of thermoregulation, there is evidence that actual control systems are even more complicated. Consequently, models should be used when they are helpful constructions for organizing observed experimental data. In most cases though, they should not be considered representations of *how* the system actually works.

A variety of simple and complex[235, 236] thermoregulatory control models have been proposed. Even the most complicated of these is simply a model, and not meant to imply a specific neurologic mechanism. The mechanisms by which the body actually controls temperature remains unknown, but certainly is extraordinarily complicated. Multiple positive and negative feedback loops interact to produce responses. Furthermore, multiple levels of excitatory and inhibitory control compete to determine responses to thermal perturbations. Nonetheless, thermoregulatory control models remain helpful because they provide a framework into which experimental data can be fit. The most sophisticated models include dynamic responses and have been validated, to greater or lesser extents, under a variety of circumstances. I will present a relatively simple model, sufficient to categorize most thermoregulatory responses. It is a compendium of various proposed systems.[225, 237, 238] Less complicated models have proven insufficient to characterize perianesthetic thermoregulatory responses.

There are three aspects to a thermoregulatory response: *threshold, gain,* and *maximum* response intensity. The threshold is the body temperature at which a specific response is initiated. In practice, thresholds are usually cited in terms of core temperature, recognizing that skin and other tissue temperatures contribute to the threshold. There is no requirement that tissue temperatures are

comparably integrated for each type of thermoregulatory response, but the autonomic responses do appear to be similarly integrated. In contrast, behavioral responses depend mostly on skin-surface temperature (Fig. 4–5).[212, 234, 239, 240]

Gain defines the rate at which a response intensity increases with further core temperature deviation from the triggering threshold. In practice, it is the slope of a plot of response intensity versus the change in core temperature. Typically, the gain of thermoregulatory responses is extremely high. It is not unusual for thermoregulatory response intensity to increase from 10 percent to 90 percent of its maximum value with a change in core temperature of only a few tenths of a degree.[241–244] Maximum response intensity is simply defined by the greatest intensity observed during core temperature perturbations far exceeding the threshold.

Temperatures *not* triggering autonomic thermoregulatory responses define the *interthreshold range.* Since arteriovenous shunt vasoconstriction is the first response to cold and sweating is the first response to warm, temperatures between these respective thresholds identify the interthreshold range. In normal humans, this range is about 0.3°C. Only slight further deviations in core temperature are necessary to trigger nonshivering thermogenesis or shivering and active vasodilation. Precise control of core temperature requires not only that the interthreshold range be small, but that the gain of thermoregulatory responses is high. The gain of thermoregulatory responses is, in fact, high: in some cases, it is so high that no gain can be identified. Vasoconstriction, for example, appears to be an "on-off" phenomenon. The gain for sweating can be detected, but is quite high (i.e., 1,500 g · m^{-2} · h^{-1} · °C^{-1}). Because the gain of vasoconstriction and sweat-

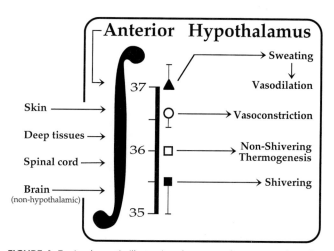

FIGURE 4–5. A schematic illustrating thermoregulatory control mechanisms. Mean body temperature is the integrated thermal input from a variety of tissues including the brain, skin surface, spinal cord, and deep central structures. However, thresholds usually are expressed in terms of core temperature. A core temperature below the thresholds for response to cold provokes vasoconstriction, nonshivering thermogenesis, and shivering. Core temperature exceeding the hyperthermic thresholds produces active vasodilation and sweating. No thermoregulatory responses are initiated when core temperature is between these thresholds; these temperatures identify the interthreshold range. (Modified from Sessler DI: Temperature monitoring. *In* Miller RD [ed]: Anesthesia, 4th ed. New York, Churchill Livingstone, 1994, p 1363, with permission.)

ing are high, and because these responses are effective, only fairly severe environmental perturbations trigger shivering or active vasodilation.

The interplay among the various thermoregulatory responses is determined in part by regulatory preference. For example, vasoconstriction normally is initiated before shivering. The result is a response requiring little in the way of nutrients and minimally impairing function is mobilized before a function that is metabolically costly. Even more complicated is the interaction between thermoregulatory and nonthermoregulatory responses. Maintenance of body temperature appears to be a high priority for mammals. Nonetheless, thermoregulatory control may be sacrificed under special conditions to maintain even more carefully regulated parameters. For example, even during water deprivation, sweating initially continues in hyperthermic humans. However, sweating stops when vascular volume depletion becomes extreme. Core hyperthermia and heat stroke typically result unless the environment is modified or the vascular volume is repleted.

Efferent Responses

By far the most important human thermoregulatory response to extreme environments is behavioral. Examples of behavioral responses include seeking shelter, donning warmer clothing, adjusting a thermostat, and assuming positions that appropriately maximize or minimize heat transferred to the environment. The overall efficacy of behavioral responses far exceeds the combined abilities of the autonomic responses. Consequently, it is behavioral responses that allow humans to exist in the most extreme environments.

The initial response to a cold environment is arteriovenous shunt vasoconstriction. In a thermoneutral condition, arteriovenous shunts are open, and peripheral cutaneous blood flow is maximal. Cold exposure decreases shunt flow without significantly altering capillary flow. In contrast, warm stress dramatically increases capillary flow without augmenting shunt flow from its thermoneutral values.

Arteriovenous shunts are 100-μm vessels located only in skin covering the most distal portions of the body, including the fingers, toes, and nose.[245] Blood flow through an arteriovenous shunt exceeds that flowing through a comparable length of 10-μm-diameter capillary by a factor of 10,000.[246] Although capillaries far outnumber shunts, even in fingers and toes, shunt flow is sufficient to increase finger blood flow more than 10-fold.[247] As a result, finger blood flow in a warm environment typically exceeds local nutritional needs by a factor of 100.

Unfortunately, heat loss is not a linear function of peripheral blood flow. Thus, even a 10-fold reduction in finger blood flow reduces heat loss to a considerably lesser extent. The effect of shunt vasoconstriction, nonetheless, is greater than might be imagined because decreased arm blood flow results in proximal arm tissue cooling, which itself reduces cutaneous heat loss. Over the entire body, thermoregulatory vasoconstriction decreases heat loss 25 to 50 percent, depending on the initial environmental temperature and the duration of vasoconstriction. Many hours of vasoconstriction are required to fully reduce pe-

ripheral tissue temperature, and thus, to maximally reduce cutaneous heat loss.

Thermoregulatory vasoconstriction is mediated by α-adrenergic nerves. Although most control originates centrally, vascular tone also is modulated by local temperature. Thus, centrally mediated vasoconstriction is more intense at low skin temperatures than it is when the local temperature is high. Within the typical clinical range of skin temperature, central control contributes far more than local control to skin blood flow.

Nonshivering thermogenesis is defined as an increase in metabolic heat production that is *not* accompanied by muscular activity. Most nonshivering thermogenesis occurs in a specialized tissue called brown fat (the tissue is grossly brown because of its enormous mitochondrial density). Brown adipose tissue is innervated by α-adrenergic nerves via a local uncoupling protein. Although activation of nonshivering thermogenesis is accompanied by a twofold increase in circulating norepinephrine, circulating catecholamines contribute little to activation of brown fat. There is some evidence that other tissues, including skeletal muscle, also contribute to nonshivering thermogenesis.

Nonshivering thermogenesis is the most important thermoregulatory response to cold stress in small mammals. For example, rats increase metabolic heat production 300 percent in a cold environment, before beginning to shiver. Nonshivering thermogenesis also is generally more important in young animals than in older ones. Nonshivering thermogenesis either does not occur in adult humans, or its magnitude is so small that it is clinically unimportant.[248, 249] In contrast, newborn infants can double metabolic heat production during cold exposure.[250, 251] Even premature infants (e.g., 1,500 g) demonstrate this response.[252] Clinically significant nonshivering thermogenesis persists for the first 2 years of life.

Infants do not shiver. Presumably, lack of shivering results from the general immaturity of the musculoskeletal system in infants. Furthermore, because infants have so little muscle mass, it is unlikely that shivering would contribute much to cold defense. The age dependence of shivering has not been fully established, but this response probably does not become important until early childhood.

There are two autonomic responses to heat stress: sweating and active precapillary vasodilation. Sweating is mediated by postganglionic, cholinergic, sympathetic nerves.[253] These nerves terminate on cutaneous sweat glands that are widely but unevenly distributed. Sweat is an ultrafiltrate of plasma, from which a large amount of electrolyte has been reabsorbed. The amount of sodium, potassium, and lactate in sweat depends on the rate of sweat production, vascular volume, and athletic conditioning.[254] Sweating starts on the chest, and then proceeds to more distal skin surfaces. Even at maximum intensity, the rate of sweating is higher on the chest than other sites. Untrained individuals can sweat nearly 1 L/hr, and the rate may be twice as great in conditioned athletes.[255, 256] Sweating is a remarkably effective defense against hyperthermia. In a dry environment, sweating can dissipate up to 10 times the basal metabolic rate. Only sweat that evaporates (as opposed to rolling off the body) dissipates heat, but each gram of evaporated water absorbs 0.58 kcal. The efficacy of sweating is illustrated by one well-hydrated scientist who remained in air that had a temperature of 250°F for 1 hour without being burned or becoming hyperthermic.

Because sweating depends on evaporation, its efficacy is completely defeated by a relative humidity approaching 100 percent. In contrast, its efficacy is substantially increased by a convective environment. Because sweating is mediated by cholinergic nerves, even a small dose of atropine (e.g., 0.5 mg) markedly impairs this response, both increasing the threshold and reducing the gain.[257, 258] Conversely, local application of cholinergic agonists, such as pilocarpine, produce vigorous sweating.

Active precapillary vasodilation can increase cutaneous blood flow enormously. This is a uniquely human response, not shared even by other primates. During severe heat stress, blood flow through the top millimeter of the skin can equal the entire resting cardiac output. The mechanism by which heat stress activates precapillary vasodilation remains unknown. However, vasodilation appears to be mediated by an unknown transmitter released from sweat glands.[253] The mediator might well be a peptide, because standard adrenergic and cholinergic blocking agents do not prevent this response. In general, active vasodilation is triggered after sweating, although distinct exceptions have been noted. In practice, active vasodilation enhances thermoregulatory responses to heat stress by transferring heat from the core to the skin surface, where it can be dissipated by evaporation.

Thermoregulation during General Anesthesia

General anesthetics increase the interthreshold range from a normal value of approximately 0.3°C to approximately 4°C (Figs. 4–6 and 4–7). It is likely that body temperature remains accurately sensed during anesthesia, but that temperatures within the interthreshold range are simply not perceived as requiring autonomic responses. However, once body temperature has deviated sufficiently from normal to trigger thermoregulatory responses, the gain and maximum intensity of these responses remains nearly normal.[241, 259]

Markedly altered thermoregulatory thresholds with relatively well preserved gain and maximum intensities is in stark contrast to anesthetic effects on most other homeostatic systems; for example, the CO_2-response curve is both "shifted to the right" and "flattened" by general anesthetics. This unusual pattern of anesthetic-induced thermoregulatory inhibition is consistent with a hierarchical thermoregulatory system in which the most precise control (i.e., thresholds) are determined by the hypothalamus and other rostral structures that are relatively sensitive to anesthetics.[225] In contrast, the "mechanical details" of these responses (i.e., gains and maximum intensities) may be largely controlled by the spinal cord and other caudal structures that are relatively resistant to anesthetics.[260]

Behavioral thermoregulation is usually of little consequence during general anesthesia because patients are unconscious and frequently paralyzed. The effects of general anesthetics on behavioral regulation in humans have not been specifically evaluated. Nonetheless, clinical observation suggests that patients in a cool environment frequently feel warmer following administration of various sedative drugs. Similarly, mice given subanesthetic concentrations of nitrous oxide choose a cooler environment than mice given only air.[261]

Cold Responses

All anesthetics so far tested significantly decrease the thermoregulatory threshold for vasoconstriction. Typical

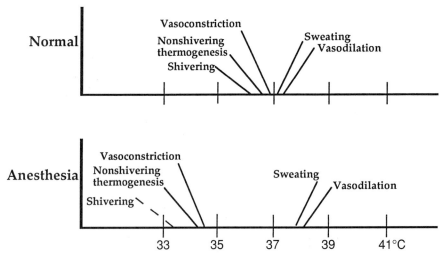

FIGURE 4–6. A schematic illustrating thermoregulatory thresholds in unanesthetized and anesthetized humans. The slanted lines represent different regulatory responses and the dark horizontal lines show core body temperature; the intersection of each line with the temperature scale is the threshold. The interthreshold range is shown as the distance between the first cold response (vasoconstriction) and the first warm response (sweating); temperatures within this range will not elicit autonomic thermoregulatory compensation. Because each thermoregulatory response has its own threshold and gain, there is an orderly progression of responses, and response intensities, in proportion to need. During general anesthesia (*bottom*), the thresholds for vasoconstriction and nonshivering thermogenesis are shifted down to ≈ 34.5°C (depending on anesthetic type and dose). Similarly, the thresholds for active precapillary vasodilation and sweating are increased ≈1°C. (Modified from Sessler DI: Temperature monitoring, *In* Miller RD [ed]: Anesthesia, 4th ed. New York, Churchill Livingstone, 1994, p 1363, with permission.)

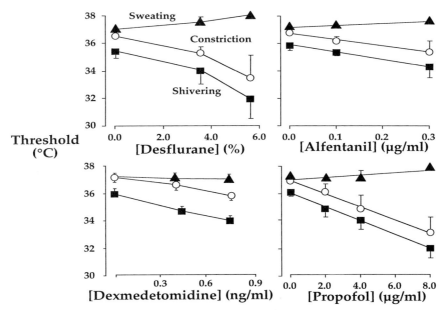

FIGURE 4–7. Anesthetic-induced inhibition of thermoregulatory control is usually the major factor determining perioperative core temperature. Concentration-dependent thermoregulatory inhibition by desflurane and isoflurane (halogenated volatile anesthetics), propofol (an intravenous anesthetic), and alfentanil (a μ-agonist opioid). The sweating (*triangles*), vasoconstriction (*circles*), and shivering (*squares*) thresholds are expressed in terms of core temperature at a designated mean skin temperature of 34°C. Anesthesia linearly (but slightly) increases the sweating threshold. In contrast, anesthesia produces substantial and comparable linear or nonlinear decreases in the vasoconstriction and shivering thresholds. Typical anesthetic concentrations thus increase the interthreshold range (difference between the sweating and vasoconstriction thresholds) approximately 20-fold from its normal value near 0.2°C. Patients do not activate autonomic thermoregulatory defenses unless body temperature exceeds the interthreshold range; surgical patients are thus poikilothermic over a 3° to 5°C range of core temperatures. Isoflurane 1 percent and desflurane 6 percent have comparable anesthetic potency. (Data obtained from Annadata et al.,[265] Xiong et al.,[371] Matsukawa et al.,[267] and Kurz et al.[372]; Error bars smaller than the data markers have been deleted.)

clinical doses of halothane (0.86 percent end-tidal),[262] enflurane,[263] nitrous oxide/fentanyl,[264] desflurane,[265] sevoflurane,[266] and propofol[267] decrease the threshold to approximately 34° to 35°C; propofol combined with nitrous oxide also produces substantial inhibition.[268] With clinical doses of most anesthetics, thermoregulatory vasoconstriction (which is usually initiated near 37°C) does not occur during typical clinical doses of isoflurane until the core temperature reaches approximately 34°C. Inhibition by the volatile anesthetics is nonlinear (being greater at higher concentratiions), whereas inhibition by propofol and opioids is linear.

Changes in thermoregulatory vasoconstriction during both halothane[269] and isoflurane[270] anesthesia are similar in infants, children, and adults (Fig. 4–8). However, the elderly constrict at core temperatures approximately 1.5°C less than those in young adults. Supramaximal painful stimulation during enflurane anesthesia increases the threshold only approximately 0.5°C when compared with unstimulated anesthetized volunteers.[263] These data suggest that thermoregulatory responses are similar in large and small surgical procedures, and in cases where surgical pain is prevented by regional or local anesthesia. Rapid skin temperature perturbations produce considerably larger thermoregulatory responses than comparable changes induced slowly.[214, 234] However, the speed of core temperature changes (within the typical clinical range) does not appear to produce higher vasoconstriction thresholds.

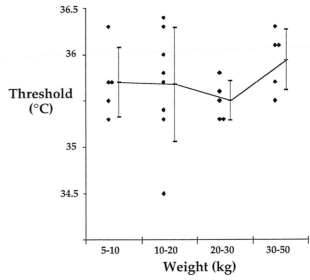

FIGURE 4–8. The core thermoregulatory threshold in 23 healthy children and infants undergoing abdominal surgery with halothane anesthesia. Differences between the groups were not statistically significant. (From Bissonnette B, Sessler DI: Thermoregulatory thresholds for vasoconstriction in pediatric patients anesthetized with halothane or halothane and caudal bupivacaine. Anesthesiology 76:387, 1992.)

Once triggered, the maximum intensity of vasoconstriction during anesthesia is similar to that in unanesthetized individuals.[259] As in unanesthetized individuals, vasoconstriction appears to be either "on" or "off." Thus, the gain of thermoregulatory vasoconstriction is extremely high in both cases.

Nonshivering thermogenesis does not increase heat production in anesthetized adults,[271] which is hardly surprising, since this response does not appear to be important in unanesthetized adults.[248, 249] However, cold exposure and core hypothermia also fail to increase metabolic rate in anesthetized infants.[272] Lack of nonshivering results in part because volatile anesthetics peripherally inhibit this response.[273]

Postanesthetic shivering frequently complicates recovery from hypothermic anesthesia in adults.[274] Infants, however, do not shiver and shivering is rare in children. Postanesthetic shivering can be prevented by maintaining intraoperative normothermia. Alternatively, it can be treated by skin-surface warming[275] or by intravenous administration of meperidine.[276]

Warm Responses

Isoflurane and the other volatile anesthetics produce a dose-dependent increase in the sweating threshold. However, the increase in the sweating threshold is far less than the decrease in the vasoconstriction threshold. For example, 1.2 percent isoflurane decreases the vasoconstriction threshold to approximately 33°C but increases the sweating threshold only to 38.2°C. Why these responses should differ so much remains unknown, but teleologically, an aggressive response to hyperthermia is appropriate because hyperthermia is far more dangerous than comparable hypothermia.

Interestingly, although the sweating threshold is increased significantly by isoflurane anesthesia, the gain of this response remains normal at all isoflurane concentrations. Similarly, maximum sweating intensity is reduced little, if at all, by isoflurane anesthesia (Fig. 4-9).[241] The sweating threshold is 0.2° to 0.5°C higher in women than in men, and this difference is preserved during isoflurane anesthesia.

Dehydration significantly decreases sweat production, particularly when dehydration is combined with physical exertion. Without adequate sweating, the body is unable to dissipate the heat of physical activity in warm environments, causing core body temperature to increase dramatically (heat stroke).

The threshold for precapillary arteriolar vasodilation increases in parallel with the sweating threshold during anesthesia.[241, 277] Although the gain and maximum intensity of cutaneous hyperemia have not been formally quantified during anesthesia, they appear relatively well preserved. Because this vasodilation is an active process, cutaneous blood flow in individuals whose core temperature exceeds the vasodilation threshold is reduced by local nerve block.[241] Consequently, maximum skin blood flow during anesthesia, as might be desired during microvascular surgery, is best produced by core hyperthermia, not regional anesthesia.

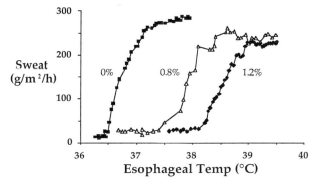

FIGURE 4-9. The sweating rate in a typical male volunteer shows the threshold, gain, and maximum intensity during hyperthermia alone (0%) and at 0.8 percent, and 1.2 percent end-tidal isoflurane concentration. The thresholds were markedly increased by anesthesia; in contrast, gains and maximum sweating rates were relatively well preserved. The thermoregulatory threshold for sweating increased linearly with increasing end-tidal isoflurane concentration. In men, the regression equation was: Threshold (°C) = 36.6°C + 1.3 · [isoflurane], r^2 = 0.94. In women, the regression equation was: Threshold (°C) = 37.1°C + 1.0 · [isoflurane], r^2 = 0.87. (From Washington D, Sessler DI, Moayeri A, et al: Thermoregulatory responses to hyperthermia during isoflurane anesthesia in humans. J Appl Physiol 74:82, 1993, with permission.)

Thermoregulatory sweating does not appear to be an important response in anesthetized infants, perhaps because heat retention and production usually is more difficult for infants than heat dissipation. The age at which sweating becomes important has yet to be determined.

Heat Balance during General Anesthesia

Thermal steady state is defined by heat loss to the environment that equals metabolic heat production. Thus, over the long term, heat loss must equal heat production if body temperature is to remain stable. The basal metabolic rate in adult humans is approximately 100 W, but increases 5 to 10-fold during exercise.

Body temperature (and therefore heat content) is not uniform. Thermoregulation maintains a nearly constant core temperature. Peripheral tissue temperature, however, is not similarly maintained, and tonic thermoregulatory vasoconstriction typically produces a 1° to 5°C core–peripheral temperature gradient. Because of their anatomic mass, the legs constitute most of the peripheral thermal buffer.

The capacity of the peripheral thermal buffering compartment is approximately 150 kcal (e.g., body heat content can change by this amount without altering core temperature). Peripheral thermal buffering allows individuals to lose heat in a cold environment or absorb heat in a warm environment without altering core temperature. This strategy minimizes need for autonomic responses, which may be costly in terms of metabolic needs, use of resources, or behavioral requirements.

Heat Transfer

Heat is lost or gained from the environment via four routes; each thermodynamic mechanism is completely reversible and may result in net heat gain or loss with equal facility. In a typical ambient environment, considerable heat is lost from the skin surface via radiation. However, the skin simultaneously absorbs considerable heat from the environment by the same mechanism. Only the difference between the loss and gain constitutes a net heat transfer. Radiative heat flux is proportional to the difference of the fourth powers of skin and mean radiant temperature of the environment. When skin and environmental temperatures do not differ excessively, little accuracy is lost by considering radiative transfer to be a linear function of the difference between these two temperatures.

Similarly, conductive heat transfer is proportional to the difference between skin and environmental temperature. However, the proportionality constant is a very strong function of the substance adjacent to the skin: good conductors such as metal and water easily transfer 50 times as much heat as air. Conductive transfer into air can be dramatically increased by destroying the barrier of still air (an excellent insulator) that collects immediately adjacent to the skin. This process is referred to as convection, and it increases heat flow by the square root of air speed.[278]

The final mechanism of cutaneous heat transfer is evaporation. Insensible loss from the skin surface (in the absence of sweating) is unimportant in adults, contributing only 10 percent to basal metabolic heat loss. In contrast, evaporative loss through thin skin can represent a substantial fraction of total heat loss in babies, and especially in premature infants.[279–281] Sweating remarkably increases cutaneous heat loss as discussed above. Evaporative heat loss during surgical skin preparation generally is small compared with other sources of hypothermia, even when large surface areas are cleaned.[282]

Evaporative heat loss also occurs in the lungs as dry inspired gases are humidified by the tracheal bronchial tree. However, evaporative heat loss via the respiratory tract is never more than a small fraction of the metabolic rate. Some additional heat is lost via respiration when cool inspired gas is warmed to body temperature; because the specific heat of air is so low, loss by this route contributes negligibly to total heat balance.[283]

Patterns of Intraoperative Hypothermia

Body temperature, which normally is well maintained even in a cold environment, decreases precipitously following induction of general anesthesia. This decrease has been attributed to undressing patients in a cool environment, anesthetic-induced vasodilation (which increases skin temperature), evaporation of surgical skin preparation solution, loss of heat from surgical incisions, and anesthetic-induced reduction in metabolic rate. However, general anesthesia reduces heat production only approximately 20 percent, and anesthetic-induced vasodilation minimally increases heat loss.[224, 284] Furthermore, hypothermia develops rapidly following induction of anesthesia even in volunteers not undergoing skin preparation[224] or surgical heat losses.[285] These data indicate that the initial rapid hypothermia results from an internal redistribution of body heat from the central core to cooler peripheral tissues.[224] In most cases, redistribution hypothermia requires approximately 40 minutes and reduces core temper-

ature 1° to 1.5°C. Because the redistribution is completely internal, body heat content and average body temperature remain constant (Fig. 4–10).

Redistribution hypothermia is followed by a slow, approximately linear decrease in core temperature usually lasting 2 to 3 hours. This linear decrease apparently results from heat loss that exceeds metabolic heat production.[286] Since heat production remains nearly constant during anesthesia, the rate at which hypothermia develops during this period is largely determined by heat loss. As mentioned above, respiratory heat loss is a small fraction of metabolic production.[283] The major factors determining heat loss are ambient temperature, insulation provided by surgical draping, and evaporative loss from within surgical incisions.[278, 282, 287, 288] Infusion of a large volume of cold intravenous fluids may also contribute.

After 3 to 4 hours of anesthesia and surgery, core temperature stops decreasing. This plateau phase may occur at a relatively high temperature (e.g., 35.5°C) in patients with minimal heat loss to the environment.[289] But more commonly, the core temperature plateau occurs at a lower temperature (e.g., 34.5°C) and is associated with peripheral thermoregulatory vasoconstriction.[290]

Development of a core temperature plateau coincident with vasoconstriction initially suggested that decreased cutaneous blood flow significantly decreased heat loss from the skin to the environment. However, subsequent evidence indicated that the decrease likely was insufficient to cause a thermal steady state.[259] Furthermore, during the hours after development of the core temperature plateau, leg heat content continues to decrease.[290, 291] These data indicate that the core temperature plateau results when thermoregulatory vasoconstriction both decreases cutaneous heat loss and constrains metabolic heat to the core thermal compartment.

During the core temperature plateau, metabolic heat production (which remains nearly constant) is largely maintained within the relatively small core thermal compartment. Because metabolic heat is constrained now to approximately half the body mass, core temperature remains nearly constant. In contrast, peripheral tissues become hypothermic at an even greater rate because heat loss to the environment is insufficiently abated and minimal heat is supplied from the core. In effect, constraint of metabolic heat to the central core reestablishes the normal

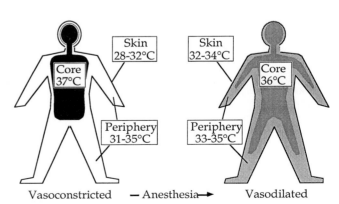

FIGURE 4–10. A cartoon illustrating internal redistribution of body heat following induction of general anesthesia.

core–peripheral temperature gradient. It is important for clinicians to realize that constant core temperature during the plateau phase may mask a continuing decrease in body heat content.

In most cases, differences between heat balance in adults and pediatric patients have not specifically been investigated. Nonetheless, several features of pediatric anatomy potentially alter perioperative heat loss. Infants and children tend to have relatively globular bodies with larger fractions of their mass in the torso than in adults. Consequently, redistribution may contribute less to intraoperative hypothermia in infants. Similarly, the head constitutes a far larger fraction of the total surface area in infants than in adults. Cutaneous heat loss from the head in adults is what would be expected from its surface area. In infants, however, heat loss from the head may be a proportionately larger fraction of the total, perhaps because the skull and scalp are thin, allowing loss of heat delivered to the brain.

Cutaneous heat loss is roughly proportional to surface area, whereas metabolic heat production is largely a function of mass. Consequently, it is relatively easy for infants and children to lose large amounts of heat (compared with production) via the skin surface. Nonetheless, as mentioned above, thermoregulatory vasoconstriction is well maintained in pediatric patients.[270, 292] Vasoconstriction, once triggered, helps prevent further hypothermia. This response is more effective in infants and children than in adults (Fig. 4–11).

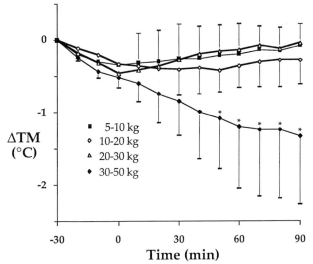

FIGURE 4–11. All patients became progressively hypothermic following induction of general anesthesia. After significant peripheral vasoconstriction was observed (defined as elapsed time zero), core temperature continued to decrease in patients weighing more than 30 kg, but remained constant or increased slightly in the others. Had the operating room been warmer, or the surgery smaller, the heavier patients would have had a core temperature plateau, and the younger ones would have become hyperthermic. Temperatures in the 30 to 50-kg group were significantly different from each of the others after 40 elapsed minutes. (From Bissonnette B, Sessler DI: Thermoregulatory thresholds for vasoconstriction in pediatric patients anesthetized with halothane or halothane and caudal bupivacaine. Anesthesiology 76:387, 1992.)

Regional Anesthesia

Hypothermia during regional anesthesia is nearly as severe as that during general anesthesia[221, 293] and produces complications, including shivering-like tremor (which unacceptably increases patients' metabolic rates),[212, 222] impaired coagulation,[294] prolonged drug action,[295] and negative postoperative nitrogen balance.[296] Comparable thermal lability occurs in patients with spinal cord transections, causing major problems in some cases.[297] Hypothermia during surgery results, in part, from environmental exposure,[285] whereas hypothermia without anesthesia occurs only during extreme exposure. These data indicate that the contribution of anesthetic-induced thermoregulatory failure to intraoperative hypothermia is substantial.

Regional anesthesia may interfere with one or more components of thermoregulation: afferent sensing, central control, or efferent responses.[237] Efferent thermoregulatory responses, including sweating, vasoconstriction, and shivering, are active neurogenic processes that certainly are obliterated in areas blocked by spinal or epidural anesthesia.[298-300] Each of these effectors produces clinically significant protection against thermal perturbations.[301-303] Anesthetic-induced inhibition of these efferent thermoregulatory responses thus contributes significantly to hypothermia during regional anesthesia. For example, inhibition of tonic thermoregulatory vasoconstriction is the major cause of core hypothermia during the first hour of epidural anesthesia.[223]

However, even restricting discussion to responses occurring above the level of anesthetic-induced sympathetic and motor block, response thresholds are abnormal. Thermoregulatory failure during regional anesthesia was first identified by Roe in 1972.[304] He observed that 1° to 3°C hypothermia was typical during spinal anesthesia, perceptively postulating that it resulted because the shivering threshold was 1°C below normal. Similar abnormal tolerance to core hypothermia also occurs during epidural anesthesia in patients[304] and volunteers.[223, 305, 306]

Regional anesthesia is unlikely to *directly* influence central thermoregulatory control. Some processing of thermal afferent signals may occur at the level of the lumbar spinal cord,[230] but evidence from animal studies suggests that nearly all integration occurs at higher levels (e.g., brain stem, midbrain, and hypothalamus).[228-230] It is unlikely that the small volumes of anesthetics injected intrathecally during spinal anesthesia diffuse rostrally in sufficient amounts to directly anesthetize higher regulatory centers. (Spinally administered opioids do diffuse rostrally, but these drugs are much more potent than local anesthetics.) There is no evidence that other cerebral regulatory systems are directly influenced by local anesthetics administered in the subarachnoid space. Moreover, epidural anesthetics are injected outside the arachnoid and dural membranes, and substantial quantities are unlikely to penetrate into cerebrospinal fluid. Nonetheless, epidural anesthesia impairs thermoregulatory responses.

Alternatively, epidural anesthesia might indirectly impair central thermoregulation via absorption of local anesthetic into the blood stream and subsequent recirculation to the central nervous system. However, intravenous administration of lidocaine sufficient to produce plasma con-

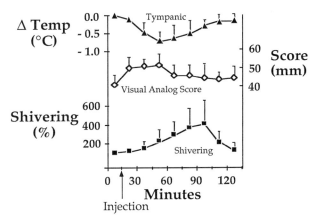

FIGURE 4–12. Changes in tympanic membrane temperatures, percentage increase in shivering intensity, and thermal comfort (millimeters on a visual analog scale) following epidural lidocaine injections in six volunteers. Zero mm on the visual analog scale was defined as worst imaginable cold; 100 mm similarly was defined as worst imaginable heat. Epidural injections were given after a 15-minute control period. Shivering started when tympanic membrane temperature decreased about 0.5°C and continued until central temperature returned to within 0.5°C of control. Thermal comfort increased following epidural injection in each volunteer; maximal comfort occurred at the lowest core temperature. Results are presented as means ± SD. (From Sessler DI, Ponte J: Shivering during epidural anesthesia. Anesthesiology 72:816, 1990, with permission.)

centrations similar to those observed during epidural anesthesia does not alter the vasoconstriction or shivering thresholds.[307] Furthermore, there is distinct thermoregulatory impairment during chloroprocaine epidural anesthesia, despite the fact that this drug is rapidly metabolized by plasma cholinesterase.[223] These data suggest that an alternative mechanism mediates thermoregulatory impairment during regional anesthesia.

Spinal and epidural anesthesia almost certainly alter afferent transmission of thermal signals. Spinal cord temperature receptors have been documented in every mammal studied,[230] and presumably also exist in humans. These receptors contribute roughly 20 percent of the total thermal information projecting to the central regulating system.[229, 308] Epidural or intrathecal injection of cold local anesthetic might thus be sufficient to initiate thermoregulatory responses. However, shivering cannot be induced in nonpregnant volunteers, even by epidural administration of large volumes of ice-cold saline.[309] Furthermore, the incidence of shivering during epidural anesthesia is comparable with cold or warm anesthetic in volunteers[222] and patients.[310]

Both skin and core temperatures contribute to thermoregulation, with skin contributing 10 to 20 percent to the total.[214, 215, 231] Most warm receptors are quiescent at skin temperatures less than or equal to 37°C.[234] Consequently, at typical ambient temperatures, predominantly cold signals converge on the central thermoregulatory system.[234] Regional anesthesia blocks all thermal information from the lower portion of the body, but tonic cold signals would be the major traffic disrupted. Accordingly, it seems likely that the central thermoregulatory system interprets their absence as warming. Supporting this hypothesis is the observation that induction of epidural anesthesia in-

creases thermal comfort, despite simultaneously decreasing core temperature.[222, 223] Therefore, regulatory responses to thermal perturbations may be impaired because regional anesthesia increases *apparent* lower body temperature far more than it increases actual tissue temperature. This theory, though, remains to be confirmed.

Although shivering-like tremor during recovery from general anesthesia contains abnormal components, involuntary muscular activity during regional anesthesia is largely normal thermoregulatory shivering. Normal shivering is preceded by core hypothermia and vasoconstriction above the level of the block, and electromyographic analysis of tremor patterns fails to detect the abnormal clonic signals sometimes occurring during recovery from general anesthesia (Fig. 4–12). There is also a nonthermoregulatory component to shivering-like tremor during epidural anesthesia that appears to be related to pain.[311]

Surprisingly, vasodilation produced by regional anesthesia only minimally increases cutaneous heat loss to the environment. In most cases, metabolic heat production either remains constant or increases after initiation of epidural anesthesia. Thus, core hypothermia results from a core-to-periphery redistribution of body heat (Fig. 4–13).[312] This mechanism is similar to that producing core hypothermia after induction of general anesthesia.[313]

Consequences of Hypothermia

Perianesthetic hypothermia produces potentially severe complications as well as distinct benefits. Thermal management, thus, deserves the same thoughtful analysis of potential risks and benefits as other therapeutic decisions.

Benefits

Hypothermia provides marked protection against tissue ischemia and hypoxia. Core temperatures between 25°

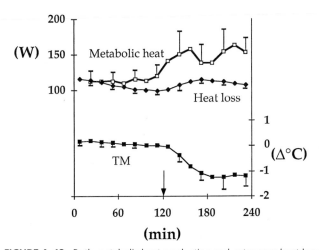

FIGURE 4–13. Both metabolic heat production and cutaneous heat loss increased following epidural injection (*arrow*); however, heat production exceeded heat loss at all times during anesthesia. Tympanic membrane (TM) temperature decreased rapidly after induction, whereas average skin temperature increased, indicating that heat was redistributed from core to peripheral tissues. (From Hynson J, Sessler DI, Glosten B, McGuire J: Thermal balance and tremor patterns during epidural anesthesia. Anesthesiology 74:680, 1991, with permission.)

and 30°C have long been used for cerebral protection during cardiopulmonary bypass. The protection provided by even lower temperatures is sufficient to permit complete circulatory arrest. However, the last decade has seen increased appreciation that just 2° to 3°C core hypothermia provides more protection against ischemia than any pharmacologic treatment.[314–316] It is clear that hypothermia provides protection far out of proportion to its reduction in metabolic rate and that numerous cellular and biochemical mechanisms contribute.

Because of its substantial protective effects, mild hypothermia is indicated in patients undergoing procedures likely to produce tissue ischemia (e.g., neurosurgery). Pediatric patients undergoing appropriate procedures should not be denied the potential benefits of mild hypothermia.

Risks

Humans sense core temperature poorly,[212] but skin temperatures roughly follows core temperature, and hypothermic postoperative patients are less comfortable than those maintained normothermic.[233, 274] Although comfort is not a life-threatening issue, it is one that clinicians perhaps should take more seriously because so many patients remember feeling cold as the *worst* part of surgery. There is no reason to believe that hypothermia produces any less discomfort in pediatric patients than in adults.

Local hypothermia decreases platelet function.[294] Since wound temperature cannot exceed core temperature, hypothermia likely contributes to surgical bleeding. In contrast, prothrombin time (PT) and partial thromboplastin time (PTT) apparently remain normal at temperatures above 33°C,[317, 318] and the euglobulin clot lysis time is prolonged by hypothermia.[319] Consistent with impaired coagulation, mild hypothermia (only 1.6°C) significantly increases blood loss and transfusion requirements during hip arthroplasty.[320, 321] Presumably, blood loss is proportionately increased during other procedures and in pediatric patients.

Mild hypothermia significantly increases the duration of action of vecuronium and atracurium.[295] The duration of vecuronium in patients with a core temperature of 34.5°C is more than twice that of patients at 36.5°C, and thus lasts nearly as long as pancuronium normally does. The duration of atracurium also is prolonged by mild hypothermia.[322] Monitoring the twitch response to ulnar nerve stimulation is therefore especially important in hypothermic patients.

One prospective[296] and several retrospective[323] studies document that postoperative nitrogen excretion is increased by intraoperative hypothermia. Although the clinical significance of this observation remains unclear, it suggests that hypothermic patients may have difficulty repairing surgical wounds. Wound infections are the most common serious complication of surgery and anesthesia, possibly causing more morbidity than all anesthetic complications combined. There is some evidence that hypothermia impairs immune response to wound infections: 3°C of core hypothermia decreases lesion size and bacterial clearance following test *Staphylococcus aureus* and *Escherichia coli* infections in guinea pigs.[324, 325] Infections

likely are aggravated mostly by impaired immune function,[326, 327] but decreased cutaneous blood flow probably also contributes.[328] Consistent with these data, mild hypothermia triples the incidence of surgical wound infection and prolongs hospitalization 20 percent.[329]

Postanesthetic tremor is not entirely normal shivering.[330] It only occurs in hypothermic volunteers,[274] but is readily detected in normothermic patients[331] and is highly correlated with surgical pain.[332] It is a serious complication, increasing oxygen consumption up to 200 percent,[333] in proportion to intraoperative heat loss.[302] Additionally, it aggravates surgical pain (by moving incisions) and increases intraocular and intracranial pressures.[334] As mentioned above, shivering can be treated by cutaneous warming[335] or meperidine administration.[276] Most studies conclude that meperidine is a more effective treatment for shivering than equianalgesic doses or other opioids.[336] The reason for this special efficacy remains unclear but may be related to the drug's κ activity.[337] It is manifested as a shivering threshold that decreases twice as much as the vasoconstriction threshold[338]—a pattern that has not been observed with any other opioid, sedative, or anesthetic.

There are some theoretical reasons to suspect that hypothermia prolongs recovery. For example, hypothermia impairs cognitive performance[339] and decreases metabolism of some drugs.[295] A number of studies suggest that mild hypothermia prolongs the duration of postanesthetic recovery.[340, 341] All suffered serious flaws, including (1) unblinded data collection, (2) temperature management not randomly assigned, (3) temperature monitored in inadequate locations, (4) unspecified discharge criteria, and (5) using temperature as a discharge criteria. A number of other studies do not confirm prolonged recovery, but did not include sufficient statistical power to rule it out.[342–344] Recently, however, the effects of mild hypothermia on recovery duration were formally evaluated in a prospective, randomized trial. The results indicate that hypothermia produces a clinically important and statistically significant prolongation of recovery duration.[345]

Maintaining Normothermia

Approximately 90 percent of metabolic heat is lost via the skin surface. Consequently, only the skin surface provides sufficient heat exchange to allow effective warming. It is relatively easy to treat hypothermia intraoperatively because anesthetic-induced vasodilation facilitates cutaneous heat transfer. In contrast, postoperative vasoconstriction markedly decreases transfer of heat from the skin surface to the core.

Airway Heating and Humidification

Less than 10 percent of metabolic heat typically is lost via the respiratory system. It thus is not surprising that airway heating and humidification has repeatedly proven ineffective in adult surgical patients. In contrast to adult patients, airway heating and humidification and heat-and-moisture exchanging filters can be effective in infants and children.[346, 347] There are two reasons for this apparent discrepancy. First, infants and children have relatively high respiratory rates and therefore lose a relatively high proportion of metabolic heat via the respiratory system. Second, the pediatric studies were undertaken in patients undergoing very small procedures, so nearly their entire skin surface was wrapped and draped. This circumstance maximizes the ratio of respiratory to total heat loss, making respiratory manipulations relatively more effective. In patients in whom core temperature maintenance is most difficult (those undergoing large operations), airway humidification is substantially less effective.[286] Given the large cost and relative inefficiency of airway heating and humidification, the technique probably is rarely indicated.

Tracheal humidification probably is helpful during prolonged procedures to prevent tracheal damage by cold, dry gasses.[348] However, passive heat and moisture–exchanging filters provide sufficient airway heating and humidification to prevent tracheal damage even when high fresh gas flows are maintained. These devices are far less expensive than the active systems and, therefore, are preferable. Furthermore, many of the passive heat and moisture exchangers incorporate bacterial and viral filters that minimize potential patient–patient cross-contamination. There are no clinically important differences in the heating and humidification properties or various brands of artificial noses[283]; consequently, clinicians should choose those having the lowest cost or the best filtration properties.

Cutaneous Warming

Approximately 90 percent of metabolic heat is lost via the skin surface. Additional heat is lost during surgery via evaporation from inside of wounds.[285] Loss from both skin and wounds is a roughly linear function of the difference between tissue and ambient temperature. Accordingly, increasing ambient temperature sufficiently will always prevent hypothermia. Typically ambient temperature is 10° to 15°C less than tissue temperature. Thus, a 1°C increase in ambient temperature decreases heat loss about 7 percent.

Typical adult operating room temperatures are near 20°C, and staff (especially gowned surgeons working under operating lights) find temperatures exceeding 23°C uncomfortable. Thus, while increasing ambient temperature is an effective way of preventing intraoperative hypothermia, it is unnecessarily stressful for the operating room staff and less sophisticated than techniques that focus application of heat on the patient.

The easiest way of decreasing cutaneous heat loss is to cover the skin with one of the passive insulators readily available in most operating rooms. These include surgical drapes, cotton blankets, and plastic bags. Additionally, several manufacturers market plastic/mylar composites purported to markedly decrease radiative heat loss. All of these devices are effective, reducing heat loss from the skin surface by approximately 30 percent.[287] However, there are no clinically important differences among the insulators, so clinicians can use whichever are readily available. The additional cost of composite "space blankets" is not warranted.

Cutaneous heat loss over the entire body is roughly proportional to surface area.[247, 259] However, heat loss from the head may be especially great in infants because the head constitutes such a large fraction of the total surface area.[349] The efficacy of cutaneous insulation thus is directly proportional to the amount of surface area covered. Far more important than the type of insulator chosen is the amount of surface area covered.[287] Combining multiple layers of passive insulators does not linearly decrease heat loss: using three cotton blankets instead of one cotton blanket reduces heat loss only from 70 percent of control values to 50 percent of control values.[288]

Circulating-water mattresses remain a popular method of intraoperative warming. However, very little heat is lost from a patient's back into the foam insulation covering most operating room tables.[259] Furthermore, it is not possible to heat the relatively small surface area adjacent to the operating room table sufficiently to transfer large amounts of heat into patients. Consequently, it is not surprising that circulating-water mattresses have repeatedly been shown ineffective in adults.[286] Circulating-water mattresses are superior to no treatment in infants weighing less than 10 kg,[350] but it is unlikely that these devices work markedly better in infants and children than in adults.

Circulating-water mattresses have been associated with burn-like tissue injuries in adults.[351, 352] The probable genesis of these injuries is "pressured/heat" necrosis.[353, 354] Even low temperatures can cause tissue injury when combined for long periods of time with high tissue pressure. Such burns are rarely reported in infants, probably because the infant's low weight minimizes tissue pressure. Furthermore, tissue perfusion tends to be better in infants than in adults. Nonetheless, water mattresses appear to be relatively ineffective. In contrast, cutaneous heat loss can be reduced to zero by positioning a circulating-water blanket *over* a patient, rather than under the patient.[355] Although such positioning is relatively easily accomplished in adults, size constraints make this approach more difficult in infants.

Forced-air warming transfers more heat than might be expected simply based on device–skin temperature gradient. This is analogous to the excess heat loss produced by a cold convective environment ("wind-chill"). In the case of modern forced-air covers, convective heat transfer augments efficacy by about 30 percent. Forced-air warming has been shown in laboratory studies to transfer considerably more heat than circulating-water or infrared systems.[355] Consequently, it is not surprising that forced-air heating is more effective than circulating-water mattresses or active airway heating and humidification in adults.[286, 356] This technique also is more effective than circulating-water in infants (Fig. 4–14).[356] Pediatric forced-air covers are designed in a tubular configuration that allows full access to the patient, yet provides adequate surface contact for heat exchange. Even during extremely extensive operations (e.g., liver transplantation), forced air maintains normothermia.[357]

Intravenous Fluids

It is not possible to warm patients by administering warmed intravenous fluids. On the other hand, it is easy to substantially decrease core temperature by administering intravenous fluids at ambient or refrigerator temperature. In adults, administration of 1 L of crystalloid at ambient

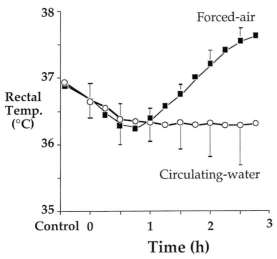

FIGURE 4–14. During maxillofacial surgery, rectal temperatures decreased in infants given forced-air (n = 10) and circulating-water (n = 10) warming after premedication and during the first 45 minutes of anesthesia. Control values were recorded just before administration of premedication, and elapsed time zero indicates induction of anesthesia. Subsequently, core temperature remained nearly constant in patients warmed with circulating water but increased in those warmed with forced air. Temperature of the forced-air warmer was decreased from the *high* to *medium* setting in all 10 patients 112 ± 13 minutes after induction of anesthesia when core temperatures reached 37°C. After 165 minutes of anesthesia, core temperatures were 1.3° C higher in the patients warmed with forced air. Differences between the groups were statistically significant after 75 minutes of anesthesia. Had the operations been larger, or the ambient temperature lower, patients warmed with circulating water would have become hypothermic, whereas those given forced air would not. (From Kurz A, Kurz M, Poeschl G, et al: Forced-air warming maintains intraoperative normothermia better than circulating-water mattresses. Anesth Analg 77:89, 1993, with permission.)

temperature or 1 U of blood at refrigerator temperature decreases mean body temperature 0.25°C. The weight- and volume-adjusted decrease in infants and children is comparable. When small volumes of fluid are administered, warming is not necessary because the resulting reduction in body temperature will be small. In contrast, large volumes administered rapidly always should be warmed. All commercially available fluid warmers heat to at least 37°C. Most of these fluid warmers are adequate for routine pediatric use.

Hyperthermia and Fever

A core body temperature exceeding normal values identifies hyperthermia. Hyperthermia thus is a generic term that does not imply a specific etiology or mechanism. In contrast, *fever* is a regulated increase in core temperature mediated by endogenous pyrogens and actively maintained by thermoregulatory responses.

Passive Hyperthermia

The most common cause of passive hyperthermia outside the operating room is heat stroke resulting from a combination of heat production and environmental conditions so extreme that even maximal thermoregulatory responses cannot dissipate sufficient heat. The environment posing

most danger of hyperthermia is a warm, humid one. Sweating is remarkably effective and nearly always can dissipate sufficient heat—so long as the humidity is low. However, heat loss decreases dramatically when the humidity increases and the body is unable to dissipate even basal metabolic heat production when ambient temperature exceeds core temperature and the humidity approaches 100 percent.

Even in a moderate environment, heat loss will be compromised when vascular volume is sufficiently reduced. Maintenance of core temperature is a high regulatory priority, but maintaining blood pressure takes distinct precedence. Thus, when vascular volume is depleted, sweating rate and active vasodilation decrease dramatically and total heat loss is correspondingly reduced. If metabolic heat production continues to exceed heat loss, hyperthermia inevitably results. The combination of vascular volume depletion and hyperthermia identifies *heat stroke*. Typically, the syndrome is accompanied by vigorous exercise.

In the perianesthetic period, hyperthermia most commonly results from excessive warming. It is considerably more common in infants and children than in adults: the same large surface area/mass ratio that allows pediatric patients to rapidly become hypothermic allows them to rapidly absorb applied cutaneous heat. Limb tourniquets increase the risk of accidental hyperthermia because restricted peripheral blood flow constrains metabolic heat to the core thermal compartment, thus increasing temperature in those tissues.[358] Consequently, reliable and frequent core temperature monitoring is essential when effective (i.e., cutaneous) warming is used in infants and children.

As mentioned above, thermoregulation most likely remains intact during malignant hyperthermia. (Although heat loss may be compromised by high circulating catecholamine concentrations, which cause cutaneous vasoconstriction, this does not represent a failure of central regulation.) Increased core temperature during this syndrome, thus, results from excessive heat production and is not a regulated fever.

Fever

Endogenous pyrogens were first identified in the 1940s, and are now known to include interleukin-1, interleukin-6, tumor necrosis factor, interferon-α, and macrophage inflammatory protein-1.[359] Mediation by circulating cytokines is in distinct contrast to normal control of body temperature, which is minimally influenced by hormones. Endogenous pyrogens cause a coordinated increase in the thermoregulatory thresholds for both warm and cold responses. The interthreshold range thus remains unchanged. Increased core temperature during fever is maintained using the same thermoregulatory responses that normally control body temperature: shivering, nonshivering thermogenesis, and vasoconstriction.

The "chills" that typically accompany development of fever result when endogenous pyrogens rapidly increase the cold response thresholds to temperatures far exceeding actual body temperature. The result is a normal core temperature that is *hypothermic* relative to the regulatory system's desired (febrile) temperature. Functionally, this is no different from being hypothermic relative to a normal threshold, and triggers the expected cold defenses including shivering. For this reason, cutaneous cooling of unsedated febrile patients makes them miserable but does little to reduce core temperature.[360]

When the fever "breaks," the thresholds rapidly return towards normal values as the effects of endogenous pyrogens fade. However, core temperature, which cannot change quickly, remains elevated. The disparity between the hyperthermic core and the now approximately normal thresholds triggers active vasodilation and sweating.

Fever is a remarkably well preserved regulatory response. Not only do all mammals and birds develop fever when infected, but reptiles and fish use behavioral regulation to increase core temperature in response to infection. There is considerable evidence that fever is an adaptive response that significantly aids response to infection.[361–365] The predominant effect appears to be a peripheral stimulation of immune function.[326, 327] Treatment of mammals with antipyretic drugs reduces resistance to test infections. In light of these data, the current practice of aggressively treating fever may not be completely appropriate.

Although many surgical patients have reason to be febrile, and many are before and after surgery, fever during anesthesia is rare. The reason is that volatile anesthetics and opioids both inhibit fever.[366–369] In contrast, epidural analgesia does not alter the febrile response.[370]

SUMMARY

Temperature disturbances are pervasive in the perioperative period. Some result from regulatory failure and others result from extreme environmental stress or excessive metabolic heat production. However, all are potentially harmful. Understanding the etiologies of these disturbances will facilitate appropriate therapeutic responses and minimize chances of serious complications.

REFERENCES

1. Wingard D: A stressful situation [editorial]. Anesth Analg 59:321, 1980.
2. Denborough M, Lovell R: Anaesthetic deaths in a family [letter]. Lancet 2:45, 1960.
3. Ludvigsen J: Muscular degeneration in hogs [preliminary report]. 15th International Veterinary Congress Stockholm, 1953, p 602.
4. Nelson T, Jones E, Henrickson R, et al: Porcine malignant hyperthermia: observations on the occurence of pale, soft, exudative musculature among susceptible pigs. Am J Vet Res 35:347, 1974.
5. Kalow W, Britt B, Terreau M, Haist C: Metabolic error of muscle metabolism after recovery from malignant hyperthermia. Lancet 2:895, 1970.
6. Britt B, Kalow W: Malignant hyperthermia: aetiology unkown. Can Anaesth Soc J 17:316, 1970.
7. Harrison G: Control of the malignant hyperpyrexic syndrome in MHS swine by dantrolene sodium. Br J Anaesth 47:62, 1975.
8. Sessler DI: Malignant hyperthermia. J Pediatr 109:9, 1986.
9. Nelson T, Flewellen E: Current concepts. The malignant hyperthermia syndrome. N Engl J Med 309:416, 1983.
10. MacLennan D, Phillips M: Malignant hyperthermia. Science 256:789, 1992.
11. Rosenberg H, Fletcher JE: An update on the malignant hyperthermia syndrome. Ann Acad Med Singapore 23:84, 1994.
12. Ruitenbeek W, Verburg P, Janssen A, et al: In vivo induced malignant hyperthermia in pigs II. Metabolism of skeletal muscle mitochondria. Acta Anaesthesiol Scand 28:9, 1984.
13. Moulds R, Denborough M: Identification of susceptibility to malignant hyperpyrexia. BMJ 2:245, 1974.
14. Fletcher J, Rosenberg H, Hilf M: Electrophoresis of soluble muscle protein from malignant hyperthermia susceptibles. Anesthesiology 61:A279, 1984.
15. Marjanen L, Denborough M: Electrophoretic analysis of proteins in malignant hyperpyrexia susceptible skeletal muscle. Int J Biochem 16:919, 1984.
16. Bennett D, Cain P, Ellis F, et al: Calcium and magnesium contents of malignant hyperpyrexia susceptible human muscle. Br J Anaesth 49:979, 1977.
17. Nelson T, Belt M, Kennamer D, Winsett O: Sudies on the Ca+2 transport function of sarcoplasmic reticulum isolated from human malignant hyperthermia skeletal muscle [abstract]. Anesthesiology 65:A243, 1986.
18. Gronert G, Heffron J, Taylor S: Skeletal muscle sarcoplasmic reticulum in porcine malignant hyperthermia. Eur J Pharmacol 58:179, 1979.
19. Moulds R: The site of the abnormality in MH muscle: a comparison of MH muscle and denervated muscle. In Aldrete JA, Britt BA (eds): Malignant Hyperthermia. New York, Grune & Stratton, 1978, p 49.
20. Lorkin P, Lehmann H: Malignant hyperthermia in pigs; a search for abnormalities in Ca2+ binding proteins. FEBS Lett 153:81, 1983.
21. Green A, Mitchell G, Heffron J: The effects of temperature, adenosine triphosphate and magnesium concentrations on the contraction of actomyosin isolated from halothane sensitive and insensitive German landrace pigs. Br J Anaesth 52:319, 1980.
22. Marjanen L, Denborough M: Effect of halothane on adenylate kinase in porcine malignant hyperpyrexia. Clin Chim Acta 122:225, 1982.
23. Bardsley M, Wheatlye A, Fowler C, et al: Metabolism of monoamines in malignant hyperthermia susceptible pigs. Br J Anaesth 54:1313, 1982.
24. Harrison G, Verburg C: Erythrocyte osmotic fragility in hyperthermia susceptible swine. Br J Anaesth 45:131, 1973.
25. Heffron J, Mitchell G: Influence of pH temperature, halothane and its metabolites on osmotic fragility of erythroctes of malignant hyperthermia susceptible and resistant pigs. Br J Anaesth 53:499, 1981.
26. Gerrard J, Duncan P, Koshyk S, et al: Halothane stimulates the aggregation of platelets of both normal individuals and those susceptible to malignant hyperthermia. Br J Anaesth 55:1249, 1983.
27. Solomons C, Bonneville M, Zsigmond E: In vitro response to halothane of human platelets in malignant hyperthermia [abstract]. Anesth Analg 66:5162, 1987.
28. Basrur P, Frombach S, McDonell W: Platelet morphology and membrane bound calcium in porcine stress syndrome. Scan Electron Microsc I:209, 1983.
29. Klip A, Ramlal T, Walker D, et al: Selective increase in cytoplasmic calcium by anesthetic in lymphocytes from malignant hyperthermia susceptible pigs. Anesth Analg 66:381, 1987.
30. Klip A, Elliott M, Frodis W, et al: Anaesthetic induced increase in ionised calcium in blood mononuclear cells from malignant hyperthermia patients. Lancet 1:463, 1987.
31. Nelson T, Denborough M: Studies on normal human skeletal muscle in relation to the pathopharmacology of malignant hyperpyrexia. Clin Exp Pharmacol Physiol 4:315, 1977.
32. Deuster P, Bockman E, Muldoon S: In vitro responses of cat skeletal muscle to halothane and caffeine. J Appl Physiol 58:521, 1985.
33. Heiman-Patterson T, Fletcher J, Rosenberg H, Tahmoush A: No realstionship between fiber type and halothane contracture test results in malignant hyperthermia. Anesthesiology 67:82, 1987.
34. Gallant E, Godt R, Gronert G: Role of plasma membrane defect of skeletal muscle in malignant hyperthermia. Muscle Nerve 2:491, 1979.
35. Bryant S, Anderson I: Mechanical activation and electrophysiological properties of intercostal muscle fibers from malignant hyperthermia susceptible (MHS) pigs. Soc Neurosci 3:213, 1977.
36. Fletcher J, Rosenberg H, Tripolitis L, Hilf M: Elevated fatty acid production in skeletal muscle from malingnant hyperthermia susceptible patients [abstract]. Anesthesiology 63:A301, 1985.

37. Fletcher JE, Tripolitis L, Erwin K, et al: Altered hormone-sensitive lipase (HSL) activity as the defect in malignant hyperthermia (MH). Anesthesiology 73:A749, 1990.
38. Cheah K, Cheah A: Malignant hyperthermia: molecular defects in membrane permeability. Experientia 41:656, 1985.
39. Cheah K: Skeletal muscle mitochondria and phospholipase A_2 in malignant hyperthermia. Biochem Soc Trans 12:358, 1984.
40. Messinco F, Rathier M, Favreau C, et al: Mechanisms of fatty acid effects on sarcoplasmic reticulum. J Biol Chem 259:1336, 1984.
41. Fletcher J, Rosenberg H, Hilf M: Possible phospholipase A2 involvement in human malignant hyperthermia [abstract]. Anesthesiology 61:A252, 1984.
42. Fletcher J, Rosenberg H, Lizzo F, Michaux K: Strontium and quinacrine antagonize contractures induced by caffeine: implications for malignant hyperthermia [abstract]. Anesth Analg 65:A238, 1986.
43. Manning BM, Quane KA, Ording H, et al: Identification of novel mutations in the ryanodine-receptor gene (RYR1) in malignant hyperthermia: genotype-phenotype correlation. Am J Hum Genet 62:599, 1998.
44. MacLennan DH, Phillips MS: The role of the skeletal muscle ryanodine receptor (RYR1) gene in malignant hyperthermia and central core disease. Soc Gen Physiol Ser 50:89, 1995.
45. Gronert GA, Heffron JJ: Skeletal muscle mitochondria in porcine malignant hyperthermia: respiratory activity, calcium functions, and depression by halothane. Anesth Analg 58:76, 1979.
46. Gronert GA, Heffron JJA, Milde JH, Theye RA: Porcine malignant hyperthermia: role of skeletal muscle in increased oxygen consumption. Can Anaesth Soc J 24:103, 1977.
47. Ohnishi S, Taylor S, Gronert G: Calcium induced Ca2+ release from sarcoplasmic reticulum of pigs susceptible to malignant hyperthermia. The effects of halothane and dantrolene. FEBS Lett 161:103, 1983.
48. Nelson T: Abnormality in calcium release from skeletal sarcoplasmic reticulum of pigs susceptible to malignant hyperthermia. J Clin Invest 72:862, 1983.
49. Niebroj-Dobosz I, Mayzner-Zawadzka E: Experimental porcine malignant hyperthermia: the activity of certain transporting enzyes and myofibrillar calcium binding protein content in the muscle fibre. Anaesthesiology 54:885, 1982.
50. Isaacs H, Heffron J: Morphological and biochemical defects in muscles of human carriers of the malignant hyperthermia syndrome. Br J Anaesth 47:475, 1975.
51. Ellis F, Halsall P, Allam P, Hay E: A biochemical abnormality found in muscle from unstressed malignant hyperpyrexia susceptible humans. Biochem Soc Trans 12:357, 1984.
52. Verburg M, Oerlemans F, van Bennekom C, et al: In vivo induced malignant hyperthermia in pigs. I. Physiological and biochemical changes and the influence of dantrolene sodium. Acta Anaesthesiol Scand 28:1, 1984.
53. Gronert G, Theye R: Halothane induced porcine malignant hyperthermia: metabolic and hemodynamic changes. Anesthesiology 44:36, 1976.
54. Fuchs F: Thermal inactivation of the calcium regulatory mechanism of human skeletal muscle actomyosin: a possible contributing factor in the rigidity of malignant hyperthermia. Anesthesiology 42:584, 1975.
55. Britt BA, Endrenyl L, Peters PL, et al: Screening of malignant hyperthermia susceptible families by creatine phosphokinase measurement and other clinical investigations. Can Anaesth Soc J 23:263, 1976.
56. Halsall P, Cain P, Ellis F: Retrospective analysis of anaesthetics received by patients before susceptibility to malignant hyperpyrexia was recognized. Br J Anaesth 51:949, 1979.
57. Hull M, Webster W, Gatz E: The effects of pentobarbital on 2,4-dinitrophenol induced malignant hyperthermia during halothane general anesthesia in dogs. J Oral Surg 29:640, 1971.
58. Hall G, Lucke J, Lister D: Porcine malignant hyperthermia. IV: Neuromuscular blockade. Br J Anaesth 48:1135, 1976.
59. Jones D, Ryan J, Taylor B, et al: Pancuronium in large doses protects susceptible swine from halothane induced malignant hyperthermia [abstract]. Anesthesiology 63:A344, 1985.
60. Nelson TE: Porcine malignant hyperthermia: critical temperatures for in vivo and in vitro responses. Anesthesiology 73:449, 1990.
61. Iaizzo PA, Kehler CH, Carr RJ, et al: Prior hypothermia attenuates malignant hyperthermia in susceptible swine. Anesth Analg 82:782, 1996.
62. Sewall K, Flowerdew R, Bromberger P: Severe muscular rigidity at birth: malignant hyperthermia sysndrome? Can Anaesth Soc J 27:279, 1980.
63. Schmitt H, Simmendinger H, Wagner H, et al: Severe morphological changes in skeletal muscles of a five month old infant dying from an anesthetic complication with general muscle rigidity. Neuropadiatrie 6:102, 1975.
64. Faust DK, Gergis SD, Sokoll MD: Management of suspected malignant hyperpyrexia in an infant. Anesth Analg 58:33, 1979.
65. Dempsey W, Mayhew J, Metz P, Southern T: Malignant hyperthermia during repair of a cleft lip in a 6-month old infant, with survival. Ann Plast Surg 1:315, 1978.
66. Mayhew J, Rudolph J, Tobey R: Malignant hyperthermia in a six month old infant: a case report. Anesth Analg 57:262, 1978.
67. Britt B, Kwong F-F, Endrenyi L: The clinical and laboratory features of malignant hyperthermia management—a review. In Henschei ED (ed): Malignant Hyperthermia: Current Concepts. East Norwalk, CT, Appleton-Century-Crofts, 1977, p 9.
68. Glassenberg R, Cohen H: Intravenous dantrolene in a pregnant malignant hyperthermia susceptible (MHS) patient [abstract]. Anesthesiology 61:A404, 1984.
69. Morison D: Placental transfer of dantrolene [letter]. Anesthesiology 59:265, 1983.
70. Britt B, Locher W, Kalow W: Hereditary aspects of malignant hyperthermia. Can Anaesth Soc J 16:89, 1969.
71. Denborough M, Forster J, Lovell R, et al: Anaesthetic deaths in a family. Br J Anaesth 34:395, 1962.
72. Lutsky I, Witkowski J, Henschel E: HLA typing in a family prone to malignant hyperthermia. Anesthesiology 56:224, 1982.
73. Mickelson JR, Gallant EM, Litterer LA, et al: Abnormal sarcoplasmic reticulum ryanodine receptor in malignant hyperthermia. J Biol Chem 263:9310, 1988.
74. Deufel T, Golla A, Iles D, et al: Evidence for genetic heterogeneity of malignant hyperthermia susceptibility. Am J Hum Genet 50:1151, 1992.
75. King JO, Denborough MA, Zapf PW: Inheritance of malignant hyperpyrexia. Lancet 1:365, 1972.
76. King JO, Denborough MA: Anesthetic-induced malignant hyperpyrexia in children. J Pediatr 83:37, 1973.
77. McPherson EW, Taylor CA Jr: The King syndrome: malignant hyperthermia, myopathy, and multiple anomalies. Am J Med Genet 8:159, 1981.
78. Kousseff BG, Nichols P: A new autosomal recessive syndrome with Noonan-like phenotype, myopathy with congenital contractures and malignant hyperthermia. Birth Defects Orig Artic Ser 21:111, 1985.
79. Saul R, Stevenson R, Roberts T: A female with the King syndrome in a family with elevated CPK levels. Proc Greenwood Genet Center 3:7, 1984.
80. Hunter A, Pinsky L: An evaluation of the possible association of malignant hyperpyrexia with the Noonan syndrome using serum creatine phosphokinase levels. J Pediatr 86:412, 1975.
81. Eng G, Epstein B, Engel W, et al: Malignant hyperthermia and central core disease in a child with congenital dislocating hips. Arch Neurol 35:189, 1978.
82. Gullotta F, Pavone L, La Rosa M, Grasso A: Minicore myopathy. Klin Wochenschr 60:1351, 1982.
83. Frank J, Harati Y, Butler I, et al: Central core disease and malignant hyperthermia. Ann Neurol 7:11, 1980.
84. Brandt A, Schleithoff L, Jurkat-Rott K, et al: Screening of the ryanodine receptor gene in 105 malignant hyperthermia families: novel mutations and concordance with the in vitro contracture test. Hum Mol Genet 8:2055, 1999.
85. Pinsky L: Birth defects and predisposition to malignant hyperthermia [letter]. J Pediatr 110:494, 1987.
86. Saidman L, Eger IE: Hyperthermia during anesthesia. JAMA 190:73, 1964.
87. Denborough M, Dennett X, Anderson RM: Central core disease and malignant hyperpyrexia. BMJ 1:272, 1973.
88. Newberg L, Lambert E, Gronert G: Failure to induce malignant hyperthermia in myotonic goats. Br J Anaesth 55:57, 1983.
89. Oka S, Igarashi Y, Takagi A, et al: Malignant hyperpyrexia and Duchenne muscular dystropy: a case report. Can Anaesth Soc J 29:627, 1982.

90. Brownell A, Paasuke R, Elash A, et al: Malignant hyperthermia in Duchenne muscular dystrophy. Anesthesiology 58:180, 1983.
91. Kelfer H, Singer W, Reynolds R: Malignant hyperthermia in a child with Duchenne muscular dystrophy. Pediatrics 113:1971, 1983.
92. Miller EJ, Sanders D, Rowlingson J, et al: Anesthesia induced rhabdomyolysis in a patient with Duchenne's muscular dystrophy. Anesthesiology 48:146, 1978.
93. Hall G, Lucke J, Lister D: Porcine malignant hyperthermia.V: Fatal hyperthermia in the Pietrain pig, associated with the infusion of α-adrenergic agonists. Br J Anaesth 49:855, 1977.
94. Lister D, Hall G, Lucke J: Pordine malignant hyperthermia. III: Adrenergic blockade. Br J Anaesth 48:831, 1976.
95. Kerr D, Wingard D, Gatz E: Prevention of porcine malignant hyperthermia by epidural block. Anesthesiology 42:307, 1975.
96. Gronert G, Milde J, Theye R: Role of sympathetic activity in porcine malignant hyperthermia. Anesthesiology 47:411, 1977.
97. Harrison G: Porcine malignant hyperthermia. Int Anesthesiol Clin 17:25, 1979.
98. Gronert G, Thompson R, Onofrio B: Human malignant hyperthermia: awake episodes and correction by dantrolene. Anesth Analg 59:377, 1980.
99. Wingard D: Malignant hyperthermia: a human stress syndrome? [letter]. Lancet 2:1450, 1974.
100. Wingard D, Gatz E: Some observations on stress susceptible patients. In Aldrete JA, Britt BA (eds): Malignant Hyperthermia. New York, Grune & Stratton, 1978, p 363.
101. Mozley P: Malignant hyperthermia following intravenous iodinated contrast media. Report of a fatal case. Diagn Gynecol Obstet 3:81, 1981.
102. Cunliffe M, Lerman J, Britt B: Is prophylactic dantrolene indicated for MHS patients undergoing elective surgery? [abstract]. Anesth Analg 66:S35, 1987.
103. Loghmanee F, Tobak M: Fatal malignant hyperthermia associated with recreational cocaine and ethanol abuse. Am J Forensic Med Pathol 7:246, 1986.
104. Caroff SN: The neuroleptic malignant syndrome. J Clin Psychiatry 41:79, 1980.
105. Guze BH, Baxter LR Jr: Current concepts. Neuroleptic malignant syndrome. N Engl J Med 313:163, 1985.
106. Caroff S, Rosenberg H, Gerber JC: Neuroleptic malignant syndrome and malignant hyperthermia [letter]. J Clin Psychopharmacol 3:120, 1983.
107. Caroff SN, Rosenberg H, Fletcher JE, et al: Malignant hyperthermia susceptibility in neuroleptic malignant syndrome. Anesthesiology 67:20, 1987.
108. Granato JE, Stern BJ, Ringel A, et al: Neuroleptic malignant syndrome: successful treatment with dantrolene and bromocriptine. Ann Neurol 14:89, 1983.
109. Goulon M, de Rohan-Chabot P, Elkharrat D, et al: Beneficial effects of dantrolene in the treatment of neuroleptic malignant syndrome: a report of two cases. Neurology 33:516, 1983.
110. Murphy AL, Conlay L, Ryan JF, Roberts JT: Malignant hyperthermia during a prolonged anesthetic for reattachment of a limb. Anesthesiology 60:149, 1984.
111. Schulte Sasse U, Hess W, Eberlein H: Postoperative malignant hyperthermia and dantrolene therapy. Can Anaesth Soc J 30:635, 1983.
112. Grinberg R, Edelist G, Gordon A: Postoperative malignant hyperthermia episodes in patients who received "safe" anesthetics. Can Anaesth Soc J 30:273, 1983.
113. Mathieu A, Bogosian AJ, Ryan JF, et al: Recrudescence after survival of an initial episode of malignant hyperthermia. Anesthesiology 51:454, 1979.
114. Gronert GA, Theye RA: Suxamethonium-induced porcine malignant hyperthermia. Br J Anaesth 48:513, 1976.
115. Schwartz L, Rockoff MA, Koka BV: Masseter spasm with anesthesia: incidence and implications. Anesthesiology 61:772, 1984.
116. Carroll JB: Increased incidence of masseter spasm in children with strabismus anesthetized with halothane and succinylcholine. Anesthesiology 67:559, 1987.
117. Smith CE, Donati F, Bevan DR: Effects of succinylcholine at the masseter and adductor pollicis muscles in adults. Anesth Analg 69:158, 1989.
118. Van der Spek AF, Fang WB, Ashton-Miller JA, et al: Increased masticatory muscle stiffness during limb muscle flaccidity associated with succinylcholine administration. Anesthesiology 69:11, 1988.
119. Nagarajan K, Fishbein WN, Carlin HM, et al: Frozen-section calcium-uptake and caffeine contracture tests on human muscle [abstract]. Anesthesiology 63:A307, 1985.
120. Larach MG, Rosenberg H, Larach DR, Broennle AM: Prediction of malignant hyperthermia susceptibility by clinical signs. Anesthesiology 66:547, 1987.
121. Rosenberg H, Fletcher JE: Masseter muscle rigidity and malignant hyperthermia susceptibility. Anesth Analg 65:161, 1986.
122. Orndahl G, Stenberg K: Myotonic human musculature: stimulation with depolarizing agents. Med Scand 172:3, 1962.
123. Lessell S, Kuwabara T, Feldman RG: Myopathy and succinylcholine sensitivity. Am J Ophthalmol 68:789, 1969.
124. Mambo NC, Silver MD, McLaughlin PR, et al: Malignant hyperthermia susceptibility. A light and electron microscopic study of endomyocardial biopsy specimens from nine patients. Hum Pathol 11:381, 1980.
125. Huckell VF, Staniloff HM, McLaughlin PR, et al: Cardiovascular manifestations of normothermic malignant hyperthermia. In Aldrete JA, Britt BA (eds): Malignant Hyperthermia. New York, Grune & Stratton, 1977, p 373.
126. Huckell VF, Staniloff HM, Britt BA, Morch JE: Electrocardiographic abnormalities associated with malignant hyperthermia susceptibility. J Electrocardiol 15:137, 1982.
127. Lucke JN, Hall GM, Lister D: Porcine malignant hyperthermia. I: Metabolic and physiological changes. Br J Anaesth 48:297, 1976.
128. Dunn CM, Maltry DE, Eggers GW Jr: Value of mass spectrometry in early diagnosis of malignant hyperthermia [letter]. Anesthesiology 63:333, 1985.
129. Baudendistel L, Goudsouzian N, Coté C, Strafford M: End-tidal CO_2 monitoring. Its use in the diagnosis and management of malignant hyperthermia. Anaesthesia 39:1000, 1984.
130. Hall GM, Lucke JN, Orchard C, et al: Effect of dantrolene on leg metabolism in porcine malignant hyperthermia. Anaesthesia 37:1167, 1982.
131. Gronert GA, Milde JH, Theye RA: Dantrolene in porcine malignant hyperthermia. Anesthesiology 44:488, 1976.
132. Gronert GA, Milde JH, Theye RA: Porcine malignant hyperthermia induced by halothane and succinylcholine: failure of treatment with procaine or procainamide. Anesthesiology 44:124, 1976.
133. Hall GM, Lucke JN, Lovell R, Lister D: Porcine malignant hyperthermia. VII: Hepatic metabolism. Br J Anaesth 52:11, 1980.
134. Gronert GA, Theye RA, Milde JH, Tinker JH: Catecholamine stimulation of myocardial oxygen consumption in porcine malignant hyperthermia. Anesthesiology 49:330, 1978.
135. Artru AA, Gronert GA: Cerebral metabolism during porcine malignant hyperthermia. Anesthesiology 53:121, 1980.
136. Huckell VF, Staniloff HM, Britt BA, et al: Cardiac manifestations of malignant hyperthermia susceptibility. Circulation 58:916, 1978.
137. Falk E, Simonsen J: The histology of myocardium in malignant hyperthermia: a preliminary report of 11 cases. Forensic Sci Int 13:211, 1979.
138. Fenoglio JJ Jr, Irey NS: Myocardial changes in malignant hyperthermia. Am J Pathol 89:51, 1977.
139. Denborough MA, Galloway GJ, Hopkinson KC: Malignant hyperpyrexia and sudden infant death. Lancet 2:1068, 1982.
140. Peterson DR, Davis N: Sudden infant death syndrome and malignant hyperthermia diathesis. Aust Paediatr J 22:33, 1986.
141. Ryan JF, Donlon JV, Malt RA, et al: Cardiopulmonary bypass in the treatment of malignant hyperthermia. N Engl J Med 290:1121, 1974.
142. Britt B: Malignant hyperthermia. In Orkin FK, Cooperman LH (eds): Complications in Anesthesiology. Philadelphia, JB Lippincott, 1983, p 291.
143. Roberts JT, Burt T, Gyulai L: Delayed recovery of intracellular skeletal muscle pH measured by phosphorus-31 nuclear magnetic resonance in malignant hyperthermic swine with partial to full recovery of arterial pH following treatment with sodium dantrolene. Anesthesiology 63:A272, 1985.
144. Rosenberg H: Trismus is not trivial. Anesthesiology 67:453, 1987.
145. Gronert GA: Management of patients in whom trismus occurs following succinylcholine. Anesthesiology 68:653, 1988.
146. Yentis SM, Levine MF, Hartley EJ: Should all children with suspected or confirmed malignant hyperthermia susceptibility be admitted after surgery? A 10-year review. Anesth Analg 75:345, 1992.
147. Tang TT, Oechler HW, Siker D, et al: Anesthesia-induced rhabdomyolysis in infants with unsuspected Duchenne dystrophy. Acta Paediatr 81:716, 1992.

148. Austin KL, Denborough MA: Drug treatment of malignant hyperpyrexia. Anaesth Intensive Care 5:207, 1977.

149. Britt BA, Kwong F, Endrenyi L: Management of malignant hyperthermia susceptible (MHS) patients—a review. In Henschei ED (ed): Malignant Hyperthermia: Current Concepts. New York, Appleton-Century-Crofts, 1977, p 63.

150. Flewellen EH, Nelson TE: Dantrolene dose response in malignant hyperthermia-susceptible (MHS) swine: method to obtain prophylaxis and therapeusis. Anesthesiology 52:303, 1980.

151. Flewellen EH, Nelson TE, Jones WP, et al: Dantrolene dose response in awake man: implications for management of malignant hyperthermia. Anesthesiology 59:275, 1983.

152. Lopez JR, Alamo L, Jones D, et al: [Ca²⁺]ᵢ reduction in skeletal muscle by dantrolene sodium prevents malignant hyperthermia [abstract]. Anesthesiology 63:A273, 1985.

153. Kolb ME, Horne ML, Martz R: Dantrolene in human malignant hyperthermia: a multicenter study. Anesthesiology 56:254, 1982.

154. Ward A, Chaffman MO, Sorkin EM: Dantrolene. A review of its pharmacodynamic and pharmacokinetic properties and therapeutic use in malignant hyperthermia, the neuroleptic malignant syndrome and an update of its use in muscle spasticity. Drugs 32:130, 1986.

155. Allen GC, Cattran CB, Peterson RG, Lalande M: Plasma levels of dantrolene following oral administration in malignant hyperthermia-susceptible patients. Anesthesiology 69:900, 1988.

156. Lerman J, McLeod ME, Strong HA: Pharmacokinetics of intravenous dantrolene in children. Anesthesiology 70:625, 1989.

157. Putney JW, Biancri CP: Site of action of dantrolene in frog sartorius muscle. J Pharmacol Exp Ther 189:202, 1974.

158. Kurihara T, Brooks JE: Excitation-contraction uncoupling. The effect of hyperosomolar glycerol solution and dantrolene sodium on mammalian muscle in vitro. Arch Neurol 32:92, 1975.

159. Morgan KG, Bryant SH: The mechanism of action of dantrolene sodium. J Pharmacol Exp Ther 201:138, 1977.

160. Allen P, Lopez JR, Jones D, et al: Measurements of [Ca²⁺]ᵢ in skeletal muscle of malignant hyperthermic swine [abstract]. Anesthesiology 63:A268, 1985.

161. Van Winkle WB: Calcium release from skeletal muscle sarcoplasmic reticulum: site of action of dantrolene sodium? Science 193:1130, 1976.

162. Roewer N, Kuck KH, Nienaber CH, et al: Electrophysiologic effects of intravenous dantrolene on dog hearts [abstract]. Anesthesiology 61:A254, 1984.

163. Roewer N, Rumberger E, Schulte am Esch J: Effects of dantrolene on excitation-contraction coupling in isolated heart muscle [abstract]. Anesthesiology 61:A255, 1984.

164. Lynch CD, Durbin CG Jr, Fisher NA, et al: Effects of dantrolene and verapamil on atrioventricular conduction and cardiovascular performance in dogs. Anesth Analg 65:252, 1986.

165. Saltzman LS, Kates RA, Norfleet EA, et al: Hemodynamic interactions of diltiazem-dantrolene and nifedipine-dantrolene [abstract]. Anesthesiology 61:A11, 1984.

166. Rubin AS, Zablocki AD: Hyperkalemia, verapamil, and dantrolene. Anesthesiology 66:246, 1987.

167. San Juan AC Jr, Wong KC, Port JD: Hyperkalemia after dantrolene and verapamil-dantrolene administration in dogs. Anesth Analg 67:759, 1988.

168. Schneider R, Mitchell D: Dantrolene hepatitis. JAMA 235:1590, 1976.

169. Roy S, Francis FT, Born CK, Hamrick ME: Interaction of dantrolene with the hepatic mixed function oxidase system. Res Commun Chem Pathol Pharmacol 27:507, 1980.

170. Abernathy CO, Utili R, Zimmerman HJ, Ezekiel M: The effects of dantrolene sodium on excretory function in the isolated perfused rat liver. Toxicol Appl Pharmacol 44:441, 1978.

171. Francis KT, Hamrick ME: Dantrolene inhibition of the hepatic mixed function oxidase system. Res Commun Chem Pathol Pharmacol 23:69, 1979.

172. Petusevsky ML, Faling LJ, Rocklin RE, et al: Pleuropericardial reaction to treatment with dantrolene. JAMA 242:2772, 1979.

173. Rosenblatt R, Tallman JRD, Weaver J, Wang Y: Dantrolene potentiates the toxicity of bupivacaine. Anesthesiology 61:A209, 1984.

174. Watson CB, Reierson N, Norfleet EA: Clinically significant muscle weakness induced by oral dantrolene sodium prophylaxis for malignant hyperthermia. Anesthesiology 65:312, 1986.

175. Wingard DW: Controversies regarding the prophylactic use of dantrolene for malignant hyperthermia [letter]. Anesthesiology 58:489, 1983.

176. Dershwitz M, Sreter FA: Azumolene reverses episodes of malignant hyperthermia in susceptible swine. Anesth Analg 70:253, 1990.

177. Harrison GG, Morrell DF: Response of mhs swine to i.v. infusion of lignocaine and bupivacaine. Br J Anaesth 52:385, 1980.

178. Wingard DW, Bobko S: Failure of lidocaine to trigger porcine malignant hyperthermia. Anesth Analg 58:99, 1979.

179. Andragna MG: Medical protocol by habit—the avoidance of amide local anesthetics in malignant hyperthermia susceptible patients. Anesthesiology 62:99, 1985.

180. Britt BA: Malignant hyperthermia. Can Anaesth Soc J 32:666, 1985.

181. Honda N, Konno K, Itohda Y, et al: Malignant hyperthermia and althesin. Can Anaesth Soc J 24:514, 1977.

182. Suresh MS, Nelson TE: Malignant hyperthermia: is etomidate safe? Anesth Analg 64:420, 1985.

183. Ellis FR, Clarke IM, Appleyard TN, Dinsdale RC: Malignant hyperpyrexia induced by nitrous oxide and treated with dexamethasone. BMJ 4:270, 1974.

184. Fitzgibbons DC: Malignant hyperthermia following preoperative oral administration of dantrolene. Anesthesiology 54:73, 1981.

185. Dolan PF: Dantrolene and malignant hyperthermia [letter]. Anesthesiology 57:246, 1982.

186. Carr AS, Lerman J, Cunliffe M, et al: Incidence of malignant hyperthermia reactions in 2,214 patients undergoing muscle biopsy. Can J Anaesth 42:281, 1995.

187. Larach MG: Standardization of the caffeine halothane muscle contracture test. North American Malignant Hyperthermia Group. Anesth Analg 69:511, 1989.

188. Islander G, Twetman ER: Comparison between the European and North American protocols for diagnosis of malignant hyperthermia susceptibility in humans. Anesth Analg 88:1155, 1999.

189. Nelson TE, Flewellen EH, Gloyna DF: Spectrum of susceptibility to malignant hyperthermia—diagnostic dilemma. Anesth Analg 62:545, 1983.

190. Fletcher JE, Rosenberg H: In vitro interaction between halothane and succinylcholine in human skeletal muscle: implications for malignant hyperthermia and masseter muscle rigidity. Anesthesiology 63:190, 1985.

191. Ellis FR, Halsall PJ, Hopkins PM: Is the "K-type" caffeine-halothane responder susceptible to malignant hyperthermia? [see comments]. Br J Anaesth 69:468, 1992.

192. Berkowitz A, Rosenberg H: Femoral block with mepivacaine for muscle biopsy in malignant hyperthermia patients. Anesthesiology 62:651, 1985.

193. Allen GC, Rosenberg H, Fletcher JE: Safety of general anesthesia in patients previously tested negative for malignant hyperthermia susceptibility [see comments]. Anesthesiology 72:619, 1990.

194. Wood DS: Human skeletal muscle: analysis of Ca2+ regulation in skinned fibers using caffeine. Exp Neurol 58:218, 1978.

195. Britt BA, Frodis W, Scott E, et al: Comparison of the caffeine skinned fibre tension (CSFT) test with the caffeine-halothane contracture (CHC) test in the diagnosis of malignant hyperthermia. Can Anaesth Soc J 29:550, 1982.

196. Ording H, Glahn K, Gardi T, et al: 4-Chloro-m-cresol test—a possible supplementary test for diagnosis of malignant hyperthermia susceptibility [see comments]. Acta Anaesthesiol Scand 41:967, 1977.

197. Mabuchi K, Sreter FA: Use of cryostat sections for measurement of Ca2+ uptake by sarcoplasmic reticulum. Anal Biochem 86:733, 1978.

198. Ohnishi ST, Waring AJ, Fang SR, et al: Abnormal membrane properties of the sarcoplasmic reticulum of pigs susceptible to malignant hyperthermia: modes of action of halothane, caffeine, dantrolene, and two other drugs. Arch Biochem Biophys 247:294, 1986.

199. Olgin J, Rosenberg H, Allen G, et al: A blinded comparison of noninvasive, in vivo phosphorus nuclear magnetic resonance spectroscopy and the in vitro halothane/caffeine contracture test in the evaluation of malignant hyperthermia susceptibility [see comments]. Anesth Analg 72:36, 1991.

200. Olgin J, Argov Z, Rosenberg H, et al: Non-invasive evaluation of malignant hyperthermia susceptibility with phosphorus nuclear magnetic resonance spectroscopy. Anesthesiology 68:507, 1988.

201. Dominguez EA, Bar-Sela A, Musher DM: Adoption of thermometry into clinical practice in the United States. Rev Infect Dis 9:1193, 1987.

202. Atkins E: Fever: the old and the new. J Infect Dis 149:339, 1984.
203. Ikeda T, Sessler DI, Marder D, Xiong J: The influence of thermoregulatory vasomotion and ambient temperature variation on the accuracy of core-temperature estimates by cutaneous liquid-crystal thermometers. Anesthesiology 86:603, 1997.
204. Iaizzo P, Zink R, Kehler C, et al: Skin and central temperature during malignant hyperthermia in swine [abstract]. Anesthesiology 77:A569, 1992.
205. Muma BK, Treloar DJ, Wurmlinger K, et al: Comparison of rectal, axillary, and tympanic membrane temperatures in infants and young children. Ann Emerg Med 20:41, 1991.
206. Yaron M, Lowenstein SR, Koziol-McLain J: Measuring the accuracy of the infrared tympanic thermometer: correlation does not signify agreement. J Emerg Med 13:617, 1995.
207. Imamura M, Matsukawa T, Ozaki M, et al: The accuracy and precision of four infrared aural canal thermometers during cardiac surgery. Acta Anaesthiol Scand 42:1222, 1998.
208. Colin J, Timbal J, Houdas Y, et al: Computation of mean body temperature from rectal and skin temperatures. J Appl Physiol 31:484, 1971.
209. Webb GE: Comparison of esophageal and tympanic temperature monitoring during cardiopulmonary bypass. Analg Anesth 52:729, 1973.
210. Stone JG, Yound WL, Smith CR, et al: Do temperatures recorded at standard monitoring sites reflect actual brain temperature during deep hypothermia? Anesthesiology 75:A483, 1991.
211. Cork RC, Vaughan RW, Humphrey LS: Precision and accuracy of intraoperative temperature monitoring. Anesth Analg 62:211, 1983.
212. Glosten B, Sessler DI, Faure EAM, et al: Central temperature changes are not perceived during epidural anesthesia. Anesthesiology 77:10, 1992.
213. Bissonnette B, Sessler DI, LaFlamme P: Intraoperative temperature monitoring sites in infants and children and the effect of inspired gas warming on esophageal temperature. Anesth Analg 69:192, 1989.
214. Wyss CR, Brengelmann GL, Johnson JM, et al: Altered control of skin blood flow at high skin and core temperatures. J Appl Physiol 38:839, 1975.
215. Benzinger TH, Pratt AW, Kitzinger C: The thermostatic control of human metabolic heat production. Proc Natl Acad Sci U.S.A. 47:730, 1961.
216. Rubinstein EH, Sessler DI: Skin-surface temperature gradients correlate with fingertip blood flow in humans. Anesthesiology 73:541, 1990.
217. Ramanathan NL: A new weighting system for mean surface temperature of the human body. J Appl Physiol 19:531, 1964.
218. Shanks CA: Mean skin temperature during anaesthesia: an assessment of formulae in the supine surgical patient. Br J Anaesth 47:871, 1975.
219. Burton AC: Human calorimetry: the average temperature of the tissues of the body. J Nutr 9:261, 1935.
220. Adragna MG: Medical protocol by habit—the avoidance of amide local anesthetics in malignant hyperthermia susceptible patients [letter]. Anesthesiology 62:99, 1986.
221. Hendolin H, Lansimies E: Skin and central temperatures during continuous epidural analgesia and general anaesthesia in patients subjected to open prostatectomy. Ann Clin Res 14:181, 1982.
222. Sessler DI, Ponte J: Shivering during epidural anesthesia. Anesthesiology 72:816, 1990.
223. Hynson J, Sessler DI, Glosten B, McGuire J: Thermal balance and tremor patterns during epidural anesthesia. Anesthesiology 74:680, 1991.
224. Sessler DI, McGuire J, Moayeri A, Hynson J: Isoflurane-induced vasodilation minimally increases cutaneous heat loss. Anesthesiology 74:226, 1991.
225. Satinoff E: Neural organization and evolution of thermal regulation in mammals—several hierarchically arranged integrating systems may have evolved to achieve precise thermoregulation. Science 201:16, 1978.
226. Ekenvall L, Lindblad LE, Norbeck O, Etzell B-M: α-Adrenoceptors and cold-induced vasoconstriction in human finger skin. Am J Physiol 255:H1001, 1988.
227. Poulos DA: Central processing of cutaneous temperature information. Fed Proc 40:2825, 1981.
228. Jessen C, Feistkorn G: Some characteristics of core temperature signals in the conscious goat. Am J Physiol 247:R456, 1984.
229. Jessen C, Mayer ET: Spinal cord and hypothalamus as core sensors of temperature in the conscious dog. I. Equivalence of responses. Pflugers Arch 324:189, 1971.
230. Simon E: Temperature regulation: the spinal cord as a site of extrahypothalamic thermoregulatory functions. Rev Physiol Biochem Pharmacol 71:1, 1974.
231. Cheng C, Matsukawa T, Sessler DI, et al: Increasing mean skin temperature linearly reduces the core-temperature thresholds for vasoconstriction and shivering in humans. Anesthesiology 82:1160, 1995.
232. Lenhardt R, Greif R, Sessler DI, et al: Relative contribution of skin and core temperatures to vasoconstriction and shivering thresholds during isoflurane anesthesia. Anesthesiology 91:422, 1999.
233. Frank S, Raja SN, Bulcao C, Goldstein D: Relative contribution of core and cutaneous temperatures to thermal comfort, autonomic, and metabolic responses in humans. J Appl Physiol 68:1588, 1998.
234. Hensel H: Thermoreception and Temperature Regulation. London, Academic Press, 1981.
235. Mekjavic IB, Morrison JB: A model of shivering thermogenesis based on the neurophysiology of thermoreception. IEEE Trans Biomed Eng 32:407, 1985.
236. Wissler EH: Comparison of computed results obtained from two mathematical models—a simple 14-node model and a complex 250-node model. J Physiologie 63:455, 1971.
237. Hammel HT: Regulation of internal body temperature. Ann Rev Physiol 30:641, 1968.
238. Brück K: Thermoregulation: Control mechanisms and neural processes. In Sinclair JC (ed): Temperature Regulation and Energy Metabolism in the Newborn. New York, Grune & Stratton, 1978, p 157.
239. Adair ER: Studies on the behavioral regulation of preoptic temperature. In Cooper KE, Lomax P, Schönbaum E (eds): Drugs, Biogenic Amines and Body Temperature. Basel, Karger, 1977, p 84.
240. Cabanac M, Dib B: Behavioural responses to hypothalamic cooling and heating in the rat. Brain Res 264:79, 1983.
241. Washington D, Sessler DI, Moayeri A, et al: Thermoregulatory responses to hyperthermia during isoflurane anesthesia in humans. J Appl Physiol 74:82, 1993.
242. Kurz A, Xiong J, Sessler DI, et al: Desflurane reduces the gain of thermoregulatory arterio-venous shunt vasoconstriction in humans. Anesthesiology 83:1212, 1995.
243. Ikeda T, Sessler DI, Tayefeh F, et al: Meperidine and alfentanil do not reduce the gain or maximum intensity of shivering. Anesthesiology 88:858, 1998.
244. Ikeda T, Kim J-S, Sessler DI, et al: Isoflurane alters shivering patterns and reduces maximum shivering intensity. Anesthesiology 88:866, 1998.
245. Rowell LB: Cardiovascular aspects of human thermoregulation. Circ Res 52:367, 1983.
246. Hales JRS: Skin arteriovenous anastomoses, their control and role in thermoregulation. In Johansen K, Burggren W (eds): Cardiovascular Shunts: Phylogenetic, Ontogenetic and Clinical Aspects. Copenhagen, Munksgaard, 1985, p 433.
247. Sessler DI, Moayeri A, Støen R, et al: Thermoregulatory vasoconstriction decreases cutaneous heat loss. Anesthesiology 73:656, 1990.
248. Jessen K: An assessment of human regulatory nonshivering thermogenesis. Acta Anaesthesiol Scand 24:138, 1980.
249. Jessen K, Rabøl A, Winkler K: Total body and splanchnic thermogenesis in curarized man during a short exposure to cold. Acta Anaesthesiol Scand 24:339, 1980.
250. Mestyan J, Jarai I, Bata G, Fekete M: The significance of facial skin temperature in the chemical heat regulation of premature infants. Biol Neonate 7:243, 1964.
251. Dawkins MJR, Scopes JW: Non-shivering thermogenesis and brown adipose tissue in the human new-born infant. Nature 206:201, 1965.
252. Hey EN, Katz G: Temporary loss of a metabolic response to cold stress in infants of low birthweight. Arch Dis Child 44:323, 1969.
253. Rowell LB: Active neurogenic vasodilation in man. In Vanhoutte P, Leusen I (eds): Vasodilatation. New York, Raven Press, 1981, p 1.
254. Falk B, Bar-Or O, Macdougall JD, et al: Sweat lactate in exercising children and adolescents of varying physical maturity. J Appl Physiol 71:1735, 1991.
255. Buono MJ, Sjoholm NT: Effect of physical training on peripheral sweat production. J Appl Physiol 65:811, 1988.

256. Roberts MF, Wenger CB, Stolwijk JAJ, Nadel ER: Skin blood flow and sweating changes following exercise training and heat acclimation. J Appl Physiol 43:133, 1977.

257. Hemingway A, Price WM: The autonomic nervous system and regulation of body temperature. Anesthesiology 29:693, 1968.

258. Ozaki M, Sessler DI, Negishi C, et al: Atropine increases the sweating threshold in humans [abstract]. Anesthesiology 85:A171, 1996.

259. Sessler DI, Hynson J, McGuire J, et al: Thermoregulatory vasoconstriction during isoflurane anesthesia minimally decreases heat loss. Anesthesiology 76:670, 1992.

260. Sessler DI: Central thermoregulatory inhibition by general anesthesia [editorial]. Anesthesiology 75:557, 1991.

261. Pertwee RG, Marshall NR, MacDonald AG: Behavioral thermoregulation in mice: effects of low doses of general anaesthetics of different potency. Exp Physiol 75:629, 1990.

262. Sessler DI, Olofsson CI, Rubinstein EH, Beebe JJ: The thermoregulatory threshold in humans during halothane anesthesia. Anesthesiology 68:836, 1988.

263. Washington DE, Sessler DI, McGuire J, et al: Painful stimulation minimally increases the thermoregulatory threshold for vasoconstriction during enflurane anesthesia in humans. Anesthesiology 77:286, 1992.

264. Sessler DI, Olofsson CI, Rubinstein EH: The thermoregulatory threshold in humans during nitrous oxide-fentanyl anesthesia. Anesthesiology 69:357, 1988.

265. Annadata RS, Sessler DI, Tayefeh F, et al: Desflurane slightly increases the sweating threshold, but produces marked, non-linear decreases in the vasoconstriction and shivering thresholds. Anesthesiology 83:1205, 1995.

266. Ozaki M, Sessler DI, Suzuki H, et al: Nitrous oxide decreases the threshold for vasoconstriction less than sevoflurane or isoflurane. Anesth Analg 80:1212, 1995.

267. Matsukawa T, Kurz A, Sessler DI, et al: Propofol linearly reduces the vasoconstriction and shivering thresholds. Anesthesiology 82:1169, 1995.

268. Hynson JM, Sessler DI, Belani K, et al: Thermoregulatory vasoconstriction during propofol/nitrous oxide anesthesia in humans: threshold and Spo2. Anesth Analg 75:947, 1992.

269. Bissonnette B, Sessler DI: Thermoregulatory thresholds for vasoconstriction in pediatric patients anesthetized with halothane or halothane and caudal bupivacaine. Anesthesiology 76:387, 1992.

270. Bissonnette B, Sessler DI: The thermoregulatory threshold in infants and children anesthetized with isoflurane and caudal bupivacaine. Anesthesiology 73:1114, 1990.

271. Hynson JM, Sessler DI, Moayeri A, McGuire J: Absence of nonshivering thermogenesis in anesthetized humans. Anesthesiology 79:695, 1993.

272. Plattner O, Semsroth M, Sessler DI, et al: Lack of nonshivering thermogenesis in infants anesthetized with fentanyl and propofol. Anesthesiology 86:772, 1997.

273. Dicker A, Ohlson KB, Johnson L, et al: Halothane selectively inhibits nonshivering thermogenesis. Anesthesiology 82:491, 1995.

274. Sessler DI, Rubinstein EH, Moayeri A: Physiological responses to mild perianesthetic hypothermia in humans. Anesthesiology 75:594, 1991.

275. Sharkey A, Lipton JM, Murphy MT, Giesecke AH: Inhibition of postanesthetic shivering with radiant heat. Anesthesiology 66:249, 1987.

276. Macintyre PE, Pavlin EG, Dwersteg JF: Effect of meperidine on oxygen consumption, carbon dioxide production, and respiratory gas exchange in postanesthesia shivering. Anesth Analg 66:751, 1987.

277. Lopez M, Ozaki M, Sessler DI, Valdes M: Physiological responses to hyperthermia during epidural anesthesia and combined epidural/enflurane anesthesia in women. Anesthesiology 78:1046, 1993.

278. English MJM, Farmer C, Scott WAC: Heat loss in exposed volunteers. J Trauma 30:422, 1990.

279. Baumgart S: Radiant energy and insensible water loss in the premature newborn infant nursed under a radiant warmer. Clin Perinatol 9:483, 1982.

280. Hammarlund K, Sedin G: Transepidermal water loss in newborn infants III. Relation to gestational age. Acta Paediatr Scand 68:795, 1979.

281. Hey EN, Katz G: Evaporative water loss in the new-born baby. J Physiol 200:605, 1969.

282. Sessler DI, Sessler AM, Hudson S, Moayeri A: Heat loss during surgical skin preparation. Anesthesiology 78:1055, 1993.

283. Bickler P, Sessler DI: Efficiency of airway heat and moisture exchangers in anesthetized humans. Anesth Analg 71:415, 1990.

284. Stevens WC, Cromwell TH, Halsey MJ, et al: The cardiovascular effects of a new inhalation anesthetic, Forane, in human volunteers at constant arterial carbon dioxide tension. Anesthesiology 35:8, 1971.

285. Roe CF: Effect of bowel exposure on body temperature during surgical operations. Am J Surg 122:13, 1971.

286. Hynson J, Sessler DI: Intraoperative warming therapies: a comparison of three devices. J Clin Anesth 4:194, 1992.

287. Sessler DI, McGuire J, Sessler AM: Perioperative thermal insulation. Anesthesiology 74:875, 1991.

288. Sessler DI, Schroeder M: Heat loss in humans covered with cotton hospital blankets. Anesth Analg 77:73, 1993.

289. Sessler DI, Rubinstein EH, Eger EI II: Core temperature changes during N2O fentanyl and halothane/O2 anesthesia. Anesthesiology 67:137, 1987.

290. Kurz A, Sessler DI, Christensen R, Dechert M: Heat balance and distribution during the core-temperature plateau in anesthetized humans. Anesthesiology 83:491, 1995.

291. Belani K, Sessler DI, Sessler AM, et al: Leg heat content continues to decrease during the core temperature plateau in humans. Anesthesiology 78:856, 1993.

292. Thornberry EA, Mazumdar B: The effect of changes in arm temperature on neuromuscular monitoring in the presence of atracurium blockade. Anaesthesia 43:447, 1988.

293. Frank SM, Beattie C, Christopherson R, et al: Epidural versus general anesthesia, ambient operating room temperature, and patient age as predictors of inadvertent hypothermia. Anesthesiology 77:252, 1992.

294. Valeri RC, Cassidy G, Khuri S, et al: Hypothermia-induced reversible platelet dysfunction. Ann Surg 205:175, 1987.

295. Hcicr T, Caldwell JE, Sessler DI, Miller RD: Mild intraoperative hypothermia increases duration of action and spontaneous recovery of vecuronium blockade during nitrous oxide-isoflurane anesthesia in humans. Anesthesiology 74:815, 1991.

296. Carli F, Emery PW, Freemantle CAJ: Effect of preoperative normothermia on postoperative protein metabolism in elderly patients undergoing hip arthroplasty. Br J Anaesth 63:276, 1989.

297. Hales JRS: Thermal physiology. In Morimoto T, Nose H, Miki K (eds): Blood Volume and Cardiovascular Function during Acute Hyperthermia and Hypothermia. New York, Raven Press, 1984, p 385.

298. Bengtsson M: Changes in skin blood flow and temperature during spinal analgesia evaluated by laser Doppler flowmetry and infrared thermography. Acta Anaesthesiol Scand 28:625, 1984.

299. Bengtsson M, Nilsson GE, Lofstrom JB: The effect of spinal analgesia on skin blood flow, evaluated by laser Doppler flowmetry. Acta Anaesthesiol Scand 27:206, 1983.

300. Benzon HT, Cheng SC, Avram MJ, Molloy RE: Sign of complete sympathetic blockade: sweat test or sympathogalvanic response? Anesth Analg 64:415, 1985.

301. Tankersley CG, Smolander J, Kenney WL, Fortney SM: Sweating and skin blood flow during exercise: effects of age and maximal oxygen uptake. J Appl Physiol 71:236, 1991.

302. Just B, Delva E, Camus Y, Lienhart A: Oxygen uptake during recovery following naloxone. Anesthesiology 76:60, 1992.

303. Belani K, Sessler D, Sessler A, et al: Thermoregulatory vasoconstriction constrains metabolic heat to the central thermal compartment [abstract]. Anesthesiology 77:A182, 1992.

304. Roe CF, Cohn FL: The causes of hypothermia during spinal anesthesia. Surg Gynecol Obstet 135:577, 1972.

305. Kurz A, Sessler DI, Schroeder M, Kurz M: Thermoregulatory response thresholds during spinal anesthesia. Anesth Analg 77:721, 1993.

306. Ozaki M, Kurz A, Sessler DI, et al: Thermoregulatory thresholds during spinal and epidural anesthesia. Anesthesiology 81:282, 1994.

307. Glosten B, Sessler DI, Ostman LG, et al: Intravenous lidocaine does not cause tremor or alter thermoregulation. Reg Anesth 16:218, 1991.

308. Mercer JB, Jessen C: Central thermosensitivity in conscious goats: hypothalamus and spinal cord versus residual inner body. Pflugers Arch 374:179, 1978.

309. Ponte J, Sessler DI: Extradurals and shivering: effects of cold and warm extradural saline injections in volunteers. Br J Anaesth 64:731, 1990.

310. Harris MM, Lawson D, Cooper CM, Ellis J: Treatment of shivering after epidural lidocaine. Reg Anesth 14:13, 1989.

311. Panzer O, Ghazanfari N, Sessler DI, et al: Shivering and shivering-like tremor during labor with and without epidural analgesia. Anesthesiology 90:1609, 1999.

312. Matsukawa T, Sessler DI, Christensen R, et al: Heat flow and distribution during epidural anesthesia. Anesthesiology 83:961, 1995.

313. Matsukawa T, Sessler DI, Sessler AM, et al: Heat flow and distribution during induction of general anesthesia. Anesthesiology 82:662, 1995.

314. Hoffman WE, Charbel FT, Portillo GG, et al: Regional tissue pO_2, pCO_2, pH and temperature measurement. Neurol Res 20:S81, 1998.

315. Neubauer RA, James P: Cerebral oxygenation and the recoverable brain. Neurol Res 20:S33, 1998.

316. Schwab S, Schwarz S, Spranger M, et al: Moderate hypothermia in the treatment of patients with severe middle cerebral artery infarction. Stroke 29:2461, 1998.

317. Bunker JP, Goldstein R: Coagulation during hypothermia in man. Proc Soc Exp Biol Med 97:199, 1958.

318. Goto H, Nonami R, Hamasaki Y, et al: Effect of hypothermia on coagulation [abstract]. Anesthesiology 63:A107, 1985.

319. Csete M, Washington DE, Sessler DI, McGuire J: Coagulopathy during hypothermia is not due to increased fibrinolysis [abstract]. Anesthesiology 77:A264, 1992.

320. Schmied H, Kurz A, Sessler DI, et al: Mild intraoperative hypothermia increases blood loss and allogeneic transfusion requirements during total hip arthroplasty. Lancet 347:289, 1996.

321. Schmied H, Schiferer A, Sessler DI, Maznik C: The effects of red-cell scavenging, hemodilution, and active warming on allogeneic blood requirement in patients undergoing hip or knee arthroplasty. Anesth Analg 86:387, 1998.

322. Leslie K, Sessler DI, Schroeder M, Walters K: Propofol blood concentration and the bispectral index predict suppression of learning during propofol/epidural anesthesia in volunteers. Anesth Analg 81:1269, 1995.

323. Carli F, Clark MM, Woollen JW: Investigation of the relationship between heat loss and nitrogen excretion in elderly patients undergoing major abdominal surgery under general anaesthetic. Br J Anaesth 54:1023, 1982.

324. Sheffield C, Sessler D, Hunt T: Mild hypothermia during anesthesia decreases resistance to S. aureus dermal infection [abstract]. Anesthesiology 77:A1106, 1992.

325. Sheffield C, Sessler D, Hunt T: Mild hypothermia impairs resistance to E. coli infections in guinea pigs [abstract]. Anesth Analg 76:S390, 1993.

326. Duff GW, Durum SK: Fever and immunoregulation: hyperthermia, interleukins 1 and 2, and T-cell proliferation. Yale J Biol Med 55:437, 1982.

327. Smith JB, Knowlton RP, Agarwal SS: Human lymphocyte responses are enhanced by culture at 40°C. J Immunol 121:691, 1978.

328. Sheffield C, Hopf H, Sessler D, et al: Thermoregulatory vasoconstriction decreases subcutaneous oxygen tension in anesthetized volunteers [abstract]. Anesthesiology 77:A96, 1992.

329. Kurz A, Sessler DI, Lenhardt RA, for the Study of Wound Infections and Temperature Group: Perioperative normothermia to reduce the incidence of surgical-wound infection and shorten hospitalization. N Engl J Med 334:1209, 1996.

330. Sessler DI, Israel D, Pozos RS, et al: Spontaneous post-anesthetic tremor does not resemble thermoregulatory shivering. Anesthesiology 68:843, 1988.

331. Horn E-P, Sessler DI, Standl T, et al: Non-thermoregulatory shivering in patients recovering from isoflurane or desflurane anesthesia. Anesthesiology 89:878, 1998.

332. Horn E-P, Schroeder F, Wilhelm S, et al: Postoperative pain facilitates non-thermoregulatory tremor. Anesthesiology 91:979, 1999.

333. Horvath SM, Spurr GB, Hutt BK, Hamilton LH: Metabolic cost of shivering. J Appl Physiol 8:595, 1956.

334. Mahajan RP, Grover VK, Sharma SL, Singh H: Intraocular pressure changes during muscular hyperactivity after general anesthesia. Anesthesiology 66:419, 1987.

335. Glosten B, Hynson J, Sessler D, McGuire J: Skin surface warming before epidural block blunts anesthetic-induced hypothermia [abstract]. Anesthesiology 75:A854, 1991.

336. Guffin A, Girard D, Kaplan JA: Shivering following cardiac surgery: hemodynamic changes and reversal. J Cardiothorac Vasc Anesth 1:24, 1987.

337. Kurz M, Belani K, Sessler DI, et al: Naloxone, meperidine, and shivering. Anesthesiology 79:1193, 1993.

338. Kurz A, Ikeda T, Sessler DI, et al: Meperidine decreases the shivering threshold twice as much as the vasoconstriction threshold. Anesthesiology 86:1046, 1997.

339. Webb P: Impaired performance from prolonged mild body cooling. In Bachrach AJ, Matzen NM (eds): Underwater Physiology VIII: Proceedings of the Eighth Symposium on Underwater Physiology. Bethesda, MD, Undersea Medical Society, 1984, p 391.

340. Gauthier R: Use of forced air warming system for intraoperative warming [abstract]. Anesthesiology 73:A462, 1990.

341. Gewolb J, Hines R, Barash P: A survey of 3,244 consecutive admissions to the post-anesthesia recovery room at a university teaching hospital [abstract]. Anesthesiology 67:A471, 1987.

342. Bissonnette B, Sessler DI: Mild hypothermia does not impair postanesthetic recovery in infants and children. Anesth Analg 76:168, 1993.

343. Morton G, Flewellen G III: Prevention of intraoperative hypothermia in geriatric patients [abstract]. Anesth Analg 68:S204, 1989.

344. Giuffre M, Finnie J, Lynam D, Smith D: Rewarming postoperative patients: lights, blankets, or forced warm air. J Postanesth Nurs 6:387, 1991.

345. Lenhardt R, Marker E, Goll V, et al: Mild intraoperative hypothermia prolongs postoperative recovery. Anesthesiology 87:1318, 1997.

346. Bissonnette B, Sessler DI: Passive or active inspired gas humidification in infants and children. Anesthesiology 71:381, 1989.

347. Bissonnette B, Sessler DI: Passive or active inspired gas humidification increases thermal steady-state temperatures in anesthetized infants. Anesth Analg 69:783, 1989.

348. Forbes AR: Temperature, humidity and mucus flow in the intubated trachea. Br J Anaesth 46:29, 1974.

349. Simbruner G, Weninge RM, Popow C, Herholdt WJ: Regional heat loss in newborn infants: Part I. Heat loss in healthy newborns at various environmental temperatures. S Afr Med J 68:940, 1985.

350. Goudsouzian NG, Morris RH, Ryan JF: The effects of a warming blanket on the maintenance of body temperatures in anesthetized infants and children. Anesthesiology 39:351, 1973.

351. Crino MH, Nagel EL: Thermal burns caused by warming blankets in the operating room. Anesthesiology 29:149, 1968.

352. Scott SM, Oteen NC: Thermal blanket injury in the operating room. Arch Surg 94:181, 1967.

353. Gendron F: "Burns" occurring during lengthy surgical procedures. J Clin Engineer 5:20, 1980.

354. Gendron FG: Unexplained Patient Burns: Investigating Iatrogenic Injuries, Brea, CA, Quest Publishing Co, Inc, 1988.

355. Sessler DI, Moayeri A: Skin-surface warming: heat flux and central temperature. Anesthesiology 73:218, 1990.

356. Kurz A, Kurz M, Poeschl G, et al: Forced-air warming maintains intraoperative normothermia better than circulating-water mattresses. Anesth Analg 77:89, 1993.

357. Kelley S, Prager M, Sessler D, et al: Forced air warming minimizes hypothermia during orthotopic liver transplantation [abstract]. Anesthesiology 73:A433, 1990.

358. Block E, Ginsberg B, Binner R, Sessler D: Limb tourniquets and central temperature in anesthetized children. Anesth Analg 74:486, 1992.

359. Davatelis G, Wolpe SD, Sherry B, et al: Macrophage inflammatory protein-1: a prostaglandin-independent endogenous pyrogen. Science 243:1066, 1989.

360. Lenhardt R, Negishi C, Sessler DI, et al: The effects of physical treatment on induced fever in humans. Am J Med 106:550, 1999.

361. Kluger MJ, Ringler DH, Anver MR: Fever and survival. Science 188:166, 1975.

362. Carmichael LE, Barnes FD, Percy DH: Temperature as a factor in resistance of young puppies to canine herpesvirus. J Infect Dis 120:669, 1969.

363. Furuuchi S, Shimizu Y: Effect of ambient temperatures on multiplication of attenuated transmissible gastroenteritis virus in the bodies of newborn piglets. Infect Immun 13:990, 1976.

364. Husseini RH, Sweet C, Collie MH, Smith H: Elevation of nasal viral levels by suppression of fever in ferrets infected with influenza viruses of differing virulence. J Infect Dis 145:520, 1982.

365. Vaughn LK, Veale WL, Cooper KE: Antipyresis: its effect on mortality rate of bacterially infected rabbits. Brain Res Bull 5:69, 1980.

366. Lenhardt R, Negishi C, Sessler DI, et al: The effect of pyrogen administration on sweating and vasoconstriction thresholds during desflurane anesthesia. Anesthesiology 90:1587, 1999.

367. Lenhardt R, Negishi C, Sessler DI, et al: Paralysis only slightly reduces the febrile response to interleukin-2 during isoflurane anesthesia. Anesthesiology 89:648, 1998.
368. Negishi C, Lenhardt R, Sessler DI, et al: Desflurane reduces the febrile response to interleukin-2 administration. Anesthesiology 88:1162, 1998.
369. Lenhardt R, Negishi C, Kim J-S, et al: Alfentanil slightly reduces the febrile response to interleukin-2 administration [abstract]. Anesthesiology 89:A1239, 1998.
370. Negishi C, Lenhardt R, Sessler DI, Ozaki M: Opioids inhibit fever in human wheras epidural analgesia does not [abstract]. Anesthesiology 91:A215, 1999.
371. Xiong J, Kurz A, Sessler DI, et al: Isoflurane produces marked and non-linear decreases in the vasoconstriction and shivering thresholds. Anesthesiology 85:240, 1996.
372. Kurz A, Go JC, Sessler DI, et al: Alfentanil slightly increases the sweating threshold and markedly reduces the vasoconstriction and shivering thresholds. Anesthesiology 83:293, 1995.

5

Pediatric Fluids, Electrolytes, and Nutrition

DANIEL SIKER

◆   ◆   ◆

Not much to offer you—
just a lotus flower floating
In a small jar of water.[1]

Ryokan

Ryokan could hardly have predicted the fluid wars of today having lived the life of a Zen Buddhist monk two centuries ago. His poems in *One Robe, One Bowl* describe the simple life possible once basic needs are met. As good physicians, we must offer our patients neither too much, too little, too early, nor too late the fluids, electrolytes, and nutrition needed to sustain life and feed the soul. Food and water fuel our metabolism. Giving children enough but not excessive fluid, salt, and calories should be the simplest way to combat the greatest worldwide killers of children, dehydration and malnutrition. Images of starving and dehydrated infants and children from countries besieged by famine and warfare remind us of the human imperative to provide nourishment and fluids. Even in industrialized countries, anesthesiologists must treat children whose medical or surgical problems include malnutrition and dehydration. The ability to manage fluids, electrolytes, and nutrition is essential in both pediatrics and anesthesiology.

The concept of intravascular fluid therapy was born after William Harvey described the fundamentally circular movement of blood in the body. He wrote in 1628, "The heart of creatures is the foundation of life, on which all vegetation does depend, from whence all vigor and strength does flow."[2] The modern science of parenteral therapy, which is based on the movement of blood, has given new meaning to Harvey's words, far beyond what he might have imagined. Failure to adequately treat fluid and electrolyte disturbances remains the leading cause of death in children worldwide.

CHOLERA AND FLUIDS

The first widely reported use of parenteral therapy occurred during the cholera epidemic of 1830 and 1831. Since cholera causes a secretory diarrhea, acute loss of water and electrolytes causes death within hours. Latta's classic description of his first subject follows: "a juvenile . . . but with a face of a hag . . . her countenance a ghastly tint; her eyes sunken deep into the sockets as though they had been driven an inch behind their natural position; her fingers shrunk, bent, and inky in their hue. In short, Sir, that face and form I can never forget." Latta then infused 10 L of an alkaline salt solution over 10 hours into her pulseless body. He reported that her "cadaverous appearance" resolved, and she was later discharged.[3] However, soon after the cholera epidemic passed, the enthusiasm for the use of parenteral fluids fell into disrepute because of many reports of sepsis.

Today, after reviewing hundreds of animal studies, Bickel et al. in the now infamous "Houston Study"[4] of immediate versus delayed fluid resuscitation in nearly 600 trauma patients, demonstrated that too much fluid too early can increase mortality in hemorrhagic shock. This important and most controversial topic is covered in the section "The Bleeding Child," below.

However, hypotension attributable to nonhemorrhagic causes such as cholera have caused us to refocus our attention on oral fluid management. The modern miracle cure has not been intravenous (IV) fluids but rather the use of carefully formulated oral rehydration solutions. The gut, even during general anesthesia, can actively absorb electrolytes when glucose is added in proper proportions to the rehydration solution. This solution more than counters the toxin-induced secretory loss of electrolytes seen with cholera. Although medical progress has enabled us to understand the mechanisms of injury and to devise accurate combinations of glucose and electrolyte solutions, we are still at the mercy of major epidemics brought about by poor sanitation techniques, war, and poverty. A record number of 300,000 cases of cholera was reported in Peru during the first 11 months of 1991. With oral WHO-UNICEF formulations and only rare use of IV rehydration, survival rates for infants and adults exceeded 99 percent,[5] compared with mortality rates during the recent cholera epidemics of greater than 30 percent.

The modern roots of parenteral therapy lie in the acceptance of Lister's germ theory of the late nineteenth century,[6] and the increased understanding of the composition of body fluids. In 1879, Claude Bernard described our body fluids as a "bit of primeval sea within us all." Bernard originated the concept of body fluid homeostasis, which he described as a delicate balance of fluids, electrolytes, and hormones that maintain a "milieu internus" or a "cosmos" protected from the external world, within which the pressures of oxygen, carbon dioxide, hydrogen ions, concentrations of essential minerals, and fluid volume are precisely maintained.[7, 8]

DIARRHEA

Pediatricians have long recognized that infantile diarrhea severely disrupts this internal environment and therefore continues to be a leading cause of mortality in children. Diarrhea illustrates the critical impact of fluid and electrolyte losses in young children and the vital role of fluid replacement therapy. In 1915, Holt and Courtney[9] directly analyzed the mineral losses associated with infantile diarrhea, which provided a rational basis for oral replacement of water and electrolytes. The next year, Howland and Marriot[10] found that tachypnea was a prominent feature of severe diarrheal dehydration. They treated this combination of hypovolemia and partially compensated metabolic acidosis with infusions of sterile water mixed with

a 4 percent solution of sodium bicarbonate, continuing this parenteral therapy until the child's urine output became adequate and alkaline. Collectively, these and other pediatricians formulated the concept that water and mineral replacement should equal the volume and content of body losses. A complete history and clinical examination were performed before initiating replacement fluid therapy, followed by direct measurement and analysis of fluid losses. These data provided a rational basis for fluid and electrolyte therapy.

Many systems have been devised to calculate the amount of water, calories, and minerals required for continuing growth, maintenance during anesthesia, replacement of fluid losses and fluid shifts, and recovery from surgical stress. These systems are usually interchangeable. Each combines clinical observations and experience, including references to basic physiology. However, at present no single system is universally accepted or applicable to all circumstances. For example, maintenance fluids can be calculated by giving so much fluid per body surface area (square meters) or per kilogram of body weight, or so much fluid per calorie expended. These systems have in common a calculation of both fluid losses, defined as *replacement* therapy, and continuing requirements, defined as *maintenance* therapy.

Although preset formulations have a place in initial plans for fluid and electrolyte management, the differing growth rates, metabolic requirements, and amount of actual lean body mass measured by skin-fold calipers[11] or more modern means such as dual-energy x-ray absorptiometry[12] must be assessed individually.

Individual responses to trauma and individual variations in sickness, healing, and health mandate a customized approach to each child's fluid and electrolyte needs. Each clinical variable requires a specific fluid and electrolyte calculation based on replacement of losses and continuing maintenance requirements. Further refinement of fluid therapy can be based only on repeated evaluation of the patient's clinical responses to therapy.

DETERMINING FLUID REQUIREMENTS

Body Surface Area

Body surface area measurements are one way to calculate the volume of water required by hospitalized children of various sizes. However, the data that have been used to devise the current body surface area nomograms are associated with wide variations. As early as 1913, Howland and Dana[13] compared two widely used surface area measures. The first was produced by Meeh, who carefully wrapped several well-nourished infants in tissue paper to measure the total body surface area. The second, produced by Lissauer, used a series of infant cadavers, many of which were severely malnourished. The two methods of determining surface area yielded an average error of 15 percent. Dubois and Dubois[14] developed a widely copied surface area nomogram that was noted by Boyd[15] to have an error of nearly 20 percent in infants under 3 kg.

Body surface area calculations require that weight and height be known and that a nomogram be used to calculate the approximate body surface area. The use of nomograms is cumbersome. Because maintenance volume calculations based solely on body surface area nomograms are so variable, their use is not recommended as the basis for determining parenteral fluid dosage.[16, 17]

The more direct and accepted method of calculating fluid requirements is based solely on body weight. Both systems (surface area and body weight) ignore variations in metabolic rates and differences in percentage of lean body mass. However, a system based on body weight is preferable because it is far easier for the examiner to obtain a consistent and accurate measurement of weight than an accurate measurement of height for a squirming infant. Plotting accurate weights is often the most reliable single method for determining changes in volume status. The introduction of beds that provide continuous weight measurements will undoubtedly simplify fluid maintenance therapy.

Calorie Consumption

Most critical in calorie measurements is to always identify any child that can be hypoglycemic. Particularly during resuscitation or acute illness, clinical signs may be unspecific.[18] Calorie expenditure[19] has become the standard for determining the fluid and calorie requirements of infants. In 1911, Howland[20] measured energy consumption in children. His data, which agree closely with currently accepted data, indicated that infants under 1 year of age (3 to 10 kg) metabolize 100 cal/kg/day, whereas older infants and adults metabolize 75 and 35 cal/kg/day, respectively. Howland concluded that infants have increased calorie requirements because of their rapid growth rate and their proportionally larger body surface area.

In 1957, Holliday and Segar[21] reviewed data on basal metabolic requirements and active energy requirements by body weight. Between the active and basal requirement curves, they extrapolated a third curve to estimate the requirements for patients at bed rest, designated "hospitalized patients" (Fig. 5–1). The slope of the curve was determined from three lines drawn between body weight curves for 3 to 10 kg, 11 to 20 kg, and more than 21 kg body weight. The calorie expenditure of hospitalized infants was approximately 100 cal/kg/day. Half of these calories were used for basal metabolic needs and the remainder were required for growth. In children weighing more than 10 kg but less than 20 kg, the growth rate slowed and the child's calorie requirements decreased to about 50 cal/kg/day. Metabolic requirements beyond 20 kg of body weight[19, 20] were substantially decreased to about 20 cal/kg/day. These data indicate that maintenance calorie rates are nonlinear. The 1-year-old, 10-kg infant requires 1,000 cal/day, whereas his 20-kg older sibling, who is twice the infant's weight, requires only 50 percent more calories,

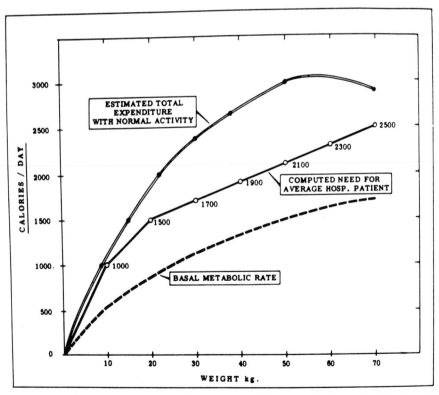

FIGURE 5–1. Using the data from Talbot et al.,[18, 19] Holliday and Segar[21] produced this figure. Talbot estimated the minimum energy required by unstressed patients (*lower graph*) and the energy required by the normal persons and stressed patients (plotted on the *upper graph*). The "computed need" is "calculated from the simple equations and is necessarily arbitrary" to estimate maintenance fluid requirements based on body weight. The computed line was derived from these now widely accepted equations:
1. 0–10 kg = 100 kcal/kg
2. 10–20 kg = 1,000 kcal + 50 kcal/kg for each kg over 10 kg but less than 20 kg
3. 20 kg and up = 1,500 kcal + 20 kcal/kg for each kg over 20 kg
(From Holliday MA, Segar WE: Maintenance need for water in parenteral fluid therapy. Pediatrics 19:823, 1957, with permission.)

1,500 cal/day. The 70-kg parent, who is about 10 times the infant's weight, requires only two to three times the number of calories required by the neonate. Metabolic rate was chosen because it is easily determined and more physiologically understandable. Increases in metabolic rates caused by hyperthyroidism, salicylism, fever, and exposure increase calorie requirements. Fever increases calorie needs by 10 to 12 percent per degree centigrade elevation from euthermia. Reductions in metabolic rate decrease caloric requirements by a similar amount.[21]

General anesthesia essentially mimics calorie requirements at closer to basal metabolic rates. Lindahl,[22] using indirect calorimetry, calculated the energy, fluid, and electrolyte needs of 31 infants and children during halothane anesthesia. In these patients, weighing up to 25 kg, his assessment of calorie and fluid requirements followed different regression equations (Table 5–1). The calorie, fluid, and electrolyte requirements are calculated according to the following four equations[22]:

$$\text{Caloric requirements} = 1.5 \times \text{kg} + 5 = \text{maintenance calories per hour (kcal/h)}$$

$$\text{Fluid requirements} = 2.5 \times \text{kg} + 10 = \text{maintenance fluid per hour (ml/h)}$$

$$\text{Sodium requirements} = 0.045 \times \text{kg} + 0.16 = \text{maintenance Na}^+ \text{ per hour (mEq/h)}$$

$$\text{Potassium requirements} = 0.03 \times \text{kg} + 0.10 = \text{maintenance K}^+ \text{ per hour (mEq/h)}$$

Maintenance Glucose

The Lindahl formula for calorie requirements during general anesthesia

$$1.5 \times \text{wt (kg)} + 5 = \text{kcal/kg/h}$$

predicts a far smaller glucose requirement than the formula suggested by Holliday and Segar[21] for hospitalized children. They proposed that calorie and fluid requirements were the same. However, Lindahl demonstrated that in anesthetized children 166 ml of fluid was required for every 100 calories metabolized. Since intraoperative hypoglycemia, even after prolonged fasting, is exceedingly

TABLE 5–1
HOURLY FLUID MAINTENANCE THERAPY

Weight (kg)	Fluid Required
0–10	4 ml/kg/h
10–20	40 ml + 2 ml/kg/h above 10 kg
>20	60 ml + 1 ml/kg/h above 20 kg
Examples	
3	12 ml/h
5	20
10	40
15	50
20	60
30	80
40	100

rare in children,[23] glucose-free balanced salt solutions are usually preferred in the operating room.

More critical for the anesthesiologist are the findings that brain, heart, and intestines may suffer greater damage during ischemic events when glucose infusions are used. The current trend of avoiding glucose-containing IV solutions in the operating room requires closer monitoring of blood glucose levels, particularly during the first 2 days of life.[24] Since as many as 2 billion home glucose measurements have been completed by diabetic patients in the United States, certainly the technology and cost should enable pediatric anesthesiologists to complete these same tests in operating room suites. This is especially important for premature infants with limited glycogen stores and for children receiving central hyperalimentation. I use a simple and relatively inexpensive bedside system (HemoCue B-Glucose, HemoCue AB, Ängelholm, Sweden) to follow intraoperative and intensive care unit variations in serum glucose. A partial drop (5 μl) of whole blood is touched by a sodium azide-containing plastic cuvette. A hand-held photometer, which utilizes a glucose dehydrogenase reaction, displays within a minute an accurate blood glucose value that is independent of sudden shifts in serum protein, a common event in cases of hemodilution or massive hemorrhage.[25]

Analyzing blood for serum glucose does have some inherent problems. Lances used to puncture fingers or toes leave scars and the wound can be painful for hours. The procedure is often messy and exposes the anesthesiologist to blood. Although urine screening for glucose has been used for years, the level is not linear with serum measurements, and there is a considerable lag in time compared with serum glucose. Urine testing to follow low blood glucose concentrations is impossible because no glucose is excreted by the normal kidney until the blood glucose exceeds 160 mg/dl. Even in the parturient, no glucose is detected in urine with serum glucose below 100 mg/dl. Other body fluids more closely aligned with the blood have been investigated, including interstitial fluid, cerebrospinal fluid, aqueous humor, lymph, sweat, and tears. Although the use of blood, sweat, and tears has a certain literary appeal, sweat and tears have poor linear correlation with serum glucose, are often more difficult to obtain, and demonstrate a significant lag time.

Maintenance Fluids

Metabolism requires substantially more water than it produces. Unlike the anesthetized child, the awake child has no net loss of water during metabolism of 100 calories. Metabolism of 1 calorie produces 0.2 ml of water and consumes 1.2 ml of water. Therefore, in the awake child calorie and water consumption are considered equal. The 1-year-old child weighing 10 kg requires 100 calories of energy and 100 ml of water per kilogram per day. Table 5–1 lists the hourly maintenance fluid requirements.

Pictured in Figure 5–2 are two infants with the same conception date. Their due date was 6 months before this photograph was taken. However, the smaller child was born at 28 weeks' gestation with a weight of 0.9 kg, whereas the larger infant was born 12 weeks later at 40 weeks'

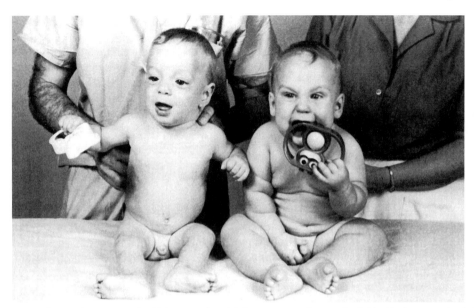

FIGURE 5–2. How fat are these 6-month-old (corrected age) infants? Count the arm fat folds. The larger 10-kg baby has five arm folds, and his wiry playmate has only one. Fat layers on the face and torso, legs, and arms of the larger baby yield a total body fat content over 40 percent versus less than 10 percent in the smaller, premature infant. This means that the more active and lean 5-kg infant may actually require the same fluid and calories as his heavier, less active 10-kg playmate.

gestation (term) with a weight of 4.2 kg. The term infant has followed a growth curve for both height and weight above the 90th percentile, and his fat content now exceeds 40 percent of total body weight. The growth of the smaller child is consistent with a curve that is two SD below normal. His fat content is about 10 percent of total body weight. Although the smaller infant is only half the weight of the larger infant, determinations of both lean body mass and calorie intake are similar. However, according to standard maintenance formulas, the larger 10-kg infant would require twice the fluids, minerals, and calories needed by the thinner 5-kg infant. Both infants at present have an almost identical intake of water and calories, approximately 250 ml (8 oz) of formula every 4 to 6 hours. If body weight is the only factor used to calculate maintenance fluid requirements and if lean body weights and metabolic rates are not taken into account, large errors in the estimated fluid requirements can occur.

Calculating the fluid deficit caused by an overnight fast can lead to administration of too much water. Take, for example, the chubby 10-kg, 6-month-old infant who has had nothing by mouth (NPO) overnight before a surgical procedure. Replacing his overnight "deficit" and supplying him with the standard maintenance volume up to lunch time would require 24 oz of fluid. Well children can tolerate large volumes of fluid, but few 6-month-old infants drink three bottles of fluid at one sitting to replace overnight deficits. Sleeping through the night, much to the parents' delight, is possible for any healthy neonate, demonstrating that infants can tolerate prolonged fasting. Therefore, no parenteral fluids may be required for short procedures in healthy infants. Conversely, infants undergoing longer, more traumatic operations and those who are toxic benefit from preoperative parenteral hydration in anticipation of large fluid losses during surgery.

Complex surgical procedures are often associated with rapid changes in fluid requirements, necessitating frequent reassessment and modification of therapy. The pediatrician carefully calculates the daily requirements for fluids and electrolytes for an individual child. In most hospitalized children, fluid, electrolyte, and metabolic needs are relatively constant over the day. In the operating room, the fluid requirements may change rapidly during the induction of anesthesia or surgery, coincident with changes in temperature, metabolism, and fluid volume shifts. The trauma, hemorrhage, and tissue exposure associated with surgery shift body fluids between compartments, necessitating fluid replacement with solutions that compensate for energy, water, blood, protein, and electrolyte losses. The anesthesiologist must determine the nature and magnitude of these losses and be alert both to the obvious fluid losses of serum and urine and to hidden fluid losses, such as can occur with evaporation or loss of body fluids into the surgical drapes.

Anesthetics blunt normal body fluid homeostatic responses, often necessitating increased administration of fluids to maintain adequate circulating blood volume. Unlike the pediatrician who can carefully plan maintenance fluid administration over a 24-hour period, the anesthesiologist must frequently modify intraoperative fluid administration in response to a series of observations. Heart rate, pulse, mean arterial pressure, capillary filling time, and urine output are important components of these observations. Monitoring the trends of these variables, as well as changes in hematocrit and urine osmolarity, is essential to planning effective replacement therapy. During major surgical procedures and in children with unstable hemodynamic function, continuous direct measurement of arterial and central venous pressures is of great assistance in perioperative fluid management (see Chapter 11).

Whatever system of fluid administration is chosen, it is essential to keep it simple. Dehydration is associated with increases in core body temperature and irritability, and rehydration increases exercise tolerance and attenuates hyperthermia.[26, 27] Calculations of fluid and electrolyte requirements must be understandable and practical to avoid mistakes that can have dire consequences in small children.

ELECTROLYTES

Late nineteenth century physiologists and chemists discovered that supplemental dietary electrolytes were essential to life. Pigeons fed an ash-free diet suffered fractured bones and died. Mice fed salt-free milk also had an early demise compared with siblings fed the same foods containing salt.[28] Ringer[29] found that the normal rhythm of an isolated heart preparation could be sustained by adding potassium to a sodium chloride solution. His early studies on ash salts led to the widely accepted parenteral solution known as Ringer's lactate.

Subsequent studies compared total body mineral mass in the developing fetus, term infant, and adult. The 4-month fetus was found to have only 1 percent ash content, whereas the total body weight of term babies and adults has 3 and 4.5 percent as ash, respectively. These data, derived from desiccation procedures, illustrate how the relative body stores of electrolytes are increased by growth, and they correlate well with our present understanding that a gradual reduction of body water content during development and growth corresponds to a proportional increase in solid mineral content. Similar analyses of electrolyte balance were also conducted by measuring the ash content of cow's milk versus human milk at oral intake and determining the ash content of urine and stool losses.[30]

MAINTENANCE FLUIDS AND ELECTROLYTES

The usual maintenance requirements for water, electrolytes, and glucose can be standardized using metabolic rates. This ratio of glucose to electrolytes has become part of currently commercial parenteral fluid preparations. The values generally accepted are found in Table 5–2.

In a parenteral fluid solution, the figures shown in Table 5–2 become 250 g of dextrose, 1.46 g of NaCl, and 1.49 g

TABLE 5–2
REPLACEMENT REQUIREMENT FOR EVERY 100 CALORIES METABOLIZED

Water	100 ml
Sodium	2.5 mEq
Potassium	2.0 mEq
Chloride	5.0 mEq
Glucose	25 g

From Hoobler BR: The role of mineral salts in the metabolism of infants. Am J Dis Child 2:107, 1911. Copyright 1911 American Medical Association, with permission.

of KCl in 1 L of water (25 percent dextrose in 0.15 percent NS plus KCl 20 mEq/L). In standard maintenance fluids, more NaCl and only 20 to 40 percent of the calculated dextrose requirement are generally used, yielding a maintenance fluid that is 5 to 10 percent dextrose and saline that is 0.2 to 0.9 percent of normality.

The 0.25, 0.33, 0.50, and 0.90 percent NS solutions contain, respectively, 38.5, 51.3, 77, and 154 mEq of sodium per liter. Ringer's lactate, a frequently used isotonic replacement solution, approximates serum concentrations of electrolytes. For each liter of water, Ringer's lactate solution contains the following: Na, 130 mEq; K, 4 mEq; Cl, 109 mEq; Ca, 3 mEq; and lactate, 28 mEq.

In 1999, Abbott initiated selling, at just twice the cost of standard lactated Ringer's (LR) solution, a balanced salt solution with enough chloride removed to add another anion, lactate, and 6 percent hetastarch (Hextend). Instead of the usual overdose of chloride in normal saline (NS), 154 mEq/L, the final solution is 124 mEq/L. This solution incorporates the advantage of the buffer in LR and the saline in NS with an additional colloid kick. With minimal experience in children but with the stated advantages, such hybrid solutions may well find themselves in common usage for large fluid-requiring operations.

When more than 5 or 10 percent dextrose is administered at rates sufficient to meet water requirements, the increased renal solute load may lead to urinary losses of both water and glucose, a glucose diuresis. Maintenance therapy with a 5 percent dextrose solution, although providing only 20 percent of the calories that are metabolized, results in decreased catabolism of endogenous protein and a lower renal solute load. This concentration of dextrose is recommended for short-term therapy, but higher concentrations of glucose are required to provide total parenteral nutrition. Total calorie requirements can usually be met by a gradual increase in dextrose concentration, which avoids the loss of glucose in the urine, and by addition of lipids and protein to an intravenous solution.

The Rebirth of Oral Rehydration

In a review of oral rehydration, Avery and Snyder[31] concluded that the evidence favoring the use of oral rehydration over IV therapy was overwhelming. She stated that the main impediment for implementation in the United States was that the use of a simple oral solution was "counterintuitive" compared with a complicated inpatient system of IV therapy technology. Now that oral rehydration has become the solution for pediatric diarrheal illnesses throughout the world, adults are also receiving this miraculous treatment.[32] The WHO-UNICEF formula is a package containing glucose (20 g/L water) and three basic salts: NaCl (3.5 g/L water), KCl (1.5 g/L water), and either trisodium citrate (2.9 g/L water) or sodium bicarbonate (2.5 g/L water). The premixed solutions available to families in the United States are given in Table 5–3.

Contraindications to the use of oral rehydration include severe gastrointestinal reflux and vomiting, ileus, and shock. Early vigorous use of oral solutions should prevent most infants and children with diarrheal dehydration from requiring hospitalization. None of the antimotility or bind-

TABLE 5-3

COMPOSITION OF SOME ORAL GLUCOSE-ELECTROLYTE SOLUTIONS AND OTHER CLEAR LIQUIDS*

Solution	Manufacturer	Na	K	Cl	Base (mmol/L)	Glucose[†]	Osmolality
Rehydration							
WHO-UNICEF oral rehydration salts	—	90	20	80	10[‡]	111 (20)	310
Rehydralyte	Ross	75	20	65	10[‡]	140 (25)	305
Maintenance							
Infalyte	Pennwalt	50	20	40	10[‡]	111 (20)	270
Lytren	Mead Johnson	50	25	45	10[‡]	111 (20)	290
Pedialyte	Ross	45	20	35	10[‡]	140 (25)	250
Resol	Wyeth	50	20	50	11[‡]	111 (20)	270
Clear liquid							
Cola	—	2	0.1	2	13[§]	730[‖]	750
Ginger ale	—	3	1	2	4[§]	500[‖]	540
Apple juice	—	3	28	30	0[§]	690[‖]	730
Chicken broth	—	250	8	250	0[§]	0	450
Tea	—	0	0	0	0[§]	0	5

* The solutions labeled "clear liquids" are inappropriate when used alone for rehydration in the presence of diarrhea. The composition of all other solutions is within acceptable ranges.
[†] Values in parentheses are grams per liter.
[‡] Citrate is used.
[§] Bicarbonate is used.
[‖] Combination of glucose and fructose.
From Avery ME, Snyder JD: Oral therapy for acute diarrhea. N Engl J Med 323:892, 1990, with permission.

ing medications was shown to decrease acute diarrheal water losses.

TOTAL BODY WATER

The perturbations of body fluid homeostasis caused by anesthesia and surgery require that certain terms be understood. A solution that causes no movement of water into or out of a cell is called *isotonic*. Fluids are of equal osmolarity on both sides of the cell membrane area. *Osmolarity* is the concentration of solute in a solution per unit of solvent and is expressed as osmoles per liter. Throughout fetal life, the solutions within and around the cells are of similar osmolarity: 280 to 300 mOsm/L. When an osmotic imbalance between compartments occurs, water and electrolytes redistribute rapidly to correct the imbalance.

Cells are suspended, supported, and provided with nourishment by the extracellular fluid. The cellular and extracellular interfaces are in osmotic and electrical balance. The electrical balance that allows potassium to be the intracellular cation and sodium to predominate as the extracellular cation is controlled by the sodium-potassium pump.[33] The small diffusion distances between extracellular and intracellular fluid allow nutrients to enter and waste products to be removed easily from the cells.

Fluid compartments within the body vary with age. Although the osmolarity of each fluid compartment is essentially constant throughout development, the fraction of fluids in each space changes. Ingestion or injection of radioactive isotopes has been used to determine the size of these spaces. However, the use of deuterium (D_2O) overestimates total body water by as much as 14 percent in growing primates compared with the water content determined by desiccation.[34] This overestimation is largely because of the rapid growth of the neonate and the incor-

poration of radioisotopes within the solid portions of the body. Studies have demonstrated a much closer agreement between body fluid compartments and desiccation. Using techniques widely used in the meat industry, body electrical conductivity,[35] and magnetic resonance imaging,[36] investigators can reliably and noninvasively measure body composition and the ratio of lean body mass to fat in human infants. A 1-kg, 28-week-gestation fetus is 80 percent water and only 1 percent total body fat. At term, total body water has decreased to 70 to 75 percent and a gradual shift of fluid from the extracellular space to the cells has occurred. One relatively anhydrous solid component, fat, has gradually increased to 17 percent of body weight by birth. At 3 months of age, the average infant has doubled in weight to 6 kg, and the total body fat content has increased to 30 percent. With these increases, total body water decreases to less than 65 percent of total body mass because the total cellular mass, including fat cells, has increased (Fig. 5–3).[37]

Extracellular Fluid

The mechanisms of extracellular fluid are discussed in a recent review.[38] The fluid includes the intravascular blood or plasma volume and the interstitial fluid and is determined by sodium and accompanying anions. These components are separated from each other by the vascular endothelium. The plasma volume and interstitial fluid volume together form the functional extracellular fluid compartment. Guyton et al.[39] described the interstitial fluid space as a gelatinous matrix that normally has a negative pressure and an elastic component. The latter allows storage of fluid that rapidly filters out of the vascular space when the plasma volume is high. Decreases in the circulating volume are corrected when fluid within the interstitium shifts to the plasma volume. Therefore, when the central venous pressure is low (i.e., when the intravascular vol-

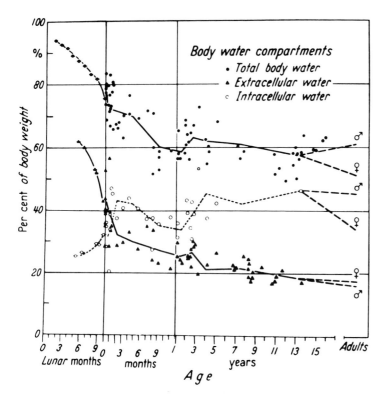

FIGURE 5–3. Body water compartments from fetal life to adult life. ●, total body water; ○, extracellular water; ▲, intracellular water. (From Venkatesh S, Schrier RW, Andreoli E: Mechanisms of tubular sodium chloride transport. Ren Fail 20:783, 1998, with permission.)

ume is low), more volume must be infused to increase central venous pressure. This situation represents an underfilled circulating volume. A rapidly increasing central venous pressure probably represents full saturation of circulatory and interstitial compartments. Oversaturation of plasma, interstitial, and cellular compartments increases transcellular fluids, causing generalized edema.

During adolescence, the volume of the interstitial space is about 20 percent of body mass. Adding the plasma volume, 7 to 10 percent of body mass, to the interstitial compartment yields a functional extracellular volume of 27 to 30 percent of the body mass. With proportionally larger plasma and interstitial compartments, the functional extracellular fluid volume of term infants may be 45 percent, whereas that of 28-week gestational age neonates may be as much as 60 percent of their total body mass. Although wide variations exist among age groups, the amount of functional extracellular fluid reserve is often insufficient to compensate for perioperative fluid losses in any size pediatric patient.

Transcellular water is nonfunctional extracellular fluid. It comprises an unavailable pool of water formed by transport of fluid from the cells and the extracellular space. It includes fluid within the lumen of the gastrointestinal tract, which increases dramatically with bowel obstruction. Surgical manipulation or other trauma also increases transcellular water volume. Ascites, pleural effusion, synovial and cerebrospinal fluid, urine, and stool are examples of transcellular water. Fluid that enters the transcellular space is essentially lost from the functional extracellular space. When plasma volume is lost directly during surgery or trauma, water, electrolytes, and protein are removed from the circulation and the interstitium.

Expansion of the extracellular fluid space (ECF) and increases in cardiac output (CO) are seen in many ill-

nesses. Ascites from any cause is related to an expansion of ECF and CO. Similar changes of high CO are seen in pregnancy, thyrotoxicosis, beriberi, and in patients with a large arteriovenous fistula.

The functional extracellular space is a reservoir for plasma and cellular fluid. Protein manufactured in the cells is stored within the extracellular tissues before it filters into the plasma compartment. Fully half of the total body plasma protein mass is located within the extracellular matrix of the skin and skeletal muscle.[40] During hemorrhage, intravascular plasma proteins are lost. Both intravascular and extracellular proteins are diluted when lost blood is replaced with crystalloid. Several days are required before extravascular plasma proteins become completely shifted into the plasma space. This is accomplished by a shift of extravascular plasma proteins into lymphatic channels to gradually replace the vascular protein deficit and is followed by an increase in protein synthesis.[41]

Most intraoperative fluid replacement is aimed at providing sufficient supplemental fluid to replace losses from the plasma and interstitial compartments. Intravenous administration of free water causes fluid to filter rapidly into the interstitium. Solutions such as 5 percent dextrose in 0.2 percent normal saline are almost 80 percent free water. Because fluid retention is a primary protective response to trauma, only balanced salt solutions should be used for preoperative maintenance fluids. Rapid filtration of free water into the extracellular fluid reduces the osmolarity and shifts water into the cells, causing anasarca.

During the early 1960s, Shires et al.[42] demonstrated that large amounts of fluid were sequestered in the "third space" during major surgical procedures. They suggested that large volumes of balanced salt solutions were required to replace fluid lost from the functional extracellular space. Intraoperative elevations in vasopressin (antidiuretic hormone) and aldosterone induce the renal tubules to avidly retain water and sodium. This fluid is distributed into the intravascular, interstitial, cellular, and transcellular compartments.

The enthusiasm for providing large volumes of supplemental fluids during surgery has been tempered by the subsequent finding that the radiolabeled sulfate used to measure extracellular fluid volume did not fully gain entrance into the functional extracellular fluid space. Therefore, the volume of extracellular fluid in the third space was overestimated. It is now generally agreed that giving excessive amounts of fluid creates a larger volume of sequestered fluid during and for a brief period after surgery. Infusion of excessive volumes of a balanced salt solution decreases the concentration of the plasma proteins within the entire functional extracellular compartment. This dilution of proteins and the excess of fluid increases transcellular fluid sequestration and cellular volume by oversaturation of the extracellular fluid compartment. Such a fluid overload delays the diuresis and protein fluxes necessary to achieve postoperative recovery of fluid balance. Conversely, major emergency operations, severe shock, hemorrhage, large burns, and other traumatic injuries cause massive loss and redistribution of fluids. Large volumes of supplemental fluids are required to avoid hypovolemia. Algorithms for diagnosing and treating some electrolyte disorders are readily available.[43]

Four major compensatory mechanisms that restore plasma volume have been reviewed[44]:

1. The neural and humoral factors that control the kidney act to decrease urine output.
2. Shifts of interstitial fluid from the skin, skeletal muscle, and bowel filter into the vascular space to augment plasma volume.
3. Hypoglycemia induced by stress decreases plasma osmolality, thus mobilizing cellular fluid to shift into the plasma space.
4. An important contribution to plasma refill is a massive increase in the absorptive capacity of the small intestine.

Intracellular Fluid

Total body water minus the extracellular fluid volume equals the intracellular fluid volume. The fluid within the cells is essentially isotonic with the surrounding interstitial fluid, because cell membranes allow free movement of water in either direction. Cell volume remains constant when isotonic fluids are administered. However, it may rapidly increase when hypotonic fluid is administered, owing to inward shifts of free water. Much of the water in the cells is bound to proteins (i.e., it does not readily participate in osmotic shifts between fluid compartments).

As previously emphasized, cells absorb or excrete water across the cell membranes in response to changes in extracellular osmolarity. Sodium is the predominant extracellular cation and potassium the predominant intracellular cation. Renal excretion of potassium in exchange for sodium increases the extracellular water space. Renal tubules conserve both water and extracellular sodium by concentrating the urine and secreting potassium. To pre-

vent intraoperative potassium losses, intraoperative fluid replacement should provide adequate supplementation of both sodium and water. It takes days to replete intracellular potassium deficits when potassium is given intravenously. Therefore, postoperative fluids should contain enough potassium to gradually replenish that lost during surgery.

Energy is required to transport potassium into and sodium out of water-permeable cells to maintain body fluid homeostasis. Cells, including cerebral cells, swell with hypotonic or shrink with hypertonic fluid administration. Rapid shifts in serum osmolarity can disrupt the fragile cerebrovascular network between the cells.

Mannitol, hypertonic saline, or infusion of any other hypertonic solution can momentarily increase cerebral blood flow by lowering viscosity. Although flow to the brain increases, intracerebral pressure rapidly decreases because these hyperosmotic solutions draw water out of cerebral cells. Such rapid shifts of fluid within the brain have been associated with central nervous system (CNS) hemorrhage in premature infants. Hypertonic solutions such as standard bicarbonate solutions and mannitol have been associated with intraventricular hemorrhage. In kittens, peritoneal injection of hypertonic saline caused an abrupt decrease in brain water.[45] On the other hand, administration of free-water-containing solutions to infants with hypernatremic dehydration causes CNS bleeding owing to rapid shifts of water into hypertonic cells.[46] Treatment of hypo- or hypernatremic dehydration is discussed below.

ANESTHETIC EFFECTS ON VASCULAR VOLUME

The ideal anesthetic would have no effect on vascular volume. However, both regional and general anesthetics decrease circulating blood volume and cause fluid shifts to occur between the plasma volume and the interstitium.[47] Interactions between anesthetics and vascular volume are only part of the many circulatory disturbances caused by anesthetics that must be understood before an anesthetic technique and fluid therapy can be chosen.

Hypotensive Effects

Inhalational anesthetics have many disruptive effects on homeostatic control of the circulation.[48] In adults, isoflurane causes hypotension because it reduces total peripheral resistance[49]; halothane causes hypotension because it depresses myocardial function. Ketamine, halothane, isoflurane, and narcotics decrease vascular resistance and cause hypotension in neonates.[50] Narcotics, barbiturates, benzodiazepines, and volatile anesthetics cause vasodilation, which increases the total vascular capacity and blunts the reflex that normally corrects hypovolemic hypotension.

Some surgeons and pediatricians are unfamiliar with the effects of anesthesia on the circulating volume. By focusing only on the retention of water coincident with trauma, elevations of vasopressin resulting from intraoperative extracellular fluid contraction, and the few postoperative days required to regain normal volume status, these physicians fail to appreciate the fact that increased amounts of fluid are required during anesthesia to correct the hypotension that is so common in infants and young children.

Venous Capacity

In normal patients, veins contain as much as 80 percent of the systemic blood volume. The remaining 20 percent is within the arteries. Changes in blood pressure or cardiac output cause veins to constrict or dilate. Baroreceptors in the carotid sinus, liver, and spleen sense pressure changes and, via the sympathetic nervous system, alter venous return to the heart. Stimulation of carotid sinus baroreceptors increased venous capacitance by 8 ml/kg before and 11 ml/kg after vagotomy.[51] The baroreceptor reflex response resulted in venous dilation and decreased venous return to the heart. Decreases in blood pressure cause reflex venous constriction and increased blood flow to the heart. The veins of the spleen, liver, and skeletal muscle store blood, and these veins participate in passive and active changes of vascular capacitance.

Changes in Venous Capacitance

Passive changes of venous volume follow Ohm's law, which states that a pressure (P) drop along the vasculature equals flow (F) times resistance (R):

$$\Delta P = F \times R$$

Veins become less elastic and passively dilate after exposure to narcotics and volatile anesthetics. With more blood sequestered in the dilated veins, less blood returns to the heart and cardiac output decreases. Children who are hypovolemic at the onset of anesthesia become effectively more hypovolemic because of this passive venous dilation. These children require less anesthesia, more intravascular volume, or both to maintain adequate cardiac output.

Active changes in venous capacity are mediated by the sympathetic nervous system. In a dose-dependent manner, halothane and isoflurane decrease the ability of the baroreceptors to mediate the capacitance changes necessary to ensure increased return of venous blood to the heart during lowered perfusion states. At increased systemic blood pressures, the normal reflex-induced increase in venous capacitance, which decreases central venous return, is also blunted. Of particular note is the fact that the gain in baroreflex capacitance during isoflurane anesthesia is significantly more preserved compared with capacitance during anesthesia with an equipotent concentration of halothane.[52] The underlying mechanism for this difference appears to be a greater sparing of sympathetic nerve activity by isoflurane than by halothane. In animals with reduced blood volumes, greater cardiac output and regional blood flows were found with isoflurane than with enflurane, halothane, and ketamine.[53] Ketamine supports the circulation of normal, volume-expanded patients but has effects similar to those of thiopental in hypovolemic patients. Both decrease cardiac output, heart rate, and

vascular resistance.[54] From the standpoint of volume control, isoflurane or sevoflurane seems to be the preferred agent in patients with moderate hypovolemia, since both maintain sympathetic nervous control in moderate doses.

Temperature and Ventilatory Effects

During anesthesia, patients often require mechanical ventilation because they are hypercarbic. Acute hypercarbia is compensated for by loss of HCO_3^- and Cl^- ions and water from the cells to the interstitium. This loss shrinks the intracellular fluid compartment while increasing the extracellular volume. Hypocarbia and hypothermia are associated with a shift of water, HCO_3^-, and Cl^- into cells. During rapid volume loss, avoidance of hypothermia and maintenance of moderate, acute hypercarbia prevents additional losses of fluid from the extracellular to the intracellular space, which can assist in maximizing the functional extracellular fluid volume. Therefore, warming replacement fluids and avoiding hyperventilation during episodes of hypovolemia are strongly advised.

FLUIDS AND ELECTROLYTES IN THE NEWBORN

Understanding the homeostasis of pediatric body fluids requires an understanding of human fetal physiology and of the rapid growth rate of the neonate. The total body mass of the term infant is expected to double between birth and 3 months of age. By 1 year of age, growth has gradually slowed. The infant is now three times birth weight, or 9 to 10 kg. Children whose fetal development is interrupted by very premature birth or severe growth retardation are termed *very low birth weight* (VLBW) infants.

The surgeon and anesthesiologist may insist on the presence of a neonatal specialist in the operating room to manage the complex fluid, mineral, and metabolic needs of these babies. Although this practice has been beneficial in some centers, it usually leads to management by committee, as no single physician understands the overall needs of the neonate. In emergencies, this may lead to delayed and inappropriate decisions. Just as the premature or VLBW neonate requires the expertise of perinatal specialists to maximize the chances of becoming a well baby, the sick, undersized, traumatized infant facing corrective or palliative surgery requires the care of physicians experienced with and knowledgeable about the effects of anesthesia and trauma on the neonate. Working together, physicians in the nursery and the operating room can continue to learn from each other. In the operating room, one physician, the anesthesiologist, must take responsibility for the child's care.

Very Low Birth Weight Infants

The decreasing morbidity and mortality of VLBW neonates is mainly because of effects by the subspecialties of perinatology and neonatology. Although the incidence of preterm and VLBW infants has not decreased, the improvement in outcome has dramatically increased. Therefore, we continue to see an ever-increasing number of nursery patients and nursery graduates for elective, emergent, and emergency operations to repair or palliate congenital and developmental defects. For the anesthesiologist who cares for these babies, an understanding of their altered fluid, electrolyte, and metabolic needs is crucial to the well-being of these infants. The following case illustrates perioperative concerns regarding fluids, electrolytes, and metabolic requirements of VLBW babies compared with term infants.

> A healthy parturient is about to deliver prematurely. At a gestational age of 26 to 28 weeks, the infant K.G. is expected to be no larger than 1 kg. The obstetrician informs you that K.G. has normal fetal heart tones and that the amniotic membranes are intact with normal amniotic fluid volume detected by ultrasound.

Fetal Fluids

An important consideration in assessing K.G.'s fluid balance is the recognition that amniotic fluid and maternal circulation function as an expanded extracellular fluid compartment.

Amniotic fluid is isotonic. It is produced from fetal urine and secretions derived from the fetal lung. Each day, 200 to 1,000 ml of urine and 200 to 400 ml of fluid from the fetal lung are excreted.[55] Other minor sources of amniotic fluid include salivary and nasal secretions. Because the skin is keratinized by 28 weeks' gestation, K.G.'s transcutaneous absorption of fluid is not significant. Therefore, K.G. absorbs amniotic fluid by swallowing. The swallowing is the "in," and the urine and tracheal secretion represent the "out"; there is a total turnover of approximately 1 L each day during the final trimester of pregnancy. The urine is slightly hypotonic because even under stress the fetal kidney cannot excrete hypertonic urine. Although a loop diuretic such as furosemide does cross the placenta, it does not increase the urine output of moderately dehydrated or stressed babies, presumably because their vasopressin concentrations are high.[56] K.G.'s renal response to vasopressin and aldosterone is similar to that of a term infant. High cortisol levels, however, result in a two- to fivefold increase in urine flow and in excretion of Na^+, Cl^-, and K^+ ions.[52] Potassium rapidly shifts from intracellular to extracellular compartments immediately after birth, leading to relatively higher serum values. With increased glomerular filtration rate and the onset of postnatal diuresis facilitating potassium excretion, plasma potassium levels generally decrease after birth.[57]

Dehydration cannot be diagnosed in fetuses, but certain stressed and most growth-retarded fetuses are relatively underhydrated after birth. Growth-retarded neonates have significantly increased water requirements compared with those who are appropriate for gestational age.[58]

Acute stress (e.g., hemorrhage, hypoxia, hypertonicity) is associated with decreased urine output and increased concentration of serum vasopressin in the fetus.[55] Fluid shifts within the mother are reflected in the fetus. After injection of hypertonic saline into pregnant ewes, fetal blood volume was reduced 11 percent owing to an increase in fetal osmolality with a shift of fluid out of the fetus. However, this effect was transient; the blood volume returned to baseline within an hour.[55] When pregnant ewes were deprived of fluids for 5 days, the fetal blood volume increased normally.[59] After 2 days of maternal Na^+ depletion, the sodium concentrations in both fetus and mother were decreased, suggesting rapid transplacental equilibration of solute.[60]

In human parturition, giving free-water-containing IV fluids in an attempt to inhibit preterm labor increases the risk of pneumothorax and pneumopericardium at birth. Stressed neonates and infants from vaginal deliveries demonstrate higher concentrations of arginine vasopressin secretion and increased urine output than nonstressed neonates and healthy infants delivered by cesarean section.[60, 61] Just as changes within the fetus parallel changes within the amniotic fluid, changes in maternal circulation can influence both fetal and amniotic fluid balance. Therefore, both the amniotic fluid and the maternal circulation function as extracellular compartments for the fetus.

Overhydration of the healthy fetus may not be possible. Brace[55] infused a balanced salt solution directly into a fetal lamb vein and measured the urine flow. He increased the infusion rates daily from 4 ml/h to a peak rate of 256 ml/h but found no edema in the fetus. Even though this IV infusion rate in the term lamb is equivalent to 80 ml/kg/h, urine output increased sufficiently to prevent changes in the fetal hematocrit. By infusing an isotonic solution of glucose, Battaglia et al.[62] were able to demonstrate parallel decreases in osmolality in both mother and fetus, presumably as a direct result of volume loading. As the women who received the infusions metabolized the glucose, both maternal and fetal osmolality decreased.

> Anesthesia is now required for an emergent cesarean section because of fetal distress and a breech presentation. Before administering a regional anesthetic, which the mother has requested, an infusion of 1.5 L of a balanced salt solution is planned to attenuate any circulatory alterations caused by the anesthetic. K.G.'s fluid balance should be unaffected if the placental circulation is not compromised and the maternal fluid, electrolyte, and metabolic status are normal.
>
> K.G. is delivered without difficulty and is vigorous and pink. After a brief moment in his mother's arms, he is whisked off to the nursery.

Fluid Balance at Birth

As summarized above, K.G. has been producing amniotic fluid from both urine and lung secretions. The latter have high chloride concentrations and are almost protein free. Before birth, the lung is filled with fluid (20 to 30 ml of isotonic fluid per kilogram). Substantial decreases in extravascular lung water occur late in gestation and during labor.[63] With the newborn's first breath, the flow of fluid into the terminal respiratory units reverses. The pulmonary interstitial space rapidly absorbs the essentially protein-free fluid to allow pulmonary gas exchange. This fluid is shifted into the pulmonary microcirculation by filtration from the interstitium toward the higher osmotic pressure of plasma. Thus, with his first breath, K.G. received a bolus of isotonic fluid. In addition, he absorbed a small volume of fluid into lung lymph channels. Subsequent breaths decreased the water pressure within the microcirculation, facilitating increases of blood flow and absorption of the interstitial fluid.

The plasma oncotic pressure is significantly lower in premature infants. K.G. and other 26- to 28-week neonates have a mean albumin concentration of 19 g/L, whereas 40-week term neonates average 31 g/L.[64] Subcutaneous edema is ubiquitous in premature infants, and the more premature the infant, the more pronounced is the edema. This degree of edema is associated with gestational age and is used in the Dubowitz scoring system for clinical determination of gestational age at birth.[65]

The severity of edema does not correlate with the plasma concentration of albumin, nor does IV infusion of human albumin reverse the edema.[64] Infused human albumin may actually increase edema in two ways. First, the additional salt load in human albumin (normal saline) may increase tissue edema. Second, capillary leakage of albumin into the interstitium increases the oncotic pressure of the interstitial space. When human albumin 0.5 mg/kg was infused into preterm neonates and transepidermal water losses were determined simultaneously, a significant inverse relation was found.[66] However, within 2 hours both water loss and intravascular albumin concentration had returned to preinfusion levels. The transient nature of this effect might be a result of the more rapid redistribution and larger volume of distribution of albumin in neonates compared to adults. In capillary leak syndromes, such as that seen in newborn infants on extracorporeal membrane oxygenation, exogenous albumin cannot measurably augment intravascular concentration.

Insensible Water Loss

In healthy children and adolescents, evaporation accounts for approximately 40 percent of total baseline water losses. However, in premature neonates, insensible water losses are several magnitudes greater because there is transepidermal water loss. Bare (exposed) premature infants have 15 times[67] more evaporative losses than naked term infants during the first few days after birth. Therefore, an exposed VLBW infant can lose 10 percent of body weight during the first day of life by this route. Evaporative losses, gestational age, and surface area are compared in Figure 5–4. Increased losses are believed to be caused by differences in skin permeability and skin water content, which are inversely related to gestational age in premature infants.

Other insensible water losses in premature neonates are caused by increased respiratory exchange. Premature infants maintain a higher respiratory rate and per-minute ventilation. K.G.'s normal respiratory rate is 80 breaths/min. The inefficient chest wall mechanics of the premature infant also increase the work of breathing, which has led some to advocate the use of tracheal intubation and mechanical ventilation for all VLBW infants to provide humidification and to spare calories needed for growth, but this suggestion has not received wide support.

Neonatologists and anesthesiologists can minimize insensible losses by wrapping infants in plastic and by providing a warm (euthermic), humid, still atmosphere. Incubators presently available offer a wide range of climate-controlled environments.[68] Humidifying the atmosphere and keeping the infant warm in a double-insulated isolette is effective in the nursery and during transport but is not practical during surgery. Babies cared for on open beds with overhead radiant heaters experience substantially increased losses of both water and energy. Despite this fact, surgeons should consider a modification of the open beds used to care for very ill neonates in the nursery. It is unclear if the infrared heater should be used when bowel is exposed, because the bowel may be injured by the heat.

In a study of VLBW babies who were cared for in open beds, oxygen consumption was constant and normal when their skin temperature was 36.5°C or more. When their skin temperature decreased by 1°C, their oxygen consumption increased significantly.[69] Just as the temperature in an incubator is adjusted to the infant's skin temperature, the output of the radiant heater should be monitored closely to prevent temperature increases (which would increase insensible water loss) or decreases (which would result in higher metabolic expenditure). Table 5–4 lists factors that increase insensible water losses.

Even in a neutral-thermal isolette, K.G. will have an evaporative loss of 60 ml during his first day of extrauterine life; after 3 weeks of age his evaporative losses will diminish to the level seen in term babies (10 ml/kg/day) because of skin changes.[70] In a warm operating room, even with room temperatures as high as 34° to 35°C, K.G.'s exposed skin temperature can rapidly decrease to 30°C because of evaporative heat loss. Wrapping his extremities and other nonoperative areas with plastic, warming all solutions (including preparation solutions), and using warm, humidified gases help to minimize the needless consumption of energy associated with increased evaporative water losses.

Neonatal Water and Electrolytes

Because sodium represents more than 90 percent of the cations and more than 90 percent of the osmotic pressure of the extracellular fluid compartment, the sodium concentration determines the size of the extracellular space. K.G.'s kidneys are less able to conserve sodium than those of term neonates, and therefore he must receive considerably more sodium than the 2 to 3 mEq/kg/day required by the latter. Early studies reported that neonatal kidneys are immature, as water and solute loads do not elicit the responses seen in adults, or at least do not elicit them to the same degree. These investigators did not know that birth caused secretion of hormones that were in part responsible for these differences. At birth, the kidney, which had a relatively passive response to stress in utero, must accommodate the rapid fluid shifts that occur after the abrupt withdrawal of the amniotic fluid and maternal circulation. The central osmoreceptors and peripheral volume receptors of infants must act to regulate water and sodium balance. The lack of renal responsiveness to a water or solute load may be a response to release of excessive effectors on both sides of the volume and so-

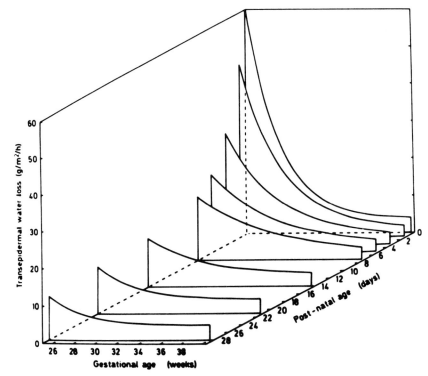

FIGURE 5–4. Transepidermal water loss (g/m²/h) plotted as a function of gestational age at birth and to 28 days of extrauterine life. Note that at birth the 26-week infant has more than 12 times the water loss of a 36- to 40-week infant. The 26-week infant at 28 days of age has only one fifth the water losses experienced during the first day of extrauterine life. (From Hammarlund K, Sedin G, Stromberg B: Transepidermal water lose in newborn infants. Acta Paediatr Scand 72:721, 1983, with permission.)

dium control system. At birth, fluid shifts required to open the lungs and maintain circulation occur coincidentally with massive elevations in the renin, aldosterone, and angiotensin system. Premature and term infants also have elevations in atrial natriuretic peptide (ANP),[71] a newly discovered hormone abundant in cardiac atrial tissue, which induces natriuresis and excretion of both water and sodium. Increases in plasma volume stretch the atria, which releases ANP and other vasoactive factors and thereby increases vascular capacitance. Premature infants with respiratory disease, especially those requiring mechanical ventilation, have higher concentrations of ANP. In these patients, ANP concentrations remained elevated despite negative water and sodium balance.[72]

It is no wonder that neonatal kidneys respond differently from those of adults: they are receiving conflicting messages. High aldosterone concentrations demand water re-

T A B L E   5 – 4
FACTORS THAT INCREASE INSENSIBLE WATER LOSS

Skin
    Decreased ambient humidity
    Increased air currents (drafts)
    Use of radiant heaters
    Increased air temperature (above neutral thermic)
    Decreased gestational age
    Increased motor activity
    Increased skin blood flow
    Phototherapy
    Increased core temperature

Respiration
    Dry inspired gas mixture
    Cool inspired gas mixture
    Increased minute ventilation
    Mouth breathing

tention via tubular sodium reabsorption, but at the same time vasopressors are constricting vessels to maintain arterial pressure. Angiotensin II signals the need for more renal sodium reabsorption, and high baseline natriuretic peptides signal the need for sodium excretion. Prostaglandins, which are present and active during the neonatal period, have differing renal effects. Their actions have been reviewed by Brenner and Stein.[73] At this time, it is unclear whether the newborn kidney is unresponsive to hormonal control or is merely confused.

Neonatal Renal Function

The term newborn kidney matures rapidly. Glomerular and proximal tubular function double in the term infant by 1 month of age,[74] whereas those of premature newborns such as K.G. mature gradually over the first few weeks. The chemical messengers, overabundant at birth, are gradually reduced and require a period of time to regenerate normal body stores.

Glomerular filtration rate is lower in premature than in term infants. After 34 weeks' gestation and the completion of nephrogenesis, the glomerular filtration rate of humans increases exponentially. However, unlike the case with adults, infusion of up to twice the volume of maintenance fluids during the first few days after birth does not increase the glomerular filtration rate in well-hydrated term infants. In one study, an increase in fluids was followed by brisk diuresis, presumably owing to decreased renal tubular reabsorption of water.[75] Other studies of preterm and term infants during the first day of extrauterine life sometimes revealed rapid changes in the glomerular filtration, corresponding to the state of hydration. This disparity in findings is further evidence that the reactivity of the renal vascular bed is increased during the perinatal period. Consequently, water and electrolyte homeostasis is difficult to predict during this period.

Water and electrolyte balance are controlled by renal structures located distal to the glomerulus. The maturation of renal tubular function lags substantially behind the maturation of glomerular function. Therefore, the neonate can produce a dilute urine but can concentrate urine to only about half as much as adults because of decreased tonicity in the medullary interstitium.[76] The function of renal tubular cells matures during the neonatal period. A 2-month-old infant can excrete urine with four times the osmolarity of plasma, whereas the term neonate can concentrate urine only to twice the osmolarity of plasma.

> An emergent procedure is planned for 3-day-old K.G. because free abdominal air is seen on the x-ray film. The baby's most notable physical feature is a toxic appearance. Vital signs are as follows: weight, 1.0 kg (up 50 g from the day before); heart rate, 180 beats/min (up from 160 beats/min); blood pressure, 45/30 mm Hg (down from 55/40 mm Hg); respiratory rate, 30 breaths/min on positive-pressure ventilator settings of 18/4 cm H_2O; temperature, 36.5°C.
>
> K.G. has a sunken anterior fontanelle, pale skin with poor turgor, and an intermittent waveform and saturation reading by pulse oximetry from his hand. His capillary filling time is prolonged to more than 5 seconds. Despite maintenance IV fluids of a balanced salt solution (150 ml/day) plus lipids, protein, and several blood transfusions, K.G. has had no urine ouput over the last 8 hours. He is "dry." His dehydration and any electrolyte imbalance, anemia, and hyperglycemia should be corrected before surgery. A careful preoperative plan that is coordinated with the neonatologist and bedside nurse is essential. With a central venous line in place, judicious boluses of a balanced salt solution can be administered and rehydration can be completed within an hour. K.G. should be well covered with cellophane and heated blankets for transport. The operating room should also be warmed before his arrival.

NEONATAL FLUID, ELECTROLYTE, AND METABOLIC HOMEOSTASIS

Sodium and Hydration

As emphasized in the case above, K.G.'s first day after birth would normally involve large fluid shifts. Owing to the expanded circulating fluid volume caused by the pulmonary interstitial fluid shifts coincident with birth, his initial fluid requirements for the first 2 days of life are about 90 and 75 ml/kg, respectively.

Serum sodium is variable in the premature infant. Therefore, it may be a relatively poor indicator of the infant's hydration status. Preterm infants have high renal and intestinal sodium losses and require additional sodium supplementation, either oral (PO) or IV, during the first 2 weeks of life.[77] The increased growth that occurs during sodium supplementation continues beyond this initial 2-week treatment period, suggesting that a positive sodium balance stimulates growth.[78] It is interesting to note that milk

from mothers who deliver a preterm infant contains two to three times more sodium than milk from mothers who deliver at term.[79]

Hyponatremia may also be caused by water retention. The use of positive-pressure ventilation and continuous positive airway pressure (CPAP), irrespective of the presence or absence of respiratory distress, is associated with natriuresis and with increased water retention and vasopressin release.[80]

Intracerebral hemorrhage and pneumothorax are also associated with acute imbalances in neonatal water homeostasis.[81, 82] Infusions of water, glucose, or hypertonic sodium have been associated with intracerebral hemorrhage in preterm infants. Rapid cerebral fluid shifts from hyper- or hypotonic solutions are thought to be the cause.[82] Marked changes in systemic blood pressure have also been associated with intracerebral hemorrhage. Continuous infusions of a balanced salt solution help to maintain circulating volume during surgery and anesthesia by preventing rapid changes in osmolarity and blood pressure.

Overhydration may cause pulmonary edema,[83] persistent patent ductus arteriosus,[84] and congestive heart failure. Therapies that lessen the likelihood of these risks include early, mild fluid and sodium restriction to decrease preload; diuretics (furosemide) to increase plasma protein concentration; cautious assisted ventilation with positive end-expiratory pressure (PEEP) to reduce supplemental oxygen requirement; adequate nutrition to promote protein synthesis and growth; and avoidance of factors that cause an increase in pulmonary blood flow, including hypoxia and painful or noxious stimuli.[63]

Because of their fear of overhydrating premature neonates, many neonatologists err on the side of underhydration in VLBW babies. The addition of anesthetics and perioperative fluid losses to this state of underhydration can lead to complete cardiovascular collapse and death. As previously emphasized, sodium requirements for VLBW infants are increased. Infants of less than 30 weeks' gestation require sodium at 5 mEq/kg/day, whereas infants of 30 to 35 weeks' gestation require 4 mEq/kg/day during the first 2 postnatal weeks.[77, 85]

Potassium

Because more than 98 percent of the total stores of potassium are intracellular, serum concentrations of potassium provide only a rough estimate of the amount of potassium in the total body. Disorders of potassium homeostasis in children have recently been reviewed.[86] Many medications used during the neonatal period induce renal potassium excretion, either directly or through their effect on pH. Such medications include diuretics (furosemide), steroids, antibiotics (aminoglycosides), and methylxanthines (theophylline). Respiratory or metabolic alkalosis signals the kidney to retain hydrogen ions at the expense of potassium ions. Extrarenal losses of potassium (e.g., gastric and intestinal fluid losses) may cause significant hypokalemia. Skin losses from perspiration constitute an additional, although minor, loss.

Glucose, insulin, calcium, and bicarbonate lower serum potassium by shifting potassium into cells. Therefore, they are clinically useful in acute management of hyperkalemia. β-Adrenergic compounds, especially albuterol, shift

TABLE 5-5
MEDICATIONS THAT INDUCE HYPERKALEMIA

Potassium supplementation
Salt substitutes
Mannitol
Indomethacin
Captopril
Heparin
Potassium-sparing diuretics
Succinylcholine
Digoxin overdose
Cyclosporin
Arginine hydrochloride
Aqueous penicillin G
Methicillin

potassium into the cells in exchange for sodium. This may explain why anxiety is associated with decreases in serum potassium.[87]

More worrisome than hypokalemia is hyperkalemia. Table 5-5 lists medications associated with increased serum potassium concentration. The serum potassium concentration increases with acidosis and decreases with alkalosis, without acutely changing total body potassium stores (Table 5-6). Cell membrane hypersensitivity to suxamethonium may cause a massive outpouring of potassium from the cells after repeated exposures. This is especially evident between 10 and 70 days after a burn, major trauma, tetanus, muscle dystrophies,[88] uremia, and in paraplegia between 14 to 28 days after the accident.[87]

Because many factors affect the serum concentration of potassium, it is essential not to treat "the number" but to seek the underlying cause of the potassium abnormality, correct it, and then carefully add or subtract potassium from IV solutions. Maintenance potassium is 2 to 3 mEq/kg/day during infancy. Because rapid potassium infusions can cause phlebitis and serious cardiac arrhythmias, bolus therapy should be avoided except in extreme emergencies. Intravenous and oral intake should provide enough potassium to meet baseline requirements and enough to replace abnormal losses. When oliguria, anuria, shock, acidosis, or renal failure is present, potassium should be withdrawn from all IV solutions. Even lactated Ringer's solution, which contains potassium at 3 to 4 mEq/L, should be discontinued and replaced with normal saline to avoid hyperkalemia associated with renal failure.

Potassium and Banked Blood

Very fresh whole blood contains less free potassium and is preferable to older whole or concentrated blood products. The infant's mother is an excellent source for fresh blood (assuming that she and the baby have compatible blood), even though she may be slightly anemic. Because neonates most often require blood replacement owing to frequent blood removal for laboratory tests, the small blood volumes required to increase the red blood cell volume can be obtained from a single acceptable donor. Our blood bank has been helpful in preparing small, concentrated frozen aliquots of mother's blood for replacement; larger, fresh volumes can be prepared for use in the operating room. This procedure has minimized donor exposures and has reduced the serum potassium of stored blood.

Calcium

Serum calcium levels of 6.5 to 8.0 mg/dl are normal for premature infants because these babies have lower serum protein concentrations and more unbound calcium than older patients. Therefore, more calcium is available to the cells. However, the body reserves of calcium are very low in preterm infants compared with those of term infants, and hypocalcemia occurs in about 90 percent of preterm infants.[89]

Daily maintenance requirements for calcium gluconate may be higher than 500 mg/kg/day for the VLBW infant. Alkalosis (caused by vigorous bicarbonate therapy or hyperventilation) decreases the ionized calcium concentration, as do infusions of albumin and citrated blood products. Hypocalcemia in the preterm neonate is associated with a decrease in myocardial function.[90] For calcium supplementation in the operating room after blood transfusion or to replace a calcium deficit, 10 percent calcium chloride 20 mg/kg (0.2 ml/kg) or an equivalent dose of 10 percent calcium gluconate 60 mg/kg (0.6 ml/kg) may be infused slowly. In these concentrations, the chloride and gluconate forms of calcium salt are equally effective for increasing ionized calcium concentrations in children.[91] Keep in mind that medications can easily precipitate in low-volume IV tubing owing to relatively slower flow rates and the use of low volumes of flush solution. Mixing of bicarbonate and calcium causes precipitation and plugging of the IV tubing and may obstruct small veins.

Management of acute hypercalcemia, although rare in children, requires immediate hydration with normal saline. Loop diuretics, bisphosphonates, plicamycin, calcitonin, gallium nitrate, steroids, phosphates, and prostaglandins all have their place in chronic and acute therapies to reduce serum calcium. Whether caused by errors in total parenteral nutrition (TPN) calculations, congenital causes, milk-alkali syndrome, cancer, or endocrine disorders, treatment is dictated by symptomatology. Gastrointestinal symptoms of hypercalcemia include anorexia, nausea, vomiting, and constipation. Hypertension, augmentation in digoxin toxicity, renal dysfunction, and CNS disturbance, including coma, are also seen during hypercalcemia.[92]

Magnesium

Magnesium deficiency is rare in the newborn. In older infants, it is associated with the prolonged use of magnesium-free hyperalimentation solutions. It is a common finding in critically ill children. Since only 1 percent

TABLE 5-6
RELATIONSHIP BETWEEN SERUM POTASSIUM CONCENTRATION AND pH

pH	K (mEq/L)
7.8	2.6
7.6	3.3
7.4	4.0
7.2	5.3
7.0	6.5

of magnesium is in the plasma, intracellular Mg^{2+} was measured in red blood cells (RBCs) by nuclear magnetic resonance. Sixty-five percent of patients in a critical care setting had total body hypomagnesemia.[93] Aldosteronism, intestinal fistulas, starvation, pancreatitis, alcoholism, catecholamine, and use of β-agonists are also associated with hypomagnesemia. Calcium deficiencies often accompany magnesium deficiencies (Mg concentrations of <1.5 mEq/L). Deficiency of either ion decreases myocardial function. Hypomagnesemia causes muscle weakness, cardiac arrhythmias, and hypokalemia.

High magnesium concentrations are often present in newborns of women who were given magnesium salts to treat toxemia of pregnancy. These salts of magnesium cause sedation and may potentiate muscle relaxants in the parturient and infant. The sedative and muscle-potentiating effects of magnesium salts can be antagonized by infusions of calcium.

Anions

Full-term and preterm infants can excrete more bicarbonate than chloride in their urine. Conversely, their kidneys can reabsorb more chloride than bicarbonate, even when the infant is acidemic. The more premature the infant, the greater the bicarbonate loss. Metabolic acidosis (pH < 7.20) should be treated with a solution containing HCO_3^- or acetate as the anion component. If sodium is given as NaCl, the term infant tolerates only 12 mEq/kg/day. However, when half the sodium is given as bicarbonate, the infant tolerates 15 mEq/kg/day.[94] Because IV solutions contain primarily NaCl, these "adult" formulations may be contraindicated for the resuscitation of preterm infants. K.G., for example, might require supplemental dilute acetate or HCO_3^- because of renal HCO_3^- wasting and acidosis. Because both normal saline and Ringer's lactate contain 50 percent more chloride than normal serum, a replacement solution for neonates can be formulated using half-strength saline plus 65 mEq of sodium bicarbonate per liter to yield a balanced salt solution of sodium with a decreased concentration of chloride. This solution should be reserved for infants with continuing metabolic acidosis. Other buffers such as tris (hydroxymethyl) aminomethane (THAM), carbicarbonate, and desoxycorticosterone acetate (DCA) have also recently been reviewed and proposed for clinical use.[95]

Chloride depletion occurs in neonates with prolonged use of diuretics, but is rarely a concern for perioperative fluid replacement. Chronic chloride deficiency, however, is associated with severe developmental delay.[96] Furthermore, metabolic alkalosis cannot be corrected without correcting the associated hypochloremia.

Plasma phosphate concentrations may decrease during surgery owing to intracellular shifts of this ion. Gastrointestinal losses from vomiting or nasogastric suctioning also contribute to perioperative hypophosphatemia. Hypophosphatemia has been associated with impaired oxygen delivery to tissues, myocardial depression, and respiratory insufficiency.[97] A rare inherited disease, hypophosphatasia, is associated with decreased mineralization of bones and teeth. The perinatal form is fatal, with fractures and convulsions being common. Infantile forms can present with mild respiratory distress, failure to thrive, hypotonia, fever, constipation, and obvious skeletal deformities.[98] Childhood forms of the disease are usually mild, with blue sclera and skeletal defects the most common findings.

Glucose

K.G. has lowered body reserves of energy substrate. Without body fat, and with few glycogen stores, he needs a continuous IV source of energy while he is ill. In addition to lower body stores of glucose, infants have significantly higher metabolic rates and oxygen consumption than older children. Healthy infants are typically made NPO for 3 to 6 hours preoperatively to lower the risk of aspirating gastric contents. Neonatal hypoglycemia, particularly pre-bypass surgery, induces a life-threatening hypoglycemia, whereas moderate replacement (2.5 mg/kg/min) is not responsible for clinically significant hyperglycemia.[99] Intraoperatively, glucose uptake by muscle is diminished.[100] In addition, the serum levels of glucose are elevated preoperatively in response to surgery, pain, and stimulation. Because glucose is not well utilized during the perioperative period, additional intraoperative glucose administration may not be necessary in older infants. In one study, children under 5 years of age were normoglycemic despite being fasted for an average of 15 hours.[94] Healthy infants and children fast for their normal overnight sleep period without becoming hypoglycemic.

K.G. has both a lower glycogen store and a lower renal threshold for glucose filtration than term infants. Infusing a 10 percent dextrose solution (100 mg of glucose per milliliter) at 6 ml/kg/h provides him with 10 mg/kg/min of glucose. A glucose administration rate of more than 7 to 10 mg/kg/min may overwhelm his renal threshold for glucose. With the stress of surgery or trauma, his serum glucose concentration may increase further and his reserve of glycogen may become severely depleted. In addition, other sugar sources, including the dextrose in banked blood, increase his serum glucose concentration. To avoid intraoperative glycosurea and osmotic diuresis, the effects of dextrose infusions should be closely monitored by determining the blood and urine concentrations with a testing kit such as Dextrostix, Chem Strips, or commercial hand-held devices such as a One Touch or HemoCue.

Hyperglycemia can be exacerbated by the impaired effectiveness of insulin during anesthesia.[101] With decreased tolerance to infused glucose and increased endogenous glucose production, fluids containing 1 percent dextrose may be preferable to 5 percent dextrose solutions for fluid replacement. To achieve this dextrose concentration, maintenance fluids can be given as a 5 percent dextrose-balanced salt solution, and fluid deficits can be alleviated and concurrent losses replaced with a plain balanced salt solution. A balanced salt solution for severely compromised premature infants can be prepared for perioperative volume replacement by removing 100 ml of solution from a 0.5-L bag of 0.5 percent normal saline and adding 40 mEq of sodium bicarbonate (2 mEq/ml = 20/ml) and 80 ml of a 5 percent dextrose-water solution. The final, well-mixed solution contains about 0.08 percent dextrose in a balanced sodium chloride and sodium bicarbonate solution. As emphasized above, all major surgical cases should undergo serum glucose monitoring.

Evidence is accumulating that solutions that prolong anaerobic metabolism in ischemic tissue (e.g., fructose 1,6-bisphosphate [FBP]), are more likely to improve clinical outcome after ischemic events. Improved survival after myocardial, bowel, and cerebral ischemia has been demonstrated in animals with this solution, suggesting that the exclusive use of glucose-containing solutions in pediatrics should be reassessed.[102–104]

Fluid Therapy for Selected Pediatric Cases

Pyloric Stenosis

Surgery is often required to relieve a bowel obstruction during the first year of life. A typical neonatal patient is one with a progressive thickening of the pyloric valve.

> A 2-week-old term infant was admitted to the hospital because of vomiting and dehydration. This baby, P.S., was toxic-appearing and had a capillary refill time of more than 6 seconds. His skin felt cool and doughy, and when pinched it took several seconds for the skin to return to its former position. He had no stool or urine in his diapers for 16 to 24 hours, and he was 10 percent below his birth weight. He had a palpable olive-sized mass 3 cm below the right costal margin. Visible gastric peristalsis waves were seen after a feed. He was admitted for medical management of dehydration and subsequent pylomyotomy.

Pyloric stenosis is a medical emergency. Rehydration is needed to correct intravascular fluid contraction. Although the repair can be classified as a minor surgical procedure, effective preoperative rehydration is imperative. Repletion of intravascular volume should precede attempts to surgically relieve the construction, even though these infants are starved. An operative repair can be performed more safely after volume and electrolyte balance are corrected, usually after 1 to 3 days of rehydration therapy.

Pyloric stenosis is caused by hypertrophy of the muscles of the pyloric sphincter. Increasing symptoms after the first or second week of extrauterine life suggest that it has a postnatal onset. Whereas newborns usually have an empty stomach 2 hours after feeding, infants with pyloric stenosis have fluid in their stomach 6 hours after their last feeding. P.S.'s admission electrolytes demonstrated a profound metabolic acidosis with mild hypernatremia.

In general, infants with pyloric stenosis present with hypochloremic, hypokalemic, metabolic alkalosis. Hypokalemia is caused by loss of potassium from the stomach and by exchange of hydrogen ions for sodium ions in the renal tubules, resulting in systemic alkalosis and a paradoxically acidic urine. Baby P.S. had become so volume depleted from vomiting and lack of water intake before arriving at the hospital that the symptoms of hypernatremic dehydration and shock obscured the contraction

alkalosis caused by dehydration and the gastric loss of sodium, potassium, and hydrogen ions.

Clinically, P.S. appeared to be 15 to 20 percent dehydrated, based on sunken eyes and fontanelles, cold skin, anuria, tachycardia and tachypnea, hypotension, and no response to stimulation. Initial management required a rapid infusion of normal saline 20 ml/kg to correct his shock. If an IV cannula cannot be inserted in such infants, normal saline 20 ml/kg can be given by an intraosseous injection with careful selection of site of placement and needle type.[105, 106] After urine output has been established and repeat electrolytes have been checked, potassium can be gradually supplemented. Severe potassium depletion is due to vomiting, inadequate potassium intake, and renal losses of this ion and may take days to become normal.

Sickle Cell Disease

Correcting the symptoms of sickle cell disease relies on minimizing the percentage of sickle cell hemoglobin (HbS) to below 40 percent by transfusion or exchange transfusion (see Chapter 6). In children with sickle cell anemia, an increase in fetal hemoglobin (HbF) also indicates normal operative recovery.[107, 108] Previous sickling episodes in the renal parenchyma may compromise renal function. Overhydration should be avoided. Adequate hydration, avoidance of hypoxemia,[108] and maintenance of euthermia helps to prevent sickling. A new option to reduce HbS concentration includes the IV use of butyrate, a natural substance used as a food flavor enhancer. Patients with both HgS and thalassemia have dramatic increases in HbF. The mechanism appears to be stimulation of gene expression.[109, 110] Identification of children at risk, but without evidence of HbS, has been achieved by most states that have mandated universal testing of all newborn with screening that includes identification of HbS by electrophoresis. Each hospital and surgical center treating children should be aware of the state laboratory phone number that reports results of newborn screening for congenital diseases.

The Scalded Child

> The surgeons have requested a surgical time for early debridement and partial-thickness skin grafting of a 5-month-old child, S.C., whose sibling pulled a pot of boiling water off the stove onto the patient. S.C. sustained full-thickness burns to her cheeks, neck, and chest. Surface area nomograms indicate that she had a 35 percent burn. She is 8 hours postinjury and has been well hydrated with crystalloids since admission to the hospital.

Fluid therapy for S.C. and other children with extensive burns requires an understanding of the damage done to tissue by heat. Whereas hot water at 150°C will cause a full-thickness burn in 0.5 second, a gasoline explosion may be far more rapid and intense. Using intrathoracic blood volume as an end point may be more accurate as an end point to resuscitation than any "canned" burn formula.[111]

Full-thickness burns have an area that is devoid of circulation because the capillaries are in spasm and lack blood. Adjacent to this tissue is a zone of stasis, a partial-thickness burn zone.[112] In this zone there is an intense inflammatory reaction and capillary leakage of fluid and proteins caused by microvascular dilation and cell injury, which lead to increased permeability and massive losses of water and proteins from both interstitial and plasma compartments. Hematocrit may be initially increased because of hemoconcentration and relative polycythemia, increasing blood viscosity and therefore increasing shunts in the microvasculature. Because much of the partial-thickness burn can recover and heal, interest has focused on maximizing microcirculatory flow in this area. The goal of therapy is to prevent these areas of partial damage from progressing to full-thickness skin loss.

Most fluid and protein is lost during the first few hours after injury, owing initially to the release of histamine followed by the loss of proteins, creating further increases in cellular permeability.[113] The amount of fluid loss is estimated by calculating the surface area burned, assessing the depth of the burn, and taking into account the age of the victim. Burns to the airway cause marked fluid losses from massive transcellular shifts of fluid. Younger children lose more fluid than older burn victims, even when the two have similar amounts of burn surface. This difference is due to the greater functional extracellular fluid volume and skin water content in young children. Separate resuscitation nomograms for children have been devised. By multiplying percentage of burn by the relative size of the patient's extracellular fluid volume, one can estimate the fluid lost. The use of invasive monitoring including intravascular saturation and pulmonary arterial pressures may also be indicated.[114]

Current controversy in burn therapy concerns whether hypertonic or isotonic saline is best and when colloids should be used as the supplemental replacement fluid. A commonly used formula provides only a Ringer's lactate type of solution at 2 to 4 ml/kg/percent burn during the first 24 hours after injury.[115] Some centers rely on data indicating that higher protein levels can be maintained with colloids as early as 6 hours after injury. All centers provide enough supplemental fluids to maintain adequate urine output. From 24 to 48 hours after injury, most centers provide colloid therapy and begin additional parenteral nutrition. Cardiac arrest is not uncommon, but at a prominent burn center, 50 percent survival has been noted.[116]

Those who advocate hypertonic solutions maintain that less fluid is needed during resuscitation and that less edema develops. This situation, they believe, leads to less stasis in the reversible zone of injury. Advocates of the early and liberal use of colloids argue that perfusion of nutrients, including oxygen, to the stasis zone is improved by administration of colloids. However, no controlled studies have proven either of these theories.[117]

S.C. gained weight secondary to liberal fluid administration. She also retained fluids as a response to trauma. Edema, respiratory problems (including pulmonary edema), prolonged gastric emptying or intestinal ileus, and signs of cerebral edema are common during early burn care. Hypertonic and protein-containing fluids are currently believed to decrease edema formation. Colloids decrease the tissue edema associated with hypoproteinemia when they are given more than 8 hours after injury.[116] It is believed that decreased edema increases oxygenation to the zone of stasis by improving microcirculatory flow.[113, 118] For advocates of vitamin C, recent evidence suggests that high doses, 66 mg/kg/h, may reduce fluid requirements, respiratory dysfunction, and edema formation.[119]

Ionized plasma calcium concentrations are low in burned patients,[120] necessitating continuous calcium infusion. Infusion of albumin and citrate-containing blood products further lowers the ionized calcium concentrations. Other electrolyte imbalances can be caused by burn dressings. For example, increased loss of sodium and potassium occur in burn eschar after the use of silver nitrate dressings.[121]

If S.C. had sustained smoke inhalation, diagnostic bronchoscopy might have been required initially. After smoke inhalation, laryngeal edema becomes evident within several hours; parenchymal injury manifests within 2 to 4 days. Wheezing, mucosal sloughing, and pulmonary edema are attributed to increased microcirculatory permeability.[122] Some investigators have advocated fluid restriction as a means of avoiding these complications. However, chronically instrumented, lung-scalded sheep that received only maintenance fluids died within 48 hours. Seventy percent of sheep resuscitated with twice the amount of maintenance fluids survived.[123]

Central venous pressure measurements help to determine the adequacy of fluid replacement. Patients who require the greatest amount of fluids to maintain central filling pressures apparently have the lowest survival rate.[124] Trauma, pain, hypovolemia, and anxiety stimulate the secretion of vasopressin, which results in water retention, concentrated urine, and oliguria in children with normal renal function. Overhydration often occurs when urine volume and urine specific gravity alone are used to determine the adequacy of hydration.

THE BLEEDING CHILD

Managing a preoperative hemorrhagic shock in infants and children mandates knowledge of recent studies demonstrating increased mortality with early and vigorous fluid replacement.[125] However, once bleeding is under control, massive and rapid fluid resuscitation, exceeding 40 ml/kg/h in the pediatric patient, is necessary in shock.[126, 127] In children, shock is usually associated with severe hypovolemia, with or without sepsis. Acute hemorrhage from trauma, severe diarrhea, peritonitis, and burns lead to loss of functional volume which, if uncorrected, leads to hypovolemia. During anesthesia, there is reduced reflex compensation for hypovolemia and surgical trauma. As functional extracellular fluid is lost, venous return is diminished and cardiac output decreases. The baroreceptor response stimulates catecholamine release and increases vascular resistance, cardiac contractility, and heart rate. It also decreases venous capacitance (by constricting the veins) and increases preload. The renin-angiotensin-aldosterone axis is switched on to conserve volume. This system interacts with other vasopressors to maintain high vascular resistance. Hypovolemia evokes compensatory responses, including intense vasoconstriction of the skin, skeletal muscle, and gastrointestinal tract. The oliguria induced by contraction of the circulatory volume can convert severely reduced renal perfusion to acute renal failure. Cellular by-products of anaerobic metabolism increase local tissue ischemia, causing metabolic acidosis. Decreased cell energy reduces activity of the sodium-potassium pump, which allows water and sodium to seep into the cells. This situation further decreases the functional extracellular volume. Ongoing blood losses should be cautiously treated to avoid increasing blood pressure whether from venous or arterial sources and treatment with narcotics to blunt a sympathetic response that may in fact increase mortality in this "Houston Study"[4] setting.

Blood is the obvious choice for fluid replacement in hemorrhagic shock. However, extensive loss of interstitial fluid is also associated with severe shock, as fluid shifts into the vascular space via transcapillary refill and into the cells. Changes in cellular permeability allow sodium and water to enter cells, causing an increase in intracellular volume and cell edema. Intravascularly administered albumin may leak into the interstitium and cause more edema fluid to accumulate. Crystalloids increase survival and prevent renal failure; they also prevent cardiovascular collapse when they are administered in addition to specific blood components.

DEHYDRATION

Treatment of severe dehydration must often begin before the results of laboratory examinations are available to indicate whether the child has hyponatremic, isonatremic, or hypernatremic dehydration. Four pertinent measurements should be made.[128]

1. Measure serum osmolarity by checking serum sodium.
2. Check acid–base status, serum pH, and base deficit.
3. Check serum potassium compared with pH.
4. Check urine output. Rule out acute tubular necrosis.

Initial fluid resuscitation is usually accomplished with a bolus of normal saline given over 10 to 20 minutes to improve circulation and restore renal perfusion. Subsequent therapy is undertaken when the serum electrolyte concentrations are known.

Even a 1 percent reduction of blood volume is associated with a rectal temperature increase of 0.3°C.[129] The mechanism for a febrile response to volume contraction may be a decrease in skin blood flow, which prevents normal skin dilation to dissipate heat. Hyperosmolarity also elevates the threshold for sweating. In each case, maintenance of blood flow to the heart and brain are maintained by shunting of blood away from other organs.

For patients with known contraction alkalosis (e.g., the infant with pylomyotomy described above), 5 percent dextrose in 0.9 percent normal saline is a reasonable first choice for fluid therapy. This solution contains 154 mEq of sodium and chloride per liter. For infants with known metabolic acidosis, a more appropriate solution can be formulated by removing 250 ml of 0.9 percent normal saline from a 1-L container and replacing it with 28 ml of a 7.5 percent sodium bicarbonate solution and 232 ml of 5 percent dextrose in 0.9 percent NS. The final solution contains approximately 1.2 percent dextrose, 140 mEq sodium, 115 mEq chloride, and 25 mEq bicarbonate. Giving solutions containing acetate or lactate to severely dehydrated infants can actually increase their acidosis if these precursors of bicarbonate cannot be metabolized to bicarbonate by the liver because of circulatory compromise. Another choice for bolus therapy might be Hextend or other hybrid solution of balanced salt solution.

The three children described below are moderately dehydrated. Each had an accurate weight charted at a recent well-baby examination.

Isotonic Dehydration

Infant I.D. has a 3-day history of vomiting and a bowel obstruction. His current weight is 9 kg, which on clinical examination is consistent with a 10 percent volume loss. I.D. has relatively normal serum electrolytes: Na, 130 mEq/L; K, 4 mEq/L; and Cl, 98 mEq/L. His fluid losses consist of Na^+ 20 to 80 mEq/L and 5 to 20 mEq/L of K^+, with variable amounts of hydrogen ion loss. Because his electrolytes are relatively normal, a balanced salt solution is indicated to replace the gastric fluid losses and expand the contracted extracellular fluid compartment. I.D.'s water deficit is calculated by a simple formula that takes into account weight change and by a clinical assessment. The patient's usual weight minus his current weight divided by his usual weight equals the percentage of fluid deficit:

$$\frac{[10\ kg-9\ kg]}{10\ kg}=\frac{[1\ kg]}{10\ kg}= 10\ percent\ volume\ deficit$$

Correction of this deficit can be initiated with two infusions of a balanced salt solution (20 ml/kg) over 10 to 20 minutes for each infusion, followed by a repeat physical examination and repeat laboratory reassessment of electrolyte balance. His maintenance fluid requirements are 4 ml/kg/h which, with his 10 kg weight, translates to 40 ml/h. Without the presence of continuing fluid losses, this child would require an additional liter of fluid to correct his calculated deficit over 24 hours. Once his shock is treated, his hourly rate of fluid administration should be adjusted to include the amount of fluid required to continue correcting the calculated deficit rather than to continue giving boluses of fluid. This step requires the infant to receive 1.5 to 2 times his maintenance rate of fluids plus enough fluid to replace continuing losses. Therefore, the fluid regimen for the first day includes two boluses equal to 2 percent of the body weight, followed by a continuous infusion at twice the maintenance rate, plus replacement of ongoing losses. Although potassium losses may equal the sodium losses, potassium should be added to the IV fluids only after renal perfusion is reestablished and acidosis is corrected. No more than 20 to 40 mEq of potassium chloride or potassium phosphate per liter should be infused because of the risk of arrhythmias and venous thrombosis associated with giving higher concentrations of parenteral potassium.

Hyponatremic Dehydration

Any child can be killed with intravenous water. The fact that hospitals still have D5W in plain sight in the emergency room, operating room, and other parenteral fluid settings continues to doom children who, when given too much free water, seize and die.[131]

> H.D. is a 1-year-old, 10-kg child with severe diarrhea of several days' duration. His serum sodium is 110 mEq/L, and he is having a seizure. Sodium losses from diarrhea are 10 to 140 mEq/L, and potassium losses are 10 to 80 mEq/L. If salt losses from diarrhea exceed the intake of salts, serious hypotonic dehydration occurs.

More salt than water is lost in hypotonic dehydration. Therefore, the extracellular fluid compartment becomes dilute and contracted, causing extracellular water to shift into the intracellular space via osmosis. Consequently, hypotonic dehydration, caused by a combination of total body water loss and relative increase in cellular water volume, leads to early signs of hypovolemia. The percentage of weight loss may be insignificant compared to the signs and symptoms of dehydration.

Although hypokalemia rarely causes symptoms in otherwise healthy infants, sodium concentrations below 120 mEq/L are often associated with seizures and death. For rapid correction of symptomatic hyponatremia, a 3 percent NaCl solution, which has 0.5 mEq of sodium per milliliter, can be rapidly infused[130] to increase the serum sodium concentration to 125 mEq/L. The formula for calculating the amount of sodium needed to increase the serum sodium to a given level is as follows: ECF × desired serum Na–actual serum Na. The extracellular fluid (ECF) (30 percent in this 5 to 10 percent dehydrated 10-kg infant is approximately 3 L) × [125 (the desired serum sodium level)–110 (the current serum sodium concentration)] indicates that 45 mEq sodium must be given to increase the sodium level from 110 to 125 mEq/L. Therapy should begin with a slow infusion at 1 to 2 ml/min; 90 ml of a 3 percent NaCl solution will raise the extracellular sodium concentration of this child to the desired level. Alternatively, 30 ml/kg (300 ml in this 10-kg infant) of a 0.9 percent NS solution should also provide 45 mEq of sodium. The addition of sodium to the extracellular space will result in further expansion of the ECF as intracellular water shifts into the extracellular space.

Hypernatremic Dehydration

> Infant H.N.D. was inadvertently fed a concentrated formula that resulted in severe hypertonic dehydration, the most worrisome form of dehydration.

As emphasized earlier, rapid shifts in osmolarity can cause seizures and cerebral damage, even though the decrease in serum sodium occurs at less than 0.5 mEq/L/h. For this reason, no entirely free-water-containing solutions should be administered to these children. Free water moves into the cells more rapidly than the kidneys can excrete sodium or water. If seizures occur owing to rapid rehydration, they may have to be treated with a 2 to 4 ml/kg bolus of a 3 percent NaCl solution. Other consequences of treating hypernatremia include pulmonary edema, congestive heart failure, hypocalcemia, and excessive water losses from a high-output isosthenuria. Treatment of these respective complications requires loop diuretics, digitalis, calcium, and modification of sodium-containing fluids.

Withdrawal of Hydration

As physicians, we are trained to diagnose, to support, and to try to cure dying children. We strive to push back the frontiers of science in hopes that our discoveries will allow such children, and many others, to survive. We are saving smaller and more severely injured infants, and we are prolonging the lives and discovering "cures" for many terminally ill children. Often more difficult is acceptance of the futility of continued medical support. The challenge is to begin to plan withdrawal of this support with the family while continuing to provide compassion to the family and the child.

Should nutrition and hydration be withheld from terminal patients, such as children in a persistent vegetative state? Should a synthetic hormone such as DDAVP (desmopressin) always be administered to children with severe central brain damage and diabetes insipidus? Diabetes insipidus may be a sign of severe irreversible central brain damage caused by inadequate pituitary function after head trauma. These children need synthetic arginine vasopressin hormone to maintain water balance. Without parenteral fluid administration and/or DDAVP, they will die rapidly. Although technology now enables us to preserve cardiac and pulmonary function, similar advances that would reverse CNS dysfunction are lacking. Must we support severely damaged or terminal infants and children who have no hope of any meaningful recovery?

The main argument proposed by hospice care workers in favor of providing ongoing hydration is that it will prevent the discomfort associated with thirst; therefore, IV or nasogastric fluids should never be withheld from a dying child. A second argument is that food and nutrition in our culture is symbolic of caring. Finally, it is argued, to deprive a child of fluids and thus actively hasten death is to devalue that child's existence. Preventing discomfort, continuing to care, and respecting life have supported the imperative to hydrate in all cases. The karma of comforting the permanently comatose child should take precedence over the dogma of "do no harm." Must we always artificially hydrate dying children? Are we always required to use DDAVP?

Responses to arguments in supporting mandatory hydration involve a closer look at comfort, caring, and dying. Oliver[132] noted that terminally ill adult patients deprived of fluids actually seemed more comfortable than patients receiving maintenance fluid. Two mechanisms have been suggested for this well-recognized sedative state. First, anesthetic effects of ketones and their natural breakdown products are seen during starvation and dehydration.[133] Second, prolonged starvation and dehydration increase endogenous opioid production.[134] Although fluid-restricted terminally ill patients may complain of thirst, this can be alleviated by frequent sips of cool water or ice chips. With respect to the argument that hydration is symbolic of caring, we can best care for dying patients by giving them adequate sedation and analgesia and not by prolonging their dying by artificially supporting nutritional requirements and maintaining adequate vascular volume. Finally, we may allow terminally ill children a better death and show them more respect by withholding hydration. In terminal patients, a "good" death may not be achieved, but a "better" death is possible by not artificially prolonging suffering.[135] This topic of study has progressed sadly through the machinations of a pathologist from Michigan to the trials of other compassionate medical personnel. Certainly, studies are urgently needed, and at least the *Journal of the American Medical Association* stands ready to encourage more investigations in this most critically needed point of life.[136]

Fluid Management in Neurologic Injury

Neurologic injury, whether from trauma or surgical intervention, must be treated cautiously by the anesthesiologist. Perioperative neurosurgical anesthesia must protect the brain by maintaining oxygenation, delivery of nutrition, and removal of metabolic waste products. The dogma of restricting fluids, long considered mandatory, must be tempered by the obvious need to maintain an adequate circulation to the brain. However, decreasing metabolism with a volatile anesthetic, such as isoflurane, or with barbiturates may be even more effective.

Blood-Brain Barrier

Fluids can pass through an intact blood-brain barrier (BBB) only if their components are less than 0.7 to 0.9 nm. By comparison, effective endothelial size in the peripheral vasculature is 4 to 5 nm.[137] Close junctions of capillary cells form a "zona occludens" that prevents even electrolytes from passing into the CNS interstitium. In addition, the CNS has no active lymphatics to help absorb electrolytes and albumin. Therefore, any rapid change in osmolarity causes a rapid shift of water towards the hyperosmotic side. With an intact BBB, mannitol actually increases cerebral blood flow (CBF) by increasing blood volume, and if it is infused at room temperature, transient cooling of the blood may vasodilate the peripheral vasculature. Decreasing the viscosity of blood (Poise units) does not seem to affect CBF. However, the CNS effects of mannitol over many minutes decrease the water content of the CNS cells, thus decreasing CNS pressure. Hyperosmotic infusions have little effect in areas with a damaged BBB. Damage to the BBB opens pores in the endothelium that can easily allow electrolytes and small protein particles into the CNS interstitium. Hyperosmotic therapy in severe brain damage probably provides little benefit, may actually increase pressure in the damaged brain cells, and may decrease

perfusion because of leakage of solute from the intravascular space. Adequate perfusion pressure, decreasing brain metabolic requirements with the judicious use of anesthesia, and using osmotic therapy when appropriate, can help to oxygenate, nourish, and cleanse the brain.

Cerebral Blood Flow

CBF in children ranges from 45 to 60 ml/100 g of brain per minute. Oxygen consumption is generally accepted to be in the range of 3 to 3.8 ml/100 g of brain per minute ($CMRO_2$). Although volatile anesthetics usually decrease cardiac output, all seem to increase CBF (see Chapter 16). General anesthesia also decreases the metabolic rate, which changes the supply and demand requirements. A planned intraoperative hypotensive technique may be well tolerated by increasing CBF and decreasing the metabolic demand of the brain. Hemodilution, which decreases intravascular oncotic pressure, has little influence on CNS pressure and CBF.

During severe hemorrhagic shock, there is some evidence that the neonate has better restored cerebral oxygenation with a hypertonic saline than lactated Ringer's solution.[138]

Subarachnoid Hemorrhage

The conditions associated with hyponatremia in children with subarachnoid hemorrhage (SAH) have not changed, but our understanding of both the pathophysiology and the treatment of this disorder has changed significantly. Hyponatremia after SAH was formerly thought to be part of a syndrome of inappropriate antidiuretic hormone (SIADH) and dilutional water retention. However, it is now known that these children have severe depletion of intravascular volume and that restricting water and salt is the opposite of what they need. SAH is now understood to be most often related to natriuresis caused by cerebrally induced salt wasting.[139] The key to managing hyponatremia after SAH is to distinguish first whether the child has dilutional hyponatremia, SIADH, or is actually intravascularly depleted of fluid and sodium because of cerebral natriuresis.[140]

After careful measurements of sodium and volume regulation following SAH, large boluses of fluid were given to prevent vasospasm and volume contraction. As expected, atrial natriuretic factor (ANF) was elevated but did not always correlate with or prevent hyponatremia. Actually, sodium balance did not correlate with arginine vasopressin (AVP), ANF, aldosterone, or renin, and fluid balance was positively correlated only with AVP.[141] Patients with SAH do excrete a digoxin-like factor[142] in addition to having elevations of catecholamines. If adequate volume status is maintained, both aldosterone and plasma renin activity are suppressed. Administering more than maintenance fluids and sodium should minimize perturbations in humoral factors that complicate the care of patients with SAH.[138]

RENAL FAILURE

Chronic renal failure in children may initially manifest as failure to thrive. The most common cause is renal dysplasia. Infants with a dysplastic or obstructed kidney in utero often have some nephrons that are normal. The adult with chronic renal failure, on the other hand, has a more uniform loss of nephron function. This difference allows greater compensatory renal responses in children.[143] Although acute renal failure is strongly suggested by a urine flow rate of less than 1 ml/kg/h, oliguria may also occur with excess vasopressin, dehydration, acute blood loss, or other causes of hypotension. Oliguria with increased urine osmolarity is not caused by renal failure. To differentiate between decreased extracellular fluid and acute renal failure as the cause for oliguria, a challenge of a balanced sodium fluid 10 to 20 ml/kg is infused. By using only a balanced salt solution, the excessive salt loads that are sometimes associated with renal insufficiency can be avoided.[144] Fluid and nutritional needs of renal failure in children have been extensively reviewed.[145]

Progression to end-stage renal disease is characterized by isosthenuria, the inability to increase the osmolarity of urine above that of plasma. In end-stage renal disease, isosthenuria is the direct result of deranged renal tubules and medullary microvasculature, which prevent the medullary interstitium from producing hypertonic urine. As the disease progresses, the renal tubules become resistant to vasopressin, causing an osmotic diuresis in the residual nephrons. As a result, the child with renal disease has decreased ability to produce a dilute urine and is unable to increase urine output when faced with excess water. In addition, solute excretion decreases and the kidney is unable to concentrate the urine.[146]

Children with renal failure may develop hyperphosphatemia as the result of decreased urinary excretion, and hypocalcemia is also associated with increased deposition of calcium phosphate salts in tissues. Solutions and enemas containing phosphate should be restricted. Magnesium or aluminum hydroxide reduces serum phosphate but may also be toxic in renal failure. Calcium carbonate treats hyperphosphatemia and raises serum calcium, but poor responses are seen if serum magnesium levels are abnormal.[145]

Soda pop with the usual sweet overdose of phosphates reverses the calcium/phosphate ratio, causing up to five times the bone fracture rate of non–soda-thriving girls.[146a]

Patients with renal failure should receive only enough fluid to replace insensible losses and most of the urine output. Surgical and trauma patients have increased metabolism and increased protein catabolism, which produces more water and further decreases maintenance fluid requirements. In such patients, it is necessary to measure and maintain the central venous pressure at the lower limits of normal.

Hypernatremia occasionally occurs when too much water is removed during dialysis. Hyponatremia occurs with water retention and diuretic-induced urinary sodium losses. If the sodium concentration falls below 120 mEq/L, a 3 percent solution of NaCl should be used to restore the sodium concentration to the desired level.

Hyperkalemia is the most worrisome electrolyte problem in renal failure. Loss of potassium in the gut and perspiration is trivial compared with the loss that normally occurs in the kidney. Patients with chronic renal failure may compensate for the loss of potassium excretion by the kidneys' increased excretion of potassium through the intestine; however, this mechanism is usually inadequate to prevent hyperkalemia in acute renal failure. Rhabdomyolysis and other conditions in which cells are broken down (e.g., burns, trauma, surgery, increased catabolism, hemolysis, and acidosis) are associated with increased serum potassium concentrations. Medications that increase serum potassium are listed in Table 5–5.

TOTAL PARENTERAL NUTRITION

The most significant advance in fluid therapy since the 1960s has been the use of total parenteral nutrition in children. Dudrick et al.[147] popularized the use of TPN by demonstrating that puppies could grow and develop normally while receiving only IV glucose and protein. Because it is so frequently used, many children with inadequate gastrointestinal function are receiving parenteral nutrition solutions when they arrive in the operating room. TPN combines high concentrations of glucose, proteins, essential fats, and trace elements. In addition to supporting cardiac and CNS requirements, addition of triacetin and triglycerides to TPN accelerates bowel healing.[148] TPN actually increases cell growth in sick neonates while increasing the metabolic rate.[149] Even in children with malignancies, TPN has been shown to improve survival.[150] Progress in TPN includes increasing and adding to the trace mineral content, especially trace metals in some VLBW infants.[151]

Starvation, trauma, premature birth, and sepsis increase extracellular volume by increasing capillary leakage of fluid and albumin. However supplemental albumin is no safer or more cost effective than other alternatives.[152] As a consequence, the concentration of albumin in the interstitium increases and the intravascular albumin concentration decreases. The net result is a large increase in total extracellular volume.[153] The extracellular compartment, not inclusive of intravascular serum, continues to expand until the microvasculature heals, allowing an increase in colloid oncotic pressure. This consideration is important when planning perioperative fluid therapy.[154] Patients requiring emergency surgery and patients with other forms of trauma have depressed rates of protein synthesis, which can lead to hypoalbuminemia.

Hypoalbuminemia is a marker for increased morbidity and mortality in hospitalized patients. It delays wound healing, extends coagulation time, and decreases gastrointestinal and renal function.[155] Providing TPN with at least 4 mg/kg/min of glucose causes more rapid protein synthesis.[156] Recent evidence indicates that the addition of IV fibronectin rapidly increases colloid oncotic pressure.[157] Even though positive nitrogen balance has been achieved, the extracellular fluid volume may remain expanded until stores of protein normalize and capillary leakage stops. Giving human growth hormone decreases weight loss, maintains total body nitrogen, potassium, and phosphorus concentrations; and increases insulin production in patients receiving only 50 percent of their estimated energy requirements.[158]

Patients often require mechanical ventilatory support. One study showed that TPN and the associated increase in serum protein permitted ventilator-dependent patients to be weaned from mechanical ventilation, whereas patients whose protein concentrations remained low continued to require mechanical ventilation.[159]

Intraoperative fluid management usually requires a reduction in the rate of parenteral nutrition administration. High-dextrose-containing solutions should not be acutely withdrawn, however, as this may cause hypoglycemia. Giving preoperative volumes of total parenteral nutrition during surgery may cause hyperglycemia and may induce an osmotic diuresis. Intraoperative glucose concentrations must be measured frequently to avoid hyper- or hypoglycemia. In a review of 36 pediatric textbooks and 178 pediatricians, the definition for hypoglycemia is less than 36 mg/dl for term infants and less than 20 mg/dl for premature infants.[160] Many people are concerned that these numbers are too low. It is safer to assume that the lower limit of normal is 40 mg/dl in all infants. Hyperglycemia is represented by glycosurea or serum values greater than 200 mg/dl.

Bacteremia and sepsis are common complications of TPN. These problems are especially common when the IV catheter through which high concentrations of dextrose are given is also used to give medications and supplemental fluids. To minimize the risk of contaminating the IV alimentation catheter, a separate IV catheter should be used to give drugs and other solutions when possible. All flushes of central lines can be accomplished with vancomycin to minimize the risk of infecting the lines.

Sodium, potassium, and water imbalances are the most common fluid and electrolyte problems in patients receiving TPN. Calcium, magnesium, and phosphate concentrations may also be low if inadequate amounts of these substances are given. Unexpected gastrointestinal or renal losses of these substances must not be overlooked. As previously emphasized, magnesium and calcium can be associated with weakness, tetany, seizures, and cardiac arrhythmias, and may alter the patient's response to muscle relaxants. Phosphate deficits can cause weakness or seizures, reduce cardiac contractility, and impair oxygen transport. Miscalculations of the amount of electrolytes required and failure to measure the blood concentrations of these electrolytes often lead to perioperative imbalances of these substances. Failure to provide adequate calories and protein to poorly nourished children during the perioperative period leads to poor wound healing, a negative nitrogen balance, and significant decreases in weight and in potassium, magnesium, and phosphorus concentrations.[161]

When TPN is the sole source of calorie intake for infants whose renal concentrating ability is less than that of older children, the increased renal solute load caused by the IV fluid may result in an osmotic diuresis and hypertonic dehydration. Additional water may be needed to enable excretion of this solute load. Ongoing fluid losses must be reversed with fluids of similar composition rather than by increasing the amount of hyperalimentation solution. Severe hyperglycemia and brain damage may occur if hyperalimentation fluid is used for this purpose. Hyperalimentation fluid should *never* be used to replace fluid losses during surgery because this will lead to severe hyperglycemia.

CONTROVERSY: CRYSTALLOID OR COLLOID?

Although there is controversy about the need for perioperative colloid administration, and although each side has strong advocates and detractors, most agree that parenteral fluid administration should begin with a crystalloid solution.[162] Blood components should be administered only when absolutely required, and each transfusion should be from the same donor, when possible, to decrease the total number of blood donors to whom the patient is exposed.

Although evidence-based studies are lacking,[163] human albumin or synthetic colloids (hetastarch, dextran, fluorocarbons) are advocated by some physicians to maintain normal intravascular osmotic pressure.[164] Since albumin has been commonly used in the pediatric operating room for volume expansion, a brief discussion of its usefulness follows.

Albumin

Nacelle, in the first volume of *Lancet* (1839), described albumin: "It is found not only in the blood but in the lymph, chyle, in the exhalations from surfaces, in the fluid of the cellular tissue, in the aqueous of the eye . . . ." He described the properties, function and usefulness of albumin.[165] The structure of albumin has been extensively studied. The primary structure is a peptide chain of 580 to 585 amino acid residues. The secondary structure contains a pattern of double loops held together by disulfide bridges. Human albumin has three "domains," each containing three loops. The structure and amino acid sequence are indicative of a common ancestry with myoglobin.

Human albumin and plasma proteins were first purified by Cohn et al.[166] in 1946. Since albumin counteracts hemorrhagic shock, the United States government requested that pharmaceutical firms produce commercially "ready-to-use" human albumin solutions for use on the battlefield. Most major industrialized nations continue to use Cohn's method of ethanol fractionation, which denatures the protein to some extent. Different methods are used to produce other protein factors, such as factor VIII, immunoglobulins, fibrinogen/fibronectin, prothrombin complex (II, VII, IX, X), activated prothrombin complex, and antithrombin III. However, because of cost considerations, Cohn's method of ethanol fractionation is used. It yields a relatively pure and safe plasma extract.

In humans, synthesis of albumin takes place in the liver. Albumin is secreted by hepatocytes within 20 minutes. When the oncotic pressure is low, nutrition is adequate, and hepatocytes are available, albumin synthesis is stimulated. Ribosomes attached to the endoplasmic reticulum produce proalbumin, which is the primary intracellular species of albumin. Although albumin is rapidly synthesized and excreted and has a life span of 3 weeks, albumin excess is rarely seen. Synthesis is stimulated by cortisol, growth hormone, and thyroid hormones. Administration of methadone is also associated with increased albumin production. Lowered albumin concentrations are most often seen with malnutrition, chronic disease, and in premature births. Synthesis is decreased by infusion of dextran or other colloids. Infusion of exogenous albumin is followed by a marked increase in albumin degradation and decreased production. Therefore, infusions of albumin to increase serum levels are rarely effective. This is especially apparent in children with capillary leak syndromes, which prevent albumin, particularly heat-treated, infused human albumin, from remaining in the intravascular space. Nephrotic syndrome, sepsis, gastrointestinal diseases,[167] (especially celiac sprue), intestinal lymphangiectasia, polyposis, and parasitic infestation are associated with severe hypoalbuminemia and are rarely treatable by exogenous administration of albumin. However, improved renal function and reduced mortality have been recently reported in the combination of bacterial peritonitis with acites in adults.[168]

The obvious clinical imperative to use human albumin infusions to treat hypoalbuminemia has been sharply criticized: IV albumin and diuretics have been used to treat the severe edema associated with nephrotic syndrome and prematurity.[169] Raising the oncotic pressure, mobilizing the cellular and interstitial fluid into the vascular space, and paralyzing the distal renal tubules would in theory resolve the edema associated with nephrotic syndrome. However, the capillary leak syndrome allows infused albumin to seep into glomerular epithelial cells. Protein nephropathy is treated by protein restriction and systemic steroids, which increase glomerular filtration rate and decrease proteinuria. In a group of children treated with IV albumin, degenerative changes persisted longer, response to steroids was inhibited, and more frequent relapses occurred compared with a matched control group of children.[170]

Albumin is most appropriately used during major corrective surgery to maintain vascular volume. When massive amounts of protein are lost acutely from burns or massive debridement procedures, the concentration of protein in the vascular space may be momentarily low; in an experimental model, when hematocrits are reduced to a fourth dilution to 5 percent, no difference in hepatic injury occurs in a comparison of albumin, Pentalyte, or Hextend.[171] With chronic hypoalbuminemia, however, use of exogenous albumin actually decreases albumin production and secretion. Since the healthy, fed liver rapidly produces massive amounts of albumin, even momentary increases in plasma oncotic pressure by infusion of albumin actually decrease its production.[172]

Loss of albumin also occurs during stress. Infection, trauma, surgery, malnutrition, and radiation alter protein synthesis. Since the skin contains between a third and half of the reservoir of exchangeable albumin, in a child with a 50 percent total body burn, as much as one third of total body albumin may be acutely lost. Other factors that decrease albumin synthesis include sustained hyperthermia and aging.

The function of albumin is twofold. It maintains osmotic and oncotic pressure, and it binds to a variety of substances. As a highly negatively charged molecule, it accumulates Na^+ molecules in the core structure, bilirubin, fatty acids, metals and ions, hormones, and medications (Table 5–7). The albumin-bound fraction of medication remains within the vascular space. However, some drugs such as sulfisoxazole (Gantricin) specifically displace other albumin-bound substances such as bilirubin, increasing the likelihood that kernicterus will develop. Other drugs that may displace bilirubin include sulfonamides, analgesics, anti-inflammatory drugs, and some radiologic contrast media.[173]

Many conditions that occur during the neonatal period are associated with high concentrations of indirect bilirubin. Prematurity and bowel obstruction are two often overlapping causes that are present before an emergency operation. Human albumin preparations are extracted from blood donors or from human placenta.[174] Increased binding potency of bilirubin in 51 sick premature infants with hyperbilirubinemia was observed. In vitro analysis of the binding of bilirubin to albumin demonstrated that the stabilizers and alcoholic fractionation used to produce albumin decrease bilirubin binding to albumin. Despite a decrease in the association constant of albumin with bilirubin, human albumin retains a high binding potency for bilirubin in vivo.[175]

Evidence from an isolated hind-limb preparation[176] demonstrated that plasma, blood, and isoproterenol decreased capillary leakage, whereas an albumin-containing solution actually increased capillary permeability. As stated earlier, albumin normally is redistributed more rapidly in neonates, and albumin infusions fail to reduce edema in hypoalbuminemic children. If albumin leaks from the circulation into the interstitium or actually increases capillary permeability, its use further decreases plasma volume. In theory, this increase in interstitial fluid would increase the amount of time required to mobilize the interstitial albumin and return it to the intravascular space.

Adverse effects of albumin include hypotension caused by vasodepressor kinins and allergic reactions to contaminants or to polymers produced during storage. Rarely, hypersensitivity reactions may be caused by inert substances such as haptens after they combine with albumin.[177] In addition, albumin may temporarily decrease ionized calcium concentrations by directly decreasing cardiac inotropic activity. Volume resuscitation with hyperon-

TABLE   5 – 7
DRUGS THAT BIND 90 PERCENT OR MORE TO ALBUMIN

CNS	Quinidine
Diazepam	Hydralazine
Amitriptyline	Renal
Imipramine	Probenecid
Chlorpromazine	Furosemide
Phenytoin	Chlorothiazide
Methadone	Ethacrynic acid
Thiopental	Anti-infective
Anti-inflammatory	Sulfa-containing antibiotics
Indomethacin	Dicloxacillin
Salicylic acid	Oxacillin
Cardiovascular	Nafcillin
Propanolol	Cefazolin
Diazoxide	

cotic infusions may lead to capillary leakage of protein and water. This may decrease renal excretion of water and sodium and thus compromise tubular function. Higher cost also is a consideration for routine use of albumin-containing solutions.

Colloids include plasma protein fraction, albumin 5 percent and 25 percent, starches (hetastarch 6 percent and pentastarch 10 percent), dextran 40, dextran 70, gelatins, blood substitutes, and blood and blood products.

Balanced salt solutions include 0.9 percent NS, Ringer's lactate, and Plasmalyte A. Their electrolyte composition and osmolarity are shown in Table 5–8.

Balanced salt solutions redistribute to all the active fluid compartments within 2 hours of infusion. Therefore, hemorrhagic losses require three to four times the volume, as opposed to whole blood replacement, to reach the same circulating blood volume.[154]

Hetastarch (hydroxyethyl [HES]) is a class of solutions similar to glycogen. Hydroxylation with amylopectin reduces its breakdown by serum amylase. The actual size of the molecules varies widely, with clinical volume expansion exceeding 3 hours and some particles remaining in the intravascular space for weeks. Hetastarch added to normal saline has an osmolarity of 310 mOsm/L. Actual doses may vary, but the manufacturers suggest giving no more than 20 ml/kg/day. Many reports have far exceeded this recommendation without untoward effects on pulmonary, hepatic, or renal function.[47] Complications of the use of hetastarch include changes in coagulation, anaphylaxis, and elevations of serum amylase. Pentastarch is more rapidly degraded by amylase and is more rapidly excreted. The 10 percent solution effectively increases intravascular volume. Active investigation is currently underway to determine if it might effectively plug leaky capillaries. Dextrans are glucose polymers produced by bacteria on a sucrose medium. The small molecules are filtered by the kidney, causing a mild diuresis. However, the large molecules in dextran 70 stay in the intravascular space for more than 24 hours and actually improve microvascular flow.[178] Adverse reactions include renal failure, significant platelet dysfunction, other bleeding diatheses, and anaphylaxis. Some reports also relate problems in crossmatching blood and measuring serum glucose. Recombinant albumin and gelatins are less likely to cause problems with anaphylactoid reactions or bleeding diatheses and have fewer effects on the kidneys. Artificial blood, consisting of perfluorochemicals, allows slightly more oxygen to dissolve in solution, which increases oxygen-carrying capacity.

Oncotic Pressure

Sodium, the major cation in the intravascular space, is responsible for osmotic pressure. Albumin, the major protein in the intravascular space, also is responsible for oncotic pressure. "Leaky membranes" created by release of histamine, complement, or other inflammatory mediators should be separated from other causes of circulating volume loss such as hemorrhage, severe burns, protein-losing enteropathy, nephropathy, and malnutrition.

Colloid Osmotic Pressure

Colloid osmotic pressure (COP) is essentially composed of circulating albumin. Although only 40 percent of total body albumin is intravascular, the small size of albumin compared with that of other circulating proteins makes its concentration equal to the COP. Patients with high globulin production, such as those with cirrhosis or multiple myeloma, may have normal total proteins but they may also be hypoalbuminemic.

Proteins are highly charged anions that trap sodium molecules within their core structures. This is described by the following equations:

$$[Na^+]A \times [Cl^-]A = [Na^+]B \times [Cl^-]B$$
$$\text{(Gibbs-Dannan equation)}$$

and

$$v = [kf(P_c - P_{if}] - \sigma(\pi_c - \pi_{if}) - Q_{lymph} \text{ (Starling's law)}$$

where $(P_c - P_{if})$ is the hydrostatic pressure within the capillary minus the hydrostatic pressure within the interstitial fluid space (Fig. 5–5). The normal pressure is 15 to 20 mm Hg. σ is the size of the capillary pore and varies from organ to tissues. Loss of lymph flow causes significant subcutaneous edema, especially in children receiving muscle relaxants or after prolonged periods of bed rest. Similar edema is not seen in constantly moving tissue, such as heart and lung tissue, and in tissue that does not possess lymph channels, such as the brain. However, even with capillary tight junctions and exercise, the lung will become edematous with severely low oncotic pressures, as seen during experimental plasmapheresis.

The kf is a filtration coefficient that may vary with the amount of albumin in the interstitium. $(\pi_c - \pi_{if})$ is the protein concentration within the circulation and interstitium. As noted above, as much as 60 percent of the total body albumin is in the interstitium. With proalbumin in the cells and rapid transport in lymph channels, significant losses in COP can be replenished rapidly. If interstitial albumin is decreased, as seen with chronic losses of circulating protein, fluid flow into the interstitium will accelerate. A better understanding of the lymphatic system may now be obtained, since lymph channels can be cannulated in humans.[180]

TABLE 5 – 8
ELECTROLYTE CONTENT AND OSMOLARITY OF BALANCED SALT SOLUTIONS

Electrolytes (mEq/L)	0.9 Normal Saline	Ringer's Lactate	Plasmalyte A
Na	154	130	140
Cl	154	109	98
K	—	4	5
Lactate	—	28	—
Acetate	—	—	27
Ca	—	3	—
Mg	—	—	3
mOsm/L	308	273	294

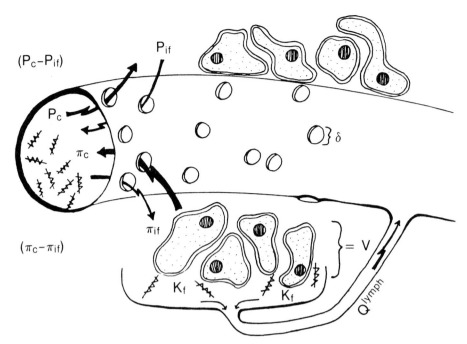

FIGURE 5–5. Starling's law illustrating that $(P_c–P_{if})$ is equal to hydrostatic pressure and $(\pi_c–\pi_{if})$ is equal to oncotic pressure. The pore membrane size is represented by δ and the lymphatic flow returning interstitial fluid and albumin back into the circulating volume is simply Q_{lymph}. (From Kaminski MV, Haase TJ: Albumin and colloid osmotic pressure implications for fluid resuscitation. Crit Care Clin 8:311, 1992, with permission.)

Low COP

Tissue variability of permeability (σ) can be seen perioperatively in the child's sclera. Low COP can form a pink spongy gelatinous mass in the dependent portion of the sclera (chemosis) with acute decreases in total protein to below 5 g/dl. Giving only crystalloid in this setting causes a greater dilution of protein, which accelerates fluid flow into the interstitium. In a recent review,[179] increased interstitial edema is said to predispose children to decubitus ulcers, to cause intestinal edema, and to weaken the ability of sutures to hold tissues together. Attempts to decrease edema by administering diuretics may decrease blood volume, compromise renal function, and fail to resolve pulmonary edema. The low COP must be evaluated carefully. If the low COP is because of low total protein, the addition of albumin to a program of parenteral nutrition is more likely to restore COP and decrease tissue edema. In general, once a child has received one blood volume of crystalloid-containing solution, some colloid must be infused to minimize critically low levels of COP.

MANAGEMENT OF PERIOPERATIVE FLUIDS

Major surgery in children causes metabolic, mineral, electrolyte, and water losses. Increases in serum concentrations of catecholamines, glucocorticoids, and antidiuretic and natriuretic hormones occur during and after surgery. The anesthesiologist must understand how these operative losses and hormone responses interact and how they can be counterbalanced to allow rapid recovery and healing in pediatric patients.

Preoperative Oral Fluids

NPO Status

Fasting, often for many hours, is recommended to ensure that patients undergoing elective surgery have a minimal amount of gastric fluid when anesthesia is induced. Mendelson[181] reviewed 44,016 pregnancies from 1932 to 1945 and found that 66 of the parturients experienced pulmonary aspiration of gastric contents. This incidence, 0.15 percent, represented mostly benign aspiration, and only six of the parturients died from "suffocation," an incidence of 0.014 percent. Mendelson completed this report by demonstrating that injecting acid vomitus into a rabbit caused death, but if the vomitus was neutralized the lungs did not suffer significant damage. The incidence of Mendelson syndrome in children is approximately 1 in 10,000, with a somewhat higher incidence in infants.[182] Solid foods remain in the stomach for long periods of time, and most children undergoing elective surgical procedures are fasted overnight.[183] Prolonged periods of fasting do predispose infants to irritability and thirst, which can increase gastric fluid volume and decrease gastric fluid pH. This reaction increases the probability that acidic gastric contents may be aspirated.

The effect of giving patients 5 oz of water PO 2 to 3 hours before the induction of anesthesia was compared with an overnight fast of up to 17 hours. Gastric fluid volume and pH were assessed after induction of anesthesia. Patients given water had less gastric fluid and a higher gastric fluid pH than those who received no fluids preoperatively.[184] Sips of clear liquids stimulate peristalsis but do not stimulate gastric acid secretion if no protein is given. Clear liquids dilute gastric acid and the resulting solution passes into the duodenum, usually within a few minutes. Large volumes of saline[185] or even tea and toast[186] are not present in the stomach of adults 2 hours after their ingestion. Children given clear liquids (e.g., water, apple juice, or crystalloid-containing solutions) 2 hours before induction of anesthesia have decreased thirst, gastric volume, and hunger compared with a control group of children fasted overnight.[187, 188] Gastric pH was the same in both groups. This is not surprising, as gastric emptying for liquid takes minutes, not hours. Maximal emptying time for solids probably correlates with the onset of thirst and hunger. The usual time between infant feedings is the most rational measurement of gastric emptying time and oral calorie deprivation.

Aspiration pneumonia is a much greater threat in children with feeding and swallowing problems, gastroesophageal reflux, seizures, or other CNS compromise (such as Guillain-Barré syndrome or myasthenia gravis).[189]

Preoperative dehydration occurs as a consequence of excessive fluid losses, lack of oral fluid intake, or insufficient maintenance fluid therapy. Although parenteral fluids may not be necessary during minor surgical procedures, preoperative rehydration can ameliorate significant morbidity in major and emergent surgical procedures. Correction of fluid and electrolyte imbalances before anesthesia induction minimizes reflex signals present during anesthesia and surgery that predispose to fluid retention. Therefore, maintaining a normal or even slightly expanded functional extracellular fluid compartment can prevent unnecessary perioperative fluid retention.

Another advantage of increasing the extracellular fluid volume preoperatively is that fewer red blood cells are lost during surgery because the additional crystalloid dilutes the blood. For example, a child whose hematocrit is 40 percent loses 40 ml of red blood cells with a 100-ml blood loss. However, if this same child, whose blood volume is 80 ml/kg, were to receive a rapid infusion of a balanced salt solution preoperatively (20 ml/kg over 10 to 20 minutes), his hematocrit would be diluted to 30 percent. Because most of the supplemental crystalloid fluid initially remains in the intravascular space, the percentage of red blood cells in the plasma space decreases to almost 30 percent. The same 100-ml blood loss would result in only a 30-ml red blood cell loss.

A child can undergo planned hemodilution by donating homologous blood before surgery and replacing that volume with crystalloid or, if scheduled in advance, by oral intake of two to three times the blood volume removed. The use of human recombinant erythropoietin has also been proposed for children able to donate blood weeks before a procedure with anticipated large blood losses.[190] The oxygen sensor that stimulates production of erythropoietin in the liver and kidney appears to be a heme protein.[191]

Homologous blood can be returned to the patient at the end of surgery or whenever additional blood is required. Although moderate hemorrhagic losses can be replaced by balanced salt solutions, severe and rapid blood loss should be replaced with whole blood. Replacement therapy can be initiated while the amount of blood loss, clinical variables, and anticipated losses are assessed.

Determination of volume status requires analysis of changes in heart rate, mean arterial pressure (MAP), capillary perfusion time, core versus extremity temperature, moistness of mucous membranes, tears, skin turgor, and weight (see Chapter 11). In emergent cases, full preoperative correction of extracellular fluid deficits may not be possible before the induction of anesthesia, but these deficits should be corrected as much as possible. Peritonitis, perforated viscus, gastroschisis, omphalocele, intussusception, bowel obstruction, and major trauma are all characterized by continuing large fluid and protein shifts that require fluid resuscitation before a general anesthetic can

be administered. Preoperative evaluation of these patients consists of a complete history of fluid intake and fluid losses. Changes in urine output and specific gravity, and a careful analysis of vital signs, must be used to assess the patient's fluid volume status.

To avoid preoperative dehydration in infants, shorter fasting times and less severe fluid restriction schedules should be used. Infants become dehydrated sooner than older patients because they have about twice the metabolic and water losses as adolescents. In addition, very young infants and some children with renal insufficiency cannot produce concentrated urine, which causes further obligate water losses. Fluid loss and the volume of fluid required to adequately replace it can be determined by a simplified deficit estimation (Table 5–9).

Replacement of fluid deficits should always begin with a balanced salt solution to increase the circulating blood volume. Hydration and the increased circulating volume increase renal blood flow and replenish the functional extravascular volume. Repeat electrolyte and urine specific gravity determinations assist in avoiding excessive salt or water administration. No single clinical or laboratory parameter should be used to assess fluid replacement. Instead, a thorough review of laboratory reports, clinical examinations, serial weights, and vital sign trends is necessary to effectively assess preoperative hydration.

Intraoperative Fluid Therapy

During surgery, maintenance fluids (see Table 5–1) are required. Breathing unhumidified gases increases fluid requirements, as does increased minute ventilation. Inhalation of warm, humidified gases causes a gain of both water and heat. Additional water is lost from exposed surface areas (e.g., abdomen and chest cavity). Losses during craniofacial surgery are proportionally larger in younger infants than in older ones, as the head represents a larger proportion of their total body surface area. Retrospective studies abound attesting to the massive amounts of replacement blood required in the perioperative period.

As previously emphasized, free-water-containing solutions rapidly filter out of the vascular compartment, expand and dilute interstitial and cellular compartments, and promote postsurgical edema. Replacing fluid losses with a balanced salt solution leads to less fluid retention, and a natriuretic response is induced. Three factors are active in the restoration of fluid homeostasis.

1. Fluid balance is sensed by volume and osmoreceptors. Infusing a balanced salt solution that contains

TABLE 5–9
ESTIMATION OF FLUID DEFICIT

Deficit	Clinical Findings
Mild (5%)	Dry mucous membranes, poor skin turgor, irritability, decreased urination
Moderate (10%)	No tears, tenting of skin, lethargy, oliguria
Severe (15%)	Sunken eyes and fontanelles, cold skin, anuria, tachycardia and tachypnea, hypotension, coma

a relative excess of sodium replaces water while increasing total body sodium.

2. This relative sodium excess helps to maintain circulation and to replete the reduced functional extracellular volume. Increases in vascular capacitance stretch the cardiac atrium and increased renal blood flow. Natriuretic hormone further increases intravascular blood volume.

3. By increasing renal blood flow and stimulating sodium secretion, body fluid homeostasis (via a diuretic [water-losing] and natriuretic [sodium-secreting] response) reequilibrates, which reduces perioperative fluid retention.

Excess water, on the other hand, dilutes the extravascular compartment, and isotonic shifts of fluid and electrolytes cause cells to absorb water. The resultant cellular edema compromises transcellular inflow of nutrients and outflow of cell wastes. The reduction of nutrients decreases cell function and retards healing and growth. The reduced outflow of waste products causes gradual poisoning. These toxic wastes, coupled with the lack of energy substrate, decrease the activity of the sodium-potassium adenosine triphosphatase–dependent pumps, which prevents the cells from maintaining normal electrolyte gradients between the cellular and extracellular compartments.

Postoperative Fluids

Tissues retain excess water postoperatively in response to increased vasopressin secretion.[192, 193] For minor operations, the use of postoperative fluids is being actively debated.[194–196] Pediatric outpatients may actually have increased nausea and vomiting after forced oral intake,[197] particularly when insufficient parenteral fluids have been infused. In some patients, blood volume contraction and hypotonic fluid intake cause an increase of several liters in the extracellular fluid. The increase in intracellular sodium concentration is associated with a decrease in serum sodium concentration. When free-water-containing solutions were used to replace the perioperative fluid losses, sodium concentration fell from 138 mEq/L to 108 mEq/L in a group of previously healthy young women.[198] This decrease was associated with seizures, respiratory arrest, and permanent brain damage or death in 15 women, possibly because of a demyelination syndrome. Rapid correction of hyponatremia is imperative,[199] although some investigators postulate that increased pontine demyelination may occur with too rapid correction of hyponatremia.[200] It is tempting to provide free water to children, but these findings in adults are a harsh reminder that giving free-water-containing solutions to patients may precipitously lower their serum sodium concentrations. This seems to be especially significant during the postoperative period, when vasopressin levels are increased. Desmopressin acetate, aqueous vasopressin, and phenothiazines may also increase water retention.

When urine output is adequate (more than 0.8 ml/kg/h), it is not necessary to increase fluid administration. Oliguria (urine flow <0.8 ml/kg/h) may be because of dehydration or renal failure. These two states can often be differentiated by measuring the serum urea nitrogen/

creatinine ratio. Decreases in intravascular volume or renal perfusion reduce urinary sodium excretion to less than 10 mEq/L and increase the serum urea nitrogen/creatinine ratio to more than 20:1. Ratios in this range are attributable to "prerenal" factors. Acute renal failure, on the other hand, is indicated by an increased renal sodium concentration (to >50 mEq/L) and increases in both serum urea nitrogen and creatinine, which leaves the ratio of the two unchanged. In both cases, enough fluid should be given to maintain renal and circulatory function.[201] Evaluation of fluid deficits often causes a delay in treatment, when the goal for a known hypovolemic child mandates a rapid correction to maintain circulating volume and renal function.[202]

The Color of Urine

Although the volume of urine output is easy to measure, the color of urine seems dependent on the turnover of bilirubin, and urochrome. However, the color of urine and specific gravity do seem to be closely related, as we have all seen from the straw-colored dilute urine rushing down the tube to the liquid gold of the slowly filling concentrated cup.[203]

Health Care Worker Risks in Parenteral Therapy

Children can seldom be counted on to give informed consent and cooperate with placement of an IV catheter. One mark of the pediatric anesthesiologist is proficiency in starting IV infusions in children and in providing secure and safe restraints for an uncooperative child to prevent injury to health care workers. Although the risk of contaminated needle sticks appears to be greatest when a syringe is recapped, the risk of serious inoculation is greater during IV puncture procedures, such as starting IV infusions or performing arterial punctures. The actual risk to pediatric anesthesiologists is difficult to assess, since most physicians do not report needle stick injuries. In addition, comparing needle stick rates between known human immunodeficiency virus (HIV) carriers and HIV-negative patients yields a needle stick rate that is essentially the same.[204]

REFERENCES

1. Stevens J: One Robe, One Bowl; The Zen Poetry of Ryokan. New York, Weatherhill, 1977.
2. Gladstone E: The lure of medical history. Calif West Med 38:432, 1933.
3. Latta T: Letter to the Secretary of the Central Board of Health London, affording a view of the rationale and the results of his practice in the treatment of cholera by aqueous and saline injections. Lancet 2:274, 1830–1832.
4. Bickel WH, Wall MJ, Pepe PE, et al: Immediate versus delayed fluid resuscitation for hypotensive patients with penetrating torso injuries. N Engl J Med 331:1105, 1994.
5. Carpenter CC: The treatment of cholera: clinical science at the bedside. J Infect Dis 166:2, 1992.
6. Lister JA: A contribution to the germ theory of putrefaction and other fermative changes, and the natural history of torulae and bacteria. Trans R Soc Edinb 27:T-2, 1875.
7. Jenkins MT: History of sequestered edema in surgery and trauma. In Brown BR (ed): Fluid and Blood Therapy in Anesthesia. Philadelphia, FA Davis, 1983, p 2.

8. Pitts RF: Physiology of the Kidney and Body Fluids. Chicago, Year Book Medical Publishers, 1963.
9. Holt E, Courtney A: The chemical composition of diarrheal as compared with normal stools in infants. Am J Dis Child 9:213, 1915.
10. Howland J, Marriot WM: Acidosis occurring with diarrhea. Am J Dis Child 1916:309, 1916.
11. Brook CG: Determination of body composition of children from skin fold measurements. Arch Dis Child 46:182, 1971.
12. Butte N, Heinz C, Hopkinson J, et al: Fat mass in infants and toddlers: comparability of total body water, total body potassium, total body electrical conductivity, and dual-energy x-ray absorptiometry. J Pediatr Gastroenterol Nutr 29:184, 1999.
13. Howland J, Dana RT: A formula for the determination of the surface area of infants. Am J Dis Child 6:33, 1913.
14. Dubois D, Dubois FF: Clinical calorimetry: formula to estimate approximate surface area if height and weight be known. Arch Intern Med 17:863, 1916.
15. Boyd E: Growth of surface area of the human body. Institute of Child Welfare, Monograph Series 10. Minneapolis, University of Minnesota Press, 1935.
16. Berry FA (ed): Anesthetic Management of Difficult and Routine Pediatric Patients. New York, Churchill Livingstone, 1986.
17. Oliver WJ, Graham BD, Wilson JL: Lack of scientific validity of body surface as a basis for parenteral fluid dosage. JAMA 167:1211, 1958.
18. Losek JD: Rapid assessment of glucose needed in children requiring resuscitation. Ann Emerg Med 35:43, 2000.
19. Talbot FB, Crawford JD, Butler AM: Medical progress; homeostatic limits to safe parenteral fluid therapy. N Engl J Med 248:1100, 1953.
20. Howland J: The fundamental requirements of an infant's nutrition. Am J Dis Child 2:49, 1911.
21. Holliday MA, Segar WE: Maintenance need for water in parenteral fluid therapy. Pediatrics 19:823, 1957.
22. Lindahl SG: Energy expenditure and fluid and electrolyte requirements in anesthetized infants and children. Anesthesiology 69:377, 1988.
23. Welborn LG, Hannallah RS, McGill WA, et al: Glucose concentrations for routine intravenous infusion in pediatric output surgery. Anesthesiology 67:427, 1987.
24. Larsson LE, Nilsson K, Niklasson A, et al: Influence of fluid regimens on perioperative blood-glucose concentrations in neonates. Br J Anaesth 64:419, 1990.
25. Karcher R, Ingram R, Kiechle F, et al: Evaluation of HemoCue B-glucose photometer for intensive care applications. Clin Chem 38:6, 1992.
26. Coyle EF, Montain SJ: Carbohydrate and fluid ingestion during exercise: are there trade-offs? Med Sci Sports Exerc 24:671, 1992.
27. Sawka MN, Greenleaf JE: Current concepts concerning thirst, dehydration, and fluid replacement: overview. Med Sci Sports Exerc 24:643, 1992.
28. Hoobler BR: The role of mineral salts in the metabolism of infants. Am J Dis Child 2:107, 1911.
29. Ringer S: Concerning the influence exercised by each of the constituents of the blood on the contraction of the ventricle. J Physiol (Lond) 3:380, 1880–1882.
30. Winters RW: Principles of Pediatric Fluid Therapy. North Chicago, Abbott Laboratories, 1970.
31. Avery ME, Snyder JD: Oral therapy for acute diarrhea. N Engl J Med 323:892, 1990.
32. Alam NH, Majumder RN, Fuchs GJ: Efficacy and safety of oral rehydration solution with reduced osmolarity in adults with cholera: a randomized double-blind clinical trial. CHOICE study group. Lancet 354:296, 1999.
33. Glynn IM, Karlish SJD: The sodium and potassium pump. Annu Rev Physiol 37:895, 1967.
34. Sheng HP, Huggins RA: A review of body composition studies with emphasis on total body water and fat. Am J Clin Nutr 32:630, 1979.
35. Cochran WJ, Klish WJ, Wong WW, et al: Total body electrical conductivity used to determine body composition in infants. Pediatr Res 20:561, 1986.
36. Lewis DS, Rollwitz WL, Bertrand HA, et al: Use of NMR for measurement of total body water and estimation of body fat. J Appl Physiol 60:836, 1986.
37. Friis-Hansen B: Water distribution in the foetus and newborn infant. Acta Paediatr Scand Suppl 305:7, 1983.

38. Venkatesh S, Schrier RW, Andreoli E: Mechanisms of tubular sodium chloride transport. Ren Fail 20:783, 1998.
39. Guyton AC, Scheel K, Murphree D: Interstitial fluid pressure: its effect on resistance to tissue fluid mobility. Circ Res 19:419, 1966.
40. Mullins RJ, Powers MR, Bell DR: Albumin and IgG in skin and skeletal muscle after plasmapheresis with saline loading. Am J Physiol 252:H71, 1987.
41. Oratz M, Rothchild MA, Schreiber SS: Albumin-osmotic function. In Rosenoer VW, Oratz M, Rothchild MA (eds): Albumin Structure, Function and Uses. New York, Pergamon Press, 1977, p 275.
42. Shires T, Williams J, Brown F: Acute changes in extracellular fluids associated with major surgical procedures. Ann Surg 154:803, 1961.
43. Fulop M: Algorithms for diagnosing and treating some electrolyte disorders. Am J Emerg Med 16:76, 1998.
44. Redfors S: Small intestinal fluid absorption in the rat during haemorrhage and its importance for plasma refill. Acta Physiol Scand 131:429, 1987.
45. Turbeville DF, Bowen FW, Killiam AP: Intracranial hemorrhage in kittens: hypernatremia versus hypoxia. J Pediatr 89:294, 1976.
46. Finberg L, Kravath R, Fleischman A: Water and Electrolytes in Pediatrics. Philadelphia, WB Saunders Company, 1982.
47. Brown DL: Anesthetic agents in trauma surgery: are there differences? In Kirby RR, Brown DL (eds): Anesthesia for Trauma. Boston, Little, Brown, 1987, p 75.
48. Seagard JL, Bosnjak ZJ, Hopp FAJ: Cardiovascular effects of general anesthetics. In Covino BG, Fozzard HA, Rehder K (eds): Effects of Anesthesia. Bethesda, MD, American Physiological Society, 1985, p 149.
49. Merin RG, Basch S: Are the myocardial functional and metabolic effects of isoflurane really different from those of halothane and enflurane? Anesthesiology 55:398, 1981.
50. Friesen RH, Henry DB: Cardiovascular changes in preterm neonates receiving isoflurane, halothane, fentanyl, and ketamine. Anesthesiology 64:238, 1986.
51. Shoukas AA, Sagawa K: Control of total vascular capacity by the carotid sinus baroreceptor reflex. Circ Res 3:22, 1973.
52. Siker D, Hoka S, Bosnjak ZB, et al: Influences of halothane and isoflurane on baroreflex control of vascular capacitance in the dog. Anesth Analg 66:S158, 1987.
53. Seyde WC, Longnecker DE: Anesthetic influences on regional hemodynamics in normal and hemorrhaged rats. Anesthesiology 60:686, 1984.
54. Weiskopf RB, Bogetz MS, Roizen MF, et al: Cardiovascular and metabolic sequelae of inducing anesthesia with ketamine or thiopental in hypovolemic swine. Anesthesiology 60:214, 1984.
55. Brace RA: Amniotic fluid volume and its relationship to fetal fluid balance: review of experimental data. Semin Perinatol 10:103, 1986.
56. Harmon CR: Maternal furosemide may not provoke urine production in the compromised fetus. Am J Obstet Gynecol 150:322, 1984.
57. Lorenz JM, Kleinman LI, Markarian K: Potassium metabolism in extremely low birth weight infants in the first week of life. J Pediatr 131:81, 1997.
58. Wiriyathian S, Rosenfield CR, Arant BSJ, et al: Urinary arginine vasopressin: pattern of excretion in the neonatal period. Pediatr Res 20:103, 1986.
59. Bell RJ, Wintour EM: The effect of maternal water deprivation on ovine fetal blood volume. Q J Exp Physiol 70:95, 1985.
60. Bell RJ, McDougal JG, Wang X, et al: Effect of maternal sodium depletion on the composition of ovine fetal fluids. J Endocrinol 107:177, 1985.
61. Kikuchi K, Shioma M, Horie K, et al: Plasma atrial natriuretic, polypeptide concentration in healthy children from birth to adolescence. Acta Paediatr Scand 77:380, 1988.
62. Battaglia F, Prystowsky H, Smisson C, et al: Fetal blood studies. XIII. The effect of the administration of fluids intravenously to mothers upon the concentrations of water and electrolytes in the plasma of the human fetuses. Pediatrics 25:2, 1960.
63. Bland RD: Dynamics of pulmonary water before and after birth. Acta Paediatr Scand Suppl 305:12, 1983.
64. Cartledge PH, Rutter N: Serum albumin concentrations and oedema in the newborn. Arch Dis Child 61:657, 1986.
65. Dubowitz KM, Dubowitz V, Goldberg C: Clinical assessment of gestational age in the newborn infant. J Pediatr 77:1, 1970.
66. Hammarlund K, Hellsing K, Sedin G, et al: Effects of human albumin infusion on transepidermal loss in newborn infants. Biol Neonate 45:112, 1984.

67. Hammarlund K, Sedin G, Stromberg B: Transepidermal water loss in newborn infants. Acta Paediatr Scand 72:721, 1983.

68. Sjors G, Hammarlund K, Oberg P, et al: An evaluation of environment and climate control in seven infant incubators. Biomed Instrum Technol 26:294, 1992.

69. Malin SW, Baumgart S: Optimal thermal management for low birth weight infants nursed under high-powered radiant warmers. Pediatrics 79:47, 1987.

70. Rutter N, Hull D: water loss from the skin of term and preterm babies. Arch Dis Child 54:558, 1979.

71. Tulassay T, Rascher W, Seyberth HW, et al: Role of atrial natriuretic peptide in sodium homeostasis in premature infants. J Pediatr 109:1023, 1986.

72. Shaffer SG, Geer PG, Goetz KL: Elevated atrial natriuretic factor in neonates with respiratory distress syndrome. J Pediatr 109:1028, 1986.

73. Brenner BM, Stein JH (eds): Body Fluid Homeostasis. New York, Churchill Livingstone, 1987.

74. Kaskel FJ, Kumar AM, Lockhart EA, et al: Factors affecting proximal tubular reabsorption during development. Am J Physiol 21:F188, 1987.

75. Aperia A, Bromberger O, Herin P, et al: Postnatal control of water and electrolyte homeostasis in pre-term and full term infants. Acta Paediatr Scand Suppl 305:61, 1983.

76. Engle WD: Development of fetal and neonatal renal function. Perinatology 10:113, 1986.

77. Al-Dahhan J, Haycock GB, Chantler C, et al: Sodium homeostasis in term and preterm neonates: renal aspects. Arch Dis Child 58:335, 1983.

78. Gross SJ: Growth and biochemical responses of preterm infants fed human milk or modified infant formula. N Engl J Med 308:237, 1983.

79. Schanler RJ, Oh W: Composition of breast milk obtained from mothers of premature infants as compared to breast milk obtained from donors. N Engl J Med 96:679, 1980.

80. Svennington NW, Andreasson B, Lindroth M: Diuresis and urine concentration during CPAP in newborn infants. Acta Paediatr Scand 73:727, 1984.

81. Garth LI, Phillips JB III, Work J, et al: Diuresis and natriuresis following acute pneumothorax in very low birthweight infants. Aust Paediatr J 21:269, 1985.

82. Coulter DM, LaPine TR, Gooch MWI: Treatment to prevent postnatal loss of brain water reduces the risk of intracranial hemorrhage in the beagle puppy. Pediatr Res 19:1322, 1985.

83. Bland RD: Edema formation in the lungs and is relationship to neonatal respiratory distress. Acta Paediatr Scand Suppl 305:92, 1983.

84. Stevenson JG: Fluid administration in the association of patent ductus arteriosis complicating respiratory distress syndrome. J Pediatr 90:257, 1977.

85. Al-Dahhan J, Haycock GB, Nichol B, et al: Sodium homeostasis in term and preterm neonates: effect of salt supplementation. Arch Dis Child 59:945, 1984.

86. Brem AS: Disorders of potassium homeostasis. Pediatr Clin North Am 37:419, 1990.

87. Vaughan RS: Potassium in the perioperative period. Br J Anaesth 67:194, 1991.

88. Tang TT, Oechler HW, Siker D, et al: Anesthesia-induced rhabdomyolysis in infants with unsuspected Duchenne dystrophy. Acta Paediatr 81:716, 1992.

89. Ventkataraman PS, Tsang RC, Streichen JJ, et al: Early neonatal hypocalcemia in extremely premature infants. Am J Dis Child 140:1004, 1986.

90. Venkataraman PS, Wilson DA, Sheldon JJ, et al: Effect of hypocalcemia on cardiac function in very low birthweight preterm neonates: studies of blood ionized calcium, echocardiography and assessment of cardiac effects of intravenous calcium therapy. Pediatrics 76:543, 1985.

91. Coté CJ, Drop LJ, Daniels AL, et al: Calcium chloride versus calcium gluconate: comparison of ionization and cardiovascular effects in children and dogs. Anesthesiology 66:465, 1987.

92. Bilezikian JP: Management of acute hypercalcemia. N Engl J Med 326:1196, 1992.

93. Ryzen E, Servis KL, Rude RK: Effect of intravenous epinephrine on serum magnesium and free intracellular red blood cell magnesium concentrations measured by nuclear magnetic resonance. J Am Coll Nutr 9:114, 1990.

94. Aperia A, Herin P, Lundin S, et al: Regulation of renal water excretion in newborn full-term infants. Acta Paediatr Scand 73:717, 1984.

95. Arieff AI: Indications for use of bicarbonate in patients with metabolic acidosis. Br J Anaesth 67:165, 1991.

96. Grossman H, Duggan E, McCamman S, et al: The dietary chloride deficiency syndrome. Pediatrics 66:366, 1980.

97. Schleien CL, Zahka KG, Rogers MC: Principles of postoperative management in the pediatric intensive care unit. In Rogers MC (ed): Textbook of Pediatric Intensive Care, Vol 1. Baltimore, Williams & Wilkins, 1987, p 440.

98. Caswell AM, Whyte MP, Russell RG: Hypophosphatasia and the extracellular metabolism of inorganic pyrophosphate: clinical and laboratory aspects. Crit Rev Clin Lab Sci 28:175, 1991.

99. Aouifi A, Neidecker J, Vedrinne C, et al: Glucose versus lactated Ringer's solution during pediatric cardiac surgery. J Cardiothorac Vasc Anesth 11:411, 1997.

100. Stjernstrom H, Jorfeldt L, Wiklund L: Influence of abdominal surgical trauma upon some energy metabolites in the quadriceps muscle in man. Clin Physiol 1:305, 1981.

101. Redfern N, Addison GM, Meakin G: Blood glucose in anesthetised children: comparison of blood glucose concentration in children fasted for morning and afternoon surgery. Anaesthesia 41:272, 1986.

102. Farias LA, Willis M, Gregory GA: Effects of fructose-1-6-diphosphate, glucose, and saline on cardiac resuscitation. Anesthesiology 65:595, 1986.

103. D'Alecy LG, Lundy EF, Barton KJ, et al: Dextrose containing intravenous fluid impairs outcome and increases death after eight minutes of cardiac arrest and resuscitation in dogs. Surgery 100:505, 1986.

104. Lanier WL, Stangland KJ, Scheithauer BW, et al: The effects of dextrose infusion and head position on neurologic outcome after complete cerebral ischemia in primates: examination of a model. Anesthesiology 66:39, 1987.

105. Ellemunter H, Simma B, Trwoger R, Mauer H: Intraosseous lines in preterm and full term neonates. Arch Dis Child 80:74F, 1999.

106. LaSpada J, Kissoon N, Melker R, et al: Extravasation rates and complications of intraosseous needles during gravity and pressure infusion. Crit Care Med 23:2123, 1995.

107. Aluoch JR: Management of sickle cell disease. East Afr Med J 68:576, 1991.

108. Charache S: Fetal hemoglobin, sickling, and sickle cell disease. Adv Pediatr 37:1, 1990.

109. Perrine SP, Ginder GD, Faller DV, et al: A short-term trial of butyrate to stimulate fetal-globin-gene expression in the beta-globin disorders. N Engl J Med 328:81, 1993.

110. Dover GJ, Smith KD, Chang YC, et al: Fetal hemoglobin levels in sickle cell disease and normal individuals are partially controlled by an X-linked gene located at Xp22.2. Blood 80:816, 1992.

111. Holm C, Melcer B, Horbrand F, et al: Intrathoracic blood volume as an end point in resuscitation of the severely burned. J Trauma 48:728, 2000.

112. Arturson G: Fluid therapy of thermal injury. Acta Anaesthesiol Scand 29:55, 1985.

113. Harms BA, Bodai BI, Kramer GC, et al: Microvascular fluid and protein flux in pulmonary and systemic circulations after thermal injury. Microvasc Res 23:77, 1982.

114. Yowler CJ, Fratianne RB: Current status of burn resuscitation. Clin Plast Surg 27:1, 2000.

115. Demling RH, Kramer G, Harms B: Role of thermal injury-induced hypoproteinemia on fluid flux and protein permeability in burned and nonburned patients. Surgery 95:136, 1984.

116. Jeschke MG, Herndon DN, Barrow RE: Long-term outcomes of burned children after in-hospital cardiac arrest. Crit Care Med 28:517, 2000.

117. Goodwin CW, Dorethy J, Pruitt BAJ: Randomized trial of crystalloid and colloid resuscitation on hemodynamic response and lung water following thermal injury. Ann Surg 197:520, 1983.

118. Kramer GC, Harms BA, Bodai BI, et al: Mechanisms for the redistribution of plasma proteins following acute protein depletion. Am J Physiol 243:803, 1982.

119. Tanaka H, Matsuda T, Miyagantani Y, et al: Reduction of resuscitation fluid volumes in severely burned patients using ascorbic acid administration: a randomized, prospective study. Arch Surg 135:326, 2000.

120. Szyfelbein SK, Drop LJ, Jeevendra-Martyn JA: Persistent ionized hypocalcemia in patients during resuscitation and recovery phases of body burns. Crit Care Med 9:454, 1981.

121. Burke JF, Bondoc CC, Morris PJ: Metabolic effects of silver nitrate therapy in burns covering more than 40% surface area. Am N Y Acad Sci 150:676, 1968.

122. Herndon DN, Traber DI, Neihaus GD, et al: The pathophysiology of smoke inhalation injury in a sheep model. J Trauma 24:1043, 1984.

123. Herndon DN, Traber DL, Traber LD: The effect of resuscitation on inhalation injury. Surgery 100:248, 1986.

124. Carlson RG, Miller SF, Finley RK, et al: Fluid retention and burn survival. J Trauma 27:127, 1987.

125. Solomonov E, Hirsh M, Yahiya A, Krausz MM: The effect of vigorous resuscitation in uncontrolled hemorrhagic shock after massive splenic injury. Crit Care Med 28:749, 2000.

126. Carcillo JA, Davis AL, Zaritsky A: Role of early fluid resuscitation in pediatric septic shock. JAMA 266:1242, 1991.

127. Falk JL, O'Brien JF, Kerr R: Fluid resuscitation in traumatic hemorrhagic shock. Crit Care Clin 8:323, 1992.

128. Ichikawa I: A bridge over troubled water . . . mixed water and electrolyte disorders. Pediatr Nephrol 12:160, 1998.

129. Morimoto T: Thermoregulation and body fluids: role of blood volume and central venous pressure. Jpn J Physiol 40:165, 1990.

130. Sarnaik AP, Meert K, Hackbarth R, et al: Management of hyponatremic seizures in children with hypertonic saline: a safe and effective strategy. Crit Care Med 19:758, 1991.

131. Jackson J, Bolte RG: Risk of intravenous administration of hypotonic fluids for pediatric patients in ED and prehospital settings: let's remove the handle from the pump. Am J Emerg Med 18:269, 2000.

132. Oliver D: Terminal dehydration. Lancet 2:631, 1984.

133. Printz L: Is withholding hydration a valid comfort measure in the terminally ill? Geriatrics 43:84, 1988.

134. Majeed N, Lawson W, Przeulocka B: Brain and peripheral opioid peptides after changes in ingestive behavior. Neuroendocrinology 46:267, 1986.

135. Printz LA: Terminal dehydration, a compassionate treatment. Arch Intern Med 152:697, 1992.

136. Winkler MA, Flanigin RN: Caring for patients at the end of life; call for papers. JAMA 282:20, 1999.

137. Sutin KM, Ruskin KJ, Kaufman BS: Intravenous fluid therapy in neurologic injury. Crit Care Clin 8:367, 1992.

138. Taylor G, Myers S, Kurth CD, et al: Hypertonic saline improves brain resuscitation in a pediatric model of head injury and hemorrhagic shock. J Pediatr Surg 31:65, 1996.

139. Wijdicks EF, Vermeulen M, Hijdra A: Hyponatremia and cerebral infarction in patients with ruptured intracranial aneurysms. Ann Neurol 17:137, 1985.

140. Swales JD: Management of hyponatremia. Br J Anaesth 67:146, 1991.

141. Diringer MN, Wu KC, Verbalis JG, et al: Hypervolemic therapy prevents volume contraction but not hyponatremia following subarachnoid hemorrhage. Ann Neurol 31:543, 1992.

142. Wijdicks EF, Vermeulen M, Van Brummelen P: Digoxin-like immunoreactive substance in patients with aneurysmal subarachnoid hemorrhage. BMJ 294:729, 1987.

143. Rodriguez-Soriano J, Arant BS, Brodehl J, et al: Fluid and electrolyte imbalances in children with chronic renal failure. Am J Kidney Dis 4:268, 1986.

144. Elema JD, Arends A: Focal and segmental glomerular hyalinosis in the rat. Lab Invest 33:554, 1975.

145. Feld LG, Cachero S, Springate JE: Fluid needs in acute renal failure. Pediatr Clin North Am 37:337, 1990.

146. Fine LG, Salehmoghaddam S: Water homeostasis in acute and chronic renal failure. Semin Nephrol 4:289, 1984.

146a. Wyshak G: Teenaged girls, carbonated beverage consumption and bone fractures [see comments]. Arch Pediatr Adolesc Med 154:610, 2000.

147. Dudrick SJ, Wilmore DW, Vars HS: Long-term total parenteral nutrition with growth, development, and positive nitrogen balance. Surgery 64:134, 1968.

148. Karlstad MD, Killeffer JA, Bailey JW, et al: Parenteral nutrition with short- and long-chain triglycerides: triacetin reduces atrophy of small and large bowel mucosa and improves protein metabolism in burned rats. Am J Clin Nutr 55:1005, 1992.

149. Sinclair JC, Driscoll JM, Heird WC, et al: Supportive management of the sick neonate. Pediatr Clin North Am 17:863, 1970.

150. Mauer AM, Burgess JB, Donaldson SS, et al: Special nutritional needs of children with malignancies: a review. JPEN J Parenter Enter Nutr 14:315, 1990.

151. Sluis KB, Darlow BA, George PM, et al: Selenium and glutathione peroxidase levels in premature infants in a low selenium community (Christchurch, New Zealand). Pediatr Res 32:189, 1992.

152. Greenough A: Use and misuse of albumin infusions in neonatal care. Eur J Pediatr 157:699, 1998.

153. Elwyn DH, Bryan-Brown CW, Shoemaker WC: Nutritional aspects of body water dislocations in post-operative and depleted patients. Ann Surg 182:76, 1975.

154. Griffel MI, Kaufman BS: Pharmacology of colloids and crystalloids. Crit Care Clin 8:235, 1992.

155. Doweiko JP, Nompleggi DJ: The role of albumin in human physiology and pathophysiology, part III: albumin and disease states. JPEN J Parenter Enter Nutr 15:476, 1991.

156. Shaw JH, Wildbone M, Wolfe RR: Whole body kinetics in severely septic patients: the response to glucose infusion and total parenteral infusion. Ann Surg 205:288, 1987.

157. Sandberg LB, Owens AJ, VanReken DE, et al: Improvement in plasma protein concentrations with fibronectin treatment in severe malnutrition. Am J Clin Nutr 52:651, 1990.

158. Manson JM, Wilmore DW: Positive nitrogen balance with human growth hormone and hypocaloric intravenous feeding. Surgery 100:188, 1986.

159. Larca L, Greenbaum DM: Effectiveness of intensive nutritional regimes in patients who fail to wean from mechanical ventilation. Crit Care Med 10:297, 1982.

160. Cornblath M, Schwartz R, Aynsley-Green A, et al: Hypoglycemia in infancy: the need for a rational definition. Pediatrics 85:834, 1990.

161. Novarini A, Borghi L, Curit A, et al: Extracellular water, electrolyte and nitrogen balance after postoperative parenteral nutrition and intracellular involvement in muscle. Acta Chir Scand 149:651, 1983.

162. Alderson P, Schierhout G, Roberts I, Bunn F: Colloids versus crystalloids for fluid resuscitation in critically ill patients. Cochrane Database Syst Rev 2:CD000567, 2000.

163. Holm C: Resuscitation in shock associated with burns. Tradition or evidence-based medicine? Resuscitation 44:157, 2000.

164. Rackow EC, Falk JL, Fein IA, et al: Fluid resuscitation in circulatory shock: a comparison of albumin, hetastarch, and saline solutions in patients with hypovolemic and septic shock. Crit Care Med 11:839, 1983.

165. Nacelle H: Course lectures on the physiology and pathology of blood and other animal fluids. Lancet 1:222, 1839.

166. Cohn EJ, Strong LE, Hughes WL: Preparation and properties of serum and plasma protein. IV. A system for the separation into fractions of the protein and lipoprotein components of biological tissues and fluids. J Am Med Soc 68:459, 1946.

167. Brinson RR, Kolts BE: Hypoalbuminemia as an indicator of diarrheal incidence in critically ill patients. Crit Care Med 15:506, 1987.

168. Sort P, Miquel N, Arroyo V, et al: Effects of intravenous albumin on renal impairment and mortality in patients with cirrhosis and spontaneous bacterial peritonitis. N Engl J Med 341:403, 1999.

169. McClure G: The use of plasma in the neonatal period. Arch Dis Child 66:373, 1991.

170. Yoshimura A, Ideura T, Iwasaki T, et al: Aggravation of minimal change nephrotic syndrome by administration of human albumin. Clin Nephrol 37:109, 1992.

171. Nielsen VG, Baird MS, Brix AE, Matalon S: Extreme, progressive isovolemic hemodilution with 5% human albumin, PentaLyte, or Hextend does not cause hepatic ischemia or histologic injury in rabbits. Anesthesiology 90:428, 1999.

172. Rothschild MA, Oratz M, Schreiber SS: Serum albumin. Hepatology 8:385, 1988.

173. Broderson R: Bilirubin transport in the newborn infant reviewed with relation to kernicterus. J Pediatr 96:349, 1980.

174. Mercatello A, Laville M, Leizorovicz A: Untoward effects of therapeutic plasma exchanges. A prospective study. Presse Med 18:325, 1989.

175. Brossard Y, Larsen M, Mesnard G, et al: Bilirubin-albumin-binding function of 2 human albumin preparations. Comparisons of their efficacy in the icteric premature infant. Arch Fr Pediatr 45:91, 1988.

176. Watson PD, Wolf MB, Beck-Montgomery IS: Blood and isoproterenol reduce capillary permeability in cat hindlimb. Am J Physiol 252:H47, 1987.

177. Doweiko JP, Nompleggi J: Use of albumin as a volume expander. JPEN J Parenter Enter Nutr 15:484, 1991.
178. Zikria BA, Subbarao C, Mehmet C, et al: Hydroxyethyl starch macromolecules reduce myocardial reperfusion injury. Arch Surg 125:930, 1990.
179. Kaminski MV, Haase TJ: Albumin and colloid osmotic pressure implications for fluid resuscitation. Crit Care Clin 8:311, 1992.
180. Castillo CE, Lillioja S: Peripheral lymphatic cannulation for physiological analysis of interstitial fluid compartment in humans. Am J Physiol 261:H1324, 1991.
181. Mendelson CL: The aspiration of stomach contents into the lungs during obstetric anesthesia. Am J Obstet Gynecol 52:191, 1946.
182. Coté CJ: NPO after midnight for children—a reappraisal. Anesthesiology 72:589, 1990.
183. Meakin G, Dingwall AE, Addison GM: Effects of fasting and oral premedication on the pH and volume of gastric aspirate in children. Br J Anaesth 59:678, 1987.
184. Maltby J, Sutherland AD, Sale JP, et al: Preoperative oral fluids: is a five-hour fast justified prior to elective surgery? Anesth Analg 65:1112, 1986.
185. Goldstein H, Boyle JD: The saline load test—a bedside evaluation of gastric retention. Gastroenterology 49:375, 1965.
186. Miller M, Wishart HY, Nimmo WS: Gastric contents at induction of anaesthesia: is a four hour fast necessary? Br J Anaesth 55:1185, 1985.
187. Splinter WM, Stewart JA, Muir JG: The effect of preoperative apple juice on gastric contents, thirst, and hunger in children. Can J Anaesth 36:55, 1989.
188. Phillips S, Hutchinson S, Davidson T: Preoperative drinking does not affect gastric contents. Br J Anaesth 70:6, 1993.
189. Khawaja IT, Buffa SD, Brandstetter RD: Aspiration pneumonia. A threat when deglutition is compromised. Postgrad Med 92:165, 1992.
190. Goodnough LT: The role of recombinant growth factors in transfusion medicine. Br J Anaesth 70:80, 1993.
191. Goldberg MA, Dunning SP, Bunn HF: Regulation of the erythropoietin gene: evidence that the oxygen sensor is a heme protein. Science 242:1412, 1988.
192. Deutsch S, Goldberg M, Dripps RD: Postoperative hyponatremia with inappropriate release of antidiuretic hormone. Anesthesiology 27:250, 1966.
193. Chung H-M, Kluge R, Schrier RW, et al: Postoperative hyponatremia: a prospective study. Arch Intern Med 146:333, 1986.
194. Raffe MR: The case for routine fluid administration. Vet Clin North Am Small Anim Pract 22:447, 1992.
195. Hellebrekers LJ: Pre- and perioperative fluid therapy guided by (arterial) blood pressure measurements. Tijdschr Diergeneeskd 117(Suppl)1:18, 1992.
196. Hubbell JA: The case against routine fluid administration. Vet Clin North Am Small Anim Pract 22:448, 1992.
197. Carabott JA, Javaheri Z, Keilty K, et al: Oral fluid intake in children following tonsillectomy and adenoidectomy. Pediatr Nurs 18:124, 1992.
198. Arieff AI: Hyponatremia, convulsions, respiratory arrest, and permanent brain damage after elective surgery in healthy women. N Engl J Med 314:1529, 1986.
199. Arieff AI, Ayus JC: Treatment of symptomatic hyponatremia: neither haste nor waste. Crit Care Med 19:748, 1991.
200. Sterns RH, Riggs JE, Schochet SS: Osmotic demyelination syndrome following correction of hyponatremia. N Engl J Med 314:1535, 1986.
201. Gold MS: Perioperative fluid management. Crit Care Clin 8:409, 1992.
202. Holliday MA, Friedman AL, Wassner SJ: Extracellular fluid restoration in dehydration: a critique of rapid versus slow. Pediatr Nephrol 13:292, 1999.
203. Fletcher SJ, Slaymaker AE, Bodenham AR, Vucevic M: Urine colour as an index of hyration in critically ill patients. Anaesthesia 54:172, 1999.
204. Berry AJ, Greene ES: The risk of needlestick injuries and needlestick-transmitted diseases in the practice of anesthesiology. Anesthesiology 77:1007, 1992.

6

Blood Transfusion and Component Therapy

LINDA STEHLING

◆   ◆   ◆

Many advances in pediatric surgery would not have been possible without concomitant developments in transfusion medicine. Among the most important was the advent of plastic tubing and blood bags in the 1950s that led to development of component therapy in the 1960s. Subsequent advances in technology and immunohematology have made it possible for transfusion services to provide more than two dozen blood components that can be tailored to specific patient needs. Anesthesiologists, who are responsible for administering a significant percentage of these components, must be familiar with the types available, the indications for their use, and the potential adverse effects of blood transfusion.

THE BLOOD SUPPLY

Approximately 13 million units of blood are collected annually in the United States. Blood centers are responsible for over 90 percent of blood collections. The American Red Cross collects approximately half of the blood, and most of the rest is collected by members of America's Blood Centers. Less than 10 percent of donated blood is collected by hospital transfusion services.

Although there are no data specific to pediatric transfusions, estimates of the total number of blood components transfused are available. Approximately 11 million red blood cell (RBC) units, 2.6 million units of fresh frozen plasma (FFP), and 0.7 million units of cryoprecipitate are administered each year. Calculations for platelet transfusions take into account the fact that platelets are obtained from two sources: platelet concentrates separated from whole blood, and single-donor platelets obtained by apheresis. Total platelet transfusions are usually reported in terms of platelet concentrates, assuming that a single-donor unit is equivalent to approximately six platelet concentrates. Thus, platelet transfusions equal the number of platelet concentrates plus six times the number of single-donor platelets transfused. Platelet transfusions peaked at slightly over 8 million units in 1992 and declined somewhat in subsequent years. In 1994, for the first time, single-donor platelets accounted for more than half of all platelet transfusions.[1]

TRANSFUSION-TRANSMITTED DISEASE

The blood supply is safer than ever because of improved donor screening and testing (Table 6–1). The primary method of preventing transfusion-transmitted disease is screening of potential donors to exclude those who, on the basis of medical or social history, are at risk of being infected with a transmissible disease. Testing of donated units provides additional safety. Donated units are currently tested for antibodies to the human immunodefi-

TABLE   6 – 1
**ESTIMATED RISK OF TRANSFUSION-
TRANSMITTED DISEASE**

Infection	Risk per Unit Transfused
Hepatitis A	1 in 1,000,000
Hepatitis B	1 in 30,000–1 in 250,000
Hepatitis C	1 in 30,000–1 in 150,000
Human immunodeficiency virus	1 in 200,000–1 in 2,000,000
Human T-cell lymphotropic virus I/II	1 in 250,000–1 in 2,000,000

Modified from Goodnough LT, Brecher ME, Kanter MH, et al: Blood transfusion. N Engl J Med 340:438, 1999.

ciency viruses (anti-HIV 1/2), hepatitis C virus (anti-HCV), hepatitis B core antigen (anti-HBc), and human T-cell lymphotrophic virus (anti-HTLV I/II). The blood is also tested for hepatitis B surface antigen (HBsAg), HIV-1 p24 antigen, and syphilis. Most collection facilities also perform alanine aminotransferase level (ALT) determinations on donated blood. The greatest remaining threat to blood safety is donation by seronegative individuals during the infectious window period when they are undergoing seroconversion and infection cannot be detected by available laboratory tests. The main goal of initiating nucleic acid amplification testing (NAT) in 1999 was to increase safety by shortening the window period of infectivity for HCV and HIV.

Human Immunodeficiency Virus

The first transfusion-associated case of acquired immunodeficiency syndrome (AIDS) was diagnosed and reported in 1982.[2] Of over 8,000 pediatric (<13 years old) AIDS cases reported to the Centers for Disease Control and Prevention (CDC) by 1998, fewer than 400 of the children acquired their infection through blood transfusion.[3] Most of the infections occurred between 1982 and 1984, prior to the availability of testing for HIV.

Testing for the antibody to HIV-1 was implemented in 1985 and for the antibody to HIV-2 in 1992. Testing for HIV-1 p24 antigen, initiated in 1996, reduced the window period by about 6 days to approximately 16 days. Testing was predicted to decrease by 25 percent the estimated 18 to 27 infectious donations not detected by antibody testing and made available for transfusion annually. However, only two donors positive for p24 antigen and negative for antibodies to HIV were identified among approximately 6 million units initially tested.[4] The current estimated risk of transfusion-transmitted HIV is between 1 in 200,000 and 1 in 2,000,000 transfusions.

Posttransfusion Hepatitis

During the late 1960s, up to one third of multiply-transfused patients developed posttransfusion hepatitis (PTH). The virtual elimination of paid donors in the 1970s led to a substantial reduction in the incidence of PTH. The introduction of screening for HBsAg in 1972 probably accounted for no more than a 25 percent decrease in the incidence of PTH, since most cases were not caused by hepatitis B, but rather were non-A, non-B hepatitis (NANBH). Since no specific test was available for NANBH, surrogate testing (ALT and anti-HBc) was introduced in 1986. Predictions that the incidence of NANBH would be reduced by 30 to 50 percent if units from donors with elevated ALT and anti-HBc were excluded proved to be correct.[5]

A new era in research related to the etiology, detection, and prevention of NANBH began when the genome of an NANBH agent, designated HCV, was cloned and a recombinant-based assay for anti-HCV was developed. Testing was begun in 1990 and an improved test was introduced in 1992. The estimated risk of transfusion-transmitted HCV is now 1 in 103,000, with a range of 1 in 30,000 to 1 in 150,000.[4] Most patients with acute HCV infection are asymptomatic. However, 75 to 85 percent of patients develop chronic HCV infection with persistent or fluctuating ALT elevations. Cirrhosis develops in 10 to 20 percent of patients over a period of 20 to 30 years and hepatocellular carcinoma in 1 to 5 percent.[6] It is likely that HCV acquired in the neonatal period or early childhood is associated with the same potential for chronic infection. The protracted course of the disease is especially important for pediatric patients infected at young ages because of their long life expectancy. Preliminary results of therapy with interferon-α in adults indicate that only 15 to 25 percent have a sustained response to therapy as measured by normalization of ALT levels and loss of detectable HCV ribonucleic acid (RNA), but that addition of ribavirin may double the response rates.[6]

Hepatitis A, for which there is no carrier state, is estimated to occur in only 1 in 1,000,000 transfusions. Hepatitis B currently accounts for about 10 percent of PTH. The estimated risk of HBV is 1 in 30,000 to 1 in 250,000. Hepatitis B virus and HCV together account for 88 percent of the aggregate risk of 1 in 34,000 for transfusion-transmitted viral infections.[7] Approximately 10 to 15 percent of patients with parenterally transmitted hepatitis are classified as having non–A-E hepatitis.[8] Studies of a recently identified virus designated hepatitis GB virus C or hepatitis G virus (HGV) indicate that it can be transmitted by transfusion, but does not appear to be implicated as a cause of non–A-E hepatitis.[9] Another newly described virus, initially termed TT virus for the initials of the patient from whom it was isolated, but now designated transfusion-transmitted virus (TTV), appears to be quite common, but no association with PTH has been demonstrated.[10] At this time, it appears that the majority of cases of non–A-E hepatitis are caused by an as yet undiscovered hepatitis agent or are due to nonviral causes.[9]

Other Transfusion-Transmitted Diseases

HTLV-I and -II can be transmitted through transfusion of cellular blood components. The risk is estimated to be 1 in 250,000 to 1 in 2,000,000 and is related to the length of time the blood is stored prior to transfusion. Units stored more than 14 days appear not to be infectious.[4] The implications of infection with HTLV-I or -II are far less clear than for the other viruses for which donated blood is tested. Infection with HTLV-I may lead to development of the chronic degenerative neurologic disease HTLV-I–associated myelopathy (HAM) or tropical spastic paraparesis (TSP) characterized by progressive spasticity, sensory deficits, lower extremity weakness, and urinary incontinence. It may also be associated with adult T-cell leukemia/lymphoma. The lifetime risk of developing neoplastic or overt neurologic disease is probably less than 4 percent.[11] Infection with HTLV-II may also cause HAM/TSP, but the association is even less certain than for HTLV-I.

Transmission of parvovirus B19, estimated to occur in 1 in 10,000 transfusions, is not usually of clinical significance. However, infection in pregnant women can cause hydrops fetalis in infants. Cytomegalovirus (CMV) infection can lead to life-threatening multisystem disease in immunocompromised patients such as low-birth-weight infants and recipients of bone marrow and solid organ transplants. Transfusion of CMV-negative blood or leukoreduced blood components is recommended for immunocompromised patients. Additional potentially transmissible viruses include Epstein-Barr virus (EBV), or human herpesvirus 4, and human herpes virus 6 (HHV-6).[12]

The causative agent of syphilis, *Treponema pallidum*, does not survive prolonged storage at 1° to 6° C, the temperature at which whole blood and RBCs are stored. Survival in stored platelets is more likely because they are stored at room temperature (22° to 24° C). Nevertheless, only two cases of transfusion-transmitted syphilis have been reported in the English literature in the last 30 years.[13] Transmission of parasitic diseases (malaria, toxoplasmosis, Chagas' disease, and babesiosis) is extremely rare in the United States. There is, however, a recent report of transmission of babesiosis to two neonates who received blood from an asymptomatic donor infected with *Babesia microti*.[14] Two additional neonates and an older child who received components from the same unit were not infected.

Considerable attention has been focused on the issue of whether Creutzfeldt-Jakob disease (CJD), an invariably fatal neurodegenerative disease, can be transmitted by transfusion. At the present time, there is no evidence for transfusion-transmitted CJD. Neither is there evidence for an increased incidence of CJD in patients at high risk for blood-borne diseases (e.g., patients with coagulation factor deficiencies such as hemophilia). Initial epidemiologic studies of almost 200 recipients of blood from donors who subsequently developed CJD have failed to demonstrate evidence of transmission.[15] The disease has, however, been transmitted through dura mater grafts, corneal transplants, reuse of surface electroencephalogram (EEG) electrodes previously used in infected patients, and injection of human pituitary-derived growth hormone. For this reason, prospective blood donors who have received tissue or tissue derivatives known to be a possible source of transmission of CJD and those with a family history of CJD are deferred indefinitely from donating blood.

Bacterial Contamination

Administration of a bacterially contaminated blood component should be part of the differential diagnosis when a child unexpectedly develops a fever within a few hours of transfusion and no other apparent cause can be found. Unsuspected asymptomatic bacteremia in the donor at the time of donation, contamination at the needle insertion site, or inadequate sterilization of blood collection bags can lead to bacterial contamination. The potential for bacterial growth is greatest in platelets because they are stored at room temperature. Patients who receive contaminated platelets may have only a mild fever or may develop fulminant sepsis, which is associated with significant mortality. The risk of platelet-related sepsis is estimated to be 1 in 12,000, and is most likely to occur in patients who receive pooled platelet concentrates.[4]

Several fatalities have been reported following transfusion of RBCs contaminated with *Yersinia enterocolitica*. Twelve of 20 recipients of *Yersinia*-contaminated RBCs reported to the CDC between 1987 and 1996 died. Symptoms were usually evident during the transfusion, and the median time to death was only 25 hours. Although the true incidence is unknown, the estimated frequency of transfusing bacterially contaminated RBCs is 1 in 500,000.[4]

NONINFECTIOUS COMPLICATIONS OF TRANSFUSION

While patients and the parents of pediatric patients are most concerned about the potential for transfusion-transmitted disease, anesthesiologists should focus their attention on transfusing blood only when indicated and appropriately identifying transfusion recipients in order to prevent serious hemolytic transfusion reactions (HTRs). The reported incidence of fatal HTRs is similar to current estimates for transfusion-transmitted HIV. However, underreporting is almost certain. Nonfatal errors resulting in administration of blood to the wrong patient are much more common. It is estimated that the administration of blood to a patient other than the intended recipient may occur as frequently as 1 in 12,000 units.[16] Most errors are clerical in nature and are preventable.

Hemolytic Transfusion Reactions

Hemolytic transfusion reactions involve the lysis of RBCs. They can be caused by immunologic incompatibility between donor and recipient RBCs or nonimmune mechanisms. The potential for immunologically mediated HTRs may be greater in pediatric patients than in adults because identifying wrist bands or leg bands are often removed during the search for intravascular cannulation sites. It is not unusual for the extremity with the identifying information to be inaccessible beneath the drapes. In any procedure where there is potential for transfusion, the anesthesiologist should verify the child's hospital number and the availability of compatible blood before induction of anesthesia. The identifying information should again be verified when blood units are checked prior to administration.

Signs and symptoms of HTRs are usually evident soon after initiation of the transfusion. In the anesthetized child, the only signs may be unexplained microvascular bleeding, hypotension, and hemoglobinuria. The severity of the reaction is usually proportional to the amount of blood transfused, and may occur following administration of only 10 to 20 mL of incompatible RBCs. When an HTR is suspected, the transfusion must be stopped and the transfusion service notified immediately. If a clerical error occurred, another patient may be at risk. Treatment of a child who sustains an HTR includes maintaining urine output at least 1 to 2 ml/kg/h with intravenous fluids and administration of furosemide and/or low-dose dopamine. Baseline coagulation studies should be obtained and therapy determined accordingly.

Although the first response of the anesthesiologist who observes unexpected red urine in the anesthetized child should be to stop the transfusion and recheck all identifying information, other causes of hemolysis also should be investigated. Nonimmune hemolysis can occur if RBCs are exposed to hypertonic solutions such as 50 percent dextrose or hypotonic solutions such as 0.45 percent sodium chloride. Thermal injury during blood storage or processing, inadequate deglycerolization of frozen RBCs, improper warming of RBCs during administration, and damage resulting from cardiopulmonary bypass or intraoperative blood recovery apparatus also can cause hemolysis.

In contrast to acute HTRs, delayed hemolytic reactions are usually not life-threatening. Most occur in previously transfused patients and are not preventable. Patients have no detectable antibodies at the time of transfusion, but develop clinically significant antibody levels in response to transfusion. The only manifestation may be a lack of expected benefit from the transfusion. The diagnosis should be considered in any child with an unexplained decrease in hemoglobin (Hb) or hematocrit (Hct) within 2 weeks following transfusion, particularly if the child is jaundiced as a result of rapid destruction of transfused RBCs. No therapy is indicated, but the child may require additional RBC transfusions.

Transfusion-Related Acute Lung Injury

Transfusion-related acute lung injury (TRALI) is a life-threatening condition characterized by severe bilateral pulmonary edema, hypoxemia, fever, tachycardia, and hypotension occurring within 1 to 6 hours following transfusion of plasma-containing blood components. Whole blood, RBC, FFP, platelet, granulocyte, and cryoprecipitate transfusions have all been implicated. The true incidence is unknown, but it has been estimated to occur as frequently as 1 in 5,000 transfusions.[4] Most patients are adults, although cases have been reported in neonates and older children. Despite the fulminant course of the presentation, most patients recover within 48 to 72 hours with appropriate ventilatory and hemodynamic support. The exact mechanism is unknown, but TRALI is believed to involve a reaction between antibodies in donor plasma and recipient leukocytes. The diagnosis is one of exclusion. If TRALI is suspected, the transfusion service should be notified, and whether investigation of implicated donors is indicated should be determined. No precautions are required if the patient requires additional transfusions.

Febrile Reactions

Although there are numerous reasons why anesthetized children develop acute temperature elevations, the possible contribution of transfusion should be considered. An increase in temperature may be the first manifestation of an HTR, administration of a bacterially contaminated blood component, or a febrile nonhemolytic transfusion reaction (FNHTR). The type blood component being administered and the timing of the temperature elevation are important diagnostic clues. If RBCs are being administered, an HTR should be considered. Bacterial contamination is more likely with platelets. With HTRs and bacterial contamination, the temperature elevation usually occurs after administration of a small volume of blood and is rarely the only manifestation of a reaction. The diagnosis of FNHTRs is usually one of exclusion. They occur most frequently in repeatedly transfused patients, particularly those requiring multiple platelet transfusions, and may be reduced by administering leukoreduced blood components.

Urticaria

Urticaria is probably the most common adverse effect of transfusion in the anesthetized patient, and the least significant. It is usually a response to foreign proteins in the transfused blood. In the absence of any manifestations of anaphylaxis, discontinuation of the transfusion is not necessary. Diphenhydramine (0.5 to 1 mg/kg) may be useful in treating the urticaria.

Allergic and Anaphylactic Reactions

Allergic and anaphylactic reactions involve the interaction of an allergen, usually a protein in the transfused plasma to which the recipient was previously sensitized, and immunoglobulin E (IgE) antibody on recipient mast cells and basophils. The antigen-antibody reaction occurs on the surface of these cells, causing release of various anaphylatoxins. The manifestations range from mild urticaria to laryngeal edema, bronchospasm, hypotension, and death. As a general principle, the shorter the interval between the initiation of transfusion and the onset of signs and symptoms, the more severe the reaction. Anaphylactic reactions are quite rare, but if suspected, the transfusion should be discontinued and therapy initiated. Treatment includes epinephrine, corticosteroids, and diphenhydramine, in addition to appropriate airway management and fluid therapy. The transfusion service also should be notified. Testing for anti-IgA may be indicated. If anti-IgA is detected, the patient is IgA deficient and should receive only IgA-deficient blood components (e.g., washed RBCs and platelets and plasma collected from IgA-deficient donors) if future transfusions are required.

Transfusion-Associated Graft-versus-Host Disease

Transfusion-associated graft-versus-host disease (TA-GVHD) occurs when immunocompetent donor lymphocytes are transfused to human leukocyte antigen (HLA)-incompatible recipients immunologically incapable of eliminating the donor cells. Children considered to be at risk include premature infants, newborns with erythroblastosis fetalis, those with congenital immunodeficiencies or

Hodgkin's disease, and recipients of bone marrow and stem cell transplants or blood from biologic relatives. Clinical manifestations include fever, a maculopapular rash, severe diarrhea, pancytopenia, and liver function abnormalities occurring within a week to 10 days after transfusion. Treatment is usually ineffective and the mortality rate high. Irradiation of blood components virtually eliminates the risk of TA-GVHD. Therefore, anesthesiologists should be familiar with the types of patients considered to be at risk and the logistics of obtaining irradiated blood.

Immunomodulation

The immunomodulatory effects of transfusion may be beneficial or detrimental. It has been recognized for over two decades that allogeneic transfusion is beneficial in improving renal allograft survival, although the explanation for the protective effect remains unclear. The association of perioperative transfusion with decreased disease-free survival in cancer patients remains controversial. Numerous studies in adults appear to support such an association, but a causal relationship has not been proven.[17, 18] Evidence for increased postoperative infection in patients transfused in the perioperative period is somewhat more convincing. In one study of patients undergoing spine surgery, several of whom were children, a fivefold increase in postoperative infection was reported in those who were transfused compared with nontransfused patients, or those who received only autologous blood.[19] Although unproved, it is hypothesized that donor-derived leukocytes are involved in the immunomodulatory effect(s) and that leukocyte reduction of blood components might be beneficial.

ADMINISTRATION OF BLOOD COMPONENTS

Pediatric transfusion practices differ in several ways from transfusions in adults. The volume of blood administered is more critical. In adults, hemotherapy is ordered by unit. Dosage in children is calculated on the basis of body weight. Methods of dispensing and administering small volumes of blood must be tailored to the child's needs. Particular attention should be given to decreasing the number of donor exposures in neonates who require repeated small-volume transfusions. In addition to being aware of hospital transfusion service policies for minimizing donor exposures, anesthesiologists should be familiar with the availability and indications for specially selected and prepared blood components.

Limiting Donor Exposures

Neonates who require transfusion support often are exposed to multiple donors. One effective method of limiting donor exposures is assigning a unit of blood to a neonate at the first transfusion episode and using the same unit until the unit or blood outdates. This system is particularly beneficial for very low birth weight (VLBW) infants, who often receive multiple 10- to 15-mL transfusions of RBCs. An early study indicated that up to 90 percent of babies

could be limited to a single donor exposure when citrate phosphate dextrose adeinine (CPDA-1) blood was utilized up to an expiration time of 35 days.[20] Subsequent studies have confirmed the efficacy of the practice and the safety of administering blood stored up to 42 days to neonates.[21]

Neonatologists often argue that there is potential for hyperkalemia and acidosis when blood stored several days to weeks is administered. Although the plasma potassium level of blood stored for 42 days may be as high as 50 mEq/L, the actual amount of bioavailable potassium administered is negligible. For example, a neonate weighing 1 kg who receives 10 mL of RBCs will receive only 2 mL of plasma if the hematocrit of the RBCs is 80 percent. The amount of potassium in a 10-mL transfusion is therefore only 0.1 mEq/L.[22] Clinical experience has shown that hyperkalemia is not a problem with small-volume transfusions. The British Committee for Standards in Haematology Blood Transfusion Task Force stated unequivocally in the *Guidelines for Administration of Blood Products: Transfusion of Infants and Neonates*[23] that the age of blood does not matter for small-volume "top-up" transfusions and that the blood can be used throughout its approved shelf life.

There is also concern about administering blood low in 2,3-diphosphoglyceric acid (2,3-DPG) with reduced ability to release oxygen to the tissues. In adults, 2,3-DPG is rapidly regenerated and the P_{50} of transfused RBCs reaches normal adult levels within about 24 hours of transfusion. Although there are no data, there is no reason to believe that neonates are incapable of regenerating 2,3-DPG in the same manner as adults. In addition, the P_{50} of older transfused RBCs is similar to the normal P_{50} value in blood of healthy preterm infants.[24] Thus, the P_{50} of older transfused RBCs is no worse than that of endogenous RBCs containing high concentrations of HbF. The dilution effect renders the 2,3-DPG content of donor blood immaterial when small-volume transfusions are administered.

Storage media used to extend the shelf life of RBCs to 42 days contain increased concentrations of dextrose and adenine for intracellular metabolism and mannitol to diminish RBC lysis. There appear to be no contraindications to administering small-volume transfusions of RBCs in additive solution, even to premature babies. Although some transfusion services wash the RBCs to remove the additive and resuspend the RBCs in saline or albumin prior to administration, it is not necessary when administering small-volume transfusions slowly. The same types of trials that have demonstrated the safety and efficacy of RBCs in additive solutions for small-volume transfusions have not been conducted in the setting of massive transfusion. Mathematical models suggest that toxicity is possible. Therefore, washing RBCs stored in additive solution prior to release would appear prudent when large volumes of blood will be administered during major procedures.[25]

Another practice to reduce donor exposures is collecting blood from a committed donor, usually a parent. A mean decrease in donor exposures of 57 percent (range, 12 to 93 percent) was demonstrated in a group of 50 pediatric patients who underwent surgery at the Mayo Clinic.[26] Committed donors provided 48 percent of the RBCs, 64 percent of platelets, and 14 percent of the FFP transfused. Another study of 73 children undergoing elective surgical procedures also demonstrated the feasibility of one committed donor providing all RBCs for a patient.[27] Of the 73 donors selected, 79 percent were able to furnish all RBCs ordered. Of the 46 children transfused, 38 (83 percent) received only single-donor RBCs.

Dispensing Techniques

Wastage of blood administered to pediatric patients is minimized by dividing units into multiple small-volume "pedi-pack" bags, usually containing 50 to 70 mL of RBCs, which can be administered to several neonates or used for multiple transfusions in the same child. Aliquots of prefiltered blood also are dispensed in syringes by some transfusion services for use in neonates.[28] A mechanical syringe pump is utilized in the neonatal intensive care unit to administer the blood. A mechanical infusion device may not be required in the operating room when blood is being administered to replace surgical blood loss.

Blood Filtration

All blood components must be filtered prior to transfusion. With the exception of aliquots filtered and drawn into syringes prior to release by the transfusion service, a blood administration set must be utilized at the time of administration. Pediatric transfusion sets incorporating volumetric devices or burettes are useful for measuring the volume of blood transfused. There are no documented benefits of using 20- to 40-μm microaggregate filters, even when large volumes of blood are administered. Microaggregate filters must not be used for transfusing platelets or granulocytes. Conventional blood administration sets incorporate a 170- to 200-μm filter.

There is ongoing debate about the appropriate indications for leukocyte reduction filters, although it is well known that leukocytes and their metabolic products, cytokines, are associated with adverse effects in some transfusion recipients. Currently available leukocyte reduction filters are capable of removing more than 99.99 percent of the leukocytes in RBCs and platelets. The blood can be filtered shortly after collection, in the laboratory after storage, or at the time of administration. Platelets collected by apheresis also can be leukocyte-reduced during the collection process. In most circumstances involving pediatric transfusion, the blood will be leukocyte-reduced prior to release by the transfusion service. If leukocyte reduction is performed at the time of blood administration, it is essential that the anesthesiologist use the appropriate filter in the manner recommended by the manufacturer. A variety of leukocyte reduction filters are available. Some are intended for use with RBCs and others with platelets; they are not interchangeable. Priming techniques and flow rates also differ. When leukocyte reduction is deemed necessary, all RBCs and platelets administered to the patient must be leukocyte-reduced.

Transfusion Apparatus

Electromechanical pumps are sometimes used for delivery of blood components. Syringe, piston, and peristaltic-type pumps have been investigated for infusion of RBCs and platelets.[29] Some pumps cause hemolysis of concentrated RBCs, although most are acceptable for use. Before any pump is used to administer cellular blood components, the manufacturer's specifications should be reviewed.

Blood can be warmed before or during transfusion. In-line blood warmers employing a water bath or electric heating plates that contact the blood tubing are most commonly used. Systems incorporating a countercurrent heat exchanger warmed by a circulating water bath are also available for rapid blood administration. Many blood warmers are not suitable for use in neonates and small children because of large priming volumes, prompting anesthesiologists to devise a number of unorthodox methods of warming small volumes of blood. These include holding the unit under the hot water tap or immersing it in a basin of warm water; inserting a blood-filled syringe in a glove and placing the glove in a basin or blood warmer containing warm water; and "sandwiching" the unit between heated IV solution bags. These techniques are to be condemned. At best, they do not work; at worst, they can cause hemolysis. Blood warmers should be equipped with a visible thermometer, a means of preventing overheating, and an audible warning system.

INDICATIONS FOR "SPECIAL" BLOOD COMPONENTS

A variety of components, collected from specially selected donors and specially processed after collection, can be provided for children with special transfusion needs. Transfusion service policies vary regarding the indications for these components. Some are in short supply and others require additional time and equipment for processing. Once prepared, the components may have a shortened shelf life. In most hospitals, such components will not routinely be provided without evaluation of the indication(s) for their use. Consultation between the ordering physician and a member of the transfusion service is usually required when patients do not appear to meet the established criteria.

Components with Reduced Risk of Transmitting Cytomegalovirus

Patients who have never been exposed to CMV are at risk for primary infection through transfusion of blood from donors infected with the virus. Some seropositive patients are at risk for clinical infection from reactivation of their own latent virus or from reinfection with a different CMV strain. Infection in immunocompetent individuals is usually not associated with disease. However, severe morbidity and mortality can result from infection in immunocompromised patients, particularly children. Manifestations may include pneumonitis, hepatitis, gastroenteritis, retinitis, meningoencephalitis, myocarditis, and pancytopenia. Infection acquired in utero can result in fetal demise or neonatal jaundice, hepatosplenomegaly, microcephaly, sensorineural hearing loss, and thrombocytopenia. Neurologic deficits occur in some apparently healthy infected neonates. Low-birth-weight (LBW) infants are the most severely affected.

Strategies for preventing CMV transmission in patients considered at risk include using blood from CMV-negative donors and leukocyte reduction of RBCs and platelets. The major drawback to using CMV-negative blood is the difficulty of maintaining an adequate inventory because the prevalence of CMV antibodies in healthy blood donors ranges from 40 to 100 percent, depending on the geographic location. Although the reason is unclear, only about 10 percent of seropositive donors transmit infection. Testing identifies previously infected donors, but does not differentiate those who are infectious. Leukocyte-reduced cellular components are now considered an acceptable alternative to CMV-negative blood.[30]

Current guidelines recommend strategies to prevent CMV infection for intrauterine transfusions, LBW (<1,200 g) neonates born to CMV-seronegative mothers, CMV-seronegative recipients of allogeneic bone marrow or solid organ transplants from seronegative donors, CMV-seronegative patients with hematologic malignancies who are likely candidates for allogeneic bone marrow transplants, CMV-seronegative patients with organ failure who are likely candidates for organ transplants, and CMV-seronegative patients with HIV.[30] It is further recommended that CMV-seronegative patients receiving immunosuppressive therapy, and those with hereditary or acquired immunodeficiencies, Hodgkin's disease, and non-Hodgkin's lymphoma also be considered for CMV-prevention strategies.

Leukocyte-Reduced Blood Components

Cellular blood components contain variable numbers of "passenger" leukocytes that can cause febrile reactions, HLA alloimmunization leading to refractoriness to platelet transfusion, TRALI, TA-GVHD, and transmission of infectious disease (e.g., CMV). Leukoreduction is not an accepted technique for preventing TRALI or TA-GVHD. Leukoreduced components are an acceptable alternative to CMV-negative blood for preventing CMV infection.[30]

Prevention of recurrent FNHTRs in repeatedly transfused patients is an accepted indication for leukocyte reduction. Administering leukocyte-depleted RBCs virtually eliminates these reactions, but is less effective in preventing FNHTRs associated with platelet transfusion. The difference is attributed primarily to different storage temperatures. Leukocytes in platelets stored at room temperature release cytokines, which are largely responsible for the FNHTRs. Prestorage leukocyte reduction, but not bedside leukocyte reduction of stored platelets, significantly reduces FNHTRs. Cytokines do not accumulate in RBCs because the low storage temperature inhibits leukocyte function and viability.

Alloimmunization leads to platelet refractoriness (i.e., failure of the recipient to achieve the expected increment in platelet count). The results of studies conducted to evaluate the effectiveness of leukocyte reduction in preventing platelet alloimmunization in chronically transfused thrombocytopenic patients have produced conflicting results.[31] Nevertheless, many institutions transfuse only leukocyte-depleted RBCs and platelets to patients with hematologic malignancies.

Several European countries have initiated universal leukocyte-reduction as a measure to reduce the theoretical risk of transfusion-transmitted CJD. Implementation of universal leukocyte reduction appears imminent in the United States.

Irradiated Blood

Irradiation of blood components is performed to prevent TA-GVHD in susceptible patients. The pathophysiology involves engraftment of viable donor lymphocytes in a susceptible host, multiplication of the engrafted lymphocytes, and mounting of an immune response against the recipient. Most irradiation is performed by blood centers or transfusion services using commercial irradiators designed for that purpose. In institutions without access to blood irradiators, the procedure can be performed in the radiation therapy department. The logistics of utilizing a radiation therapy department can result in delays in obtaining irradiated blood components.

Whole blood, RBCs, platelets, granulocytes, and fresh plasma must be irradiated. It is not necessary to irradiate FFP or cryoprecipitate. Irradiated blood is recommended for intrauterine and neonatal exchange transfusions and during extracorporeal membrane oxygenation (ECMO). Immunocompromised marrow and organ transplant recipients, patients with hematologic disorders anticipating imminent allogeneic marrow transplant, those with Hodgkin's disease, those with congenital cell-mediated immunodeficiencies, and recipients of directed blood donations from biologic relatives or donations from HLA-matched donors also should receive irradiated blood. Possible indications include LBW neonates, individuals receiving immunosuppressive therapy, cancer patients immunosuppressed from chemotherapy or irradiation, and AIDS patients with opportunistic infections.[32]

Anesthesiologists should be familiar with the recommendations for irradiation of blood components for several reasons. First, it is important for children to receive irradiated components when indicated. Second, the logistics of irradiating blood at a blood center or radiation treatment center are such that the anesthesiologist cannot expect to receive irradiated blood components within the usual time period. Finally, blood should not be irradiated in anticipation of use when the likelihood of transfusion is remote. Although lymphocytes are the target cells of the irradiation process, radiation effects are not confined to lymphocytes. The shelf-life of irradiated RBCs is reduced to 28 days because 24-hour recovery is reduced and extracellular potassium and plasma Hb levels are increased. The biochemical changes that occur during the 28-day shelf-life are insignificant for most patients, but may present a hazard to neonates and patients susceptible to hyperkalemia.

FRESH WHOLE BLOOD

Conceptually, the use of fresh whole blood is appealing; logistically, it presents tremendous problems. Only a limited number of controlled studies have evaluated the use of fresh whole blood. Interestingly, the definition of "fresh" is not consistent, making comparison of the few studies difficult. Some investigators refer only to blood less than 6 hours old as "fresh." Others consider blood less than 48 hours old fresh. Neonatologists traditionally have defined fresh as less than 7 days old.

Although whole blood is not altered by removal of any constituents, it is drawn into plastic bags containing anticoagulant and stored between 1° and 6°C. Metabolic changes begin almost immediately and continue throughout the storage period. The most significant early changes affect platelet function. Storage at 1° to 6°C for even a few hours alters the hemostatic effects of platelets. It is for this reason that platelets are stored at room temperature. Refrigerated blood is intact, but it is not functionally whole.

One group of investigators studied postoperative blood loss in 161 children undergoing open heart surgery in relation to the storage time of the transfused blood.[33] The children received either whole blood stored at room temperature for less than 6 hours; refrigerated whole blood 24 to 48 hours old; or reconstituted blood consisting of RBCs less than 5 days old, platelets, and FFP. The surgical blood loss in children over 2 years of age did not differ among the treatment groups. Storage time had no effect on blood loss for procedures classified as simple or intermediate in complexity. Blood loss was, however, significantly less in children under 2 years of age who underwent complex surgery in which fresh rather than reconstituted blood was administered. The results were comparable with blood less than 6 hours and that 24 to 48 hours old. Although the authors concluded that the beneficial effects of fresh blood may be due in part to better platelet function, it is difficult to believe that this is the only explanation, because the 24- to 48-hour-old blood was refrigerated. It should be emphasized that the beneficial effects were seen only in the subgroup of approximately 70 children under 2 years of age who underwent complex procedures. Additional studies are indicated to define the mechanism whereby "fresh whole" blood may improve hemostasis and to identify which patients may benefit.

Although whole blood may be useful in some children who undergo cardiac surgery, thousands who do not receive fresh whole blood have cardiac surgery each year without apparent evidence of coagulopathy. Provision of fresh blood for all of them, even for all pediatric patients, would be impossible because of the logistics of blood collection and the time required for infectious disease testing.

RED BLOOD CELL TRANSFUSION

Pediatricians and anesthesiologists have been accused of administering RBC transfusions on the basis of custom rather than indication. Neonatologists traditionally have maintained the Hb of neonates with severe respiratory distress or symptomatic heart disease above 13 g/dl,[23, 34] although there is little evidence to substantiate this practice. Equally doubtful is the administration of RBCs to premature infants to treat tachypnea, dyspnea, apneic episodes, feeding difficulties, lethargy, decreased activity, and poor weight gain.[35]

Recent guidelines specifically addressing neonatal transfusion,[23] as well as those dealing with older patients,[36, 37] emphasize the importance of the patient's overall physical status, not just the Hb level, in the transfusion decision. Nevertheless, the Hb concentration remains the primary criterion for RBC transfusion. The normal variations in Hb with age, determinants of tissue oxygenation, compensatory mechanisms activated in response to acute and chronic anemia, and the expected physiologic responses to RBC transfusion are factors that should be considered, in addition to the patient's Hb level.

Physiologic Anemia

Hemoglobin levels normally decrease in infants during the first weeks of life. In term neonates, the Hb level declines to approximately 11 g/dl between 8 and 12 weeks of age. The rapidity with which the Hb decreases and the nadir vary inversely with gestational age. The decline is more rapid and greater in premature infants. Levels of 7 g/dl are not unusual between 6 and 8 weeks in babies weighing less than 1,000 g at birth.

There are multiple causes of the so-called physiologic anemia of infancy. The most important is decreased erythropoiesis, which virtually ceases shortly after birth. A dilutional effect secondary to increased plasma volume also contributes. In addition, RBC survival is somewhat shorter in neonates than in older children. All of these effects are accentuated in premature infants because of diminished erythropoietin production in response to anemia.

Red Blood Cell Transfusion in Critically Ill Patients

It has been estimated that 38,000 premature infants with birth weights less than 1,500 g receive in excess of 300,000 RBC transfusions each year in the United States.[24, 38] Replacement of blood withdrawn for laboratory studies accounts for approximately 90 percent of transfusions administered to premature infants in some intensive care units.

There is considerable variation in transfusion practices among institutions. This was confirmed in a six-site prospective study of transfusion rates in infants with birth weights less than 1,500 g.[39] Although the number of transfusions and the volume transfused varied significantly, clinical outcomes (incidence of intraventricular hemorrhage, necrotizing enterocolitis, bronchopulmonary dysplasia, growth, and length of hospital stay) were no different. The authors speculated that applying phlebotomy and transfusion guidelines could result in fewer transfusions, fewer complications, and reduced cost. Indeed, adoption of transfusion guidelines for treating preterm infants with birth weights less than 1,250 g and gestational age less than 32 weeks decreased the mean number of transfusions per infant in the first 2 weeks of life from 4.7 to 2.7.[40]

The rationale for transfusing stable critically ill prematures to arbitrary Hb levels has been questioned by many clinicians and studied by few. One group of investigators evaluated the effects of prophylactic small-volume RBC transfusions in 56 prematures randomly assigned to either a prophylactic transfusion group in which the Hb was maintained above 10 g/dl or a control group in which RBCs were administered only for symptomatic anemia.[41]

The Hb values differed significantly at discharge (9.1 ± 1.6 g/dl and 11.7 ± 1.7 g/dl, respectively), but the two groups were comparable in length of stay, as well as frequency and severity of clinical problems.

Doppler echocardiography has been employed to evaluate the effects of anemia in premature infants and their responses to RBC transfusion.[42] In babies transfused from a mean Hb of 7.5 ± 0.4 g/dl to a mean Hb of 15 ± 1.6 g/dl, myocardial function indexes, as well as weight gain and metabolic demands, were normal both before and after transfusion. The investigators concluded that premature infants with no cardiopulmonary complications can tolerate low Hb levels in excess of 6.5 g/dl. However, they cautioned that the findings should not be extrapolated to all infants with anemia of prematurity. Similar studies were conducted in anemic (Hb range, 6.5 to 8.8 g/dl) preterm infants with bronchopulmonary dysplasia (BPD) who were oxygen dependent, but did not require mechanical ventilation.[43] Although RBC transfusion to a mean Hb of 12.5 ± 1.6 g/dl resulted in decreased cardiac output, oxygen consumption remained unchanged. The investigators concluded that the infants with BPD were able to tolerate Hb levels as low as 7 g/dl, and questioned the practice of transfusing at Hb levels of 10 g/dl.

Several studies have been performed in critically ill older children and adults to evaluate the effects of RBC transfusion. One group of pediatric patients was studied during the postresuscitation stage of septic shock, at a time of relative hemodynamic stability.[44] The mean Hb was 10.2 ± 0.8 g/dl before transfusion and 13.2 ± 1.4 g/dl after transfusion of 8 to 10 ml/kg RBCs. Oxygen delivery increased, but oxygen consumption did not change. The oxygen extraction ratio decreased from 28 to 22 percent. In an adult study, one unit of RBCs administered to critically ill postoperative patients raised the mean Hb from 9.4 to 10.4 g/dl, as expected. There was an increase in oxygen delivery, no change in oxygen consumption, and the oxygen extraction ratio decreased from 31 percent to 28 percent.

The results of a large, multicenter, randomized, controlled clinical trial of transfusion requirements in critically ill adults were recently reported.[45] A total of 838 patients with Hb concentrations less than 9 g/dl within 72 hours of intensive care unit (ICU) admission were randomly assigned either to a restrictive or a liberal transfusion strategy. In the restrictive group, RBCs were transfused if the Hb declined below 7 g/dl and Hb levels were maintained between 7 and 9 g/dl. In the liberal transfusion group, RBCs were administered when the Hb fell below 10 g/dl and Hb levels were maintained between 10 and 12 g/dl. Overall 30-day mortality rates were similar in the two groups, but were significantly lower in the restrictive transfusion group of patients who were less acutely ill. The mortality rate during hospitalization was significantly lower in the restrictive than in the liberal group. The investigators concluded that the restrictive transfusion strategy was at least as effective, and possibly superior, to a liberal transfusion strategy in critically ill adult patients.

Alternatives to Red Blood Cell Transfusion

Allowing patients to remain at lower Hb levels is the simplest method of avoiding RBC transfusion. Administration of recombinant human erythropoietin (r-HuEPO) is another option. The drug has been administered extensively to adults with chronic anemia of multiple etiologies, as well as pre- and postoperatively in surgical patients. While experience is more limited in children, several studies have demonstrated the efficacy of r-HuEPO and iron in stimulating erythropoiesis in premature infants. The efficacy of r-HuEPO in reducing RBC transfusion requirements, while statistically significant, is clinically modest. In the European multicenter trial involving more than 240 VLBW infants, subcutaneous administration of r-HuEPO three times a week from day 3 to day 42 reduced the mean transfusions from 1.25 to 0.87.[46] In the multicenter, randomized trial conducted in the United States,[38] either r-HuEPO or a placebo was administered to over 150 VLBW infants during the 6-week study period. The results were similar to the European study: the mean number of RBC transfusions in the r-HuEPO-treated babies was 1.1, whereas babies in the placebo group received a mean of 1.6 transfusions. The investigators concluded that employing conservative transfusion criteria, minimizing phlebotomy losses, and treatment with r-HuEPO are complementary strategies to reduce RBC transfusions in VLBW infants.

Physiologic Response to Blood Loss

Little information is available regarding physiologic responses to acute blood loss in pediatric patients. It is assumed that the newborn is less able to compensate for anemia than the older child or adult because of the newborn's high resting cardiac output (CO) and oxygen consumption. Animal studies have demonstrated age-related differences in the cardiovascular responses to hypoxia. However, it is unclear why younger animals do not compensate as well as older animals.

The physiologic responses to acute anemia depend on the rate of RBC loss, the degree of anemia, the patient's ability to compensate, and tissue oxygen requirements. Compensatory mechanisms activated by acute blood loss include stimulation of the adrenergic nervous system, release of vasoactive hormones, hyperventilation, resorption of fluid from the interstitium into the vascular space, a shift of fluid from the intracellular to the extracellular compartment, and renal conservation of body water and electrolytes. Unless the blood loss exceeds the patient's compensatory ability, the combination of these physiologic alterations restores CO to or toward normal within a few minutes of acute blood loss. The shift of interstitial fluid into the vascular compartment can restore up to 50 percent of intravascular volume.[47] Somewhat slower, but no less important, is the shift of fluid from the intracellular compartment to the intravascular space.

Hypovolemia, rather than reduced oxygen-carrying capacity, is the most important aspect of acute blood loss. Therefore, administration of asanguinous fluid is the primary initial therapy. The infused fluid, together with fluid mobilized from the interstitial space, can lead to significant hemodilution. The clinician must decide, on the basis of the child's overall physical condition and whether additional blood loss is anticipated, the degree of anemia that presumably can be tolerated without impairing tissue oxygen delivery. Such decisions are not easy.

Animal studies and a wealth of clinical experience indicate that a Hb of 10 g/dl is not required and that the ability to compensate tends to be lost at a Hb of approximately 3 g/dl. Extrapolating data from numerous studies of acute normovolemic hemodilution supports the safety of Hb values of 6 to 7 g/dl.[48] Limited studies of extreme hemodilution in teenage patients indicate that a Hb of 5 g/dl is safe in appropriately selected and monitored children free of systemic disease.[49] A very small study of invasively monitored healthy children and adolescents undergoing spine surgery and hemodiluted to a mean Hb level of 3 ± 0.8 g/dl demonstrated that global oxygen consumption could be maintained at that level during the intraoperative period.[50] The investigators cautioned that the effects on regional organ oxygen delivery and organ specific functions were unknown. Although the children sustained no discernible adverse effects, the investigators were not implying that the very low Hb values in their patients should be adopted as the threshold values for transfusion.

Determining the Amount to Transfuse

In addition to calculating the dosage of medications preoperatively for infants and children, the anesthesiologist also should calculate the child's estimated blood volume (EBV) and allowable blood loss (ABL) before any procedure in which blood loss is expected. The EBV of prematures is 90 to 100 ml/kg, and that of term newborns is 80 to 90 ml/kg. Children less than 1 year old have an EBV of 75 to 80 ml/kg. The EBV of older children is 70 to 75 ml/kg. The child's weight, initial Hct (Hct_i), estimated RBC mass (ERCM), and the lowest allowable perioperative Hct (Hct_p) are used to calculate permissible blood loss. For example, in a 20-kg child with a Hct of 40 percent in whom an intraoperative Hct of 25 percent is considered safe:

$$EBV: 20 \text{ kg} \times 70 \text{ ml/kg} = 1,400 \text{ ml}$$

$$ERCM_{40}: 1,400 \text{ ml} \times 0.40 = 560 \text{ ml}$$

$$ERCM_{25}: 1,400 \text{ ml} \times 0.25 = 350 \text{ ml}$$

$$ARL: 560 - 350 \text{ ml} = 210 \text{ ml}$$

Using an average Hct of 30 percent, the ABL would be approximately 660 ml. A similar ABL is estimated by using the Hct_i, Hct_p, and the average of the two (Hct_{av}):

$$ABL = EBV \times \frac{(Hct_i - Hct_p)}{Hct_{av}}$$

$$ABL = 1,400 \times \frac{(40 - 25)}{32.5} = \sim650 \text{ ml}$$

Estimation of blood loss is critical but grossly inaccurate. Suction containers used to measure blood loss in pediatric patients should have a capacity of 50 to 250 ml, depending on the child's size. Suction tubing deadspace between the operative field and the container should be minimized. The weight of sponges not moistened with saline is relatively reliable. When saline-soaked sponges are used, weighing is virtually useless. As a very general rule, a saturated 4 × 4-inch sponge holds 10 to 15 ml of blood. Laparotomy packs may hold as much as 100 to 150 ml.

The increase in Hct with RBC administration approximates the milliliters per kilogram administered. Using the previous example, if the 20-kg child had a Hct of 20 percent, 100 ml of RBCs would raise the Hct to approximately 25 percent. However, once the child is exposed to the potential risks of transfusion, it is often preferable to administer somewhat more than the calculated amount of blood to allow for additional operative blood loss and losses from phlebotomy for laboratory tests. In the older child, it may be wise to administer the entire unit unless there is danger of fluid overload.

The information available at the time of transfusion should be documented on the anesthesia record. This includes, at a minimum, the estimated blood loss (EBL), and vital signs. Most operating rooms have equipment for determining Hct or Hb values in the operating room, rather than relying on a remote laboratory. Any values obtained should be recorded. Just as the indications for pharmacologic agents such as antiarrhythmics are documented, the indications for blood components should be recorded. Blood is sometimes administered when, in retrospect, the child would have done well without transfusion. Blood loss can be overestimated or hemostasis achieved more quickly than anticipated. Such situations are inevitable, just as underestimation of blood loss occurs in some cases. Careful documentation of the information available at the time of transfusion is the best indication of the thought process leading to transfusion.

Nonindications for Red Blood Cell Transfusion

Neonatologists and anesthesiologists are not the only specialists guilty of administering RBCs without scientific evidence of benefit; so are surgeons. Wound healing, well-being, and an improved postoperative clinical course are used as indications for RBC transfusion. Animal studies, confirmed by observations in postoperative adult surgical patients, indicate that normovolemic anemia is not detrimental to wound healing. Collagen deposition is directly proportional to wound oxygen tension and perfusion. The oxygen extraction ratio of healing tissue is only about 3 percent, and oxygen delivered in the plasma alone begins to satisfy that need when the Pao_2 rises toward 300 mm Hg. The critical Hct at which anemia influences tissue repair in physiologically normal surgical patients appears to be approximately 15 percent.[51]

Studies in adult patients evaluating exercise capacity after cardiac surgery[52] and the duration of hospitalization in orthopedic patients[53] have failed to show that transfused patients did better than controls who were not transfused. No comparable studies have been conducted in pediatric patients. However, if elderly adults with cardiovascular disease and other systemic diseases do not benefit from postoperative RBC transfusion in terms of well-being, can any benefit be expected in young, otherwise healthy children?

It is crucial that the anesthesiologist, in the zeal to avoid potential transfusion-related complications, not err on the side of unnecessarily exposing children to the risks of inadequate oxygen delivery. Statements such as that of the American College of Physicians[54] that in the absence of risks, transfusion is not indicated, independent of Hb level in anesthetized patients with stable vital signs, cannot be condoned. Although vital signs are one parameter to consider, the stress response associated with anesthesia and surgery and the pharmacologic agents employed significantly alter the normal physiologic responses to acute blood loss. In addition, optimal anesthetic management is based on therapeutic intervention before physiologic decompensation, not afterward. It is impossible to reliably predict the occurrence of acute intraoperative hemorrhage, decreases in cardiac output, or abnormalities of ventilation that may impair oxygen delivery. Therefore, some margin of safety is indicated. Although not specifically addressing the pediatric patient, the recommendation in the Practice Guidelines for Blood Component Therapy published by the American Society of Anesthesiologists[36] can serve as a useful guideline: transfusion is rarely indicated when the Hb concentration is greater than 10 g/dl and is almost always indicated when it is less than 6 g/dl, especially when the anemia is acute.

HEMOSTASIS AND THROMBOSIS

Control of bleeding is achieved through a series of interrelated processes involving the vasculature, platelets, and coagulation proteins. Fibrinolysis, the process by which fibrin clots are removed, also is initiated when coagulation begins. The balance between the two systems is designed to ensure that interruption of vascular integrity is followed by clot formation and that clot dissolution occurs after an appropriate interval so that blood flow through occluded vessels is restored.

In the primary phase of hemostasis, vasoconstriction follows vessel injury, platelets adhere to damaged endothelium, and a platelet plug is formed. Secondary hemostasis is mediated by the coagulation proteins. The sequence of events leading to generation of thrombin and formation of a fibrin clot is usually considered a biochemical cascade composed of two distinct pathways (intrinsic and extrinsic) that converge into a common pathway. This scheme is useful for describing in vitro clot formation and laboratory testing, but in vivo coagulation is a far more complex process.

The Vascular Component of Hemostasis

The vascular system is more than an inert conduit for blood flow. Vasoconstriction and diversion of blood flow away from damaged vessels is an immediate response to vascular injury. A number of physiochemical reactions also occur. Disruption of the endothelium exposes the underlying collagen and basement membrane, leading to activation of platelets and plasma coagulation factors and resulting in platelet adhesion and thrombus formation. The extrinsic coagulation pathway also is activated by the released tissue thromboplastin. Adenosine diphosphate (ADP), liberated by the endothelium, induces platelet aggregation. The vascular phase of hemostasis usually lasts less than a minute. Fibrinolysis is initiated simultaneously by release of tissue plasminogen activators from the vascular wall.

The Role of Platelets in Hemostasis

Platelets are both morphologically and functionally complex. The platelet membrane serves as a substrate for the interaction of plasma proteins involved in coagulation. It also contains the mechanism responsible for platelet adhesion and aggregation. When platelets are stimulated, contraction of microtubules in their cytoskeletons leads to internal structural changes and formation of peripheral pseudopods. The inner organelle zone is responsible for the metabolic activities of platelets. The most numerous organelles in this area are the dense bodies and α granules. The contents of these granules are extruded during the platelet release reaction. The dense tubular system, also in the organelle zone, is the site of prostaglandin synthesis and calcium sequestration.

Platelets perform several distinct functions in response to vascular damage. They are responsible for the initial control of bleeding by platelet plug formation. The steps involved in formation of the platelet plug are adhesion, aggregation, and the release reaction. Platelet adhesion involves the interaction of platelet surface glycoproteins with subendothelial connective tissue, and is dependent on the presence of von Willebrand factor (VIII:vWF). The precise sequence of reactions that follows is not defined, but the platelets undergo a change in shape, release their granular contents, and interact with each other, or aggregate.

Platelet aggregation is promoted by several substances released from platelets and the vascular endothelium. A potent initiator of aggregation, ADP, is released from both sites. Binding of ADP to platelet membranes also triggers a series of reactions leading to formation of thromboxane A_2. In addition to promoting platelet aggregation, thromboxane A_2 mediates the platelet release reaction and induces vasoconstriction. Thrombin generated through the coagulation system also enhances platelet aggregation.

The final stage in the formation of the platelet plug is the release reaction, which involves the release or extrusion of substances stored in platelet granules. The activated platelets provide an environment or "meeting place" for fibrin formation. Conversion of fibrinogen to fibrin by thrombin results in the formation of a stable hemostatic plug of aggregated, activated platelets enmeshed in fibrin strands.

The Coagulation Phase of Hemostasis

Secondary hemostasis is mediated by coagulation factors normally present in blood in the inactive state. All, with the possible exception of factor VIII, are produced in the liver. The nomenclature used to describe the factors is confusing because the numbers were assigned in the order of discovery and do not reflect their point of interaction in the coagulation cascade. Activated factors are designated by the letter "a" after the Roman numeral identifying the factor. The coagulation factors are divided into substrate, cofactors, and enzymes on the basis of their hemostatic function. Fibrinogen is the substrate, since the goal of coagulation is conversion of fibrinogen to fibrin. Factors III (tissue thromboplastin), V, VIII, and Fitzgerald factor, or high-molecular-weight kininogen (HMWK), are cofactors. Their purpose is to accelerate the enzymatic reactions of the coagulation system. The remaining factors are enzymes.

Coagulation involves a series of interrelated biochemical reactions classically divided into three pathways: intrinsic, extrinsic, and common (Fig. 6–1). Although convenient, the cascade theory is a vast oversimplification and minimizes the multiple effects of components of each pathway.

The extrinsic coagulation pathway is initiated when tissue thromboplastin (factor III) enters the vascular system. The term extrinsic is used because the pathway is initiated by a substance not normally found in the blood. Factor VII is activated to VIIa in the presence of tissue thromboplastin and calcium. Factor VIIa in turn activates factor X to Xa. This is a rapid process that produces small quantities of thrombin for conversion of fibrinogen to fibrin. Thrombin generated by the extrinsic pathway can accelerate the intrinsic pathway by enhancing the activity of factors V and VIII. The prothrombin time (PT) is used to monitor the extrinsic pathway.

The intrinsic pathway is so named because all factors involved are normally present in the blood. Factor XII is activated to XIIa when exposed to subendothelial collagen. Factor XIIa then activates factor XI to XIa. The reactions are enhanced by HMWK and Fletcher factor (prekallikrein). In the presence of calcium, factor XIa activates factor IX to IXa. Further activation requires not only calcium, but also interaction with the platelet membrane. Platelet factor 3 (PF$_3$), a phospholipoprotein produced on platelet membranes, facilitates activation of factor X to Xa. Calcium and factor VIII also must be present. Factor VIII is the largest protein involved in the coagulation cascade. However, a small subunit, VIII:C, is actually responsible for the coagulant activity. The activated partial thromboplastin time (aPTT) measures the activity of the intrinsic coagulation pathway.

The common pathway begins when factor X is activated to Xa. In the presence of factor V that functions as a cofactor, calcium, and PF$_3$, Xa converts prothrombin (factor II) to the active enzyme thrombin. Thrombin then converts fibrinogen to fibrin. Thrombin also activates factor XIII to XIIIa, enhances the activity of factors V and VIII, and promotes platelet aggregation.

Fibrinogen is composed of three pairs of polypeptide chains. Thrombin cleaves fibrinogen to produce fibrinopeptides A and B and a fibrin monomer. The fibrin monomers rapidly polymerize to form fibrin. Factor XIIIa forms covalent linkages between the fibrin monomers, converting the initial friable fibrin clot to a stable clot. Both the PT and aPTT are prolonged when the common pathway does not function properly.

Again, it must be emphasized that the coagulation process is not simply the result of two separate pathways coming together to form a common pathway. There is ample evidence of interaction between the pathways. For example, factor VIIa (extrinsic pathway) can activate factor IX (intrinsic pathway) and factor VII can be activated by factors XIIa, IXa, Xa, and thrombin.

Inhibition of Coagulation

A parallel series of reactions designed to limit the extent of fibrin deposition and thrombus formation begins at the

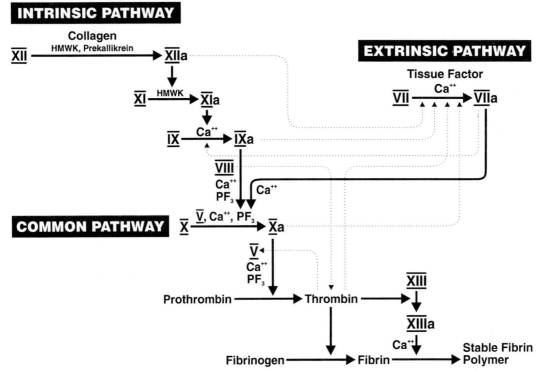

FIGURE 6–1. The coagulation pathways. The classic intrinsic, extrinsic, and common pathways are indicated by the *solid lines.* The interaction between pathways is illustrated by the *dotted lines.* Abbreviations: Ca^{++}, calcium; PF$_3$, platelet factor 3; HMWK, high-molecular-weight kininogen.

time clot formation is initiated. The fibrinolytic system is mediated primarily by the enzyme plasmin, which lyses fibrin clots. Plasminogen, an inactive circulating zymogen, is activated to plasmin via two pathways. Factor XIIa initiates intravascular activation. Tissue plasminogen activator (t-PA), released from vascular endothelium and other injured tissue, initiates extravascular activation. Plasminogen also can be activated by thrombin, kallikrein, and exogenous substances such as urokinase, streptokinase, and staphylokinase.

The proteolytic activity of plasmin is not limited to degradation of fibrin. Plasmin also cleaves fibrinogen, factors V and VII, and some components of the complement system. The initial cleavage of fibrinogen results in the production of X monomers that are subsequently split into Y and D fragments. The Y fragments are then converted to E and additional D fragments. The X monomer, Y, D, and E fragments are termed fibrin-split products (FSPs), or fibrin-degradation products (FDPs). The FDPs are normally removed by the reticuloendothelial system. If not removed, they can interfere with clot formation by inhibiting cross-linking of fibrin monomers, affect platelet function, and increase vascular permeability. A rapid latex agglutination test can be used to detect FDPs.

Antithrombin III (AT-III) is a naturally occurring inhibitor of coagulation synthesized in the liver. Referred to as heparin cofactor and factor Xa inhibitor, AT-III inactivates thrombin; factors Xa, XIIa, XIa, IXa, and VIIIa; kallikrein; and plasmin. Although AT-III is a slow inhibitor of coagulation, it acts almost instantaneously in the presence of heparin. In fact, the effect of heparin is entirely dependent on the level of AT-III. Individuals who lack the inhibitor do not respond to heparin administration. Congenital AT-III deficiency is associated with thrombotic disorders.

Protein C is a vitamin K–dependent protein that inactivates factors V and VIII, inhibits Xa, and promotes fibrinolysis by stimulating release of t-PA from endothelial cells. Another vitamin K–dependent cofactor, protein S, appears necessary for protein C function. Individuals deficient in proteins C or S are prone to thrombosis.

The Kinin and Complement Systems

The coagulation and fibrinolytic systems interact with the kinin and complement systems. Although the kinin system plays a central role in the inflammatory process, it also is involved in coagulation and fibrinolysis. The enzymes prekallikrein and kallikrein and the cofactor HMWK are essential components of the coagulation pathway, and HMWK also is involved in the fibrinolytic system.

The complement system, important in immune and allergic reactions, also influences coagulation and fibrinolysis. Platelet aggregation is enhanced by C5a. The activity of plasmin and thrombin is inhibited by C1 esterase inhibitor. Plasmin, on the other hand, is an important activator of complement. Both complement and kinin are involved in the coagulopathy associated with hemolytic transfusion reactions.

EVALUATION OF HEMOSTASIS

Four general types of clinical situations related to hemostasis may confront the anesthesiologist: (1) the child with a personal or family history of bleeding; (2) the preoperative patient with a negative history but abnormal laboratory tests; (3) the surgical patient who is not bleeding but has abnormal laboratory studies; and (4) the child who is actively bleeding. The diagnosis and management must be individualized and based on the history, clinical evaluation, and laboratory studies.

History and Physical Examination

A useful approach for the anesthesiologist evaluating a child's bleeding history is to think in terms of the three components of the hemostatic system: the vascular system, platelets, and the coagulation system. Vascular and platelet disorders are usually associated with petechiae and mucosal bleeding, although ecchymoses can occur. Easy and apparently spontaneous bruising is characteristic. Bleeding occurs immediately after injury in children with platelet disorders, whereas the onset may be delayed in patients with coagulation factor abnormalities. Factor deficiencies are characterized by large ecchymoses, bleeding into deep tissues such as muscle and joints, and moderate to severe mucosal bleeding.

Bleeding disorders are categorized on the basis of etiology as inherited or acquired. In general, the inherited disorders are confined to one hemostatic component, often one coagulation protein. The acquired disorders are more common, frequently involve several hemostatic defects, and are usually more difficult to diagnose and treat.

In evaluating a child's history, the anesthesiologist should attempt to determine if bleeding occurred at birth, particularly whether there was bleeding from the umbilical cord. It is often helpful to ask the parents to compare the child's history of bruising and bleeding with that of their other children. Information about previous surgery, especially minor procedures such as circumcision, dental extractions, and tonsillectomy, is particularly important. Was transfusion required? Have similar bleeding episodes occurred in relatives, especially male members of the family?

In eliciting a medication history, questions must be asked about over-the-counter medications. Aspirin inhibits the enzyme cyclooxygenase and blocks formation of prostaglandins by platelets, thereby inhibiting platelet aggregation. It exerts an irreversible effect on platelets circulating at the time of drug ingestion. The effect persists for the life of the platelet (approximately 9 days), and diminishes as new platelets, not affected by the drug, enter the circulation. When aspirin is administered on a regular basis, 7 to 10 days may be required for production of an adequate number of platelets to return the bleeding time to normal. Nonsteroidal anti-inflammatory drugs (NSAIDs) (e.g., indomethacin and ibuprofen) affect platelet function, but only as long as the drug is present in the circulation.

The review of systems may identify disorders associated with coagulopathies. For example, a qualitative platelet defect occurs in patients with uremia. The exact mechanism is unknown, but platelet aggregation studies are abnormal and the bleeding time prolonged. Both platelets and the coagulation pathway may be affected in children with severe hepatic disease. A variety of disorders (Table 6–2) are associated with disseminated intravascular coagulation (DIC).

TABLE 6 – 2
DISORDERS ASSOCIATED WITH DISSEMINATED INTRAVASCULAR COAGULATION

Septicemia	Heat stroke
Leukemia	Hypothermia
Disseminated malignancy	Snakebite
Viral infection	Necrotizing enterocolitis
Liver disease	Acute pancreatitis
Massive trauma	Kasabach-Merritt syndrome
Extensive burns	Extracorporeal circulation
Brain tissue destruction	Hemolytic transfusion reactions
Fat embolism	Freshwater near-drowning

An important component of the physical examination is evaluation of the skin for petechiae, purpura, or ecchymoses. The insertion sites of intravascular cannulas should be inspected for oozing or unusually large hematomas. Vascular abnormalities such as telangiectases on the mucous membranes or skin should be noted. On the basis of the history and the physical findings, the anesthesiologist may choose to order laboratory tests to evaluate hemostasis.

Laboratory Evaluation

Evaluation of hemostasis in children whose history or physical examination suggests a hemostatic abnormality should be undertaken in an organized manner by physicians familiar with laboratory tests and their limitations. A pediatric hematologist should be involved in the perioperative management of children with congenital coagulopathies.

The necessity for routine preoperative hemostatic evaluation of children not considered to be at risk for excessive intraoperative and postoperative bleeding is somewhat controversial. Some surgeons continue to order preoperative coagulation studies for children with no history suggestive of a bleeding tendency. Proponents of routine testing argue that many patients and parents give unreliable histories. Others consider testing a protection against the physician's failure to take an adequate history. Another rationale is that the tests provide a baseline for comparison if excessive intraoperative bleeding should occur. It is reasoned that any laboratory values obtained at the time of bleeding might be uninterpretable if blood components had been administered or if consumption or dilution of coagulation factors is responsible for the coagulopathy. However, the laboratory value at the time of bleeding, not the baseline value, is the one used to determine the need for administration of blood components.

In addition to being expensive, routine preoperative testing can lead to poor history taking, substitution of numbers for clinical evaluation, and unnecessary cancellation of procedures. The low prevalence of clinically unsuspected coagulopathies results in a high ratio of false-positive to true-positive test results. Blood components may unnecessarily be administered to treat clinically insignificant laboratory abnormalities.

Preoperative hemostatic evaluation generally is considered indicated in children who are to undergo cardiac surgery. Although most data are relatively old, there is evidence that children with cyanotic heart disease frequently have quantitative and qualitative platelet abnormalities and low factor levels. The occurrence of these abnormalities appears to correlate with the degree of polycythemia and inversely with age. Preexisting hemostatic abnormalities may be exacerbated by the detrimental effects of cardiopulmonary bypass (CPB) on platelet function and dilutional coagulopathy secondary to the pump prime.

Although problems with coagulation should be anticipated, it is not possible to reliably predict which children will develop them. In one study of 30 neonates 1 to 30 days old undergoing CPB, neither initial diagnosis, age, use of prostaglandin E_1, nor the need for preoperative inotropic support were predictive of preoperative coagulation defects.[55] Over half of the children had factor levels significantly below reported normal values for neonates. A recent small study comparing infants less than 2 months of age and children greater than 12 months of age undergoing CPB found that the platelets of young infants were less reactive than those of older children, as determined by CPB-induced alterations in platelet membrane adhesive receptors. In neonates, there was an absence of CPB-induced increase of p-selectin and a smaller decrease of glycoprotein Ib.[56]

A prospective study of over 400 consecutive children undergoing open heart procedures also confirmed the association between patient age, blood loss, and transfusion requirements.[57] Thirty-eight percent of the children studied were less than 1 year at the time of surgery. Neonates more often had abnormal preoperative coagulation test results. Postoperative blood loss and the amount of blood transfused were inversely related to age. Per kilogram of body weight, neonates bled more and received more transfusions than any other age group.

Principles of Hemostasis Testing

Proper collection of the blood sample for coagulation testing is essential. The appropriate volume of blood must be placed in the correct tube and sent promptly to the laboratory. The usual ratio of anticoagulant to specimen is 1:9. The tube labels are conventionally marked to indicate the level to which the tube should be filled. Blood is collected in citrate (blue-top tube) for determination of PT, aPTT, and thrombin time (TT). A lavender-top tube containing ethylenediaminetetra-acetic acid (EDTA) is used when a blood smear, platelet count, Hb, or Hct is performed. A clotted specimen (red-top tube) is required for typing and cross-matching, free Hb determination, and detection of FDPs.

In the operating room, blood samples are usually obtained from an indwelling vascular cannula with a heparin flush system. Withdrawing an aliquot twice the deadspace volume of the system before obtaining the specimen is adequate to remove all flush solution.[58] Use of specially designed reservoirs for withdrawing blood before the specimen allows the blood to be reinfused without contamination. When both a central venous and arterial catheter are in situ, it is preferable to use the central venous site because the larger caliber catheter facilitates sample withdrawal and minimizes damage to cellular elements. In addition, the potential for heparin contamination may be less, since the catheter tip is in a larger vascular compartment, where dilution of the infused heparin occurs more readily than in a small peripheral artery.

Anesthesiologists and surgeons traditionally have relied on coagulation tests performed in the laboratory. However, there are numerous reports of the benefits of point-of-care testing in the operating room. Use of transfusion algorithms based on point-of-care measurements of whole blood PT, aPTT, platelet count,[59] and thromboelastography[60] can be effective in decreasing transfusions in patients undergoing CPB. More recently, a platelet-activating clotting test (PACT) has been introduced for use in the operating room. It assesses the acceleration of the activated clotting time (ACT) by platelet-activating factor (PAF). Conflicting results have been reported regarding usefulness of the test in adult cardiac surgery,[61-63] and studies in pediatric patients have not been reported.

Whole blood viscoelastic testing devices that examine the entire process of coagulation from the time of initial platelet-fibrin interaction through platelet aggregation, clot strengthening, and fibrin cross-linkage to eventual clot lysis have been utilized for several years, particularly during liver transplantation and cardiac surgery. Data on thromboelastography in over 200 children less than 2 years of age were recently published.[64] Clinicians who are proponents of utilizing these devices report they are useful in identifying and treating coagulopathies in the perioperative period.

Platelet Evaluation

The platelet count is easily and rapidly determined with electronic particle counters. Normal values range from 150 to 450×10^9/L. When abnormally low platelet counts are obtained, examination of a blood film is necessary to ensure that the apparent thrombocytopenia is not because of inappropriate techniques of sample collection. A spuriously low platelet count can be caused by clotting in the collection tube because of inadequate or inactive anticoagulant. Clotting may be visible in the tube and platelet clumping will be evident when the blood film is examined.

Platelet function is much more difficult to assess than platelet number. Platelet aggregation studies are performed by specialized laboratories and are not suitable for rapid evaluation and treatment of surgical patients. Various substances (epinephrine, ADP, collagen) are added to a suspension of platelets in plasma and light transmission is measured with a spectrophotometer. As platelets aggregate in response to the reagents, more light is transmitted through the suspension. The pattern of light transmission is recorded on a chart recorder. Various disorders of platelet function have specific aggregation patterns. It has been suggested that the PACT may be useful in identifying patients at risk of excessive blood loss after CPB who might benefit from platelet transfusion or administration of DDAVP (desmopressin).[61] The validity of this approach in pediatric patients awaits confirmation.

The bleeding time (BT), defined as the time for a standardized skin wound to cease bleeding, assesses both platelet function and the vascular component of hemostasis. It is a crude in vivo test, lacks specificity, and is highly technique dependent. There are several methods of performing a BT, but the most common employs a sterile, disposable spring-loaded device designed to make uniform incisions. The volar surface of the forearm is usually used, although the incisions also can be made on the lower leg.[65] A blood pressure cuff is inflated to 40 mm Hg, the skin incisions are made, and the blood is blotted from the incisions with filter paper at 30-second intervals. When commercially available devices are appropriately used for the skin incisions, the normal BT is less than 10 minutes. If bleeding continues for 15 minutes, the blotting procedure is discontinued and pressure is applied to the wound.

The BT is prolonged with platelet counts less than 100 $\times 10^9$/L. In general, the BT increases proportionately to the decrease in platelet count. Aspirin and aspirin-containing medications, as well as many congenital and acquired qualitative platelet disorders, prolong the BT. Although still used preoperatively by some clinicians, the BT is not a good screening test.[66, 67] It has not been demonstrated that a prolonged BT correlates with excessive surgical bleeding or that bleeding from the test skin incision predicts bleeding elsewhere in the body. Drugs that prolong the BT in a statistically significant manner often have no clinically significant effect. Conversely, the BT cannot be used to reliably identify patients who recently ingested aspirin or NSAIDs or who have a platelet defect attributable to such drugs. As stated in the College of American Pathologists' and American Society of Clinical Pathologists' position article entitled "The Preoperative Bleeding Time Test Lacks Clinical Benefit," the bleeding time fails as a screening test and is, therefore, not indicated as a routine preoperative test.[68]

Evaluation of the Coagulation Pathway

The coagulation phase of hemostasis is conventionally evaluated with the PT, aPTT, TT, and fibrinogen level. Abnormalities are determined as prolongations of the clotting time beyond normal compared with results obtained when pooled plasma from normal subjects is tested. The PT measures factors of the extrinsic coagulation pathway (I, II, V, VII, and X). It is especially useful in detecting early vitamin K deficiencies because factor VII, a vitamin K–dependent factor, has the shortest half-life of the coagulation factors. Factor VII is the only factor restricted to the extrinsic pathway; the others are part of the common pathway. Variations in testing methodologies among laboratories can result in significantly different levels of clinical anticoagulation despite seemingly comparable PT ratios. The international normalized ratio (INR) allows standardization of PT reporting worldwide. The INR is useful for following patients receiving warfarin therapy, but is not used for evaluation of coagulopathies.

The aPTT assesses factors of the intrinsic pathway (I, II, V, VIII, IX, X, XI, XII, Fletcher, and Fitzgerald). Factors VIII, IX, XI, XII, Fletcher, and Fitzgerald are limited to the intrinsic pathway. Both the PT and aPTT are prolonged by abnormalities of factors of the common pathway (I, II, V, and X). Factor deficiencies can be caused by decreased synthesis, synthesis of abnormal factors, excessive destruction, or inactivation of factors by circulating inhibitors.

Among the inhibitors are heparin, lupus-like anticoagulant, FDPs, and antibodies to specific coagulation factors.

To determine whether a prolonged PT or aPTT occurs because of a factor deficiency or an inhibitor, an aliquot of the patient's plasma is mixed with an equal volume of normal pooled plasma and the tests are repeated. If the test results on the mixture of patient and normal plasma are normal, the diagnosis is most likely a factor deficiency that was corrected by the normal plasma. Persistence of the abnormal PT and aPTT usually indicates the presence of a coagulation inhibitor that also neutralized or interfered with the coagulation factors in the normal plasma.

The TT is a measure of the ability of thrombin to convert fibrinogen to fibrin when purified thrombin is added to a plasma sample. The TT does not measure defects in the intrinsic or extrinsic pathways because these steps are bypassed when the test is performed. The TT is prolonged in three circumstances: (1) a deficiency of or structurally abnormal fibrinogen; (2) the presence of heparin; and (3) the presence of FDPs. To differentiate an abnormality of fibrinogen from the presence of inhibitors, an aliquot of the patient's plasma is mixed with control plasma and the TT is repeated. If the resulting TT approximates that of the control plasma, a deficiency or abnormality of fibrinogen is the most likely diagnosis. If the TT is still abnormal, a circulating inhibitor (e.g., heparin or FDP) is present. The normal value is approximately 15 seconds. A reptilase time, which is not affected by heparin and only minimally prolonged by FDPs, is performed by some laboratories to differentiate the etiology of a prolonged TT. A fibrinogen level and tests for FDPs also should be performed.

Fibrinogen usually is measured by a modification of the TT using dilute plasma. Normal values range from 200 to 400 mg/dl. Low levels occur in children with congenital hypofibrinogenemia. Acquired deficiencies are seen with liver disease, DIC, and fibrinolysis. Since fibrinogen is an acute-phase reactant, elevated levels may be seen in association with acute infection, neoplasia, and collagen disorders.

FDPs can be detected by a simple semiquantitative latex agglutination test. The test is sensitive, but is associated with a high incidence of false-positive results. The more specific D-dimer test can be used to confirm that both thrombin generation and fibrinolysis have occurred. An elevated D-dimer level is usually indicative of DIC. Other characteristics of DIC are a low platelet count; prolonged PT, aPTT, and TT; and a low fibrinogen level.

Laboratory testing reveals quantitative deficiencies in the coagulation system of healthy babies for at least the first 6 months, but these laboratory abnormalities are not associated with increased bleeding.[64] In both term and premature neonates, factors XII, XI, prekallikrein, HMWK, the vitamin K–dependent factors (II, VII, IX, and X), and many of the coagulation inhibitors (proteins C and S, AT-III, and heparin cofactor II) are present in lower concentrations than in adults. Nevertheless, PT and TT values are similar to adult values in healthy babies. The aPTT is initially somewhat prolonged but by 3 to 6 months of age is similar to adult values.

In addition to taking into consideration the age of the patient when evaluating laboratory test results, the anesthesiologist must recognize that there is variability among laboratories and test results. A recent study evaluating several PT and aPTT tests in patients sustaining significant blood loss during extensive spine surgery revealed marked variations in the results of the tests.[69] The variability among tests was most marked when PT and aPTT were increased 1.5 to 2.0 times the mean reference range values—the range in which most guidelines specify that transfusion of FFP is indicated. It is essential that laboratory values be correlated with clinical findings when determining whether coagulopathy is present and treatment is indicated.

Making the Diagnosis

The child's history, current clinical situation, and laboratory values must all be considered. Although the anesthesiologist should be familiar with general patterns of laboratory values associated with specific types of bleeding disorders (Table 6–3), patients, not numbers, should be treated. Some children with markedly abnormal laboratory values are not at risk for bleeding and should not receive blood components. For example, prophylactic administration of platelets is not indicated in a child with immune thrombocytopenic purpura (ITP) and a platelet count of 20×10^9/L. The pathophysiology of the disorder involves immune destruction of platelets, and transfused platelets are subject to the same reduction in life span as the patient's own platelets. Children with ITP usually do not bleed intraoperatively, even with very low platelet counts. On the other hand, a child with diffuse bleeding after CPB and a platelet count of 75×10^9/L may well benefit from platelet transfusion because CPB induces a qualitative platelet defect.

Realistically, there are times when patients are bleeding excessively in the operating room and, in the anesthesiologist's judgment, delaying transfusion would compromise the child's well-being. In such circumstances, a blood sample should be sent for coagulation studies, but treatment can be initiated. The anesthesiologist should document on the anesthesia record the clinical circumstances and any available laboratory data.

PLATELET TRANSFUSION

Platelets are prepared by two methods: centrifugation of whole blood and apheresis. Storage at room temperature (20° to 24°C) and constant agitation are necessary for maximum platelet viability. Exposure to refrigerated temperatures for even a few hours induces changes in platelet properties and affects viability. Although platelets stored at room temperature remain viable up to 7 days, the shelf-life is limited to 5 days because of concerns about bacterial growth at that temperature in the event of bacterial contamination.

Testing for ABO compatibility is not required. Although platelets do not have to be ABO compatible, there is evidence that platelet survival is greater when ABO-compatible platelets are administered. Platelet components contain few RBCs, but adherence to recipient Rh compatibility is important when transfusing females of

┌T A B L E   6 – 3┐
TABLE 6 – 3
TESTS OF HEMOSTASIS AND BLEEDING DISORDERS

	Platelet Disorders		Heparin Effect	DIC	Hypo-/Dys-fibrinogenemia	Common Pathway Factor Disorder or Inhibitor	Hemophilia	von Willebrand's Disease
	Quantitative	*Qualitative*						
Platelet Count	↓	N	N	↓	N	N	N	N
PT	N	N	N/↑	↑	N/↑	↑	N	N
aPTT	N	N	↑	↑	N/↑	↑	↑	↑
TT	N	N	↑	↑	↑	N	N	N
Fibrinogen	N	N	N	↓	N/↓	N	N	N
BT	↑	↑	N	↑	N	N	N	↑
Reptilase time	N	N	N	N	↑	N	N	N

PT, prothrombin time; aPTT, activated partial thromboplastin time; TT, thrombin time; BT, bleeding time; N, normal; ↑ prolonged; ↓, low.

childbearing potential. If Rh-positive platelets are administered to an Rh-negative female of childbearing potential, the administration of Rh immune globulin should be considered.

Platelets prepared from whole blood are referred to as "random-donor" platelets or platelet concentrates. Each unit should contain at least 5.5×10^{10} platelets in 50 to 70 ml plasma. The usual dose for infants is 10 ml/kg and for older children 1 unit/10 kg body weight. The required number of units may be combined in one bag by the transfusion service as a pooled product. Pooled platelets have a shelf-life of only 4 hours. Therefore, it is important that the anesthesiologist not request pooled platelets when there is little likelihood of administration.

Single-donor platelets are collected by apheresis. Each unit contains at least 3×10^{11} platelets and is considered approximately equivalent to six random-donor platelets. Several types of apheresis devices are available, several of which produce a leukocyte-reduced platelet product. The primary advantage of single-donor platelets is reduction of donor exposures in patients who would otherwise require several random-donor platelet units.

Indications for Platelet Transfusion

Platelets may be administered prophylactically or therapeutically. The appropriate threshold for administration of platelets to children considered to be at risk of bleeding because of thrombocytopenia or impaired platelet function varies with the patient's underlying condition and is influenced by previous responses to platelet transfusion. The anesthesiologist should be familiar with institutional guidelines regarding platelet transfusions in premature infants, oncology patients, and patients refractory to platelet transfusion.

The major concern in thrombocytopenic premature infants is the potential for intracranial hemorrhage. Thrombocytopenia is usually defined as a platelet count less than 150×10^9/L, but the level of thrombocytopenia at which platelet transfusion is indicated is not generally agreed on. The results of a multicenter, prospective, randomized, controlled trial conducted in premature infants with platelet counts less than 150×10^9/L within 72 hours

of birth provides some guidance.[70] The investigators evaluated whether administration of platelet concentrates (10 ml/kg) reduced the incidence or extension of intracranial hemorrhage. Although platelet transfusion increased platelet counts and shortened bleeding times, neither the incidence nor extent of intracranial hemorrhage was reduced. It was concluded that nonbleeding premature infants with platelet counts greater than approximately 60×10^9/L do not require prophylactic platelet transfusion.

Many recommendations regarding prophylactic platelet transfusion are based on studies conducted in patients with acute leukemia. The patients initially studied often also were receiving aspirin because the research was performed prior to recognition of the effects of aspirin on platelet function. For many years, a platelet count less than 20×10^9/L was considered an indication for prophylactic platelet transfusion.[71] Recently, a platelet count of 10×10^9/L has been suggested as an appropriate threshold, at least during induction chemotherapy in adolescents and adults with acute leukemia.[72, 73] The recommendations do not apply to patients undergoing surgical procedures.

Management of patients refractory to platelet transfusion can be challenging. The definition of platelet refractoriness varies, but the concept of the corrected count increment (CCI), which adjusts the observed raw increment in platelet count for the platelet content of the transfusion and the body surface area of the patient, is useful. A CCI less than 7.5×10^9/L measured within 1 hour after platelet transfusion is usually considered a platelet failure, and consistent failures represent refractoriness. Management of refractory patients varies somewhat among institutions, but may initially include provision of ABO-compatible and "fresh" platelets, followed by HLA-matched or crossmatch-compatible platelets in patients documented to be alloimmunized.[74] Identification of factors other than alloimmunization that can cause platelet refractoriness is essential. Fever, infection, sepsis, DIC, splenomegaly, and multiple medications are all known to affect platelet recovery and survival. Treatment of the infection or elimination of the offending medication may be all that is required.

Management of massively transfused patients, conventionally defined as the transfusion of one or more blood volumes within a few hours, ranges from administering platelets by formula according to the number of RBC units transfused to transfusing platelets only if there is laboratory and clinical evidence of coagulopathy. Prophylactic formula-defined platelet transfusion cannot be condoned. Neither is awaiting the occurrence of clinical coagulopathy in the presence of predictable, ongoing, large-volume blood loss an acceptable approach. When the need for platelet transfusion is anticipated, the transfusion service should be notified of the expected platelet requirements, particularly if platelet shortages are frequent.

Limited studies in pediatric patients have demonstrated that changes in serial platelet counts with massive transfusion are similar to those in adults, when related to blood volumes transfused. In a study of 26 children who lost at least one blood volume, it was found that the preoperative platelet count was a reliable predictor of platelet transfusion requirements.[75] The investigators concluded that children with initial platelet counts greater than 150×10^9/L may require platelet transfusion after only one blood volume exchange, but those with higher counts may not require platelet administration until more than two blood volumes are lost. As in adult studies, platelet counts were above predicted values, presumably because of release of platelets from the spleen, which normally sequesters about one third of the platelets.

The need for platelet transfusion is determined by more than the platelet count. It is also influenced by the type and extent of surgery, the rate and magnitude of bleeding, the ability to surgically control bleeding, and additional factors that adversely affect platelet function (e.g., CPB, uremia, or medications with antiplatelet activity).[36] As a general guideline, children with platelet counts greater than or equal to 100×10^9/L rarely require platelet transfusion, in the absence of factors influencing platelet function. Even with normal platelet function, children with platelet counts less than 50×10^9/L undergoing surgical procedures may benefit from platelet transfusion. If abnormal bleeding occurs with a platelet count greater than 50×10^9/L, other causes of bleeding, such as DIC or inadequate surgical hemostasis, should be sought.

Prophylactic platelet administration has not been studied in children undergoing cardiac surgery. However, studies in adults have demonstrated no value of prophylactic platelet administration.[76] Since blood loss has been shown to vary inversely with patient age, it may be anticipated that neonates undergoing cardiac surgery are more likely to require platelet transfusion than other children.

Regardless of whether platelets are administered prophylactically or therapeutically, the response to transfusion should be determined. Unless point-of-care testing is available in the operating room, it is necessary to send a specimen to the laboratory. The results of the platelet count are usually available prior to a full coagulation profile. Anesthesiologists may request that platelet count results be phoned to the operating room as soon as they are available. Ideally, the platelet count should be determined between 15 minutes and 1 hour after platelet transfusion. In the absence of significant ongoing blood loss, it is easy to differentiate a normal response from platelet refractoriness or the presence of DIC (Fig. 6-2). Patients who are refractory will not show the expected increase

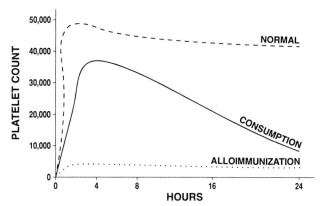

FIGURE 6-2. Responses to platelet transfusion in the normal patient and in the presence of DIC or alloimmunization causing platelet refractoriness.

in platelet count. With DIC, the count will initially increase, but then decrease.

TRANSFUSION OF FRESH FROZEN PLASMA

FFP is most often prepared from whole blood by separating and freezing the plasma within 8 hours of phlebotomy. The FFP units contain approximately 220 ml. Units of 600 ml prepared by apheresis also are available in some institutions. Both products are stored at −18°C and have a 1-year shelf life. The plasma is prepared for administration by thawing at 30° to 37°C in a water bath or a microwave oven designed for that purpose. Once thawed, FFP may be stored at 1° to 6°C for up to 24 hours.

A recently licensed product, pooled plasma, solvent/detergent treated (S/D-P), is prepared by incubating up to 2,500 units of ABO group-specific plasma with an organic solvent and a nonionic detergent. After removal of the S/D reagents, the plasma is sterile-filtered and refrozen in standardized 200-ml bags. The process has been demonstrated to effectively inactivate lipid-enveloped viruses, including HIV, HCV, and HBV.[77] It does not, however, affect nonenveloped virus such as hepatitis A virus (HAV) and parvovirus B19. Although the advantages in terms of the lipid-enveloped viruses are obvious, serious concerns have been raised about potential transmission of nonenveloped viruses in view of the large number of donor units used for each lot of S/D-P.

As an alternative to S/D-P, some blood centers are making available FFP, donor retested (FFP-DR). The plasma is produced from single whole blood or apheresis donations by the usual methods. It is then held in quarantine until the donor returns at least 112 days later and again tests negative.

Institutions may elect to make available all three products: FFP, S/D-P, and FFP-DR. Others, on the basis of scientific and economic considerations, may stock only one or two products. The term FFP will be used to refer to all types of FFP, since the therapeutic implications (but not potential complications) are similar.

Indications for Fresh Frozen Plasma

Over 2 million units of FFP are transfused annually in the United States. A significant percentage of FFP is administered without apparent justification. In the surgical population, FFP is most frequently administered to patients who are massively transfused, those having cardiac surgery, and patients with severe liver disease, including those undergoing liver transplantation. In medical patients, large volumes of FFP are used during therapeutic plasma exchange procedures. In an occasional patient receiving warfarin and requiring urgent surgery, FFP will be indicated to acutely reverse the effects of the drug.

The once-prevalent practice of administering FFP in a fixed ratio of FFP/RBC units has declined. Dilutional coagulopathy can develop when large numbers of RBC units are administered, but blood usually coagulates appropriately when coagulation factor concentrations are at least 20 to 30 percent of normal. Replacement of an entire blood volume leaves the patient with approximately one third of the original concentration of coagulation factors.

Clinical assessment must be combined with laboratory evaluation. Although laboratory values for PT and aPTT may be outside the normal range, clinical coagulopathy from dilution does not ordinarily occur until the values are greater than or equal to 1.5 times control. This correlation of increased surgical bleeding and abnormal laboratory tests was confirmed by a study of 32 children (mean age, 15.6 ± 2.3 years) who lost more than 50 percent of their blood volumes during spine surgery.[78] Patients with increased surgical bleeding had greater increases in PT and aPTT (> 1.5 times mean control) than patients without evidence of increased bleeding. As expected, patients with increased clinical bleeding sustained greater blood volume loss than patients without increased bleeding (1.14 ± 0.28 and 0.87 ± 0.22 blood volumes, respectively). Administration of FFP (10 ml/kg) was judged to correct the increased surgical bleeding in 14 of the 17 children. The authors of the study speculated that the reason they saw a dilutional coagulopathy, rather than the DIC previously described in patients having emergency surgical procedures, was that their patients did not experience shock or acidosis, which are associated with development of DIC.

On the basis of the foregoing study and others, it is suggested that FFP administration be considered for patients with PT and aPTT values greater than or equal to 1.5 times the laboratory's normal values. There is significant variability among laboratory tests, especially when the PT and aPTT are 1.5 to 2 times normal[69]; therefore, institutional guidelines should be based on local laboratory testing procedures.

Fresh frozen plasma is sometimes administered prophylactically to premature babies considered to be at risk of intracranial hemorrhage. A large randomized study, involving over 700 babies of gestational age at birth less than 32 weeks, recently evaluated this practice.[79] The babies were randomly allocated within 2 hours of birth to receive FFP (20 ml/kg initially and an additional dose of 10 ml/kg after 24 hours) or serve as controls. There was no difference in the number of babies who died or who survived with severe disability. The survivors had similar mean developmental quotients at 2 years of age. It was concluded that there was no basis for the routine early use of FFP to prevent intraventricular hemorrhage in premature infants.

Another clinical circumstance during which FFP is used prophylactically is open heart surgery. In a recent study of 75 children undergoing CPB, it was found that FFP administration offered no benefit in correcting post-CPB coagulopathies.[80] In children with ongoing bleeding despite platelet administration, administration of FFP actually seemed to worsen coagulation parameters and was associated with greater chest tube drainage.

When indicated, FFP should be administered in doses calculated to achieve a minimum of 30 percent of plasma factor concentrations. This is usually achieved with the administration of approximately 10 ml/kg. Plasma should be ABO compatible and a filter must be used during administration. It should be kept in mind that patients receiving platelets, such as massively transfused patients with thrombocytopenia, also will be receiving plasma. Four or five platelet concentrates or a single-donor apheresis platelet unit contain approximately the same volume of plasma as 1 unit of FFP.

CRYOPRECIPITATE ADMINISTRATION

Cryoprecipitate is a concentrated source of certain plasma proteins (factors VIII:vWF, VIII:C, XIII, and fibrinogen) prepared by thawing FFP at 4°C. The white precipitate formed when FFP is thawed is the cryoprecipitate. The supernatant plasma is removed, leaving the cold precipitated protein in 10 to 15 ml plasma, which is then refrozen at −18°C. Cryoprecipitate is thawed at 30° to 37°C prior to use.

There are few uses for cryoprecipitate. Once the treatment of choice for patients with hemophilia A and von Willebrand's disease, cryoprecipitate has been replaced by safer therapies. The recent licensure of a commercially prepared fibrin sealant or "glue" has obviated the need for allogeneic or autologous cryoprecipitate for that use.

Cryoprecipitate may be indicated in the setting of massive transfusion, clinical bleeding, and a fibrinogen level less than 80 to 100 mg/dl.[36] The dose is approximately 1 unit/7 kg body weight. Administration of ABO-compatible units is preferable, and they must be transfused through a filter.

AUTOLOGOUS TRANSFUSION

Children are often appropriate candidates for preoperative blood donation, acute normovolemic hemodilution, and intra- and postoperative blood recovery techniques. Although one technique may not eliminate the need for allogeneic transfusion, a combination of methods can reduce or, in some circumstances, eliminate the need for allogeneic blood.

Preoperative Blood Donation

The concept of donating blood prior to surgery has been advocated since the 1930s. However, the inclusion of children in predonation programs is relatively recent. Factors limiting preoperative autologous donation by pediatric patients are patient cooperation; vascular access; and commitment of surgeons, parents, and blood center personnel. The amount of blood that can be withdrawn at each donation is determined by the child's weight. A conventional unit is drawn from children weighing 50 kg or more. Proportionate units are drawn in smaller children so that no more than 15 percent of the estimated blood volume is removed at one time. The Hct must be at least 33 percent prior to each phlebotomy. Donations may be scheduled more than once a week, and the last should occur no less than 72 hours before surgery to allow time for restoration of intravascular volume and for transport and testing of the donated blood. Donation is contraindicated if the child has, or is being treated for, bacteremia or has a bacterial infection that can be associated with bacteremia.

A predonation program for children scheduled for orthopedic surgery was established at the Alfred I. Du Pont Institute in 1967, and data on over 200 procedures were reported in 1974.[81] Patients ranged in age from 7 to 21 years (mean, 14 years). Complete data were available for 147 patients who had 155 procedures. Only autologous blood was required for two thirds of the procedures. The only serious complication was a nasal fracture in a child who fainted during donation.

Experience with 180 children between 8 and 18 years of age who participated in a blood center–based predonation program was reported in 1987.[82] The children, weighing as little as 27 kg, donated between 1 and 5 proportionate units. Eighty-eight percent of the patients were able to provide all of their own blood. Numerous reports attest to the safety and efficacy of predonation by older children and adolescents. In fact, predonation has become so routine for procedures such as scoliosis surgery that clinicians no longer document and publish their experience.

More recently, predonation by very young children has been reported. In one study, blood was withdrawn at the time of cardiac catheterization and stored for use during cardiac surgery.[83] A total of 27 children anesthetized with thiopental had blood (10 ml/kg) removed approximately 2 weeks prior to cardiac surgery. The children ranged in age from 6 months to 6 years of age (average, 1.9 ± 2.1 years) and weighed 5.8 to 20.2 kg (average, 9.7 ± 5.5 kg). Acyanotic children received intravenous r-HuEPO on day 1 and day 7 following phlebotomy. Cyanotic children were not treated with r-HuEPO, but all children received oral ferrous sulfate daily. The predonated blood was used as pump prime or administered during or after CPB. Nineteen (76 percent) of the patients required no allogeneic blood during surgery. In another study, 80 children as young as 3 years (mean, 8.6 ± 3.9 years) weighing as little as 12.3 kg (mean, 29.2 ± 14.5 kg) donated 735 ± 388 ml during an average of 3.1 ± 1.5 phlebotomies before cardiac surgery.[84] Seventy-five (94 percent) of the children did not require allogeneic transfusion during surgery. It should be noted that both of these study sites used a combination of blood conservation strategies, making the contribution of predonation impossible to quantitate.

Very young children also have donated blood prior to other types of surgery, including procedures for Hirschsprung's disease[85] and craniosynostoses.[86, 87] In the latter case, children were anesthetized and blood withdrawn via an arterial catheter. Babies as young as 6 months of age were included. Administration of r-HuEPO, acute normovolemic hemodilution, and intraoperative blood salvage also were utilized where appropriate. With this protocol, 11 of 13 babies had surgery without receiving allogeneic blood.

Although few would question the merits of predonation by teenagers scheduled for scoliosis surgery, the benefits of predonation by very young children are less certain. The number of cases reported is small and the contribution of predonation to avoidance of allogeneic transfusion cannot be determined when several blood conservation techniques are employed. Administration of r-HuEPO is effective in increasing the amount of blood that can be donated, but it is expensive and several injections are required. Some patients sustain reactions, mostly vasovagal episodes requiring no treatment, during the donation process. Finally, transfusion of preoperatively donated blood is not without potential hazard.

The greatest potential hazard associated with transfusion of predonated blood is administration of an autologous unit to an unintended recipient. Such errors do occur. One analysis of autologous donations by 175 pediatric orthopedic patients revealed 13 errors.[88] Three children received allogeneic blood when autologous units were available. Several units expired and some were destroyed because of problems with storage, necessitating allogeneic transfusion. One patient received the wrong type of allogeneic blood. The anesthesiologist's index of suspicion for a transfusion reaction may be low when the patient is receiving blood thought to be autologous, reducing the probability of early diagnosis and intervention. In addition to hemolysis related to administration of the wrong unit of RBCs, there is potential for administration of contaminated blood. Two of 10 cases of sepsis caused by *Yersinia enterocolitica* reported in the United States between 1991 and 1996 were in patients who received autologous RBCs.[89] Acute intravascular hemolysis also has been reported caused by transfusion of inadequately deglycerolized previously frozen RBCs.[90]

A point of frequent controversy is whether all predonated blood should be reinfused, regardless of surgical blood loss or the patient's Hct. Approximately 50 percent of units donated by adults are not reinfused. Comparable data are not available for pediatric patients, but the discard rate is probably lower. Children scheduled for procedures during which transfusion is rarely necessary should not donate. However, it is preferable to discard units, rather than administer them when there is no indication. It may be appropriate to utilize somewhat more liberal criteria for transfusing autologous than allogeneic RBCs in situations where the indications for transfusion are equivocal. The *Practice Guidelines for Blood Component Therapy* of the American Society of Anesthesiologists[36] state that the indications for transfusion of autologous RBCs may be more liberal because of the lower (but still significant) risks associated with autologous blood. On the other hand, the *Guidelines for Red Blood Cell and Plasma Transfusion for Adults and Children*[37] published by the Canadian Medical

Association state that the indications for transfusion of autologous and allogeneic blood should be the same.

Acute Normovolemic Hemodilution

Acute normovolemic hemodilution (ANH) is the removal of blood immediately before or after induction of anesthesia and replacement with acellular fluid.[48] Limited or moderate hemodilution is the term applied when the Hct is reduced to approximately 28 percent. Extreme hemodilution refers to reduction of the Hct below 20 percent. Augmented acute normovolemic hemodilution (AANH) is the term coined by the author to refer to administration of a temporary oxygen-carrying RBC substitute in addition to other replacement fluids.

The major advantage of ANH is reduction in RBC loss. As a general guideline, if a child with a Hct of 45 percent loses 500 ml of blood, the RBC loss is 225 ml. If the Hct is 25 percent, the RBC loss is only 125 ml. In addition, ANH provides the only available source of fresh, whole autologous blood. Some parents of the Jehovah's Witnesses faith will allow ANH for their children.

The amount of blood that can be withdrawn (V) depends on the child's estimated blood volume (EBV), initial Hct (Hct$_o$), the lowest Hct desired (Hct$_f$), and the average of the two (Hct$_{av}$). For a 30-kg child with an EBV of 2.1 L, Hct 45 percent, and desired Hct of 27 percent, using the formula:

$$V = EBV \times \frac{[(Hct_o) - (Hct_f)]}{Hct_{av}}$$

approximately 1 L of blood can be withdrawn and stored for later reinfusion:

$$V = 2.1 \times \frac{(0.45 - 0.27)}{0.36} = 1.05 \text{ L}$$

Crystalloid, colloid, or both are infused as the blood is withdrawn. When crystalloid is used, the amount administered must be approximately three times the volume of blood removed because about two thirds of the crystalloid leaks into the extravascular space. Since colloids are retained within the intravascular space, the amount of albumin, hydroxyethyl starch, or other colloid required to maintain normovolemia is approximately equal to the amount of blood withdrawn. The primary advantage of using crystalloid, aside from cost, is that excess fluid can be excreted if a diuretic such as furosemide (0.5 to 1 mg/kg) is administered prior to reinfusion of the blood.

The blood can be withdrawn from a central or antecubital vein or radial artery. Use of a vein distal to the antecubital area is not recommended because poor blood flow often results in clotting. The blood is drawn into bags containing an anticoagulant, usually citrate-phosphate-dextrose (CPD). Hemodilution kits containing bags with anticoagulant, a Y-type connection set with Luer-lock adapter, and a blood recipient identification band are available (Autologous Blood Collection Kit 4R5012, Fenwal Division, Baxter Healthcare, Deerfield, IL). A scale should be used to weigh the bags to ensure they contain the appropriate amount of blood relative to anticoagulant. Use of an automated blood collection and mixing device, or blood "shaker," permits continuous monitoring of collection volumes and prevents clotting (Blood Shaker/Flow and Weight Monitor Model 1040, Sebra, Tucson, AZ). Each unit should be labeled with the child's name, hospital number, and time of blood withdrawal, and should be numbered sequentially. The blood is usually kept in the operating room with the patient and maintained at room temperature to preserve platelet function. If it is anticipated that more than 8 hours will elapse prior to reinfusion, refrigeration of the blood is required. The blood is reinfused after major blood loss ceases, or sooner if necessary. Estimation of blood loss and serial Hct determinations are used to guide transfusion.

The minimal safe Hct during ANH depends on the child's ability to compensate for decreased arterial oxygen content. Hematocrits of approximately 20 percent are well tolerated by most children. Extreme ANH in children and adolescents has been reported by several investigators. Children hemodiluted to Hb levels of 3 ± 0.8 g/dl have been shown to maintain global oxygen consumption.[50] The oxygen extraction ratio increased from 17 to 44 percent and mixed venous oxygen saturation decreased from 90.8 ± 5.4 percent to 72.3 ± 7.7 percent. In children of the Jehovah's Witnesses faith in whom the Hct was reduced to 16 percent, the oxygen extraction ratio increased from 22 to 33 percent and mixed venous oxygen saturation declined from 80 to 70 percent.[91] The safety of extreme ANH to Hct values of 12 to 14 percent in combination with mild hypothermia and controlled hypotension to mean arterial pressures of 40 to 50 mm Hg has been demonstrated in patients undergoing spinal fusions.[92] While global oxygenation is preserved at very low Hct levels in healthy, properly selected, invasively monitored children, it is not known whether there are adverse effects on regional oxygen delivery and specific organ functions.

Although used most often in adolescents, ANH has been employed in children less than 1 year of age. Between 1974 and 1983, ANH was used in more than 300 children at one pediatric hospital.[93, 94] When the procedure is performed in small children, the amount of blood to be withdrawn must be carefully calculated, the volume of anticoagulant in the bag reduced if necessary to provide an appropriate ratio of blood to anticoagulant, and the blood removal process meticulously monitored. The transfusion service can provide information about the amount of anticoagulant for the volume of blood to be withdrawn.

Intraoperative and Postoperative Blood Recovery

A double-lumen aspiration set that delivers a citrate or heparin solution at a controlled rate is utilized when blood is aspirated from the surgical field. Anticoagulated blood is collected in a rigid disposable reservoir. Use of a small (e.g., 125 ml) centrifuge bowl is preferable when devices that process or "wash" the blood prior to reinfusion are utilized in pediatrics. Alternatively, a device that continuously processes small volumes of blood for reinfusion may be used. With conventional processing devices, the blood is pumped into the bowl, washed with saline, and the RBCs suspended in saline are pumped into a reinfusion bag. The supernatant solution containing debris from the surgical field, white blood cells (WBCs), platelets, activated clotting factors, free Hb, and anticoagulant is eliminated into a waste bag.

The Hct of processed blood is usually between 50 and 60 percent. The oxygen transport properties and survival of recovered RBCs are equal to or better than those of stored RBCs, and 2,3-DPG levels are higher.[95-97] When citrate is used as an anticoagulant, it is metabolized by the liver. Processed RBCs do not contain clinically significant amounts of residual heparin when it is used as the anticoagulant.[98] The blood is depleted of coagulation proteins and functional platelets.

Spine and cardiac surgery and orthotopic liver transplantation are the procedures during which blood recovery is most often employed in children. Use of the technique is generally considered contraindicated when the wound is contaminated with intestinal contents. The presence of tumor cells in the operative field traditionally has been considered a relative contraindication to intraoperative blood recovery, but there is evidence that leukocyte-reduction[99] or irradiation[100] of the salvaged blood prior to reinfusion may render it tumor free. Blood should not be aspirated during application of topical hemostatic agents such as thrombin or while the wound is being irrigated with antibiotics not intended for parenteral use.

The literature is replete with reports of use of the technique in adults, and some reports combine pediatric and adult patients. One study of 218 patients included 139 children with a mean age of 14.5 years.[96] It was estimated that 54 percent of the RBC loss in children was recovered, whereas 68 percent was retrieved in adults. Studies in children having spine surgery have demonstrated that 50 to 80 percent of shed RBCs could be recovered and reinfused.[101, 102]

Blood also can be collected and transfused in the postoperative period. Cardiac surgeons long have advocated reinfusion of mediastinal drainage after cardiac surgery. Blood within the mediastinum undergoes coagulation and subsequent fibrinolysis. It contains virtually no fibrinogen, and no anticoagulation is required prior to reinfusion. The Hct of the blood usually averages 20 to 25 percent. Transfused RBCs have normal survival and oxygen delivery capacity. FDPs are detected in the majority of patients when unwashed shed mediastinal blood is reinfused. The presence of FDPs should not be interpreted as indicative of DIC in the absence of clinical bleeding.[103] Caution also must be exercised when interpreting cardiac enzyme levels in patients who receive shed mediastinal blood because elevations can mimic laboratory evidence of a myocardial infarction.[104]

Postoperative blood recovery also is utilized following orthopedic surgery, primarily in adults having total hip or knee replacements. In pediatric patients, the technique may be used following spine surgery. A prospective study conducted in 16 children undergoing Cotrel-Dubousset instrumentation and posterior spinal fusion demonstrated the usefulness of recovery and processing of shed blood.[105]

The average volume of blood reinfused was 354 ml (range, 200 to 900 ml).

Potential complications of reinfusion of shed blood include hemoglobinuria (with or without renal damage), coagulopathy from infusion of residual anticoagulant or dilution of coagulation factors, air or fat embolism, and sepsis. These complications should not occur if the devices are utilized according to the manufacturers' instructions. Proper use of the suction device and maintaining vacuum levels within the recommended range ($\leq$100 to 150 mm Hg) will minimize hemolysis during the collection process.

PHARMACOLOGIC AGENTS TO DECREASE SURGICAL BLOOD LOSS

The role of pharmacologic agents to decrease surgical blood loss is still evolving. The initial enthusiasm for use of DDAVP in cardiac surgery waned when subsequent studies failed to demonstrate beneficial effects of the drug in decreasing allogeneic transfusion requirements. Studies in children undergoing spinal fusion for idiopathic or neuromuscular scoliosis also have not shown a reduction in allogeneic transfusion with DDAVP.[106, 107]

Aprotinin, a serine protease inhibitor, has been shown to decrease bleeding and transfusion in pediatric cardiac surgery patients. In a prospective, randomized, placebo-controlled, double-blind study evaluating two dose levels of aprotinin in 61 children (median age, 3.7 years) undergoing reoperative open heart surgery, both high- and low-dose treatment was superior to placebo in reducing transfusion requirements.[108] In addition to decreasing the number of units of blood administered during the first 24 hours postoperatively, aprotinin administration was associated with decreased operating room time and duration of hospitalization. In another study of 31 children undergoing repair of congenital heart defects, transfusion was not required in 64 percent of aprotinin-treated patients, whereas only 25 percent of the placebo group did not receive blood postoperatively.[109] In yet another study of 80 pediatric patients who received aprotinin at the time of repair of congenital cardiac defects, the drug was shown to be effective in decreasing chest tube drainage, time to skin closure, and transfusion requirements.[110] A retrospective review of 46 consecutive children undergoing single-ventricle palliation demonstrated that aprotinin was associated with decreased thoracic drainage, as well as evidence of lowered pulmonary vascular resistance.[111]

At this time, aprotinin is approved in the United States for use in patients undergoing cardiopulmonary bypass in the course of coronary artery bypass grafting (CABG) procedures. A consideration in all patients, but perhaps most relevant in children with congenital heart disease who may require several surgical procedures, is the potential for anaphylactic reactions with administration of aprotinin. The estimated overall risk is 0.5 percent, but may increase to 6 to 9 percent when reexposure occurs within 6 months.[112] The optimal dose regimen also remains to be determined. Cost considerations favor low-dose regimens. In adults, ε-aminocaproic acid and tranexamic acid have been shown to be cost-effective alternatives to aprotinin.[113, 114]

CONGENITAL HEMATOLOGIC DISORDERS

The perioperative management of the child with a congenital hematologic disorder should be coordinated with the child's hematologist. While some diseases have a predictable clinical course, many do not. It is important to know the severity of the individual patient's disease and previous response to therapy. If the child has had a surgical procedure in the past, the records should be reviewed. Therapeutic approaches that were previously successful may be repeated, and an alternative should be sought for those that were not. Many children with congenital hematologic disorders are quite sophisticated and knowledgeable about their disease and can appropriately be involved in decisions about perioperative management.

Congenital Coagulopathies

The management of children with congenital coagulopathies, particularly hemophilia A, hemophilia B, and von Willebrand disease (vWD) has changed significantly in recent years. Virus-attenuated plasma-derived clotting factor concentrates, recombinant products, and synthetic agents such as DDAVP have made treatment much safer. Prophylactic regimens have decreased the incidence and severity of debilitating joint disease in patients with hemophilia. Perhaps of greatest significance, transmission of viral diseases, which once decimated the hemophilia community, is now rare.

Hemophilia A

Hemophilia A (factor VIII deficiency) and hemophilia B (factor IX deficiency, Christmas disease) are inherited as X-linked recessive traits and affect males almost exclusively. In approximately one third of newly diagnosed infants and young children, there is no family history, and the disease represents spontaneous mutation in the factor VIII or factor IX gene.[115] The clinical presentation of the disorders is similar and specific factor assays are required to make the initial diagnosis. Severity differs, but as a general rule, the severity is similar in affected members of a family. Approximately two thirds of patients with hemophilia have severe disease, 15 percent have moderate disease, and 20 percent have mild disease. Severity is based on levels of factor VIII and factor IX in hemophilia A and hemophilia B, respectively.

Several plasma-derived and recombinant factor VIII products are available for treating patients with hemophilia A. Dosage is determined by the type and severity of bleeding and the desired circulating factor VIII level. In general, 1 U/kg will increase the plasma level by 2 percent. For example, to raise a child's factor VIII level by 50 percent, a dose of 25 U/kg would be infused. The factor VIII level is raised to 80 to 100 percent for surgery. If bolus doses are administered, they are usually repeated every 12 hours. In the perioperative period, continuous infusion of factor VIII is often utilized. Children with inhibitor antibodies do not respond to appropriate doses of factor VIII. Those with low titers may respond to increased doses of factor VIII, but most require alternative agents.

For individuals with mild disease, as well as female carriers who have low levels of factor VIII, DDAVP is the treatment of choice.[115] The drug acts by causing rapid release of factor VIII and vWF from storage sites. The initial intravenous dose is 0.3 μg/kg. The response is variable but usually reproducible in a given patient. Tachyphylaxis may occur when doses are repeated at frequent intervals. The anesthesiologist should be alert for signs of hyponatremia and water intoxication because DDAVP is a potent antidiuretic. It may be necessary to decrease the amount of intravenous fluid administered perioperatively.

Hemophilia B

Several types of plasma-derived and recombinant factor IX products are available for treating patients with hemophilia B. Fortunately, the thrombotic complications previously reported in surgical patients treated with prothrombin complex concentrates (e.g., Konyne, Proplex) do not seem to occur when factor IX products are administered. There is no equivalent of DDAVP for treating patients with mild hemophilia B. The percentage of patients who develop inhibitors is less than with hemophilia A, and alternative therapies are available.

Von Willebrand's Disease

vWD is the most common hereditary disorder of coagulation, affecting an estimated 1 to 2 percent of the population.[115] The true incidence is unknown because mild forms of the disease go undiagnosed. It should be suspected in patients with a history of abnormal bleeding beginning in childhood. Epistaxis, prolonged bleeding after trauma or surgery, ecchymoses from minimal injury, menorrhagia, and bleeding from the gums are characteristic. A family history of bleeding and worsening of bleeding episodes in association with ingestion of aspirin are clues to the diagnosis. The disorder is usually transmitted as an autosomal dominant trait, but penetrance is variable. The severity of the disease, as well as the response to treatment, may fluctuate in a given patient.

The basic defect in vWD is in vWF, a large multimeric plasma glycoprotein synthesized in endothelial cells and megakaryocytes. Von Willebrand's factor is essential for platelet adhesion to injury sites in the vessel wall. It also protects factor VIII from proteolytic degradation in the circulation by forming a complex with factor VIII, thereby stabilizing it. Either a quantitative or qualitative defect occurs in patients with vWD. The disease is classified by type, based on structural differences in the vWF molecule.

Approximately 80 percent of patients have type 1 disease characterized by vWF that is structurally and functionally normal, but present in low levels. Patients with type 2 disease produce vWF that is structurally and functionally abnormal. The levels may be normal or decreased. There are several variants of type 2 disease, which accounts for about 20 percent of cases of vWD. Type 3 disease is rare, and the most severe form of vWD. It is essential to know the type of disease an individual has because treatment differs.

The treatment of choice for children with type 1 vWD is DDAVP.[115] In the outpatient setting, an intranasal spray formulation is used. The drug is given intravenously in the perioperative period. The recommended dose is 0.3 μg/kg every 12 to 24 hours. The antidiuretic effects of the drug can cause hyponatremia and water intoxication. Therefore, the volume of intravenous fluids administered may need to be decreased in the intra- and postoperative period and electrolytes should be monitored.

DDAVP may be somewhat effective in type 2A vWD. A test dose is administered when the patient is in a nonbleeding state to see if the bleeding time is corrected. For patients with type 2A disease who do not respond to DDAVP, and those with types 2B and 3, the usual treatment is plasma-derived factor VIII concentrate.[115]

It cannot be overemphasized that the management of children with congenital coagulation disorders must be coordinated with the child's hematologist. Knowledge of the specific type of coagulopathy and the patient's previous response to therapy are essential for optimal management. The most common coagulopathies have been outlined, but there are other more rare congenital disorders of coagulation that may be encountered by the anesthesiologist.

Sickle Cell Disease

Sickle cell Hb (HbS) results from the substitution of valine for glutamic acid at the sixth position of the β-globin chain of Hb. Fully oxygenated HbS causes no problems. However, when the oxygen tension is reduced, the Hb molecules aggregate into large polymers within the RBCs, distorting them into classic sickle shapes and reducing their deformability. The sickled cells cannot pass readily through small vessels, adhere to the endothelium, and cause vaso-occlusion. The cells also are easily hemolyzed and have a markedly reduced half-life. In vitro studies indicate that intracellular polymerization of Hb begins when the oxygen saturation is less than 85 percent.[116]

Patients who are homozygous (i.e., both β-globin genes have the mutation characteristic of HbS) have sickle cell anemia (SS disease). When the abnormal HbS gene is complemented by the normal HbA gene, both HbS and HbA are produced. Electrophoresis usually reveals approximately 60 percent HbA and 40 percent HbS. Such individuals have sickle cell trait, a benign condition not ordinarily associated with morbidity.[117] Patients with sickle cell trait are asymptomatic because the concentration of HbS is not high enough to cause sickling. The RBC survival is normal and patients are not anemic. Additional alterations in the β-globin chain and reduced synthesis of one or more globin chains produce a variety of additional disorders with varying clinical manifestations.

Children with sickle cell anemia (SS disease) usually have severe anemia that is diagnosed at an early age. Newborns are not, however, anemic because they have high concentrations of fetal hemoglobin (HbF), which prevents formation of HbS polymers. Anemia becomes evident by approximately 4 months of age as the HbF production diminishes. The Hb level is usually 6 to 9 g/dl in children with SS disease and the reticulocyte count 10 to 25 percent. Electrophoresis demonstrates 80 to greater than 90 percent HbS.

Sickle cell anemia is characterized by episodic exacerbations or crises. Aplastic crises are transient periods of bone marrow aplasia that often are associated with infection. Vaso-occlusive crises occur because of intravascular sickling and tissue infarction. The most common involve bone and are characterized by severe pain. Children with painful crises often require hospitalization and parenteral narcotics. However, a double-blind, randomized study comparing oral controlled-release morphine with intravenous morphine demonstrated comparable efficacy of the two preparations, suggesting that outpatient treatment may more often be feasible.[119] Patient-controlled analgesia is often utilized, even in relatively young children.

Episodes of acute chest pain (acute chest syndrome) may be difficult to differentiate from pulmonary infection because infiltrates, fever, hypoxia, cough, and leukocytosis are features of both. It is usually assumed that the acute chest syndrome is caused by vaso-occlusion in the pulmonary vascular bed, but infection may be superimposed.[120] Acute abdominal pain, believed to be caused by sickling in the mesenteric vessels, may be indistinguishable from an acute surgical abdomen. Acute splenic sequestration crisis, characterized by rapidly progressive, massive enlargement of the spleen, a falling Hct, and thrombocytopenia, may be a life-threatening emergency. Treatment includes prompt restoration of intravascular volume and RBC administration.

Stroke occurs in about 11 percent of patients with sickle cell anemia. The incidence of the first stroke is highest between the ages of 2 and 5 years. A recent randomized study of 130 children (mean age, 8.3 ± 3.3 years) considered by transcranial Doppler studies to be at high risk for stroke evaluated the benefits of transfusion in preventing a first stroke.[121] Transfusion to reduce the HbS concentrations to less than 30 percent significantly reduced the incidence of stroke. There were 10 cerebral infarctions and 1 intracerebral hematoma in the standard-care group, compared with 1 infarction in the transfusion group, a 92 percent difference in the risk of stroke. Although the results were dramatic, serious unresolved questions remain. First, is it reasonable to subject children, the overwhelming majority of whom will not have a stroke, to monthly transfusions for several years? Second, how long should such treatment be continued?

The life expectancy of patients with sickle cell anemia has improved considerably in the last 40 years. Death prior to age 5 used to be relatively common. The primary cause was infection, predominantly sepsis caused by *Streptococcus pneumoniae*. Such deaths have virtually been eliminated by placing all children on prophylactic penicillin.[120]

Many children with sickle cell anemia will require surgical procedures. The most frequent procedures related to SS disease are cholecystectomy and splenectomy.[122] The most controversial aspect of perioperative management is the transfusion regimen. Until relatively recently, it was common practice to transfuse patients preoperatively to lower HbS levels to less than 30 to 50 percent and raise the Hct to approximately 36 percent. This was accomplished by exchange transfusion or "simple" transfusion. With the "simple" method, RBCs (10 ml/kg) were transfused every 3 to 4 days, beginning 10 to 14 days prior to surgery.

The results of a large multicenter study comparing the rates of perioperative complications among patients randomly assigned to receive either an aggressive transfusion regimen designed to decrease the HbS level to less than 30 percent or a conservative regimen designed to increase the Hb level to 10 g/dl form the basis of current transfusion recommendations.[123] A total of 551 patients underwent 604 operations. Most of the patients were adults, but children were included in the study. Cholecystectomy was the most frequent procedure, followed by head and neck surgery and orthopedic procedures. With the exception of transfusion-related complications, which occurred in 14 percent of the aggressive group and 7 percent of the conservative group, the frequency of serious complications was similar in the two groups (31 percent and 35 percent, respectively). The acute chest syndrome developed in 10 percent of patients and painful crises prolonged hospitalization in 5 percent. Seventy-seven percent of the patients in the conservative group received a single preoperative transfusion. In contrast, 57 percent of the aggressively treated patients underwent exchange transfusions and 30 percent were repeatedly transfused. Children in the aggressive group received an average of 3.8 units, whereas those in the conservative group received an average of 1.5 units. It was concluded that a conservative transfusion regimen is as effective as an aggressive regimen in preventing perioperative complications, and the conservative approach reduced the risk of transfusion-associated complications by 50 percent.

The same group of investigators also compared the results of patients in the study who had cholecystectomies ($n = 230$) with patients not in the study ($n = 134$) who had the same operative procedure.[124] Open cholecystectomies were performed in 58 percent and laparoscopic procedures in 42 percent. Laparoscopic procedures took longer, but patients were discharged more quickly. Perioperative outcomes were similar with both approaches. Patients who were not transfused had the highest incidence of vaso-occlusive pain episodes and acute chest syndrome.

A conservative regimen of RBC transfusion to a preoperative Hb of approximately 10 g/dl without reducing the percentage HbS to a specific percentage appears to be the currently accepted approach, at least for major surgical procedures. The necessity for preoperative transfusion of children having minor procedures has been questioned.[125] The concept that there may be minor surgery, but no minor anesthetics, might well apply.

Appropriate preoperative evaluation and preparation, administration of a flawless anesthetic, and continued observation and oxygen administration in the postoperative period are essential. Dehydration, hypoxemia, acidosis, and decreased tissue perfusion promote RBC sickling and must be prevented. Children should be allowed to ingest clear fluids until a few hours before surgery. Intravenous hydration also should be considered. Ideally, surgery should be scheduled in the early morning to avoid delays and prolonged periods without oral intake. Preoperative medication can be omitted or administered in the preoperative holding area so the child can be continuously observed to ensure that oversedation and hypoventilation do not occur.

Preoxygenation and administration of an inspired oxygen concentration adequate to prevent hypoxemia are mandatory. Hypothermia should be prevented by raising the ambient temperature, warming fluids and inspired gases, and using warming blankets or other devices to maintain body temperature. Standard monitoring should be employed and consideration given to monitoring arterial blood gases during major procedures, particularly intra-abdominal and intrathoracic surgery.

Regional anesthesia is not contraindicated. Although a previous report suggested a higher rate of complications in patients receiving regional anesthesia,[122] the complication rate may have been related to the types of surgical procedures for which regional anesthesia was employed. If the child is also sedated, the dose of medication must be carefully titrated and the patient monitored for signs of oversedation.

If the surgical procedure necessitates a bloodless field, a pneumatic tourniquet can be used. Neither acidosis nor an increase in irreversibly sickled cell count have been demonstrated when tourniquets were used in patients with SS disease.[126] Careful exsanguination of the limb prior to tourniquet inflation is recommended. Although moderate hyperventilation before tourniquet deflation has been recommended, there is no documentation that it is beneficial.

Experience with autologous transfusion in patients with sickle cell disease is limited. Preoperative donation of blood is not an option in patients with sickle cell anemia, but is acceptable for patients with sickle cell trait.[127] There is a case report of sickling of salvaged and processed blood in a patient with sickle cell trait.[128] Samples from the patient and reservoir of the cell-processing unit showed no evidence of sickling, but 50 percent of the processed RBCs were sickled. In contrast, favorable experiences have been reported for both children and adults with sickle cell trait undergoing CPB.[116] On the basis of this experience, it seems unreasonable to avoid use of blood recovery devices in patients with sickle cell trait. Blood recovery also can be used in patients with SS disease who are transfused preoperatively and have low concentrations of HbS.[129] It has been suggested that smears of processed blood be examined to assess sickling before reinfusion, but the practicality of that approach is questionable.

Children with sickle cell trait require little or no modification of anesthetic technique, since their RBCs do not ordinarily sickle until the oxygen saturation is less than 40 percent. However, the same meticulous attention to detail as provided for patients with sickle cell anemia is advisable. Indeed, the anesthetic management of children with sickle cell anemia can serve as a model for all anesthetics.

Most serious complications (vaso-occlusive crises and the acute chest syndrome) in patients with sickle cell anemia occur in the postoperative period. Pulse oximetry and supplemental oxygen administration should be continued postoperatively. Adequate oral and/or intravenous hydration is important. Postoperative pain management, including patient-controlled analgesia and, where appropriate, epidural analgesia, can be provided by the anesthesiologist. Anesthesiologists also can play an important role in pain management for children with painful vaso-occlusive crises unrelated to surgery.[130]

FUTURE TRANSFUSION PRACTICES

Concerns regarding transfusion-transmitted disease will undoubtedly continue to influence transfusion practices. Screening of blood donors and testing of donated blood have led to the safest blood supply in history, and additional testing procedures are currently being implemented. Research on blood substitutes and viral inactivation methods continues. The role of pharmacologic agents to increase production of blood cells and decrease surgical blood loss and autologous transfusion techniques continue to evolve.

Blood transfusion remains a lifesaving treatment for the foreseeable future. It should be employed wisely, properly documented, and the effects monitored with appropriate laboratory tests and clinical evaluations. Transfusion guidelines should, whenever possible, be based on controlled studies such as those conducted by the Perioperative Transfusion in Sickle Cell Disease Study Group. Unrealistic fears about the risks of transfusion-transmitted disease must not lead to withholding of indicated blood transfusions.

REFERENCES

 1. Wallace EL, Churchill WH, Surgenor DM, et al: Collection and transfusion of blood components in the United States, 1994. Transfusion 38:625, 1998.
 2. Curran JW, Lawrence DL, Jaffe H, et al: Acquired immunodeficiency syndrome (AIDS) associated with transfusions. N Engl J Med 310:69, 1984.
 3. Centers for Disease Control and Prevention: HIV/AIDS Surveillance Report 10:1, 1998.
 4. Goodnough LT, Brecher ME, Kanter MH, et al: Blood transfusion. N Engl J Med 340:438, 1999.
 5. Donahue JG, Munoz A, Ness PM, et al: The declining risk of post-transfusion hepatitis C virus infection. N Engl J Med 327:369, 1992.
 6. Centers for Disease Control and Prevention: Recommendations for prevention and control of hepatitis C virus (HCV) infection and HCV-related chronic disease. MMWR Morb Mortal Wkly Rep 47(No. RR-19):1, 1998.
 7. Schreiber GB, Busch MP, Kleinman SH, et al: The risk of transfusion-transmitted viral infections. N Engl J Med 334:1685, 1996.
 8. Alter MJ, Gallagher M, Morris TT, et al: Acute non-A-E hepatitis in the United States and the role of hepatitis G virus infection. N Engl J Med 336:741, 1997.
 9. Naoumov NV, Petrova EP, Thomas MG, et al: Presence of a newly described human DNA virus (TTV) in patients with liver disease. Lancet 352:195, 1998.
10. Alter HJ, Nakatsuji Y, Melpolder J, et al: The incidence of transfusion-associated hepatitis G virus infection and its relation to liver disease. N Engl J Med 336:747, 1997.
11. Centers for Disease Control and Prevention and the U.S.P.H.S. Working Group: Guidelines for counseling persons infected with human T-lymphotropic virus type I (HTLV-I) and type II (HTLV-II). Ann Intern Med 118:448, 1993.
12. Sayers MH: Transfusion-transmitted viral infections other than hepatitis and human immunodeficiency virus infection. Cytomegalovirus, Epstein-Barr virus, human herpesvirus 6, and human parvovirus B19. Arch Pathol Lab Med 118:346, 1994.
13. Herrera GA, Lackritz EM, Janssen RS, et al: Serologic test for syphilis as a surrogate marker for human immunodeficiency virus infection among United States blood donors. Transfusion 37:836, 1997.
14. Dobroszycki J, Herwaldt BL, Boctor F, et al: A cluster of transfusion-associated babesiosis cases traced to a single asymptomatic donor. JAMA 281:927, 1999.
15. Murphy MF: New variant Creutzfeldt-Jakob disease (nvCJD): the risk of transmission by blood transfusion and the potential benefit of leukocyte-reduction of blood components. Transfus Med Rev 13:75, 1999.
16. Linden JV, Kaplan HS: Transfusion errors: causes and effects. Transfus Med Rev 8:169, 1994.
17. Vamvakas EC: Transfusion-associated cancer recurrence and postoperative infection: meta-analysis of randomized, controlled clinical trials. Transfusion 36:175, 1996.
18. Landers DF, Hill GE, Wong KC, et al: Blood transfusion-induced immunomodulation. Anesth Analg 82:187, 1996.
19. Triulzi DJ, Vanek K, Ryan DH, et al: A clinical and immunologic study of blood transfusion and postoperative bacterial infection in spinal surgery. Transfusion 32:517, 1992.
20. Patten E, Robbins M, Vincent J, et al: Use of red blood cells older than five days for neonatal transfusion. Am J Perinatol 11:37, 1991.
21. Lee DA, Slagle TA, Jackson TM, et al: Reducing blood donor exposures in low birth weight infants by the use of older, unwashed packed red blood cells. J Pediatr 126:280, 1995.
22. Strauss RG, Sacher RA, Blazina JF, et al: Commentary on small-volume red cell transfusions for neonatal patients. Transfusion 30:565, 1990.
23. British Committee for Standards in Haematology Blood Transfusion Task Force: Guidelines for administration of blood products: transfusion of infants and neonates. Transfus Med 4:63, 1994.
24. Hume H, Bard H: Small volume red blood cell transfusions for neonatal patients. Transfus Med Rev 9:187, 1995.
25. Luban NLC: Massive transfusion in the neonate. Transfus Med Rev 9:200, 1995.
26. Brecher ME, Taswell HF, Clare DE, et al: Minimal exposure transfusion and the committed donor. Transfusion 30:599, 1990.
27. Strauss RG, Wieland MR, Randels MJ, et al: Feasibility and success of a single-donor red cell program for pediatric elective surgery patients. Transfusion 32:747, 1992.
28. Chambers LA: Evaluation of a filter-syringe set for preparation of packed cell aliquots for neonatal transfusion. Am J Clin Pathol 104:253, 1994.
29. Ciavarella D, Snyder E: Clinical use of blood transfusion devices. Transfus Med Rev 2:95, 1988.
30. Przepiorka D, LeParc GF, Werch J, et al: Prevention of transfusion-associated cytomegalovirus infection. Practice Parameter. Am J Clin Pathol 106:463, 1996.
31. Sirchia G, Rebullla P: Evidence-based medicine: the case for white cell reduction. Transfusion 37:543, 1997.
32. Przepiorka D, LeParc GF, Stovall MA, et al: Use of irradiated blood components. Practice parameter. Am J Clin Pathol 106:6, 1996.
33. Manno CS, Hedberg KW, Kim HC, et al: Comparison of the hemostatic effects of fresh whole blood, stored whole blood, and components after open heart surgery in children. Blood 77:930, 1991.
34. Simon TS, Alverson DC, AuBuchon J, et al: Practice parameter for the use of red blood cell transfusions. Developed by the Red Blood Cell Administration Practice Guideline Development Task Force of the College of American Pathologists. Arch Pathol Lab Med 122:130, 1998.
35. Keyes WG, Donohue PK, Spivak JL, et al: Assessing the need for transfusion of premature infants and role of hematocrit, clinical signs, and erythropoietin level. Pediatrics 84:412, 1989.
36. American Society of Anesthesiologists Task Force on Blood Component Therapy: Practice guidelines for blood component therapy. Anesthesiology 84:732, 1996.
37. Expert Working Group: Guidelines for red blood cell and plasma transfusion for adults and children. Can Med Assoc J 156(Suppl): S1, 1997.
38. Shannon KM, Keith JF, Mentzer WC, et al: Recombinant human erythropoietin stimulates erythropoiesis and reduces erythrocyte transfusions in very low birth weight preterm infants. Pediatrics 95:1, 1995.
39. Bednarek FJ, Weisberger S, Richardson DK, et al. Variations in blood transfusions among newborn intensive care units. J Pediatr 133:601, 1998.
40. Alagappan A, Shattuck KE, Malloy MH: Impact of transfusion guidelines on neonatal transfusions. J Perinatol 18:92, 1998.

41. Blank JP, Sheagren TG, Vajaria J, et al: The role of RBC transfusion in the premature infant. Am J Dis Child 138:831, 1984.
42. Lachance C, Chessex P, Fouron J-C, et al: Myocardial, erythropoietic, and metabolic adaptations to anemia of prematurity. J Pediatr 125:278, 1994.
43. Bard H, Fouron J-C, Chessex P, et al: Myocardial, erythropoietic, and metabolic adaptations to anemia of prematurity in infants with bronchopulmonary dysplasia. J Pediatr 132:630, 1998.
44. Mink RB, Pollack MM: Effect of blood transfusion on oxygen consumption in pediatric septic shock. Crit Care Med 18:1087, 1990.
45. Hebert PC, Wells G, Blajchman MA, et al: A multicenter, randomized, controlled clinical trial of transfusion requirements in critical care. N Engl J Med 340:409, 1999.
46. Maier RF, Obladen M, Scigalla P, et al: The effect of epoetin beta (recombinant human erythropoietin) on the need for transfusion in very-low-birth-weight infants. N Engl J Med 330:1173, 1994.
47. Stehling L, Zauder HL: How low can we go? Is there a way to know. Transfusion 30:1, 1990.
48. Stehling L, Zauder HL: Acute normovolemic hemodilution. Transfusion 31:857, 1991.
49. Martin E, Ott E: Extreme hemodilution in the Harrington procedure. Bibl Haematol 47:322, 1981.
50. Fontana JL, Welborn L, Mongan PD, et al: Oxygen consumption and cardiovascular function in children during profound intraoperative normovolemic hemodilution. Anesth Analg 80:219, 1994.
51. Jonsson K, Jensen JA, Goodson WH, et al: Tissue oxygenation, anemia, and perfusion in relation to wound healing in surgical patients. Ann Surg 214:605, 1991.
52. Johnson RG, Thurer RL, Kruskall MS, et al: Comparison of two transfusion strategies after elective operations for myocardial revascularization. J Thorac Cardiovasc Surg 104:307, 1992.
53. Kim DM, Brecher ME, Estes TJ, et al: Relationship of hemoglobin level and duration of hospitalization after total hip arthroplasty: implications for the transfusion target. Mayo Clin Proc 68:37, 1993.
54. American College of Physicians: Practice strategies for elective red blood cell transfusion. Ann Intern Med 116:403, 1992.
55. Kern FH, Morana NJ, Sears JJ, et al: Coagulation defects in neonates during cardiopulmonary bypass. Ann Thorac Surg 54:541, 1992.
56. Ichinose F, Uezono S, Muto R, et al: Platelet hyporeactivity in young infants during cardiopulmonary bypass. Anesth Analg 88:258, 1999.
57. Williams GD, Bratton SL, Riley EC, et al: Association between age and blood loss in children undergoing open heart operations. Ann Thorac Surg 66:870, 1998.
58. Palermo LM, Andrews RW, Ellison N: Avoidance of heparin contamination in coagulation studies drawn from indwelling lines. Anesth Analg 59:222, 1980.
59. Despotis GJ, Santoro SA, Spitznagel E, et al: Prospective evaluation and clinical utility of on-site monitoring of coagulation in patients undergoing cardiac operations. J Thorac Cardiovasc Surg 107:271, 1994.
60. Shore-Lesserson L, Manspeizer HE, DePerio M, et al: Thromboelastography-guided transfusion algorithm reduces transfusions in complex cardiac surgery. Anesth Analg 88:312, 1999.
61. Despotis GJ, Levine V, Filos KS, et al: Evaluation of a new point-of-care test that measures PAF-mediated acceleration of coagulation in cardiac surgical patients. Anesthesiology 85:1311, 1996.
62. Ereth MH, Nuttall GA, Santrach PJ, et al: The relation between the platelet-activated clotting test (HemoSTATUS) and blood loss after cardiopulmonary bypass. Anesthesiology 88:962, 1998.
63. Ereth MH, Nuttall GA, Klindworth JT, et al: Does the platelet-activated clotting test (HemoSTATUS®) predict blood loss and platelet dysfunction associated with cardiopulmonary bypass? Anesth Analg 85:259, 1997.
64. Miller BE, Bailey JM, Mancuso TJ, et al: Functional maturity of the coagulation system in children: an evaluation using thromboelastography. Anesth Analg 84:745, 1997.
65. Hertendorf LR, Stehling L, Kurec AS, et al: Comparison of bleeding times performed on the arm and the leg. Am J Clin Pathol 87:393, 1987.
66. Lind SE: The bleeding times does not predict surgical bleeding. Blood 77:2547, 1991.
67. Rodgers RPC, Levin J: A critical reappraisal of the bleeding time. Semin Thromb Hemost 16:1, 1990.
68. Peterson P, Hayes TE, Arkin CF, et al: The preoperative bleeding time test lacks clinical benefit. College of American Pathologists'

and American Society of Clinical Pathologists' position article. Arch Surg 133:134, 1998.
69. Murray D, Pennell B, Olson J: Variability of prothrombin time and activated partial thromboplastin time in the diagnosis of increased surgical bleeding. Transfusion 39:56, 1999.
70. Andrew M, Vegh P, Caco C, et al: A randomized, controlled trial of platelet transfusions in thrombocytopenic premature infants. J Pediatr 123:285, 1993.
71. Beutler E: Platelet transfusions: the 20,000/μL trigger. Blood 81:1411, 1993.
72. Wandt H, Frank M, Ehninger G, et al: Safety and cost effectiveness of a 10×10^9/L trigger for prophylactic platelet transfusions compared with the traditional 20×10^9/L trigger: a prospective comparative trial in 105 patients with acute myeloid leukemia. Blood 91:3601, 1998.
73. Rebulla P, Finazzi G, Marangoni F, et al: The threshold for prophylactic platelet transfusions in adults with acute myeloid leukemia. N Engl J Med 337:1870, 1997.
74. Slichter SJ: Algorithm for managing the platelet refractory patient. J Clin Apheresis 12:9, 1997.
75. Cote CJ, Liu LMP, Szyfelbein SK, et al: Changes in serial platelet counts following massive blood transfusion in pediatric patients. Anesthesiology 62:197, 1985.
76. Simon TL, Bechara F, Akl BF, et al: Controlled trial of routine administration of platelet concentrates in cardiopulmonary bypass surgery. Ann Thorac Surg 37:359, 1984.
77. Bianco C: Choice of human plasma preparations for transfusion. Transfus Med Rev 13:84, 1999.
78. Murray DJ, Pennell BJ, Weinstein SL, et al: Packed red cells in acute blood loss: dilutional coagulopathy as a cause of surgical bleeding. Anesth Analg 80:336, 1995.
79. Northern Neonatal Nursing Initiative Trial Group: Randomised trial of prophylactic early fresh-frozen plasma or gelatin or glucose in preterm babies: outcome at 2 years. Lancet 348:229, 1996.
80. Miller BE, Mochizuki T, Levy JL, et al: Predicting and treating coagulopathies after cardiopulmonary bypass in children. Anesth Analg 85:1196, 1997.
81. Cowell HR, Swickard JW: Autotransfusion in children's orthopaedics. J Bone Joint Surg Am 54:908, 1974.
82. Silvergleid AJ: Safety and effectiveness of predeposit autologous transfusions in preteen and adolescent children. JAMA 257:3403, 1987.
83. Fukahara K, Murakami A, Ueda T, et al: Scheduled autologous blood donation at the time of cardiac catheterization in infants and children. J Thorac Cardiovasc Surg 114:504, 1997.
84. Masuda M, Kawachi Y, Inaba S, et al: Preoperative autologous blood donation in pediatric cardiac surgery. Ann Thorac Surg 60:1694, 1995.
85. Kemmotsu H, Joe K, Nakamura H, et al: Predeposited autologous blood transfusion for surgery in infants and children. J Pediatr Surg 30:659, 1995.
86. Velardi F, Di Chirico A, Di Rocco D, et al: "No allogeneic blood transfusion" protocol for the surgical correction of craniosynostoses. I. Rationale. Childs Nerv Syst 14:722, 1998.
87. Velardi F, Di Chirico A, Di Rocco D, et al: "No allogeneic blood transfusion" protocol for the surgical correction of craniosynostoses. II. Clinical application. Childs Nerv Syst 14:732, 1998.
88. Simpson MB, Georgopoulos G, Orsini E, et al: Autologous transfusions for orthopaedic procedures at a children's hospital. J Bone Joint Surg Am 74:652, 1992.
89. Centers for Disease Control and Prevention: Red blood cell transfusions contaminated with Yersinia enterocolitica—United States, 1991–1996, and initiation of a national study to detect bacteria-associated transfusion reactions. MMWR Morb Mortal Wkly Rep 46:553, 1997.
90. Cregan P, Donegan E, Gotelli G: Hemolytic transfusion reaction following transfusion of frozen and washed autologous red cells. Transfusion 31:172, 1991.
91. van Iterson M, van der Waart FJM, Erdmann W, et al: Systemic haemodynamics and oxygenation during haemodilution in children. Lancet 346:1127, 1995.
92. Haberkern M, Dangel P: Normovolaemic haemodilution and intraoperative autotransfusion in children: experience with 30 cases of spinal fusion. Eur J Pediatr Surg 1:30, 1992.

93. Schaller RT, Schaller J, Morgan A, et al: Hemodilution anesthesia: a valuable aid to major cancer surgery in children. Am J Surg 146:79, 1983.
94. Schaller RT, Schaller J, Furman EB: The advantages of hemodilution anesthesia for major liver resection in children. J Pediatr Surg 19:705, 1984.
95. McShane AJ, Power C, Jackson JF, et al: Autotransfusion: quality of blood prepared with a red cell processing device. Br J Anaesth 59:1035, 1987.
96. Ray JM, Flynn JC, Bierman AH: Erythrocyte survival following intraoperative autotransfusion in spinal surgery: an in vivo comparative study and 5-year update. Spine 11:879, 1986.
97. O'Hara PJ, Hertzer NR, Santilli PH, et al: Intraoperative autotransfusion during abdominal aortic reconstruction. Am J Surg 14:215, 1983.
98. Rouge P, Fourquet D, Depoix-Joseph JP, et al: Heparin removal in three intraoperative blood savers in cardiac surgery. Appl Cardiopulm Pathophysiol 5:5, 1993.
99. Elelman MJ, Potter P, Mahaffey KG, et al: The potential for reintroduction of tumor cells during intraoperative blood salvage: reduction of risk with use of the RC-400 leukocyte-depletion filter. Urology 47:179, 1996.
100. Hansen E, Altmeppen J, Talger K: Practicability and safety of intraoperative autotransfusion with irradiated blood. Anaesthesia 53(Suppl 2):42, 1998.
101. Flynn JC, Metzger CG, Csencsitz TA: Intraoperative autotransfusion (IAT) in spinal surgery. Spine 7:432, 1982.
102. Kruger LM, Colbert JM: Intraoperative autologous transfusion in children undergoing spinal surgery. J Pediatr Orthop 5:332, 1985.
103. Griffith LD, Billman GF, Daily PO, et al: Apparent coagulopathy caused by infusion of shed mediastinal blood and its prevention by washing of the infusate. Ann Thorac Surg 47:400, 1989.
104. Wahl GW, Feins RH, Alfieres G, et al: Reinfusion of shed blood after coronary operation causes elevation of cardiac enzyme levels. Ann Thorac Surg 53:625, 1992.
105. Flynn JC, Price CT, Zink WP: The third step of total autologous blood transfusion in scoliosis surgery. Spine 16:S328, 1991.
106. Guay J, Reinberg C, Poitras B, et al: A trial of desmopressin to reduce blood loss in patients undergoing spinal fusion for idiopathic scoliosis. Anesth Analg 75:405, 1992.
107. Theroux MC, Corddry DH, Tietz AE, et al: A study of desmopressin and blood loss during spinal fusion for neuromuscular scoliosis. A randomized, controlled, double-blinded study. Anesthesiology 87:260, 1997.
108. D'Errico CC, Shayevitz JR, Martindale SJ, et al: The efficacy and cost of aprotinin in children undergoing reoperative open heart surgery. Anesth Analg 83:1193, 1996.
109. Herynkopf F, Lucchese F, Pereira E, et al: Aprotinin in children undergoing correction of congenital heart defects. A double-blind pilot study. J Thorac Cardiovasc Surg 108:517, 1994.
110. Penkoshe PA, Entwistle LM, Marchak E, et al: Aprotinin in children undergoing repair of congenital heart defects. Ann Thorac Surg 60:S529, 1995.
111. Tweddell JS, Berger S, Frommelt PC, et al: Aprotinin improves outcome of single-ventricle palliation. Ann Thorac Surg 62:1329, 1996.
112. Slaughter TE, Greenberg CS: Antifibrinolytic drugs and perioperative hemostasis. Am J Hematol 56:32, 1997.
113. Laupacis A, Fergusson D, for the International Study of Perioperative Transfusion (ISPOT) Investigators: Drugs to minimize perioperative blood loss in cardiac surgery: meta-analyses using perioperative blood transfusion as the outcome. Anesth Analg 85:1258, 1997.
114. Bennett-Guerrero E, Sorohan JG, Gurevich ML, et al: Cost-benefit and efficacy of aprotinin compared with ε-aminocaproic acid in patients having repeated cardiac operations. A randomized, blinded clinical trial. Anesthesiology 87:1373, 1997.
115. Lusher JM: Treatment of congenital coagulopathies. In Mintz PD (ed): Transfusion Therapy: Clinical Principles and Practice. Bethesda, MD, AABB Press, 1999, p 97.
116. Esseltine DW, Baxter MRN, Bevan JC: Sickle cell states and the anaesthetist. Can J Anaesth 35:385, 1988.
117. Steinberg MH: Management of sickle cell disease. N Engl J Med 340:1021, 1999.
118. Bunn HF: Pathogenesis and treatment of sickle cell disease. N Engl J Med 337:762, 1997.
119. Jacobson SH, Kopecky EA, Joshi P, et al: Randomized trial of oral morphine for painful episodes of sickle-cell disease in children. Lancet 350:1358, 1997.
120. Rosse WF, Telen M, Ware RE: Transfusion Support for Patients with Sickle Cell Disease. Bethesda, MD, AABB Press, 1998.
121. Adams RJ, McKie VC, Hsu L, et al: Prevention of a first stroke by transfusions in children with sickle cell anemia and abnormal results of transcranial Doppler ultrasonography. N Engl J Med 339:5, 1998.
122. Koshy M, Weiner SJ, Miller ST, et al: Surgery and anesthesia in sickle cell disease. Blood 86:3676, 1995.
123. Vichinsky EP, Haberkern CM, Neumayer L, et al: A comparison of conservative and aggressive transfusion regimens in the perioperative management of sickle cell disease. N Engl J Med 333:206, 1995.
124. Haberkern CM, Neumayr LD, Orringer EP, et al: Cholecystectomy in sickle cell anemia patients: perioperative outcome of 364 cases from the National Preoperative Transfusion Study. Blood 89:1533, 1997.
125. Griffin TC, Buchanan GR: Elective surgery in children with sickle cell disease without preoperative blood transfusion. J Pediatr Surg 28:681, 1993.
126. Adu-Gyamfi Y, Sankarankutty M, Marwa S: Use of a tourniquet in patients with sickle-cell disease. Can J Anaesth 40:24, 1993.
127. Romanoff ME, Woodward DG, Bullard WG: Autologous blood transfusion in patients with sickle cell trait. Anesthesiology 68:820, 1988.
128. Brajbord D, Johnson D, Ramsay M, et al: Use of the cell saver in patients with sickle cell trait. Anesthesiology 70:878, 1989.
129. Cook A, Hanowell LH: Intraoperative autotransfusion for a patient with homozygous sickle cell disease. Anesthesiology 73:177, 1990.
130. Yaster M, Tobin JR, Billett C, et al: Epidural analgesia in the management of severe vaso-occlusive sickle cell crisis. Pediatrics 93:310, 1994.

7

Cardiopulmonary Resuscitation

DONALD H. SHAFFNER
CHARLES L. SCHLEIEN
MARK C. ROGERS

◆ ◆ ◆

In the late 1950s, children suffering cardiac arrest during anesthesia received 1.5 minutes of knee-to-chest "artificial respiration,"[1] followed by a thoracotomy for internal cardiac massage. In 1958, closed-chest compressions were successfully performed on a 2-year-old child.[2] The resuscitation of this child, along with several successful resuscitations of subsequent patients (many undergoing anesthesia), led to the reporting of closed-chest compressions.[3] The high rate of successful resuscitation after cardiac arrest in the operating room (42 percent)[4] helped establish closed-chest compression as the standard for cardiopulmonary resuscitation (CPR).

Forty-four percent of the cardiac arrests reported in 1961 occurred in the operating room.[4] Today, cardiac arrests during anesthesia occur less often, but children, especially infants, appear to be at highest risk. Cardiac arrests during anesthesia in the pediatric age group occur at a rate that is three times higher than that of adults.[5, 6] The risk is highest in children less than 1 year of age.[7, 8] The reasons for the increased risk of cardiac arrest during anesthesia with children are unknown.

The etiologies of cardiac arrest during anesthesia are similar for adults and children and include difficult airway management, inhalational agent overdose, succinylcholine-induced arrhythmia, and inappropriate volume administration.[5, 6, 8, 9] A recent report indicates that cardiovascular events during the maintenance phase of the anesthetic remain the most likely causes of cardiac arrest during anesthesia in children.[10] Unanticipated difficult airway, succinylcholine-related hyperkalemia, malignant hyperthermia, aspiration, and latex allergy were less frequently reported as causes of cardiac arrest than in the past.[10] A summary of causes and their prevention is provided in Table 7–1.

Resuscitation from cardiac arrest appears to be more successful in the operating room than outside of it (42 vs. 9 percent, respectively).[4] The most recent report of survival in children who suffer cardiac arrest during anesthesia is that 53% survive.[10] Many factors contribute to the increased resuscitation rate from arrests during anesthesia including the resuscitation skills of the anesthesiologist, the preparation by the anesthesiologist for emergencies, the reversibility of the causes of cardiac arrest in the operating room, and the increased monitoring during anesthesia to provide early recognition of problems. Progressive bradycardia precedes many arrests during anesthesia and may alert the anesthesiologist to the impending danger.[5] Whatever the success rate of resuscitation during anesthesia, the potential for disaster and the increased likelihood of arrests in children require that pediatric anesthesiologists

145

T A B L E   7 – 1
COMMON ETIOLOGIES OF CARDIAC ARREST DURING ANESTHESIA

Etiology	Prevention
Airway difficulty	Identification of anatomic problems from history and physical and appropriate preparation
	Continuous monitoring of oxygen delivery and saturation to prevent hypoxia
	Continuous monitoring of P_{ETCO_2} to detect tracheal extubation or disconnection
	Continuous monitoring of airway pressure to recognize leaks or obstructions
Inhalation agent overdose	Continuous monitoring of agent concentration to prevent inadvertent high concentrations
	Frequent monitoring of blood pressure for early recognition
Sux arrhythmias	Identification of muscular disease from history and physical—muscle pain with exercise, Gower's sign, calf muscle pseudohypertrophy, red urine with previous anesthetic
	Continuous ECG monitoring for early recognition
	Atropine premedication as needed
	Appropriate use of Sux
Inappropriate volume	Good assessment of preoperative status, intraoperative requirements, and ongoing losses
	Appropriate vascular access and available fluids

Sux, succinylcholine; ECG, electrocardiogram.

have a complete understanding of the physiology and pharmacology of CPR.

PHYSIOLOGY OF CARDIOPULMONARY RESUSCITATION

All successful resuscitations require recognition of the need for CPR, reestablishment of respiration, reestablishment of circulation, and the maintenance of both respiration and circulation until the underlying pathology can be corrected. These steps are the same for every resuscitation whether it occurs on the street or in the operating room. The earlier these steps are implemented, the better the outcome should be.

Recognition of the Need for CPR

The decision to begin CPR in a pediatric patient requires the recognition that the patient's vital signs are inadequate. An understanding of the cerebral and cardiac perfusion requirements in children is necessary to determine the adequacy of the vital parameters. Data are lacking to address these requirements for the wide range of patients in the pediatric anesthesiologist's care. Therefore, experience and specific pediatric training provide the background necessary to make decisions about these perfusion requirements. Knowledge of the appropriate values for these hemodynamic variables in children may reduce the need for resuscitation. The evidence for this statement is

the lower rate of CPR required in children who receive anesthetics from pediatric anesthesiologists, as opposed to those cared for by general anesthesiologists.[8]

CPR should be started immediately when the circulation is inadequate to deliver oxygen, metabolites, or resuscitative drugs to the heart and brain. The presence of inadequate respiration or circulation should be evident in the patient undergoing invasive monitoring in the operating room. In infants, chest auscultation and brachial or femoral artery palpation are the most reliable ways to confirm the presence of pulses or to detect heart rate abnormality without invasive monitoring.[11, 12] In children and adults, the carotid artery is most reliable to confirm pulses. The presence of either a heart rate or a blood pressure alone is not sufficient to provide adequate perfusion, as both an appropriate heart rate and blood pressure are necessary.

Reestablishment of Respiration

Exhaled air from the rescuer (16 percent oxygen) provides adequate oxygenation of the victim (Sao_2 of 90 percent or greater).[13] This finding is the basis for bystander CPR when supplemental oxygen is not available. The delivery of 100 percent oxygen via endotracheal intubation during CPR will help to maximize oxygen delivery to the vital organs. The need to optimize oxygen delivery outweighs the risk of oxygen toxicity during resuscitation, and 100 percent oxygen should be used when available.

Initially, researchers believed that closed-chest compressions alone provided adequate ventilation to the victim requiring CPR.[3] Unfortunately, soft tissue obstruction prevents adequate ventilation in humans without intubation and positive-pressure ventilation.[14] Airway adjuvants are not currently recommended in children to replace endotracheal intubation.[15] The endotracheal tube (ETT) remains the airway of choice, and appropriate placement can be verified by the presence of end-tidal CO_2 (P_{ETCO_2}).

The incidence of accidentally intubating the esophagus of a child is greater during an arrest (19 to 26 percent inadvertent esophageal intubations vs. 3 percent in nonarrest situations).[16, 17] The demonstration of P_{ETCO_2} after intubation is extremely reliable to confirm correct placement of the ETT in children with spontaneous circulation.[16] After cardiac arrest, the lower pulmonary blood flow produced during CPR causes P_{ETCO_2} to be falsely low or absent in correctly placed endotracheal tubes (14 to 15 percent of tracheal tubes had no P_{ETCO_2} in arrested children receiving CPR).[16, 17] Measurable P_{ETCO_2} is proof of endotracheal intubation. In its absence, ETT placement should be visually inspected to discriminate esophageal intubation and to avoid removal of a correctly placed ETT. The ETT also provides access to the circulation for drug administration (Table 7–2).

A comparison of different patterns of ventilation during chest compression revealed differences in oxygenation, ventilation, and hemodynamics.[18] Both oxygen administration without pressure and continuous positive airway pressure produce adequate oxygenation, but not ventilation or hemodynamic effects. Ventilation independent of compression, ventilation interposed between compressions, and ventilation synchronized with compression allow both adequate oxygenation and ventilation, but their ef-

T A B L E   7 – 2
VASCULAR ACCESS DURING CPR

Route	Characteristics
Peripheral venous access	Route of first choice because of ease in obtaining
	All drugs and fluids may be given by this route
	Need to flush each drug with 0.25 ml/kg normal saline to ensure central delivery (20 ml in adults)
Intraosseous access	Easy to obtain in children less than 6 years old
	All drugs and fluids may be given by this route
	Use flush as with peripheral venous access
Endotracheal route	Use only if no IV or IO access
	Only give lidocaine, atropine, naloxone, and epinephrine by ETT
	Deliver distal into bronchial tree and use 1 to 2 ml of saline to increase distribution (10 ml in adults)
	ETT drug administration requires 2 to 10 times IV dose
Cutdown saphenous or central line	Use if no IV or IO line
	Central access first choice if already in place

ETT, endotracheal tube; IV, intravenous; IO, intraosseous.

fects on hemodynamic pressures vary. Delivery of ventilation has hemodynamic impact because of the changes in intrathoracic pressure. Simultaneous compression and ventilation yielded improvement in blood flow and survival in dogs but remains an experimental mode of CPR. The current recommendations are that in unintubated patients ventilations should be interposed between compressions, but it is unnecessary to coordinate ventilations with compressions in intubated patients.[19]

Reestablishment of Circulation
Mechanisms of Blood Flow During CPR

Kouwenhoven et al.[3] proposed that external chest compressions squeeze the heart between the sternum and the vertebral column, forcing blood to be ejected. This assumption of direct cardiac compression during external CPR became known as the *cardiac pump mechanism* of blood flow. The cardiac pump mechanism implies that the atrioventricular valves close during ventricular compression and that ventricular volume decreases during ejection of blood. During chest relaxation, ventricular pressures fall below atrial pressures, enabling the atrioventricular valves to open and the ventricles to fill. This sequence of events resembles the normal cardiac cycle and occurs during cardiac compression when open-chest CPR is performed.

Several observations of the hemodynamics during external CPR are inconsistent with the cardiac pump mechanism for blood flow (Table 7–3). First, similar elevations in the arterial and venous intrathoracic pressures during closed-chest CPR suggest a generalized increase in intrathoracic pressure.[20] Second, reconstructing the integrity of the thorax in patients with flail sternums improves the

blood pressure during CPR (unexpected, since a flail sternum should allow direct cardiac compression during closed-chest CPR).[21] Third, patients who develop ventricular fibrillation produce enough blood flow to maintain consciousness by repetitive coughing or deep breathing.[22–25] The assumption that changes in intrathoracic pressure without direct cardiac compression (i.e., a cough) produce blood flow characterizes the *thoracic pump mechanism* of blood flow during CPR. Extensive research has addressed the involvement of the cardiac and thoracic pump mechanisms in blood flow.

Thoracic Pump Mechanism

Chest compressions during CPR generate almost equal pressures in the left ventricle, aorta, right atrium, pulmonary artery, airway, and esophagus.[21, 25–31] Since all intrathoracic vascular pressures are equal, the suprathoracic arterial pressures must be higher than the suprathoracic venous pressures for a cerebral perfusion gradient to exist. Venous valves, either functional or anatomic, prevent the direct transmission of the elevation in intrathoracic pressure to the suprathoracic veins. These jugular venous valves are present in animals[21, 26, 32–37] and humans.[30, 31, 33, 38–40] This unequal transmission of the intrathoracic pressure to the suprathoracic vasculature establishes the gradient necessary for blood flow to the brain during this mechanism of CPR.

During normal cardiac function, the low pressure on the atrial side of the atrioventricular valves allows venous return to the pump. The extrathoracic shift of this low-pressure area to the cephalic side of the jugular venous valves during the thoracic pump mechanism of blood flow implies that the heart is merely a conduit during this mechanism. Angiographic studies show blood passing from the venae cavae, through the right heart, to the pulmonary artery, and from the pulmonary veins, through the left heart, to the aorta during a single chest compression.[28, 33] Unlike the findings in normal cardiac activity and open-chest CPR, echocardiographic studies during closed-chest CPR in dogs[28, 33] and humans[41–43] show that the atrioventricular valves are open during blood ejection. In addition, unlike native cardiac activity and open-chest CPR, aortic diameter decreases instead of increasing during blood ejection.[33, 42] These findings during closed-chest CPR support the thoracic pump theory and suggest that the heart becomes a passive conduit for blood flow.

Cardiac Pump Mechanism

Despite mounting evidence for the thoracic pump mechanism of blood flow during external chest compressions, there are specific situations in which the cardiac pump mechanism predominates during closed-chest CPR. First, applying more force during chest compressions increases the likelihood of direct cardiac compression. Increasing the force of chest compressions in animals undergoing CPR increases the closure of the atrioventricular valves, implying more direct cardiac compression.[44, 45] Second, a smaller chest size seems to allow more direct cardiac compression. Adult dogs with small chests have better hemodynamics during closed-chest CPR than dogs with

T A B L E　7 – 3
COMPARISON OF MECHANISMS OF BLOOD FLOW DURING CLOSED-CHEST COMPRESSIONS

	Cardiac Pump Mechanism (Sternum and Spine Compress Heart)	Thoracic Pump Mechanism (General Increase in Intrathoracic Pressure)
Findings during compression		
AV valves	Closed	Open
Aortic diameter	Increases	Decreases
Blood movement	Left ventricle to aorta	Pulmonary veins to aorta
Ventricular volume	Decreases	Little change
Compression rate	Dependent	Little effect
Duty cycle	Little effect	Dependent
Compression force	Increases role	Decreases role
Clinical situations	Small chest	Large chest
	High compliance	Low compliance

AV, atrioventricular.

large chests.[46] Third, the very compliant infant chest should permit more direct cardiac compression. During closed-chest CPR in an infant swine model, excellent blood flows are produced compared with most adult models.[47] Unlike the adult model, the addition of simultaneous ventilation with compression (SCV) does not augment the flow produced during piglet CPR.[48] This failure of SCV CPR to augment already high flows also occurs in small dogs.[46] The lack of contribution of SCV CPR in the infant or small adult animal models implies that excellent compression (probably direct cardiac) occurs and that the additional intrathoracic pressure is of no benefit.

Recent transesophageal echocardiography studies demonstrated closing of the atrioventricular valves during the compression phase of CPR in humans.[49, 50] In addition, atrioventricular valve closure occurs even in thoracic pump animal models of CPR.[51] These findings support the occurrence of cardiac compression during CPR.

Distribution of Blood Flow During CPR

The distribution of blood flow during CPR is altered from the normal physiologic state. The total blood flow decreases during CPR and is redistributed to optimize perfusion to the heart and brain. This redistribution toward the vital organs should improve outcome. Maintenance of myocardial blood flow during CPR is necessary for the return of spontaneous circulation, and maintenance of cerebral blood flow determines the quality of the eventual outcome.

The distribution of blood flow to the brain depends on the development of three gradients. The intrathoracic–suprathoracic, intracranial–extracranial, and caudal–rostral gradients influence the distribution of blood destined for the cerebral circulation.

The first gradient, intrathoracic–suprathoracic, provides the flow of oxygenated blood from the chest to the upper extremities and head. Either venous collapse, secondary to the elevated intrathoracic pressure, or closure of anatomic valves in the jugular system prevents the transmission of intrathoracic pressure to the suprathoracic venous system.[21, 33, 34] Arterial collapse does not occur and elevated intrathoracic pressure results in a gradient that promotes suprathoracic blood flow.

The second gradient for blood flow distribution to the brain involves movement away from the extracranial suprathoracic vessels and toward the intracranial vessels. Vasoconstrictors have little effect on the intracranial vessels but do constrict the extracranial vessels, increasing intracranial blood flow. Use of the vasoconstrictor epinephrine increases intracranial blood flow while decreasing flow in the cephalic skin, muscle, and tongue.[47]

The third gradient for the distribution of blood flow occurs within the intracranial vessels. CPR alone seems to increase the distribution of flow to caudal areas of the brain, and ischemia preceding CPR significantly increases the distribution of flow to these areas.[52-54] This pattern of greater flow to the caudal areas also occurs in other models of global ischemia.[55]

Myocardial blood flow does not have the advantage of the large extrathoracic pressure gradient that augments cerebral flow. The thoracic pump generates equal increases in all intrathoracic structures. This lack of a gradient causes poor myocardial blood flow during external chest compressions. Many studies show much lower blood flows for the myocardium compared with cerebral flows during closed-chest CPR.[47, 52, 56]

The type of CPR influences the production of myocardial blood flow. Studies of methods that are more likely to cause direct cardiac compression, such as high-impulse CPR, report unusually high myocardial blood flows.[56, 57] The method of CPR applied impacts not only the amount of direct cardiac compression but also the phase of compression during which myocardial flow occurs. Myocardial blood flow may be present only during relaxation of chest compression,[57] correlating with a "diastolic" pressure,[28] or, in some instances, during compression, correlating with a "systolic" pressure.[47, 52]

Regional flows within the heart appear to change during CPR, with a shift in the ratio of subendocardial to subepicardial blood flow from the normal 1.5:1 to 0.8:1.[47] This ratio reverts to normal with epinephrine administration.

Blood flow to organs other than the heart or brain falls dramatically during CPR. The lack of valves in the infrathoracic veins causes retrograde transmission of venous pressure and decreases the gradient for blood flow below the diaphragm in animals.[58] Regional blood flows for infrathoracic organs during CPR are usually less than 20 percent of prearrest rates and often close to zero.[52,59–61] The addition of abdominal compressions does not alter the infrathoracic organ blood flow.[59,61] Administration of epinephrine during closed-chest CPR almost eliminates flow to the subdiaphragmatic organs, with the exception of the adrenal glands.[62]

Few data are available regarding pulmonary blood flow during CPR. Pulmonary blood flow occurs primarily at times of low intrathoracic pressure during closed-chest CPR.[28] High extrathoracic venous pressure builds up during compression and results in pulmonary filling during relaxation as intrathoracic pressure falls. Resuscitation methods that lower intrathoracic pressure may augment pulmonary vascular filling.

Rate and Duty Cycle

In 1986, the American Heart Association Guidelines for CPR and Emergency Cardiac Care recommended increasing the rate of chest compressions from 60 per minute to 100 per minute.[63] This change represents a compromise between advocates of the thoracic pump mechanism and those of the cardiac pump mechanism.[64] The mechanics of these two theories of blood flow differ, but a faster compression rate could augment both. It is necessary to understand the concepts of *compression rate, duty cycle,* and *compression force* to understand the mechanics of CPR.

Compression rate is the number of cycles per minute. *Duty cycle* is the ratio of the duration of the compression phase to the entire compression–relaxation cycle expressed as a percent. For example, at a rate of 60 compressions per minute (total cycle, 1 second), a 0.6-second compression time produces a 60 percent duty cycle. The impact of duty cycle differs between the two mechanisms of blood flow (Table 7–3). *Compression force* is the pressure and the acceleration applied to the chest.

If direct cardiac compression generates blood flow (cardiac pump), then the force of the compression determines the stroke volume. Prolonging the compression (increasing the duty cycle) beyond the time necessary for full ventricular ejection fails to produce any additional increase in stroke volume in this model. In contrast, increasing the rate of compressions increases cardiac output, since a fixed ventricular blood volume ejects with each cardiac compression. Therefore, in the cardiac pump mechanism, blood flow is rate sensitive but duty cycle insensitive.

If the thoracic pump produces blood flow, the reservoir of blood to be ejected is the large capacitance of the thoracic vasculature. With the thoracic pump mechanism, increasing both the force of compression and the duty cycle enhances flow. Changes in compression rate do not affect flow over a wide range of rates.[65] Blood flow in the thoracic pump mechanism is duty cycle sensitive but rate insensitive.

Mathematical models of the cardiovascular system have confirmed that both the applied force and the compression duration determine blood flow with the thoracic pump mechanism.[66,67] It appears from the experimental animal data that either the thoracic pump or the cardiac pump mechanism can effectively generate blood flow during closed-chest CPR. Discrepancies among the results of various studies can be attributed to differences in CPR models and in compression techniques. These differences may involve issues of chest compliance and geometry, maturity of different animal species, or chest-compression techniques. For example, either mechanism may come into play in an infant with a very compliant chest wall. Differences in techniques may include the magnitude of sternal displacement, compression force, compression rate, and duty cycle.

Several studies in dogs show a benefit of a fast compression rate (120 per minute) over slower rates during conventional CPR.[57,64,68] Studies in piglets,[69] puppies,[70] and humans[38,71,72] find no difference in the effectiveness of conventional CPR at various rates. A piglet CPR study found that the duty cycle was the major determinant of cerebral perfusion pressure.[68] The duty cycle at which venous return becomes limited varies with age. Increasing the duty cycle is more effective in younger piglets and more likely to limit venous return in the adult models.

The discrepancy between the importance of rate and duty cycle in various models by different investigators generates confusion. Increasing the rate of compressions during conventional CPR to 100 per minute satisfies both those who prefer the faster rates and those who support a longer duty cycle. This is true because it is physically easier for a rescuer to produce a 50 percent duty cycle at a rate of 100 than at 60 compressions per minute (holding compression is physically difficult at slow rates). This is the reason behind the rate change in the 1986 American Heart Association guidelines for CPR. This increased rate continues to be recommended.[73]

Chest Geometry

Chest geometry plays an important role in the ability of extrathoracic compressions to generate intrathoracic pressures. *Shape, compliance,* and *deformability* are significant chest characteristics during CPR. The age of the patient affects each of these characteristics, which may explain some differences in CPR between the pediatric and adult animal models.

Chest Shape

During anterior to posterior-delivered compressions, the change in cross-sectional area of the chest relates to its shape.[70] The thoracic index refers to the ratio of the anteroposterior diameter to the lateral diameter. A keel-shaped chest, as in an adult dog, has a greater anteroposterior diameter and thus a thoracic index greater than 1. A flat chest, as in a thin human, has a greater lateral diameter and thus a thoracic index of less than 1. A circular chest would have a thoracic index of 1. A circular chest also has a larger cross-sectional area than either of these elliptical chests. As an anteroposterior compression flattens a circle, it decreases the cross-sectional area and compresses the contents. In contrast, as a keel-shaped chest approaches a circular shape, the cross-sectional area increases during the application of anteroposterior compression. The cross-sectional area of the keel-shaped chest does not decrease until the compression continues past the circular shape to flatten the chest. This implies a threshold distance past which the compression must proceed before the intrathoracic contents are compressed.[74] Therefore, the rounded, flatter chests of small dogs and pigs may require less displacement than the keel-shaped chests of adult dogs to generate thoracic ejection of blood. The rounded chest of small dogs improves the efficacy of external thoracic compression compared to the keel-shaped adult dog.[46]

Chest Compliance

With increasing age, the cartilage in the chest becomes calcified and the compliance changes. The stiffer, or less compliant, older chest may require greater compression force to generate the same anteroposterior displacement. Three-month-old swine require a much greater pressure for anteroposterior displacement than their 1-month-old counterparts.[74] The compliance of the chest affects not only the amount of displacement but also the structures compressed. Direct cardiac compression is more likely to occur in the more compliant chests of younger animals. Cerebral blood flow production in a piglet model of external CPR was much greater than expected compared with the usual findings in adult animals.[47] The more compliant infant chest may allow more direct cardiac compression, accounting for the high flows that resemble those produced by open-chest cardiac massage.

Chest Deformation

Chest deformation occurs as CPR becomes prolonged. The chest assumes a flatter shape as compressions continue, producing larger decreases in cross-sectional area at the same displacement. Progressive deformation may be beneficial if it leads to more direct cardiac compression. Unfortunately, too much deformation may decrease the recoil of the chest wall during release of compression. Decreased chest recoil with progressing deformation will limit the displacement and produce less effective compression. A pediatric model of conventional CPR shows a progressive decrease over time in the effectiveness of chest compressions to produce blood flow.[47, 75] The permanent deformation of the chest in this model approaches 30 percent of the original anteroposterior diameter. Attempting to limit the deformation by increasing intrathoracic pressure from within during compression with SCV CPR was ineffective.[48] Neither the amount of deformation nor the time to deterioration of flow was different. In an attempt to limit the production of deformation, investigators used a third mode of infant animal CPR with a vest to deliver compressions. The vest distributes compression force diffusely around the thorax and greatly decreases permanent deformation (3 percent vs. 30 percent).[76] Unfortunately, the deterioration of blood flows with time still occurs and appears to be unrelated to the amount of deformation in this model.

The relevance to humans of chest geometry characteristics found in animal studies is unclear. Body weight, surface area, chest circumference, and chest diameter did not correlate with the aortic pressure produced during CPR in a study of nine adults already declared dead.[30] There has not been a direct comparison of adult and pediatric human CPR. The increased compliance and deformability of the infant chest make it likely that CPR would be more effective in children than in adults (as seen in animal models).

Maintenance of Circulation
Efficacy of Blood Flow During CPR

Blood flows produced by conventional closed-chest CPR without pharmacologic support are disappointingly low. The range of cerebral blood flow in dogs is 3 to 14 percent of prearrest levels.[61, 77–80] Cerebral perfusion pressures are also low, 4 to 24 percent of prearrest levels in animals[61, 77, 78] and only 21 mm Hg in humans.[40] Myocardial blood flows in this basic CPR mode are also discouragingly low at 1 to 15 percent of prearrest levels in dogs.[26, 59, 65, 76, 80] Myocardial perfusion pressures correlate with myocardial blood flow. Plotting myocardial blood flow in milliliters per minute per gram versus myocardial perfusion pressure in millimeters of mercury gives a slope of 0.01 to 0.015.[59, 62] These data imply a one-to-one relationship between myocardial blood flow (when measured in milliliters per minute per 100 g) and myocardial perfusion pressure (millimeters of mercury).

In addition to pharmacologic support, several other factors affect cerebral and myocardial blood flow during CPR. These factors include the victim's age, intracranial pressure, duration of CPR, and duration of preresuscitation ischemia.

Age appears to affect cerebral blood flow during closed-chest CPR. Two-week-old piglets have substantially higher cerebral blood flows (50 percent of prearrest) and slightly higher myocardial flows (17 percent of prearrest) than those reported for adult models.[47] Two studies on slightly older pigs yielded opposing results. Cerebral blood flows in these two studies were 26 to 95 percent and 1 to 4 percent of prearrest values, with corresponding myocardial values of 2 to 8 percent and 1 to 6 percent.[58, 60] The cerebral blood flow in the first of these two studies was markedly higher than in adults during closed-chest CPR, and neither of the myocardial flows was different from adult models.

Intracranial pressure can represent the downstream pressure for cerebral blood flow and, if elevated, can inhibit cerebral perfusion. Increasing intrathoracic pressure with closed-chest CPR contributes to intracranial pressure increases.[81] This relationship is linear, and one third of the increase in intrathoracic pressure is transmitted to the intracranial pressure.[35] The carotid arteries and jugular veins do not appear to be involved in the transmission of intrathoracic pressure to the intracranial contents. The transmission can be partially blocked by occluding the cerebrospinal fluid or vertebral vein flow.[35] The rise in intracranial pressure with chest compressions becomes more significant in the setting of baseline increased intracranial pressure (two thirds of the intrathoracic pressure is transmitted to the intracranial pressure). Clinicians need to be aware that the efficacy of CPR deteriorates markedly in the face of elevated intracranial pressure and that when possible the intracranial pressure should be lowered early in the resuscitation (i.e., shunt tapped, hematoma drained).

Increased duration of CPR has a negative effect on cerebral blood flow and seems to be most detrimental in the infant preparation.[47, 60] The length of the ischemic period before CPR begins also has a negative effect on cerebral blood flow.[53, 82] Forebrain blood flow during subsequent CPR is reduced more than brain stem as the preceding ischemic interval is increased.[53, 54] Hypothermia has some protective effect and prevents this reduction in the ischemic intervals tested in dogs.[54] The cause of these detrimental effects on cerebral blood flow is unclear. It remains obvious that a short ischemic period and quick resuscitation improve eventual outcome.

There appear to be thresholds for minimal vital organ blood flow during CPR. The inability to maintain blood flow above these thresholds during CPR results in organ malfunction. A myocardial blood flow of 20 ml/min/100 g or greater is necessary for successful defibrillation in dogs.[35, 83] A cerebral blood flow of greater than 15 to 20 ml/min/100 g is necessary to maintain normal electrical activity during CPR.[52]

Monitoring the Effectiveness of CPR

Monitoring the effectiveness of CPR can be difficult. An adequate myocardial perfusion pressure is necessary to allow the heart to be restarted during CPR. The above data suggest that a myocardial blood flow of 20 ml/min/ 100 g is necessary for return of spontaneous circulation. This flow would correlate with a myocardial perfusion pressure (MPP) of 20 mm Hg (aortic relaxation pressure minus right atrial relaxation pressure). Data from CPR in humans show that a MPP of 15 mm Hg was necessary for, but did not guarantee, return of spontaneous circulation.[84] Often, right atrial relaxation pressure is low and the aortic "diastolic" pressure represents the myocardial perfusion pressure. In clinical practice, detection of this "diastolic" pressure is difficult without an arterial line.

Measurement of venous oxygen saturation has been described as a method to monitor the effectiveness of CPR. In humans, the level of venous oxygen saturation correlated with the return of spontaneous circulation.[85, 86] This observation may be of use during CPR in victims with central venous access.

Another method to monitor the effectiveness of myocardial perfusion during CPR is to follow the production of P_{ETCO_2}. The amount of CO_2 exhaled relates to the amount of pulmonary blood flow. In general, P_{ETCO_2} levels decrease as pulmonary blood falls during CPR. Therefore, as blood flow to the heart and lungs improves during CPR, P_{ETCO_2} should return toward arterial levels.

A P_{ETCO_2} measured at 20 minutes of CPR of less than 10 mm Hg predicts an inability to restore spontaneous circulation.[87–89] Alternatively, a P_{ETCO_2} greater than 15 mm Hg during CPR predicts resuscitation.[17, 90, 91] These studies imply that P_{ETCO_2} monitoring is useful in determining the effectiveness of CPR and that the production of P_{ETCO_2} of less than 10 to 15 mm Hg suggests a need to modify CPR to improve blood flow. P_{ETCO_2} may also detect cardiac output during electromechanical dissociation,[91] the return of spontaneous circulation during CPR,[92] and the presence

of spontaneous circulation during cardiopulmonary bypass.[93]

The measurement of P_{ETCO_2} in patients receiving CPR without tracheal intubation appears useful to determine the effectiveness of cardiac compressions at producing blood flow.[94] In patients receiving CPR with a face mask or a laryngeal mask airway, the level of P_{ETCO_2} correlated with the rate of return of spontaneous circulation. The correlation was not as close as reports from studies of intubated patients. More patients with a low P_{ETCO_2} had return of spontaneous circulation and fewer with higher P_{ETCO_2} had return of spontaneous circulation than in studies with intubated patients.

There are pitfalls in the monitoring of P_{ETCO_2} during CPR. Administration of bicarbonate increases CO_2 production and may elevate P_{ETCO_2} without a corresponding increase in pulmonary blood flow. Administration of epinephrine may decrease P_{ETCO_2} despite an increase in the myocardial perfusion, causing a misinterpretation that CPR has become less effective.[95] Contamination of disposable P_{ETCO_2} detectors by resuscitation medications (epinephrine, atropine, or lidocaine) or gastric acid may decrease their accuracy in the assessment of CPR effectiveness or the detection of esophageal intubation.[96]

METHODS OF CARDIOPULMONARY RESUSCITATION

Conventional CPR: Manual Versus Mechanical

Conventional CPR consists of closed-chest compressions delivered manually with ventilations interposed after every fifth compression (Table 7–4). This system of CPR can be delivered in any setting without additional equipment and with a minimum of training. Present investigations fail to consistently demonstrate the superiority of any alternative mode of CPR over conventional CPR in humans in a large randomized study.

Conventional CPR is usually performed with sternal compressions applied to a supine patient. There is a report of two patients who required CPR while undergoing anesthesia in the prone position and who were successfully resuscitated.[97] The closed-chest compressions were delivered with one hand under the sternum and compression delivered to the back. These patients were undergoing posterior cranial and cervical spine surgery and could not be repositioned quickly. When possible, patients should be turned supine for CPR.

Fatigue is a major problem with manual CPR in the field. Individual variation among rescuers performing manual CPR can be a problem in the field and in the lab. To overcome fatigue and to standardize compression delivery, mechanical devices are available to deliver chest compressions. The most common of these is a pneumatic, piston-driven compression device. Piston and manual CPR appear to be comparable in animals[98] and humans.[99] A mechanical device that actively expands the chest during the relaxation phase of CPR exists. The rescuer applies compression force to the device as with manual CPR, but the chest is reexpanded actively by suction as the rescuer

T A B L E   7 – 4
BASIC LIFE SUPPORT PROCEDURES

	Newlyborn (<12 hr)	Infant (<1 yr)	Child (1–8 yr)	Adult (>8 yr)
Breathing	30 breaths/min	20 breaths/min	20 breaths/min	12 breaths/min
Pulse check	Umbilical cord	Brachial/femoral	Carotid	Carotid
Compress area	Below nipples	Lower half of sternum	Lower half of sternum	Lower half of sternum
Compress with	2 fingers/encircle	2 fingers/encircle	Heel of hand	Two hands
Depth	0.5–0.75 inch*	0.5–1 inch*	1–1.5 inches*	1.5–2 inches*
Rate	90/min	100/min	100/min	100/min
Ratio	3:1	5:1	5:1	15:2

Data from American Heart Association: Circulation 102:I-253, 2000.
* 1/3 to 1/2 of anteroposterior diameter.

pulls on the device during relaxation. Mechanical devices are presently limited to adult CPR and are not recommended for pediatric patients.[100]

The overall low efficacy of conventional CPR has led to investigations of multiple CPR modalities. These methods usually reflect attempts to enhance the contribution of the thoracic pump or cardiac pump to blood flow during CPR (Table 7–5). For example, the use of both hands to encircle the chest of an infant while the thumbs apply sternal compressions attempts to both raise intrathoracic pressure and compress the heart.[101, 102]

Simultaneous Compression–Ventilation CPR

Simultaneous compression–ventilation CPR (SCV CPR) represents an attempt to augment conventional CPR by increasing the contribution of the thoracic pump mechanism to blood flow. Delivering ventilation simultaneously with every compression (instead of interposed after every fifth compression) adds to the intrathoracic pressure and should augment blood flow produced by conventional closed-chest CPR.

Several studies suggest that SCV CPR increases the carotid blood flow compared with conventional CPR.[26, 32, 46, 78, 103] Subsequent studies confirm the physiologic advantages of SCV CPR in canine models.[61, 104] In contrast, SCV CPR offers no advantage over conventional CPR in infant pigs[48] and small dogs.[46, 105, 106] In these small animals, the compliance and geometry of the chest may allow more

direct cardiac compression and thus achieve higher intravascular pressure than with conventional CPR.[47, 69, 74] Animal studies also show the detrimental impact of excessive airway pressure during SCV CPR and the resulting arterial collapse.[32] Human studies comparing SCV with conventional CPR show that coronary perfusion pressure increases minimally (3.6 mm Hg increased to 6.6 mm Hg)[103] or decreases (11 mm Hg to 6 mm Hg).[107] Survival is worse in both animals[106] and humans[108] when SCV CPR is compared with conventional CPR. No study has shown an increased survival with this CPR technique.

Abdominal Binding

Researchers have used abdominal binders and military antishock trousers (MAST) to augment closed-chest CPR. Both methods apply continuous compression circumferentially below the diaphragm. There are three proposed mechanisms for the augmentation of CPR by these binders. First, binding the abdomen decreases the compliance of the diaphragm and raises intrathoracic pressure. Second, squeezing blood out of the subthoracic structures increases the circulating blood volume (autotransfusion effect). Third, applying pressure to the subdiaphragmatic vasculature and increasing resistance should increase suprathoracic blood flow. The increases in intrathoracic pressure and blood volume lead to increased aortic pressure and carotid blood flow in both animals[61, 109, 110] and humans.[111, 112] Unfortunately, as the aortic pressure increases, the right atrial "diastolic" pressure increases to a greater extent (the downstream component of the coronary perfusion pressure), resulting in a decrease in the coronary perfusion pressure.[106, 109] This deterioration of coronary perfusion pressure is coincidental with a decreased myocardial blood flow.[109] This technique also adversely influences the cerebral perfusion pressure. Transmission of the intrathoracic pressure to the intracranial vault raises the intracranial pressure (the downstream component of the cerebral perfusion pressure), with a resulting decrease in the cerebral perfusion pressure.[35] This fall in cerebral perfusion pressure with the increase in ICP may not be detected in studies using jugular venous pressure as the downstream pressure. The use of abdominal binders or MAST suits to augment CPR does not increase survival in clinical studies.[106, 113, 114] Liver laceration from abdominal binder CPR has been reported[103] but is no more frequent than with conventional CPR.[21, 109, 113, 115]

T A B L E   7 – 5
CONTRIBUTION OF CARDIAC OR THORACIC PUMP TO VARIOUS METHODS OF CPR

	Cardiac Pump	Thoracic Pump
Open chest	++	0
High impulse	++	+
Conventional	0/+	+
Abdominal binding	0/+	++
IAC CPR*	0/+	++
SCV CPR	0/+	++
Vest CPR	0	++
Cough CPR	0	++

* Also moves blood by abdominal compression alone.
SCV, simultaneous compression ventilation; IAC, interposed abdominal compression.

Abdominal Compression

Interposed abdominal compression CPR (IAC CPR) consists of delivery of an abdominal compression during the relaxation phase of chest compression. IAC CPR may augment conventional CPR in several ways. First, IAC CPR may push venous blood back into the chest during the abdominal compression/chest relaxation phase and "prime the pump"[59, 116] (resembling the atrial contribution to ventricular filling). Second, IAC CPR causes increased intrathoracic pressure and adds to the duty cycle of the compression delivered to the chest.[117] Third, IAC CPR may compress the aorta and send blood retrograde to the carotids or coronaries[116] (similar to cross-clamping applied to the aorta to improve supradiaphragmatic flow).

Several studies have shown hemodynamic improvements secondary to IAC CPR. In animal experiments, cardiac output and cerebral and coronary blood flow improved when IAC CPR was compared with conventional CPR in adult models[59, 116–118] but not in an infant swine model.[119] Human studies have also shown an increase in aortic pressure and coronary perfusion pressure during IAC CPR compared with conventional CPR.[38, 120–124] Although one study reports a 10 percent aspiration rate,[118] most report no aspiration or liver lacerations.[59, 117, 120, 123–126] Clinically, IAC CPR requires extra manpower or equipment and remains experimental. Outcome studies have mixed results, showing no increase in survival with prehospital arrests but increased survival with in-hospital arrests.[125, 126]

Vest CPR

Vest CPR uses an inflatable bladder that is wrapped circumferentially around the chest (resembling a blood pressure cuff) and cyclically inflated. This method of delivering chest compressions by diffuse application of pressure has two unique characteristics. First, chest dimensions change minimally and direct cardiac compression is unlikely (an almost pure thoracic pump technique). Second, the diffuse distribution of pressure decreases the likelihood of trauma.

Vest CPR in dogs improves the hemodynamic data, as shown by better cerebral and myocardial blood flows, more than conventional CPR.[65, 104, 127] Survival was also significantly improved in dogs with vest or vest and binder CPR compared with conventional closed-chest CPR.[36, 127] In a pediatric model of vest CPR, only a 3 percent permanent chest deformation occurred after 50 minutes of vest CPR[76] compared with almost 30 percent deformation produced by an equivalent period of conventional CPR.[47] In humans, vest CPR increases aortic systolic pressure but does not significantly increase diastolic pressure compared with conventional CPR.[30] In a preliminary study of vest CPR in victims of out-of-hospital arrest, an increased aortic and coronary perfusion pressure were demonstrated, and there was a trend toward a greater return of spontaneous circulation compared with standard CPR.[128] A large clinical trial is underway to determine if these benefits improve outcome.

The lack of metallic parts has allowed vest CPR to be used experimentally during nuclear magnetic resonance spectroscopy to study brain intracellular pH.[129] In addition, the vest has been used as an external cardiac assist device in nonarrested dogs with heart failure.[130, 131] Clinically, the use of vest CPR depends on sophisticated equipment, and the technique remains experimental at this time.

High-Impulse CPR

High-impulse CPR involves the application of greater than usual force during chest compression. This increase in force can be in the form of greater mass, greater velocity, or both. It is hypothesized that the larger impulses result in greater chest deflection, causing more contact with the heart.[132] Direct cardiac compression is more likely with this form of closed-chest CPR, which would cause the technique to be more rate dependent and less duty cycle dependent, as predicted by the cardiac pump mechanism of blood flow. This rate dependence found in high-impulse CPR supports the cardiac pump hypothesis.[57, 133]

Hemodynamic improvement occurs when this CPR technique augments conventional closed-chest CPR. Dog studies demonstrate significant improvements in myocardial and cerebral blood flow with high-impulse compared with low-impulse CPR.[56] High-impulse CPR can generate myocardial blood flows as high as 60 to 75 percent of prearrest values.[57] In humans, high-impulse CPR generates increased aortic pressures.[30] An outcome study in dogs compared high-impulse CPR with conventional closed-chest CPR and found no significant improvement in resuscitation, survival, or neurologic outcome.[133]

Active Compression–Decompression CPR

Active compression–decompression (ACD) CPR requires a device that attaches to the chest and allows the rescuer to pull up on the sternum and decompress the thorax between compressions. The theoretical advantages of decompressing the chest between compressions include restoring chest wall shape, actively pulling gas into the lungs, and actively pulling blood into the intrathoracic vessels. These characteristics allow for more effect from the compression, as more intrathoracic pressure can be generated and more blood ejected with the compression.

Preliminary studies in humans showed that after advanced cardiac life support failed, ACD CPR was more effective than standard CPR at improving hemodynamic variables.[134] Following a witnessed in-hospital arrest, more patients had return of spontaneous circulation, survival at 24 hours, and had a better Glasgow Coma scale score when they received ACD CPR than when standard CPR was given.[135] A larger study of in-hospital cardiac arrest victims failed to show any difference in the resuscitation or outcomes between patients receiving ACD or standard CPR.[136] Several large studies of patients who suffered an out-of-hospital cardiac arrest did not find a difference in the effectiveness of ACD or standard CPR for improving the incidence of return of spontaneous circulation, hospital admission, hospital discharge, or short-term neurologic outcome.[136–140]

Complication rates following CPR were not different following ACD CPR or standard CPR in most studies.[137–139] It is interesting that the same study that showed that ACD had more complications than standard CPR (hemoptysis and sternal dislodgment) was also one of the few large studies that found ACD CPR more effective than standard CPR for out-of-hospital arrests.[141]

Phased Chest Abdominal Compression–Decompression CPR

A new manual method of phased chest and abdominal compression–decompression (PCACD) cardiopulmonary resuscitation has been described.[142] PCACD CPR resembles a combination of active compression–decompression CPR and interposed abdominal compression CPR. It offers the theoretical advantages of both methods because chest shape is restored and blood and gas are pulled into the thorax during active decompression of the chest and blood flow augmented because of the compression, and active decompression, of the abdomen. Coronary perfusion pressure, return of spontaneous circulation, short-term survival, and neurologic outcome were improved in a porcine model of fibrillatory cardiac arrest resuscitated using PCACD CPR.[142]

Open-Chest CPR

Open-chest CPR involves a thoracotomy, and direct compression of the heart generates blood flow. The application of this technique requires a high level of sophistication and training as well as special equipment and facilities. These requirements limit open-chest CPR to certain hospital settings.

Open-chest CPR represents a model of the cardiac pump mechanism for generation of blood flow. In theory, this model eliminates the production of intrathoracic pressure which, if transmitted, could reduce the gradients for blood flow. This enhanced gradient combined with directly applied compression could result in near-normal blood flows.

Open-chest CPR produces cardiac outputs of 25 to 61 percent of prearrest values.[78, 143, 144] These studies and others demonstrate cardiac outputs two to three times larger than with conventional closed-chest CPR.[78, 143–146] Increases in cerebral perfusion pressure have been significant in some studies[145] but not in others.[78, 146] Myocardial perfusion pressures are significantly increased compared with closed-chest CPR.[145, 147] Cerebral blood flow in dogs of 150 percent of prearrest values could be produced with open-chest CPR.[79] Cross-clamping the descending aorta during open-chest CPR further increases carotid blood flow.

Survival in dogs can be improved by use of open-chest CPR after inadequate closed-chest CPR.[148] Dogs with myocardial perfusion pressure of less than 30 mm Hg after 15 minutes of closed-chest external CPR received 2 to 4 minutes of either open-chest or closed-chest external CPR before defibrillation was attempted. The dogs that received open-chest CPR had significantly greater myocardial perfusion pressures and survival rates.

The length of time of closed-chest CPR affects the success of subsequent open-chest CPR.[149] After 20 and 25 minutes of closed-chest CPR, the success rate of open-chest CPR dropped to 38 and 0 percent, respectively. This implies that the benefits from open-chest CPR are time limited and that early application is crucial. There are no data to recommend the routine use of open-chest CPR in the pediatric patient.[150]

Cardiopulmonary Bypass

Cardiopulmonary bypass (CPB) is a very effective way to restore circulation after cardiac arrest. Animal studies show that CPB increases 72-hour survival and recovery of consciousness, and preserves myocardium better than conventional CPR.[151, 152] In dogs, CPB results in better neurologic outcome than continued conventional CPR after a 4-minute ischemic period (neurologic outcome was dismal in both groups when the ischemic period lasted for 12 minutes).[151, 152] Twenty-four-hour survival is possible for at least 90 percent of dogs after 15 or 20 minutes of cardiac arrest but for only 10 percent of dogs after 30 minutes of arrest with CPB stabilization during defibrillation.[153] CPB decreases myocardial infarct size in a model involving coronary artery occlusion, compared with conventional CPR.[154] In most animal models, CPB facilitates resuscitation and improves success compared with conventional CPR.

There is little experience with CPB for cardiac arrest in humans outside the operating room. Timely application of percutaneous femoral artery and vein bypass has been successful in resuscitating patients with "refractory" cardiac arrest. Unfortunately, many patients who are stabilized on CPB after failing standard CPR cannot be weaned off CPB or have a low likelihood of long-term survival or of good neurologic outcome.[155–159] There are reports of patients with cardiac arrest in the operating room or catheterization suite who have cardiac arrest under anesthesia and fail to respond to conventional CPR but benefit from the institution of CPB. These patients are reported to have good neurologic outcomes despite over 30 minutes (even over 2 hours) of failed conventional resuscitation efforts.[160, 161]

Cardiopulmonary bypass requires considerable technical support and sophistication. It is impressive that the procedure can be fully operational in less than 10 minutes after it is requested.[155, 156] Despite rapid availability and restoration of circulation, the lack of effective resuscitation before institution of CPB limits the ability to preserve neurologic or cardiac function. Because of these limitations, CPB may have limited value for patients who suffer out-of-hospital cardiac arrest or require more than 30 minutes of conventional CPR.[157, 159, 162]

PHARMACOLOGY OF CARDIOPULMONARY RESUSCITATION

Adrenergic Agonists

Almost since the inception of closed-chest compression in 1960, adrenergic agonists, such as epinephrine, have been in use for CPR. Redding and Pearson[163] in 1963 first described the use of adrenergic agonists during CPR, demonstrating that early administration of epinephrine in a canine model of cardiac arrest improved the success rate. They also demonstrated that the increase in diastolic pressure produced by administration of adrenergic agonist drugs was responsible for the success of resuscitation.[164]

They theorized that vasopressors such as epinephrine were of value because they increased systemic vascular resistance. Since that time, epinephrine continues to be the drug of choice during CPR, without compelling evidence for a change in that role.

Yakaitis et al.[165] investigated the relative importance of α- and β-adrenergic agonist actions during resuscitation. Only one in four dogs receiving both the pure β-adrenergic agonist isoproterenol and an α-adrenergic antagonist were successfully resuscitated. In contrast, all the dogs treated with both an α-adrenergic agonist drug and a β-adrenergic antagonist were successfully resuscitated. These data suggest that the α-adrenergic agonist receptor action of epinephrine is responsible for successful resuscitation after cardiac arrest.

More recent studies have reconfirmed this notion. Michael et al.[52] demonstrated that the effects of epinephrine during CPR are mediated by selective vasoconstriction of peripheral vessels, excluding those supplying the brain and heart. During an epinephrine infusion, higher aortic pressures are maintained, resulting in higher perfusion pressure to the heart and brain.[52] Despite the increase in both mean and diastolic aortic pressures, flow to other "nonvital" organs, such as the kidneys and small intestine, decreases markedly because of intense vasoconstriction of the vessels supplying those organs.[47, 52, 166]

Coronary Blood Flow

The increase in aortic diastolic pressure associated with epinephrine or other α-adrenergic agonist drugs administered during CPR is critical for maintaining coronary blood flow and improving the rate of successful resuscitation. In the beating heart, the contractile state of the myocardium is increased by β-adrenergic receptor agonist action. During CPR, these drugs may stimulate spontaneous myocardial contractions and increase the intensity of ventricular fibrillation. In the fibrillating heart, the inotropic effect of β-adrenergic agonists might be deleterious by increasing intramyocardial wall pressure.[167] This increased wall pressure causes decreased coronary perfusion pressure and diminished myocardial blood flow. In addition, β-adrenergic stimulation could increase myocardial oxygen demand by increasing cellular metabolism and oxygen consumption. The superimposition of an increased oxygen demand on the low myocardial blood flow available during CPR could cause ischemia.

In normally beating hearts, subendocardial blood flow occurs almost entirely during diastole. During ventricular fibrillation, intramyocardial wall pressure simulates a period of sustained contraction.[168] As above, the high intramyocardial wall pressure and low diastolic pressure results in a decreased coronary perfusion pressure and the risk of further damage to an already ischemic heart.

Other α-adrenergic agonist drugs have been used successfully during CPR. As expected, drugs such as methoxamine and phenylephrine cause peripheral vasoconstriction. As with epinephrine, the increase in aortic diastolic pressure results in an increased coronary blood flow. However, the absence of direct β-adrenergic stimulation avoids an increase in oxygen uptake by the myocardium, resulting in a more favorable oxygen demand-to-supply ratio in the ischemic heart. These nonepinephrine α-adrenergic agonists have been used successfully for resuscitation,[163–165, 169] and maintain myocardial blood flow during CPR as effectively as epinephrine.[165] Schleien et al.[169] found that high aortic pressures can be sustained in a canine model of CPR with the α-adrenergic agonist phenylephrine. The high levels of myocardial perfusion pressure and coronary blood flow produced were equivalent in the phenylephrine- and epinephrine-treated animals, yielding a resuscitation rate of 75 percent with the use of both drugs. In that study, the ratio of endocardial to epicardial blood flow did not differ between the two drug groups. The debate continues about the merits of pure α-adrenergic agonist drugs for resuscitation because of the confusion regarding the benefit versus detriment of the β-adrenergic effects of epinephrine.[170–172]

Cerebral Blood Flow

During CPR, the generation of cerebral blood flow, like coronary blood flow, depends on the vasoconstriction of peripheral vessels. This vasoconstriction is enhanced by administration of α-adrenergic agonists. Epinephrine and other α-agonist drugs produce selective vasoconstriction of noncerebral peripheral vessels to areas of the head and scalp (i.e., tongue, facial muscle, and skin) without causing cerebral vasoconstriction in adult[51, 61] and infant models of CPR.[47] Infusion of either epinephrine or phenylephrine maintained cerebral blood flow and oxygen uptake at prearrest levels for 20 minutes in a canine model of CPR. This implies that blood flow was higher than that needed to maintain adequate cerebral metabolism.[169] There were no differences in neurologic outcome 24 hours after resuscitation when either epinephrine or phenylephrine was administered 9 minutes after ventricular fibrillation.[173] Other investigators found epinephrine to be more beneficial in generating vital organ blood flow.[170, 171, 174] This may have been due to the use of drug dosages that were not equipotent in generating vascular pressure and subsequent blood flow.

Cerebral oxygen uptake may be increased by a central β-adrenergic receptor effect if sufficient amounts of epinephrine cross the blood–brain barrier during or after resuscitation.[175, 176] In addition, epinephrine may have a vasoconstricting or vasodilating effect on cerebral vessels, depending on the balance between α- and β-adrenergic actions.[177] When cerebral ischemia is very brief, epinephrine and phenylephrine have similar effects on cerebral blood flow and metabolism. In this situation, the blood–brain barrier most likely is not disrupted.[169] Catecholamines may cross the blood–brain barrier when mechanical disruption occurs or when enzymatic barriers to vasopressors (i.e., monoamine oxidase inhibitors) are overwhelmed during tissue hypoxia.[178, 179] During CPR, the blood–brain barrier may be disrupted owing to the generation of large fluctuations in cerebral venous and arterial pressures during chest compressions. In addition, the permeability of the barrier may increase because of the arterial pressure surge that occurs in a maximally dilated vascular bed after resuscitation.[180] An increase in cerebral oxygen demand when cerebral blood flow is limited could affect cerebral recovery adversely. In an infant model of

CPR producing 8 minutes of cardiac arrest, disruption of the blood–brain barrier was present 4 hours after defibrillation.[181] In similar protocols involving 8 minutes of cardiac arrest, endothelial vacuolization has been shown, with extravasation of protein through the blood–brain barrier.[182]

Dosage

The correct dose of epinephrine during CPR remains controversial. The dose currently recommended by the American Heart Association's Guidelines for CPR and Emergency Cardiac Care has been modified because of newer research suggesting increased survival when doses larger than previously recommended are administered after cardiac arrest.[183] More recent studies, however, are not as optimistic about this improvement in outcome.

Recent studies have examined the physiologic response of animals and humans to higher doses of epinephrine. Cerebral blood flow increases further in response to administration of larger doses of epinephrine.[173, 184, 185] In animals, several investigators have shown that high-dose epinephrine increases myocardial and subendocardial blood flow, with improvement of oxygen delivery over oxygen consumption.[57, 79, 186, 187] However, increased myocardial oxygen consumption and decreased left ventricular subendocardial blood flow with epinephrine administration have been demonstrated in fibrillating dog models.[167, 188] In a swine model, high-dose epinephrine failed to increase myocardial blood flow to levels achieved with lower doses.[184]

Recent studies in humans have been contradictory regarding survival of patients who were given high-dose epinephrine after cardiac arrest. In earlier studies, investigators were optimistic that higher doses of epinephrine would increase aortic diastolic pressure and therefore improve the return to spontaneous circulation compared with standard epinephrine doses. Gonzalez et al.[189, 190] demonstrated a dose-dependent increase in aortic blood pressure in patients who failed to respond to prolonged resuscitation efforts. Also, Paradis et al.[84] showed increased aortic diastolic pressure and successful resuscitation in patients who failed advanced cardiac life support (ACLS) protocols. They also reported on seven pediatric patients treated successfully with 0.2 mg/kg of epinephrine.[191] Other investigators have also reported higher aortic diastolic pressures and an improvement in return of spontaneous circulation.[84, 192, 193] In these nonrandomized, unblinded studies there were few survivors, although three patients survived in the pediatric study.

Subsequently, three large multicenter studies were published that dampened the enthusiasm for the use of high-dose epinephrine. Stiell et al.[194] reported on 650 adult patients who suffered cardiac arrest. These patients were randomly assigned to either a standard or a high-dose (7 mg) epinephrine protocol. High-dose epinephrine did not improve survival (18 percent vs. 23 percent 1-hour survival; 3 percent vs. 5 percent hospital discharge) or alter neurologic outcome. In a multicenter prospective study, Brown et al.[195] reported on 1,280 adult patients who received either standard (0.02 mg/kg) or high-dose (0.2 mg/kg) epinephrine after cardiac arrest. Again, no differences

were seen between groups in return to spontaneous circulation, short-term survival, survival to hospital discharge, or neurologic outcome between patients treated with a standard dose of epinephrine and those treated with a high dose. Callaham et al., in a study of 816 adults, reported a higher rate of spontaneous circulation in the high-dose epinephrine group. However, there were no differences in the rate of hospital discharge or survival of these patients.[196]

High doses of epinephrine may account for some of the adverse effects that occur after resuscitation. High doses may worsen myocardial ischemia and result in tachyarrhythmias, hypertensive crisis, pulmonary edema, digitalis toxicity, hypoxemia, and cardiac arrest.[183, 195, 197] Tang et al.[198] showed that epinephrine induced a decrease in PaO_2 and an increase in alveolar dead space ventilation, thought to be due to a redistribution of pulmonary blood flow, compared with an α-agonist.

The differences in the results of these studies account for the ambivalence in recommendations from the 1992 American Heart Association Standards and Guidelines for CPR and Emergency Cardiac Care.[183] The present guidelines recommend shortening the epinephrine dosing interval for adult patients from 5 minutes to 3 to 5 minutes. Higher dose epinephrine is neither recommended nor discouraged. An intermediate dose of 2 to 5 mg IV, escalating doses from 1 to 3 to 5 mg, and a high dose of 0.1 mg/kg IV are all possible regimens. In children, the dosing scheme is more explicit. Higher doses are preferred when epinephrine is given through the endotracheal tube because of its decreased bioavailability. To treat a pulseless arrest in children, the first intravenous (IV) or intraosseous (IO) dose is 0.01 mg/kg (1 : 10,000). All endotracheal (ET) doses are 0.1 mg/kg (1 : 1,000); second and subsequent IV/IO/ET doses are 0.1 mg/kg (1 : 1,000) administered every 3 to 5 minutes during arrest (Table 7–6).

Vasopressin

Recent, renewed interest for the vasoconstrictor vasopressin has brought it into the CPR literature and possibly into the CPR cart of medications. Studies in both animals and humans show its efficacy in restoring a life-sustaining

T A B L E 7 – 6
EPINEPHRINE ADMINISTRATION DURING CPR

Actions
  Decreases perfusion to nonvital organs—α-adrenergic effect
  Better coronary perfusion (aortic diastolic pressure)—α-adrenergic effect
  Increases intensity of ventricular fibrillation—β-adrenergic effect
  Stimulates cardiac contractions—β-adrenergic effect
  Intensifies cardiac contractions—β-adrenergic effect
Indications
  Bradyarrhythmia with hemodynamic compromise
  Asystole or pulseless arrest
Dosage
  Bradycardia—0.01 mg/kg IV/IO or 0.1 mg/kg ETT
  Repeat every 3–5 min at the same dose
  Pulseless
    First dose—0.01 mg/kg IV/IO or 0.1 mg/kg ETT
    Subsequent—0.1–0.2 mg/kg IV/IO/ETT
    Repeat every 3–5 min

Data from American Heart Association.[150]

rhythm in patients who present in cardiac arrest with ventricular fibrillation[199–202] but not those presenting with asystole or pulseless electrical activity.[203]

During CPR for ventricular fibrillation, vasopressin has a theoretical advantage compared with epinephrine. This stems from the absence of β-adrenergic activity, which may result in a lower myocardial (and other organ) oxygen consumption at a time when oxygen delivery is limited, resulting in less ischemia and less hyperadrenergic-related ventricular ectopy and tachycardia in the postresuscitation period. This may be offset, however, by intense vasoconstriction following return of spontaneous circulation, resulting in worsening of myocardial ischemia.[204, 205]

No study has shown improved survival with vasopressin compared with epinephrine. One study showed improved return of spontaneous circulation with vasopressin. In an uncontrolled trail, vasopressin (40 units IV) was administered to 8 adults with in-hospital ventricular fibrillation, in whom conventional resuscitation, including epinephrine, had failed. All eight patients recovered spontaneous circulation and three were eventually discharged with intact neurologic function.[206] In an out-of-hospital randomized controlled trial comparing epinephrine to vasopressin (40 units IV) after an initial unsuccessful defibrillation attempt, there was a trend (14 of 20 vs. 7 of 20, $p = 0.06$) toward more successful resuscitation with vasopressin. However, survival to hospital discharge was not different ($p = 0.16$) between the groups.[207] Ultimately, the role that vasopressin will play in patients with ventricular fibrillation is to be determined.

Sodium Bicarbonate

Clinical Effects

Sodium bicarbonate use during CPR is one of the most controversial issues in the cardiac arrest literature. This stems from its potential side effects and the lack of evidence that neither laboratory animals nor humans actually benefit from receiving bicarbonate during CPR.[208–210] Administration of sodium bicarbonate results in an acid–base reaction in which bicarbonate combines with hydrogen ion to form water and carbon dioxide, resulting in an elevated blood pH:

$$HCO_3^- + H^+ \rightarrow H_2CO_3 \rightarrow H_2O + CO_2$$

Since bicarbonate generates carbon dioxide, adequate alveolar ventilation must be present before its administration.

Indications

Sodium bicarbonate is indicated for correction of significant metabolic acidosis, especially when cardiovascular compromise is present. Acidosis depresses myocardial function by decreasing spontaneous cardiac activity, the electrical threshold for ventricular fibrillation, the inotropic state of the myocardium, the cardiac responsiveness to catecholamines, and by prolonging diastolic depolarization.[211–214] Acidosis also decreases systemic vascular resistance and blunts the vasoconstrictive response of peripheral vessels to catecholamines.[215] The resultant vasodilation is contrary to the desired effect of vasoconstriction during CPR. In addition, pulmonary vascular resistance increases with acidosis in patients with a reactive pulmonary vascular bed. Rudolph and Yuan[216] observed a twofold increase in pulmonary vascular resistance in calves by lowering pH from 7.4 to 7.2 under normoxic conditions. Therefore, correction of acidosis may be of help in resuscitating patients who have the potential for right-to-left shunting. Sodium bicarbonate is also indicated in hyperkalemic arrest because the increase of pH causes potassium to go intracellularly, resulting in a lowered serum concentration.

Dosage

When the $Paco_2$ and pH are known, the dose of bicarbonate needed to correct the pH to 7.0 can be calculated from the formula $(0.3 \times \text{weight [kg]} \times \text{base deficit}) = \text{mEq bicarbonate}$. Because of the possible side effects of bicarbonate and the large arterial-to-venous carbon dioxide gradient that develops during CPR, we recommend giving half the dose based on a volume of distribution of 0.6. If blood gases are not available, the initial dose is 1 mEq/kg, followed by 0.5 mEq/kg every 10 minutes of ongoing arrest.[217] The importance of alveolar ventilation cannot be overemphasized, as well as the need for repeated arterial blood gas analyses.

Adverse Effects

The multiple side effects that are seen with bicarbonate administration include metabolic alkalosis, hypercapnia, hypernatremia,[218] and hyperosmolarity,[219] all of which are associated with an increased mortality rate. Metabolic alkalosis causes a leftward shift of the oxyhemoglobin dissociation curve that impairs the release of oxygen from hemoglobin to tissues at a time of low cardiac output and low oxygen delivery.[220] Hypernatremia and hyperosmolarity may decrease organ perfusion by increasing interstitial edema in microvascular beds. There are many theoretical aspects of bicarbonate administration that may preclude its frequent use. It may produce a paradoxical intracellular acidosis because of the rapid entry of carbon dioxide into the cell with the slower egress of the hydrogen ion out of the cell. A marked hypercapnic acidosis in both systemic venous and coronary sinus blood develops during cardiac arrest and may be worsened by administration of bicarbonate.[221, 222] Hypercapnic acidosis in the coronary sinus may cause decreased myocardial contractility.[211, 212, 223] Falk et al.[224] measured the mean venoarterial difference of $Paco_2$ as 23.8 ± 15.1 mm Hg in five patients during CPR. In one patient, the difference increased from 16 mm Hg to 69 mm Hg after administration of sodium bicarbonate. In another study of 16 patients during CPR, the venoarterial gradient for carbon dioxide was 42 mm Hg.[222] In the central nervous system, however, intracellular acidosis probably does not occur unless overcorrection of the pH occurs. Sessler et al.[225] demonstrated that after administration of two doses of bicarbonate of 5 mEq/kg to neonatal rabbits recovering from hypoxic acidosis, the arterial pH increased to 7.41 and the intracellular brain pH increased to prehypoxic levels.[225] They did not observe a paradoxical intracellular acidosis. Cohen et al.[226] showed that the intracellular brain adenosine triphosphate (ATP) concentration did not change during 70 minutes of extreme hypercarbia in rats, despite a decrease in the intracellular brain pH to 6.5. After hypercarbia, these animals could not be distinguished from normal controls and their brains were not morphologically different from those of control animals. Eleff et al.,[227] using nuclear magnetic resonance spectroscopy to measure brain pH in dogs during CPR, showed that brain pH decreased to 6.29 after 6 minutes of ventricular fibrillation, with total depletion of brain ATP. After 6 minutes of effective CPR, the ATP level returned to 86 percent of prearrest levels, and after 35 minutes of CPR brain pH had returned to normal despite ongoing peripheral arterial acidosis[227] (Table 7–7).

Other Alkalinizing Agents

Several other alkalinizing agents have been used experimentally in animals and humans to avoid the real and theoretical side effects of sodium bicarbonate. Unfortunately, to date none has demonstrated real advantages over sodium bicarbonate. Carbicarb (International Medication Systems, Ltd.), a recently developed solution of equimolar amounts of sodium bicarbonate and sodium carbonate, works by consuming carbon dioxide and water to generate bicarbonate ion and sodium:

$$(Na_2CO_3 + CO_2 + H_2O \rightarrow 2HCO_3^- + 2Na^+)$$

In animal models, Carbicarb administration resulted in a higher elevation of pH and a lesser increase in Pa_{CO_2}, lactate, and serum osmolarity compared with sodium bicarbonate use.[228–230]

Dichloroacetate (DCA), another alkalinizing agent, works by stimulating the activity of pyruvate dehydrogenase, which facilitates the conversion of lactate to pyruvate.[231] Initial studies have shown that DCA decreased lactate concentration by half and increased bicarbonate concentration and pH when administered to humans.[232]

T A B L E   7 – 7
SODIUM BICARBONATE ADMINISTRATION DURING CPR

Indications
  Hyperkalemia
  Preexisting metabolic acidosis
  Long CPR time without blood gas availability
  Pulmonary hypertensive crisis
Dose
  1 mEq/kg intravenous/intraosseous empirically, or calculated from base deficit
  Ensure adequate ventilation when administering bicarbonate
Complications
  Metabolic alkalosis
    Impairs O_2 delivery by shift of oxyhemoglobin dissociation
    Decreases cardiac contractility
    Decreases fibrillation threshold
    Decreases plasma K^+ and Ca^{2+} by intracellular shift
  Hypernatremia
  Hyperosmolarity
  Hypercapnia
  Paradoxical intracellular acidosis

It was also shown to improve cardiac output, possibly by enhancing myocardial metabolism of lactate and carbohydrate.[233, 234] Unfortunately, in a multicenter trial that studied patients with lactic acidosis, DCA did not improve outcome or survival compared with standard alkalinizing agents.[235]

Tromethamine (THAM), or tris-[hydroxymethyl]aminomethane, is an organic amine that attracts and combines with hydrogen ions. It is available as a 0.3 M solution adjusted to a pH of 8.6. A dose of 3 ml/kg should raise the bicarbonate concentration by 3 mEq/L. Side effects of this drug include hyperkalemia, hypoglycemia, acute hypocarbia, and apnea. Most importantly, it also acts as a peripheral vasodilator when administered during CPR, which may worsen myocardial perfusion. THAM is contraindicated in patients with renal failure.

Calcium
Clinical Effects

Indications for the administration of calcium during CPR are now limited to a few specific areas. This is primarily due to the possibility that in the setting of ischemia–reperfusion injury, calcium administration may worsen postischemic hypoperfusion and hasten the development of intracellular cytotoxic events that lead to cell death. Intracellular calcium overload occurs in many pathologic conditions, including ischemia, and may be a part of the final common pathway of cell death.[236, 237] Nevertheless, no study has shown that transient elevation of plasma calcium concentration worsens the outcome after cardiac arrest.

The calcium ion is essential in myocardial excitation-contraction coupling and myocardial contractility, and it enhances ventricular automaticity during asystole.[238] Therefore, calcium should be useful in the setting of asystole or electromechanical dissociation. Ionized hypocalcemia leads to decreased ventricular performance, peripheral vasodilation, and blunting of the hemodynamic response to catecholamines.[239–243] Severe ionized hypocalcemia (mean, 0.67 mmol/L) was present in adult patients who experienced out-of-hospital cardiac arrest.[244] Evidence for beneficial clinical effects of calcium during these clinical situations is lacking.[245–247]

Calcium channel blockers improve blood flow and function after ischemia to the heart,[248] kidney,[249] and brain.[250] Calcium channel blockers also raise the threshold of the ischemic heart to ventricular fibrillation.[251] Therefore, the use of calcium in these settings seems incongruous.

Indications

The few firm indications for calcium use during CPR include cardiac arrest secondary to total or ionized hypocalcemia, hyperkalemia, hypermagnesemia, and an overdose of a calcium channel blocker. Hypocalcemia occurs in patients with a vast array of conditions that predispose to low total body calcium stores, including the long-term use of loop diuretics. Ionized hypocalcemia may coexist with a normal total plasma calcium concentration. This occurs

---

T A B L E   7 – 8
CALCIUM CHLORIDE ADMINISTRATION DURING CPR

Indications
  Hyperkalemia
  Hypocalcemia
  Hypermagnesemia
  Calcium channel blocker overdose
Dose
  20 mg/kg intravenous/intraosseous; given slowly

---

in the presence of severe alkalosis, which may be seen in the operating room secondary to iatrogenic hyperventilation. Ionized hypocalcemia also follows massive or rapid transfusion of citrated blood products into patients during surgery. The degree of hypocalcemia caused by citrated products depends on the rate of administration, the total dose, and the hepatic and renal function of the patient. Administration of 2 ml/kg/min of citrated whole blood causes a significant but transient decrease in the ionized calcium in anesthetized patients.[252] Because calcium administration is not a first-line treatment during CPR, hypocalcemia must be considered as a cause of cardiac arrest, particularly in the operating room, and if present, must be treated aggressively.

Dosage

The adult dose of calcium chloride is 200 mg given as 2 ml of the 10 percent solution. The pediatric dose is 20 mg/kg or 0.2 ml/kg of the 10 percent calcium chloride solution. Calcium gluconate is as effective as calcium chloride in raising ionized calcium concentration during CPR.[253] Calcium gluconate can be given as a dose of 30 to 100 mg/kg, with a maximal dose of 2 g in pediatric patients.

Adverse Effects

Calcium should be given slowly through a large-bore, free-flowing IV line, preferably a central venous line. Severe tissue necrosis can occur when calcium infiltrates into subcutaneous tissue. When administered too rapidly, calcium may cause severe bradycardia, heart block, or ventricular standstill (Table 7–8).

Atropine
Clinical Effects

Atropine is a parasympatholytic agent that acts by reducing vagal tone to the heart. This, in turn, increases the discharge rate of the sinus node, enhances atrioventricular (AV) conduction, and activates latent ectopic pacemakers.[254] Atropine has minimal effects on systemic vascular resistance, myocardial perfusion, and myocardial contractility.[255]

Indications

Atropine is indicated for treatment of asystole, electromechanical dissociation, bradycardia associated with hypotension,[256] ventricular ectopy, second- and third-degree

heart block, and slow idioventricular rhythms.[257] Atropine, therefore, may be a useful drug in clinical states associated with excessive parasympathetic tone. Acute myocardial infarction may augment parasympathetic tone and lead to arrhythmias (including asystole) that are responsive to atropine. In pediatric patients who present in cardiac arrest, bradycardia or asystole is commonly the initial rhythm and atropine is therefore a first-line drug for such patients. In infants, during the perioperative period, any type of stress (i.e., laryngoscopy), may result in severe bradycardia or even asystole secondary to enhanced parasympathetic tone. These conditions should be treated with atropine.

Dosage

The recommended adult dose of atropine is 0.5 mg IV given every 5 minutes until a desired heart rate is obtained or to a maximal dose of 2.0 mg. Full vagal blockade occurs in adults who receive a dose of 2.0 mg. For asystole, 1.0 mg IV should be given and repeated every 5 minutes if asystole persists. The pediatric dose for atropine is 0.01 to 0.02 mg/kg, with a minimal dose of 0.15 mg and a maximal dose of 2.0 mg. A minimal dose is necessary because of the possible occurrence of paradoxical bradycardia resulting from a central stimulating effect on the medullary vagal nuclei.[258] Atropine may be given via any route: intravenous, endotracheal, intraosseous, intramuscular, or subcutaneous. Onset of action occurs within 30 seconds and the peak effect occurs 1 to 2 minutes after an IV dose.

Adverse Effects

Atropine should not be used in patients in whom tachycardia is undesirable. In patients after myocardial infarction or ischemia with persistent bradycardia, atropine should be used in the lowest dose possible to increase the heart rate. Tachycardia, which increases myocardial oxygen consumption and can lead to ventricular fibrillation, is common after large doses of atropine in these patients. In patients with pulmonary or systemic outflow tract obstruction or idiopathic hypertrophic subaortic stenosis, tachycardia can decrease ventricular filling and lower cardiac output (Table 7–9).

T A B L E   7 – 9
ATROPINE ADMINISTRATION DURING CPR

Indications
  Symptomatic bradycardia with AV node block
  Vagal bradycardia during intubation attempts
  After epinephrine for bradycardia with poor perfusion
Dose
  0.02 mg/kg IV/IO/ETT after ensuring oxygenation (2.5 times dose if given ETT)
  Repeat every 3–5 min at the same dose
  Maximum single dose 0.5 mg in a child and 1.0 mg in an adolescent
  Maximum total dose 1.0 mg in a child and 2.0 mg in an adolescent

Data from American Heart Association.[150]

Glucose

Glucose use during CPR should be restricted to patients with documented hypoglycemia because of the possible detrimental effects of hyperglycemia on the brain during ischemia. Myers[259] first hypothesized that hyperglycemia worsens the neurologic outcome after cardiac arrest. Siemkowicz and Hansen[260] confirmed this finding when they found that after 10 minutes of global brain ischemia the neurologic recovery of hyperglycemic rats was worse than in normoglycemic control animals. Hyperglycemia exaggerates ischemic neurologic injury by increasing the production of lactic acid in the brain by anaerobic metabolism. During ischemia under normoglycemic conditions, brain lactate concentration reaches a plateau. However, when hyperglycemia is present, the brain lactate concentration continues to rise for the duration of the ischemic period.[261] The severity of intracellular acidosis during brain ischemia is directly proportional to the preischemic plasma glucose concentration.[262] These negative effects of hyperglycemia during brain ischemia are based on the existence of at least a small amount of blood flow to brain tissue. In one study, collaterally perfused but not end-arterial brain tissue had greater neuronal damage during hyperglycemic focal ischemia.[263] Clinical studies have shown a direct correlation between the initial serum glucose concentration and a poor neurologic outcome.[264–267] Longstreth et al.[268] suggested that a higher admission plasma glucose concentration may be an endogenous response to severe stress and not the cause of more severe brain injury. Given the likelihood of additional ischemic events during the postresuscitation period, it may be wise to maintain serum glucose in the normal range. Voll and Auer[269] showed that administration of insulin to hyperglycemic rats after global brain ischemia improved the neurologic outcome. It is not known if active treatment of hyperglycemia enhances the clinical outcome after an ischemic episode. This effect of insulin may be independent of its glucose-lowering properties, since normoglycemic-treated rats had a better outcome than placebo-treated controls.[270] Before any surgical procedure, when the possibility of brain ischemia exists, tight pre- and intraoperative control of the serum glucose level is desirable.[271]

Infants, patients with hepatic disease, and debilitated patients with low endogenous glycogen stores are prone to hypoglycemia when stressed. This may occur during surgery. In these patients, bedside monitoring of the serum glucose level is critical during the perioperative period. In cardiac arrest, glucose is administered to the hypoglycemic patient to maintain normal substrate delivery to vital organs. To treat hypoglycemia, an IV dose of 1 ml/kg of 50 percent dextrose for adults, 2 ml/kg of 25 percent dextrose in children, or 3 to 5 ml/kg of 10 percent dextrose for infants can be administered.

Defibrillation

Physiology

Ventricular fibrillation is a sustained burst of multiple, uncoordinated regional ventricular depolarizations and contractions, resulting in an ineffective cardiac output and cessation of myocardial blood flow. Reentrant impulses, generated within the ventricles with multiple, shifting circuits, maintain ventricular fibrillation. Several physiologic conditions lower the threshold for fibrillation, including hypoxia, hypercapnia, myocardial ischemia, hypothermia, metabolic acidosis, and electrolyte disturbances including those of potassium, calcium, sodium, and magnesium.

Ventricular tachycardia and fibrillation are relatively uncommon rhythms during cardiac arrest in children. Typically, an initial electrocardiographic (ECG) finding of a bradyarrhythmia, which progresses to asystole, is found. However, with increasing numbers of children with congenital heart disease (especially those with a history of cardiac surgery) or toxic ingestions in older children and adolescents, ventricular fibrillation appears to be more frequent in children. A recent study showed ventricular fibrillation as the initial rhythm in 19 percent of children presenting with cardiac arrest.[272] The etiology of ventricular fibrillation in that study was medical illness, toxic overdose, drowning, trauma, and congenital heart defect.

When ventricular tachycardia or fibrillation with hypotension or absent pulses is present, electric countershock is the treatment of choice. Drug treatment by itself cannot be relied on to terminate ventricular fibrillation. High-voltage electric countershock, when correctly applied, sends more than 2 A through the heart and can terminate ventricular fibrillation by simultaneously depolarizing and causing a sustained contraction of the myocardium. This allows spontaneous cardiac contractions to commence if the myocardium is in a well-oxygenated environment with a normal acid–base status. Modern defibrillators deliver only direct current (DC) shocks. The amount of myocardial damage produced by the countershock relates proportionally to the amount of energy delivered.[273, 274] In addition, the incidence of postdefibrillation arrhythmias increases as the energy dose increases.[275] Frequent, concentrated, high-density electric current can damage the myocardium, decrease the likelihood of successful defibrillation, and lead to postdefibrillation arrhythmias.[276] These arrhythmias are thought to be associated with prolonged depolarization of the myocardial cell membrane, which increases with the intensity of the stimulus[277, 278] and provides an ideal setting for reentrant arrhythmias.[278] In humans after synchronized cardioversion, the frequency of arrhythmias and the degree of ST-segment displacement relate directly to the energy level used.[251]

In most adult patients, energy levels of 100 to 300 J are successful when shocks are delivered with minimal delay. There is no need for higher voltages (500 to 1,000 J) even in obese adults.[276, 279] In an in-hospital group of adults, 95 percent were successfully defibrillated with 200 J of stored energy, even in patients weighing more than 100 kg.[279] Another study compared the use of 175- to 320-J shocks in 249 adult patients with ventricular fibrillation. Survival did not relate to the energy level used or the weight of the patient, which ranged up to 102 kg.[276] One study showed no differences in heart weight or energy per gram of heart weight in patients who ultimately underwent autopsy.[280] The goal of defibrillation is to deliver a minimum of electrical energy to a critical mass of ventricular muscle (but not to every cell) and to avoid an overdose of current that could further damage the heart. Zipes et al.[281] found that a critical amount of myocardial tissue must be depolarized to terminate ventricular fibrillation.

The optimal dose of electrical energy required to defibrillate the hearts of infants and children is not conclusively established, but available data suggest an initial dose of 2 J/kg.[282] If the initial dose is unsuccessful, then a dose of 4 J/kg should be used on the second and subsequent attempts at defibrillation.

Several clinical factors affect the success rate of ventricular defibrillation in humans. Success decreases with an increased duration of ventricular fibrillation. Short fibrillation time is the most accurate predictor for successful defibrillation.[280, 283] Defibrillatory attempts were successful in patients shocked within 8 minutes of fibrillation, whereas attempts were unsuccessful in patients shocked at an average of 17 minutes after the onset of ventricular fibrillation.[280] A brief period of myocardial perfusion in dogs before electric countershock improves cardiac resuscitation outcome after prolonged ventricular fibrillation.[284] Acidosis and hypoxia also decrease the success of defibrillation.[280] The temperature of the patient does not alter the energy dose required for successful defibrillation.[285] Patients with terminal illness are more resistant to successful defibrillation,[286] as are those who fibrillate later in the course of a myocardial infarction.

Correct paddle size and position are also important to the success of defibrillation. Three paddle sizes are available for external defibrillation: 13 cm in diameter for adults, 8 cm for older children, and 4.5 cm for infants. The largest paddle size appropriate for the patient should be used because large size reduces the density of current flow, which reduces myocardial damage. If the entire paddle does not rest firmly on the chest wall, a high-density current will be delivered to a small contact point on the skin. The paddles should be positioned on the chest wall with most of the myocardium included between them. If for some reason two paddles cannot be placed on the anterior chest, an alternate approach is to place one paddle anteriorly over the left precordium and the other paddle posteriorly between the scapulae.

The interface between the paddle and chest wall can be electrode cream, saline, paste, soap, or moist gauze pads. The cream produces lower impedance than the paste. Care should be taken not to allow the substance from one paddle to touch that from the other paddle, as electric current follows the path of least resistance. This is especially important in infants, in whom the distance between electrodes is very small.

When the onset of ventricular fibrillation is observed, common in the in-hospital perioperative period, defibrillation should be attempted when possible. If a second defibrillation attempt is unsuccessful, basic life support should be continued, epinephrine administered, and sodium bicarbonate given (if metabolic acidosis is documented or if the duration of cardiac arrest warrants its administration). If a third defibrillatory attempt is necessary, 360 J of delivered energy to adults or 4 J/kg in children should be used. If ventricular fibrillation is recurrent, an antiarrhythmic can be used (see below). It is not necessary to increase the energy dose for each successive defibrillation attempt. On the contrary, ventricular fibrillation threshold often increases with CPR and the administration of resuscitation medications.

Open-chest defibrillation should be performed when the chest is already open during surgery. To perform open-chest defibrillation, a dose of 5 to 20 J of delivered energy should be used, beginning with the lower energy level. Paddles made specifically for this purpose are applied directly to the heart. Open-chest paddles have a diameter of 6 cm for adults, 4 cm for children, and 2 cm for infants. The handles should be insulated. The paddles are applied with saline-soaked pads. One electrode is placed behind the left ventricle and the other over the right ventricle on the anterior surface of the heart.

Automated External Defibrillation

Automated external defibrillation (AED) is now becoming the standard therapy for ventricular fibrillation in the out-of-hospital environment, due to the awareness that early defibrillation is the key to successful resuscitation in most adult patients.[287] Low-energy, 150-J, impedance-adjusted shocks for adults appears to be clinically safe and effective.[288] These AED units continue to improve, with smaller, lighter, cheaper, easier-to-use, and more accurate, with improved waveform units being manufactured.[289]

Use of AED has generally been limited to adults because of the lower incidence of ventricular fibrillation in children. These units are automated and deliver a higher than usual dose to children. However, with the increasing frequency of ventricular fibrillation as a cause of cardiac arrest in children, the use of AED for children would be beneficial. A retrospective review of 18 adolescents and children aged 5 to 15 years receiving AED by Emergency Medical Services crews, showed accurate rhythm detection and shock delivery.[290]

Lidocaine
Chemistry

Lidocaine, a class 1B antiarrhythmic, depresses the fast inward sodium channel, which results in an increased refractory period and shortening of the total action potential. The drug is metabolized primarily in the liver by the microsomal enzyme system.[291] Up to 10 percent of the drug is excreted unchanged in the urine. The amount excreted unchanged increases in acid urine. There is no biliary excretion or intestinal absorption in humans.

Electrophysiology

Lidocaine causes a decrease in automaticity and in spontaneous phase 4 depolarization of pacemaker tissue. The drug increases the ventricular fibrillation threshold while having essentially no effect on the ventricular diastolic threshold for depolarization. It decreases the duration of the action potential of Purkinje fibers and ventricular muscle while increasing the effective refractory period of these fibers. Lidocaine does not affect conduction time through the AV node or intraventricular conduction time. By decreasing automaticity, lidocaine prevents or terminates ventricular arrhythmias caused by accelerated ectopic foci. Lidocaine abolishes reentrant ventricular arrhythmias by decreasing action potential duration and conduction time of Purkinje fibers, thus reducing the nonuniformity of action. The effect on ischemic tissues in which lidocaine delivery may be limited is unknown.[291]

Hemodynamic Effects

In animal models, rapid IV delivery of lidocaine causes a decrease in stroke work, blood pressure, systemic vascular resistance,[292] and left ventricular contractility,[293] and a slight increase in heart rate. In healthy adults, the drug does not appear to cause any change in heart rate or blood pressure[294, 295]; awake patients with cardiac disease have a slight decrease in ventricular function.[294] In most patients, even in those who have sustained a recent myocardial infarction, a 1- to 2-mg/kg bolus of lidocaine does not alter cardiac output, heart rate, or blood pressure.[295] Excessive doses of lidocaine given by rapid infusion may decrease cardiac function in patients with cardiac disease, especially in those suffering an acute myocardial infarction. Therefore, slow IV administration, no greater than 50 to 100 mg/min in adults, is recommended.[291] When given to a patient with a normal heart, lidocaine usually causes few, if any, hemodynamic changes.

Antiarrhythmic Effects

Lidocaine is effective in terminating ventricular premature beats (VPBs) and ventricular tachycardia in humans during the perioperative period of general or cardiac surgery, after an acute myocardial infarction, and in patients with digitalis intoxication. Treatment of VPBs after myocardial infarction is indicated if they occur at a rate of more than five per minute and are of unifocal origin, they occur on a normal T-wave, are multifocal, or if runs of VPBs occur (ventricular tachycardia). Lidocaine is also effective in preventing and treating ventricular arrhythmias during cardiac catheterization. The drug is indicated after cardioversion from ventricular fibrillation, especially when ventricular fibrillation or tachycardia recurs. Lidocaine is not effective in the treatment of atrial or AV junctional arrhythmias.

Pharmacokinetics

To achieve and maintain therapeutic levels of lidocaine, a bolus dose should be given at the initiation of a constant infusion. If an infusion is begun without an initial bolus, approximately five half-lives are required to approach a plateau serum concentration.[291] Therefore, with a half-life of 108 minutes, a 9-hour infusion would be required to reach a plateau concentration. When a bolus administration is used alone, ventricular arrhythmias often return within 15 to 20 minutes because of its rapid clearance.[143]

Lidocaine toxicity with serum concentration greater than 7 to 8 μg/kg, occurs most commonly in patients with severe hepatic disease or severe congestive heart failure. Decreased cardiac output results in decreased hepatic blood flow, which in turn leads to decreased lidocaine clearance. During CPR, lidocaine clearance is decreased because of the inherent decrease in cardiac output and very low hepatic blood flow. In dogs, with the use of conventional CPR to obtain a blood pressure of 20 percent of control values, an IV lidocaine bolus of 2 mg/kg resulted in very elevated blood and tissue concentrations. During CPR, distribution of the drug, which is usually complete in 20 minutes, was still not complete after 1 hour. In addition, lidocaine clearance and distribution may be altered owing to changes in protein binding and metabolism during CPR.[296] In humans, high peak blood and tissue concentrations of lidocaine occur during CPR, with a delay in the time to peak concentration. Comparison of the peripheral, central, and intraosseous routes of administration of lidocaine during open-chest CPR in dogs revealed no difference in time to peak serum concentration.[297]

Dosage

In patients with normal cardiac and hepatic function, an initial IV bolus of lidocaine 1.5 to 2 mg/kg is given, followed by a constant IV infusion at a rate of 55 μg/kg/min (Table 7–10). If the arrhythmia recurs, a second IV bolus of the same dose can be given.[238] Patients with a moderate decrease in cardiac output or those suffering an acute myocardial infarction should receive an IV bolus of 1 to 1.5 mg/kg with an infusion rate of 30 μg/kg/min. In patients with severe diminution of cardiac output, a bolus no greater than 0.75 mg/kg should be administered, followed by an infusion at a rate of 10 to 20 μg/kg/min. In patients with hepatic disease, dosages should be decreased by 50 percent of normal. Patients with chronic renal disease on hemodialysis have normal lidocaine pharmacokinetics. Drug interactions with lidocaine are common. Phenobarbital increases lidocaine metabolism, requiring increased doses. Isoniazid and chloramphenicol decrease lidocaine metabolism, so a decreased dosage should be used. Any drug that decreases cardiac output (i.e., β-blockers) increases the serum concentration of lidocaine, whereas drugs (such as isoproterenol) that increase cardiac output and hepatic blood flow cause the serum concentration to be lower than predicted.

Adverse Effects

The toxic effects of lidocaine generally involve the central nervous system and include seizures, psychosis, drowsi-

T A B L E   7 – 1 0
LIDOCAINE AND BRETYLIUM ADMINISTRATION DURING CPR

Lidocaine indications
  Ventricular arrhythmias (not ventricular escape rhythm)
  Suppress ventricular ectopy
  Raise threshold for fibrillation
Dose
  1.0 mg/kg IV/IO/ETT bolus (2.5 times dose if ETT)
  30–50 μg/kg/min IV/IO infusion
  Reduce infusion rate if low cardiac output or liver failure
Bretylium indications
  Ventricular arrhythmias not responsive to lidocaine
Dose
  5.0 mg/kg IV/IO bolus
  Repeat with 10 mg/kg IV/IO

Data from American Heart Association.[150]

ness, paresthesias, disorientation, muscle twitching, agitation, and respiratory arrest. Treatment for seizures and psychosis consists of a benzodiazepine or a barbiturate. True allergic reactions to lidocaine are extremely rare. Cardiovascular side effects (discussed above) are usually observed in patients whose myocardial function is already decreased. Conversion of second-degree heart block to complete heart block has been described.[298] Further slowing of sinus bradycardia has also been observed. These effects are infrequent and occur with large-dose administration. These potential side effects do not prohibit the use of lidocaine in these patients.

Amiodarone
Chemistry

Amiodarone is a di-iodinated benzofuran derivative containing a diethylated tertiary amine chain. It is strongly lipophilic and has extensive tissue distribution. The drug is metabolized in the liver with mainly bile elimination. There is little renal elimination. Amiodarone has a long elimination half-life ranging from 20 to 47 days.[299]

Pharmacologic Effects

Amiodarone has a broad range of pharmacologic effects, including all four antiarrhythmic classes.[300] It has K^+ channel blocking action, blocks the fast inward Na^+ current, is a noncompetitive β-blocker, and has Ca^{2+} channel blocking properties. Interestingly, its major electrophysiologic effect is dependent on the route (and duration) of administration.[301] With long-term treatment, its predominant activity is in its ability to increase the action potential duration in most cardiac tissue, a class III effect. When used acutely by the intravenous route, the drug increases AV node refractoriness and intranodal conduction interval time, class II antiadrenergic effect, or class IV calcium-channel blocker effect.[302]

Additionally, amiodarone causes both coronary and systemic vasodilation.[303] It does have phosphodiesterase inhibition[304] and is a selective inhibitor of thyroid hormone metabolism.[300]

Clinical Indications

Amiodarone has been studied as both a prophylactic long-term medication for patients with high arrhythmogenic potential due to organic heart disease and for the use of acute life-threatening arrhythmias. It has been shown to be effective when lidocaine or bretylium were not for ventricular tachycardia or fibrillation, in over 15 studies.[299, 305-308] When IV amiodarone was compared with placebo in a randomized trial (ARREST trial), there was significant improvement in the number of patients surviving to the emergency department following an out-of-hospital arrest.[309]

Amiodarone has been studied in children with generally favorable outcome. Perry et al. showed arrhythmia resolution in 6 of 10 children (mean age, 6.8 years) who had failed with multiple other antiarrhythmics.[310] Figa et al. studied 30 infants and children with life-threatening ar-

rhythmias, including supraventricular and ventricular tachycardia. Arrhythmias were eliminated in 71 percent of patients, and an additional 23 percent experienced a significant improvement in clinical status and rhythm.[311]

A number of studies have shown its effectiveness in treating patients chronically with a high risk of arrhythmia-related sudden death. A number of randomized, prospective studies are underway.

Adverse Effects

All of the adverse effects of amiodarone appear to be less frequent at lower dosages.[312] Cardiovascular effects appear to be the most common and include hypotension due to the acute vasodilation and negative inotropic effects of the drug. Bradyarrhythmias, congestive heart failure, cardiac arrest, and ventricular tachycardia have all been reported. Proarrhythmias, although possible, are seen less frequently than with other class III antiarrhythmics. The incidence is thought to be approximately 2 percent. Torsades de pointes occurs in one third of these cases.[310]

The most common noncardiovascular-related toxicity is related to pulmonary complications. A hypersensitivity pneumonitis can occur early in the course of treatment. Interstitial pneumonitis is more frequent, usually associated with oral long-term treatment. Symptoms include cough, low-grade fever, dyspnea, weight loss, respiratory-associated chest pain, and bilateral interstitial infiltrates. These symptoms are usually reversible upon cessation of the drug.[313]

Hepatotoxicity also occurs more commonly with oral use. Thyroid dysfunction may occur in as many as 10 percent of patients resulting in either hypo- or hyperthyroidism. Optic neuritis or neuropathy resulting in decreased acuity or blurred vision can progress to permanent blindness. Neurologic symptoms include ataxia, tremor, peripheral neuropathy, malaise or fatigue, sleep disturbance, dizziness, and headache. Dermatologic reactions include allergic rash, photosensitivity, and blue-gray skin discoloration.[314]

Sotalol
Chemistry

Sotalol HCl is a racemic compound consisting of equimolar concentrations of l- and d-isomers. The l-isomer possesses the majority of the β-blocking activity. Both isomers have similar class III effects.[315]

Pharmacologic Effects

Sotalol is a noncardioselective β-blocker. Besides these class II effects, sotalol also has class III antiarrhythmic effects. The β-blocker effects include prolongation of sinus cycle length, the AH interval, and the effective refractory period of the AV node. These effects are dose-dependent. Its class III effects consist of an increase in the action potential duration and lengthening of the effective and absolute refractory periods of all cardiac tissue. Prolongation of the action potential duration by sotalol is rate-dependent, being more pronounced at low heart rates.[316]

At the cellular level, these effects on the action potential are caused by inhibition of the outward potassium current, which is activated during the plateau phase of the action potential.[317] Some age-dependent effects have been observed with sotalol. QT interval and action potential duration prolongation was more pronounced in neonates than in adult dogs.[318] As a result of prolonging repolarization, the PQ and QT interval are prolonged and the sinus cycle length is increased.

Pharmacokinetics

Oral sotalol is almost completely absorbed from the gastrointestinal tract and does not undergo hepatic first-pass metabolism. Peak plasma levels are observed 2 to 4 hours after ingestion. Elimination of sotalol is almost entirely renal without detectable metabolites. As the drug is hydrophilic, its effects on the central nervous system are minimal compared with other β-blockers.[319]

Following an intravenous dose of sotalol, there is a rapid onset of electrophysiologic effects with a significant increase in the right ventricular effective refractory period after either bolus or infusion doses.[320] The IV dose is 0.5 to 1.5 mg/kg over 1 to 5 minutes.[320]

Clinical Use

Sotalol is used for the treatment of the various forms of supraventricular reentrant tachyarrhythmias with an overall success rate of approximately 90 percent.[315] The drug has also been used with moderate success for patients with atrial ectopic tachycardias and atrial flutter.[315, 318, 321]

The use of sotalol for ventricular tachyarrhythmias is not as extensive as in adults, and also shows it to be a moderately effective drug for patients with life-threatening ventricular arrhythmias.[315, 318]

Side Effects

Clinical side effects of sotalol are mostly due to its β-blocking properties, and include fatigue, dizziness, and bradycardia.[322] Other effects including left ventricular dysfunction and congestive heart failure are seen mostly in patients with ischemic heart disease.[323] Proarrhythmic effects by sotalol are probably due to the induction of early after-depolarizations.[324] Proarrhythmia manifests mainly as torsades de pointes or as nonsustained ventricular tachycardias in adults. In children, the incidence of proarrhythmia is probably lower and includes exacerbation of bradycardia and ventricular ectopy.[315, 318]

Bretylium

Chemistry

Bretylium, a class III antiarrhythmic (prolongs phase 3 repolarization, prolonging the refractory period), is a bromobenzyl quaternary ammonia compound not structurally related to lidocaine. Its half-life gradually increases over time, with a mean elimination half-life of 9.8 hours.[325] The drug is 80 percent excreted unchanged in the urine over the first 24 hours. An additional 10 percent of the drug is excreted in the urine during the next 72 hours.[326]

Mechanism of Action

The mechanism of action of bretylium is still controversial, but it appears to act by adrenergic stimulation. There is an initial release of norepinephrine from adrenergic nerve endings, with subsequent inhibition of norepinephrine release.[327] There is also blockade of the reuptake of norepinephrine and epinephrine by adrenergic nerve endings, thereby potentiating the action of these agonists on adrenal receptors.

Bretylium also appears to have direct cardiac effects that pretreatment with reserpine or denervation of the heart do not abolish.[328] Bretylium increases the action potential duration of cardiac muscle and increases the effective refractory period of Purkinje and ventricular muscle fibers. In dogs, bretylium decreases the disparity in action potential duration between normal and infarcted areas of the heart, probably the major physiologic explanation for its antiarrhythmic actions.[329] Bretylium also increases the ventricular fibrillation threshold in normal and infarcted myocardium. It has been known to defibrillate a heart without electric countershock.[330]

Clinical Effects

Bretylium is effective in suppressing ventricular arrhythmias when other antiarrhythmics are not, including ventricular fibrillation resistant to electric countershock.[281] At present, it is indicated for the treatment of life-threatening ventricular arrhythmias, principally ventricular fibrillation and tachycardia that have failed to respond to adequate doses of the first-line agents lidocaine and procainamide.[331] Electrocardioversion is still the first line of treatment when ventricular fibrillation or ventricular tachycardia associated with hypotension is present. The drug is not used to suppress asymptomatic VPBs, nor is it used to treat atrial arrhythmias. There was no difference between lidocaine and bretylium as the initial treatment for ventricular fibrillation in one study.[332] There was no difference in out-of-hospital resuscitation of ventricular fibrillation when the number of patients achieving a stable rhythm, the time needed to achieve that rhythm, the number of defibrillation shocks required, and the numbers of patient discharged from the hospital were compared. In that study, none of the patients were defibrillated with electrocardioversion.[330]

Dosage

The dose of bretylium used to treat ventricular fibrillation or tachycardia is 5 to 10 mg/kg given by rapid IV bolus. If the drug can be given less urgently, 500 mg should be diluted in not less than 50 ml of fluid given over 10 minutes. The slower regimen decreases the incidence of nausea in the awake patient. Close monitoring, including an ECG and blood pressure, is critical during bretylium administration. Its onset of action in suppressing ventricular fibrillation and facilitating electrocardioversion is within minutes, although it can be delayed by up to 10 to 15 minutes. After an intramuscular injection, the drug is effective in 20 to 60 minutes. Its duration of action is 6 to 12 hours.[332]

After an IV dose of bretylium is given, an electric countershock should be administered. If the arrhythmia then persists, the drug can be repeated every 15 to 30 minutes, up to a total dose of 30 mg/kg. If the arrhythmia is abolished, a maintenance dose, the same as the initial dose, can be given every 6 to 8 hours. In treating ventricular tachycardia, the second dose should be repeated in 1 to 2 hours and then for maintenance every 6 to 8 hours. The drug can also be given by constant infusion at 1 to 2 mg/min in adults.

Adverse Effects

Hypertension due to norepinephrine release is the most commonly seen side effect due to bretylium. Sixteen percent of patients who received bretylium had an increase in blood pressure.[333] A slight increase in heart rate or an increase of the frequency of VPBs may be observed. In addition, bretylium appears to have an inotropic effect.[327]

After the initial hypertensive response, more than half of the patients subsequently show a mild decrease in blood pressure including orthostatic changes,[331] due to the adrenergic blocking effects of bretylium. If hypotension is severe, fluids and vasopressors should be given.[327] After receiving bretylium, a patient may have an exaggerated response to dopamine, norepinephrine, and epinephrine because of the impaired uptake of those drugs. When kept on maintenance doses, patients appear to be tolerant of the hypotensive effects of bretylium within days. With rapid infusions of the drug, nausea and vomiting are common. Parotid swelling and pain are complications of oral use of bretylium[331] (see Table 7–10).

CORRECTION OF UNDERLYING PATHOLOGY

CPR is not a definitive treatment for cardiac arrest but rather is a means of maintaining respiration and circulation until the underlying pathology can be corrected. In children, the inciting event is often related to the airway, and restoring the airway by initiating CPR can be therapeutic. Because of the limited efficacy of CPR, it is important to identify the underlying pathology as early as possible and correct it so that spontaneous circulation can be restored. During anesthesia, this often means restoring the airway, reducing the anesthetic level, or correcting vascular volume deficits. If electromechanical dissociation is present, hypovolemia, tension pneumothorax, and pericardial tamponade must be considered if no improvement occurs with restoration of the airway. If ventricular fibrillation is present, then electrolyte disorders, hypoglycemia, hypothermia, and digitalis or tricyclic antidepressant overdose must be considered. A list of precipitating and contributing factors is shown in Table 7–11.

T A B L E   7 – 1 1
CARDIAC ARREST DURING ANESTHESIA: PRECIPITATING AND CONTRIBUTING FACTORS

Acidosis
Adrenal insufficiency
Airway compromise (hypoxia, hypercarbia)
Anaphylaxis (latex or drug allergy)
Anesthetic overdose
Arrhythmias
   Primary
   Secondary (succinylcholine, central lines)
Drug intoxication
Electrolyte abnormality (hypocalcemia from citrate intoxication, hyperkalemia with release of vascular clamps)
Embolism (air, clot, fat)
Hemorrhage
Hypoglycemia
Hypothermia
Hypovolemia
Malignant hyperthermia
Myocardial ischemia
Pneumothorax
Seizures
Sepsis
Tamponade

REFERENCES

1. Rainer EH: Respiratory and cardiac arrest during anaesthesia in children. BMJ 2:1024, 1957.
2. Sladen A: Closed-chest massage. JAMA 251:3137, 1984.
3. Kouwenhoven WB, Jude JR, Knickerbocker GG: Closed-chest cardiac massage. JAMA 173:1064, 1960.
4. Jude JR, Kouwenhoven WB, Knickerbocker GG: Cardiac arrest: report of application of external cardiac massage on 118 patients. JAMA 178:1063, 1961.
5. Keenan RL, Boyan CP: Cardiac arrest due to anesthesia: a study of incidence and causes. JAMA 253:2373, 1985.
6. Olsson GL, Hallen B: Cardiac arrest during anaesthesia. A computer-aided study in 250543 anaesthetics. Acta Anaesthesiol Scand 32:653, 1988.
7. Cohen MM, Cameron CB, Duncan PG: Pediatric anesthesia morbidity and mortality in the perioperative period. Anesth Analg 70:160, 1990.
8. Keenan RL, Shapiro JH, Dawson KD: Frequency of anesthetic cardiac arrests in infants: effect of pediatric anesthesiologists. J Clin Anesth 3:433, 1991.
9. Crone RK: Frequency of anesthetic cardiac arrests in infants: effect of pediatric anesthesiologists. J Clin Anesth 3:431, 1991.
10. Flick R, Martin LD: Twelfth annual meeting of the Society for Pediatric Anesthesia, Orlando, Florida, October 16, 1998. Anesth Analg 88:955, 1999.
11. Lee CJ, Bullock LJ: Determining the pulse for infant CPR: time for a change? Mil Med 156:190, 1991.
12. Cavallaro DL, Melker RJ: Comparison of two techniques for detecting cardiac activity in infants. Crit Care Med 11:189, 1983.
13. Elam JO, Brown ES, Elder JD: Artificial respiration by mouth-to-mask method. N Engl J Med 250:749, 1954.
14. Safar P, Brown TC, Holtey WJ, Wilder RJ: Ventilation and circulation with closed-chest cardiac massage in man. JAMA 176:92, 1961.
15. American Heart Association's Guidelines for Cardiopulmonary Resuscitation and Emergency Cardiac Care. JAMA 268:2202, 1992.
16. Bhende MS, Thompson AE, Cook DR, Saville AL: Validity of a disposable end-tidal CO_2 detector in verifying endotracheal tube placement in infants and children. Ann Emerg Med 21:142, 1992.
17. Bhende MS, Thompson AE: Evaluation of an end-tidal CO_2 detector during pediatric cardiopulmonary resuscitation. Pediatrics 95:395, 1995.
18. Wilder RJ, Weir D, Rush BF, Ravitch MM: Methods of coordinating ventilation and closed chest cardiac massage in the dog. Surgery 53:186, 1963.
19. American Heart Association's Guidelines for Cardiopulmonary Resuscitation and Emergency Cardiac Care. JAMA 268:2200, 1992.
20. Weale FE, Rothwell-Jackson RL: The efficiency of cardiac massage. Lancet 1:990, 1962.
21. Rudikoff MT, Maughan WL, Effron M, et al: Mechanism of blood flow during cardiopulmonary resuscitation. Circulation 61:345, 1980.

22. Criley JM, Blaufuss AH, Kissel GL: Cough-induced cardiac compression: self-administered form of cardiopulmonary resuscitation. JAMA 236:1246, 1976.
23. Niemann JT, Rosborough JP, Hausknecht M, et al: Cough-CPR: documentation of systemic perfusion in man and in an experimental model: a "window" to the mechanism of blood flow in external CPR. Crit Care Med 8:141, 1980.
24. Harada Y, Fuxeno H, Ohtomo T, et al: Self-administered hyperventilation cardiopulmonary resuscitation for 100 s of cardiac arrest during Holter monitoring. Chest 99:1310, 1991.
25. MacKenzie GJ, Taylor SH, McDonald AH, Donald KW: Haemodynamic effects of external cardiac compression. Lancet 1:1342, 1964.
26. Chandra N, Weisfeldt ML, Tsitlik J, et al: Augmentation of carotid flow during cardiopulmonary resuscitation by ventilation at high airway pressure simultaneous with chest compression. Am J Cardiol 48:1053, 1981.
27. Niemann JT, Rosborough JP, Hausknecht M, et al: Blood flow without cardiac compression during closed chest CPR. Crit Care Med 9:380, 1981.
28. Cohen JM, Chandra M, Alderson PO, et al: Timing of pulmonary and systemic blood flow during intermittent high intrathoracic pressure cardiopulmonary resuscitation in the dog. Am J Cardiol 49:1883, 1982.
29. Raessler KL, Kern KB, Sanders AB, et al: Aortic and right atrial systolic pressures during cardiopulmonary resuscitation: a potential indicator of the mechanism of blood flow. Am Heart J 115:1021, 1988.
30. Swenson RD, Weaver WD, Niskanen RA, et al: Hemodynamics in humans during conventional and experimental methods of cardiopulmonary resuscitation. Circulation 78:630, 1988.
31. Paradis NA, Martin GB, Goetting MG, et al: Simultaneous aortic, jugular bulb, and right atrial pressures during cardiopulmonary resuscitation in humans: insights into mechanisms. Circulation 80:361, 1989.
32. Chandra N, Rudikoff M, Weisfeldt ML: Simultaneous chest compression and ventilation at high airway pressure during cardiopulmonary resuscitation. Lancet 1:175, 1980.
33. Niemann JT, Rosborough JP, Hausknecht M, et al: Pressure-synchronized cineangiography during experimental cardiopulmonary resuscitation. Circulation 64:985, 1981.
34. Fisher J, Vaghaiwall F, Tsitlik J, et al: Determinants and clinical significance of jugular venous valve competence. Circulation 65:188, 1982.
35. Guerci AD, Shi A, Levin H, et al: Transmission of intrathoracic pressure to the intracranial space during cardiopulmonary resuscitation in dogs. Circ Res 56:20, 1985.
36. Criley JM, Niemann JT, Rosborough JP, Hausknecht M: Modification of cardiopulmonary resuscitation based on the cough. Circulation 74(Suppl IV):IV-42, 1986.
37. Gudipati CV, Weil MH, Deshmukh HG, et al: Right atrial-jugular venous pressure gradients during experimental CPR. Chest 89:443s, 1986.
38. Chandra N, Tsitlik J, Halperin HR, et al: Observations of hemodynamics during human cardiopulmonary resuscitation. Crit Care Med 18:929, 1990.
39. Goetting MG, Paradis MA: Right atrial-jugular venous pressure gradients during CPR in children. Ann Emerg Med 20:27, 1991.
40. Goetting MG, Paradis NA, Appleton TJ, et al: Aortic-carotid artery pressure differences and cephalic perfusion pressure during cardiopulmonary resuscitation in humans. Crit Care Med 19:1012, 1991.
41. Rich S, Wix HL, Shapiro EP: Clinical assessment of heart size and valve motion during cardiopulmonary resuscitation by two-dimensional echocardiography. Am Heart J 102:368, 1981.
42. Werner JA, Greene HL, Janko CL, Cobb LA: Visualization of cardiac valve motion in man during external chest compression using two-dimensional echocardiography: implications regarding the mechanism of blood flow. Circulation 63:1417, 1981.
43. Clements FM, De Bruijn NP, Kisslo JA: Transesophageal echocardiographic observations in a patient undergoing closed-chest massage. Anesthesiology 64:826, 1986.
44. Feneley MP, Maier GW, Gaynor JW, et al: Sequence of mitral valve motion and transmitral blood flow during manual cardiopulmonary resuscitation in dogs. Circulation 76:363, 1987.
45. Hackl W, Simon P, Mauritz W, Steinbereithner K: Echocardiographic assessment of mitral valve function during mechanical cardiopulmonary resuscitation in pigs. Anesth Analg 70:350, 1990.
46. Babbs CF, Tacker WA, Paris RL, et al: CPR with simultaneous compression and ventilation at high airway pressure in 4 animal models. Crit Care Med 10:501, 1982.
47. Schleien CL, Dean JM, Koehler RC, et al: Effect of epinephrine on cerebral and myocardial perfusion in an infant animal preparation of cardiopulmonary resuscitation. Circulation 73:809, 1986.
48. Berkowitz ID, Chantarojanasiri T, Koehler RC, et al: Blood flow during cardiopulmonary resuscitation with simultaneous compression and ventilation in infant pigs. Pediatr Res 26:558, 1989.
49. Higano ST, Oh JK, Ewy GA, Seward JB: The mechanism of blood flow during closed chest cardiac massage in humans: transesophageal echocardiographic observations. Mayo Clin Proc 65:2, 1990.
50. Kuhn C, Juchems R, Frese W: Evidence for the 'cardiac pump theory' in cardiopulmonary resuscitation in man by transesophageal echocardiography. Resuscitation 22:275, 1991.
51. Beattie C, Guerci AD, Hall T, et al: Mechanisms of blood flow during pneumatic vest cardiopulmonary resuscitation. J Appl Physiol 70:454, 1991.
52. Michael JR, Guerci AD, Koehler RC, et al: Mechanisms by which epinephrine augments cerebral and myocardial blood perfusion during cardiopulmonary resuscitation in dogs. Circulation 69:822, 1984.
53. Shaffner DH, Eleff SM, Brambrink AM, et al: Effect of arrest time and cerebral perfusion pressure during cardiopulmonary resuscitation on cerebral blood flow, metabolism, ATP recovery, and pH in dogs. Crit Care Med 27:1335, 1999.
54. Shaffner DH, Eleff SM, Koehler RC, Traystman RJ: Effect of the no-flow interval and hypothermia on cerebral blood flow and metabolism during cardiopulmonary resuscitation in dogs. Stroke 29:2607, 1998.
55. Jackson DL, Dole WP, McGloin J, Rosenblatt JI: Total cerebral ischemia: application of a new model system to studies of cerebral microcirculation. Stroke 12:66, 1981.
56. Ditchey RV, Winkler JV, Rhodes CA: Relative lack of blood flow during closed-chest resuscitation in dogs. Circulation 66:297, 1982.
57. Maier GW, Tyson GS, Olsen CO, et al: The physiology of external cardiac massage: high-impulse cardiopulmonary resuscitation. Circulation 70:86, 1984.
58. Brown CG, Werman HA, Davis EA, et al: The effects of graded doses of epinephrine on regional myocardial blood flow during cardiopulmonary resuscitation in swine. Circulation 75:491, 1987.
59. Voorhees WD, Niebauer MJ, Babbs CF: Improved oxygen delivery during cardiopulmonary resuscitation with interposed abdominal compressions. Ann Emerg Med 12:128, 1983.
60. Sharff JA, Pantley G, Noel E: Effect of time on regional organ perfusion during two methods of cardiopulmonary resuscitation. Ann Emerg Med 13:649, 1984.
61. Koehler RC, Chandra N, Guerci AD, et al: Augmentation of cerebral perfusion by simultaneous chest compression and lung inflation with abdominal binding after cardiac arrest in dogs. Circulation 67:266, 1983.
62. Ralston SH, Voorhees WD, Babbs CF: Intrapulmonary epinephrine during prolonged cardiopulmonary resuscitation: improved regional blood flow and resuscitation in dogs. Ann Emerg Med 13:79, 1984.
63. American Heart Association's Guidelines for Cardiopulmonary Resuscitation and Emergency Cardiac Care. JAMA 255:2921, 1986.
64. Feneley MP, Maier GW, Kern KB, et al: Influence of compression rate on initial success of resuscitation and 24 hour survival after prolonged manual cardiopulmonary resuscitation in dogs. Circulation 77:240, 1988.
65. Halperin HR, Tsitlik JE, Guerci AD, et al: Determinants of blood flow to vital organs during cardiopulmonary resuscitation in dogs. Circulation 73:539, 1986.
66. Beyar R, Kishon Y, Sideman S, Dinnar U: Computer studies of systemic and regional blood flow mechanisms during cardiopulmonary resuscitation. Med Biol Eng Comput 22:499, 1984.
67. Halperin HR, Tsitlik JE, Beyar R, et al: Intrathoracic pressure fluctuations move blood during CPR: comparison of hemodynamic data with predictions from a mathematical model. Ann Biomed Eng 15:385, 1987.
68. Sanders AB, Kern KB, Fonken S, et al: The role of bicarbonate and fluid loading in improving resuscitation from prolonged cardiac arrest with rapid manual chest compression CPR. Ann Emerg Med 19:1, 1990.

69. Dean JM, Koehler RC, Schleien CL, et al: Age-related effects of compression rate and duration in cardiopulmonary resuscitation. J Appl Physiol 68:554, 1990.

70. Fleisher G, Delgado-Paredes C, Heyman S: Slow versus rapid closed-chest cardiac compression during cardiopulmonary resuscitation in puppies. Crit Care Med 15:939, 1987.

71. Taylor GJ, Tucker WM, Greene HL, et al: Importance of prolonged compression during cardiopulmonary resuscitation in man. N Engl J Med 296:1515, 1977.

72. Ornato JP, Gonzalez ER, Garnett AR, et al: Effect of cardiopulmonary resuscitation compression rate on end-tidal carbon dioxide concentration and arterial pressure in man. Crit Care Med 16:241, 1988.

73. American Heart Association's Guidelines for Cardiopulmonary Resuscitation and Emergency Cardiac Care. JAMA 268:2256, 1992.

74. Dean JM, Koehler RC, Schleien CL, et al: Age-related changes in chest geometry during cardiopulmonary resuscitation. J Appl Physiol 62:2212, 1987.

75. Dean JM, Koehler RC, Schleien CL, et al: Improved blood flow during prolonged cardiopulmonary resuscitation with 30% duty cycle in infant pigs. Circulation 84:896, 1991.

76. Shaffner DH, Schleien CL, Koehler RC, et al: Cerebral and coronary perfusion with vest cardiopulmonary resuscitation in piglets. Crit Care Med 18:S243, 1990.

77. Luce JM, Rizk NA, Niskanen RA: Regional blood flow during cardiopulmonary resuscitation in dogs. Crit Care Med 12:874, 1984.

78. Bircher N, Safar P: Comparison of standard and "new" closed-chest CPR and open-chest CPR in dogs. Crit Care Med 9:384, 1981.

79. Jackson RE, Joyce K, Danosi SF, et al: Blood flow in the cerebral cortex during cardiac resuscitation in dogs. Ann Emerg Med 13:657, 1984.

80. Koehler RC, Michael JR, Guerci AD, et al: Beneficial effect of epinephrine infusion on cerebral and myocardial blood flow during CPR. Ann Emerg Med 14:744, 1985.

81. Rogers MC, Nugent SK, Stidham GL: Effects of closed-chest cardiac massage on intracranial pressure. Crit Care Med 7:454, 1979.

82. Lee SK, Vaagenes P, Safar P, et al: Effect of cardiac arrest time on cortical cerebral blood flow generated by subsequent standard external cardiopulmonary resuscitation in rabbits. Ann Emerg Med 13:385, 1984.

83. Sanders AB, Atlas M, Ewy GA, et al: Expired PCO_2 as an index of coronary perfusion pressure. Am J Emerg Med 3:147, 1985.

84. Paradis NA, Martin GB, Rivers EP, et al: Coronary perfusion pressure and the return of spontaneous circulation in human cardiopulmonary resuscitation. JAMA 263:1106, 1990.

85. Snyder AV, Salloum LJ, Barone JE, et al: Predicting short-term outcome of cardiopulmonary resuscitation using central venous oxygen tension measurements. Crit Care Med 19:111, 1991.

86. Rivers EP, Martin GB, Smithine H, et al: The clinical implications of continuous central venous oxygen saturation during human CPR. Ann Emerg Med 21:1094, 1992.

87. Callaham M, Barton C: Prediction of outcome of cardiopulmonary resuscitation from end-tidal carbon dioxide concentration. Crit Care Med 19:358, 1990.

88. Wayne MA, Levine RL, Miller CC: Use of end-tidal carbon dioxide to predict outcome in prehospital cardiac arrest. Ann Emerg Med 25:762, 1995.

89. Levine RL, Wayne MA, Miller CC: End-tidal carbon dioxide and outcome of out-of-hospital cardiac arrest. N Engl J Med 337:301, 1997.

90. Sanders AB, Kern KB, Otto CW, et al: End-tidal carbon dioxide monitoring during cardiopulmonary resuscitation: a prognostic indicator for survival. JAMA 262:1347, 1989.

91. Barton C, Callaham M: Lack of correlation between end-tidal carbon dioxide concentrations and $PaCO_2$ in cardiac arrest. Crit Care Med 19:108, 1991.

92. Garnett AR, Ornato JP, Gonzales ER, Johnson EB: End-tidal carbon dioxide monitoring during cardiopulmonary resuscitation. JAMA 257:512, 1987.

93. Gazmuri RJ, Weil MH, Bisera J, Rackow EC: End-tidal carbon dioxide tension as a monitor of native blood flow during resuscitation by extracorporeal circulation. J Thorac Cardiovasc Surg 101:984, 1991.

94. Nakatani K, Yukioka H, Fujimori M, et al: Utility of colorimetric end-tidal carbon dioxide detector for monitoring during prehospital cardiopulmonary resuscitation. Am J Emerg Med 17:203, 1999.

95. Martin GB, Gentile NT, Paradis NA, et al: Effect of epinephrine on end-tidal carbon dioxide monitoring during CPR. Ann Emerg Med 19:396, 1990.

96. Muir JD, Randalls PR, Smith GB: End tidal carbon dioxide detector for monitoring cardiopulmonary resuscitation. BMJ 301:41, 1990.

97. Sun W, Huang F, Kung K, et al: Successful cardiopulmonary resuscitation of two patients in the prone position reversed precordial compression. Anesthesiology 77:202, 1992.

98. Kern KB, Carter AB, Showen RL, et al: Manual versus mechanical cardiopulmonary resuscitation in an experimental canine model. Crit Care Med 13:899, 1985.

99. Taylor GJ, Rubin R, Tucker M, et al: External cardiac compression: a randomized comparison of mechanical and manual techniques. JAMA 240:644, 1978.

100. American Heart Association's Guidelines for Cardiopulmonary Resuscitation and Emergency Cardiac Care. JAMA 268:2204, 1992.

101. Todres ID, Rogers MC: Methods of external cardiac massage in the newborn infant. J Pediatr 86:781, 1975.

102. David R: Closed chest cardiac massage in the newborn infant. Pediatrics 81:552, 1988.

103. Harris LC, Kirimli B, Safar P: Ventilation-cardiac compression rates and ratios in cardiopulmonary resuscitation. Anesthesiology 28:806, 1967.

104. Luce JM, Ross BK, O'Quin RJ, et al: Regional blood flow during cardiopulmonary resuscitation in dogs using simultaneous and non-simultaneous compression and ventilation. Circulation 67:258, 1983.

105. Babbs CF, Fitzgerald KR, Voorhees WD, Murphy RJ: High-pressure ventilation during CPR with 95% O_2:5% CO_2. Crit Care Med 10:505, 1982.

106. Sanders AB, Ewy GA, Alferness CA, et al: Failure of one method of simultaneous chest compression, ventilation, and abdominal binding during CPR. Crit Care Med 10:50913, 1982.

107. Martin GB, Carden DL, Nowak RM, et al: Aortic and right atrial pressures during standard and simultaneous compression and ventilation CPR in human beings. Ann Emerg Med 15:125, 1986.

108. Krischer JP, Fine EF, Weisfeldt ML, et al: Comparison of prehospital conventional and simultaneous compression-ventilation cardiopulmonary resuscitation. Crit Care Med 17:1263, 1989.

109. Niemann JT, Rosborough JP, Ung S, Criley JM: Hemodynamic effects of continuous abdominal binding during cardiac arrest and resuscitation. Am J Cardiol 53:269, 1984.

110. Lee HR, Wilder RJ, Downs P, et al: MAST augmentation of external cardiac compression: role of changing intrapleural pressure. Ann Emerg Med 10:560, 1981.

111. Chandra N, Snyder LD, Weisfeldt ML: Abdominal binding during cardiopulmonary resuscitation in man. JAMA 246:351, 1981.

112. Lilja GP, Long RS, Ruiz E: Augmentation of systolic blood pressure during external cardiac compression by use of the MAST suit. Ann Emerg Med 10:182, 1981.

113. Mahoney BD, Mirick MJ: Efficacy of pneumatic trousers in refractory prehospital cardiopulmonary arrest. Ann Emerg Med 12:8, 1983.

114. Niemann JT, Rosborough JP, Pelikin PCD: Hemodynamic determinants of subdiaphragmatic venous return during closed-chest CPR in a canine cardiac arrest model. Ann Emerg Med 19:1232, 1990.

115. Redding JS: Abdominal compression in cardiopulmonary resuscitation. Anesth Analg 50:668, 1971.

116. Ralston SH, Babbs CF, Niebauer MJ: Cardiopulmonary resuscitation with interposed abdominal compression in dogs. Anesth Analg 61:645, 1982.

117. Einagle V, Bertrand F, Wise RA, et al: Interposed abdominal compressions and carotid blood flow during cardiopulmonary resuscitation. Chest 93:1206, 1988.

118. Walker JW, Bruestle JC, White BC, et al: Perfusion of the cerebral cortex by use of abdominal counterpulsation during cardiopulmonary resuscitation. Am J Emerg Med 2:391, 1984.

119. Eberle B, Schleien CL, Shaffner DH, et al: Effects of three modes of abdominal compression on vital organ blood flow in a piglet CPR model. Anesthesiology 73:A300, 1990.

120. Berryman CR, Phillips GM: Interposed abdominal compression-CPR in human subjects. Ann Emerg Med 13:226, 1984.

121. Howard M, Carruba C, Guiness M, et al: Interposed abdominal compression CPR: its effects on coronary perfusion pressure in human subjects. Ann Emerg Med 13:989, 1984.

122. Howard M, Carruba C, Foss F, et al: Interposed abdominal compression-CPR: its effects on parameters of coronary perfusion in human subjects. Ann Emerg Med 16:253, 1987.

123. Ward KR, Sullivan RJ, Zelenak RR, Summer WR: A comparison of interposed abdominal compression CPR and standard CPR by monitoring end-tidal PCO$_2$. Ann Emerg Med 18:831, 1989.
124. Barranco F, Lesmes A, Irles JA, et al: Cardiopulmonary resuscitation with simultaneous chest and abdominal compression: comparative study in humans. Resuscitation 20:67, 1990.
125. Mateer JR, Stueben HA, Thompson BM, et al: Pre-hospital IAC-CPR versus standard CPR: paramedic resuscitation of cardiac arrests. Am J Emerg Med 3:143, 1985.
126. Sack JB, Kesselbrenner MB, Bregman D: Survival from in-hospital cardiac arrest with interposed abdominal counterpulsation during cardiopulmonary resuscitation. JAMA 267:379, 1992.
127. Halperin HR, Guerci AD, Chandra N, et al: Vest inflation without simultaneous ventilation during cardiac arrest in dogs: improved survival from prolonged cardiopulmonary resuscitation. Circulation 74:1407, 1986.
128. Halperin HR, Tsitlik JE, Gelfand M, et al: A preliminary study of cardiopulmonary resuscitation by circumferential compression of the chest with use of a pneumatic vest. N Engl J Med 329:762, 1993.
129. Eleff SM, Schleien C, Koehler RC, et al: Brain bioenergetics during cardiopulmonary resuscitation. Anesthesiology 76:77, 1992.
130. Beyar R, Halperin HR, Tsitlik JE, et al: Circulatory assistance by intrathoracic pressure variations: optimization and mechanisms studied by a mathematical model in relation to experimental data. Circ Res 64:703, 1989.
131. Chandra NC, Beyar R, Halperin HR, et al: Vital organ perfusion during assisted circulation by manipulation of intrathoracic pressure. Circulation 84:279, 1991.
132. Kernstine KH, Tyson GS, Maier GW, et al: Determinants of direct cardiac compression during external cardiac massage in intact dogs. Crit Care Med 10:231, 1982.
133. Kern KB, Carter AB, Showen RL, et al: Twenty-four hour survival in a canine model of cardiac arrest comparing three methods of manual cardiopulmonary resuscitation. J Am Coll Cardiol 7:859, 1986.
134. Cohen TJ, Tucker KJ, Lurie KG, et al: Active compression-decompression. A new method of cardiopulmonary resuscitation. Cardiopulmonary Resuscitation Working Group. JAMA 267:2916, 1992.
135. Cohen TJ, Goldner BG, Maccaro PC, et al: A comparison of active compression-decompression cardiopulmonary resuscitation with standard cardiopulmonary resuscitation for cardiac arrests occurring in the hospital. N Engl J Med 329:1918, 1993.
136. Stiell IG, Hebert PC, Wells GA, et al: The Ontario trial of active compression-decompression cardiopulmonary resuscitation for in-hospital and prehospital cardiac arrest. JAMA 275:1417, 1996.
137. Lurie KG, Shultz JJ, Callaham ML, et al: Evaluation of active compression-decompression CPR in victims of out-of-hospital cardiac arrest. JAMA 271:1405, 1994.
138. Schwab TM, Callaham ML, Madsen CD, Utecht TA: A randomized clinical trial of active compression-decompression CPR vs standard CPR in out-of-hospital cardiac arrest in two cities. JAMA 273:1261, 1995.
139. Mauer D, Schneider T, Dick W, et al: Active compression-decompression resuscitation: a prospective, randomized study in a two-tiered EMS system with physicians in the field. Resuscitation 33:125, 1996.
140. Nolan J, Smith G, Evans R, et al: The United Kingdom pre-hospital study of active compression-decompression resuscitation. Resuscitation 37:119, 1998.
141. Plaisance P, Adnet F, Vicaut E, et al: Benefit of active compression-decompression cardiopulmonary resuscitation as a prehospital advanced cardiac life support. A randomized multicenter study. Circulation 95:955, 1997.
142. Tang W, Weil MH, Schock RB: Phased chest and abdominal compression-decompression. A new option for cardiopulmonary resuscitation. Circulation 95:1335, 1997.
143. Bartlett RL, Stewart NJ, Taymond J, et al: Comparative study of three methods of resuscitation: closed-chest, open chest manual, and direct mechanical ventricular assistance. Ann Emerg Med 13:773, 1984.
144. Weiser FM, Adler LN, Kuhn LA: Hemodynamic effects of closed and open chest cardiac resuscitation in normal dogs and those with acute myocardial infarction. Am J Cardiol 10:555, 1962.
145. Bircher N, Safar P, Stewart R: A comparison of standard, "MAST"-augmented, and open-chest CPR in dogs: a preliminary investigation. Crit Care Med 8:147, 1980.
146. Del Guercio LR, Feins NR, Cohn JD, et al: Comparison of blood flow during external and internal cardiac massage in man. Circulation 32(Suppl I):I-171, 1965.
147. Sanders AB, Ewy GA, Taft TV: Prognostic and therapeutic importance of the aortic diastolic pressure in resuscitation from cardiac arrest. Crit Care Med 12:871, 1984.
148. Sanders AB, Kern KB, Ewy GA, et al: Improved outcome from cardiac arrest with open-chest massage. Ann Emerg Med 13:672, 1984.
149. Sanders AB, Kern KB, Ewy GA: Time limitations for open-chest cardiopulmonary resuscitation from cardiac arrest. Crit Care Med 13:897, 1985.
150. American Heart Association's Guidelines for Cardiopulmonary Resuscitation and Emergency Cardiac Care. JAMA 268:2171, 1992.
151. Levine R, Gorayeb M, Safar P, et al: Cardiopulmonary bypass after cardiac arrest and prolonged closed-chest CPR in dogs. Ann Emerg Med 16:620, 1987.
152. Pretto E, Safar P, Saito R, et al: Cardiopulmonary bypass after prolonged cardiac arrest in dogs. Ann Emerg Med 16:611, 1987.
153. Reich H, Angelos M, Safar P, Leonov Y: Cardiac resuscitability with cardiopulmonary bypass after increasing ventricular fibrillation times in dogs. Ann Emerg Med 19:887, 1990.
154. Angelos MG, Gaddis ML, Gaddis GM, Leasure JE: Improved survival and reduced myocardial necrosis with cardiopulmonary bypass reperfusion in a canine model of coronary occlusion and cardiac arrest. Ann Emerg Med 19:1122, 1990.
155. Phillips SJ, Ballentine B, Slonine D, et al: Percutaneous initiation of cardiopulmonary bypass. Ann Thorac Surg 36:223, 1983.
156. Mattox KL, Beall AC: Resuscitation of the moribund patient using portable cardiopulmonary bypass. Ann Thorac Surg 22:436, 1976.
157. Hartz R, LoCicero J, Sanders JH, et al: Clinical experience with portable cardiopulmonary bypass in cardiac arrest patients. Ann Thorac Surg 50:437, 1990.
158. Reichman RT, Joyo CI, Dembitsky WP, et al: Improved patient survival after cardiac arrest using a cardiopulmonary support system. Ann Thorac Surg 49:101, 1990.
159. Martin GB, Rivers EP, Paradis NA, et al: Emergency department cardiopulmonary bypass in the treatment of human cardiac arrest. Chest 113:743, 1998.
160. Lee G, Antognini JF, Gronert GA: Complete recovery after prolonged resuscitation and cardiopulmonary bypass for hyperkalemic cardiac arrest. Anesth Analg 79:172, 1994.
161. Cochran JB, Tecklenburg FW, Lau YR, Habib DM: Emergency cardiopulmonary bypass for cardiac arrest refractory to pediatric advanced life support. Pediatr Emerg Care 15:30, 1999.
162. Tisherman SA, Safar P, Abramson NS, et al: Feasibility of emergency cardiopulmonary bypass for resuscitation from CPR-resistant cardiac arrest—a preliminary report. Ann Emerg Med 20:491, 1991.
163. Redding JS, Pearson JW: Evaluation for drugs for cardiac resuscitation. Anesthesiology 24:203, 1963.
164. Pearson JW, Redding JS: Influence of peripheral vascular tone on resuscitation. Anesth Analg 44:746, 1965.
165. Yakaitis RW, Otto CW, Blitt CD: Relative importance of alpha and beta adrenergic receptors during resuscitation. Crit Care Med 7:293, 1979.
166. Koehler RC, Michael JR: Cardiopulmonary resuscitation, brain blood flow, and neurologic recovery. Crit Care Clin 1:205, 1985.
167. Livesay JJ, Follette DM, Fey KH, et al: Optimizing myocardial supply/demand balance with alpha-adrenergic drugs during cardiopulmonary resuscitation. J Thorac Cardiovasc Surg 76:244, 1978.
168. Downey J, Chagrasulis RW, Hemphill V: Quantitative study of intramyocardial compression in the fibrillating heart. Am J Physiol 237:H191, 1979.
169. Schleien CL, Koehler RC, Gervais H, et al: Organ blood flow and somatosensory evoked potentials before and after cardiopulmonary resuscitation with epinephrine and phenylephrine. Circulation 79:1332, 1989.
170. Brown CG, Werman HA, Davis EA, et al: The effect of high-dose phenylephrine versus epinephrine on regional cerebral flow during CPR. Ann Emerg Med 16:743, 1987.
171. Brown CG, Davis EA, Werman RL: Methoxamine versus epinephrine on regional cerebral blood flow during cardiopulmonary resuscitation. Crit Care Med 15:682, 1987.
172. Holmes HR, Babbs CF, Voorhees WD, et al: Influence of adrenergic drugs upon vital organ perfusion during CPR. Crit Care Med 8:137, 1980.

173. Brillman JA, Sanders AB, Otto CW, et al: Outcome of resuscitation from fibrillatory arrest using epinephrine and phenylephrine in dogs. Crit Care Med 13:912, 1985.
174. Brown CG, Birinyi F, Werman HA, et al: The comparative effects of epinephrine versus phenylephrine on regional cerebral blood flow during cardiopulmonary resuscitation. Resuscitation 14:171, 1986.
175. Carlsson C, Hagerdal M, Kaasid AE, Siesjo BK: A catecholamine-mediated increase in cerebral oxygen uptake during immobilization stress in rats. Brain Res 119:223, 1977.
176. MacKenzie ET, McCulloch J, O'Keane M, et al: Cerebral circulation and norepinephrine: relevance of the blood-brain barrier. Am J Physiol 231:483, 1976.
177. Winquist RJ, Webb RC, Bohr OF: Relaxation to transmural nerve stimulation and exogenously added norepinephrine in porcine vessels. A study utilizing cerebrovascular intrinsic tone. Circ Res 51:769, 1982.
178. Edvinsson L, Hardebo JE, MacKenzie ET, Owman C: Effect of endogenous noradrenaline on local cerebral blood flow after osmotic opening of the blood-brain barrier in the rat. J Physiol (Lond) 274:149, 1978.
179. Lasbennes F, Sercombe R, Seylaz J: Monoamine oxidase activity in brain microvessels determined using natural and artificial substances: relevance to the blood-brain barrier. J Cereb Blood Flow Metab 3:521, 1983.
180. Arai T, Watanabe T, Nagaro T, Matsuo S: Blood-brain barrier impairment after cardiac resuscitation. Crit Care Med 9:444, 1981.
181. Schleien CL, Koehler RC, Shaffner DH, et al: Blood-brain barrier disruption after cardiopulmonary resuscitation in immature swine. Stroke 22:477, 1991.
182. Schleien CL, Caceres MJ, Kuluz JW, et al: Light and electron microscopic blood-brain barrier (BBB) changes following cardiopulmonary resuscitation in young piglets. Anesthesiology 77(Suppl IIIA):712, 1992.
183. American Heart Association's Guidelines for Cardiopulmonary Resuscitation and Emergency Cardiac Care. JAMA 268:2268, 1992.
184. Berkowitz ID, Gervais H, Schleien CL, et al: Epinephrine dosage effects on cerebral and myocardial blood flow in an infant swine model of cardiopulmonary resuscitation. Anesthesiology 75:1041, 1991.
185. Brown CG, Werman HA, Davis EA, et al: Comparative effects of graded doses of epinephrine on regional brain blood flow during CPR in a swine model. Ann Emerg Med 15:1138, 1986.
186. Brown CG, Taylor RB, Werman HA, et al: Effect of standard doses of epinephrine on myocardial oxygen delivery and utilization during cardiopulmonary resuscitation. Crit Care Med 16:536, 1988.
187. Brown CG, Taylor RB, Werman HA, et al: Myocardial oxygen delivery/consumption during cardiopulmonary resuscitation: a comparison of epinephrine and phenylephrine. Ann Emerg Med 17:302, 1988.
188. Ditchey RV, Lindenfeld J: Failure of epinephrine to improve the balance between myocardial oxygen supply and demand during closed chest resuscitation in dogs. Circulation 78:382, 1988.
189. Gonzalez ER, Ornato JP, Levine RL: Vasopressor effect of epinephrine with and without dopamine during cardiopulmonary resuscitation. Drug Intell Clin Pharm 22:868, 1988.
190. Gonzalez ER, Ornato JP, Garnett AR, et al: Dose-dependent vasopressor response to epinephrine during CPR in human beings. Ann Emerg Med 18:920, 1989.
191. Goetting MG, Paradis NA: High dose epinephrine in refractory pediatric cardiac arrest. Crit Care Med 17:1258, 1989.
192. Martin D, Werman HA, Brown CG: Four case studies: high dose epinephrine in cardiac arrest. Ann Emerg Med 19:322, 1990.
193. Cipolotti G, Paccagnella A, Simini G: Successful cardiopulmonary resuscitation using high doses of epinephrine. Int J Cardiol 33:430, 1991.
194. Stiell IG, Hebert PC, Weitzman BN, et al: High-dose epinephrine in adult cardiac arrest. N Engl J Med 327:1045, 1992.
195. Brown CG, Martin DR, Pepe PE, et al: A comparison of standard-dose and high-dose epinephrine in cardiac arrest outside the hospital. N Engl J Med 327:1051, 1992.
196. Callaham M, Madsen CD, Barton CW, et al: A randomized clinical trial of high-dose epinephrine and norepinephrine vs standard-dose epinephrine in prehospital cardiac arrest. JAMA 268:2667, 1992.
197. Schleien CL, Kuluz JW, Shaffner DH, Rogers MC: Cardiopulmonary resuscitation. In Rogers MC (ed): Textbook of Pediatric Intensive Care. 2nd ed. Baltimore, Williams & Wilkins, Baltimore, 1992, p 52.
198. Tang W, Weil MH, Gazmuri RJ, et al: Pulmonary ventilation/perfusion defects induced by epinephrine during cardiopulmonary resuscitation. Circulation 84:2101, 1991.
199. Lindner KH, Brinkmann A, Pfenninger EG, et al: Effect of vasopressin on hemodynamic variables, organ blood flow, and acid-base status in a pig model of cardiopulmonary resuscitation. Anesth Analg 77:427, 1993.
200. Lindner KH, Prengel AW, Pfenninger EG, et al: Vasopressin improves vital organ blood flow during closed-chest cardiopulmonary resuscitation in pigs. Circulation 91:215, 1995.
201. Prengel AW, Lindner KH, Keller A: Cerebral oxygenation during cardiopulmonary resuscitation with epinephrine and vasopressin in pigs. Stroke 27:1241, 1996.
202. Strohmenger HU, Lindner KH, Keller A, et al: Effects of graded doses of vasopressin on median fibrillation frequency in a porcine model of cardiopulmonary resuscitation: results of a prospective, randomized, controlled trial. Crit Care Med 24:1360, 1996.
203. Morris DC, Dereczyk BE, Grzybowski M, et al: Vasopressin can increase coronary perfusion pressure during human cardiopulmonary resuscitation. Acad Emerg Med 4:878, 1997.
204. Prengel AW, Lindner KH, Keller A, et al: Cardiovascular function during the postresuscitation phase after cardiac arrest in pigs: a comparison of epinephrine versus vasopressin. Crit Care Med 24:2014, 1996.
205. Prengel AW, Lindner KH, Wenzel V, et al: Splanchnic and renal blood flow after cardiopulmonary resuscitation with epinephrine and vasopressin in pigs. Resuscitation 38:19, 1998.
206. Lindner KH, Prengel AW, Brinkmann A, et al: Vasopressin administration in refractory cardiac arrest. Ann Intern Med 124:1061, 1996.
207. Lindner KH, Dirks B, Strohmenger HU, et al: Randomised comparison of epinephrine and vasopressin in patients with out-of-hospital ventricular fibrillation. Lancet 349:535, 1997.
208. Stacpoole PAW: Lactic acidosis: the case against bicarbonate therapy. Ann Intern Med 105:276, 1986.
209. Guerci AD, Chandra N, Johnson E, et al: Failure of sodium bicarbonate to improve resuscitation from ventricular fibrillation in dogs. Circulation 74:IV-75, 1986.
210. Graf H, Leach W, Arieff AI: Evidence for a detrimental effect of bicarbonate therapy in hypoxic lactic acidosis. Science 227:754, 1985.
211. Cingolani HE, Mattiazi AR, Blesa ES: Contractility in isolated mammalian heart muscle after acid-base changes. Circ Res 26:269, 1970.
212. Pannier JL, Leusen I: Contraction characteristics of papillary muscle during changes in acid-base composition of the bathing fluid. Arch Int Physiol Biochem 76:624, 1968.
213. Steinhart CR, Permutt S, Gurtner GH, Traystman RJ: Beta-adrenergic activity and cardiovascular response to severe respiratory acidosis. Am J Physiol 244:H46, 1983.
214. Orlowski JP: Cardiopulmonary resuscitation in children. Pediatr Clin North Am 27:495, 1980.
215. Wood WB, Manley ES Jr, Woodbury RA: The effects of CO_2 induced respiratory acidosis on the depressor and pressor components of the dog's blood pressure to epinephrine. J Pharmacol Exp Ther 139:238, 1963.
216. Rudolph AM, Yuan S: Response of the pulmonary vasculature to hypoxia and hydrogen ion concentration changes. J Clin Invest 45:399, 1966.
217. Martinez LR, Holland S, Fitzgerald J, Kountz S: pH homeostasis during cardiopulmonary resuscitation in critically ill patients. Resuscitation 7:109, 1979.
218. Worthley LS: Sodium bicarbonate in cardiac arrest. Lancet 2:903, 1976.
219. Mattar JA, Weil MH, Shubin H, Stein L: Cardiac arrest in the critically ill: II. Hyperosmolal states following cardiac arrest. Am J Med 56:162, 1974.
220. Bishop RL, Weisfeldt ML: Sodium bicarbonate administration during cardiac arrest: effect on arterial pH, PCO_2, and osmolality. JAMA 235:506, 1976.
221. Grundler W, Weil MH, Rackow EC: Arteriovenous carbon dioxide and pH gradients during cardiac arrest. Circulation 77:234, 1988.
222. Weil MH, Rackow EC, Trevino R, et al: Differences in acid-base state between venous and arterial blood during cardiopulmonary resuscitation. N Engl J Med 315:153, 1986.

223. Desmukh HG, Gudipati CV, Weil MH, et al: Myocardial respiratory acidosis during CPR. Crit Care Med 14:433, 1986.
224. Falk JL, Rackow EC, Weil MH: End-tidal carbon dioxide concentration during cardiopulmonary resuscitation. N Engl J Med 318:607, 1988.
225. Sessler D, Mills P, Gregory G, et al: Effects of bicarbonate on arterial and brain intracellular pH in neonatal rabbits recovering from hypoxic lactic acidosis. J Pediatr 111:817, 1987.
226. Cohen Y, Chang LH, Litt L, et al: Stability of brain intracellular pH during prolonged hypercapnia in rats. J Cereb Blood Flow Metab 10:277, 1990.
227. Eleff SM, Schleien CL, Koehler RC, et al: Brain bioenergetics during cardiopulmonary resuscitation in dogs. Anesthesiology 76:77, 1992.
228. Gazmuri RJ, Planta M, Weil MH, Rackow EC: Cardiac effects of carbon dioxide-consuming and carbon dioxide-generating buffers during cardiopulmonary resuscitation. JAMA 15:482, 1990.
229. Sun JH, Filley GF, Hord K, et al: Carbicarb: an effective substitute for NaHCO$_3$ for the treatment of acidosis. Surgery 102:835, 1987.
230. Bersin RM, Arieff AI: Improved hemodynamic function during hypoxia with Carbicarb, a new agent for the management of acidosis. Circulation 77:227, 1988.
231. Stacpoole PAW: The pharmacology of dichloroacetate. Metab Clin Exp 38:1124, 1989.
232. Stacpoole PAW, Lorenz AC, Thomas RG, Harman EM: Dichloroacetate in the treatment of lactic acidosis. Ann Intern Med 108:58, 1988.
233. Wargovich TJ, MacDonald RG, Hill JA, et al: Myocardial metabolic and hemodynamic effects of dichloroacetate in coronary artery disease. Am J Cardiol 61:65, 1988.
234. Stacpoole PAW, Gonzalez MG, Vlasak J, et al: Dichloroacetate derivatives. Metabolic effects and pharmacodynamics in normal rats. Life Sci 41:2167, 1987.
235. Stacpoole PAW, Wright EC, Baumgartner TG: A controlled clinical trial of dichloroacetate for treatment of lactic acidosis in adults. N Engl J Med 327:1564, 1992.
236. Katz AM, Reuter M: Cellular calcium and cardiac cell death. Am J Cardiol 44:188, 1979.
237. White BC, Winegar CD, Wilson RF, et al: Possible role of calcium blockers in cerebral resuscitation: a review of the literature and synthesis for future studies. Crit Care Med 11:202, 1983.
238. Greenblatt DJ, Gross PL, Bolognini V: Pharmacotherapy of cardiopulmonary arrest. Am J Hosp Pharm 33:379, 1976.
239. Bristow MR, Schwartz HD, Binetti G, et al: Ionized calcium and the heart. Elucidation of in vivo concentration-response relationships in the open chest dog. Circ Res 41:565, 1977.
240. Drop LJ, Scheidegger D: Plasma ionized calcium concentration: important determinant of the hemodynamic response to calcium infusion. J Thorac Cardiovasc Surg 79:425, 1980.
241. Marquez J, Martin D, Virja MA, et al: Cardiovascular depression secondary to ionic hypocalcemia during hepatic transplantation in humans. Anesthesiology 65:457, 1986.
242. Scheidegger D, Drop LJ, Laver MB: Interaction between vasoactive drugs and plasma ionized calcium. Intensive Care Med 3:200, 1977.
243. Urban P, Scheidegger D, Buchmann B, Skarvan K: The hemodynamic effects of heparin and their relation to ionized calcium levels. J Thorac Cardiovasc Surg 91:303, 1986.
244. Urban P, Scheidegger D, Buchmann B, Barth D: Cardiac arrest and blood ionized calcium levels. Ann Intern Med 109:110, 1988.
245. Dembo DH: Calcium in advanced life support. Crit Care Med 9:358, 1981.
246. Stueven HA, Thompson BM, Aprahamian C, et al: The effectiveness of calcium chloride in refractory electromechanical dissociation. Ann Emerg Med 14:626, 1985.
247. Stueven HA, Aprahamian C, Tonsfeldt DJ, Kastenson EH: Lack of effectiveness of calcium chloride in refractory asystole. Ann Emerg Med 14:630, 1985.
248. Clark RE, Kristlieb IY, Henry PD: Nifedipine: a myocardial protective agent. Am J Cardiol 44:825, 1979.
249. Burke TJ, Arnold PE, Gordon JA, et al: Protective effect of intrarenal calcium membrane blockers before or after renal ischemia: functional, morphological, and mitochondrial studies. J Clin Invest 74:1830, 1984.
250. Holthoff V, Beil C, Hartmann-Klosterkotter U, et al: Effect of nimodipine on glucose metabolism in stroke patients. Stroke 21:IV95, 1990.
251. Resnekov L: Calcium antagonist drugs—myocardial preservation and reduced vulnerability to ventricular fibrillation during CPR. Crit Care Med 9:360, 1981.
252. Denlinger JK, Nahrwold MLL, Gibbs PS, Lecky JH: Hypocalcemia during rapid blood transfusion in anaesthetized man. Br J Anaesth 48:995, 1976.
253. Heining MPD, Band DM, Linton RAF: Choice of calcium salt: a comparison of the effects of calcium chloride and gluconate on plasma ionized calcium. Anaesthesia 39:1079, 1984.
254. Gillette PC, Garson A: Pediatric Cardiac Dysrhythmias, 1981. New York, Grune & Stratton, 1981.
255. Gilman AG, Rall TW, Nies AS, Taylor P: Goodman and Gilman's The Pharmacological Basis of Therapeutics. 8th ed. Elmsford, NY, Pergamon Press, 1990.
256. Goldberg AH: Cardiopulmonary arrest. N Engl J Med 290:381, 1974.
257. Scheinman MM, Thorburn D, Abbott JA: Use of atropine in patients with acute myocardial infarction and sinus bradycardia. Circulation 52:627, 1975.
258. Kottmeier CA, Gravenstein JS: The parasympathomimetic activity of atropine and atropine methylbromide. Anesthesiology 29:1125, 1968.
259. Myers R: Lactic acid accumulation as a cause of brain edema and cerebral necrosis resulting from oxygen deprivation. In Korbin R, Gilleminault C (eds): Advances in Perinatal Neurology. New York, Spectrum, 1979, p 84.
260. Siemkowicz E, Hansen AJ: Clinical restitution following cerebral ischemia in hypo-, normo- and hyperglycemic rats. Acta Neurol Scand 58:1, 1978.
261. Siesjo BK: Cerebral circulation and metabolism. Neurosurgery 60:883, 1984.
262. Chopp M, Welch KMA, Tidwell CD, Helpern JA: Global cerebral ischemia and intracellular pH during hyperglycemia and hypoglycemia in cats. Stroke 19:1383, 1988.
263. Prado R, Ginsberg MD, Dietrich WD, et al: Hyperglycemia increases infarct size in collaterally perfused but not end-arterial vascular territories. J Cereb Blood Flow Metab 8:186, 1988.
264. Pulsinelli WA, Levy DE, Sigsbee B, et al: Increased damage after ischemic stroke in patients with hyperglycemia with or without established diabetes mellitus. Am J Med 74:540, 1983.
265. Longstreth WT, Inui TS: High blood glucose level on hospital admission and poor neurological recovery after cardiac arrest. Ann Neurol 15:59, 1984.
266. Ashwal S, Schneider S, Tomasi L, Thompson J: Prognostic implications of hyperglycemia and reduced cerebral blood flow in childhood near-drowning. Neurology 40:820, 1990.
267. Woo E, Chan YW, Yu YL, Huang CY: Admission glucose level in relation to mortality and morbidity outcome in 252 stroke patients. Stroke 19:185, 1988.
268. Longstreth WT, Diehr P, Cobb LA, et al: Neurologic outcome and blood glucose levels during out-of-hospital cardiopulmonary resuscitation. Neurology 36:1186, 1986.
269. Voll CL, Auer RN: The effect of postischemic blood glucose levels on ischemic brain damage in the rat. Ann Neurol 24:638, 1988.
270. Voll CL, Auer RN: Insulin attenuates ischemic brain damage independent of its hypoglycemic effect. J Cereb Blood Flow Metab 11:1006, 1991.
271. Sieber FE, Traystman RJ: Special issues: glucose and the brain. Crit Care Med 20:104, 1992.
272. Mogayzel C, Quan L, Graves JR, et al: Out-of-hospital ventricular fibrillation in children and adolescents: causes and outcomes. Ann Emerg Med 25:484, 1995.
273. Dahl CF, Ewy GA, Warner ED, Thomas ED: Myocardial necrosis from direct current countershock: effect of paddle electrode size and time interval between discharges. Circulation 50:956, 1974.
274. DiCola VC, Freedman GS, Downing SE, Zaret BL: Myocardial uptake of technetium-99m stannous pyrophosphate following direct current transthoracic countershock. Circulation 54:980, 1976.
275. Peleska B: Cardiac arrhythmias following condenser discharges and their dependence upon strength of current and phase of cardiac cycle. Circ Res 13:21, 1963.
276. Weaver WD, Cobb LA, Copass MK, Hallstrom AP: Ventricular defibrillation—a comparative trial using 175-J and 320-J shocks. N Engl J Med 307:1101, 1982.
277. Jones JL, Lepeschkin E, Jones RE, Rush S: Response of cultured myocardial cells to countershock-type electrical field stimulation. Am J Physiol 235:H214, 1978.
278. Anderson GJ, Reiser J, McAllister H, Likoff W: Electro-physiological characterization of myocardial injury induced by defibrillation shocks. Med Instr 14:54, 1980.

279. Campbell NPS, Webb SW, Adgey AA, Pantridge JF: Transthoracic ventricular defibrillation in adults. BMJ 2:1379, 1977.
280. Kerber RE, Sarnat W: Factors influencing the success of ventricular defibrillation in man. Circulation 60:226, 1979.
281. Zipes DP, Fischer J, King RM, et al: Termination of ventricular fibrillation in dogs by depolarizing a critical amount of myocardium. Am J Cardiol 36:37, 1975.
282. Gutgesell HP, Tacker WA, Geddes LA, et al: Energy dose for ventricular defibrillation of children. Pediatrics 58:898, 1976.
283. Pionkowski RS, Thompson BM, Gruchow HW, et al: Resuscitation time in ventricular fibrillation—a prognostic indicator. Ann Emerg Med 12:733, 1983.
284. Niemann JT, Cairns CB, Sharma J, Lewis RJ: Treatment of prolonged ventricular fibrillation: immediate countershock versus high-dose epinephrine and CPR preceding countershock. Circulation 85:281, 1992.
285. Tacker WA Jr, Babbs CF, Abendschein DR, Geddes LA: Transchest defibrillation under conditions of hypothermia. Crit Care Med 9:390, 1981.
286. Gascho JA, Crampton RS, Cherwek ML, et al: Determinants of ventricular defibrillation in adults. Circulation 60:231, 1979.
287. Weaver WD, Hill D, Fahrenbruch CE, et al: Use of the automatic external defibrillator in the management of out-of-hospital cardiac arrest. N Engl J Med 319:661, 1988.
288. Cummins RO, Eisenberg MS, Litwin PE, et al: Automatic external defibrillators used by emergency medical technicians. A controlled clinical trial. JAMA 257:1605, 1987.
289. Niskanen RA: Automated external defibrillators—experiences with their use and options for their further development. New Horiz 5:137, 1997.
290. Atkins DL, Hartley LL, York DK: Accurate recognition and effective treatment of ventricular fibrillation by automated external defibrillators in adolescents. Pediatrics 101:393, 1998.
291. Collingsworth KA, Kalman SM, Harrison DC: The clinical pharmacology of lidocaine as an antiarrhythmic drug. Circulation 50:1217, 1974.
292. Constantino RT, Crockett SE, Vasko JS: Cardiovascular effects and dose response relationships of lidocaine. Circulation 36:89, 1967.
293. Austen WG, Moran JM: Cardiac and peripheral vascular effects of lidocaine and procainalol. Am J Cardiol 16:701, 1965.
294. Schunacher RR, Lieberson AD, Childress RH, Williams JF: Hemodynamic effects of lidocaine in patients with heart disease. Am J Cardiol 24:191, 1969.
295. Jewitt DE, Kishow Y, Thomas M: Lidocaine in the management of arrhythmias after myocardial infarction. Circulation 37:965, 1968.
296. Chow MSS, Ronfeld RA, Hamilton RA, et al: Effect of external cardiopulmonary resuscitation on lidocaine pharmacokinetics in dogs. J Pharmacol Exp Ther 224:531, 1983.
297. Chow MSS, Ronfeld RA, Ruffett D, Fieldman A: Lidocaine pharmacokinetics during cardiac arrest and external cardiopulmonary resuscitation. Am Heart J 102:799, 1981.
298. Lichstein E, Chadda KD, Gupta PK: Atrioventricular block with lidocaine therapy. Am J Cardiol 31:277, 1973.
299. Chow MS: Intravenous amiodarone: pharmacology, pharmacokinetics, and clinical use. Ann Pharmacother 30:637, 1996.
300. Singh BN, Venkatesh N, Nademanee K, et al: The historical development, cellular electrophysiology and pharmacology of amiodarone. Prog Cardiovasc Dis 31:249, 1989.
301. Bauman JL: Class III antiarrhythmic agents: the next wave. Pharmacotherapy 17:76S, 1997.
302. Nattel S: Comparative mechanisms of action of antiarrhythmic drugs. Am J Cardiol 72:13F, 1993.
303. Cote P, Bourassa MG, Delaye J, et al: Effects of amiodarone on cardiac and coronary hemodynamics and on myocardial metabolism in patients with coronary artery disease. Circulation 59:1165, 1979.
304. Harris L, Kimura Y, Shaikh NA: Phospholipase inhibition and the electrophysiology of acute ischemia: studies with amiodarone. J Mol Cell Cardiol 25:1075, 1993.
305. Bauman JL, Berk SI, Hariman RJ, et al: Amiodarone for sustained ventricular tachycardia: efficacy, safety, and factors influencing long-term outcome. Am Heart J 114:1436, 1987.
306. Helmy I, Herre JM, Gee G, et al: Use of intravenous amiodarone for emergency treatment of life-threatening ventricular arrhythmias. J Am Coll Cardiol 12:1015, 1988.
307. Podrid PJ: Amiodarone: reevaluation of an old drug. Ann Intern Med 122:689, 1995.
308. Roberts SA, Viana MA, Nazari J, et al: Invasive and noninvasive methods to predict the long-term efficacy of amiodarone: a compilation of clinical observations using meta-analysis. Pacing Clin Electrophysiol 17:1590, 1994.
309. Gonzalez ER, Kannewurf BS, Ornato JP: Intravenous amiodarone for ventricular arrhythmias: overview and clinical use. Resuscitation 39:33, 1998.
310. Perry JC, Knilans TK, Marlow D, et al: Intravenous amiodarone for life-threatening tachyarrhythmias in children and young adults. J Am Coll Cardiol 22:95, 1993.
311. Figa FH, Gow RM, Hamilton RM, et al: Clinical efficacy and safety of intravenous amiodarone in infants and children. Am J Cardiol 74:573, 1994.
312. Singh BN: Antiarrhythmic actions of amiodarone: a profile of a paradoxical agent. Am J Cardiol 78:41, 1996.
313. Jessurun GA, Boersma WG, Crijns HJ: Amiodarone-induced pulmonary toxicity. Predisposing factors, clinical symptoms and treatment. Drug Saf 18:339, 1998.
314. Hilleman D, Miller MA, Parker R, et al: Optimal management of amiodarone therapy: efficacy and side effects. Pharmacotherapy 18:138S, 1998.
315. Pfammatter JP, Paul T: New antiarrhythmic drug in pediatric use: sotalol. Pediatr Cardiol 18:28, 1997.
316. Woosley RL, Barbey JT, Wang T, Funck-Brentano C: Concentration/response relations for the multiple antiarrhythmic actions of sotalol. Am J Cardiol 65:22A, 1990.
317. Carmeliet E: Electrophysiologic and voltage clamp analysis of the effects of sotalol on isolated cardiac muscle and Purkinje fibers. J Pharmacol Exp Ther 232:817, 1985.
318. Pfammatter JP, Paul T, Lehmann C, Kallfelz HC: Efficacy and proarrhythmia of oral sotalol in pediatric patients. J Am Coll Cardiol 26:1002, 1995.
319. Schnelle K, Klein G, Schinz A: Studies on the pharmacokinetics and pharmacodynamics of the beta-adrenergic blocking agent sotalol in normal man. J Clin Pharmacol 19:516, 1979.
320. Ho DS, Zecchin RP, Cooper MJ, et al: Rapid intravenous infusion of d-l sotalol: time to onset of effects on ventricular refractoriness, and safety. Eur Heart J 16:81, 1995.
321. Tipple M, Sandor G: Efficacy and safety of oral sotalol in early infancy. Pacing Clin Electrophysiol 14:2062, 1991.
322. MacNeil DJ, Davies RO, Deitchman D: Clinical safety profile of sotalol in the treatment of arrhythmias. Am J Cardiol 72:44A, 1993.
323. Kehoe RF, Zheutlin TA, Dunnington CS, et al: Safety and efficacy of sotalol in patients with drug-refractory sustained ventricular tachyarrhythmias. Am J Cardiol 65:58A, 1990.
324. Singh BN: When is QT prolongation antiarrhythmic and when is it proarrhythmic? Am J Cardiol 63:867, 1989.
325. Romhilt DW, Bloodfield SS, Lipicky RJ: Evaluation of bretylium tosylate for the treatment of premature ventricular contractions. Circulation 45:800, 1972.
326. Kuntzman R, Tsai I, Chang R: Disposition of bretylium in man and rat: a sensitive chemical method for its estimation in plasma and urine. Clin Pharmacol Ther 11:829, 1970.
327. Markis JE, Koch-Weser J: Characterizations and mechanisms of inotropic and chronotropic actions of bretylium tosylate. J Pharmacol Exp Ther 178:94, 1971.
328. Bigger JT Jr, Jaffe CC: The effect of bretylium tosylate on the electrophysiologic properties of ventricular muscle and Purkinje fibers. Am J Cardiol 27:82, 1971.
329. Chatterjee K, Mandel WJ, Vyden JK, et al: Cardiovascular effects of bretylium tosylate in acute myocardial infarction. JAMA 223:757, 1973.
330. Bacaner MB: Bretylium tosylate for suppression of induced ventricular fibrillation. Am J Cardiol 17:528, 1966.
331. Koch-Weser J: Drug therapy-bretylium. N Engl J Med 300:473, 1979.
332. Haynes RE, Chinn TL, Copass MK, Cobb LA: Comparison of bretylium tosylate and lidocaine in management of out-of-hospital ventricular fibrillation: a randomized clinical trial. Am J Cardiol 48:353, 1981.
333. Bernstein JG, Koch-Weser J: Effectiveness of bretylium tosylate against refractive ventricular arrhythmias. Circulation 45:1024, 1972.

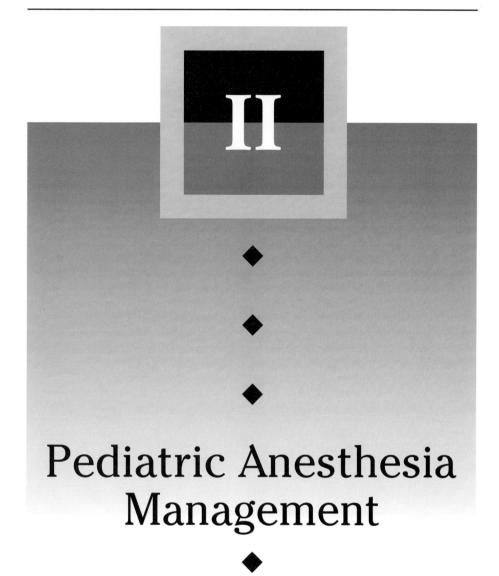

Pediatric Anesthesia
Management

8

Preoperative Evaluation and Preparation for Surgery

DAVID J. STEWARD

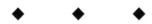

PREOPERATIVE EVALUATION

The primary objective of the anesthesiologist during the preoperative period is to establish whether the child is fit for the proposed procedure. In addition, it is necessary to identify any disease present that might need preoperative treatment or that could affect the course of anesthesia and surgery and to determine which anesthesia care regimen is optimal for the child. The evaluation period also provides an excellent opportunity for the anesthesiologist to establish a good relationship with the child and his family and to allay their anxieties. At this time, the child's state of psychological preparation can be assessed and can perhaps be further improved. The need for preoperative sedation or any other medication (e.g., antibiotics, corticosteroids) should also be determined.

The recent trend is increasingly toward either outpatient surgery or "admit day of surgery" for pediatric surgical patients. These practices tend to limit the anesthesiologist's opportunity for preoperative interaction with the child and the parents, but every effort should be made to ensure that enough time is available to assess the child fully and to establish whatever rapport is possible. In some cases, this may require an additional outpatient visit to the hospital to meet with the anesthesiology team. Prefera-

bly, the child can be seen at the time of a preoperative surgical visit.

A major objective of the anesthesiologist in planning the perioperative care of pediatric patients is to minimize any adverse psychological effects of the entire experience. This can only be achieved if the anesthesiologist understands the potential problems, carefully assesses each child, and arranges an individualized perioperative management plan. It is most important that the anesthesiologist play a leading and dynamic role in the team that plans for preoperative preparation and medication, operating room care, and postoperative recovery with optimal pain management.

PSYCHOLOGICAL ASPECTS OF HOSPITALIZATION, SURGERY, AND ATTENDANT PROCEDURES

Children who are admitted to the hospital for a surgical procedure may suffer lasting psychological effects.[1] Usually, however, after a brief period of hospitalization for a relatively minor procedure such effects are negligible and difficult to detect. Day surgery is particularly free of lasting emotional upset in most children.[2] A longer duration of hospitalization associated with more major surgery does result in persisting, readily measurable psychological difficulties. It has been suggested that anesthesiologists, because of the nature of their interventions, are particularly likely to contribute to these adverse effects.[3] Several studies have also suggested that individual anesthesiologists vary considerably in how well they avoid generating emotional upset in their pediatric patients.[4]

To provide the best possible care for pediatric patients, the anesthesiologist must clearly understand the factors affecting the child's emotional responses. In addition, the anesthesiologist must strive to develop a natural ease and good communication skills with which to gain the confidence of each young patient. This demands a knowledge of things that interest children of all ages. It is most important that every technical manipulation that must be performed before the induction of anesthesia should be completed with gentleness and consummate skill.

Factors that Affect the Psychological Response of the Child

Age

Age is obviously a most important determinant. Neonates and infants under 6 months of age do not appear to be greatly upset by separation from parents and admission to the hospital. A nurse is readily accepted as a substitute parent. Prolonged separation of parent and child may, however, have a detrimental effect on parental bonding and thus lead to later problems with parent–child relationships.[5] To prevent such problems, frequent visiting and constant participation of parents in the hands-on care of their infant must be promoted; during visits, physical contact between parents and infant should be encouraged. If consistent with optimal medical care, the first 6 months of life might be considered the most favorable time to complete necessary major surgery.

Because two-way verbal communication with young babies is not possible, there is no way to assess their needs or prepare them for surgery. We assume, however, that their lack of comprehension at this age obviates the need for psychological preparation or sedative premedication. However, infants do feel pain and should therefore receive optimal analgesia for all potentially painful procedures. They usually respond very favorably to appropriate general nursing and comforting measures. Premedication for this age group is limited to drugs intended to modify the physiologic or pharmacologic responses to anesthesia and surgery (e.g., anticholinergic drugs).

Infants more than 6 months of age are usually upset when separated from their parents. At this age they also recognize a particularly threatening situation (e.g., being placed on the operating room table) but are too young to understand explanations and reassurances. Therefore, it is not surprising that the period from 6 months until 4 or 5 years of age is associated with the greatest degree of posthospitalization emotional upset and regression of behavior.[1] This regression usually includes greatly increased fear of separation (clinging to mother), poor sleeping and possible nightmares, poor feeding, fear of strangers, and sometimes loss of toilet training.

Children 4 to 6 years of age are slightly easier to communicate with. Having commenced school, they become more independent and more readily accept a period of separation from home, although it is still a major source of anxiety. However, at this age, the surgical procedure itself becomes more of a threat. Children in this age group have a great concern for the integrity of their bodies; every little cut must be covered by a Band-Aid. They may also harbor the wildest misconceptions about the surgery, and fears of mutilation are prominent. For example, the child undergoing a strabismus operation may believe that the eye will be taken out and turned around. Indeed, one child after his operation reported, "I was one of the lucky ones; I got my own eye back after they took it out and turned it around."[6]

After the age of 6 years the child attends school, and the problems of separation from home and family begin to diminish. Children learn to make new friends at school and can do so in the hospital. Although they may be frightened by the prospect of surgery, they can function more independently of their parents and are much more amenable to assessment and reassurance.

As children grow into adolescence, many new problems emerge. Adolescents fear the process of narcosis and worry about any loss of control that might occur. They may be very concerned about their ability to cope with the various challenges of their illness and its treatment and may worry about breaking down and losing face. The adolescent's self-esteem and body image are especially vulnerable. They fear that the treatment may fail, that they may awaken during surgery, or even that they may die while anesthetized. Teenaged patients have many problems, and the added stresses of hospitalization, anesthesia, and surgery inevitably accentuate and compound these problems. However, a teenager who has successfully coped with a serious illness may show many positive effects of the experience and may gain additional self-esteem.[7]

Parental, Ethnic, and Socioeconomic Influences

Some children are much more upset by hospitalization and surgery than others of a similar age. The influence of the parents undoubtedly has a major effect. Parental anxiety is readily communicated to the child and has a major influence on behavior. Some parents may be concerned that they are in some way responsible for their child's illness, which leads to feelings of guilt and confusion. Some children have been much more closely mothered than others; some have been excessively pampered, some encouraged to be more independent and stoic. These differences in upbringing are commonly linked to the different customs of various ethnic groups and may obviously affect the behavior of the child during a medical procedure. How the parent prepares the child for hospitalization or operation is very important. Failure to explain the situation (or even worse, deliberately misleading the child about the truth of hospitalization) leads to confusion, distrust, and feelings of abandonment. Parents vary in their ability to influence their child's fear and coping behavior, and this ability may be difficult to assess before the actual stressful medical situation occurs. Children of separated parents show a high incidence of posthospitalization emotional disturbance and require special consideration.

The socioeconomic status of the child also affects the response to a period of hospitalization. Children from lower socioeconomic backgrounds show much less regression of behavior than others and may even appear to benefit from a stay in the hospital. This is probably because they are more accustomed to the "hard knocks" of life and because the hospital environment and companionship may represent an improvement over the conditions at home.[1]

Nature of the Illness: Repeated Hospitalization

The severity of the disease and the extent of the proposed surgery influence the degree of anxiety of the child. In some instances (e.g., a planned amputation), the procedure may be an overriding focus of anxiety, and special psychiatric assistance should be provided to coordinate the care of the patient. Elective surgery of the genitalia may also have significant psychological implications for the young child.[8] Patients with cryptorchidism or hypospadias appear to have an increased tendency toward emotional disturbance, which is heightened by parental anxiety. The degree of disturbance is more severe in older children, and it has been suggested that the optimal time for elective genital surgery is between 6 and 18 months of age.[8]

Although previous experience may sensitize many children, repeated hospitalization does not always increase the severity of the emotional response. Indeed, some well-prepared children may exhibit less fear on the next occasion. The unfortunate child who must undergo repeated surgical procedures does require special consideration and careful preparation for each operation.

Hospital Environment

The planning and routine of the hospital environment are important. It is easier to provide optimal complete care for infants and children in a specialized pediatric hospital. It is essential to provide appropriate play and educational therapy facilities suitable for each child. The decor of the wards, corridors, and procedure rooms should be warm and appealing to children. Television, computer games, and other age-appropriate distractions should be readily available. Visiting hours should be liberal and flexible, and when possible the parents should be permitted to stay in the room with the young child. If parents cannot visit, other relatives should be encouraged to visit regularly. When no relatives are available, many pediatric hospitals arrange for a "foster visitor" to visit the child regularly.

The contribution of the medical, nursing, and other staff of the hospital to the child's emotional disturbance may be considerable. All staff members in contact with the child must appreciate their potential to cause upset. Providing staff who are well versed in the emotional needs of children is easier to achieve in a pediatric hospital but must nevertheless be the objective for all hospitals in which children are treated. In a unit that cares for seriously ill patients, it is advantageous to have one nurse specifically responsible for coordinating the emotional care of the child and family.

Specific Anxieties of Children

Separation from parents and the familiar home environment is the principal focus of anxiety in very young children (1 to 3 years of age). The slightly older child (4 to 6 years) is concerned about the operation, and might also be afraid, as are older children, of awakening during the operation or not waking up when it is over. Older children and adolescents may fear the process of induced loss of consciousness. They are concerned about what they might do or say while under anesthesia. They are also afraid of not being able to cope with the challenge of their disease and their operation. Older children and teenagers worry about the possibility of death. They may have heard of anesthesia or surgical misadventures and are concerned that they might die or be otherwise harmed during an operation.

Some of the procedures associated with the operation worry children. Undressing and putting on strange clothes is disturbing to young children. Restrictions of food and fluid intake upsets many patients and should be sensibly planned to minimize emotional upset (see below).

Needles are a focus of anxiety for almost every child but are usually not the overwhelming fear.[9] Careful preparation and an empathic approach may reduce the fear of the needle considerably.[10] The use of EMLA cream (Astra Pharmaceutical Products, Inc., Westborough, MA), a eutectic mixture of prilocaine and lidocaine, can remove the pain associated with venipuncture,[11] but will not remove the child's aversion to the procedure. Therefore, appropriate distraction should be provided and needles and other materials should be concealed during any procedure.

The insertion of rectal thermometers, rectal administration of drugs, and administration of enemas are usually objectionable to children over 3 years of age. In addition, young children do not like to have solutions squirted into their nose.

Relating to Parents and Understanding their Anxieties

Parents also have their anxieties and these are readily communicated to the child and may in turn adversely affect their responses. The anesthesiologist should understand the nature of parental anxieties, recognize those parents who are over-anxious, and whenever possible allay these anxieties. A particular dilemma for the anesthesiologist is to obtain a proper informed consent for his interventions without increasing the level of parental anxiety.

Being unable to chose parents for your patients, you must make do with those who come with the child . . . it would be abnormal if they showed no anxiety.

Mellish, 1969

There are many factors that influence the extent of parental anxiety when their child requires an operation. Many parents of children with only minor problems may initially be very anxious. However, full explanations and very good communication with the medical/nursing team will usually do much to reduce this anxiety level.

The anesthesiologist is frequently placed in a difficult situation when obtaining informed consent for general anesthesia; providing information on all the potential risks before a minor surgical procedure might well be expected to increase the level of anxiety of the parents. In fact, it has been demonstrated that parents appear to benefit from an appropriate discussion of the risks of anesthesia in that this fulfills their own needs of responsibility and understanding. The parents should preferably be permitted to dictate the extent of the information that they wish to be provided. Most parents of children having minor procedures accept that there are risks, including death, and prefer to have the opportunity for discussion of these risks.[12, 13]

The overanxious parent requires special consideration. The anxiety of overanxious parents is usually of multifactorial origin, and may not be necessarily entirely related to this child or the present surgical condition. Such parents may not gain much reduction in their anxiety level from further information regarding their child's forthcoming procedure.[14]

In general, the anesthesiologist should rely on well-established general priciples in dealing with anxious parents. An approach that is found most helpful in decreasing parental anxiety is one built on genuine warmth and friendliness, empathy, understanding, and a cooperative plan for the child. The anesthesiologist must listen carefully to the parent's concerns for their child, and must respect their opinion as to how that child may respond to anesthesia interventions.

The question of the parent accompanying the child during induction of anesthesia may be considered during the preoperative evaluation. Many parents express a strong wish to be present and many facilities have routinely allowed them to stay with their child. Studies are confusing as to the extent that parents can positively affect the child and help during induction. Certainly, the parents of the older handicapped child can frequently be of great assistance. Most parents are calm and supportive of their child, and appear to benefit from participating in the induction process. However, the anxious parent who insists in remaining with the child may do more harm than good and may increase the anxiety level in the child.[15] It is suggested that such anxious parents should be counseled and excluded if possible. Good effective preoperative sedation calms both parent and child and lessens the desire of the parent to remain with the child at induction.[16] Parents of an only child, health care workers, and those with an anxious spouse are often most anxious.[17] If the parents are to attend induction, good preparation is essential, or they may become alarmed. Parents should be informed that the child will fall asleep quite rapidly, become limp, and may look strange.

Psychological Preparation for Surgery

The age of the child is the most important determinant of the potential for psychological preparation and the form that it should take. Generally speaking, any child old enough to understand a simple conversation can benefit from such preparation. In practice, much of this psychological preparation becomes the responsibility of the parents, who will need advice on when and how to proceed.

When first to tell a child of an impending hospitalization or operation also depends on the age. It is unwise to tell the very young child too far in advance. Young children have little appreciation of time and will worry constantly about when they will be going to the hospital. They should be told of the planned procedure only a short time (i.e., 24 hours) before. Older children should be prepared some days ahead of the event. Adolescents must participate in the plans for their operation from the beginning, and often have many questions that require consideration.

In helping parents with advice about how to prepare their child, two important principles must be emphasized. First, under no circumstances should they deceive the child: children become very upset and lose all their trust if they discover that they have not been told the truth. Second, parents may need to be convinced that their child is old enough to understand and benefit from being told what is going to happen. Many parents underestimate their child's powers of comprehension. It should also be stressed that although the broad truth should be stated, it is unwise to include potentially disturbing minor details. Certainly, the child should be told that he is going to the hospital, will have his own bed, and is going to have an operation. As stated previously, parents vary greatly in their potential to reduce anxiety and assist their child to cope. Some become agitated and anxious themselves at times of stress. This increases anxiety in the child and reduces their ability to cope. It is suggested[18] that parents should be encouraged to engage in active coping methods (e.g., providing information and distraction). They should avoid "emotion-focused coping," such as becoming agitated, ignoring the child, or merely providing restraint and reassurance. Parents can be greatly helped by ensuring that they have all the information and reassurance needed to prepare themselves for their child's surgical procedure.

Security objects (e.g., blankets or dolls) are often important to the young, and sometimes also to older patients. Such objects should be carefully labeled and should accompany the child to the hospital. It is extremely important not to mislay a precious security object during the operation. Television has become an invaluable distraction for the hospitalized child, and reassurance before admission that this will be available is worthwhile. Portable computer games (Nintendo, etc.) also provide great distraction for the older child who is able to participate.

Special preadmission programs, including hospital tours and parties, slide or puppet shows, and video presentations, can be used to prepare children. These have been generally demonstrated to reduce anxiety effectively before induction of anesthesia and to reduce posthospitalization behavior problems. A variety of programs have been designed, some more labor intensive and expensive than others. A videotape is the simplest method to deliver a message but may be more effective when combined with a hospital tour and a question-and-answer session. Individual training of the child and parents in coping strategies to deal with anxieties and discomfort has been proven effective but is very labor intensive and expensive. It has been suggested that preparation for hospitalization and medical procedures should not be limited to children presently scheduled for hospital care. Rather, children and families in the community should be provided with some instruction before they are faced with the need for pediatric medical or surgical care. In this way, primary prevention of medical fears in a population of children at risk could be attempted. This might be achieved by the use of videotape presentations on community television channels and by appropriate booklets and pamphlets.

Some children, especially those with previous experience, may become sensitized by such routine preadmission programs, resulting in increased anxiety.[19] This reemphasizes that all children deserve individual consideration and should have programs tailored to their special needs.

When the anesthesiologist sees the child before surgery, it is helpful to have the parents present, although this is not always possible. If the parents are present, the child can witness their acceptance of the anesthesiologist into the group. Attention should be directed primarily at the child while a complete assessment is being made and the child's confidence is gained.

It is sometimes very difficult to identify the fearful child. Some children appear nonchalant and self-possessed, only to become very upset at the induction of anesthesia. Children who exhibit such nonchalance or, alternatively, the "silent child", deserve special attention, as they are especially likely to be anxious and to become very upset at the time of induction. It should be recognized that children, like adults, vary in their ability to cope when faced with a medical procedure. In broad terms, two patterns or coping emerge: an active, information-seeking pattern and an avoidant, information-denying pattern.[20] Children who use the former pattern of coping benefit from preparation and are usually better adjusted during hospitalization and less distressed by procedures. Those who use the latter pattern of coping are much more difficult to deal with and are likely to be much more upset. A crucial and controversial question is whether attempts at preparation by providing what may be unwanted information may increase the anxiety of these children and their degree of emotional upset.[20] Some have suggested that they should be allowed to pursue their strategy of avoidance and might be helped by the addition of further distraction techniques rather than by any other form of preparation.

When talking to children, the anesthesiologist should explain in simple, reassuring terms exactly what will happen during induction of anesthesia. A warm, friendly, empathic approach is necessary. It should be openly accepted that the child may be anxious and afraid, and may even cry. Moreover, the anesthesiologist should admit that what must be done may be unpleasant but will soon be over. This "empathic approach" induces fewer adverse responses from children than does the "directive approach." The latter approach, which is generally condemned, typically directs the child to "be brave, not cry, hold still, and cooperate."

Children should be told that they will sleep soundly and pleasantly during the operation and will not awaken until it is over, but will then awaken in bed in the recovery room or intensive care unit (ICU). The parent(s) should be allowed to come to the bedside of the child in the recovery room as soon as vital signs have been taken, and the the child's condition is stable. The presence of the parent will usually reduce the distress of the young child, and will establish which children are crying because they want their parents and which children have persisting pain. The latter group should receive whatever additional analgesic therapy is appropriate.

PREOPERATIVE MEDICAL EVALUATION

Infants and children do not suffer from the chronic degenerative diseases seen in many older patients who present for anesthesia; in fact, most pediatric surgical patients are in otherwise excellent general health. There is, however, the possibility in every patient of an unrecognized abnormality that could give rise to a serious anesthesia complication. Some children have diseases that demand very special perioperative management. Because congenital abnormalities tend to be multiple, the presence of one lesion should prompt a search for others. Multiple defects are found clustered in many familiar syndromes, and certain other well-recognized associations may occur (e.g., Down syndrome and congenital heart disease). Therefore, every patient must undergo a meticulous and thorough assessment, the extent of which will be determined by the findings.

The History

Most children are not capable of giving a medical history, and the parents must therefore be questioned. In the case of a healthy child, the history will be quite short. However, it is essential to obtain a concise overview of the child's progress since birth, including physical and emotional development. The antenatal and birth history may also be significant in some instances; it is therefore appropriate to determine whether there were problems during the pregnancy, whether this was a term birth, and whether there were any perinatal complications. A history of premature birth is particularly important, as infants born prematurely may have an increased incidence of important diseases during the first months and years of life. It is also essential to question the parents specifically concerning any history of problems with the heart, lungs, nervous system, kidneys, or other serious disease. A history of allergy, the results of previous anesthesia experiences, and family problems with anesthetic drugs must always be carefully sought. Current medication must be documented, as some drugs may have significant implications for the anesthesiologist (Table 8–1). The anesthesiologist should ask specifically whether the child is taking any medicines; parents often forget to mention that their child has been taking medication. Obtaining such a history takes very little time and provides the foundation for a complete preoperative evaluation.

Unfortunately, the parents of the child with a complex disease may not be able to provide a comprehensive and clear account of their child's health problems. In such cases, the anesthesiologist must rely heavily on a review

```
 T A B L E    8 - 1
```
CONCURRENT MEDICATIONS AND ANESTHESIA IMPLICATIONS

Drug	Anesthesia Implications
Analgesic, anti-inflammatory	
Acetylsalicylic acid (ASA, aspirin)	Prolonged bleeding time because of platelet inactivation. Check bleeding time if ASA given within 10 days
Nonsteroidal anti-inflammatory drugs (NSAIDs) (e.g., ibuprofen, ketorolac)	Affect platelet aggregation and prolong bleeding time
Antibiotics	Many of the "mycins" may potentiate neuromuscular blockade. Monitor neuromuscular block carefully
Aminoglycosides	May potentiate succinylcholine and nondepolarizing relaxant drugs; renal toxicity
Clindamycin	Cardiac depression when given rapidly
	May potentiate nondepolarizing relaxant drugs
Erythromycin	May prolong the effect of alfentanil
Gentamycin	May prolong the effect of succinylcholine
	Potentiates nondepolarizing relaxant drugs
Vancomycin	Potentiates nondepolarizing relaxant drugs
	Cardiac depression and "red man" syndrome with rapid administration
Anticancer agents	All may cause blood dyscrasia, coagulopathy, anorexia, nausea and vomiting, stomatitis, and reduced resistance to infection
Doxorubicin (Adriamycin), daunorubicin (Cerubidine)	Severe cardiac depression with halothane, especially likely when cumulative dose exceeds 250 mg/m² (or 150 mg/m² with mediastinal radiation). Check echocardiogram required
Bleomycin	Pulmonary fibrosis, which may be exacerbated by excess oxygen. Control F_{IO_2} carefully
Busulfan	Inhibits plasma cholinesterases
Cyclophosphamide (cytoxan)	Inhibits plasma cholinesterases
Anticonvulsants	
Phenytoin, mephenytoin	May cause blood dyscrasia, hypotension, bradycardia, arrhythmia
	May increase requirements for nondepolarizing relaxants and fentanyl
	May cause peripheral neuropathy
Valproic acid	May cause hypotonia
	Hepatotoxic
Antihypertensive drugs	Severe hypotension may occur with potent anesthetics
Clonidine	Must not be abruptly withdrawn—severe hypertension may result
	Interaction with β-blockers—hypotension
Hydralozine (Apresoline)	May cause SLE-type syndrome
	Decreases tachycardia with atropine
Labetolol	May prolong spinal analgesia with tetracaine
Prazosin (Minipress)	May potentiate effects of ketamine
Antiviral agents	
Acyclovir	Nephrotoxic
	Bone marrow depression
β-Agonist agents (e.g., Albuterol, alupent)	May cause tachycardia, hypertension, arrhythmia
	Interact with tricyclic antidepressants or MAO inhibitors
β-Blocking drugs	May cause bronchospasm, potentiate cardiac depression of halothane
	May cause bradycardia with anticholinesterase drugs (e.g., neostigmine)
Calcium channel blockers (verapamil, nifedipine)	Potentiate nondepolarizing relaxant drugs
Corticosteroid preparations	Chronic therapy may lead to depression of the hypothalamic–pituitary–adrenal axis; severe collapse may occur perioperatively
	Supplemental steroid therapy should be ordered preoperatively
Digoxin	May potentiate bupivacaine toxicity
	Hypokalemia, if induced (e.g., by hyperventilation) predisposes to arrhythmias
Diuretics	All may result in electrolyte disturbances
Acetazolamide (Diamox)	Produces hyperchloremic metabolic acidosis
Furosemide	May prolong effect of d-tubocurarine
	Hypokalemia, if present, may prolong action and delay reversal of relaxants
Ophthalmic topical drugs	
Echothiopate (anticholinesterase)	Inhibits plasma cholinesterases. Prolonged apnea with succinylcholine
Phenylephrine	May cause tachycardia and hypertension
Timolol (β-blocker)	May exacerbate asthma
Theophylline	Severe arrythmias may occur with halothane

of all the available medical records. It is useful to review these records *before* approaching the parents and child. This ensures that appropriate questions can be asked and also reassures the parents that the anesthesiologist is very thoroughly investigating all available data. Throughout the assessment process, the child's medical history should be reviewed by body system and then, with each significant fact elicited, the possible implications for anesthesia can be considered (Table 8–2).

When the history is taken, the child's emotional state should be assessed. Although many parents will be forthcoming with concerns about their child's special needs, others may have to be questioned to establish the requirements for optimal preoperative and anesthesia management. Every opportunity should be taken to interact with the child and, while doing so, to assess the potential of the parents to assist in achieving a smooth anesthesia experience.

TABLE 8–2
ANESTHESIA IMPLICATIONS RELATING TO REVIEW OF THE PATIENT'S HISTORY

System	History	Concerns for the Anesthesiologist
Central nervous system	Seizures	Adequacy of seizure medication, ? Recent convulsions
		Phenytoin increases nondepolarizing relaxant and fentanyl requirements
		Produces gingival hyperplasia and bleeding, plus ? hepatic dysfunction
		Ketamine, enflurane, methohexital relatively contraindicated
	Hydrocephalus	Possible raised intracranial pressure
		? Need for prophylactic antibiotics to prevent shunt infection
	Head injury	Possible raised intracranial pressure
		? Danger of hyperkalemia with succinylcholine
	Cerebral tumor	Possible raised intracranial pressure
		? Chemotherapeutic agents and possible interactions
	Cerebral palsy	Nutritional status, presence of chronic infections
		? History of chronic aspiration
		? Difficulties with positioning
		Intelligence may be normal—careful psychological preparation needed
	Down syndrome	How can we obtain optimal cooperation at induction (? with parent)
		? Airway (large tongue, subglottic stenosis)
		? Heart disease
		? Evidence of joint hypermobility, indications of atlanto-axial instability
	Neuromuscular disease	Hyperkalemia with succinylcholine
		Altered response to nondepolarizing relaxants
	Meningomyelocele	? Associated hydrocephalus
		? History suggesting latex allergy
		? Renal infections
		? Impaired renal function
		Difficulty positioning
		? Repeated surgery—careful psychological preparation
Cardiovascular system	Heart murmur	Is this an innocent murmur or a significant lesion?
		? Need for prophylactic antibiotics
		? Risk of paradoxical embolism
	Cyanosis	? Hemoconcentration—risk of hyperviscosity with fluid restriction
		? Coagulopathy secondary to hyperviscosity
		Reduced response to hypoxemia—caution with premedication
		Risk of air embolism via IV routes
	Dyspnea, tachypnea Sweating	? Is there evidence of congestive cardiac failure. ? Has the patient been on digoxin
		If so, ? digoxin level. ? History of diuretic therapy. ? electrolyte levels
	Previous heart surgery	Need for prophylactic antibiotics. ? Cardiac conduction defects. ? history of arrhythmias
	Hypertension	Renal disease, coarctation of the aorta, endocrine disease
Respiratory system	Prematurity	? Risk of perioperative apnea
	Respiratory distress syndrome	? Present postconceptual age. ? Gestational age at birth. ? Anemia
		? History of apnea. ? Residual chronic respiratory disease, impaired gas exchange
		? History of prolonged ventilation. ? Residual subglottic stenosis
	Recent URTI	? Evidence of acute infection. ? Pyrexia. ? Lower respiratory infection
		? Reactive airways prone to secondary infection
	Bronchiolitis	? Reactive airways. ? Evidence of bronchospasm
	Croup	? Possible subglottic stenosis ? Avoid intubation
	Asthma	? Reactive airways ? Current status ? Theophylline therapy (blood level)
		? β-drug therapy ? History of corticosteroid therapy (Rx supplements)
		Develop a plan to ensure optimal status preoperatively
	Cystic fibrosis	? Present pulmonary function ? Any acute infection
		Can condition be improved? Can regional analgesia be used?
		Present drug therapy
		Nutritional status

Table continued on following page

T A B L E   8 – 2
ANESTHESIA IMPLICATIONS RELATING TO REVIEW OF THE PATIENT'S HISTORY *Continued*

System	History	Concerns for the Anesthesiologist
Gastrointestinal system	Gastroesophageal reflux	? Evidence of aspiration pneumonia. ? Reactive airways and bronchospasm ? Recent food intake, risk of regurgitation, and need for antacid and H_2 histamine-blocking drugs
	Vomiting	Nutritional and hydration status. Electrolyte values. Urine output ? Immediate full stomach danger
	Diarrhea	Nutritional, fluid, and electrolyte status.
	Liver disease	Risk of hypoglycemia. ? Drug metabolism ? Increased requirements for nondepolarizing relaxants
Genitourinary system	Renal failure	Anemia and coagulopathy, electrolyte abnormality, volume status Acid–base status. Hypertension and incipient congestive cardiac failure ? History of infection. ? Impaired immunity ? Psychological status
	Bladder surgery Exstrophy	? History suggestive of latex allergy
Endocrine system	Diabetes mellitus	? Current status and therapy ? Plans for perioperative management Need for planning with surgeon and endocrinologist
	Thyroid disease	? Current status and medication. ? Euthyroid. ? Enlarged thyroid effect on the airway
	Pituitary disease	? Intracranial pressure ? Adrenal insufficiency, ? Diabetes insipidus
	Adrenal disease	? Need for corticosteroid therapy ? Volume and electrolyte status
Hemopoietic system	Anemia	Cause ? Can this be improved by medical therapy? Will this affect the course of anesthesia? Is transfusion indicated?
	Bruising or bleeding	? Coagulopathy ? Further tests ? Preoperative therapy
	Sickle cell disease	? Trait or disease ? Other abnormal hemoglobins (Hb electrophoresis) ? Preoperative preparation
Muscular system	Muscular dystrophy	? History of malignant hyperpyrexia ? Risk of hyperkalemia with succinylcholine. Avoid relaxants if possible. ? Postoperative ICU admission

Modified from Cote CJ, Todres ID, Ryan JF: Preoperative evaluation of pediatric patients. *In* Ryan JF, Todres ID, Cote CJ, Goudsouzian NG (eds): A Practice of Anesthesia for Infants and Children. 2nd ed. Orlando, FL, Grune & Stratton, 1993, p 42, with permission.

Physical Examination

The extent of the physical examination will be dictated by the findings in the medical history. There are, however, some general considerations and some important examinations that must be made in every patient.

First, it is necessary to respect the modesty of the older child, who may be quite distressed at having to undress. Infants and children should be undressed only to the extent required for an efficient and complete examination; infants lose heat rapidly when uncovered. Some children are very upset at being examined, and it is necessary to balance the need for each step of the examination against the degree of distress. The examination usually proceeds more smoothly when the child is allowed to sit with a parent.

Each patient should be observed for nutritional and conscious state, color, and the presence of respiratory distress or nasal discharge. The temperature should be taken and the heart and respiratory rate recorded. The nose, mouth, pharynx, lungs, and heart should always be examined. The teeth should be examined and the position of any loose teeth carefully noted. Primary teeth that are very loose should be removed after induction of anesthesia, but this should be discussed with child and parents beforehand and the tooth carefully saved to give to the child afterwards. The airway should be assessed for the probable ease of tracheal intubation. When possible, the surgical lesion should be viewed so that the extent of the procedure can be accurately estimated. Furthermore, additional extensive examination or laboratory or radiologic tests may be required, depending on individual findings.

Some children deserve special consideration. Among these, one of the most common problems is the child with the symptoms and signs of an upper respiratory infection (URI). There are many causes for runny noses in small children, and each patient must be considered carefully. How should we handle each of these patients and decide whether to proceed with anesthesia? The key is to make an exact diagnosis of the cause of the symptoms, ascertain the real urgency of the surgery, and understand the risks associated with proceeding with anesthesia. The first important step is to take a complete history. Sometimes the parents will state that their child "always has a runny nose." On other occasions, the history will clearly point to an acute onset of coryza. Examination of the nose and throat should identify the type of secretions present and other evidence of acute infection. The temperature should be taken and the chest carefully examined for any evidence of lower respiratory disease. An elevated temperature or any signs of pulmonary disease would be considered reason enough to postpone all purely elective surgery. The more difficult decisions are when to proceed with necessary surgery (e.g., myringotomy) in the child with otitis and the symptoms and signs of a URI, or how long to wait after a URI before scheduling more major surgery (e.g., thoracotomy).

In children, the symptoms of coryza do not appear to be exacerbated by a brief period of anesthesia,[21] and there is no good evidence that postoperative pulmonary complications will be precipitated. However, there may be an increased incidence of intraoperative and postoperative airway complications.[22] Infants appear to be at special risk for such perioperative complications,[23] and endotracheal intubation is suggested to further increase the incidence of postoperative airway problems.[22] It may therefore be appropriate to be especially conservative in accepting infants under 1 year of age with a URI for anesthesia in elective surgery. In addition, it may be preferable to use mask anesthesia for appropriate short procedures. The laryngeal mask airway has also been reported to be preferable to endotracheal intubation in the child with an URI.[24] Episodes of destauration during and after anesthesia may be more common in children with URI.[25, 26] Children with symtomatic URI desaturate more rapidly during apnea,[27] and laryngospasm is more likely to occur.[28] Thus, care should be taken to ensure that all airway events are rapidly corrected and that supplemental oxygen is administered postoperatively. The risks versus the benefits of proceeding with general anesthesia in the child with a URI should be discussed with the parents. There are economic and emotional implications to cancellation of surgery,[29] and the decision to cancel should be very carefully considered. While complications are more likely, these are usually easy to manage, and when efficiently managed do not result in serious morbidity. Infants and children scheduled for more major surgery should have this deferred, if possible, for 2 to 4 weeks after an acute URI, as the risk for pulmonary complications may be increased during this period.[30] It has been suggested that changes throughout the respiratory tract during the period after a viral infection may predispose to atelectasis and bacterial infection.

Heart murmurs are not uncommon in infants and young children and require careful assessment.[31] In the neonate, murmurs are quite common and may have little clinical significance, but, conversely, serious heart defects may be present when no audible signs of cardiac disease are heard. The transitional circulation of the neonate may tend to mask the clinical signs of congenital heart disease. For example, the high pulmonary vascular resistance of the neonate limits left-to-right shunting via septal defects, and a persistant ductus arteriosus may provide for systemic flow to the lower body in the presence of aortic arch defects. The diagnosis of congenital heart disease by clinical and radiologic evidence may be quite difficult even for the cardiologist.[32] Hence, in all infants with lesions commonly associated with congenital heart disease (e.g.,

congenital diaphragmatic hernia), an echocardiogram is usually performed.[32] If there is a history of a heart murmur in an older child, or if a new murmur is found, a full medical history should first be obtained. If the child is completely asymptomatic, it is unlikely that the murmur results from a lesion that will significantly complicate the course of anesthesia; however, prophylactic antibiotics may be indicated.[33] Innocent murmurs are soft, systolic, and variable.[31] Murmurs that are loud, constant, or transmitted are likely to be because of structural heart defects, as are all diastolic murmurs. A cardiology consultation should be obtained when there is doubt about the presence of cardiovascular disease, a question that can usually be rapidly decided by an echocardiographic examination.

Prophylactic antibiotics should be ordered for all patients with suspected or proven cardiac defects, including those with mitral valve prolapse accompanied by a murmur.[34] Patients who have had previous surgery for congenital heart disease require prophylactic antibiotics, except for those who have had suture ligation of a patent ductus arteriosus or suture closure of a secundum atrial septal defect. Patients with prosthetic valves, conduits, or pulmonary/systemic shunts and those with tetralogy of Fallot or aortic stenosis are at the greatest risk. The recommendations for endocarditis prophylaxis of the American Heart Association should be followed[34] (Table 8–3).

The child with a history of asthma should be carefully assessed to determine the severity of the illness, and the

T A B L E   8 – 3
RECOMMENDATIONS FOR PROPHYLACTIC ANTIBIOTIC THERAPY IN CHILDREN WITH HEART LESIONS

Prophylactic Regimens for Dental, Oral, Respiratory Tract or Esophageal Procedures

Standard general prophylaxis:	Amoxicillin 50 mg/kg orally 1 h before procedure
Unable to take oral medications:	Ampicillin 50 mg/kg IM or IV within 30 min before procedure
Allergic to penicillin:	Clindamycin 20 mg/kg orally 1 h before procedure
Allergic to penicillin and unable to take oral medications:	Clindamycin 20 mg/kg

Prophylactic Regimens for Genitourinary Gastrointestinal (Excluding Esophageal) Procedures

High risk patients*	Ampicillin 50 mg/kg (max 2 g) + Gentamycin 1.5 mg/kg IM or IV 30 min before starting the procedure. Ampicillin 25 mg/kg IM or IV or Amoxicillin 25 mg/kg orally 6 h later
Allergic to ampicillin or amoxicillin	Vancomycin 20 mg/kg IV over 1 to 2 h plus gentamycin 1.5 mg/kg IV/IM. Complete infusion and injection within 30 min before commencing procedure
Moderate risk patients	Amoxicillin 50 mg/kg orally 1 h before procedure or Ampicillin 50 mg/kg IM/IV within 30 min of starting the procedure
Moderate risk patients allergic to ampicillin/ amoxicillin.	Vancomycin 20 mg/kg IV over 1 to 2 h complete infusion within 30 min of starting procedure

* High risk patients include those with prosthetic valves, shunts or conduits, complex cyanotic congenital heart disease, or a previous history of subacute bacterial endocarditis.

current status of the child's asthma. Children with clinical evidence of significant bronchospasm should not be accepted for elective surgery, and it is preferable to defer surgery on those who have had an acute asthma attack within the past 4 weeks. A history of a previous ICU admission or systemic corticosteroid therapy should be sought. Supplemental steroid therapy should be ordered for those who have had recent or prolonged corticosteroid therapy. Patients receiving theophylline therapy should have a blood level determined preoperatively; elevated theophylline levels may cause serious intraoperative arrhythmias. Asthmatic children can usually be effectively prepared for elective surgery by optimizing their maintenance therapy and adding preoperative inhalations of β_2-adrenergic agonist agents (e.g., albuterol) as necessary. The anesthesia technique should be carefully designed to include bronchodilator agents (e.g., sevoflurane) and to avoid histamine-releasing drugs (e.g., d-tubocurarine, atracurium, or morphine).[35]

ROUTINE PREOPERATIVE LABORATORY STUDIES

In recent years, the value of routine preoperative screening tests for healthy infants and children has been questioned, and consequently less testing is now performed. Routine chest radiographs have never been considered a part of the evaluation process of the healthy child. Routine urinalysis has not been found useful in detecting important diseases in a population of healthy pediatric surgical patients,[36] and most hospitals and surgical centers now omit this test. Routine preoperative hemoglobin or hematocrit determinations have been recommended in the past, and have been or still are required by law in some jurisdictions. However, there are few data to support the practice of subjecting every healthy child to a painful fingerprick or venipuncture. Recent studies[36, 37] indicate that the incidence of serious anemia is very low in "healthy" pediatric surgical patients. Mild degrees of anemia do not usually affect the decision to proceed with the operation or result in any modification of the anesthesia management.[37, 38] Significant anemia, when present, is usually found in young infants or in older children with chronic diseases. There is a growing movement to omit all routine testing and to test only those patients at risk for more severe and physiologically important anemia. These would include all infants under the age of 1 year, patients with a chronic disease, all those at risk of having a hemoglobinopathy (e.g., sickle cell disease), those with symptoms or signs of anemia, and those who "just don't look well." In addition, patients with the potential for significant intraoperative blood loss should undergo baseline hematologic studies.

The present consensus, therefore, is that routine screening tests are of little value. When these are omitted, however, the place of a careful and thorough preoperative assessment, considering all aspects of the child's health, assumes great importance.[38]

The child who is found to be anemic should be carefully assessed but, as stated above, mild degrees of anemia are usually not contraindications to necessary minor surgery. There is no justification for preoperative transfusion unless the anemia is severe and symptomatic, or significant cardiorespiratory disease is present. Unexpected anemia should be investigated to determine its cause, and suitable medical therapy can then be applied. In some cases it may be appropriate to defer purely elective surgery until the medical treatment of anemia is completed. In cases of nutritional anemia, oral iron therapy can be expected to increase the hemoglobin level within a few weeks.

PREOPERATIVE FASTING: WHAT IS NECESSARY?

It is now well recognized that withholding fluids preoperatively is distressing to a child and may result in significant fluid depletion. In the past, children have often suffered through many hours of fluid restriction. Over the past few years, a much more liberal approach to the matter of preoperative fasting has emerged. This is based on a number of good studies that clearly demonstrate that prolonged periods of fluid deprivation are unnecessary.[39] The volume and acidity of the stomach contents of healthy children are not increased in those who have reasonable amounts of clear fluid 2 hours preoperatively compared with those who are fasted for 6 to 8 hours.[40] Therefore, most authorities now favor allowing reasonable amounts (3 ml/kg) of clear fluids orally (PO) until 2 hours before induction of anesthesia.[41]

Solid and semisolid foods are of more concern, as they may remain in the stomach for longer periods. In general, it is common practice to omit food on the day of surgery for morning cases and to allow only a small, soft breakfast for afternoon cases.

Infants who are being breast-fed should complete their last preoperative feeding at a time preoperatively that is equal to the usual interval between feedings. Thus, if the infant is being fed every 4 hours, the last feeding should be completed 4 hours before operation. Such infants may be offered clear fluids, if they will take them, until 2 hours preoperatively.

Children who are not otherwise healthy and those who present for emergency surgery require special consideration. Those with gastrointestinal disease or history of gastroesophageal reflux are at special risk for regurgitation during induction of anesthesia. The volume and acidity of the stomach contents of children who present for emergency surgery may constitute a significant hazard. Gastric emptying is delayed after trauma; even 6 to 8 hours later, large volumes of acid contents may be present.[42] The volume and acidity of gastric contents are similar in children with orthopedic or urologic disease to those with abdominal emergencies.[43] Children about to undergo emergency surgery should receive no further fluids PO and may benefit from intravenous fluids and therapy to reduce the volume and acidity of the gastric contents. Glycopyrrolate (0.1 mg/kg intramuscularly [IM]) reduces the volume and acidity of the stomach contents of children.[44] Cimetidine (5 mg/kg PO) reduces gastric acidity, and when given to children by the rectal route in a dose of 40 mg/kg also reduces the volume of gastric contents.[45] Cimetidine also may be infused intravenously (IV) over 15 to 30 minutes in a dose of 5 to 10 mg/kg. Metoclopramide 0.15 mg/kg

IV hastens gastric emptying and may also increase the tone of the lower esophageal sphincter. However, it should be noted that atropine antagonizes both of these effects. Metoclopramide should not be given to patients with intestinal obstruction. Sodium citrate PO will reduce the acidity of gastric contents. Every child at any risk for acid regurgitation and aspiration should be carefully assessed preoperatively and a decision made about the need for prophylactic therapy. Children at special risk (e.g., those with a history of gastroesophageal reflux, hiatus hernia, or an acute abdomen) require special preoperative attention.

PHARMACOLOGIC PREPARATION: PREMEDICATION

The introduction of new drugs over the past decade has facilitated a more rational approach to premedication for pediatric patients. Suitable premedication eases separation from the parents, if this is necessary, and facilitates smooth induction of anesthesia. It has also been demonstrated that postoperative emotional disturbances may be reduced by effective preoperative medication.[46, 47] The value of a well-chosen premedication should not be underestimated as a means to reduce distress. It has been suggested that sedative premedication may be more effective in reducing anxiety during induction of anesthesia than is the presence of a parent.[48]

Clearly, premedicant drugs should be ordered for children only after careful consideration of every aspect of each patient and of the operation he or she is about to undergo. There is no place for routine premedication schedules for children. When such drugs are ordered, their effects should be borne in mind, as well as the possibility that an initial supposedly beneficial effect may be negated if it is followed later by a side effect that increases the patient's discomfort. The nausea and vomiting that may follow the use of the narcotic analgesic premedicant drugs is a good example of such an effect.

The route of administration for premedicants should also be carefully considered. Intramuscular injections are painful and not a good way to induce tranquility; they should be avoided whenever possible. The oral route is most pleasant and is appropriate for most infants and children.

Premedication has been given with the following objectives:

1. To block possibly harmful vagal reflexes.
2. To dry secretions in the respiratory tract.
3. To produce sedation, ease separation, and facilitate induction of anesthesia.
4. To supplement analgesia and reduce the requirements for general anesthetic drugs.

The first two objectives are achieved with the use of anticholinergic drugs. The others may be effected with a variety of narcotic, hypnotic, or tranquillizing drugs.

Anticholinergic Drugs

Anticholinergic drugs are commonly omitted when premedication for adults is ordered. The tachycardia caused by atropine may be deleterious to patients with cardiovascular disease. Modern potent anesthetic vapors are generally less irritating and do not stimulate excessive airway secretions. Despite the absence of profuse secretions, however, there is some evidence that in adults the course of anesthesia induction is smoother when an anticholinergic is administered to dry up secretions.[49] Therefore, I recommend administration of an anticholinergic before induction of anesthesia in the child with a difficult airway, to minimize the possibility of coughing or breath-holding.

Infants and children must be considered separately from adults. The brisk nature of their vagal reflexes on instrumentation of the airway, especially during light levels of anesthesia, may lead to serious bradycardia.[50] Merely inserting a gastric tube in the neonate can significantly slow the heart rate.[51] An initial intravenous dose of succinylcholine usually causes bradycardia in infants and children unless preceded by an anticholinergic drug.[52] Halothane administration produces a progressive decrease in myocardial contractility, heart rate, and cardiac output. Atropine administration increases heart rate, and hence tends to restore cardiac output, but does not affect the reduced contractility.[53]

Autonomic innervation of the heart in infants is predominantly parasympathetic because of the relatively sparse sympathetic innervation.[54] Therefore, a variety of physiologic stimuli that might occur during anesthesia and surgery may produce serious bradycardia. Because the infant's stroke volume is relatively constant, a slow heart rate is invariably accompanied by decreased cardiac output and decreased systemic blood pressure.

Because of these multiple factors that may cause bradycardia and hypotension during anesthesia, many pediatric anesthesiologists have favored a more liberal use of anticholinergics for infants and children. Anesthesiologists who usually withhold anticholinergic drugs from adult patients have cautioned that infants and children must be considered differently.[55]

In recent years, the trend in North America has been to use both halothane and succinylcholine less frequently, and this has reduced the indications for anticholinergic premedication.

If, in the absence of any indication for their use, anticholinergics are withheld, they should be readily available for immediate use during anesthesia if necessary. In infants, bradycardia delays the action of intravenous atropine on the heart rate.[56] This effect is presumably because of the longer circulation time that accompanies the decrease in cardiac output secondary to bradycardia. Therefore, if bradycardia occurs because of vagal hyperactivity (e.g., during halothane anesthesia), it should be corrected by administration of intravenous atropine before the heart rate slows excessively. If the intravenous route is not available, atropine can be given by the intratracheal route and will be effective with similar rapidity.[57]

Anticholinergics in common use are atropine, hyoscine, and glycopyrrolate (Robinul).

Atropine

Many consider atropine the most useful drug for pediatric patients. It can be given by the oral,[58] rectal,[59] subcutaneous, intramuscular, intravenous, or intratracheal route.[57] In a dose of 0.02 mg/kg IM or IV, it is effective in preventing the bradycardia that follows intravenous administration of succinylcholine,[60] instrumentation of the airway, or traction on the eye muscles. When atropine is given IM, the peak plasma concentrations and the maximal chronotropic effect of the drug occur 30 minutes after injection.[61] After intravenous injection, a high initial plasma level rapidly decreases to concentrations similar to the peak that follows intramuscular injection. From this concentration, the decline in plasma concentration is similar, whatever the route of administration.[61]

It is usually accepted that atropine produces a more effective block of the cardiac vagus nerve and less drying effect than hyoscine.[62] It has been suggested, however, that the drugs have not been compared at clinically equivalent dose levels.[63] The cardiac effects of atropine are as follows. An intramuscular dose of the drug is followed within a few minutes by a transient slowing of the heart rate and sinus arrhythmia.[64] This slowing, which is replaced by an acceleration within 2 to 3 minutes, is considered to be because of central stimulation of the vagal centers before a block of the postganglionic nerve endings is complete,[65] although other mechanisms may also be involved.[66]

After intravenous atropine administration to healthy young patients, the heart rate and cardiac output increase, with a slight decrease in the systemic vascular resistance.[66] Infants and young children show less cardiac acceleration than older patients when the atropine dose is titrated according to body weight.[67] It is therefore suggested that the higher doses of atropine usually ordered for this age group are appropriate.

Patients with certain types of congenital heart disease may be adversely affected by atropine, especially if it is given intravenously; the resulting tachycardia may cause a decrease in cardiac output in patients with obstructive valvular disease, and the shortened diastolic period may seriously compromise myocardial perfusion. When an anticholinergic drug is required for such patients, a small intramuscular dose of hyoscine is more appropriate.

The drying effect of atropine on the secretions in the respiratory tract reduces intraoperative complications but might contribute to postoperative pulmonary complications. Mucociliary clearance is slowed for a period of several hours.[68] However, at least one study of adult patients has failed to demonstrate any increased incidence of postoperative pulmonary complications when the drug was used.[69] Nonetheless, many pediatric anesthesiologists try to limit the use of atropine for children with impaired muciliary clearance, as typified by those with cystic fibrosis.

Atropine also inhibits activity of the sweat glands and may compromise thermoregulation, especially in a hot environment or when the child has a fever. In such cases, the drug, if given at all, should be withheld until induction of anesthesia and then should be given IV. Once anesthesia is established, temperature control can be more readily effected.

Children with Down syndrome are reportedly more sensitive to the mydriatic and chronotropic effects of atropine. This effect may be because of the altered sensitivity of the cholinergic receptors, to an imbalance between the

cholinergic and adrenergic receptors, or to altered distribution of the drug.[70] However, studies have shown that the effect of atropine on the heart rates of children with Down syndrome was similar to that in age- and weight-matched control patients.[71, 72] Therefore, it is now suggested that children with Down syndrome be given atropine in doses similar to those recommended for other children.[72]

Atropine causes relaxation of the lower esophageal sphincter and may therefore predispose to gastroesophageal reflux of stomach contents and subsequent pulmonary aspiration. The effect on the lower esophageal sphincter occurs rapidly after intravenous injection, simultaneously with the onset of tachycardia.[73] In children at risk for gastroesophageal reflux, atropine should be withheld until induction of anesthesia has occurred. During a rapid-sequence intubation, cricoid pressure should be applied immediately after thiopentone, atropine, and succinylcholine have been injected. Metoclopramide may antagonize the effect of atropine on the lower esophageal sphincter.[74]

An erythematous rash often develops after atropine administration and is especially visible over the chest and neck. This is believed to be a result of histamine release. Parents who have seen this rash may report that their child is "allergic to atropine," but true allergy to the drug is extremely rare, if indeed it exists. Accidental overdosage with large amounts of atropine, with subsequent full recovery of the children, has been described,[75] and atropine has justifiably been termed a "safe drug" for children.[76]

Hyoscine

Hyoscine is less frequently used than atropine for pediatric patients. It is less effective in blocking the cardiac vagus nerve, but it has a greater drying effect on secretions, which is unnecessary and undesirable. Hyoscine also causes greater inhibition of sweat gland activity and may cause more problems with temperature control than atropine.[77]

Hyoscine, unlike atropine, produces sedation and amnesia, which has been a reason for its use as a premedicant. Hyoscine is 10 times more potent than atropine in its effects on the central nervous system.[78] Small children, however, may be excessively sedated, may demonstrate confused and irrational behavior, and may experience hallucinations, as occurs in the elderly.

Glycopyrrolate

Glycopyrrolate has also been used as an anticholinergic agent for premedication of children. It is a synthetic quaternary ammonium compound that does not cross the blood-brain barrier to the same extent as atropine and hyoscine. Therefore, its central effects are minimal. It has been reported to cause less tachycardia than atropine[79] and to have a greater drying effect on secretions.[80] It is also more effective in reducing the volume and acidity of the gastric contents.[44] Glycopyrrolate 0.01 mg/kg is as effective as atropine for blocking the oculocardiac reflex.[81]

Sedative Drugs

Infants under 6 months of age do not usually require sedative premedication. They do not comprehend the situation and therefore are not apprehensive or anxious. In addition, they may be more sensitive to depressant drugs, whose use may cause respiratory depression and/or delayed recovery from anesthesia. Older children may benefit from the use of sedative premedication, but serious consideration must be given to selecting the most appropriate drugs and route of administration. Sedative and depressant drugs should not be given to children with airway problems or central nervous system disease. When preoperative sedation is administered to children with cardiac or other significant systemic disease, appropriate monitoring, including pulse oximetry, should be instituted. The child should be retained in a supervised area with facilities for resuscitation.

Midazolam

A wide variety of drugs have been used over the years in an attempt to produce tranquillity and sedation of the pediatric patient before surgery and at induction of anesthesia. None was ideal. When midazolam became available, many pediatric anesthesiologists found that this drug was perhaps closer to the ideal than all others, and consequently it has become the drug of choice.[82] It is not perfect, but its rapid and widespread adoption indicates that it is probably better than most of the alternative drugs available at this time. It may be given by the oral, nasal, intravenous, intramuscular, or rectal route. It rapidly produces sedation, axiolysis, and some anterograde amnesia.[83] Separation from parents is facilitated, the induction of anesthesia is less distressing,[84] and postoperative emotional and behavioral disturbance may be reduced.[46, 47] The oral transmucosal (sublingual) route of administration is as effective and much less distressing than the nasal route.[85] Many infants and children may be given midazolam by the oral route. The bitter flavor of the drug may be effectively masked by a cherry syrup. A dose of 0.5 mg/kg PO will usually result in effective sedation and anxiolysis within 20 to 30 minutes, after which the effects diminish. Larger doses may result in respiratory depression. The administration of oral midazolam has little effect on the volume or acidity of the gastric contents.[86]

Patients who cannot take oral premedication may be given midazolam by the intravenous or the rectal route. A dose of 0.1 mg/kg IV rapidly induces sedation and anxiolysis. If the intravenous route is chosen, facilities for the administration of oxygen and artificial ventilation should be on hand in case excessive sedation and respiratory depression occur. By the rectal route, a dose of 3 mg/kg of midazolam diluted in 5 ml saline has been found to produce effective sedation in 20 to 30 minutes.[87]

The postoperative effects of preoperative sedation with midazolam have been the subject of some studies and the results are conflicting. It has been noted that some children seem to be disturbed when awakening in the postanesthasia care unit (PACU) after short procedures. It has also been reported that children given midazolam experienced an increased incidence of adverse behaviors, including nightmares, fearfulness, and food rejection during the 2 to 4 weeks following their surgery.[88, 89] On the other hand, other reports suggest that children premedi-

cated with midazolam exhibit less anxiety and emotional disturbance in the weeks following their surgery.[46, 47]

Lorazepam

Lorazepam (Ativan) has been used to sedate adults and has been reported to produce good sedation and better retrograde amnesia than other benzodiazapines. Unfortunately, in children the doses required to produce sedation and amnesia result in a high incidence of nausea and vomiting. Hallucinations have occurred in children prone to nightmares.[90] Lorazepam is therefore not recommended for pediatric premedication. However, older adolescents may benefit from the preoperative use of this drug in a dose of 1 or 2 mg with a sip of water 1 hour preoperatively.

Narcotic Analgesics

Narcotic analgesics were widely used for pediatric premedication for many years. It has been stated that morphine is unsurpassed for its analgesic and euphoriant actions as well as its predictability.[91] Narcotic analgesics, however, produce significant respiratory depression, especially in younger infants, and increase the incidence of postoperative vomiting in all patients.[92, 93] A major additional disadvantage of these drugs is that they have commonly been given by intramuscular injection, a painful procedure not likely to produce tranquility and cooperation in a child.

In recent years, the narcotic analgesic fentanyl has become available in the form of a lozenge on a stick, much like a lollipop, but sold under the name Oralet to avoid the "candy connotation." The presence of the stem on the Oralet provides for its removal from the mouth of the child once the desired drug effect has been achieved. The use of the Oralet formulation ensures that, provided the patient does not chew and swallow the drug, it will be dissolved in the saliva and delivered via the oral mucous membrane. This results in a more rapid and reliable elevation of the blood level of the drug than if the drug is swallowed and absorption occurs through the stomach.[94] It also avoids the first-pass metabolism in the liver. Plasma fentanyl levels are found to peak at about 20 to 30 minutes and are lower in children than in adults given the same dose; this may be a result of a larger volume of distribution or more of the drug being swallowed.[95] The fentanyl Oralet, in a dose of 15–20 μg/kg, has been studied as a preoperative medication and found to produce sedation and reduce anxiety. Respiratory rate was decreased, but the hemoglobin/oxygen saturation level was not significantly reduced. Pruritis and vomiting were increased.[96] Nausea, vomiting, and pruritis limit the usefulness of the fentanyl Oralet as a preoperative sedative. In some patients, preoperative vomiting occurred, an especially alarming complication.[97] The high incidence of nausea and vomiting is not significantly reduced by prophylactic droperidol[98] or by infusions of propofol.[97] All of this makes it unlikely that oral transmucosal fentanyl will gain wide acceptance as a routine premedicant. In summary, the oral transmucosal route for medication is very attractive for the pediatric patient, but fentanyl is not the optimal drug to use as a preoperative sedative.

Ketamine, Barbiturates, and Other Hypnotics

Oral ketamine has been used as a premedicant[99]; 6 mg/kg in a small volume of soft drink was accepted well by young children and was effective in producing sedation. However, compared with midazolam, ketamine was more likely to prolong recovery and delay discharge from the postanesthesia room in ambulatory surgery patients.[100] Oral ketamine (2 mg/kg) may also be combined with oral midazolam (0.5 mg/kg) and had been found most useful in the management of the uncooperative child. Ketamine via the oral route does not usually produce any adverse effects (e.g., hallucinations).

The "short-acting" barbiturate drugs (e.g., pentobarbital) have been extensively used in pediatric premedication. Pentobarbital (2 to 4 mg/kg) has been given orally, rectally, or intramuscularly. The latter route is not recommended, as intramuscular pentobarbital is followed by persistent pain at the injection site.[101] Barbiturate premedication is not usually ordered for infants under 1 year of age. It is unnecessary, and these drugs are metabolized more slowly, especially in neonates, so a prolonged effect may result.[102]

For children up to 2 to 3 years of age, the rectal route of administration may be preferred; suitable older patients may be given the drug by mouth 1 to 1.5 hours before surgery. Oral premedication cannot, of course, be ordered for children with gastrointestinal disorders. It is well known that barbiturates have no analgesic properties, and hence when these drugs are given to children who have pain, they may develop restlessness, excitation, and irrational behavior.

Trichloroethanol (Trichlorfos) given PO at a dose of 70 mg/kg has been reported to produce good sedation.[103] It has probably been the most popular of the nonbarbiturate hypnotics for pediatric use. Trichloroethanol produces good "anxiolysis" and permits smooth induction of anesthesia, especially in children under 5 years of age, being superior to diazepam or flunitrazepam.[104] Trichloroethanol also has an antisialogogue effect that is superior to these other drugs given in combination with oral atropine.[104] Children given trichloroethanol were also found to have a significantly higher gastric pH than those given diazepam or flunitrazepam.

COMMENTARY

Is sedative premedication of value, and when should it be ordered? In recent years, midazolam has become very widely used in pediatric premedication. Most studies suggest that its use may confer continuing benefit to the child by reducing postoperative emotional upset. The use of preoperative sedation facilitates separation from the parents (when necessary) and a smooth induction of anesthesia.

In view of the foregoing facts, the pediatric anesthesiologist should carefully plan all the aspects of the preoperative care of each patient and may include in this plan a suitable premedicant when it is not contraindicated. First, optimal psychological preparation should be ensured whenever

this is possible. Next, it should be planned so that the operating room environment can accommodate the requirements for appropriate induction of anesthesia. Third, the anesthesiologist should carefully consider the mode of induction of anesthesia for each patient and also the possible role of the parent in this process. Finally, a suitable premedicant may be appropriate to complement these first three steps. This medication can be selected according to the following general guidelines:

1. Children under 6 months of age do not need sedation.
2. Children do not like intramuscular injections, nor do they like having solutions squirted into their nose. Older children (over 3 years) do not like rectal administrations of drugs.
3. Sedative premedication should not be given to those with problems of the airway or ventilation or those with central nervous system disease.

The introduction of midazolam has provided us with a drug that can be pleasantly administered, produces considerable tranquility, and does not unduly prolong recovery. When the requirement is to calm a troubled child, to ease separation, and/or to facilitate induction of anesthesia, it appears that midazolam may, at present, be the drug of choice.

REFERENCES

1. Vernon DTA, Schulman JL, Foley JM: Changes in children's behavior after hospitalization. Am J Dis Child 111:581, 1966.
2. Steward DJ: Experiences with an outpatient anesthesia service for children. Anesth Analg 52:877, 1973.
3. Geist H: A child goes to hospital. Springfield, IL, Charles C Thomas, 1965.
4. Rita L, Cox JM, Seleny FL, Tolentino RL: Ketamine hydrochloride for pediatric premedication: comparison to pentazocine. Anesth Analg 53:375, 1974.
5. Korsch BM: The child in the operating room. Anesthesiology 43:251, 1975.
6. Vaughan GF: Children in hospital. Lancet 1:1117, 1957.
7. Hoffman AD, Becker RD, Gabriel HP: The Hospitalised Adolescent. New York, Free Press, 1976.
8. Manley CB: Elective genital surgery at one year of age: psychological and surgical considerations. Surg Clin North Am 62:941, 1982.
9. Jessner L, Blom GE, Waldfogel S: Emotional implications of tonsillectomy and adenoidectomy in children. Psychoanal Study Child 7:126, 1952.
10. Fassler D: The fear of needles in children. Am J Orthopsychiatry 55:371, 1985.
11. Hopkins CS, Buckley CJ, Bush GH: Pain free injection in infants. Anaesthesia 43:198, 1988.
12. Waisel DB, Truog RD: The benefits of explanation of the risks of anesthesia in the day surgery parent. J Clin Anesth 7:200, 1995.
13. Littman DO, Perkons FM, Dawson SC: Parental knowledge and attitudes toward discussing the risk of death from anesthesia. Anesth Analg 77:256, 1993.
14. Poole SR: The "over anxious" parent: Clin Pediatr 19:557, 1980.
15. Bevan JC, Johnston C, Tousignant G, et al: Preoperative parental anxiety predicts behavioural and emotional responses to induction of anaethesia in children. Can J Anaesth 37:177, 1990.
16. Braude N, Ridley SA, Sumner E: Parents and paediatric anaesthesia: a prospective study of parental attitudes to their presence at induction. Ann R Coll Surg Engl 72:41, 1990.
17. Vessey JA, Bogetz MS, Caserza CL, et al: Parental upset associated with participation in induction of anaesthesia in children. Can J Anaesth 41:276, 1994.

18. Bush JP, Melamed BG, Sheras PL, Greenbaum PE: Mother-child patterns of coping with anticipatory medical stress. Health Psychol 5:137, 1986.
19. Melamed BG, Dearborn M, Hermecz DA: Necessary considerations for surgery preparation: age and previous experience. Psychosom Med 45:517, 1983.
20. Peterson L: Coping by children undergoing stressful medical procedures: some conceptual, methodological, and therapeutic issues. J Consult Clin Psychol 57:380, 1989.
21. Tait AR, Knight PR: Intraoperative respiratory complications in patients with upper respiratory tract infections. Can J Anaesth 34:300, 1987.
22. Cohen MM, Cameron CB: Should you cancel the operation when a child has an upper respiatory tract infection. Anesth Analg 72:282, 1991.
23. Liu LMP, Ryan JF, Cote CJ, Goudsouzian NG: Influence of upper respiratory infections on critical incidents in children during anesthesia. Abstracts World Congress of Anesthesiology, 1988.
24. Tait AR, Pandit UA, Voepel-Lewis T, et al: Use of the laryngeal mask airway in children with upper respiratory tract infections: a comparison with endotracheal intubation. Paediat Anaesth 86:706, 1998.
25. Desoto H, Patel RI, Soliman I, Hannalah RS: Changes in oxygen saturation following general anesthesia in children with upper respiratory infection signs and symptoms undergoing otolaryngological procedures. Anesthesiology 68:276, 1988.
26. Rolf N, Cote CJ: Frequency and severity of desaturation events during general anesthesia in children with and without upper respiratory infections. J Clin Anesth 4:200, 1992.
27. Kinouchi K, Tanigami H, Tashiro C, et al: Duration of apnea in anesthetized infants and children required for desaturation of hemoglobin to 95%: The influence of upper respiratory infection. Anesthesiology 77:1105, 1992.
28. Schreiner MS, O'Hara I, Markakis DA, Politis GD: Do children who experience laryngospasm have an increased risk of upper respiratory infection. Anesthesiology 85:475, 1996.
29. Tait AR, Voepel-Lewis T, Munro HM, et al: Cancellation of pediatric outpatient surgery: emotional and financial consequences to patients and their families. J Clin Anesth 9:213, 1997.
30. Tait AR, Ketcham TR, Klein MJ, Knight PR: Perioperative complications in patients with upper respiratory tract infections. Anesthesiology 59:A433, 1983.
31. Rosenthal A: How to distinguish between innocent and pathologic murmurs in childhood. Pediatr Clin North Am 31:1229, 1984.
32. Tulloh RMR, Tansey SP, Parashar K, et al: Echocardiographic screening in neonates undergoing surgery for selected gastrointestinal malformations. Arch Dis Child 70:F206, 1994.
33. Child JS: Infective endocarditis: risks and prophylaxis. J Am Coll Cardiol 18:337, 1991.
34. Dajani AS, Bisno AL, Chung KJ, et al: Prevention of bacterial endocarditis: recommendations by the American Heart Association. JAMA 277:1794, 1997.
35. Kingston HGG, Hirshman CA: Perioperative management of the patient with asthma. Anesth Analg 63:844, 1984.
36. O'Connor ME, Drasner K: Preoperative laboratory testing of children undergoing elective surgery. Anesth Analg 70:176, 1990.
37. Hackmann T, Steward DJ, Sheps SB: Anemia in pediatric day-surgery patients: prevalence and detection. Anesthesiology 75:27, 1991.
38. Steward DJ: Screening test before surgery in children. Can J Anaesth 38:693, 1991.
39. Splinter WM, Schaefer JD, Zunder IH: A 2-hour fluid fast is safe for children. Anesth Analg 70:S386, 1990.
40. Splinter WM, Stewart JA, Muir JG: Large volumes of apple juice preoperatively do not affect gastric pH and volume in children. Can J Anaesth 37:36, 1990.
41. Cote CJ: NPO after midnight for children—a reappraisal. Anesthesiology 72:589, 1990.
42. Bricker SR, McLuckie A, Nightingale DA: Gastric aspirates after trauma in children. Anaesthesia 44:721, 1989.
43. Schurizek BA, Rybro L, Boggild-Madsen NB, Juhl B: Gastric volume and pH in children for emergency surgery. Acta Anaesthesiol Scand 30:404, 1986.
44. Salem MR, Wong AY, Mani M, et al: Premedicant drugs and gastric juice pH and volume in pediatric patients. Anesthesiology 44:216, 1976.
45. Tryba M, Yildiz F, Kuhn K, et al: Rectal and oral cimetidine for prophylaxis of aspiration pneumonitis in paediatric anaesthesia. Acta Anaesthesiol Scand 27:328, 1983.
46. Payne KA, Coetzee AR, Mattheyse FJ, Heydenrych JJ: Behavioural changes in children following minor surgery—is premedication benificial. Acta Anaesthesiol Belg 43:173, 1992.
47. Kain ZN, Mayes L, Wang SM, et al: Effect of premedication on postoperative behavioral outcomes in children. Anesthesiology 87:A1032, 1997.
48. Kain ZN, Wang SM, Mayes L, Hofstadter MB: Parental presence during induction of anesthesia vs sedative premedication: which is most effective? Anesthesiology 89:A1266, 1998.
49. Leighton KM, Sanders HD: Anticholinergic premedication. Can Anaesth Soc J 23:563, 1976.
50. Sargaminaga J, Wynands JE: Atropine and electrical activity of the heart during induction of anesthesia in children. Can Anaesth Soc J 10:328, 1963.
51. Lipton EL, Steinschneider A, Richmond JB: Autonomic function in the neonate VIII. Cardiopulmonary observations. Pediatrics 33:212, 1964.
52. Digby-Leigh M, McCoy DD, Belton MK, Lewis GB: Bradycardia following intravenous administration of succinylcholine to infants and children. Anesthesiology 18:698, 1957.
53. Barash PG, Glanz S, Katz JK, et al: Ventricular function in children during halothane anesthesia: an echocardiographic evaluation. Anesthesiology 49:79, 1978.
54. Rogers MC, Richmond JB: The autonomic nervous system. In Stave U, Weech AA (eds): Perinatal Physiology. New York, Plenum, 1978, p 727.
55. Kessel J: Atropine premedication. Anesth Intensive Care 2:77, 1974.
56. Zimmerman G, Steward DJ: Bradycardia delays the onset of action of intravenous atropine in infants. Anesthesiology 65:320, 1986.
57. Howard RF, Bingham RM: Endotracheal compared with intravenous administration of atropine. Arch Dis Child 65:449, 1990.
58. Binning R, Watson WR, Samrah M, Martin E: Premedication for adenotonsillectomy. Br J Anaesth 34:812, 1962.
59. Goresky GV, Steward DJ: Rectal methohexital for induction of anaesthesia in children. Can Anaesth Soc J 26:213, 1979.
60. Lambert TF: Heart rate changes in anesthetized children following suxamethonium. In Proceedings of the Association of Paediatric Anaesthetists of Great Britain and Ireland. Belfast, Abbott Laboratories, 1977.
61. Burghem L, Bergman U, Schildt B, Sorbo B: Plasma atropine concentrations determined by radioimmune assay after single dose IV and IM administration. Br J Anaesth 52:597, 1980.
62. Eger EI: Atropine, scopolamine and related compounds. Anesthesiology 23:365, 1962.
63. Rackow H, Salanitre E: Modern concepts in pediatric anesthesiology. Anesthesiology 30:208, 1969.
64. Hayes AH, Copelan HW, Ketchum JS: Effects of large intramuscular doses of atropine on cardiac rhythm. Clin Pharmacol Ther 12:482, 1971.
65. Heinekamp WJR: The central influence of atropine and hyoscine on the heart rate. J Lab Clin Med 164:104, 1922.
66. Shutt LE, Bowes JB: Atropine and hyoscine. Anesthesia 34:476, 1979.
67. Dauchot P, Gravenstein JS: Effects of atropine on the electrocardiogram in different age groups. Clin Pharmacol Ther 12:274, 1971.
68. Yeates DB, Aspin N, Leveson H, et al: Mucociliary transport rates in man. J Appl Physiol 39:487, 1975.
69. Jones GC, Drummond GB: Effect of atropine premedication on respiratory complications. Br J Anaesth 53:441, 1981.
70. Harris WS, Goodman RM: Hyperreactivity to atropine in Down's syndrome. N Engl J Med 279:407, 1968.
71. Wark HJ, Overton JH, Marian P: The safety of atropine premedication in children with Down's syndrome. Anaesthesia 38:871, 1983.
72. Kobel M, Creighton RE, Steward DJ: Anaesthetic considerations in Down's syndrome: experience with 100 patients and a review of the literature. Can Anaesth Soc J 29:593, 1982.
73. Opie J, Steward DJ: Intravenous atropine very rapidly reduces lower esophageal sphincter pressure in children. Anesthesiology 67:989, 1987.
74. Brock-Utne JG, Rubin J, Downing JW, et al: The administration of metoclopramide with atropine. Anaesthesia 31:1186, 1976.
75. MacKenzie AL, Piggott JFG: Atropine overdose in three children. Br J Anaesth 43:1088, 1971.

76. Arthurs JG, Davies R: Atropine—a safe drug. Anaesthesia 35:1077, 1980.
77. Eger EI, Kraft ID, Keasling HH: Comparison of atropine or scopolamine plus phenobarbital, meperidine, or morphine as pediatric preanesthetic medication. Anesthesiology 22:962, 1961.
78. Longo VG: Behavioural and electroencephalographic effects of atropine and related compounds. Pharmacol Rev 18:965, 1966.
79. McCubbin TD, Brown JH, Dewar KMS, et al: Glycopyrrolate as a premedicant: comparison with atropine. Br J Anaesth 51:885, 1979.
80. Wyant GM, Kao E: Glycopyrrolate methobromide. I. Effect on salivary secretion. Can Anaesth Soc J 21:230, 1974.
81. Meyers EF, Tomeldan SA: Glycopyrrolate compared to atropine in the prevention of the oculocardiac reflex during eye muscle surgery. Anesthesiology 51:350, 1979.
82. Kain ZN, Bell C, Rimar S, et al: Use of premedication in the United States: status report on pediatric patients. Anesthesiology 85:A1070, 1996.
83. Feld LH, Negus JB, White PF: Oral midazolam preanesthetic medication in pediatric outpatients. Anesthesiology 73:831, 1990.
84. Twersky RS, Hartung J, Berger BJ, et al: Midazolam enhances anterograde but not retrograde amnesia in pediatric patients. Anesthesiology 78:51, 1993.
85. Karl HW, Rosenberger JL, Larach MG, Ruffle JM: Transmucosal administration of midazolam for premedication of pediatric patients. Anesthesiology 78:885, 1993.
86. Riva J, Lejbusiewicz G, Papa M, et al: Oral premedication with midazolam in paediatric anaesthesia. Effects on sedation and gastric contents. Paediatr Anaesth 7:191, 1997.
87. Saint-Maurice C, Meistelman C, Rey E, et al: The pharmacokinetics of rectal midazolam for premedication in children. Anesthesiology 65:536, 1986.
88. McGraw T: Oral midazolam and postoperative behaviour in children. Can J Anaesth 40:682, 1993.
89. McGraw T, Kendrick A: Oral midazolam premedication and postoperative behaviour in children. Paediatr Anaesth 8:117, 1998.
90. Peters CG, Brunton T: Comparative study of lorazepam and trimeprazine for oral premedication in paediatric anaesthesia. Br J Anaesth 54:623, 1982.
91. Vivori E: Preparation for surgery and premedication. In Gray TC, Rees GJ (eds): Modern Trends in Paediatrc Anaesthesia. London, Butterworths, 1981, p 101.
92. Booker PD, Chapman DH: Premedication in children undergoing day care surgery. Br J Anaesth 51:1083, 1979.
93. Smith BL, Manford MLM: Postoperative vomiting after paediatric adenotonsillectomy. Br J Anaesth 46:373, 1974.
94. Streisand JB, Varvel JR, Stanski DR, et al: Absorption and bioavailability of oral transmucosal fentanyl citrate. Anesthesiology 75:223, 1991.
95. Preston RA, Csontos ER, East KA, et al: Plasma fentanyl concentraions after oral transmucosal fentanyl citrate: children versus adults. Anesthesiology 79:A370, 1993.
96. Feld LH, Champeau MW, van Steennis CA, Scott JC: Preanesthetic medication in children: a comparison of oral transmucosal fentanyl versus placebo. Anesthesiology 71:374, 1989.
97. Epstein RH, Mendel HG, Witkowski TA, et al: The safety and efficacy of oral transmucosal fentanyl citrate for preoperative sedation in young children. Anesth Analg 83:1200, 1996.
98. Friesen RH, Lockhart CH: Oral transmucosal fentanyl citrate for preanesthetic medication of pediatric day surgery patients with and without droperidol as a prophylactic anti-emetic. Anesthesiology 76:46, 1992.
99. Gutstein HB, Johnson KL, Heard MB, Gregory GA: Oral ketamine preanesthetic medication in children. Anesthesiology 76:28, 1992.
100. Alderson PJ, Lerman J: A comparison of ketamine and midazolam as oral premedicants for ambulatory anesthesia in children. Anesthesiology 77:A42, 1992.
101. Dundee JW, Nair SG, Assaf RAE, et al: Pentobarbitone premedication for anaesthesia. Anaesthesia 31:1025, 1976.
102. Kraver B, Draffan GH, Williams FM: Elimination kinetics of amobarbital in mothers and their newborn infants. Clin Pharmacol Ther 14:442, 1973.
103. Boyd JD, Manford ML: Premedication in children. A controlled trial of oral triclofos and diazepam. Br J Anaesth 45:501, 1973.
104. Lindgren L, Saarnivaara L, Himberg JJ: Comparison of oral triclofos, diazepam, flunitrazepam as premedicants in children undergoing otolaryngological surgery. Br J Anaesth 52:283, 1980.
105. Dupre LJ, Stieglitz P: Extrapyramidal syndromes after premedication with droperidol in children. Br J Anaesth 52:831, 1980.
106. Cote CJ, Todres ID, Ryan JF: Preoperative evaluation of pediatric patients. In Ryan JF, Todres ID, Cote CJ, Goudsouzian NG (eds): A Practice of Anesthesia for Infants and Children. 2nd ed. Orlando, FL, Grune & Stratton, 1993, p 42.

Anesthesia Equipment
for Pediatrics

DENNIS M. FISHER

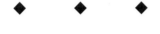

The anesthesia . . . nevertheless left much to be desired. Some babies did very well, but often rapid, "sighing" respirations, accompanied by ashy pallor and sweating, presented anything but a satisfactory picture of anesthesia, while dark congested oozing at the site of operation made it difficult for the surgeon to see what he was doing. After the operation, varying degrees of shock were present: some babies were very ill for days, and nearly all seemed exhausted and "knocked out" by the operation.[1]

Ayre

Ayre's 1937 description of cyanosis and venous congestion in children undergoing anesthesia illustrates the anesthetic hazards of that era. Today, the anesthetic management of children has improved greatly and we are unlikely to witness the scenario described by Ayre. The improvements in anesthetic practice can be credited to several factors, including an increased knowledge of physiology and the availability of better inhaled and intravenous anesthetic drugs. In addition, the equipment used in pediatric anesthesia has been improved. The modern anesthesiologist is offered a choice of nonrebreathing circuits, "adult" and "pediatric" circle systems, "adult" and "pediatric" mechanical ventilators, and other pieces of equipment. The multitude of options makes choosing the best equipment difficult. This chapter discusses the equipment available for pediatric anesthesia, focusing on principles governing the function of equipment used in clinical practice. Its purpose is to enable the clinician to select the most appropriate pediatric anesthesia equipment for a given situation and to use it with confidence.

VENTILATORY REQUIREMENTS AND WORK OF BREATHING

The equipment used in pediatric anesthesia should enable the anesthesiologist to provide adequate oxygenation and the desired quantity of ventilation (i.e., arterial carbon dioxide tensions [Pa_{CO_2}] should be within the range desired by the anesthesiologist, whether low, normal, or high) without imposing a significant workload or toxicity on the patient. Many factors influence arterial oxygenation, including the inspired oxygen concentration, the patient's functional residual capacity, and the quantity of ventilation. The latter is addressed in this section; the other issues are addressed later in this and other chapters.

There are various ways to measure ventilation. The most important of these is alveolar ventilation ($\dot{V}_A$) because of its relationship to carbon dioxide production ($\dot{V}_{CO_2}$) and alveolar carbon dioxide tension (Pa_{CO_2} which, under normal circumstances, is similar to Pa_{CO_2}):

$$Pa_{CO_2} \propto \dot{V}_{CO_2}/\dot{V}_A \qquad (1)$$

that is, for any quantity of alveolar ventilation, an increase in CO_2 production increases P_{ACO_2} and, for any $\dot{V}_{CO_2}$ production, an increase in alveolar ventilation decreases P_{ACO_2}.

Alveolar ventilation is seldom measured in the clinical environment. Instead, we measure total ventilation (usually exhaled ventilation, $\dot{V}_E$, rather than inspired ventilation, $\dot{V}_I$, although these values differ little if we ignore leaks and humidification). Because each tidal breath can be divided into alveolar and dead space components ($V_T = V_A + V_{DS}$), $\dot{V}_E$ is a function of alveolar ventilation and dead space ventilation. To assess alveolar ventilation, we must consider the factors that influence the volume of the physiologic dead space and, if our measurements include the breathing circuit, factors that influence the dead space of the circuit.

Clinical estimation of alveolar ventilation is further confounded in that measurements are typically made at a remote part of the breathing circuit, such as the expiratory valve, rather than at the patient's airway. As a result, measured values for ventilation include the compression volume of the circuit (defined later). Consequently, there are three measured values for ventilation: alveolar ventilation, minute ventilation, and ventilation measured in the breathing circuit. For example, for a child weighing 5 kg, a minute ventilation of 2 L/min measured at the expiratory valve may result in a minute ventilation of 1 L/min measured at the tracheal tube (TT). In turn, this may result in an alveolar ventilation of 0.7 L/min and, if CO_2 production is normal, a P_{CO_2} of 40 mm Hg. Because of the role of CO_2 production in determining P_{CO_2} and the great disparity between the different values for ventilation, the clinician should understand the factors that influence CO_2 production, dead space, and compressible volume. In turn, the quantity of ventilation determines the patient's work of breathing during anesthesia.

Carbon Dioxide Production

Carbon dioxide production in anesthetized subjects, normalized for body weight, decreases markedly with age.[2] For example, infants anesthetized with nitrous oxide and paralyzed with a muscle relaxant had a CO_2 production of 8 ml/kg/min, whereas in patients weighing 60 kg it was 4 ml/kg/min (Fig. 9–1). Similar age-related differences have been found during anesthesia with nitrous oxide and both halothane and enflurane.[3] Therefore, infants produce twice as much CO_2 per kilogram of body weight as adults (a result of their higher metabolic rate) and require twice as much weight-normalized alveolar ventilation.

During anesthesia, several factors influence carbon dioxide production.

Anesthetic Technique

Bain and Spoerel[4] found that during halothane anesthesia, CO_2 production of adults remained constant at a mean value of 87 ml/m²/min. In contrast, during anesthesia with nitrous oxide and opioids, CO_2 production was higher initially (100 ml/m²/min) and increased an additional 30 percent during the next 30 minutes.

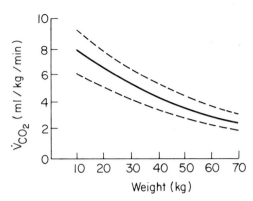

FIGURE 9–1. Age-related changes in CO_2 production. The x axis represents weight in kilograms and the y axis represents measured CO_2 production during anesthesia with nitrous oxide and halothane. The *solid line* is the mean value for each age; 95 percent of the values fell between the dashed lines. (From Nightingale DA, Lambert TF: Carbon dioxide output in anaesthetised children. Anaesthesia 33:594, 1978, with permission.)

Temperature

Changes in body temperature alter CO_2 production by approximately 7 percent per degree Centigrade.[5]

Nutritional Status

The influence of nutritional status on CO_2 production has been appreciated only recently.[6] Malnutrition, even for brief periods, decreases CO_2 production.[7] Conversely, parenteral nutrition increases CO_2 production by as much as 70 percent above normal values,[4] the magnitude of increase depending on the composition of the parenteral fluids. Because the respiratory quotient (the ratio of CO_2 production to oxygen consumption) is lower for the metabolism of lipid than for carbohydrate, a diet in which 50 percent of the calories are provided by intravenous fat emulsions results in a CO_2 production of approximately 20 percent less than that resulting from a diet consisting entirely of carbohydrates.[8] In addition, when large quantities of dextrose are administered acutely to a starved patient, some glucose is converted to fat; because the conversion of glucose to fat has a high respiratory quotient (~8), CO_2 production increases markedly.

Normal Variability

Even in normal subjects there is marked variability in CO_2 production: Approximately 5 percent of subjects differ from the mean value by more than 25 percent.[4]

Rebreathing (Dead Space)

Normally, there is almost no CO_2 in inspired gas; consequently, P_{CO_2} is inversely proportional to minute ventilation. However, during anesthesia (depending on the anesthetic equipment and fresh gas flows) there may be CO_2 in the inspired gas reaching the alveoli and, if minute ventilation remains constant, P_{CO_2} will increase. (CO_2 inspired during the terminal portion of inspiration reaches the tracheal dead space but not the alveoli; therefore, it is not considered to be a source of rebreathing.) Inspiration of expired gas, termed rebreathing, may be advantageous during anesthesia as long as exhaled CO_2 is absorbed from the breathing circuit: both closed-circuit and low-flow anesthesia require breathing of exhaled oxygen and anesthetic gases. In addition, rebreathing of expired gas may increase both the temperature and humidity of the inspired gases, depending on the flow rate of gases in the breathing circuit. However, rebreathing of exhaled CO_2 must be limited to ensure adequate alveolar ventilation. The extent of CO_2 rebreathing differs with each anesthesia circuit and will be discussed later.

Resistance of Anesthesia Airway Equipment

Gas enters and exits the lung as a result of pressure gradients. Because the work of breathing is the product of gas flow and the pressure difference across the airways, anything that increases the pressure gradient increases work of breathing, possibly inducing fatigue and compromising the patient's ability to maintain adequate alveolar ventilation. Smooth and orderly gas flow parallel to the walls of a tube, known as laminar flow, obeys the Hagen-Poiseuille equation.[9]

$$\text{Gas flow rate} \propto \frac{(\text{Pressure difference}) \cdot (\text{Radius of tube})^4}{(\text{length of tube}) \cdot (\text{gas viscosity})} \quad (2)$$

However, breathing passages are not necessarily smooth, straight tubes. As the flow through a tube exceeds its ability to maintain a laminar pattern, it becomes irregular and disorderly. This pattern, known as turbulent flow, requires a larger pressure drop to move gas. Breathing circuits, masks, and tracheal tubes (TTs) contribute to the overall resistance through which the patient breathes, and the anesthesiologist must consider the contribution of each.

Valves

Unidirectional and overflow (popoff) valves are employed in many anesthesia breathing circuits. Because most valves are spring-loaded or contain disks, their resistance can be separated into two components; that of opening the valve and that of the inflow and outflow tubes.[10, 11] When the valve is closed, the disk must be lifted from its seat before gas can flow. The pressure required to do so is given by the following equation[10]:

$$\text{Pressure required to lift the disk} \propto \frac{(\text{weight of the disk})}{(\text{diameter of the disk})^2} \quad (3)$$

Substituting $\rho \cdot r^2 \cdot h$ (where ρ is the disk's density, r is its radius, and h its thickness) for the disk's weight, Equation 3 can be rewritten as:

$$\text{Pressure required to lift the disk} \propto \rho \cdot h \quad (4)$$

Therefore, resistance to opening a valve is least if the disk is thin and is made of a lightweight material. With the valve open, the size of its orifice and the contour of the inflow and outflow tubes each contribute to the resistance. The contribution of these components to valve resistance is seen in Figure 9–2: at low flows, resistance is constant; at high flows, it increases with increasing flow. Consequently, resistance resulting from valves is known as *threshold resistance.* If humidification of anesthetic gases causes water to condense on the bottom of the disk, the pressure required to open the valve increases by approximately 0.25 cm H_2O,[10] regardless of flow.

Canisters, Connectors, and Tracheal Tubes

Canisters, connectors, and TTs each contribute to the resistance of anesthesia equipment. For example, the acute angulation of a right-angled adapter markedly increases resistance compared with a curved connector with the same lumen.[11] The resistance of canisters is generally low, ranging from 0.25 to 0.8 cm H_2O at a flow of 40 L/min. This varies with the degree of packing (packing the absorbant tightly may double its resistance[12]), the type of granule (large, irregular granules have lower resistance than fine, regular ones[10]), and the configuration of the canister (a short, wide canister minimizes resistance).

The majority of the resistance of a breathing circuit is because of the TT (known as *tubular resistance*) because its lumen is markedly smaller than that of the other parts of the breathing system.[13] In an adult, the resistance of the nasopharynx is comparable to that of a TT with an internal diameter (ID) of 10 mm.[11] The common practice of using a 7- or 8-mm-ID TT for an adult increases airway resistance by 300 percent or 150 percent, respectively, compared with that of the nasopharynx. Should anatomic abnormalities of the larynx or other problems necessitate using a smaller TT, resistance will increase further. Changing the TT size from 8 to 7.5 mm increases airway resistance by 29 percent. For a child, selecting a 4.5-mm rather than a 5-mm tube increases airway resistance by 52 percent. Similarly, a 3.5-mm TT has a resistance 71 percent greater than that of a 4-mm tube. These calculations assume that flow is laminar with the two tubes; in

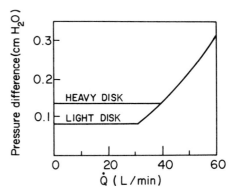

FIGURE 9–2. Flow-pressure measurements of a unidirectional disk valve. The *x* axis represents flow in L/min. The *y* axis represents the pressure drop across the valve (resistance) in cm H_2O. At low flows, resistance of the valve is constant, whereas at higher flows resistance increases with increasing flows. Note that at low flows the resistance of a heavy disk is greater than that of a light disk; however, these differences are small. (Adapted from Hunt KH: Resistance in respiratory valves and canisters. Anesthesiology 16:190, 1955, with permission.)

fact, the smaller tube is more likely to result in turbulent flow, increasing resistance further.

Cole,[14] observing that the larynx and trachea restrict the dimensions of a TT, designed a tube whose narrow portion was limited to the area below the glottis; the proximal portion was wider. Resistance of these tubes was assumed to be lower than that of nontapered tubes, although dead space was approximately 1 ml larger.[15] However, turbulence at the point of narrowing makes resistance of these tubes similar to that of uniform bore tubes.[16] In addition, the tube's shoulder can injure the vocal cords.[17] Consequently, this tube is no longer in common use, except for neonatal resuscitation.

An alternative approach to minimizing resistance of the TT is to reinforce the walls with wires, permitting the walls to be one third as thick as in conventional TTs.[18] For a given external diameter, the lumen of these tubes is larger than that of conventional TTs, decreasing resistance. These tubes have not become popular, perhaps because of their expense. Another simple means to decrease the resistance contributed by the TT is to decrease its length to the minimum necessary.

The resistance of other devices added to the anesthesia breathing circuit must also be considered. The volume-measuring device on the expiratory limb of Ohmeda anesthesia machines has little resistance, producing a pressure drop of less than 0.5 cm H_2O at a flow rate of 30 L/min (A. Berssenbrugge, PhD, personal communication, Ohmeda, Madison, WI). Artificial noses (heat-moisture exchangers) add minimal resistance to the circuit (e.g., the Servo Humidifier, Siemens-Elema, Schaumburg, IL, has a resistance of only 0.4 cm H_2O at a flow rate of 30 L/min) unless mucus accumulates on the device.[19]

Ventilatory Response During Anesthesia

The resistance of anesthesia breathing circuits and the increased ventilatory requirement resulting from rebreathing expired CO_2 increase the work of breathing in the anesthetized patient. The effects of increased resistance and dead space have been examined in both pediatric patients and in adults. Olsson and Lindahl[20, 21] added CO_2 to the inspired gas of spontaneously breathing infants and children anesthetized with nitrous oxide and halothane 1 to 1.5 percent. Patients older than 6 months increased their minute ventilation by 16 percent with 2.2 percent CO_2 and by 34 percent with 3.7 percent CO_2, accomplished entirely by an increase in tidal volume. In contrast, patients younger than 6 months did not increase their minute ventilation in response to the same CO_2 challenge. Infants less than 6 months of age anesthetized with lower concentrations of halothane (0.8 to 0.9 percent) did increase their minute ventilation (by an average of 61 percent) during inhalation of 4 percent CO_2, a response deemed adequate. These findings suggest that in infants, the ventilatory response to CO_2 may be preserved with light anesthesia but is abolished with deeper anesthesia. Consequently, a deeply anesthetized infant breathing spontaneously is likely to hypoventilate. Although the ventilatory response to CO_2 has not been examined in anesthetized human neonates, studies in rats suggest that it is markedly depressed. Rats anesthetized with ketamine or pentobarbital did not increase minute ventilation when challenged with 5 percent CO_2; in contrast, unanesthetized animals increased their minute ventilation by 70 percent during inhalation of CO_2.[22]

The ventilatory effects of increased dead space were examined by Charlton et al.[23] by increasing dead space volume from 2 ml to 16 ml in infants and children anesthetized with nitrous oxide and halothane. In subjects weighing more than 10 kg, minute ventilation increased by 40 percent (a result of an increase in tidal volume rather than respiratory rate) and end-tidal Pco_2 ($PETCO_2$) changed minimally. Subjects weighing less than 10 kg increased their minute ventilation by 49 percent to maintain the same $PETCO_2$. These investigators felt that subjects weighing less than 10 kg would be compromised by this increased work and concluded that apparatus dead space should be minimized in the equipment used for pediatric anesthesia.

The ventilatory effects of both threshold (i.e., valve-like) and tubular resistance have been investigated in adults.[24] The effects of threshold resistance were assessed by having anesthetized patients inspire or exhale through a water column ranging from 2 to 17 cm in depth. As soon as resistance was introduced, tidal volume decreased markedly, some patients becoming apneic for as long as 45 seconds; within 90 seconds, tidal volume recovered but remained below the control value. For example, an expiratory resistance of 12 cm H_2O resulted in tidal volumes (measured 2 to 3 minutes after adding the resistance to the circuit) decreasing 20 to 45 percent. As a result, unidirectional valves in common clinical use (such as the Ohio adult and pediatric valves with resistances of 2 and 3.5 cm H_2O, respectively, at a flow of 5 L/min[13]) may decrease minute ventilation significantly.

The effects of tubular resistance were assessed by having adults inspire and exhale through a tube 25 mm in length with an internal diameter of either 4.5 or 3 mm.[24] Although this form of resistance never produced apnea, ventilation decreased by an average of 7 percent with the 4.5-mm resistor and 21 percent with the 3-mm resistor. The response of children aged 1 to 12 years to tubular resistance was studied by adding connectors with internal diameters of 3.5 and 3 mm to their breathing circuits.[25] Immediately after these connectors were inserted, minute ventilation decreased by 17 percent and 22 percent, respectively. Within 5 minutes, minute ventilation returned to the control value. A similar study was performed in infants 2 to 11 months of age who were anesthetized with nitrous oxide and halothane and in whom inspiratory and expiratory resistances were increased by more than 200 percent by inserting a smaller TT.[26] After the smaller tube had been in place for 10 minutes, tidal volume increased by 12 percent, respiratory rate decreased by 16 percent, and minute ventilation decreased by 8 percent. Despite a threefold increase in the work of breathing, $Paco_2$ increased by an average of less than 2 mm Hg and decreased in 4 of 10 patients.

Long periods of increased airway resistance may not be well tolerated by neonates and infants because their diaphragms differ from those of adults. Fatigue-resistant, high-oxidative (type I) fibers constitute only 10 percent of the diaphragm of the premature neonate and 25 percent in the full-term neonate; the adult value of 55 percent is reached at approximately 1 year of age (Fig. 9–3).[27] As a consequence, neonates and infants are readily susceptible to diaphragmatic fatigue, particularly when the work of breathing is increased.[28] As the diaphragm fatigues, these patients are likely to hypoventilate or develop apnea. In addition, because an adult's respiratory muscles consume only 2 percent of total metabolic rate,[9] doubling or tripling the work of breathing increases oxygen consumption minimally. In contrast, because breathing consumes a larger portion of total oxygen consumption of an infant,[29] an increase in work of breathing may increase oxygen consumption beyond that tolerated.

Extensive clinical experience[30–32] supports the belief that infants do not tolerate long periods of spontaneous ventilation during anesthesia. Whether this can be attributed to resistance of the anesthesia equipment or to other anesthetic effects has not been determined. Nevertheless, many clinicians recommend that infants not breathe spontaneously during anesthesia.[23,33] Although neonates and infants may tolerate spontaneous ventilation without immediate evidence of respiratory fatigue or of metabolic or circulatory effects, the increased work of breathing associated with spontaneous ventilation during anesthesia may lead to postoperative respiratory compromise.

Wasted Ventilation (Compression Volume)

One of the more confusing aspects of ventilation during pediatric anesthesia concerns the relationship between minute ventilation measured in the breathing circuit and minute ventilation measured at the patient's airway. During positive-pressure ventilation (either manual or mechanical), pressure within the breathing circuit increases by approximately 20 cm H_2O, causing two important changes to the gas contents in the circuit. First, the 2 percent increase in pressure within the circuit (pressure increases from atmospheric, approximately 760 mm Hg, to atmospheric plus 20 cm H_2O, approximately 775 mm Hg) increases the number of molecules of gas in the same

volume 2 percent. If the volume of the circuit is 5 L, 100 ml of gas may be compressed; this is known as *compression volume*. As soon as exhalation starts, the circuit returns to atmospheric pressure, the compressed gas reexpands, and the excess compressed gas passes through the expiratory valve. Although this quantity of gas will be measured by a spirometer on the inspiratory or expiratory limbs of a circuit, it does not contribute to the volume of gas entering or leaving the patient.

The second change that occurs to the gas content of the breathing circuit results from the distensibility of the circuit tubing. With the increase in pressure, the tubing stretches, increasing its volume. On exhalation, as the circuit returns to atmospheric pressure, it returns to its unstretched state. The change in gas volume of the circuit that results from distending the tubing (known as *compliance volume*) will be measured in the inspiratory or expiratory limbs but not at the patient's airway. The change in circuit volume varies as a result of the distensibility of the tubing (e.g., metal or thick-walled plastic tubing would not distend, whereas flexible plastic or rubber breathing circuits used in clinical anesthesia are highly distensible).

Typically, compression volume and compliance volume are combined and called *compression volume*. The compression volume of anesthesia breathing circuits can be large. For example, a typical adult circle system with narrow-bore disposable tubing may have a compression volume of 4 ml/cm H_2O; adding a humidifier, a second set of hoses, or other components to the breathing circuit may increase the compression volume to as much as 10 ml/cm H_2O.[34] For an adult ventilated with airway pressures of 20 cm H_2O, compression volume may be 80 to 200 ml, a small fraction of the typically large tidal volumes administered during anesthesia. However, because compression volume for a given breathing circuit is a function of airway pressures rather than the patient's size, its effects are more significant for an infant or child. For example, to deliver a tidal volume of 10 ml/kg at a peak inspired pressure of 20 cm H_2O to a 5-kg infant using a circuit with a compression volume of 5 ml/cm H_2O, 150 ml must be delivered to the breathing circuit: 50 ml for the patient

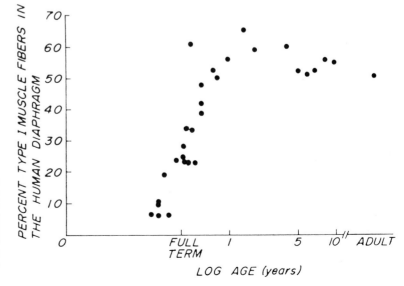

FIGURE 9–3. The percentage of type I muscle fibers in the diaphragm is plotted against age. Type I muscle fibers constitute a smaller portion of the diaphragm in patients under 1 year of age. Consequently, neonates and infants are readily susceptible to diaphragmatic fatigue if the work of breathing is increased. (From Keens TG, Bryan AC, Levison H, Ianuzzo CD: Developmental pattern of muscle fiber types in human ventilatory muscles. J Appl Physiol 44:909, 1978, with permission.)

plus 100 ml compression volume. If compression volume were 10 ml/cm H_2O, the delivered volume would be 250 ml, of which only 50 ml would be destined for the patient's lungs. The difference between the volume measured in the circuit and the volume that actually reaches the patient, compression volume, can also be thought of as wasted ventilation.[34] Because compression volume is a direct function of the magnitude of pressure changes within the breathing circuit, it is important only during controlled ventilation: during spontaneous ventilation, airway pressure fluctuations are small, minimizing compression volume.

The anesthetist can estimate a breathing circuit's compression volume by closing the overflow valve, turning off all gas flows, occluding the patient end of the circuit (with a finger), and delivering a small ($\sim$100 ml) volume of gas to the circuit (using a calibrated "super syringe" or, more practically, adjusting the ventilator to deliver that volume). The compression volume will be the volume of gas delivered to the circuit divided by the peak pressure. For example, a 100-ml volume may yield a 20 cm H_2O peak pressure, indicating a compression volume of 5 ml/cm H_2O. Therefore, during positive-pressure ventilation, if peak pressure is 18 cm H_2O, 90 ml of gas (5 ml/cm H_2O is $\times$ 18 cm H_2O) is "wasted" during each breath.

ANESTHESIA BREATHING CIRCUITS

Many anesthesia breathing circuits were introduced to anesthesia practice during the twentieth century. Some, such as the adult circle and the Mapleson D, continue in clinical practice, whereas others, such as nonrebreathing valves and the to-and-fro canister, are no longer in common use. Others, such as the Johannesburg A-D circuit (see below) never became popular. There are many classification schemes for anesthesia breathing circuits based on the presence or absence of rebreathing or a reservoir[35] or a summary of the components of the system and fresh gas flow.[36] In this chapter, breathing systems are categorized according to the presence or absence of valves.

Circuits Without Valves

The circuit of greatest historical importance to pediatric anesthesia is the T-piece. Although a T-piece was described before the twentieth century,[37] introduction of the circuit to clinical anesthesia is generally credited to Ayre.[38] Intended initially for spontaneous ventilation for infants undergoing cleft lip and palate repairs, the circuit consisted of a lightweight metal tube 1 cm in diameter (Fig. 9–4). Nitrous oxide, oxygen, and ether entered the tube through a small inlet at right angles to the main limb. To prevent dilution of inspired gas with room air, a fresh gas flow equal to peak inspiratory flow (approximately three times the patient's minute volume) was required. Because this flow would be excessive, Ayre added a reservoir (a corrugated tube) whose volume approximated one third of the patient's tidal volume. During the expiratory pause, a continuous flow of fresh gas flushed alveolar gas from the corrugated tube. Then, if inspiratory flow exceeded fresh gas flow, the patient would inspire the fresh gas

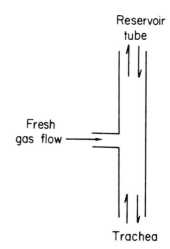

FIGURE 9–4. The original T-piece proposed by Ayre. (From Ayre P: The t-piece technique. Br J Anaesth 28:520, 1956, with permission.)

remaining in the reservoir. In clinical practice, fresh gas flow of 1.5 to 2 times the minute volume could be used without rebreathing or dilution of inspired gas.[39] Ayre monitored spontaneous ventilation by observing the movement of a piece of gauze placed over the opening of the corrugated tube; to control ventilation, he occluded the corrugated tube intermittently. He observed that there was no venous congestion and that ventilation was quiet during neurosurgical procedures. This can be attributed to the minimal resistance, 1 cm H_2O at a flow of 50 L/min, of the circuit.[40] Since Ayre's original description, many modifications of the T-piece have appeared, each with connectors of different diameters, new Y-attachments, or reservoirs of various capacities.[40] Ayre criticized these modifications and requested "an appraisal of the situation before the essential simplicity of the original technique becomes irretrievably lost in a tangled web of expiratory valves and corrugated tubing."[39] Of the many modifications, one became popular. Jackson-Rees[41] altered Ayre's T-piece by adding "a double-ended bag. . . to the exhaust tube, the open end of which is fitted with a vulcanite tap." During spontaneous ventilation, the tap is open and the circuit functions identically to a T-piece; in addition, ventilation can be monitored by observing the reservoir bag. During controlled ventilation, the tap is partially closed, acting as an expiratory valve; the circuit then functions as a Mapleson D (see below).

Circuits with Overflow ("Popoff") Valves

The next phase in circuit design was the addition of an overflow valve and reservoir bag to the T-piece. With the overflow valve partially closed, ventilation could be controlled by manually compressing the reservoir bag, an improvement over the occlusion of the T-piece's corrugated tube. Mapleson[42] categorized these circuits as the A, B, C, D, and E circuits (Fig. 9–5) depending on the locations of the fresh gas inflow, overflow valve, and reservoir bag, as well as the size of the corrugated tube. Because of the differing locations of these components, each circuit behaves differently. The E circuit lacks an expiratory valve;

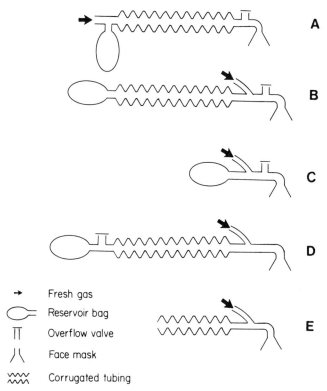

→   Fresh gas
⊂⊃   Reservoir bag
⊓   Overflow valve
⋀   Face mask
⋁⋁⋁   Corrugated tubing

FIGURE 9–5. Mapleson's classification of circuit. Note the difference in the location of the fresh gas inlet, the overflow valve (circuit A–D), and the reservoir bag. (Adapted from Mapleson WW: The elimination of rebreathing in various semi-closed anaesthetic systems. Br J Anaesth 26:323, 1954, with permission.)

therefore, it is identical to Ayre's T-piece. Of the valved systems, the A and D remain in common clinical use.

Mapleson A Circuits

With the Mapleson A system (also known as the Magill attachment[43]), fresh gas enters at or near the reservoir bag and an overflow valve is located at the patient end of the circuit (Fig. 9–6). When this system is used for spontaneous ventilation, dead space gas, followed by alveolar gas, enters the corrugated tube during exhalation while the reservoir fills with gas from both the corrugated limb and fresh gas hose. As the reservoir bag fills, pressure increases, forcing open the overflow valve and venting alveolar gas. During the expiratory pause, fresh gas continues to enter the reservoir bag, directing alveolar, dead space and fresh gas through the overflow valve. As a result, only fresh gas remains in the corrugated hose and the patient inspires only fresh gas. Mapleson[42] predicted that rebreathing would be prevented if fresh gas flow equalled or exceeded minute ventilation. In adults, laboratory[44] and clinical studies[45, 46] documented that rebreathing does not occur until fresh gas flow rate falls below 70 percent, or even 50 percent, of minute ventilation.

During controlled ventilation, the circuit is inefficient. At the beginning of exhalation, the reservoir bag is collapsed and dead space and alveolar gas enter the corrugated tube while fresh gas fills the reservoir bag. On inspiration, as pressure is applied to the reservoir bag, the patient inspires alveolar gas from the proximal corrugated tube. As

airway pressure increases at end inspiration, the overflow valve opens, discharging a mixture of dead space and fresh gas. The patient inspires gas rich in CO_2 while fresh gas is vented through the overflow valve. In adults, a fresh gas flow larger than 20 L/min is necessary to prevent rebreathing during controlled ventilation.[47] Comparable data are not available for children; however, for controlled ventilation there are other circuits with rebreathing characteristics better than the Mapleson A.

Mapleson D Circuits

The circuit identified most commonly with pediatric anesthesia is the Mapleson D. With the D circuit, fresh gas enters the circuit at the patient end and the overflow valve is located near the reservoir bag. Despite the existence of the circuit for many years, there is disagreement regarding optimal flow and ventilatory requirements and new recommendations appear regularly. For many anesthetists, both novice and experienced, the use of the circuit seems confusing, a situation well summarized by Ayre: "How it

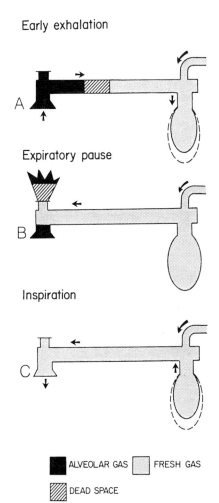

Early exhalation

Expiratory pause

Inspiration

■ ALVEOLAR GAS   □ FRESH GAS
▨ DEAD SPACE

FIGURE 9–6. Mapleson A circuit. During spontaneous ventilation, the overflow valve is open. During exhalation, dead space and alveolar gas enter the corrugated tube while fresh gas enters the reservoir bag. When the reservoir bag fills, alveolar gas, followed by dead space gas, exits from the overflow valve, leaving only fresh gas in the corrugated tube. On inspiration, the patient receives only fresh gas. Function of the circuit during controlled ventilation is described in the text.

works, or what exactly goes on inside its lumen is still something of a mystery even after 30 years."[48] The D system functions differently during controlled and spontaneous ventilation. When it is used for controlled ventilation (Fig. 9–7), the overflow valve is partially closed and opens only during the higher pressures toward the end of inspiration. During exhalation, dead space gas, alveolar gas, and fresh gas enter the corrugated limb. During the expiratory pause, fresh gas continues to enter the circuit, moving the mixed contents of the corrugated tube toward the reservoir bag. As the next breath is initiated, the patient inspires the contents of the corrugated tube, a mixture of fresh, dead space, and alveolar gas. As the pressure in the system increases, the overflow valve opens, discharging the contents of the reservoir bag.

During spontaneous ventilation, the overflow valve is open and gas is exhausted from the circuit when airway pressure is maximal, at the end of exhalation. Early in exhalation, dead space, alveolar, and all fresh gas enter

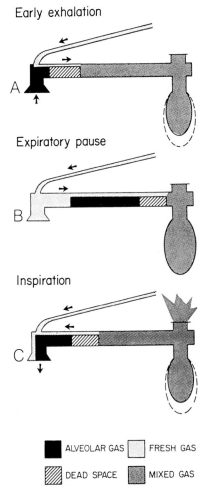

Early exhalation

A

Expiratory pause

B

Inspiration

C

■ ALVEOLAR GAS   □ FRESH GAS

▨ DEAD SPACE   ▨ MIXED GAS

FIGURE 9–7. Mapleson D circuit. During controlled ventilation, the overflow valve is partially closed. During exhalation, dead space, alveolar, and all fresh gas enter the corrugated tube. During the expiratory pause, fresh gas continues to enter the circuit, moving the mixed contents of the corrugated tube toward the reservoir bag. On inspiration, the patient receives the contents of the corrugated tube as well as all fresh gas. The ratio of fresh to alveolar gas in the inspired mixture results from many factors described in the text. The function of the circuit during spontaneous ventilation is also described in the text.

the corrugated limb, as they did during controlled ventilation. As the reservoir bag fills, pressure within the system increases, opening the overflow valve and allowing some of this mixture to exit. On inspiration, the patient receives fresh gas as well as mixed gas from the corrugated tube.

Many factors influence the gas content of the corrugated tube and, therefore, the inspired gas mixture. The influence of these on alveolar ventilation must be considered.

Carbon Dioxide Production

As discussed earlier, the amount of ventilation that the patient requires is a function of CO_2 production. Ventilation must be adjusted to the size and temperature of the patient and the anesthetic technique, and allowances must be made for individual variation.

Respiratory Rate

In breathing circuits in which no rebreathing occurs, changes in minute ventilation are matched by changes in alveolar ventilation and, therefore, P_{CO_2}. With the Mapleson D circuit, the effect of respiratory rate on CO_2 elimination is more complex. During both spontaneous and controlled ventilation, inspired gases derive from both the fresh gas hose and the corrugated tube. At the beginning of exhalation, the gas in the corrugated tube nearest the patient is the fresh gas that accumulated during the expiratory pause. If the expiratory pause is long (e.g., the respiratory rate is slow), the flow of fresh gas will flush alveolar gas toward the reservoir bag; during the next breath, the contents of the inspired gas will be predominantly fresh gas. If the expiratory pause is short (e.g., the respiratory rate is fast), there is insufficient time for fresh gas to flush alveolar gas down the corrugated tube unless the inflow rate of fresh gas is high. As the next breath begins, there is alveolar gas at the patient end of the corrugated hose and the patient inspires both fresh gas from the fresh gas hose and mixed gas from the corrugated tube. In practice, changes in respiratory rate may produce a decrease, no change (Fig. 9–8), or an increase[49] (Fig. 9–9) in P_{CO_2}, depending on the extent of rebreathing.

Fresh Gas Flow

The gas that the patient receives on inspiration derives from the fresh gas hose and the corrugated tube. If the proximal end of the corrugated tube contains fresh gas, the patient will receive mostly fresh gas; conversely, if the alveolar gas has not been flushed toward the reservoir bag, the patient inspires some portion of the previous exhaled breath. Changes in the fresh gas flow affect the contents of the corrugated tube: as flow is increased, alveolar gas is flushed farther from the patient and the inspired gas consists largely of fresh gas (Fig. 9–10). If flows are sufficient to completely eliminate rebreathing, further increases in flow do not affect inspired P_{CO_2}. As fresh gas flow is decreased, less alveolar gas is flushed from the patient end of the circuit and rebreathing is more likely.

Alveolar ventilation is ultimately limited by fresh gas flow (i.e., for any fresh gas flow, P_{CO_2} asymptotes as ventilation increases). Consider the composition of inspired gas

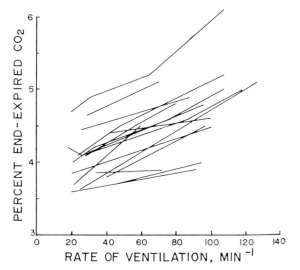

FIGURE 9–8. The effect of changes in respiratory rate on P_{ETCO_2} during controlled ventilation with the Mapleson D circuit. Nightingale et al. administered fresh gas flows of 220 ml/kg and found that P_{CO_2} increased as the respiratory rate increased. (From Nightingale DA, Richards CC, Glass A: An evaluation of rebreathing in a modified t-piece system during controlled ventilation in anesthetized children. Br J Anaesth 37:762, 1965, with permission.)

as ventilation is increased. First, as ventilation is increased, the contribution of fresh gas to each breath decreases (i.e., each breath consists increasingly of contents of the corrugated tube). Second, when ventilation exceeds three times fresh gas flow, the content of the corrugated tube becomes homogeneous and must be equivalent to that exhausted through the overflow valve: assuming a steady state and no leaks (and ignoring small differences between oxygen uptake and CO_2 elimination and the effects of humidification), the P_{CO_2} of this gas must equal CO_2 production divided by the fresh gas flow. Third, P_{ACO_2} must always exceed inspired P_{CO_2}. As a result, once mixing in the corrugated tube is complete, further increases in ventilation do not decrease P_{CO_2}. For example, if CO_2 production were 5 ml/kg/min and fresh gas flow were 100 ml/kg/min, complete mixing of the contents of the corrugated tube would result in an inspired P_{CO_2} of 5 percent; in turn, P_{ACO_2} could never fall below 35 mm Hg, despite high levels of ventilation.

Tidal Volume

Although the effect of changes of tidal volume on gas exchange within the Mapleson D circuit has received little study, knowledge of the rebreathing characteristics of the circuit allows certain predictions. As tidal volume increases, the volume of alveolar gas reaching the corrugated tube increases. If the expiratory pause or the fresh

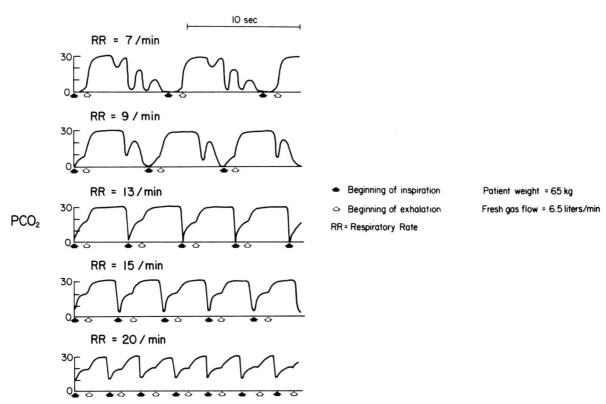

FIGURE 9–9. The effect of changes in respiratory rate on P_{ETCO_2} during controlled ventilation with the Mapleson D circuit. These are an artist's drawing of actual capnographs obtained during anesthesia of a 65-kg child. The x axis represents time in seconds and the y axis P_{CO_2} in mm Hg. The beginnings of inspiration and of exhalation are marked. Tidal volume was 650 ml/breath and the fresh gas flow was 6.5 L/min. Note that an increase in respiratory rate from 7 breaths/min to 20 breaths/min did not change P_{ETCO_2}. At the low respiratory rate, there is no CO_2 in the inspired gas; as the respiratory rate is increased, progressively more CO_2 is present in inspired gas.

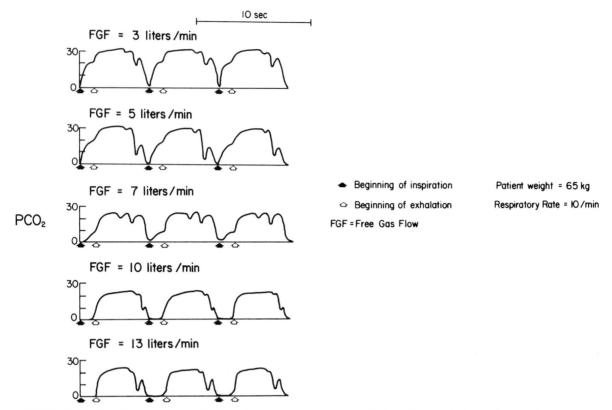

FIGURE 9–10. The effect of changes in fresh gas flow on P_{ETCO_2} during controlled ventilation with the Mapleson D circuit. These are an artist's drawing of actual capnographs obtained during anesthesia of a 65-kg child. The x axis represents time in seconds and the y axis P_{CO_2} in mm Hg. The beginnings of inspiration and of exhalation are marked. Tidal volume was 650 ml/breath and respiratory rate was 10 breaths/min. Increasing fresh gas flow from 3 L/min to 13 L/min decreased P_{ETCO_2} from 32 mm Hg to 24 mm Hg. At the fresh gas flow rate, there is no CO_2 in the inspired gas; as the fresh gas flow rate is decreased, there is progressively more CO_2 in inspired gas.

gas flow is sufficient to allow the corrugated tube to be flushed of alveolar gas, no rebreathing occurs and P_{CO_2} decreases. However, if fresh gas flow or the expiratory pause is not sufficient to flush the additional alveolar gas from the corrugated tube, rebreathing will increase and P_{CO_2} may not decrease. Thus, with high fresh gas flows, an increase in tidal volume may result in a lower P_{CO_2}; with lower fresh gas flows, changes in tidal volume may not affect carbon dioxide exchange.

The complexity of factors affecting rebreathing within the Mapleson D circuit has resulted in a variety of recommendations for fresh gas flow and minute ventilation. Because of the differences in rebreathing with spontaneous and controlled ventilation, there are recommendations for each.

Recommendations for Fresh Gas Flow and Ventilation During Controlled Ventilation. Nightingale et al.[49] varied the fresh gas flow and respiratory rate of children anesthetized with nitrous oxide and measured P_{ETCO_2}. They noted that "carbon dioxide retention is prevented by using a minimum total gas flow of 3 l/min for children under 30 lb. (13.5 kg) body weight and by a fresh gas flow of 100 ml/lb. (220 ml/kg) body weight per minute for larger children." They also encouraged users "to stay within the range of 20 to 60 breaths per minute, regardless of the size of the child."

Rose and Froese,[50] using a lung model, varied fresh gas flow, minute ventilation, and the volume of dead space to define the relationship of these variables to P_{ETCO_2}. These results were then used to determine optimal requirements for fresh gas flow and minute ventilation for the circuit. To achieve normocarbia, they recommended a flow of 1,000 ml/min plus 100 ml/kg/min for patients weighing 10 to 30 kg and 2,000 ml/min plus 50 ml/kg/min for children larger than 30 kg. Using a minute ventilation equal to twice the fresh gas flow, P_{CO_2} averaged 44 mm Hg and ranged from 30 to 48 mm Hg. To achieve hypocarbia (P_{CO_2} of 30 mm Hg), they recommended increasing flow to 1,600 ml/min plus 100 ml/kg/min for smaller patients and 3,200 ml/min plus 50 ml/kg/min for larger subjects. With minute ventilation set at twice the fresh gas flow, P_{CO_2} averaged 34 mm Hg and ranged from 27 to 41 mm Hg.

Rayburn and Graves,[51] using the alveolar gas equation and Bain and Spoerel's values for CO_2 production, calculated that a fresh gas flow of 2,000 ml/m²/min would be necessary to maintain normocarbia during anesthesia with nitrous oxide, halothane, and d-tubocurarine. In practice, a fresh gas flow of 2,500 ml/m²/min was required to maintain a P_{CO_2} of 40 mm Hg, a discrepancy they explained by variability in CO_2 production, anesthetic uptake, and alveolar dead space.

Baraka et al.[52] evaluated the D circuit during controlled ventilation in patients 2 months to 4 years of age anesthetized with halothane. Using a fresh gas flow of 5 L/m²/min, a tidal volume of 15 ml/kg, and a respiratory rate of 19 to 26 breaths/min, P_{CO_2} averaged 37 mm Hg and ranged from 32 to 42 mm Hg. They concluded that normocarbia could be achieved using this fresh gas flow and a calculated minute volume equal to 1.5 times fresh gas flow.

Bain and Spoerel,[53] using the circuit in adults, initially recommended a fresh gas flow of 5.5 L/min and a minute ventilation exceeding fresh gas flow to maintain normocarbia. Later, these recommendations were revised to a fresh gas flow of 70 ml/kg/min, a tidal volume of 10 ml/kg/breath, and a respiratory rate of 12 to 14 breaths/min.[54] For patients under 50 kg, they recommended a fresh gas flow of 3.5 L/min. Subsequently, observing that infants weighing less than 10 kg ventilated with a fresh gas flow of 3.5 L/min were always hypocapnic, they recommended using fresh gas flows of 2 L/min for smaller infants.[3]

Ramanathan et al.[55] acknowledged that normocapnia could be maintained using the fresh flows proposed by Bain and Spoerel. However, using these flows in a lung model, they found that the inspired concentration of carbon dioxide was as high as 2.4 percent, considerably above the 1 percent limit they considered acceptable. Consequently, they recommended that the circuit always be used with flows of 8 L/min to ensure that CO_2 retention would not result from rebreathing.

Seeley et al.[56] performed a theoretical analysis of the relationship between Pa_{CO_2}, CO_2 production, alveolar ventilation, and fresh gas flow. These analyses resulted in nomograms from which Pa_{CO_2} could be predicted on the basis of fresh gas flow and minute ventilation. However, the nomograms were not tested in humans.

To establish requirements for use of the Mapleson D circuit in newborns, Gwilt et al.[57] studied rabbits weighing 2 to 4 kg. They found that a fresh gas flow of 3 L/min, a tidal volume of 10 ml/kg, and a respiratory rate of 40 breaths/min consistently resulted in hypocapnia (mean P_{CO_2}, 27 mm Hg). They concluded that these settings were directly applicable to human neonates.

The anesthetist who uses the Mapleson D circuit with controlled ventilation has available many recommendations for fresh gas flow and minute ventilation, each of which has been shown to provide predictable alveolar ventilation. How, then, can the user select the most appropriate recommendations? Several recommendations require special attention on the part of the anesthesiologist: Rayburn and Graves' proposal requires the anesthetist to consult a nomogram to determine body surface area, whereas the recommendations of Seeley et al. require use of their nomogram. Of the remaining proposals, those by Rose et al. and by Bain and Spoerel are simplest (Table 9–1). Use of the recommendations of Rose et al. requires knowledge of two formulas for fresh gas flow; ventilation is set at twice this fresh gas flow. Even simpler is Bain and Spoerel's recommendation of the fresh gas flow of 70 ml/kg/min with a minimal flow of 3.5 L/min; in infants weighing less than 10 kg, a flow of 2 L/min is used. Ventilation is identical for all patients: a respiratory rate of 12 to 14 breaths/min and a tidal volume of 10 ml/kg. The simplicity of these settings is apparent to users of time-cycled mechanical ventilators such as the Ohmeda 7800. With inspiratory rate set to 12 to 14 breaths/min, inspiratory gas flow can be adjusted until peak airway pressure in approximately 20 cm H_2O; this typically results in the desired tidal volume of 10 ml/kg.

Recommendations for Fresh Gas Flow and Ventilation During Spontaneous Ventilation.

Mapleson[42] determined that during spontaneous ventilation a fresh gas flow exceeding twice the patient's minute volume was necessary to prevent rebreathing of expired gas. Harrison[58] examined patterns of respiratory flow and demonstrated that rebreathing can be avoided completely if fresh gas flow exceeds peak inspiratory flow. However, peak flows varied greatly and, in infants, exceeded three times minute volume. He concluded that fresh gas flows of 2.5 times minute volume were generally sufficient to prevent rebreathing. For many years, it was believed that the circuit could be used with spontaneous ventilation only if rebreathing was avoided completely; therefore, high fresh gas flows were necessary and the circuit was deemed inefficient for use during spontaneous ventilation beyond infancy.

Spoerel et al.[59] subsequently demonstrated that, despite rebreathing, normocapnia can be achieved during spontaneous ventilation with the D circuit using fresh gas flows of less than twice minute volume. They studied adults anesthetized with nitrous oxide and halothane who breathed spontaneously. Pet_{CO_2} increased from 36 ± 3 (mean $\pm$ SD) to 42 ± 4 mm Hg as fresh gas flow decreased from 140 ml/kg/min to 70 ml/kg/min. Despite the presence of inspired CO_2, all patients maintained normal alveolar ventilation by increasing their minute ventilation markedly. Minute volume was 4.7 L/m^2/min through the circle system, not significantly different from the value of 5.3 L/m^2/min in patients breathing through the Mapleson D at high fresh gas flows (140 ml/kg/min). As fresh gas flow in the D circuit was decreased to 100 and then to 70 ml/kg/min, minute ventilation increased to 5.7 and then 7.5 L/m^2/min, respectively. Thus, Pet_{CO_2} remained normal despite significant rebreathing; this was accomplished by a marked increase in minute ventilation. Based on these findings, Spoerel et al. advocated that the Mapleson D circuit could be used with spontaneous ventilation in anesthetized adults with a fresh gas flow of 100 ml/kg/min. They also suggested that rebreathing could be advantageous because it stimulated the patient to hyperventilate, "contributing to better oxygenation and the prevention of alveolar collapse."

This recommendation was criticized by Byrick,[60] who observed that low fresh gas flows increased respiratory rate rather than tidal volume. In addition, the ventilatory response to inspired CO_2 was highly variable in adults anesthetized with 1 percent halothane. When he decreased fresh gas flows in a Mapleson D circuit from 150 ml/kg/min to 70 ml/kg/min, some patients increased their minute ventilation; as a result, Pet_{CO_2} changed minimally. However, in others, the decrease in fresh gas flow did not result in an increase in minute ventilation and Pet_{CO_2} increased. These "poor responders" depended on the absence of rebreathing to maintain normal alveolar ventilation. Byrick also questioned the benefit of hyperpnea. Rose et al.,[61] using a lung model, found that the lower fresh gas flow increased minute ventilation and, in turn, increased the inspired concentration of CO_2. They questioned whether patients would be able to sustain high levels of minute ventilation without fatiguing.

Fresh gas requirements during spontaneous ventilation in children have received less attention. Soliman and

TABLE 9 – 1			
TWO SETS OF RECOMMENDATIONS FOR FRESH GAS FLOW AND MINUTE VENTILATION TO PRODUCE NORMOCAPNIA DURING VENTILATION WITH THE MAPLESON D CIRCUIT			
Recommendations by Bain and Spoerel[3, 53, 54]			
Weight (kg)	**Fresh Gas Flow (ml/min)**	**Tidal Volume (ml/kg)**	**Respiratory Rate (breaths/min)**
<10	2,000 ml/min	10	12–14
10–50	3,500 ml/min	10	12–14
>50	70 ml/kg/min	10	12–14
Recommendations by Rose and Froese[50]			
Weight (kg)	**Fresh Gas Flow**		**Minute Ventilation**
10–30	1,000 ml/min + 100 ml/kg/min		2 × fresh gas flow
> 30	2,000 ml/min + 50 ml/kg/min		2 × fresh gas flow

Laberge[62] studied children aged 1 to 5 years anesthetized with nitrous oxide and halothane. Fresh gas flow was set to 50 percent more than the desired alveolar ventilation based on body surface area. A fresh gas flow of 206 ± 42 (mean ± SD) ml/kg/min resulted in normocapnia. However, Soliman and Laberge measured neither inspired CO_2 nor minute ventilation, and their suggestions are subject to the same criticisms as those of Spoerel and colleagues.

Lindahl et al.[63] evaluated several formulas for fresh gas flow during spontaneous ventilation to determine which formulas ensured that there was no rebreathing. They anesthetized infants and children with nitrous oxide and halothane and permitted them to breathe spontaneously. Fresh gas flow was then decreased until inspired CO_2 could be detected. The fresh gas flow at the time that rebreathing occurred was then compared with the fresh gas flow requirements that had been predicted using several formulas. A fresh gas flow equal to twice minute ventilation consistently resulted in rebreathing, whereas a flow equal to three times minute ventilation usually eliminated rebreathing. A third formula, fresh gas flow = 15 × patient's weight × respiratory rate, underestimated fresh gas flow requirements in only one subject (whose respiratory rate was less than 15 breaths/min). The fourth formula, a fresh gas flow of 3 × (1,000 + 100 × weight in kilograms), never underestimated fresh gas flow requirements.

As with controlled ventilation, the anesthesiologist must select among several recommendations for fresh gas flow during spontaneous ventilation. In infants, a fresh gas flow (approximately 4.5 L/min for a 10-kg infant) of three times predicted minute ventilation can be used without polluting the operating room; however, expense may be large. In larger children, fresh gas flows of three times predicted minute ventilation are likely to be expensive. Using the recommendations by Spoerel et al. of 100 ml/kg/min, normocapnia can probably be achieved but at the expense of a marked increase in minute ventilation. If the clinician monitors alveolar ventilation with blood gases or capnography, these lower fresh gas flows can probably be used safely. However, if the clinician is unable to monitor end-tidal (and inspired) P_{CO_2}, higher fresh gas flows may be advisable to ensure that rebreathing is not excessive. Finally, in most (and possibly all) patients, a circle system with a CO_2 absorber can be used with lower fresh gas flows than those necessary in the Mapleson D circuit. As newer but more expensive inhalational anesthetics have

become available, increasing emphasis on cost reduction may limit the clinician's opportunity to use high fresh gas flows during anesthesia, further limiting the utility of the Mapleson D circuit.

Bain Circuit

The Bain circuit is a variant of the Mapleson D in which the fresh gas flow is placed coaxial with the expiratory limb (Fig. 9–11).[53] Developed originally for the evaluation of life jackets,[12] this circuit was introduced to anesthesia in 1972 by Bain and Spoerel.[53] Despite the placement of the fresh gas hose within the expiratory limb, fresh gas enters the circuit directly at the patient end of the circuit and alveolar gas is exhausted through the expiratory limb to the overflow valve. Therefore, the circuit functions identically to the Mapleson D. Bain and Spoerel's suggestion that this was a universal anesthesia circuit, applicable with both spontaneous and controlled ventilation and with patients of all sizes, led to renewed interest in the use of the Mapleson D circuit.

The Bain circuit has some advantages over other Mapleson D circuits. Because the fresh gas hose is internal, the circuit is streamlined and may interfere less with the operating field during neurosurgical and other head and neck procedures. Made of lightweight plastic, the circuit is less likely to cause kinking of the TT or accidental extubation. In addition, because the Bain circuit can be mounted on the anesthesia machine, expired gases are

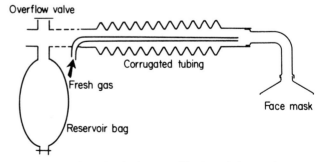

FIGURE 9–11. The Bain circuit, a modification of the Mapleson D in which the fresh gas hose is coaxial with the corrugated tube. Because fresh gas enters the circuit at the patient end and the overflow valve is located near the reservoir, the Bain circuit functions identically to the Mapleson D.

more readily scavenged than with many older Mapleson circuits. However, the belief that placing the fresh gas hose inside the corrugated tube increases heat and humidity in the inspired gas[64] is not valid for pediatric patients. For example, the anesthesiologist might use a fresh gas flow of 2.0 L/min for an infant weighing 5 kg. If minute ventilation were 150 ml/kg/min, then only 37.5 percent (750/2,000) of the fresh gas would ever enter the patient and be warmed and humidified. The remaining larger percentage of inspired gas would be cold and dry. Decreasing the fresh gas flow would increase the temperature and humidity of inspired gas but would also increase rebreathing of exhaled CO_2. The anesthesiologist concerned about temperature and humidity of inspired gas should probably add a humidifier or artificial nose to the breathing circuit.

One problem with the Bain circuit concerns the potential for unacceptable levels of rebreathing if the fresh gas hose fractures or disconnects within the expiratory limb. If this occurs, fresh gas enters the corrugated tube near the reservoir (rather than near the patient), the entire volume of the circuit between the fracture and the patient becomes dead space, and marked hypercarbia is inevitable.[65] To assess the integrity of the fresh gas hose, Pethick[66] recommended that a high flow of gas (i.e., oxygen flush) be passed through the circuit. If the fresh gas hose is intact, a Venturi effect decreases the pressure in the expiratory limb, causing the reservoir bag to collapse. If the fresh gas hose is fractured, gas enters the expiratory limb, causing the reservoir bag to fill. This maneuver requires only seconds and is recommended as part of the preanesthetic check for this circuit.

Another coaxial circuit, the CPRAM (Controlled Partial Rebreathing Anesthesia Method) Breathing System (KHI Anesthesia and Resuscitation, Frazer, PA) differs from the Bain circuit by having two side-holes at the patient end of the inner hose. The manufacturer claimed (although they provide no documentation) that this results in "vortex dynamics," which provides better humidification of fresh gases and efficient removal of CO_2. Unfortunately, these side-holes prevent the clinician from performing Pethick's maneuver because gas exits through the side-holes and the reservoir bag always fills. Although the manufacturer claims that the corrugated design of the inner hose makes it less likely to fracture, the clinician cannot determine whether a problem exists. Pethick's maneuver was modified for the CPRAM circuit by Robinson and Fisher,[67] who occluded the side-holes by placing a 1.5-cm segment of a 6.5-mm ETT over the patient end of the inner hose (Fig. 9–12). However, if this segment of tubing is not removed from the circuit before its use, the tubing may be lost in the patient's airway.[68] Consequently, I recommend against using the CPRAM circuit.

Circuits Combining Features of the Mapleson A and D

When both controlled and spontaneous ventilation are required during the same anesthetic (e.g., if a muscle relaxant is given to facilitate tracheal intubation, a period of controlled ventilation is required until spontaneous ventilation resumes), a circuit incorporating features of both the A and the D might be desirable. Several breathing

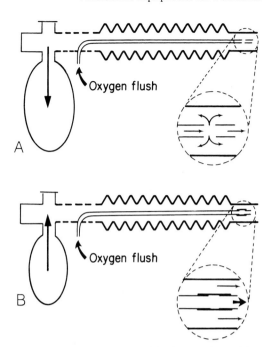

FIGURE 9–12. Checking the integrity of the fresh gas hose of the CPRAM circuit. A, With the CPRAM circuit, Pethick's maneuver results in gas exiting through the side-holes of the fresh gas hose and the reservoir bag fills. B, Occluding the side-holes with a short segment of a 6.5-mm TT permits the user to assess the integrity of the fresh gas hose. (From Robinson S, Fisher DM: Safety check for the CPRAM circuit. Anesthesiology 59:488, 1983, with permission.)

circuits have been described that function as the A circuit during spontaneous ventilation and as the D circuit during controlled ventilation.

Waters[69] described a circuit with overflow valves at both ends and a rotating valve that directed fresh gas into either end of the circuit. By adjusting the overflow valves and directing the fresh gas appropriately, the circuit could be interchanged rapidly between the A and D configurations. Baraka et al.[70] described a circuit that contained two T-pieces, one at the reservoir and the other at the patient end of the circuit. If the fresh gas hose was attached at the patient end, the circuit functioned as a D; attaching the fresh gas hose to the other T-piece resulted in the A configuration.

Several coaxial versions of these circuits have been described.[71-73] In one, Manicom and Schoonbee[73] added a valve to the Bain circuit near the reservoir bag. With the valve in the D position, the circuit is identical to the Bain circuit, with fresh gas entering the inner hose and exhaled gas exiting at the relief valve. By revolving the valve to the A position, fresh gas now enters the outer tube at the machine end and exhaled gas is transported via the inner tube to the overflow valve. Because all expired gas passes through the narrow inner tube during spontaneous ventilation, expiratory resistance is high, 2.6 cm H_2O at a 30-L/min gas flow. Despite theoretical advantages of gas economy with these circuits, none of them has become popular.

Circuits with Inspiratory, Expiratory, and Overflow (Popoff) Valves

The breathing circuit most widely used for adults is the circle system. The circuit consists of a fresh gas source, undirectional inspiratory and expiratory valves, an over-flow valve, inspiratory and expiratory tubes, a reservoir bag, a Y-shaped airway adapter, and a canister containing CO_2 absorbant (Fig. 9–13). The circuit functions similarly during controlled and spontaneous ventilation. The inspiratory valve is opened by negative intrapleural pressure or compression of the reservoir bag. Fresh gas is then directed into the inspiratory limb and, as inspiratory flow exceeds fresh gas flow, gas that has passed through the canister follows. On exhalation, pressure within the circuit increases, closing the inspiratory valve and opening the expiratory valve. This directs alveolar gas down the expiratory limb towards the overflow valve and canister. During the expiratory pause, the inspiratory valve is closed and fresh gas flows retrograde through the canister. If the valves are competent and the absorbant is functioning, gas flow through the patient's part of the circuit is unidirectional and there is no inspired CO_2. Although valves may appear competent, large quantities of expired gas could enter the inspiratory limb (and be rebreathed) if the inspiratory valve does not close immediately during exhalation. In adults with normal lung compliance, as much as 150 ml of gas leaked through the inspiratory value during manual ventilation.[74] Dead space of the circle system is only from the Y-piece to the patient's airway and does not include the volume of the breathing hoses.[75] Circle systems differ from the circuits previously described by having unidirectional valves and a canister, each of which contributes to the resistance of the circuit.

During the 1950s, the circle system was believed to be undesirable for pediatric anesthesia. Stephen and Slater[76] noted "early fatigue of the patient and undesirable upset in body metabolism," and Adriani and Griggs[77] observed that the breathing of infants was "laborious and deep." This was attributed to excessive dead space and resistance. These experiences might have limited use of the circle system to adult anesthesia. However, cyclopropane had been demonstrated to be a versatile and potent anesthetic for children and its excessive cost and flammability mandated its use in semiclosed systems such as the circle. This led to alterations of the adult circle designed to lower dead space and decrease resistance. Similar considerations of the cost of new inhaled anesthetics (desflurane and sevoflurane) has once again propeled clinicians towards using circle systems for pediatric patients.

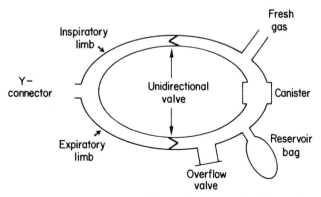

FIGURE 9–13. Components of the circle system and their usual arrangement.

Conventional Adult Circle Systems

The unfavorable experiences of Adriani and Griggs and of Stephen and Slater suggested that respiratory compromise was the result of excessive dead space and resistance. The introduction of improved valves and canisters and connectors of lower resistance renewed interest in using adult circle systems for pediatric anesthesia. Graff et al.[78] anesthetized infants with nitrous oxide and halothane and alternated between an Ayre's T-piece and an adult circle. Arterialized capillary blood obtained after the infants had breathed through each circuit for 15 minutes demonstrated no difference in pH or P_{CO_2}. There was no evidence of cardiovascular or other clinical compromise with either breathing circuit.

Van Steeg and Stevens[79] compared the respiratory efforts of infants anesthetized with nitrous oxide and halothane and breathing through T-piece and several infant and adult circle systems. Although respiratory work was least with the T-piece and infant circles, minute ventilation was not compromised with any circuit.

The circle system is now commonly used for pediatric anesthesia. If a circle system is used, the anesthesiologist must be sure that the equipment will not injure the patient. Valves must have low resistance and must use nonsticking disks. Canisters and connectors must be designed to offer minimal resistance to the movement of anesthetic gases. If equipment that satisfies these criteria is available, it appears that infants and children tolerate periods of spontaneous ventilation without compromise. If ventilation is controlled, as is becoming increasingly common, there is little advantage of Mapleson circuits compared with the circle system.

Pediatric Circles

Several circle systems specific for pediatric patients have been described. Each contains the basic components of the adult circle; however, these components are reduced in size. With the Bloomquist Pediatric Circle Absorber, the anesthesiologist can assemble the circuit with the canister on either the inspiratory or expiratory limb.[80] Bloomquist suggested that placing the canister on the inspiratory limb permitted the anesthesiologist to assist ventilation to overcome resistance of the canister. The Ohio Infant Circle Absorber[75] differs from the usual circle configuration because the fresh gas inlet is placed downstream from the inspiratory valve, ensuring a constant flow of fresh gas to flush the dead space of the mask. At a fresh gas flow of 3 L/min, dead space under the mask was less than 5 ml compared with 7 to 19 ml with other breathing systems.[81] Both of these pediatric circle systems incorporated smaller inspiratory and expiratory tubing, reservoirs, and canisters as well as a divided Y-connector (see below) to minimize dead space. Resistance of these circuits is low, less than 0.3 cm H_2O at a flow of 10 L/min with the Ohio system.

Clinical experience with these circuits was favorable. McDonald[82] found the circuits to be acceptable for children less than 30 kg, and Van Steeg and Stevens[79] found that respiratory effort with the infant circle was no different from that with the valveless T-piece. Podlesch et al.[31] measured P_{ETCO_2} in infants who were anesthetized with nitrous oxide and halothane and breathing spontaneously through pediatric circle systems and T-pieces: no difference in P_{ETCO_2} was noted.

Although the value of the pediatric circle has been demonstrated, it did not become popular. Smith[33] noted that there is a "considerable nuisance factor in . . . (the) complete changeover from adult systems." Adriani and Griggs[77] noted that many parts of these pediatric circles are not interchangeable with standard anesthesia equipment. They believed that, unless carefully maintained, the pediatric circles are unlikely to be readily available for use in children. In institutions where adult circles are used and special equipment is desired for children, a T-piece or Mapleson D circuit can be used with less difficulty than an infant circle.

Special Devices for Use with Circle Systems

Divided Airway Adapter

The dead space of the circle system includes the volume of the Y-connector; with older circuits, this may be as large as 40 ml.[77] Although this volume is of minor consequence to an adult, it represents a large portion of the tidal volume of an infant and results in excessive rebreating. One means to reduce this dead space was to substitute "divided chimney piece." The Columbia Pediatric Circle Valve (Fig. 9–14) consisted of an 8.5-mm tube placed

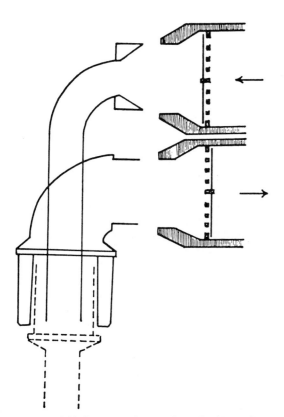

FIGURE 9–14. Divided airway adapter. The Columbia pediatric circle valve. Dead space is 0.5 ml, markedly less than the 40-ml dead space of conventional airway adapters used in earlier eras. (From Rackow H, Salanitre E: A new pediatric circle valve. Anesthesiology 29:833, 1968, with permission.)

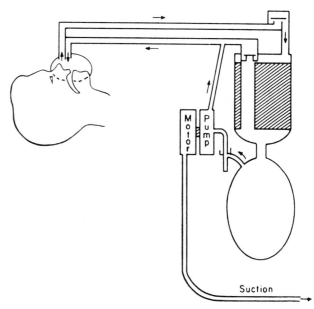

FIGURE 9–15. Circulator for circle system. The Revell circulator consists of two automobile windshield wiper pumps joined, so that one, driven by wall suction, powers the other, which circulates gas through the circle system. Beneath the circulator is a water trap. (From Revell DG: A circulator to eliminate mechanical dead space in circle absorption system. Can Anaesth Soc J 6:98, 1959, with permission.)

concentric to a curved 15-mm airway adaptor.[83] This separated inspiratory and expiratory gas, decreasing the connector's dead space to 0.5 ml. Because the cros-sectional areas of the inspiratory and expiratory pathways were similar, resistance was low, 1 cm H_2O at a flow of 15 L/min.[83]

Circulators

The volume of gas under the face mask also contributes to the apparatus dead space of the circle system. With contoured masks, this may be only 7 ml,[81] but for an infant this represents a large portion of the tidal volume and may results in excessive rebreathing. This dead space could be reduced by removing exhaled gas from the mask during the expiratory pause, using devices known as circulators. Adriani and Griggs[77] mounted a 50-ml rubber bulb with unidirectional valves on the inspiratory limb. During spontaneous ventilation in a 5-year-old, P_{CO_2} under the mask fell from 2.4 mm Hg to 0.6 mm Hg when the bulb was manipulated. Unfortunately, this manually operated device required constant attention.

Revell[84] added a power source, thereby minimizing the burden for the anesthesiologist. To avoid electrical hazards he drove his device with suction. The shafts of two automobile windshield wiper motors were attached. One, driven by suction, operates as the motor; the other, connected to the anesthesia circuit, becomes a pump (Fig. 9–15). The pump consists of two chambers: while one is filling, the other is discharging. As a result, the gas content of the circuit remains constant so that the volume of the reservoir bag is not disturbed. Another source of driving power for the circulator, fresh gas entering the circuit at low flows through parallel jets, was proposed by Neff et al.[85] Because of the Venturi principle, this results in a continuous flow of 18 to 20 L/min and the inspiratory and expiratory valves float in the open position. Functionally, this modification resembles the Revell circulator.

These devices offer an additional advantage. At high flows, the valves are kept open and the patient need not exert any energy to open them. Despite the efficiency of these devices in decreasing apparatus dead space, they have not become popular. In addition to the nuisance of additional equipment, continuous flow within the circle system magnifies the effects of small leaks and may result in loss of anesthetic gas or entrainment of room air. Although circulators are now largely of historical interest, they may be incorporated into revolutionary future anesthetic breathing circuits (A. Berssenbrugge, personal communication, PhD, Ohmeda).

Selecting a Breathing Circuit

Several anesthesia breathing circuits and their advantages and disadvantages have been reviewed. The simplest of these, Ayre's T-piece, is now used infrequently and has been replaced by circuits that permit monitoring of spontaneous ventilation and facilitate control of ventilation. The Mapleson A circuit has limited utility (during spontaneous ventilation) and is used rarely. In contrast, the Mapleson D circuit, because it lacks inspiratory and expiratory valves, has been popular for pediatric anesthesia. With this circuit, alveolar ventilation is a function of fresh gas flow, respiratory rate, and CO_2 production; although these factors appear complex, their effect on rebreathing can be learned. A coaxial version of the Mapleson D circuit, the Bain circuit, led to renewed interest in the use of these circuits.

The other circuit commonly used for pediatric anesthesia is the adult circle. The presence of inspiratory and expiratory valves increases resistance compared with the Mapleson D circuit; however, the resistance of modern breathing circuits is less than that imposed by the TT.[86] Ideally, work of breathing should be measured in anesthetized children breathing spontaneously through modern circle systems or Mapleson D circuits. These data do not exist. However, work of breathing determined in a lung model (using a tidal volume of 500 ml; therefore, applicability to infants is questionable) was similar with the circle system and the circuits corresponding to the Mapleson A and D.[87] In addition, Conterato et al.[88] studied halothane-anesthetized children aged 1 to 3 years breathing alternatively through Mapleson D and circle systems. Minute ventilation was slightly higher with the circle system, but PETCO2 was similar with the two circuits, suggesting a larger dead space with the circle system (possibly a result of differences in lung volume). Both dynamic compliance and total pulmonary resistance were similar with the two circuits. These findings suggest that there is little functional difference between circuits when used for children older than 1 year. Additional data are necessary to assess the relative advantages of the circuits for spontaneous ventilation in younger patients. Finally, if ventilation is controlled (as has become common practice for infants and children and should probably always be done for neonates), there is little difference between the Mapleson D and the circle system.

As newer inhaled anesthetics are adopted into clinical practice, the increased expense of these drugs necessitates that clinicians consider using equipment that permits lower fresh gas flows. In that the Mapleson D circuit (and its variants) offers little advantage over the circle system but requires a larger fresh gas flow to prevent hypercarbia, it is likely that the use of Mapleson D circuits will decrease in future decades.

Finally, the anesthesiologist should be aware of the factors that influence work of breathing, alveolar gas exchange, and adequacy of oxygenation. However, modern monitoring devices including pulse oximetry and capnography afford the anesthesiologist assurance that his or her patient's oxygenation and ventilation are adequate.

ENDOTRACHEAL TUBES

Selecting a TT for the pediatric patient requires the anesthesiologist to consider several issues. The tube must be sufficiently large to permit spontaneous or controlled ventilation but not so large as to damage the trachea. It must also seal the trachea against aspiration; this can be accomplished either by inflating a cuff or by selecting a tube whose external diameter nearly fills the trachea. In addition, the tube must be composed of materials that do not elicit an inflammatory response.

The increased resistance of a small TT typically leads the anesthesiologist to select the largest tube that will enter the patient's trachea. Additional reasons for selecting a large tube include the lesser likelihood of secretions plugging a larger tube, the ability to pass a larger suction catheter should suctioning be necessary, and the lesser likelihood that a large tube will permit aspiration of foreign material into the lung. However, placing a large TT may damage the trachea by applying excessive pressure to the tracheal mucosa. Therefore, the anesthesiologist must select a tube that is sufficiently large, but not too large.

Tracheal damage occurs when pressure from the TT against the wall of the trachea exceeds the capillary pressure of the tracheal mucosa. This pressure is believed to be 25 to 35 mm Hg in adults.[89] No values are available for children, but the mean arterial pressure of term neonates is one third to one half that of adults. The anesthesiologist can estimate pressure against the tracheal wall in the intubated patient by slowly inflating the reservoir bag. The pressure at which a leak is audible (listening over the neck or mouth) is believed to approximate the pressure against the tracheal wall.[90] However, several factors in addition to the size of the TT may influence the pressure at which a leak occurs. Turning the patient's head to the side or making the measurement when the patient has not been paralyzed with a muscle relaxant increases the pressure required to cause a leak; in contrast, leak pressure is not influenced by the depth of insertion of the tube into the trachea or the fresh gas flow rates.[90] The influence of depth of anesthesia on leak pressure has not been determined.

If the leak occurs at a high pressure, it is likely that the tube is too large for that patient's trachea[91] and may induce ischemic damage. In contrast, if the leak occurs at a very low pressure, the patient may not be protected from aspiration and it may be difficult to ventilate the lungs with positive pressure, particularly if compliance is abnormal. Unfortunately, there is no information regarding the leak pressure at which tracheal damage will occur in pediatric patients. A leak at less than 10 cm H_2O suggests that the TT is inappropriately small, whereas a leak pressure exceeding 40 cm H_2O is probably excessive. Whether a leak pressure of 15, 20, 25, or 30 cm H_2O is most appropriate remains to be determined. My approach is to aim for a higher leak pressure (25 to 35 cm H_2O) when higher peak inspiratory pressures or increased minute ventilation may be required during anesthesia (e.g., during a throacotomy, craniotomy, or a procedure in the upper abdomen, or when the patient has abnormal pulmonary compliance). When high airway pressures will not be required during anesthesia, a leak pressure of 10 to 25 cm H_2O appears not to be associated with morbidity.

Several methods are available to aid in the selection of the appropriate TT. Two techniques, measuring the diameter of the distal joint of the index finger or the lumen of the external naris,[33] are popular but have not been evaluated formally. Clinical experience has resulted in a number of tables and formulas for tube size based on age and weight.[33, 92–96] The variability of these recommendations led Chodoff et al.[97] to question whether tube size should be based on physical characteristics or age. By inserting progressively larger tubes until they found the largest tube that could be gently inserted into the trachea, they found that the best correlate of tube size was age rather than height, weight, or body surface area. Penlington[98] suggested two formulas to estimate tracheal tube size:

Tube size (mm ID) for children younger than 6 years
$$= \frac{\text{Age (years)}}{3} + 3.75$$

Tube size (mm ID) for children older than 6 years
$$= \frac{\text{Age (years)}}{4} + 4.5$$

For practical reasons, Levin[99] recommended a single formula based on age:

$$\text{Tube size (mm ID)} = \frac{\text{Age (years)} + 18}{4}$$

When Lee et al.[100] used this formula, leak pressure exceeded 40 cm H_2O in 30 percent of the patients, and in 23 percent the leak occurred at less than 20 cm H_2O. This suggests that use of a single formula based on age frequently leads to selection of an excessively large or small TT. This is corroborated by Mostafa,[101] who found that for children in each age range, 15 percent required a tube one size smaller, 1 percent two sizes smaller, and 11 percent one size larger than that predicted for age.

The rapid growth during the first months of postnatal life makes these formulas invalid for neonates. The larynx of a full-term neonate usually accommodates a 3-mm[33] or 3.5-mm[102] TT, and infants weighing 1,500 to 3,500 g tolerate a 3-mm tube.[103] In infants weighing less than 1,500 g, a 2.5-mm tube is usually recommended.[33] However, autopsy measurements in these infants suggest that the diameter of the cricoid ring is often less than 3.8 mm, the external diameter of a 2.5-mm TT.[104] This may explain why subglottic stenosis occasionally occurs after prolonged intubation in small neonates.

Although no formula or table guarantees selection of the appropriate tube, the anesthesiologist must recognize that a tight TT might traumatize the trachea, whereas a loose tube may not protect against aspiration. If the leak test indicates that the size of the tube is inappropriate, the TT should probably be changed to one of an appropriate size.

Cuffed Tubes

Cuffed TTs are used routinely for adults, whereas uncuffed tubes are generally used in infants and young children. The common use of uncuffed tubes in pediatric patients results from two factors. First, the cuff increases the external diameter of the TT and may necessitate using a smaller tube, increasing airway resistance and the work of breathing. The second factor is less widely appreciated. The narrowest portion of the airway of the adult, at the glottis or the vocal cords,[105] is rarely circular.[106] Therefore, a round TT that passes through the glottis will not seal the trachea. In contrast, the smallest portion of the trachea of the infant is the rounded cricoid ring,[107, 108] and a tube whose outer diameter approximates the diameter of the cricoid ring seals the trachea without applying excessive pressure to the tracheal wall. Therefore, in children, uncuffed TTs of the appropriate size can be used to seal the trachea.

When a cuffed TT is used in children and adults, the cuff must be inflated cautiously. If a cuff is inflated to the "just seal" point, lateral wall pressures may reach 75 mm Hg.[89] If nitrous oxide is administered, the volume and pressure of both low- and high-pressure cuffs increases as nitrous oxide diffuses into the cuff,[109] possibly damaging the trachea. Tracheal damage can be minimized by selecting a tube whose cuff seals the trachea before the cuff is filled to its residual volume. Periodic deflation and careful reinflation of the cuff may protect against tracheal damage. However, this is not proven.

Recently, Khine et al.[110] challenged the traditional assumption that cuffed TTs should not be used in pediatric anesthesia. Children ($n = 488$) aged 0 to 8 years were randomized to receive either uncuffed TTs (ID [mm] of 4 + age/4; age in years) or cuffed TTs (ID of 3 + age/4). With cuffed tubes, the cuff was inflated using a device that limited its pressure to 25 mm Hg. With both TTs, if there was not an audible leak around the TT when the lungs were inflated to a pressure of 20 to 30 cm H_2O, a smaller tube was placed.

Replacement of the TT initially selected for intubation was necessary more often with uncuffed TTs (23 percent of patients) than with cuffed TTs (1 percent). Postextubation croup was infrequent (2.4 percent and 2.9 percent of patients with cuffed and uncuffed TTs, respectively) and there was no evidence of tracheal damage. Khine et al. recommended that cuffed TTs, sized appropriately and with care taken to prevent overinflation of the cuff, were safe for pediatric patients. Although I adopted their recommendations into my clinical practice, several cautions are warranted. First, a larger clinical series or extensive clinical experience may be needed to ensure that cuffed tubes do not induce tracheal damage. Second, most clinicians will not use a pressure-limiting device similar to that used by Khine et al. to ensure that cuff pressure is not excessive. Third, should the patient remain intubated after anesthesia, nonanesthesia clinicians caring for the patient (e.g., neonatologists) may not be familiar with issues related to overinflation of the cuff. The study by Khine et al. did not determine if subglottic stenosis occurred at a later age.

Materials

TTs have traditionally been available in several materials. Polyvinyl chloride (PVC) is the most widely used and silicone rubber (Silastic) has become increasingly popular; use of red rubber has decreased markedly. The finding in the 1960s that certain materials were toxic to tracheal mucosa, producing an inflammatory response, led to testing to evaluate toxicity.[111] The most common procedure requires implanting a sliver of TT material into the paravertebral muscle of a rabbit and examining for tissue toxicity, both macroscopically and microscopically, in 3 or 7 days. If there is no inflammatory response, tubes made from that batch of material can be marked IT (implant-tested) or Z79 (the symbol of the Z79 committee of the American Society for Testing of Materials). However, passing the implant test does not ensure that mucosal damage will not occur. If the trachea is abused by inserting too large an TT or the vocal cords are traumatized during laryngoscopy, damage may occur despite the use of a nontoxic material.

Configuration of the Tracheal Tube

Tracheal tubes with special configurations may be of benefit during certain surgical procedures, particularly those involving the head and neck. For example, preformed tubes, such as those described by Ring, Adair, and Elwyn[112] (RAE tubes) or Morgan and Steward,[113] may fit better into an oral gag and may be easier to secure to the lower portion of the face without distorting the upper lip; the latter is of particular importance for patients undergoing cleft lip repairs. During oral surgery, a preformed nasal tube may interfere less with the surgeon's field. Despite the potential advantages of these tubes, they have a major limitation: for each internal diameter, the tubes are available in only one length (as measured from the "bend" to the tip). If a patient with a narrowed cricoid ring requires a tube that is smaller than usual for age, the tube may be too short and may become dislodged accidentally during surgery. I have seen this occur on two occasions when the surgeons extended and flexed the head repeatedly. In addition, if a larger TT is used for a patient with an unusually large trachea, the tube may be too long and its tip may enter the bronchus. Therefore, I use preformed TTs only when I can use the usual size for the patient's age.

Selecting A Tracheal Tube

The anesthesiologist must select a TT that does not compromise ventilation by being too small and does not damage the trachea because of its material, size, or the presence of a cuff. With the wide choice of materials available for clinical use, the anesthesiologist is advised to select tubes marked IT or Z79. Until recently, I routinely used uncuffed TTs for all patients less than 6 years of age. However, in many instances I found myself replacing tubes that leaked at low pressures (<10 cm H_2O) and in other instances I found that "appropriately sized" tubes (as documented by leak test) did not permit adequate ventilation when compliance decreased or inflating pressures increased intraoperatively. To avoid this situation, I now typically insert a cuffed tracheal tube, sized as shown in Table 9–2, and measure the leak with the cuff deflated. If the leak pressure is appropriate (i.e., <30 cm H_2O), I leave the tube in place and check periodically that the cuff has not inflated during administration of nitrous oxide. If the leak pressure exceeds 30 cm H_2O, I select either a smaller cuffed tube or an uncuffed tube. If the leak pressure is less than 10 cm H_2O, I typically add air to the cuff until the leak pressure exceeds 10 cm H_2O, seeking a higher leak pressure for certain types of surgery. If higher inflating pressures are required during surgery, the cuff can then be inflated. Although not commonly used, cuffed tubes with internal diameters as small as 2.5 mm are available commercially.

LARYNGEAL MASKS

The laryngeal mask airway (LMA) can be used to manage the airway of infants and children. The LMA consists of a mask—a silicone inflatable cuff that seals the perimeter of the larynx—and a wide-bore tube that connects to the anesthesia circuit (Fig. 9–16).[114, 115] Although early reports suggested that the pressure in the cuff is low, a recent study shows that the pressure is similar to that of high-pressure TT cuffs.[116] Therefore, in infants, whose arterial pressures are lower than in adults, inflation of the cuff for long periods of time might produce ischemic injury to the pharynx and larynx. If so, this would prevent this device from being used to wean infants from mechanical ventilation.

There has been relatively little investigation of the mechanics of infants and children breathing through an LMA.

T A B L E   9 – 2
RECOMMENDATIONS FOR SIZE (INTERNAL DIAMETER) AND TYPE OF TRACHEAL TUBE

Patient Age	Size (Internal Diameter, mm)	Type*
Premature neonate	2.5–3.0	Uncuffed
Full-term neonate	3.0–3.5	Cuffed or uncuffed
3 mo–1 year	4.0	Cuffed or uncuffed
2 year	4.5	Cuffed or uncuffed
4 year	5.0	Cuffed or uncuffed
6 year	5.5	Cuffed
8 year	6.0	Cuffed
10 year	6.5	Cuffed
12 year	7.0	Cuffed

* Although uncuffed tubes are traditionally used in neonates and younger children, cuffed tubes may be appropriate under certain circumstances. See text for explanation. When a cuffed tube is used, it may be necessary to choose one with a smaller internal diameter.

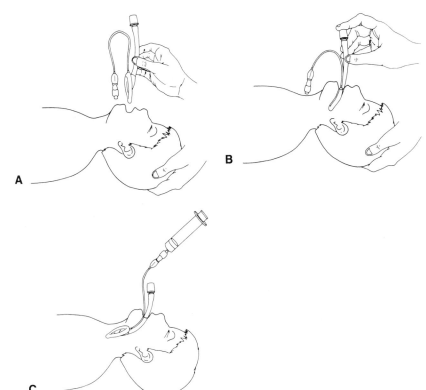

FIGURE 9–16. The laryngeal mask airway (LMA). *A* and *B,* To insert the LMA, the neck is extended and the lubricated, deflated LMA is passed into the pharynx with firm backward and downward pressure until it fails to advance further. *C,* The cuff of the LMA is then inflated. (From Marjot R: Pressure exerted by the laryngeal mask airway cuff upon the pharyngeal mucosa. Br J Anaesth 70:25, 1993.)

Reignier et al.[117] anesthetized children aged 6 to 24 months with halothane and permitted them to breathe spontaneously through either an LMA or an TT. Tidal volume and minute ventilation were larger and various measures of inspiratory airway obstruction were better with the LMA. However, there was no difference in P_{ETCO_2}. These findings suggest that LMAs have a larger dead space but less resistance than TTs.

Before an LMA is inserted, the mask is inflated to ensure the absence of leaks, and then is deflated and lubricated, preferably with a water-soluble lubricant. The patient's neck is extended and the mask is inserted into the pharynx with firm backward and downward pressure until the mask fails to advance farther. It may be helpful to pull the tongue forward by grasping it with gauze. Occasionally, before the LMA can be inserted, it is necessary to insert a laryngoscope to separate the tongue from the pharyngeal wall. Some clinicians inflate the cuff during insertion of the LMA.

Once the mask is in place, the cuff is inflated; values for typical gas volumes required to inflate the cuff are shown in Table 9–3. When the mask is inflated, the tube recedes slightly from the mouth and the submental triangle and neck bulge slightly. If the mask is positioned correctly, the anesthesia bag moves with each inspiration, there is no evidence of airway obstruction, and breath sounds are normal. Oxygenation should remain normal.

After insertion, an LMA provides an adequate airway in more than 90 percent of infants and children,[118, 119] but changes in position may compromise airway patency during anesthesia. Usually, this can be corrected by slight repositioning of the head or jaw. In one study, correct positioning of the LMA was observed in only 44 percent

of infants, and delayed airway obstruction occurred in 12 of 50 patients.[120] In infants, the epiglottis frequently lies within the mask; however, this seldom causes airway obstruction and will be detected only by radiographic or fiberoptic examination.[119] Laryngospasm has been reported when the mask was inserted during light anesthesia.[121]

LMAs are useful in many situations. One is to manage the airway of infants with the Robin (Pierre-Robin) sequence. Markakis et al.[122] recommend spraying the larynx of these patients with 2 percent lidocaine, applying 2 percent viscous lidocaine to the mask, inserting the mask while the patient is awake, then inducing anesthesia. They used this sequence successfully in three infants weighing less than 5 kg, after which they inserted a fiberoptic laryngoscope (with the appropriate size TT over it) through the LMA. Once the larynx was visualized, an TT was advanced into the trachea. The patient must be adequately anesthetized

T A B L E   9 – 3
VOLUME OF GAS REQUIRED TO INFLATE THE CUFF OF A LARYNGEAL MASK AIRWAY

Mask Size	Patient Size	Gas Volume (ml)*
1	<5	2–4
1.5	5–10	4–6
2	6.5–25 kg	5–10
2.5	20–30 kg	12–15
3	25 kg–small adult	20
4	Large adult	20–30

* These volumes may have to be altered in some patients.

during this latter maneuver to prevent coughing and laryngospasm.

LMAs also have been used for airway management during tonsillectomies and adenoidectomies.[121] Compared with patients in whom a TT was used, those managed with an LMA had less blood in the trachea, less postoperative coughing, and a less eventful recovery from anesthesia. In most instances, the mask and its large tube did not interfere with surgery; however, if the pharyngeal tonsils were very large, insertion of the mask was compromised. Despite there being less blood in the trachea of these patients, the LMA does not prevent aspiration of gastric contents: if the patient has residual gastric contents, an incompetent gastroesophageal junction, or other risk factors for aspiration of gastric contents, a TT should be inserted using the appropriate precautions.

LMAs have little effect on intraocular pressure.[123] Therefore, they may be useful for airway management of patients undergoing examination of the eye under anesthesia: the absence of a face mask may facilitate the examination.

MECHANICAL VENTILATORS

Using a mechanical ventilator can simplify the workload of the anesthesiologist and may improve ventilation by delivering breaths with a rate and volume more constant than can be accomplished manually. However, a ventilator that works well for adults under a variety of anesthetic conditions may function poorly when used for infants and children. Therefore, the anesthesiologist must understand under what conditions ventilators used routinely for adults can be used without alteration for pediatric patients.

Potential problems related to the use of adult ventilators for pediatric patients can be seen with a commonly used ventilator, the Ohmeda 7800 (or its free-standing relative, the 7810), whose inspiratory flow can be varied from 10 to 100 L/min. Ventilating a 1-kg neonate with a tidal volume of 10 ml using a theoretical circuit with zero compression volume, the lowest inspiratory flow would yield an inspiratory time of less than 0.1 second (assuming a negligible fresh gas flow; a higher fresh gas flow or inspiratory flow would further shorten inspiratory time). This short inspiratory time does not permit adequate ventilation, particularly if compliance is altered by surgical manipulation. Although the anesthesiologist may respond to this inadequate ventilation by increasing tidal volume, peak airway pressure measured at the TT might then be excessive. The existence of compression volume permits a longer inspiratory time. For example, if compression volume were 2 ml/cm H_2O (a reasonable target value for a pediatric breathing circuit) and peak airway pressure were 20 cm H_2O, then each machine-delivered breath would be 50 ml (of which 40 ml was "wasted") and inspiratory time would be 0.5 second. Increasing compression volume to 4.5 ml/cm H_2O (a typical value for some ventilator/circuit combinations[124]) permits an inspiratory time of approximately 1 second. Therefore, a larger compression volume permits a longer inspiratory time.

This larger compression volume represents a mixed blessing. This can be seen by comparing the relative effects of compression volume in adults and children. With a compression volume of 4.5 ml/cm H_2O and a 20-cm H_2O peak pressure, 90 ml is lost to compression volume. If the ventilator is set to deliver a 600-ml tidal volume to an adult, the patient receives 510 ml, not markedly different from the machine-delivered volume. In contrast, to ventilate a 3-kg infant with a 30-ml tidal volume at the same airway pressure, the ventilator must deliver 120 ml. Although the volume lost to compression is still 90 ml, it now represents three fourths of the machine-delivered breath. As a result, any attempt to correlate tidal volumes measured in the breathing circuit to actual ventilation is useless; instead, ventilation must be adjusted by observation of chest excursion and measurement of P_{ETCO_2}.

The problem is further confounded if compliance changes. For example, if compliance decreases by 50 percent (as might happen during surgery in the thorax or upper abdomen), peak inspiratory pressure approximately doubles for the same inspired volume. For the 3-kg infant to receive the same 30-ml tidal volume, a peak pressure of 40 cm H_2O would be required. However, if the ventilator still delivers 120 ml per breath, 103 ml is now lost to compression volume and the patient receives only 17 ml. Although inspiratory pressure increases to 23 cm H_2O, actual tidal volume decreases. Therefore, the anesthesiologist cannot depend on mechanical ventilators with large compression volumes to deliver consistent ventilation to infants and children (or, to a lesser extent, to adults) during changing compliance.

Compression volume of pediatric bellows for adult ventilators as well as ventilators designed for pediatric anesthesia is lower than that for adult ventilators, ranging from 1.1 to 2.6 ml/cm H_2O.[125] However, with the exception of a research ventilator with a compression volume of 0.03 ml/cm H_2O,[126] the compression volume of all pediatric and adult ventilators is too large to ensure that ventilation remains constant if compliance changes during anesthesia. An additional problem will occur if there is a leak around the TT: if the leak varies with the patient's position and pulmonary compliance, volume delivered to the patient will not be constant.

For a ventilator to be practical in pediatric anesthesia, it should be designed so that the anesthesiologist can adjust either tidal volume, inspiratory time, or respiratory rate with minimal difficulty. The controls of most ventilators permit the ventilator to be preset before induction of anesthesia. For example, the Ohmeda 7000 has controls for minute ventilation, respiratory rate, and inspiratory time to expiratory time (I:E) ratio. If the anesthesiologist presets a respiratory rate of 12 to 15 breaths/min and an I:E ratio of 1:2, tidal volume can then be selected rapidly by adjusting the control of minute ventilation. A newer model, the Ohmeda 7800, also has three controls: tidal volume, inspiratory flow, and respiratory rate. If the anesthesiologist presets an appropriate inspiratory flow (for neonates and infants, I almost always select the lowest inspiratory flow, 10 L/min) and a ventilator rate of 12 to 15 breaths/min, tidal volume can then be adjusted readily. Because the compression volume of these ventilators is large (5 to 10 ml/kg), displacement of the bellows or volume reported by a measuring device within the breathing circuit does not correspond to actual tidal volume delivered to the patient.

The difference in the versatility of the controls of these two machines can be seen by considering the steps necessary to deliver the same tidal volume at a slower rate at the end of surgery. With the Ohmeda 7800, the anesthesiologist decreases the respiratory rate and need not adjust the remaining controls; the inspiratory portion of the breath is unchanged. However, with the Ohmeda 7000, changing the minute ventilation control decreases tidal volume rather than respiratory rate; to maintain tidal volume, the respiratory rate control must also be changed. Although tidal volume can now be restored to its original value, the slower respiratory rate now results in a longer, and possibly excessive, inspiratory time. To maintain an appropriate inspiratory time, the I:E ratio must also be adjusted. Therefore, changing respiratory rate with this ventilator requires adjusting all three controls to deliver an appropriate breath.

The anesthesiologist must also recognize that when the patient is ventilated mechanically, changing the fresh gas flow alters minute ventilation. Because the overflow valve is closed throughout inspiration, tidal volume is a function of fresh gas flow during inspiration (i.e., fresh gas flow per unit time times the duration of inspiration) plus the excursion of the bellows minus compression volume. Therefore, if inspiratory time is 1 second and fresh gas flow is increased from 3 L/min to 6 L/min, tidal volume will increase by approximately 50 ml.

The anesthesiologist must recognize that changes in compliance during anesthesia and surgery limit the ability of most mechanical ventilators to maintain constant ventilation. Consequently, during surgery in which compliance is not likely to be altered by surgical interventions (i.e., procedures not involving the thorax or upper abdomen), a mechanical ventilator can be used effectively. However, when compliance varies markedly, most ventilators will not deliver constant ventilation.

The Educated Hand

The use of mechanical ventilators during anesthesia has often been discouraged, the belief being that manual ventilation permitted the clinician to "assess subtle changes in compliance" and adjust ventilation accordingly. Personal experience suggests that the "educated hand" claimed by several experts is not prevalent. For example, I have often asked clinicians manually ventilating neonates and infants if I could clamp the patient's TT briefly (for < 15 seconds) so that they could report when compliance was compromised. In no instance was a clinician able to report complete occlusion of the TT; therefore, it is unlikely that they could detect subtle changes in compliance. A study using models corresponding to the lungs of full-term and premature neonates demonstrates that anesthesiologists (ranging in expertise from the first year of anesthesia residency to more than 10 years of experience as pediatric anesthesiologists) rarely can detect even complete airway occlusion.[127] Heneghan[128] suggests (and I agree[129]) that the inability to detect changes in compliance results from the large compressible volume of the breathing circuits commonly used in the United States. However, unless clinicians are willing to modify their choice of breathing circuits for pediatric patients, the "educated hand" should probably be categorized as a myth.

An alternative approach to ventilation of infants and neonates is to use a mechanical ventilator. Although the ventilator delivers the same volume to the breathing circuit with each breath, the actual tidal volume varies as a function of compliance. Significant decreases in compliance may be recognized visually (e.g., by seeing the surgeon compress the upper abdomen or the lung) or aurally (by hearing changes in breath sounds) or may be detected by changes in P_{ETCO_2} or Sp_{O_2}. Using this approach, the clinician responds to actual sequelae of changes in compliance rather than attempting to respond to perceived changes.

OTHER DEVICES FOR THE ANESTHESIA MACHINE

Although much special equipment is necessary or desirable for pediatric anesthesia, the anesthesia machine can generally be used without alteration. However, several modifications may assist in the anesthetic management of infants and children.

Compressed Air Flowmeters

Improved neonatal intensive care has increased the number of sick neonates who require surgical intervention. These neonates may not tolerate even the myocardial depressant effects of nitrous oxide.[130] In addition, nitrous oxide may worsen pneumatosis intestinalis in neonates with necrotizing enterocolitis.[131] In adults, if nitrous oxide is avoided, the majority of the anesthetic mixture is typically oxygen; however, in premature neonates, the risk of retinopathy of prematurity may necessitate limiting the inspired oxygen concentration.[132] The appropriate F_{IO_2} can be achieved by adding compressed air, from cylinders or via the hospital gas delivery system,[75] to the inspired gas. Contaminants must be eliminated by using a filter and condensed water eliminated by drying. If an inspired oxygen concentration of between 21 and 100 percent is desired, compressed air and oxygen can be combined using a nomogram.[133] If the use of nitrous oxide is desired in conjunction with both compressed air and oxygen, flow requirements are available in a table.[134]

Ratiometers

As described earlier, when a patient is ventilated with a Mapleson D circuit, P_{CO_2} varies as a function of fresh gas flow. Therefore, the anesthesiologist must first select a total fresh gas flow, then determine appropriate flows for oxygen and nitrous oxide. Should it be necessary to increase fresh gas flow to decrease rebreathing, the anesthesiologist must recalculate the required flows for oxygen and nitrous oxide to maintain the same F_{IO_2}. This task can be simplified by using a ratiometer (MDM, Fraser Harlake, Orchard Park, NY; Ohio 30/70 Proportioner, Ohmeda). These devices contain two controls, one to select total flow, the other to select an F_{IO_2} between 30 and 100 percent. The anesthesiologist first selects a fresh gas flow by setting the FIO_2 to 100 percent and adjusting the flowmeter until the oxygen flow is correct. When an FIO_2 is selected, the device delivers the appropriate flows of nitrous oxide and oxygen. Should higher flows be necessary to decrease rebreathing, the anesthesiologist can increase the fresh gas flows without being concerned about altering the FIO_2.

Positive End-Expiratory Pressure Valves

Induction of anesthesia changes the position and motion of the chest wall and diaphragm, decreasing functional residual capacity (FRC). This may result in mismatching of ventilation and perfusion and cause arterial hypoxemia.[135] These changes are particularly important for pediatric patients because of the small difference between FRC and closing volume, even in normal children.[136] During anesthesia, should the decrease in FRC compromise oxygenation, FRC can be increased using positive end-expiratory pressure (PEEP). The improvement in oxygenation and FRC with PEEP has been demonstrated in both children[137] and adults.[138] The use of PEEP during anesthesia has been simplified by the introduction of valves that can be added to the anesthesia circuit.[139, 140] With a circle system, these valves are placed between the patient and the expiratory valve. A commonly used valve (Boehringer Laboratories, Wynnewood, PA) consists of a plastic housing containing a weighted ball calibrated to provide 2.5 to 15 cm H_2O of PEEP. Higher levels of PEEP can be achieved by connecting two or more valves in series.

Using PEEP valves with Mapleson D circuits is more complicated. Because the valves are unidirectional, placing them on the corrugated hose obstructs inspiratory flow from the corrugated hose. Erceg[141] modified the Bain circuit to permit use of a conventional PEEP valve (Fig. 9–17). The modification requires several connectors and two unidirectional valves but adds no dead space to the circle. This modification may be used with both coaxial and noncoaxial D circuits. Another modification of the Bain circuit was proposed by Arandia and Byles.[142] They

placed an Emerson water column PEEP valve (J.H. Emerson Co., Cambridge, MA) between the Bain circuit and the manifold (the device to which the overflow valve and reservoir bag are attached). During positive-pressure ventilation, PEEP equals the depth of the water column. However, this valve had to be removed during spontaneous ventilation, decreasing its practical value.

Devices to Scavenge Waste Anesthetic Gas

In recent decades, there has been increasing concern about pollution of operating rooms and risks to exposed personnel. Chronic exposure to low levels of anesthetic gases has been associated with spontaneous abortions, congenital anomalies, and alterations in intellectual function.[143] These concerns led to the use of scavenging devices to collect and remove excess anesthetic gas from the operating room.

Scavengers can be effective for adults because anesthetic gases are typically delivered through a TT or a tightly applied face mask so that excess gas is collected as it exits the overflow valve. Operating room exposure is then limited to minor leaks from the anesthesia machine and breathing circuit as well as anesthetic gas exhaled from the patient during recovery.[144] Even an inexpensive scavenging system, consisting of a plastic jug, pieces of breathing hose, and several connectors,[145] can maintain nitrous oxide levels at 16 parts per million (ppm), better than the standard of 25 ppm recommended by the National Institute of Occupational Safety and Health (NIOSH).[146] The pediatric anesthesiologist faces a more difficult problem. To minimize psychic trauma, the anesthesia mask is usually not applied tightly to the child's face. Even more extreme, in a "steal" induction, a sleeping child is not disturbed while nitrous oxide and a potent anesthetic agent are directed towards the face; the mask is not applied until the child has lost consciousness. During a several-minute induction period in which gas flows of at least 5 L/min are used, 10 or more L of nitrous oxide enters

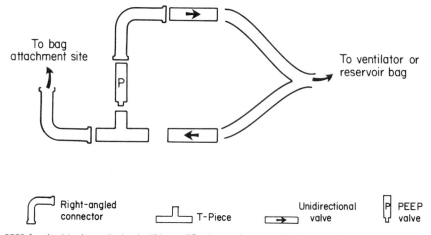

FIGURE 9–17. PEEP for the Mapleson D circuit. This modification makes possible the use of a conventional PEEP valve with the Mapleson D circuit. Two unidirectional valves, two right-angled connectors, a T-piece, a Y-connector, and several pieces of breathing hose are assembled with one right-angled connector at the bag attachment site and the Y-connector leading to the reservoir bag or anesthesia ventilator, (From Wu W-H, Turndorf H: PEEP valve for an anesthesia machine. Anesthesiology 43:667, 1975, with permission.)

the operating room. In an average operating room of 4,000 cubic feet, this results in nitrous oxide concentrations of 100 ppm, well above the NIOSH standard. The constant circulation of air through the operating room causes nitrous oxide concentrations to decrease to acceptable levels within 10 minutes after induction of anesthesia. However, in a busy pediatric operating room with multiple brief procedures, pollutant levels may remain high. Pollution can be minimized if the use of the "steal" or "mask" induction without a tightly applied mask is limited or if anesthesia is induced with nongaseous agents.

An additional problem arises with the Mapleson D circuit. Because many of these circuits are connected to the anesthesia machine only by the fresh gas hose, the overflow valve is not attached to the anesthesia machine and can be vented to the atmosphere. Fresh gas flows of 3.5 L/min introduce 2 to 2.5 L/min of nitrous oxide to the atmosphere. In a typical operation room, nitrous oxide levels remain at 100 to 200 ppm, well above NIOSH standards.

Several attempts have been made to scavenge anesthetic gas from the Mapleson D circuits. Jackson-Rees' modification of Ayre's T-piece, in which excess gas leaves the circuit through the tail of the reservoir bag, can be scavenged by using a series of connectors between the reservoir bag and wall suction.[147] Waste gas can be scavenged with one of several commercially available devices (Dupaco, American Hospital Supply Corp., San Marcos, CA) or by venting excess gas into a modified circle system and through its scavenger.[148] Excess gas vented through a hole in the side of the reservoir bag (as in the Montreal Infant Set[149]) can be scavenged using a pediatric urine collection bag (U-Bag, Pediatric Size, Hollister Incorporated, Libertyville, IL) placed over the hole in the reservoir bag and connected to wall suction.

These devices are awkward and may result in the reservoir bag overinflating if their outflow is obstructed. This dangerous situation can be averted by using a Mapleson D circuit modified for use with a conventional machine-mounted scavenging system. The Bain circuit and several noncoaxial D circuits (Vital Signs, Inc., East Madison, NJ) can be machine-mounted (Boehringer Labs, Inc.; Vital Signs, Inc.) and thereby integrated with conventional scavenging devices. For those accustomed to the great mobility offered by the freestanding D circuits, these anesthesia machine-mounted circuits are available in several lengths, enabling the anesthesiologist to reach the patient easily. These devices enable comparable scavenging of excess anesthetic gas during pediatric cases to the practice during adult anesthesia.

MASKS

The ideal anesthesia face mask should permit optimal management of the patient's airway, should not be offensive to the patient, and should be comfortable for the anesthesiologist to use for brief or extended periods. To satisfy these needs, the mask should be easy to apply to the patient's face and should fit the face well enough to prevent leaks with usual airway pressures. The dead space of the mask should be minimal and should not increase either work of breathing or P_{CO_2}. In addition, the mask should not have an odor and should not obstruct the patient's view. Finally, it should not cause discomfort for the patient or the anesthesiologist.

Although no face mask satisfies all these criteria, some are better than others. For example, the dead space of the Rendall-Baker mask is less than that of some other masks[150, 151] However, this mask does not easily fit all faces and, on occasion, significant pressure must be applied to obtain a good fit. Many reusable masks made of black rubber acquire the smell of halogenated anesthetics, and masks made of black or other nontransparent materials may appear threatening to a child.

Recently, disposable, clear plastic masks have been marketed by several manufacturers (Vital Signs, Inc.). These masks are better accepted by children, as evidenced by the requests of several patients for these, rather than conventional black rubber masks. The masks conform well to the faces of most children and can be held comfortably by the anesthetist. Although these masks have a larger dead space than the Rendell-Baker masks, the clinical significance of this dead space is probably minor: studies in animals suggest that the dead space of a mask (as measured by water displacement) markedly overestimates the increase in physiologic dead space that results from that mask.[152] Therefore, clear masks appear to offer advantages over other masks available for pediatric anesthesia.

SUMMARY

The anesthetic management of pediatric patients requires that the anesthesiologist consider many issues beyond those relating to the choice of anesthetic equipment. However, if the anesthesiologist selects equipment appropriate for the pediatric patient and understands the proper use of that equipment, the anesthetic course should be markedly smoother than that described by Ayre at the beginning of this chapter.

REFERENCES

1. Ayre P: Endotracheal anesthesia for babies with special reference to hare-lip and cleft lip operations. Anesth Analg 16:330, 1937.
2. Nightingale DA, Lambert TF: Carbon dioxide output in anaesthetised children. Anaesthesia 33:594, 1978.
3. Bain JA, Spoerel WE: Carbon dioxide output and elimination in children under anesthesia. Can Anaesth Soc J 24:533, 1977.
4. Bain JA, Spoerel WE: Carbon dioxide output in anaesthesia. Can Anaesth Soc J 23:153, 1976.
5. Michenfelder JD, Theye RA: Hypothermia: effect on canine brain and whole body metabolism. Anesthesiology 29:1107, 1968.
6. Askanazi J, Weissman C, Rosenbaum S, et al: Nutrition and the respiratory system. Crit Care Med 10:163, 1982.
7. Doekel RC, Zwillich CW, Scoggin CH, et al: Clinical semi-starvation. Depression of hypoxic ventilatory response. N Engl J Med 295:358, 1976.
8. Askanazi J, Nordenstrom J, Rosenbaum SH, et al: Nutrition for the patient with respiratory failure: glucose vs. fat. Anesthesiology 54:373, 1981.
9. Nunn JF: Applied Respiratory Physiology. London, Butterworths, 1977.

10. Hunt KH: Resistance in respiratory valves and canisters. Anesthesiology 16:190, 1955.
11. Smith WDA: The effects of external resistance to respiration. II: Resistance to respiration due to anesthetic apparatus. Br J Anaesth 33:610, 1961.
12. Robson JG, Pask EA: Some data on the performance of Waters canister. Br J Anaesth 36:333, 1954.
13. Brown ES, Hustead RF: Resistance of pediatric breathing systems. Anesth Analg 48:842, 1969.
14. Cole F: A new endotracheal tube for infants. Anesthesiology 6:87, 1945.
15. Glauser EM, Cook CD, Bougas TP: Pressure-flow characteristics and dead spaces of endotracheal tubes used in infants. Anesthesiology 22:339, 1961.
16. Hatch DJ: Tracheal tubes and connectors used in neonates—dimensions and resistance to breathing. Br J Anaesth 50:959, 1978.
17. Brandstater B: Dilatation of the larynx with Cole tubes. Anesthesiology 31:378, 1969.
18. Boretos JW, Battig CG, Goodman L: Decreased resistance to breathing through a polyurethane pediatric endotracheal tube. Anesth Analg 51:292, 1972.
19. Weeks DB: Evaluation of a disposable humidifier for use during anesthesia. Anesthesiology 54:337, 1981.
20. Olsson AK, Lindahl SGE: Ventilation, dynamic compliance and ventilatory response to CO_2. Effects of age and body weight in infants and children. Anaesthesia 40:229, 1985.
21. Olsson AK, Lindahl SGE: Pulmonary ventilation, CO_2 response and inspiratory drive in spontaneously breathing young infants during halothane anaesthesia. Acta Anaesthesiol Scand 30:431, 1986.
22. Saetta M, Mortola JP: Breathing pattern and CO_2 response in newborn rats before and during anaesthesia. J Appl Physiol 58:1988, 1985.
23. Charlton AJ, Lindahl SGE, Hatch DJ: Ventilatory responses of children to changes in deadspace volume. Br J Anaesth 57:562, 1985.
24. Nunn JF, Ezi-Ashi TI: The respiratory effects of resistance to breathing in anesthetized man. Anesthesiology 22:174, 1961.
25. Lindahl SGE, Charlton AJ, Hatch DJ, Phythyon JM: Ventilatory responses to inspiratory mechanical loads in spontaneously breathing children during halothane anaesthesia. Acta Anaesthesiol Scand 30:122, 1986.
26. Graff TD, Sewall K, Lim HS, et al: The ventilatory response of infants to airway resistance. Anesthesiology 27:168, 1966.
27. Keens TG, Bryan AC, Levison H, Ianuzzo CD: Developmental pattern of muscle fiber types in human ventilatory muscles. J Appl Physiol 44:909, 1978.
28. Muller N, Gulston G, Cade D, et al: Diaphragmatic muscle fatigue in the newborn. J Appl Physiol 46:688, 1979.
29. Polgar G: Mechanical properties of the lung and chest wall. In Thibeault DW, Gregory GA (eds): Neonatal Pulmonary Care. Menlo Park, CA, Addison-Welsey, 1979, p 25.
30. Reynolds RN: Acid-base equilibrium during cyclopropane anesthesia and operation in infants. Anesthesiology 27:127, 1966.
31. Podlesch I, Dudziak R, Zinganell K: Inspiratory and expiratory carbon dioxide concentrations during halothane anesthesia in infants. Anesthesiology 27:823, 1966.
32. Freeman A, St Pierre M, Bachman L: Comparison of spontaneous and controlled breathing during cyclopropane anesthesia in infants. Anesthesiology 25:597, 1964.
33. Smith RM: Anesthesia for Infants and Children, 4th ed. St Louis, CV Mosby, 1980.
34. Coté CJ, Petkau AJ, Ryan JF, Welch JP: Wasted ventilation measured in vitro with eight anesthetic circuits with and without inline humidification. Anesthesiology 59:442, 1983.
35. Moyers J: A nomenclature for methods of inhalation anesthesia. Anesthesiology 14:609, 1953.
36. Hamilton WK: Nomenclature of inhalation anesthetic systems. Anesthesiology 25:3, 1964.
37. Keys TE: The History of Surgical Anesthesia. New York, Shuman, 1945.
38. Ayre P: Anaesthesia for intracranial operation. A new technique. Lancet 1:561, 1937.
39. Ayre P: The t-piece technique. Br J Anaesth 28:520, 1956.
40. Brooks W, Stuart P, Gabel PV: The t-piece technique in anesthesia: an examination of its fundamental principle. Anesth Analg 37:191, 1958.
41. Rees GJ: Anaesthesia in the newborn. BMJ 2:1419, 1950.
42. Mapleson WW: The elimination of rebreathing in various semi-closed anaesthetic systems. Br J Anaesth 26:323, 1954.
43. Magill IW: Endotracheal anaesthesia. Proc R Soc Med 22:83, 1929.
44. Woolmer R, Lind B: Rebreathing in a semi-closed system. Br J Anaesth 26:316, 1954.
45. Norman J, Adams AP, Sykes MK: Rebreathing with the Magill attachment. Anaesthesia 23:75, 1968.
46. Kain ML, Nunn JF: Fresh gas economics of the Magill circuit. Anesthesiology 29:964, 1968.
47. Sykes MK: Rebreathing during controlled respiration with the Magill attachment. Br J Anaesth 31:247, 1959.
48. Ayre P: Theme and variations (on a t-piece). Anaesthesia 22:359, 1967.
49. Nightingale DA, Richards CC, Glass A: An evaluation of rebreathing in a modified t-piece system during controlled ventilation in anesthetized children. Br J Anaesth 37:762, 1965.
50. Rose DK, Froese AB: The regulation of Pa_{CO_2} during controlled ventilation of children with a t-piece. Can Anaesth Soc J 26:104, 1979.
51. Rayburn RL, Graves SA: A new concept in controlled ventilation of children with the Bain anesthetic circuit. Anesthesiology 48:250, 1978.
52. Baraka A, Maktabi M, Haroun S, et al: Fresh gas flow per surface area in children anesthetized with the t-piece circuit. Middle East J Anaesthesiol 8:249, 1985.
53. Bain JA, Spoerel WE: A streamlined anaesthetic system. Can Anaesth Soc J 19:426, 1972.
54. Bain JA, Spoerel WE: Flow requirements for a modified Mapleson D system during controlled ventilation. Can Anaesth Soc J 20:629, 1973.
55. Ramanathan S, Chalon J, Capan L, et al: Rebreathing characteristics of the Bain anesthesia circuit. Anesth Analg 56:822, 1977.
56. Seeley HF, Barnes PK, Conway CM: Controlled ventilation with the Mapleson D circuit. Br J Anaesth 49:107, 1977.
57. Gwilt DJ, Goat VA, Maynard P: The Bain system: gas flows in small subjects. Br J Anaesth 50:127, 1978.
58. Harrison GA: Ayre's t-piece: a review of its modifications. Br J Anaesth 36:115, 1964.
59. Spoerel WE, Aitken RR, Bain JA: Spontaneous respiration with the Bain breathing circuit. Can Anaesth Soc J 25:30, 1978.
60. Byrick RJ: Respiratory compensation during spontaneous ventilation with the Bain circuit. Can Anaesth Soc J 27:96, 1980.
61. Rose DK, Byrick RJ, Froese AB: Carbon dioxide elimination during spontaneous ventilation with a modified Mapleson D system: studies in a lung model. Can Anaesth Soc J 25:353, 1978.
62. Soliman MG, Laberge R: The use of the Bain circuit in spontaneously breathing paediatric patients. Can Anaesth Soc J 25:276, 1978.
63. Lindahl SGE, Charlton AJ, Hatch DJ: Accuracy of prediction of fresh gas glow requirements during spontaneous breathing with the T-piece. Eur J Anaesthesiol 1:269, 1984.
64. Weeks DB: Provision of endogenous and exogenous humidity for the Bain breathing circuit. Can Anaesth Soc J 23:185, 1976.
65. Hannallah R, Rosales JK: A hazard connected with re-use of the Bain's circuit: a case report. Can Anaesth Soc J 21:511, 1974.
66. Pethick SL: Letter to the editor. Can Anesth Soc J 22:115, 1975.
67. Robinson S, Fisher DM: Safety check for the CPRAM circuit. Anesthesiology 59:488, 1983.
68. Knepshield WR: Safety check for the CPRAM circuit. Anesthesiology 59:489, 1983.
69. Waters DJ: A composite semiclosed anaesthetic system suitable for controlled or spontaneous respiration. Br J Anaesth 33:417, 1961.
70. Baraka A, Brandstater B, Muallem M, Seraphim C: Rebreathing in a double t-piece system. Br J Anaesth 41:47, 1969.
71. Burchett KR, Bennett JA: A new coaxial breathing system. Anaesthesia 40:181, 1985.
72. Humphrey D: A new anaesthetic breathing system combining Mapleson A, D and E principles. A simple apparatus for low flow universal use without carbon dioxide absorption. Anaesthesia 38:361, 1983.
73. Manicom AW, Schoonbee CG: The Johannesburg A-D circuit switch. Br J Anaesth 51:1185, 1979.
74. Loehning RW, Davis G, Safar P: Rebreathing with "nonrebreathing" valves. Anesthesiology 25:854, 1964.
75. Dorsch JA, Dorsch SE: Understanding Anesthesia Equipment: Construction, Care and Complications. 2nd ed. Baltimore, Williams & Wilkins, 1984.

76. Stephen CR, Slater HM: Agents and techniques employed in pediatric anesthesia. Anesth Analg 29:254, 1950.

77. Adriani J, Griggs T: Rebreathing in pediatric anesthesia: recommendations and descriptions of improvements in apparatus. Anesthesiology 14:337, 1953.

78. Graff TD, Holzman RS, Benson DW: Acid-base balance in infants during halothane anesthesia with the use of an adult circle-absorption system. Anesth Analg 43:583, 1964.

79. Van Steeg J, Stevens WC: A comparison of respiratory effort of infants anesthetized with several adult and pediatric systems. Anesthesiology 27:229, 1966.

80. Bloomquist ER: Pediatric circle absorber. Anesthesiology 18:787, 1957.

81. Brown ES, Hustead RF: Rebreathing in pediatric anesthesia systems. Anesthesiology 28:241, 1967.

82. McDonald I: A circle absorber for infants. Br J Anaesth 33:58, 1961.

83. Rackow H, Salanitre E: A new pediatric circle valve. Anesthesiology 29:833, 1968.

84. Revell DG: A circulator to eliminate mechanical dead space in circle absorption system. Can Anaesth Soc J 6:98, 1959.

85. Neff WB, Burke SF, Thompson R: A Venturi circulator of anesthetic systems. Anesthesiology 29:838, 1968.

86. Rasch DK, Bunegin L, Ledbetter J, Kaminskas D: Comparison of circle absorber and Jackson-Rees systems for paediatric anaesthesia. Can J Anaesth 35:25, 1988.

87. Kay B, Beatty PCW, Healy TEJ, et al: Change in the work of breathing imposed by five anaesthetic breathing systems. Br J Anaesth 55:1239, 1983.

88. Conterato JP, Lindahl SGE, Meyer DM, Bires JA: Assessment of spontaneous ventilation in anesthetized children with use of a pediatric circle or a Jackson-Rees system. Anesth Analg 69:484, 1989.

89. Tonneson AS, Vereen L, Aren JF: Endotracheal tube cuff residual volume and lateral wall pressure in a model trachea. Anesthesiology 55:680, 1981.

90. Finholt DA, Henry DB, Raphaely RC: Factors affecting leak around tracheal tubes in children. Can Anaesth Soc J 32:326, 1985.

91. Finholt DA, Audenaert SM, Stirt JA, et al: Endotracheal tube leak pressure and tracheal lumen size in swine. Anesth Analg 65:667, 1986.

92. Cole F: Pediatric formulas for the anesthetist. Am J Dis Child 94:672, 1957.

93. Corfield HMC: Orotracheal tubes and the metric system. Br J Anaesth 35:34, 1963.

94. Mayer BW: Pediatric Anesthesia: A Guide to Its Administration. Philadelphia, JB Lippincott, 1981.

95. Slater HM, Sheridan CA, Ferguson RH: Endotracheal tube sizes for infants and children. Anesthesiology 16:950, 1955.

96. Keep PJ, Manford MLM: Endotracheal tube sizes for children. Anaesthesia 29:181, 1974.

97. Chodoff P, Helrich M: Factors affecting pediatric endotracheal tube size: a statistical analysis. Anesthesiology 28:779, 1967.

98. Penlington GN: Endotracheal tube sizes for children. Anaesthesia 29:494, 1974.

99. Levin RM: Pediatric Anesthesia Handbook. New York, Medical Examination Publishing Company, 1980.

100. Lee KW, Templeton JJ, Dougal R: Tracheal tube size and postoperative croup in children [abstract]. Anesthesiology 53:S325, 1980.

101. Mostafa SM: Variation in subglottic size in children. Proc R Soc Med 69:793, 1976.

102. Gregory GA: Pediatric anesthesia. In Miller RD (ed): Anesthesia. New York, Churchill Livingstone, 1981, p 1198.

103. Thibeault DW, Nelson P: Pulmonary care of infants with endotracheal tubes. In Thibeault DW, Gregory GA (eds): Neonatal Pulmonary Care. Menlo Park, CA, Addison-Wesley, 1979, p 242.

104. Lane GA, Pashley NRT, Fishman RA: Tracheal and cricoid diameters in the premature infant [abstract]. Anesthesiology 53:S326, 1980.

105. Rees GJ: Pediatric anaesthesia. Br J Anaesth 32:132, 1960.

106. Mackenzie CF, McAslan TC, Shin B, et al: The shape of the human adult trachea. Anesthesiology 49:48, 1978.

107. Eckenhoff JR: Some anatomic considerations of the infant larynx influencing endotracheal anesthesia. Anesthesiology 12:401, 1951.

108. Butz RO: Length and cross-section growth patterns in the human trachea. Pediatrics 42:336, 1968.

109. Stanley TH: Nitrous oxide and pressures and volumes of high- and low-pressure endotracheal-tube cuffs in intubated patients. Anesthesiology 42:637, 1975.

110. Khine HH, Corddry DH, Kettrick RG, et al: Comparison of cuffed and uncuffed endotracheal tubes in young children during general anesthesia. Anesthesiology 86:627, 1997.

111. Guess WL, Stetson JB: Tissue reactions to organotin-stabilized polyvinyl chloride (PVC) catheters. JAMA 204:580, 1968.

112. Ring WH, Adair JC, Elwyn RA: A new pediatric endotracheal tube. Anesth Analg 54.273, 1974.

113. Morgan GAR, Steward DJ: A pre-formed paediatric orotracheal tube design based on anatomical measurements. Can Anaesth Soc J 29:9, 1982.

114. Brain AI: The laryngeal mask—a new concept in airway management. Br J Anaesth 55:801, 1983.

115. Brain AI, McGhee TD, McAteer EJ, et al: The laryngeal mask airway. Development and preliminary trials of a new type of airway. Anaesthesia 40:356, 1985.

116. Marjot R: Pressure exerted by the laryngeal mask airway cuff upon the pharyngeal mucosa. Br J Anaesth 70:25, 1993.

117. Reignier J, Ben Ameur M, Ecoffey C: Spontaneous ventilation with halothane in children. A comparative study between endotracheal tube and laryngeal mask airway. Anesthesiology 83:674, 1995.

118. Grebenik CR, Ferguson C, White A: The laryngeal mask airway in pediatric radiotherapy. Anesthesiology 72:474, 1990.

119. Goudsouzian NG, Denman W, Cleveland R, Shorten G: Radiologic localization of the laryngeal mask airway in children. Anesthesiology 77:1085, 1992.

120. Mizushima A, Wardall GJ, Simpson DL: The laryngeal mask airway in infants. Anaesthesia 47:849, 1992.

121. Williams PJ, Bailey PM: Comparison of the reinforced laryngeal mask airway and tracheal intubation for adenotonsillectomy. Br J Anaesth 70:30, 1993.

122. Markakis DA, Sayson SC, Schreiner MS: Insertion of the laryngeal mask airway in awake infants with the Robin sequence. Anesth Analg 75:822, 1992.

123. Watcha MF, White PF, Tychsen L, Stevens JL: Comparative effects of laryngeal mask airway and endotracheal tube insertion on intraocular pressure in children. Anesth Analg 355, 1992.

124. Robbins L, Crocker D, Smith RM: Tidal volume losses of volume limited ventilators. Anesth Analg 46:428, 1967.

125. Binda RE, Cook DR, Fischer CG: Advantages of infant ventilators over adapted adult ventilators in pediatrics. Anesth Analg 55:769, 1976.

126. Epstein RA, Hyman AI: Ventilatory requirements of critically ill neonates. Anesthesiology 53:379, 1980.

127. Spears RS Jr, Yeh A, Fisher DM, Zwass MS: The "educated hand." Can anesthesiologists assess changes in neonatal pulmonary compliance manually? Anesthesiology 75:693, 1991.

128. Heneghan C: The educated hand. Anesthesiology 76:1063, 1992.

129. Fisher DM, Zwass MS: Reply to "the educated hand." Anestheisology 76:1063, 1992.

130. Price HL: Myocardial depression by nitrous oxide and its reversal by Ca^{++}. Anesthesiology 44:211, 1976.

131. Dierdorf SF, Krishna G: Anesthetic management of neonatal surgical emergencies. Anesth Analg 60:204, 1981.

132. Phibbs RH: Oxygen therapy: a continuing hazard to the premature infant. Anesthesiology 47:486, 1977.

133. Yost LC, Bernhard WN, Merrill C, Turndorf H: Oxygen-air blending nomogram. Anesth Analg 56:290, 1977.

134. Teeple E, Pavlov I: The use of compressed air made easy—a table. Anesthesiology 55:696, 1981.

135. Schmid ER, Rehder K: General anesthesia and the chest wall. Anesthesiology 55:668, 1981.

136. Mansell A, Bryan C, Levison H: Airway closure in children. J Appl Physiol 33:711, 1972.

137. Gregory GA, Edmunds LH, Kitterman JA, et al: Continuous positive pressure and pulmonary and circulatory function in infants less than three months of age. Anesthesiology 43:426, 1975.

138. Wyche MQ, Teichner RL, Kallos T, et al: Effect of continuous positive-pressure breathing on functional residual capacity and arterial oxygenation during intra-abdominal operations: studies in man during nitrous oxide and d-tubocurarine anesthesia. Anesthesiology 38:68, 1973.

139. Wu W-H, Turndorf H: PEEP valve for an anesthesia machine. Anesthesiology 43:667, 1975.
140. Weeks DB, Comer PB: A PEEP device for anesthesia circuits. Anesth Analg 56:578, 1977.
141. Erceg GW: PEEP for the Bain breathing circuit. Anesthesiology 50:542, 1979.
142. Arandia HY, Byles PH: PEEP and the Bain circuit. Can Anaesth Soc J 28:467, 1981.
143. Cohen EN: Inhalational anesthetics may cause genetic defects absorptions and miscarriages in operating room personnel. *In* Eckenhoff JE (ed): Controversy in Anesthesia. Philadelphia, WB Saunders, 1979, p 45.
144. Lecky JH: The mechanical aspects of anesthetic pollution control. Anesth Analg 56:769, 1977.
145. Meyers EF: An effective low-cost scavenging system. Anesthesiology 52:277, 1980.
146. National Institute of Occupational Safety and Health, DHEW: Criteria for a recommended standard—Occupational exposure to waste anesthetic gases and vapors. Publication 77-141, 1977.
147. Cullen BF: An anesthetic gas scavenging device for use with the modified Ayre's t-piece. Anesthesiol Rev 1:19, 1974.
148. Albert CA, Kwan A, Kim C, et al: A waste gas scavenging valve for pediatric systems. Anesth Analg 56:291, 1977.
149. Anonymous: Infant anaesthesia set. Anesthesiology 21:776, 1960.
150. Rendell-Baker L, Soucek DH: New paediatric face masks and anaesthetic equipment. BMJ 5293:1690, 1962.
151. Harrison GG, Ozinsky J, Jones CS: Choice of an anaesthetic facepiece. Br J Anaesth 31:269, 1959.
152. Haskins SC, Patz JD: Effects of small and large face masks and translaryngeal and tracheostomy intubation on ventilation, upper-airway dead space, and arterial blood gases. Am J Vet Res 47:945, 1986.

Induction, Maintenance, and Emergence

CHARLES B. CAULDWELL

◆ ◆ ◆

PREINDUCTION

Equipment

Before a child is brought to the operating room, the anesthesiologist must prepare the equipment necessary to anesthetize the child safely and quickly. There are mnemonics to help the anesthesiologist to ensure that crucial equipment is always available. One of these mnemonics is SOAP, which stands for *s*uction, *o*xygen, *a*irway, and *p*harmacy.

Suction should always be immediately available to the anesthetist and should be located where the suction can be reached without the anesthesiologist having to take his/her eyes off of the patient. The Yankauer suction is the standard device used because it has large holes, can be used for all but the smallest infants, and is particularly useful for removing large volumes or particulate emesis. Alternatively, a 14- to 18-Fr suction catheter or a 10- or 14-Fr oxygen catheter can be used for this purpose. Oxygen catheters are softer, but they are shorter than suction catheters. Catheters also can be used to aspirate the patient's stomach after the induction of anesthesia is completed and at the end of surgery. Suction must always be turned on and immediately available to the anesthesiologist.

Oxygen is delivered to the patient via an anesthesia circuit. There are usually two alternative circuits for children. Some anesthesiologists use Mapleson D or Jackson-Rees nonrebreathing circuits when anesthetizing neonates and small infants to minimize the work of breathing and decrease rebreathing of exhaled gases. Nonrebreathing circuits can be used on most anesthesia machines with some minor modifications. The alternative to the nonrebreathing circuit is the semiclosed circle system commonly used for adults. The valves currently used in anesthesia machines require minimal effort to open, even for the smallest infants. Moreover, breathing will be controlled during the operation in most cases. There are choices in the size of circuit tubing available. Pediatric anesthetic circuits have small hoses and lower compliance, which ensure that less volume is lost through expansion of the hoses during positive-pressure ventilation and may allow more consistent tidal volumes. Some anesthetic machines have a choice of bellows as well. While the pediatric bellows often can deliver more accurate tidal volumes for small infants, many anesthesiologists find that the bellows designed for adults work quite adequately for infants and children. The integrity of the circuit, the function of the inspiratory and expiratory valves, and the function of the ventilator must be checked by the anesthesiologist during the preanesthetic machine check.

After ensuring that oxygen can be delivered with positive pressure, the anesthesiologist should determine whether air and nitrous oxide are available. Being able to add air to the gas mixture prevents excessive arterial oxygen partial pressures, which have been associated with retinopathy of prematurity (see Chapter 14).[1] Nitrous oxide is a useful anesthetic agent because it has minimal effects on cardiac performance. Tanks (E-cylinders) of these gases should be attached to the anesthesia machine for emergency use or for use when anesthetizing patients in locations outside the operating room. The anesthesiologist must ensure that the tanks are sufficiently full so they can be used for a period of time if the central source of nitrous oxide and oxygen fail. The anesthetic vaporizers should be filled and checked during the routine preanesthetic check.

Airway equipment comes in a variety of sizes to accommodate different sized children. Masks with a soft air-filled cuff come in many sizes, enclose the nose and mouth, conform to the contours of the face, and allow positive-pressure ventilation. However, the anesthesiologist should ensure that the soft air-filled cuffs do not compress the nasal alae and occlude the airway. It is important to ensure that the mask is placed on the bridge of the nose and not lower. A Rendall-Baker-Soucek mask will often allow better access to the eyes for ophthalmologic examinations. The correct size mask is generally one that comfortably fits from the bridge of the nose to the chin. The anesthesiologist should have a choice of masks and oral and nasal airways readily available.

Other airway adjuncts, such as appropriately sized oral and nasal airways, should be available, particularly the former (see Chapter 9). Nasal airways are less commonly used for children because there is a tendency to cause bleeding when adenoidal tissue is traumatized during insertion of a nasal airway. If a nasal airway is to be used, it should be well lubricated before it is inserted. A laryngeal mask airway (LMA) of the correct size also is a valuable device when the anesthetic can be performed using a mask.

Equipment needed for endotracheal intubation should always be available to the anesthesiologist, even if endotracheal intubation is not part of the anesthetic plan. Laryngoscope handles come in several sizes, and there is no particular reason to choose one over the other as long as the available handle provides adequate light. Straight laryngoscope blades are usually used for children, especially infants, because of the small size of their oropharynx, the relatively large size of the tongue, and the difficulty in manipulating the epiglottis with a curved blade. An appropriate sized straight blade allows better control of the tongue to improve visualization of the glottis. Blades that are too short afford an inadequate view of the glottis. Blades that are too long are hard to control and can damage tooth buds. Blades that are too narrow allow the tongue to protrude over the edge of the blade and obscure the view of the larynx. If the blade is too wide, there will be inadequate room for the endotracheal tube (ETT). The Miller 0 blade is suitable for premature infants and is often used for newborns. However, it may be too small for some term neonates. The Miller 1 blade works well for most term neonates. The Miller 2 blade can be used for children over 1 to 2 years of age, but a significant portion of the blade protrudes from the mouth, making it more difficult to control the blade. Choice of laryngoscope blade is often a matter of familiarity. In many situations, several different blades will work equally well. Macintosh blades are seldom used in infants but are used successfully in older children.

A selection of appropriately sized endotracheal tubes must be readily available whenever a child is brought to the operating room. For infants and children, uncuffed endotracheal tubes are frequently used. A leak around the tube at 10 to 30 cm H_2O pressure allows adequate ventilation of the lungs and prevents mucosal ischemia. A general rule for choosing the appropriate size uncuffed endotracheal tube is

$$\frac{Age + 16}{4}$$

However, this rule breaks down for children under 2 to 3 years of age. Most newborns have an appropriate gas leak with a 3.0 ETT. By a few months of age, a 3.5 tube can be used. Another way to choose the correct tube size in about 85 percent of patients is to select a tube that has the same external diameter as the distal phalanx of the patient's smallest finger.[2] Since the wrong ETT size will be chosen a certain percentage of the time, the size predicted and one size larger and one size smaller ETT should be readily available. A recent study examined the use of cuffed ETTs in infants and young children.[3] Using the formula

$$\frac{Age}{4 + 3}$$

for the size of a cuffed ETT, a better fit, avoidance of repeated laryngoscopy, use of lower gas flows, and reduction of operating room contamination by nitrous oxide were demonstrated. However, there is no long-term follow-up of these patients to know if any of them developed subsequent subglottic stenosis. The use of a stylet for tracheal intubation is a matter of personal preference.[2] A stylet stiffens a small, soft endotracheal tube, making intubation of the neonatal trachea easier. It also may improve the chance of successful tracheal intubation during rapid sequence induction of anesthesia for patients who have a full stomach. If the end of the stylet is prevented from projecting beyond the end of the endotracheal tube, there should be no increased risk of tracheal damage. The ETT is secured to the child's face, usually with tape. To ensure a stickier surface, liquid adhesive may be painted on the patient's face prior to applying the tape. There are a variety of ways to tape an endotracheal tube. Whichever approach is used, it should prevent movement of the tube. It has been suggested by some, only partly in jest, that one should be able to lift the child's head off the bed by the ETT without removing it.

Pharmacy refers to the drugs required during the anesthetic. These fall into two broad categories: anesthetic drugs and nonanesthetic drugs. The anesthetic drugs include intravenous (IV) induction agents (e.g., sodium thiopental, propofol), muscle relaxants, opioids, and any local anesthetics that will be used for peripheral nerve blocks. Nonanesthetic drugs include those that restore the heart rate or blood pressure to normal when nonpharmacologic means have been unsuccessful. Examples include atropine for bradycardia and epinephrine for hypotension. Ephedrine or phenylephrine are other useful vasoactive agents. Only the dose of drug required for a particular patient should be drawn into the syringe. For example, the dose of thiopental needed for a neonate might be slightly less than 1 ml, so a 1-ml syringe filled with pentothal would be appropriate to have available. This reduces the likelihood of delivering an overdose of drug to a small child. Estimating body weight is often a problem. However, most newborns weigh about 3 kg, double their weight by 6 months, and triple it by 1 year of age. Each year thereafter, for the next 4 years, weight gain is about 2½ kg. Therefore, a 3-year-old weighs about 15 kg.

The mnemonic SOAP leaves out several important additional pieces of equipment required during induction of anesthesia, including the monitors. The American Society of Anesthesiologists (ASA) Standards for Basic Intraoperative Monitoring state that: "the patient's oxygenation, ventilation, circulation, and temperature shall be continually evaluated."[4] Oxygenation should be monitored by (1) an inspired O_2 analyzer with a low oxygen concentration alarm, and (2) a pulse oximeter. Ventilation is continuously evaluated by both observation and by monitoring for the presence of expired carbon dioxide, including quantitative analysis when an endotracheal intubation or an LMA is used. There must be a functioning ventilator-disconnect monitor with alarm when the ventilator is in use. An electrocardiogram (ECG) should be displayed continuously and the heart rate and blood pressure recorded at least every 5 minutes. Finally, temperature should be monitored when significant changes are expected. Early changes in temperature are difficult to detect unless the infant's body temperature is monitored continuously. These monitors should be present in the operating room and should be functioning correctly, before the patient is brought into the room.

Finally, IV fluids and the material needed to obtain intravenous access should be prepared. For infants and small children, the IV set should include a buretrol that contains about 1 hour's worth of fluid (50 ml for infants and 100 ml for older patients) in the chamber to prevent fluid overload if the IV accidentally runs wide open. A selection of IV catheters, skin cleansing solutions, and tape should be available.

The room temperature should be elevated for all but the largest pediatric patients. For premature neonates, the room temperature should be at least 32°C and an overhead warmer also may be required to minimize radiant heat loss (see Chapter 4).

Preoperative Review

A final check of the patient's status should be made immediately before going into the operating room by reviewing the chart and examining the patient, as something may have changed overnight or since the preoperative visit. NPO status should be checked and new signs or symptoms of disease should be elicited. Upper respiratory infections (URIs) may easily develop overnight. A URI may herald a concomitant lower respiratory infection with airway secretions and the potential for airway obstruction, atelectasis, bronchospasm, and hypoxia, that could present in the operating room.[5] A fever or productive cough should make the anesthetist suspicious of an acute illness that might well delay the planned procedure. There is some evidence that general anesthesia can be performed on children with active upper respiratory infections without undue risk,[6, 7]

but that conclusion has been disputed.[8, 9] Recent laboratory results should be reviewed as well. The surgical consent should be in the chart and signed. If an anesthesia consent is routinely obtained, it should be in the chart and signed as well. If blood products have been ordered for the operation, their availability should be ensured before the child enters the operating room. If the child has an IV line in place, any changes to the solutions should be made in the preoperative holding area. Finally, if the plan is to administer some form of premedication before going to the operating room, it is wise to remember that for any route other than parenteral, it will take several minutes to have the desired effect. Therefore, the earlier premedication is administered, the more likely it will be that the child will separate easily and calmly from parents when it is time to go to the operating room.

Parental Involvement

With the recent increase in the incidence of same-day surgery, many hospitals have established preoperative clinics and programs that allow children and their parents to visit the hospital and receive information about what to expect on the day of surgery, as well as to familiarize themselves with the location and personnel. In an informal setting they can talk to representatives of the anesthesia and nursing departments, see and touch some of the equipment used, and have their questions answered. It is usually not possible, however, to meet the anesthesiologist who will be responsible for the child during the operation. A recent study examined one preoperative preparation program and found that anxiety alleviation extended only to the preoperative period but not to the intraoperative or postoperative periods.[10]

A number of studies by Kain and his colleagues have addressed the issues surrounding parental presence during induction of anesthesia in children.[11] There are several predictors of preoperative anxiety, among them the parents' and child's anxiety, the age of the child, and the quality of previous medical encounters.[12] There are minimal significant differences between a parent being present or absent in terms of behavior or physiologic measures. Parental presence has been compared with premedication for induction of anesthesia.[13] Oral premedication with midazolam was significantly better in reducing the child's or the parent's anxiety during the preoperative and the postoperative periods, but the advantages may only extend for the first postoperative week.

Despite these studies, it is common for parents to be present during induction, especially in Great Britain,[14] and parents seem grateful for the opportunity to be present and would want to accompany their child again in the future.[15]

INDUCTION OF ANESTHESIA

There are a variety of ways to induce a level of anesthesia suitable for surgery in children, but they all have potential hazards, and there must be alternate plans in case the original approach fails.

The induction technique used should be safe, rapid, and one with which the anesthesiologist is familiar and feels comfortable. It is helpful for the child to be in physical contact with someone during the induction of anesthesia. This can be a parent, a nurse, or the anesthesiologist. A calm, soothing voice and an unhurried manner contribute to a successful induction of anesthesia.

Monitoring During Induction of Anesthesia

Because induction of anesthesia involves a transition from an awake state to an anesthetized state, with potential hemodynamic and respiratory consequences, careful monitoring of the patient's condition is mandatory. If the child is awake, calm, and cooperative, it should be possible to place all the monitors, including the blood pressure cuff, prior to beginning the induction of anesthesia. However, some children will lose control if the anesthesiologist spends time applying the monitors before the induction of anesthesia. The agitation that ensues can subvert an otherwise smooth transition from a preoperative holding area to the operating room or induction room. Therefore, the anesthesiologist must decide which monitors are the most important (i.e., which can be sacrificed to maintain the trust and cooperation of the patient). The anesthesiologist is the most important monitor because observation of the patient provides valuable clues to the patient's status. Skin color, chest wall movement, and breath sounds give the anesthesiologist important information about how well the child is doing. However, these observations are not infallible, and they should be supplemented as soon as practical with other monitors. Probably the most valuable monitor, and fortunately one that most children will allow, is the pulse oximeter. Hypoxia is detrimental if it persists too long and often is an early sign that something is wrong during the induction of anesthesia. The pulse oximeter probe can be applied quickly to any extremity, especially if the child's attention is distracted by the red light. This allows the presence of hypoxia and the heart rate and peripheral perfusion to be assessed quickly. Hypovolemic or vasoconstricted children may not have adequate distal peripheral perfusion to give an oximeter signal.[16] An inadequate oximeter signal should not be ignored by the anesthesiologist! A prewarmed precordial stethoscope can often be placed on the child's chest without disturbing the child if the chest piece is first warmed. Precordial chest pieces will adhere to the chest, even to that of a sitting child, and give information about airway, ventilation, and cardiac response during the induction of anesthesia. The latter is particularly important for young infants who may be quite sensitive to the depressant effects of volatile anesthetic agents. If the child is struggling, application of a blood pressure cuff is not very useful because the values obtained do not reflect the patient's normal blood pressure. Because normal children rarely have dysrhythmias, except those associated with hypoxia, the ECG also is not vital during the transition to unconsciousness. However, when the child becomes unconscious and relaxes, the ECG monitor and blood pressure cuff should be applied. The oxygen analyzer and an inspired/expired gas analyzer also should be functioning during the induction of anesthesia. *For any child who is ill, all monitors should be applied before induction of anesthesia begins.*

Techniques of Induction
Hypnosis

Webster's Dictionary defines hypnosis as "a state that resembles sleep but is induced by a hypnotizer whose suggestions are readily accepted by the subject."[17] Though it is unlikely that hypnosis can be the only anesthetic induction agent, it can be a valuable adjunct and assist in a smooth induction and emergence from anesthesia. The hypnotic state is one of heightened awareness, not somnolence, and the patient is in a state of concentrated attention to the suggestions of the hypnotizer.[18] Typical suggestions would include amnesia for the events; feelings of general well-being; and absence of postoperative nausea, vomiting, or pain.

A major requirement for hypnosis to be successful is a patient who is capable of concentrating. Children should be at least 4 years of age, calm, and able to understand the words that the hypnotist will use. The hypnotist will usually start by asking the patient to concentrate. Subjects can fix their eyes on an object above their head, close their eyes and relax, or look into the eyes of the hypnotist. Eye fixation probably works best for children in the operating room. The hypnotist must be the only person talking in the room and must use a calm, even voice. Hypnosis begins by telling the child that their eyes are getting heavier, and that they will not be able to keep them open. Once the patient's eyes close, the hypnotist tells the child to imagine an object (e.g., a leaf) and concentrate on it for a few seconds. Then the hypnotist will describe a change occurring to the object (e.g., the leaf falling to the ground), and during the change the child will feel more and more relaxed, all the while being told by the hypnotist that they cannot open their eyes. The hypnotist tells the child that when the leaf hits the ground, they will feel completely relaxed and comfortable and will not want to move. Posthypnotic suggestions can now be placed. The hypnotist tells the patient that they will drift into a pleasant deep sleep and then the hypnotist/anesthesiologist begins the induction of anesthesia. The hypnotist also can suggest that at the end of the operation, the patient will awaken without pain or nausea and will do very well postoperatively.

Induction of Anesthesia Using Drugs Administered Rectally

Several drugs have been administered rectally to induce anesthesia. The advantages to this approach include (1) the induction can be done with the patient in a parent's arms, minimizing separation anxiety; (2) the onset of sleep is smooth, takes place over several minutes, and doesn't require needles; and (3) rectal administration of drugs is similar to taking the child's temperature, which most young children have had done. A disadvantage of this technique is the patient's urge to defecate due to distention of the rectum. Consequently, it is helpful for someone to hold the child's buttocks together for a few minutes after the drug is administered to ensure adequate absorption of the drug across the rectal mucosa. For older, toilet-trained children, or those who might require large volumes of solution, the rectal route of drug administration may not be suitable.

Since rectal drug administration is usually performed in a holding area outside the operating room, and because many of these drugs are respiratory depressants, oxygen and a means of delivering positive-pressure ventilation should be available before the drug is administered. An anesthesiologist or someone skilled in airway management should be continuously present once the drug is administered.

Several drugs have been investigated for induction of anesthesia by the rectal route (see Chapter 3). The most common is methohexital. This oxybarbiturate comes as a powder and can be made in a variety of concentrations. When 25 to 30 mg/kg of the drug is given, sleep is produced in about 7 to 8 minutes.[19] Peak plasma concentrations of the drug occur in about 15 minutes.[20] If the concentration is kept at or below 10 percent, the incidence of mucosal irritation is low. A number of studies have looked at the use of different concentrations and volumes of the drug, and concentrations between 2 percent and 10 percent are the most common. Lower concentrations of methohexital lead to higher plasma concentrations of drug and may be slightly more effective at inducing anesthesia, but they do not take effect more rapidly and may not produce a clinically noticeable difference.[21] When rectal methohexital is given after an inadequate premedication, the dose of methohexiatal should be decreased. Once asleep, the child can be transported to the operating room and the induction of anesthesia continued with volatile anesthetics. There is no evidence that administering rectal methohexital slows emergence from anesthesia or delays discharge from the recovery room. The correct dose of methohexital is placed in a syringe with a soft plastic or red rubber catheter attached to the end of the syringe. By having 2 to 3 ml of air in the syringe, all of the drug can be cleared from the catheter. After the parents are informed about the procedure, the soft catheter tip is inserted, preferably not beyond the dentate line. Drug deposited above this line enters the portal circulation and much of the drug is removed by the liver and metabolized. If the drug is deposited below the dentate line, the drug is taken up by the vena caval circulation and delivered to the effector site, the brain, before any of it is circulated to and removed by the liver. Rectal methohexital appears not to have a significant effect on cardiac index.[22] Thiopental also has been administered rectally. A dose of 40 mg/kg produces the same effect as 25 to 30 mg/kg of methohexital, but recovery from anesthesia is not as rapid and stay in the recovery room may be prolonged.[23,24] If premedication has been given before thiopental is administered rectally, the thiopental dose should be reduced.

Ketamine also has been administered rectally. An average of 8.7 mg/kg of a 5 percent solution caused sleep in 7 to 15 minutes, and recovery occurred 36 minutes after a 35-minute operation.[25]

Both diazepam and midazolam have been given rectally. They produce acceptance of a face mask, but rarely produce sleep. Therefore, they are more similar to preinduction medications than drugs for induction of anesthesia.[26]

Induction of Anesthesia with Drugs Given Nasally

Sufentanil and midazolam have been given nasally to children. Sufentanil administered in doses of 1.5 to 4.5 μg/kg intranasally caused most patients to become calm or drowsy.[27] Only 4 percent were asleep. A significant percentage of patients exhibited some decrease in pulmonary compliance, especially when the highest dose was used. Discharge from the recovery room was not prolonged, and the patients recovered normally.

Intranasal midazolam, 0.1 to 0.6 mg/kg, caused peak plasma levels in about 11 minutes, and produced noticeable sedation in 5 to 10 minutes.[28-30] Recovery from anesthesia was not prolonged.

Though both drugs have a definite salutary effect on the induction of anesthesia, neither reliably produces sleep and should be thought of as preinduction agents.

Intramuscular Induction of Anesthesia

In rare circumstances, anesthesia may be induced by intramuscular (IM) injection. Such situations include children with severe developmental delay who are incapable of cooperating, children who refuse all other methods of premedication or induction, and children with severe congenital heart disease.

Advantages of using IM drugs for the induction of anesthesia are the rapid onset of action and a more predictable effect than with drugs administered rectally or nasally. The disadvantages of this technique include pain for the patient, unpredictable onset compared with IV induction, and the potential for sterile abscess formation.

Ketamine, methohexital, and midazolam have been administered IM.[31-33] Ketamine is probably the most widely used agent given by this route, and the dose used varies depending on the effect sought. If complete induction of anesthesia is desired, 6 to 10 mg/kg of ketamine is appropriate. Grant et al.[34] showed that 6 mg/kg IM ketamine gave plasma levels similar to 2 mg/kg of IV ketamine. Peak drug levels occurred in less than 5 minutes. If IM ketamine is used as a preinduction drug to achieve cooperation in an uncooperative patient, 4 to 6 mg/kg is usually adequate.

IM barbiturates can be used for induction or preinduction agents, but this approach has not found much favor, due in part to the severe pain on injection.[32] IM midazolam produces sedation and acceptance of a face mask, but there is little information on the use of IM midazolam as a true induction agent.[33]

Intravenous Induction of Anesthesia

Children do not like needles, and most pediatric anesthesiologists do not like to cause children pain. Starting an IV for induction of anesthesia in a small child meets with a great deal of resistance. Nevertheless, IV induction of anesthesia has some advantages. The process is rapid, can eliminate the use of a face mask, and can lessen the risk of an excitement phase and the risk of laryngospasm. In general, if an IV is present prior to the induction of anesthesia, it is reasonable to use it to induce anesthesia.

If an IV is not in place, most pediatric anesthesiologists in the United States induce anesthesia with a vapor, and start the IV after the child is unconscious. However, there may be situations where an IV induction is preferred (e.g., known propensity for malignant hyperthermia).

There are two approaches to IV induction of anesthesia. One is to insert a small butterfly needle into an obvious vein, usually in the hand, and inject a drug to produce unconsciousness quickly. After the child is asleep, a volatile agent is delivered and an indwelling IV catheter is placed and the anesthetic proceeds. The alternative is to insert an IV line before the induction of anesthesia. The choice of where to place the IV and what catheter to use is usually a matter of experience and personal preference. Popular sites for inserting IVs in children are the dorsum of the hand and the saphenous vein. The volar surface of the wrist also can be used, but the veins are small and the hand must be immobilized in a dorsiflexed position if this IV is to be used for more than just the surgical procedure. IVs are often placed in the scalp of newborns in nurseries. Though they can be used subsequently in the operating room, the veins are fragile, the IV easily infiltrates, and insertion of an IV in the scalp is quite painful. The scalp usually is not a first choice for an IV site. The external jugular vein can sometimes be seen in infants where few other veins are visible, and a catheter can be inserted into it. Usually, a 22-gauge catheter is adequate for infants and young children and a 20-gauge catheter is adequate for most older children. In young infants, a 24-gauge catheter may be the only access available. I have used a 24-gauge catheter as part of the vascular access during a liver transplant for an infant, and this catheter performed quite well.

Some anesthesiologists decide that all patients beyond a certain age (e.g., 10 to 12 years of age) will undergo IV induction of anesthesia unless they specifically request that anesthesia be induced with an inhaled agent. Some children, even fairly young ones, will occasionally ask for an IV induction of anesthesia. This happens most often with children who have had multiple experiences with anesthesia and dislike the mask and the smell of the agent more than they fear needles. Several steps can be taken to maximize the success of starting an IV in an awake child. First, likely IV sites should be quickly surveyed during conversation with the child who should be reassured that no needles will be used while a site is being considered. When a likely site is identified, it can be prepared. If alcohol is used it should be dried or wiped off before the needle is inserted, or there will be more pain when the needle pierces the skin. When a 20-gauge or larger IV is used, the skin should first be anesthetized with a small amount of lidocaine, using the smallest needle possible. Insertion of the catheter should be painless, although the patient may feel some pressure. A mixture of local anesthetics (EMLA cream) can be applied to the dorsum of the hands of patients while they are being checked into the preoperative area. Ideally, by the time it is necessary to start the IV, the skin is numb.[35] Unfortunately, EMLA requires 45 to 60 minutes for complete effectiveness, making it impractical in situations when the child is brought to the preoperative area shortly before the operation. EMLA also may cause some venoconstriction, making it more

difficult to see the vein when it is time to start the IV. Recently, another technique for anesthetizing the skin has been developed. Iontophoresis produces anesthesia by the transdermal delivery of local anesthetic by means of a low-level electric current.[36, 37] The child's attention can be distracted and the IV can be started with a minimum of fuss. The skin of children tends to be very loose and must be stretched to anchor the vein while the IV catheter is being inserted. When a small plastic catheter traverses the skin, it may shred away from the needle, making it very difficult to slide the catheter into the vein. It is helpful to first make a small nick in the skin with a larger needle (19 gauge) at the proposed insertion site to make passage of the catheter through the skin smoother. After the catheter is in place, a dry dressing should be applied to cover the insertion site to minimize the risk of infection. Peripheral IV sites should ideally be changed every 2 to 3 days.

Just before induction of anesthesia, the child's lungs should be preoxygenated, by blowing O_2 toward the child's face or by applying a face mask if the child will tolerate it.

Several drugs have been used for IV induction of anesthesia in children. Sodium thiopental is the most commonly used drug for this purpose because it has a rapid onset of action and a short duration of effect. In normal, euvolemic patients it causes few hemodynamic effects. The dose of drug required for loss of the lid reflex and acceptance of a face mask is greater in children than in adults, and averages 6 to 7 mg/kg.[38, 39] If the patient has received premedication and is sedated, a smaller dose of drug should be used. Methohexital 1 to 2 mg/kg can also be used as an IV induction agent, but it offers no particular benefits in children.[40]

Ketamine 1 to 2 mg/kg is used as an intravenous induction agent in certain situations, especially for children with compromised cardiovascular systems or severe reactive airway disease. Ketamine, a sympathomimetic agent, causes a slight increase in heart rate, arterial blood pressure, and brochodilation in normovolemic patients. It has been associated with prolonged emergence reactions, even in children.[41] Coadministration of a benzodiazepine may decrease the development of bad dreams.[42] Ketamine does increase the amount of oral secretions and it may be helpful to administer an antisialogogue.

Over the last few years, propofol has been used frequently in children to induce anesthesia. Higher doses of the drug are required for induction of anesthesia in children than for adults; at least 2.5 to 3.0 mg/kg are required to produce unconsciousness.[43] Propofol can cause pain on injection. Preadministration of lidocaine or an opioid, mixing propofol with lidocaine, or slow administration of the drug may decrease the amount of pain.

Midazolam can be used for IV induction of anesthesia, but it offers very few advantages over the above-mentioned drugs.

Inhalation Induction of Anesthesia

Induction of anesthesia by inhalation of nitrous oxide and volatile anesthetic agents is the most common technique for induction of general anesthesia in pediatric patients. The status of the patient at the beginning of induction dictates how the induction will be done. The anesthesiologist must be flexible. If the patient is already asleep, a "steal" induction can be done. Without moving the patient from his bed, the anesthesiologist holds the end of the circuit close to the patient's nose and mouth without touching the patient. After the patient breathes nitrous oxide for a minute or two, the anesthesiologist determines whether a face mask can be placed on the bridge of the nose without awakening the patient. If so, the patient can be moved to the operating room table, the monitors applied, and the induction of anesthesia continued with a volatile agent. If the child doesn't tolerate the mask, low concentrations of agent can be added before the child is moved. Monitors should be applied as soon as possible. If the child is awake on arrival in the operating room, the anesthesiologist should do everything possible to make the child feel secure. Open-ended questions such as, "What do you want to do?" should be avoided in favor of offering acceptable choices (e.g., "Do you want to sit or lie down?"). Some children prefer to be held in the arms of a parent, the anesthesiologist, or a nurse. Others do not want to be held but want to sit up rather than lie down on the table. If the child is afraid of the mask, the end of the circuit can be held near her or his face (although this leads to some contamination of the room with anesthetic gases). When the child is asleep, the mask can be moved onto the face. For the child who tolerates a mask, it may help to place a few drops of food flavoring on the mask to hide the smell of the volatile agent. Favorite smells are bubble gum and strawberry. If a child who had a preoperative visit with someone from the anesthesia department may already be familiar with the mask. One technique is to place the mask lightly on the patient's face and to administer only nitrous oxide for the first minute or two. Then a volatile agent, sevoflurane or halothane, is slowly added by increasing the concentration of the gas by no more than 0.5 to 1 percent every three to five breaths until unconsciousness is achieved. The maximum concentration administered to a young infant should be lower than that administered to an older child to prevent negative hemodynamic responses, especially when halothane is used. Obviously, at higher concentrations the risk of anesthetic overdose is greater and very close monitoring is necessary. As soon as the child is unconscious, the anesthetic concentration can be turned down and the IV inserted. Occasionally, patients are initially cooperative and calm but become quite upset when the mask is applied. Rather than stopping the process, the concentration of agent should be increased to the maximum until the child is unconscious. The child will be asleep in a few seconds. This is not very elegant, but it is expeditious.

Cooperative children can be allowed or even encouraged to hold the mask themselves. Clear masks are much superior to black or opaque masks because they allow the child to see more clearly and not feel suffocated.

When a mask is held on a child's face it is better not to place the fingers in the submental triangle because this forces the child's tongue up into the airway. It is preferable either to place the fingers on the mandible alone or to cup the hand under the entire jaw and pull the soft tissue of the neck and chin forward. Be aware of the position of the hand. It is not necessary to have part of the hand

over the patient's eyes. This may only increase the child's anxiety.

While the child is going to sleep, a single person should talk in a soft, nonthreatening voice. Extraneous noise in the room should be discouraged. The child can be told a story or be told about favorite items, such as a pet or a toy brought along to the operating room. Words that stimulate anxiety or words with negative connotations should be avoided. In general, a calm, unhurried manner and the expectation that everything will be fine is most helpful for the patient.

Inhalation induction of anesthesia can be performed with several volatile agents. Despite the irritation that isoflurane can cause, anesthesia can be successfully induced with this drug if the concentration of the drug is increased slowly. A study comparing the induction of and emergence from anesthesia with three volatile agents demonstrated that halothane, despite its greater solubility and theoretically slower onset of anesthesia, was faster than either isoflurane or enflurane because it caused fewer episodes of coughing and breath holding than the other agents.[44] A new agent, desflurane, is even more irritating to the airway and is not recommended as an agent for induction of anesthesia.[45] Sevoflurane has become widely used for the induction of anesthesia in children over the last few years. It is nonirritating to the airway and is taken up rapidly. Induction of anesthesia proceeds slightly more quickly than with halothane.[46] Because of its low blood-gas solubility and the increased speed of induction, sevoflurane may be an acceptable induction agent for older or larger patients to whom only an IV induction would have been offered in the past. There may be an increased incidence of excitement, both with induction and with emergence.[47]

Maintenance of the Airway

Obviously, it is of utmost importance to maintain a patent airway throughout anesthesia. This can be accomplished in several ways. The least invasive way is with a face mask. Once anesthesia is induced, no instrumentation of the airway is performed. For some operations, such as myringotomies and insertion of tympanostomy tubes, this approach is very common and effective. Anesthetics that can be administered via a mask alone usually are short, minimally invasive, and usually do not involve the head and neck. Herniorrhaphy, cast changes, and cystoscopy are other typical examples. In general, because of changes in pulmonary mechanics (loss of functional residual capacity [FRC] and, possibly, distal airway collapse) that occur in children during general anesthesia, it is better to reserve mask anesthesia for children over 1 year of age except for very short procedures. There will be less atelectasis and oxygen desaturation if the anesthesiologist maintains 2 to 3 cm H_2O continuous positive airway pressure (CPAP) during spontaneous ventilation. This technique is unsuitable for children at risk for aspiration of gastric contents. If there are difficulties maintaining a patent airway during mask anesthesia, the tongue may be obstructing the airway. Insertion of an oral or nasopharyngeal airway may alleviate the problem. Nasopharyngeal airways occasionally may cause trauma to the adenoids and produce bleeding.

Nasal insufflation of oxygen and inhaled anesthetic is a useful technique for short procedures in which the anesthesiologist must be away from the patient (e.g., during radiation therapy).[48] Inhalation induction of anesthesia is performed. When the child is anesthetized, a well-lubricated, soft catheter is placed through one nare until resistance is felt at the back of the nasopharynx, and the catheter is advanced about 1 cm farther so that the catheter tip lies in the posterior pharynx above the epiglottis. A suitable catheter can be made from a red rubber urethral catheter that has been cut to the appropriate length (nose to tragus length plus at least 5 to 10 cm extra). The appropriate size catheter should comfortably fit into the nare. An alternative is a nasopharyngeal airway. The nasal end of the catheter is fitted with an endotracheal tube connector and connected to the anesthesia circuit. The pop-off valve is closed sufficiently to distend the anesthesia bag and a mixture of oxygen and volatile agent is insufflated into the child's pharynx. This technique is particularly suitable for patients who must undergo repeated anesthetics (e.g., daily radiation therapy treatments) for which the use of an anesthesia mask is impractical. It is crucial that the patient have an adequate airway after induction of anesthesia for this technique to be effective and safe.

The LMA is an alternative to endotracheal intubation or nasal insufflation (see Chapter 9).[49] This device is designed to sit in the pharynx and seat itself over the epiglottis. It comes in a variety of sizes suitable for children of all ages.[50] Its advantages are ease of introduction into the airway, lack of stimulation of the glottis, and absence of need to instrument the larynx. When it is placed appropriately, positive pressure can be applied to the airway. The laryngeal mask is potentially useful for operations in which evaluation of the vocal cords may be useful (thyroidectomy) or when it is advantageous to avoid tracheal intubation (severe reactive airway disease). The disadvantages of the LMA are that it does not prevent aspiration of regurgitated gastric contents or laryngospasm, and the amount of positive pressure that can be applied is limited to about 20 cm H_2O. It can also be used as a guide for flexible fiberoptic laryngoscopy and is part of the ASA Practice Parameter for the difficult airway.[51, 52]

Endotracheal Intubation

The most secure means of maintaining a patent airway is intubation of the trachea. Intubation of the trachea of older children does not differ significantly from intubation of the trachea of adults. Small children and infants, however, have anatomic differences that make tracheal intubation more challenging. Their oropharynx is small relative to the size of the tongue. Their epiglottis is floppy and more difficult to manipulate. Their larynx lies at the level of C3-C4 as opposed to the adult, where it lies at C4-C5. The anterior attachment of the vocal cords is more caudal so they are not perpendicular to the airway as they are in adults. These factors make it necessary to displace the tongue and mandible more in order to visualize the infant's vocal cords. Therefore, straight laryngoscope blades

are used more commonly to intubate the tracheas of children.

Correct head positioning is the first step to successful endotracheal intubation. Children have relatively large heads and large occiputs, which tend to flex the head when the infant is placed supine and may cause partial airway obstruction. A roll or lift under the shoulders will keep the head in a more neutral position and promote an open airway. Overextension of the head also can displace the larynx anteriorly and can partially collapse the trachea.

The mouths of children are relatively small and their tongues are relatively large, making adequate exposure of their larynx more difficult. The laryngoscope blade should be inserted in the right side of the mouth and the tongue displaced to the left. The blade of the laryngoscope is gradually advanced down the pharynx until the epiglottis is seen. The tip of the blade is placed into the vallecula and the blade is lifted up and out at a 45-degree angle. Most of the time, the vocal cords are easily visualized. The endotracheal tube is inserted into the right side of the mouth, not down the channel of the laryngoscope blade. Placing the tube in the channel obscures the view of the vocal cords. Sometimes, the epiglottis is quite floppy and lifting the vallecula does not expose the vocal cords. It may be necessary to lift the tip of the epiglottis with the tip of the laryngoscope blade to expose the vocal cords. Levering the laryngoscope blade against the upper teeth or gums must be avoided because teeth can be broken or dislodged and may be aspirated. If the view of the vocal cords is inadequate, hyoid pressure can be applied to move the larynx posteriorly. Occasionally, the larynx is not midline. When this occurs, it is often useful to apply pressure on the lateral aspect of the hyoid bone and move the glottic opening to the midline.

The endotracheal tube is advanced until its tip is positioned at least 2 cm below the vocal cords. There are often marks on the tube that assist in ensuring the correct location of the tip of the tube. Most term newborns need the ETT taped at about 9 cm at the gums. (Often the correct position of the tip of the ETT can be achieved by remembering that the tip of the ETT will be in the midtrachea for a 1, 2, 3, and 4 kg infant if the tip of the tube is 7, 8, 9, or 10 cm from the gums, respectively.) Another way to correctly position the tip of the ETT is to advance it just until breath sounds are no longer heard or are markedly diminished on the left (i.e., when the ETT is presumably just in the right mainstem bronchus) and then pull the ETT back 2 or 3 cm. Another method of placing the tip of the endotracheal tube in the correct position is to place the tip of the ETT a distance from the teeth or gums that is about about 30 times the internal diameter of the tube. For example, a 5.0 mm inside diameter (ID) ETT should be taped with its tip about 15 cm from the teeth. After the tube is in place, it is fixed with the right hand against the teeth or alveolar ridge and the laryngoscope blade carefully removed from the mouth. Next, the anesthesiologist should perform several maneuvers to ensure correct placement of the ETT. The apices of the lungs should rise equally with ventilation. Auscultation of both sides of the chest, at the apices and in the axillae, should confirm equal breath sounds bilaterally. The right lung field should be auscultated first to establish a baseline for comparison to the left. If breath sounds are not heard over the left lung, the ETT may be placed endobronchially or esophageally. If breath sounds are absent or markedly reduced over the right side of the chest, it is likely that the ETT tube is in the esophagus. In addition, one should listen over the stomach. It is quite possible in children to have good chest movement, hear good breath sounds over the chest, and still have an esophageal intubation. However, the breath sounds over the stomach should never be as loud as over the chest when the ETT is in the trachea. A capnograph provides the most reliable means of detecting an endotracheal intubation. If the ETT is in the trachea, end-tidal carbon dioxide ($PETCO_2$) will be detected. To determine if the ETT is too large or too small, the anesthesiologist should pressurize the circuit and listen for a gas leak from the mouth. Ideally, the leak should occur between 10 and 30 cm H_2O. If the leak occurs below 10 cm H_2O pressure, the tube may be too loose to effectively ventilate the child's lungs. If the leak occurs above 30 cm H_2O, the risk of postextubation stridor is increased. If the leak is outside these limits, it is reasonable to reintubate the trachea with a larger or smaller ETT.

After intubation of the trachea, the stomach should be aspirated with a nasogastric tube or suction catheter to remove any air introduced during the induction of anesthesia and to remove any liquid present in the stomach.

Occasionally, patients arrive in the operating room with a tracheostomy in place. It usually is easy to attach the tracheostomy device to the anesthesia circuit and perform an inhalation induction of anesthesia. The anesthesiologist should discuss with the surgeon the need to replace the tracheostomy tube with an ETT for the operation. After the operation, a new or cleaned tracheostomy tube should be reinserted through the stoma.

Problems During Induction of Anesthesia

During induction of general anesthesia of children, a number of potentially life-threatening problems can occur.

Airway Obstruction

As a child is anesthetized, the muscles of the airway, including those of the tongue, submental triangle, and the upper pharynx, lose their tone, which predisposes young children to upper airway obstruction. As airway muscle tone is lost, the tongue falls backward and obstructs the airway. This usually can be recognized by lack of air movement (monitored by the precordial stethoscope) and paradoxical movement of the chest wall. Owing to a higher oxygen consumption and the greater loss of FRC in children during general anesthesia, hypoxia develops in a matter of seconds.[53]

The first step in correcting airway obstruction is to place the head of a young child in a neutral position, or to place towels under the head of the older child to put the head in a sniffing position. Placing towels under the shoulders of an infant also may help. The position of the mask should be reassessed. If adjusting the head and mask position does not relieve the airway obstruction, the jaw should be pulled forward to remove the tongue from the pharynx. The help of a second person may be required if it is necessary to control ventilation at the same time. If these maneuvers do not correct the airway the obstruction, apply a CPAP of at least 10 cm H_2O. If this fails to relieve the obstruction, an oral or nasal airway should be inserted. Oral airways should fit between the alveolar ridge or teeth and the back of the pharynx. The purpose of an oral airway is to pull the tongue away from the pharyngeal wall. If an oral airway is too small, the tongue may be forced backward and this will increase the obstruction. If the airway is too long, it can cause laryngospasm and emesis. It is often useful to depress the tongue with a tongue depressor to make insertion of the oral airway easier. The airway should not be inserted upside down and rotated to its normal position, as is commonly done in adults. Doing so may dislodge teeth and traumatize the palate. Oral airways should not be left in place as a bite block during the operation because they are hard, they irritate the palate and cause pain, and they can damage or loosen teeth if the child bites down. A soft gauze bite block placed between the molars is more appropriate. A soft rubber nasal airway also can be used, but this can injure the adenoidal tissue of children and cause bleeding.

Children often have pathologic processes that can lead to upper airway obstruction (e.g., epiglottitis, croup) and that require tracheal intubation (see Chapter 23). These children usually can be identified before the induction of anesthesia takes place. It is important to keep these children calm, because anxiety leads to hyperpnea, which increases airway resistance and airway obstruction. It is usually dangerous to administer a premedication that depresses respiration. Although there are circumstances that might make IV rapid-sequence induction preferable; a slow, controlled inhalation induction of anesthesia with halothane or sevoflurane and maintenance of spontaneous ventilation is probably the best choice. If the airway obstruction worsens, it is possible to discontinue an inhaled anesthetic. A surgeon capable of performing a tracheostomy should be scrubbed and available in the operating room during the induction of anesthesia. Once the child loses consciousness, an IV can be started. When the child is deeply anesthetized, laryngoscopy can take place. The use of muscle relaxants for laryngoscopy has its proponents.[54]

Inadequate Access to the Airway

Some children have anatomic abnormalities of the upper airway (e.g., Pierre Robin syndrome, Treacher Collins syndrome, Goldenhar's syndrome, and temporomandibular joint problems) that make maintenance of a patent airway and successful laryngoscopy and tracheal intubation difficult or impossible without special preparation and backup plans.

The question of whether to perform an awake tracheal intubation or to induce general anesthesia first still arises. The choice depends on whether the anesthesiologist feels the airway can be maintained after anesthesia is induced. Some clinicians prefer to do an awake tracheal intubation when a child has a difficult airway. However, children seldom cooperate, require extensive topical anesthesia, and may need sedatives to prevent tracheal intubation from becoming a test of strength between the anesthesiologist and the patient. Beyond the newborn period, awake tracheal intubation is quite challenging. If laryngoscopy is attempted after general anesthesia has been induced, patency of the airway must be ensured. Blind nasotracheal intubation, use of an LMA, either by itself or as an aid in fiberoptically guided tracheal intubation, fiberoptic laryngoscopy, a lighted stylet, or use of a retrograde wire to guide tracheal intubation can be utilized. A vasoconstrictor/anesthetic agent(s) should be applied to the nasal passages using pledgets or cotton-tipped applicators before a blind nasotracheal intubation is attempted. An appropriately sized, well-lubricated ETT is inserted through a nare into the posterior pharynx. The anesthesia circuit is attached to the end of the tube and the tube is advanced slowly. If a bulge appears on one side of the neck or the other, the tip of the tube is lateral to the glottis. If the tube meets resistance and no sign of it is seen in the neck, it probably is in the esophagus. The head should be extended to bring the tip of the tube anterior. Blind nasal intubations are more difficult in children than in adults because of the tilt of the larynx and the more cephalad position of the vocal cords.

The flexible fiberoptic bronchoscope dramatically improves the chances of successfully intubating the tracheas of children who have difficult airways. A 2.1-mm bronchoscope will pass through a 3.0-mm ID ETT. A connector can be attached to a face mask and the bronchoscope can be inserted through a diaphragm in the mask while the mask is held in place and anesthesia and oxygenation are continued. Alternatively, anesthesia can be delivered by insufflation through the contralateral nare while the other nare is instrumented. (It is important to keep the posterior pharynx as free as possible of secretions and blood to improve visualization of the airway.) A fiberoptic bronchoscope with an ETT over it is advanced through the vocal cords and the tube is advanced over the scope and into the trachea. The scope is removed and the circuit is connected to the ETT. An LMA can be inserted under general anesthesia. When the mask is in the proper location, it lies directly above the glottis. An ETT threaded over a fiberoptic scope can be placed through the mask. Once the vocal cords are visualized, the ETT can be advanced into the trachea.[52] If none of the above techniques works, a retrograde wire or a plastic IV catheter can be inserted through the cricothyroid membrane and advanced in a cephalad direction into the mouth. The wire should exit either the mouth or nose. A red rubber catheter is then advanced through the nose into the mouth and pulled out the mouth. The ends of the wire and catheter are tied together and pulled out a nare. An endotracheal tube then is threaded over the wire into the trachea. Occasionally, the tube catches on the epiglottis. Rotating the tube often allows the end of the tube to enter the trachea. The wire is then removed in the cephalad direction while downward pressure is applied to the ETT. If all attempts to intubate the trachea fail, the options are to cancel the operation and return another day, or to perform a tracheostomy.

Laryngospasm

Laryngospasm occurs during induction of anesthesia if the vocal cords are stimulated during light anesthesia. The stimulation can be as minor as adjustment of the airway, the presence of secretions or blood on the vocal cords, or attempted intubation of the trachea before the patient is adequately anesthetized. Laryngospasm is more likely to occur during inhalation induction of anesthesia because the patient goes through stage II much more slowly than during an IV induction of anesthesia. Laryngospasm presents as loss of air movement (detected by the precordial stethoscope) and paradoxical movement of the chest (outward movement of the abdomen and collapse of the chest during attempted inspiration). As soon as laryngospasm is recognized, the anesthesiologist should apply the face mask tightly to the face and exert positive-pressure ventilation. At the same time, marked forward pressure should be exerted on the angles of the jaw. It is rare that CPAP, forward pressure on the jaw, and 100 percent oxygen do not break the laryngospasm, although a high level of CPAP may be necessary. If the oxygen saturation continues to decrease and the laryngospasm is not relieved, a small dose of succinylcholine can be administered.

Bronchospasm

Children with reactive airways frequently come to the operating room for procedures, including former premature infants with bronchopulmonary dysplasia and children with asthma. Their tracheas are very sensitive to stimuli and react to the presence of a foreign body (e.g., an ETT) by increasing bronchomotor tone. Narrowing of medium and small airways leads to an increase in ventilation–perfusion mismatching and possible hypoxia. The degree of bronchospasm may be severe enough to prevent effective ventilation of the lungs. The best treatment for bronchospasm is prevention.

If a child with a history of well-controlled reactive airway disease is scheduled for elective surgery and has just begun to wheeze again, it is probably best to postpone the operation until the bronchospasm is resolved. If the operation is urgent or emergent, the patient should be treated preoperatively with a nebulized bronchodilator (e.g., albuterol) before going into the operating room. If the patient is on a regular schedule of bronchodilators, it is important to continue these on the day of surgery. To reduce the incidence and severity of bronchospasm in children with reactive airway disease, deep anesthesia is critical before instrumentation of the airway is attempted. This is most easily accomplished by inhalation induction of anesthesia with a volatile agent, halothane or sevoflurane. Although all of the volatile agents are believed to be bronchodilators, there is some evidence that isoflurane may increase bronchomotor tone.[55] Because deep levels of anesthesia are required to decrease the potential for bronchospasm, careful attention must be paid to cardiovascular responses during the induction of anesthesia. Although a fluid bolus given early in the induction of anesthesia may prevent hypotension, excessive fluid may increase interstitial edema in patients who have bronchopulmonary dysplasia. If an IV induction of anesthesia is chosen, many anesthesiologists use ketamine as the induction agent of choice because its weak sympathomimetic actions tend to cause bronchodilation. Thiopental, on the other hand, may cause brochoconstriction.[56]

If a child begins to wheeze during surgery, mechanical causes of airway obstruction should be quickly sought (e.g., kinked ETT, mucous plugs in the ETT) by inspecting the circuit and inserting a suction catheter carefully down the ET tube without inserting its tip beyond the end of the tube. If these measures do not reveal the problem, increasing the level of anesthesia and administering bronchodilators directly through the ETT may be helpful. As a general rule, wheezing during or after induction of anesthesia usually indicates a light level of anesthesia.

Pulmonary Disease

The pediatric anesthesiologist must occasionally anesthetize children with active pulmonary disease (e.g., pneumonia). These diseases are characterized by a loss of FRC. Children without lung disease may lose as much as 45 percent of their FRC.[57,58] Children with pulmonary diseases may lose even more of their FRC, exposing them to increasing ventilation–perfusion mismatch and hypoxia. Several principles are helpful when such children are anesthetized. An increased inspired oxygen concentration helps overcome ventilation perfusion mismatch and application of positive end-expiratory pressure (PEEP) may partially restore FRC. This is particularly true in infants under 1 year of age whose FRC loss is greater with general anesthesia. All infants should have their ventilation controlled during anesthesia because hypoventilation exacerbates their tendency toward hypoxia. However, PEEP must be applied carefully. Excessive PEEP reduces venous return and cardiac output. Pulmonary blood flow also is reduced because some alveoli become overdistended and alveolar pressure exceeds pulmonary capillary pressure.

Cardiovascular Problems

Children with congenital heart disease often require surgery and present with cyanosis and/or congestive heart failure.

The amount of pulmonary blood flow in children who have cyanotic heart disease depends on the balance between pulmonary vascular resistance and systemic vascular resistance. Because decreased systemic or increased pulmonary vascular resistance may increase hypoxia and oxygen desaturation, it is important to use anesthetics that maintain these resistances close to normal. One such combination is ketamine 4–8 mg/kg and succinylcholine 1–2 mg/kg, given either IM or IV. As long as the patient is not hypovolemic, ketamine maintains near-normal blood pressure and can either maintain or increase oxygenation. Control of ventilation, if it leads to hyperventilation, may lower pulmonary arterial pressure and increase pulmonary blood flow. An alternative method for inducing anesthesia is to use inhaled anesthetics, although right-to-left shunting of blood may prolong induction of anesthesia and may cause greater myocardial depression, especially with halothane (see Chapter 3).

Patients with congestive heart failure usually have volume overload of the heart, commonly because of a large left-to-right shunt that produces pulmonary overcirculation. The effects of pulmonary overcirculation can be ameliorated by inducing anesthesia in a way that does not decrease the pulmonary vascular resistance further (e.g., normocapnia, maintaining the F_IO_2 as close to that of room air as possible). Drugs used for IV and inhaled induction of anesthesia should be given carefully and in small doses because they can depress myocardial contractility. Very careful fluid management is also paramount. To provide adequate anesthesia for surgery, it may be necessary to use an inotropic agent(s) to support cardiac output.

Hypovolemia

Some patients coming to the operating room will be hypovolemic (e.g., premature neonates on diuretics, patients who have had bowel preparation, patients with pyloric stenosis, and those with bleeding from a recent tonsillectomy). Because they have a relative lack of circulating intravascular volume, such patients should have a functioning IV catheter of adequate size inserted *before* the induction of anesthesia. Except in the most unusual circumstances, the operation can be delayed while a bolus of fluid is administered to correct the fluid deficit. If the procedure is a true emergency, high doses of narcotics plus a muscle relaxant can be given while a bolus of fluid is being infused.[60] An alternative is to give ketamine and pancuronium IV. Ketamine will increase circulating catecholamines and increase sympathetic tone. However, in hypovolemic patients, hypotension may develop with the injection of ketamine. Smaller doses of all drugs that depress the myocardium or cause vasodilation should be used, and the volume deficit should be replaced as quickly as possible.

Hypotension

Decreases of up to 20 percent of arterial blood pressure are common during the induction of general anesthesia in children and are well tolerated by healthy children. However, sick children may not tolerate these changes. Since it may be difficult to measure arterial blood pressure before induction of anesthesia, it is often better to do so as soon as the patient becomes unconscious. In one study, the arterial blood pressure responses of premature infants undergoing repair of a patent ductus arteriosus decreased 25 percent after induction of anesthesia with halothane, but returned to normal with 5 to 10 ml/kg of isotonic crystalloid given IV over 5 minutes.[61] There were no intraoperative sequelae from the hypotension. In the same study, induction of anesthesia with high-dose narcotics (30 to 50 μg/kg of fentanyl) produced no hemodynamic changes for the same population and operation.

Full Stomach

It is often necessary to anesthetize pediatric patients who have a full stomach. There are two ways of dealing with this situation. The first is to wait until the patient has been NPO long enough. However, waiting does not guarantee that the stomach will be empty, especially if the patient has a process that slows gastric emptying (e.g., pain). There may still be significant fluid in the stomach 18 hours after the child was made NPO. If the surgery cannot be delayed or if the patient has one of the known risks for aspiration (e.g., neurologic disorders or medications that prolong gastric emptying time), anesthesia must proceed. The second is to do a rapid-sequence induction of anesthesia with cricoid pressure.

When possible, the stomach should be emptied by inserting an orogastric or nasogastric suction tube and removing as much of the gastric contents as possible before the induction of anesthesia begins. Although it is rarely possible to remove all of the fluid from the stomach, suctioning the stomach may lessen the risk for serious aspiration. Whether IV or inhalation induction of anesthesia is chosen, and despite removing as much of the stomach contents as possible, cricoid pressure (the Sellick maneuver) should be used to occlude the esophagus and prevent movement of gastric contents into the pharynx.[62] This maneuver is effective even when a gastric suction tube is in place. Unless excessive ventilation pressures are used, the lungs can be ventilated despite the cricoid pressure. Before induction of anesthesia is begun, the lungs should be preoxygenated for several minutes. A functioning Yankauer suction device should be immediately at hand. Reverse Trendelenburg position may help to reduce the risk of passive regurgitation of fluid but can also lead to hypotension in hypovolemic patients. It is unlikely that positioning will be of much benefit for small children. For older, larger children, tilting the bed can increase the difference in height between the gastroesophageal junction and the pharynx by approximately 20 cm.[54] Use of positive-pressure ventilation in excess of 10 to 15 cm H_2O should be avoided during the induction of anesthesia because higher pressures increases the passage of air into the stomach. Lower pressures may reduce passive regurgitation. Finally, completing the induction of anesthesia and gaining rapid control of the airway is always advisable.

If a functioning IV catheter is in place, IV induction of anesthesia is often appropriate. There is debate about the most suitable muscle relaxant to use for these cases. Although succinylcholine causes the most rapid onset of muscle paralysis, succinylcholine administration is associated with a number of side effects and risks, and in many hospitals, it is seldom administered to pediatric patients. Instead, the intermediate acting nondepolarizing muscle relaxants are used and the lungs are ventilated while cricoid pressure is held until adequate muscle relaxation occurs to facilitate intubation of the trachea.

MAINTENANCE OF GENERAL ANESTHESIA

Pediatric anesthesiologists have several goals during maintenance of general anesthesia, including provision of adequate anesthesia and operating conditions for the surgeon, maintaining physiologic homeostasis, and providing appropriate fluid administration to maintain adequate circulating blood volume.

Anesthesia should render a patient unconscious, amnestic, pain-free, and immobile. A number of agents and techniques can be used to accomplish this: volatile agents, IV agents, or more commonly, a combination of both. The use of light general anesthesia with an inhaled anesthetic agent plus opioids, supplemented by muscle relaxation, is a common method of maintaining anesthesia for pediatric patients. This method allows relatively quick awakening from anesthesia and adequate immobility for the surgeon during the operation. It also avoids the use of deeper levels of inhaled anesthetics that cause myocardial depression, especially in young infants.

Inhaled Anesthetic Agents

The primary anesthetic agents used in pediatric anesthesia are nitrous oxide and the volatile anesthetic agents, especially sevoflurane, halothane, and isoflurane because of the rapid uptake and elimination of these agents in children (Table 10–1).

Nitrous Oxide

Nitrous oxide (N_2O) has a number of features that make it attractive for use in pediatric anesthesia. Because of its low blood–gas solubility coefficient of 0.47, uptake and elimination of this gas by the body are rapid. This favorable pharmacokinetic profile is augmented in children by their higher minute ventilation/FRC ratio, higher cardiac output, and higher percentage of vessel-rich tissues.[64] Because of its low solubility and the second gas effect, nitrous oxide reaches equilibrium in the brain within a few minutes, significantly faster than the volatile agents. Since the minimum alveolar concentration (MAC) of nitrous oxide is over 100 percent, it is not possible to deliver a complete anesthetic solely with nitrous oxide. However, it can be used as an analgesic agent at concentrations up to 50 percent, for instance, in pediatric dentistry. For general anesthesia, N_2O is used to supplement other inhaled or intravenous agents. The effect of nitrous oxide appears to be additive with some anesthetic agents (i.e., 0.5 MAC of nitrous oxide plus 0.5 MAC of halothane seems to be equivalent to 1.0 MAC of halothane alone). However, this additivity may not be true for some of the newer volatile agents.[65] In theory, nitrous oxide reduces the concentration of volatile agents needed to produce anesthesia, which decreases the time to endotracheal extubation at the end of surgery.

Nitrous oxide causes minimal respiratory depression and is a mild stimulant of the sympathetic nervous system. However, when N_2O is combined with volatile anesthetics, it has the same circulatory depressant effects as an equianesthetic dose of volatile anesthetic, which may offset its proposed advantages.[66] Nitrous oxide also antagonizes methionine synthetase, the enzyme responsible for vitamin B_{12} synthesis. Nitrous oxide probably should not be used to anesthetize children with bone marrow suppression or those who have had a bone marrow transplant to avoid the possible risk of megaloblastic anemia, though single short exposures to nitrous oxide probably pose minimal risks to the patients. Nitrous oxide was formerly believed to increase pulmonary arterial pressure, but it was shown to have little effect on the pulmonary artery pressures of pediatric intensive care unit (ICU) patients.[67, 68] Finally, because nitrous oxide is about 30 times more soluble than nitrogen, it can diffuse into closed spaces of the body more rapidly than nitrogen can exit from the space, leading to expansion of the space. Examples of situations where this can be clinically significant are pneu-

TABLE 10 – 1					
INHALATIONAL ANESTHETIC AGENTS					
Agent	Blood–Gas Solubility	MAC (%)				
		0–1 Mo	1–6 Mo	6 Mo–1 Yr	1–12 Yr	Adult
Nitrous oxide	0.47					105
Halothane	2.4	0.87	1.2	0.97	0.89	0.76
Enflurane	1.9					1.6
Isoflurane	1.4	1.6	1.87	1.8	1.6	1.2
Sevoflurane	0.69		3.1	2.7	2.55	1.7
Desflurane	0.42	9.2	9.4	9.9	8–8.7	7.3

Data from Gregory et al.,[71] Lerman et al.,[75] Cameron et al.,[103] Lerman,[177] and Taylor and Lerman.[113]

mothorax and tympanoplasty. In the former, rapid accumulation of nitrous oxide can lead to circulatory and respiratory compromise. In the latter, it can cause the graft to lift off of the tympanic membrane. Other situations in which there is increased theoretic risk of gas accumulation include long abdominal surgery procedures that might lead to bowel distention and procedures in children with bronchopulmonary dysplasia or obstructive pulmonary disease who have pulmonary blebs. The latter may expand and rupture over the course of anesthesia. When venous air embolism is present, nitrous oxide can increase the size of the embolus. There was no difference in the outcome of adult patients who underwent sitting craniotomies if they did or did not receive nitrous oxide, as long as the nitrous oxide was discontinued as soon as signs of embolism occurred.[69]

Halothane

Halothane has a slightly sweet smell and is relatively nonirritating to airways. Therefore, less coughing and breath holding accompany its inhalation than occurs with other potent inhaled agents. Despite the highest blood–gas and tissue–blood solubilities of the commonly used volatile anesthetic agents, uptake of halothane is rapid in children due to their high minute ventilation/FRC ratio (5:1 vs. 1.5:1 for adults), higher cardiac index, and greater percentage of vessel-rich tissues than in adults.[64] In addition, current vaporizers allow a higher MAC multiple for halothane than for other agents, notably sevoflurane. Table 10-2 shows the time constants for halothane in various

TABLE 10 – 2		
TIME CONSTANTS FOR HALOTHANE (MIN)*		
Tissue	Adult	Infant
Brain	3.4	2.2
Heart	2.3	1.4
Splanchnic	5.0	2.5
Kidney	0.35	0.30
Muscle	49.0	8.4
Fat	2,000	540

* Tissue time constants = LV/Q.
From Brandom BW, Brandom RB, Cook DR: Uptake and distribution of halothane in infants: in vivo measurements and computer simulations. Anesth Anlag 62:404, 1983, with permission.

tissues in adults and children.[70] Note that the time constant for halothane in the brains of children is more than 30 percent less than in adults. Therefore, the induction of anesthesia occurs more quickly. Despite its higher solubility, induction of anesthesia with halothane is faster than with other volatile agents due to its lack of side effects (e.g., coughing, breath holding).[44] Emergence from anesthesia, however, was more closely related to the relative tissue–blood solubilities, but the differences in emergence times were not clinically significant. To achieve more rapid equilibration of the agent with the blood and tissues, the inspired concentration of halothane usually is increased during induction of anesthesia to a level that is much higher than the final concentration of halothane needed to maintain anesthesia (overpressuring). This allows the partial pressures of anesthetic required to cause loss of consciousness to be attained quickly, thus avoiding a prolonged second stage of anesthesia. The safety of this technique depends on the anesthesiologist decreasing the concentration of anesthestic as soon as the patient is asleep. In very healthy, well-hydrated patients, the anesthesia circuit can be filled with 5 percent halothane and the patient can be asked to exhale to residual volume before taking a vital capacity breath of 5 percent halothane. With this single-breath technique, unconsciousness can be induced very rapidly.

Halothane's effect on the brain produces unconsciousness, amnesia, and mild analgesia. MAC is age dependent, being highest in infants (1.08 percent) and lower (0.76 percent) in young adults (see Chapter 3).[71] Children, especially infants, are prone to anesthetic dose-dependent circulatory depression during halothane anesthesia.[72] Newborn animals develop cardiac failure at lower concentrations of halothane.[73] A number of clinical observations have noted the greater cardiac depression in infants during inhalation induction of anesthesia.[74] Subsequent work by Lerman et al.[75] showed that neonates had a lower MAC than infants 1 to 6 months of age (see Fig. 10–1). These results demonstrate that there is only a small margin for error in the use of halothane or other inhaled anesthetics. If the trachea is intubated using deep concentrations of halothane without muscle relaxants, the patient's condition must be scrupulously monitored throughout the procedure. An alternative technique uses halothane to produce unconsciousness. When this is achieved, an IV is started, muscle relaxants and narcotics are administered,

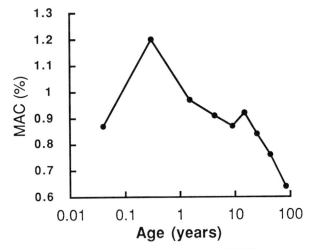

FIGURE 10–1. The minimum alveolar concentration (MAC) for halothane as a function of age in man. (Data from Gregory et al.,[71] and Lerman et al.[75])

and a relatively light level of inhaled anesthesia is maintained during maintenance of surgery. This avoids using deep levels of volatile agent.

More than 2 μg/kg of epinephrine sensitizes the adult halothane-exposed myocardium to dysrhythmias. Children, however, have received up to 15 μg/kg of epinephrine in the presence of halothane without developing arrhythmias.[76] Arrhythmias do occur with spontaneous ventilation and hypercarbia. Junctional rhythms and bi- and trigeminy are the most common arrhythmias seen in these children.

Halothane maintains a normal to increased respiratory rate and decreased tidal volume.[77] As a consequence, minute ventilation decreases and the $Paco_2$ increases. The effect is dose dependent. Ventilation is decreased both by central ventilatory depression and by decreased intercostal muscle tone.[78] The response to exogenous CO_2 remains, but the CO_2 response curve is shifted to the right.[79] Halothane does possess some weak neuromuscular relaxing properties and potentiates the action of nondepolarizing muscle relaxants. It also increases dead space ventilation and ventilation–perfusion mismatching, probably through alterations in hypoxic pulmonary vasoconstriction. Because of halothane's multiple effects on pulmonary gas exchange, controlled ventilation usually is recommended when halothane is a major component of the anesthetic. Halothane is a potent bronchodilator in both animals and humans and often is helpful when anesthetizing patients with reactive airway disease.[80, 81] This effect is dose related.

Halothane also increases cerebral blood flow, cerebral blood volume, and intracranial pressure (ICP).[82, 83] At higher concentrations, halothane abolishes cerebral vascular autoregulation. Therefore, its use is probably contraindicated as the only anesthetic agent in children with elevated ICP. Low-dose halothane, in conjunction with hyperventilation, should not significantly increase ICP. However, the use of a nitrous oxide, narcotic-based anesthetic and avoiding the use of high concentrations of halothane is recommended if there is concern about ICP. There are occasions when a child with potentially increased ICP

and no IV (e.g., a blocked ventriculoperitoneal shunt) requires surgery. Crying and breath holding during attempts to start an IV may increase ICP as much as halothane. Therefore, anesthesia is often induced with halothane, the lungs are hyperventilated to reduce the $Petco_2$ to approximately 25 mm Hg, and an IV is started. Narcotics and muscle relaxants can then be administered and the concentration of halothane can be reduced greatly.

Up to 20 percent of absorbed halothane may undergo metabolism by the liver versus 2 to 5 percent of sevoflurane and 0.2 percent of isoflurane. Biotransformation can be either oxidative or reductive. During normoxic conditions, halothane is oxidized and produces trifluoroacetic acid and bromide, neither of which cause significant problems. Under hypoxic conditions, halothane can produce free fluoride ions, which may cause defects in renal concentration. However, no increase occurred in renal or hepatic dysfunction in children with cyanotic congenital heart disease when they were exposed to halothane.[84]

In adults, halothane-caused hepatitis occurs at a rate of 1 in 6,000 to 1 in 35,000 cases.[85, 86] It is more common with female patients, obese patients, and those who have had multiple exposures to halothane over a short time period. In the pediatric population, however, it is difficult to implicate halothane as the sole cause of hepatitis, even when halothane is administered every day. Recent retrospective studies suggest halothane hepatitis occurs in 1 in 80,000 to 1 in 200,000 exposures in infants and children.[87, 88] It is postulated that metabolic intermediates of halothane are converted to haptens by binding to serum proteins or lipoproteins and that the subsequent antigens elicit an autoimmune response that damages the liver.[89] There is no compelling evidence that administration of halothane to patients with liver disease is associated with hepatitis.[90]

Sevoflurane

In the last few years, the use of sevoflurane has dramatically increased in pediatric anesthesia. It may be less irritating to airways than halothane, even when a maximum concentration of 8 percent is used for the induction of anesthesia. The low blood–gas solubility (0.69) of sevoflurane predicts that uptake of the drug will be rapid. Indeed, in most but not all comparison studies, induction of anesthesia with sevoflurane was significantly faster than with halothane.[46] There may be more excitement during the induction of anesthesia with sevoflurane, especially without nitrous oxide.[47] However, a recent study in young infants did not demonstrate a difference.[91] Emergence from anesthesia is also more rapid with sevoflurane, which may be associated with more agitation during emergence, especially if postoperative pain control has not been adequately dealt with intraoperatively.[92]

The MAC for sevoflurane is age-dependent, as occurs with other volatile agents. The MAC for neonates and young infants is 3.3 percent, and decreases with age.[92] Like desflurane, the contribution of nitrous oxide to MAC is attenuated.[92]

Studies on the hemodynamic effects of sevoflurane have been inconsistent. One study showed minimal changes in blood pressure with a small rise in heart rate.[93] Another showed a decrease in blood pressure with preservation of heart rate.[94]

The respiratory effects of sevoflurane and halothane have been compared and small differences were found at 1 MAC, although differences in the flow waveform suggest differences in the mechanisms of these respiratory effects.[95] Studies in adults have demonstrated greater respiratory depression with sevoflurane at 1.4 MAC.[96] Anecdotally, we have observed a high incidence of apnea and marked hypoventilation during the induction of anesthesia with 6 to 8 percent sevoflurane.

Although studies in adults showed little difference in the response of cerebral blood flow to sevoflurane and isoflurane, there are few studies in children. Berkowitz et al. showed no difference in the cerebral blood flow velocity during sevoflurane and halothane anesthesia.[97]

The metabolism of sevoflurane has been a controversial issue. Two metabolic products of sevoflurane have potential toxicities. They are the fluoride ion and a vinyl ether called Compound A. Fluoride ion has been identified as a product of several volatile agents. Methoxyflurane was shown to produce significantly increased concentrations of fluoride ion secondary to metabolism, and these high concentrations of fluoride were shown to be associated with renal concentrating defects. Sevoflurane also produces fluoride but at lower concentrations and for shorter times. These low concentrations of fluoride have not been associated with clinically significant renal damage.[98] Studies on Compound A have yielded contradictory results,[99–101] but the potential for damage led the Food and Drug Administration (FDA) to originally recommend that sevoflurane not be used with total gas flows of less than 2 L/min. Studies in children are limited but are consistent with its safe use.[102] The original recommendation to limit fresh gas flows have been altered slightly and the currently approved package insert reads: "To minimize exposure to Compound A, sevoflurane exposure should not exceed 2 MAC-hours at flow rates of 1 to 2 L/min. Fresh gas flows of less than 1 L/min are not recommended."

Isoflurane

Isoflurane, like enflurane, has more qualitative than quantitative differences from halothane. Its blood–gas solubility is 1.4, but because of its very pungent and irritating odor, inhalation induction of anesthesia is associated with a high incidence of airway problems, including laryngospasm.[44] Nevertheless, if isoflurane is administered slowly and after pretreatment with atropine to reduce secretions, isoflurane can be used to provide safe inhalation induction of anesthesia. The MAC in adults is 1.2 percent, and it has an age dependency similar to halothane.[103, 104] Its MAC has been determined for premature infants (Fig. 10–2).[105] In clinical studies, isoflurane led to a slower induction of anesthesia than halothane.[44] Emergence from anesthesia is similar to halothane, despite halothane's greater solubility. This may be related to isoflurane's virtual lack of metabolism (0.2 percent) and halothane's high metabolism (20 percent).

The respiratory depression produced by isoflurane is intermediate between that caused by halothane (the least) and enflurane (the greatest).[106] Ventilation still should be

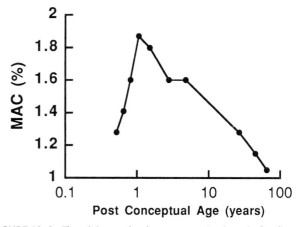

FIGURE 10–2. The minimum alveolar concentration (MAC) of isoflurane as a function of postconceptual age. The postconceptual age is calculated by adding 40 weeks to the mean postnatal age for each age group. (Data from Cameron et al.,[103] LeDez et al.,[105] and Stevens et al.[107])

controlled during isoflurane anesthesia. Isoflurane decreases brochomotor tone, although there is some contradictory evidence.[80]

Isoflurane preserves heart rate and cardiac output while decreasing arterial blood pressure. Unlike halothane, isoflurane has little direct effect on the myocardium, but instead causes peripheral vasodilation and a decrease in systemic vascular resistance, although this result has been challenged.[107, 108] When compared with halothane and enflurane, isoflurane is least likely to sensitize the heart to arrhythmias. Similar studies have not been done in children.

Isoflurane has less effect on cerebral blood flow than enflurane or halothane.[109, 110] At concentrations below 1.1 MAC, there are minimal increases in cerebral blood flow in normocapneic adults that can be prevented by hyperventilation. Furthermore, isoflurane is associated with a greater decrease in the cerebral metabolic rate for oxygen.[111]

Despite some attractive features (e.g., no association with hepatic necrosis, less circulatory depression, and more favorable cerebral hemodynamics) isoflurane is used in pediatric anesthesia primarily for maintenance of anesthesia because emergence from anesthesia may be slightly faster than with halothane and less stormy than with sevoflurane.

Desflurane

Desflurane has a blood–gas solubility coefficient of 0.42, similar to that of nitrous oxide, and should provide rapid induction and awakening from anesthesia.[112] Its MAC in children is about 9 percent, higher than in adults.[113] It is unsuitable as an inhalation agent for the induction of anesthesia because desflurane is associated with a high incidence of coughing, breath holding, and laryngospasm.[45] When halothane is used to induce anesthesia and desflurane is used for maintenance of anesthesia, patients emerge very rapidly from anesthesia and are often excited and/or in pain.[114] This is presumably related to the rapid disappearance of desflurane from the brain and consequent loss of analgesic and sedative properties of low levels of volatile agent. Therefore, use of desflurane promotes the use of regional anesthesia or narcotics to prevent the immediate onset of postoperative pain. The respiratory, circulatory, and cerebral blood flow effects of desflurane in adults are similar to isoflurane.

Routine use of desflurane is complicated by the need for special vaporizers and the fact that at more than 1 MAC (6 to 9 percent) the inspired oxygen concentration is reduced. Although desflurane probably will not replace halothane for routine use in pediatric anesthesia, it may find a use in long cases where rapid awakening from anesthesia is desirable. It should be remembered that if narcotics are administered during anesthesia, awakening from anesthesia is not shorter than with halothane. Discharge from the recovery room occurs sooner with desflurane than with halothane.[114]

Parenteral Agents

Several classes of parenteral agents are used in pediatric anesthesia that can be combined to provide complete anesthesia (total intravenous anesthesia [TIVA]) or used as adjuncts in a balanced anesthetic.

Opioids

Opioids are the basis for the high-dose opioid–oxygen anesthetic frequently used to anesthetize critically ill premature infants, part of a nitrous oxide–narcotic–low-dose volatile agent anesthetic often used for neuroanesthesia and other surgery, or they are used to provide postoperative pain control.

Morphine, when used in high doses, can cause histamine release, vasodilation, and hypotension. However, 0.1 to 0.2 mg/kg of morphine provides intraoperative and postoperative analgesia and usually leads to a smoother awakening from anesthesia in most patients. Lower doses of morphine are appropriate for sick patients. Like all opioids, morphine can cause respiratory depression. Neonates are more sensitive to morphine than meperidine because the neonate's blood–brain barrier is less well developed, and water-soluble morphine crosses the barrier easily.[115] This leads to increased respiratory depression relative to analgesic potency. In addition, elimination and clearance of morphine are prolonged in neonates, although both approach adult values by 1 month of age.[116] Great caution should be used when administering morphine to neonates; mechanical ventilation may be necessary postoperatively in some neonates given morphine.

Meperidine has clinical properties similar to morphine, although it is about 10 times less potent. Because it is very lipid soluble, it readily crosses the blood–brain barrier. Consequently, the dose-dependent respiratory depression caused by meperidine does not change with age (i.e., it is not exaggerated in neonates). A disadvantage of meperidine is that its major metabolite, normeperidine, may accumulate and cause central nervous system excitation (e.g., seizures). Nevertheless its more rapid onset and shorter half-life may make it useful for postoperative pain control in same-day surgery patients.

Fentanyl is a synthetic opioid widely used to supplement inhaled anesthetics in pediatric patients. It causes few hemodynamic changes, even in high doses. It has been particularly useful for anesthetizing critically ill premature infants and children. Studies by Robinson and Gregory[60, 61] showed that ligation of a patent ductus arteriosus could be safely performed in premature infants and that there were far fewer hemodynamic changes with 30 to 50 μg/kg of fentanyl than with halothane if the intravascular volume was adequate. Doses of 12.5 to 15 μg/kg of fentanyl also prevent hemodynamic changes in newborns who must undergo major surgery in the first few days of life.[117] Fentanyl is commonly used in high doses for surgical correction of congenital heart disease. The potential for respiratory depression exists with fentanyl, especially in higher doses, because its clearance is prolonged in both term or premature infants.[118, 119] The two major factors that influence clearance of highly extracted drugs like fentanyl are the hepatic blood flow and the volume of distribution (see Chapter 3). Delayed clearance of opioids prolongs their respiratory depressant effects and may increase the need for postoperative mechanical ventilation. A study by Hertzka et al. examined the respiratory effects of fentanyl in infants, children, and adults.[120] Infants and children had similar partial pressures of carbon dioxide as a function of plasma fentanyl concentration and less variability of respiratory rate and less apnea in the recovery room than adults. Major side effects of fentanyl include bradycardia and chest wall rigidity. The former is related to a vagotonic effect of the drug and can be prevented by the simultaneous administration of atropine or pancuronium. Chest wall rigidity may be due to changes in the extrathoracic airway, and can be minimized by slow administration of the drug and not giving high doses of fentanyl before administering muscle relaxants.[121] Because of its high lipid solubility, fentanyl crosses the blood–brain barrier quickly. Thus, its analgesic and respiratory effects begin shortly after the drug is administered. Because it is highly extracted by the liver, fentanyl's metabolism is very dependent on liver blood flow. Conditions that decrease hepatic blood flow would be expected to decrease the clearance of fentanyl, but this has not been confirmed in animal studies.[122] Fentanyl is delivered in intermittent boluses or by continuous infusion. In theory, the latter ensures a consistent blood level of drug. However, difficulty in identifying a therapeutic end point makes titration of the infusion difficult and can lead to accumulation of the drug and delayed recovery. Theoretic and clinical studies demonstrate the difficulty of predicting a drug's pharmacodynamic behavior based solely on the redistribution and elimination half-lives.[123]

Sufentanil is 5 to 10 times more potent than fentanyl. Pharmacokinetic studies performed with sufentanil in pediatric patients undergoing open heart surgery demonstrate lower clearance and longer elimination of the drug than occurred in older children.[124] The side effects of bradycardia and chest wall rigidity are similar to those seen with fentanyl. A recent comparison of sufentanil to halothane/morphine anesthesia for repair of congenital heart disease claimed that sufentanil was better at preventing hemodynamic changes intraoperatively and led to a better outcome than the other drugs.[125] However, the numbers of patients studied was small and the groups were unequal.

Alfentanil has a rapid onset of action and the drug is rapidly eliminated from the system, owing to its smaller volume of distribution. These properties may make alfentanil useful for procedures where quick awakening is desired. However, during prolonged infusions of alfentanil, the drug may accumulate and be associated with a slower awakening.[123]

Remifentanil is a new synthetic opioid that is hydrolyzed in plasma and tissues by esterases, which cause the drug to be rapidly eliminated from the body.[126] Pharmacokinetic studies have shown that the context-sensitive half-life, regardless of the duration of an infusion, is 3 minutes. All the other opioids show dose-related accumulation in the serum, especially with longer infusions. Remifentanil has about the same potency as fentanyl and the same side effects as other opioids (e.g., respiratory depression, chest wall rigidity, nausea). There is little information about pharmacokinetic or clinical studies in children.[127]

Sedative-Hypnotics

As a class of drugs, sedative-hypnotics have not been particularly useful for the maintenance of general anesthesia because they often are associated with prolonged postoperative sleepiness, they are not analgesic, and other agents, especially volatile anesthetic agents, are easy and safe to use in children. However, there are specific instances where they may be useful (e.g., during laryngoscopy when inhaled anesthetics cannot easily be used). Propofol has become particularly popular in these situations because of its rapid onset and offset of action. It is usually delivered as an infusion and, unless the procedure is painless, requires concomitant use of an analgesic agent for complete anesthesia. Administration of a muscle relaxant is helpful during propofol infusion because patients anesthetized with propofol have a tendency to move, either involuntarily or in response to stimulation if the level of anesthesia is inadequate. Propofol is useful for nonpainful radiologic procedures. Though this is often described as conscious sedation, in reality, it is unconscious sedation and requires the same close monitoring as general anesthesia.[128]

Although ketamine does not formally belong to the class of sedative hypnotics, and has been used as the sole anesthetic agent for children, it can be useful as an analgesic and amnestic agent for short painful procedures, such as burn debridement or suturing lacerations in the emergency department. As part of a general anesthetic, it offers little, but is occasionally useful as an IM anesthesia induction agent for handicapped older children and for children with cyanotic heart disease.

TIVA has not been used widely in pediatric anesthesia,[129] in part because the pharmacokinetics and pharmacodynamics of the volatile agents are much better understood in children than are the parenteral agents used for TIVA. Furthermore, there is significant variability in response to parenteral agents across the first two decades of life, from premature infants to adolescents, because of differences in distribution and elimination of these drugs in developing children. These differences make it more challenging, but not impossible, to provide a complete anesthetic to a child using only parenteral agents.

Muscle Relaxants

Muscle relaxants are used to facilitate tracheal intubation, to maintain muscle relaxation during surgery, or to prevent movement during a light general anesthetic. There are two choices, depolarizing muscle relaxants (succinylcholine is the only one available in this country) or nondepolarizing muscle relaxants.

As discussed in Chapter 3, succinylcholine has the quickest onset and the shortest duration of action of currently used muscle relaxants. Therefore, when it is necessary to quickly intubate the trachea and establish a patent airway to reduce the risk of gastric aspiration (e.g., in cases of full stomach, trauma, bulbar palsy), succinylcholine is indicated. Unfortunately, succinylcholine administration is associated with some serious side effects: jaw stiffness, masseter spasm, hyperkalemia, arrhythmias, myoglobinemia, and malignant hyperthermia. For this reason, succinylcholine is rarely used in some pediatric centers. Instead, a modified rapid-sequence IV induction with a nondepolarizing muscle relaxant and cricoid pressure is used, even for patients with full stomachs.

The nondepolarizing muscle relaxants have a variety of onsets, durations of action, and side effects. The choice of drug is dictated by the patient's clinical situation and the drug's intended use. The dose of drug required for tracheal intubation and the time to onset of effective muscle relaxation depends in part on the type of general anesthetic used (i.e., inhalational vs. N_2O–narcotic) and the age of the patient.

Nondepolarizing muscle relaxants are categorized by their duration of action as short, intermediate, or long acting. The only short-acting nondepolarizing muscle relaxant currently in use is mivacurium.[130] Its onset of action is similar to vecuronium, 2 to 4 minutes. Recovery from the effects of this drug is rapid, about 10 to 20 minutes, which makes it attractive for short procedures like bronchoscopy for removal of foreign bodies, or when muscle relaxation during surgery is not desired. The rapid recovery from paralysis caused by this drug may mean that if the adductor pollicis is used to monitor relaxation, maximal relaxation of the respiratory muscles may already have occurred and tracheal intubation may be more challenging. Mivacurium also may be administered as an infusion when muscle relaxation is required for a significant portion of the operation and rapid reversal of paralysis is desirable (e.g., during spinal fusion where a wake-up test is needed). Since the drug is metabolized by pseudocholinesterase, patients with abnormal pseudocholinesterase may have quite prolonged recovery times. A new short-acting nondepolarizing muscle relaxant is now available called rapacuronium, which has a pharmacokinetic profile like succinylcholine, with both rapid onset and recovery.[131]* It also has similar responses at both the laryngeal muscles and the adductor pollicis. Intermediate-acting drugs such as atracurium, cis-atracurium, vecuronium, and rocuronium have onset times of 2 to 4 minutes and durations of action of 20 to 45 minutes. The muscle relaxation is reversible within 15 to 30 minutes after administering

---

* Rapacuronium has been withdrawn from the market due to the occurrence of severe bronchospasm.

an intubating dose of drug. Although atracurium can cause histamine release, hypotension, and flushing, when it is given slowly and in the correct dose this is usually not a problem. Its great advantage is that its elimination is independent of renal or hepatic metabolism. Therefore, it is useful for patients with renal or hepatic failure. *Cis*-atracurium is a stereoisomer of atracurium that has been available for a few years. It has the same clinical properties as atracurium without the histamine release and has replaced its sibling in most formularies. Vecuronium has no cardiovascular effects. Its elimination depends on hepatic clearance and secretion in bile. In infants, the duration of action of vecuronium is significantly longer than in children, and resembles that of pancuronium.[132] Rocuronium, a relative of vecuronium, has a rapid onset of action that approaches that of succinylcholine.[133] Its duration of action approximates that of vecuronium. There is usually a slight rise in heart rate with its administration, as well as some pain associated with injection.

Long-acting nondepolarizing muscle relaxants have a slower onset of action than intermediate duration drugs, about 3 to 5 minutes, and their duration of action is an hour or more. Older drugs in this category are *d*-tubocurare, metocurine, and pancuronium, all of which have some cardiovascular effects. Of these drugs, pancuronium is the most widely used. Two new drugs in this class, doxacurium and pipecuronium, do not have cardiovascular effects, but have durations of action at least as long as those of the previously existing drugs in this class.

Since infants are very dependent on heart rate to sustain cardiac output because of their relatively thicker walled, somewhat stiff ventricles, maintenance of a normal heart rate is important for maintaining organ perfusion. Therefore, pancuronium, which often causes tachycardia, is commonly used as a muscle relaxant for neonates. It tends to offset the bradycardia caused by high doses of volatile anesthetics and narcotics.

Antagonism of every case of muscle relaxation is controversial. When a long-acting muscle relaxant is used, its effects should be antagonized. When a single dose of an intermediate-acting muscle relaxant is used, there is some question whether reversal of its action is needed in every case. Whether reversal drugs are given or not, one must ensure that the patient has return of full strength before leaving the operating room. This can be done by noting a full train-of-four response and no apparent fade with 50-Hz tetanus. (However, neonates normally have a slight fade in the train-of-four without exposure to muscle relaxants.) An alternative to nerve stimulation is clinical assessment of the patient's muscle strength. Bilateral hip flexion against gravity has been reported to be equivalent to a 5-second head lift in an adult.[134]

Regional Anesthesia

It is rare to use only regional anesthesia for surgery in pediatric patients. Occasionally, the motivated older adolescent undergoing knee arthroscopy may wish to view the operation, but as a general rule, children don't want to be awake during their operation. On the other hand, regional anesthesia, as a supplement to general anesthesia, lowers the concentration of volatile agents required and helps to alleviate postoperative pain.

Physiologic Homeostasis

In addition to providing adequate anesthesia, the pediatric anesthesiologist must monitor and maintain the vital signs of the patient. The depressant effects of the anesthetic must be balanced against the noxious stimuli provided by the surgery. For each parameter monitored (e.g., heart rate, blood pressure, temperature) there are limits within which the anesthesiologist will be comfortable and outside of which action must be taken to bring the value back to the safe range.

Before surgery is begun, the anesthesiologist must ensure that the child is ready for surgery, since access to the child is limited once the patient is covered with drapes. The ETT must be securely taped in place and equal bilateral breath sounds ensured. Patients are often moved from the position in which their trachea was intubated. During the process, the endotracheal tube can become dislodged easily (i.e., either removed from the trachea or advanced into a mainstem bronchus). Monitoring devices (i.e., the electrocardiograph [ECG] leads, blood pressure cuff, and pulse oximeter probe) must be secured away from the surgical field. The IV catheter should be securely taped in place and should be infusing well before the child is covered with drapes. Many IVs in pediatric patients are positional and run intermittently. This problem also should be corrected before the child is covered with drapes. All pressure points should be padded. A functioning warming/cooling blanket should be in place. Either a precordial or esophageal stethoscope should be in place, and there should be a means of measuring temperature. Finally, all the lines, leads, and tubes should be supported so that nothing is being pulled and the lines are not under or on top of the patient. This is especially true of the circuit hoses, which can pull the endotracheal tube out of the trachea. The hoses should be fixed with tape to the bed or a "Christmas tree." After the child is draped, the anesthesiologist should recheck to ensure that nothing has changed. Constant monitoring of the child for accidental pressure by the surgeons or by equipment, and appropriate positioning of the extremities, should take place. Slight pressure on an extremity of a baby often causes the pulse oximeter to cease functioning. The anesthesiologist should have visual and physical access to the head of the patient and the ETT as soon as possible.

Ventilation and Oxygenation

Ventilation and oxygenation must be evaluated continuously during general anesthesia by observing a number of parameters that provide indirect or direct evidence of the adequacy. Respiratory rate and tidal volume in spontaneously breathing patients give an estimate of the minute ventilation and depth of anesthesia. Lightly anesthetized children tend to breathe more deeply. Respiratory rate and volume can be assessed by feeling the reservoir bag of the anesthesia machine, observing chest movement, listening to the precordial or esophageal stethoscope, and monitoring expired gases. Volatile anesthetics tend to increase respiratory rate and decrease tidal volume, leading to decreased minute volume, hypoventilation, and hypercarbia. Whereas the stimulus of surgery can increase the respiratory rate and tidal volume towards normal, anesthesia almost inevitably decreases respiratory drive and shifts the CO_2 response curve to the right. When spontaneous ventilation is required for infants and small children during anesthesia, PEEP should be provided to maintain FRC. Children lose a larger percentage (as much as 70 percent) of their FRC during general anesthesia.[58] The resultant atelectasis leads to ventilation–perfusion mismatching and hypoxia. During controlled ventilation the respiratory rate is set slightly below normal for the age of the patient and tidal volume is set to make the chest rise. The peak inspiratory pressure resulting from a 10 to 12 ml/kg tidal volume breath in a child who has normal lung and chest wall compliance should be less than 20 cm H_2O. Subsequent changes in ventilator settings are dictated by the values obtained by monitoring expired gases and blood gases.

Assessment of oxygenation is done best by continuous arterial pulse oximetery. Changes in oxygenation can be detected quickly, and the problem can be rapidly corrected (see Chapter 11). Because the monitor works only when there is a good pulse, the monitor also is an indirect monitor of the adequacy of distal perfusion. In certain circumstances, it may be the only monitor that consistently works (e.g., during magnetic resonance imaging [MRI] scanning). For neonates and sick children, it is always good to place a second oximeter probe as a backup device.

The second useful monitor is capnography or mass spectrometery, which measures expired gases. In the most recently published Standards for Basic Intra-operative Monitoring, monitoring CO_2 is now a standard of care; this includes quantitative monitoring of CO_2 during endotracheal intubation and LMA use.[4] The most recent ASA recommendation for this type of monitoring has been changed to "strongly encouraged." Respiratory gas monitors provide information about the inspired and expired concentrations of CO_2, O_2, nitrous oxide, anesthetic agents, and N_2 in some cases. Accurate $PETCO_2$ monitoring may be difficult in small infants, because of their small tidal volumes and the gas aspiration rate of the individual monitor. If there are any concerns about the validity of the information received from the monitors, the results should be corroborated by analyzing an arterial blood gas sample. The presence of fetal hemoglobin shifts the hemoglobin–oxygen dissociation curve of neonates to the left, making it necessary to think in terms of the fetal oxygen saturation curve when PaO_2 is derived from SaO_2 (e.g., P_{50} in adults is 27 mm Hg, but in neonates P_{50} is 19 mm Hg). Children with lung diseases and large amounts of wasted ventilation make it much more difficult to predict the arterial carbon dioxide from $PETCO_2$ measurements. Oximetry and end-tidal gas monitoring are useful guides to oxygenation and ventilation, but arterial blood gas measurements are still the standard to which these values must be compared.

Hemodynamics

The circulation must be assessed frequently by the anesthesiologist during anesthesia. Heart rate and blood pressure are semiquantitative guides to cardiovascular performance. Evaluation of the heart tones via a precordial or esophageal stethoscope and observation of the capillary refill time also provide useful information about the circulation. The cardiac output of infants is relatively dependent on heart rate, which makes continuous measurement of heart rates important. Because their sympathetic nervous system is not well developed at birth and because their parasympathetic nervous system is well developed, children show a distressing tendency to develop bradycardia during physiologic perturbations. Early recognition of bradycardia is obviously an advantage. Blood pressure is a relative index of adequate cardiac output in children, especially mean arterial pressure. Hypotension may reflect inadequate venous return, hypovolemia, or cardiac depression from an anesthetic overdose, and should never be ignored. Pulse oximetry is also a qualitative estimate of peripheral perfusion. Loss of the oximeter signal may be due to poor peripheral perfusion. Continuous manual palpation of an axillary or other peripheral pulse provides valuable information about the circulation. Loss of the pulse or a reduced pulse volume suggests circulatory changes are occurring. Invasive monitoring is usually reserved for cases in which it is suspected that major changes in the circulation will occur. Arterial and central venous pressure catheters give beat-to-beat information about the circulating volume and cardiovascular function. However, insertion of these catheters can be time consuming and can be associated with serious complications.

Temperature

Temperature regulation in the child is discussed in more detail in Chapter 4. Measurement of temperature during surgery is part of the Basic Anesthesia Monitoring Standards of the ASA when it is expected that significant changes in temperature may occur.[4] Even for short cases, infants may lose significant amounts of heat and develop hypothermia, metabolic acidosis, and pulmonary hypertension. Every effort should be made during both induction and maintenance of anesthesia to preserve core temperature in children. Prewarming the room, covering the patients with warm blankets, and using radiant heat warmers will help prevent hypothermia in infants. Humidifiers prevent heat loss by warming and humidifying inspired gases. When dry gas is inspired, water must be evaporated to humidify alveolar gas, and 540 calories of body heat per gram of water are used to humidify the gas.

Temperature can be measured in many places in a child, including the rectum, axilla, mouth, nasopharynx, and ear. Normal values in each location may be slightly different, but all will provide useful trends. The American Academy of Pediatrics recommends not measuring rectal temperatures in neonates to avoid perforating the rectum. The efforts made to preserve temperature occasionally raise body temperature above normal. It also is common for the body temperature to increase during genitourinary, bowel, and oral surgery, presumably because the circulation is seeded with bacterial pyrogens during manipulation of the tissues. Temperatures that exceed 38.5° to 39.0°C must suggest the possibility of malignant hyperthermia (see Chapter 4).

Fluids

A third major responsibility of the pediatric anesthesiologist is the administration of fluids and blood products during surgery. General aspects of fluid and electrolyte management are discussed more fully in Chapter 5.

Several factors must be considered when determining the amount of fluid replacement required during surgery (Table 10–3). The first factor is the child's fluid deficit upon entering the operating room. This deficit is derived from two sources. The first source is that the child has been NPO for a number of hours. This deficit is quickly calculated by the following:

<10 kg	(4 ml/kg) × number of hours NPO
10 to 20 kg	(40 ml + 2 ml/kg over 10 kg) × number of hours NPO
>20 kg	(60 ml + 1 ml/kg over 20 kg) × number of hours NPO

Most children do not awaken in the morning and immediately consume their entire fluid deficit. Therefore, their fluid deficit should be replaced in the operating room over several hours. Fluid deficit also can be the result of pathologic processes (e.g., vomiting, diarrhea) or of iatrogenic causes (e.g., bowel preparation). These deficits can often be estimated in terms of percent body weight lost (e.g., 5 percent, 10 percent) and replaced with isotonic crystalloid over several hours. One recommendation is to replace half the deficit over the first hour of the operation and one quarter of the deficit over each of the next 2 hours.

Maintenance fluid also must be provided during surgery. The volume of fluid required is calculated in the same manner as above. Again, maintenance fluid usually can be replaced with isotonic crystalloid.

Significant blood loss should be replaced during surgery. As long as there is adequate oxygen delivery to vital organs, small blood losses are usually replaced with isotonic crystalloid solutions. There has been much discussion recently about the minimum hematocrit required by patients during surgery. Because of fears about the safety of blood, most clinicians now accept lower hematocrits to avoid blood transfusions. In general, if the hematocrit

is or is likely to be less than 20 percent during or immediately after surgery, it is reasonable to transfuse the child. If not, transfusion can be delayed or avoided. Transfusion should be discussed with the family prior to surgery and with the surgeon before blood or blood products are administered. A recent task force has made recommendations about the use of blood products (see Chapter 6).[135]

Finally, translocated fluid (i.e., third-space losses) should be replaced intraoperatively. This is the fluid lost from extravascular and extracellular spaces due to evaporation or as the result of tissue trauma. It is difficult to estimate the amount of fluid lost, so fluid replacement is often guided by the response to therapy. General guidelines are that at least 8 to 10 ml/kg/h are necessary to replace third-space losses during major abdominal cases. For minor cases, such as hernia repairs, maintenance fluid plus 2 to 4 ml/kg/h is adequate. Intermediate cases require amounts of fluid between these two values. However, there are cases like neonatal gastroschisis repair for which truly extraordinary amounts of fluid are required, predominantly to replace third-space losses. Fluid replacement probably is guided best during surgery by arterial blood pressure, central venous pressure, heart rate, and base deficit.

Two issues must be considered when deciding what kind of fluid to give intraoperatively. The first is glucose. The risks of hypoglycemia are well known. Unfortunately, during anesthesia the ability to monitor the premonitory signs of hypoglycemia (e.g., dizziness, change in mentation) is lost. Studies by Welborn et al.[136] demonstrated that administering 5 percent glucose solutions as the sole source of fluid, even to children who have been NPO for many hours, commonly produces hyperglycemia. Hyperglycemia may be as injurious as hypoglycemia if there is a period of cerebral hypoperfusion. Hyperglycemia also produces an osmotic diuresis that can cause severe dehydration in some children. Welborn et al. recommended the use of 2.5 percent glucose solutions to avoid causing hyperglycemia during surgery.[137] If 2.5 percent glucose solutions are not available, there are several alternatives. One can administer 5 percent glucose or non–glucose-containing solutions and intermittently measure blood glucose intraoperatively. Another solution to this problem is to administer D_5 lactated Ringer's solution as maintenance fluid and a second solution without glucose for volume replacement. The latter option is particularly useful for premature infants, neonates, or any critically ill child. For children already receiving increased concentrations of glucose preoperatively (via total parenteral nutrition), it is important to continue to administer significant amounts of glucose during the operation at a rate that maintains the glucose concentration normal. *These solutions should not be used to replace blood loss and third-space losses.* Blood glucose concentrations should be measured frequently to ensure that the child does not develop hyper- or hypovolemia.

A second issue is when to administer non–blood-containing colloid solutions (e.g. albumin, hetastarch) during surgery. One clear indication is during preoperative intentional hemodilution (see Chapter 13). Other indications remain matters of individual judgment. In the short term, colloids increase intravascular volume more than crystal-

T A B L E   1 0 – 3
FLUID MANAGEMENT

Category	Volume	Type
Maintenance	4 ml/kg/h for 0–10 kg 2 ml/kg/h for 10–20 kg 1 ml/kg/h for >20 kg	Isotonic crystalloid + glucose (see text)
Deficit	No. hours × maintenance Replace ½ in 1st h, ¼/h × next 2 h	Isotonic crystalloid
Blood loss	3 ml of crystalloid/ml blood loss	Isotonic crystalloid (or blood products)
Third space	2–10 ml/kg/h, depending on extent of surgery and vital signs	Isotonic crystalloid

loid solutions. Theoretically, colloids remain in the interstitial space and are mobilized more slowly postoperatively. As long as euvolemia is maintained, oxygen delivery to tissues is the same with crystalloid or colloid. Most trauma literature shows that crystalloid is as effective as colloid for the initial fluid resuscitation if both solutions are given in adequate volumes. Crystalloids are cheaper and more readily available. There are no studies that have evaluated the use of hypertonic saline for resuscitation of children.

EMERGENCE AND RECOVERY FROM GENERAL ANESTHESIA

Emergence and recovery from anesthesia are the transition from anesthesia (i.e., unconscious, amnestic, analgesic, and weak) to the baseline state. Recovery has been described as occurring in three stages.[138] The first stage, or immediate recovery, takes minutes; includes the resumption of respiration, the return of airway reflexes, stabilization of hemodynamics, and a return of consciousness; and begins in the operating room. It usually ends in the postanesthesia care unit (PACU) or in the ICU. The second stage, or intermediate recovery, takes minutes to hours after surgery, involves the return of coordination and clearing of the sensorium, and usually occurs in the PACU. The third stage, or long-term recovery, may take hours to days, involves the return to baseline function (both motor and mental), and occurs on the ward or at home. As with most transitions, vigilance and attention to detail will prevent many of the potential problems that can occur at this time.

Routine Recovery

Recovery from general anesthesia depends to a great extent on the type of anesthetic delivered to the child. Some premedication may make the child quite sleepy during emergence from anesthesia, particularly if the surgery was short. For example, oral premedication with midazolam or diazepam-meperidine may have little effect, but oral pentobarbital-meperidine may cause children to be somnolent for some time after surgery. The type of general anesthetic also may affect the speed of emergence, the amount of emergence delirium, and patient comfort. Emergence from a pure inhalation anesthetic is more often associated with excitement and disorientation than is a nitrous oxide–narcotic-based anesthetic.[139] Other drugs or supplementation of general anesthesia with regional anesthesia also affects emergence from anesthesia. Administration of droperidol prevents postoperative nausea and vomiting, but droperidol also may cause somnolence in the PACU. Caudal blocks or peripheral nerve blocks with local anesthetics may dramatically decrease postoperative pain and delirium.

At the end of an operation, the anesthesiologist must decide whether to extubate the trachea in the operating room and whether to do so when the patient is awake or deeply anesthetized. Ultimately, the choices one makes about these issues are individual, and there is often no right or wrong answer.

The two common locations for tracheal extubation to occur after surgery are the operating room and the PACU.

In any given hospital, one or the other location is usually the routine. Wherever the trachea is extubated (i.e., operating room, PACU, or ICU), it must be done in a controlled environment with equipment and facilities available to reestablish control of the airway if there are complications. In my opinion, the preferred location is the operating room, because the means for reestablishing control of the airway (i.e., oxygen, suction, and airway equipment) are already present, along with ancillary personnel needed to rapidly reestablish a patent airway. There also is only one patient on whom attention must be focused. In the recovery room, several patients may demand intervention simultaneously. The primary argument for extubating the trachea in the PACU is to decrease time in the operating room and facilitate turnover of the operating room. As experience with children is gained, it should be possible to time the emergence of the pediatric patient from anesthesia to cause minimal delay in operating room turnover. In addition, transport of an intubated patient is associated with more problems (e.g., accidental tracheal extubation) than transport of a patient with a stable, extubated airway.

Extubating the trachea, both while deeply anesthetized and when awake, have their proponents. One study demonstrated that extubating the trachea of patients while they were still deeply anesthetized is associated with fewer complications.[140] However, extubating the trachea during light levels of anesthesia is associated with increased complications, especially laryngospasm. Removing the endotracheal tube while the patient is still deeply anesthetized leaves the child's airway unprotected during emergence from general anesthesia. In practice, aspiration of gastric contents occurs infrequently.[140] There is, however, the possibility of laryngospasm occurring during transport to the PACU. If this happens, little equipment will be immediately available to the anesthesiologist. For these reasons, I prefer to extubate the trachea when the patient is awake in the operating room when he or she has intact reflexes.

Criteria for extubation of the trachea include adequate return of strength, regular respirations, and an empty stomach. If the child received nondepolarizing neuromuscular relaxing agents, their effects should have fully dissipated or be antagonized before the trachea is extubated. If the train-of-four has completely returned to normal and there is no fade to a 50-Hz 5-second tetanus, the patient probably has adequate strength to resume normal ventilation. However, if the patient has received a long-acting nondepolarizing relaxant, it is probably prudent to antagonize the effects of the muscle relaxant, regardless of the time that has elapsed since the last dose of muscle relaxant was given. Neonates demonstrate fade to tetanic stimulation even when they have not received muscle relaxants, so assessment of strength in this case must be clinical (see above). With very rare exceptions, return of regular respirations should be present before the trachea is extubated. This implies that either the patient is still deeply anesthetized or is in stage I and not in stage II, because coughing and breath holding are more common during these two stages of anesthesia. Rarely, it is beneficial to extubate the trachea of a patient who is still paralyzed and then antagonize the effects of muscle relaxants to avoid having the ETT cause coughing. Surgery on the larynx may be one reason for this unusual approach. Emptying the stomach probably should be routine for all cases, either shortly after tracheal intubation or before tracheal extubation (preferably at both times), but removing all of the fluid possible through a orogastric tube does *not* guarantee that the stomach will be empty. Although complete emptying of the stomach is unlikely, decreasing the gastric volume reduces the risk of a serious aspiration and may reduce postoperative nausea.

There also is a choice in the drugs appropriate for antagonism of muscle relaxation. Several children's hospitals routinely use the combination of neostigmine 0.04 to 0.07 mg/kg and atropine 0.02 mg/kg. Glycopyrrolate can also be used as an anticholinergic agent in doses of 0.01 mg/kg. Edrophonium has the advantage of a more rapid onset of action and the cardiovascular effects of the anticholinesterase can be prevented by a smaller dose of atropine (0.01 mg/kg) given 30 seconds before the edrophonium is administered.[141]

The major difference beween awake and deep tracheal extubation, therefore, is that in the former, one waits until the patient displays some purposeful movement. The assumption is that a purposefully responding patient can protect his or her airway, which is not necessarily the case. Eye opening has sometimes been related to the ability to protect the airway. Even though a patient appears to be conscious and is responding to their surroundings, that patient is most likely still in stage I anesthesia and is still amnestic and sedated. Once the criteria for tracheal extubation are satisfied, the patient's mouth is suctioned free of secretions that might fall onto the vocal cords and cause larygospasm, and the ETT is removed. It is helpful to give a large positive-pressure breath during tracheal extubation to cause the patient to cough as the ETT is removed. This helps clear the airway of secretions and reduce the likelihood of aspirating any secretions that have accumulated around the ETT; it may also help reexpand the FRC. Lung expansion also provide a little extra oxygen reserve in the event of subsequent airway obstruction. During the next few seconds, the airway must be evaluated because many children are apneic for a few seconds after removal of the ETT. If, after tracheal extubation, the chest and abdomen move in concert and breath sounds are heard over the sternal notch or lung fields, the airway is open and the child is ready for transfer to the PACU. If, despite efforts by the patient to ventilate their lungs, no breath sounds are heard and there are paradoxical chest movements, it must be assumed that the patient has laryngospasm. The first maneuver is to apply the face mask tightly to the face, apply continuous positive pressure, and lift the mandible and tongue by pulling on the angles of the jaw. It often takes airway pressures of 20 cm H_2O to break the spasm. The potential for laryngospasm is the reason why patients should breath 100 percent oxygen immediately before tracheal extubation. In the majority of circumstances, positive airway pressure and jaw pressure resolve the problem quickly and breath sounds are heard. Positive pressure should be applied for a few minutes more, however, as long as the circulation is stable, because the patient is still in stage II anesthesia and needs to lower the brain concentration of anesthetic agent farther. If continued positive pressure does not break the laryngospasm or if the oxygen saturation decreases to unacceptable levels,

a small dose of muscle relaxant should be given IV. This does not need to be a full intubating dose of muscle relaxant; a partial dose is usually enough to resolve the laryngospasm. A patient who has been breathing adequately for several minutes and is hemodynamically stable is ready to move to the PACU.

Transport to the PACU

During transport to the PACU, the trachea must either be extubated and the airway must be adequate, or an ETT must be firmly taped in place. The patient also must be hemodynamically stable. If there is any question about either of these factors, the patient should remain in the operating room for close observation. Intravenous and invasive monitoring lines should be untangled. A full portable oxygen tank and a circuit capable of providing positive-pressure ventilation should be available to administer oxygen during transport. Because of the loss of FRC that occurs during anesthesia, the tendency toward atelectasis, and a high oxygen consumption, the oxygen saturation of children decreases very quickly, even when the airway is patent. Consequently, supplemental oxygen should be provided during transport. It is probably best to transport children lying on their side, because their tongues are less likely to occlude the airway and because emesis and secretions will tend to fall away from the larynx.

If the patient is awake with stable respiratory and circulatory systems, it usually is unnecessary to use any monitors for transport to the PACU, other than a precordial stethoscope and careful observation. If the respiratory system is less stable than described above, pulse oximetry is advisable. If the patient's hemodynamics are potentially unstable, a blood pressure and ECG monitor should be used. All of these monitors should be present for critically ill children being transported to the ICU. In addition, if the trachea is intubated, equipment for reestablishing the airway and emergency drugs also should go with the patient.

In addition to the anesthesiologist, two other people should also go to the PACU or ICU: a nurse from the operating room and a member of the surgical team. If a problem occurs, two of these people can attend to the patient's needs and the third can go for help.

The decision to transport the patient to an ICU is usually made before the end of the case. Recovery from certain operations traditionally takes place in the ICU, including cardiothoracic, craniofacial, neurosurgical, organ transplant, and airway surgery. In general, if the patient needs intensive observation postoperatively for more than a few hours, or if there is the potential for instability of the cardiorespiratory system, it is probably best to transport the patient directly to a pediatric ICU from the operating room.

The Postanesthesia Care Unit

Ideally, the PACU should be located near the operating room complex. It has been recommended that the PACU have two to three bed spaces for each operating room.[142, 143] The number depends on the duration of cases and average recovery times. PACU nurses should have no more than three patients at the most, preferably two patients at a time. Critically ill patients may require the care of two nurses for short periods of time, as in the ICU.

Each recovery space should have immediate access to monitoring and resuscitation equipment. Every spot should have oxygen and a means of delivering positive-pressure ventilation and/or PEEP (e.g., a Jackson-Rees circuit with a suitable mask). Every recovering pediatric patient should receive oxygen during transport and until awake. Oxygen delivery can be delivered by nasal prongs (usually not well tolerated), a mask, or some apparatus for blow-by oxygen. Effective suction must be available. A pulse oximeter should be used for each patient to give an early indication of airway problems. There should be a means of measuring arterial blood pressure. ECG monitoring is optional because myocardial ischemia is very rare in children and even the incidence of arrhythmias is low. An ECG monitor should be available, however, in the event one is needed. A respiratory monitor should be available for the child who is at risk for airway obstruction or apnea (e.g., the ex-premature infant following general anesthesia). Finally, a monitor that can measure and display continuous arterial, central venous, and ICP pressures should be available for children with more complex problems. Although patients who require such measurements often go the ICU postoperatively, it is occasionally necessary for them to stay in the PACU until a bed is available for them in the ICU.

Emergency equipment (including face masks, airways [oral and nasal], laryngoscopes and blades of different sizes, a selection of endotracheal tubes, stylets, a device to deliver positive pressure, and equipment to perform emergent cricothyroidotomy) must be immediately available in the PACU for cardiopulmonary resuscitation. For cardiac resuscitation, there should be a defibrillator, appropriate drugs, equipment for venous or arterial cannulation, a thoracostomy tray, and sterile gloves, gowns, and towels. It is most efficient to have this equipment on a cart that can be rolled to any bedside within a few seconds.

Children with contagious infections (e.g., chickenpox) often require surgery. Spreading their infection to other patients in the PACU is potentially devastating. Each recovery area should have a separate room in which infected patients can be physically isolated from other patients. Preferably, this room should be at negative pressure with a good exhaust system. Nurses caring for the child should have known immunity to the disease. Immunocompromised children should be recovered in reverse isolation when possible.

Traditionally, parents have not been allowed into recovery rooms, but this situation is changing. In many PACUs, parents are not only allowed, they are encouraged to be with their children once report has been given by the anesthesiologist and the patient's condition is stable. An alternative, especially for day surgery patients, is to have a second-stage recovery room where the patient completes awakening, begins to ambulate, and takes oral fluids. Having a parent present during awakening from anesthesia often prevents much of the excitement that occurs in children with emergence from anesthesia (see below). For children with special needs (e.g., deafness, mental retardation), parents know the child's needs better than the PACU staff and can assist with care of the child in the PACU.

Patients in the PACU are still the responsibility of the anesthesia department and should not be discharged from the PACU without the consent of an anesthesiologist, either the anesthesiologist who anesthetized the child or someone assigned to the PACU. An alternative for busy PACUs is to have a set of criteria developed by the anesthesia department that can guide the nursing staff. The patient's surgeon obviously cooperates in the child's care.

As soon as the patient arrives in the PACU, assessment of his or her airway and oxygen saturation, and provision of supplemental oxygen should occur. The anesthesiologist can help by straightening out the IV and monitoring lines. The nurse who will care for the patient should determine vital signs before the anesthesiologist provides his or her report. This report usually includes age, weight, preoperative hematocrit, preoperative vital signs, allergies, the operation, anesthetic agents and adjunct drugs, lines, drains, intraoperative events, and a thumbnail sketch of pertinent medical/surgical history. The nurse in the recovery room now assumes minute-to-minute care for this child until the child is ready to go home or to be transferred to the ward. However, an anesthesiologist is still responsible for the child's overall care. For the remainder of the recovery time, vital signs are determined at least every 15 minutes, fluids are delivered as ordered, medications (including pain medications) are given, and any laboratory examinations requested are obtained.

In addition to measuring vital signs, the nurse assesses the child for return of normal function. There are several scoring systems that attempt to quantify recovery from anesthesia. The system devised by Aldrete and Kroulik assesses five functions: respiration, circulation, activity, consciousness, and color.[144] Each function is scored from 0 to 2 points, with a maximum of 10 points (Table 10–4). At a predetermined number of points, usually 9 or 10, the patient can be discharged from the PACU. Because the Aldrete scale is oriented toward adults, Steward developed a more suitable scale for children.[145] This scale again scores airway, consciousness, and movement from 0 to 2 points (Table 10–5). The maximum number of points is 6. As a general rule, day surgery patients should have equal or higher scores for discharge from the PACU than patients who will spend the night of surgery in the hospital.

Discharge from the PACU depends on the patient's overall functional status. From a physiologic standpoint, there is no minimal length of time required for recovery from anesthesia. Patients undergoing very short minor procedures with a volatile anesthetic may be ready for discharge from the PACU 10 to 15 minutes after arrival, whereas those undergoing long operations and receiving parenteral drugs may require hours to recover from anesthesia. Each institution may have its own guidelines for the appropriate minimal duration of stay in the PACU for certain operations and procedures. For example, if the trachea has been intubated, if opioids were given intra- or postoperatively, or in the case of certain operations (tonsillectomy or cleft palate repair, in which postoperative bleeding may compromise the airway for several hours) the patient may have to remain in the PACU a certain length

TABLE 10 – 4
ALDRETE RECOVERY SCORE

Criterion	Score
Activity	
Moves 4 extremities voluntarily or on command	2
Moves 2 extremities voluntarily or on command, or moves weakly	1
Does not move any extremities voluntarily or on command	0
Respiration	
Able to deep breathe, cough, and/or cry	2
Dyspneic or limited in breathing	1
Apneic	0
Circulation	
BP ± 20% of preanesthetic value	2
BP ± 20–50% of preanesthetic value	1
BP ± 50% of preanesthetic value	0
Consciousness	
Fully awake	2
Arousable to stimuli	1
Unresponsive	0
Color	
Pink	2
Pale, dusky, blotchy, other	1
Cyanotic	0

Modified from Aldrete JA, Kroulik D: A postanesthetic recovery score. Anesth Analg 49:924, 1970, with permission.

of time. Where the patient is going after leaving the PACU determines how much recovery is needed before discharge. If the child's condition becomes unstable or progressively deteriorates, the patient should be transferred to the ICU as soon as their condition stabilizes. If the patient will be cared for postoperatively on the ward, the general criteria for discharge are stable vital signs, a clear airway with intact airway reflexes, awake or easily arousable, and an acceptable level of activity. The child's oxygen saturation must be evaluated carefully, since Soliman et al.[146] showed that recovery room scores correlated poorly with oxygen saturation. The proportion of children with oxygen saturations below 95 percent was the same for children with low and high recovery room scores. A child who has achieved an appropriate score for transfer to the ward who still has an oxygen saturation below 95 percent should continue to receive oxygen on the ward, and the oxygen saturation should be checked on a regular basis until the oxygen saturation is acceptable while breathing room air.

Children going home from the PACU must recover more fully than children remaining in the hospital. The vital sign of the former group should be stable and near normal for that child; they should have normal gag, cough, and swallow reflexes; they should have normal coordination, minimal nausea and vomiting; and they should be alert, oriented, and comfortable. Voiding is not necessary prior to discharge from the PACU unless the urinary tract has been instrumented.[147] There is no difference in outcome if children do not drink before discharge from the PACU as long as they receive adequate IV fluid to replace their fluid deficit and enough fluid is provided for maintenance requirements and fluid losses during the operation.[148] Before discharge home, the parents and child, if old enough,

should be told what to expect. They must understand that the child will be sleepy or groggy and may have some problems with coordination and that there may be some nausea or vomiting and a sore throat or hoarse voice for a few hours. Oral intake should be reestablished slowly. Finally, there may be some pain related to the operation, and children should be allowed to regulate their activity accordingly. The family should be sent home with a phone number to call if they have any problems or questions. Finally, a follow-up call should be made to the family the next day to ascertain whether there are any ongoing problems.

Occasionally, a day surgery patient must be admitted to the hospital for vomiting, bleeding, pain, or postextubation croup.[142, 149, 150] If any of these events occur during the child's stay in the PACU, the surgical service must be notified and admission to the hospital arranged.

Complications

Most children do very well postoperatively and recover quickly from anesthesia and surgery and return to full function faster than adults. Since recovery from anesthesia is a time of transition, a number of potential complications may occur and require immediate attention in the PACU.

Emergence Delirium

Occasionally, a child will emerge from general anesthesia restless, disoriented, crying, combative, and communicate poorly. Such children can pose a danger to themselves or others. Emergence delirium occurs most often following premedication with scopolamine and barbiturates or with the use of pure inhalational anesthetics, or ketamine.[139] In one study, 13 percent of children between 3 and 9 years of age were disoriented during recovery from anesthesia. When disorientation occurs it can be very disconcerting to the recovery room staff, other recovering patients, and to the child's parents. Fortunately, disorientation resolves relatively quickly. Until it does, the child should be gently restrained as necessary, comforted, and reassured. Because disorientation can resemble the effects of hypoxia,

TABLE 10 – 5
STEWARD RECOVERY SCORE

Criterion	Score
Consciousness	
Awake	2
Responding to stimuli	1
Not responding	0
Airway	
Coughing on command or crying	2
Maintaining good airway	1
Airway requires maintenance	0
Movement	
Moving limbs purposefully	2
Nonpurposeful movements	1
Not moving	0

From Steward DJ: A simplified scoring for the post-operative recovery room. Can Anaesth Soc J 22:111, 1975, with permission.

pain, or hypoglycemia, these more serious conditions must be ruled out before it is assumed that the child's behavior is due to emergence delirium.

Pain

There are a number of myths about children and pain that have caused children to be chronically undermedicated for pain.[151, 152] In the past, it was felt that children, especially infants, did not feel or remember pain, because their nervous systems were immature. Consequently, anesthetic techniques developed that included virtually no analgesia. Narcotics were not used out of fear that they would depress respiration. Some people felt that pain was beneficial for children. Fortunately, we now have better information. Children, even premature infants, do respond to painful stimuli.[153] Tachycardia and hypertension are early signs that the patient is having pain. Serum catecholamine, glucocorticoid, glucagon, and growth hormone concentrations increase after painful stimuli. Children do remember pain. When given in appropriate doses, narcotics reduce or eliminate pain, while causing little respiratory depression. It has been suggested that patient outcome is worse if pain is inadequately treated.[125]

The most challenging part of treating pain in children is determining if the patient is indeed having pain. Children often cannot or do not complain. However, they may exhibit other behaviors that may not be identified by the staff as representing pain. It is the responsibility of the PACU staff to communicate with the child or, if that is not possible, to assess whether or not the child has pain. This task is complicated by the fact that the recovering child is still under the influence of the anesthetic and has a depressed sensorium.

Scales have been developed to assess pain in children.[154] The visual analogue scale (VAS) is used in both adults and older children, but its use requires fairly sophisticated abstract thinking. The results of using this scale is improved by using scales with faces that range from sad to happy. The children identify the face that represents the way they feel. Other scales use numbers, thermometers, or colors. Effective use of these scales presumes that the patient has intact cognitive function. This is unlikely to be the case for children in the PACU. Consequently, the staff must interpret the child's behavioral and physiologic signs of pain as a basis for treatment.

Pain increases sympathetic nervous system discharge and causes tachycardia, hypertension, and diaphoresis. If the operation involved the thorax or the abdomen, the breathing pattern may be altered and the child may splint during a deep breath or may adopt a shallow, rapid pattern of breathing.

Behaviors consistent with pain are crying, restlessness, groaning, or grimacing. Crying, however, can indicate hunger or desire for the parents rather than the presence of pain. The other behavior patterns may be seen with emergence from anesthesia or with hypoxia, but it must be considered that the child is acting unusually because he or she is experiencing pain.

Adequate treatment for pain should return the child's behavior and vital signs toward baseline. If pain was the cause of hypertension, administration of an analgesic should decrease the heart rate and blood pressure toward normal.

The anesthesiologist should always include a plan for postoperative analgesia as part of the anesthetic plan of children. This often includes starting postoperative pain therapy in the operating room by administering IV opioids or regional anesthesia. Day surgery patients require postoperative pain relief that allows the patient to be comfortable until oral medications are tolerated and does not delay discharge from the recovery room.

Acetaminophen 10 to 15 mg/kg orally and 25 to 40 mg/kg rectally may be the only analgesic needed following uncomplicated surgery. Acetaminophen is widely available and has few side effects. Codeine 0.5 to 1.0 mg/kg or codeine with acetaminophen can be given orally for more significant postoperative pain. However, codeine may upset the stomach of some patients and cause constipation. Parenteral use of codeine is not recommended because it can cause histamine release. The use of oral medications is often limited because they cause nausea and vomiting. Oral methadone, a long-acting opioid, 0.1 mg/kg is well absorbed through the gastrointestinal system and often gives 6 to 9 hours of postoperative pain relief. It also can cause preoperative sedation and make the induction of anesthesia easier.

Parenteral analgesics, primarily opioids, are used widely to relieve the postoperative pain of children. In most instances, intravenous administration of opioids is the preferred route because administering these or any other drug IM is painful. Morphine 0.05 to 0.1 mg/kg and fentanyl 1 to 2 μg/kg are common choices for pain relief in the PACU. Fentanyl has a rapid onset of action and can be used for outpatients prior to discharge home, although discharge may be delayed. Morphine has a slower onset of action, 5 to 10 minutes, but a longer duration of action due to its limited lipid solubility. This may make it less suitable for day surgery patients. However, it is quite suitable for intraoperative administration to smooth the transition to the awake state without the patient experiencing severe pain. Many clinicians are concerned that administering narcotics will cause respiratory depression in infants and children. However, it is uncommon for this to occur if the patient has pain and is given small, repeated doses of opioids. Hertzka et al.[120] demonstrated that, if anything, infants and children were less sensitive to alterations in breathing patterns than adults following IV opioid administration. Nonsteroidal anti-inflammatory drugs (NSAIDs) have not been used widely in pediatric anesthesia, but ketorolac, which can be administered IM or IV, has proven effective in children for postoperative pain relief without causing significant side effects.[155, 156]

Regional analgesia can be used very effectively to provide postoperative pain relief for children (see Chapter 25). For outpatient surgery, caudal blocks and peripheral nerve blocks are used intraoperatively to reduce the requirement for general anesthesia, and if a long-acting local anesthetic such as bupivacaine is injected, the block can provide analgesia well into the postoperative period. The duration of postoperative pain relief is unaffected by whether the block is placed at the beginning or the end of the surgery.[157] For patients staying in the hospital postoperatively, caudal blocks with opioids, such as morphine, prolong analgesia. For major surgery, epidural catheters can be placed intraoperatively, to provide intraoperative anesthesia and postoperative analgesia. Epidural opioids can cause urinary retention, nausea, and pruritus, and these complications require treatment. Therefore, someone must be available to follow and manage the postoperative course of patients given intrathecal or epidural opioids. A pain service effectively provides this service (see Chapter 25).

Nausea and Vomiting

Nausea and vomiting occur in 11 to 34 percent of children who receive general anesthesia.[158] These complications are more common after longer anesthetics, opioid administration, and certain operations. Steward found that the incidence of vomiting increased from 10 percent to 23 percent when surgery lasted less than 10 minutes or more than 20 minutes.[159] Abramowitz et al.[160] found that 85 percent of children vomited after strabismus repair and that 75 μg/kg of droperidol decreased the incidence of vomiting to 43 percent. Lerman et al.[161] found that droperidol administration decreased the incidence of vomiting after strabismus to 10 percent. Lower doses of the drug have not been shown to be as effective. Extrapyramidal symptoms have not been reported, despite the use of large doses of droperidol. Somnolence is a side effect of droperidol, but it does not delay discharge from the recovery room as much as prolonged vomiting. Droperidol 75 μg/kg was compared with metoclopromide: 0.25 mg/kg of metoclopromide was equally effective as an antiemetic.[162] However, 0.15 mg/kg of metoclopromide was less effective than droperidol. Ondansetron was the first of the serotonin antagonists used for postoperative nausea and vomiting.[163] Its use has not been universally adopted because of its cost, though studies have demonstrated that it is more effective than either droperidol or metoclopromide. In a number of institutions, ondansetron is used only for treatment of nausea and vomiting rather than for prophylaxis. A new serotonin antagonist has been released, dolasetron, which is less expensive and may find wider use.

Vomiting also may be secondary to inadequate pain relief after a hernia repair or orchidopexy and will be ameliorated by analgesics.

Respiratory Complications

Extrathoracic Obstruction

Extrathoracic airway obstruction is among the more serious problems that occur in the PACU. The characteristics of this complication include inspiratory stridor, intercostal retractions, paradoxical chest movement, and oxygen desaturation. In patients who are still somnolent, the tongue is the most likely cause of the obstruction, and a chin lift or jaw thrust usually restores the airway. Alternatively, the child can be turned on the side to allow the tongue to fall away from the pharynx. If the airway remains obstructed, mask CPAP is often helpful. If it is not, placing an oral or nasal airway may relieve the obstruction. However, an oral airway that is too small may push the tongue backwards and further compromise ventilation. An oral airway that is too large can cause gagging and vomiting, or it may depress the epiglottis and obstruct the pharynx. A nasal airway usually is better tolerated, but, in children, this may traumatize the adenoids and cause bleeding—sometimes, a lot of bleeding! Children with Pierre Robin, Treacher Collins, and Goldenhar's syndromes have small mandibles and often have postoperative airway obstruction. It is usually best to ensure that these patients are fully awake before removing the ETT.

Children who have undergone tonsillectomy and adenoidectomy and have a history of snoring consistent with partial airway obstruction and children who have undergone cleft palate repair often have continued airway obstruction postoperatively. Swelling and bleeding from the airway may compromise airway patency. In most instances, these patients also should be completely awake when their trachea is extubated.

Secretions in the pharynx may result in gurgling sounds and cause what appears to be upper airway obstruction. Listening with a stethoscope over the trachea usually differentiates secretions from anatomic obstruction. Removal of the secretions usually solves the problem.

Laryngospasm, tight adduction of the vocal cords, presents as a complete airway obstruction and is more common in children than in adults. It most commonly occurs in patients who are in a lightly anesthetized, excited state. It rarely occurs in the PACU in patients who were extubated awake in the operating room. However, it occasionally occurs in patients whose trachea was extubated without adequate suctioning of the airway while the patient was deeply anesthetized. During emergence from anesthesia, secretions fall onto the vocal cords and cause laryngospasm. With laryngospasm, breath sounds are either nonexistent or very high pitched and squeaky. As described earlier, a face mask should be applied tightly to the face, positive pressure with 100 percent oxygen should be provided, and the jaw should be firmly pulled forward. If this does not break the laryngospasm, or the oxygen saturation decreases to unacceptable levels, a small dose of succinylcholine (25 to 50 percent of an intubating dose) should relieve the spasm quickly and provide a patent airway. Operations like tonsillectomy/adenoidectomy or cleft palate repair also are associated with an increased incidence of laryngospasm because they are associated with blood in the airway during emergence from anesthesia. Thorough suctioning of the airway at the end of surgery and attention to the airway in the PACU should prevent most episodes of laryngospasm.

Postextubation croup occurs in about 1 percent of children following tracheal intubation during general anesthesia. The classic study by Koka et al.[164] showed that croup occurs most commonly in patients between 1 and 4 years of age who have had traumatic tracheal intubation, repeated attempts at tracheal intubation, a tight ETT (leak above 30 cm H_2O), a change in body position while the trachea is intubated, or tracheal intubation lasting longer than 1 hour. The presence of an upper respiratory infection did not correlate with postoperative croup. Stridor usually appears within an hour of tracheal extubation and the severity of the stridor peaks at 4 hours; occasionally, both stridor and croup appear much later. Treatment of postextubation croup is to administer 100 percent oxygen and mist. If the croup does not improve, racemic epinephrine 0.5 ml in 2.5 to 3 ml saline is delivered over 10 to 15 minutes by face mask. If a day surgery patient requires racemic epinephrine, the patient should be observed for several hours after the treatment because the croup may be worse (rebound phenomenon) after the effect of the drug subsides. He or she may have to be admitted to hospital for observation.

Bronchospasm

Children with a history of reactive airway disease may develop bronchospasm in the PACU as they emerge from anesthesia. Because the volatile anesthetic agents are relatively good bronchodilators, wheezing in the operating room is relatively uncommon. However, as the child emerges from anesthesia, the salutary effect of the anesthetic is lost and bronchospasm may develop. Bronchospasm can be differentiated from extrathoracic obstruction because the wheezing associated with the former occurs primarily during expiration. Furthermore, there is often a history of bronchospasm and previous treatment with bronchodilators. In the PACU, bronchospasm is treated with a bronchodilator (e.g., albuterol) nebulized with 100 percent oxygen. Albuterol is a relatively specific β_2-agent that quite effectively treats brochospasm. The usual dose is 0.25 ml of albuterol in 2.5 ml of saline delivered via face mask over 10 minutes. If wheezing is not relieved, another treatment can be administered in 30 minutes. If the bronchospasm is still not relieved, blood gases should be analyzed and consideration should be given to initiating IV aminophylline, epinephrine, and steroids. Plans should be made to transfer the patient to a monitored care unit and pediatric consultation should be sought.

Hypoventilation

Occasionally, patients arrive in the PACU with patent airways and hypoventilation. There are a number of possible reasons for this failure of respiratory drive, and the therapy for each is different.

Patients who have inadequate antagonism of neuromuscular blocking drugs hypoventilate because of muscle weakness. Whereas the degree of muscle relaxation can be determined with a peripheral nerve stimulator, inadequate antagonism of muscle paralysis often can be diagnosed simply by observing the child's breathing pattern, noting his or her inability to move his extremities as expected, and his or her or his failure to maintain bilateral hip flexion or head lift for 5 seconds. If weakness persists, more antagonism of muscle paralysis may be required in the PACU prior to tracheal extubation, or ventilation can be controlled until muscle strength has returned.

Excessive amounts of opioids will depress respiration (i.e., near-normal tidal volumes and decreased respiratory rates). Small doses of naloxone 0.5 to 1 μg/kg should significantly increase ventilation if the lack of breathing is due to opioids. If the dose of naloxone is titrated carefully to the point where breathing is normal, there is little danger of suddenly reversing the analgesic effects of the narcotics.

Pain itself can cause patients to hypoventilate, particularly after abdominal or thoracic surgery. Thoracic and abdominal incisions can be very painful and cause the patient to splint and hypoventilate. Giving insufficient analgesics to relieve pain usually allows the child to breathe more easily. Studies in adults have shown that the pulmonary mechanics are abnormal for several weeks after abdominal or thoracic operations, even when pain is controlled.

Preterm infants often demonstrate an extreme form of postoperative hypoventilation. They develop apnea. Children born at less than 37 weeks' gestation are at risk for apnea and periodic breathing following a general anesthetic.[165] The risk of developing apnea is inversely proportional to the postconceptual age at the time of surgery, and seems to be present until the child is between 50 and 60 weeks postconceptual age.[166] If apnea does not occur in the first 12 hours after surgery, it is unlikely to do so. However, if apnea does occur during this time, it may continue for several days. This has led to the recommendation that all infants who are less than 50 to 60 weeks postconceptual age remain in the hospital overnight and be monitored for apnea after general anesthesia. An alternative to general anesthesia is spinal anesthesia (see Chapter 12). Welborn et al.[167] found no apnea occurring after spinal anesthesia, whereas 30 percent of the patients who received general anesthesia developed apnea. Attempts to determine the appropriate minimal age for outpatient surgery for ex-premature infants generated a meta-analysis of all data collected to date,[168] but the results of that analysis have been questioned.[169]

The apnea of premature infants is both central and obstructive in nature.[170] Furthermore, the response of preterm infants to hypoxia and hypercarbia is different from that of older children. Hypercarbia causes a smaller increase in ventilation in neonates and infants than occurs in older children.[171] Hypoxia causes a biphasic response.[172] Initially, hypoxia causes a slight increase in ventilation, which is quickly followed by hypoventilation. If the infant is hypothermic, hypoxia only reduces ventilation. Hypothermia is a well-known inducer of apnea in premature infants. Anemia also increases the incidence of apnea in former premature infants.[173]

The incidence of apnea occurring in term neonates following general anesthesia is unknown, although it certainly exists.[174] The general feeling among many pediatric anesthesiologists is that if general anesthesia can be avoided until after the child is 1 month old, it is best to do so. If surgery is required in the first month, the child should be kept overnight.

Alternatively, the child can be watched in the PACU for several hours (e.g., 4 to 6 hours). If there is no evidence of apnea or periodic breathing, the child can be sent home. There are insufficient data at this time to support either decision. Consequently, most surgeons and anesthesiologists have patients who are less than 50 weeks' gestation remain in hospital for at least 12 hours postoperatively.

Pulmonary Edema

Pulmonary edema is uncommon during pediatric anesthesia. When it occurs, it is due to excess extravascular water in the lungs that fills alveoli, reduces lung compliance, and produces hypoxia. Pulmonary edema can occur because of a relative increase in total body fluid in a child with poor cardiac reserve. Usually, these children are recognized preoperatively and attempts are made in the operating room to avoid giving excessive fluid. Pulmonary edema also can be caused by absolute fluid overload in a normal child. Treatment of pulmonary edema includes providing supplemental oxygen and positive-pressure ventilation if necessary. Pulmonary edema from fluid overload usually resolves quickly if the cardiovascular system is normal.

Pulmonary edema also may occur after relief of an upper airway obstruction (e.g., laryngospasm).[175] Pulmonary edema from this cause is thought to be due to the extreme negative intrathoracic pressure developed during attempts to breathe while the airway is obstructed. Therapy is the same as that for edema caused by fluid overload.

Atelectasis

Though their FRC is similar to that of adults while awake, children may lose more than half of their FRC during general anesthesia.[58] These atelectatic areas may not reexpand fully during the next breath. Atelectasis may occur in mechanically ventilated children during surgery, but is much more likely to occur in children who breathe spontaneously. Measures to prevent atelectasis include PEEP and several sustained vital capacity breaths delivered just before tracheal extubation. In the PACU, atelectasis is manifested as a need for supplemental oxygen, tachypnea, and intercostal retractions. Physiotherapy or vigorous crying often reexpands atelectatic portions of the lungs.

Aspiration

It is not common for children to vomit during emergence from general anesthesia. However, when vomiting occurs in a somnolent child, aspiration of gastric contents may occur. A number of routine precautions can reduce the incidence of aspiration in anesthetized patients. Adherence to a strict NPO policy, suctioning the stomach after induction of anesthesia and before extubation of the trachea, and extubating the trachea of patients awake can reduce the risk of serious aspiration. Transporting patients on their side helps prevent vomited gastric contents from entering the pharynx. A child suspected of aspirating gastric material must be watched carefully. If after 2 hours there are no symptoms of clinically apparent aspiration, significant respiratory sequelae are unlikely to develop.[176] In extreme cases of aspiration, it may be necessary to intubate the trachea and mechanically ventilate the lungs.

Cardiovascular Complications

Due to the absence of coronary artery disease, children seldom have cardiac complications in the PACU, unless they have congenital heart disease.

Hypotension

Hypotension is uncommon in the PACU if fluid management was appropriate during surgery. Although hypoten-sion may be caused by decreased venous return, decreased myocardial contractility, decreased afterload, or bradycardia, the most common cause of hypotension in children in the PACU is decreased venous return, or hypovolemia that is caused by underestimating the volume of blood lost, or inadequate replacement of the fluid deficit during surgery. The resulting hypovolemia leads to inadequate circulating blood volume and hypotension. The diagnosis of hypovolemia is made clinically by the presence of tachycardia, decreased pulses, delayed capillary refill (more than 3 seconds) in the extremities, and low urine output (<1 ml/kg/h). Hypovolemia is treated with isotonic crystalloid, albumin, or hetastarch, if the hematocrit is adequate. If the child is anemic, red blood cells are an excellent volume expander. Fluid boluses of 5 to 10 ml/kg should be given until the arterial blood pressure is appropriate for age and the central venous pressure (if measured) is 3 to 8 cm H_2O.

Bradycardia can reduce cardiac output in infants, since cardiac output is dependent on heart rate. Bradycardia is usually secondary to something else. The presence of bradycardia should lead to a search for its cause (e.g., hypoxia or vagal stimulus). Treatment of bradycardia is to remove the cause and, on occasion, to administer atropine 0.02 mg/kg.

Hypertension

Hypertension occurring in the PACU is almost always due to pain and is associated with tachycardia and other other pain-related behaviors. Treatment of hypertension initially is treated by administering analgesic agents. Occasionally, hypertension is due to fluid overload.

Children in renal failure or those who have undergone a previous solid organ (liver, kidney, pancreas) transplant often have hypertension and may be taking several antihypertensive medications. In the PACU, they may have an elevated arterial blood pressure despite good pain control. Children who are undergoing dialysis for renal failure are very sensitive to fluid administration. If they receive a large amount of IV fluid during surgery, they may become hypervolemic and hypertensive and require postoperative dialysis to correct the hypertension.

Arrhythmias

With the exception of children who have congenital heart disease, arrhythmias are uncommon in the PACU. Bradycardia, either sinus or junctional, is often secondary to hypoxia or vagal stimuli and usually resolves when the stimulus is removed. Sinus tachycardia is common and usually is secondary to pain, emergence delirium, hypovolemia, hypercarbia, or atropine. Arrhythmias usually are caused by hypoxia, hypercarbia, metabolic, or acid–base disturbances; removing the stimulus usually resolves the arrhythmia.

Some children have cardiac conduction abnormalities. Many of these children have had surgery to correct or palliate congenital heart defects. These children should undergo ECG monitoring during their stay in the PACU. If problems arise, consultation with a pediatric cardiologist should be sought. Antiarrhythmic drugs and a defibrillator should be close at hand in the event that life-threatening arrhythmias occur.

Abnormalities of Temperature

Small children lose heat rapidly (see Chapter 4). Hypothermia can develop rapidly in the PACU, particularly in small infants, and normothermia in the operating room does not guarantee normothermia in the PACU. Hypothermic neonates are more prone to apnea, bradycardia, acidosis, hypotension, and aspiration of gastric contents. They may need prolonged ventilatory support. Neuromuscular blockade is prolonged in hypothermic patients. Oxygen consumption rises markedly as the baby attempts to regenerate the heat lost. Normothermia can be maintained with warm blankets and warming lights. Caution should be used, as *infants can be burned by overly vigorous warming*.

Hyperthermia develops often in the operating room as a result of efficient prevention of heat loss and provision of heat to the child by the use of heated humidifier circuits and warming blankets on the bed. When the child arrives in the PACU, he or she may still be hyperthermic. This usually resolves quickly when the heat sources are removed and the child is uncovered. Hyperthermia, however, may be an indicator of infection or underlying disease and may require specific diagnosis and treatment with antipyretics or antibiotics. Finally, malignant hyperthermia may not develop until the postoperative period. This condition, discussed in Chapter 4, requires immediate diagnosis and therapy.

Postoperative Bleeding

Excessive bleeding in the PACU may be due either to inadequate surgical hemostasis or a coagulopathy. Treatment for the former is to return to the operating room. Treatment for the latter begins with investigation of the possible causes. Determination of the prothrombin time, the partial thromboplastin time, fibrinogen level, and the platelet count help differentiate among a dilutional thrombocytopenia, a lack of coagulation factors, or disseminated intravascular coagulation, and can direct therapy appropriately (see Chapter 6). Platelets, plasma, or cryoprecipitate can be used to correct the deficits.

REFERENCES

1. Quinn GE, Betts EK, Diamond GR: Neonatal age (human) at retinal maturation. Anesthesiology 55:A326, 1981.
2. Gregory GA: Induction of anesthesia. In Gregory GA (ed): Pediatric Anesthesia. 2nd ed. New York, Churchill Livingstone, 1989, p 540.
3. Khine HH, Corddry DH, Kettrick RTG, et al: Comparison of cuffed and uncuffed endotracheal tubes in young children during general anesthesia. Anesthesiology 86:627, 1997.
4. American Society of Anesthesiologists: Standards for basic intraoperative monitoring. American Society of Anesthesiologists: 1999 Directory of Members. 64th ed. Park Ridge, IL, ASA, 1999, p 462.
5. McGill WA, Coveler LA, Epstein BS: Subacute respiratory infections in small children. Anesth Analg 58:331, 1979.
6. Miller BE, Betts EK, Jorgenson JJ, et al: URI and perioperative desaturation in children. Anesthesiology 71:A1170, 1989.
7. Tait AR, Knight PR: Intraoperative respiratory complications in patients with upper respiratory tract infections. Can J Anaesth 34:300, 1987.
8. Jacoby DB, Hirshman CA: General anesthesia in patients with viral respiratory infections: an unsound sleep? Anesthesiology 74:969, 1991.
9. Cohen MM, Cameron CB: Should you cancel the operation when a child has an upper respiratory infection? Anesth Analg 72:282, 1991.
10. Kain ZN, Caramico LA, Mayes LC, et al: Preoperative preparation programs in children: a comparative examination. Anesth Analg 87:1249, 1998.
11. Kain ZN, Mayes LC, Caramico LA, et al: Parental presence during induction of anesthesia: a randomized controlled trial. Anesthesiology 84:1060, 1996.
12. Kain ZN, Mayes LC, O'Connor TZ, et al: Preoperative anxiety in children. Predictors and outcomes. Arch Pediatr Adolesc Med 150:1238, 1996.
13. Kain ZN, Mayes LC, Wang SM, et al: Parental presence during induction of anesthesia versus sedative premedication: which intervention is more effective? Anesthesiology 89:1147, 1998.
14. Kain ZN, Farris CA, Mayes LC, et al: Parental presence during induction of anesthesia: practical differences between the United States and Great Britain. Paediatr Anaesth 6:187, 1996.
15. McEwen AM, Caldicott LD, Barker I: Parents in the anaesthesia room—parents' and anaesthetists' views. Anaesthesia 49:987, 1994.
16. Severinghaus JW, Kelleher JF: Recent developments in pulse oximetry. Anesthesiology 76:1018, 1992.
17. Webster's New Collegiate Dictionary. Springfield, IL, G & C Merriam Co., 1979.
18. Gregory GA: Induction of anesthesia. In Gregory GA (ed): Pediatric Anesthesia. 2nd ed. New York, Churchill Livingstone, 1989, p 544.
19. Liu LMP, Goudsouzian NG, Liu P: Rectal methohexital premedication in children: a dose comparison study. Anesthesiology 53:343, 1980.
20. Liu LMP, Gaudreault P, Friedman PA, et al: Methohexital concentrations in children following rectal administration. Anesthesiology 62:567, 1985.
21. Forbes RB, Vandewalker GE: Comparison of two and ten per cent methohexitone for induction of anaesthesia in children. Can J Anaesth 35:345, 1988.
22. Audenaert SM, Lock R, Pedigo NW, et al: Rectal methohexital's cardiac effects. J Clin Anesth 4:116, 1992.
23. Whitwam JG, Manners JM: Clinical comparison of thiopentone and methohexitone. BMJ 1:1663, 1962.
24. Barry LT, Lawson R, Davidson DGD: Recovery from methohexitone and thiopentone. Anaesthesia 22:228, 1967.
25. Idvall J, Holasek J: Rectal ketamine for induction of anaesthesia in children. Anaesthesia 38:60, 1983.
26. Spear R, Yaster M, Berkowitz I: Preinduction of anesthesia in children with rectally administered midazolam. Anesthesiology 74:670, 1991.
27. Henderson JM, Brodsky DA, Fisher DM, et al: Pre-induction of anesthesia in pediatric patients with nasally administered sufentanil. Anesthesiology 68:671, 1988.
28. Walbergh EJ, Wills RJ, Eckhert J: Plasma concentrations of midazolam in children following intranasal administration. Anesthesiology 74:233, 1991.
29. Wilton NCT, Leigh K, Rosen DR: Preanesthetic sedation of preschool children using intranasal midazolam. Anesthesiology 69:972, 1988.
30. Slover R, Dedo W, Schlesinger T, et al: Use of intranasal midazolam in preschool children. Anesth Analg 70:S377, 1990.
31. Wyant GM: Intramuscular ketalar (CI-581) in paediatric anaesthesia. Can Anaesth Soc J 18:72, 1971.
32. Miller JR, Stoelting VK, Dann MV: A preliminary report of the use of methohexital sodium (Brevital) for pediatric anesthesia. Anesth Analg 40:573, 1961.
33. Rita L, Seleny FL, Mazurek A, et al: Intramuscular midazolam for pediatric pre-anesthetic sedation: a double blind controlled study with morphine. Anesthesiology 63:528, 1985.
34. Grant IS, Nimmo WS, McNichol LR, et al: Ketamine disposition in children and adults. Br J Anaesth 55:1107, 1983.
35. de Waard-vander Spek FB, Van den Berg GM, Oranje AP: EMLA cream: an improved local anesthetic. Review of current literature. Pediatr Dermatol 9:126, 1992.
36. Irsfeld S, Klement W, Lipfert P: Dermal anaesthesia: comparison of EMLA cream with iontophoretic local anaesthesia. Br J Anaesth 71:375, 1993.

37. Zampsky WT, Anand KJS, Sullivan KM, et al: Lidocaine iontophoresis for topical anaesthesia before intravenous line placement in children. J Pediatr 132:1061, 1998.
38. Liu LMP, Cote CJ, Goudsouzian NG, et al: The dose response of intravenous thiopental for the induction of general anesthesia in unpremedicated children. Anesthesiology 55:703, 1981.
39. Brett CM, Fisher DM: Thiopental dose-response relations in unpremedicated infants, children, and adults. Anesth Analg 66:1024, 1987.
40. Liu LMP, Cote CJ, Goudsouzian NG, et al: Response to intravenous induction doses of methohexital in children. Anesthesiology 55:A330, 1981.
41. Perel A, Davidson JT: Recurrent hallucinations following ketamine. Anaesthesia 31:1081, 1976.
42. Meyers EF, Charles P: Prolonged adverse reactions to ketamine in children. Anesthesiology 49:39, 1978.
43. Patel DK, Leeling PA, Newman GB, et al: Induction doses of propofol in children. Anaesthesia 43:949, 1988.
44. Fisher DM, Robinson S, Brett CM, et al: Comparison of enflurane, halothane, and isoflurane for diagnostic and therapeutic procedures in children with malignancies. Anesthesiology 63:647, 1985.
45. Zwass MS, Fisher DM, Welborn LG, et al: Induction and maintenance characteristics of anesthesia with desflurane and nitrous oxide in infants and children. Anesthesiology 76:373, 1992.
46. Lerman J, Davis PJ, Welborn LG, et al: Induction, recovery, and safety characteristics of sevoflurane in children undergoing ambulatory surgery: a comparison with halothane. Anesthesiology 84:1332, 1996.
47. Sarner JB, Levine M, Davis PJ, et al: Clinical characteristics of sevoflurane in children. Anesthesiology 82:38, 1995.
48. Brett CM, Wara WM, Hamilton WK: Anaesthesia for infants during radiotherapy: an insufflation technique. Anesthesiology 64:412, 1986.
49. Brain AI: The laryngeal mask—a new concept in airway management. Br J Anaesth 55:801, 1983.
50. Mason DG, Bingham RM: The laryngeal mask in children. Anaesthesia 45:760, 1990.
51. Benumof JL: Management of the difficult airway. With special emphasis on awake tracheal intubation. Anesthesiology 75:1087, 1991.
52. Benumof JL: Use of the laryngeal mask to facilitate fiberscope-aided tracheal intubation. Anesth Analg 74:313, 1992.
53. Peabody JL, Gregory GA, Willis MM, et al: Transcutaneous oxygen monitoring in sick infants. Ann Rev Respir Dis 118:83, 1978.
54. Berry FA: Management of the pediatric patient with croup or epiglottitis. In 41st Annual Refresher Course Lectures. Park Ridge, IL, ASA, 1990.
55. Rehder K, Mallow JE, Fibuch EE, et al: Effects of isoflurane anesthesia and muscle paralysis on respiratory mechanics in normal man. Anesthesiology 41:477, 1974.
56. Lenox WC, Mitzner W, Hirshman CA: Mechanism of thiopental-induced constriction of guinea pig trachea. Anesthesiology 72:921, 1990.
57. Hatch D, Fletcher M: Anaesthesia and the ventilatory system in infants and young children. Br J Anaesth 68:398, 1992.
58. Motoyama EK, Brinkmeyer SD, Mutich RL, et al: Reduced FRC in anesthetized infants: effects of low PEEP. Anesthesiology 57:A418, 1982.
59. Hickey PR, Hansen DD, Cramolini MD: Pulmonary and systemic hemodynamic responses to ketamine in infants with normal and elevated pulmonary vascular resistnace. Anesthesiology 62:287, 1985.
60. Robinson S, Gregory GA: Fentanyl-air-oxygen anesthesia for ligation of patent ductus arteriosus in preterm infants. Anesth Analg 60:331, 1981.
61. Robinson S, Gregory GA: Urine specific gravity as a predictor of hypovolemia and a hypotensive response to halothane anesthesia in the newborn. In Abstracts of Scientific Papers, Annual Meeting. American Society of Anesthesiologists, 1977, p 57.
62. Salem MR, Wong AY, Fizzotti GF: Efficacy of cricoid pressure in preventing aspiration of gastric contents in paediatric patients. Br J Anaesth 44:401, 1972.
63. Salem MR, Wong AY, Collins VJ: The pediatric patient with a full stomach. Anesthesiology 39:435, 1973.
64. Salanitre E, Rackow H: The pulmonary exchange of nitrous oxide and halothane in infants and children. Anesthesiology 30:388, 1969.

65. Fisher DM, Zwass MS: MAC of desflurane in 60% nitrous oxide in infants and children. Anesthesiology 76:354, 1992.
66. Murray D, Forbes R, Murphy K, et al: Nitrous oxide: cardiovascular effects in infants and small children during halothane and isoflurane anesthesia. Anesth Analg 67:1059, 1988.
67. Schulte-Susse U, Hess W, Tarnow J: Pulmonary responses to nitrous oxide in patients with normal and high pulmonary vascular resistance. Anesthesiology 57:9, 1982.
68. Hickey PR, Hansen DD, Stafford M, et al: Pulmonary and systemic hemodynamic effects of nitrous oxide in infants with normal and elevated pulmonary vascular resistance. Anesthesiology 65:374, 1986.
69. Losasso TJ, Muzzi DA, Dietz NM, et al: Fifty percent nitrous oxide does not increase the risk of venous air embolism in neurosurgical patients operated upon in the sitting position. Anesthesiology 77:21, 1992.
70. Brandom BW, Brandom RB, Cook DR: Uptake and distribution of halothane in infants: in vivo measurements and computer simulations. Anesth Anlag 62:404, 1983.
71. Gregory GA, Eger EI, Munson ES: The relationship between age and halothane requirements in man. Anesthesiology 30:488, 1969.
72. Rao CC, Boyer MS, Krishna G, et al: Increased sensitivity of the isometric contraction on the neonatal isolated rat atria to halothane, isoflurane, and enflurane. Anesthesiology 64:13, 1986.
73. Cook DR, Brandom BW, Shen G, et al: The inspired median effective dose, brain concentration at anesthesia, and cardiovascular index for young rats. Anesth Analg 60:182, 1981.
74. Diaz JH, Lockhart CH: Is halothane really safe in infancy? Anesthesiology 51:S313, 1979.
75. Lerman J, Robinson S, Willis MM, et al: Anesthetic requirements for halothane in young children 0-1 month and 1-6 months of age. Anesthesiology 59:421, 1983.
76. Karl HW, Swedlow MD, Lee KW, et al: Epinephrine-halothane interactions in children. Anesthesiology 58:142, 1983.
77. Podlesch I, Dudziak R, Zinganell K: Inspiratory and expiratory carbon dioxide concentrations during halothane anesthesia in infants. Anesthesiology 27:823, 1966.
78. Murat I, Delleur MM, MacGee K, et al: Changes in ventilatory patterns during halothane anaesthesia in children. Br J Anaesth 57:569, 1985.
79. Murat I, Chaussain M, Saint-Maurice C: Ventilatory responses to carbon dioxide in children during nitrous oxide-halothane anaesthesia. Br J Anaesth 57:1197, 1985.
80. Kingston HGG, Hirshman CA: Perioperative management of the patient with asthma. Anesth Analg 63:844, 1984.
81. Hirshman CA, Edelstein G, Peetz S, et al: Mechanism of action of inhalational anesthesia on airways. Anesthesiology 56:107, 1982.
82. Smith AL, Wollman H: Cerebral blood flow and metabolism: effects of anesthetic drugs and techniques. Anesthesiology 36:378, 1972.
83. Shapiro HM: Intracranial hypertension: therapeutic and anesthetic considerations. Anesthesiology 43:445, 1975.
84. Moore RA, McNicholas KW, Gallagher JD, et al: Halothane metabolism in acyanotic and cyanotic patients undergoing open heart surgery. Anesth Analg 65:1257, 1986.
85. Mushin WW, Rosen M, Jones EV: Post-halothane jaundice in relation to previous administration of halothane. BMJ 3:18, 1971.
86. Summary of the National Halothane Study: A study of the possible association between halothane anesthesia and post-operative hepatic necrosis. JAMA 197:775, 1966.
87. Wark HJ: Post-operative jaundice in children. The influence of halothane. Anaesthesia 38:237, 1983.
88. Warner LO, Beach TP, Garvin JP, et al: Halothane and children: the first quarter century. Anesth Analg 63:838, 1984.
89. Kenna JG, Neuberger J, Mieli-Vergani G, et al: Halothane hepatitis in children. BMJ 294:1209, 1987.
90. Cote CJ: Practical pharmacology of anesthetic agents, narcotics, and sedatives. In Cote CJ, Ryan JF, Todres ID, et al (eds): A Practice of Anesthesia for Infants and Children. 2nd ed. Philadelphia, WB Saunders Company, 1993, p 105.
91. O'Brien CM, Robinson DN, Morton NS: Induction and emergence in infants less than 60 weeks post-conceptual age: comparison of thiopental, halothane, sevoflurane, and desflurane. Br J Anaesth 80:456, 1998.
92. Lerman J: Sevoflurane in pediatric anesthesia. Anesth Analg 81:S4, 1995.

93. Piat V, Dubois M, Johanet S, et al: Induction and recovery characteristics and hemodynamic responses to sevoflurane and halothane in children. Anesth Analg 79:840, 1994.
94. Lerman J, Sikich N, Kleinman S, et al: The pharmacology of sevoflurane in infants and children. Anesthesiology 80:814, 1994.
95. Brown K, Aun C, Stocks J, et al: A comparison of the respiratory effects of sevoflurane and halothane in infants and young children. Anesthesiology 89:86, 1998.
96. Green WB Jr: The ventilatory effects of sevoflurane. Anesth Analg 81(Suppl 6):S23, 1995.
97. Berkowitz RA, Hoffman WE, Cunningham F, et al: Changes in cerebral blood flow velocity in children during sevoflurane and halothane anesthesia. J Neurosurg Anesthesiol 8:194, 1996.
98. Levine MF, Sarner J, Lerman J, et al: Plasma inorganic fluoride concentrations after sevoflurane anesthesia in children. Anesthesiology 84:348, 1997.
99. Eger EI, Koblin DD, Bowland T, et al: Nephrotoxicity of sevoflurane versus desflurane anesthesia in volunteers. Anesth Analg 84:160, 1997.
100. Kharasch ED, Frink EJ Jr, Zager R, et al: Assessment of low-flow sevoflurane and isoflurane effects on renal function using sensitive markers of rubular toxicity. Anesthesiology 86:1238, 1997.
101. Mazze RI, Jamison RL: Low flow (1 L/min) sevoflurane: is it safe? Anesthesiology 86:1225, 1997.
102. Frink EJ Jr, Green WB Jr, Brown EA, et al: Compound A concentration during sevoflurane anesthesia in children. Anesthesiology 84:566, 1996.
103. Cameron CB, Robinson S, Gregory GA: The minimum anesthetic concentration of isoflurane in children. Anesth Analg 63:418, 1984.
104. Stevens WC, Dolan WM, Gibbons RT, et al: Minimum alveolar concentration (MAC) of isoflurane with and without nitrous oxide in patients of varying ages. Anesthesiology 42:197, 1975.
105. Le Dez KM, Lerman J: The minimum alveolar concentration (MAC) of isoflurane in preterm neonates. Anesthesiology 67:301, 1987.
106. Eger EI: Isoflurane: a review. Anesthesiology 55:559, 1981.
107. Wolf WJ, Neal MB, Peterson MD: The hemodynamic and cadiovascular effects of isoflurane and halothane in children. Anesthesiology 64:328, 1986.
108. Murray D, Vandewalker G, Matherne GP, et al: Pulsed Doppler and two dimensional echocardiography: comparison of halothane and isoflurane on cardiac function in infants and small children. Anesthesiology 67:211, 1987.
109. Julien RM, Kavan EM, Elliott HW: Effects of volatile anesthetic agents on EEG activity recorded in limbic and sensory systems. Can Anaesth Soc J 19:263, 1972.
110. Wade JG, Stephen WC: Isoflurane: anesthetic for the eighties? Anesth Analg 60:666, 1981.
111. Newberg LA, Michenfelder JD: Cerebral protection by isoflurane during hypoxemia or ischemia. Anesthesiology 59:29, 1983.
112. Yasuda N, Targ AG, Eger EI: Solubility of I-653, sevoflurane, isoflurane, and halothane in human tissues. Anesth Analg 69:370, 1989.
113. Taylor RH, Lerman J: Minimum alveolar concentration of desflurane and hemodynamic responses in neonates, infants, and children. Anesthesiology 75:975, 1991.
114. Welborn LG, Hannallah RS, Norden JM, et al: Comparison of emergence and recovery characteristics of sevoflurane, desflurane, and halothane in pediatric ambulatory patients. Anesth Analg 83:917, 1996.
115. Way WL, Costley EC, Way EL: Respiratory sensitivity of the newborn infant to morphine and meperidine. Clin Pharmacol Ther 6:454, 1965.
116. Dahlstrom B, Bolme P, Feychting H, et al: Morphine kinetics in children. Clin Pharmacol Ther 26:354, 1979.
117. Yaster M: The dose response of fentanyl in neonatal anesthesia, Anesthesiology 66:433, 1987.
118. Collins C, Koren G, Crean P, et al: Fentanyl pharmacokinetics and hemodynamic effects in preterm infants during ligation of patent ductus arteriosus. Anesth Analg 64:1078, 1985.
119. Koehntop DE, Rodman JH, Brundage DM, et al: Pharmacokinetics of fentanyl in neonates. Anesth Analg 65:227, 1986.
120. Hertzka RE, Gauntlett IS, Fisher DM, et al: Fentanyl-induced ventilatory depression: effects of age. Anesthesiology 70:213, 1989.
121. Arandia HY, Patil VU: Glottic closure following large doses of fentanyl. Anesthesiology 66:574, 1987.
122. Gauntlett IS, Fisher DM, Hertzka RE, et al: Pharmacokinetics of fentanyl in neonatal humans and lambs: effects of age. Anesthesiology 69:683, 1988.
123. Shafer SL, Stanski DR: Improving the clinical utility of anesthetic drug pharmacokinetics. Anesthesiology 76:327, 1992.
124. Greely WJ, de Bruijn NP: Changes in sufentanil pharmacokinetics within the neonatal period. Anesth Analg 67:86, 1988.
125. Anand KJ, Hickey PR: Halothane-morphine compared with high-dose sufentanil for anesthesia and postoperative analgesia in neonatal cardiac surgery. N Engl J Med 326:1, 1992.
126. Michelson LG, Hug CC Jr: The pharmacokinetics of remifentanil. J Clin Anesth 8:679, 1996.
127. Lynn AM: Remifentanil: the paediatric anaesthetists' opiate. Paediatr Anaesth 6:433, 1996.
128. Cauldwell CB, Fisher DM: Sedating pediatric patients: is propofol a panacea? Radiology 186:9, 1993.
129. Morton NS: Total intravenous anaesthesia (TIVA) in paediatrics: advantages and disadvantages. Paediatr Anaesth 8:189, 1998.
130. Goudsouzian NG, Alifimoff JK, Eberly C, et al: Neuromuscular and cardiovascular effects of mivacurium in children. Anesthesiology 70:237, 1989.
131. Wright PMC, Brown R, Lau M, et al: A pharmacodynamic explanation for the rapid onset/offset of rapacuronium bromide. Anesthesiology 90:16, 1999.
132. Meretoja OA: Is vecuronium a long-acting neuromuscular blocking agent in neonates and infants? Br J Anaesth 62:184, 1989.
133. Witkowski TA, Bartkowski RR, Azad SS, et al: ORG 9426 onset of action: a comparison with atracurium and vecuronium. Anesthesiology 77:A964, 1992.
134. Mason LJ, Betts EK: Leg lift and maximal inspiratory force: clinical signs of neuromuscular blockade reversal in neonates and infants. Anesthesiology 52:441, 1980.
135. Practice guidelines for blood component therapy: A report by the American Society of Anesthesiologists' Task Force on Blood Component Therapy. Anesthesiology 84:732, 1996.
136. Welborn LG, McGill WA, Hannallah RS, et al: Perioperative blood glucose concentration in pediatric outpatients. Anesthesiology 65:543, 1986.
137. Welborn LG, Hannallah RS, McGill WA: Glucose concentration for routine intravenous infusion in pediatric outpatient surgery. Anesthesiology 67:427, 1987.
138. Steward DJ, Volgyesi G: Stabilometry: a new tool for the measurement of recovery following general anesthesia for outpatients. Can Anaesth Soc J 25:4, 1978.
139. Eckenhoff JE, Kneale DH, Dripps RD: The incidence and etiology of postanesthetic excitement: a clinical survey. Anesthesiology 22:667, 1961.
140. Pounder DR, Blackstock D, Steward DJ: Tracheal extubation in children: halothane versus isoflurane, anesthetized versus awake. Anesthesiology 74:653, 1991.
141. Fisher DM, Cronnelly R, Sharma M, et al: Clinical pharmacology of edrophonium in infants and children. Anesthesiology 61:428, 1984.
142. Wetchler BV: Problem solving in the postanesthesia care unit. In Wetchler BV (ed): Anesthesia for Ambulatory Surgery. 2nd ed. Philadelphia, JB Lippincott, 1991, p 375.
143. Practice advisory for the recovery room. American Society of Anesthesiologists Newsletter, 1978.
144. Aldrete JA, Kroulik D: A postanesthetic recovery score. Anesth Analg 49:924, 1970.
145. Steward DJ: A simplified scoring for the post-operative recovery room. Can Anaesth Soc J 22:111, 1975.
146. Soliman IE, Patel RI, Ehrenpreis MB, et al: Recovery scores do not correlate with postoperative hypoxemia in children. Anesthesiology 67:53, 1988.
147. Fisher GA, McComiskey CM, Hill JL, et al: Postoperative voiding interval and duration of analgesia following peripheral or caudal nerve blocks in children. Anesth Analg 76:173, 1993.
148. Schreiner MS, Nicolson SC, Martin T, et al: Drinking before discharging children from day surgery: is it necessary? Anesthesiology 76:528, 1992.
149. Steward DJ: Outpatient pediatric anesthesia. Anesthesiology 43:268, 1975.
150. Natof HE, Gold B, Kitz DS: Complications. In Wetchler BV (ed): Anesthesia for Ambulatory Surgery. 2nd ed. Philadelphia, JB Lippincott, 1991, p 437.

151. Beyer JE, De Good DE, Ashley LC, et al: Patterns of postoperative analgesic use with adults and children following cardiac surgery. Pain 17:71, 1983.
152. Loeser JD: Pain in children. *In* Tyler DC, Krane EJ (eds): Advances in Pain Research and Therapy. Vol 15: Pediatric Pain. New York, Raven Press, 1990, p 1.
153. Anand KJS, Hickey PR: Pain and its effects in the human neonate and fetus. N Engl J Med 317:1321, 1987.
154. Maunuksela E, Olkkola KT, Korpela R: Measurement of pain in children with self-reporting and behavioral assessment. Clin Pharmacol Ther 42:137, 1987.
155. Watcha MF, Jones MB, Lagueruela RG, et al: Comparison of ketorolac and morphine as adjuvants during pediatric surgery. Anesthesiology 76:368, 1992.
156. Houck CS, Wilder RT, McDermott JS, et al: Safety of intravenous ketorolac therapy in children and cost savings with a unit dosing system. J Pediatr 129:292, 1996.
157. Rice LJ, Pudimat MA, Hannallah RS: Timing of caudal block placement in relation to surgery does not affect duration of postoperative analgesia in pediatric ambulatory patients. Can J Anaesth 37:429, 1990.
158. Jerome EH: Recovery of the pediatric patient from anesthesia. *In* Gregory GA (ed): Pediatric Anesthesia. 2nd ed. New York, Churchill Livingstone, 1989, p 619.
159. Steward DJ: Experiences with an outpatient anesthesia service for children. Anesth Analg 52:877, 1973.
160. Abramowitz MD, Oh TH, Epstein BS, et al: The antiemetic effect of droperidol following outpatient strabismus surgery in children. Anesthesiology 59:579, 1983.
161. Lerman K, Eustis S, Smith DR: Effect of droperidol pretreatment on postanesthetic vomiting in children undergoing strabismus surgery. Anesthesiology 65:322, 1986.
162. Lim DM, Furst SR, Rodarte A: A double-blinded comparison of metoclopramide and droperidol for prevention of emesis following strabismus surgery. Anesthesiology 76:357, 1992.
163. Alon E, Himmelscher S: Ondansetron in the treatment of postoperative vomiting: a randomized double-blind comparison with droperidol and metoclopramide. Anesth Analg 75:561, 1992.
164. Koka BV, Jeon IS, Andre JM, et al: Postintubation croup in children. Anesth Analg 56:501, 1977.
165. Gregory GA, Steward DJ: Life-threatening perioperative apnea in the ex-"premie." Anesthesiology 59:495, 1983.
166. Kurth CD, Spitzer AR, Broennle AM, et al: Postoperative apnea in preterm infants. Anesthesiology 66:483, 1987.
167. Welborn LG, Rice LJ, Hannallah RS, et al: Postoperative apnea in former preterm infants: prospective comparison of spinal and general anesthesia. Anesthesiology 72:838, 1990.
168. Cote CJ, Saslavsky A, Downes JJ, et al: Postoperative apnea in former preterm infants after inguinal herniorraphy. A combined analysis. Anesthesiology 82:809, 1995.
169. Fisher DM: When is the ex-premature infant no longer at risk for apnea? Anesthesiology 82:807, 1995.
170. Kurth CD, LeBard SE: Association of postoperative apnea, airway obstruction, and hypoxemia in former preterm infants. Anesthesiology 75:22, 1991.
171. Frantz ID, Adler SM, Thatch BT, et al: Maturational effects on respiratory responses to carbon dioxide in premature infants. J Appl Physiol 41:41, 1976.
172. Brady JP, Ceruit E: Chemoreceptor reflexes in the newborn infant: effects of varying degrees of hypoxia on heart rate and ventilation in a warm environment. J Physiol (Lond) 184:631, 1966.
173. Welborn LG, Hannallah RS, Luban NLC, et al: Anemia and postoperative apnea in former preterm infants. Anesthesiology 74:1003, 1991.
174. Noseworthy J, Duran C, Khine HH: Postoperative apnea in a full term infant. Anesthesiology 70:879, 1989.
175. Lee KWT, Downes JJ: Pulmonary edema secondary to laryngospasm in children. Anesthesiology 59:347, 1983.
176. Warner MA, Warner ME, Weber JG: Clinical significance of pulmonary aspiration during the perioperative period. Anesthesiology 78:56, 1993.
177. Lerman J: New inhalational agents in pediatric anaesthesia, sevoflurane and desflurane. *In* Society for Pediatric Anesthesia. 6th Annual Meeting, 1992.

Monitoring During Surgery

GEORGE A. GREGORY

◆ ◆ ◆

Advances in microelectronics and bioengineering have made it possible to monitor infants and children effectively to obtain early warning of potential problems. However, monitors are of little value unless the meaning and limitations of the information they provide are understood. This chapter reviews some of the monitoring techniques available and discusses their advantages and disadvantages.

OVERALL MONITORING GOALS

The purpose of monitoring is to detect potential problems. It is not a substitute for close observation of the patient by the anesthesiologist, who must maintain constant contact with the patient and continuously evaluate and integrate all incoming information. Electronic monitoring enables us to do this more efficiently.

Unfortunately, most anesthesiologists were not trained to understand monitoring equipment in depth, which has led to unreal expectations of what monitors do. Our expectations can be made more realistic by trying equipment in a clinical setting before buying it. Equipment should never be purchased from a company that does not allow such a trial. Reputable companies always allow a device to be tried and provide the names of others who have purchased it. The anesthesiologist should first call the company to confirm that a particular piece of equipment does

the job desired. No equipment should be purchased unless there is a dependable service representative in the area who can repair the instrument quickly. Nothing is more frustrating than sending a monitor away for weeks or months to get it repaired. If there is no local 24-hour repair service, it is probably better not to buy that particular piece of equipment no matter how good it sounds. If a service agreement is available, it should be purchased at the same time as the instrument. All devices break down.

Monitors are of no value unless they are attached to the patient. Often, expensive monitoring equipment is purchased but sits unused in a corner because it is "too much trouble" to use. Taking the time to understand the basic principles, operation, and information coming from the machine ensures that the anesthesiologist will feel comfortable with the monitor and will use it.

In this day of high technology it is easy to forget that the person who processes information received from a monitor is still the most important link in the chain. Monitors sometimes give false information. If information from a monitor disagrees with clinical information, the cause of this difference should be investigated. It is unwise to blindly believe or disbelieve a machine. If a piece of equipment "stops working" (e.g., the electrocardiogram [ECG] "disappears"), it should be independently confirmed that the patient is all right before it is assumed that the monitor or the electrodes are at fault. The patient may

TABLE 11–1
HEART RATE ACCORDING TO AGE

Age	Heart Rate (beats/min)
Preterm	150 ± 20
Term	133 ± 18
6 mo	120 ± 20
12 mo	120 ± 20
2 y	105 ± 25
5 y	90 ± 10
12 y	70 ± 17
23 y	77 ± 5

really have had a cardiac arrest. A quick check of the pulse, arterial blood pressure, and heart tones will confirm whether the problem is with the patient or the monitor.

CARDIOVASCULAR MONITORING

Heart Rate: Monitoring by Auscultation and ECG

The most direct way to monitor heart rate and rhythm continuously is with a chest piece or esophageal stethoscope attached by a tube to the anesthesiologist's ear. This allows constant contact with the patient and frees the anesthesiologist's hands to do other things. It also allows early detection of changes in heart tones, which Cullen[1] found to be associated with changes in myocardial contractility. Because myocardial contractility decreases with the first few breaths of halothane,[2] it is important to monitor every aspect of the cardiovascular system as well as possible. A child's heart tones usually become "mushy" before the arterial blood pressure and peripheral perfusion decrease, especially when the blood volume is borderline. An esophageal stethoscope is useful only if the person using it hears and processes the information it is providing.[3] Cooper and Cullen.[3] found that 87 percent of surreptitious occlusions of the stethoscope were detected in less than 60 seconds. However, 2.3 percent went undetected for more than 240 seconds. Sick premature infants have significantly decreased long-term variability of heart rate while they are ill.[4] Consequently, significant changes in cardiac output may occur in some patients without a response in heart rate.

The ECG is an important adjunct to cardiac monitoring in the operating room because anesthesia often causes bradycardia in infants and children. Other dysrhythmias are uncommon unless the child is hypoxemic, acidotic, or alkalotic. Young children depend primarily on heart rate for cardiac output.[5] The slower the heart rate, the lower their cardiac output. Therefore, bradycardia should be detected as early as possible. ECG monitors should be set to alarm when the child's heart rate exceeds or falls below predetermined rates. It is difficult to watch the monitor continuously, especially if it is located behind or beside the anesthesiologist. Monitors designed for adults may not work well for small children because they sometimes fail to track rapid heart rates adequately. This is especially true when small pediatric chest electrodes are used to interface the machine with the patient.

All electronic monitoring equipment should be isolated from stray currents to prevent electric shocks or burns.[6] Even though they are electrically safe, monitors may pick up electrical noise from the environment and make the output of the machine unreadable. Good grounding and patient isolation circuits prevent both problems. Electrical noise is especially a problem when monitors designed for use in the intensive care unit (ICU) are used in the operating room with an electrocautery. Even very expensive monitors designed for use in the operating room may not eliminate interference from an electrocautery. This is one reason why all monitors should be used in the operating room before they are purchased.

The most difficult part of ECG monitoring is obtaining a proper patient–machine interface. A poor interface usually occurs when there is poor contact between the chest pads and chest. Contact can be improved by cleaning the chest with alcohol, allowing the alcohol to dry, and then applying the pads. If the electrode paste is dry, more paste should be added before the pads are applied; dry pads do not conduct. Table 11–1 shows the normal heart rates for patients of various ages.

Blood Pressure Monitoring

Arterial Pressure

Anesthetics decrease the blood pressures of infants and children more than those of adults (Table 11–2),[7-9] because anesthetics more effectively reduce the peripheral vascular resistance and myocardial contractility of pediatric patients than of adults. Because children tend to lose blood relatively more rapidly than adults, blood pressure should be monitored in all patients (Fig. 11–1). Table 11–3 lists the normal arterial blood pressures of pediatric patients. To obtain accurate blood pressures, the blood pressure cuff must be an appropriate size for the patient. The width of the cuff must be two thirds the distance from the acromion process to the olecranon,[10] or the diameter of the cuff bladder must be 20 percent greater than the diameter of the extremity and should encircle one half to three fourths of the extremity.[11] If the cuff is too small (15 to 20 percent less than the appropriate size), the blood pressure determination will be falsely high.[12] If the cuff is too large (15 to 20 percent larger), the pressure reading will be falsely low. Cuffs that encompass the unlar condyle may compress and damage the ulnar nerve. The bladder of the cuff must be over the artery or it may be difficult to obtain an aterial blood pressure. Aneroid blood pressure manometers always should be available in case the elec-

TABLE 11–2
BLOOD PRESSURE CHANGES
WITH HALOTHANE ANESTHESIA

Patient	% Change with Halothane	
	1.0 MAC	*1.5 MAC*
Newborn	27 ± 8	38 ± 11
Adult	5 ± 5	15 ± 5

MAC, minimum anesthetic concentration.

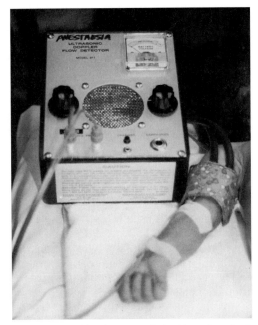

FIGURE 11–1. Doppler blood pressure device. Transducer is placed over the radial artery at the wrist. Inflating the blood pressure cuff occludes the blood flow under the transducer. As the cuff pressure is decreased, flow occurs under the transducer, producing an amplified sound.

TABLE 11 – 4
ARTERIAL BLOOD PRESSURE DETERMINED BY DOPPLER AND DIRECT METHODS

	Systolic Blood Pressure	
Age	Doppler (mm Hg)	Direct (mm Hg)
Preterm	57 ± 4	50 ± 3
Term	76 ± 9	67 ± 3
3 mo	72 ± 13	70 ± 8
6 mo	88 ± 18	89 ± 29

mean) correlate well with intra-arterial pressures.[14] The correlation is much better than with Korotkoff sounds. With care and the appropriate cuff, arterial pressures can be obtained in very small infants with this device.[15] However, there is a wide variation in the pressures of infants of similar size. The correlation with intra-arterial pressures usually is relatively good. Table 11–4 shows the poor correlation between arterial pressures measured by oscillometry and from an intra-arterial catheter in small premature infants. Note that oscillometry tends to give higher pressures, which while comforting, are inaccurate and overestimate the true arterial pressure of the patient. This is potentially a serious problem for these children.

Oscillometers can be set to give a blood pressure reading every 1 to 5 minutes in the operating room, and alarms can be set to sound if the arterial pressure is less than the preset limits. One disadvantage of these devices is their sensitivity to position, especially in small infants. Unless the cuff is aligned exactly over the artery, it will be difficult to measure the arterial pressure. In infants who weigh less than 1,000 g it is often easier and far less frustrating to place a Doppler device over the radial or brachial artery to determine arterial pressure rather than to use an oscillometer apparatus during surgery.

Doppler devices detect sound waves that are "bounced" off moving arterial walls. When the cuff pressure exceeds arterial pressure, the artery beneath the cuff ceases to move and sound is absent. When the cuff pressure falls below the pressure that occludes the artery, arterial movement and sound return. This is the systolic pressure. When the diastolic pressure is reached, the strength and quality of the sound decrease. The Doppler head must be placed directly over the artery to ensure accurate pressures. The correlation between Doppler blood pressures and those from intravascular catheters, even during shock or cardiopulmonary bypass, is good.[16, 17]

Doppler devices that automatically measure arterial pressure at preset intervals are available. The pressures attained correlate well with directly measured pressures in older infants but are falsely high in the neonate (Table 11–4). The transducer must be placed directly over the artery, especially in neonates and preterm infants, or no blood pressure will be measured. A slight movement of the arm can move the transducer off the artery. The anesthesiologist should determine that pressure is being measured appropriately just before the patient is draped and when the patient's position is changed. On occasion the cuff fails to deflate. If so, the extremity may become ischemic and muscles and nerves may be damaged. Failure

tronic blood pressure monitor fails, as it does sometimes. However, aneroid manometers are difficult to read in the lower pressure ranges, especially below 50 mm Hg, and may be inaccurate unless they have large faces and have been accurately calibrated. All manometers should be calibrated periodically against a mercury manometer to ensure accuracy.

Oscillometry is the most common method of measuring arterial blood pressure in neonates and children. Blood flow through an artery causes the arterial wall to oscillate, and this oscillation is transmitted to a blood pressure cuff that encircles the extremity.[13] As the cuff pressure decreases, a characteristic change in the magnitude of oscillation occurs at the systolic, diastolic, and mean pressures. The systolic pressure is denoted by a rapid increase in the oscillation amplitude, and this occurs when the arterial pressure first exceeds the cuff pressure. The mean pressure is denoted by the maximal oscillation, and the diastolic pressure is denoted by a sudden decrease in oscillation as the pressure decreases. These pressures (systolic, diastolic,

TABLE 11 – 3
ARTERIAL BLOOD PRESSURE ACCORDING TO AGE

	Arterial Blood Pressure	
Age	Systolic (mm Hg)	Diastolic (mm Hg)
Preterm	50 ± 3	30 ± 2
Term	67 ± 3	42 ± 4
6 mo	89 ± 29	60 ± 10
12 mo	96 ± 30	66 ± 25
2 y	99 ± 25	64 ± 25
5 y	94 ± 14	55 ± 9
12 y	109 ± 16	58 ± 9
23 y	122 ± 30	75 ± 20

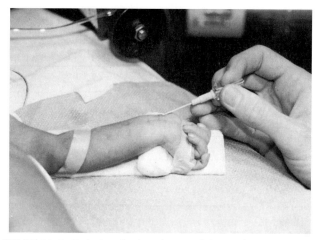

FIGURE 11–2. Technique for inserting a radial artery line in an infant. The angle of insertion is approximately 45 degrees with the skin. The patient's hand is extended over a sponge and taped to an arm board.

of the cuff to deflate is indicated by persistent cyanosis of the extremity.

If large fluid shifts or blood losses are expected, the arterial pressure should be continuously measured with an arterial line and strain gauge.[18] The catheter can usually be inserted percutaneously if the patient weighs more than 400 g (Fig. 11–2).[19] Arterial catheters are very helpful in the care of patients, but they often are associated with complications. Insertion of an arterial catheter can injure vessels and cause vascular occlusion. Flushing the arterial catheter may cause retrograde flow and emboli may be showered into remote locations, including the brain.[20]

In infants weighing less than 1 kg, it may be necessary to transfix the artery with the catheter and then withdraw it slowly until there is good blood return. In larger patients, the catheter can usually be inserted without penetrating the back wall of the artery. In either case, as soon as there is good blood return the catheter should be advanced up the arterial lumen and fixed in place. Catheters can also be inserted into arteries by cutting off the plastic tubing from a 21-guage butterfly catheter and inserting the needle into the artery. As soon as there is good blood return, an 0.018-inch wire can be inserted through the needle and advanced up the artery. The needle is then withdrawn and the catheter is advanced over the wire. This maneuver is useful in small infants.

Pearse[19] described locating the radial arteries of preterm infants by shining a bright, *cold,* fiberoptic light through the wrist from below. This makes it possible to visualize the artery as it pulsates in the wrist. The catheter tip can then be inserted into the artery and advanced up the lumen, which is especially useful when attempting to cannulate the radial, ulnar, and posterior tibial arteries. Recently, a catheter with a Doppler probe in its tip has been developed to insert venous catheters. When the vessel is under the catheter and the flow signal is maximal, the catheter is advanced into the vessel. The closer the needle is to the vessel, the louder the flow signal. When the needle enters the vessel the sound becomes very loud. These devices are expensive but may allow cannulation of small vessels that otherwise would be difficult to cannulate.

Before any attempt to insert an arterial catheter, the extremity should be placed on a board and taped securely to it. The wrist should be hyperextended to immobilize the artery. It is often useful to inject 0.1 to 0.2 ml of 1 percent lidocaine into the skin and around the artery to reduce pain and arteriospasm. An adequate incision should be made in the skin with a needle tip to enable the catheter to penetrate the skin easily. If this is not done, the tips of small catheters may shred as they pass through the skin. The catheter should enter the artery at a 45-degree angle or less to allow the bevel of the catheter to be completely within small arteries rather than partly in and partly out, as occurs when the needle is inserted at right angles to the artery (Fig. 11–3).

A 22-gauge catheter is usually appropriate for an infant who weighs more than 1,500 g. A 24-gauge catheter is more appropriate for an infant who weighs less than 1,500 g. A 20-gauge catheter is usually appropriate for older children. Longer catheters are apparently less likely to cause arterial occlusion than short catheters.[21] Catheter sepsis is uncommon and is not reduced by frequently changing the arterial catheter. The catheter should be fixed firmly with tape and benzoin and the hub supported. If arterial lines are securely fixed in place, prevented from moving in the artery, and kept open by a continuous infusion of saline 0.5 to 1.0 ml/h, the catheters usually function in infants for 2 to 3 weeks or more. Radial nerve palsy has been reported in infants after prolonged radial arterial catheterization.[22] There is a 63 percent rate of radial artery occlusion after cannulation of this artery in infants.[23] The occlusion was present for 1 to 29 days, was directly related to the duration of arterial catheterization, and was inversely related to birth weight. Normal saline should be infused at 1 to 2 ml/kg/h to prevent occlusion of the artery. Infusion of glucose into these catheters increases the likelihood of causing local injury and of occluding the catheters.[24] A small-dead-space, stiff tube should connect the arterial catheter to a strain gauge. The response time of the intravascular catheter, connecting tubing, and strain gauge must be adequate to allow faithful pressure wave transmission at high heart rates.[25] The internal volume of the tubing should be small (< 0.5 ml).

Three times the volume of the tubing, catheter, and stopcock must be removed and discarded (or injected into a venous catheter) before the blood sample adequately

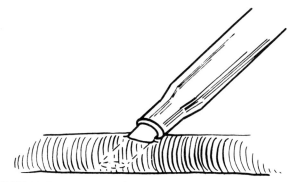

FIGURE 11–3. Penetration of the arterial needle into the artery. Care must be taken to advance the plastic cannula off the needle. Withdrawing the needle before advancing the cannula often withdraws the catheter from the artery.

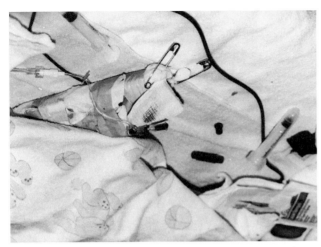

FIGURE 11–4. Abbott T-connector attached to a radial artery line. A 25-gauge needle is inserted into the rubber bung and three drops of blood are allowed to come out before the blood sample is drawn.

reflects arterial pH, electrolytes, and blood gases.[26] Reinjecting withdrawn blood into the radial artery catheter may occlude small blood vessels of the forearm.[27] Discarding this small amount of blood eventually necessitates a blood transfusion. These problems can be avoided, or at least reduced, by using a T-connector (Fig. 11–4). The tubing leading to the connector is clamped. A 25-gauge needle is inserted into the rubber bung, three drops of blood and fluid are allowed to drip from the needle, and the sample is withdrawn. The tubing is unclamped and flushed over 5 to 10 seconds to avoid transient arterial hypertension and flushing of thrombi into the central circulation.[20] This technique reduces both blood loss and red blood cell clumping in the syringe and tubing. Failure to wedge the connector tightly into the catheter and to tighten the Luer-lock adequately allows hemorrhage to occur. The extremity and connector must be kept in plain view at all times and should never be covered. If the tubing becomes disconnected from the catheter and the catheter is covered, the patient may exanguinate before the catheter-disconnect is detected, especially if the patient is small. Arterial catheters placed in an emergency room have an inordinate number of complications and must be replaced frequently.[28]

Arterial lines should be flushed with care. It is possible to inject clots and damaged cells not only into extremity vessels but into the cerebral vessels as well, as demonstrated by Lowenstein et al.,[29] who visualized the carotid arteries of children with 1 ml of dye rapidly injected into a radial artery. The cerebral and pulmonary arteries also can be visualized by rapidly injecting dye into umbilical arterial catheters, even when the catheter tip is at the L3–L4 vertebral level.[30] Injecting as little as 0.2 ml of air through an umbilical artery catheter can occlude blood flow to the lower extremities for several hours. Umbilical artery catheters are associated with higher incidences of intracranial hemorrhage, possibly because emboli are showered to the brain.[31] Umbilical artery catheters should be positioned at the body of L3 or L4 to prevent vascular occlusion and gastrointestinal and renal problems.[32]

Monitors to which strain gauges are attached should be designed for pediatric use. Those designed for adults often give falsely high arterial blood pressures, especially when the arterial pressure is low. To ensure accuracy, all pressure channels should periodically be calibrated against a mercury manometer. (The monitor is disconnected form the patient while it is being calibrated.[33]) Devices designed for both pediatric and adult use have several scales to accommodate the various pressure levels. Care must be taken to ensure that the strain gauge is positioned at the level of the heart. If it is below the level of the heart, the pressure reading will be too high. If it is above the heart, the pressure reading will be too low. The position of the strain gauge can make a great difference in the arterial pressure reading in small premature infants.

There is more information in the arterial blood pressure tracing than merely the systolic, diastolic, and mean pressures (Fig. 11–5). The normal tracing has a sharp upstroke, a narrow peak, a dicrotic notch that is one third of the way down the descending limb of the wave in older children and one half the way down the waveform in infants and neonates, and a slow runoff. A damped tracing is wider, the upstroke more horizontal, and the dicrotic notch absent, and the peak is rounded. Damping is usually caused by an air bubble in the line or by myocardial dysfunction. Each pressure wave can be divided into systolic and diastolic areas. Normally, the ratio of the two areas is greater than 0.65 to 0.80.[34] Lower ratios are associated with subendocardial ischemia.

The position of the dicrotic notch on the pressure wave is an indication of peripheral vascular resistance. Normally, the notch appears one third the distance down the descending limb of the pressure wave in older children. In young infants, the dichrotic notch will be in the upper half of the pressure wave. When the peripheral vascular resistance is relatively low (e.g., arteriovenous malformations, patent ductus arteriosus, hypovolemia), the position of the dicrotic notch is lower on the descending limb of the waveform. The slope of the diastolic pressure is steeper than normal because there is insufficient time for the aorta and other arteries to constrict before a major portion of the blood runs out of the systemic arteries into the low-pressure circuit. A similar blood pressure tracing is seen in patients whose blood volumes are inadequate. Figure

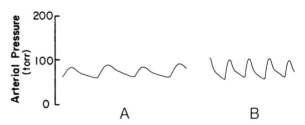

FIGURE 11–5. A damped and a normal arterial blood pressure tracing. *A,* Damped tracing has a more flattened upstroke, a rounded peak, and a more flattened downstroke to the pressure wave. *B,* The normal pressure tracing has a rapid upstroke and a dicrotic notch that occurs about one third the distance down the descending limb of the pressure wave. The rapid upstroke is indicative of good myocardial contractility. The normal position of the dicrotic notch is suggestive of a normal intravascular volume and peripheral vascular resistance. (Compare with Fig. 11–6, an arterial pressure tracing from a hypovolemic patient.)

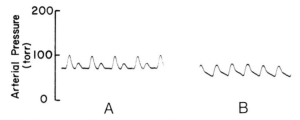

FIGURE 11–6. Arterial pressure tracing from a hypovolemic patient before (A) and after (B) blood volume replacement. The patient was able to maintain a normal blood pressure (A) by vasoconstriction, but note that the dicrotic notch was absent. Replacing blood, 10 ml/kg, returned the arterial blood pressure tracing to normal.

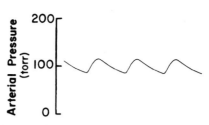

FIGURE 11–8. Arterial pressure tracing from an infant with myocarditis. Note the poor upstroke of the pressure wave, the narrow pulse pressure, the absence of a dicrotic notch, and the slow runoff of blood during diastole.

11–6 shows the effect of blood volume on the position of the dicrotic notch and the shape of the arterial pressure waveform.

Figure 11–7 shows the effects of breathing on the arterial blood pressure tracing. During spontaneous or mechanical breathing, the systolic and diastolic pressures vary slightly. When patients are hypovolemic and mechanically ventilated, these changes are magnified. Initially, the positive airway pressure forces blood out of the pulmonary circulation into the left atrium and ventricle, which raises the arterial pressure for two to three beats. At the same time, the positive pressure in the lung interferes with venous return, which reduces the arterial pressure of subsequent beats. During exhalation, the airway pressure decreases, and the venous return, cardiac output, and arterial blood pressure increase. A normal blood volume minimizes these changes. Similar blood pressure changes can occur when a pneumothorax or other pulmonary gas leak is present.

The upstroke of the pressure wave is an indication of left ventricular contractility (i.e., dp/dt). Under normal conditions, it is nearly vertical. When contractility is decreased (myocardial dysfunction, hypotension), the upstroke becomes more horizontal (Fig. 11–8). In some infants, initiation of effective mechanical ventilation reduces fluctuations in arterial blood pressure because of a reduction in spontaneous breathing.[35]

Central Venous Pressure

The central venous pressure (CVP) of infants and children is normally 3 to 12 cm H_2O. Pressures higher than this suggest abnormal right heart filling pressure.[36] CVP is easily measured with a strain-gauge whose diaphragm is at the level of the right atrium or with a fluid-filled column. However, the latter should not be used repeatedly in infants because each measurement infuses an additional 1 to 2 ml of fluid. Over the course of several hours the patient may become overhydrated. Because small blood and fluid losses significantly decrease the atrial filling pressure of children, CVP should be measured continuously, not intermittently. The rapidity with which the CVP decreases in young children following blood loss is impressive (Fig. 11–9). Central venous lines usually are inserted into the subclavian, the external jugular, or the internal jugular vein. For long-term monitoring, subclavian vein catheters are usually more comfortable for the patient because they allow greater freedom of movement. However, insertion of subclavian vein catheters can be associated with a relatively high complication rate in infants and children,[37] although this has not been my experience. One life-threatening complication is cardiac tamponade caused by a catheter perforating the vena cava or the atrium. Central venous lines placed in the operating room may be associated with a significant number of complications including arterial puncture, pneumothoraces, hemothoraces, and superior venal cava syndrome.[38] Catheters placed in the subclavian vein were less likely to cause complications than those inserted into the internal jugular vein. It is often useful to use the Site-Rite, an ultrasonic device that allows the vein to be visualized before a catheter is inserted.

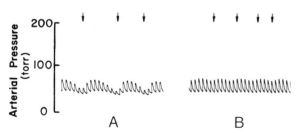

FIGURE 11–7. Effects of positive-pressure ventilation on the arterial pressure tracing before (A) and after (B) administering whole blood (15 ml/kg) to a hypovolemic infant. Arrows mark inspiration. Note the marked decrease in pressure (A) when the patient was hypovolemic. The decrease in arterial pressure with each breath was considerably less after the blood transfusion (B).

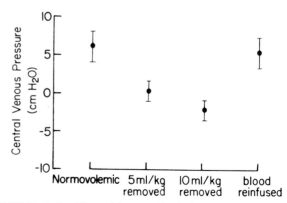

FIGURE 11–9. Rapidity and degree with which the central venous pressure decreases in young children during phlebotomy and reinfusion of blood.

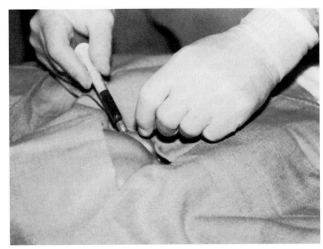

FIGURE 11-10. Technique for inserting a subclavian line in a small child. The index finger of the operator's left hand is on the child's chin. The needle has entered just under the clavicle. It is important to start more laterally in the young child than one does in the adult or it will be difficult to get the needle under the clavicle. Care must be taken to avoid cannulating the subclavian artery because injecting small amounts of air or clot into this artery may cause cerebral ischemia.

Figure 11-10 shows the technique for inserting subclavian catheters. If for some reason it is not feasible to insert a catheter into the subclavian vein, one can usually be inserted into an external or internal jugular vein (Fig. 11-11).[39] In my experience, internal jugular vein punctures are more likely to cause a pneumothorax because the cupula of the infant's lung rises higher in the neck. If the needle is inserted too medially, the trachea or carotid artery can be punctured. The complication rate of inserting either a subclavian or internal jugular line decreases as experience inserting these lines increases. The CVP tracing from an infant has the same components as that of adults, including "a" and "v" waves.

Pulmonary Artery Pressure

Many desperately ill surgical patients require pulmonary artery pressure (PAP) monitoring.[40] A 3.5-, 5.0-, or 7.0-Fr catheter is used, depending on the size of the patient. All three catheters have two lumens and can be used to measure cardiac output. The catheter should be connected to a strain-gauge to measure phasic and mean pressures continuously. Figure 11-12 shows normal phasic and wedge pulmonary artery pressure tracings from a 3-kg infant. It is not wedged. This picture of a normal tracing should be permanently etched in the memory of everyone who uses these catheters, because a catheter that remains wedged for more than a few minutes may infarct all or part of a lung. *Permanent wedging* is more likely to occur in small children because the catheter occupies most of the main pulmonary artery in which it is located, and movement of the catheter by less than 2 cm may move it into the wedge position. To avoid permanently wedging pulmonary artery catheters in infants, the catheter tip should be kept in the main pulmonary artery and the balloon should not be inflated. Pulmonary artery catheters are inserted in the same sites and manner as central venous catheters. Thermodilution car-

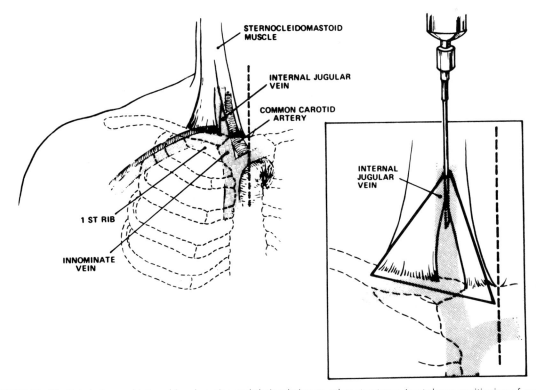

FIGURE 11-11. Subclavian and internal jugular veins and their relation to other structures. *Inset* shows positioning of needle for insertion into an internal jugular vein. The needle tip should be directed toward the right nipple. (From Prince S, Sullivan L, Hackel A: Percutaneous catheterization of the internal jugular vein in infants and children. Anesthesiology 44:170, 1976.)

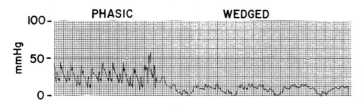

FIGURE 11–12. Pulmonary artery pressure tracing from an infant. Note the phasic changes on the left. They disappear when the catheter is in the wedge position (*right*).

diac output can be measured in patients who weigh more than 3 kg. These measurements correlate well with cardiac outputs determined by Fick or dye-dilution methods.[41–44] Repeated measurements of cardiac output may cause overhydration of small children because 3 to 10 ml of fluid is required for each determination.

Cardiac Output

The clinical estimation of cardiac output and peripheral perfusion is not a science but an art, and is one of the most important skills in all of medicine. Cardiac output provides tissue perfusion. Therefore, tissue perfusion is used as evidence of cardiac output. If tissue perfusion is adequate, the skin temperature is warm all the way to the fingers and toes (Fig. 11–13). If blood volume is reduced by 5 percent, the extremity becomes cold at midforearm or midcalf. This change in temperature is circumferential and of the glove-and-stocking type. If the skin becomes cool at midthigh or midupper arm, approximately 10 percent volume depletion is present. If the trunk is warm and the entire extremity is cool from the axilla and groin outward, there is 15 percent or more volume depletion.

These are imperfect estimates of blood volume but are clinically quite useful.

Pulses are also good indicators of peripheral perfusion. The pulses in the feet and wrists of most pediatric patients are 2+ to 3+. With 5 percent volume depletion, the pulses in the wrists and feet decrease to 0 to 1+. Brachial pulses are usually present. With 10 percent volume depletion the brachial pulses are absent or severely reduced, but groin and axillary pulses are still present. With 15 percent volume depletion, axillary and groin pulses are weak and thready.

Urine output decreases early with volume loss. Five percent volume depletion decreases urine volume slightly below the lower limits of normal (more than 0.75 ml/kg/h). With 10 percent volume depletion, the patient is oliguric. He or she is anuric when the blood volume is reduced by 15 percent.

The arterial blood pressure is often within normal limits despite 10 percent volume depletion. The heart rate may be constant and within the normal range. Rudolph et al.[45] showed that sick infants have fixed heart rates of approximately 150 bpm. As they recover, their heart rates vary. Infants and young animals lose their baroreceptor

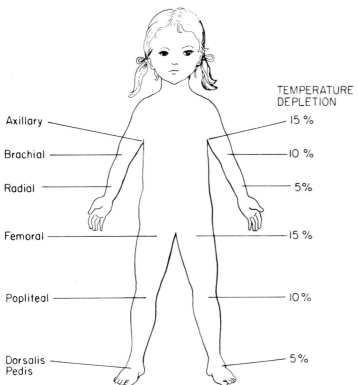

Pulses	Temperature Depletion
Axillary	15 %
Brachial	10 %
Radial	5 %
Femoral	15 %
Popliteal	10 %
Dorsalis Pedis	5 %

FIGURE 11–13. Relation between skin temperature (*right*) and pulses (*left*) and the percentage of blood volume depletion (percent). See text for explanation.

responses with approximately 0.5 minimum anesthetic concentration (MAC) halothane.[46, 47] The baroresponses are also significantly attenuated by fentanyl 10 μg/kg.[48] Therefore, a heart rate within the normal range does not necessarily indicate normal blood volume.

Urine specific gravity of more than 1.009 is associated with hypotension (systolic pressure decrease > 30 percent of control) in more than 50 percent of neonates.[49]

RESPIRATORY MONITORING

Blood Gases and pH

The blood gases and pH of sick children should be determined during surgery because these variables are often abnormal. Monitoring of oxygenation is especially important in preterm infants who are susceptible to retinopathy of prematurity (ROP)[50] (see Chapter 14). Although it is unknown what Pao_2 causes ROP, the retinal vessels of these neonates certainly constrict maximally with a Pao_2 of 100 mm Hg.[51] To reduce the likelihood of ROP, the Pao_2 should be maintained in the normal range (50 to 70 mm Hg) or the oxygen saturation (Sao_2) between 87 percent and 93 percent when infants less than 44 weeks' gestation are anesthetized.[52] This Pao_2 provides adequate oxygenation, but even these levels of oxygenation may represent hyperoxia in premature infants. Their Pao_2 in utero should be 30 to 40 mm Hg.

Blood gas samples are usually not obtained from the brachial or femoral arteries, because the former has been associated with nerve damage and the latter has been associated with femoral head necrosis and limb shortening. If only one or two blood gas determinations are required, blood usually can be obtained from a radial artery with a 1-ml syringe and 25-gauge needle or with a heparin-filled butterfly needle. An arterial line should be inserted (see above) if more than two or three blood gas determinations are required during surgery or the postoperative period. Table 11–5 shows the normal blood gas and pH values for pediatric patients.

It has become possible to measure blood gases continuously with small Clark or Severinghaus electrodes attached to the skin with a double-backed sticky electrode ring (Fig. 11–14).[53–55] The electrodes are heated to 44°C to dilate underlying capillaries, increase their blood flow, and shift the oxygen dissociation curve to the right, thus displacing oxygen from hemoglobin. This increases the oxygen concentration on the skin surface. The oxygen diffuses into the electrode, where it is reduced and converted to an

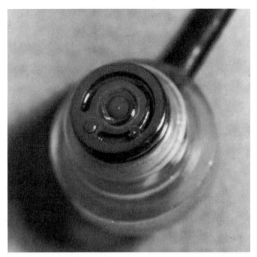

FIGURE 11–14. Combined skin oxygen and carbon dioxide electrode. (Courtesy of Dr. John W. Severinghaus.)

electrical signal. The 95 percent response to a step change in oxygen occurs in about 15 seconds. The amount of heat required to maintain the electrode and skin at a constant temperature is a function of blood flow under the electrode. The greater the flow, the more rapidly heat is carried away, and vice versa. To maintain the temperature constant, heat must be added to the system.

These electrodes are more accurate in infants less than 1 year of age because they have a greater capillary density per cubic centimeter of skin than older patients. The more capillaries, the more oxygen there is to be released. As infants grow older, their skin cornifies, the distance oxygen molecules must travel to reach the electrode increases, and the skin's oxygen consumption increases. For these reasons, $TcPo_2$ is a better trend monitor than a true indicator of Pao_2 in older patients.[54]

$TcPo_2$ electrodes are most accurate when the Pao_2 is 30 to 150 mm Hg (Fig. 11–15).[55] Their accuracy can be improved outside this range by calibrating the electrode

TABLE 11–5
BLOOD GASES AND pH IN PEDIATRIC PATIENTS

Age	Pao_2 (mm Hg)	$Paco_2$ (mm Hg)	pH (mm Hg)
Preterm	60 ± 8	37 ± 6	7.37 ± 0.03
Term	70 ± 11	39 ± 7	7.40 ± 0.02
1 mo	95 ± 8	40 ± 6	7.41 ± 0.04
1 y	93 ± 10	41 ± 7	7.39 ± 0.02

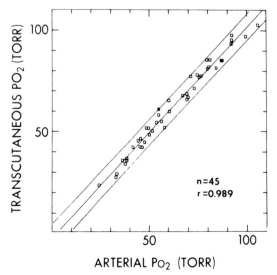

FIGURE 11–15. Relation between transcutaneous Po_2 and arterial Pao_2.

in the expected range of Pa_{O_2}. Calibration is simple and rapid. In most instances, it is done by placing the electrode in humidified room air and setting the P_{O_2} to the atmospheric P_{O_2} (150 mm Hg at sea level). Failure to create an airtight seal between skin and electrode allows air to insinuate itself under the electrode, which makes the TcP_{O_2} greater than the Pa_{O_2} if the Pa_{O_2} is lower than 150 mm Hg. If the Pa_{O_2} is higher than that of air (150 mm Hg), the TcP_{O_2} will be lower than the Pa_{O_2}.

If the body temperature is less than 35.5°C or the mean arterial pressure is more than 2 SD below the average for patients of that age, the electrode does not accurately reflect the Pa_{O_2}.[55] Both of these conditions constrict large proximal arteries and arterioles. This constriction cannot be overcome by local heating. When a vasodilator such as tolazoline (Priscoline) is infused, skin blood vessels dilate maximally and local heating cannot further increase flow.[56] In effect, blood is "stolen" from under the electrode and TcP_{O_2} is lower than Pa_{O_2}.

Transcutaneous electrodes also can be used for continuous monitoring of the P_{CO_2} on the skin surface (TcP_{CO_2}).[56] These miniature Severinghaus electrodes are attached in the same manner as TcP_{O_2} electrodes. Unlike TcP_{O_2} electrodes, TcP_{CO_2} electrodes are unaffected by arterial pressure, body temperature, or drugs, but they are affected by air leaks. They are easily calibrated with known CO_2 concentrations and have a 95 percent response time of approximately 2 minutes. At 44°C, TcP_{CO_2} tends to be high by an amount equal to the skin's metabolic rate. This factor can easily be taken into account by the electronic design of the device.

Anesthesia affects the accuracy of TcP_{O_2} but not the accuracy of TcP_{CO_2} electrodes.[57] Halothane and nitrous oxide are reduced by TcP_{O_2} electrodes, which falsely elevate TcP_{O_2}. This effect can be overcome by polishing the electrode, offsetting the applied voltage to 500 mV, and changing the electrolyte.[58, 59] Another solution is to use an anesthetic that is not reduced. Forane has less effect on TcP_{O_2} than halothane and nitrous oxide, although it does have some effect (J. W. Severinghaus, personal communication). Any hypotension or hypothermia caused by the anesthetic affects the accuracy of the electrode (see above). Both sources of inaccuracy can be reduced or eliminated by anesthetizing infants, especially preterm infants, with fentanyl (Sublimaze) 10 to 50 $\mu g/kg$.[60]

Pulse oximetry allows continuous monitoring of oxygenation.[61, 62] Arterial oxygen saturation compares pulsatile changes in two wavelengths of light transmitted through the finger, ear, hand, nose, or other tissue; one wavelength is at about 660 μm (red) and the other at 940 μm (infrared). The pulsating vascular bed expands and relaxes, which creates a change in the light path length and modifies the amount of light detected. The amplitude of the detected light depends on the size of the arterial pulse change, the wavelength of light used, and the oxygen saturation of arterial hemoglobin. Because the detected waveform is from arterial blood, the amplitude at each wavelength and Beer's law (with factors derived from in vitro measurement of oxygen saturation) allow measurement of arterial blood oxygen saturation without interference from venous blood, skin, connective tissue, or bone. Pulse oximeters require no heating and no user calibration. There is good correlation between measurement of oxygen saturation made in vitro and in vivo and these values are similar between 70 and 100 percent saturation. Below this range, most of these devices fail to reliably detect and display the Sa_{O_2}.[63] Failures occur in both directions. Sometimes the displayed Sa_{O_2} is lower than the true Sa_{O_2},[64] and sometimes it is higher.[65] Some machines deal with rapidly falling Sa_{O_2} by defaulting to zero Sa_{O_2}. Vasoconstriction of the arm or hand causes a lag in the time it takes the Sa_{O_2} to reach a plateau. Therefore, the displayed Sa_{O_2} may not reflect beat-to-beat Sa_{O_2} during rapid changes in oxygenation.

Pulse oximetry accurately reflects the Sa_{O_2} of infants and children of all ages when the Sa_{O_2} is above 70 percent. It is much less accurate in severely hypoxic infants.[66] Under certain circumstances the devices may show a normal Sa_{O_2} when the patient is hypoxic.[67] Because there is a wide standard deviation for Pa_{O_2} versus Sa_{O_2} in premature infants, it is best to keep the Sa_{O_2} between 87 and 92 percent to reduce the likelihood of ROP.

Sa_{O_2} is valuable for detecting hypoxemic episodes during anesthesia. Cote et al.[68] showed that experienced anesthesiologists detected oxygen desaturation much sooner by pulse oximetry than by other means.

A significant problem with pulse oximeters is the difficulty of ensuring that the two diodes are aligned opposite one another in neonates, especially premature neonates. Slight movement of the diode on the skin causes the device to fail, as does the electrocautery. Because these devices fail so often, there is a tendency to disbelieve them when they indicate that the Sa_{O_2} is low. The appropriate response is to believe the oximeter and to determine if the patient is hypoxemic by some other means. The pulse oximeter is also a valuable tool for detecting hyperoxia in infants.[69] In a small percentage of patients the oximeter suggested that the patient was hyperoxic when this was not the case. Fetal hemoglobin, carbon monoxide, or methemoglobinemia have no effect on the accuracy of the pulse oximeter, but inotropes increase the difference between Sp_{O_2} and Sa_{O_2}.[70]

Pulse oximeters can injure the skin of some infants.[65, 71, 72] In at least one study, injury occurred when the probe was placed on the pulp of the toe. Placing the probe over the nail resulted in no further injury. Severe burns have been reported when standard pulse oximeters were used during magnetic resonance imaging (MRI).[65] This usually occurs when the oximeter cable is coiled inside the magnet, which induces current and heat. This problem is best prevented by using a fiberoptic pulse oximeter (Nellcor, Hayward, CA), but it may be difficult to apply this device to the extremity of small children. It often takes persistence to obtain accurate measurements.

End-Tidal Gases

Monitoring end-tidal gases gives early warning of changes in inspired oxygen, expired carbon dioxide, and anesthetic concentrations (see Chapter 9). The characteristics of these systems and their uses have been reviewed elsewhere.[73] The response time of the system must be rapid enough to obtain end-tidal samples in spontaneously breathing babies. If the end-tidal CO_2 (ET_{CO_2}) tracing has a plateau during expiration (Fig. 11–16), the response of the catheter and system is usually adequate. The flow rate of the catheter should equal approximately 60 percent of the tidal volume. If the flow rate is too high, inspired gas is entrained, and the measured concentration is a mixture of both inspired and expired gas. There is usually a 2- to 10-mm Hg (average, 5 mm Hg) difference between end-tidal and arterial $PaCO_2$ during anesthesia. The larger differences result from increased wasted ventilation. $ETCO_2$ measurements are especially useful for patients undergoing sitting craniotomy, in whom a sudden decrease in $ETCO_2$ is usually indicative of an air embolus. When the decrease is first detected, the surgery should be stopped and the site of air entry sought (see Chapter 16). The decrease in $ETCO_2$ often occurs before a murmur is heard, the blood pressure decreases, or changes are noted in the ECG.

Measurement of the end-tidal and inspired anesthetic gas concentrations enables the anesthesiologist to follow the rapidity with which these parameters approach each other. It is surprising how quickly this difference narrows in small infants.[74]

The accuracy of $ETCO_2$ measurements depends on whether the gas sample is obtained from the tracheal or ventilator end of the endotracheal tube (ETT), especially when the patient weighs less than 12 kg.[75] Samples obtained from the tracheal end of the ETT are more reliable than those obtained from the proximal end.[61] This also is true during mechanical ventilation.

Correlation between end-tidal and arterial $PaCO_2$ is especially poor in sick infants.[76] The correlation between $PaCO_2$ and $ETCO_2$ is best when otherwise normal neonates are ventilated with rates below 20 breath/min, tidal volumes of 15 ml/kg, and the gas sample is obtained from the tracheal end of the ETT. These slow ventilation rates often require the application of a positive end-expiratory pressure (PEEP) of 2 to 5 cm H_2O to avoid atelectasis. Because $ETCO_2$ is an important adjunct in the detection of malignant hyperthermia,[77, 78] we should attempt to obtain the best end-tidal samples possible. However, it is the rapid increase in $ETCO_2$, not the absolute level of CO_2, that is important. Therefore, even poorly correlated end-tidal and arterial $PaCO_2$ values still would be useful.

METABOLIC MONITORING

Metabolic changes are common in infants and children during surgery, but frequently are not appreciated because we fail to look for them. Some intraoperative "sinking spells" and cardiac arrests are related to metabolic events, especially hypocalcemia or hypoglycemia. Sick infants, especially those who have been hypoxemic, are frequently hypocalcemic (< 8.0 mg/dl), but this seldom manifests in the form of ECG changes.[79–82] The primary effects of hypocalcemia are reduction of arterial blood pressure and cardiac output (decreased peripheral perfusion, capillary filling, and pulses) and development of cardiomegaly. Alkalosis (hyperventilation) worsens the effects of hypocalcemia because it reduces the ionized calcium fraction. Administration of calcium gluconate 100 to 200 mg/kg over 2 to 3 minutes raises the serum calcium concentration, but this effect may last only 10 to 15 minutes. If

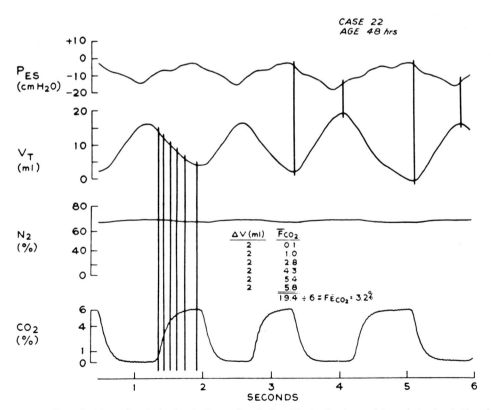

FIGURE 11–16. Carbon dioxide tracing during inspiration and expiration. The tracing has a plateau during inspiration. (Courtesy of Dr. W. H. Tooley.)

so, another dose and a continuous infusion of calcium gluconate 100 to 400 mg/kg/day may be needed. After the initial calcium bolus, it is usually better to infuse calcium continuously than to give repeated boluses of the drug, because infusion maintains a more constant serum calcium concentration. When calcium is added to solutions, they should be infused at a constant rate and should never be used to replace third-space losses. Other fluids and blood should be infused separately. Calcium should be infused into scalp or other small veins only if the infusion site is in plain view at all times. Inadvertent infusion of calcium into the skin or subcutaneous tissue causes tissue necrosis.[83] An infant who was hypocalcemic preoperatively is likely to be hypocalcemic during surgery. Therefore, the serum calcium concentration should be redetermined if the procedure lasts more than an hour or if the patient is hypotensive for unknown reasons. Determination of the ionized calcium concentrations is easily done on most modern blood gas machines.

Hypoglycemia (< 40 mg/dl) also is a common occurrence in small infants, especially in those who are preterm, small for gestational age, or hypoxemic. Although some authors have considered a serum glucose of 20 mg/dl normal, better feeding regimens have shown this belief to be incorrect.

Hypoglycemia is also common in sick infants and children.[84, 85] As pointed out by Berry (see Chapter 21), the infant's maximum renal tubular clearance (TM) for glucose, especially that of the preterm infant, is low. Therefore, a serum glucose level of 125 to 150 mg/dl often causes glycosuria and dehydration. In some infants, hyperglycemia occurs even when as little as 2.5 percent glucose is infused. Table 11–6 shows the blood and urine glucose concentrations of term and preterm infants during surgery and anesthesia. Note that few of these infants were actually hypoglycemic, which confirms the findings of others.[86] Most infants were hyperglycemic and had a good urine output despite the fact that some of them were hypotensive. To detect hyper- or hypoglycemia during anesthesia, blood glucose concentrations should be measured periodically with a glucometer, a blood gas machine, or Dextrostix. Blood for this test should not be drawn from intravenous (IV) lines that contain glucose because doing so will cause falsely high values. Glucose that has "stuck" to the walls of the tubing is released if blood with a lower glucose concentration is withdrawn through the tubing. Blood for this test should be obtained by fingerstick or from an arterial line if possible. Attempts should be made to maintain the infant's blood glucose between 45 and 90 mg/dl

by infusing the daily fluid requirements, including the glucose requirements of 5 to 7 mg/kg/min, and piggybacking other fluids and blood into this line or giving them through a separate IV line. However, even this amount of glucose may increase the blood glucose to unacceptable concentrations. Because of the concern about the adverse effects of hyperglycemia on the ischemic brain,[87–89] glucose should only be administered during surgery to normal infants and children if their blood glucose concentration is low. If the procedure lasts more than 1 hour, measure the blood glucose concentration. Only if the glucose concentration is below normal for age should glucose be added to the IV fluid (Table 11–7). Glucose *is* given to neonates and to sick infants (as described above), and the glucose concentration is measured intermittently to determine if more or less glucose is needed.

Infants and children coming to surgery may be hypoglycemic if they have been given nothing by mouth (NPO) for many hours. However, when they are fed up to 4 hours before surgery the glucose concentration remains within the normal range.[90–92] Some anesthetics (halothane, thiopental, ketamine) increase the blood glucose concentration in young patients and cause hyperglycemia.[92] Therefore, it is necessary to measure the patient's blood glucose concentration to be sure that it is adequate.

URINE OUTPUT

Urine output should be monitored during surgery when large blood loss or extracellular fluid shifts are expected or when the surgery is expected to last more than 4 to 6 hours. This is usually done in infants with either a straight catheter or a 5- or 8-Fr feeding tube. Beyond the newborn period, a Foley catheter can be used. The catheter should be connected to a sterile closed drainage system to reduce infection. Urine collecting bottles should be graduated finely enough to allow measurement of 1 ml of urine. Urine output should normally exceed 0.75 ml/kg/h. In most instances, it exceeds 1 ml/kg/h. If the urine glucose concentration exceeds 2+, the blood glucose concentration should be determined.

BLOOD LOSS

It is difficult to determine blood loss accurately in infants and small children, but it can be done. Suction tubing should be kept as short and narrow as possible. The col-

TABLE 11 – 6
BLOOD AND URINE GLUCOSE CONCENTRATIONS IN TERM AND PRTERM INFANTS DURING SURGERY (% OF PATIENTS)

Age	% of Patients by Urine* Results				% of Patients by Blood[†] Results (mg/dl)		
	Negative	*2+*	*3+*	*4+*	*45–90*	*130–175*	*≥250*
Preterm	50	20	15	15	40	50	10
Term	70	14	10	6	66	20	25

* Labstix
[†] Dextrostix

TABLE 11 – 7

EFFECT OF ADDING GLUCOSE TO INTRAVENOUS FLUID OF INFANTS AND CHILDREN DURING SURGERY*

Age	Glucose Concentration (mg/dl)			
	Ringer's Lactate		D-5 Ringer's Lactate	
	Infants	Children	Infants	Children
Preoperative Anesthesia	78 ± 12	95 ± 13	76 ± 9	87 ± 13
20 min	88 ± 20	122 ± 17	143 ± 18	147 ± 38
60 min	78 ± 12	93 ± 18	201 ± 39	186 ± 37
120 min	81 ± 15	93 ± 12	213 ± 41	158 ± 32

* Glucose was added when the intravenous infusion was started in those receiving glucose. Infants were 1 week to 1 year of age. Children were 1 to 7 years of age.

lecting bottle should be small. The amount of fluid used to clear suction tubing and to irrigate the wound should be measured, recorded, and subtracted from the total volume of liquid in the bottle. The gradations on the bottle used for blood collection from neonates and infants should be small enough to estimate a 1-ml volume change.[93] The amount of blood on sponges and laparotomy drapes can be estimated by weighing the drapes or sponges when dry and again after use. The difference in weight is because of blood. If laparotomy drapes are wetted before use, the added weight must be taken into account. It is often difficult to estimate accurately the blood lost in the drapes, but a constant attempt should be made. The volumes of blood lost and of fluid administered should be determined and recorded at least every 15 minutes (more often if the blood loss is rapid), to avoid getting ahead or behind on either. It is helpful to write the blood loss on the wall or some other convenient place so that it is available to all members of the team. The nurse can usually do this each time the sponges are weighed.

TEMPERATURE

The temperature of infants and children should be measured to prevent hypo- or hyperthermia. Hyperthermia is now more common during surgery than hypothermia because the "holy grail" of pediatric anesthesia has been to prevent hypothermia. This is the correct thing to do, as it turns out (see Chapter 4). Temperature should be measured continuously via the axilla, skin, esophagus, and tympanic membrane and kept between 36° and 37°C.[94] There appears to be no clinically important difference among the temperatures measured in the rectum, esophagus, tympanic membrane, or axilla.[95] Rectal temperatures should not be measured in infants weighing less than 3 kg because their bowel can be perforated by the temperature probe or thermometer. This has occurred so often in the past that the American Academy of Pediatrics recommends against it. When esophageal temperatures are measured, the probe must be soft and flexible to avoid esophageal perforation and ulcers. Tympanic membrane temperature monitoring has proven useful.[96] However, inserting the probe too far can perforate the eardrum.

Infants maintain their body temperature by metabolizing brown fat under the influence of norepinephrine.[97, 98] Mitochondrial uncoupling protein and a form of iodothy-

ronine are also important in this process.[99] Infants seldom shiver, and they lose heat more readily than adults because the ratio of their surface area to body weight is high (see Chapter 4). Anesthesia with fentanyl and propofol allow peripheral vasoconstriction to occur when the core temperature decreases to 36°C. There is no effective increase in metabolism of brown adipose tissue.[100] Neonates who suffer birth asphyxia have less ability to initiate nonshivering thermogenesis than nonasphyxiated neonates.[101]

Hypothermia slows awakening and recovery from anesthesia and increases $Paco_2$ because anesthetic solubility is increased at lower temperatures and the patients hypoventilate. Metabolic acidosis develops as the result of atelectasis and hypoxemia. Hypoxemia reduces the ventilation of young patients rather than increases it, as occurs in older patients. This leads to apnea or periodic breathing,[102] especially in preterm infants who are less than 3 months beyond term. Infants who have been or are hypothermic have more difficulty eating than patients who are normothermic.[103] They are more apt to vomit or regurgitate food and to aspirate it into their lungs, and they are also more prone to dehydration because they drink inadequately and develop a diuresis. Bissonnette and Sessler[104] reported that mild hypothermia, about 35.5°C, was not associated with delayed recovery from anesthesia or with apnea or hypoxia. They also showed that active or passive warming of the inspired gases tended to maintain normal body temperatures during anesthesia.[105, 106] The thermo-regulatory thresholds differed between halothane and isoflurane in 5- to 50-kg children.[107, 108] These studies were done in larger infants and children rather than in neonates. The results of similar studies may differ in younger patients. Recent data suggest that hypothermia is associated with increased infections.[109]

To avoid hypothermia, the room should be warmed to 30° to 37°C, depending on the size of the infant. The smaller the patient, the higher the room temperature should be. Infants should be placed under an infrared heater (Fig. 11–17).[110] The infant's head also should be covered with a thermal cap[111] and the extremities wrapped with sheet wadding (Fig. 11–18). Preparation solutions should be warmed to body temperature. Covering the patient with plastic drapes maintains the body temperature better because it traps the body heat in a much smaller space and prevents it from radiating to the environment. Placing a heating pad under the patient and setting the pad at 36° to 37°C reduces conductive heat loss. Warming and fully

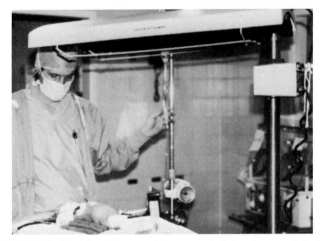

FIGURE 11–17. Infrared heater with servo control placed over an infant to monitor body temperature during induction of anesthesia.

humidifying the inspired gases at 32° to 37°C significantly reduces heat loss during anesthesia[103–117] and prevents damage to the tracheal mucosa as well.[118] If all of these measures are used, the body temperature remains normal or, as often happens, rises. It is usually possible to decrease the room temperature so that it is comfortable for the staff after the patient is draped for surgery. Care also must be taken to maintain the infant's body temperature normal in the recovery room.

INTRACRANIAL PRESSURE

Surgery is commonly performed on infants and children who have increased intracranial pressure. This necessitates measuring the intracranial pressure to avoid potentially dangerous increases in pressure (see Chapter 16).

TRANSESOPHAGEAL ECHOCARDIOGRAPHY

In the past few years transesophageal echocardiography (ECHO) monitoring has become well established in adults and has proven to be very useful for infants undergoing cardiac surgery.[119] Improvement in equipment has made this possible. The primary use of TEE has been during cardiac surgery, where it is used to detect whether the repair is complete. However, it also has been shown to provide relatively accurate indications of cardiac index.[120] When more anesthesiologists are trained to use TEE and the probes are made smaller and easier to insert, the use of TEE will increase in patients who will have marked changes in their blood volumes and cardiac output during other types of surgery. Uniplane probes of 6.9 to 9.0 mm are now available and are used in infants and children to provide information about ventricular function and the structure of the heart. TEE is especially useful during surgery to corroborate the preoperative diagnosis, detect inadequate surgical repairs, and evaluate patients postoperatively in the intensive care unit (ICU). There are several excellent reviews of TEE and its uses in pediatric patients.[121–123]

Most TEE studies in children are performed in anesthetized or heavily sedated patients. The head is usually placed in the midline, and the lubricated transducer tip is advanced through the hypopharynx into the esophagus. The tip of the probe is positioned correctly by using real-time imaging as the probe is advanced. TEE is superior to transthoracic echocardiography for identifying normal and abnormal systemic and pulmonary venous connections[124–126] and can be used to diagnose anomalous pulmonary venous drainage in infants[126] or for performing Rashkind procedures in the neonatal intensive care unit.[121] Single-plane TEE poorly detects residual pulmonic insufficiency or stenosis because it inadequately images the right ventricular outflow tract.[127, 128] This problem is solved by biplanar TEE.[121]

Few complications of TEE have been reported. Bleeding, esophageal rupture or injury, hoarseness or aphonia, and other complications are rare. Bronchial obstruction has been reported,[128] as has severe bronchospasm.[120] With the advent of more sophisticated devices, TEE is likely to become as widely used in infants as it is in adults. The most important development is a commercially available biplanar probe of sufficiently small size for routine use in infants and children.

Hickey[129] raised a very important question. Is it appropriate for anesthesiologists to decide whether a cardiac repair is adequate on the basis of interpretation of TEE? How much training is required for competency? Most hospitals have solved this problem by having a cardiologist and/or echocardiographer present in the operating room or available on call to determine if there are residual lesions.

BISPECTORAL INDEX

Bispectoral index (BIS) is a relatively new method of monitoring the depth of anesthesia. The review by Ira Rampil is excellent for understanding the use of this device.[130] This device is applied to the scalp. There is a good correlation between the depth of anesthesia and BIS.[131] Using sufficient inhaled anesthetics to produce low BIS values is

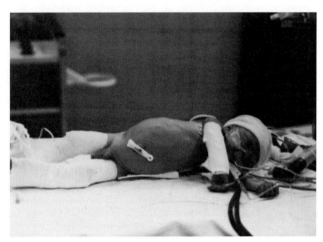

FIGURE 11–18. Arms and legs of an infant are wrapped with sheet wadding and the head is covered with a stockinette cap to reduce heat loss during anesthesia and surgery.

associated with a low incidence of movement in response to stimulation.[132] There was no difference in the BIS values between infants 0 to 2 years of age and children 2 to 12 years of age.[132] The sevoflurane concentration for a BIS of 50 was significantly higher in the infants than in the children studied. BIS also has been shown to correlate well with oxygenation associated with interruption of cerebral blood flow in infants and adults.[133] This promising method of monitoring anesthetic depth deserves much more study in infants and children.

REFERENCES

1. Cullen SC: Anesthesia. Year Book Med Anesthesiol 28:396, 1967.
2. Eisselle J, Trenchard D, Stubbs J, et al: The immediate cardiac depression by anaesthetics in conscious dogs. Br J Anaesth 41:86, 1969.
3. Cooper JO, Cullen BF: Observer reliability in detecting surreptitious random occlusions of the monaural esophageal stethoscope. J Clin Monit 6:271, 1990.
4. Van R, Arts CM, Hopman JC, et al: The influence of respiratory distress syndrome on heart rate variability in very preterm infants. Early Hum Dev 27:207, 1991.
5. Rudolph AM: Congenital Heart Disease. Chicago, Year Book Medical Publishers, 1974.
6. Bruner JMR: Hazards of electrical apparatus. An improved standard blood pressure cuff size. Clin Pediatr 15:784, 1976.
7. Nicodemus HF, Nassiri-Rahimi C, Bachman L, Smith TC: Median effective dose (ED$_{50}$) of halothane in adults and children. Anesthesiology 31:344, 1969.
8. Dias JH, Lockhart CH: Is halothane really safe in infancy? Anesthesiology 51:S313, 1979.
9. Friesen RH, Henry DB: Cardiovascular changes in preterm neonates receiving isoflurane, halothane, fentanyl, and ketamine. Anesthesiology 64:238, 1986.
10. Myung K, Kawabori I, Guntheroth WG: Need for an improved standard blood pressure cuff size. Clin Pediatr 15:784, 1976.
11. Burch GE, Shewey L: Sphygmomanometric cuff size and blood pressure recording. JAMA 225:1215, 1973.
12. Hill GE, Machin RH: Doppler determined blood pressure recordings: the effect of varying cuff sizes in children. Can Anaesth Soc J 73:323, 1976.
13. Ramsey M III: Noninvasive blood pressure monitoring methods and validation. In Gravenstein JS, Newbauer RS, Ream AK, et al (eds): Essential Noninvasive Monitoring in Anesthesia. Orlando, FL, Grune & Stratton, 1980, p 37.
14. Park MK, Menard SM: Accuracy of blood pressure measurement by the Dinamap monitor in infants and children. Pediatrics 79:907, 1987.
15. Spinazzola RM, Harper RG, de Soler M, Lesser M: Blood pressure values in 500- to 750-gram birthweight infants in the first week of life. J Perinatol 11:147, 1991.
16. Hochberg HM, Saltzman MB: Accuracy of an ultrasound blood pressure instrument in neonates, infants and children. Curr Ther 13:482, 1971.
17. Waltemath CL, Preuss DD: Determination of blood pressure in low-flow states by the Doppler technique. Anesthesiology 34:77, 1971.
18. Kitterman JA, Phibbs RH, Tooley WH: Catheterization of umbilical vessels in newborn infants. Pediatr Clin North Am 17:895, 1970.
19. Pearse RG: Percutaneous catheterization of the radial artery in newborn babies using transillumination. Arch Dis Child 53:549, 1978.
20. Butt WW, Gow R, Whyte H, et al: Complications resulting from use of arterial catheters: retrograde flow and rapid elevation of blood pressure. Pediatrics 76:250, 1985.
21. Dahl MR, Smead WL, McSweeney TD: Radial artery cannulation: a comparison of 1.52- and 4.45-cm catheters. J Clin Monit 8:193, 1992.
22. Tollner U, Bechinger D, Pohlandt F: Radial nerve palsy in a premature infant following long-term measurement of blood pressure. J Pediatr 96:921, 1980.
23. Hack WW, Vos A, van der Lei J, Okken A: Incidence and duration of total occlusion of the radial artery in newborn infants after catheter removal. Eur J Pediatr 149:275, 1990.
24. Rais-Bahrami K, Karna P, Dolanski EA: Effect of fluids on life span of peripheral arterial lines. Am J Perinatol 7:122, 1990.
25. Gardner RM: Direct blood pressure measurements—dynamic response requirements. Anesthesiology 54:227, 1981.
26. Brown DR, Fenton LJ, Tsang RC: Blood sampling through umbilical catheters. Pediatrics 55:227, 1975.
27. Miyasaka K, Edmonds JF, Conn AW: Complications of radial artery lines in the paediatric patient. Can Anaesth Soc J 23:9, 1976.
28. Saladino R, Bachman D, Fleischer G: Arterial access in the pediatric emergency department. Ann Emerg Med 19:382, 1990.
29. Lowenstein E, Little JW, Lo HH: Prevention of cerebral embolization from flushing radial artery cannulas. N Engl J Med 285:1414, 1971.
30. Thibeault DW, Emmanuilides GC: Patent ductus arteriosus complicating the respiratory distress syndrome in preterm infants. J Pediatr 86:120, 1975.
31. Schick JB, Beck AL, DeSilva HN: Umbilical artery catheter position and intraventricular hemorrhage. J Perinatol 9:382, 1989.
32. Kemply ST, Gamsu HR: Randomised trial of umbilical arterial position: Doppler ultrasound findings. Arch Dis Child 67:855, 1992.
33. Kitterman JA: Fatal air embolism through an umbilical venous catheter. Eur J Pediatr 131:71, 1979.
34. Hoffman JIE, Buckberg GD: The myocardial supply-demand ratio: a critical review. Am J Cardiol 41:327, 1978.
35. Goldstein RF, Brazy JE: Fluctuations of arterial blood pressure decrease with mechanical ventilation in premature infants with respiratory distress syndrome. J Perinatol 10:267, 1990.
36. Rudolph AM, Drorbaugh JE, Auld PAM, et al: Studies on the circulation in the neonatal period: the circulation in the respiratory distress syndrome. Pediatrics 27:551, 1961.
37. Groff DB, Ahmed N: Subclavian vein catheterization in the infant. J Pediatr Surg 9:171, 1974.
38. Johnson EM, Saltzman DA, Suh G, et al: Complications and risks of central venous catheter placement in children. Surgery 124:911, 1998.
39. Prince S, Sullivan L, Hackel A: Percutaneous catheterization of the internal jugular vein in infants and children. Anesthesiology 44:170, 1976.
40. Archer G, Cobb LA: Long term pulmonary artery pressure monitoring in the management of the critically ill. Ann Surg 180:747, 1974.
41. Moodie DS, Feldy RH, Kaye MP, et al: Measurement of cardiac output by thermodilution: development of accurate measurements at flows applicable to the pediatric patient. J Surg Res 25:305, 1978.
42. Freed MD, Keane JF: Cardiac output measured by thermodilution in infants and children. J Pediatr 92:39, 1978.
43. Mathur M, Harris EA, Barratt-Boyes BG: Measurement of cardiac output by thermodilution in infants and children after open-heart operations. J Thorac Cardiovasc Surg 72:221, 1976.
44. Notterman DA, Castello FV, Steinberg C, et al: A comparison of thermodilution and pulsed Doppler cardiac output measurement in critically ill children. J Pediatr 115:554, 1989.
45. Rudolph AJ, Vallbona C, Desmond MM: Cardiodynamic studies in the newborn. III. Heart rate patterns in infants with idiopathic respiratory distress syndrome. Pediatrics 36:551, 1965.
46. Ware R, Robinson S, Gregory GA: The effect of halothane on the baroresponses of adult and baby rabbits. Anesthesiology 56:28, 1982.
47. Gregory GA: The baroresponses of preterm infants during halothane anesthesia. Can Anaesth Soc J 29:105, 1982.
48. Murat I, Levron JC, Berg A, Saint-Maurice C: Effects of fentanyl on baroreceptor reflex control of heart rate in newborn infants. Anesthesiology 68:717, 1988.
49. Robinson S, Gregory GA: Urine specific gravity as a predictor of hypovolemic and hypotensive response to halothane anesthesia in the newborn [abstract]. Am Soc Anesth Abst 37:123, 1978.
50. Stark DJ, Manning LM, Lenton L: Retrolental fibroplasia today. Med J Aust 1:275, 1981.
51. Lucey JF, Dongman B: A reexamination of the role of oxygen in retrolental fibroplasia. Pediatrics 73:82, 1984.
52. Koch G, Wendel H: Adjustment of arterial blood gases and acid base balance in the normal newborn infant during the first week of life. Biol Neonate 12:136, 1968.
53. Huch R, Huch A, Albani M, et al: Transcutaneous PO$_2$ monitoring in routine management of infants and children with cardiorespiratory problems. Pediatrics 57:681, 1976.

54. Gothgen I, Jacobsen E: Transcutaneous oxygen tension measurements. I. Age variation and reproducibility. Acta Anaesthesiol Scand Suppl 67:71, 1978.
55. Peabody JL, Gregory GA, Willis MM, Tooley WH: Transcutaneous oxygen tension in sick infants. Am Rev Respir Dis 118:83, 1978.
56. Hansen T, Tooley WH: Skin surface carbon dioxide tension in sick infants. Pediatrics 63:942, 1979.
57. Gothgen I, Jacobsen E: Transcutaneous oxygen measurement. II. The influence of halothane and hypotension. Acta Anaesthesiol Scand Suppl 67:71, 1978.
58. Severinghaus JW, Weiskopf RB, Nishimura M, Bradley AF: Oxygen electrode errors due to polarographic reduction of halothane. J Appl Physiol 31:640, 1971.
59. Thunstrom AM, Severinghaus JW: Problems of calibration and stabilization of tcPO$_2$. Acta Anaesthesiol Scand Suppl 68:55, 1978.
60. Robinson S, Gregory GA: Fentanyl-air-oxygen anesthesia for ligation of patent ductus arteriosus in preterm infants. Anesth Analg 60:331, 1981.
61. Payne JP, Severinghaus JW (eds): Pulse Oximetry. Berlin, Springer-Verlag, 1986.
62. Severinghaus JW, Naifeh KH: Accuracy of response of six pulse oximeters to profound hypoxia. Anesthesiology 67:551, 1987.
63. Francone S: Reliability of pulse oximetry in hypoxic infants. J Pediatr 112:424, 1988.
64. Severinghaus JW, Naifeh KH, Koh SO: Errors in 14 pulse oximeters during profound hypoxia. J Clin Monit 5:72, 1989.
65. Poets CF, Wilken M, Seidenberg J, et al: Reliability of a pulse oximeter in the detection of hyperoxemia. J Pediatr 122:87, 1993.
66. Costarino AT, Davis DA, Kean TP: Falsely normal saturation reading with the pulse oximeter. Anesthesiology 67:830, 1987.
67. Wasuna A, Whitlaw AGL: Pulse oximetry in preterm infants. Arch Dis Child 62:957, 1987.
68. Cote CJ, Goldstein EA, Cote MA, et al: A single blind study of pulse oximetry in children. Anesthesiology 68:184, 1988.
69. Canet J, Ricos M, Vidal F: Early postoperative arterial oxygen desaturation. Determining factors and response to oxygen therapy. Anesth Analg 69:207, 1989.
70. Rajadurai VS, Walker AM, Yu VY, Oates A: Effect of fetal haemoglobin on the accuracy of pulse oximetry in preterm infants. J Paediatr Child Health 28:43, 1992.
71. Pettersen B, Kongsgaard U, Aune H: Skin injury in an infant with pulse oximetry. Br J Anaesth 69:204, 1992.
72. Sobel DB: Burning of a neonate due to a pulse oximeter: arterial saturation monitoring. Pediatrics 89:154, 1992.
73. Kirpalani H, Kechagias S, Lerman J: Technical and clinical aspects of capnography in neonates. J Med Eng Technol 15:154, 1991.
74. Salanitre E, Rakow H: The pulmonary exchange of nitrous oxide and halothane in infants and children. Anesthesiology 30:388, 1969.
75. Badgwell JM, McLeod ME, Lerman J, Creighton RE: End-tidal PCO$_2$ measurements sampled at the distal and proximal ends of the endotracheal tube in infants and children. Anesth Analg 66:959, 1987.
76. Watkins HMC, Weindling AM: Monitoring of end tidal CO$_2$ in neonatal intensive care. Arch Dis Child 62:837, 1987.
77. Neubauer KR, Kaufman RD: Another use for mass spectrometry: detection and monitoring of malignant hyperthermia. Anesth Analg 64:837, 1985.
78. Dunn CM, Maltry DE, Eggers GWN Jr: Value of mass spectrometry in early diagnosis of malignant hyperthermia. Anesthesiology 63:333, 1985.
79. Tsang RC, Donovan EF, Steichen JJ: Calcium physiology and pathology in the neonate. Pediatr Clin North Am 23:611, 1976.
80. Baltrop D: Neonatal hypocalemia. Postgrad Med 51:7, 1975.
81. Robertson NRC, Smith MA: Early neonate hypocalcemia. Arch Dis Child 50:604, 1975.
82. Peterson AW, Jacker LM: Neonatal tetany during anesthesia: a case report. Anesth Analg 52:555, 1973.
83. Brown AS, Hoelzer DJ, Piercy SA: Skin necrosis from extravasation of intravenous fluids in children. Plast Reconstr Surg 64:145, 1979.
84. Pagliara AS, Karl I, Haymond M, Kapnis DM: Hypoglycemia in infancy and childhood. I. J Pediatr 82:365, 1973.
85. Pagliara AS, Karl I, Haymond M, Kapnis DM: Hypoglycemia in infancy and childhood. II. J Pediatr 82:558, 1973.
86. Stafford M, Jean A, Pascucci R: Pre- and post-induction blood glucose concentrations in healthy, fasting children [abstract]. Anesthesiology 63A:350, 1985.
87. Pulsinelli WA, Levy DE, Sigsbee B, et al: Increased damage after ischemic stroke in patients with hyperglycemia with or without established diabetes mellitus. Am J Med 74:540, 1983.
88. Ginsberg MD, Welsh FA, Budd WW: Local cerebral blood flow and glucose utilization. Stroke 11:347, 1980.
89. Welsh FA, Ginsberg MD, Rieder W, Budd WW: Deleterious effect of glucose pretreatment on recovery from diffuse cerebral ischemia in the cat. Stroke 11:355, 1980.
90. Thomas DKM: Hypoglycemia in children before operation: its incidence and prevention. Br J Anaesth 46:66, 1974.
91. Morrice JJ, Taylor KM, Blair JI, Young DG: Preoperative plasma glucose level. Arch Dis Child 49:898, 1974.
92. Kaniaris P, Kyoniatis LM, Kastanas E: Serum free fatty acid and blood sugar levels in children under halothane, thiopentone, and ketamine anaesthesia (comparative study). Can Anaesth Soc J 22:509, 1975.
93. Jones JF: Measuring blood loss in the pediatric patient. Anesthesiology 39:462, 1973.
94. Benzinger TH: Clinical temperature. JAMA 209:1200, 1969.
95. Bissonnette B, Sessler DI, LaFlamme P: Intraoperative temperature monitoring sites in infants and children and the effect of inspired gas warming on esophageal temperature. Anesth Analg 69:192, 1989.
96. Benzinger M: Tympanic thermometry in surgery and anesthesia. JAMA 209:1207, 1969.
97. Silverman WA, Sinclair JC: Temperature regulation in the newborn. N Engl J Med 274:92, 1966.
98. Sinclair JC: Heat production and thermoregulation in the small-for-date infant. Pediatr Clin North Am 17:147, 1970.
99. Houstek J, Vizek K, Pavelka S, et al: Type II iodothyronine 5'-deiodinase and uncoupling protein in brown adipose tissue of human newborns. J Clin Endocrinol Metab 77:382, 1993.
100. Plattner O, Semsroth M, Sessler DI, et al: Lack of nonshivering thermogenesis in infants anesthetized with fentanyl and propofol. Anesthesiology 86:772, 1997.
101. Schubring C: Temperature regulation in healthy and resuscitated newborns immediately after birth. J Perinat Med 14:27, 1986.
102. Chernick V, Heldrich F, Avery ME: Periodic breathing in premature infants. J Pediatr 64:330, 1964.
103. Hacket PR, Crosby RMN: Some effects of inadvertent hypothermia. Anesthesiology 21:356, 1960.
104. Bissonnette B, Sessler DI: Mild hypothermia does not impair postanesthetic recovery in infants and children. Anesth Analg 76:168, 1993.
105. Bissonnette B, Sessler DI: Passive or active inspired gas humidification increases thermal steady-state temperatures in anesthetized infants. Anesth Analg 69:783, 1989.
106. Bissonnette B, Sessler DI, LaFlamme P: Passive and active inspired gas humidification in infants and children. Anesthesiology 71:350, 1989.
107. Bissonnette B, Sessler DI: Thermoregulatory thresholds for vasoconstriction in pediatric patients anesthetized with halothane or halothane and caudal bupivacaine. Anesthesiology 76:387, 1992.
108. Bissonnette B, Sessler DI: The thermoregulatory threshold in infants and children anesthetized with isoflurane and caudal bupivacaine. Anesthesiology 73:1114, 1990.
109. Hollyoak MA, Ong TH, Leditschke JF: Critical appraisal of surgical venous access in children. Pediatr Surg Int 12:177, 1997.
110. Levison H, Linsao L, Swyer PR: A comparison of infra-red and convective heating for newborn infants. Lancet 2:1346, 1966.
111. Marks KH, Devenyi AG, Bello ME, et al: Thermal head wrap for infants. J Pediatr 107:956, 1985.
112. Chalon J, Simon R, Ramanathan S, et al: A high-humidity circle system for infants and children. Anesthesiology 49:205, 1978.
113. Rashad K, Benson DW: Role of humidity in prevention of hypothermia in infants and children. Anesth Analg 46:712, 1967.
114. Berry FA Jr, Hughes-Davies DI, Di Fazio CA: A system for minimizing respiratory heat loss in infants during operation. Anesth Analg 53:170, 1973.
115. Bennett EJ, Patel KP, Grundy EM: Neonatal temperature in surgery. Anesthesiology 46:303, 1977.
116. Gard GP: Humidification of the Rees-Ayre T-piece system for anesthesia. Anesth Analg 52:207, 1973.
117. Baker JD, Wallace CT, Brown CS: Maintenance of body temperature in infants during surgery. Anesth Rev 4:21, 1977.
118. Chalon J, Leow DA, Malebranche J: Effects of dry anesthetic gases on tracheobronchial ciliated epithelium. Anesthesiology 37:338, 1972.

119. Lam J, Neirotti RA, Lubbers WJ, et al: Usefulness of biplane trans-esophageal echocardiography in neonates, infants and children with congenital heart disease. Am J Cardiol 73:625, 1994.

120. Murdoch IA, Marsh MJ, Tibby SM, McLuckie A: Continuous haemo-dynamic monitoring in children: use of transesophageal Doppler. Acta Paediatr 84:761, 1995.

121. Ritter SB: Transesophageal real-time echocardiography in infants and children with congenital heart disease. J Am Coll Cardiol 18:569, 1991.

122. Weintraub R, Shiota T, Elkadi T, et al: Transesophageal echocardiog-raphy in infants and children with congenital heart disease. Circula-tion 86:711, 1992.

123. Chaliki HP, Click RL, Abel MD: Comparison of intraoperative trans-esophageal echocardiographic examinations with the operative findings: prospective review of 1918 cases. J Am Soc Echocardiogr 12:237, 1999.

124. Nanda NC, Pinheiro L, Sanyal R, et al: Transesophageal echocardio-graphic examination of left-sided superior vena cava and azygos and hemiazygos veins. Echocardiography 8:73, 1991.

125. Strumper OFW, Seeram N, Elzenga NJ, Sutherland G: Diagnosis of atrial sinus by transesophageal echocardiography. J Am Coll Cardiol 16:442, 1990.

126. Stumper O, Vargus-Barron J, Rijilaarsdam M, et al: Assessment of anomalous systemic and venous connections by transesophageal echocardiography in infants and children. Br Heart J 66:411, 1991.

127. Muhiudeen IA, Roberson DA, Silverman NH, et al: Intraoperative echocardoigraphy for evaluation of congenital heart defects in in-fants and children. Anesthesiology 76:165, 1992.

128. Stumper OF, Elzenga NJ, Hess J, Sutherland GR: Transesophageal echocardiography in children with congenital heart disease: an initial experience. J Am Coll Cardiol 16:433, 1990.

129. Hickey PR: Transesophageal echocardiography in pediatric cardiac surgery [letter]. Anesthesiology 77:610, 1992.

130. Rampil IJ: A primer for EEG signal processing in anesthesia. Anesthe-siology 89:980, 1998.

131. Denman WT, Swanson EL, Rosow D, et al: Pediatric evaluation of the bispectral index (BIS) monitor and correlation of BIS with end-tidal sevoflurane concentration in infants and children. Anesth Analg 90:872, 2000.

132. Sebel PS, Lang E, Rampil IJ, et al: A multicenter study of bispectral electroencephalogram analysis for monitoring anesthetic effect. Anesth Analg 84:891, 1997.

133. Pithan C, Mazariegos M, Solomons NW, Furst P: Monitoring of fluid changes in hospitalized, malnourished, Guatemalan children using bioelectrical impedance spectroscopy (BIS). Appl Radiat Isot 49:615, 1998.

12

Pediatric Regional Anesthesia

NAVIL F. SETHNA
CHARLES B. BERDE

◆   ◆   ◆

In the past two decades, there has been considerable progress in the understanding of infants' and children's perception of pain and responses to pain.[1] A parallel noteworthy advancement has occurred in the knowledge of anatomy, physiology, and pharmacology of regional anesthetic techniques in infants and children. Some of these techniques are now an integral part of perioperative and procedure-related pain management in children of all ages.[2]

Regional anesthesia has been used for children since the beginning of the 20th century. Early enthusiasts published accounts of their success with the use of regional anesthesia in infants and children who were considered poor risk and unfit for general anesthetics available then.[3,4] Pediatric regional anesthesia was thus used originally in high-risk situations with insufficient understanding of its physiologic and pharmacologic effects. This led to a significant incidence of complications and consequent disfavor.[5] The advent of safer general anesthetic agents and techniques in 1950s led to further reluctance in considering regional anesthesia for children. In the late 1970s, the interest in pediatric regional anesthesia in the United States was renewed after reintroduction of spinal anesthesia as a safe alternative to general anesthesia in high-risk premature infants,[6] and with the realization that peripheral nerve blocks and epidural single-shot injections or infu-

sions provided postoperative analgesia with an excellent safety profile.

Wide application and increased experience with regional anesthetic techniques in children in the last two decades have earned these techniques a central place in pediatric anesthetic care. As with adults, a major impetus for use of regional anesthesia is to improve postoperative pain management, to reduce opioid-related side-effects, and to accelerate recovery.

In the adult literature, there are several situations in which prospective studies have shown regional techniques to improve outcome relative to general anesthesia and systemic analgesics.[7-10] Controlled outcome studies in children are more limited, though several studies that suggest benefit in clinical outcomes will be summarized below.

Pediatric regional blockade is frequently used as an adjunct to general anesthesia or administered as a sole anesthetic in awake or sedated patients for short peripheral surgical procedures of less than 2 hours. For more extensive procedures, it is now common practice to use general anesthesia supplemented with continuous epidural infusions of local anesthetics, either alone or in combination with an opioid or other additives such as clonidine.

Although most of the available regional techniques used in adults have been tried in children, individual techniques should be selected for a particular child based on consideration of risks and benefits.

INDICATIONS AND CONTRAINDICATIONS

Indications

There are relatively few absolute indications for regional anesthesia in children, and the decision to employ these techniques in particular cases will be influenced greatly by local technical expertise; expectations of patients, parents, and surgical colleagues; and other factors. Situations in which we frequently utilize regional anesthesia without a general anesthetic or under light sedation include the following:

1. Children and adolescents who dread being made unconscious or the loss of self-control under general anesthesia (though some of these children will also become distressed when they experience sensory and motor blockade).
2. Children with a family history of malignant hyperthermia.[11]
3. Hypotonic infants and children with neuromuscular diseases who may have reduced respiratory reserve and weakened pharyngeal or laryngeal reflexes.
4. Premature infants with a history of apnea undergoing inguinal hernia repair or other procedures below the T10 dermatome.
5. Children and adolescents with chronic airways diseases including asthma and cystic fibrosis.
6. Cooperative older children and adolescents for emergency peripheral procedures following recent intake of food.

Contraindications

Assuming that the anesthesiologist has sufficient expertise in the particular block, the age of the child does not pose limitation to the performance of regional anesthesia safely. Absolute contraindications include the following:

1. Lack of parental consent.
2. Infection at the site of injection.

Relative contraindications include the following:

1. Lack of rapport or patient cooperation in older children. While it is legally sanctioned to perform regional block against a child's wishes but with parental consent, this course is almost never indicated. In children who are old enough to discuss matters (e.g., age 5 to 6 and above), it should be performed with prior discussion and agreement on the part of the patient.
2. Poorly controlled seizures.
3. Difficult airway. It has been argued that employment of a regional anesthetic implies the capacity to take control of the airway in the event of toxic reactions, and thus a difficult airway is a relative contraindica-

tion to performance of neural block. This issue depends on several factors, including the nature of the airway difficulty (i.e., presumed difficulty with mask ventilation vs. presumed difficult intubation), whether there is the possibility of a full stomach, the operative procedure planned, and the regional techniques under consideration. For example, the risk of loss of airway control is probably greater for spinal anesthesia for upper abdominal surgery than for an ankle block, caudal block, or "saddle" block for foot surgery.
4. Coagulopathy. In general, regional techniques are avoided in the presence of clinically significant coagulopathy. Experience with lumbar puncture in the presence of mild thrombocytopenia in oncology patients has a very low complication rate. In selected cases, it may be appropriate to use regional anesthesia in the presence of mild clotting abnormalities, or to consider infusion of platelets, frozen plasma, or other blood products immediately prior to performing the block.
5. Anatomic anomalies at the site of the injection such as spina bifida or other spinal defects. We found that the presence of congenital lumbosacral spinal anomalies does not preclude performance of safe epidural analgesia, provided that the preoperative neurologic status is documented and radiographs confirm normal vertebral anatomy at the level of entry into the epidural space. Local anesthetic spread in these patients may be unpredictable; carefully incremental dosing is recommended.[12]
6. Hypovolemia. Moderate hypovolemia can usually be corrected prior to undertaking regional block. Severe hypovolemia and ongoing blood loss are contraindications to major regional block.
7. Neurologic diseases. There is no evidence that properly conducted regional anesthesia worsens the progression of neurologic disorders. The consideration for avoiding regional anesthesia in certain of these states that are characterized by unpredictable exacerbations and remissions of the disease state, is that subsequent neuralgic deterioration occurring following neural block may be attributed to the block.[13] Where there is proper patient selection and patient education, conduction block can be used advantageously in patients with many stable and progressive neurologic or neuromuscular disorders, including cerebral palsy, myopathies, and neuropathies.

PHARMACOLOGY OF LOCAL ANESTHETICS IN INFANT AND CHILDREN

General Considerations

Pharmacology

Uptake, distribution, and elimination of local anesthetics in infants and children has received increasing study in recent years.[14-16] Only recently have attempts been made to objectively measure the clinical level of anesthesia and analgesia in children. Measurement of the extent of anesthetized spinal dermatomal segments is made difficult (1) intraoperatively, because most regional anesthetic techniques are performed in anesthetized, heavily sedated children; and (2) postoperatively, because reporting on the extent and quality of sensory block is not feasible for infants and preverbal children. Therefore, the determination of dose or volume response of local anesthetics for most regional techniques is based on either the maximal allowable safe dose in adults (milliliters or milligrams per kilogram body weight) or individual investigator's clinical experience in a subset of pediatric patients (Table 12–1).

The systemic absorption of local anesthetics varies with the regional blood flow and the magnitude of the fat content at the site of local anesthetic deposition and the administered dose of local anesthetic; absorption is very rapid from upper airway respiratory mucosa, interpleural space, and intercostal spaces. Sparse epidural fat in infants and children may be one factor in the rapid absorption and faster attainment of plasma peak level compared to adults; the larger the injected dose the greater the peak plasma levels (Table 12–1).[17–19]

The extracellular space is larger in neonates and infants than in adults (40 percent vs. 20 percent of the body weight); consequently, the initial dose of a local anesthetic is diluted in a larger volume of distribution, resulting in a relatively lower initial plasma peak concentration as compared to adults. Since most local anesthetic agents' pKa values are close to plasma pH 7.4, a considerable fraction of these agents are ionized and distributed in body water.[20]

PROTEIN BINDING

Neonates have lower concentrations of albumin and α_1-acid glycoprotein. This may lead to reduced protein binding of local anesthetics and dramatic increases in the concentration of free drug, which may potentially predispose to central nervous system (CNS) and cardiac toxicity.[14, 21, 22] The free fraction of bupivacaine in plasma is significantly higher in infants under the age of 2 months compared to older infants. The serum concentration of α_1-acid glycoprotein is even lower in preterm neonates, 50 percent less than that in term neonates.[23, 24] α_1-Acid glycoprotein is an acute phase protein, and its plasma concentration generally increases by two-fold following surgery. This increase in α_1-acid glycoprotein concentrations leads to increased protein binding, and may partially offset the risks associated with local anesthetic accumulation with prolonged infusions.[16, 25]

Hepatic degradation of amide-type local anesthetics is slower in newborns and reaches adult functional capacity by approximately 3 to 6 months of life. The elimination half-life is a function of volume of distribution and clearance. Thus, alteration in the half-life of elimination of a local anesthetic agent may be due to change in one or both of these parameters. Bupivacaine and lidocaine, the most commonly used local anesthetics in children, have prolonged elimination half-lives in infants below the age of 3 months (Table 12–2).

Duration of both spinal anesthesia and peripheral blocks appears shorter in infants compared with adults, and larger weight-scaled doses are required in infants to achieve the same extent of blockade. This could be due to a number of factors, including age-related changes in regional blood flow, changes in tissue fat content, and the effects of scaling for body size per se.[26, 27]

Infants, in comparison to adults, eliminate local anesthetics more slowly, have shorter duration of blockade, and require larger doses of anesthetic per kilogram to achieve blockade. Therefore, infants have a narrow therapeutic index for local anesthetics compared with adults: repeated administration of doses sufficient to achieve effective blockade poses a greater risk of systemic toxicity in infants compared with adults.[14, 28]

Spatial Disposition

The local anesthetics spread more freely in the epidural space of infants and young children than adults, presumably due to less dense epidural fat. This may also explain the ease with which the caudal-to-epidural catheters is threaded in this age group.[29, 30]

Neurodevelopmental Differences

Developmental changes in myelination of neural tracts may alter the action of local anesthetic in premature as well as full-term infants, although there are no specific clinical data regarding this point. Incomplete myelination of nerves could theoretically lead to greater susceptibility to neural block by local anesthetic agents. In vitro studies of excised mammalian nerves and sciatic nerves of newborn puppies give some support for this hypothesis.[31, 32] One recent study in infant and adolescent rats suggests that a specific antihyperalgesic (as opposed to conduction-blocking) effect of epidural bupivacaine occurs with more dilute concentrations in infant animals compared with adolescent animals.* However, in vivo studies of peripheral blockade and clinical studies of epidural infusions in rats do not consistently support the hypothesis that newborns and infants achieve blockade with either more dilute solutions or smaller volumes.[26]

Ester Local Anesthetics

Ester local anesthetics, especially chloroprocaine, have the attractive feature of rapid hydrolysis by plasma cholinesterases, with elimination half-lives of only minutes in adults. Neonates and infants up to 6 months of age have lower plasma cholinesterase activity, averaging approximately half of adult values.[33] Clearance of procaine and chloroprocaine may therefore be diminished somewhat in neonates, but even with half of adult cholinesterase activity, the rapid clearance of chloroprocaine makes it attractive for epidural infusions in neonates. An older paper recommended maximal doses of 7 mg/kg of chloroprocaine and 5 mg/kg of procaine.[34] Subsequently, we reported that 2-chloroprocaine can be used safely and effectively for continuous caudal anesthesia in much

---

*Richard Howard et al., Anesthesiology (in press).

T A B L E   1 2 - 1
RECOMMENDED DOSES AND VOLUMES OF LOCAL ANESTHETIC SOLUTIONS AND THEIR PHARMACOKINETIC PROFILES IN CHILDREN

Age	Route	Agent Concentration (%, w/v)	Dose (mg/kg)	Epinephrine	Maximum Plasma Levels (mean plasma level µg/ml)*	Peak Time (min)	βt 1/2 Hours**	References
4 months–12 years	Caudal	Bupivacaine 0.25%	3	—	1.6 (1.4)	15	NA	334
3.5–9 years	Caudal	Lidocaine 1%	5	—	2.5 (2)	28 ± 3	2.6 ± 0.5	37
5.5–10 years	Caudal	Bupivacaine 0.25%	2.5	—	1.6 (1.2)	29 ± 3	4.6 ± 0.5	43
1–6 months	Caudal	Bupivacaine 0.25%	2.5	—	1.9 (1.0)	28 ± 1	7.7 ± 2.4	22
2–11 years	Lumbar	Bupivacaine 0.5%	3	—	2.9 (1–2)†	12–30	NA	335
1.6–11.3 years	Lumbar	Bupivacaine 0.25%	1.7 ± 0.2	1:200,000	0.8 (0.64)	10–20	3.8 ± 0.6	336
3 months–4 years	Lumbar/thoracic	Lidocaine 1%	5 mg bolus 2.5 mg/kg/h for 5 h	—	<5	—	—	38
34–50 weeks postconceptual age	Intrathecal	Bupivacaine 0.5% (isobaric)	1 1	— 1:200,000	0.31 ± 0.2 0.25 ± 0.1	10 10	—	82
2–12 years	Paravertebral thoracic block	Lidocaine 1% bolus infusion	0.5 0.25 mg/kg/h	1:200,000	1.7–3.0 2.1–3.2 (steady state levels)	15–30 min at 8–10 h	—	209
2 days–5 months	Paravertebral thoracic block	Bupivacaine 0.25% Bupivacaine 0.125%	1.25 bolus 0.25 mg/kg/h	1:400,000	1.6 ± 0.7 at 48 h after infusion (3.1–3.3 in three infants)	—	—	216
3 months–16 years	Intercostal	Bupivacaine 0.5%	2 3 4	1:200,000 1:200,000 1:200,000	1.2 (0.8) 1.7 (1.4) 2.4 (2)	5–10 5–10 <5–10	2.5 ± 1.3	18
10.8 ± 6 years	Interpleural	Bupivacaine 0.25%	1.25–2.5 mg/kg/h	1:200,000	7 (1–2) (2.4–4)	12 h 24 h	NA	17
2–15 years	Axillary block	Bupivacaine 0.33% Bupivacaine 0.5%	2 3	—	2.7(1.4 ± 0.4) (1.8 ± 0.5)	22 ± 8 22 ± 11	NA NA	228

Age	Block/procedure	Local anesthetic	Dose (mg/kg)	Epinephrine	Peak plasma concentration	Time (min)		Reference
1–10 years	Ilioinguinal-iliohypogastric nerve block	Bupivacaine 0.25% or 0.5%	2	—	2.9 (1.4 ± 0.4)	26 ± 10	NA	249
1–10 years	Ilioinguinal-iliohypogastric nerve block	Bupivacaine 0.5%	1.25 (0.25 ml/kg)	—	1.5 ± 1 (10–15 kg) / 1 ± 0.3 (15–30 kg)	18 ± 5 / 16 ± 5		250
3–11 years	Dorsal penile nerve block	Bupivacaine 0.25%	0.5	—	0.27 ± 0.1	23 ± 5	—	337
1–14 years	Fascia iliacus block	Bupivacaine 0.25%	0.8 / 0.8	— / 1 : 200,000	Median 1.1 / Median 0.4	20 / 45		240
2–7 years	Femoral nerve block	Bupivacaine 0.5%	2	—	(0.9 ± 0.4)	24.4 ± 12.6	NA	236
1–5 years	Tracheal spray	Lidocaine 4%	4	—	10.3 (5.2–5.9)	Mean 6–11	NA	333
5 days–15 years	Subcutaneous	Bupivacaine 0.5% / Lidocaine 1%	2 / 4	— / —	0.5 / 2	15–20 / 10–20	NA / NA	19
Mean 6 years	Topical on skin lacerations	Tetracaine 0.5%, epinephrine 0.05%, and cocaine 11.8% (TAC)	3 ml		274 ng/ml-1	45–60‡		319
3–12 months	Topical on intact skin	Lidocaine and prilocaine cream (5% EMLA)	2 ml		131 ng/ml-1 (in 3–6 months) / 127 ng/ml-1 (in 6–12 months)	240‡		298
3 months–3 years	Laryngeal spray	Lidocaine 5%	0.9–2.6 (8 mg for < 10 kg and 16 mg for 10–20 kg body weight)		1 ± 0.6	12.6 ± 9		331
1.5 months–16 years	Nebulization via mask	Lidocaine 2%	4–8 mg/kg		0.24 ± 0.1 (less than 3 years) / 0.39 ± 0.1 (older than 3 years)			332

* Estimated venous blood concentration range potential for CNS toxicity is 2–4 μg/ml for bupivacaine and > 10 μg/ml for lidocaine.[20]

** $\beta t1/2$; elimination half-life

† Significant positive correlation between the peak plasma concentration and age > 3 years.

‡ Time at which the plasma concentrations of local anesthetics were measured.

TABLE 12–2
COMPARISON OF MEAN ELIMINATION HALF-LIVES (HOURS) OF LIDOCAINE AND BUPIVACAINE IN PEDIATRIC PATIENTS

Local Anesthetic Agents	Neonates	Infants (1–6 mo)	Children (3.5–10 yr)	Adults
Lidocaine	3.2	NA	2.5	1.6
Bupivacaine	8.1	7.7	4.5	3.5

NA, not available.
Data from Mazoit et al.,[22] Ecoffey et al.,[37] Mihaly et al.,[338] and Morgan et al.[339]

larger doses (loading doses of 30 mg/kg; 1 ml/kg of the 3 percent solution) given over 15 minutes, infusions of 30 to 60 mg/kg/h in a series of conscious former preterm infants undergoing inguinal hernia repair.[35] Despite the low plasma cholinesterase activity in some of our infants, no evidence of systemic toxicity was detected, and plasma chloroprocaine concentrations were uniformly low. Further studies in a large population of infants are warranted to assess the safety of epidural 2-chloroprocaine in neonates. The high infusion rates cited above in Henderson et al.'s study apply to awake caudal anesthesia to provide dense abdominal motor and sensory blockade; more dilute solutions and lower hourly dosing is recommended for postoperative use. We are unaware of toxicity data in infants and children for these two agents, nor are we aware of any incidence data regarding true allergies to these agents in children. We recommend use of preservative-free chloroprocaine formulations.

Tetracaine is mainly used for spinal anesthesia. Newborns and infants require larger doses on a kilogram basis than adults and the duration of action is shorter (see below).

Amide Local Anesthetics

Lidocaine

The effects of lidocaine in children (administered via several routes) have been studied. Finholt and co-workers[36] observed no difference in the distribution and elimination of intravenous lidocaine in children ages 0.5 to 3 years compared to adults. Neonates have an increased volume of distribution, a slight decrease in hepatic clearance (normalized per kilogram body weight), and a slight increase in urinary excretion of both metabolized and unmetabolized lidocaine. However, lidocaine administered via the epidural space has much longer terminal elimination half-life (mean value, 3.2 hours) in newborns relative to adults (1.8 hours).[37] Recommended initial maximum doses for lidocaine in newborns are slightly less than those for adults on a kilogram basis: 4 mg/kg without epinephrine, 5 mg/kg with epinephrine.[20] Preliminary data on short-term continuous epidural infusion of lidocaine in children 3 months to 4 years showed that the plasma concentration of lidocaine increased at a slower rate than its active metabolite MEGX, but remained below the toxic level of 5 μg/ml at the end of 5-hour infusion. During prolonged infusion of lidocaine, its metabolites may accumulate to produce tox-

icity even when total plasma lidocaine concentration remains within a safe range. Reduced protein binding may further predispose to systemic toxicity in neonates.[38, 39] Therefore, prolonged epidural lidocaine infusions in neonates and younger infants should be used with caution. Our provisional recommendation is that maximum infusion rates in neonates should not exceed 0.8 mg/kg/h.

Clinicians who employ topical lidocaine ointments, jellies, or sprays for topical use should limit total dosage to the recommended safe amounts for regional blockade, as there are reports of convulsions in children following their use.[40] For infants, this may require use of more dilute preparations for mucosal use (1 percent) or for infiltration (0.3 to 0.5 percent). Toxicity, as a function of age, has been studied systematically in a sheep model.[18] Issues related to pediatric local anesthetic toxicity are discussed elsewhere.[28, 41]

Bupivacaine

Bupivacaine has achieved great popularity for neural block for postoperative pain because of its prolonged duration of action and because of the ability to use concentrations (approximately 0.125 to 0.25 percent) that produce greater sensory than motor block.

Eyres et al.[42] and Ecoffey et al.[43] studied plasma concentrations of bupivacaine following caudal epidural administration of bupivacaine. Bupivacaine doses up to 3 mg/kg produced total plasma concentrations in a range generally regarded as safe (mean, < 2 μg/ml). In infants under age 6 months, the terminal half-life of bupivacaine following caudal epidural block with 2.5 mg/kg is significantly longer than that reported in older children (7.7 vs. 4.6 hours). In the younger infants, the maximum free plasma concentration was just below the range regarded as toxic in adults. Thus, we recommend restricting bupivacaine bolus dosing to 2 to 2.5 mg/kg. Bupivacaine's clearance is reduced in neonates. Epidural infusions of 0.4 mg/kg/h appear safe in children. Based on studies by Larsson et al.[16] and Mazoit et al.,[22] we recommend that infusions in neonates and infants less than 3 months of age should not exceed 0.2 mg/kg/h. Even at this low infusion rate, it is possible that infusions lasting more than 72 hours could result in accumulation of the drug and delayed toxicity.

Levobupivacaine

Levobupivacaine is an enantiomer of bupivacaine with slightly less arrhythmogenic and CNS toxicity than the same dose range of racemic bupivacaine in healthy volunteers. It produces a sensory and motor block for surgery similar to that of racemic bupivacaine, though some adult studies suggest a slightly longer duration of postoperative analgesia.[44, 45] Studies of levobupivacaine pharmacology in infants and children are ongoing; a preliminary study in children demonstrated that levobupivacaine is safe and effective for inguinal and iliohypogastric nerve blocks for pain management after hernia repair.[46]

Ropivacaine

Ropivacaine was recently introduced as a new amide local anesthetic with evidence for slightly less cardiotoxicity and a suggestion of slightly greater sensory selectivity in some studies, though not in others (see below).[47-51] Ropivacaine in infants and toddlers shows comparatively slow uptake from the epidural space into the circulation; measured clearances were slightly lower than those reported for bupivacaine. Our study of ropivacaine and bupivacaine in infant and adult rats supported the greater safety margin for ropivacaine, but found no difference in the durations of sensory versus motor blockade for the two agents in any age group.[27]

Local Anesthetic Test Dosing

Since regional anesthesia is commonly performed while children are anesthetized or sedated, symptoms of impending systemic toxicity may not be apparent. Accidental intravascular injection of local anesthetics under general anesthesia remains a significant risk.[52, 53] Negative aspiration does not always exclude intravascular placement of a needle or catheter because of the tendency of veins to collapse upon gentle aspiration. Hemodynamic changes following co-injection of epinephrine are the primary indicator of intravascular injection, and a series of studies have examined sensitivity and specificity of test dosing in children anesthetized with halothane, sevoflurane, and isoflurane.[54-56] Earlier work showed some false-negatives (lack of heart rate increase) among children anesthetized with halothane who were receiving a simulated intravenous test dose of 1 percent lidocaine 1 mg/kg and epinephrine 0.5 μg/kg dose (0.1 ml/kg lidocaine 1 percent with epinephrine 1:200,000); fewer false-negatives were found when the test doses was preceded by intravenous atropine. More recent studies suggest that the reliability of test dosing is improved by use of isoflurane or sevoflurane instead of halothane, by pretreatment with atropine, and by increasing the test dose of epinephrine from 0.5 to 0.75 μg/kg.[55-57] Combined consideration of sensitivity, specificity, and prevalence estimates leads to the conclusion that the reliability of a negative test (no heart rate increase) is high, but that a high percentage of positive tests (heart rate increases) will be false-positive indicators of intravascular placement.[58]

The lack of increase in heart rate in some cases of intravascular epinephrine injection has been ascribed to a baroreceptor-mediated slowing of heart rate in response to the blood pressure increase evoked by epinephrine. Intravascular injection of epinephrine can result in a significant blood pressure increase in those conditions where heart rate increases are dampened.[59] Thus, very frequent monitoring of blood pressure along with heart rate (HR) may increase the reliability of test dosing compared with monitoring heart rate alone.

Increases in T-wave amplitude of greater than or equal to 25 percent may be an indicator of intravascular placement and local anesthetic injection.[57, 60] The T-wave amplitude increase preceded an increase in HR by 10 seconds and was inversely related to age of the child.[57] Further controlled trials are needed to evaluate the ability to detect T-wave changes on routine electrocardiogram (ECG) monitor before T-wave changes can be recommended as a reliable marker.

Despite all of the above, there remains a small but unavoidable risk of false-negative test dosing and failure to detect an intravascular local anesthetic injection. Therefore, test dosing does not obviate the need for repeated aspiration and slow incremental dosing of local anesthetics in all major nerve blocks. With infiltration blockade or field blockade, constant movement of the needle through the field during injection helps to ensure that the needle does not remain in a vein long enough to administer a significant intravascular dose of drug.

Peripheral Nerve Stimulator

Accurate placement of a nerve block needle requires familiarity with regional anatomy and landmarks. However, difficulty arises when there is anatomic variation, deeply placed nerves, the anesthesiologist is unfamiliar with the block, or the child is uncooperative. An electrical nerve stimulator can be useful in finding any peripheral nerve that has a motor component. Eliciting paresthesias (mechanical nerve stimulation) and motor response to nerve stimulation (electrical stimulation) are aids to ensure close proximity of the needle tip to the neural tissue. Both procedures have limitations in adults as well as in children.[61]

Seeking a paresthesia is painful and may be frightening to an awake child who may not understand the concept of paresthesia. Lack of the child's cooperation and undue movement during the procedure may theoretically result in nerve tissue damage.

The use of a nerve stimulator allows localization of a nerve by electrical stimulation of the motor component only and is not associated with discomfort. Therefore, the child's cooperation is unnecessary and is suitable for an awake as well as a heavily sedated, developmentally impaired or anesthetized child. Since a smaller current is needed to depolarize a motor nerve than a sensory nerve, the evoked muscle contraction is pain-free. A high current should be avoided because it can depolarize nerves distant from the exploring needle and through thin fascial sheaths, particularly in infants. Therefore, an optimal current is essential for precise localization of the nerves and to achieve a successful block with minimum volume and dose of an anesthetic solution.

The desirable features in a nerve stimulator unit are the ability to provide a low constant current output. The motor fibers (large diameter) require a small current (usually 0.5 mA or less) and a lower frequency pulse (1 Hz of less than 1 msec duration) to initiate painless stimulation when the stimulating needle is as close as possible to the nerve.[62, 63]

Insulated needles are recommended because they deliver current density more selectively to the tip of a needle, affording more precise nerve localization.[64, 65] Standard noninsulated needles allow a part of the stimulating current to disperse along the shaft of the needle, depolarizing muscles or nerves along the course of the needle rather than at the tip, producing false localization and unpleasant direct muscle contraction.

Specialized nerve stimulator instruments are available, and some standard neuromuscular function (twitch) monitor units have a dual output capability, the low-output outlet serves for guiding peripheral nerve blockade. A peripheral nerve is stimulated when it lies in the path of the electrical current (positive and negative terminals). The negative polarity of a low-output socket of the standard neuromuscular monitor is connected to the metal hub or the shaft of a nerve-finding needle by an alligator clamp. The positive polarity is connected to the skin electrode (ground) away from the block field. The initial current used to locate a nerve is 1 to 2 mA. As the needle is advanced in the direction of the nerve, the current dial is gradually turned down to a minimum current of 0.5 mA and to produce a maximum motor response in the distribution of the nerve (i.e., optimal current). Injection of 1 to 2 ml of a local anesthetic should abolish the muscle contractions within seconds if the needle is in the precise vicinity of the nerve.

Our experience has been most favorable with Stimuplex-S Nerve Stimulator (Burron Medical Inc., Bethlehem, PA) which meets most requirements for an ideal nerve stimulator. It is capable of delivering a constant current of 0 to 10 mA (adjustable at 0.1-mA increments) and low-frequency rectangular impulse at a frequency of 0.5 to 2 Hz with a short pulse duration of 0.1 second. Conveniently, a wide range of needles of different sizes and lengths are available in individual packages or in procedural trays. These needles are of short bevel (45 degrees), Teflon-coated, disposable needle sizes (24-, 22-, 21-, and 20-gauge, 25 to 150 mm) and with preattached extension set and sterile cable connector to fit to the Stimuplex-S Nerve Stimulator (Burron Medical). A major disadvantage of specifically designed nerve stimulators is the higher cost as compared to the standard neuromuscular function monitors; but this could be viewed as a trade-off for greater electrophysiological accuracy, safety, and as an aid for teaching (Fig. 12–1).[66] A novel use of nerve stimulation for epidural catheter advancement is described below in the section Epidural Analgesia.

SPINAL ANESTHESIA

Spinal anesthesia has gained considerable acceptance among pediatric anesthesiologists and surgeons because,
unlike other regional techniques, its benefits are supported by randomized controlled trials in a small number infants. When spinal anesthesia is used alone, it provides satisfactory surgical anesthesia and lowers the incidence of postoperative bradycardia, desaturation, and apnea in preterm and former preterm infants.[67–69]

Indications

Indications include (1) surgical procedures involving extraperitoneal sites below the T10 dermatome such as inguinal hernia, circumcision, hypospadias repair, perineal surgery, and lower extremity procedures; (2) short procedures that do not exceed 1.5 to 2 hours; (3) preterm and former preterm infants under age 56 to 60 weeks postconceptional age, who are prone to develop apnea, bradycardia, and desaturation after general anesthesia[67, 68]; and (4) term infants younger than 44 weeks postconceptional age who are occasionally at risk for apnea after general anesthesia.[70–72] More recent case series report use of spinal anesthesia in more complex procedures in neonates including repair of meningomyelocele and primary closure of gastroschisis, as well as routine day-case surgery.[73–75]

The incidence of apnea after inguinal herniorrhaphy has been investigated in a small number of controlled trials. The incidence of apnea has varied widely among institutions probably because of different monitoring patterns used to detect the rate of apnea, as well as differences in anesthetic technique and drug selection.[76] Cote et al. conducted a pooled analysis of eight prospective studies of spinal anesthesia in infants to predict which infants are at risk.[76] The probability of apnea in nonanemic (hematocrit [Hct] >30 percent) infants with a postconceptual age of 48 weeks and a gestational age of 35 weeks or less at birth was estimated to be 5 percent. This estimated risk decreases to 1 percent at a postconceptual age of 54 weeks and a gestational age of 35 weeks or at postconceptual age of 56 weeks with a gestational age of 32 weeks. Anemia (Hct < 30 percent) was identified as an independent risk factor. The relative risk associated with factors such as

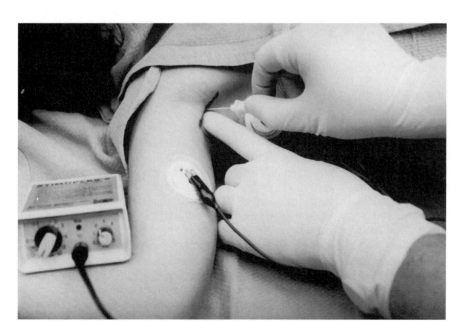

FIGURE 12–1. Axillary nerve block in a child using the Stimuplex-S Nerve Stimulator.

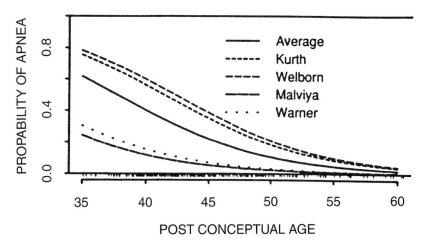

FIGURE 12–2. Predicted probability of apnea in recovery room and postrecovery room by weeks postconceptual age for all patients for each investigator. Bottom marks indicate the number of data points versus postconceptual age. (From Cote CJ, Zaslavsky A, Downes JJ, et al: Postoperative apnea in former preterm infants after inguinal herniorrhaphy. Anesthesiology 82:809, 1995.)

history of necrotizing enterocolitis, neonatal apnea, respiratory distress syndrome, bronchopulmonary dysplasia, or operative use of opioids and/or muscle relaxants could not be determined (Fig. 12–2).[76]

Anesthetic Solutions, Volumes, and Doses

As with adults, the most frequently administered solutions are hyperbaric tetracaine, bupivacaine, and lidocaine. Isobaric and hypobaric solutions have received less attention. Spinal anesthetic doses for infants and children are calculated safely on a body weight basis.[11,77] The local anesthetic dose requirement is much higher in infants and toddlers than in adults to achieve anesthesia of a given spinal segment. In our experience, 0.8 to 1 mg/kg of hyperbaric tetracaine in newborns gives a sensory spinal level ranging from T2 to T4, without hemodynamic instability or significant respiratory compromise.[78,79] Lower doses of tetracaine (≤0.65 mg/kg) are associated with a higher incidence of failure, due to insufficient cephalad spread of the drug and shorter duration of anesthesia. Inadequate spinal anesthesia may require repeat lumbar puncture, supplemental infiltration of local anesthetic, or intravenous analgesia

and general anesthesia.[6, 78–81] In older children, comparison of similar doses of hyperbaric and isobaric bupivacaine (0.5 percent) reported significantly higher success rate of motor and sensory block with a hyperbaric (96 percent) compared with isobaric solution (82 percent), although both solutions produced a similar initial median sensory block of T4.[73]

Several investigators have used isobaric and hyperbaric spinal bupivacaine with variable surgical durations and satisfactory level of spinal anesthesia (Table 12–3).[82–84]

The reasons for the higher requirement and the shorter duration of action of local anesthetics in infants compared to adults is unclear. Age-dependent differences in dose requirement has previously been ascribed to (1) a larger volume of cerebrospinal fluid (CSF) (≥4 mg/kg body weight in infants vs. ≤2 mg/kg in adults), and (2) a higher height to body weight ratio compared to body weight in infancy is seemingly a better predictor of dose requirement (Fig. 12–3).[85, 86]

There is only one study that measured the total plasma bupivacaine concentration after a spinal anesthetic dose of 1 mg/kg in infants with postconceptual ages of 34 to 50 weeks. The plasma concentrations were measured at 10 minutes after bupivacaine administration and were be-

	T A B L E 1 2 – 3			
LOCAL ANESTHETIC DOSES FOR INFANT SPINAL ANESTHESIA

Local Anesthetic Agent	Mean Dose (mg/kg)	Mean Sensory Block	Anticipated Mean Duration of Surgery (min)	References
Tetracaine 0.5% with 5% dextrose	0.4*	NA	86 ± 4	6,344
Tetracaine 0.5% with 5% dextrose and epinephrine (10–40 μg)	0.4–0.8†	T2-4	80–128	6,78,79,341
Bupivacaine 0.5% (isobaric) with epinephrine 1 : 200,000	0.8‡	T3.2 ± 1	80 (complete motor recovery)	
Bupivacaine 0.75% with dextrose 8.25% with epinephrine 20 μg	0.6‡	T3	< 75	83
Lidocaine 5% with dextrose 0.75% with epinephrine	3*	NA	56 ± 2.5	84
Bupivacaine 0.5% (isobaric)	0.3–0.5	T4 (T1-12)§ T4 (T1-7)§	125 (55–420)‖	340
Bupivacaine 0.5% with 8% dextrose	0.3–0.5		110 (53–270)‖	73

* For infants < 12 months.
† The higher dose is recommended for infants ≤ 5 kg body weight.
‡ For infants < 6 months.
§ Median (range).
‖ Median (range) time to first dose of rescue analgesic.

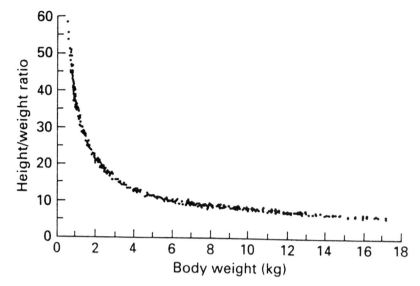

FIGURE 12–3. Change in height (cm) to body weight (kg) ratio in premature infants as they gain weight. (From Yamashita M, Kumagai M, Miyazono Y: Height to body weight ratio and spinal anaesthesia for ex-premature infants. Paediatr Anaesth 4:397, 1994. Blackwell Scientific Ltd, with permission.)

low the toxic levels. The mean concentration without epinephrine was 0.25 and with epinephrine 1:200,000 was 0.31 μg/ml. The free unbound maximum individual bupivacaine concentration was also below the acceptable values in adults (0.11 vs. 0.2 μg/ml).[82]

Duration of Spinal Anesthesia

Duration of spinal anesthesia in infants and young children is much shorter than in adults for a given weight-scaled dose. The duration is longer with larger doses of local anesthetics in infants and varies directly with the age of the child. In children younger than 1 year, the motor function returns in approximately 20 percent of the time needed for adults (Fig. 12–4). Addition of epinephrine to tetracaine increases the duration of the block by an average of 32 percent.[6] Similar correlation has been observed between duration of motor block and dose of spinal bupivacaine scaled to body weight (Table 12–3).[77, 83]

A prospective, double-blind, randomized study in older children reported no difference in the median duration of time to two-segment regression of block with isobaric and hyperbaric bupivacaine 0.5 percent, 80 minutes (30 to 190) in patients ages 2 to 115 months.[73]

Ventilatory Response

Careful monitoring of infants receiving spinal anesthesia is imperative, particularly among preterm infants with

bronchopulmonary dysplasia (BPD). A large dose of hyperbaric tetracaine (1 mg/kg) for spinal anesthesia in preterm infants with BPD produces a spinal dermatomal blockade of T2-4. This produces loss of lower intercostal muscle activity and paralysis of abdominal muscles, which increases reliance on diaphragm for tidal breathing; despite this, tidal volume is generally maintained, and respiratory rate is generally not increased (Fig. 12–5).[79] Vigilance is necessary at all times during spinal anesthesia for early detection of breathing difficulties that can arise from total spinal anesthesia, or restriction of diaphragmatic motion by the surgeon's hands and surgical instruments pushing down on the paralyzed abdominal muscles.

Cephalad spread of local anesthetics may be influenced by the baricity of the solution, posture of the patient, dose, volume, and speed of injection. Care should be taken to avoid elevating the lower body (e.g., when placing the electrocautery pad).

Cardiovascular Response

Despite the large weight-scaled doses and sensory block levels ranging up to T2 to T4, most studies report no hypotension or bradycardia in children under the age of 5 years.[6, 77, 80, 81] Two factors seem responsible for the lack of hypotension and bradycardia in infants: (1) there is less vasodilatation in infants than in older children and adults, and (2) infants respond to high thoracic spinal anesthesia by reflex withdrawal of vagal parasympathetic tone to

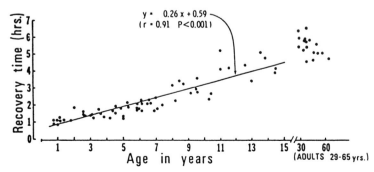

$y = 0.26 x + 0.59$
$(r = 0.91 \quad P < 0.001)$

FIGURE 12–4. Relation between the time required to recover from motor block and age in children. (From Dohi S, Naito H, Takahashi T: Age-related changes in blood pressure and duration of motor block in spinal anesthesia. Anesthesiology 50:319, 1979.)

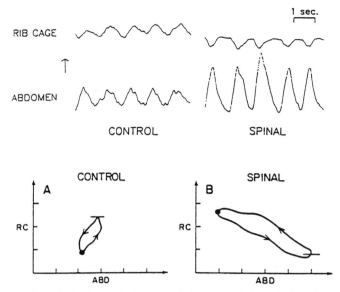

FIGURE 12–5. *Top,* Typical tracing of rib cage and abdominal motion before (control) and 10 minutes after induction of spinal anesthesia (spinal). *Bottom,* Rib cage versus abdominal displacement (Konno-Mead) respiratory loops before (*A*) and during spinal anesthesia (*B*). *Closed circles,* end expiration; *short horizontal lines,* end inspiration. After spinal anesthesia, rib cage moves paradoxically and abdominal displacements increase. (From Pascucci RC, Hershenson MB, Sethna NF, et al: Chest wall motion of infants during spinal anesthesia. J Appl Physiol 68:2087, 1990. The American Physiological Society, with permission.)

with local anesthetic. A 25-gauge 1-inch or 22-gauge 1.5-inch spinal needle is inserted in the sagittal plane in the midline between the spinous processus and advanced to less than 1 inch in neonates and to 1 inch or greater in infants and older children. A free flow of CSF confirms that the needle tip is in the subarachnoid space. The local anesthetic is then injected slowly. Loss of resistance before dural puncture may not be felt in an infant owing to softness of the ligamentum flavum and the dura. The child is then placed in the supine position and the cephalad spread of spinal anesthetic is monitored by testing the response to gentle pin-prick or cold stimulus and observing changes in respiratory rate, heart rate, and blood pressure. If a hyperbaric solution is used, and cephalad ascent of nerve blockade appears to be progressing rapidly, reverse Trendelenburg position (15- to 20-degree head up) may minimize excessive cephalad spread. Conversely, if after 45 to 60 seconds the block does not appear to extend above T10, then cautious return to a neutral supine position may aid in the spread.

The depth of lumbar puncture necessary to clear CSF varies with the size of the infants. This distance at L3-4 correlates best with body surface area ($r = 0.93$) and is consistent throughout ages of 1 to 18 years, mean 22 months.[91]

the heart. (Adults receiving high spinal anesthesia with marked vasodilatation often show a maladaptive persistence of vagal tone.) This interpretation is supported by a study of spinal anesthesia in former preterm infants undergoing herniorrhaphy. This study analyzed heart rate variability to estimate effects of spinal anesthesia on sympathetic and parasympathetic modulation of heart rate (Fig. 12–6).[78]

Experiments in newborn animals suggest that functional immaturity of adrenergic neurotransmission may cause less dependence of venous capacitance or systemic vascular resistance on sympathetic outflow in newborns.[87, 88]

Technique

The technique of spinal anesthesia in infants and children is similar to that in adults, easy to perform, and safe, provided anatomic differences are observed. In newborns, the conus medullaris ends at the body of L3 and the dural sac ends at approximately S3. During the first year of life, the dural sac retracts to its adult level at S1-2, and the spinal cord recedes to the adult level of L1. Thus, dural puncture is recommended at the L5-S1, L4-5 or L3-4 interspaces, but not at more cephalad interspaces. The child may be positioned either sitting or in the lateral decubitus position. When performed in the lateral decubitus position, the infant is held with the back, hips, and knees flexed and neck unflexed. When performed in sitting position, the head is held in an upright position to avoid airway obstruction and hypoventilation (Fig. 12–7).[89, 90] Contrary to common practice and belief, flexion of the cervical spine provides no benefit to successful lumbar dural puncture. Under aseptic condition, the skin is first infiltrated

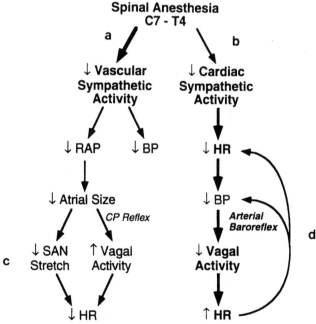

FIGURE 12–6. Effect of spinal anesthesia in infants. The mean arterial blood pressure (BP) remained constant without volume loading and without an increase in heart rate (HR), suggesting that either the overall effect of decreased sympathetic activity was minimal (*c*) or the effect of decreased sympathetic activity was offset by an arterial baroreflex-mediated vagal withdrawal (*d*). These observations may be supported by partial or incomplete cardiac sympathetic block in infants who have less sympathetic control over vascular tone or less dependence of the neonate on sympathetic vasoconstriction at rest. CP reflex, cardiopulmonary mediated reflex; SAN, sinoatrial node stretch. (From Oberlander TF, Berde CB, Lam KH, et al: Infants tolerate spinal anesthesia with minimal overall autonomic changes: analysis of heart rate variability in former premature infants undergoing hernia repair. Anesth Analg 80:20, 1995.)

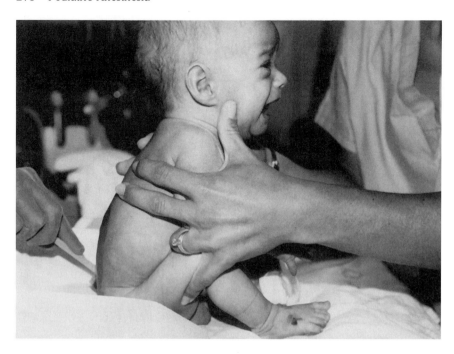

FIGURE 12–7. Sitting position of an infant for performance of spinal anesthesia.

Linear regression of the body surface area reveals the following relation: depth of lumbar puncture = 0.77 cm + 2.56 (m²).

A variety of needle sizes and types of are employed for performing spinal tap. A styleted needle should be used to prevent the remote possibility of implanting skin tissue into the subarachnoid tissue that may over time grow into a dermoid tumor.[92, 93] If freely flowing CSF is not obtained, it is advisable to try another intervertebral space or place the patient in sitting position to increase the CSF hydrostatic pressure.[94]

Management of the Patient during Spinal Anesthesia

Infants are often soothed with a pacifier, by shielding their eyes from the operating room lights, and by minimizing noise; they frequently fall asleep, probably due to sensory deafferentation. A restless and crying infant represents anesthetic failure to the surgical team even if spinal anesthesia is technically successful. Inadequate anesthesia or difficulty breathing from high spinal anesthesia should be considered in an agitated and restless infant.

Older children receptive to spinal anesthesia may benefit from preparation for the spinal anesthesia and surgical procedure, supportive operative room staff, frequent reassurances, distraction with music and video player, storytelling, engaging the child in an imaginative conversation, and other distracting activities. An anxious cooperative child may benefit from anxiolytic-amnesic (e.g., midazolam) or sedative (e.g., low-dose propofol infusion) agent (Fig. 12–8).

Monitoring after Spinal Anesthesia

How long a former preterm infant should be monitored after spinal anesthesia is uncertain. The potential for postoperative apnea occurrence in former preterm infants can-

not be completely eliminated, even after spinal anesthesia. Therefore, most pediatric centers monitor former preterm infants under the postconceptual age of 56 weeks overnight or a minimum of 12 apnea-free hours after surgery. The safe duration of postoperative monitoring is ultimately determined by an individual physician's and institution's decision as what is an acceptable risk of postoperative apnea for different subsets of former preterm infants.[68, 76, 95, 96]

Apnea is a multifactorial phenomenon and may be precipitated by a variety of perioperative stresses unrelated to type of anesthetics; pain, excessive handling, postoperative opioid analgesics, hypothermia, hypoglycemia, dehydration, and so forth.

Complications

Technical failure may be related to anatomic differences, vigorous infant movement, epidural venous bleeding, low CSF pressure, improper positioning of the infant, and an inexperienced operator. The failure incidence is less than 4 percent in experienced hands.[81, 97, 98] In skilled hands, spinal puncture is achieved with one to two attempts and completed within 3 minutes in 96 percent of children.[99]

Total spinal anesthesia has been reported with moderate doses of hyperbaric tetracaine 0.4 to 0.6 mg/kg when head-down position is assumed even for a brief time and with rapid injection of anesthetics.[98, 100–102] Other complications include postspinal apnea (concomitant administration of CNS depressants; sedative, hypnotics, and nitrous oxide is associated with an increased incidence of apnea[67, 98, 103]) and post–lumbar puncture headache.

It is a common belief among pediatricians and pediatric subspecialists that post–dural puncture headache (PDPH) is uncommon among infants and children. Clinicians may fail to diagnose PDPH in infants and preverbal children. A diagnosis of PDPH should be considered if an infant or child consistently cries and becomes distressed when

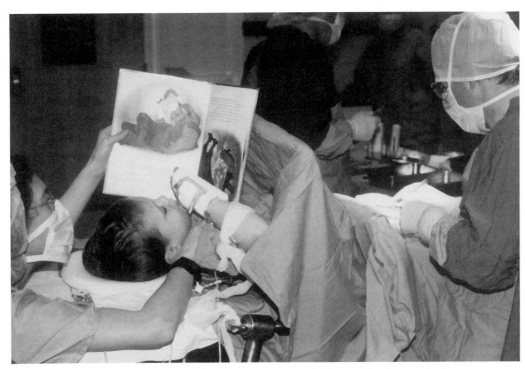

FIGURE 12–8. A 5-year-old child undergoing muscle biopsy with spinal anesthesia.

sitting upright, but not when placed supine. Three recent prospective studies in infants and children undergoing diagnostic or therapeutic spinal taps with a variety of needle types reported incidences of PDPH ranging from 4 to 17 percent, depending on the age group, needle type, and clinical context.[99, 104, 105] A more recent report, a prospective randomized and parallel group study in 215 children ages 1 to 18 years demonstrated that PDPH is as common in children (incidence of 4 percent) as in adults with use of 25- and 27-gauge cutting needles. None of the children required an epidural blood patch.[73]

Our pain service performs roughly five to eight epidural blood patches annually for infants and children who have PDPH following lumbar puncture for diagnostic purposes or for instillation of intrathecal chemotherapy. These children are referred to us by pediatric oncologists, pediatric neurologists, and other specialists. We usually employ a 22-gauge 1.5-inch spinal needle for neonates and children up to the age of 1.5 to 2 years, primarily to ensure clear flow of CSF. For older children and adolescents, a 25- to 27-gauge Whitacre or Sprotte spinal needle is used.

Other complications include back pain and neurologic symptoms. A large series in a prospective controlled trial of spinal block in 200 children age 2 months and older reported low back pain in 5 percent and transient radicular irritation in 1.5 percent lasting less than 5 days with complete recovery. Paresthesia during needle insertion was not reported by children, probably due to premedication or difficulty with verbal reporting of the symptom (Table 12–4).[73]

EPIDURAL ANALGESIA

Epidural analgesia is an extremely versatile form of regional anesthesia for infants and children. In the majority of cases, it is performed under general anesthesia. Placement following sedation or general anesthesia requires more indirect means for determining catheter tip position.

Identification of the Epidural Space

Identification of the epidural space is most commonly accomplished by the use of loss of resistance to injection of saline. Saline is preferred to air because unintentional intravascular injection of even small amounts of air in infants can result in significant venous air embolism and transient cardiorespiratory compromise.[106, 107] Blunt needles may reduce the risk of dural puncture.[108, 109]

Single-Shot Caudal Epidural Analgesia

Caudal epidural anesthesia/analgesia is the most widely employed technique for management of pain following a vast range of surgical procedures within the distribution of T10-S5 dermatomes for young children. Wide acceptance of caudal block attests to the technical simplicity, reliability, safety, and rapid performance in a large series of infants and children.[108] Single-shot caudal blocks are commonly used for ambulatory procedures and more minor procedures; continuous catheter techniques are commonly used for inpatients undergoing more extensive procedures. A common approach is to administer the caudal block before the surgical incision and immediately after induction of general anesthesia. Advocates of this approach cite the following potential benefits: (1) it permits maintenance of anesthesia with lower concentrations of potent vapor anesthetics; (2) it permits rapid, comfortable emergence from anesthesia; (3) in many cases it permits use of spontaneous breathing with near-normal end-tidal carbon dioxide and minute ventilation; (4) it reduces the

T A B L E   1 2 – 4
PARENTS' REPORT OF NEUROLOGIC COMPLAINTS AT HOME AFTER DAY SURGERY SPINAL BLOCK IN CHILDREN*

| | Study Groups | | | |
| | Cutting Point Needle | | Non–Cutting Point Needle | |
	25G Quincke	26G Atraucan	26G Sprotte	27G Whitacre
N	50	50	50	50
Positional headache	3	4	3	0
Nonpositional headache[†]	2	1	2	2
Stiffness of the neck	1	2	2	0
Low back pain	3	3	2	2
Vertigo	2	2	0	3
Photophobia[†]	0	2	2	0
Nausea/vomiting	5	4	4	2
Difficulties in passing urine[‡]	6	3	5	1
Muscle weakness in legs[†]	3	1	3	4
Transient radicular irritation[‡]	0	0	2	1

* Data are expressed as number of cases.
[†] Unrelated to spinal block. Symptoms attributed to ongoing cold and aggravation of preexisting migraine.
[‡] Transient complaints resolved without treatment.
From Kokki H, Hendolin H, Turunen M: Postdural puncture headache and transient neurologic symptoms in children after spinal anaesthesia using cutting and pencil point paediatric spinal needles. Acta Anaesthesiol Scand 42:1076, 1998.

need for endotracheal intubation in many cases; and (5) it may facilitate early discharge from the postanesthesia care unit (PACU) to home.[110]

While caudal blocks are generally used in conjunction with general anesthesia, awake caudal-epidural anesthesia has been used as an alternative to spinal anesthesia in infants undergoing lower extremity and perineal procedures. The primary advantage of this technique is a high technical success rate: the success rate in achieving analgesia with caudal block varies from 95 to 98 percent, whereas the success rate with achieving lumbar puncture is approximately 75 to 96 percent.[6, 98, 108] However, the success rate of achieving surgical anesthesia in awake infants with single-shot caudal blockade is probably much lower.

Published series on caudal bupivacaine anesthesia (concentrations ranging from 0.25 to 0.375 percent) for surgery among infants with a high risk for apnea from general anesthesia have reported variable success rates.[108, 111] In these series, the level of sensory block was variable, motor block of the lower extremities was rarely dense, and many infants received supplementation of the block with local anesthetic infiltration through the operative field and use of systemic analgesics and sedatives. Use of supplemental local anesthetic increases the risk of systemic toxicity, while use of systemic analgesics and sedatives increases the risk of intraoperative hypoventilation and postoperative apnea.[111, 112] Because bupivacaine has a long plasma elimination half-life (mean, 7.7 hours) in infants and a relatively short anesthetic duration, it is not suitable for frequent supplementation lest systemic toxicity occur.[22] An alternative is to use continuous caudal anesthesia with chloroprocaine, as described below.

Anatomy

The anatomy of the infant's sacral hiatus is similar to that of the adult, but the landmarks are more easily identifiable, because they are more superficial. The sacral hiatus is formed by nonfusion of the S5 vertebral arch. The remnants of the arch are represented by the prominences, known as sacral cornua, on either side of the hiatus. They are easily palpable and are usually more proximal in relation to the natal cleft than in adults. The hiatus extends from the sacral cornua (at the sacrococcygeal junction) to the fused arch of the S4. The sacrococcygeal membrane (or ligament) covers the sacral hiatus, isolating the sacral canal from the subcutaneous tissue. There is considerable variation in the anatomy of the sacral hiatus, mainly owing to developmental defects of the sacral canal roof, and this may account for the small percentage of caudal block failures. These anatomic abnormalities and their relevance to performance of the caudal block are extensively reviewed elsewhere.[113]

Technique

Caudal epidural block is easily performed in the lateral decubitus position or in the prone position (either in a knee-chest position or with a roll under the hip) (Fig. 12–9A). The sacral hiatus is readily felt with the thumbnail as a depression between the sacral cornua bound proximally by a bony edge (i.e., fused arch of the S4 vertebra). Under sterile conditions, the needle is directed at approximately 60 to 70 degrees to the skin and is advanced until it pierces the sacrococcygeal ligament. Loss of tissue resistance is felt as the needle enters the epidural space (Fig. 12–9B). The angle of the needle is reduced, and the needle is then advanced 2 mm into the space. Placement of the needle in the epidural space is confirmed by the loss of resistance to injection of saline and absence of subcutaneous swelling with injection.

The needle should not be advanced more than 2 to 4 mm after loss of resistance in younger infants because the dural sac and the epidural veins may terminate at about S3-S4. Once the needle position is confirmed and no blood or CSF is obtained by aspiration, a test dose of local anesthetic with epinephrine 1:200,000 is administered to rule

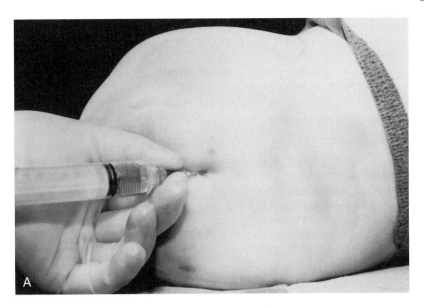

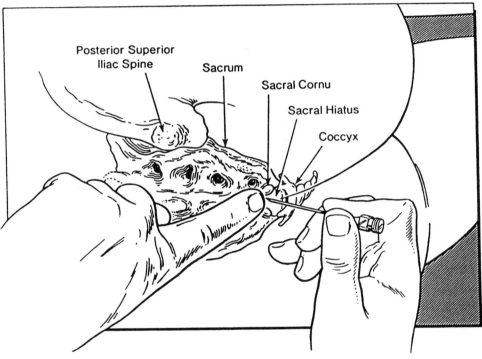

FIGURE 12–9. *A,* Caudal epidural blockade in a child. The child is in a lateral position. *B,* Caudal epidural blockade. Note the landmarks and the needle position. (From Willis RJ: Caudal epidural blockade. *In* Causins MJ, Bridenbaugh PO [eds]: Neural Blockade in Clinical Anesthesia and Management of Pain. Vol 3. Philadelphia, Lippincott-Raven, 1998, p 323, with permission.)

out inadvertent intravascular injection (cf, epidural test dose).

This is followed by slow injection of the calculated dose of the local anesthetic to avoid excessive cephalad spread. If accidental puncture of a sacral epidural vein occurs, the needle must be withdrawn and redirected until there is no blood flow spontaneously or on gentle aspiration. Subsequent injection of local anesthetic should be done very slowly and in small aliquots with monitoring for systemic toxic reactions. A variety of sizes (19- to 23-gauge) and types of hypodermic needles and intravenous cannulas with hollow stylets are favored by investigators. The

incidence of accidental vascular puncture can be reduced to 1.6 percent with the use of a short-bevel needle to identify the caudal space in children.[108]

Technical Difficulties

Recent papers have reported failure rates of less than 4 to 11 percent. Most failures occurred in children over the age of 7 years, presumably because of the development of a presacral fat pad.[108, 114]

Unilateral and uneven spread of local anesthetic solution occurs occasionally irrespective of the volume used and usually occurs in older children due to denser areolar connective tissue and compartmentalization of the epidural space.[108, 115] Inadequate caudal anesthesia after apparently successful caudal injection of local anesthetic is reported to occur in 3 to 7 percent of cases.[115–117]

Anesthetic Solutions, Dosage, Volume, and Concentration

Bupivacaine is the most commonly employed local anesthetic for regional blocks in pediatric patients because of its prolonged duration and mild degree of sensory selectivity, particularly in more dilute concentrations. Bupivacaine 0.25 percent at a dose of 2.5 mg/kg produces satisfactory anesthesia (i.e., suppression of autonomic responses) when used with light general anesthesia, and produces effective postoperative pain relief after inguinal hernia repair and lower extremity surgery.

A large number of formulas based on weight, age, number of spinal segments, and the length from C7 to the sacral hiatus have been proposed to calculate the dose of local anesthetic.[118] Nomograms are also suggested to serve as a guide to calculate caudal anesthetic dose, but they remain, like many other difficult-to-remember formulas and correction factors, impracticable in daily busy practice and tend to introduce the potential for errors in calculations.[119] Our belief is that the primary guide to dosing of local anesthetics should be to avoid any combination of concentration and volume that yields doses in excess of 2.5 mg/kg; with 0.25 percent solutions this gives the readily remembered limit of 1 ml/kg. For procedures below T10 level, a volume of 0.75 ml/kg is generally sufficient.

The spread of the local anesthetic best correlates well with age and body weight. While the weight is a better predictor in children younger than 7 years, age is a better guide in children 8 to 13 years.[119, 120] A significant linear correlation ($r = 0.93$) is demonstrated between body weight and segment volume of local anesthetic requirement for infants and children less than 7 years and body weight 20 kg or less (Fig. 12–10). This regression equation predicts that the volume dose (ml) = 0.65 ml × number of segments × body weight in kilograms. The accuracy of determining the level of analgesia based on age is high.[121]

Based on this relationship, the total dose of bupivacaine 0.25 percent calculated is well below the maximum allowable dose.[120] Volumes of bupivacaine 0.25 percent in excess of 1 ml/kg should be avoided in both anesthetized and awake children, both because of the potential for systemic toxicity and because in unanesthetized children these higher doses of drug may on rare occasions produce excessive cephalad spread of the anesthetic and cause airway difficulty. All dosing should be fractionated. Rapid inadvertent intravascular administration of bupivacaine can lead to cardiac arrest with a potential for difficult or impossible resuscitation.[108, 112]

Optimal Concentration of Bupivacaine

Bupivacaine in concentration of 0.25 percent is suitable for a single caudal epidural injection when used as an adjunct to general anesthesia. Increasing the concentration to 0.30 percent and 0.375 percent does not offer any additional advantage in analgesic effect, may produce undesirable degrees of motor blockade,[122] and because smaller volumes of anesthetic are required to keep within safe dose limits, there may be insufficient cephalad spread of the drug for surgical procedures in the inguinal region. Lower concentrations of bupivacaine ranging from 0.125 to 0.18 percent (0.75 to 1 ml/kg) appear equally effective to 0.25 percent bupivacaine when the drug is administered at the conclusion of the surgery, and these more dilute solutions produce significantly less motor weakness.[123] Similarly, a slightly lower volume (0.7 ml/kg) of bupiva-

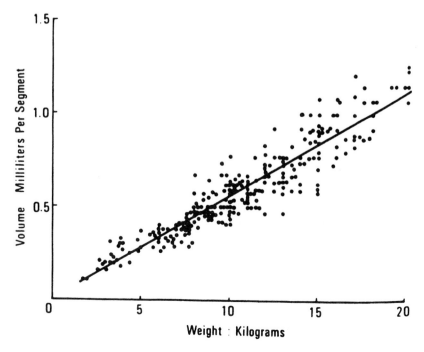

FIGURE 12–10. Scattergram of the relationship of body weight and dose requirement per spinal segment. The regression equation is y = 0.05608 × –0.00204 ($r = 0.932$, $p < 0.001$). (From Takasaki M, Dohi S, Kawabata Y, Takahashi T: Dosage of lidocaine for caudal anesthesia in infants and children. Anesthesiology 47:527, 1977.)

caine 0.175 percent was reported to produce optimal analgesia for outpatient surgical procedures.[124]

Duration of Analgesia

The median duration of analgesia produced by a single caudal dose of bupivacaine 0.25 percent, 1 ml/kg, with epinephrine 1:200,000 is 5 hours when the drug is administered at the end of the surgery; however, there is some degree of motor and sensory block in most patients following the administration of this dose and volume of drug.[125] A comparable analgesic duration is reported with a single injection of bupivacaine 0.25 percent or 0.125 percent and a smaller dose of 0.75 ml/kg in children. Approximately 60 percent and 50 percent of children did not require further analgesia 6 and 12 hours postoperatively, respectively (Table 12–5).[123]

The duration of analgesia has varied widely in previous studies of caudal blockade. The block has lasted as short as 4 hours and as long as 18 hours. The variation is due to a larger number of factors, including the choice of solution, the type of surgery, and the measures used to determine analgesic duration. Our impression is that some of the earlier studies were probably overly optimistic in their estimates of analgesic duration from caudal blocks with bupivacaine alone. It should be emphasized that single-shot caudal blockade with bupivacaine does not guarantee absence of postoperative pain for the entire first postoperative day. It is essential to provide parents with specific guidance on when to administer oral analgesics and how much to give to prevent rapid progression of severe pain when the block wears off.[126]

Addition of Epinephrine

Addition of epinephrine 1:200,000 to bupivacaine 0.25 percent (0.75 ml/kg) produces small increases in the mean duration of analgesia and only prolongs the mean time to first voiding by 60 minutes (202 vs. 262 minutes) after surgery. However, considerable variation in time to first void is observed; 8.5 percent of well-hydrated children void spontaneously for the first time after surgery 8 or more hours after caudal block was done.[115] Incidence of urinary retention is difficult to assess from current reports because of variable practice in preoperative fasting regimens, extent of intraoperative hydration, and definition of duration of urinary retention.

TABLE 12–5
DURATION OF POSTOPERATIVE ANALGESIA AFTER CAUDAL ANESTHESIA

Bupivacaine Concentration	Dose (ml/kg)	Time of Assessment Postblock	Percentage or Patients Requiring No Analgesia
0.25% or 0.125%	0.75	1, 2, 3, 4, 5, 6, and 12 hours	95, 80, 80, 75, 65, 60, and 50
0.25%	0.75–1	5 hours	97
0.25%	0.75*	4 hours	75

* With and without epinephrine.
Data from Dalens and Hasnaoui,[108] Fisher et al.,[115] and Wolf et al.[123]

Addition of Clonidine

Clonidine is an attractive additive to caudal local anesthetics because, unlike opioids, clonidine enhances and prolongs the analgesic effect of local anesthetics without causing respiratory depression, motor block, urinary retention, nausea, or pruritus. Clonidine alone is ineffective unless it is used in large doses that may also produce excessive sedation and hemodynamic instability. Addition of clonidine to caudal-epidural local anesthetics in children may improve analgesic efficacy and duration of analgesia. The optimal dose remains undetermined.[127-134]

Controlled trials of a single injection of caudal-epidural clonidine in children over the age of 1 year show wide variation in analgesic duration and sedation. The discrepancy among trials arises from differences in study design; type and volume of local anesthetics (bupivacaine, lidocaine, mepivacaine); assessment of pain (CHEOPS, facial pain scales, OPS, modified OPS, Broadman OPS, analgesic requirement, etc.); and inclusion of wide age range, and surgical procedures invoking variable pain intensity.[127, 131-136] In general, caudal blocks with bupivacaine plus clonidine appear to provide analgesia that lasts one-half to two times longer than bupivacaine alone.

Comparison of a single dose of clonidine 1 to 5 μg/kg combined with bupivacaine or mepivacaine to local anesthetics alone in children over the age of 1 year demonstrated (1) similar intensity and significantly longer duration of block with better quality of analgesia, (2) significant reduction in mean arterial blood pressure and heart rate with higher dose (5 μg/kg) but clinically insignificant, (3) no motor weakness or respiratory depression but significantly greater transient sedation, and (4) a pharmacologic profile similar to that reported in adults.[135]

Comparison of clonidine 1.5 μg/kg to fentanyl 1 μg/kg and clonidine 1 μg/kg to morphine 30 μg/kg as adjuncts to caudal-epidural local anesthetic show comparable postoperative analgesic duration but a higher incidence of vomiting and oxyhemoglobin desaturation with fentanyl.[127, 133]

Our practice for single-shot caudal blocks, particularly in outpatients, is to add clonidine 1 to 1.5 μg/kg to bupivacaine in children over age one year, up to a maximum of 30 μg in older children and adolescents. Increasing the dose to 2 μg/kg appears generally safe, but may increase the incidence of sedation postoperatively. Doses in excess of 2 μg/kg may occasionally produce prolonged sedation or mild degrees of hypotension or bradycardia.

The pharmacokinetics of a single epidural clonidine dose (2 mg/kg) has been examined in a small number of children ages 1 to 9 years.[135] The venous plasma concentration varied widely between patients. Similarly, the time to 95 percent clonidine absorption from the epidural space widely ranged from 36 minutes to 7.6 hours. Sedation developed at a 50 percent lower plasma concentration compared to adults, but none of the children developed excessive sedation or respiratory depression. The analgesic effect of clonidine outlasted its sedative effect, and the postoperative pain scores showed no correlation with plasma clonidine concentrations. These observations support the conclusion from animal studies that epidural clonidine exerts its analgesic action predominantly at spinal sites rather than via systemic uptake and transfer to brain-stem sites.

Caudal Ropivacaine

Ropivacaine is a new long-acting amino-amide local anesthetic with similar structure to bupivacaine that has been claimed to reduce cardiac and CNS toxicity and to provide slightly greater sensory selectivity.[137–139] In healthy human adult volunteers, intravenous ropivacaine caused fewer CNS and cardiovascular symptoms compared to bupivacaine. Subjects tolerated a 25 percent higher ropivacaine than bupivacaine dose before exhibiting CNS toxicity symptoms.[140–142] Similar toxicity data on ropivacaine are not available in children; it would not be feasible to perform such a study on ethical grounds. As a surrogate indicator of relative toxicity in infants, an infant and adult rat model was developed to assess efficacy and systemic toxicity. Work by Kohane and others in our group showed that the LD_{50} of both ropivacaine and bupivacaine was higher in infant animals than in adult animals. In both infant and adult rats, the LD_{50} of ropivacaine was roughly 50 percent higher than the LD_{50} for bupivacaine. In both infant and adult rats, ropivacaine and bupivacaine showed equal durations of sensory and motor blockade.[27] These data support the view of a slightly greater therapeutic index for ropivacaine compared with bupivacaine, but they do not find support for ropivacaine having either greater sensory selectivity or longer analgesic duration.

Preliminary studies of ropivacaine's pharmacokinetic profile following a single injection of drug via lumbar and caudal routes in children over the age of 3 months is similar to that described in adults, except for the fact that the time to peak plasma concentration is longer.[143, 144] Pharmacokinetic data after a single injection of caudal ropivacaine (2.5 mg/kg) in children ages 1 to 6 years old showed that the time to peak venous plasma concentration occurred later in children (median, 90 minutes) than in adults (median, 25 minutes).[143, 145] The mean clearance of 7.6 ml/min/kg in children is similar to mean values of 5.5 and 7.7 ml/min/kg reported in adults receiving epidural ropivacaine.[138, 140, 143, 146] Elimination half-life of the drug in children (mean, 3.9 hours) were similar to the mean values reported in adults after epidural ropivacaine (mean, 4.3 and 5.5 hours).[137, 139, 145]

A number of studies in children show that a single injection of caudal ropivacaine provides analgesia that is similar to that for bupivacaine. The side-effects are also comparable at similar doses (2 mg/kg) or concentrations (ropivacaine, 0.2 to 0.25 percent vs. 0.25 percent bupivacaine). A recent study found that ropivacaine produced a longer duration of postoperative analgesia but a significantly shorter duration of motor block than bupivacaine when compared at a concentration of 0.375 percent.[48–50] Motor block is dose and concentration dependent, and a higher ropivacaine concentration of 0.5 percent produces significantly greater duration of analgesia than 0.25 percent, longer time to first voiding, and significantly longer time to ambulation.[148] These studies of caudal ropivacaine are promising, and may suggest advantages in terms of both safety and efficacy. Additional studies are needed to confirm the clinical significance of differences in either analgesic duration or duration of motor blockade between ropivacaine and bupivacaine.

Caudal Opioids

Even longer duration of caudal analgesia can be provided by giving repeated injections of local anesthetics or by injecting opioids into the caudal space. Caudal morphine provides longer analgesia than bupivacaine alone and extends analgesia beyond the lumbosacral dermatomes; it can also be used for thoracic and upper abdominal procedures.[149] Injection of caudal morphine has the further advantages of not causing motor and autonomic blocks. Caudal morphine was found to be superior to systemic opioid administration in a study of children undergoing penile surgery.[150]

Although epidural morphine dose of 50 μg/kg provides effective and prolonged analgesia (mean, 19 hours) in children over the age of 2 years, the ventilatory response to carbon dioxide remained depressed for 22 hours after injection of the drug. Patients receiving caudal morphine should be closely monitored during this vulnerable period because sporadic respiratory depression is reported with this and lower doses.[151–154] Because of concerns for respiratory depression, itching, nausea, and urinary retention, we generally do not recommend use of caudal opioids in outpatients.

Other Drugs for Caudal Administration

There are a growing number of case series on use of other agents added to local anesthetics for caudal analgesia, including ketamine S(+).[155–157] Many of these drug combinations appear to provide good analgesia and a good side-effect profile. We would encourage clinicians to use considerable caution in introducing new neuraxial analgesics for children in their general practice. In our opinion, new neuraxial agents for children should be introduced in clinical trials only when (1) there are published clinical trials for their use in adults and (2) there is a sufficient body of animal histopathologic neurotoxicity data to suggest that the agent has a very low risk for neurotoxicity.[158]

Continuous Epidural Infusions

Continuous epidural infusions are an extremely versatile method for analgesia for infants and children undergoing major thoracic, abdominal, pelvic, and lower extremity procedures. Specific aspects of caudal, lumbar, and thoracic epidural infusions will be discussed below.

Pharmacokinetics, Choice of Drugs, and Dosing Guidelines

Early reports described cases of convulsions in infants and children receiving continuous epidural infusions of bupivacaine.[159, 160] In reviewing these cases, it was apparent that these convulsions were due to accumulation of toxic plasma concentrations of bupivacaine. Consideration of clearances derived from single-dose studies and from considerations regarding the slower clearance in neonates and very young infants led to provisional recommendations to keep infusion rates below 0.4 mg/kg/h for older infants and children, and to keep infusion rates below 0.2 mg/kg/h for neonates and infants in the first few months of life.[28] Subsequent pharmacokinetic studies of infants and children receiving infusions for several days have tended to confirm these recommendations, with some qualifiers as described below.

Infants over the age of 6 months and children tolerate bupivacaine infusion rates of 0.3 to 0.4 mg/kg/h with plasma concentrations in a safe range of less than 2 to 3 μg/ml following an initial priming dose of 2 to 2.5 mg/kg.[15, 161]

Studies of repeated intermittent dosing or continuous lumbar and thoracic epidural infusion of bupivacaine 0.25 percent (1.25 to 6 mg/24 h) reported good safety in children older than 3 months of age. Although the bupivacaine levels obtained at steady-state infusion reached 2.2 μg/ml, no systemic toxicity was observed.[147, 162, 163]

In a study in neonates receiving continuous infusions of bupivacaine, the total bupivacaine plasma concentration was noted to continually rise in five of nine patients after 48 hours. However, in four patients the free fraction of plasma bupivacaine remained stable during the first 24 hours of infusion, probably due to the corresponding increase in α_1-glycoprotein induced by the stress of surgery. The plasma concentration of bupivacaine ranged from 0.2 to 3.0 μg/ml with considerable interindividual variability. The maximum plasma concentrations occurred in patients with increased intra-abdominal pressure and was thought to be caused by compromised hepatic flow.[16]

A subsequent study measured total and free bupivacaine plasma concentrations during continuous epidural infusion in infants and children and observed that in infants younger than 5 months of age, the maximum plasma concentrations of free bupivacaine were significantly higher than in older children, and this difference was markedly higher with elapse of epidural infusion time. Unlike the previous study, plasma protein binding was also significantly lower in infants than in children, and jitteriness and irritability occurred in four infants after 7 hours of bupivacaine infusion (Fig. 12–11).[14]

These pharmacokinetic studies have implications for choice of drugs for infusions. Our view is that, because of the scaling considerations for efficacy, metabolism, and toxicity listed earlier, there will be a high incidence of inadequate analgesia using plain bupivacaine solutions at the maximum safe infusion rates, namely, less than 0.2 mg/kg/h for infants 3 months or less and less than 0.4 mg/kg/h for children and infants older than 6 months of age. Analgesic failures with plain bupivacaine will be particularly frequent if the catheter tip is sited lower than the dermatomes involved in the surgery (e.g., lumbar placement for thoracic or upper abdominal surgery). Our preference, therefore, is to add either opioid or clonidine or both to local anesthetic in almost all epidural infusions. The rationale for coadministration of either opioids or clonidine or both is that these agents provide additive or synergistic analgesic effects achievable with safe bupivacaine infusion rates. Infusion of lidocaine offers no wider therapeutic index than bupivacaine.

Our general practice is to use dilute bupivacaine solutions (i.e., 0.1 percent, in combination with either fentanyl

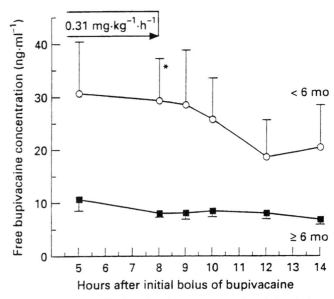

FIGURE 12–11. Total bupivacaine plasma concentrations during the last 3 hours of continuous bupivacaine infusion (5 and 8 hours after bolus) and after termination of infusion (9, 10, 12, and 14 hours after bolus). Values are means ± SEM. (From Luz G, Wieser C, Innerhofer P, et al: Free and total bupivacaine plasma concentrations after continuous epidural anaesthesia in infants and children. Paediatr Anaesth 8:473, 1998. Blackwell Scientific Ltd, with permission.)

2 μg/ml or fentanyl 2 μg/ml plus clonidine 0.8 μg/ml, or hydromorphone 10 μg/ml). (Other groups prefer lower hydromorphone concentrations, e.g., 3 to 5 μg/ml.) For infants or children with a high risk of apnea, or with severe opioid side-effects (e.g., persistent itching or nausea), our practice is to infuse bupivacaine 0.1 percent with clonidine 0.4 to 0.8 μg/ml with no epidural opioid. Details regarding maximum infusion rates are given in Table 12–6. In general, lower starting infusion rates should be used when catheter tips are at thoracic levels than when catheter tips are at lumbar or caudal levels. This recommendation for lower starting infusion rates is particularly relevant when hydrophilic opioids are used.

Caudal Epidural Infusions

Caudal epidural infusions may involve catheters left at sacral levels or catheters that have been advanced cephalad to lumbar or thoracic levels. The considerations regarding dosing and choice of infusions will be reviewed in the sections on lumbar and thoracic epidural infusions. One specific consideration for continuous caudal infusions is the increased chance for fecal soiling compared with lumbar or thoracic placement. Different approaches to this problem have included (1) use of plastic barrier drapes immediately caudad to the skin entry site, (2) routinely tunneling all caudal catheters with a more cephalad skin exit site, and (3) limiting the duration of caudal catheter use to no more than 2 to 3 days.

Continuous Caudal Anesthesia for Former Preterm Neonates

To circumvent the limitation of prolonged clearance of amide local anesthetic in infants, and to provide sufficient

T A B L E   1 2 - 6
EPIDURAL INFUSION REGIMENS

Patient Age	Local Anesthetic Agent	Initial Dose (mg/kg)	Steady-State Infusion Rate (mg/kg/h)	Plasma Levels (mg/ml)	Reference
11 months–15 years	Bupivacaine	1.25	0.2	< 1.2	Desparmet et al.[162]
≤ 4 months	Bupivacaine	1.9*	0.31	< 1[†]	Luz et al.[15]
> 9 months	Bupivacaine	1.9*	0.31	< 0.6	
3 months–4 years	Lidocaine	5	2.5	< 5[‡]	Miyabe et al.[38]
6 days–5.2 months	Bupivacaine	1.9*	0.31	< 1.5[†§]	Luz et al.[14]
1.5–9 years	Bupivacaine	1.9*	0.31	< 0.9	

* Initial dose of 1.25 mg/kg was given over 5 min followed by 0.63 mg/kg/h for an hour followed by infusion at 0.31 mg/kg/h.
† Progressively rising concentrations at steady-state infusion.
‡ Five-hour infusion, both lidocaine and it's metabolite MEGX increased significantly as a function of time.
§ Progressively rising concentrations at 7 hours of steady-state infusion. Four infants developed jitteriness and irritability probably due to significant increase in the free fraction of plasma bupivacaine.

doses of local anesthetic to give dense sensory and motor blockade of the lower extremities and lower abdomen, we previously evaluated the feasibility of continuous caudal anesthesia in awake former preterm neonates using 3 percent 2-chloroprocaine (2-CP), which is rapidly metabolized in the plasma, and has an elimination half-life of less than 6.5 minutes. The initial dose of 2 ml/kg (60 mg/kg) was administered over 10 minutes in increments of no more than 0.3 ml to establish a T2-4 dermatomal level of sensory block. Subsequent infusion of 2-CP 3 percent was started at 1 ml/kg/h to maintain the desired anesthetic level during inguinal hernia repairs lasting 60 to 170 minutes. If this infusion rate was insufficient, incremental doses of 0.3 ml were given up to a repeat loading dose of 0.5 to 1 ml/kg of the same solution if the infant appeared to be in pain and responded to surgical manipulations.[35] More studies are needed to determine whether these high doses can be given safely for the rare patient with cholinesterase deficiency. Although no cases of neurotoxicity have been identified either in the Henderson et al. study, in our subsequent clinical experience, or in the subsequent study by Tobias, further prospective investigation is needed to better determine a confidence limit on the incidence of neurotoxic sequelae, especially in the case of unanticipated intrathecal injection of large doses of the drug.[35, 164] We recommend use of preservative-free formulations.

Combining caudal with general anesthesia significantly suppresses the neuroendocrine response (adrenocorticotropic hormone, β-endorphin, antidiuretic hormone, and cortisol) compared to halothane anesthetic alone.[161, 165, 166] Regional anesthesia exerts an antistress effect by preventing surgically induced noxious afferent neural input from reaching the central nervous system; this minimizes the establishment of spinal cord hyperexicitibility.[167]

LUMBAR AND THORACIC EPIDURAL ANALGESIA

Lumbar and thoracic epidural analgesia are used with increasing prevalence in pediatric centers both intraoperatively as a component of a "balanced" anesthetic technique, particularly for thoracic, abdominal, and major pelvic surgery and for postoperative analgesia.[147, 162, 163, 168–171] Several series suggest that this technique provides effective analgesia, facilitates early postoperative extubation, and in some case series appears to result in improved postoperative pulmonary function.[147, 168, 172, 173] Epidural anesthesia/analgesia effectively controls the nociceptive afferent input from major abdominal procedures and thereby favorably modifies the neuroendocrine and metabolic responses intraoperatively and postoperatively.[161, 174]

Technique

Despite the short distance from skin to lumber and thoracic epidural spaces,[169, 175] easy identification of the intervertebral space and ligamentum flavum and easy placement of lumbar and thoracic epidural catheters are reported in infants and children by standard loss of resistance technique; the children are positioned in the lateral decubitus position and 18- or 19-gauge Tuohy needles and 20- or 21-gauge catheters are used.[169, 175] Our preference is generally to use 18-gauge needles and 20-gauge catheters. One of us (N.F.S.) prefers incremental two-handed advancement of the needle with frequent checking for loss of resistance, whereas the other author (C.B.B.) prefers continuous needle advancement and constant thumb pressure on the plunger using Bromage's grip.[176]

In children, epidural catheters are often placed either after induction of general anesthesia or after administration of intravenous sedation. Which method is used depends on the level of the child's cooperation and whether the anesthesiologist feels the patient will be immobile and calm. Although the placement of *lumbar* epidural catheters in heavily sedated or anesthetized children is generally regarded as a safe procedure, there remains a small but nonzero risk of neurologic complications. There is greater disagreement regarding the risk/benefit ratio of direct *thoracic* epidural needle placement in anesthetized infants and children (see section Side Effects and Complications of Epidural Single-Shot Injections and Continuous Infusions, below).

Cephalad Advancement of Catheters from Caudal or Lumbar Needle Entry Sites

In general, epidural infusions are most effective when catheter tips are in the dermatomes involved in the surgery. Local anesthetics are essential to permit pain relief with movement as well as at rest, and local anesthetics do not spread far cephalad from their infusion sites. If catheter tips are left at caudal or lumbar levels for upper abdominal or thoracic surgery, then it is more reasonable to include a hydrophilic opioid, such as hydromorphone, because of its cephalad spread.

Because dermatomal placement of epidural catheter tips is desirable, and because of the above-mentioned concerns regarding direct thoracic needle placement, several investigators have examined advancement of catheters to thoracic levels following caudal or lumbar needle entry into the epidural space. Early studies by Bosenberg and by Schulte-Steinberg indicated good success, particularly among infants, in caudal to thoracic placement. Subsequent studies have produced variable success rates. Variability in success of thoracic placement of the catheter tip may relate in part to patient age (higher success rates in infants than children), to choice of catheters (higher success rates with styletted catheters), and to different criteria for determining sufficiently high placement of the catheter tip.[29, 30, 177, 178] Force must not be applied when the catheter is advanced. Using force may injure nerves or the spinal cord.[30] Reported procedural difficulties and misplacement of the epidural catheter are shown in Table 12-7.

Lumbar to thoracic placement has been reported to have a lower success rate than caudal to thoracic placement of the catheter tip.[177] It is more likely to succeed if the epidural space is entered at high lumbar levels (i.e., L1-2 rather than L3-4 or L4-5), and if the epidural needle is angled in a cephalad direction rather than directly perpendicular to the axis of the spine. It is important to note that the distance from skin to epidural space is shorter at the T12-L1 and L1-L2 interspaces than at L3-L4 or L4-L5. Failure to recognize this fact may predispose to inadvertent dural puncture at these levels.

To ensure a high success with thoracic advancement of the catheter tip, two alternatives to blind placement can be considered: fluoroscopic guidance and nerve-stimulation guidance. Fluoroscopic guidance of cephalad advancement produces high success rates. Wire-wrapped, styletted, 20-gauge catheters are readily visible with fluoroscopy; alternatively, standard nonradiopaque catheters can be visualized by repeated injection of very small volumes of nonionic, myelographic contrast agents. Disadvantages of fluoroscopy include expense, radiation exposure, and lack of ready availability in many operating rooms. We routinely use fluoroscopic confirmation for placement of catheters for extended periods, as in palliative care of oncology patients.

Recently, Tsui and co-workers have developed a novel approach to confirm cephalad advancement of catheters by use of electrical nerve stimulation directly through the catheter.[179-181] A wire-wrapped, styletted, saline-filled epidural catheter is equipped with a special ECG-lead connector to permit delivery of current at the tip of the epidural catheter. They have shown very good sensitivity and specificity and an improved success rate in guiding catheters from caudal entry to thoracic tip placement. There are a number of technical points needed to ensure success of this approach, including (1) avoidance of neuromuscular blockade to permit visualization of motor responses; (2) meticulous elimination of bubbles from the catheter and connectors, to ensure current delivery through the entire course of the catheter; (3) use of nonmetal or shielded epidural needles to minimize dispersion of current; and (4) making the ECG-lead on the catheter negative and the lead on the skin positive. If these results can be confirmed by other groups with an acceptably rapid learning curve, then this approach may dramatically improve the safety and effectiveness of placing epidural catheters into the thoracic epidural space.

Monitoring of Patients with Continuous Epidural Infusions

At our institution, standing orders are written by the pain treatment service physicians and initiated in the postoperative care unit. The orders outline the recording of vital signs, degree of sedation, and pain scores every 4 hours. Depth and rate of respiration and level of sedation are recorded hourly for the first 24 hours. Infants younger than 6 to 12 months of age and those patients who are at increased risk for ventilatory compromise from preexisting disorders or use of hydrophilic opioids are monitored with electronic monitors that record chest wall impedance, ECG and, in some cases, pulse oximetry. Our view is that

TABLE 12-7
PROBLEMS ENCOUNTERED WITH THORACIC PLACEMENT OF EPIDURAL CATHETERS VIA CAUDAL AND LUMBAR ROUTES IN INFANTS AND CHILDREN

Age	Epidural Approach	No. of Complications/ Total No. of Patients Studied	Untoward Effects	Reference
1–10 years	Caudal	3/20	Vascular placement Coiled catheter Failure to thread to desired level	Gunter and Eng[29]
1–60 days premature infants	Caudal	3/20	Vascular placement Intrathecal placement Coiled catheter	van Niekerk et al.[178]
4–22 weeks	Caudal	2/20	Vascular placement Failure to thread to desired level	Bosenberg et al.[30]
Neonates–8 years (mean, 3.4 ± 2.8 years)	Lumbar	1/39*	Vascular placement	Blanco et al.[177]

* In 32 of 39 children, the epidural catheter failed to reach the desired thoracic level.

electronic monitors should alarm throughout the hallway and at the nurses' station, not simply in the patient's room. Alarms that only sound in the patient's room are likely to be ignored. Protocols for both human and electronic monitoring will depend in part on local staffing conditions and nursing expertise; what is crucial is that assessment of the recorded variables should be systematic. Premonitory clinical signs or alarms on electronic monitors should trigger protocols for immediate responses. The epidural dressing is periodically inspected by the nurses each shift for dressing disruption, local anesthetic leakage, and skin infection. Secure sufficient heel padding and 4-hourly position change prevent pressure ischemia. In general, systemic opioids are not administered simultaneously with epidural opioids. If systemic opioids are considered desirable, for example, to treat incident-related pain, one alternative is to administer local anesthetic and clonidine, but no opioid, in the epidural infusion, and then to permit intravenous opioid boluses by the nurses for rescue medication or incident-related pain. Epidural analgesia requires a high degree of physician attention. An acute pain service that is staffed by physicians and nurses can help create an ideal system for regular assessment. In any case, there should be formal daily rounds on each patient by an anesthesiologist or other experienced pain management physician, and there must be 24-hour, 7-days-per-week immediate availability of anesthesiologists or other physicians specifically trained in acute care of infants and children.

Side Effects and Complications of Epidural Single-Shot Injections and Continuous Infusions

Dilute solutions of bupivacaine and other local anesthetics usually provides good autonomic and sensory blocks with only a mild motor block. The incidence of postoperative vomiting, lower extremity muscle weakness, and urinary retention and delayed micturition is difficult to ascertain, because different investigators employed various concentrations of bupivacaine, as well as different systemic agents. Most investigators agree that the incidence of postoperative vomiting after caudal analgesia with local anesthetic agents is approximately 0 to 30 percent,[108, 182–184] which is lower than that reported with administration of single-dose intravenous morphine during inguinal herniorrhapy in children.[185, 186] Vomiting is also significantly less frequent after caudal anesthesia than with intramuscular administration of morphine for postoperative pain relief for comparable patients.[187]

Motor block and inability to walk occurred for up to 6 hours after caudal block in 31 percent of children who received caudal bupivacaine 0.5 percent for postcircumcision analgesia.[121, 184, 187] The incidence of motor weakness in the first postoperative hour is significantly less and the ability to stand unaided is greater with 0.125 percent than 0.25 percent bupivacaine but of equal postoperative analgesic effect; these solutions are suitable for procedures in the day surgery unit.[123] In our view, there are few if any indications to use bupivacaine concentrations in excess of 0.25 percent for epidural analgesia in infants and children.

Difficulties in locating the sacral hiatus is reported and vary with the experience of the anesthesiologist (see section on caudal technique).

Unilateral and uneven spread of local anesthetic solution after single-injection caudal anesthesia occurs occasionally, irrespective of the volume of solution used. This usually occurs in older children, most likely because of compartmentalization of the epidural space and denser areolar connective tissue with increasing age.[108]

Accidental intravascular injection of local anesthetics occurs most commonly when sharp-point needles are advanced cephalad more than 1 to 2 cm beyond the entry point of the sacral canal. Unintentional vessel puncture occurs with a significantly greater frequency when sharp long-bevel needles (10.6 percent) rather than blunt short-bevel needles (1.6 percent) are used.[108]

Failure to aspirate blood through the needle diminishes but does not eliminate the possibility of intravascular needle placement.[108, 114] In one study, accidental intravascular injection of local anesthetics was practically eliminated when blunt short-bevel needles were used.[108] The overall incidence of accidental puncture of epidural vessels also seems to be influenced by the experience of the person performing the block, the type of technique, and the difficulties encountered in locating the sacral hiatus.[114]

If blood is aspirated, the needle should be repositioned. The child should be closely monitored after administration of a test dose, since addition of epinephrine to an anesthetic solution sometimes does not herald a systemic toxic reaction in the anesthetized child.[114] Therefore, repeated aspiration and injection of a small fraction of the total anesthetic dose may allow early detection of systemic toxicity.

Dural puncture is rare in most recent series of caudal blocks in infants and children, and is attributable either to excessive cranial advancement of the needle or to use of sharp-tipped needles (Table 12–8). Unrecognized dural puncture and subsequent injection of anesthetic solution could lead to respiratory arrest and total spinal anesthesia.[188, 189] The incidence of this complication can be reduced by avoiding cephalad advancement of the needle and by aspiration for CSF before injecting the anesthetic solution.[190, 191] It may be possible to detect a high subarachnoid block early by monitoring for apnea in a spontaneously breathing child who is lightly anesthetized.

Sacral marrow puncture and injection of local anesthetic may result in systemic toxicity. The signs of toxicity

---

┌─────────────────────────────┐
│ T A B L E   1 2 – 8 │
└─────────────────────────────┘

INCIDENCE OF ACCIDENTAL DURAL PUNCTURE DURING PERFORMANCE OF PEDIATRIC CAUDAL BLOCK

Reference	No. of Dural Tap	Total No. of Caudal Block
Armitage[342]	6	4,000
Brown and Schulte-Steinberg[333]	3	3,500
Broadman[343]	1	3,500
Dalens and Hasnaoui[108]	1	750
Gunter[344]	2	160,000
Veyckemans et al.[114]	1	1,100
Gaufré et al.[165]	4	15,013

may appear nearly as rapidly as with intravenous injection of local anesthetics. Placement of the needle in the marrow can be recognized by the presence of resistance to injection and by the systemic effects of a test dose.[116]

In our view, the rare but nonzero risk for inadvertent intravenous or intrathecal injection of local anesthetics mandates that caudal blocks be performed with standard monitors (ECG, blood pressure, oximeter, capnograph) in place, with intravenous access established, and with ready access to drugs and equipment for resuscitation.

Penetration of pelvic organs with the needle is extremely rare but has been reported with use of sharp-tipped needles.[116, 192]

Sympathetic block to the T10 level has not led to symptomatic hypotension or bradycardia in a large number of children receiving caudal epidural blocks. Caudal anesthesia to T5 in infants aged 6 months produces minimal sympathetic denervation in the lower extremity and no significant changes in heart rate, cardiac index and blood pressure.[108, 193, 194] Accidental internal caudal catheter shearing has occurred.[195]

In adults, infectious complications associated with epidural catheter are rare, but cases of epidural abscess, deep-tissue infection, and meningitis have been reported after short-term epidural infusion for pain management.[196] In children, available information indicates that the incidence of clinically significant infection with postoperative epidural infusions appears very low. A retrospective review of short-term epidural infusion in a large series of pediatric patients reports no cases of epidural infection with short-term postoperative use; cases of infection were limited to prolonged infusion of solutions in patients with compromised immunity.[197] Recently, two studies examined the incidence of bacterial colonization of caudal and lumbar epidural catheters and skin insertion sites.[198, 199] In one prospective series, 45 caudal and 46 lumbar epidural catheters placed for postoperative analgesia in children showed a high incidence of colonization. Colonization is significantly higher with caudal catheter tips (20 percent) than lumbar catheter tips (4 percent). However, both groups had similar rates of skin colonization (caudal 66 percent vs. lumbar 52 percent).[199] In both groups, *Staphylococcus epidermidis* was the predominant skin and catheter tip microorganism, but gram-negative bacteria also colonized four caudal catheter tips.

A second prospective series of 210 children, ages 1 to 21 years, documented a 35 percent incidence of catheter tip colonization. A similar incidence of gram-positive colonization was reported in caudal (25 percent) and lumbar catheter tips (23 percent). Gram-negative colonization was more frequent with the caudal (16 percent) than lumbar (3 percent) catheter tips. Local cellulitis was noted at the skin insertion sites in 11 percent of patients with similar incidence in all age groups.[198] Despite the presence of significant bacterial colonization with short-term (<5 days) indwelling caudal and epidural catheter tips in both series, serious local and systemic infection did not ensue. In both these studies, the culture results and risk of infection may be influenced by prophylactic concurrent administration of antibiotics in most of the surgical patients. Nevertheless, a few cases of serious infectious complications have been reported in children and infants.[198, 200–202]

Acute skin abscess is reported in two infants after 5 days of continuous lumbar epidural analgesia and delayed recurrent skin abscess in a third 4-year-old child after 29-hour continuous caudal analgesia.[200, 202] Surgical drainage was necessary in the latter case. Extensive epidural abscess is reported in a fourth 1-year-old infant after repeated lumbar and thoracic catheter placement within a short time. The abscess resolved after antibiotic therapy.[201] These reports underscore the importance of strict aseptic technique, avoidance of local tissue trauma, daily inspection of skin entry sites, and use of styleted epidural needles and closed infusion system.

The frequency of neurologic deficits following epidural anesthesia or analgesia in children is unknown. The largest prospective, uncontrolled multicenter study consisted of 14,507 caudal and lumbar epidural blocks; these authors reported only two cases of transient paresthesia.[203] Although the overall risk seems very low, some clinicians suggest that, in circumstances where there is a peripheral block or wound infiltration, it is likely to be at least as safe and effective, and the peripheral approach should be preferred over the neuraxial approach. Larger prospective controlled trials of efficacy and neurologic complications are needed to properly define these relative risks and benefits.

There is somewhat more controversy regarding the risk/benefit ratio of direct thoracic epidural catheter placement in anesthetized infants and children.[204, 205] Several series have reported good efficacy and safety, but the cumulative number of cases is too small to make a quantitative estimate of the risk of neurologic injury. Adverse events can occur. We make selective use of direct thoracic placement of catheters for extensive thoracic and abdominal procedures in selected infants and children who are at increased risk of postoperative pulmonary complications. We would urge caution for routine use, particularly among occasional practitioners or in healthy patients undergoing less extensive surgery. The decision to insert high lumbar and thoracic epidural catheters in anesthetized children should involve consideration of benefit/risk ratios, and should be performed by anesthesiologists with extensive experience in pediatric regional anesthesia.[165, 205]

PERIPHERAL NERVE BLOCKADE AND PLEXUS BLOCKADE

Paravertebral Thoracic Block

Paravertebral thoracic block (PVTB) is extensively studied in adults and only recently received attention among pediatric anesthesiologists for management of postthoracotomy pain because of several benefits.[206–213] When compared to thoracic epidural catheterization, percutaneous catheterization of paravertebral space has the potential advantages of a reduced risk of neurologic injury, hypotension, urinary retention, or motor blockade of the abdomen or hip flexors; these features may facilitate early mobilization after surgery. The main disadvantage of percutaneous PVTB is the risk of pneumothorax; direct catheterization of the paravertebral space before closure of a thoracotomy incision further improves the reliability of this technique and eliminates the potential for neurologic injury, pneumothorax, and unintentional vascular cannulation. In adults, PVTB has been shown to significantly improve pain relief, reduce opioid requirements and its side effects, and reduce pulmonary complications.[214] Similar benefits of PVTB have been reported in infants and children.

Indications

Local anesthetics deposited in the paravertebral space usually spread longitudinally within the paravertebral gutter and laterally along the intercostal spaces, thereby effecting ipsilateral neural blockade of both sympathetic and somatic nerves. PVTB is used in adults for procedures such as cholecystectomy, renal surgery, and unilateral thoracotomy.

Anatomy

The thoracic paravertebral space contains somatic nerves, sympathetic chain, vessels, and loose connective tissue. It is a wedge-shaped space that separates the parietal pleura from the bony structures of ribs, vertebral transverse process, and vertebral body. It communicates with the epidural space medially via the intervertebral foramen and the intercostal space laterally. Local anesthetic solution usually spreads up and down the midline, but large volumes of the drug may spread laterally along the intercostal space or medially into the epidural space.[215]

Technique

In children, the PVTB catheter is placed either percutaneously or under direct vision through a thoracotomy incision. Percutaneous insertion of the catheter is generally performed in the lateral position with the side to be blocked facing up. The site of catheter insertion depends on the desired level of intercostal nerve blockade. A 18- or 20-gauge Tuohy needle is inserted approximately 2 to 3 cm lateral to the spinous processes and advanced at 90 degrees to the skin to strike the transverse process or the rib. The needle is attached to air or normal saline-filled syringe and redirected cephalad, "walked" off the bone, and advanced through the costotransverse ligament (Fig. 12–12). A slight "pop" may be felt (which is less distinct than that occurring when the epidural space is identified), and there is loss of resistance and easy injection of the fluid when the needle tip is within the paravertebral space. After negative aspiration for blood, CSF, and air, an epidural catheter is threaded to the desired level. Unlike epidural space cannulation, manipulation of the catheter may be necessary to facilitate passage of the catheter to the desired position.

Anesthetic Solution, Dose, Concentration, and Volume

Both bupivacaine and lidocaine have been safely used for continuous infusion of PVTB in a small numbers of infants and children. In anesthetized children who are more than 1 month of age, PVTB is accomplished by injecting a bolus of lidocaine 1 percent with epinephrine

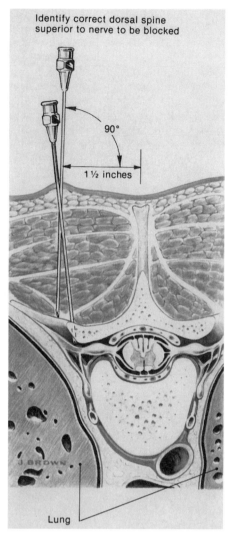

FIGURE 12–12. Midthoracic paravertebral nerve block. After contacting transverse process, the needle is withdrawn and redirected medially and inferiorly until loss of resistance to saline injection is identified or paresthesia of the thoracic nerve is elicited in an wake patient. (From Katz J: Thoracic paravertebral nerve block. *In* Atlas of Regional Anesthesia. Norwalk, CT, Appleton-Century-Crofts, 1989, p 95. The McGraw-Hill Companies, with permission.)

1:200,000, 0.5 ml/kg (5 mg/kg) followed by infusion of 0.25 ml/kg/h (2.5 mg/kg/h) 2 hours after the bolus. Safe peak plasma concentrations occurred at 15 to 30 minutes after a bolus injection of drug and ranged between 1.7 and 3.0 μg/ml. Steady-state concentrations of lidocaine were reached by 8 to 10 hours and remained below levels reported for systemic toxicity.[209]

In infants less than 5 months of age, an initial dose of bupivacaine of 0.5 ml/kg (1.25 mg/kg) is used followed an hour later by an infusion of 0.2 ml/kg (0.5 mg/kg/h) for 24 hours. The peak serum bupivacaine concentration occurred at a mean time of 10 minutes and the concentration progressively increased during the infusion period. Mean peak serum concentrations of bupivacaine after the initial bolus and during the infusion were low, 1 ± 0.6 and 2 ± 6, respectively. No patient showed clinical evidence of systemic drug toxicity.[212] We do not recommend prolonged infusion of bupivacaine at rates greater than 0.4 mg/kg/h using this technique. A longer infusion time of

36 to 48 hours and lower infusion dose of bupivacaine 0.125 percent, 0.25 mg/kg/h (0.2 ml/kg/h) with epinephrine 1:400,000 in infants less than 5 months produced comparable analgesia and mean serum concentration 1.6 ± 0.7 μg/ml (maximum, 3 μg/ml in three infants).[216] No systemic toxicity was observed in either regimen. The use of a safer local anesthetic such as 2-chloroprocaine, ropivacaine, or levobupivacaine, rather than racemic bupivacaine, may improve analgesia and reduce the risk of potential systemic toxicity.

Complications

The paravertebral space communicates medially with the epidural space; consequently, there is a significant risk of inadvertent epidural and spinal anesthesia.[215, 217] Other potential complications include pneumothorax and inadvertent intravascular injection of local anesthetics.[208] In a multicenter prospective study of percutaneous insertion of PVTB in 48 children ages 1 month to 15 years, the reported failure rate was 6.2 percent (3 of 48); one pleural puncture occurred, which did not result in a pneumothorax.[218] Inadvertent vascular puncture was recognized in two instances. There were no reports of hypotension or inadvertent subarachnoid puncture. These complications and failure rates can be minimized further by insertion of catheters into the paravertebral space under direct vision via thoracotomy incision.[212, 216] Such a technique is believed by its advocates to be inherently safer than thoracic or caudal-to-thoracic epidural catheter insertion in neonates and infants.

UPPER EXTREMITY BLOCK

Brachial Plexus Block

The axillary approach to brachial plexus block in children has gained favor because of its safety and ease of performance.[219] However, other techniques of brachial plexus block can be applied safely to children.[220–222] These techniques are utilized for elective and emergency procedures on the hand and forearm and for postoperative sympathetic block and pain control.

Axillary Brachial Plexus Block

Technique

The axillary artery is easily palpated in children at the junction of the pectoralis major and coracobrachialis muscles when the arm is abducted and externally rotated but not hyperextended. The artery and the plexus are more superficial in children than in adults. Once pulsation of the axillary artery is felt, a 22- or 23-gauge short-bevel needle is advanced superior and parallel to the artery until a distinct fascial click is felt as the needle enters the perivascular sheath. Confirmation of correct needle placement is manifested either by eliciting a paresthesia (not recommended because of increased potential for nerve injury and usually not tolerated by children) by using a nerve stimulator, or by simply observing the lateral

pulsation of the needle (Fig. 12–1).[223] In infants and toddlers, the axillary neurovascular sheath is superficial, located easily with a high success rate using a small cannula (e.g., 22-gauge cannula over the needle) and without the need to confirm proximity to the nerves.[224]

The supraclavicular approach for brachial plexus block is infrequently utilized in children because of the concern of producing a pneumothorax. Dalens and associates[225] described a modified parascalene supraclavicular approach to brachial plexus block in children. They based this approach on anatomic studies and designed it to avoid injuring the dome of the lung and other vital structures of the neck. The exploring needle approaches the brachial plexus in a strict anteroposterior direction. The child is positioned supine, the shoulders are propped up, and the head is turned to the side opposite the block. The needle enters the skin at the junction of the lower third and upper two thirds of a line joining the midclavicle to the C6 transverse process. An insulated block needle is inserted at 90 degrees to the skin and is advanced through the sternocleidomastoid and anterior scalene muscles to enter the interscalene space where the brachial plexus is located. The use of a nerve stimulator confirms correct placement of the needle (Fig. 12–13).

When the parascalene approach was compared with the classical supraclavicular approach, both techniques produced conduction blockade of almost all the infraclavicular branches of the brachial plexus. However, the complications (subclavian vessel puncture, phrenic nerve palsy, and Horner's syndrome) were observed significantly less often with the parascalene approach.[225] In children aged 0.5 to 12 years, a single injection of bupivacaine 0.25 percent 0.5 ml/kg via parascalene approach provides effective pain control in the first 12 postoperative hours.[226]

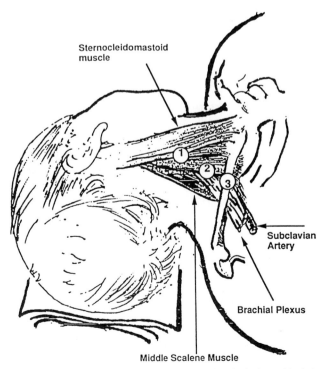

FIGURE 12–13. Parascalene approach to the brachial plexus block in a child.

Other techniques for brachial plexus block in children are similar to those frequently used in adults and should be applied in children with the same attention, precautions, and awareness of the anatomic landmarks used in adults. These techniques are well described by Dalens.[227]

Local Anesthetic Dose, Volume, and Concentration

The choice of local anesthetic solution depends on the expected duration of the surgical procedure. Long-acting local anesthetic solutions are preferred if the intention is to provide postoperative analgesia. The volume of anesthetic solution injected is crucial to the success of perivascular plexus block. It has been suggested that 0.6 to 0.7 ml/kg body weight or a volume based on the child's height will produce adequate anesthesia.[228, 229] The relationship of volume of anesthetic to degree of anesthesia has not been evaluated in infants and children. However, since a large volume of local anesthetic solution enhances the chances of anesthetizing all branches of the brachial plexus in adults, the largest volume of a local anesthetic solution permissible (i.e., giving a safe milligram per kilogram dose) is therefore employed in children for brachial plexus block (Table 12–9).

Recently, Campbell and colleagues[228] measured venous plasma bupivacaine concentrations in 41 children 2 to 15 years old after axillary block. These investigators compared two doses of bupivacaine 2 mg/kg and 3 mg/kg administered as 0.6 ml/kg. Absorption of the drug was very rapid, and mean peak plasma concentrations were reached by 22 minutes. They were below toxic levels for both doses: 1.4 ± 0.4 μg/ml after 2 mg/kg and 1.8 ± 0.5 μg/ml after 3 mg/kg. The highest individual plasma concentration of 2.7 μg/ml occurred in a patient who received 3 mg/kg without clinical manifestation of systemic toxicity. With infusions or repeated injections, maximum hourly dosing should not exceed the guidelines prescribed for epidural infusions in the previous section.[230]

Complications

The serious adverse reactions of this technique, convulsions and dysrhythmias, result from accidental intravascular injection. Puncturing the axillary artery may produce a hematoma and direct trauma to nerves may cause painful neuralgia or neuropathy.

Continuous Brachial Plexus Analgesia

Placement of an indwelling catheter into the brachial plexus sheath can now be done as the result of develop-

ment of the appropriate equipment and the use of the modified Seldinger technique. This technique is particularly useful in infants and children because it allows the the dose of anesthetic to be individualized, to provide prolonged postoperative analgesia, and to produce long-lasting sympathetic blockade after microvascular and reconstructive procedures of the hand. Successful continuous axillary analgesia with bupivacaine has been reported in teenagers with traumatic hand injury.[230, 231] Easy cannulation and threading of the catheter into the axillary sheath in children provides the advantage of promoting better proximal spread of the local anesthetic and greater opportunity of anesthetizing musculocutaneous nerve before it leaves the sheath. On occasion, we have employed continuous axillary infusion of bupivacaine to control pain after painful limb-lengthening (Ilizarov) procedures, which use multiple long-bone osteotomies and application of an external fixation frame that is fastened to the bones by many pins. These children undergo daily painful and vigorous physical therapy and bone distraction by stepwise elongation of the frame (Fig. 12–14).

Cervical Plexus Block

The cervical plexus arises from cervical nerves C2-4. They emerge between the tubercles of the cervical transverse processus, divide, and form loops that lie on the scalenus medius and beneath the prevertebral fascia. The posterior primary rami of the cervical nerves supply the cutaneous innervation to the back of the skull as high as the vertex, and the anterior rami supply the sensory innervation of the neck. The superficial cervical plexus emerges from the midpoint of the posterior border of the sternocleidomastoid muscle and fans out. These nerves include lesser occipital (C2), greater auricular (C2-3), transverse cervical (C2-3), and supraclavicular nerves (C3-4) (Fig. 12–15). Superficial cervical plexus block results in analgesia of the neck from the mandible to the clavicle anterolaterally. The deep cervical plexus provides motor innervation to strap muscles and the sternocleidomastoid muscle. The thyroid gland receives sympathetic innervation via the deep cervical nerve plexus.

The deep cervical plexus (C2-4 spinal nerves) is formed by paravertebral nerves that supply the prevertebral muscles, strap muscles of the neck, and the diaphragm (phrenic nerve).

A combination of superficial cervical plexus and local infiltration or deep cervical plexus block alone, with or without anxiolysis, is a safe alternative to general anesthesia for unilateral diagnostic cervical lymph node biopsy in older children and adolescents with mediastinal masses and potentially compromised airways.[232]

Technique

The technique of both the superficial and deep cervical plexus block is similar to that described in adults.

Superficial Plexus

The patient is positioned supine with head turned away from the side of the block. The sternocleidomastoid mus-

---

T A B L E   1 2 – 9
VOLUMES OF LOCAL ANESTHETIC SOLUTION FOR AXILLARY BRACHIAL PLEXUS BLOCK IN CHILDREN

Age (years)	Volume (ml)
< 1	3
1–15	0.6 ml/kg

Data from Eriksson,[220] Niesel et al.,[223] and Campbell et al.[228]

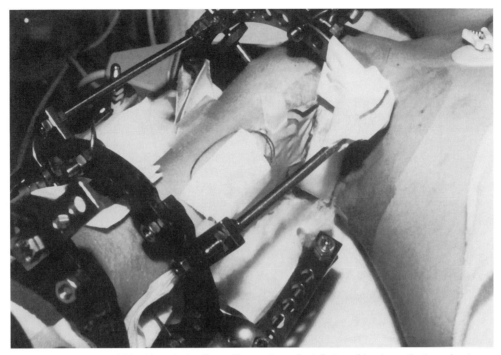

FIGURE 12–14. A child with an indwelling axillary catheter for infusion of local anesthetic analgesia.

cle is identified and a 22-gauge short bevel blunt needle is inserted at the midpoint of the posterior border of the muscle (C4 level at the upper border of the thyroid cartilage) and advanced into the interscalene groove and 2 to 5 ml of lidocaine 1 percent or bupivacaine 0.25 percent is injected depending on the size of the child.

Deep Cervical Plexus

The deep cervical plexus block is performed by blocking the C2-4 spinal nerves as they exit the intervertebral foramina and lie in the groove between the transverse processus. The tips of the cervical transverse processus are readily identified along a line drawn between the tip of the mastoid process and insertion of the sternocleidomastoid on the clavical. The C2 transverse process is first felt below the tip of the mastoid process. A 25-gauge, short-bevel, 1.5-inch, blunt needle is advanced medial and caudad to contact the transverse process and avoid inadvertent entry into the intervertebral foramina or slipping between the transverse processus and puncturing the vertebral artery. Proper needle positioning can be verified by the use of a nerve stimulator to elicit sternocleidomastoid and strap muscle contraction. Paresthesias should not be sought because they are painful and can be frightening to a child. A local anesthetic such as lidocaine 1 percent, usually 4 to 8 ml, depending on the size of the child, is usually adequate to spread along the paravertebral fascial plane and produce deep cervical plexus anesthesia.

Complications

Because of the proximity of the deep cervical plexus to the carotid and vertebral arteries, inadvertent intravascular injection of even a small volume of a local anesthetic can result in seizures and unconsciousness. Inadvertent injection of a local anesthetic into dural sleeves or extension of the local anesthetic into the intervertebral foramina may produce high epidural, subdural, and spinal anesthesia. Other potential complications include phrenic nerve block and sympathetic block if the needle is placed anterior to the prevertebral fascia. Bilateral deep cervical plexus blocks should be avoided because of the potential for serious respiratory compromise in the event both phrenic nerves are inadvertently blocked.

LOWER EXTREMITY BLOCK

Femoral Nerve Block

The femoral nerve (L2, L3, and L4) supplies motor innervation to the quadriceps muscle and sensory innervation to the overlying skin in the anterior aspect of the thigh, and sensory innervation to the periosteum of most of the femoral shaft. Grossbard and Love[233] and Tondare and Nadkarni[234] used femoral nerve blocks to relieve quadriceps muscle spasm and to allow pain-free manipulation of femoral shaft fractures in children, particularly fractures of the middle third of the shaft.

Technique

Landmarks for this block are the same as described for adults.[235] Femoral artery pulsation is identified about 1 to 1.5 cm below the middle of the inguinal ligament. A 22-gauge short-bevel needle is directed perpendicular to the skin just lateral to the femoral artery pulsation. A distinct pop is felt as the needle pierces the fascia surrounding the femoral neurovascular bundle. Local anesthetic is then

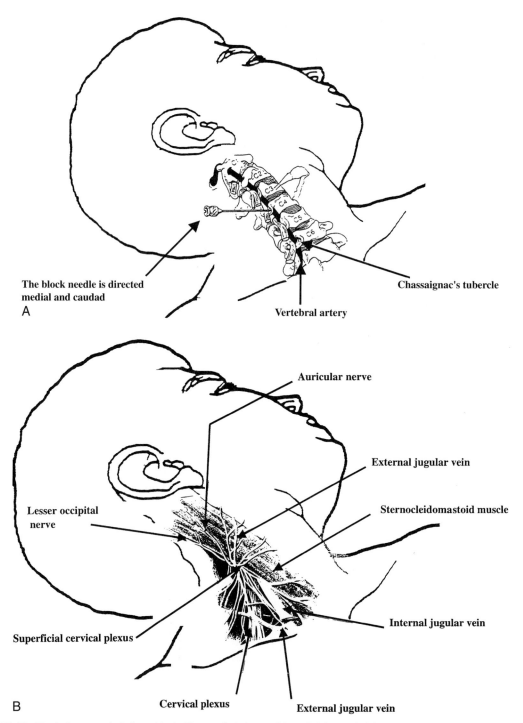

The block needle is directed medial and caudad

A

Chassaignac's tubercle

Vertebral artery

Auricular nerve

External jugular vein

Sternocleidomastoid muscle

Lesser occipital nerve

Internal jugular vein

Superficial cervical plexus

B

Cervical plexus

External jugular vein

FIGURE 12–15. *A,* Deep cervical plexus block. The needle is inserted in a slightly caudad direction until the tip of the transverse process is contacted. *B,* Superficial cervical plexus block. The needle is inserted along the posterior border and at midway between sternocleidomastoid muscle origin on the clavicle and insertion on the mastoid.

injected. Electrical nerve stimulation can be used to confirm proper positioning.

Khoo and Brown[235] described an alternative technique for blocking the femoral nerve. This block is based on the fact that the femoral nerve lies just lateral and slightly deep to the femoral artery but is separated from it by fascia iliaca. Loss of resistance is felt twice as the needle penetrates the two fascial layers of lata and iliaca (Fig. 12–16).

Anesthetic Solution, Dose, Volume, and Concentration

Selection of the anesthetic solution depends on the duration of neural block desired. Although the volumes re-

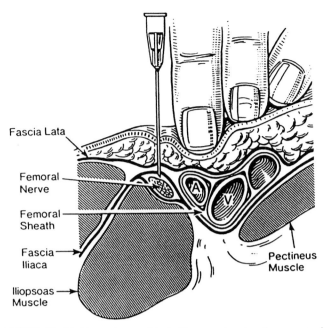

FIGURE 12–16. Femoral nerve block. Diagram showing the course of the needle piercing fascia lata and iliaca. (From Bridenoaugh PO: The lower extremity: somatic blockade. *In* Cousins MJ, Bridenbaugh PO [eds]: Neural Blockade in Clinical Anesthesia and Management of Pain. 2nd ed. Philadelphia, JB Lippincott Company, 1988, p 421, with permission.)

Labels on figure:
Fascia Lata
Femoral Nerve
Femoral Sheath
Fascia Iliaca
Iliopsoas Muscle
Pectineus Muscle

quired to block the femoral nerve at different ages have not been determined, Grossbard and Love[233] reported effective analgesia in children with femoral shaft fractures with 0.2 ml/kg (1 mg/kg) of bupivacaine 0.5 percent up to a maximum of 10 ml. This block lasted up to 4 hours.

One study used 0.4 ml/kg (2 mg/kg) of bupivacaine 0.5 percent for femoral nerve block in seven children aged 2 to 10 years old, which resulted in mean peak plasma levels of 0.9 ± 0.4 μg/ml at mean 24.4 ± 12.6 minutes and was below toxic levels. However, the analgesia lasted for only 3 hours.[236] We use 0.2 ml/kg (2 mg/kg) of lidocaine 1 percent without epinephrine for short procedures such as muscle biopsy. Onset of anesthesia occurs within 10 minutes and lasts for 40 to 50 minutes (Table 12–10). For prolonged analgesia for femur surgery or femur fracture, our preference would be to use bupivacaine 0.25 to 0.375 percent (or alternatively ropivacaine or levobupivacaine) with epinephrine in a larger volume (e.g., 0.6 ml/kg, up to a maximum of 30 ml). Fascia iliaca block (see below) is a useful alternative to femoral or inguinal perivascular nerve blockade.

Continuous femoral block via an indwelling catheter in the femoral sheath of children is an effective means of providing effective analgesia and continuous sympathectomy of a limb after major vascular and nerve injury repair

as well as for femoral fracture traction.[237] Continuous infusion of bupivacaine is commonly used, and the dosage is similar to the hourly maximum permissible rate of epidural analgesia (Table 12–6).

Lateral Femoral Cutaneous Nerve Block

Technique

The lateral femoral cutaneous nerve is anesthetized easily as the nerve emerges just below the inguinal ligament, medial and inferior to the anterior superior iliac spine. A 25- or 22-gauge needle is used to deposit local anesthetic solution in a fanwise manner deep and superficial to the fascia lata. Injection is continued as the needle is withdrawn to the skin. The lateral femoral cutaneous nerve can also be blocked before it leaves the pelvis, behind the anterior superior iliac spine at the iliac crest. The needle is advanced until it touches the inner side of the iliac crest and the local anesthetic is deposited at multiple angles. Suggested adequate block can be achieved with 0.25 mg/kg of 0.25 percent bupivacaine for prolonged block and 1 mg/kg of lidocaine 1 percent for short-duration block.

Inguinal Paravascular Block

In theory, this technique blocks the femoral, lateral femoral cutaneous, and obturator nerves (L1-L5). It provides excellent analgesia for surgical procedures on the anterior thigh. The technique is very similar to that for a femoral nerve block, except that the needle is directed cephalad 30 to 45 degrees. The position of the needle tip within the femoral fascial sheath is entered by the methods mentioned above. Once in place, the needle is immobilized and the desired volume of local anesthetic solution is injected while digital pressure is applied distal to the needle entry site to promote cephalad flow of the anesthetic solution.

Anesthetic Solution, Dose, Volume, and Concentration

The volume of anesthetic required to produce the block has not been established in children. Winnie[238] showed that a volume of 20 ml or greater is required to block all three nerves in adults. Dalens[227] suggested that 1 ml/kg of anesthetic is required for inguinal paravascular block in children ages 2 to 10 years. Any agent and concentration can be used for peripheral nerve block, as long as the maximal dose limit is not exceeded. If bupivacaine 0.5 percent is chosen, 0.5 ml/kg achieves the maximal allow-

TABLE 12 – 10
RECOMMENDED DOSES FOR FEMORAL NERVE BLOCK

Age	Bupivacaine Concentrations	Dose (ml/kg)	Duration	References
2–10 years	0.5%	0.4	~3 hours	Ronchi et al.[236]
≤1 year	0.5%	0.2	~3 hours	Bosenberg[65] and Tondare and Nadkarni[234]
15 months–5 years	0.125%	0.3 ml/kg/h (0.4 mg/kg/h)	2–5 days	Johnson[237]

able dose of 2.5 mg/kg. The study of Dalens et al.[239] suggests that the obturator and lateral femoral cutaneous nerves will not be reliably blocked with this approach (cf, below).

Complications

Accidental intravascular injection of local anesthetic may produce serious systemic toxicity, or a hematoma may occur if the femoral artery is injured. Nerve injury can produce sensory deficits, motor deficits, or pain.

Fascia Iliaca Compartment Block

This is a new single-injection technique whereby femoral, lateral femoral cutaneous, and obturator nerve blocks can be accomplished. These nerves lie on the anterior surface of the iliacus muscle and are enclosed by iliacus fascia.

Technique

The iliacus compartment is easily approached by inserting a needle at the junction of the lateral one third and the medial two thirds of the inguinal ligament. The needle is inserted 0.5 to 1 cm below the inguinal ligament and directed at a right angle to the skin. A short-bevel, blunt, 22- or 24-gauge needle is advanced until two "pops" are felt as the needle pierces the fascia lata and the iliacus fascia to enter the iliacus compartment. As the iliacus fascia is pierced, there is a distinct loss of resistance, analogous to that with entry into the epidural space. Local anesthetic is administered if there is no resistance to injection (Fig. 12–17).

A prospective comparison of the fascia iliacus block with the classic three-in-one femoral compartment block in children aged 0.7 to 17 years demonstrated that the iliacus block is easy to perform, does not require nerve location, and is effective in more than 90 percent of children. Fascia iliaca block is also likely to be safer than femoral or inguinal perivascular approaches, because with fascia iliaca block the needle is inserted centimeters away from major neurovascular structures. All children received the same mixture of anesthetic solution (lidocaine 1 percent and bupivacaine 0.5 percent, both with epinephrine 1:200,000). The volumes of the solution were based on body weights: 0.7 ml/kg for children weighing less than 20 kg, and 0.5 ml/kg for children weighing 20 kg and greater. The mean duration of postoperative analgesia was 5 hours.[239] In our experience, when bupivacaine is used as the sole local anesthetic in a dose of 2.5 mg/kg (up to a maximum of 100 mg), and epinephrine is added, the duration of analgesia is generally 10 to 12 hours, and occasionally as long as 18 hours.

The pharmacologic profile of bupivacaine 0.25 percent (2 mg/kg; 0.8 ml/kg) administered for fascia iliaca compartment block in children ages 1 to 14 years appears to be safe and similar to that for pediatric caudal anesthesia.[240] The median maximum plasma concentration of bupivacaine did not exceed 1.29 μg/ml with the plain solution and 0.96 μg/ml with addition of epinephrine (1:200,000) (Table 12–1).

Sciatic Nerve Block

The sciatic nerve (L4-L5, S1-S3) supplies motor innervation to extensor muscles of the hip and to flexors of the knee and ankle. It also supplies sensory innervation to the skin over the back of the thigh and leg to the dorsum of the foot. Sciatic nerve block is performed either in conjunction with saphenous nerve block for foot surgery and lower leg surgery or with femoral, obturator, and lateral femoral cutaneous nerve block (or fascia iliaca block) for lower extremity surgery around or above the knee.

Technique

Anterior and posterior approaches to sciatic nerve block have been safely and reliably employed in children.[241]

Posterior Approach

The child is placed in Sim's position. The landmarks for sciatic nerve block are the greater trochanter and the posterior superior iliac spine (Fig. 12–18). A line is drawn to connect these two points, and from its midpoint a perpendicular line is dropped to meet a line drawn from the greater trochanter medially to either the sacral hiatus or the tip of the coccyx. The points of intersection are the two alternative needle entry points, for the block. A 22-gauge, 3-inch spinal needle is inserted perpendicular to the skin and is advanced through the gluteal muscles until a paresthesia radiating down to the foot is elicited. Alternatively, a nerve stimulator connected to the needle will produce movement of the foot as the needle tip nears the nerve.

Anterior Approach

The patient is positioned supine with the lower extremy in a neutral position. A line representing the inguinal ligament is divided into three equal parts. A perpendicular line is drawn from the junction of the middle and medial thirds to meet a parallel line drawn from the greater trochanter that is extended medially. Intersection of these lines represents the needle entry point. A 22-gauge, 3.5-inch spinal needle is inserted at a right angle to the skin and is advanced until bone is contacted (lesser trochanter). The needle point is slipped off the bone medially and advanced to seek a paresthesia radiating to the foot or to elicit dorsal or plantar flexion of the foot when a nerve stimulator attached to the exploring needle is used. The distance from the skin to the sciatic nerve varies with the age and size of the child. McNicol[241] described a distinct sudden loss of resistance on entering the sciatic neurovascular compartment when a large-bore needle (16-gauge Medicut-Argyle) was used. A reliable block of the sciatic nerve occurred in 95 percent of children without complications. Despite that very positive report, the use of such a large-bore, sharp, long-bevel needle is a bit worrisome, given the relatively small diameter of the sciatic nerve in children and the blind nature of this technique. Aspiration for blood and injection of a test dose of local anesthetic will avoid intravascular injection of the calculated amount of local anesthetic solution.[241]

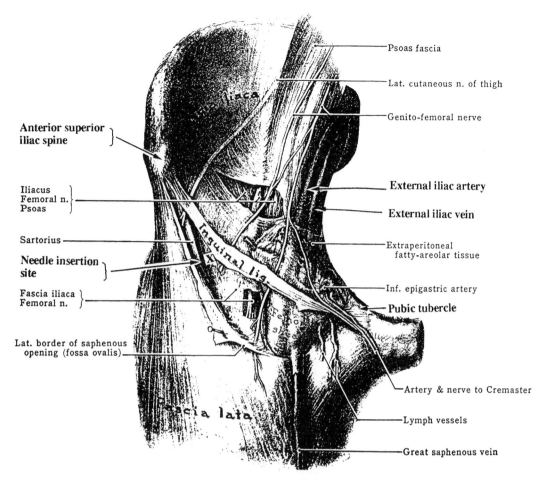

FIGURE 12–17. Fascia iliaca compartment block. Diagram showing the iliacus muscle compartment anatomy, landmarks, and the block needle entry site. (From Grant JCB: An Atlas of Anatomy. 5th ed. Baltimore, Williams & Wilkins, 1962, p 256, with permission.)

Labels in figure:
- Psoas fascia
- Lat. cutaneous n. of thigh
- Genito-femoral nerve
- External iliac artery
- External iliac vein
- Extraperitoneal fatty-areolar tissue
- Inf. epigastric artery
- Pubic tubercle
- Artery & nerve to Cremaster
- Lymph vessels
- Great saphenous vein
- Anterior superior iliac spine
- Iliacus / Femoral n. / Psoas
- Sartorius
- Needle insertion site
- Fascia iliaca / Femoral n.
- Lat. border of saphenous opening (fossa ovalis)

Single-Position Supine Sciatic Approach (Raj's Technique)

We prefer Raj's technique[242] for sciatic nerve block because the patient is placed in a tolerable lithotomy position, the landmarks are readily palpable, no special measurement is necessary, and the procedure can be performed readily with a high rate of success (Fig. 12–19).

The hip is fully flexed to 90 to 120 degrees and the leg is supported. This position flattens the gluteus maximus, decreasing the distance from skin to sciatic nerve. The sciatic nerve lies midway between the ischial tuberosity and the greater trochanter. A long 25- to 22-gauge needle is inserted perpendicular to the skin at the midpoint of a line drawn between the ischial tuberosity and the greater trochanter and is advanced until maximal ankle flexion-extension is elicited by a nerve stimulator.

Complications

As with all major nerve blocks, the complications include systemic toxicity that is caused by accidental intravascular injection of anesthetic solution or administration of a large amount of the anesthetic agent, and injury to the sciatic nerve and transient dysesthesia or delayed neuropathy.

Local Anesthetic Dose, Volume, and Concentration

The anesthetic agent and the concentration used for this block depend on the desired duration of the block. The suggested volume of bupivacaine 0.5 percent in children 3 months to 15 years is 0.2 ml/kg, or the dose regimen of lidocaine and bupivacaine combination recommended for fascia iliaca compartment block may also be employed for the sciatic nerve block.[242]

Sciatic Nerve Blockade in the Popliteal Fossa

The popliteal fossa is a diamond-shaped area filled with fat, delineated superiorly by long head of the biceps femoris and semitendinosus laterally and inferiorly by the medial and lateral heads of the gastrocnemius muscles. The sciatic nerve branches into two nerves in the popliteal fossa. The larger of the two nerves is the tibial and the smaller nerve is the common peroneal nerve. The tibial nerve descends caudally in the midline of the popliteal fossa. The sciatic nerve supplies cutaneous branches to popliteal fossa and back of the leg as well as muscular innervations to muscles of the posterior compartment of

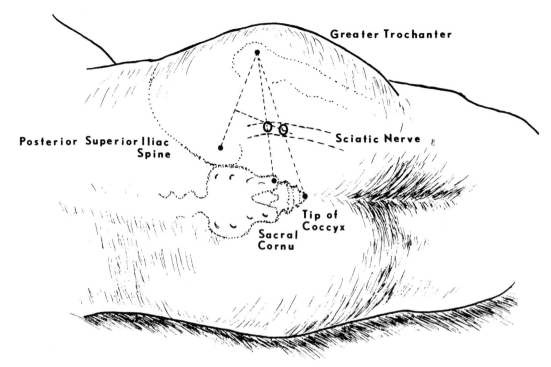

FIGURE 12–18. Sciatic nerve block. (From Sethna NF, Berde CB: Pediatric regional anesthesia. *In* Gregory GA [ed]: Pediatric Anesthesia. 2nd ed. New York, Churchill Livingstone, 1990, p 647, with permission.)

the leg. In the foot, the tibial nerve innervates the heel via medial calcanean branches and small muscles of the foot and the planter skin via medial and lateral plantar branches. The common peroneal nerve supplies articular nerves to the knee, muscular branches to the anterior compartment of the leg, and cutaneous innervation to the anterolateral aspect of the leg, foot, and heel.

Technique

The block is performed after aseptic skin preparation. The knee is extended while the patient is either prone or in the lateral decubitus position. The affected extremity is in

nondependent position. The popliteal fossa is outlined and divided into two upper and lower triangles by a horizontal line at the popliteal crease (intercondylar line) formed by flexing the leg. The upper triangle is further divided into two equal medial and lateral triangles by a vertical midline that is drawn from the apex. The nerves are anesthetized in the upper triangle, where the they lie superficial and lateral to the popliteal vessels. The needle is inserted as close to the apex of the upper triangle as possible, because at this point either the sciatic nerve or its two branches (tibial and common peroneal nerves) can be blocked with a single injection of local anesthetic. A short-beveled, blunt tip, 25- or 22-gauge needle is in-

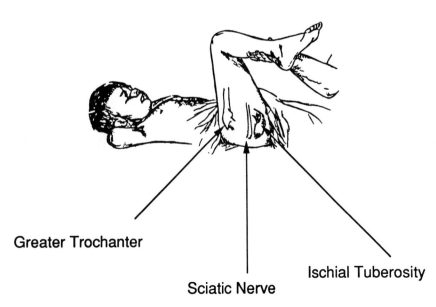

Greater Trochanter

Sciatic Nerve

Ischial Tuberosity

FIGURE 12–19. Landmarks for supine approach to sciatic nerve block.

serted 45 to 60 degrees to the skin just lateral to the midline vertical line and advanced through skin, subcutaneous fat, and popliteal fascial membrane. A nerve stimulator is used to locate the sciatic, peroneal, or tibial nerve; stimulation of either nerve results in twitching of the calf muscles and/or ankle flexion or extension. Very little resistance is encountered to injection of local anesthetic if the needle tip is in the correct place (Fig. 12–20).

Two approaches to locate the sciatic nerve and its branches have been described in children.[243, 244] In the first approach, the tibial and common peroneal nerves were blocked separately in 50 children. The block needle was placed just lateral to the popliteal artery pulsation at a point midway between the intercondylar line and the apex to block the tibial nerve. The needle was redirected laterally to block the common perineal nerve. In this study, the saphenous nerve block was also employed, using subcutaneous infiltration of local anesthetic at the medial aspect of the leg just below the knee where the nerve travels along with the saphenous vein.[243] The success rate with this technique was not stated, but a similar approach in adults has a 92 to 95 percent success rate.

In the second approach, the sciatic nerve was blocked at the apex of the popliteal diamond-shaped fossa wherein either the sciatic nerve or its two branches lie. Fifty children were prospectively studied and the block was successful in all patients. The successful block was defined as no significant change in hemodynamics (< 20 percent change in response to surgical stimulation). The latter technique has the distinct advantage that sciatic nerve blockade can be accomplished with a single injection. The depth of the insertion of the point of the needle to successfully locate the sciatic nerve with minimal nerve stimulation (0.4 mA, 1 msec) correlated with age, weight, and height of the patients, but weight was the best predictor. The minimal depth was 13 mm in a 2-month-old child.[244]

Saphenous Nerve Block

This nerve was blocked by subcutaneous infiltration of local anesthetic around the saphenous vein below the medial aspect of the knee, where it travels along with the saphenous vein.

Complications

Although no neural or cardiovascular complications were reported in the studies cited above when either of these approaches were used, the potential for these complications must be considered. Repeated aspiration is advised to avoid accidental entry of the needle into the popliteal vessels.

Local Anesthetic Dose, Volume, and Concentration

Bupivacaine 0.25 to 0.5 percent is used for sciatic nerve blockade in children. A single injection of 1 ml/kg of bupivacaine 0.25 percent was adequate for successful intraoperative blockade in children ages 2 months to 18 years.[244] Neural blockade of the tibial, common peroneal, and saphenous nerves around the knee in children with bupivacaine 0.5 percent, a total dose of 2.5 mg/kg (0.5 ml/kg), has produced complete analgesia of the lower extremity below the knee and provided postoperative analgesia of 12 hours.[243]

Ilioinguinal and Iliohypogastric Block

The ilioinguinal (L1) and iliohypogastric (T12, L1) nerves are major branches of the lumbar plexus. These nerves run in a plane between the transversus abdominus and the internal oblique muscles. The ilioinguinal nerve becomes superficial as it approaches the superficial inguinal ring

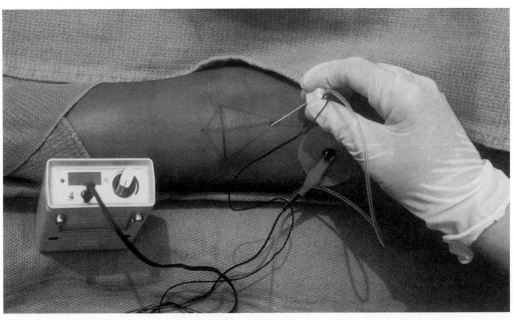

FIGURE 12–20. Popliteal fossa block. Skin markings outline the popliteal fossa. The needle is inserted close to the apex of the upper triangle and lateral to the midline.

and supplies cutaneous sensory innervation to the scrotum and the inner part of the thigh. The iliohypogastric nerve becomes superficial earlier in its course and supplies cutaneous innervation above the inguinal ligament.

Ilioinguinal and iliohypogastric (II-IH) nerve blocks are easy to perform and are widely used for postoperative pain relief after inguinal herniotomy, varicocele ligation, and orchidopexy. They are inadequate for operative anesthesia to explore and manipulate the spermatic cord and for testicular surgery. However, performing this block before surgery substantially decreases the requirement for deep levels of general anesthesia. Consequently, emergence from anesthesia is rapid, the requirement for postoperative analgesia is significantly reduced, and ambulation is possible earlier than with caudal and opioid analgesia.[245, 246]

Technique

Ilioinguinal and iliohypogastric nerve block are easily and readily accomplished by one of the following approaches: (1) percutaneous infiltration of bupivacaine into the fascial planes surrounding the nerves before the surgical incision is made, (2) direct infiltration of bupivacaine in proximity to the nerves after the incision is made, and (3) instillation of bupivacaine into the fascial and skin wounds (Fig. 12–21).[247, 248]

Local Anesthetic Dose, Volume, and Concentration

Various doses and concentrations of bupivacaine have been used successfully and without untoward effects. Shandling and Steward[246] recommended 2 mg/kg of bupivacaine 0.5 percent with epinephrine 1 : 200,000 for infants and children. This dose was effective and without clinical evidence of toxicity. Epstein et al.[249] used the same dose of bupivacaine 2 mg/kg for II-IH block in children over the age of 13 months and reported a mean maximal plasma bupivacaine concentration of 1.4 $\mu g/ml$, which is well below the concentration that causes minor CNS toxicity in adults. Peak venous plasma concentration were obtained in 26 minutes.

Much higher and near toxic plasma concentrations of bupivacaine are reported at 15 to 20 minutes after percutaneous II-IH nerve block in children with body weight less than 15 kg.[250] The mean venous plasma concentrations of bupivacaine in children with body weight less than 15 kg was 1.5 ± 0.9 (range, 0.43 to 4 $\mu g/ml$), while the mean plasma concentrations in children 15 to 30 kg was 0.9 ± 0.3 (range, 0.35 to 1.34 $\mu g/ml$). Although none of the children manifested systemic toxicity under general anesthesia, based on these findings, the investigators recommend not giving more than 1.25 mg/kg of bupivacaine in children with body weights of less than 15 kg (Table 12–1).

Casey and associates[247] prospectively compared the postoperative pain relief provided by simple instillation by bupivacaine into the hernia wound with that provided by infiltrating bupivacaine in the vicinity of the II-IH nerves. Both techniques were performed by the surgeon under direct vision at the end of inguinal herniorrhaphy in children. All blocks were performed with plain bupivacaine 0.25 percent (0.25 ml/kg). After irrigation of the surgical wound and skin, a 2-minute period was allowed for fixation of bupivacaine to the nerves. Although the instillation technique is simple and devoid of complications, unlike the percutaneous infiltration block, instillation cannot be utilized to supplement surgical anesthesia.[247] Moreover, the study design did not optimally detect differences in analgesia from 2 to 8 hours postoperatively. Recently, Conroy et al.[251] observed a significantly shorter emergence time from general anesthesia, less postoperative pain-related behavior, and less requirement for opioids after inguinal hernia repair in children who had received caudal analgesia compared with children who had received local anesthetic instilled into the wound.

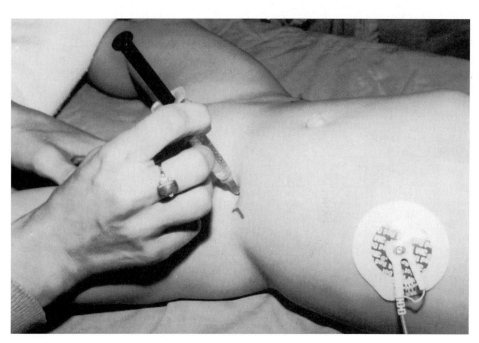

FIGURE 12–21. Ilioinguinal and iliohypogastric nerve block in a child.

Comparison of two regional anesthetic techniques of II-IH nerve block with subcutaneous infiltration to caudal anesthesia using bupivacaine with epinephrine demonstrated similar postoperative pain scores, opioid consumption, incidence of vomiting, and time to first micturition, but the discharge time was slightly longer with caudal injection.[117]

A rare effect of II-IH block is transient paresis of the quadriceps muscle group and/or numbness over the cutaneous distribution of the femoral nerve, which results from unintentional femoral nerve block. This occurs if the local anesthetic injection diffuses and tracks between fascial planes to reach the femoral nerve. This complication has been reported with the maximal recommended dose of bupivacaine 2 mg/kg, as well as with smaller doses of 1.25 mg/kg.[245, 252] No special treatment is required other than observation and avoidance of weight-bearing until the femoral nerve block dissipates.

Postoperative vomiting after pediatric herniorrhaphy is a common and distressing occurrence. The incidence of vomiting with II-IH nerve block is similar to that in children who receive codeine and fentanyl for postoperative analgesia.[245, 246, 253]

Percutaneous Infiltration Block of II-IH Nerves

Both II-IH nerves are blocked at a point 0.5 to 1 cm medial and 0.5 to 1 cm inferior to the anterior superior iliac spine above the inguinal ligament where the nerves converge (Fig. 12–22). A 22- or 23-gauge, short-bevel, blunt-tipped needle is directed at right angle to the skin and advanced through the skin, subcutaneous tissue, Scarpa's fascia, and the external oblique aponeurosis. A click is felt as the needle pierces the fascia and then the aponeurosis. The local anesthetic solution is injected, and the injection is continued as the needle is withdrawn. The latter maneuver ensures block of the T11 and T12 cutaneous innervation of the overlying skin.

Penile Block

The penis is innervated by the pudendal nerves (S2-S4) via two dorsal penile nerves. These nerves emerge from the pelvis under the symphysis pubis and run alongside the dorsal arteries and veins, deep to Buck's fascia. The dorsal nerves provide sensory innervation for the glands and most of the penile shaft except for the proximal and scrotal portions, which are innervated by branches of the genitofemoral and ilioinguinal nerves.[254]

Dorsal Penile Nerve Block

Dorsal penile nerve block (DPNB) is a reliable means of managing pain and distress in infants and children undergoing circumcision or correction of distal hypospadias.[255, 256] These surgical procedures are commonly performed in obstetrics wards, neonatal intensive care units, and pediatric surgical day-care units. Many studies have demonstrated that the DPNB is safe and effective, but it requires skill to perform. It is often used as the sole anesthetic during neonatal circumcision and appears to reduce the discomfort and distress incurred by the surgical pain.[257] Although DPNB may not completely block all the pain of circumcision (incomplete analgesia in 4 to 6 percent), it significantly mitigates the physiologic (heart rate, blood

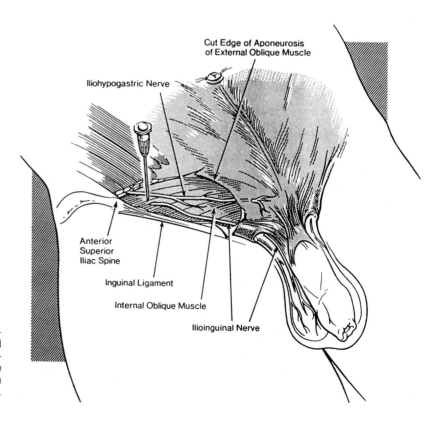

FIGURE 12–22. Diagram showing the course of ilioinguinal and iliohypogastric nerve, the landmarks, and the block needle insertion site. (From Brown T, Schulte-Steinberg O: Neural blockade for pediatric surgery. *In* Cousins MJ, Bridenbaugh PO [eds]: Neural Blockade in Clinical Anesthesia and Management of Pain. 2nd ed. Philadelphia, JB Lippincott Company, 1988, p 687.)

pressure, respiratory rate, transcutaneous oxygen tension, oxygen saturation, palmar sweating) and behavioral responses (crying, awake-sleep state, motor activity, grimace and other facial expressions) and modifies the adrenocortical stress responses of neonates undergoing circumcision.[258] The advantages of employing DPNB in conjunction with general anesthesia for circumcision and hypospadias repair in older children are the reduced requirement for inhalation anesthetic agents, quick emergence from anesthesia, less agitation during emergence, shorter recovery times, and earlier discharge from hospital. The postoperative analgesic requirement is also diminished when a long-acting local anesthetic solution is used.[254, 259] Caudal analgesia has also been employed to alleviate postcircumcision pain and is more effective than parenteral opioids or DPNB during the early postoperative period.[183, 260] Nevertheless, DPNB may afford a longer duration of analgesia when bupivacaine is used, and is free of undesirable effects that may be associated with caudal analgesia (e.g., delayed ambulation and micturition, vomiting, and lower extremity numbness). Moreover, in one study the analgesic requirement during the first 6 to 24 hours after PDNB was less than with caudal block.[184]

A recent randomized double-blind study showed that additional anesthesia of cutaneous perineal nerves (branches of pudendal nerve at the ventral aspect of penile shaft root) that innervates the base of the penis can improve the success of DPNB to 100 percent.[261]

The recommended local anesthetic doses and duration of analgesia vary, depending on how the volumes of anesthetic are calculated (weight vs. age) (Table 12–11). Maxwell et al.[262] measured the serum concentration of lidocaine after penile block with 0.8 ml of lidocaine 1 percent in 30 healthy term neonates and demonstrated serum concentrations considerably below accepted toxic concentrations in adults.

Although penile block is easy to perform, serious complications can result nevertheless, from inadvertent puncture either of the dorsal penile artery or the corpus cavernosum, which may produce a localized hematoma or from accidental injection of anesthetic solution into these structures, which can lead to systemic toxicity.[263] The use of large volumes of local anesthetic solutions is not recommended because they may cause pressure-induced compression of the penile blood vessels.

Penile Subcutaneous Ring Block

Penile cutaneous analgesia also can be achieved merely by infiltrating local anesthetic subcutaneously around the base of the penile shaft. Such a block produces effective and prolonged postcircumcision analgesia when a long-acting local anesthetic is used. It does not require specialized training, and it avoids injection of a local anesthetic deep in the vicinity of major penile neurovascular structures. Broadman et al.[264] demonstrated that, compared with placebo, a subcutaneous circumferential block of the penis with bupivacaine 0.25 percent in children 18 months to 10 years of age provided effective postoperative analgesia after circumcision, significantly reduced the postoperative analgesic requirement, shortened postanesthetic care unit stay, and allowed early discharge from the hospital.

Subpubic Penile Block

Recently, Dalens et al.[265] described a simple two-injection technique of penile nerve block via the subpubic space. They prospectively evaluated this technique in 100 children aged 3 months to 16 years undergoing penile shaft surgery. The technique consists of inserting a needle 0.5 to 1 cm on either side of midline, directing the needle approximately 70 degrees to the skin, and advancing it mesiad and caudad at approximately 20 degrees. Two injections are necessary because the two subpubic compartments are noncommunicating. The advantages of this technique compared with other penile nerve block techniques are that it is easy to perform and that there is less risk of damaging neurovascular or other penile structures. An effective block can be accomplished within 15 minutes of injecting a small volume of local anesthetic 0.1 ml/kg on each side (Fig. 12–23). Either lidocaine 1 percent or bupivacaine 0.5 percent can be used with a reported 100 percent reliability. Up to 24 hours of analgesia can be obtained with the latter solution. No complications were reported.[265]

Topical Penile Analgesia

Tree-Trakarn and Pirayavaraporn[266] have demonstrated the effectiveness of a single local application of lidocaine to produce topical analgesia for postcircumcision wound pain in children of ages 1 to 13 years. The topical lidocaine was used in the form either of a spray (10 to 20 mg of 10 percent solution), and ointment (0.5 ml of 5 percent preparation), or a jelly (0.5 to 1 ml of 2 percent preparation). The analgesia achieved with these topical preparations was highly effective in relieving pain in 95 percent of the children, compared with 72.7 percent of children given intramuscular morphine and 93.3 percent of those

---

T A B L E   1 2 – 11
RECOMMENDED DOSES FOR DORSAL PENILE NERVE BLOCK IN INFANTS AND CHILDREN*

Reference	Age	No. of Patients	Plain Anesthetic Solution	Dose	Plasma Concentrations (μg/ml)	Duration of Analgesia	Success Rate (%)
Sfez et al.[337]	3–11 years	12	Bupivacaine 0.25%	0.1 ml/kg	0.27 ± 0.1	6.7 ± 1.7 h	100
Kirya and Werthmann[257]	2–3 days	52	Lidocaine 1%	0.5 ml	NA	30 min	93
Maxwell et al.[262]	Newborns	30	Lidocaine 1%	0.8 ml	0.5 ± 0.2	NA	94

* No adverse effects or complications reported in these studies.

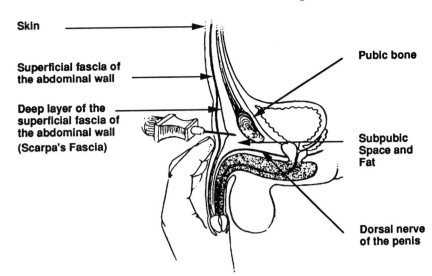

Skin

Superficial fascia of
the abdominal wall

Deep layer of the
superficial fascia of
the abdominal wall
(Scarpa's Fascia)

Pubic bone

Subpubic
Space and
Fat

Dorsal nerve
of the penis

FIGURE 12–23. Penile nerve block via the subpubic space approach in children. (From Dalens B, Vanneuville G, Dechelotte P: Penile block via the subpublic space in 100 children. Anesth Analg 69:41, 1989, with permission.)

having DPNB. The pain-free period following general anesthesia was significantly shorter (1 hour) compared with groups receiving topical lidocaine, intramuscular morphine, or DPNB (4 to 5 hours). No complications were reported, but plasma lidocaine concentrations were not measured. The absorption and safety of these preparations for neonatal circumcision sites have not as yet been determined. Despite the similarity in effectiveness of all the topical preparations of lidocaine, the spray appeared to be the most acceptable to the children, since it could be applied repeatedly without wound contact.

Topical Anesthesia for Circumcision

Numerous studies have described the benefits of DPNB. This technique has been recently compared to anesthetic infiltration of the foreskin and to topical anesthesia. The effectiveness of these techniques to blunt the physiologic, behavioral, and endocrine responses to neonatal circumcision is variable, and none is capable of entirely abolishing all the markers of the stress response.[262, 267–273]

Topical Analgesic EMLA Cream

Several investigators have examined the efficacy of 5 percent EMLA cream (Eutectic Mixture of 2.5 percent lidocaine and 2.5 percent prilocaine cream) in neonates and infants for a variety of superficial cutaneous and invasive medical procedures. A potential concern with the use of EMLA in newborns and infants is prilocaine toxicity. Prilocaine's metabolite ortho-toluidine can oxidize significant amount of hemoglobin to methemoglobin. Neonates and preterm infants are at increased risk for prilocaine toxicity for two reasons. First, the stratum corneum is thinner leading to high plasma levels. Second, the NADH-dependent methemoglobin reductase enzyme is 40 percent less active compared to adults. Normally, this enzyme reduces the methemoglobin to hemoglobin. Other possible risk factors that may predispose neonates to systemic toxicity are presence of anemia, sepsis, metabolic acidosis, hypoxemia, glucose-6-phosphate dehydrogenase (G6PD) deficiency, and the concomitant administration of

sulfonamides, acetaminophen, phenytoin, phenobarbital, nitroglycerin, nitroprusside, benzocaine, and other methemoglobin-inducing agents.[274] Despite this concern, clinical trials and case series indicate that the incidence of methemoglobinemia is very low among neonates receiving EMLA.

Effectiveness of EMLA cream is determined by dose, size of skin area over which it is applied, and duration of application. The estimated absorption rate in children (>1 month) and adults is 0.045 ± 0.016 for lidocaine and 0.077 ± 0.036 mg/cm^2/h for prilocaine. One study suggested that there might be racial differences in effectiveness of EMLA cream. The skin permeability is lower in adult black patients compared with adult Caucasian patients due to increased stratum corneum thickness, and therefore the dose and duration requirement may be higher.[275]

Cutaneous Side Effects

Local skin reactions associated with EMLA cream are related to prilocaine. Initial blanching is presumably caused by vasoconstriction at lower doses and redness is due to vasodilation when higher concentrations of the drug are used. Transient purpuric lesions have been described in areas of repeated applications within the first 4 days of life in preterm infants.[277]

Clinical experience has confirmed the safety and effectiveness of EMLA cream for dermal anesthesia in children. However, EMLA cream is not recommended for use in traumatized or inflamed skin and mucous membranes because of the potential risk for rapid absorption of the drug and systemic toxicity.

Use of EMLA in Neonatal Circumcision

Safe and effective method of topical analgesia produced by EMLA has been investigated in prospective, placebo-controlled, randomized trials for control of circumcision pain in full-term male neonates.[276, 278, 279] The largest of these trials included 68 neonates; 38 received EMLA cream and 30 received placebo.[279] The circumcision was effectively performed 60 to 80 minutes after EMLA cream application.

To ensure even spread of the cream over the penile skin, one third of a total dose of 1 ml (1 g) was applied to the lower abdomen, and the penis was extended upward and gently pressed against the abdomen. The remainder of the dose was applied to a transparent occlusive dressing that was placed over the penis and taped to the abdomen. No adverse effects were observed clinically. Plasma lidocaine and prilocaine concentrations were detectable in 61 percent and 55 percent of the infants, respectively. Neither drug was detectable 18 hours after the EMLA cream application. The prilocaine metabolite ortho-toluidine was undetectable in all infants. The apparent safety of similar dose of EMLA cream (1 g) has been confirmed in a smaller series of full-term infants undergoing circumcision. Blood methemoglobin concentration increased in these infants but did not exceed the normal baseline range.[280]

Although EMLA cream effectively decreases the pain associated with neonatal circumcision, as assessed by decreased facial activity, the duration of crying, and heart rate increases, it is less effective than dorsal penile nerve block and subcutaneous foreskin infiltration with local anesthetic.[279] Nevertheless, the demonstrated safety, efficacy, and simplicity of EMLA cream application is likely to prompt widespread implementation by general practitioners in an attempt to minimize the pain and distress of neonatal circumcision. Future studies are needed to examine whether longer application times and/or larger doses of the drug will yield safe plasma local anesthetic concentrations, low methemoglobin concentrations, and improved efficacy.

In view of the imperfections of all the available anesthetic techniques, other measures of supplemental analgesia and comfort should also be considered, such as use of acetaminophen, sucrose, pacifier, and maternal consolation.[278]

Use of EMLA in Preterm Infants

Application of a single dose of EMLA cream 0.5 g for 60 min/day on normal intact skin of preterm infants older than 30 gestational weeks appears to be safe and effective. The blood methemoglobin concentrations obtained at 4, 8, and 12 hours after application were not significantly different from baseline. These infants did not have any additional risk factors that predisposed them to methemoglobinemia.[276] Uncontrolled trials suggest repeated application of EMLA cream in term and preterm infants during the first week of life can result in high blood methemoglobin concentration and, although no clinical evidence of methemoglobin toxicity was observed, caution is advised.[276, 277]

INTERCOSTAL NERVE BLOCK

Intercostal nerve blocks are very useful for the relief of severe somatic pain caused by surgical procedures on the thorax and upper abdominal wall and by rib fractures. They can also be used to diagnose pain syndromes. In children, intercostal nerve blocks have been used for postthoracotomy incisional analgesia. In adults undergoing thoracotomy, intercostal nerve blocks are superior to systemic opioids for management of postoperative pain and improvement of pulmonary function.[282]

Technique

Intercostal nerve block can be accomplished by the anterior, lateral, and posterior approaches. The posterior approach is most suitable for relief of postthoracotomy incisional pain because the block is performed proximal to the surgical wound and the sympathetic chain is occasionally blocked when the anesthetic solution spreads dorsally. A sympathetic block may prevent conduction of nociceptive stimuli from the viscera. To perform the block, the child is positioned in the lateral decubitus position with the side to be blocked nondependent and the upper arm flexed and pulled forward. The block is performed just lateral to the sacrospinalis muscles at the angle of the rib. After the skin is prepared, a 22-gauge, short-bevel needle is advanced perpendicular to the skin until it touches the lower edge of the rib. With the other hand, the skin is moved caudally over the ribs so that the needle tip is walked off the lower edge of the rib (Fig. 12–24). The needle is advanced slowly 1 to 2 mm deeper until a pop is felt. The needle is fixed in place and is aspirated for air or blood. If aspiration is negative, 2 to 3 ml of anesthetic solution is injected. For each intercostal space that is to be blocked, the space on either side of this intercostal space is also blocked.

Caution must be exercised not to nick the pleura with the needle when the posterior approach is used. The internal intercostal muscles extend dorsally as far as the angles of the ribs, and the intercostal space beyond the rib angles is separated from the pleura by a thin aponeurosis of the internal intercostal muscle.[283] The distance from the skin to the intercostal space increases from lateral to posterior due to changes in the configuration of the rib from oval to trapezoidal shape and due to the size of the child and the thickness of the subcutaneous fat.

Intercostal nerve block can be performed percutaneously at the conclusion of the surgery or the surgeon can inject anesthetic solution into the intercostal spaces while the chest is open.

We usually avoid doing repeated percutaneous intercostal nerve blocks because most children object to the pain associated with multiple injections. To avoid this, we have employed continuous intercostal block by inserting epidural-type catheters via the thoracotomy incision space into the spaces on either side of the incision to allow intermittent injection of local anesthetic. The surgeon places these catheters percutaneously through a Tuohy needle at the termination of surgery before closing the thoracic cavity. Alternatives for prolonged postthoracotomy pain relief include thoracic or lumbar epidural infusions or interpleural catheter infusions. One alternative under investigation is the use of single-injection, sustained-release local anesthetics for prolonged intercostal blockade.[284, 285]

Anesthetic Solution, Dose, Volume, and Concentration

Bupivacaine is the most commonly used local anesthetic for intercostal nerve blocks because it typically relieves

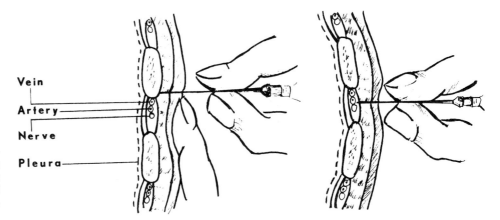

FIGURE 12–24. Technique of posterior intercostal nerve block. (From Bonica JJ: Local anesthetic and regional blocks. *In* Wall PD, Melzack R [eds]: Textbook of Pain. New York, Churchill Livingstone, 1980, p 551, with permission.)

pain for 4 to 10 hours, with the relief occasionally lasting for 24 hours in adults. Either 0.25 percent or 0.5 percent bupivacaine 1 to 5 ml can be used for intercostal nerve blocks in children. The maximal recommended dose of bupivacaine with 1:200,000 epinephrine should not exceed 3 mg/kg in anesthetized children. Absorption of local anesthetic from the intercostal spaces appears to be more rapid in children than in adults; consequently, children may achieve higher mean peak blood concentrations of bupivacaine than adults after being given comparable doses of the drug (Table 12–1).[18]

Complications

Inadvertent Pleural Puncture

Pleural puncture can cause pneumothorax with any of the three techniques. The incidence of pneumothorax in adults is very low when the block is done correctly. Most of these pneumothoraces in spontaneously ventilating patients are small and do not cause significant problems.[286] Data regarding technical aspects of performing intercostal block percutaneously by the three techniques and the associated complications in children are lacking.

Systemic Toxicity

The absorption of anesthetic solution from the intercostal space is much more rapid and the peak blood level is attained sooner than when the same amount of local anesthetic is deposited in other locations for regional anesthesia. Systemic absorption of local anesthetic from the intercostal space is even more rapid in children than in adults. Therefore, it is important not to exceed the maximal allowable dose of anesthetic solution and to add vasoconstrictors to delay the absorption of anesthetic from the intercostal space.

Accidental Subarachnoid Injection of Local Anesthetics

Subarachnoid injection of local anesthetic can occur if the needle is placed too close to the vertebral column while using the posterior approach for intercostal nerve block, because the dura usually extends anteriorly over the intercostal nerves before finally adhering to the nerve

sheaths. High spinal anesthesia may also result.[286] If it does, cardiopulmonary support should be instituted and continued until the effect of the local anesthetic wears off.

INTRAVENOUS REGIONAL ANESTHESIA (BIER BLOCK)

Intravenous regional anesthesia (IVRA) is effective for brief surgical procedures involving soft tissue, distal bony fracture reduction, and metacarpophalangeal pinning. Clinical and pharmacologic data on the use of IVRA in children are limited, despite the reliability and ease of this technique. IVRA should be used only when the child is able to understand the preblock preparation and the procedure. The onset of the block is rapid and recovery is prompt. IVRA provides satisfactory muscle relaxation and a bloodless field.

This technique is not suitable for surgical procedures exceeding 90 minutes. Intermediate-acting local anesthetics, such as lidocaine, are used. It is not advisable to use IVRA in children with seizure disorders or cardiac arrhythmias, nor is it appropriate in patients for whom tourniquet ischemia may aggravate disorders of peripheral nerves or circulation (e.g., Raynaud's phenomenon) or unstable hemoglobin (e.g., sickle hemoglobinopathy).

Simple equipment is adequate for safe and reliable induction of IVRA. A small-bore intravenous catheter (20 or 22 gauge), syringes, cotton padding (Webril), elastic bandage (Esmarch), inflatable cuffs appropriate for age and the child's limb circumference, and a calibrated standard sphygmomanometer or an automatic pneumatic tourniquet system are required. We often use an automatic pneumatic tourniquet system with high- and low-pressure alarms. This system compensates for minor cuff leaks by continually adding air. If the leak is substantial, a pressure alarm sounds within a few seconds to alert the operator. Nevertheless, the operator must periodically check for spontaneous deflation of the cuff.

In children younger than 12 years of age, elevation of the limb for 3 to 5 minutes is adequate to exsanguinate the limb and may spare the child the discomfort of applying an elastic bandage, particularly in the presence of a painful injury. Inflation of a single-cuffed tourniquet to 50 mm Hg above the child's measured systolic blood pressure satisfactorily occludes the blood flow to the limb.[287] Higher inflation pressures that are similar to those used in adults are applied to upper (180 to 240 mm Hg) and lower extremities (350 to 500 mm Hg) of children over the age of 3 years. Lower tourniquet pressures may be sufficient to occlude arterial blood flow in younger children who have lower systolic blood pressures.[288] However, it is always prudent to confirm the absence of peripheral pulses before injecting a local anesthetic, irrespective of the occlusion pressure used.

The safety and reliability of this technique are solely dependent on the completeness of arterial blood flow occlusion to the limb and adequate volume of local anesthetic agent. This seemingly easy technique has the potentially lethal hazard of tourniquet system failure and leak of a toxic dose of local anesthetic into the systemic circulation. The volume and speed with which a local anesthetic solution is injected into the veins determines the intravenous pressure generated distal to the correctly inflated tourniquet. Sufficient pressure can build up from injecting a large volume of a local anesthetic rapidly and cause leakage of local anesthetic into a large proimal vein, which may cause drug to escape past the tourniquet.[289] Injection of the local anesthetic over 60 seconds is safe in children.[290]

Although these safety measures for IVRA in adults have not been systematically evaluated in children of various ages, IVRA with lidocaine 0.5 percent has been employed successfully in children for both the upper and lower extremities.[288]

Olney and colleagues[290] recently reported their experience in 400 children aged 3 to 16 years with IVRA for emergency closed reduction of fractures and dislocation injuries distal to the elbow. Most children cooperated and tolerated IVRA very well when they had been prepared, received premedication, and were given an ongoing explanation of the various steps of the procedure. The limb was elevated for 30 to 60 seconds before the tourniquet cuff was inflated to 200 to 250 mm Hg; 3 mg/kg of preservative-free lidocaine 0.5 percent was injected slowly. The cuff was kept inflated for at least 20 minutes. The quality of anesthesia was graded as good in 90.3 percent of the children, fair in 3.5 percent, and poor in 6.2 percent, but only 2.3 percent had unacceptable analgesia and required general anesthesia for acceptable reduction of the fracture.

Of interest was the demonstration of lidocaine in the systemic circulation despite a functional tourniquet in 2 of 15 children. The plasma concentrations of lidocaine were below the toxic range. A third child, the only child who experienced a complication, developed myoclonic muscle contractions approximately 25 to 30 minutes after the cuff was deflated, probably because lidocaine was released after mobilization of forearm muscles, which produced a sudden rise in the peak plasma lidocaine concentrations.

The volume of local anesthetic required for a successful lower extremity IVRA block is less well defined. Good success has been reported with lidocaine 0.5 percent or 0.25 percent using 60 to 100 ml of drug, depending on the size of the lower extremity. There was no major CNS toxicity. The doses were calculated from body weights

and were approximately 5.4 mg/kg for the lower extremity, which exceeds the safe recommended dose of 3 mg/kg for the upper extremity.[288, 291]

Local Anesthetic Dose, Volume, and Concentration

Although many local anesthetic agents have been used for IVRA block, lidocaine is the most popular. It usually produces analgesia and muscle paralysis within 10 minutes. The cuff must not be deflated within 15 minutes of injection of the anesthetic solution because peak plasma levels of lidocaine can reach toxic levels greater than 5 μg/ml when 3 mg/kg of lidocaine is used. Peak concentrations of lidocaine after tourniquet release decline inversely with tourniquet time to subtoxic levels (Table 12–12).[292]

Complications

The major feared complications of this technique are unintentional leak of anesthetic from under the tourniquet or accidental deflation of the tourniquet cuff. Both can release toxic quantities of anesthetic solution into the systemic circulation. Therefore, all patients receiving IVRA must be monitored closely during and for an hour after the release of the tourniquet cuff. Neuropathy from tourniquet pressure may occur transiently but is a rare complication.[290]

ANKLE NERVE BLOCK

Neural block at the ankle is indicated for surgery on the plantar and dorsal aspect of the foot for removal of a foreign body or ingrowing toenail or for closure of lacerations. This block is of great value in children with recent intake of food. Unfortunately, the discomfort associated with the multiple injections necessary to block several nerves makes this procedure objectionable to many pediatric patients.

Five nerves innervate the foot. The dorsum of the foot is innervated by the saphenous, deep peroneal, and superficial nerves. The plantar aspect of the foot is mainly supplied by medial and lateral branches of the posterior tibial nerve. The lateral aspect of the foot, including the fifth toe, is innervated by the sural nerve.

The saphenous nerve is the only branch of the femoral nerve distal to the knee. It runs subcutaneously and innervates the proximal medial aspect of the foot. It is easily blocked by infiltration of anesthetic solution around the saphenous vein anterior to the medial malleolus.

The remaining four nerves are branches of the sciatic nerve. The deep peroneal nerve (anterior tibial nerve) runs deep to the extensor retinaculum and is next to the anterior tibial artery on the anterior surface of the distal end of the tibia. It runs between the tibialis anterior and the extensor hallucis longus tendons at the level of the medial malleolus. It innervates the adjacent joints and the skin between the first and second toes. A 25-gauge needle is advanced lateral to the extensor hallucis longus until

T A B L E 1 2 – 12					
RECOMMENDED LIDOCAINE DOSES FOR UPPER EXTREMITY IVRA IN CHILDREN					
Reference	Concentration (%)	Dose (mg/kg)	Fair–excellent Anesthesia (%)	CNS Complications (%)	
				Minor	Major
Carrel and Eyring[288]	0.25–0.5	2.4	82	8	None
FitzGerald[287]	0.5	4	94	None	None
Turner et al.[345]	0.5	3	80	0.5	None
Olney et al.[290]	0.5	3	94	0.2	None

the tibial bone is contacted, and anesthetic solution is deposited just superficial to the bone.

The posterior tibial nerve lies deep under the flexor retinaculum and posterior to the pulsation of the posterior tibial artery at the upper level of the medial malleolus. It innervates the skin and muscles of the plantar surface of the foot. The needle is inserted posterior to the pulsation of the posterior tibial artery and the local anesthetic is deposited in a fan-shaped distribution.

The sural nerve is a cutaneous nerve that supplies sensation to the lateral side of the foot and the lateral side of the little toe. The sural nerve is blocked by injecting a cuff of anesthetic subcutaneously from the lateral malleolus to the Achilles tendon.

The superficial peroneal nerve provides sensory innervation to the dorsum of the foot and is easily blocked by placing a subcutaneous wheal from the lateral malleolus to the extensor hallucis longus tendon.

After an ankle block, sufficient time (at least 15 minutes) should be allowed for adequate analgesia to develop.

Anesthetic Solution, Dose, Volume, and Concentration

Lidocaine and bupivacaine are commonly recommended solutions for ankle block. Lidocaine 1 or 1.5 percent provides a block of intermediate duration, whereas bupivacaine 0.25 to 0.5 percent provides long-lasting analgesia. These solutions can be used with epinephrine. To avoid toxic serum anesthetic concentrations, the total volume of drug administered must not exceed the maximal recommended dose (Table 12–1).

Singler[34] suggested using lower concentrations of local anesthetic for infants and children. He suggested that lidocaine 1 percent or bupivacaine 0.25 percent with epinephrine be used for infants under 1 year of age and lidocaine 1 or 1.5 percent or bupivacaine 0.25 or 0.375 percent with epinephrine 1:200,000 for children between 1 and 5 years of age.

Complications

Pressure ischemia is a theoretical concern when a large volume of anesthetic solution is injected around the anterior aspect of the ankle between the two malleoli. Other potential but rare complications are infection, neuropathy, and hematoma. The latter two complications can result from direct needle injury to a nerve or an artery, respectively.

INTERPLEURAL ANALGESIA

Preliminary studies suggested that continuous interpleural analgesia in children provided excellent analgesia with a high success rate after thoracotomy. Infusions of 0.5 to 1 ml/kg/h of bupivacaine 0.25 percent with epinephrine 1:200,000 were used. Although the peak plasma concentration in some patients exceeded 2 μg/ml and in a few greater than 7 μg/ml after 24 hours of drug infusion, none of the children exhibited CNS toxicity.[293] Many children in this study also received benzodiazepines and hypnotics during the infusion period. Although no convulsions were reported in this study, we are aware of anecdotal reports of convulsions from other clinicians. As with infusions in other sites, we would recommend not exceeding bupivacaine infusion rates of 0.2 mg/kg/h for infants less than 6 months of age, and not exceeding rates of 0.4 mg/kg/h for older infants and children.

For management of subcostal incisional pain, the recommended initial dose is 0.5 ml/kg (2.5 mg/kg) of bupivacaine 0.5 percent with epinephrine 1:200,000. This can be followed by 0.15 ml/kg/h of bupivacaine 0.25 percent with epinephrine.[17, 293]

Additional studies are warranted to evaluate the pharmacokinetics of continuous infusions lasting more than 24 hours in children and the safety of this technique compared with continuous epidural analgesia. It is our view that epidural analgesia is safer and more efficacious than interpleural analgesia.

INFILTRATION OF THE SURGICAL WOUND WITH ANESTHETIC

Incisional pain and tenderness in adults have been effectively alleviated by infiltrating local anesthetic around the wound edges, application of topical anesthetics, or perfusion of local anesthetic into the wound and the surrounding fascial planes.[266, 294]

Fell and colleagues[295] injected local anesthetic into inguinal herniotomy incisions in children and produced analgesia comparable to that of caudal analgesia. The effective dose of bupivacaine 0.25 percent used for wound edge infiltration was 0.5 ml/kg.

The absorption of bupivacaine 0.25 percent after subcutaneous infiltration is considerably slower, and the plasma concentrations measured are far below toxic ranges (see Table 12–1).[19]

The extent and duration of analgesia provided by local anesthetic solution, whether by infiltration or topical application, are contingent on the dose and concentration of the solution used (see Table 12–1).

TOPICAL ANALGESIA OF CUTANEOUS OR MUCOSAL SURFACES

Clinicians have long been aware of the potential psychological trauma to pediatric patients from hospitalization and medical procedures. Painful medical procedures increase their emotional distress, and fear often renders them uncooperative.[296] Topical local anesthetics are now available to alleviate the pain and distress associated with needle insertion and performance of simple procedures such as venipuncture, lumbar puncture, minor wound suturing, laryngoscopy, and bronchoscopy.[297]

EMLA (Eutectic Mixture of Local Anesthetics)

A eutectic mixture of local anesthetics with equal amounts of lidocaine and prilocaine (5 percent EMLA) provides analgesia by penetration through intact skin when applied for 60 minutes or more, making it useful for venipuncture and other needle procedures, and some minor superficial types of cutaneous surgery. A double-blind comparison of 5 percent EMLA cream with placebo in 102 children aged 1 to 5 years showed significantly less pain associated with venipuncture in the group receiving cutaneous EMLA analgesia.[298] Although similar results have been demonstrated in older children, some of these children exhibited anxiety because they anticipated needle-induced pain.[299, 300]

The minimal application time for 5 percent EMLA to become effective has been reported to range from 45 minutes in children under 5 years compared with 60 minutes in older children aged 4 to 15 years.[299, 301] The reliability of EMLA is increased if it is applied for at least 70 to 90 minutes before the painful stimulus is initiated.

Venous plasma concentrations of lidocaine and prilocaine after dermal application of 5 percent EMLA cream (2 ml applied over a 16-cm^2 area for 4 hours) in 22 infants aged 3 to 12 months were below the toxic level; the maximum peak plasma concentration in children greater than 6 months was 155 ng/ml for lidocaine and 79 ng/ml for prilocaine; in infants ages 3 to 6 months, it was 127 ng/ml for lidocaine and 131 ng/ml for prilocaine. The doses used were 5 to 12 mg/kg for both lidocaine and prilocaine. The plasma concentrations of methemoglobin 4 hours after cutaneous application of EMLA cream were below toxic levels. The highest individual concentration of methemoglobin was 2 percent of the total hemoglobin.[298]

Prilocaine-lidocaine cream should be used with caution in infants less than 3 months old and in infants and children receiving other methemoglobin-inducing medications. Combining these drugs increases the risk for clinically significant methemoglobinemia.[274, 298]

Halperin et al.[302] evaluated 5 percent EMLA cream to relieve the pain of venipuncture, subcutaneous medication reservoir injection, and lumbar subarachnoid tap in 18 children with cancer, aged 6 to 12 years, in a double-blind, placebo-controlled trial. Application of EMLA significantly alleviated the pain associated with repeated needle sticks in these children.

EMLA may facilitate other painful procedures, such as caudal, lumbar, and spinal anesthesia. It may also facilitate other peripheral nerve blocks in infants and children who may not otherwise cooperate without sedation. A recent report suggests that EMLA is safe and effective as the sole anesthetic for circumcision in neonates.

Amethocaine Gel

Amethocaine (tetracaine) gel is a newly introduced topical local anesthetic available in the British Isles and Australia for anesthetizing intact skin surfaces. It contains tetracaine as a free base (4 percent w/w) in an aqueous gel, and 1g of the gel provides a dose of 40 mg of amethocaine. Amethocaine is a highly lipophilic aminoester type local anesthetic that easily penetrates stratum corneum, resulting in faster and prolonged duration onset of action compared to other percutaneous topical anesthetics.[305, 306] Tetracaine is rapidly metabolized by nonspecific esterases locally in the skin and circulation and therefore produces low systemic toxicity.

The onset of cutaneous anesthesia occurs within 45 minutes after application for venous cannulation and lasts for 4 to 6 hours.[307] When compared to EMLA cream, amethocaine produced significantly greater acceptable analgesia (defined as pain scores of 0 to 1 on Visual Analogue Scale of 10 points) for venous cannulation in 85 percent of children receiving amethocaine for 40 minutes in contrast to 67 percent of those who were treated with EMLA.[308, 309] Another advantage of amethocaine gel over EMLA cream is vasodilatation, which facilitates visualization of the veins.

Adverse effects with amethocaine are primarily at the site of application and presumably due to vasodilatation. The reported incidence of erythema is 30 percent (not necessarily an adverse effect), and edema and itching in less than 5 percent of the patients.[308, 310] Because of rapid tissue hydrolysis of amethocaine, little or no systemic absorption is reported in an adult preliminary trial, even when the drug was applied for prolonged periods of time.[311] To date, no systemic toxicity has been reported with application of amethocaine onto intact skin in adults or children. Amethocaine is not presently recommended for use on damaged or inflamed skin and mucosal surfaces because of risk of rapid absorption and systemic toxicity. No data are available on the safety of amethocaine in term infants under the age of 1 month or in preterm infants. The safety of amethocaine gel use in patients with quantitative or qualitative pseudocholinesterase deficiencies has not been reported, but it is generally considered safe given the negligible amount of amethocaine absorbed from intact skin. The risk of sensitization reactions from repeated application, contact by health care providers, and accidental mucosal contact remains unknown and deserves further investigation.[312] Further studies are needed to assess efficacy of amethocaine use in many clinical settings in which EMLA cream is used.

Amethocaine appears to be an attractive alternative to EMLA because of its safety, shorter onset time, prolonged duration of action, and relatively lower cost.

Other Topical Anesthetic Agents

Successful topical analgesia with tetracaine-epinephrine-cocaine (TAC) for nonintact skin, such as lacerations of the skin of the face and scalp, has been widely used in pediatric patients. TAC, when applied to lacerated wounds, produces profound cutaneous anesthesia. The standard formulation of TAC consists of tetracaine 0.5 percent, epinephrine 1:2,000, and cocaine 11.8 percent.[313, 314] It is usually applied to the dermal lacerations via a gauze and moistened with TAC. The pad is held gently against the wound surface to promote spread of the TAC solution. Local analgesia is achieved after a minimum of 10 minutes or when visible blanching of the wound is observed.[315]

Variations of the original TAC preparation have efficacy similar to the original solution. One half the standard concentration (half-strength), standard TAC formulation without tetracaine, and TAC mixture containing different concentrations of tetracaine 1 percent, epinephrine 1:4,000, and cocaine 4 percent have all been used successfully.[316–318]

The anesthetic efficacy of TAC for facial and scalp wounds in children ranges from 75 to 98 percent; the success rate is greater in preadolescent children.[315] The optimal dose of TAC in children has not been determined. Consequently, some investigators have recommended using diluted solution and lower volumes of the standard TAC mixture.[318, 319] Terndrup et al.[319] recently measured the plasma concentrations of the local anesthetic components of TAC after applying 3 ml of the standard solution to the wounds of children under the age of 16 years. No tetracaine was found in the plasma. Cocaine was measurable in 75 percent of the children, but its presence was not associated with clinical evidence of systemic toxicity.[308, 309] The plasma concentrations of these drugs were highest after the drugs were applied to facial wounds.

Despite its short elimination half-life (40 to 150 minutes), cocaine and its metabolites have been detected in the blood and urine of patients for many hours after the application of TAC mixture. Prolonged elimination of cocaine by these patients is presumed to be due to slow release of the drug from subcutaneous deposits and/or to delayed elimination of cocaine that is caused by competition between tetracaine and cocaine for hydrolysis by cholinesterases.[315, 320]

Systemic cocaine toxicity has been reported in children after misuse of TAC. Excessive TAC doses, accidental contact of TAC with mucous surfaces, and application of TAC to burns all have resulted in deaths, seizures, agitation, and hemodynamic instability.[321–323]

Cocaine and norepinephrine are vasoconstrictors and should not be used on distal body tissues that lack collateral circulation, such as the digits, nose, and penis. Since tetracaine and cocaine are hydrolyzed by serum cholinesterase, a history of cholinesterase deficiency should be sought before TAC anesthesia is used. TAC is also inadvisable in the presence of cardiac arrhythmias, coronary disease, and seizures.[315]

TAC has been used widely in pediatric practice because it is effective, easy to apply, and causes minimal discomfort. Because of the lack of data on the optimal formulation and minimal effective dose, as well as the potential life-threatening side effects that may result from accidental misapplication of this mixture, TAC should be used only by physicians familiar with the toxicity of local anesthetics and its treatment. Personnel skilled in pediatric resuscitation should be readily available.[315, 324] Replacement of aqueous cocaine with viscous cocaine in the TAC solution significantly reduces the cocaine absorption from small lacerations (a mean length of 2.2 cm) in children ages 3 to 13 years.[325]

Recently, a combination of lidocaine, epinephrine, and tetracaine (LET) (4 percent lidocaine, 1:2,000 epinephrine, and 0.5 percent tetracaine) has been introduced as a safer alternative to TAC for repair of simple lacerations of the face and scalp in children. It has replaced TAC in many pediatric emergency departments because of its effectiveness for dermal lacerations, lower cost, lack of requirement for a controlled substance with abuse potential, and significantly lower systemic toxicity, even when applied close to mucous membranes.[326]

Many new combinations of topical anesthetic preparations have been introduced and designed for open skin wounds and are currently under investigation for application on the broken skin and mucosal surfaces and for safety and efficacy relative to TAC and lidocaine infiltration.[327–330]

Topical Lidocaine Anesthesia

The absorption kinetics of topical lidocaine to the nasopharynx, supraglottis and glottis, and tracheobronchial tree have received limited attention in children.

Many factors influence the absorption characteristics of lidocaine, such as the age of the child; concentration of lidocaine; mode of delivery via spray, jell, or neubulization; site of delivery (highly absorptive surface in the distal respiratory tract); and mucosal moisture (faster from dry mucosa).

A controlled trial of spraying the glottis and supraglottis of spontaneously breathing children with lidocaine 5 percent, 0.8 mg/kg in less than 10 kg and 1.6 to 0.8 mg/kg in children 10 to 20 kg produced safe maximum plasma concentration of 1 ± 0.5 μg/ml (Table 12–1).[331]

Wilson and associates[324] have reported experience with 575 bronchoscopic and/or bronchographic procedures in infants and children utilizing lidocaine 1 percent as a spray to anesthetize the respiratory mucosa. More than 99 percent of patients tolerated bronchoscopy with minimal discomfort. Only 0.5 percent of the patients felt that the procedure was unsatisfactory. The dose of lidocaine ranged from 1.4 to 2.3 mg/kg body weight. Although plasma concentrations of lidocaine were not determined, lidocaine toxicity was not observed clinically. Absorption of topical laryngeal and tracheal lidocaine in children is rapid, and the peak plasma levels are widely variable and much higher than with other regional techniques (see Table 12–1). A recent controlled, randomized, double-blind trial in a small number of children (1.5 months to 16 years) found that nebulization of lidocaine 4 to 8 mg/kg via a face mask was safe (mean plasma levels, 1.2 ± 0.5 μg/ml) and moderately effective in producing anesthesia in 50 percent of the children for flexible bronchoscopy.[332] A major disadvantage of nebulization is that a substantial amount of the lidocaine dose is lost to the room and oropharynx (Table 12–1).

REFERENCES

1. Anand KJ, Coskun V, Thrivikraman KV, et al: Long-term behavioral effects of repetitive pain in neonatal rat pups. Physiol Behav 66:627, 1999.
2. Dalens B: Regional Anesthesia in Infants, Children, and Adolescents. 2nd ed. London, Baltimore, Williams & Wilkins, Waverly Europe, 1995.
3. Gray HT: A study of spinal anaesthesia in children and infants. Lancet 913, 1909.
4. Bainbridge WS: A report of twelve operations on infants and young children during spinal analgesia. Arch Pediatr 18:510, 1901.
5. Amster L: Spinal anesthesia for poor pediatric surgical risks. N Y Med Rec 213, 1936.
6. Abajian JC, Mellish RWP, Browne AF, et al: Spinal anesthesia for surgery in the high-risk infant. Anesth Analg 63:359, 1984.
7. Liu SS, Carpenter RL, Mackey DC, et al: Effects of perioperative analgesic technique on rate of recovery after colon surgery. Anesthesiology 83:757, 1995.
8. Kehlet H: Multimodal approach to control postoperative pathophysiology and rehabilitation [Review]. Br J Anaesth 78:606, 1997.
9. Yeager MP, Glass DD, Neff RK, Binck-Johnsen T: Epidural anesthesia and analgesia in high-risk surgical patient. Anesthesiology 66:729, 1987.
10. Basse L, Hjort Jakobsen D, Billesbolle P, et al: A clinical pathway to accelerate recovery after colonic resection. Ann Surg 232:51, 2000.
11. Berkowitz A, Rosenberg H: Femoral block with mepivacaine for muscle biopsy in malignant hyperthermia patients. Anesthesiology 62:651, 1985.
12. Cooper MG, Sethna NF: Epidural analgesia in patients with congenital lumbosacral spinal anomalies. Anesthesiology 75:370, 1991.
13. Vandam LD, Dripps RD: Exacerbation of pre-existing neurologic disease after spinal anesthesia. N Engl J Med 255:843, 1956.
14. Luz G, Wieser C, Innerhofer P, et al: Free and total bupivacaine plasma concentrations after continuous epidural anaesthesia in infants and children. Paediat Anaesth 8:473, 1998.
15. Luz G, Innerhofer P, Bachmann B, et al: Bupivacaine plasma concentrations during continuous epidural anaesthesia in infants and children. Anesth Analg 82:231, 1996.
16. Larsson BA, Lonnqvist PA, Olsson GL: Plasma concentrations of bupivacaine in neonates after continuous epidural infusion. Anesth Analg 84:501, 1997.
17. McIlvaine WB, Chang HT, Jones M: The effective use of intrapleural bupivacaine for analgesia after thoracic and subcostal incisions in children. J Pediatr Surg 23:1184, 1988.
18. Rothstein P, Arthur CR, Feldman HS, et al: Bupivacaine for intercostal nerve blocks in children: blood concentrations and pharmacokinetics. Anesth Analg 65:625, 1986.
19. Eyres RK, Kidd J, Oppeneim R, Brown TCK: Local anaesthetic plasma levels in children. Anaesth Intensive Care 6:243, 1978.
20. Tucker GT: Parmacokinetics of local anaesthetic agents. Br J Anesth 58:717, 1986.
21. Wood M: Plasma binding and limitation of drug access to site of action. Anesthesiology 75:721, 1991.
22. Mazoit JX, Denson DD, Samii K: Pharmacokinetics of bupivacaine following caudal anesthesia in infants. Anesthesiology 68:387, 1988.
23. Lerman J, Strong HA, LeDez KM, et al: Effects of age on the serum concentration of alpha 1-acid glycoprotein and the binding of lidocaine in pediatric patients. Clin Pharmacol Ther 46:219, 1989.

24. Lerman J, Strong A, LeDez KM, et al: Effects of age on the serum concentration of alpha-acid glycoprotein and the binding of lidocaine in pediatric patients. Clin Pharmacol Ther 46:219, 1989.
25. Booker PD, Taylor C, Saba G: Perioperative changes in alpha 1-acid glycoprotein concentrations in infants undergoing major surgery. Br J Anaesth 76:365, 1996.
26. Hu D, Hu R, Berde CB: Neurologic evaluation of infant and adult rats before and after sciatic nerve blockade. Anesthesiology 86:957, 1997.
27. Kohane DS, Sankar WN, Shubina M, et al: Sciatic nerve blockade in infant, adolescent, and adult rats: a comparison of ropivacaine with bupivacaine. Anesthesiology 89:1199, 1998.
28. Berde CB: Toxicity of local anesthetics in infants and children. J Pediatr 122:S14, 1993.
29. Gunter JB, Eng C: Thoracic epidural anesthesia via the caudal approach in children. Anesthesiology 76:935, 1992.
30. Bosenberg AT, Bland BA, Schulte SO, Downing JW: Thoracic epidural anesthesia via caudal route in infants. Anesthesiology 69:265, 1988.
31. Heavner JE, Racz GB: Conduction block by lidocaine and bupivacaine: neonate versus adult. In Tyler DC, Krane EJ (eds): Pediatric Pain. Vol 15. New York, Raven Press, 1990, p 181.
32. Benzon HT, Strichartz GR, Gissen AJ, et al: Developmental neurophysiology of mammalian peripheral nerves and age-related differential sensitivity to local anaesthetic. Br J Anaesth 61:754, 1988.
33. Zsigmond EK, Downs JR: Plasma cholinesterase activity in newborns and infants. Can Anaesth Soc J 18:278, 1971.
34. Singler RC: Pediatric regional anesthesia. In Gregory GA (ed): Pediatric Anesthesia. New York, Churchill Livingstone, 1980, p 487.
35. Henderson K, Sethna NF, Berde CB: Continuous caudal anesthesia for inguinal hernia repair in former preterm infants. J Clin Anesth 5:129, 1993.
36. Finholt DA, Stirt JA, DiFazio CA, Moscicki JC: Lidocaine pharmacokinetics in children during general anesthesia. Anesth Analg 65:279, 1986.
37. Ecoffey C, Desparmet J, Berdeaux A, et al: Pharmacokinetics of lignocaine in children following caudal anaesthesia. Br J Anaesth 56:1399, 1984.
38. Miyabe M, Kakiuchi Y, Kihara S, et al: The plasma concentration of lidocaine's principal metabolite increases during continuous epidural anaesthesia in infants and children. Anesth Analg 87:1056, 1998.
39. Resar LM, Helfaer MA: Recurrent seizures in a neonate after lidocaine administration. J Perinatol 18:193, 1998.
40. Rothstein P, Dornbusch J, Shaywitz BA: Prolonged seizures associated with the use of viscous lidocaine. J Pediatr 101:461, 1982.
41. Eyres RL: Local anaesthetic agents in infancy. Paediatr Anaesth 5:213, 1995.
42. Eyres RL, Brown TCK, Hastings C: Plasma level of bupivacaine during convulsion. Anaesth Intensive Care 11:385, 1983.
43. Ecoffey C, Desparmet J, Maury M, et al: Bupivacaine in children: pharmacokinetics following caudal anesthesia. Anesthesiology 63:447, 1985.
44. McClellan KJ, Spencer CM: Levobupivacaine. Drugs 56:355, 1998.
45. Bardsley H, Gristwood R, Baker H, et al: A comparison of the cardiovascular effects of levobupivacaine and rac-bupivacaine following intravenous administration to healthy volunteers. Br J Clin Pharmacol 46:245, 1998.
46. Gunter JB, Gregg T, Varughese AM, et al: Levobupivacaine for ilioinguinal/iliohypogastric nerve block in children. Anesth Analg 89:647, 1999.
47. Ivani G, Mereto N, Lampugnani E, et al: Ropivacaine in paediatric surgery: preliminary results. Paediatr Anaesth 8:127, 1998.
48. Ivani G, Lampugnani E, Torre M, et al: Comparison of ropivacaine with bupivacaine for paediatric caudal block. Br J Anaesth 81:247, 1998.
49. Da Conceicao MJ, Coelho L, Khalil M: Ropivacaine 0.25% compared with bupivacaine 0.25% by the caudal route. Paediatr Anaesth 9:229, 1999.
50. Da Conceicao MJ, Coelho L: Caudal anaesthesia with 0.375% ropivacaine or 0.375% bupivacaine in paediatric patients. Br J Anaesth 80:507, 1998.
51. Khalil S, Campos C, Farag AM, et al: Caudal block in children: ropivacaine compared with bupivacaine. Anesthesiology 91:1279, 1999.

52. Fried E, Bailey A, Valley R: Electrocardiographic and hemodynamic changes associated with unintentional intravascular injection of bupivicaine with epinephrine in infants. Anesthesiology 79:394, 1994.

53. Ved SA, Pinosky M, Nicodemus H: Ventricular tachycardia and brief cardiovascular collapse in two infants after caudal anesthesia using a bupivacaine-epinephrine solution. Anesthesiology 79:1121, 1993.

54. Desparmet J, Mateo J, Ecoffey C, Mazoit X: Efficacy of an epidural test dose in children anesthetized with halothane. Anesthesiology 72:249, 1990.

55. Tanaka M, Nishikawa T: Simulation of an epidural test dose with intravenous epinephrine in sevoflurane-anesthetized children. Anesth Analg 86:952, 1998.

56. Sethna NF, Sullivan LJ, Retik A, et al: Efficacy of simulated epinephrine-containing epidural test-dose after intravenous atropine in children anesthetized with Isoflurane. Reg Anesth Pain Manage 25:566, 2000.

57. Tanaka M, Nishikawa T: Evaluating T-wave amplitude as a guide for detecting intravascular injection of a test dose in anesthetized children. Anesth Analg 88:754, 1999.

58. Toledano A, Roizen MF, Foss J: When is testing the test dose the wrong thing to do? [Editorial; comment]. Anesth Analg 80:861, 1995.

59. Guinard JP, Mulroy MF, Carpenter RL, Knopes KD: Test dose: optimal epinephrine content with and without acute beta-adrenergic blockade. Anesthesiology 73:386, 1990.

60. Tanaka M, Nishikawa T: The efficacy of a simulated intravascular test dose in sevoflurane-anesthetized children: a dose-response study. Anesth Analg 89:632, 1999.

61. Selander D, Edshage S, Wolff T: Paresthesiae or no paresthesiae? Acta Anaesthiol Scand 23:27, 1979.

62. Kaiser H, Niesel HC, Hans V: Basic considerations and requirements of peripheral nerve stimulation. Reg Anesth 13:143, 1990.

63. Pither CE, Raj PP, Ford DJ: The use of a peripheral nerve stimulator for regional anesthesia: a review of experimental characteristics, technique, and clinical applications. Reg Anesth 10:49, 1985.

64. Montogomery SJ, Raj P, Nettles D, Jenkins MT: The use of the nerve stimulator with standard unsheathed needles in nerve blockade. Anesth Analg 52:827, 1973.

65. Bosenberg A: Lower limb nerve blocks in children using unsheathed needles and a nerve stimulator. Anaesthesia 50:206, 1995.

66. Sethna NF, Berde CB: Pediatric regional anesthesia equipment. Int Anesthesiol Clin 30:163, 1992.

67. Welborn LG, Rice LJ, Hannallah RS, et al: Postoperative apnea in former preterm infants: prospective comparison of spinal and general anesthesia. Anesthesiology 72:838, 1990.

68. Krane EJ, Haberkern CM, Jacobson LE: Postoperative apnea, bradycardia, and oxygen desaturation in formerly premature infants: prospective comparison of spinal and general anesthesia. Anesth Analg 80:7, 1995.

69. Somri M, Gaitini L, Vaida S, et al: Postoperative outcome in high-risk infants undergoing herniorrhaphy: comparison between spinal and general anaesthesia. Anaesthesia 53:762, 1998.

70. Cote CJ, Kell DH: Postoperative apnea in a fulll-term infant with a demonstrable respiratory pattern abnormality. Anesthesiology 72:559, 1990.

71. Noseworthy J, Duran C, Khine HH: Postoperative apnea in a full-term infant. Anesthesiology 70:880, 1989.

72. Tetzlaff JE, Annand DW, Pudimat MA, Nicodemus HF: Postoperative apnea in a full-term infant. Anesthesiology 69:426, 1988.

73. Kokki H, Tuovinen K, Hendolin H: Spinal anaesthesia for paediatric day-case surgery: a double-blind, randomized, parallel group, prospective comparison of isobaric and hyperbaric bupivacaine. Br J Anaesth 81:502, 1998.

74. Vane DW, Abajian JC, Hong AR: Spinal anesthesia for primary repair of gastroschisis: a new and safe technique for selected patients. J Pediatr Surg 29:1234, 1994.

75. Viscomi CM, Abajian JC, Wald SL, et al: Spinal anesthesia for repair of meningomyelocele in neonates. Anesth Analg 81:492, 1995.

76. Cote CJ, Zaslavsky A, Downes JJ, et al: Postoperative apnea in former preterm infants after inguinal herniorrhaphy. Anesthesiology 82:809, 1995.

77. Dohi S, Naito H, Takahashi T: Age-related changes in blood pressure and duration of motor block in spinal anesthesia. Anesthesiology 50:319, 1979.

78. Oberlander TF, Berde CB, Lam KH, et al: Infants tolerate spinal anesthesia with minimal overall autonomic changes: analysis of heart rate variability in former premature infants undergoing hernia repair. Anesth Analg 80:20, 1995.

79. Pascucci RC, Hershenson MB, Sethna NF, et al: Chest wall motion of infants during spinal anesthesia. J Appl Physiol 68:2087, 1990.

80. Harnik EV, Hoy GR, Potolicchio S, et al: Spinal anesthesia in premature infants recovering from respiratory distress syndrome. Anesthesiology 64:95, 1986.

81. Blaise GA, Roy WL: Spinal anaesthesia for minor paediatric surgery. Can Anaesth Soc J 33:227, 1986.

82. Beauvoir C, Rochette A, Desch G, D'Athis F: Spinal anaesthesia in newborns: total and free bupivacaine plasma concentration. Paediatr Anaesth 6:195, 1996.

83. Mahe V, Ecoffey C: Spinal anesthesia with isobaric bupivacaine in infants. Anesthesiology 68:601, 1988.

84. Parkinson SK, Little WL, Malley RA, et al: Use of hyperbaric bupivacaine with epinephrine for spinal anesthesia in infants. Reg Anesth 15:86, 1990.

85. Gouveia MA: Raquianestesia para pacientes pediatricos. Rev Bras Anestesiol 20:503, 1970.

86. Yamashita M, Kumagai M, Miyazono Y: Height to body weight ratio and spinal anaesthesia for ex-premature infants. Paediatr Anaesth 4:397, 1994.

87. Assali NS, Brinkman CRI, Woods JRJ, et al: Development of neurohumoral control of fetal, neonatal, and adult cardiovascular functions. Am J Obstet Gynecol 129:748, 1977.

88. Duckles SP, Banner WJ: Changes in vascular smooth muscle reactivity during development. Annu Rev Pharmacol Toxicol 24:65, 1984.

89. Gleason CA, Martin RJ, Anderson JV, et al: Optimal position for a spinal tap in preterm infants. Pediatrics 71:31, 1983.

90. Weisman LE, Merenstein GB, Steenburger JR: The effect of lumbar puncture position in sick neonates. Am J Dis Child 137:1077, 1983.

91. Bonadio WA, Smith DS, Metrou M, Dewitz B: Estimating lumbar puncture depth in children. N Engl J Med 319:952, 1988.

92. Batnitzky S, Keucher TR, Mealey J, Campbell RL: Iatrogenic intraspinal epidermoid tumors. JAMA 237:148, 1977.

93. Tabadorr K, Lamorgese UR: Lumbar epidermoid cyst following single spinal puncture. J Bone Joint Surg 57:1168, 1975.

94. Darson H, Welch K, Segal M: Physiology and Pathophysiology of the Cerebral Spinal Fluid. New York, Churchill Livingstone, 1987, p 733.

95. Kurth CD, Spitzer AR, Broennle AM, Downes JJ: Postoperative apnea in preterm infants. Anesthesiology 66:483, 1987.

96. Malviya S, Swartz J, Lerman J: Are all preterm infants younger than 60 weeks postconceptual age at risk for postanesthetic apnea? Anesthesiology 78:1076, 1993.

97. Gallagher TM, Crean PM: Spinal anaesthesia in infants born prematurely. Anaesthesia 44:434, 1989.

98. Sartorelli KH, Abajian JC, Kreutz JM, Vane DW: Improved outcome utilizing spinal anesthesia in high-risk infants. J Pediatr Surg 27:1022, 1992.

99. Kokki H, Hendolin H, Turunen M: Postdural puncture headache and transient neurologic symptoms in children after spinal anaesthesia using cutting and pencil point paediatric spinal needles. Acta Anaesthesiol Scand 42:1076, 1998.

100. Bailey A, Valley R, Peacock J: Regional anaesthesia in high-risk infants [Letter]. Can J Anaesth 39:203, 1992.

101. Tobias JD, Burd RS, Helikson MA: Apnea following spinal anaesthesia in two former pre-term infants. Can J Anaesth 45:985, 1998.

102. Wright TE, Orr RJ, Haberkern CM, Walbergh EJ: Complications during spinal anesthesia in infants: high spinal blockade. Anesthesiology 73:1290, 1990.

103. Cox RG, Goresky GV: Life-threatening apnea following spinal anesthesia in former premature infants. Anesthesiology 73:345, 1990.

104. Ramamoorthy C, Geiduschek JM, Bratton SL, et al: Postdural puncture headache in pediatric oncology patients. Clin Pediatr 37:247, 1998.

105. Burt N, Dorman BH, Reeves ST, et al: Postdural puncture headache in paediatric oncology patients. Can J Anaesth 45:741, 1998.

106. Schwartz N, Eisenkraft JB: Probable venous air embolism during epidural placement in an infant. Anesth Analg 76:1136, 1993.

107. Guinard J-P, Borboen M: Probable venous air embolism during caudal anesthesia in a child. Anesth Analg 76:1134, 1993.

108. Dalens B, Hasnaoui A: Caudal anesthesia in pediatric surgery: success rate and adverse effects in 750 consecutive patients. Anesth Analg 68:83, 1989.
109. Sethna NF, Berde CB: Venous air embolism during identification of the epidural space in children [Editorial; comment]. Anesth Analg 76:925, 1993.
110. Hatch D, Hulse M, Lindahl G: Caudal analgesia in children. Influence on ventilatory efficiency during halothane anaesthesia. Anaesthesia 39:873, 1984.
111. Gunter JB, Watcha MF, Forestner JE, et al: Caudal epidural anesthesia in conscious premature and high-risk infants. J Pediatr Surg 26:9, 1991.
112. Spear R, Deshpande J, Maxwell L: Caudal anesthesia in the awake, high-risk infant. Anesthesiology 69:407, 1988.
113. Willis RJ: Caudal epidural blockade. In Cousins MJ, Bridenbaugh PO (eds): Neural Blockade in Clinical Anesthesia and Management of Pain. Vol 3. Philadelphia, Lippincott-Raven, 1998, p 323.
114. Veyckemans F, Van Obbergh LJ, Gouverneur JM: Lessons from 1100 pediatric caudal blocks in a teaching hospital. Reg Anesth 17:119, 1992.
115. Fisher QA, McComiskey CM, Hill JL, et al: Postoperative voiding interval and duration of analgesia following peripheral or caudal nerve blocks in children. Anesth Analg 76:173, 1993.
116. McGown RG: Caudal analgesia in children. Anaesthesia 37:806, 1982.
117. Splinter WM, Bass J, Komocar L: Regional anaesthesia for hernia repair in children: local vs caudal anaesthesia. Can J Anaesth 42:197, 1995.
118. Sethna NF, Berde CB: Pediatric regional anesthesia. In Gregory GA (ed): Pediatric Anesthesia. 2nd ed. New York, Churchill Livingstone, 1990, p 647.
119. Busoni P, Andruccetti T: The spread of caudal analgesia in children: a mathematical model. Anaesth Intensive Care 14:140, 1986.
120. Takasaki M, Dohi S, Kawabata Y, Takahashi T: Dosage of lidocaine for caudal anesthesia in infants and children. Anesthesiology 47:527, 1977.
121. Schulte SO, Rahlfs VW: Caudal anaesthesia in children and spread of 1 per cent lignocaine. A statistical study. Br J Anaesth 42:1093, 1970.
122. Broadman LM, Hannallah RS, Norrie WC, et al: Caudal analgesia in pediatric outpatient surgery: a comparison of three different bupivacaine concentrations [Abstract]. Anesth Analg 66:S191, 1987.
123. Wolf AR, Valley RD, Fear DW, et al: Bupivacaine for caudal analgesia in infants and children: the optimal effective concentration. Anesthesiology 69:102, 1988.
124. Gunter JB, Dunn CM, Bennie JB, et al: Optimum concentration of bupivacaine for combined caudal–general anesthesia in children. Anesthesiology 75:57, 1991.
125. Krane EJ, Jacobson LE, Lynn AM, et al: Caudal morphine for postoperative analgesia in children: a comparison with caudal bupivacaine and intravenous morphine. Anesth Analg 66:647, 1987.
126. Finley GA, McGrath PJ, Forward SP, et al: Parents' management of children's pain following 'minor' surgery. Pain 64:83, 1996.
127. Constant I, Gall O, Gouyet L, et al: Addition of clonidine or fentanyl to local anaesthetics prolongs the duration of surgical analgesia after single shot caudal block in children. Br J Anaesth 80:294, 1998.
128. Cook B, Grubb DJ, Aldridge LA, Doyle E: Comparison of the effects of adrenaline, clonidine and ketamine on the duration of caudal analgesia produced by bupivacaine in children. Br J Anaesth 75:698, 1995.
129. Dupeyrat A, Goujard E, Muret J, Ecoffey C: Transcutaneous CO_2 tension effects of clonidine in paediatric caudal analgesia. Paediatr Anaesth 8:145, 1998.
130. Ivani G, Mattioli G, Rega M, et al: Clonidine-mepivacaine mixture vs plain mepivacaine in paediatric surgery. Paediatr Anaesth 6:111, 1996.
131. Jamali S, Monin S, Begon C, et al: Clonidine in pediatric caudal anesthesia. Anesth Analg 78:663, 1994.
132. Klimscha W, Chiari A, Michalek-Sauberer A, et al: The efficacy and safety of a clonidine/bupivacaine combination in caudal blockade for pediatric hernia repair. Anesth Analg 86:54, 1998.
133. Luz G, Innerhofer P, Oswald E, et al: Comparison of clonidine 1 microgram kg^{-1} with morphine 30 micrograms kg^{-1} for postoperative caudal analgesia in children. Eur J Anaesthesiol 16:42, 1999.
134. Motsch J, Bottiger BW, Bach A, et al: Caudal clonidine and bupivacaine for combined epidural and general anaesthesia in children. Acta Anaesthesiol Scand 41:877, 1997.
135. Ivani G, Bergendahl HT, Lampugnani E, et al: Plasma levels of clonidine following epidural bolus injection in children. Acta Anaesthesiol Scand 42:306, 1998.
136. Lee JJ, Rubin AP: Comparison of a bupivacaine-clonidine mixture with plain bupivacaine for caudal analgesia in children. Br J Anaesth 72:258, 1994.
137. Concepcion M, Arthur GR, Steele SM, et al: A new local anesthetic, ropivacaine. Its epidural effects in humans. Anesth Analg 70:80, 1990.
138. Katz JA, Bridenbaugh PO, Knarr DC, et al: Pharmacodynamics and pharmacokinetics of epidural ropivacaine in humans. Anesth Analg 70:16, 1990.
139. Morrison LM, Emanuelsson BM, McClure JH, et al: Efficacy and kinetics of extradural ropivacaine: comparison with bupivacaine. Br J Anaesth 72:164, 1994.
140. Emanuelsson BM, Persson J, Sandin S, et al: Intraindividual and interindividual variability in the disposition of the local anesthetic ropivacaine in healthy subjects. Ther Drug Monit 19:126, 1997.
141. Knudsen K, Beckman Suurkula M, Blomberg S, et al: Central nervous and cardiovascular effects of i.v. infusions of ropivacaine, bupivacaine and placebo in volunteers. Br J Anaesth 78:507, 1997.
142. Scott DB, Lee A, Fagan D, et al: Acute toxicity of ropivacaine compared with that of bupivacaine. Anesth Analg 69:563, 1989.
143. Habre W, Bergesio R, Johnson C, et al: Pharmacokinetics of ropivacaine following caudal analgesia in children. Paediatr Anaesth 10:143, 2000.
144. McCann M, Sethna N, Sullivan L, et al: Pharmacokinetics of lumbar epidural ropivacaine in children and adolescents. Anesthesiology 3A:1251, 1998.
145. Emanuelsson BM, Persson J, Alm C, et al: Systemic absorption and block after epidural injection of ropivacaine in healthy volunteers. Anesthesiology 87:1309, 1997.
146. Emanuelsson BM, Zaric D, Nydahl PA, Axelsson KH: Pharmacokinetics of ropivacaine and bupivacaine during 21 hours of continuous epidural infusion in healthy male volunteers. Anesth Analg 81:1163, 1995.
147. Meignier M, Souron R, Le Neel J: Postoperative dorsal epidural analgesia in the child with respiratory disabilities. Anesthesiology 59:473, 1983.
148. Koinig H, Krenn CG, Glaser C, et al: The dose-response of caudal ropivacaine in children. Anesthesiology 90:1339, 1999.
149. Rosen KR, Rosen DA: Caudal epidural morphine for control of pain following open heart surgery in children. Anesthesiology 70:418, 1989.
150. Wolf AR, Hughes D, Wade A, et al: Postoperative analgesia after paediatric orchidopexy: evaluation of a bupivacaine-morphine mixture. Br J Anaesth 64:430, 1990.
151. Krane EJ, Tyler DC, Jacobson LE: The dose response of caudal morphine in children. Anesthesiology 71:48, 1989.
152. Attia J, Ecoffey C, Sandouk P, et al: Epidural morphine in children: pharmacokinetics and CO_2 sensitivity. Anesthesiology 65:590, 1986.
153. Vila R, Miguel E, Montferrer N, Barat G, et al: Respiratory depression following epidural morphine in an infant of three months of age. Paediatr Anaesth 7:61, 1997.
154. Karl HW, Tyler DC, Krane EJ: Respiratory depression after low-dose caudal morphine. Can J Anaesth 43:1065, 1996.
155. Findlow D, Aldridge LM, Doyle E: Comparison of caudal block using bupivacaine and ketamine with ilioinguinal nerve block for orchidopexy in children. Anaesthesia 52:1110, 1997.
156. Semple D, Findlow D, Aldridge LM, Doyle E: The optimal dose of ketamine for caudal epidural blockade in children. Anaesthesia 51:1170, 1996.
157. Marhofer P, Krenn CG, Plochl W, et al: S(+)-ketamine for caudal block in paediatric anaesthesia. Br J Anaesth 84:341, 2000.
158. Yaksh TL: Epidural ketamine: a useful, mechanistically novel adjuvant for epidural morphine? [Editorial; comment]. Reg Anesth 21:508, 1996.
159. Agarwal R, Gutlove DP, Lockhart CH: Seizures occurring in pediatric patients receiving continuous infusion of bupivacaine. Anesth Analg 75:284, 1992.
160. McCloskey JJ, Haun SE, Deshpande JK: Bupivacaine toxicity secondary to continuous caudal epidural infusion in children. Anesth Analg 75:287, 1992.

161. Wolf AR, Eyres RL, Laussen PC, et al: Effect of extradural analgesia on stress responses to abdominal surgery in infants. Br J Anaesth 70:654, 1993.
162. Desparmet J, Meistelman C, Barre J, Saint-Maurice C: Continuous epidural infusion of bupivacaine for postoperative pain relief in children. Anesthesiology 67:108, 1987.
163. Ecoffey C, Dubousset AM, Samii K: Lumbar and thoracic epidural anesthesia for urologic and upper abdominal surgery in infants and children. Anesthesiology 65:87, 1986.
164. Tobias JD, Rasmussen GE, Holcomb GW 3rd, et al: Continuous caudal anaesthesia with chloroprocaine as an adjunct to general anaesthesia in neonates. Canad J Anaesth 43:69, 1996.
165. Gaufré E, Dalens B, Gombert A: Epidemiology and morbidity of regional anesthesia in children: a one-year prospective survey of the French-language society of pediatric anesthesiologists. Anesth Analg 83:904, 1996.
166. Nakamura T, Takasaki M: Metabolic and endocrine responses to surgery during caudal analgesia in children. Can J Anaesth 38:969, 1991.
167. Kehlet H: The stress response to anaesthesia and surgery: release mechanisms and modifying factors. Clin Anesthesiol 2:314, 1984.
168. Bosenberg AT, Hadley GP, Wiersma R: Oesophageal atresia: caudo-thoracic epidural anaesthesia reduces the need for post-operative ventilatory support. Pediatr Surg Int 7:289, 1992.
169. Dalens B, Tanguy A, Haberer JP: Lumbar epidural anesthesia for operative and postoperative pain relief in infants and young children. Anesth Analg 65:1069, 1986.
170. Kart T, Walther-Larsen S, Svejborg TF, et al: Comparison of continuous epidural infusion of fentanyl and bupivacaine with intermittent epidural administration of morphine for postoperative pain management in children. Acta Anaesthesiol Scand 41:461, 1997.
171. Lovstad RZ, Halvorsen P, Raeder JC, Steen PA: Post-operative epidural analgesia with low dose fentanyl, adrenaline and bupivacaine in children after major orthopaedic surgery. A prospective evaluation of efficacy and side effects. Eur J Anaesthesiol 14:583, 1997.
172. Isakov Y, Geraskin G, Koshernikov V: Long term peridural anaesthesia after operations on the organs of the chest in children. Grudnaja Chir 13:104, 1971.
173. Cass LJ, Howard RF: Respiratory complications due to inadequate analgesia following thoracotomy in a neonate. Anaesthesia 49:879, 1994.
174. Murat I, Walker J, Esteve C, et al: Effect of lumbar epidural anaesthesia on plasma cortisol levels in children. Can J Anaesth 35:20, 1988.
175. Kosaka Y, Sato Y, Kawaguchi R: Distance from skin to epidural space in pediatric patients. Jpn J Anesthesiol 23:874, 1974.
176. Cousins M, Bromage P: Epidural blockade. In Cousins MJ, Bridenbaugh PO (eds): Neural Blockade in Clinical Anesthesia and Management of Pain. 2nd ed. Philadelphia, Lippincott-Raven, 1998, p 324.
177. Blanco D, Llamazares J, Rincon R, et al: Thoracic epidural anesthesia via the lumbar approach in infants and children. Anesthesiology 84:1312, 1996.
178. van Niekerk J, Bax-Vermeire BMJ, Geurts JWM, Kramer PPG: Epidurography in premature infants. Anaesthesia 45:722, 1990.
179. Tsui BC, Gupta S, Finucane B: Confirmation of epidural catheter placement using nerve stimulation. Can J Anaesth 45:640, 1998.
180. Tsui BC, Gupta S, Finucane B: Confirmation of epidural catheter placement using nerve stimulation. Thoracic epidural analgesia via the caudal approach using nerve stimulation in an infant with CATCH22. Can J Anaesth 45:640, 1998.
181. Tsui BC, Seal R, Entwistle L, et al: Thoracic epidural analgesia via the caudal approach using nerve stimulation in an infant with CATCH22. Can J Anaesth 46:1138, 1999.
182. Martin LV: Postoperative analgesia after circumcision in children. Br J Anaesth 54:1263, 1982.
183. Vater M, Wandless J: Caudal or dorsal nerve block? A comparison of two local anaesthetic techniques for postoperative analgesia following day care circumcision. Acta Anaesthesiol Scand 29:175, 1985.
184. Yeoman PM, Cooke R, Hain WR: Penile block for circumcision. A comparison with caudal blockade. Anaesthesia 38:8628, 1983.
185. Weinstein MS, Nicolson SC, Schreiner MS: A single dose of morphine sulfate increases the incidence of vomiting after outpatient inguinal surgery in children. Anesthesiology 81:572, 1994.
186. Jensen BH: Caudal block for post-operative pain relief in children after genital operations. A comparison between bupivacaine and morphine. Acta Anaesthesiol Scand 25:373, 1981.
187. Lunn JN: Postoperative analgesia after circumcision. Anaesthesia 34:552, 1979.
188. Afsan G, Khan FA: Total spinal anaesthesia following caudal block with bupivacaine and buprenorphine. Paediatr Anaesth 5:101, 1996.
189. Desparmet J: Total spinal anaesthesia after caudal anesthesia in an infant. Anesth Analg 70:665, 1990.
190. Desparmet JF: Total spinal anesthesia after caudal anesthesia in an infant. Anesth Analg 70:667, 1990.
191. Lumb AB, Carli F: Respiratory arrest after a caudal injection of bupivacaine. Anaesthesia 44:324, 1989.
192. Casta A: Attempted placement of a thoracic epidural catheter via the caudal route in a newborn [Letter]. Anesthesiology 91:1965, 1999.
193. Payen D, Ecoffey C, Dubousset AM: Pulsed Doppler ascending aortic, carotid, brachial, and femoral artery blood flows during caudal anesthesia in infants. Anesthesiology 67:681, 1987.
194. Tsuji MH, Horigome H, Yamashita M: Left ventricular functions are not impaired after lumbar epidural anaesthesia in young children. Paediatr Anaesth 6:405, 1996.
195. De Armendi AJ, Ryan JF, Chang HM, et al: Retained caudal catheter in a paediatric patient. Paediatr Anaesth 2:325, 1992.
196. Pegues DA, Carr DB, Hopkins CC: Infectious complications associated with temporary epidural catheters. Clin Infect Dis 19:970, 1994.
197. Strafford MA, Wilder RT, Berde CB: The risk of infection from epidural analgesia in children: a review of 1620 cases. Anesth Analg 80:234, 1995.
198. Kost-Byerly S, Tobin JR, Greenberg RS, et al: Bacterial colonization and infection rate of continuous epidural catheters in children. Anesth Analg 86:712, 1998.
199. McNeely JK, Trentadue NC, Rusy LM, Farber NE: Culture of bacteria from lumbar and caudal epidural catheters used for postoperative analgesia in children. Reg Anesth 22:428, 1997.
200. Emmanual ER: Post-sacral extradural catheter abscess in a child. Br J Anaesth 73:548, 1994.
201. Larsson BA, Lundeberg S, Olsson GL: Epidural abscess in a one-year-old boy after continuous epidural analgesia. Anesth Analg 84:1245, 1997.
202. Meunier JF, Norwood P, Dartayet B, et al: Skin abscess with lumbar epidural catheterization in infants: is it dangerous? Report of two cases. Anesth Analg 84:1248, 1997.
203. Flandin-Blety C, Barrier G: Accidents following extradural analgesia in children. Paediatr Anaesth 5:41, 1995.
204. Bromage PR, Benumof JL: Paraplegia following intracord injection during attempted epidural anesthesia under general anesthesia. Reg Anesth Pain Med 23:104, 1998.
205. Krane EJ, Dalens BJ, Murat I, Murrell D: The safety of epidurals placed during general anesthesia [Editorial]. Reg Anesth Pain Med 23:433, 1998.
206. Downs CS, Cooper MG: Continuous extrapleural intercostal nerve block for post thoracotomy analgesia in children. Anaesth Intensive Care 25:390, 1997.
207. Eng J, Sabanathan S: Continuous paravertebral block for postthoracotomy analgesia in children. J Pediatr Surg 27:556, 1992.
208. Lonnqvist PA: Continuous paravertebral block in children. Initial experience. Anaesthesia 47:607, 1992.
209. Lonnqvist PA: Plasma concentrations of lignocaine after thoracic paravertebral blockade in infants and children. Anaesthesia 48:958, 1993.
210. Lonnqvist PA, Olsson GL: Paravertebral vs epidural block in children. Effects on postoperative morphine requirement after renal surgery. Acta Anaesthesiol Scand 38:346, 1994.
211. Shah R, Sabanathan S, Richardson J, et al: Continuous paravertebral block for post thoracotomy analgesia in children. J Cardiovasc Surg 38:543, 1997.
212. Karmakar MK, Booker PD, Franks R, Pozzi M: Continuous extrapleural paravertebral infusion of bupivacaine for postthoracotomy analgesia in young infants. Br J Anaesth 76:811, 1996.
213. Cooper MG: Continuous extrapleural intercostal nerve block for post thoracotomy analgesia in children. Anaesth Intensive Care 25:390, 1997.
214. Sabanathan S, Mearns AJ, Bickford Smith PJ, et al: Efficacy of continuous extrapleural intercostal nerve block on post-thoracotomy pain and pulmonary mechanics. Br J Surg 77:221, 1990.

215. Conacher ID, Kokri M: Postoperative paravertebral blocks for thoracic surgery. A radiological appraisal. Br J Anaesth 59:155, 1987.
216. Cheung SLW, Booker PD, Franks R, Pozzi M: Serum concentrations of bupivacaine during prolonged continuous paravertebral infusion in young infants. Br J Anaesth 79:9, 1997.
217. Purcell-Jones G, Pither CE, Justins DM: Paravertebral somatic nerve block: a clinical, radiographic, and computed tomographic study in chronic pain patients. Anesth Analg 68:32, 1989.
218. Lonnqvist PA, MacKenzie J, Soni AK, Conacher ID: Paravertebral blockade. Failure rate and complications. Anaesthesia 50:813, 1995.
219. DePablo JS, Deiz-Mallo J: Experience with 3000 cases of brachial plexus block: its dangers, report of a fatal case. Ann Surg 128:956, 1948.
220. Eriksson E: Axillary brachial plexus anaesthesia in children with citanest. Acta Anaesthiol Scand 16:291, 1965.
221. Neill RS: Postoperative analgesia following brachial plexus block. Br J Anaesth 50:379, 1978.
222. Small GA: Brachial plexus block anesthesia in children. JAMA 147:1648, 1951.
223. Niesel HC, Rodriguez P, Wilsmann I: Regional anaesthesie der oberen extremitat bei kindern. Anaesthesist 23:178, 1974.
224. Fisher WJ, Bingham RM, Hall R: Axillary brachial plexus block for perioperative analgesia in 250 children. Paediatr Anaesth 9:435, 1999.
225. Dalens B, Vanneuville G, Tanguy A: A new parascalene approach to the brachial plexus in children: comparison with the supraclavicular approach. Anesth Analg 66:1264, 1987.
226. McNeely J, Hoffman G, Eckert J: Postoperative pain relief in children from the parascalene injection technique. Reg Anesth 16:20, 1991.
227. Dalens BJ: Proximal blocks of the upper extremity. *In* Dalens BJ (ed): Regional Anesthesia in Infants, Children, and Adolescents. London and Baltimore, Waverly Europe, Williams & Wilkins, 1995, p 275.
228. Campbell RJ, Ilett KF, Dusci L: Plasma bupivacaine concentrations after axillary block in children. Anaesth Intensive Care 14:343, 1986.
229. Winnie AP: Interscalene brachial plexus block. Anesth Analg 49:455, 1970.
230. Rosenblatt R, Pepitone-Rockwell F, McKillop MJ: Continuous axillary analgesia for traumatic hand injury. Anesthesiology 51:565, 1979.
231. Vatashsky E, Aronson HB: Continuous interscalene brachial plexus block for surgical operations on the hand. Anesthesiology 53:356, 1980.
232. Brownlow RC, Berman J, Brown RE Jr: Superficial cervical block for cervical node biopsy in a child with a large mediastinal mass. J Ark Med Soc 90:378, 1994.
233. Grossbard GD, Love BRT: Femoral nerve block: a simple and safe method of instant analgesia for femoral shaft fractures in children. Aust N Z J Surg 49:592, 1979.
234. Tondare AS, Nadkarni AV: Femoral nerve block for fractured shaft of femur. Can Anaesth Soc J 29:270, 1982.
235. Khoo ST, Brown TCK: Femoral nerve block—the anatomical basis for a single injection technique. Anaesth Intensive Care 11:40, 1983.
236. Ronchi L, Rosenbaum D, Athouel A, et al: Femoral nerve blockade in children using bupivacaine. Anesthesiology 70:622, 1989.
237. Johnson CM: Continuous femoral nerve blockade for analgesia in children with femoral fractures. Anaesth Intensive Care 22:281, 1994.
238. Winnie AP, Ramamurthy S, Durrani Z: The inguinal perivascular technique of lumbar plexus anaesthesia: 3-in-1 block. Anesth Analg 52:989, 1973.
239. Dalens B, Vanneuville G, Tanguy A: Comparison of the fascia iliaca compartment block with the 3-in-1 block in children. Anesth Analg 69:705, 1989.
240. Doyle E, Morton NS, McNicol LR: Plasma bupivacaine levels after fascia iliaca compartment block with and without adrenaline. Paediatr Anaesth 7:121, 1997.
241. McNicol LR: Sciatic nerve block for children. Anaesthesia 40:410, 1985.
242. Raj PP, Parks RI, Watson TD, Jenkins MT: A new single-position supine approach to sciatic-femoral nerve block. Anesth Analg 54:489, 1975.
243. Kempthorne PM, Brown TC: Nerve blocks around the knee in children. Anaesth Intensive Care 12:14, 1984.
244. Konrad C, Johr M: Blockade of the sciatic nerve in the popliteal fossa: a system for standardization in children. Anesth Analg 87:1256, 1998.
245. Langer JC, Shandling B, Rosenberg M: Intraoperative bupivacaine during outpatient hernia repair in children: a randomized double blind trial. J Pediatr Surg 22:267, 1987.
246. Shandling B, Steward DJ: Regional analgesia for postoperative pain in pediatric outpatient surgery. J Pediatr Surg 15:477, 1980.
247. Casey WF, Rice LJ, Hannallah RS, et al: A comparison between bupivacaine instillation versus ilioinguinal-iliohypogastric nerve block for postoperative analgesia following inguinal herniorrhaphy in children. Anesthesiology 72:637, 1990.
248. Hinkle AJ: Percutaneous inguinal block for the outpatient management of post-herniorrhaphy pain in children. Anesthesiology 67:411, 1987.
249. Epstein RH, Larijani GE, Wolfson PJ, et al: Plasma bupivacaine concentrations following ilioinguinal-iliohypogastric nerve blockade in children. Anesthesiology 69:773, 1988.
250. Smith T, Moratin P, Wulf H: Smaller children have greater bupivacaine plasma concentrations after ilioinguinal block. Br J Anaesth 76:452, 1996.
251. Conroy JM, Othersen HB Jr, Dorman BH, et al: A comparison of wound instillation and caudal block for analgesia following pediatric inguinal herniorrhaphy. J Pediatr Surg 28:565, 1993.
252. Roy-Shapira A, Amoury RA, Ashcraft KW, et al: Transient quadriceps paresis following local inguinal block for postoperative pain control. J Pediatr Surg 20:554, 1985.
253. Hannallah RS, Broadman LM, Belman AB, et al: Comparison of caudal and ilioinguinal/iliohypogastric nerve blocks for control of post-orchiopexy pain in pediatric ambulatory surgery. Anesthesiology 66:832, 1987.
254. Lau JTK: Penile block for pain relief after circumcision in children. A randomized, prospective trial. Am J Surg 147:797, 1984.
255. Blaise G, Roy W: Postoperative pain relief after hypospadias repair in pediatric patients: regional analgesia versus systemic analgesics. Anesthesiology 65:84, 1986.
256. Soliman MG, Tremblay NA: Nerve block of the penis for postoperative pain relief in children. Anesth Analg 57:495, 1978.
257. Kirya C, Werthmann MW: Neonatal circumcision and penile dorsal nerve block: a painless procedure. J Pediatr 96:998, 1978.
258. Williamson PS, Williamson ML: Physiologic stress reduction by a local anesthetic during newborn circumcision. Pediatrics 71:36, 1983.
259. Carlsson P, Svensson J: The duration of pain relief after penile block to boys undergoing circumcision. Acta Anaesthesiol Scand 28:432, 1984.
260. May AE, Wandless J, James RH: Analgesia for circumcision in children. A comparison of caudal bupivacaine and intramuscular buprenorphine. Acta Anaesthesiol Scand 26:331, 1982.
261. Serour F, Mori J, Barr J: Optimal regional anesthesia for circumcision. Anesth Analg 79:129, 1994.
262. Maxwell LG, Yaster M, Wetzel RC, Niebyl JR: Penile nerve block for newborn circumcision. Obstet Gynecol 70:415, 1987.
263. Sara CA, Lowry CJ: A complication of circumcision and dorsal nerve block of the penis. Anaesth Intensive Care 13:79, 1985.
264. Broadman LM, Hannallah RS, Belman B, et al: Post-circumcision analgesia—A prospective evaluation of subcutaneous ring block of the penis. Anesthesiology 67:399, 1987.
265. Dalens B, Vanneuville G, Dechelotte P: Penile block via the subpubic space in 100 children. Anesth Analg 69:41, 1989.
266. Tree-Trakarn T, Pirayavaraporn S: Postoperative pain relief for circumcision in children: comparison among morphine, nerve block, and topical analgesia. Anesthesiology 62:519, 1985.
267. Dixon S, Snyder J, Holve R, Bromberger P: Behavioral effects of circumcision with and without anesthesia. J Dev Behav Pediatr 5:246, 1984.
268. Holve RL, Bromberger PJ, Groveman HD, et al: Regional anesthesia during newborn circumcision. Effect on infant pain response. Clin Pediatr 22:813, 1983.
269. Lander J, Brady-Fryer B, Metcalfe JB, et al: Comparison of ring block, dorsal penile nerve block, and topical anesthesia for neonatal circumcision: a randomized controlled trial. JAMA 278:2157, 1997.
270. Masciello AL: Anesthesia for neonatal circumcision: local anesthesia is better than dorsal penile nerve block. Obstet Gynecol 75:834, 1990.
271. Stang HJ, Gunnar MR, Snellman L, et al: Local anesthesia for neonatal circumcision. Effects on distress and cortisol response. JAMA 259:1507, 1988.

272. Taddio A, Katz J, Ilersich AL, Koren G: Effect of neonatal circumcision on pain response during subsequent routine vaccination. Lancet 349:599, 1997.

273. Williamson PS, Evans ND: Neonatal cortisol response to circumcision with anesthesia. Clin Pediatr 25:412, 1986.

274. Jakobson B, Nilsson A: Methemoglobinemia associated with prilocaine-lidocaine cream and trimethoprim sulfamethoxazole. A case report. Acta Anaesthesiol Scand 29:453, 1985.

275. Hymes JA, Spraker MK: Racial difference in the effectiveness of a topically applied mixture of local anesthetics. Reg Anesth 11:11, 1986.

276. Gourrier E, Karoubi P, el Hanache A, et al: Use of EMLA cream in a department of neonatology. Pain 68:431, 1996.

277. Gourrier E, Karoubi P, el Hanache A, et al: Use of EMLA cream in premature and full-term newborn infants. Study of efficacy and tolerance [in French]. Arch Pediatr 2:1041, 1995.

278. Marchette L, Main R, Redick E, et al: Pain reduction interventions during neonatal circumcision. Nurs Res 40:241, 1991.

279. Taddio A, Stevens B, Craig K, et al: Efficacy and safety of lidocaine-prilocaine cream for pain during circumcision. N Engl J Med 336:1197, 1997.

280. Taddio A, Goldbach M, Ipp M, et al: Effect of neonatal circumcision on pain responses during vaccination in boys. Lancet 345:291, 1995.

281. EMLA full prescription. Astra USA, Inc. Westborough, MA 01581-4500.

282. Kopacz D, Thompson GE: Celiac and hypgastric plexus, intercostal, intrapleural, and peripheral neural blockade of the thorax and abdomen. In Cousins MJ, Bridenbaugh PO (eds): Neural Blockade in Clinical Anesthesia and Management of Pain. 3rd ed. Philadelphia, Lippincott-Raven Publishers, 1998, p 451.

283. Tucker GT, Moore DC, Bridenbaugh PO, et al: Systemic absorption of mepivacaine in commonly used regional block procedures. Anesthesiology 37:277, 1977.

284. Curley J, Castillo J, Hotz J, et al: Prolonged regional nerve blockade. Injectable biodegradable bupivacaine/polyester microspheres. Anesthesiology 84:1401, 1996.

285. Drager C, Benziger D, Gao F, Berde CB: Prolonged intercostal nerve blockade in sheep using controlled-release of bupivacaine and dexamethasone from polymer microspheres. Anesthesiology 89:969, 1998.

286. Otto CW, Wall CL: Total spinal anesthesia: a rare complication. Surgery 22:289, 1976.

287. FitzGerald B: Intravenous regional anaesthesia in children. Br J Anaesth 48:485, 1976.

288. Carrel ED, Eyring EJ: Intravenous regional anesthesia for childhood fractures. J Trauma 11:301, 1971.

289. Grice SC, Morell RC, Balestrieri FJ, et al: Intravenous regional anesthesia: evaluation and prevention of leakage under the tourniquet. Anesthesiology 65:316, 1986.

290. Olney BW, Lugg PC, Turner PL, et al: Outpatient treatment of upper extremity injuries in childhood using intravenous regional anesthesia. J Pediatr Orthop 8:576, 1988.

291. Mazze RL, Dunbar RW: Plasma lidocaine concentrations after caudal, lumbar epidural, axillary block and intravenous regional anesthesia. Anesthesiology 27:574, 1966.

292. Van Niekerk JP, Tonkin PA: Intravenous regional analgesia. S Afr Med J 40:165, 1966.

293. McIlvaine WB, Knox RJ, Fennessey PV, Goldstein M: Continuous infusion of bupivacaine via intrapleural catheter for analgesia after thoracotomy in children. Anesthesiology 69:261, 1988.

294. Hashemi K, Middleton MD: Subcutaneous bupivacaine for postoperative analgesia after herniorrhaphy. Ann R Coll Surg Engl 65:38, 1983.

295. Fell D, Derrington MC, Wandless JG: Caudal and ilioinguinal/iliohypogastric nerve blocks in children [Letter]. Anesthesiology 67:1020, 1987.

296. Weisman SJ, Bernstein B, Schechter NL: Consequences of inadequate analgesia during painful procedures in children. Arch Pediatr Adolesc Med 152:147, 1998.

297. Koplin LM: Topical anesthesia in pediatric lacerations or putting away the papoose. Plast Reconstr Surg 79:669, 1987.

298. Engberg G, Danielson K, Henneberg S, Nilsson A: Plasma concentrations of prilocaine and lidocaine and methaemoglobin formation in infants after epicutaneous application of a 5% lidocaine-prilocaine (EMLA). Acta Anaesthesiol Scand 31:624, 1987.

299. Maunuksela EL, Korpela R: Double-blind evaluation of a lignocaine-prilocaine cream (EMLA) in children. Effect on the pain associated with venous cannulation. Br J Anaesth 58:1242, 1986.

300. Soliman IE, Broadman LM, Hannallah RS, McGill WA: Comparison of the analgesic effects of EMLA (eutectic mixture of local anesthetics) to intradermal lidocaine infiltration prior to venous cannulation in unpremedicated children. Anesthesiology 68:804, 1988.

301. Hallen B, Olsson GL, Uppfeldt A: Pain-free venipuncture. Effect of timing of application of local anaesthetic cream. Anaesthesia 39:969, 1984.

302. Halperin DL, Koren G, Attias D, et al: Topical skin anesthesia for venous, subcutaneous drug reservoir and lumbar punctures in children. Pediatrics 84:281, 1989.

303. Sethna NF: Regional anesthesia and analgesia. Semin Perinatol 22:380, 1998.

304. Taddio A, Shennan AT, Stevens B, et al: Safety of lidocaine-prilocaine cream in the treatment of preterm neonates. J Pediatr 127:1002, 1995.

305. Fisher R, Hung O, Mezei M, Stewart R: Topical anaesthesia of intact skin: liposome-encapsulated tetracaine vs EMLA. Br J Anaesth 81:972, 1998.

306. Woolfson AD, McCafferty DF, McClelland KH, Boston V: Concentration-response analysis of percutaneous local anaesthetic formulations. Br J Anaesth 61:589, 1988.

307. McCafferty DF, Woolfson AD, Boston V: In vivo assessment of percutaneous local anaesthetic preparations. Br J Anaesth 62:17, 1989.

308. Doyle E, Freeman J, Im NT, Morton NS: An evaluation of a new self-adhesive patch preparation of amethocaine for topical anaesthesia prior to venous cannulation in children. Anaesthesia 48:1050, 1993.

309. Lawson RA, Smart NG, Gudgeon AC, Morton NS: Evaluation of an amethocaine gel preparation for percutaneous analgesia before venous cannulation in children. Br J Anaesth 75:282, 1995.

310. O'Connor B, Tomlinson AA: Evaluation of the efficacy and safety of amethocaine gel applied topically before venous cannulation in adults. Br J Anaesth 74:706, 1995.

311. Mazumdar B, Tomlinson AA, Faulder GC: Preliminary study to assay plasma amethocaine concentrations after topical application of a new local anaesthetic cream containing amethocaine. Br J Anaesth 67:432, 1991.

312. Sanchez-Perez J, Cordoba S, Cortizas CF, Garcia-Diez A: Allergic contact balanitis due to tetracaine (amethocaine) hydrochloride. Contact Dermatitis 39:268, 1998.

313. Pryor G, Kilpatrick W, Opp D: Local anesthesia in minor lacerations: topical TAC vs lidocaine infiltration. Ann Emerg Med 9:568, 1980.

314. Vinci RJ, Fish SS, Blackburn RE, et al: Efficacy of topical anesthesia in children: comparison of tetracaine-adrenaline-cocaine (TAC) with topical lidocaine-epinephrine (TLE): efficacy and cost. Arch Pediatr Adolesc Med 150:466, 1996.

315. Grant SAD, Hoffman RS: Use of tetracaine, epinephrine, and cocaine as a topical anesthetic in the emergency department. Ann Emerg Med 21:987, 1992.

316. Smith S, Barry R: A comparison of three formulations of TAC (tetracaine, adrenalin, cocaine) for anesthesia of minor lacerations in children. Pediatr Emerg Care 6:266, 1990.

317. Bonadio WA, Wagner V: Efficacy of tetracaine-adrenaline-cocaine topical anesthetic without tetracaine for facial laceration repair in children. Pediatrics 86:856, 1990.

318. Bonadio W, Wagner V: Half-strength TAC topical anesthetic. For selected dermal lacerations. Clin Pediatr (Phila) 27:495, 1988.

319. Terndrup TE, Walls HC, Mariani PJ, Karatay CM: Plasma cocaine and tetracaine levels following application of topical anesthesia in children. Ann Emerg Med 21:162, 1992.

320. Tucker G, Mather L: Properties, absorption, and disposition of local anesthetic agents. In Cousins MJ, Bridenbaugh PO (eds): Neural Blockade in Clinical Anesthesia and Management of Pain. 3rd ed. Philadelphia, New York, Lippincott-Raven Publishers, 1998, p 55.

321. Jacobsen S: Errors in emergency practice. Emerg Med 19:109, 1987.

322. Dailey R: Fatality secondary to misuse of TAC solution. Ann Emerg Med 17:159, 1988.

323. Tipton G, DeWitt G, Eisenstein S: Topical TAC (tetracaine, adrenaline, cocaine) solution for local anesthesia in children: prescribing inconsistency and acute toxicity. South Med J 82:1344, 1989.

324. Wilson JF, Peters GN, Fleshman K: A technique for bronchography in children. An experience with 575 patients using topical anesthesia. Am Rev Respir Dis 105:564, 1972.

325. Vinci RJ, Fish S, Mirochnick M: Cocaine absorption after application of a viscous cocaine-containing TAC solution. Ann Emerg Med 34:498, 1999.

326. Schilling CG, Bank DE, Borchert BA, et al: Tetracaine, epinephrine (adrenalin), and cocaine (TAC) versus lidocaine, epinephrine, and tetracaine (LET) for anesthesia of lacerations in children. Ann Emerg Med 25:203, 1995.

327. Smith GA, Strausbaugh SD, Harbeck-Weber C, et al: Tetracaine-lidocaine-phenylephrine topical anesthesia compared with lidocaine infiltration during repair of mucous membrane lacerations in children. Clin Pediatr 37:405, 1998.

328. Keyes PD, Tallon JM, Rizos J: Topical anesthesia. Can Fam Physician 44:2152, 1998.

329. Resch K, Schilling C, Borchert BD, et al: Topical anesthesia for pediatric lacerations: a randomized trial of lidocaine-epinephrine-tetracaine solution versus gel. Ann Emerg Med 32:693, 1998.

330. Smith GA, Strausbaugh SD, Harbeck-Weber C, et al: Prilocaine-phenylephrine and bupivacaine-phenylephrine topical anesthetics compared with tetracaine-adrenaline-cocaine during repair of lacerations. Am J Emerg Med 16:121, 1998.

331. Sitbon P, Laffon M, Lesage V, et al: Lidocaine plasma concentrations in pediatric patients after providing airway topical anesthesia from a calibrated device. Anesth Analg 82:1003, 1996.

332. Gjonaj ST, Lowenthal DB, Dozor AJ: Nebulized lidocaine administered to infants and children undergoing flexible bronchoscopy. Chest 112:1665, 1997.

333. Brown T, Schulte-Steinberg O: Neural blockade for pediatric surgery. In Cousins MJ, Bridenbaugh PO (eds): Neural Blockade in Clinical Anesthesia and Management of Pain. 2nd ed. Philadelphia, JB Lippincott Company, 1988, p 687.

334. Eyres RL, Bishop W, Oppenheim RC, Brown TCK: Plasma bupivacaine concetrations in children during caudal epidural analgesia. Anesth Intensive Care 11:20, 1983.

335. Eyres RL, Hastings C, Brown TC, Oppenheim RC: Plasma bupivacaine concentrations following lumbar epidural anaesthesia in children. Anaesth Intensive Care 14:131, 1986.

336. Murat I, Montay G, Delleur MM, et al: Bupivacaine pharmacokinetics during epidural anaesthesia in children. Eur J Anaesthesiol 5:113, 1988.

337. Sfez M, Le MY, Mazoit X, Dreux BH: Local anesthetic serum concentrations after penile nerve block in children. Anesth Analg 71:423, 1990.

338. Mihaly GW, Moore RG, Thomas J, et al: The pharmacokinetics and metabolism of the anilide local anaesthetics in neonates. Eur J Clin Pharmacol 13:143, 1978.

339. Morgan D, McQuillan D, Thomas J: Pharmacokinetics and metabolism of the anilide local anaesthetics in neonates. II Etidocaine. Eur J Clin Pharmacol 13:365, 1978.

340. Rice LJ, DeMars PD, Whalen TV, et al: Duration of spinal anesthesia in infants less than one year of age. Comparison of three hyperbaric techniques. Reg Anesth 19:325, 1994.

341. Abajian J, Sethna N: Regional and topical anesthesia. In Anand K, McGrath P (eds): Pain Research and Clinical Management. Vol 5. Amsterdam, Elsevier Science Publishers, 1993, p 199.

342. Armitage EN: Regional anaesthesia in pediatrics. Clin Anesthesiol 3:553, 1985.

343. Broadman LM: Regional anesthesia for pediatric patients. Annual Meeting of the American Society of Anesthesiologists, Las Vegas, October 19–23, 1990.

344. Gunter J: Caudal anesthesia in children: a survey. Anesthesiology 75:A936, 1991.

345. Turner PL, Batten JB, Hjorth D, et al: Intravenous regional anaesthesia for the treatment of upper limb injuries in childhood. Aust N Z J Surg 56:153, 1986.

13

Special Techniques

ACUTE NORMOVOLEMIC HEMODILUTION, CONTROLLED HYPOTENSION AND HYPOTHERMIA, AND ECMO

JERROLD LERMAN

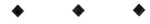

ACUTE NORMOVOLEMIC HEMODILUTION

Acute normovolemic hemodilution (ANH) is a technique used to reduce or completely obviate the need for homologous blood transfusions during surgery. Up to 50 percent of the patient's blood volume may be replaced with asanguinous colloid or crystalloid solutions (thereby maintaining the normal circulating blood volume) to provide a reserve of autologous blood for reinfusion at a later time. Hemodilution has been used effectively in patients of all ages (from infancy to middle age) and for all types of surgery.[1–9] Acute normovolemic hemodilution also has been used for Jehovah's Witnesses patients who refuse homologous blood or blood product transfusions. It also has been used for patients who are difficult to cross-match, and for patients who prefer to minimize the risks of complications associated with homologous blood and blood product transfusion (i.e., hepatitis, acquired immunodeficiency syndrome [AIDS], and transfusion reactions).[10–12] Fresh autologous blood has several advantages over banked homologous blood, including a greater concentration of both clotting factors and active, functioning platelets and a significantly reduced risk of transfusion reactions associated with homologous blood transfusion (e.g., ABO and Rh incompatibilities, leukocyte reactions, and

temperature and metabolic disturbances). These advantages, however, must be balanced against the major risk of hemodilution: a reduction in the oxygen-carrying capacity of blood that reduces oxygen reserves during anesthesia and surgery.[13] The reduction in oxygen-carrying capacity, which may be moderate (hematocrit of 25 to 30 percent) or extreme (hematocrit <10 to 15 percent) is compensated for by several physiologic mechanisms.[10, 13]

Recent evidence has questioned the value of ANH in clinical care. Although hemodilution is reported to decrease the need for allogenic transfusions in some studies,[8] in others there have been no clear benefits.[14–16] This section discusses the physiology of hemodilution, the choice of diluent solutions, contraindications to hemodilution, and an anesthetic protocol for hemodilution.

Physiology

The primary physiologic advantage of acute normovolemic hemodilution is a reduction in blood viscosity.[10, 13] The *viscosity* (resistance to flow) of a fluid is defined as the ratio of the shear stress (force applied) to the shear rate (velocity of flow). Newtonian fluids (e.g., plasma and crystalloid solutions) are those in which the shear rate varies linearly and directly with the shear stress (i.e., viscosity is constant). In contrast, nonnewtonian fluids (e.g., whole blood) are those in which the shear stress varies inversely with the shear rate (i.e., viscosity increases as shear rate decreases). Because blood is a nonnewtonian fluid, nonnewtonian fluid mechanics are particularly relevant to a complete understanding of the physiologic effects of hemodilution.

The viscosity of blood is the sum of the viscosities of the red blood cell fraction (hematocrit) and the plasma fraction. The relationship between hematocrit and viscosity has been well described[13] (Fig. 13–1). As the shear rate decreases, changes in hematocrit have a greater effect on the apparent viscosity. In the postcapillary venules, where blood flow is slow, the apparent viscosity decreases by 50 percent when the hematocrit is reduced from 40 percent to 20 percent, whereas in the precapillary bed viscosity decreases by less than 25 percent. This pattern suggests that hemodilution has its most profound effect on decreasing the viscosity of blood in the postcapillary venules.

The contribution of plasma to the viscosity of blood depends primarily on the concentrations of fibrinogen and α_2-globulins.[13] These proteins determine the extent of cell-to-cell interaction in vivo (i.e., the tendency toward rouleaux formation). Lowering the plasma concentrations of these two proteins decreases the viscosity of blood.

Hemodilution reduces blood viscosity by diluting the red blood cells and by decreasing the concentration of plasma proteins. The former may be attributed in part to a decrease in rouleaux formation and to an increase in deaggregation, particularly at low shear rates. The latter may be attributed to the properties of the fluids administered during hemodilution.[10, 13] In vitro, 5 percent albumin and dextran 40, 60, and 70 increase the viscosity of plasma, whereas lactated Ringer's solution decreases the serum concentration of plasma proteins and the viscosity of

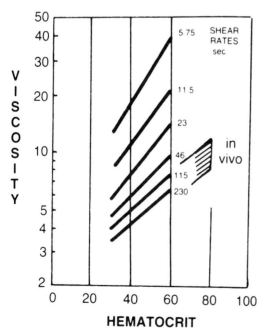

FIGURE 13–1. Relation between hematocrit and viscosity at varying shear rates. In vivo shear rates range from 50 to 250/s, and in this range changes in viscosity and hematocrit are almost linearly related. (Adapted from Dormandy JA: Clinical significance of blood viscosity. Ann R Coll Surg Engl 47:211, 1970, with permission.)

plasma. In vivo, the increase in plasma viscosity after colloid administration is offset by a decrease in rouleaux formation. Dextran increases plasma viscosity less in vivo than in vitro. The latter discrepancy can be attributed in part to the increase in intravascular water that results from an increase in colloid oncotic pressure and a decrease in protein concentration.[10, 13]

The flow characteristics of fluids during laminar flow (Reynold's number less than 2,000) is described by the Hagen-Poiseiulle equation:

$$Q = \frac{\pi}{8} \cdot \frac{\Delta P \cdot r^4}{\mu \cdot L}$$

where Q = flow rate, ΔP = pressure gradient, r = radius of the vessel, μ = viscosity, and L = length of the vessel. This equation indicates that the flow rate through a vessel decreases by the fourth power of the decrease in vessel radius. This decrease in flow is magnified by an increase in viscosity (which occurs in nonnewtonian fluid as the velocity decreases). Hence, hemodilution may exert a beneficial effect in the slow-flow regions of the vascular bed.

During acute normovolemic hemodilution, decreases in shear rate exert decreasing effects on the shear stress. Therefore, net flow may actually increase in the smaller vessels. This increase in blood flow increases both venous return[17] and cardiac output.[5, 6] In addition, hemodilution decreases afterload, thereby increasing cardiac output by yet another mechanism. When the hematocrit is between 5 and 70 percent, cardiac output varies inversely with the hematocrit.[10] The increase in cardiac output is the single most important physiologic compensatory mechanism for maintaining the tissue oxygen supply during acute normovolemic hemodilution.

The increase in cardiac output (i.e., in stroke volume) that occurs during acute normovolemic hemodilution has been attributed to an increase in venous return, a decrease in afterload, and an increase in myocardial contractility[10, 13] (Fig. 13–2). The increase in venous return can be attributed in part to an increase in flow in the smaller vessels and to a reduction in the capacitance of the venous system. The reduction in venous capacitance depends on stimulation of the aortic chemoreceptors by the reduced oxygen content of blood. The decrease in afterload is a direct result of the decrease in systemic vascular resistance (Fig. 13–2).

The etiology of the increase in myocardial contractility during hemodilution is unclear. The most likely explanation is a reduction in left ventricular afterload,[10] although other explanations including increased sympathetic stimulation have been proposed. Studies in rats suggest that the increase in cardiac output during hemodilution can be attributed to an improved efficiency of cardiac mitochondria.[17] The contribution of catecholamines to the increase in myocardial contractility is probably small. Local tissue hypoxia (and lactic acidosis) is unlikely to contribute to the increased myocardial contractility, as hypoxemia rarely occurs when the hematocrit exceeds 15 percent.

Total organ blood flow, including flow to the brain, kidney, and liver, increases in parallel with the increase in cardiac output during acute normovolemic hemodilu-

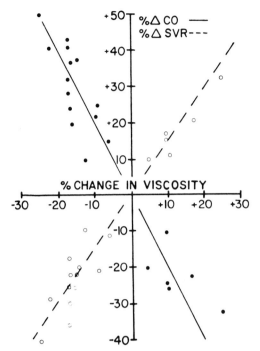

FIGURE 13-2. Changes in cardiac output (CO) and systemic vascular resistance (SVR) with changes in blood viscosity. (Adapted from Dormandy JA: Clinical significance of blood viscosity. Ann R Coll Surg Engl 47:211, 1970, with permission.)

tion. In contrast, coronary blood flow increases out of proportion to the increase in cardiac output.[10, 13] Normovolemic hemodilution increases cerebral blood flow to regions with normal and low blood flow.[18] The decrease in blood viscosity and the decrease in the oxygen content of blood each account for approximately half of the increase in cerebral blood flow during hemodilution.[19] Studies in dogs have shown that the cerebral vasculature is reactive to CO_2 during limited hemodilution but is impaired during extreme hemodilution. Normovolemic hemodilution with crystalloid solutions increases intracranial pressure and brain water content of rabbits, whereas hemodilution with hydroxyethyl starch does not.[20] In a study of monkeys anesthetized with halothane in oxygen, spontaneous and evoked electrical brain activity were reduced during normovolemic hemodilution with lactated Ringer's solution (hematocrit, 14 percent).[21] However, there was no histologic evidence of ischemic brain damage. Similar data in humans are lacking.

Both renal and hepatic blood flows increase during hemodilution. Urine output increases up to 100 to 150 ml/h in adults who are hemodiluted with 5 percent albumin. This can be attributed in part to the reduced viscosity and a redistribution of renal blood flow to the renal cortex.

Coronary blood flow increases out of proportion to the increase in cardiac output because of a decrease in blood viscosity and coronary vasodilation.[10, 13, 22] Studies in dogs suggest that the increase in coronary blood flow is evenly distributed throughout the subendocardium and epicardium except during extreme hemodilution, when subendocardial ischemia may occur.[22]

The reduced oxygen content of blood may reduce the tissue oxygen supply/demand ratio in hemodiluted pa-

tients. This decrease in the tissue oxygen supply/demand ratio is compensated for, in part, by an increase in tissue blood flow, an increase in the amount of dissolved oxygen, an improved oxygen extraction (lower venous Po_2), and a rightward shift of the oxyhemoglobin dissociation curve.[13, 23] Nutritional blood flow and tissue Po_2 remain normal and adequate for the metabolic rate at hematocrit values of 25 percent or more in many organs (skeletal muscle, pancreas, kidney, liver). The increase in dissolved oxygen results from an increase in the volume of plasma and a decrease in the concentration of proteins (Fig. 13–3). If hypothermia is added, the amount of dissolved oxygen further increases. Oxygen extraction at the tissue level is unchanged until the hematocrit is less than 20 percent. At an hematocrit less than 20 percent, venous Po_2 decreases and oxygen extraction increases. Although a rightward shift of the oxyhemoglobin dissociation curve does not occur with hematocrits 20 percent or greater in humans and animals,[23] the P_{50} increases from 26.9 mm Hg to 28.4 mm Hg at a hematocrit less than 20 percent (at normothermia) within 30 minutes of a stepwise dilution with dextran. In animals, a further rightward shift of the P_{50} to 31 mm Hg occurs within 10 days of hemodilution. This rightward shift of the oxyhemoglobin dissociation curve has been attributed to an increase in plasma 2,3-diphosphoglycerate (2,3-DPG).

Two additional factors that attenuate the decrease in the oxygen demand during acute hemodilution are hypothermia and general anesthesia. Mild to moderate hypothermia (30° to 32°C) reduces the oxygen requirements by 5 to 9 percent per degree centigrade,[24, 25] although this is offset in part by a leftward shift of the oxyhemoglobin dissociation curve. In this temperature range, the risk of arrhythmias is small (see "Hypothermia," below). This degree of hypothermia can be achieved by passive cooling. However, to limit the decrease in temperature, heating devices should be introduced when 60 to 75 percent of the desired decrease in temperature is achieved. Anesthesia may further attenuate the oxygen supply/demand ratio by reducing the total body oxygen consumption. Therefore, by reducing oxygen demand, both hypothermia and general anesthesia increase the supply/demand ratio, moving it closer to normal values. These factors combine to maintain a reasonable tissue oxygen supply/demand ratio during moderate hemodilution.

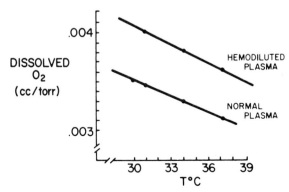

FIGURE 13-3. Dissolved oxygen-carrying capacity versus temperature.

Moderate hypotension (mean arterial pressure [MAP] of 40 to 50 mm Hg) has been used as an adjunct to acute normovolemic hemodilution to further reduce left ventricular afterload (myocardial work) and to decrease surgical blood loss. Hypotension combined with hemodilution may compromise tissue oxygen supply critically.[26, 27] In dogs, the combination of either trimethaphan or adenosine-induced hypotension and hemodilution decreased brain, retinal, and renal cortical blood flows.[27, 28]

In adult humans, preliminary data indicate that the combination of nitroprusside-induced hypotension and hemodilution decreases the need for homologous blood transfusions compared to either technique individually. Furthermore, the nitroprusside requirements are reduced in patients who are hemodiluted. The combination of isoflurane/epidural-induced hypotension and hemodilution has been evaluated electroencephalographically and electrocardiographically in adults and is considered to be safe during orthopedic and general surgeries.[29] In children, the combination of hypotension and hemodilution has been used clinically, although several cases of ischemic optic neuritis have been reported.[30–32] Therefore, I recommend avoiding this combination in children until further studies establish the safety of this technique.

Acute normovolemic hemodilution does not adversely affect the lung. In animals, hemodilution has no significant effect on pulmonary gas exchange despite significant increases in lung water.[33] In humans, hemodilution with colloid-containing solutions neither increases lung water nor causes deterioration of arterial blood gases. The effect of hemodilution on intrapulmonary shunt is variable: in zone 3 areas (i.e., areas with a low ventilation-perfusion [V̇/Q̇] ratio during hemodilution), intrapulmonary shunting may increase to 15 percent of the cardiac output because the reduced viscosity increases regional blood flow. On the other hand, the increase in pulmonary blood flow during hemodilution more than offsets the increase in shunt when V̇/Q̇ ratios are normal; that is, intrapulmonary shunt actually decreases.

Perioperative clinical coagulopathies have not been reported in association with moderate hemodilution,[34] although transient intraoperative disturbances of coagulation have been reported. Although hemodilution to a hematocrit of 25 percent is associated with a decrease in the concentration of fibrinogen and the platelet count to approximately 30 percent of control values, the prothrombin, partial thromboplastin, and clotting times are unchanged. Acute normovolemic hemodilution to a hematocrit of 20 percent or more is not associated with coagulation defects, provided the diluent does not specifically inhibit clotting. However, hemodilution to a hematocrit of less than 20 percent dilutes clotting factors and platelets and may inhibit the clotting process.

Diluent Solution

Two types of diluent solution, colloid and crystalloid, may be used to maintain normovolemia during acute hemodilution. It is imperative that normo- or hypervolemia be maintained at all times to maintain adequate cardiac output and tissue perfusion.[4, 7, 21] Hypovolemia must be avoided during acute hemodilution lest it interfere with

the primary compensatory mechanism for reduced blood oxygen content, an increase in cardiac output, and lead to tissue hypoxia.[21, 35] The recent controversy over the use of colloid and crystalloid solutions in resuscitations has rekindled the controversy regarding the salient differences between the two solutions, with no clear resolution in sight.[36, 37]

Crystalloid solutions (e.g., lactated Ringer's solution) are commonly used for hemodilution. Because these solutions rapidly distribute throughout the extracellular fluid space, it is acceptable practice to transfuse three times the volume of crystalloid as blood removed. Although the increase in lung water associated with hemodilution using crystalloid solutions is not normally associated with a decrease in lung function, accumulation of large volumes of fluid in the bowel has been reported in two patients.[38] This resulted in difficulty closing the abdomen. Despite this report, the low cost, low risk, and availability of crystalloid solutions have contributed to the popularity of their use.

Colloid solutions such as 5 percent human albumin, dextran 70, hydroxyethyl starch, and pentastarch have been used successfully for hemodilution.[38–40] These solutions remain in the intravascular space for approximately 6 hours and maintain colloid oncotic pressure (and therefore minimize tissue edema). Recent evidence suggests that if 5 percent albumin is used for volume replacement during hemodilution, then the volumetric replacement should exceed a 1:1 volumetric ratio with blood as albumin and fluid extravasate slowly into the interstitium during prolonged surgery.[41] Albumin 5 percent and pentastarch do not interfere with coagulation apart from their dilutional effects.[40] Dextran is unique in that it has antithrombotic activity in normal doses and anticoagulant properties if the total dose exceeds 1.5 g/kg. Hetastarch may interfere with fibrin clot formation and increase fibrinolysis. When the maximum daily dose of hetastarch exceeds the daily limit of 20 ml/kg, clinically significant coagulopathies have been reported. Several authors have combined albumin and dextran 70 for hemodilution to reduce the cost and minimize the volume of dextran 70 (to avoid coagulopathies). Hydroxyethyl starch has also been used in pediatric patients without complications.[38] In adults, the intravascular half-life of pentastarch (2.5 hours) is approximately one half that of hydroxyethyl starch (25.5 hours).[40, 42] Similar data in children are lacking. There is currently no optimal solution for hemodilution nor is there an optimal fluid regimen for hemodilution in children.[36, 37]

Contraindications

Acute normovolemic hemodilution is contraindicated in the presence of end-organ dysfunction (pulmonary, cardiac, renal, neurologic, or hepatic diseases), when there are significant hemoglobinopathies (sickle-cell or sickle cell hemoglobin C disease), and in clotting disorders.

Indications for Hemodilution

Acute normovolemic hemodilution has become a widely accepted practice for infants and older children for whom the anticipated blood loss is expected to exceed 15 percent of their blood volume, for patients who refuse blood transfusion (i.e., Jehovah's Witnesses), for patients who have a rare blood type and are therefore difficult to cross-match, and for those patients who are concerned about complications of homologous transfusions. When the blood loss is less than or equal to 15 percent of the patient's blood volume, blood transfusions are not normally required. However, blood may be required if the initial hematocrit is low or organ perfusion is compromised. If so, the blood loss can be replaced with crystalloid (three times the volume lost) or an equivalent volume of colloid. Blood loss in excess of 50 percent of the circulating blood volume usually requires homologous blood transfusions, as the minimal acceptable hematocrit for acute hemodilution even in the presence of moderate hypothermia (32° to 35°C) is approximately 15 to 20 percent. Therefore, when the anticipated blood loss exceeds 50 percent of the circulating blood volume, hemodilution may reduce but not preclude the need for homologous blood transfusions.

Protocol for Hemodilution

Before surgery, the parents must be fully informed of the risks and harms of the proposed blood conservation strategies. These risks include reduced oxygen delivery to tissues, unanticipated need for homologous blood transfusions; the physiologic effects of administering large volumes of asanguinous fluids on the brain, retina, and upper airway; and the risk of end-organ damage (brain and cardiac ischemic injury). A complete preoperative history, with particular attention to a history of decreased cardiorespiratory reserve and impaired neurologic and renal function, should be obtained preoperatively.

Members of the Jehovah's Witnesses faith commonly refuse transfusions of homologous and autologous blood as well as blood products. However, some members of the Jehovah's Witnesses faith accept some of the following:

1. Autologous blood transfusions
2. Hemodilution
3. Blood from a cell-saver
4. Albumin and other fractionated blood products

Members who accept hemodilution or blood from a cell-saver may accept them only if the blood or blood products have been in continuous contact with the patient's circulation. Blood that must be in continuous contact with the patient is withdrawn from one limb continuously and reinfused into another. On the basis of this practice, some members of the Jehovah's Witnesses faith will consent to hemodilution. Less commonly, they may accept blood products completely de novo.

Physical examination must include identification of sites for venous and arterial access. Laboratory investigations should include hematocrit; serum electrolytes; blood urea nitrogen and serum creatinine concentrations; platelet count; and prothrombin, partial thromboplastin, and bleeding times. A chest radiograph and an electrocardiogram (ECG) should also be obtained, particularly if the child has a history of cardiorespiratory dysfunction.

To maximize the preoperative hemoglobin concentration when hemodilution is planned, oral iron therapy and parenteral recombinant erythropoietin (Epogein) should be considered.[43-45] Oral iron therapy (300 mg/kg/day in divided doses) should begin 4 weeks before surgery to prevent or correct iron deficiency during the reticulocytosis. Parenteral erythropoietin (100 to 600 U/kg) subcutaneously should be administered twice weekly for 2 to 3 weeks before surgery. Baseline and weekly hematocrit, iron stores, and reticulocyte count should be followed. Erythropoietin should be withheld if the hematocrit reaches or exceeds 50 vol%.

The volume of blood to be removed during hemodilution can be estimated by the following formula[46]:

$$V_I = EBV \times [H_o - H_F / H_{AV}]$$

where V_I = volume of blood to be removed, EBV = estimated blood volume, H = hematocrit or hemoglobin concentration, H_o = initial hematocrit, H_F = minimum allowable hematocrit after dilution, and H_{AV} = average of initial and minimal hematocrits. The estimated normal blood volume depends on the patient's age: 85 to 100 ml/kg for preterm infants, 80 to 85 ml/kg for neonates, 70 to 75 ml/kg for children, and 65 to 70 ml/kg for young adults. The maximal discrepancy between the hematocrit estimated by this equation and the logarithmic solution to this equation is 7.5 percent, which is acceptable for clinical purposes.[46] Based on this equation, for an H_F/H_o of 0.6, the V_I/EBV is approximately 0.55, which suggests that 55 percent of the patient's blood volume can be replaced with an asanguinous solution to obtain a final hematocrit that is about 60 percent of the original value.

Although the concentration of hemoglobin has been the variable that limits the extent of hemodilution, in some instances the concentrations of coagulation factors and clotting indices may limit the extent of hemodilution. This may be especially relevant for patients with high hematocrits and low plasma volumes. In these patients, hemodilution to an acceptable concentration of hemoglobin might decrease the concentrations of coagulation factors below the acceptable minimal values. It therefore seems prudent to monitor coagulation indices during hemodilution.

Several factors contribute to the adequacy of tissue oxygen delivery during extreme hemodilution. The increase in cardiac output discussed in the preceding section is the primary factor, although two additional factors are also important: an increase in the amount of dissolved oxygen (Fig. 13-3) and a decrease in the oxygen requirements of tissues.

The amount of dissolved oxygen increases when the plasma concentration of proteins decreases and the body temperature decreases. The protein concentration decreases when crystalloid solutions, such as lactated Ringer's solution, are used to maintain normovolemia during hemodilution. During extreme hemodilution with lactated Ringer's solution and hypothermia (30° to 33°C), the amount of dissolved oxygen may increase by 30 percent (Fig. 13-3).

Anesthetic Protocol

Children scheduled for acute normovolemic hemodilution may be premedicated according to customary practice in the institution. Vagolytic drugs are contraindicated in these patients, as tachycardia may significantly increase myocardial oxygen demand. Children should be fasted preoperatively as per standard protocols.

After application of the routine monitors, anesthesia can be induced with either intravenous (IV) (thiopental or propofol)[47] or inhaled agents (halothane or sevoflurane).[48] Tracheal intubation may be facilitated by a nondepolarizing muscle relaxant such as rocuronium or pancuronium. In adults, hemodilution increases the potencies of all relaxants: d-tubocurarine, pancuronium, vecuronium by 20 percent,[49] and rocuronium by 40 percent.[50] This shift of the dose–response curve to the left has been attributed to an increase in cardiac output and decrease in the protein binding of muscle relaxants during hemodilution. Succinylcholine should be avoided during hemodilution to obviate the need for a vagolytic drug. Pancuronium and the benzylisoquinolonium series of relaxants are avoided, as they may cause tachycardia. If anesthesia is induced with inhaled drugs, oxygen, nitrous oxide, and halothane or sevoflurane can be used alone or with one of the recommended muscle relaxants to facilitate tracheal intubation. Because nitrous oxide limits oxygen reserves, it is relatively contraindicated during acute normovolemic hemodilution. Therefore, 100 percent oxygen (with up to 5 percent nitrogen) should be used throughout the period of hemodilution to maximize the dissolved fraction of oxygen. After tracheal intubation, ventilation should be controlled to maintain normocapnia ($Paco_2$ 35 to 40 mm Hg). Hyperventilation should be avoided for two reasons: one, because it reduces cerebral blood flow and therefore the cerebral oxygen supply, and two, because it shifts the oxyhemoglobin dissociation curve to the left, thereby reducing release of oxygen in the tissues. Anesthesia can be maintained either with an inhaled agent and a narcotic or with an amnestic drug and high-dose narcotic to maintain a normal MAP (60 to 75 mm Hg) during the period of hemodilution. Any of the three inhaled agents, isoflurane, sevoflurane, or desflurane, can be used because all three preserve cardiac output to a greater extent than halothane.[48, 51]

Additional monitors should include nasopharyngeal and rectal temperatures, continuous arterial and central venous pressures (or, less commonly, pulmonary arterial pressures), pulse oximetry, $Petco_2$ and hourly urine output. Electroencephalographic (EEG) monitoring is recommended during hemodilution when possible.

IV access must be established with two large-bore cannulas for administration of crystalloid or colloid solutions. These solutions should be maintained at room temperature to passively reduce the body temperature to 32° to 34°C. Blood warmers may be required during surgery to prevent a temperature decrease below the desired value.

Rapid and accurate laboratory analyses must be available when hemodilution is performed. Arterial and central venous samples should be analyzed for blood gases every 30 to 60 minutes during hemodilution and whenever unexpected hypo- or hypertension occurs. Serum glucose and electrolyte concentrations also should be determined regularly. The serum concentration of ionized calcium should be determined during hemodilution, during reinfusions of autologous blood, and after surgery. If the serum concentration of ionized calcium is below the lower accepted limit (0.80 mg/dl), IV calcium chloride (10 to 20 mg/kg) should be infused to maintain myocardial contractility. Cardiac output can be determined by dye dilution or thermodilution if a pulmonary artery catheter is in place.

Hemodilution can begin as soon as a stable level of anesthesia has been established and baseline hemodynamic and metabolic indices have been obtained and recorded.

Hemodilution is achieved by phlebotomizing the patient through the central venous pressure catheter or the arterial catheter while simultaneously infusing crystalloid (3 ml crystalloid per milliliter blood removed) or colloid (1 to 2 ml colloid per milliliter blood removed) solutions through an IV cannula. The blood is collected in a sterile citrate-phosphate-dextrose bag (with or without adenine). The volume of blood removed is monitored by weighing the bag continuously. The removed blood is assumed to have a density of 1 g/ml. The phlebotomized blood is gently mixed and maintained at room temperature.

Hemodilution should be completed before surgery commences because surgical blood loss during the period of hemodilution may result in acute hypovolemia, which can cause profound hypotension, end-organ tissue hypoxia, and tissue damage. Furthermore, the circulatory and metabolic responses to hemodilution can be difficult to differentiate from those caused by surgical blood loss.

Heart rate and central venous pressure should not change significantly from control values during hemodilution unless hypovolemia develops. If tachycardia occurs during acute hemodilution, hypovolemia must be suspected and corrected immediately.

Intraoperative surgical blood loss is replaced with asanguinous fluid (3 ml crystalloid per milliliter blood or 1 to 2 ml colloid per milliliter blood) or autologous blood. Autologous blood should be infused to maintain the minimal acceptable hematocrit for that patient or to raise the hematocrit after blood loss has ceased.[52] In children of the Jehovah's Witnesses faith, premature transfusion of autologous blood depletes the only available source of blood, leaving none to replace subsequent losses. However, failure to transfuse the patient early enough may result in a very low hematocrit (and low oxygen supply), albeit in an anesthetized, mildly hypothermic patient whose tissue oxygen requirements are already reduced. Although the decision as to when to transfuse the Jehovah's Witnesses patient may be difficult, I recommend withholding blood until after the surgical bleeding has subsided, if it is possible. If bleeding continues after all available blood has been transfused, surgery may have to be terminated prematurely. The parents should be fully informed of the risk/benefit ratio of hemodilution, including central nervous system damage and death.

Intraoperative fluid management must include maintenance and third-space fluid replacement. Lactated Ringer's solution is used to replace both types of fluids, except in infants and other patients at risk for hypoglycemia.[53] Third-space fluid losses are replaced in accordance with the extent of surgical dissection (lactated Ringer's solution 2 to 15 ml/kg/h or colloid 2 to 10 ml/kg/h). I restrict the volume of crystalloid solution transfused to 75 to 100 ml/kg. Crystalloid volumes approaching 100 ml/kg or more increase the risk of a coagulopathy. Despite the large volumes of lactated Ringer's solution used for hemodilution, blood replacement, and replacement of third-space losses, neither hyperlactatemia nor postoperative respiratory alkalosis has been reported.

Because infusion of large volumes of crystalloid solutions causes generalized edema, normovolemic hemodilution to hemocrits less than 20 percent should be restricted to 4 hours or less. If colloid solutions are used instead of crystalloid solutions, the duration of hemodilution may be extended.

Early detection of hypotension is critical to prevent end-organ hypoxia. Tissue hypoperfusion (increase in serum lactate concentration or central venous oxyhemoglobin desaturation) occurs when cardiac output is inadequate for total body oxygen requirements. Under these circumstances, the central venous oxygen saturation decreases below 60 percent. Normal central blood volume and cardiac output must therefore be maintained at all times. Therefore, a stable cardiac output, systemic blood pressure, filling pressure, and central venous oxygen saturation of more than 60 percent must be maintained throughout the period of hemodilution. If the serum lactate concentration increases, inadequate tissue perfusion must be corrected.

Interstitial pulmonary edema is an uncommon cause of increased alveolar-arterial oxygen difference [$(A-a)Do_2$] and intraoperative hypoxemia during hemodilution. A tidal volume of at least 10 ml/kg with positive end-expiratory pressure (PEEP), when appropriate, is required to maintain adequate ventilation. PaO_2 should be maintained at 400 mm Hg or more during hemodilution. An increasing $(A-a)Do_2$ requires immediate investigation of the cause and prompt institution of therapy.

Reversal of Hemodilution

Reinfusion of autologous blood should commence as soon as the surgical blood loss has ceased, or earlier if the hematocrit decreases below the minimal acceptable value for the patient. When autologous blood is reinfused, central venous pressure and serum ionized calcium, with or without cardiac output measurements, should be followed serially. As soon as evidence of hypervolemia is detected (increased central venous pressure, rales, decreased lung compliance, and enlarged liver span), low-dose furosemide (Lasix) 0.1 mg/kg should be administered intravenously. Additional doses of furosemide can be administered as necessary to maintain a diuresis. Extensive increases in interstitial fluid volume are uncommon when the period of fluid accumulation is brief. Electrolyte imbalance is also uncommon unless massive transfusions of old homologous blood are required. When the excess total body water is reduced to 10 percent of the total volume of fluid administered, tracheal extubation can be considered.

During recovery, it is essential to monitor the child very carefully. Because ventilation may be controlled for 4 to 12 hours or more after surgery, a nasotracheal tube may be easier to manage in infants and children. Adequate tissue oxygenation must be maintained during this period, as transient tissue edema may be severe. Venous oxyhe-

moglobin desaturation may occur during this time, as hematocrit and viscosity increase rapidly after reversal of hemodilution; the core temperature increases more slowly. The desaturation of venous blood may become critical if the metabolic rate is allowed to increase too rapidly. The metabolic rate can be reduced in intubated patients by adequate sedation (morphine 0.05 to 0.25 mg/kg/h and midazolam 0.05 to 0.2 mg/kg every 8 hours), and/or paralysis with rocuronium (Zemuron), to prevent shivering and to control ventilation.

Fluid management during the postoperative period includes replacement of ongoing third-space fluid losses with lactated Ringer's solution (4 to 10 ml/kg/h or more). Administration of colloid solutions during this period may lead to protein accumulation in edematous tissues, thereby delaying the mobilization of excess fluid and the resultant diuresis. Supplemental parenteral iron therapy and recombinant erythropoietin can be resumed during the postoperative period to stimulate bone marrow production of red cells.

In summary, acute normovolemic hemodilution is an effective technique in children to minimize or obviate blood transfusions. Meticulous perioperative preparation and management of patients are crucial for a successful outcome. The combination of hemodilution, mild hypothermia, and general anesthesia reduces the need for homologous blood transfusions. Careful monitoring of end-organ function should minimize the risks of end-organ damage associated with this technique.

CONTROLLED HYPOTENSION

During controlled hypotension, systemic arterial blood pressure is reduced in a controlled and deliberate manner to reduce blood loss and improve visibility in the surgical field.[54, 55] This technique has been used in pediatric patients of all ages and for many surgical procedures.[56-58] This section discusses the indications, contraindications, physiology, pharmacology, and anesthetic management of controlled hypotension.

Indications

The indications for controlled hypotension include surgery for neurosurgical[56] or orthopedic[55, 58-60] problems; major vascular abnormalities[61]; ear, nose, and throat disorders[62]; burns[63]; and craniofacial reconstruction.[54, 57] In fact, it is appropriate for most surgical procedures where a "bloodless" field, small blood loss,[55, 59] and less operating time are desirable.[55] Studies in young adults indicate that controlled hypotension does not cause long-term neuropsychological changes.[64]

Contraindications

The contraindications to controlled hypotension must be weighed carefully when this technique is contemplated (Table 13–1). Any one of these contraindications precludes its use, as the inappropriate use of controlled hypotension can result in irreversible cardiac or brain dam-

T A B L E   1 3 – 1
CONTRAINDICATIONS TO CONTROLLED HYPOTENSION
Physician's lack of understanding of the technique, lack of technical expertise, or inability to monitor the patient's condition adequately
Inadequate postoperative care
Focal or generalized decreased organ blood flow
Elevated intracranial pressure
Anemia/hemoglobinopathies
Polycythemia
Allergy or sensitivity to the hypotensive agent

age.[54, 65] Furthermore, significant deviations from the management described below may cause organ damage.

Physiology

The physiologic changes that accompany controlled hypotension depend in part on the type of hypotensive agent used. Hypotensive agents can be divided into two types: volatile anesthetic agents and vasodilators. The vasodilators can be subdivided into those that act directly on vessels (e.g., sodium nitroprusside and nitroglycerin), those that act indirectly through the sympathetic ganglia (e.g., pentolinium), and those that act both directly and indirectly (e.g., trimethaphan).

Central Nervous System

The control of cerebral blood flow and cerebral oxygen demand during anesthesia and controlled hypotension in pediatric patients is poorly understood. Furthermore, the minimum cerebral blood flow that prevents cerebral dysfunction in pediatric patients is unknown. Most data on cerebral blood flow and metabolism in young patients have been extrapolated from studies in adults. Nevertheless, the arterial blood pressure that is recommended for pediatric patients undergoing controlled hypotension should not increase the risk of cerebral ischemia. This fact, together with the difficulty of monitoring cerebral function during anesthesia, has led clinicians to adopt conservative guidelines for managing controlled hypotension in pediatric patients.

Both volatile anesthetic drugs and vasodilators affect the ratio of cerebral blood flow to metabolic rate of oxygen consumption of the brain. All volatile anesthetic drugs attenuate or abolish the autoregulation of cerebral blood flow in a dose-dependent manner; the effect of halothane > enflurane > isoflurane > desflurane.[66, 67] The relative potency of these inhaled anesthetics on the cerebral metabolic rate of oxygen follows the reverse order (i.e., isoflurane > enflurane > halothane).[67] Studies with isoflurane-induced hypotension indicate that the decrease in cerebral blood flow is less than or equal to the decrease in the cerebral metabolic rate for oxygen, regardless of whether or not the patient is hypocapnic.[68–71] These effects may be regionally specific.[72] Therefore, isoflurane is proba-

bly the volatile anesthetic of choice for controlled hypotension.

Vasodilators such as sodium nitroprusside and nitroglycerin dilate cerebral vessels directly without affecting the cerebral metabolic rate for oxygen, and attenuate the autoregulation of cerebral blood flow in a manner not dissimilar to that of volatile anesthetics. In addition, nitroprusside affects the blood-brain barrier to a greater extent than trimethaphan, although the clinical significance of this finding is unclear.[73] In contrast, trimethaphan does not interfere with autoregulation of cerebral blood flow except at very high doses, but it does interfere with regional cerebral blood flow and regional oxygen supply to a greater extent than nitroprusside.[74] In normocapnic dogs, a MAP of 40 mm Hg induced with sodium nitroprusside or halothane or a pressure of 40 to 50 mm Hg induced with trimethaphan decreases cerebral blood flow without affecting the cerebral metabolic rate for oxygen.[75] Furthermore, electrical cortical activity and cortical blood flow are preserved to a greater extent during nitroprusside- or oligemia-induced hypotension than during trimethaphan-induced hypotension.[76–78] In monkeys, nitroprusside-induced hypotension reduces cerebral blood flow and the cerebral metabolic rate for oxygen to similar degrees, whereas trimethaphan reduces cerebral blood flow to a greater extent than the metabolic rate.[79]

Whether it is wise to combine hypocapnia and controlled hypotension remains a contentious issue. Hypocapnia decreases the cerebral blood flow in normotensive subjects by 2 percent per millimeter of mercury decrease in $PaCO_2$.[80] In hypotensive subjects, this effect is attenuated[81] or abolished,[82, 83] depending on the hypotensive agent. In hypocapnic dogs, nitroprusside-, nitroglycerin-, and trimethaphan-induced hypotension reduce cerebral blood flow relative to the cerebral metabolic rate for oxygen.[84, 85] Although it has been suggested that isoflurane uncouples the cerebral oxygen supply/demand ratio,[81, 86] data from dogs indicate that during hypocapnia ($PaCO_2$ 20 to 40 mm Hg) and isoflurane-induced hypotension (MAP 40 to 60 mm Hg), cerebral blood flow decreases in proportion to the decrease in the cerebral metabolic rate for oxygen. This combination of hypocapnia and isoflurane had no adverse effects on cerebral metabolism or function.[70, 87] These data indicate that cerebral metabolism and function in animals are preserved as follows: isoflurane > nitroprusside = nitroglycerin > trimethaphan.[70, 84, 85] On the basis of these animal studies, when hypocapnia is combined with hypotension, isoflurane is the preferred hypotensive agent. However, until the effects of this combination are studied in children, it seems prudent to avoid it.

If the reduction in cerebral blood flow exceeds the reduction in cerebral metabolic rate for oxygen, cerebral ischemia may develop. EEG changes occur when the cerebral blood flow is reduced by 40 to 50 percent below control values and is isoelectric when the cerebral blood flow is reduced by 60 percent or more below control values. To minimize the risks of cerebral ischemia during controlled hypotension, I recommend that hypotension be limited to a minimal MAP of 55 mm Hg, that hypotension be induced with isoflurane (using sodium nitroprusside or nitroglycerin as an adjunct if necessary), and that normocapnia be maintained.

The position of the head during hypotensive anesthesia, in particular the head-up tilt, may decrease cerebral perfusion pressure. This pressure decreases 2 mm Hg for every 2.5 cm the head is raised above the level of the arterial transducer.[88]

Controlled hypotension decreases the anesthetic requirements for volatile anesthetics. In dogs, nitroprusside-, trimethaphan-, and pentolinium-induced hypotension decreased the anesthetic requirements for halothane by 30 percent.[89] The reason is not understood.

Respiratory System

Controlled hypotension affects the respiratory system by increasing the alveolar dead space, and increasing the intrapulmonary shunt.[54, 90, 91] Head-up tilt and an increase in zone 1 increase dead space ventilation (V_D) and may increase $Paco_2$. Although head-up tilt increases V_D/V_T (V_T is the tidal volume) by as much as threefold in adults, it does not increase V_D/V_T in pediatric patients. This discrepancy can be attributed to the lesser gravitational effect on the lung in these smaller (pediatric) patients.

In patients with normal lungs, intrapulmonary shunt increases during controlled hypotension. This increase has been attributed to a decrease in pulmonary artery pressure, an increase in blood flow through dependent regions of the lung (increasing preexisting shunts), and a reversal of hypoxic pulmonary vasoconstriction. This reversal occurs with nitroprusside,[91–93] nitroglycerin[93] and, to a lesser extent, with isoflurane.[94]

Arterial blood gases, together with serum lactate concentrations, must be monitored frequently during controlled hypotension to ensure the adequacy of ventilation and oxygenation. Baseline blood gas and pH values should be obtained after induction of anesthesia, before and after head-up tilt, and after every 30 to 60 minutes of controlled hypotension. Normocapnia ($Paco_2$ of 35 to 45 mm Hg) and hyperoxia ($Pao_2 > 300$ mm Hg) must be maintained. Hypocapnia should be avoided during hypotension because it may reduce cerebral blood flow and cardiac output, thereby decreasing the cerebral oxygen supply/demand ratio. Similarly, hyperoxia should be provided to compensate for intrapulmonary shunts during general anesthesia and hypotension.

$Petco_2$ is now commonly used to estimate the arterial Pco_2 in pediatric patients during anesthesia.[95] However, the relation between arterial and $Petco_2$ values should be established during each of the maneuvers described above before relying on serial or continuous $Petco_2$ measurements. Previous studies suggest that the arterial to end-tidal Pco_2 gradient in pediatric patients remains stable for up to 2 hours after induction of hypotension.

Cardiovascular System

Hypotensive agents decrease afterload and, to a lesser extent, decrease preload.[96] The decrease in afterload usually improves left ventricular function, as long as exaggerated decreases in preload do not compromise the left ventricular filling volume, particularly in the newborn.[54, 97]

Coronary blood flow is rarely compromised in the pediatric patient. Therefore, factors that increase myocardial oxygen demand (e.g., an increase in heart rate) should not precipitate myocardial ischemia even when the patient is hypotensive.

Pharmacology

Drugs used to induce hypotension affect one or more factors that control blood pressure: systemic vascular resistance, sympathetic tone, and myocardial contractility. A reduction in heart rate should not be used to reduce arterial pressure in children. An increase in heart rate during induced hypotension may indicate drug toxicity or organ hypoperfusion and may require immediate intervention.

Sodium Nitroprusside

Sodium nitroprusside, a commonly used hypotensive agent in children, is a direct-acting, potent arterial and, to a lesser extent, venous vasodilator with a rapid onset of action (within 1 to 2 minutes), a brief duration of action, and no direct myocardial depression.[96] Likely mediators responsible for the vasodilating properties of nitroprusside include endothelium-derived relaxing factor or a nitrosothiol compound.[98] Despite these favorable characteristics, nitroprusside must be administered carefully and monitored continuously, as fatal cyanide toxicity has been reported previously.[99] The safe use of nitroprusside requires continuous arterial pressure monitoring, a dedicated IV cannula for the infusion of nitroprusside, the means to regulate the infusion rate of the drug precisely, and periodic blood gas analyses.

Dose

Sodium nitroprusside (50 mg/bottle) is available as a lyophilized powder that is recommended for reconstitution in 5 percent dextrose in water (500 ml) to give a 0.01 percent solution (0.1 mg/ml).[96] Because nitroprusside decomposes spontaneously in the presence of light, it must be shielded from light by wrapping the IV bag with aluminum foil. The IV tubing need not be shielded, as spontaneous degradation of nitroprusside is insignificant within the first 8 hours.[100, 101] Once dissolved, a shielded nitroprusside solution is stable for up to 24 hours,[100] after which it should be discarded. If a solution of nitroprusside turns blue, it should also be discarded. Nitroprusside should be administered by continuous infusion through a separate IV catheter. Careful adjustment of the infusion rate with an infusion pump is essential to minimize large swings in arterial pressure. Direct infusion of the drug into a central venous cannula or into the hub of an IV catheter minimizes dead space and prevents delayed responses to changes in the infusion rate. The infusion rate of nitroprusside should begin at 0.1 μg/kg/min and can be increased up to a maximal rate of 8 to 10 μg/kg/min.[102–104] Nitroprusside requirements can be reduced by the coadministration of volatile anesthetics,[105] β-blockers,[106] aminophylline, or captopril,[107] or coadministration of trimethaphan (in a ratio of 1:2.5 to 1:5 nitroprusside to trimethaphan).[108] If the infusion rate of nitroprusside approaches the maximum rate, nitroprusside toxicity must be considered. Measures must be taken to verify the diagnosis and to treat the toxicity. The maximal recommended dosage of nitroprusside is approximately 2 to 3 mg/kg/day.[96, 99, 101]

Physiology

Sodium nitroprusside is a direct-acting vascular smooth muscle relaxant that rapidly decreases afterload, preload, and myocardial oxygen consumption without depressing myocardial contractility. Cardiac output may increase,[96, 99, 105] decrease,[96, 109] or remain unchanged[91, 92, 110–112] during nitroprusside-induced hypotension. Tachycardia, a common response to nitroprusside,[109] may attenuate the hypotensive effects[111] and necessitate increasing doses of nitroprusside with or without incremental doses of β-blocker such as IV propranolol 0.015 mg/kg up to a maximal dose of 0.150 mg/kg or esmolol 0.2 to 0.3 mg/kg/h.[106] Tachycardia may also herald the onset of tachyphylaxis (i.e., resistance to nitroprusside that requires increasing doses of nitroprusside to maintain the desired level of hypotension).

Nitroprusside is a direct cerebral vasodilator that increases intracranial pressure slightly in healthy patients.[113] However, if the intracranial pressure is already increased, it could increase pressure significantly. It shifts the cerebral autoregulation curve to the left in a dose-dependent manner. Nitroprusside has no effect on the cerebral metabolic rate for oxygen.

Sodium nitroprusside directly relaxes the pulmonary vascular smooth muscle, which may decrease right ventricular afterload. It attenuates hypoxic pulmonary vasoconstriction, which may increase venous admixture (intrapulmonary shunt), particularly in normal lungs.[91, 92] Therefore, oxygenation must be monitored intermittently with arterial blood gases and continuously with pulse oximetry.

In the isolated kidney, sodium nitroprusside decreases renovascular resistance and increases renal blood flow. In the intact kidney, nitroprusside-induced hypotension transiently decreases creatinine clearance, which returns to normal after the arterial blood pressure returns to normal.[114] In the dog, renal blood flow remains normal despite a 15 to 50 percent decrease in systolic arterial pressure.[115, 116]

Catecholamines and the renin-angiotensin system are activated to a greater extent during nitroprusside-induced hypotension than during trimethaphan-induced hypotension.[117] However, the greater release of vasopressin in response to hypotension in the ewe suggests that vasopressin is more important than renin for attenuating nitroprusside-induced hypotension.[118] Whether the same holds true for children remains to be established.

Nitroprusside-induced hypotension during halothane anesthesia has not been associated with liver dysfunction.[90, 119] However, nitroprusside-induced hypotension may inhibit platelet aggregation after surgery for at least 24 hours.[120]

Sodium nitroprusside is contraindicated when continuous arterial pressure monitoring is not available, resuscitation equipment is not available, or the oxygen content of the blood is reduced (i.e., in anemia). Relative contraindications include the presence of Leber's optic atrophy,

tobacco amblyopia, renal and hepatic failure, or an unstable cardiovascular system. It has been suggested that in the presence of hepatic insufficiency, the rhodanase enzyme system (see below) in organs other than the liver is capable of metabolizing nitroprusside.[96] It has also been suggested that renal insufficiency does not impair short-term detoxification of cyanide, although thiocyanate could accumulate and lead to thiocyanate toxicity.[96]

Tachyphylaxis, which is defined as an increased need for nitroprusside to maintain a desired level of hypotension, occurs occasionally in patients. Early signs of tachyphylaxis include failure to maintain hypotension with a previously effective dose of nitroprusside (resistance) and unexplained tachycardia.[121] Tachyphylaxis has been attributed in part to stimulation of the baroreflex, which occurs in response to induced hypotension. This reflex can be attenuated with β-blocking drugs. However, tachycardia also may be the first sign of cyanide toxicity.[99, 121, 122] An unexplained metabolic acidosis should raise further suspicion of cyanide toxicity.[101] If tachyphylaxis is suspected, nitroprusside *must* be stopped. Alternate techniques for maintaining the desired level of hypotension should be instituted.

Rebound systemic and pulmonary hypertension may occur after nitroprusside is discontinued[110] and require treatment with direct vasodilators and β-blocking drugs.

Toxicity

Cyanide is the primary toxic metabolite of nitroprusside.[96] Five cyanide ions are released from each molecule of nitroprusside metabolized (Fig. 13–4). Cyanide is detoxified by both the rhodanase enzyme system (80 percent) and the methemoglobin pathway (20 percent). Both detoxification systems require a sulfur atom donor (thiosulfate) and vitamin B_{12}. Thiocyanate, the detoxified cyanide moiety, is excreted via the kidneys. However, if the amount of cyanide present exceeds the capacity of these detoxification pathways, cyanide irreversibly binds mitochondrial cytochrome oxidases and causes cytotoxic hypoxia. This reaction increases the mixed venous Po_2, increases venous and arterial serum lactate concentrations, and decreases venous and arterial pH. Persistent hypotension after discontinuation of nitroprusside administration suggests that cyanide (and thiocyanate) toxicity may be present.[96]

Immediate treatment of cyanide toxicity includes stopping the infusion of nitroprusside and administering 100 percent oxygen. Venous and arterial blood samples are obtained for blood gas analyses and serum lactate and cyanide concentrations. Initial therapy is aimed at increasing the availability of methemoglobin, which has a greater affinity for cyanide than does the cytochrome oxidase enzyme. Methemoglobin concentration can be increased rapidly by administering sodium nitrite[123] (10 mg/kg initially and then 5 mg/kg over 30 minutes) by infusion.[99, 102] To facilitate transfer of cyanide from cyanmethemoglobin to thiocyanate, sodium thiosulfate 150 mg/kg should also be administered intravenously.[99, 102, 124] This dose of thiosulfate can be repeated several times if necessary, as thiosulfate is rapidly excreted by the kidneys, with an elimination half-life of 23 minutes.[125] Amyl nitrite may be administered by inhalation (for 30 seconds every 2 minutes) to increase

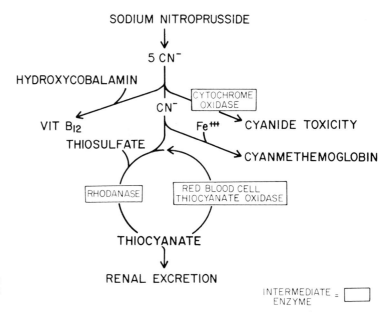

FIGURE 13–4. Metabolic degradation of sodium nitroprusside in the human. Enzymatic pathways are identified with boxes enclosing intermediate enzymes.

methemoglobin levels. As cyanide is transferred from cyanmethemoglobin to thiocyanate and hydrogen cyanide, methemoglobin is reformed. Methemoglobin is then converted back to hemoglobin by the glutathione reductase enzyme system. One note of caution should be added: overzealous administration of nitrites may produce excessive quantities of methemoglobin, which itself can cause hypoxia.

Hydroxycobalamin (vitamin $B_{12\alpha}$) 0.1 mg/kg has been recommended as a second-line treatment for cyanide toxicity and as a means of minimizing the effect of thiocyanate on hematopoiesis because it forms cyanocobalamin (vitamin B_{12}).[102, 103] However, its lack of potency, short shelf-life, and high cost have precluded further studies in humans.[124]

Nitroglycerin

Nitroglycerin is a direct-acting vasodilator that acts primarily on the venous capacitance and secondarily on the arterial smooth muscle. It induces hypotension smoothly and gradually, with minimal danger of precipitous hypotension.[126] Nitroglycerin is available in solution (5 mg/ml) for infusion. The dose of nitroglycerin required to induce hypotension ranges from 1 to 10 μg/kg/min, although larger doses have been used. Nitroglycerin, like sodium nitroprusside, should be infused through a separate IV line that has minimal dead space. Nonpolyvinylchloride tubing should be used to minimize adsorption of nitroglycerin to the tubing wall. Continuous arterial pressure monitoring is mandatory during nitroglycerin infusions.

Nitroglycerin is metabolized by reductive hydrolysis by the glutathione organic nitrate reductase hepatic enzyme system. The water-soluble nitrate and inorganic nitrite metabolites of nitroglycerin are considerably less potent vasodilators than the parent compound.[127]

Toxicity from nitroglycerin is rare, although tachyphylaxis is relatively common. Some patients show resistance to the hypotensive effects of nitroglycerin.[102, 128]

Nitroglycerin is a potent coronary vasodilator that increases myocardial oxygen supply. It may decrease cardiac output and pulmonary artery pressure.[128] Unlike nitroprusside, rebound hypertension has not been reported after abrupt cessation of nitroglycerin. Nitroglycerin is a direct cerebral vasodilator that increases cerebral blood flow and may increase intracranial pressure if intracranial compliance is low.[129] Cerebral metabolism (as determined by lactate, pyruvate, and lactic dehydrogenase activity) during nitroglycerin-induced hypotension (MAP, 33 mm Hg) is undisturbed in healthy young patients.[130] Nitroglycerin increases capillary blood flow and oxygen tension in striated muscle to a greater extent than nitroprusside.[131] Nitroglycerin also increases plasma renin activity, although this reaction is not related to resistance to the drug.[128]

In a controlled double-blind study of the effects of nitroprusside and nitroglycerin in children, nitroprusside 6 to 8 μg/kg/min was administered without an inhalational anesthetic. It reliably induced hypotension without any side effects apart from small increases in the $(A-a)Do_2$ and a slight metabolic acidosis (base excess was -6 mEq/L).[104] Nitroglycerin was significantly less effective than nitroprusside for producing hypotension. During spine surgery, intravenous nitroglycerin has proven to be as effective as halothane in reducing blood loss and surgical time.[132]

Trimethaphan

Trimethaphan is a rapid-acting vasodilator that decreases systolic blood pressure by decreasing systemic vascular resistance. This decrease in vascular resistance has been attributed to ganglionic blockade (arterial and venular),[99, 133] direct vasodilation, histamine release, and, when used in high doses, α-adrenergic blockade.[133, 134] The role of histamine in the hypotensive effect of trimethaphan has been questioned.[135]

Trimethaphan is available as a white powder that has a bitter taste and a slight odor. It has a pH of 5 to 6 when prepared as a 1 percent solution. Trimethaphan should be prepared as a 0.1 or 0.2 percent solution in 5 percent dextrose in water.[133] This solution is stable for up to 24 hours. Because of its rapid onset and brief duration of action, trimethaphan must be given by continuous infusion through a separate IV line. The infusion dose ranges from 10 to 200 μg/kg/min. Continuous arterial blood pressure monitoring is required when trimethaphan is infused. Arterial pressure begins to decrease within 5 minutes after the infusion is started and reaches minimal values within 10 minutes.[135, 136] The reverse Trendelenburg position facilitates the hypotension induced by ganglionic blockade. The patient should be monitored carefully when the dose being administered approaches the recommended upper range.

Trimethaphan decreases cardiac output by either ganglionic blockade or a negative inotropic effect,[136, 137] although the latter may depend on the rate of induction of hypotension.[91, 135] Intracranial pressure is unchanged during trimethaphan-induced controlled hypotension.[113] Trimethaphan causes a transient reduction in the glomerular filtration rate similar to that caused by nitroprusside; it returns to normal after discontinuation of the drug.[138] Trimethaphan has no effect on the renin-angiotensin system.[117] Supplemental techniques for hypotension must often be used to maintain the desired level of hypotension, as tachyphylaxis is common.[139]

The disadvantages of trimethaphan include tachyphylaxis, tachycardia, histamine release, inhibition of pseudocholinesterase activity, tachycardia-induced resistance to hypotension, mild myoneural blockade, urinary retention, and gastrointestinal disturbances.[133] Fixed, dilated pupils may persist for as long as 24 hours after the drug is discontinued.

Contraindications to trimethaphan include asthma, pseudocholinesterase deficiency, liver disease, and chronic malnutrition.

Pentolinium

Pentolinium (Ansolysen), a ganglion-blocking drug, has a relatively slow onset of action (5 minutes), maximal hypotensive effect approximately 30 minutes after its administration, and a prolonged duration of action (1 to 4 hours).[133] It is available as a 0.5 percent solution (5 mg/ml). Pentolinium 0.1 mg/kg can be administered intravenously over 5 to 10 minutes; the same dose can be repeated up to a maximum of 0.3 mg/kg.[133] Pentolinium is rarely used in pediatric anaesthesia today and has been supplanted by other agents.

The mechanism of action of pentolinium is direct ganglionic blockade. Peripheral vascular resistance decreases. Reflex tachycardia is common.[99] These effects tend to increase cardiac output.[140] IV propranolol, given in increments of 0.015 mg/kg, or an infusion of esmolol (100 to 300 μg/kg/min), may be required to control the heart rate and restore cardiac output to normal.

Pentolinium should be administered after induction of anaesthesia but before surgery commences.[141] As the hypotension develops, it can be augmented by placing the child in a head-up position and/or by increasing the concentration of volatile anesthetic. Although a transient increase in heart rate is common in pediatric patients, few other side effects have been reported. Histamine release,

serum cholinesterase-blocking action, neuromuscular blocking properties, and (to a lesser extent) tachyphylaxis are uncommon.[134, 141] Mydriasis and cycloplegia may last several hours.

The duration of a single dose of pentolinium (1 to 4 hours) is usually sufficient for most surgical procedures. Hypotension can be reversed by returning the patient to the horizontal position, stopping the inhaled anesthetic, or by infusing balanced salt solutions or colloids. In an emergency, α-agonists (phenylephrine or methoxamine) are effective, as there is no α-blockade.

Adenosine

Adenosine is a hypotensive agent that is currently available for use for this indication in Europe but not in North America. The obstacle to adenosine's approval in North America rests primarily with its effects on the α_1-receptor in the myocardium and the kidney as outlined below.

The infusion dose recommended for adults is 100 to 800 μg/kg/min.[142-148] Studies in animals and humans indicate that it is a direct systemic and pulmonary vasodilator that compares favorably with nitroprusside in ability to rapidly induce easily controllable hypotension without inducing tachyphylaxis, rebound hypertension, or the accumulation of toxic metabolites.[111, 112, 142-148] During adenosine-induced hypotension, right atrial pressure and preload are unchanged, and cardiac output is unchanged or increased.[111, 112, 142, 144-146, 148] There is no evidence that myocardial ischemia occurs.[111, 144, 148] In addition, cerebral blood flow and oxygen utilization are maintained during adenosine-induced hypotension in contrast to nitroprusside.[142, 143, 147] In the presence of hypocapnia, adenosine-induced hypotension maintains CO_2 reactivity in the cerebral vasculature and does not reduce cerebral blood flow to ischemic levels.[143] Hypotensive doses of adenosine have been shown to decrease the minimum alveolar concentration (MAC) of halothane in dogs by 50 percent.[149] There is no published experience to date with the use of this drug in children.

The effects of adenosine are mediated via two receptors: α_1 and α_2. α_1-Receptors are located in the cardiac conduction system (sinoatrial [SA] and atrioventricular [AV] nodes) and in the preglomerular arterioles in the kidney. Activation of α_1-receptors in the cardiac conduction system may result in bradycardia and transient AV block. Activation of the receptors in the kidneys may lead to renal vasoconstriction. α_2-Receptors mediate systemic arterial vasodilation. Although adenosine, an α_1/α_2-receptor agonist, may not achieve widespread use, selective α_2-receptor agonists are currently being developed for clinical use.

Miscellaneous Medications

Other medications have been investigated for use as hypotensive agents during anesthesia. Clonidine, an α_2-agonist, is available in some countries for parenteral use as a sedative, vasodilator, and hypotensive agent. Clonidine may be an effective adjunct to isoflurane/metoprolol hypotensive anesthesia,[150] although clonidine's postoperative sedative effects require careful consideration. Magnesium sulphate, which has been used to control hypertension in preeclamptic patients, is under investigation as a hypotensive agent during general anaesthesia.[151] However, its use may be limited by side effects including postoperative sedation, weakness, and abnormal coagulation. Further studies are required to confirm the safety of this technique.[151] β-Blockers and calcium channel blockers have been used as adjuncts to anesthesia and vasodilator agents to facilitate hypotensive anesthesia.[106, 152–156] Propofol also has been investigated as an hypotensive agent to limit blood loss during surgery.[157]

Volatile Anesthetics

A potent volatile anesthetic (halothane, isoflurane, or sevoflurane) can be used as the sole hypotensive agent or in combination with the aforementioned drugs.[105, 132, 137] Volatile anesthetics act by several dose-dependent mechanisms to cause hypotension; these include myocardial depression, dilation of the vascular beds, and depression of central and peripheral sympathetic nerves.[158, 159] Isoflurane decreases systemic vascular resistance, depresses the myocardium to a lesser extent than halothane, and attenuates sympathetic responses.[68, 160] The effect of sevoflurane on the circulation is intermediate between those of halothane and isoflurane.[161] Induced hypotension with all of these drugs is enhanced by the reverse Trendelenburg position, avoidance of vagolytic drugs, and administration of β-blockers.[154] Atropine and pancuronium are best avoided when hypotension is required.

Anesthetic Management

The decision to use controlled hypotension is based on a risk–benefit analysis. This decision should be made before induction of anesthesia so that the anesthetic management and monitoring strategies can be properly planned.

Preoperative Management

Routine laboratory data, including hemoglobin level, urinalysis, and serum glucose concentration, are essential. A minimal hemoglobin level of 10 g/dl is recommended before hypotensive anesthesia is begun, although there is evidence that patients may tolerate hypotension in combination with hemodilution.[8] Premedication may include a venodilator or ganglion-blocking drug such as morphine, droperidol, or chlorpromazine. Premedication with vagolytic drugs should be avoided.

Intraoperative Management

Hypotension should not be induced before induction of anesthesia. After an IV infusion is started, balanced salt or colloid solutions should be infused to restore the intravascular volume. A large-bore IV cannula is strongly recommended to facilitate rapid administration of fluids during periods of rapid blood loss. A second IV line should be available for infusing the hypotensive agent.

Meticulous monitoring of the patient's condition is essential for the safe conduct of controlled hypotension. An indwelling arterial cannula is mandatory, as rapid and profound changes in arterial pressure may require immedi-

ate intervention as well as determination of arterial blood gases, serum electrolytes, and glucose levels (particularly when labetalol, metoprolol, or esmolol is given) every 30 to 60 minutes.[54] Noninvasive blood pressure monitors may overestimate or underestimate the arterial blood pressure during hypotension.[162] A radial or axillary arterial catheter is preferable to a dorsalis pedis catheter because the latter overestimates arterial pressure during nitroprusside-induced hypotension and underestimates arterial pressure during isoflurane-induced hypotension.[163] The use of a pulse oximeter is recommended during hypotensive anesthesia, although the reduced pulse size may obscure the oximeter signal.

Central venous pressure monitoring is recommended to maintain atrial filling pressure during induced hypotension. Because right-sided filling pressures parallel left-sided filling pressures in children, central venous pressure is a good indication of left ventricular filling pressures. Therefore, pulmonary artery catheters are not routinely used.

Organ perfusion is most accurately assessed by organ function. Lactic acid accumulation suggests on-going anerobic metabolism but is not specific for any organ. Urine output is indicative of renal perfusion in the absence of renal and urologic dysfunction. Therefore, a urinary catheter should be inserted after induction of anesthesia but before hypotension is induced, and care should be taken to maintain a urine output of 0.5 to 2 ml/kg/h throughout the anesthetic. If urine output is less than 0.5 ml/kg/h, the patency of the catheter system should be checked before administering a fluid challenge (crystalloid or colloid).

Body temperature must be carefully monitored, as drug-induced generalized vaso- and venodilation may increase heat losses. Normothermia should be maintained.

Anesthesia should be induced smoothly with either IV (thiopental or propofol) or inhaled (halothane or sevoflurane) drugs to minimize hypertension, tachycardia, and increased venous pressures. IV lidocaine 1.5 mg/kg or opioids may be used to maintain hemodynamic stability during induction. Muscle relaxants can be used to facilitate endotracheal intubation. Rocuronium (0.5 to 1.0 mg/kg) is preferable to pancuronium because the former does not increase heart rate.[164] Anesthesia should be maintained with a potent inhalational agent in 60 percent nitrous oxide/40 percent oxygen (see below), an opioid (preferably morphine for its venodilating properties), and a muscle relaxant (see above). Ventilation should be controlled to maintain normocapnia. After arterial and central venous catheters are inserted, the patient is positioned for surgery. Care must be taken to ensure that positioning does not obstruct venous return. If the patient is positioned head up, the arterial pressure transducer should be adjusted to the level of the head and the central venous pressure transducer at the level of the right atrium. Both transducers should then be rezeroed. The effects of body position (head-up tilt) and positive-pressure ventilation should be evaluated before controlled hypotension is induced.

Before inducing hypotension, the hemoglobin, arterial blood gases, serum concentrations of electrolytes, and the serum concentration of glucose should be determined. The hemoglobin concentration should be greater than or equal to 10 g/dl, although this guideline has not been confirmed in humans.[165] The arterial P_{O_2} should be maintained above 300 mm Hg at all times during hypotension, which may require discontinuation of nitrous oxide.[115, 166] In this circumstance, the concentration of inhalational agent should be increased to maintain an adequate depth of anesthesia. To minimize the risk of cerebral hypoperfusion, hypocapnia should be avoided during controlled hypotension.

Hypotension should be induced gradually with incremental increases in the concentration of isoflurane or sevoflurane. If the degree of hypotension is insufficient after appropriate positioning and general anesthesia, an adjunctive hypotensive agent is administered (see above).

Postoperative Management

In one study, death after controlled hypotension was caused by postoperative complications in 97 percent of cases.[54] Therefore, in addition to routine recovery room or intensive care unit care after general anesthesia, meticulous care must be directed to properly positioning the patient (particularly when long-acting vasodilators were used), providing a normal central blood volume, and maintaining normal circulatory and respiratory function. If attention is paid to these factors during the postoperative period, the morbidity and mortality associated with controlled hypotension should approximate zero.

Risks and Complications

In addition to the need for appropriate postoperative care after hypotensive anesthesia, several other strategies should be considered to avoid or attenuate the severity of complications. A sudden and dramatic decrease in blood pressure may occur during occult blood loss. Euvolemia or hypervolemia should be restored promptly to preclude end-organ hypoxia. Several recent reports of blindness have been associated with severe hemodilution and hypotension in children undergoing scoliosis surgery.[30-32] The blindness has been attributed to an ischemic optic neuritis that is believed to be associated with severe anemia, hypotension, and head dependency.

CONTROLLED HYPOTHERMIA

Temperature homeostasis is a prime concern in pediatric anesthesia. Indeed, accidental hypothermia may be associated with metabolic acidosis, vasoconstriction, decreased myocardial contractility, and cardiorespiratory collapse. However, the benefits of a decreased oxygen requirement during controlled hypothermia in patients with circulatory stability and an adequate oxygen supply can be substantial. When combined with total circulatory arrest, controlled hypothermia facilitates certain surgical procedures that would otherwise be impossible.[167-171] This section deals with the physiology and methods of inducing and controlling hypothermia. Hypothermia as an adjunct to cardiopulmonary bypass is discussed in detail in Chapter 18.

Okamura[172] defined five levels of hypothermia.

Mild hypothermia: 30° to 37°C

Moderate hypothermia: 25° to 30°C
Deep hypothermia: 20° to 25°C
Profound hypothermia: 10° to 20°C
Severe hypothermia: less than 10°C

At each of these levels, the physiologic considerations, risks, and potential complications are different.

Mild Hypothermia

In adults, mild hypothermia occurs frequently in operating rooms that are maintained at temperatures between 15.5° and 21.0°C. In these patients, mild hypothermia is seldom of concern. In pediatric patients, however (as in the adult patient with atherosclerotic cardiovascular disease), the response to even mild hypothermia can be striking. During the postoperative period, older children shiver to increase heat production, which in turn increases oxygen consumption two- to fourfold above that present in the resting, awake state. This increase in oxygen consumption may result in end-organ damage, particularly if congenital heart disease, congestive heart failure, or anemia is present.

Temperature homeostasis in the neonate is different from that in the older child. During the first month of life the neonate is relatively poikilothermic (i.e., is less able than older children to actively alter core body temperature in response to changes in environmental temperature). However, studies in fetal and neonatal sheep indicate that neonates are capable of mounting catecholamine and cardiovascular responses to mild hypothermia.[173, 174] Neonates use norepinephrine-dependent brown fat metabolism to produce heat and maintain their core temperature. Brown fat is stored in the interscapular, back, and neck regions in the neonate. This metabolic pathway increases the total body oxygen consumption in an effort to maintain core temperature.

As core temperature decreases, changes in the cardiovascular system may be dramatic. Mild hypothermia causes vasoconstriction, by increasing systemic vascular resistance, which in turn increases arterial blood pressure, afterload, and myocardial oxygen consumption. At temperatures below 28° to 30°C, however, myocardial contractility decreases. Together with a slowing of the heart rate, this decrease can cause hypotension. Central neural input into cardiac rate and rhythm decreases significantly with hypothermia. At 25°C, cardiac rate and rhythm are governed almost solely by local automatic phenomena. It is not surprising, therefore, that cardiac dysrhythmias occur with increasing frequency as the body temperature decreases below 28°C. Typical ECG changes (bradycardia or atrial fibrillation, prolongation of the PR interval, a widened QRS complex, and elevation of the ST segment) occur below 28°C. Osborn (J) waves are pathognomonic of hypothermia, occurring in 30 percent of patients with accidental hypothermia (below 30°C).[175] Ventricular fibrillation occurs with increasing frequency below 28°C. Although these ECG changes are often associated with irreversible myocardial injury in the normothermic state, they are common during hypothermia and disappear without residual myocardial damage after restoration of normothermia, provided that ischemia has not occurred.

Hypothermia globally depresses the central nervous system (CNS). Cerebral blood flow decreases in proportion to the reduction in the cerebral metabolic rate for oxygen consumption ($CMRO_2$). Cerebral oxygen consumption and that of other highly perfused organs decreases by approximately 5 to 9 percent per degree centigrade decrease in temperature.[24, 25] If vasoconstriction does not occur during hypothermia, the oxygen supply exceeds the oxygen demand. The MAC of potent inhalational agents also decreases about 5 percent per degree centigrade decrease in temperature,[176] although the MAC of nitrous oxide is minimally affected.[177]

Hypothermia affects pulmonary function and the pulmonary circulation.[178] As the metabolic rate decreases during hypothermia, CO_2 production decreases. To maintain normocapnia, ventilation must be reduced. Hypoxic pulmonary vasoconstriction is attenuated by 50 percent when the temperature decreases from 40°C to 30°C.[179] The latter effect may increase intrapulmonary shunt.

Mild hypothermia (34.5°C) increases the duration of action of vecuronium by approximately twofold.[180] This effect is more likely attributable to an effect of hypothermia on the pharmacokinetics of vecuronium than on its pharmacodynamics.[181]

The use of mild hypothermia requires that facilities for active rewarming be available as the body temperature decreases to 31° or 32°C. At these temperatures, the incidence of cardiac dysrhythmias remains low. However, temperature often continues to decrease below 30°C in spite of warming blankets and a heated humidifier. Provided direct, myocardial irritation does not occur, arrhythmias generally do not occur and rewarming is effective. If dysrhythmias do occur, it may be necessary to institute immediate cardiopulmonary bypass to rewarm the patient. This measure can be lifesaving. During thoracotomy or upper abdominal surgery, ventricular fibrillation may occur when the temperature reaches 30°C. If facilities for immediate cardiopulmonary bypass are not available, mild hypothermia is best limited to 33°C or above. At this temperature, it is usually possible to reverse ventricular fibrillation with electrical direct-current countershock.

Moderate and Deep Hypothermia

When the body temperature decreases below 30°C, it is likely that cardiac arrhythmias will occur and that immediate cardiopulmonary bypass will be required. Although bypass increases the myocardial temperature, thereby facilitating defibrillation, it does not attenuate some of the other problems that occur during moderate and severe hypothermia.

As temperature decreases, blood viscosity increases and flow decreases.[178] The viscosity of blood increases 2 to 3 percent per degree centigrade decrease in temperature. A further increase in viscosity may occur as the temperature approaches 25°C, as fluid moves from the intravascular space to the interstitium, causing hypovolemia and polycythemia. This may be particularly important for children with cyanotic heart disease, whose blood viscosity is already increased secondary to polycythemia. Modest hemodilution is indicated during cardiopulmonary bypass in these children to maintain cardiac output and systemic

oxygen transport. However, shear stress increases in children whose hematocrits exceed 50 percent when the temperature is between 27°C and 38°C.[182]

Coagulation may be affected during moderate hypothermia. Below 25°C the platelet count decreases and the tendency to bleeding increases. The enzymatic clotting cascade is also depressed, although it returns to normal during rewarming. Auhdi et al.[183] were unable to detect a significant alteration in coagulation after cardiopulmonary bypass, although fibrinolysis may be activated after bypass. Antifibrinolytic drugs such as ε-aminocapoic acid, aprotinin, or cyclocapron may attenuate the bleeding after bypass, particularly if administered before the skin incision occurs.[184]

During hypothermia, skeletal muscle, renal, and splanchnic blood flows decrease, whereas myocardial and cerebral blood flows increase by 300 percent and 200 percent, respectively.[185, 186] Renal blood flow decreases significantly during hypothermia, reflecting the reduced oxygen consumption. Renal function also decreases during hypothermia. Glomerular filtration rate and tubular cellular function, including active ionic secretion and resorption, decrease.

There has been considerable discussion about acid–base equilibrium during hypothermia.[187] CO_2 production decreases during moderate hypothermia, whereas the solubility of CO_2 in blood and tissues increases. As a result, the $Paco_2$ of cold blood measured at 37°C (the operating temperature of the blood gas machine) increases, suggesting the presence of marked respiratory acidosis. If CO_2 production does not change, the $Paco_2$ should decrease to 23 mm Hg at 25°C, solely as a result of the increased solubility in blood. If decreases in CO_2 production are taken into account, the "normal" $Paco_2$ at 25°C may in fact be even lower than 23 mm Hg. As a result of the direct effect of cold temperature on both the hydrogen ion dissociation and the pK of the Henderson-Hasselbach equation, cooling increases the measured pH. This reaction, along with the decreased $Paco_2$, leads to respiratory alkalosis. CO_2 can be added to the inspired gas to restore the pH toward 7.4.

It has been suggested that autoregulation of cerebral blood flow is affected by the $Paco_2$ during hypothermia.[188] Whether to temperature-correct (the pH STAT value) or not to temperature-correct (α-STAT) the $Paco_2$ values during controlled hypothermia is unclear.[187, 189] Studies suggest, however, that α-STAT $Paco_2$ maintains autoregulation of cerebral blood flow during hypothermia and is the preferred method of Pco_2 determination.[188]

The effect of temperature-correcting the acid–base status on myocardial function is poorly understood. In one study, there were fewer dysrhythmias and improved myocardial contractility in patients whose $Paco_2$ values were not temperature corrected (α-STAT) compared to those whose $Paco_2$ values were temperature corrected (pH STAT).[190] This finding supports the view that α-STAT is preferred.

The ideal acid–base status during deep hypothermia remains unclear. CO_2 is commonly added to the inspired gas mixture or to the cardiopulmonary bypass gases to maintain the α-STAT $Paco_2$ at 35 to 40 mm Hg, while the pH STAT $Paco_2$ at 18°C is as low as 15 to 20 mm Hg.

Therefore blood samples warmed to 37°C are used to establish the "normal," or α-STAT, Paco₂.

Profound Hypothermia

In infants, profound hypothermia is often used during cardiopulmonary bypass to allow brief periods of total circulatory arrest, to facilitate difficult surgical procedures (e.g., hepatic lobectomy, removal of hemangiomas, excision of intracranial aneurysms) and unusual reconstructive procedures on the heart.[167, 169, 171, 178, 191] Reducing the temperature to 16°C permits 40 minutes or more of circulatory arrest, during which time a bloodless field and the absence of arterial or venous bypass cannulas allow optimal operating conditions[192] (Table 13–2). Reducing the temperature to 13°C permits 60 minutes of circulatory arrest in dogs without neurologic deficit or neuropathologic changes at autopsy.[192] If a safe arrest period has not been exceeded, the characteristic changes in the EEG that are present during cooling and circulatory arrest return to normal during rewarming and usually return to their preoperative state before discharge from hospital.[193] Although the safe maximum duration of circulatory arrest during hypothermia has not been established,[168, 172, 194–196] the consensus is that young infants tolerate prolonged circulatory arrest better than older children.

Brunberg et al.[197] noted that circulatory arrest times of 10 to 57 minutes were tolerated by infants cooled to 14° to 23°C. Those who had postoperative neurologic injury consistently demonstrated continuous low-voltage EEG activity during circulatory arrest. In contrast, the postoperative EEG was normal in patients who had electrical silence on the EEG during circulatory arrest. Evidence suggests that the EEG changes attributable to hypothermia during rewarming can be distinguished from those attributable to cerebral ischemia.[198, 199] Therefore, electrical silence during circulatory arrest may be a reasonable indicator of the adequacy of cooling and brain protection during ischemia.

Somatosensory evoked potentials have been studied in infants undergoing profound hypothermic circulatory arrest. Preliminary evidence indicates that evoked potentials may be used to assess neurophysiologic function.[200] Visual evoked potentials disappear at temperatures of 19°C

and do not reappear until 22 minutes after circulatory arrest.[201] Increases in anterior fontanel pressure correlate with the absence of visual evoked potentials and may predict neurophysiologic dysfunction.[201]

The safe periods of circulatory arrest based on data from dogs are shown in Table 13–2. These observations are consistent with data in humans. The authors observed a mean oxygen consumption at 30°C that was 48 percent of the predicted value in humans at 37°C and a decrease of 26 percent as temperature decreased from 34°C to 30°C. These values are consistent with a 5 to 9 percent reduction in oxygen consumption per degree centigrade decrease in body temperature. Despite the decreased oxygen consumption, recent evidence suggests that oxygen consumption continues during the first 40 minutes of circulatory arrest.[203] This may have relevance for the etiology of brain injury after circulatory arrest.

In a study of 180 patients, Bailey et al.[168] found small but consistent differences in the relationship between total times of circulatory arrest and survival. The survivors were ischemic for a shorter period of time. These differences, however, were not large enough to identify the single most important determinant of mortality: length of ischemic arrest, complexity of the lesion, or preoperative status.

In 1976, Barratt-Boyes et al. reported a 93 percent survival for repair of ventricular septal defects in infants with a mean core temperature of 20°C and a mean ischemic arrest of 40 minutes.[204] Psychometric studies of these patients at 3 to 4 years of age failed to demonstrate any relationship between cerebral damage and ischemic arrest time. Evidence indicates that infants and young children who are less than 2 years of age at the time of surgery tolerate circulatory arrest for up to 74 minutes with no difference in developmental quotient at 2 to 4 years of age compared with normal children.[195] In the same study, older children (mean age 2 years) undergoing cardiac surgery without circulatory arrest had a high incidence of abnormalities. Current evidence indicates that the circulatory arrest time should be limited to 60 minutes to minimize neurologic sequelae but may be safe for up to 74 minutes in infants and children under specific conditions.[195, 205, 206]

Severe Hypothermia

Severe hypothermia is almost always used for local applications only. Isolated perfusion of the heart to temperatures as low as 7°C enables surgeons to perform procedures that take longer than would be feasible under total circulatory arrest. This degree of hypothermia is attained by directly perfusing the heart with a cooled mixture or by immersing it in an ice-saline slush. The use of severe hypothermia is generally restricted to surgery involving the heart and is used for the repair of complex cardiac defects and the revascularization of coronary arteries.

Methods of Cooling

Deliberate hypothermia is induced with surface cooling and core cooling. For surface cooling, a gradient is established between the outside and inside of the body or organ so that temperature gradually decreases over time. With

TABLE 13–2
ESTIMATED TIME LIMITS FOR CIRCULATORY ARREST IN DOGS AT VARIOUS BODY TEMPERATURES

Temperature	Oxygen Consumption (% of Normal)	Time Limits for Circulatory Arrest (min)
37°C	100	—
28°C	50	8–10
22°C	25	16–20
16°C	12	32–40
10°C	6	64–80

Adapted from Gordon AS, Jones SC, Luddington LG, et al: Deep hypothermia for intracardiac surgery: experimental and clinical use without an oxygenator. Am J Surg 100:332, 1960, with permission.

core cooling (e.g., cardiopulmonary bypass), organ temperature is reduced directly by a cold perfusate. Both surface cooling and core cooling have been applied to whole-body systems as well as to the isolated myocardium. Surface cooling satisfactorily induces mild hypothermia. However, the combination of surface cooling and core cooling is the preferred method for inducing deep or profound hypothermia.

Surface cooling can be undertaken in several ways. Immersing the whole body in an iced saline bath is efficient, but is seldom used today. Instead, hypothermia may be effected by placing cooling blankets either below or above and below the child. Hypothermia can be induced more rapidly by placing bags of iced saline in the axillae and groins as well. This reduces body temperature by approximately 1°C every 15 minutes. Although surface cooling is simple, body temperature still decreases slowly compared with other techniques. The primary risk of surface cooling is crystallization of intracellular water from contact with the cooling blanket or ice bag. Crystallization can be avoided by keeping the cooling medium above 4°C or by placing a towel between the cooling surface and the body. Care must be taken during surface cooling to protect thin, dependent cutaneous areas from becoming ischemic and developing pressure-induced necrosis. During surface cooling, the temperature gradient between the outside and the inside of the body causes core temperature to drift 2° or 3°C, below the lowest temperature measured at the time rewarming is started. Therefore active cooling should stop approximately 2°C above the desired minimal temperature. The cold solution is removed from the cooling blanket and is replaced with fluid having a temperature at or above the desired minimal temperature. In fact, one may begin rewarming while the body temperature is still 2°C above the minimal level desired, as the core temperature will continue to decrease after cooling techniques have been withdrawn.

Core cooling is achieved much more rapidly and with much more precision than surface cooling. However, core cooling adds the risks of cardiopulmonary bypass. The advantage of using bypass is that rewarming can be accomplished evenly and rapidly at the completion of the surgical procedure. A temperature gradient exists between the core and surface temperature during core cooling and warming. Temperature afterdrop during rewarming has been attributed to mobilization of cold peripheral blood to the central circulatory compartment, but more recent evidence suggests that afterdrop may actually represent the effect of thermal gradients between the core and the surface of the body that act as a heat sink from warm to cool tissues, respectively.[207]

Liquid ventilation with a cold oxygenated fluorocarbon has been used in neonatal lambs to minimize the duration of cooling and rewarming by using the high surface area of the lung for heat transfer.[208] This technique is not currently available for use in humans.

EXTRACORPOREAL MEMBRANE OXYGENATION

The first membrane oxygenators used polyethelene or Teflon membranes,[209] but long-term use of these devices caused significant lung and blood injury. Silicone rubber membranes improved the efficiency of gas exchange and prolonged the duration of safe treatment with extracorporeal membrane oxygenation (ECMO).[210–212] However, a controlled trial of ECMO showed no difference in survival over mechanical ventilation,[213, 214] except in infants with reversible respiratory failure.[215–217] Bartlett and others found that they could reverse the mortality of infants with some types of acute respiratory failure.[218] However, like all new therapies, ECMO has produced problems, some of which require surgery and anesthesia.

Criteria for ECMO

Infants with severe pulmonary or cardiac disease who are expected to improve in 10 days or less are candidates for ECMO. Most of them have pulmonary hypertension caused by meconium aspiration, persistent fetal circulation, diaphragmatic hernia, or sepsis. They are usually more than 34 weeks' gestational age and weigh more than 2,000 g. Most have failed conventional therapy, including 100 percent oxygen, muscle paralysis, standard mechanical ventilation, high-frequency ventilation, and inotropic and vasodilator therapy. Mechanical ventilation usually has been used for less than 8 days because longer periods of ventilation lead to chronic lung disease that will not improve in 10 days or less. The patients should be free of congenital defects that are incompatible with a meaningful life, there should be no significant congenital heart disease, and there should be no intracranial hemorrhage in excess of grade II.[219] The patient should be free of bleeding disorders and have a greater than 80 percent expected mortality with standard therapy in that hospital.

Many clinicians use an (A–a)Do_2 of greater than 610 for 12 hours[220] or greater than 620 for 4 to 8 hours,[221, 222] or a Ventilation Index of 40 or more [Ventilation Index = (mean airway pressure × Fio_2)/Pao_2 × 100] as indications for ECMO because more than 80 percent of infants with a ventilation index of 40 or more die with conventional therapy. Some centers also use a Pao_2 of less than 55 mm Hg for 3 hours, a pH of less than 7.4, and hypotension, or they use an acute deterioration of oxygenation with the Pao_2 less than 40 mm Hg and the pH less than 7.15 for 2 hours.[218] the myocardial function of patients who require ECMO is more often abnormal than that of patients treated successfully with standard therapy alone. Overall survival of ECMO-treated patients exceeds 80 percent[223] (see below).

Disease Processes

ECMO is usually initiated because the patient has pulmonary hypertension (PH), a common problem of neonates and a major cause of extrauterine death in term or near-term infants. PH is the cause of most deaths of patients with diaphragmatic hernias. Patients with PH usually have suprasystemic pulmonary artery pressures and right-to-left shunting of blood through the ductus arteriosus, the foramen ovale, or both. The resulting hypoxia and acidosis further increase pulmonary vasoconstriction and worsen pulmonary hypertension.

In normal infants, about half of the pulmonary arteries contain muscle and constrict in response to hypoxia and acidosis. In neonates with PH, small pulmonary arteries also contain muscle. Even though pulmonary vascular resistance is normal at birth, it can increase over a few days if the pericytes and intermediate cells (precursors of smooth muscle) are exposed to hypoxia, acidosis, elevated pulmonary arterial pressures, or increased blood flow, or if endothelial cells are injured.[224, 225] Both constriction of the vessels and platelet aggregation reduce the cross-sectional area of the vessels.[226] Most infants with PH are fall- or postterm, and many have normal lung function by pulmonary function testing. Many have experienced meconium aspiration (66 percent); others have diaphragmatic hernias, pneumonia, or sepsis. A small percentage of these patients have none of these predisposing factors.[227-230]

Because there is no single etiology for PH, no single form of therapy is universally effective. Antibiotics are given because approximately 20 percent of patients with PH have sepsis and/or pneumonia. The blood volume is normalized with blood and plasma, and metabolic acidosis is corrected with bicarbonate or tris(hydroxymethyl)aminomethane (THAM). Respiratory alkalosis is frequently induced, but the amount of mechanical ventilation required to induce alkalosis often causes a pneumothorax (45 percent) and/or chronic lung disease (31 percent).[218] Hyperventilation (pH > 7.5) decreases cerebral and renal blood flow.

Drug therapy for PH has had variable success because the nature of the disease is multifactorial. Muscle relaxants, narcotics, and sedatives are used to prevent "fighting the ventilator" and to reduce oxygen consumption.[231] Pulmonary vasodilators are helpful in about 50 percent of cases. Priscoline (Tolazoline), the most frequently used drug, is nonspecific in its actions,[232] frequently causes severe systemic hypotension, and increases right-to-left shunting of blood. Arachidonic acid metabolites are important regulators of the pulmonary vascular bed in normal patients and may be important in the initiation of nonhypoxic PH. However, prostaglandin (PG)E_1,[233] PGI_2,[234] and PGD_2[235] have not consistently reduced pulmonary arterial pressures in patients with PH.

An increase in the free calcium concentration of cytoplasm (>0.1 mmol/L) constricts vascular smooth muscle. However, calcium channel blockers seldom improve the survival of patients with PH, despite the fact that they bring about a decrease in pulmonary vascular resistance.

Patients who have failed medical management of PH are candidates for ECMO. Gas exchange improves and pulmonary vascular resistance decreases after several days of ECMO. Anesthesiologists are often asked to provide anesthesia for patients on ECMO, and therefore, should have a working knowledge of ECMO and its problems.

ECMO Circuit and Cannulation

The ECMO circuit in general use is shown in Figure 13–5. It consists of a venous reservoir, a silicone membrane oxygenator (Sci Med Life Systems, Inc., Minneapolis, MN), a heat exchanger, and polyvinyl chloride tubing, all of which are disposable. The roller pump, a bladder box

assembly with its return volume monitor, gas flow meters, and the water heater are nondisposable. Oxygen and CO_2 delivery systems are also required. Monitoring equipment includes a means of continuously measuring oxygen saturation of "venous" and "arterial" blood in the circuit and a device for measuring the activated clotting time.

The circuit is flushed with CO_2 and primed with albumin (to coat the membranes) and crystalloid. The primer is replaced with blood and the blood pH is normalized with bicarbonate or THAM. In most cases, *venoarterial* bypass is used. A large-bore catheter placed in the right internal jugular vein provides adequate blood return to the pump in most instances. Occasionally, it is necessary to insert more than one venous catheter to provide adequate venous return. A roller pump circulates blood through the oxygenator, where oxygen is added and CO_2 is removed. The blood then is warmed to 37°C in the heat exchanger and returned to the infant via a carotid artery cannula whose tip is in the ascending aorta. Thus, the coronary and carotid arteries are perfused with fully oxygenated blood. *Venovenous* bypass uses the femoral and jugular veins to accomplish ECMO. Although successful, it does not achieve the same degree of oxygenation as arteriovenous bypass and it requires normal myocardial function, which is often lacking in these patients. Another form of venovenous bypass utilizes a single jugular venous catheter and a push-pull system. This system offers promise for the future but still requires good myocardial function.

Management of ECMO

ECMO flow is started at approximately 50 ml/min and is increased to 60 to 80 percent of the patient's predicted cardiac output. In practice, this is 300 to 400 ml/min. PaO_2 is maintained above 60 mm Hg and venous oxygen saturation above 70 percent by a combination of pump flow and oxygen supplied to the oxygenator. $PaCO_2$ is maintained in the normal range by adding or subtracting CO_2 from the oxygenator. Once ECMO is established, the ventilator pressures are reduced to 20/5 cm H_2O and the FIO_2 of the ventilator is decreased to 0.21 to reduce lung injury. The reduction in ventilator pressures, plus the use of ECMO, results in severe atelectasis and small tidal volumes (<0.5 ml/kg). The lung reexpands in 3 to 4 days. If ECMO must be discontinued before reexpansion occurs, adequate oxygenation and ventilation may be difficult to achieve. High, sustained (2- to 3-second) inflation pressures, exogenous surfactant administration, and 5 to 10 cm H_2O PEEP are often required to reinflate the lungs. Once they have reexpanded, ventilation of the lungs can usually be accomplished with more normal pressures and inspiratory times.

Muscle relaxants are usually discontinued once ECMO is begun so that neurologic function can be evaluated. However, the patient should be sedated (usually with a continuous infusion of narcotics) to prevent the vascular catheters from being dislodged. If fentanyl is used, its dose often must be increased daily to maintain the same level of sedation,[236] and at times more than 25 μg/kg/h is required. Some physicians infuse morphine instead of fentanyl to decrease cost and to reduce drug tolerance, although

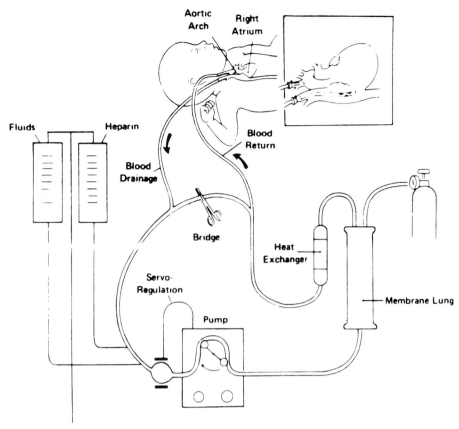

FIGURE 13–5. The circuit used to provide ECMO in neonates. (From Bartlett RH, Roloff DW, Cornell RG, et al: Extracorporeal circulation in neonatal respiratory failure: a prospective randomized study. Pediatrics 76:479, 1985, with permission.)

the latter is questionable. Patients sedated with high-dose fentanyl often require as much as 200 μg/kg of fentanyl to provide adequate anesthesia during surgery.

Clotting of the circuit interferes with oxygenator function and poses a danger to the patient. Consequently, all patients are heparinized while on ECMO and the activated clotting time (ACT) is kept between 190 and 260 seconds. The lower the ECMO flow rate, the higher the ACT must be. Obviously, prolonged ACTs are a problem for patients on ECMO who are undergoing surgery. The platelet counts of patients on ECMO usually decrease and platelet transfusions are required to maintain the platelet concentration above 100,000/mm^3. The fibrinogen concentration decreases during ECMO, and fresh frozen plasma and/or cryoprecipitate transfusions are required to keep it above 100 mg/dl. Administration of platelets, fresh frozen plasma, and cryoprecipitate often shortens the ACT and increases the likelihood of clot formation. Therefore, the ACTs must be measured shortly after these blood components are administered, and the heparin administration must be altered appropriately.

When flow of blood in the circuit has been reduced to 50 ml/min and oxygenation and ventilation are adequate, ECMO is discontinued. If mechanical ventilation with low pressures and normal ventilator rates maintains adequate gas exchange for 2 hours, the cannulas are removed. Usually the trachea can be extubated 2 to 3 days later. Heparinization is discontinued once the vessels are decannulated.

Complications of Treatment with ECMO

There are many potential technical problems associated with ECMO, including clot formation in the circuit, failure of the oxygenator or pump, hemorrhage from a ruptured raceway or tubing, or dislodged cannulae. Therefore, adequate personnel, including a nurse to care for the patient, a nurse or technician to run the ECMO machine, and a physician who is fully trained in the treatment of patients on ECMO must be immediately available.

Recent data from the National Registry of the Extracorporeal Life Support Organization[223] indicate that hemorrhage continues to be a problem. Of the almost 7,000 patients treated with ECMO throughout the world, hemorrhage occurred from the gastrointestinal system, cannula and surgical sites, and from hemolysis in 4 to 13 percent of patients. Central nervous system hemorrhage occurred in approximately 15 percent. Pulmonary hemorrhage was relatively uncommon. Survival after hemorrhage occurred in 50 to 85 percent of the patients, depending on the bleeding site. Fifteen percent of patients had seizures, but it is unclear if the seizures were related to the severe hypoxia present before ECMO or to ECMO itself. Brain death occurred in about 1 percent of patients. Approximately 10 percent had some element of renal failure (creatinine concentration >1.5). A small number of patients experienced cardiac problems during ECMO, including myocardial stun, cardiac arrhythmias, and patent ductus arteriosus. During ECMO, 10 percent of patients had significant hypertension, which is often exaggerated in patients undergoing surgery (see below). The incidence and severity of complications are similar in patients who require ECMO after cardiac surgery to those treated with ECMO for other reasons.

The neurologic outcome of patients treated with ECMO is generally good. However, in one nursery, 26 percent of patients treated with ECMO had nonhemorrhagic intracranial abnormalities on computed tomographic (CT) scan.[237] Half of these abnormalities were not visible with head ultrasound studies. Of the 42 patients treated with ECMO, 75 percent were normal neurologically and 19 percent exhibited increased tone and mild asymmetry of tone. Five percent showed developmental delay but were socially appropriate. No infant was profoundly impaired and there was no preponderance of right-sided functional asymmetry, a concern because the right carotid artery usually is ligated when the arterial cannula is removed. Nine infants were delayed in both mental and motor development. Significant delay (score <70) occurred in 10 percent of the patients. Factors related to poor outcome included sepsis on admission to the hospital, chronic lung disease, and an intracranial abnormality by ultrasound or CT scan. Intracranial hemorrhage occurred twice as often in the delayed group as in those who were not developmentally delayed. However, long-term follow-up of these infants may reveal significant improvement.

The overall survival of noncardiac, ECMO-treated infants is good.[223] This includes congenital diaphragmatic hernia (60 percent), meconium aspiration syndrome (93 percent), persistent fetal circulation (85 percent), pneumonia (77 percent), air leak (64 percent), and others (78 percent).[223] Overall survival for patients with congenital heart disease is less than 60 percent and is decreasing yearly as sicker and less salvageable patients are treated with ECMO. Survival of patients after cardiac surgery is 45 percent; after cardiac transplant, about 30 percent; and after myocarditis and myocardiopathy, is approximately 60 percent. It should be remembered that all of these patients had a greater than 80 percent risk of dying with conventional therapy.

Anesthesia and ECMO

The anesthesiologist is often asked to anesthetize infants who are undergoing or about to undergo treatment with ECMO. In most instances, surgery will take place in the neonatal intensive care unit (NICU) because the problems associated with transporting patients on ECMO are often life threatening. However, performing surgery in the NICU has its own set of problems. The NICU is not an operating room and most of its staff are not familiar with the operating room environment. Therefore, the entire operating room team (nurses and physicians) must go to the nursery with their equipment and must interact with the nurses and physicians in a foreign environment. The surgery area must be screened off from the rest of the NICU and someone must ensure that people not directly involved in the care of the patient do not wander in and out during sur-

gery. Everyone must be constantly vigilant to prevent contamination of the sterile field.

Preoperative Evaluation

Preoperatively, the anesthesiologist must speak with the physicians and nurses caring for the patient to determine how this patient has responded to ECMO. The anesthesiologist must clearly understand why ECMO is being discontinued. Is it because there is a problem (e.g., hemorrhage, pump failure)? If so, ventilation and oxygenation of the patient may be difficult. If ECMO is being discontinued because the patient no longer needs it, oxygenation and ventilation will be accomplished easily. The clotting status of the patient should be known, and adequate blood and fresh frozen plasma must be available in the ICU (in ice chests) to treat unexpected hemorrhage. Usually the patient's intravascular volume is adequate at the time ECMO is discontinued. However, ongoing third-space fluid loses, a marginal intravascular volume, or myocardial dysfunction can lead to severe hypotension when ECMO is withdrawn. The serum electrolytes are usually normal, with the exception of the serum bicarbonate concentration. The latter is often elevated and can be a problem if hyperventilation occurs and reduces the arterial blood pressure and cerebral blood flow.

Types of Surgery

All patients require surgery to place the ECMO catheters. In many centers this is accomplished with pancuronium and small doses of fentanyl because these patients are so hypoxic and acidotic that they usually cannot tolerate deep levels of anesthesia. When anesthesia is required, the anesthesiologist should be prepared to infuse volume and high concentrations of vasopressors if hypotension and decreased cardiac output occur. If dissection of the carotid artery induces arterial hypertension, intracranial hemorrhage may occur because of absent or decreased cerebral vascular autoregulation.[238] Occasionally, a pneumothorax is produced during the neck dissection and catheter placement and is heralded by a sudden deterioration in the patient's condition.[239] Blood loss is usually minimal unless one of the vessels is lacerated or there is difficulty inserting the catheters, especially the carotid artery catheter.

Congenital diaphragmatic hernias are frequently repaired during ECMO. Bleeding is a major problem, even though the ACT is shortened to approximately 180 to 190 seconds before surgery. Blood loss must be replaced immediately to maintain intravascular volume and to prevent the ECMO machine from shutting off in response to inadequate venous return. If this happens, pump flow is reduced, blood or plasma is added to the ECMO circuit, and the flow is returned to its former level. Pump flow rates are kept high during surgery because the ACT is short. ACTs should be determined frequently (every 15 to 30 minutes) during surgery and the rate of heparin infusion adjusted to maintain the desired ACT.

Intra-abdominal catastrophes occasionally occur during ECMO and require anesthesia and surgery. Bleeding is the major problem during surgery, and is the result of

TABLE 13 – 3
**ARTERIAL BLOOD PRESSURE
DURING NECK DISSECTION AND
MANIPULATION OF THE CAROTID ARTERY**

	Neck Dissection	Manipulation of Carotid Artery
Mean arterial pressure (mm Hg)	56 ± 6	79 ± 10

From Gregory GA: What every anesthesiologist needs to know about ECMO. Semin Anesth 3:147, 1993.

heparinization and diffuse intravascular coagulation (DIC). Care must be taken to replace third-space fluid losses, which may exceed 30 ml/kg/h.

When the patient no longer needs ECMO, the catheters are removed and, in some centers, the jugular vein and carotid artery are reconstructed. Because the patient is still heparinized, bleeding often occurs. Systemic hypertension is a major problem during reconstruction of the carotid artery, especially when the vessels are manipulated (Table 13–3). Systolic blood pressures of greater than 80 mm Hg should be treated, as Sell et al.[240] demonstrated an increased incidence of intracranial hemorrhage in hypertensive patients on ECMO. The hypertension is related to increased concentrations of angiotension and responds well to captopril.

During ECMO, anesthesia can be accomplished with either inhaled or IV agents, or both. Because inhaled anesthetics are more likely to cause hypotension, narcotics (usually fentanyl) are used. Large quantities of the drug (based on heart rate and arterial blood pressure) are often required (150 to 200 μg/kg) because tolerance to fentanyl has developed and because no other anesthetic agent is being administered. Administering small quantities of barbiturates reduces the need for narcotic (Table 13–4).

The postoperative course of these patients is often complicated by hemorrhage and third-space fluid losses. ECMO appears to increase rather than decrease the third-space fluid losses during and after abdominal surgery. Consequently, large volumes of crystalloid, blood, and plasma are often required to maintain intravascular volume and provide adequate venous return to the ECMO machine. Most patients can be weaned from mechanical ventilation a few days after ECMO is discontinued. However, patients who have undergone diaphragmatic hernia repair while on ECMO frequently require mechanical ventilation for weeks because of their hypoplastic lungs. In the past, such patients died. Now, with ECMO, they survive

TABLE 13 – 4
**EFFECT OF BARBITURATES ON
FENTANYL REQUIREMENT DURING ECMO
DECANNULATION AND CAROTID ARTERY REPAIR**

	Fentanyl	Fentanyl + Nembutal*
Dose (μg/kg)	186 ± 28	105 ± 31

* The dose of nembutal was 4 mg/kg.
From Gregory GA: What every anesthesiologist needs to know about ECMO. Semin Anesth 3:147, 1993.

but have inadequate alveolar surface area to sustain life without mechanical ventilation. Several weeks to months may be required for the lungs to grow sufficiently to support spontaneous ventilation.

CONCLUSION

ECMO has reduced the mortality of infants with severe hypoxia but has been associated with problems, some of which require surgery. Anesthesia can be accomplished with relative safety if we understand ECMO, its problems, and the solutions to these problems. Future developments in the treatment of patients with pulmonary hypertension will, we hope, reduce or eliminate the need for ECMO, but until then, ECMO is with us, and increasing numbers of patients will require our help.

REFERENCES

1. Schaller RT, Schaller J, Morgan A, Furman EB: Hemodilution anesthesia: a valuable aid to major cancer surgery in children. Am J Surg 146:79, 1983.
2. Olsfanger D, Jedeikin R, Metser U, et al: Acute normovolaemic haemodilution and idiopathic scoliosis surgery: effects on homologous blood requirements. Anaesth Intensive Care 21:429, 1993.
3. van Iterson M, van der Waart FJ: Systemic haemodynamics and oxygenation during haemodilution in children. Lancet 346:1127, 1995.
4. Fontana JL, Welborn L, Mongan PD, et al: Oxygen consumption and cardiovascular function in children during profound intraoperative normovolemic hemodilution. Anesth Analg 80:219, 1995.
5. Kreimeier U, Messmer K: Hemodilution in clinical surgery: state of the art 1996. World J Surg 20:1208, 1996.
6. Johnson LB, Plotkin JS, Kuo PC: Reduced transfusion requirements during major hepatic resection with use of intraoperative isovolemic hemodilution. Am J Surg 176:608, 1998.
7. Copley LA, Richards BS, Safavi FZ, Newton PO: Hemodilution as a method to reduce transfusion requirements in adolescent spine fusion surgery. Spine 24:219, 1999.
8. Karakaya D, Ustun E, Tur A, et al: Acute normovolemic hemodilution and nitroglycerin-induced hypotension: comparative effects on tissue oxygenation and allogeneic blood transfusion requirement in total hip arthroplasty. J Clin Anesth 11:368, 1999.
9. Goodnough LT, Monk TG, Despotis GJ, Merkel K: A randomized trial of acute normovolemic hemodilution compared to preoperative autologous blood donation in total knee arthroplasty. Vox Sang 77:11, 1999.
10. Spahn DR, Leone BJ, Reves JG, Pasch T: Cardiovascular and coronary physiology of acute isovolemic hemodilution: a review of nonoxygen-carrying and oxygen-carrying solutions. Anesth Analg 78:1000, 1994.
11. Robblee JA, Crosby E: Transfusion medicine issues in the practice of anesthesiology. Trans Med Rev 9:60, 1995.
12. Van Hemelen G, Avery CM, Venn PJ, et al: Management of Jehovah's Witness patients undergoing major head and neck surgery. Head Neck 21:80, 1999.
13. Messmer K: Hemodilution. Surg Clin North Am 55:659, 1975.
14. Schmied H, Schiferer A, Sessler DI, Meznik C: The effects of red-cell scavanging, hemodilution, and active warming on allogenic blood requirements in patients undergoing hip or knee arthroplasty. Anesth Analg 86:387, 1998.
15. Bryson GL, Laupacis A, Wells GA, International Study of Perioperative Transfusion: Does acute normovolemic hemodilution reduce perioperative allogeneic transfusion? A meta-analysis. Anesth Analg 86:9, 1998.
16. Zohar E, Fredman B, Ellis M, et al: A comparative study of the postoperative allogeneic blood-sparing effect of tranexamic acid versus acute normovolemic hemodilution after total knee replacement. Anesth Analg 89:1382, 1999.

17. Weinstein ES, Hampton WW, Yokum MD, Fry DE: Isovolemic hemodilution: correlations of mitochondrial and myocardial performance. J Trauma 26:620, 1986.
18. Bruder N, Cohen B, Pellisier D, Francois G: The effect of hemodilution on cerebral blood flow velocity in anesthetized patients. Anesth Analg 86:320, 1998.
19. Tomiyama Y, Jansen K, Brian JE Jr, Todd MM: Hemodilution, cerebral O2 delivery, and cerebral blood flow: a study using hyperbaric oxygenation. Am J Phys 276:H1190, 1999.
20. Tommasino C, Moore S, Todd MM: Cerebral effects of isovolemic hemodilution with crystalloid or colloid solutions. Crit Care Med 16:862, 1988.
21. Dong W, Bledsoe S, Chadwick H, et al: Electrical correlates of brain injury resulting from severe hypotension and hemodilution in monkeys. Anesthesiology 65:617, 1986.
22. Buckberg G, Brazier J: Coronary blood flow and cardiac function during hemodilution. Bibl Haematol 41:173, 1975.
23. Sunder-Plassmann L, Kessler M, Jesch F, et al: Acute normovolemic hemodilution. Bibl Haematol 41:44, 1975.
24. Michenfelder JD, Uihlein A, Daw EF, Theye RA: Moderate hypothermia in man: haemodynamic and metabolic effects. Br J Anaesth 37:738, 1965.
25. Prakash O, Johnson B, Bos E, et al: Cardiorespiratory and metabolic effects of profound hypothermia. Crit Care Med 6:340, 1978.
26. Crystal GJ, Salem MR: Myocardial and systemic hemodynamics during isovolemic hemodilution alone and combined with nitroprusside-induced controlled hypotension. Anesth Analg 72:227, 1991.
27. Plewes JL, Farhi LE: Cardiovascular responses to hemodilution and controlled hypotension in the dog. Anesthesiology 62:149, 1985.
28. Crystal GJ, Rooney MW, Salem MR: Regional hemodynamics and oxygen supply during isovolemic hemodilution alone and in combination with adenosine-induced controlled hypotension. Anesth Analg 67:211, 1988.
29. Shapira Y, Gurman G, Artru AA, et al: Combined hemodilution and hypotension monitored with jugular bulb oxygen saturation, EEG, and ECG decreases transfusion volume and length of stay for major orthopedic surgery. J Clin Anesth 9:643, 1997.
30. Brown RH, Schauble JF, Miller NR: Anemia and hypotension as contributors to perioperative loss of vision. Anesthesiology 80:222, 1994.
31. Williams EL, Hart WM Jr, Tempelhoff R: Postoperative ischemic optic neuropathy. Anesth Analg 80:1018, 1995.
32. Roth S, Nunez R, Schreider BD: Unexplained visual loss after lumbar spinal fusion. J Neurosurg Anesth 9:346, 1997.
33. Cooper JD, Maeda M, Lowenstein E: Lung water accumulation with acute hemodilution in dogs. J Thorac Cardiovasc Surg 69:957, 1975.
34. Laks H, Handin RI, Martin V, Pilon RN: The effects of acute normovolemic hemodilution on coagulation and blood utilization in major surgery. J Surg Res 20:225, 1976.
35. Schou H, Kongstad L, Perez V, et al: Uncompensated blood loss is not tolerated during acute normovolemic hemodilution in anesthetized pigs. Anesth Analg 87:786, 1998.
36. Schierout G, Roberts I: Fluid resuscitation with colloid or crystalloid solutions in critically ill patients: a systematic review of randomized trials. BMJ 316:961, 1998.
37. Choi PT, Yip G, Quinonez LG, Cook DJ: Crystalloids vs. colloids in fluid resuscitation: a systematic review. Crit Care Med 27:200, 1999.
38. Adzick NS, deLorimier AA, Harrison MR, et al: Major childhood tumour resection using normovolemic hemodilution anesthesia and hetastarch. J Pediatr Surg 20:372, 1985.
39. Aly Hassan A, Lochbuehler H, Frey L, et al: Global tissue oxygenation during normovolaemic haemodilution in young children. Paediatr Anaesth 7:197, 1997.
40. London MJ, Ho JS, Triedman JK, et al: A randomized clinical trial of 10% pentastarch (low molecular weight hydroxyethyl starch) versus 5% albumin for plasma volume expansion after cardiac operations. J Thorac Cardiovasc Surg 97:785, 1989.
41. Payen JF, Vuillez JP, Geoffray B, et al: Effects of preoperative intentional hemodilution on the extravasation rate of albumin and fluid. Crit Care Med 25:243, 1997.
42. Yacobi A, Stoll RG, Sum CY, et al: Pharmacokinetics of hydroxyethyl starch in normal subjects. J Clin Pharmacol 22:206, 1982.
43. Faulds D, Sorkin EM: Epoetin (recombinant human erythropoietin): a review of its pharmacodynamic and pharmacokinetic properties and therapeutic potential in anemia and the stimulation of erythropoiesis. Drugs 38:863, 1989.
44. Goodnough LT, Rudnick S, Price TH, et al: Increased preoperative collection of autologous blood with recombinant human erythropoietin therapy. N Engl J Med 321:1163, 1989.
45. Rothstein P, Roye D, Verdisco L, Stern L: Preoperative use of erythropoietin in an adolescent Jehovah's Witness. Anesthesiology 73:568, 1990.
46. Gross JB: Estimating allowable blood loss: correction for dilution. Anesthesiology 58:277, 1983.
47. Hannallah RS, Britton JT, Schafer PG, et al: Propofol anaesthesia in paediatric ambulatory patients: a comparison with thiopentone and halothane. Can J Anaesth 41:12, 1994.
48. Lerman J, Davis PJ, Welborn LG, et al: Induction, recovery and safety characteristics of sevoflurane in children undergoing ambulatory surgery: a comparison with halothane. Anesthesiology 84:1332, 1996.
49. Xue FS, Liu JH, Liao X, et al: The influence of acute normovolemic hemodilution on the dose-response and time course of action of vecuronium. Anesth Analg 86:861, 1998.
50. Xue FS, Liao X, Tong SY, et al: Influence of acute normovolaemic haemodilution on the relation between the dose and response of rocuronium bromide. Eur J Anaesth 15:21, 1998.
51. Taylor RH, Lerman J: Minimum alveolar concentration (MAC) of desflurane and hemodynamic responses in neonates, infants and children. Anesthesiology 75:975, 1991.
52. Cassady JF, Patel RI, Epstein BS: Calculations for predicting blood transfusion needs. Anesthesiology 59:491, 1983.
53. Payne K, Ireland P: Plasma glucose levels in the perioperative period in children. Anaesthesia 39:868, 1984.
54. Edwards MW, Flemming DC: Deliberate hypotension. Surg Clin North Am 55:947,1975.
55. Thompson GE, Miller RD, Stevens WC, Murray WR: Hypotensive anesthesia for total hip arthroplasty: a study of blood loss and organ function (brain, heart, liver and kidney). Anesthesiology 48:91, 1978.
56. Diaz JH, Lockhart CH: Hypotensive anesthesia for craniectomy in infancy. Br J Anaesth 51:233, 1979.
57. Precious DS, Splinter W, Bosco D: Induced hypotensive anesthesia for adolescent orthognathic surgery patients. J Oral Maxillofac Surg 54:680, 1996.
58. Fox HJ, Thomas CH, Thompson AG: Spinal instrumentation for Duchenne's muscular dystrophy: experience of hypotensive anaesthesia to minimise blood loss. J Pediatr Orthop 17:750, 1997.
59. Grundy BL, Nash CL, Brown RH: Deliberate hypotension for spinal fusion: prospective randomized study with evoked potential monitoring. Can Anaesth Soc J 29:452, 1982.
60. Malcolm-Smith NA, MacMaster MY: The use of induced hypotension to control bleeding during posterior fusion and Harrington-rod instrumentation. J Bone Joint Surg Br 65:255, 1983.
61. Viguera MG, Terry RN: Induced hypotension for extensive surgery in an infant. Anesthesiology 27:701, 1966.
62. Fairbairn ML, Eltringham RJ, Young PN, Robinson JM: Hypotensive anaesthesia for microsurgery of the middle ear: a comparison between isoflurane and halothane. Anaesthesia 41:637, 1986.
63. Szyfelbein SK, Ryan JF: Use of controlled hypotension for primary surgical excision in an extensively burned child. Anesthesiology 41:501, 1974.
64. Townes BD, Dikman SS, Bledsoe SW, et al: Neuropsychological changes in a young, healthy population after controlled hypotensive anesthesia. Anesth Analg 65:955, 1986.
65. Lindop MJ: Complications and morbidity of controlled hypotension. Br J Anaesth 47:799, 1975.
66. Brüssel T, Fitch W, Brodner G, et al: Effects of halothane in low concentrations on cerebral blood flow, cerebral metabolism, and cerebrovascular autoregulation in the baboon. Anesth Analg 73:758, 1991.
67. Strebel S, Lam AM, Matta B, et al: Dynamic and static cerebral autoregulation during isoflurane, desflurane and propofol anesthesia. Anesthesiology 83:66, 1995.
68. Van Aken H, Fitch W, Graham DI, et al: Cardiovascular and cerebrovascular effects of isoflurane-induced hypotension in the baboon. Anesth Analg 65:565, 1986.
69. Seyde WC, Longnecker DE: Cerebral oxygen tension in rats during deliberate hypotension with sodium nitroprusside, 2-chloroadenosine, or deep isoflurane anesthesia. Anesthesiology 64:480, 1986.

70. Artru AA: Cerebral metabolism and EEG during combination of hypocapnia and isoflurane-induced hypotension in dogs. Anesthesiology 65:602, 1986.

71. Newman B, Gelb AW, Lam AM: The effect of isoflurane-induced hypotension on cerebral blood flow and cerebral metabolic rate for oxygen in humans. Anesthesiology 64:307, 1986.

72. Hoffman WE, Edelman G, Kochs LS, et al: Cerebral autoregulation in awake versus isoflurane-anesthetized rats. Anesth Analg 73:753, 1991.

73. Ishikawa T, Funatsu N, Okamoto K, et al: Blood-brain barrier function following drug-induced hypotension in the dog. Anesthesiology 59:526, 1983.

74. Maekawa T, McDowall DG, Okuda Y: Brain-surface oxygen tension and cerebral cortical blood flow during hemorrhagic and drug-induced hypotension in the cat. Anesthesiology 51:513, 1979.

75. Michenfelder JD, Theye RA: Canine systemic and cerebral effects of hypotension induced by hemorrhage, trimethaphan, halothane or nitroprusside. Anesthesiology 46:188, 1977.

76. Magness A, Yashon D, Locke G, et al: Cerebral function during trimethaphan-induced hypotension. Neurology 23:506, 1973.

77. Ishikawa T, McDowall DG: Electrical activity of the cerebral cortex during induced hypotension with sodium nitroprusside and trimethaphan in the cat. Br J Anaesth 53:605, 1980.

78. Thomas WA, Cole PV, Etherington NJ, et al: Electrical activity of the cerebral cortex during induced hypotension in man: a comparison of sodium nitroprusside and trimethaphan. Br J Anaesth 57:134, 1985.

79. Sivarajan M, Amory DW, McKenzie SM: Regional blood flows during induced hypotension produced by nitroprusside or trimethaphan in the rhesus monkey. Anesth Analg 64:759, 1985.

80. Harp JR, Wollman H: Cerebral metabolic effects of hyperventilation and deliberate hypotension. Br J Anaesth 45:256, 1973.

81. Artru AA: Partial preservation of cerebral vascular responsiveness to hypocapnia during isoflurane-induced hypotension in dogs. Anesth Analg 65:660, 1986.

82. Artru AA, Colley PS: Cerebral blood flow response to hypocapnia during hypotension. Stroke 15:878, 1984.

83. Artru AA: Cerebral vascular responses to hypocapnia during nitroglycerin-induced hypotension. Neurosurgery 16:468, 1985.

84. Artru AA, Wright K, Colley PS: Cerebral effects of hypocapnia plus nitroglycerin-induced hypotension in dogs. J Neurosurg 64:924, 1986.

85. Artru AA: Cerebral metabolism and the electroencephalogram during hypocapnia plus hypotension induced by sodium nitroprusside or trimethaphan in dogs. Neurosurgery 18:36, 1986.

86. Drummond JC, Todd MM: The response of the feline cerebral circulation to Pa_{CO_2} during anesthesia with isoflurane and halothane, and during sedation with nitrous oxide. Anesthesiology 62:268, 1985.

87. Newberg LA, Milde JH, Michenfelder JD: Systemic and cerebral effects of isoflurane-induced hypotension in dogs. Anesthesiology 60:541, 1984.

88. Salem MR: Therapeutic uses of ganglionic blocking drugs. Int Anesthesiol Clin 16:171, 1978.

89. Rao TLK, Jacobs Salem MR, Santos P: Deliberate hypotension and anesthetic requirements of halothane. Anesth Analg 60:513, 1981.

90. Eckenhoff JE, Enderby GEH, Larson A, et al: Pulmonary gas exchange during deliberate hypotension. Br J Anaesth 35:750, 1963.

91. Casthely PA, Lear S, Cottrell JE, Lear E: Intrapulmonary shunting during induced hypotension. Anesth Analg 61:231, 1982.

92. Colley PS, Cheney FW: Sodium nitroprusside increases Qs/Qt in dogs with regional atelectasis. Anesthesiology 47:388, 1977.

93. Hales C, Slate J, Westphal D: Blockade of alveolar hypoxic pulmonary vasoconstriction by sodium nitroprusside and nitroglycerin [abstract]. Am Rev Respir Dis 115:335, 1978.

94. Carlsson AJ, Bindslev L, Hedenstierna G: Hypoxia-induced pulmonary vasoconstriction in the human lung: the effect of isoflurane anesthesia. Anesthesiology 66:312, 1987.

95. Badgwell JM, McLeod ME, Lerman J, Creighton RE: End-tidal P_{CO_2} measurements sampled at the distal and proximal end of the endotracheal tube in infants and children. Anesth Analg 66:959, 1987.

96. Friederich JA, Butterworth JF IV: Sodium nitroprusside: twenty years and counting. Anesth Analg 81:152, 1995.

97. Kuipers JRG, Sidi D, Heymann MA, Rudolph AM: Effects of nitroprusside on cardiac function, blood flow distribution, and oxygen consumption in the conscious young lamb. Pediatr Res 18:618, 1984.

98. Moncada S, Palmer RM, Higgs EA: Nitric oxide: physiology, pathophysiology, and pharmacology. Pharmacol Rev 43:109, 1991.

99. Davies DW, Kadar D, Steward DJ, Munro IR: A sudden death associated with the use of sodium nitroprusside for induction of hypotension during anaesthesia. Can Anaesth Soc J 22:547, 1975.

100. Ikeda S, Schweiss JF, Frank PA, Homan SM: In vitro cyanide release from sodium nitroprusside. Anesthesiology 66:381, 1987.

101. Ikeda S, Frank PA, Schweiss JF, Homan SM: In vitro cyanide release from sodium nitroprusside in various intravenous solutions. Anesth Analg 67:360, 1988.

102. Bennett NR, Abbott TR: The use of sodium nitroprusside in children. Anaesthesia 32:456, 1977.

103. Vesey CJ, Cole PV: Blood cyanide and thiocyanate concentrations produced by long-term therapy with sodium nitroprusside. Br J Anaesth 57:148, 1985.

104. Yaster M, Simmons RS, Tolo VT, et al: A comparison of nitroglycerin and nitroprusside for inducing hypotension in children: a double-blind study. Anesthesiology 65:175, 1986.

105. Bedford RF: Increasing halothane concentrations reduced nitroprusside dose requirement. Anesth Analg 57:457, 1978.

106. Edmondson R, Del Valle O, Shah N, et al: Esmolol potentiation of nitroprusside-induced hypotension: impact on the cardiovascular, adrenergic and renin-angiotensin systems in man. Anesth Analg 69:202, 1989.

107. Woodside J, Garner L, Bedford RF, et al: Captopril reduces the dose requirement for sodium nitroprusside-induced hypotension. Anesthesiology 60:413, 1984.

108. Nakazawa K, Taneyama C, Benson KT, et al: Mixtures of sodium nitroprusside and trimethaphan for induction of hypotension. Anesth Analg 73:59, 1991.

109. Wang HH, Liu LMP, Katz RL: A comparison of the cardiovascular effects of sodium nitroprusside and trimethaphan. Anesthesiology 46:40, 1977.

110. Todd MM, Morris PJ, Moss J, Philbin DM: Hemodynamic consequences of abrupt withdrawal of nitroprusside or nitroglycerin following induced hypotension. Anesth Analg 61:261, 1982.

111. Bloor BC, Fukunaga AF, Ma C: Myocardial hemodynamics during induced hypotension: a comparison between sodium nitroprusside and adenosine triphosphate. Anesthesiology 63:517, 1985.

112. Kien ND, White DA, Reitan JA, Eisele JH: Cardiovascular function during controlled hypotension induced by adenosine triphosphate or sodium nitroprusside in the anesthetized dog. Anesth Analg 66:103, 1987.

113. Turner JM, Powell G, Gibson RM, McDowall DG: Intracranial pressure changes in neurosurgical patients during hypotension induced with sodium nitroprusside or trimethaphan. Br J Anaesth 49:419, 1977.

114. Behnia R, Siqueira EB, Brunner EA: Sodium nitroprusside-induced hypotension: effect on renal function. Anesth Analg 57:521, 1978.

115. Leighton KM, Bruce C, MacLeod BA: Sodium nitroprusside-induced hypotension and renal blood flow. Can Anaesth Soc J 24:637, 1977.

116. Bagshaw RJ, Cox RH, Campbell KB: Sodium nitroprusside and regional arterial haemodynamics in the dog. Br J Anaesth 49:735, 1977.

117. Knight PR, Lane GA, Hensinger RN, et al: Catecholamine and renin-angiotensin response during hypotensive anesthesia induced by sodium nitroprusside or trimethaphan camsylate. Anesthesiology 59:248, 1983.

118. Zubrow AB, Daniel SS, Stark RI, et al: Plasma renin, catecholamine, and vasopressin during nitroprusside-induced hypotension in ewes. Anesthesiology 58:245, 1983.

119. Gelman S, Ernst EA: Hepatic circulation during sodium nitroprusside infusion in the dog. Anesthesiology 49:182, 1978.

120. Dietrich GV, Heesen M, Boldt J, Hempelmann G: Platelet function and adrenoreceptors during and after induced hypotension using nitroprusside. Anesthesiology 85:1334, 1996.

121. Perschau RA, Modell JH, Bright RW, Shirley PD: Suspected sodium nitroprusside-induced cyanide intoxication. Anesth Analg 56:533, 1977.

122. Tremblay NAG, Davies DW, Volgyesi G, et al: Sodium nitroprusside: factors which attenuate its action; studies with the isolated gracilis muscle of the dog. Can Anaesth Soc J 24:641, 1977.

123. Berlin CM: The treatment of cyanide poisoning in children. Pediatrics 46:793, 1970.

124. Vesey CJ, Krapez JR, Varley JG, Cole PV: The antidotal action of thiosulfate following acute nitroprusside infusion in dogs. Anesthesiology 62:415, 1985.

125. Ivankovich AD, Braverman B, Shulman M, Klowden AJ: Prevention of nitroprusside toxicity with thiosulfate in dogs. Anesth Analg 61:120, 1982.

126. Fahmy NR: Nitroglycerin as a hypotensive drug during general anesthesia. Anesthesiology 49:17, 1978.

127. Robertson RM, Robertson D: Drugs used for the treatment of myocardial ischemia. In Hardman JG, Limbird LE (eds): 9th ed. Goodman & Gilman's The Pharmacological Basis of Therapeutics. New York, McGraw-Hill, 1996, p 760.

128. Guggiari M, Dagreou F, Lienhart A, et al: Use of nitroglycerine to produce controlled decreases in mean arterial pressure to less than 50 mmHg. Br J Anaesth 57:142, 1985.

129. Rogers MC, Hamburger C, Owen K, Epstein MH: Intracranial pressure in the cat during nitroglycerin-induced hypotension. Anesthesiology 51:227, 1979.

130. Ryba M, Johansson K, Cybulska A: Brain metabolism in deep controlled hypotension in neurological patients. Eur Neurol 24:392, 1985.

131. Endrich B, Franke N, Peter K, et al: Induced hypotension: action of sodium nitroprusside and nitroglycerin on the microcirculation: a micropuncture investigation. Anesthesiology 66:605, 1987.

132. Kadam PP, Saksena SG, Jagtap SR, Pantavaidya SM: Hypotensive anaesthesia for spine surgery—nitroglycerin vs halothane. J Postgrad Med 39:26, 1998.

133. Klowden AJ, Ivankovich AD, Miletich DJ: Ganglionic blocking drugs—general considerations and metabolism. Int Anesthesiol Clin 16:113, 1978.

134. Harioka T, Hatano Y, Mori K, Toda N: Trimethaphan is a direct arterial vasodilator and an α-adrenoceptor antagonist. Anesth Analg 63:290, 1984.

135. Fahmy NR, Soter NA: Effects of trimethaphan on arterial blood histamine and systemic hemodynamics in humans. Anesthesiology 62:562, 1985.

136. Stoyka WW, Schutz H: The cerebral response to sodium nitroprusside and trimethaphan controlled hypotension. Can Anaesth Soc J 22:275, 1975.

137. Scott DB, Stephen GW, Marshall RL, et al: Circulatory effects of controlled arterial hypotension with trimethaphan during nitrous oxide halothane anaesthesia. Br J Anaesth 44:523, 1972.

138. Behnia R, Martin A, Koushanpour E, Brunner EA: Trimethaphan-induced hypotension: effect on renal function. Can Anaesth Soc J 29:581, 1982.

139. Anderson SM: Controlled hypotension with Arfonad in paediatric surgery. BMJ 2:103, 1955.

140. Fahmy NR, Laver MB: Hemodynamic response to ganglionic blockade with pentolinium during $N_{20}O$-halothane anesthesia in man. Anesthesiology 44:6, 1976.

141. Salem MR, Toyama T, Wong AY, et al: Haemodynamic responses to induced arterial hypotension in children. Br J Anaesth 50:489, 1978.

142. Kassel NF, Boarini DJ, Olin JJ, Sprowell JA: Cerebral and systemic circulatory effects of arterial hypotension induced by adenosine. J Neurosurg 58:69, 1983.

143. Boarini DJ, Kassell NF, Sprowell JA, et al: Cerebrovascular effects of hypocapnia during adenosine-induced arterial hypotension. J Neurosurg 63:937, 1985.

144. Owall A, Sollevi A, Rudehill A, Sylven C: Effect of adenosine-induced controlled hypotension on canine myocardial performance, blood flow and metabolism. Acta Anaesthesiol Scand 30:167, 1986.

145. Owall A, Gordon E, Lagerkranser M, et al: Clinical experience with adenosine for controlled hypotension during cerebral aneurysm surgery. Anesth Analg 66:229, 1987.

146. Owall A, Jarnberg P-O, Brodin L-A, Sollevi A: Effects of adenosine-induced hypotension on myocardial hemodynamics and metabolism in fentanyl anesthetized patients with peripheral vascular disease. Anesthesiology 68:416, 1988.

147. Lagerkranser M, Bergstrand G, Gordon E, et al: Cerebral blood flow and metabolism during adenosine-induced hypotension in patients undergoing cerebral aneurysm surgery. Acta Anaesth Scand 33:15, 1989.

148. Owall A, Sollevi A: Myocardial effects of adenosine- and sodium nitroprusside-induced hypotension: a comparative study in patients anaesthetized for abdominal aortic aneurym surgery. Acta Anaesth Scand 35:216, 1991.

149. Seitz PA, Riet M, Rush W, Merrell J: Adenosine decreases the minimum alveolar concentration of halothane in dogs. Anesthesiology 73:990, 1990.

150. Lee J, Lovell AT, Parry MG, et al: IV clonidine: does it work as a hypotensive agent with inhalation anaesthesia? Br J Anaesth 82:639, 1999.

151. Sanders GM, Sim KM: Is it feasible to use magnesium sulphate as a hypotensive agent in oral and maxillofacial surgery? Ann Acad Med Singapore 27:780, 1998.

152. Jakobsen C-J, Grabe N, Christensen B: Metoprolol decreases the amount of halothane required to induce hypotension during general anaesthesia. Br J Anaesth 58:261, 1986.

153. Goldberg ME, McNulty SE, Azad SS, et al: A comparison of labetolol and nitroprusside for inducing hypotension during major surgery. Anesth Analg 70:537, 1990.

154. Pilli G, Guzeldemir ME, Bayhan N: Esmolol for hypotensive anesthesia in middle ear surgery. Acta Anaesthesiol Belg 47:85, 1996.

155. Sum DC, Chung PC, Chen WC: Deliberate hypotensive anesthesia with labetalol in reconstructive surgery for scoliosis. Acta Anaesthesiol Sin 34:203, 1996.

156. Tobias JD, Hersey S, Mencio GA, et al: Nicardipine for controlled hypotension during spinal surgery. J Pediatr Orthop 16:370, 1996.

157. Valtonen M, Kuttila K, Kanto J, et al: Hypotensive anaesthesia for middle ear surgery: a comparison of propofol infusion and isoflurane. Exp Clin Pharmacol 14:383, 1992.

158. Bosnjak ZJ, Seagard JL, Wu A, Kampine JP: The effects of halothane on sympathetic ganglionic transmission. Anesthesiology 57:473, 1982.

159. Jordan D, Shulman SM, Miller ED Jr: Esmolol hydrochloride, sodium nitroprusside, and isoflurane differ in their ability to alter peripheral sympathetic responses. Anesth Analg 77:281, 1993.

160. Wolf WJ, Neal MB, Peterson MD: The hemodynamic and cardiovascular effects of isoflurane and halothane anesthesia in children. Anesthesiology 64:328, 1986.

161. Goa KL, Spencer CM: Sevoflurane in paediatric anaesthesia: a review. Paediatr Drugs 1:134, 1999.

162. Gourdeau M, Martin R, Lamarche Y, Tetreault L: Oscillometry and direct blood pressure: a comparative clinical study during deliberate hypotension. Can Anaesth Soc J 33:300, 1986.

163. Abou-Madi M, Lenis S, Archer D, et al: Comparison of direct blood pressure measurements at the radial and dorsalis pedis arteries during sodium nitroprusside- and isoflurane-induced hypotension. Anesthesiology 65:692, 1980.

164. Meretoja OA, Taivainen T, Erkola O, et al: Dose-response and time-course of effect of rocuronium bromide in paediatric patients. Eur J Anaesth 11(Suppl 11):19, 1995.

165. Plewes JL, Farhi LE: Cardiovascular responses to hemodilution and controlled hypotension in the dog. Anesthesiology 62:149, 1985.

166. Salem MR, Kim Y, Shaker MH: The effect of alteration of inspired oxygen concentration of jugular-bulb oxygen tension during deliberate hypotension. Anesthesiology 33:358, 1970.

167. Ward CF, Arkin DB, Benumof JL: The use of profound hypothermia and circulatory arrest for hepatic lobectomy in infancy. Anesthesiology 47:473, 1977.

168. Bailey LL, Takeuchi Y, Williams WG, et al: Surgical management of congenital cardiovascular anomalies with the use of profound hypothermia and circulatory arrest: analysis of 180 consecutive cases. J Thorac Cardiovasc Surg 71:485, 1976.

169. Ein SH, Shandling B, Williams WG, Trusler G: Major hepatic tumor resection using profound hypothermia and circulation arrest. J Pediatr Surg 16:339, 1981.

170. Milligan NS, Edwards JC, Monro JL, Atwell JD: Excision of giant haemangioma in the newborn using hypothermia and cardiopulmonary bypass. Anaesthesia 40:875, 1985.

171. Little KET, Cywes S, Davies MRQ, Louw JH: Complicated giant hemangioma: excision using cardiopulmonary bypass and deep hypothermia. J Pediatr Surg 11:533, 1976.

172. Okamura H: Inhalation anesthesia for simple deep hypothermia induced by surface cooling. Med J Osaka Univ 20:29, 1969.

173. Sidi D, Kuipers G Jr, Heymann MA, Rudolph AM: Effects of ambient temperature on oxygen consumption and the circulation in newborn lambs at rest and during hypoxemia. Pediatr Res 17:254, 1983.

174. Gunn TR, Johnston BM, Iwamoto HS, et al: Haemodynamic and catecholamine responses to hypothermia in the fetal sheep in utero. J Dev Physiol 7:241, 1985.

175. Osborn JJ: Experimental hypothermia: respiratory and blood pH changes in relation to cardiac function. Am J Physiol 175:389, 1953.

176. Vitez TS, White PF, Eger EI II: Effects of hypothermia on halothane MAC and isoflurane MAC in the rat. Anesthesiology 41:80, 1974.

177. Antagonini JF, Lewis BK, Reitan JA: Hypothermia minimally decreases nitrous oxide anesthetic requirements. Anesth Analg 79:980, 1994.

178. Sessler DI: Temperature monitoring. *In* Miller RM (ed): Anesthesia 4th ed. New York, Churchill Livingstone, 1994, p 1363.

179. Benumof JL, Wahrenbrock EA: Dependency of hypoxic pulmonary vasoconstriction on temperature. J Appl Physiol 42:56, 1977.

180. Heier T, Caldwell JE, Sessler DI, Miller RD: Mild intraoperative hypothermia increases duration of action and spontaneous recovery of vecuronium blockade during nitrous oxide-isoflurane anesthesia in humans. Anesthesiology 74:815, 1993.

181. Heier T, Caldwell JE, Sharma ML, et al: Mild intraoperative hypothermia does not change the pharmacodynamics (concentration-effect relationship) of vecuronium in humans. Anesth Analg 78:973, 1994.

182. Marty AT, Eraklis AJ, Pelletier GA, Merrill EW: The rheologic effects of hypothermia on blood with high hematocrit values. J Thorac Cardiovasc Surg 61:735, 1971.

183. Auhdi N, Carey JM, Greer AE: Hemodilution and coagulation factors in extracorporeal circulation. J Thorac Cardiovasc Surg 43:816, 1962.

184. Carrel TP, Schwanda M, Vogt PR, Turina MI: Aprotinin in pediatric cardiac operations: a benefit in complex malformations and with high-dose regimen only. Ann Thorac Surg 66:153, 1998.

185. Delin NA, Kjartansson KB, Pollock L, Schenk WG: Redistribution of regional blood flow in hypothermia. J Thorac Cardiovasc Surg 49:511, 1965.

186. Anzai T, Turner MD, Gibson WH, Neely WA: Blood flow distribution in dogs during hypothermia and posthypothermia. Am J Physiol 234:H706, 1978.

187. Prough DS, Stump DA, Troost BT: $PaCO_2$ management during cardiopulmonary bypass: intriguing physiologic rationale, convincing clinical data, evolving hypothesis? [Editorial]. Anesthesiology 72:3, 1990.

188. Murkin JM, Farrar JK, Tweed WA, et al: Cerebral autoregulation and flow/metabolism coupling during cardiopulmonary bypass: the influence of $Paco_2$. Anesthesiology 66:825, 1987.

189. Bashein G, Townes BD, Nessly ML, et al: A randomized study of carbon dioxide management during hypothermic cardiopulmonary bypass. Anesthesiology 72:7, 1990.

190. Svadjian E, Goldiner PL, Limjoco R: Ectothermic inheritance suggests abandoning temperature correction of pH and Pco_2 during hypothermic cardiopulmonary bypass [abstract]. Anesthesiology 65:A527, 1986.

191. Connolly JE, Boyd RJ, Calvin JW: The protective effect of hypothermia in cerebral ischemia: experimental and clinical application by selective brain cooling in the human. Surgery 52:15, 1962.

192. O'Connor JV, Wilding T, Farmer P, et al: The protective effect of profound hypothermia on the canine central nervous system during one hour of circulatory arrest. Ann Thorac Surg 41:255, 1986.

193. Cohen ME, Olszowka JS, Subramanian S: Electroencephalographic and neurological correlates of deep hypothermia and circulatory arrest in infants. Ann Thorac Surg 23:238, 1977.

194. Weiss M, Weiss J, Cotton J, et al: A study of the electroencephalogram during surgery with deep hypothermia and circulatory arrest in infants. J Thorac Cardiovasc Surg 70:316, 1975.

195. Clarkson PM, MacArthur BA, Barratt-Boyes BG, et al: Developmental progress after cardiac surgery in infancy using hypothermia and circulatory arrest. Circulation 62:855, 1980.

196. Blackwood MJA, Haka-Ikse K, Steward DJ: Developmental outcome in children undergoing surgery with profound hypothermia. Anesthesiology 65:437, 1986.

197. Brunberg JA, Reilly EL, Doty DB: Central nervous system consequences in infants of cardiac surgery using deep hypothermia and circulatory arrest. Circulation 50(Suppl II):II-60, 1974.

198. Levy WJ: Quantitative analysis of EEG changes during hypothermia. Anesthesiology 60:291, 1984.

199. Russ W, Kling D, Sauerwein G, Hempelmann G: Spectral analysis of the EEG during hypothermia cardiopulmonary bypass. Acta Anaesthesiol Scand 31:111, 1987.

200. Coles JG, Taylor MJ, Pearce JM, et al: Cerebral monitoring of somatosensory evoked potentials during profoundly hypothermic circulatory arrest. Circulation 70(Suppl I):1, 1984.

201. Burrows FA, Hillier SC, McLeod ME, et al: Anterior fontanel pressure and visual evoked potentials in neonates and infants undergoing profound hypothermic circulatory arrest. Anesthesiology 73:632, 1990.

202. Gordon AS, Jones SC, Luddington LG, et al: Deep hypothermia for intracardiac surgery: experimental and clinical use without an oxygenator. Am J Surg 100:332, 1960.

203. Kurth CD, Steven JM, Nicolson SC, et al: Kinetics of cerebral deoxygenation during deep hypothermic circulatory arrest in neonates. Anesthesiology 77:656, 1992.

204. Barratt-Boyes BG, Neutze JM, Clarkson PM, et al: Repair of ventricular septal defect in the first two years of life using profound hypothermia-circulatory arrest techniques. Ann Surg 184:376, 1976.

205. Wells FC, Coghill S, Caplan HL, Lincoln C: Duration of circulatory arrest does influence the psychological development of children after cardiac operation in early life. J Thorac Cardiovasc Surg 86:823, 1983.

206. Molina JE, Einzig S, Mastri AR, et al: Brain damage in profound hypotension. J Thorac Cardiovasc Surg 87:596, 1984.

207. Webb P: Afterdrop of body temperature during rewarming: an alternative explanation. J Appl Physiol 60:385, 1986.

208. Forman DL, Bhutani VK, Tran N, Shaffer TH: A new approach to induced hypothermia. J Surg Res 40:36, 1986.

209. Clowes GHA Jr, Hopkin AL, Neville WE: An artificial lung dependent upon diffusion of oxygen and carbon dioxide through plastic membranes. J Thorac Surg 32:630, 1956.

210. Kolobow T, Bowman RL: Construction and evaluation of an alveolar membrane artificial heart lung. Trans Am Soc Artif Intern Organs 9:238, 1963.

211. Pierce EC II: Modification of the Clowes membrane lung. J Thorac Cardiovasc Surg 39:438, 1960.

212. Lande AJ, Dos SJ, Carlson RG, et al: A new membrane oxygenator-dialyzer. Surg Clin North Am 47:1461, 1967.

213. Zapol WM, Snider MT, Hill DJ, et al: Extracorporeal membrane oxygenation in severe acute respiratory failure, a randomized prospective study. JAMA 242:2193, 1979.

214. Gille JP, Bagniewski AM: Ten years of extracorporeal membrane oxygenation (ECMO) in the treatment of acute respiratory insufficiency (ARI). Trans Am Soc Artif Intern Organs 22:102, 1976.

215. Bartlett RH, Gazzaniga AB, Huxtable RF, et al: Extracorporeal circulation (ECMO) in neonatal respiratory failure. J Thorac Cardiovasc Surg 74:826, 1977.

216. Bartlett RH, Andrews AF, Toomasian JM, et al: Extracorporeal membrane oxygenation for newborn respiratory failure: forty-five cases. Surgery 92:425, 1982.

217. Bartlett RH, Toomasian JM, Roloff DW, et al: Extracorporeal membrane oxygenation (ECMO) in neonatal respiratory failure: 100 cases. Ann Surg 204:236, 1986.

218. Bartlett RH, Roloff DW, Cornell RG, et al: Extracorporeal circulation in neonatal respiratory failure: a prospective randomized study. Pediatrics 76:479, 1985.

219. Volpe JJ: Intraventricular hemorrhage and brain injury in the premature infant. Neuropathology, pathogenesis, diagnosis, prognosis and prevention. Clin Perinatol 6:361, 1989.

220. Kirkpatrick BV, Krummel TM, Mueller DG, et al: Use of extracorporeal oxygenation for respiratory failure in term infant. Pediatrics 72:872, 1983.

221. Beck R, Anderson KD, Pearson GD, et al: Criteria for extracorporeal membrane oxygenation in a population of infants with persistent pulmonary hypertension of the newborn. J Pediatr Surg 2:297, 1986.

222. Short BL, Miller JK, Anderson KD: Extracorporeal membrane oxygenation in the management of respiratory failure in the newborn. Clin Perinatol 14:737, 1987.

223. Extracorporeal Life Support Organization National Registry: Data summary. Ann Arbor, MI, September 1992.

224. Haworth SG, Reid L: Persistent fetal circulation: newly recognized structural features. J Pediatr 88:614, 1976.

225. Rudolph AM: Fetal and neonatal pulmonary circulation. Annu Rev Physiol 41:383, 1979.

226. Levin D, Weinberg A, Perkin R: Pulmonary microthrombi syndrome in newborn infants with unresponsive persistent pulmonary hypertension. J Pediatr 102:299, 1983.

227. Fox WW, Duara S: Persistent pulmonary hypertension of the neonate: diagnosis and clinical management. J Pediatr 103:505, 1983.

228. Krummel TM, Greenfield LJ, Kirkpatrick BV, et al: Alveolar-arterial oxygen gradients versus the neonatal pulmonary insufficiency index

for prediction of mortality in ECMO candidates. J Pediatr Surg 19:380, 1984.

229. Davis JM, Spitzer AR, Cox C, Fox WW: Predicting survival in infants with persistent pulmonary hypertension of the newborn. Pediatr Pulmonol 5:609, 1988.

230. Anonymous: Persistent fetal circulation and extracorporeal membrane oxygenation. Lancet 2:1289, 1988.

231. Palmisano BW, Fisher DM, Willis M, et al: The effect of paralysis on oxygen consumption on normoxic children after cardiac surgery. Anesthesiology 61:518, 1984.

232. Weiner N: Drugs that inhibit adrenergic nerves and block adrenergic receptors. In Gilman AG, Goodman LS, Gilman A (eds): The Pharmacological Basis of Therapies. New York, Macmillan, 1980, p 183.

233. Philips JB III: Prostaglandin and related compounds in the perinatal pulmonary circulation. Pediatr Pharmacol 4:129, 1983.

234. Kaapa P, Koivisto M, Ylikorkala O, Kouvalainen K: Prostacyclin in the treatment of neonatal pulmonary hypertension. J Pediatr 107:951, 1985.

235. Phillips JB III, Lyrene RK, McDevitt M, et al: Prostaglandin D_2 inhibits hypoxic pulmonary vasoconstriction in neonatal lambs. J Appl Physiol 54:1585, 1983.

236. Arnold JH, Truog RD, Orav EJ, et al: Tolerance and dependence in neonates sedated with fentanyl during extracorporeal membrane oxygenation. Anesthesiology 73:1136, 1990.

237. Griffin MP, Minifee PK, Landry SH, et al: Neurodevelopmental outcome in neonates after extracorporeal membrane oxygenation: cranial magnetic resonance imaging and ultrasonography correlation. J Pediatr Surg 27:33, 1992.

238. Lou HC, Lassen NA, Fuiis-Hansen B: Impaired autoregulation of cerebral blood flow in the distressed newborn infant. Pediatrics 94:1188, 1979.

239. Ogata ES, Gregory GA, Kitterman JA, et al: Pneumothorax in respiratory distress syndrome: incidence and effects on vital signs, blood gases and pH. Pediatrics 58:177, 1976.

240. Sell EJ, Gaines JA, Guckman C, et al: Persistent fetal circulation. Neurodevelopmental outcome. Am J Dis Child 139:25, 1985.

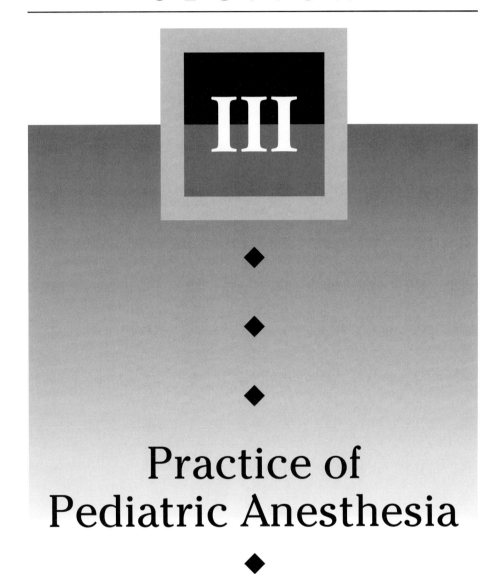

SECTION

III

Practice of
Pediatric Anesthesia

Anesthesia for Premature Infants

GEORGE A. GREGORY

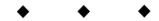

Six percent of infants are born prematurely. The more immature they are, the more likely they are to die during the neonatal period and the more likely they are to require surgery. Great strides have been made in reducing this mortality rate, even in very small infants (Fig. 14–1). However, with this increased survival has come a host of complications, many of which are partly or wholly iatrogenic (e.g., patent ductus arteriosus, retinopathy of prematurity [ROP], necrotizing enterocolitis).

Infants are considered premature if they are born before 37 weeks' gestation or if they are born within 259 days of the mother's last menstrual period. In the past, infants weighing less than 2,500 g at birth were considered premature. However, some term infants weigh less than 2,500 g depending on their race, maternal diet, and fetal infections. The incidence of morbidity or mortality does not necessarily increase just below this age. However, the smaller the neonate, the more likely it is that serious problems will occur. During the last 3 months' gestation, most body organs undergo continuous structural and functional development. When infants are born prematurely, their inadequately developed organs are called on to function fully, which they frequently cannot do. As a result, preterm infants are less able to maintain their body temperature, suck, swallow, eat, and sustain ventilation. Many experience asphyxia at or just before birth, which predisposes them to central nervous system injury, intraventricular

hemorrhage, necrotizing enterocolitis, and the respiratory distress syndrome (RDS).

LEVEL OF PREMATURITY

Preterm infants can be divided into three groups: borderline premature (36 to 37 weeks' gestation); moderately premature (31 to 36 weeks' gestation); and severely premature (24 to 30 weeks' gestation).

Borderline Prematurity

Sixteen percent of all live births fall into the category of borderline prematurity, with the newborns weighting 2.5 to 3.2 kg at birth. As a result, they are usually cared for in the normal neonatal nursery. However, they should be observed closely for the first 12 hours of life, because they have more difficulty maintaining their body temperature without external heat and they may not suck well. They also may require gavage feedings for a few days and may be slower to regain their birth weight, especially if they have respiratory distress.

Eight percent of borderline premature infants who are delivered by cesarean section have RDS; 1 percent of those born vaginally have this problem.[1] Infants born per vagina more effectively remove water from their lungs.[2, 3]

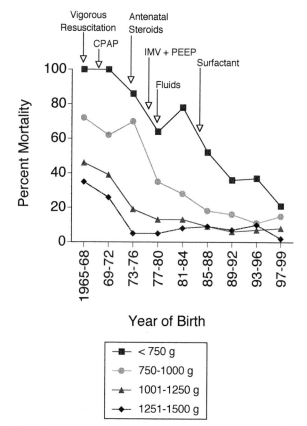

FIGURE 14–1. Mortality by birth weight at the University of California, San Francisco, from 1965 to 1999.

Because of their predisposition to respiratory distress, the respiratory system of near-term infants should be carefully evaluated during the preoperative visit. Intercostal retractions, tachypnea, and cyanosis suggest RDS but also may be signs of meconium aspiration, pneumothorax, or pneumonia in these large preterm infants. Temperature instability and hyperbilirubinemia suggest sepsis but are usually only manifestations of prematurity.

Preterm infants can be differentiated from term infants by the absence of creases on the posterior two thirds of the soles of their feet (38-weeks-gestation infants have some creases on their arches). The 40-week-gestation infant (term) has creases over the entire foot. Preterm infants also have absent or small breast buds, fuzzy hair on their heads, lanugo, and less-developed genitalia.

Moderate Prematurity

Moderately premature infants (31 to 36 weeks' gestation) account for 6 to 7 percent of all births. Approximately half of these infants weigh less than 2.5 kg at birth. Those at the lower end of this group weigh as little as 1.5 kg. The neonatal mortality of those born at 31 weeks' gestation is less than 5 percent, whereas it is nearly zero at 36 weeks. The major causes of death are intracranial hemorrhage, sepsis, and RDS.

Extremely Premature Infants

Infants of 24 to 30 weeks' gestation (400 to 1,500 g) make up approximately 1 percent of all live-born infants. How-

ever, these infants account for more than 70 percent of neonatal mortality. They also account for a major portion of infants who have neurologic damage later in life. The causes of death include birth asphyxia, acidosis, and respiratory failure (congestive heart failure, patent ductus arteriosus, RDS, infections [especially β-Streptococcus and Listeria]), necrotizing enterocolitis (NEC), and intracranial hemorrhage.

As pointed out by Usher,[4] "the major therapeutic challenge in managing these very immature infants is not so much the specific treatment of disease entities as it is the control of the many pathophysiologic derangements resulting from marked immaturity itself." All of the problems of prematurity are exaggerated in very immature infants. It is just as important, or maybe more important, to prevent iatrogenic complication.

ASPHYXIA

Asphyxia is common in preterm fetuses and is often the cause of prematurity. Preterm infants are more prone to asphyxia because their hemoglobin concentration and, therefore, their oxygen-carrying capacity is reduced. Slight degrees of stress lead to anaerobic metabolism and metabolic acidosis, which in turn reduce cardiac output and increase cerebral blood flow. The latter may damage the central nervous system (CNS).[5,6] Neonatal asphyxia occurs in 1 out of 20 moderately premature infants, 1 out of 200 term infants, and 1 out of 2 infants weighing less than 1 kg at birth. The causes of asphyxia include antepartum hemorrhage, intrauterine infections, breech delivery, and RDS. The treatment of birth asphyxia has been described elsewhere.[7]

Most premature infants are asphyxiated at birth and require tracheal intubation and assisted ventilation as part of resuscitation. They frequently have both metabolic and respiratory acidosis, which should be quickly corrected by hyperventilation, blood volume expansion and, if necessary, a slow, cautious infusion of enough sodium bicarbonate or tris(hydroxymethyl)aminomethane (THAM) to correct the pH to 7.3. Sodium bicarbonate should *never* be infused more rapidly than 1 mEq/kg/min because it may cause intracranial hemorrhage by rapidly expanding the intravascular volume and increasing the $Paco_2$. It also may reduce cerebral blood flow to dangerous levels.[8] Fifty milliliters of sodium bicarbonate produces 1,250 cc of CO_2 when fully reacted with hydrogen ions. Therefore, artificial ventilation should be continued until it is clear than the patient can sustain his or her ventilation and maintain a relatively normal $Paco_2$.

In the past, hypoglycemia was partly responsible for the high incidence of CNS damage in small preterm infants.[9] To prevent such damage, these infants should receive enough glucose to maintain their blood glucose concentrations between 45 and 90 mg/dl as indicated by a glucometer. They should not be made hyperglycemic, however, because it might worsen CNS damage if they were to have a cardiac arrest.[10–12]

BACKGROUND INFORMATION

The following are some of the basic problems associated with prematurity. They may be covered more fully in other chapters, but they are presented here to give an overview of the problems and to provide a basis for organizing one's thoughts when it becomes necessary to anesthetize a preterm infant.

Temperature Regulation

Exposure to cold or hypothermia greatly increases the metabolic rate and oxygen consumption of preterm infants (see Chapter 4) and causes hypoxemia, acidosis, apnea, or respiratory distress. Hypothermia is a risk factor for infant mortality.[13] The minimal oxygen consumption of preterm infants is 4.3 to 5.4 ml/kg/min on day 1 and increases to 8 or 9 ml/kg/min by 2 weeks of age.[14] As the oxygen consumption increases, so do the ventilatory and caloric requirements. Body heat is dissipated by conduction, convection, radiation, and evaporation. In the steady state, heat production equals heat loss. The surface/volume ratio of preterm infants is high. Their flaccid, open posture tends to increase heat loss rather than conserve it, whereas the flexed, curled-up position of the older infant tends to conserve heat. The lack of insulating fat reduces the surface-air insulation and the absolute amount of tissue through which heat must be transferred. In this situation, heat is transferred more readily from the core to the surface. Infants maintain temperature regulation during sleep.[15]

Day[16] and others[17] observed that preterm infants exposed to heat stress experience dilation of the peripheral vessels if their rectal temperature is 36.6° to 37.3°C. Hey and Koty[18] noted that term infants sweat when their rectal temperature exceeds 37.2°C. Those born more than 3 weeks before term do not. Sweating appears to be related to gestational age rather than body size; babies who are small for gestational age sweat appropriately. Evaporative heat loss accounts for approximately 25 percent of the heat lost in term neonates and adults.

Bruck[9] showed that preterm neonates experience vasoconstriction when they are exposed to cold, but they still lose heat because their insulation is decreased. He also demonstrated that preterm neonates can increase heat production when exposed to a cold environment, but the increase is less than that of term neonates. The rise in metabolic rate in preterm neonates is approximately linear between 28° and 36°C (Fig. 14–2).[14]

Young infants are agitated and increase their muscle movement in response to cold. Increased serum norepinephrine concentrations stimulate brown fat metabolism and increase heat production, which warms the CNS and vital organs.[20] Primitive brown fat cells begin to differentiate from reticular cells at 26 to 30 weeks' gestation[21] and increase in size and number for 3 to 6 weeks after birth. Infants born before these cells develop are less able to maintain their body temperature when exposed to cold environments. Hypoglycemic infants and those with CNS damage also have difficulty maintaining their body temperature, probably on a central basis.

Small premature infants lose heat and water through their thin, transparent skin and therefore easily become dehydrated, especially when they are cared for under radiant warmers and their fluid intake is restricted. The magnitude of the water loss is inversely related to body size and directly related to the radiant power density required to maintain body temperature.[22] Covering the premature infant's body with plastic wrap (SaranWrap) and his or her head with a cap significantly reduces both heat and water loss. In addition, the inspired gases should be warmed and fully humidified at 34° to 37°C.

The clinical consequences of chilling are described in Chapter 4. In brief, they are periodic breathing or apnea, bradycardia, metabolic acidosis, hyperglycemia, and aspiration of gastric contents. The survival of infants nursed in less than neutral thermal environments is decreased. Those who survive gain weight more slowly. Tympanic

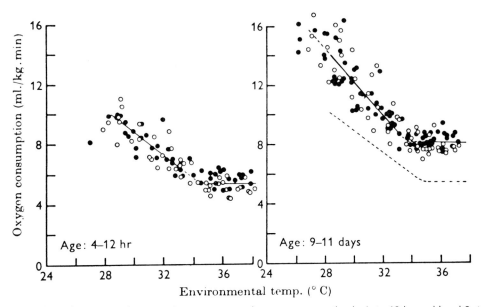

FIGURE 14–2. Relation between environmental temperature and oxygen consumption in 4- to 12-hour-old and 9- to 11-day-old babies weighing 2.0 and 2.5 kg at birth. (From Hey EN: The relation between environmental temperature and oxygen consumption in the newborn baby. J Physiol [Lond] 200:589, 1965, with permission.)

membrane temperature increases after 38 weeks' gestation.[23]

Maternal anesthesia may cause hypothermia in infants[24] as does fentanyl anesthesia after birth.[25] Patients receiving morphine or conduction anesthesia maintained normal body temperatures.

Respiratory Manifestations

Respiratory Distress

Respiratory distress is common in preterm infants. It occurs three times more often in infants born by cesarean section than in infants born vaginally. The less mature the infant, the more severe the diseases tends to be, although some very immature infants escape this affliction. Moderately premature babies with respiratory distress require more ventilatory support and have a lower survival rate than larger preterm infants. However, survival of the former group should still exceed 95 percent. The survival of very small preterm infants depends on their size. Eighty-five percent of those weighing less than 1,000 g survive, whereas about 80 percent of those weighing less than 750 g survive (Fig. 14–1). Recently, an increase in survival and a decrease in serious complications have been associated with administration of surfactant into the lungs at birth.[26, 27] This may improve their lung function to near normal. Consequently, failure to decrease ventilation pressures and tidal volumes as the compliance of the lung improves will increase the likelihood of pulmonary gas leaks and lung injury. It also is easy to hyperoxygenate these patients, increasing the likelihood of their developing ROP (see below).

Bronchopulmonary Dysplasia

Many preterm infants develop chronic lung disease (bronchopulmonary dysplasia [BPD]) as a result of mechanical ventilation, oxygen, infection, or a combination of these factors. The number of such patients is increasing because of the marked increase in survival of 500- to 750-g infants. BPD usually progresses through four stages (Table 14–1).

The end result is maldistribution of ventilation and perfusion, hypercarbia, hypoxemia, and occasionally prolonged mechanical ventilation. Positive end-expiratory pressure (PEEP) and large doses of furosemide (Lasix) 5 to 10 mg/kg every 6 hours are often required to decrease pulmonary edema and improve gas exchange. Furosemide therapy induces metabolic alkalosis unless adequate amounts of potassium and chloride are administered along with the drug. The alkalosis is compensated for by retention of CO_2. Care must be taken not to hyperventilate patients with compensated metabolic alkalosis because they may develop hypotension from severe alkalosis (Fig. 14–3). During surgery, some of these patients require increased ventilator pressures and oxygen concentrations, but in some of them ventilation is improved and oxygen requirements are decreased. In fact, some patients must be ventilated with room air during surgery to keep their oxygen saturation between 87 and 92 percent and their PaO_2 between 50 and 70 mm Hg. Although these oxygen concentrations are felt to be safe, they may represent hyperoxygenation because these patients would have a PaO_2 of 30 to 40 mm Hg if they were still in utero. The newer anesthesia machines do not allow delivery of room air without some added oxygen. This often prevents the anesthesiologist from maintaining the SaO_2 in the desired range and may increase the likelihood of ROP in some infants.

Apnea

Periodic breathing and apnea are common in preterm infants,[28–30] especially after the first week of life. The causes are multiple and include hypo- and hyperthermia, hypo- and hyperglycemia, hypo- and hypercalcemia, hypo- and hypervolemia, anemia, decreased functional residual capacity, patent ductus arteriosus, constipation, hypothyroidism, poorly developed control of respiration, and excessive handling. Repeated apnea increases the likelihood of CNS damage because it is associated with repeated bouts of hypoxemia. Infants who have apneic spells do *not* breathe or breathe inadequately during anesthesia and must be ventilated, from the time of anesthesia induction.

	T A B L E 1 4 – 1		
	BRONCHOPULMONARY DYSPLASIA		
Stage	Onset (Days of Age)	X-Ray Findings	Pathology
I	2–3	"Classic" respiratory distress syndrome	Atelectasis, hyaline membranes, hyperemia, lymphatic dilation, metaplasia, and necrosis of bronchiolar mucosa
II	4–10	Obscure cardiac borders: nearly complete opacification of lung fields	Necrosis and repair of epithelium, persisting hyaline membranes, emphysematous coalescence of alveoli, thickening of alveolar and capillary membranes
III	10–20	Small rounded areas of radiolucency (sponge-like)	Few hyaline membranes, regeneration of clear cells, bronchiolar metaplasia, mucous secretion, emphysematous alveoli, focal thickening of basement membrane
IV	>30	Enlargement of radiolucent areas seen in stage III alternating with thin strands of radiodensity	Emphysematous alveoli, marked hypertrophy of epithelium

Adapted from Northway WH Jr, Rosan R, Porter D: Pulmonary disease following respiratory therapy of hyaline membrane disease: bronchopulmonary dysplasia. N Engl J Med 276:357, 1967, with permission.

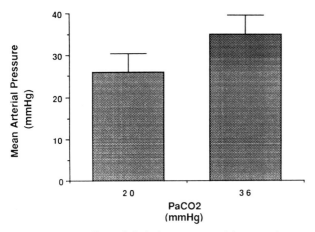

FIGURE 14–3. The effects of alkalosis on mean arterial pressure in premature infants. Ventilation was maintained constant and CO_2 was added to raise the Pa_{CO_2} to normal.

It is unwise to have these patients attempt to breathe spontaneously during surgery.

Moderately premature infants, especially those recovering from RDS and those who required mechanical ventilation, may have chronic lung disease. If they do, the Pa_{CO_2} is often elevated and the Pa_{O_2} or Sa_{O_2} decreased when they breathe room air. They occasionally require some increased oxygen and mechanical ventilation for months to years. Care should be taken not to overexpand the lungs of premature infants, as this may lead to severe lung injury.[31]

Patent Ductus Arteriosus

Fifty percent of full-term infants close their ductus arteriosus by 24 hours of age and almost all of them do so by 72 hours of age.[32] Most preterm infants of 30 weeks' gestation or more have a closed ductus arteriosus by 96 hours of age.[33] However, smaller preterm infants often have a patent ductus arteriosus,[32] which often appears on the third to fifth day after birth in patients not treated with surface active material.[34] It can occur in the first few hours of life in infants who receive surfactant at or near birth. Its appearance often coincides with the decrease in pulmonary vascular resistance that accompanies recovery from RDS.[35] The murmur is usually heard at the left upper sternal border, is often described as a "machinery" murmur, and is often continuous. It is loudest during apnea or exhalation, and its intensity can be increased by hyperventilation. The patient's pulses are bounding and the pulse pressure widened (Fig. 14–4). A gallop rhythm is often present.

As the left-to-right shunt increases, so does the pulmonary blood flow, and the heart is unable to keep up with the demand for cardiac output. This leads to congestive heart failure (CHF), manifested by increased respiratory failure (intercostal retractions, diminished breath sounds, poor air entry, rales), tachycardia, and a gallop rhythm. The Pa_{O_2} decreases and the Pa_{CO_2} rises. Apnea and increasing ventilatory requirements, along with a widened pulse pressure, are often the earliest signs of a patent ductus arteriosus, and frequently occur before a murmur is heard.[36] In fact, the ductus arteriosus may be so large that there is no murmur heard and the patency of this structure is only detected by echocardiogram.

The initial treatment of patent ductus arteriosus is medical.[37] It includes fluid restriction[38] (often to the point of severe dehydration) and administration of diuretics and indomethacin (Indocin).[39,40] Indomethacin administration has greatly reduced the number of patients who require surgical closure of a ductus arteriosus. Digitalis should *not* be given to small preterm infants because it does not effectively improve stroke volume or ventricular emptying.[41] It does, however, decrease the heart rate. Because tachycardia is a major means by which premature infants increase their cardiac output, decreasing the heart rate may be detrimental. We have anesthetized more than 1,000 infants who weighed less than 1,500 g at the time their patent ductus arteriosus was ligated and have had only two deaths related to anesthesia and surgery. One infant weighed 630 g, the other 580 g; both were moribund at the time of transfer to us. During the same period we had six infants die of digitalis toxicity before surgery. Consequently, we no longer administer digitalis to preterm infants, nor do we dehydrate them with potent diuretics. If we must restrict their fluids to the point that we cannot provide adequate calories, we first attempt to close the ductus arteriosus with indomethacin. If this fails, we surgically ligate the ductus arteriosus. Earlier closure of the ductus arteriosus (either with indomethacin or surgically) has reduced the morbidity and mortality (NEC, pulmonary hemorrhage, and intraventricular hemorrhage) associated with patent ductus arteriosus and has allowed the patients to be weaned from assisted ventilation and fed within a few days. Recently, there has been a trend to close the PDA thorascopically or to close the PDA with a transcatheter closure.[42] Both require anesthesia. There is a significant number of patients whose PDAs are incompletely closed following transcatheter closure of the PDA.

A second reason to close a patent ductus arteriosus early is to reduce the incidence of necrotizing enterocolitis.[43] A large patent ductus arteriosus shunts as much as 80 per-

FIGURE 14–4. Aortic blood pressure of a preterm infant during periods when the murmur of a ductus arteriosus was and was not present. Note the widening of the pulse pressure and elevated arterial pressure when the murmur was present. (Courtesy of Dr. Joseph A. Kitterman.)

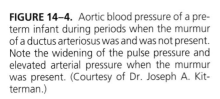

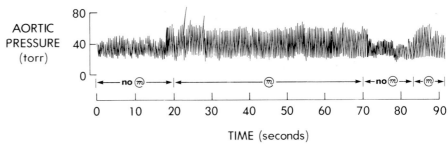

cent of the cardiac output away from the systemic circulation and into the lungs, leaving little blood for the remaining body. Because the gut is one of the first organs to be deprived of blood, it is the shock organ in the neonate. The resulting ischemia causes abdominal distention; a discolored, blue, tender abdomen; bloody stools; and, occasionally, intestinal perforation and peritonitis. If dilated loops of bowel and bloody stools are persistently present or if there is air in the bowel wall, the ductus arteriosus should be closed surgically. This policy has significantly reduced the need to resect bowel because of this disease. The use of prostaglandin synthetase inhibitors does not seem to have increased the incidence of necrotizing enterocolitis.

Infection

Infections (e.g., pneumonia, sepsis, and meningitis) are common in preterm infants, especially those who are moderately or severely preterm, because the cellular and tissue immunity of these patients is reduced. Although the signs of sepsis are often subtle, sepsis should be suspected if the infant becomes hypo- or hyperthermic (despite a neutral thermal environment), lethargic, mottled, gray, or apneic. An increase in the serum glucose concentration, despite a constant infusion of glucose, should lead one to suspect sepsis. Laboratory examinations may be helpful, but preterm infants can develop sepsis in the absence of a positive blood culture, an elevated white blood cell (WBC) count, or a fever. In fact, this is more often true than not. The presence of an abnormal WBC count, whether increased or decreased, is diagnostically helpful (Table 14–2). A shift to the left is also helpful, but this is not always present. Band counts in excess of 15 percent are abnormal and are a good indicator of infection in preterm infants.[44] Cerebral spinal fluid (CSF) should contain fewer than 1 WBC per 200 red blood cells (RBCs), although an absolute count of 70 WBCs/mm^3 may be normal in the neonate.[45] The CSF glucose concentration should be at least 50 to 60 percent of that in the blood. The urine should contain fewer than 5 WBCs per high-power field. A bladder tap urine specimen should be devoid of WBCs.

Preterm infants respond appropriately to antibiotics, although the dosage and interval between doses may have to be altered (see Chapter 3). The aminoglycosides may cause muscle weakness or paralysis and act synergistically with nondepolarizing muscle relaxants to increase their effect.

Necrotizing Enterocolitis

NEC (see Chapter 20) is more common in tiny preterm infants than in any other age group[46] and usually occurs after gastric feedings have been instituted.[47, 48] The cause of NEC is multifactorial and difficult to determine in most infants. An infant who usually has been doing well and suddenly develops abdominal distention, vomiting, bloody stools, reducing substances in the stool, and shock should be suspected of having NEC. Shock occurs because large amounts of fluid move into the peritoneal cavity, gut, and other tissues. Radiographs of the abdomen show distended loops of bowel, air in the bowel wall and, if the gut has perforated, free air in the peritoneal cavity. Such infants are extremely ill (often moribund) and require fluid resuscitation with blood, colloid, and large volumes of lactated Ringer's solution before surgery if they are to survive. However, administration of this amount of fluid usually worsens their respiratory failure and increases their need for assisted ventilation. They should be started on intravenous (IV) broad-spectrum antibiotics preoperatively. Most of these neonates survive, although some of them do so with short gut syndrome.

Hematologic Manifestations

Anemia is common in preterm infants because their ability to produce RBCs is reduced. Their anemia is worsened by frequent blood sampling. Failure to provide iron in the diet also worsens this condition. So long as these infants have respiratory or cardiovascular problems, their hemoglobin levels should be maintained between 10 and 15 g/dl by blood transfusions. A hemoglobin of 14 to 15 g/dl is more likely than one of 8 to 10 g/dl to prevent apneic spells and the CHF associated with a patent ductus arterio-

TABLE 14 – 2
WBC COUNT AND DIFFERENTIAL COUNT DURING THE FIRST 2 WEEKS OF LIFE

Age	Leukocytes	Neutrophils			Eosinophils	Basophils	Lymphocytes	Monocytes
		Total	Segs.	Bands				
Birth								
Mean	18,100	11,000	9,400	1,600	400	100	5,500	1,050
Range	9.0–30.0	6.0–26			20–850	0–640	2.0–11.0	0.4–3.1
Mean %	—	61	52	9	2.2	0.6	31	5.8
7 Days								
Mean	12,200	5,500	4,700	830	500	50	5,000	1,100
Range	5.0–21.0	1.5–10.0			70–1,100	0–250	2.0–17.0	0.3–2.7
Mean %	—	45	39	6	4.1	0.4	41	9.1
14 Days								
Mean	11,400	4,500	3,900	630	350	50	5,500	1,000
Range	5.0–20.0	1.0–9.5			70–1,000	0–230	2.0–17.0	0.2–2.4
Mean %	—	40	34	5.5	3.1	0.4	48	8.8

From Avery GB (ed): Neonatology, 4th ed. Philadelphia, JB Lippincott, 1994, with permission.

sus. However, this does not replace the need for transfusion for acute blood loss. The WBC count of normal preterm infants is shown in Table 14–2. Usually, the WBC count is elevated at birth and decreases during the first week of life. Stress tends to elevate the WBC count, often to 40,000 to 50,000/mm³.

Infants who are deficient in vitamin E have increased RBC destruction, jaundice, anemia, lethargy, apnea, and occasionally CHF. This picture is usually seen in infants born before 30 weeks' gestation.

In the growing fetus, there is a high level of erythropoiesis, a relatively high hematocrit, and predominant synthesis of hemoglobin F. Erythropoietin (EPO) is produced in the liver and regulates erythropoiesis. Fetal EPO concentrations are high at birth in full-term infants but decline relatively rapidly. In preterm infants, the hemoglobin concentration decreases farther than in full-term infants, causing premature infants to become anemic. Phibbs et al.[49] showed that recombinant human erythropoietin 100 U/kg given intravenously twice weekly for 6 weeks to infants with anemia of prematurity produced an earlier increase in reticulocyte counts compared with placebo. Exogenous EPO did not suppress subsequent release of endogenous EPO. Subsequent studies by this group have shown a decrease in the necessity for blood transfusions in premature infants treated with exogenous EPO (see Chapter 6).

Rarely, premature infants are polycythemic. If the hematocrit is greater than 60 percent, it may have to be reduced by exchange transfusion before surgery. Failure to do so may lead to vascular occlusion of the renal vein, portal vein, or cerebral veins if the patient becomes dehydrated (hypovolemic) or develops hypotension during surgery. Care must be taken to provide sufficient fluid during surgery and to use anesthetic techniques that are least likely to cause hypotension.

Nutrition and Growth

Moderately premature infants have difficulty sucking effectively for some time after birth and usually require intermittent or continuous gavage feedings. Their gastric capacity and gastrointestinal motility are adequate to accept the instilled food, but their respiratory distress and need for assisted ventilation somehow decreases their ability to absorb feedings. As a result, it often is necessary to give fluids intravenously. Infants who cannot be fed 3 or 4 days after birth should receive intravascular feedings with 12.5 percent glucose, protein (amino acids) 2 to 3 g/kg, and lipids 3 g/kg (see Chapter 20). From this diet they can derive 80 to 100 kcal/kg/day, depending on the volume of fluid infused. Early attempts at oral feeding of infants who were asphyxiated at birth increase the occurrence of necrotizing enterocolitis or abdominal distention and regurgitation. It usually is best to delay oral feeding for 5 to 6 days after birth in these patients.

Sufficient free water is required to maintain normal intra- and extravascular fluid volumes. However, administering large volumes of fluid (> 130 to 150 ml/kg/day) increases the likelihood that a patent ductus arteriosus and congestive heart failure will occur. Electrolytes (3 mEq/kg sodium, 2 mEq/kg potassium, 200 to 500 mg/kg calcium gluconate), and vitamins (including vitamin E) should be added to the maintenance fluids. Because antibiotics kill gut flora, vitamin K 1 mg should be administered twice weekly as long as the patient is receiving antibiotics.

Metabolic Concentration Determinations

Metabolic disorders are common in preterm infants because they have decreased protein intake and decreased ability to reabsorb sodium bicarbonate (renal tubular acidosis) and to secrete ammonia (see Chapter 21). The respiratory rate and work increase in moderately preterm infants in response to acidosis, but they may not increase in small preterm infants. Acidosis also reduces weight gain. Late metabolic acidosis of prematurity should be suspected if (1) the weight gain is inadequate despite adequate calorie intake, (2) lethargy or apneic spells occur, or (3) pallor or tachypnea is present. It may be necessary to correct the acidosis with sodium bicarbonate before surgery (0.6 times base deficit times weight in kilograms). Moderate or small preterm infants may have a relative respiratory acidosis ($Paco_2 > 35$ mm Hg) despite a pH below 7.3 because their chest walls limit their ability to increase minute ventilation sufficiently.

Blood Level Determinations

Calcium

The serum calcium concentration of preterm infants is normally lower than that of term infants because preterm infants have diminished concentrations of serum proteins (3 to 4.5 g/dl). It probably is not necessary to maintain the serum calcium concentration above 7 mg/dl if the ionized-calcium concentration is normal.[50] The ionized-calcium concentrations of preterm neonates are lower on days 1 through 5 of life than those of term infants but are still above 1 mM and are within the lower range of normal for older patients. The ionized calcium concentration increases with gestational age. Phosphate and magnesium concentrations are similar in the two age groups.

If symptoms of hypocalcemia occur (e.g., twitching, seizures, hypotension), the infant should be treated with calcium gluconate 100 to 200 mg/kg. Hyperventilation may reduce the unbound fraction of calcium, which can lower the seizure threshold. Despite hypocalcemia, the electrocardiogram (ECG) is usually normal.

Sodium

The serum sodium concentration of tiny preterm infants is labile. It rises quickly with dehydration and decreases just as quickly with overhydration. Care must be taken to keep the sodium concentration of the blood normal because hypernatremia may damage the CNS or hyponatremia (< 120 mEq/L) may induce seizures. Persistent hyponatremia is usually associated with water intoxication. It seldom is necessary to infuse hypertonic saline to correct hyponatremia; fluid restriction will usually suffice.

Glucose

Preterm infants tolerate a glucose load poorly. Most unanesthetized preterm infants tolerate an infusion of 5 to

7 mg/kg/min of glucose without developing hyperglycemia, glucosuria, polyuria, and dehydration (see Chapter 5), but some small premature infants will not tolerate 2 mg/kg/min without becoming hyperglycemic. Excessively high serum glucose concentrations (> 200 mg/dl) can be deleterious to the CNS and can cause an osmotic diuresis and hypovolemia. Failure to gain 25 to 30 g/day and to increase head growth by 0.8 to 1 cm/wk is usually caused by undernutrition. It may, however, be difficult to provide sufficient nutrition to achieve this growth before 5 to 10 days of age because of a myriad of factors. The level of nutrition and weight gain should be determined carefully before surgery because infants with poor preoperative nutritional states tolerate anesthesia and surgery less well.

A blood glucose concentration below 40 mg/dl is common in preterm infants and is abnormal. This hypoglycemia should be corrected with a bolus of 10 to 20 percent glucose 2 to 5 ml/kg given over 5 minutes and by a continuous infusion of sufficient glucose to maintain the serum glucose concentration above 40 mg/dl. Continued severe hypoglycemia (glucose < 10 mg/dl) may damage the CNS. On the other hand, marked hyperglycemia should be avoided for the reasons stated above and because hypoximia or ischemia (combined with hyperglycemia) increases the incidence of CNS injury after resuscitation.[51, 52]

Bilirubin

The bilirubin concentration is higher in preterm than in term infants because preterm infants have a lesser ability to conjugate substances. Infants who are bruised, polycythemic, and those with intracranial, gastrointestinal, or pulmonary hemorrhage have greater hyperbilirubinemia. The relative hypoproteinemia of prematurity, the decreased effectiveness of the blood-brain barrier, and the often present acidemia increase the susceptibility of premature infants to kernicterus. Even low concentrations of bilirubin (10 to 15 mg/dl) may cause kernicterus if the infant is acidotic.[53–55] Therefore, a two-volume exchange transfusion should be performed before surgery if the patient has an elevated indirect bilirubin concentration and if time permits, because intraoperative hypoxemia and acidosis may prove disastrous (Table 14–3).

Retinopathy of Prematurity (Retrolental Fibroplasia)

Some degree of ROP occurs in about 50 percent of infants weighing 1,000 to 1,500 g at birth.[56] Seventy-eight percent of those weighing 750 to 999 g have ROP, whereas more than 90 percent of those weighing less than 750 g have some degree of ROP. ROP rarely occurs in term infants. Most stage 4 and 5 ROP occurs in infants who weigh less than 750 g at birth.[57] ROP begins with retinal vascular obliteration and is followed by increased vascularity, hemorrhage and, in the worst cases, retinal detachment. Oxygen is a major contributing factor to the development of ROP, but it is unclear whether the culprit is oxygen content or PaO$_2$. Nor is it known what level of oxygenation causes ROP, but a PaO$_2$ of 150 mm Hg for as short a time as 1 to 2 hours can do so. It is also possible that ROP might

TABLE 14 – 3
SERUM CONCENTRATIONS FOR EXCHANGE TRANSFUSION*

Birth Weight (g)	Serum Bilirubin Concentrations for Exchange Transfusion (mg/dl)	
	Normal Infants[†]	Abnormal Infants[‡]
<1,000	10.0	10.0[§]
1,001–1,250	13.0	10.0[§]
1,251–1,500	15.0	13.0
1,501–2,000	17.0	15.0
2,001–2,500	18.0	17.0
>2,500	20.0	18.0

* These guidelines have not been validated.
[†] There have been case reports of basal ganglion staining at concentrations considerably lower than 10 mg.
[‡] Normal infants are defined for this purpose as having none of the problems listed below.
[§] Abnormal infants have one or more of the following problems: perinatal asphyxia, prolonged hypoxemia, acidemia, persistent hypothermia, hypoalbuminemia, hemolysis, sepsis, hyperglycemia, elevated free fatty acids or presence of drugs that compete for bilirubin binding, and signs of clinical or central nervous system deterioration.
Data from American Academy of Pediatrics, Committee on Fetus and Newborns: Standards and Recommendations for Hospital Care of Newborn Infants, 6th ed. Evanston, IL, American Academy of Pediatrics, 1977.

develop at considerably lower PaO$_2$ levels because premature infants are normally exposed to PaO$_2$ levels of 30 to 40 mm Hg in utero, not the PaO$_2$ levels of 50 mm Hg or more found during the neonatal period. Although oxygen is an important cause of ROP, it is not the only one.[58] This disease appears to be multifactorial in nature, with oxygen being only one of the factors involved.

Normally, the retinal vasculature spreads outward from the optic disk as the fetus matures. It reaches the nasal side of the retinal periphery by 36 weeks' gestation and the temporal side at 40 weeks. Hyperoxia constricts the retinal arterioles and causes swelling and degeneration of the endothelium of the arterioles and the capillaries.[59–61] Retinal ischemia is present despite systemic hyperoxia. The presence of fetal hemoglobin (HbF) may protect against retrolental fibroplasia, and patients transfused with adult blood may be at greater risk for developing this condition.

Kretzer et al.[62] proposed that spindle cells normally migrate and canalize to form inner retinal vessels, but when they are stressed by one of several factors (including oxygen) they secrete angiogenic factor. When these cells are removed from the relative hypoxic environment at birth, they are bombarded with oxygen free radicals. Since the premature infant's ability to scavenge these radicals is reduced, there is extensive membrane lipid peroxidation. The spindle cells form intracellular linkages via gap junctions, and the cells fail to migrate and canalize. The secretion of angiogenic factor by these cells causes vascular proliferation between the vascular and avascular portions of the retina. Immature infants have a large number of spindle cells.

Vitamin E may protect against ROP through the membrane-stabilizing and antioxidant actions of vitamin E,[63, 64] but this is far from proven. Vitamin E concentrations decrease rapidly after birth owing to inadequate intake of vitamin E and lack of adipose tissue. Many studies have attempted to determine the efficacy of giving vitamin E to premature infants. Unfortunately, these studies provide no clear evidence that giving more than physiologic amounts of vitamin E is of value. Vitamin E reduces the severity of ROP but not its incidence.[65] Giving high enough concentrations of vitamin E to induce supranormal serum concentrations has resulted in increased incidences of necrotizing enterocolitis[66, 67] and infection.[67] At present, most clinicians give only enough vitamin E to maintain normal physiologic levels of the drug.

Retinopathy of prematurity is divided into five stages.[68]

Stage 1: A thin white line separates the posterior vascularized portion of the retina from the anterior avascular retina.

Stage 2: The demarcation line increases in volume and elevates. At this point it is known as the "ridge." The changes in stage 1 and 2 regress in 80 percent of patients. Between 5 and 10 percent of premature infants with stage 1 and 2 disease progress to stage 3.[69]

Stage 3: Tissue proliferation develops from the ridge, usually posteriorly. Stage 3 can be mild, moderate, or severe, depending on the volume of the extraretinal tissue.

Stage 4: Partial retinal detachment occurs with the macula still attached (stage 4a). The macula is detached in stage 4b.

Stage 5: Total retinal detachment occurs.

The appearance of the retinal vessels in the posterior pole changes during the acute proliferative phase. These vessels may become congested, increase in caliber, and develop increased tortuosity. This is referred to as *plus disease.* The retina also is divided into three zones. Zone 1 is the posterior pole, zone 2 is the midperiphery, and zone 3 is the far periphery. The division into zones is important because cryotherapy of zone 1 effectively reduces the seriousness of ROP, whereas similar therapy of zones 2 and 3 does not.[70]

Approximately 85 percent of acute cases of ROP undergo spontaneous regression.[71] Grades 1 and 2 regress in 2 to 3 months and grade 3 in 6 months or more. Most grade 4 and 5 ROP results in blindness or limited vision. Patients with ROP come to the attention of the anesthesiologist because the patient requires eye examination, photocoagulation, or scleral buckling procedures under anesthesia.

It is not known if exposure to increased concentrations of oxygen worsens preexisting ROP. Therefore, it is wise to maintain the SaO_2 within normal limits during anesthesia and to monitor the SaO_2 during surgery with a pulse oximeter (see Chapter 11). If the infant is less than 44 weeks' gestation (some say 50 weeks), it may be appropriate to keep the SaO_2 between 87 and 92 percent.[72] Because it is often necessary to inject air into the eye during surgery, nitrous oxide should be avoided or turned off 30 minutes before the air is injected. Air can be used as the carrier gas for the inhaled anesthetic. Enough oxygen should be added to maintain the PaO_2 at a normal level.

Hypoxemia may occur during anesthesia in those patients who also have chronic lung disease. The SaO_2 may fall precipitously when anesthesia is induced, due to maldistribution of ventilation and perfusion. Adding a small amount of PEEP (2 to 3 cm H_2O) often improves the match of ventilation–perfusion and improves oxygenation. Excessive PEEP may overdistend the ventilated portions of the lung and further decrease oxygenation.

ANESTHESIA

Anesthesia for premature infants is often difficult because they often have multisystem disease and respond poorly to anesthesia. It is important to garner as much information and help preoperatively as possible, in the hope of reducing the incidence of complications. A common mistake, especially among beginning anesthesiologists, is to ignore the fact that those caring for the infant in the neonatal intensive care unit have considered the patient's problems over an extended time and have come to a plan of therapy based on an understanding of these problems. It is neither appropriate nor sensible to alter this plan without thorough discussions with the neonatologists without a very good reason.

Preoperative Preparation

History

Preoperative evaluation of preterm infants must be based on a clear understanding of the preceding sections of this chapter. The patient's chart must be read, understood, and thoroughly discussed with the physicians and nurses caring for the patient. It is the nurses who stand at the bedside all day and who provide the patient's minute-to-minute care. They know the quirks of each individual patient, things of which the physician may not be aware. For example, the nurses may know that very brief periods of apnea cause severe hypoxemia and cyanosis or that the patient's perfusion decreases when the blood glucose concentration is below 40 mg/dl or the calcium concentration is below 7 mg/dl.

Both the past history and the birth history are important when planning an anesthetic for preterm infants. If the infant was asphyxiated at birth, the effects of asphyxia may still be present and autoregulation of the cerebral circulation may be absent.[6, 73] If so, sudden increases in arterial pressure may cause intracranial hemorrhage.[74] Myocardial function may still be depressed and the heart may show signs of hypoxic strain, or there may be insufficiency of the tricuspid valve. Gut blood flow may be decreased and the blood volume and hemoglobin may be low. All of these abnormalities can persist for several days after birth.

A maternal drug history should be sought in every case because most pregnant women take drugs during pregnancy. Many, especially middle-class women, use illicit drugs. Infants born to heroin-addicted mothers may be withdrawing from the drug at the time of surgery. The symptoms of withdrawal include agitation, tremors, poor feeding, and occasionally seizures. Infants withdrawing from barbiturates, diazepam, or methadone have the same symptoms, but the symptoms may not appear until 5 to 10 days of age. Many fetuses are now exposed to cocaine, which is associated with an increased incidence of premature delivery, pulmonary hypertension, and bowel perforation. Infants born after maternal ingestion of large doses of aspirin or acetaminophen are more likely to exhibit pulmonary hypertension and persistent fetal circulation during the first few days of life.[75] This possibility must be considered in any severely hypoxemic infant.

Systems Review and Examination

Head, Eyes, Ears, Nose, and Throat

Congenital anomalies of the face and mouth are common, either as part of a syndrome or as a single entity. A cleft palate is often missed in infants who are mechanically ventilated from birth. This condition poses no problem for the anesthesiologist unless it is necessary to reintubate the patient's trachea. The presence of a cleft palate makes tracheal intubation more difficult in small babies because the tongue cannot be fixed against the palate and tends to flop over the laryngoscope blade and obstruct vision. The small mouth and the relatively large tongue of preterm infants frequently obstruct breathing, especially when pressure is applied to the submental triangle while an anesthesia mask is held on the patient's face. Even slight pressure in this area can completely obstruct the airway. Anesthesia masks that have a large air-filled cuff can be dangerous if they are allowed to slip off the bridge of the nose and compress the nares. This is especially true if the mouth is held closed at the same time. A nasogastric tube usually obstructs half of the infant's upper airway when the trachea is not intubated and the mouth is closed. The tube increases respiratory work, which may cause apnea during induction of anesthesia. In such cases, the nasogastric tubes should be removed and reinserted orally if possible.

It should be determined if the patient has ROP (see above), cataracts, or glaucoma. The intraocular pressure may increase significantly and there may be further damage to the eye if atropine is administered to patients with some types of glaucoma (see Chapter 23).

Pulmonary System

As stated above, pulmonary dysfunction is common in preterm infants. Therefore, the pulmonary system must be carefully evaluated preoperatively. Answers should be sought to the following questions. Does the patient now have or is he or she recovering from RDS? If so, how much ventilatory support is required? What is the ventilator rate, pressure (peak inspiratory and end-expiratory), inspired oxygen concentration (it will probably be higher during anesthesia), and inspiratory time? Is the patient breathing spontaneously? If so, how often is he or she breathing? What SaO_2, blood gas, and pH values do spontaneous breathing or the ventilator settings occasion? How labile are the blood gases? Do the blood gases and pH change when the patient is moved from side to side, when the trachea is suctioned, or when the chest is percussed?[76]

The latter point may be important if the patient is to be turned into the lateral position and this position is the one in which the blood gas concentrations are the worst. Has the patient had a pulmonary hemorrhage? If so, has the bleeding stopped? Is pneumonia present? Pneumonia may be difficult to discern when it is associated with RDS or pulmonary edema. A WBC count, a differential WBC count, and a smear of the tracheal secretions may be helpful, but they also may be unhelpful. If the infant has pneumonia, the tracheal smear will show both WBCs and bacteria. Either finding alone is seldom significant. Is the endotracheal tube (ETT) fixed securely in place? Having the ETT come out of the trachea on the way to the operating room is disconcerting. The tape used to hold the tube in place should not completely encircle the infant's head because this may cause brain stem hemorrhage.[77] Does the infant have intercostal retractions? Most preterm infants have grade 1 out of 4 to 2 out of 4 retractions because of their weak chest walls. Those with pulmonary disease have grade 3 out of 4 to 4 out of 4 retractions. Retractions are indicative of decreased lung compliance, increased airway resistance, or both. Are rales heard on auscultation? Most preterm infants have occasional rales. Moist rales indicate intra-alveolar fluid, usually from pulmonary edema or infection. Dry rales are usually associated with atelectasis. Rhonchi are also common in infants after several days of tracheal intubation. There are few tracheal secretions for the first 48 hours of tracheal intubation, but thereafter they increase in volume and tonicity. White or clear secretions seldom mean anything. Yellow or greenish secretions are often indicative of infection. Frothy, pink, or blood-tinged secretions are usually indicative of pulmonary edema.

The preterm infant normally breathes 30 to 60 times per minute. However, the respiratory rate can be as much as 100 to 150 breaths/min, depending on how severely the lung compliance is decreased. Babies "choose" to breathe rapidly and shallowly rather than slowly and deeply, probably because the metabolic cost is less. In addition, rapid respirations tend to maintain functional residual capacity by not allowing time for complete exhalation. Slow respiratory rates decrease functional residual capacity unless a PEEP is used (Fig. 14–5).[78]

Preoperative evaluation of blood gas data is important. The preterm infant's PaO_2 is normally lower than that of term babies (Tables 14–4 and 14–5). Therefore, small

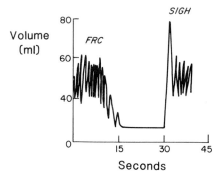

FIGURE 14–5. Changes in functional residual capacity (FRC) with bradypnea and apnea. (From Gregory GA: Respiratory care of the child. Crit Care Med 8:582, 1980, with permission.)

T A B L E   1 4 – 4
ARTERIAL BLOOD GASES IN NORMAL TERM INFANTS

Parameter	Birth	1 Hour	5 Hours	1 Day	5 Days	7 Days
Pao$_2$ (mm Hg)						
x̄	46.6	63.3	73.7	72.7	72.1	73.1
SD	9.9	11.3	12.0	9.5	10.5	9.7
Paco$_2$ (mm Hg)						
x̄	46.1	36.1	35.2	33.4	34.8	35.9
SD	7.0	4.2	3.6	3.1	3.5	3.1
pH						
x̄	7.207	7.332	7.339	7.369	7.371	7.37
SD	0.051	0.031	0.028	0.032	0.031	0.02

x̄, mean; SD, standard deviation.
From Koch G, Wendel H: Adjustment of arterial blood gases and acid base balance in the normal newborn infant during the first week of life. Biol Neonate 12:136, 1968, with permission.

changes in Pao$_2$ cause large changes in oxygen saturation and oxygen content.[79] Brief periods of apnea cause significant hypoxemia.

Is the patient having apneic spells (see above)? Apneic spells often are indicative of other problems. Figure 14–6 shows the chest radiograph of a normal infant and one of a patient with hyaline membrane disease.

CARDIOVASCULAR SYSTEM

Preterm infants often have cardiovascular problems, but they seldom have congenital heart disease. They have less muscle in their pulmonary arteries and their ductus arteriosus than older infants. As a consequence, blood tends to shunt from left to right through the ductus arteriosus or through a ventricular septal defect (if one exists). Shunting occurs earlier (3 to 5 days) in preterm infants than it does in term infants (7 to 14 days). The net result is increased pulmonary blood flow, pulmonary edema, congestive heart failure, and reduced lung compliance. With the administration of surfactant, left-to-right shunting may occur shortly after birth.

CHF is usually caused by a patent ductus arteriosus or fluid overload in preterm infants and is seldom heralded

T A B L E   1 4 – 5
ARTERIAL BLOOD GASES IN NORMAL PRETERM TERM INFANTS

Parameter	Birth	3–5 Hours	13–24 Hours	5–10 Days
Pao$_2$				
x̄		59.5	67.0	80.3
SD		7.7	15.2	12.0
Paco$_2$				
x̄		47.0	27.2	36.4
SD		8.5	8.4	4.2
pH				
x̄	7.32	7.329	7.464	7.3780
SD		0.38	0.064	0.043

x̄, mean; SD, standard deviation.
From Orzalesi MM, Mendicini M, Bucci G, et al: Arterial oxygen studies in premature newborns with and without mild respiratory disorders. Arch Dis Child 42:174, 1967, with permission.

by tachycardia as it is in older patients. In fact, the heart rate is often monotonously regular and usually within normal limits (120 to 160 beats/min) (Table 14–6). A third heart sound (gallop) is usually present but may be difficult to hear because of the rapid heart rate or because of environmental noise (e.g., mechanical ventilators, alarms, monitors). Murmurs also may be difficult to hear for the same reason. Two murmurs are commonly heard in preterm infants, that of a patent ductus arteriosus and that of tricuspid insufficiency. The murmur of a patent ductus arteriosus is a systolic ejection murmur that is best heard along the upper left sternal border when the ductal flow is small. When the ductal flow is large, the murmur extends into diastole, is continuous, and is heard throughout the chest. The "machinery murmur" described in older patients is seldom heard. The murmur of tricuspid insufficiency is systolic in nature and is best heard along the right sternal border. It seldom radiates far, and it disappears after several days of life.

CHF reduces the peripheral perfusion of preterm infants. Capillary filling is slow. The pulses are decreased except in patients with a patent ductus arteriosus (their pulses are increased). Peripheral edema is also common, in part because of the low serum protein concentrations (see above). Edema usually occurs first in the eyelids. Pitting edema of the feet and shins is less common and usually is present only in the sickest babies. However, puffiness of the feet is common.

The chest radiographs of preterm infants with CHF are often difficult to differentiate from those of infants with RDS. The former usually shows central fluffiness and the markings are slightly larger than those seen with respiratory distress (Fig. 14–7).

The infant's liver size is an important indicator of CHF, since the liver is a *very* distensible organ in the neonate. Its inferior margin is normally sharp and is located 1 to 2 cm below the right costal margin; when CHF occurs, the liver can distend into the pelvis in a matter of minutes. With appropriate therapy it will ascend to its normal position in the same amount of time. Excessive pressure should not be exerted on the abdomen when the liver is examined because the pressure may push the liver up into the thoracic cavity and make the organ appear smaller than it really is. In addition, the liver may be ruptured, or blood

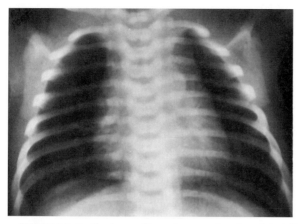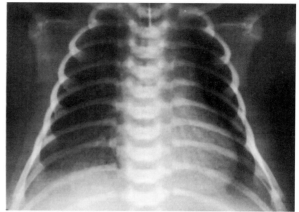

FIGURE 14–6. Chest x-ray films of a normal preterm infant (*left*) and one with respiratory distress syndrome (*right*). Note the air bronchograms, the loss of lung volume, and the heart border in the latter. (Courtesy of Dr. Robert C. Brasch.)

may be forced into the central circulation, elevating the central venous pressure. The position of the liver edge can usually be felt by gently running the fingertips over the right upper abdomen or by percussing the abdomen. The latter technique is especially helpful when the abdomen is distended. When enlarged, the liver may extend across the midline and be difficult to differentiate from the spleen, which also can be enlarged during CHF.

Abdomen

The preterm infant's abdomen is normally protuberant and soft because the abdominal wall has little muscle tone, and a diastasis rectus is usually present. The venous pattern is prominent over the abdominal wall, and this pattern becomes exaggerated when the liver is diseased. The intra-abdominal organs are usually easy to palpate. The spleen is often enlarged and palpable below the left costal margin in patients with CHF, erythroblastosis fetalis, systemic infections, or fluid overload. Erythroblastotic infants often have enough ascites to interfere with ventilation, and sometimes it is necessary to remove some of this fluid to enable adequate ventilation of the infant's lungs. The kidneys of preterm infants are easily palpable as small masses in the retroperitoneal space. If they are enlarged, is it because of renal vein thromboses or of renal, ureteral, or bladder anomalies? Is the enlargement caused by hypoxemia? Renal vein thrombosis is more likely in infants born by breech delivery. The urinary bladder can be felt as a round mass extending above the pelvic rim. However, it may distend up to or above the umbilicus if the urethra is obstructed. The ureters are occasionally palpable as cords running longitudinally in the retroperitoneal space.

T A B L E 1 4 – 6 HEART RATE IN PRETERM INFANTS WITH PATENT DUCTUS ARTERIOSUS	
Condition	Heart Rate (bpm)
Normal cardiac function	150 ± 18
Congestive heart failure	148 ± 22
Postligation ductus arteriosus	146 ± 18

Loops of bowel are often visible through the abdominal wall, especially if the bowel is dilated. Despite being distended, the abdomen is seldom tender unless the infant has peritonitis. Then it becomes tender, rigid, and edematous. Intraperitoneal fluid often distends the inguinal canals and scrotums of male infants. Redness around the umbilicus is often a sign of systemic or intra-abdominal infections.

One should always ascertain if the anus is patent before the infant goes to surgery. Nothing should be inserted more than 0.5 cm into the rectum, to avoid perforating the bowel.

The incidence of CNS damage increases with increasing degrees of prematurity and asphyxia (see Chapter 16). CNS injury is usually manifested as flaccidity, hypertonia, or a difference in tone between the upper and lower body or the right and left sides. Deep tendon reflexes and the grasp reflex are often absent. Preterm infants normally have a positive Babinski sign. The back, neck, and sacral area should be examined for evidence of a meningomyelocele. These problems are occasionally missed because sick infants are placed on their backs and left in this position for days.

State of Hydration

The state of hydration must be assessed in these infants during the preoperative visit. Their large surface/volume ratio and thin skin allow increased evaporative water losses, as do their rapid respiratory rate and their relatively large minute volume.[80] Infrared warmers increase evaporative water loss and the daily water requirement.[81] Failure to supply this extra water leads to progressive dehydration. Covering the baby with SaranWrap or a plastic shield significantly reduces these losses. The discovery that reducing fluid intake below 130 ml/kg/day reduces the incidence of patent ductus arteriosus in preterm infants has led to severe fluid and calorie restriction in many instances.[38] These infants may therefore be dehydrated when they are scheduled for surgery. Administration of potent diuretics dehydrates them further. Preterm infants lose fluid to the third space more easily than do older patients, and their capillaries leak more. In addition, they have lower levels of serum proteins and a reduced oncotic

RDS   CHF

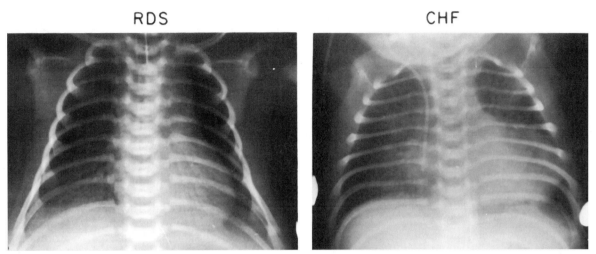

FIGURE 14–7. Chest x-ray films of a normal preterm infant with respiratory distress syndrome (*left*) and one with a patent ductus arteriosus and congestive heart failure (*right*). Note the enlarged heart, the central fluffiness, and the loss of clear vascular shadows in the latter. (Courtesy of Dr. Robert C. Brasch.)

pressure.[82, 83] Therefore, infants with sepsis or shock are prime candidates for large amounts of fluid loss to the peritoneal cavity. Such patients commonly gain 20 to 50 percent of their body weight despite intravascular volume depletion.

Laboratory Findings

Most sick preterm infants have undergone a multitude of laboratory tests. The results of these tests should be reviewed and understood before anesthesia is induced.

Hematology

The hemoglobin concentration should exceed 10 g/dl to ensure adequate oxygen-carrying capacity if the infant has cardiorespiratory disease. In a well infant, the hemoglobin concentration is usually adequate if it is above 7 g/dl. As discussed above, the hemoglobin concentration decreases rapidly after birth, frequently because large volumes of blood are taken for tests.

Electrolytes

The serum electrolyte concentrations of preterm infants vary more than those of older patients because the electrolyte concentrations of infants are more affected by small changes in fluid and electrolyte intake and by their environment. A single electrolyte value can be misleading; serial values are much more helpful. A rise in serum sodium is caused by either dehydration or excessive sodium administration. The latter is associated with peripheral edema. Although hyperkalemia is common, it seldom affects the ECG. Hypokalemia (< 3 mEq/L) is also common, especially in preterm infants who received potent diuretics. Hyperventilation further decreases the serum potassium value. The serum chloride concentration is normally higher in preterm infants (105 to 115 mEq/L) than in older children, which in part accounts for their metabolic acidosis. The total calcium concentration is usually lower than that of term infants, but the ionized calcium concentration is about the same as that of older patients. Hyperventilation may reduce the ionized calcium concentration to unacceptable levels. The tendency of most neonatologists is to maintain the total serum calcium concentration above 8 mg/dl, although many neonates do perfectly well with concentrations below this level. Ionized calcium concentrations are probably a more useful measure of the infant's calcium status. The normal ionized calcium concentrations vary with age.[50]

Clotting Status

Does the infant have a bleeding diathesis? Infants who are asphyxiated at birth have depression of factors V, VII, and VIII. Those who are quickly resuscitated, have these factors return to normal within 3 to 4 days.[84] In infants with more prolonged hypoxia, these values may not return to normal for a week or more. Such infants frequently exhibit thrombocytopenia, often below 10,000/mm³. Even at these levels, bleeding seldom occurs in the absence of surgery. Therefore, premature infants are seldom transfused with platelets unless they require surgery or their platelet count falls below 5,000/mm³ if their other clotting parameters are normal. When surgery is required, enough platelets should be administered to raise the concentration to 50,000/mm³ or greater. If the surgical procedure lasts for several hours, more platelets may be required during the procedure. If the patient has not received vitamin K after birth, has been NPO, or has received IV antibiotics, vitamin K 1 mg should be administered preoperatively.

Bleeding disorders, such as diffuse intravascular coagulation (DIC), must be corrected preoperatively with fresh frozen plasma or cryoprecipitate. If both the clotting factors and the platelets are decreased, the patient will benefit from fresh whole blood. Fresh donor blood contains all of the clotting factors, platelets, proteins, and RBCs required.

Preoperative Plan

It is usually advisable to have a second anesthesiologist in the operating room to help during surgery. It is difficult for one person to ventilate the patient's lungs, give fluids and blood, watch the surgical field and monitors, and keep the anesthesia record at the same time. The operating room should be warmed to 35° to 37°C before the patient arrives, and a servo-controlled infrared heater should be placed over the operating table. A water-circulated heating blanket should be placed under the table sheet and a thermometer placed on top of the heating blanket. The blanket's temperature should be kept at 37° to 38°C. Strain gauges for monitoring arterial and central venous pressure are set up and calibrated when they are to be used. IV solutions are set up if they are different from those being infused in the nursery. The latter is often 5 percent dextrose in 0.2 normal saline, which is *inappropriate* for replacement of third-space losses during surgery. Third-space losses should be replaced with Ringer's lactate. All fluid should be delivered through an infusion pump when possible. The drip chamber should never contain more fluid than is safe to give in 1 hour, in case the IV infusion accidentally runs wide open.

Transporting preterm infants to and from the operating room can be dangerous. To reduce this risk, the anesthesiologist should always accompany sick infants. To improve safety during transport, the patient is *not* disconnected from the monitors. Battery-operated monitors should be used to monitor arterial pressure, ECG, and oxygen saturation continuously. Heart tones should be continuously monitored with a chest piece or an esophageal stethoscope. Infusion pumps should continue to infuse fluids, especially vasoactive drugs. Ventilation must be supported during transport, usually with a Jackson-Reese device (see Chapter 9). The inspired oxygen should be sufficient to keep the oxygen saturation between 87 and 92 percent.[72] The inspired oxygen concentration should be 100 percent only if that concentration is required to maintain the desired oxygen saturation. Therefore, the transport cart must provide air and oxygen and a means of blending them to give the desired oxygen concentration. Keeping the patient warm is a major problem during transport unless a transport incubator that runs off batteries is available. Unfortunately, these incubators are expensive and usually not available.

Table 14–7 shows the changes in body temperature of preterm infants being transported to and from the operating room for ligation of a ductus arteriosus. Note that they lost nearly a degree of body temperature during this short period. Their body temperature increased to normal in the operating room and decreased again during the trip back to the nursery. We now prevent these heat losses

TABLE 14–7
BODY TEMPERATURE OF PRETERM INFANTS DURING TRANSPORT TO AND FROM THE OPERATING ROOM

Time	Body Temperature (°C)
Preoperative—nursery	36.4 ± 0.5
Preoperative—operating room	35.7 ± 0.7
End of surgery	36.4 ± 1.0
Postoperative—nursery	35.9 ± 1.7

by covering the baby's body with SaranWrap and warm blankets, by putting a cap on the head, and by placing a chemically activated heating pad under the patients (Porta-Warm, Allegiance Health Care Corp.). Elevators should be waiting for the patient, not vice versa. The operating room should be warm and the infant should be taken directly into the operating room and placed under a radiant warmer immediately on arrival in the operating suite.

We use the patient's intensive care bed as both a transport bed and an operating room table. As a result, the same monitors are used during transport and during anesthesia and surgery; we use the built-in warmer to maintain body temperature during preparation for surgery. Transport time to and from the operating room is shortened, and induction of anesthesia is begun as soon as the patient arrives in the operating room. We also bring the patient's oxygen saturation monitor and use it during surgery.

In some instances, it is better to do the surgery in the neonatal intensive care unit (NICU) to avoid all of the problems that can occur during transport of the patient to and from the operating room. In addition, there is no need to discontinue use of the patient's mechanical ventilator. This works well for patients requiring ligation of a patient ductus arteriosus, insertion of a Broviac catheter, or treatment of necrotizing enterocolitis. In some hospitals, all surgery in premature infants is performed in the NICU. Many older infants also undergo repair of a diaphragmatic hernia in the NICU while on extracorporeal membrane oxygenation (ECMO).

Induction of Anesthesia

Although preterm infants do require anesthesia,[85] their requirement is lower than that of older patients.[86-88] Failure to provide adequate anesthesia predisposes them to hypertension and intracranial hemorrhage if they lack the ability to autoregulate cerebral blood flow. An increase or decrease in arterial blood pressure increases or decreases cerebral blood flow. Adequate anesthesia prevents or attenuates these increases. On the other hand, deep anesthesia reduces the arterial blood pressure of infants and children more than it does that of adults.[89, 90] Therefore, an attempt should be made to provide the smallest amount of anesthesia possible that still prevents increases in blood pressure. Increases in heart rate and blood pressure are signs of light anesthesia. When the blood pressure decreases, heart rate usually does not increase because even light levels of anesthesia obtund the baroreceptors in preterm infants.[87] Nitrous oxide (70 percent) reduces the baroresponse to the same extent as 0.5 minimum alveolar concentration (MAC) halothane (Fluothane).[91] Fentanyl (Sublimaze), even at a concentration of 10 μg/kg, also significantly depresses the baroreceptor reflex,[92] although this dose does not cause hypotension. Anand and his associates have shown that preterm infants are capable of mounting a stress response if given inadequate anesthesia for surgery.[85]

If the ETT is not in place before surgery, one must be inserted. If it is inserted without anesthesia, the arterial and intracranial pressure may rise.[93] Obviously, some patients are too ill to anesthetize before an ETT is inserted, but this is uncommon after the immediate neonatal period.

Anesthesia can be induced with inhaled anesthetics (usually halothane or sevoflurane). However, ventilation should be controlled during the induction of anesthesia only if the infant develops apnea and bradycardia. Ventilation should be controlled throughout surgery. It is necessary to use the correct dose of anesthetic to avoid sudden, severe hypotension.[94] An alternative anesthetic technique employs thiopental sodium (Pentothal) 1 to 2 mg/kg or fentanyl (Sublimaze) 10 to 30 μg/kg intravascularly over 1 to 2 minutes. When the eyelid reflexes are lost, an ETT is inserted, usually without the need for muscle relaxants. The lungs can then be ventilated with an inhaled anesthetic if so desired. As the ETT is being inserted, an assistant should place a finger in the suprasternal notch and tell the intubator when the tip of the tube hits the assistant's finger. When it does, the tube should not be advanced any farther and should be fixed and taped in this position. This technique reduces the incidence of inadvertent endobronchial intubation. If necessary, the patient can be paralyzed with pancuronium bromide (Pavulon) 0.1 mg/kg, curare 0.3 mg/kg, or rocuronium 0.3 to 1.0 mg/kg. However, all but the latter may alter arterial blood pressure and, as a result, affect cerebral blood flow and pressure.

Maintenance of Anesthesia

There are few data on the anesthetic requirements of preterm infants. However, experience suggests that they require less anesthesia than their healthy full-term counterparts. The halothane requirement for infants undergoing ductus arteriosus ligation is approximately 0.57 to 0.80 percent end-tidal. At that dosage, no change occurs in either heart rate or arterial pressure with a skin incision. This requirement is significantly lower than that of term infants.[88, 95] The reason for this difference is unknown.

Inhaled anesthetics cause more hypotension in preterm infants than in older patients,[90] probably because their peripheral responses to catecholamines are reduced,[96] their myocardial depression is greater, and their baroresponse is nearly absent.[91] Because preterm infants depend primarily on increases in heart rate to maintain cardiac output, loss of baroresponses makes it difficult for them to respond to hypotension. Table 14–8 shows the heart rate and arterial pressures of preterm infants anesthetized with halothane for ligation of a patent ductus arteriosus. Note the failure to increase heart rate when the blood pressure decreased or increased.

TABLE 14–8
RELATION BETWEEN HEART RATE AND SYSTOLIC BLOOD PRESSURE IN PRETERM INFANTS ANESTHETIZED WITH HALOTHANE FOR PATENT DUCTUS ARTERIOSUS LIGATION

Condition	Heart Rate (bpm)	Systolic Pressure (mm Hg)
Preinduction	146 ± 20	62 ± 16
Before ductal ligation	143 ± 17	48 ± 16
After ductal ligation	145 ± 16	66 ± 15

To avoid problems of hypotension caused by inhaled anesthetics, we and others have used fentanyl to anesthetize preterm infants.[86, 97] The dose premature infants require is lower than that required by adults: 10 to 30 μg/kg prevents an increase in either heart rate or arterial pressure when the skin is incised, strongly suggesting that the patient is anesthetized. Hypotension is uncommon if the blood volume is adequate (this is not true when inhaled anesthetics are used). These patients may require much more fentanyl if they have received fentanyl regularly in the NICU. In this case, the dose of fentanyl must be titrated to produce the desired clinical effect. Often, more than 50 μg/kg of fentanyl will be required.

Muscle relaxants are used to prevent movement and reduce the concentrations of anesthetics, especially when morphine 0.1 mg/kg or meperidine (Demerol) 1 mg/kg is used as the primary anesthetic agent. Patients are not anesthetized with either of these drugs in these doses and are awake and paralyzed. The addition of nitrous oxide to the inspired gases significantly helps this situation, but it should be remembered that 70 percent nitrous oxide is only 0.5 MAC in term infants. It is probably greater in preterm infants. However, nitrous oxide is not without cardiovascular effects in preterm infants. It can decrease arterial pressure and can cause cardiac arrest if the patient is hypovolemic.

The ventilation of preterm infants must be controlled during surgery because these infants are incapable of effective pulmonary ventilation when anesthetized. Neonatal ventilators do not allow the administration of inhaled anesthetics. Fentanyl anesthesia avoids this problem. Also, neonatal ventilators cannot adequately compensate for the changes in compliance and resistance caused by retractors and packs. Apparently, neither can the human hand, although this study was done very artificially.[98]

The patient probably should be ventilated by hand while the anesthesiologist watches the surgical field and ensures that the chest and lungs rise with inspiration. Ventilation can be accomplished with a Jackson-Reese device,[99] which permits instantaneous compensation for changes in lung compliance and resistance. It also allows the use of PEEP. Because most neonates require PEEP in the NICU, they also require it in the operating room. The physicians and nurses in the NICU will have spent a considerable amount of time finding the ventilator settings that produce the best blood gas concentrations with the least pressure for each individual patient. These values should be used as the initial ventilation pressures, rates, and oxygen concentrations in the operating room. They should be adjusted as needed to maintain the Pao_2 between 50 and 70 mm Hg, the $Paco_2$ between 35 and 50 mm Hg, the pH between 7.30 and 7.45, and the oxygen saturation between 87 and 92 percent.[72] It is often necessary to ventilate premature infants with room air to maintain oxygen saturations in this range and to increase the inspired oxygen concentration as needed. Ventilation by hand is often more effective than with a mechanical ventilator, and this results in marked improvement of oxygen saturation.

It must be possible to provide an inspired oxygen concentration of 21 to 100 percent during surgery. If nitrous oxide is not part of the anesthetic technique, air should be used as the carrier gas and enough oxygen added to maintain the desired Pao_2 or oxygen saturation. Giving 100 percent oxygen to a preterm infant who does not need it unnecessarily exposes the baby to the risk of ROP (see above). Only by measuring the patient's Pao_2 or oxygen saturation (see Chapter 11) do we know if we are giving too much or too little oxygen. Transcutaneous Po_2 devices are adversely affected by halothane and nitrous oxide,[100] hypotension (a mean arterial pressure > 2.5 SD below normal for this patient), and hypothermia (temperature < 35.5°C). Fentanyl anesthesia causes less hypotension than inhaled agents and does not affect the transcutaneous oxygen electrode. If a transcutaneous monitor is not available, Pao_2 should be measured during the surgery.

Replacement of blood and fluid is critical in small preterm infants because their total blood volume is small (85 to 100 ml/kg). In a 1-kg infant, loss of 8 to 10 ml/kg of blood is equivalent to a 10 percent loss of blood volume. Blood loss should be replaced as it occurs.

It is difficult to determine blood losses accurately, but weighing the used sponges provides a relatively accurate measurement. A 1-mg increase in the weight of the sponge equals 1 ml of blood. Suctioned blood should be collected in a small suction bottle. Blood loss into the drapes and tissues is more difficult to estimate. To compensate, therefore, the measured losses should be increased by 25 to 50 percent and that amount of blood or an appropriate volume of crystalloid (three times the amount of blood loss) given for replacement. Adequacy of blood and fluid replacement is verified by arterial and central venous pressure and hematocrit measurements. If the hematocrit is low to begin with, blood losses are replaced with packed RBCs. Care must be taken to avoid causing polycythemia, because it interferes with tissue blood flow.

The volume of fluid administered depends on the amount of tissue trauma occurring. Abdominal or thoracic surgical procedures are more traumatic than peripheral surgical procedures and therefore require lactated Ringer's solution 8 to 12 ml/kg/h or more. Dilute saline (0.2 or 0.3 N) is not what is being lost. Its use in the operating room leads to hyponatremia and water overload.

Approximately 5 to 7 mg/kg/min (300 to 420 mg/kg/h) of glucose should be provided as long as the blood sugar concentration is less than 120 mg/dl. Giving more glucose than this to these patients often causes hyperglycemia (Table 14–9). It should be remembered that 5 percent dextrose in water contains 50 mg glucose per milliliter of fluid. Hyperglycemia can be avoided by infusing sufficient glucose to keep the blood sugar concentration normal without inducing hyperglycemia. The remaining fluid should consist of plain lactated Ringer's solution, albumin, blood, or a combination of these. IV alimentation fluid is *never* used to replace fluid losses during surgery because it is certain to cause severe hyperglycemia and possibly CNS damage. Instead, the hyperalimentation fluid should be infused at its preoperative rate and the fluid losses replaced with plain lactated Ringer's solution. Glucose concentrations should be measured repeatedly throughout long surgical procedures (e.g., with Dextrostix or Acu Check), and attempts should be made to maintain the infant's blood glucose concentration in the desired range.

The adequacy of fluid and blood replacement can be determined in several ways. First, mean arterial blood pressure is a good indicator of intravascular volume in preterm infants. A pressure more than 2 SD below normal for that age group[101] usually means that the infant is hypovolemic (Fig. 14–8). Infusing fluids usually returns the blood pressure to normal. Second, a central venous pressure (CVP) below 3 cm H_2O is indicative of hypovolemia. CVP can be measured from percutaneously inserted subclavian lines (see Chapter 11) connected to a strain gauge. A water column should not be used to measure CVP because repeated measurements may overload the infant with fluid. Third, an adequate urine output (> 0.75 mg/kg/h) is also indicative of adequate intravascular volume if there is not significant glucosuria. The urine specific gravity is usually less than 1.005. A specific gravity value greater than 1.009 usually indicates that the patient is hypovolemic (see above). Fourth, a fontanel that is below the inner table of the skull indicates volume depletion in an anesthetized infant.

Body temperature must be maintained between 36° and 37°C to avoid the postoperative complications of hypoventilation, atelectasis, respiratory and metabolic acidosis, infection, and poor feeding. This is best done by warming the operating room. IV fluids and blood should be warmed by placing the IV tubing under the heating blanket, which is set at 37° to 38°C, and leading a short tube to the catheter. Care must be taken to keep the short segment of tubing in view so that no air bubbles are infused. Even small air bubbles can be lethal if they enter the left heart and lodge in a coronary or cerebral artery. The inspired gases should be warmed and fully humidified to 35° to 37°C. The extremities should be wrapped with sheet wadding and the head should be covered with a cap to help maintain body heat.

Recovery from Anesthesia

Emergence from anesthesia can be equally as dangerous as the induction of anesthesia. There is often pressure to remove the patient from the operating room quickly so that the next case can start. This pressure must be resisted while careful preparation is made to transport the patient to the recovery area, usually the NICU. Before the patient leaves the operating room, it must be ascertained that the intensive care nurses are ready to receive and care for the patient. There is a great deal of confusion and unhappiness if the patient arrives in the NICU from the operating room while the baby's nurse is at lunch. The NICU should be called before leaving the operating room. It is better to wait in the operating room, with complete control of

---

TABLE 14–9
SERUM AND URINE GLUCOSE VALUES AND URINE VOLUME IN A 1-kg INFANT

Assay	Time (h)			
Serum glucose (mg/dl)	45–90	90	175	130
Urine glucose	1+	2+	4+	4+
Fluid intake (ml/kg/h)	4	7	15	12
Glucose infused (mg/h)	400	700	1,500	1,200

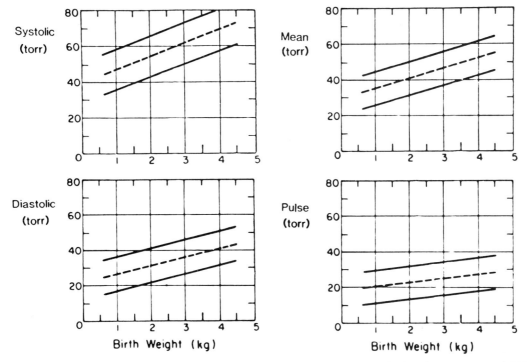

FIGURE 14-8. Systolic, diastolic, and mean arterial blood pressures and pulse pressures of infants between 610 and 4,200 g. (From Versmold HT, Kitterman JA, Phibbs RH, et al: Aortic blood pressure during the first 12 hours of life in infants with birth weight 610–4200 grams. Pediatrics 67:607, 1981, with permission.

the situation, than to stand around in the nursery or hall waiting for the nurse to return.

The infant's lungs should be ventilated on the way to the nursery. After arriving in the nursery, it can be decided whether the child requires mechanical ventilation postoperatively or whether the trachea can safely be extubated. If it is decided that the ETT can be removed (which is rare), muscle relaxants must be reversed.

Many preterm neonates who are less than 44 weeks postconceptual age develop apnea postoperatively.[102–108] Although the cause of this apnea is unknown, it may be because of persistence of small amounts of anesthetic in the CNS that alter the autonomic nervous system.[109] Or it might be related to an incompletely developed CNS.[110] Infants with postoperative apnea were usually apneic earlier in life. Postoperative apnea can occur as long as 4 hours or more after surgery.[111] Therefore, all of these patients probably should be monitored for 24 hours after surgery to detect apnea or periodic breathing. Infants who develop apnea postoperatively require mechanical ventilation for several hours to several days. Therefore, anesthesia probably should *not* be given on an outpatient basis for patients who are less than 44 weeks postconceptual age. This has been disputed in one study.[112]

Welborn and associates have demonstrated an increased incidence of apnea in patients with low hematocrits.[113] If the hematocrit was below 30 percent, 89 percent of the infants were apneic, whereas only 21 percent of those with a hematocrit above that level developed apnea.

These same authors also showed a difference in the incidence of apnea in infants anesthetized with general anesthesia and those anesthetized with spinal anesthesia.[114] There were no instances of apnea in patients in whom a spinal anesthetic was given without sedation. However, eight of nine infants premedicated with ketamine had significant apnea, and 5 of 16 infants treated with general anesthesia had postoperative apnea. Although spinal anesthesia appears to cause fewer instances of postoperative apnea,[115] there are reported cases of apnea[116] and of total spinal anesthesia occurring.[117] Kunst et al. found no difference in incidence of apnea in patients who received general or spinal anesthesia.[118] Krane et al. found that patients receiving general anesthesia were more likely to have oxygen desaturation and bradycardia than those who received a spinal anesthetic.[119] Tashiro and associates[120] found that gestational age, birth weight, postconceptual age, and use of aminophylline correlated with the need for postoperative ventilation. Kurth et al.[121] determined the incidence of apnea in two groups of premature infants. One group consisted of infants undergoing hernia repairs and the other consisted of patients undergoing other procedures. Apnea occurred in approximately one third of the patients. In group 1, the apnea was central in origin in 73 percent of patients, obstructive in 6 percent, and mixed in 21 percent. In the other group, the distribution of apnea type was very similar. Oxygen saturation below 80 percent occurred more often in patients with mixed or central apnea. Welborn et al. have shown that giving IV caffeine 5 mg/kg prevented life-threatening postoperative apnea but did not prevent lesser degrees of apnea.[122] A larger dose of caffeine also may have eliminated the latter. Even the dose used eliminated the need for mechanical ventilation and the expense of the ICU. If surgery can be delayed until the patient is more than 44 weeks postconceptual age, most postoperative apnea can be avoided. If surgery must be done before 44 weeks' gestation, giving the patient caffeine intravenously should be considered.

Anesthesia for Micropremies

There has been a marked improvement in the survival of very premature infants ("micropremies," i.e., 400 to 1,000 g at birth) over the past few years. However, these patients can require a considerable amount of surgery before they are discharged from the hospital. Of concern is the neurologic and developmental outcome of such small premature infants. Recent evidence[123, 124] suggests that 67 to 71 percent of 24- to 25-week-gestation infants are neurologically normal at 24 to 25 weeks' gestation, whereas 89 percent of those born at 26 weeks' gestation are normal (Table 14–10). An additional 22 percent of 24-week-gestation infants have suspicious neurologic examinations. Only 28 percent of neonates born at 24 weeks' gestation have normal cognitive development at 4.5 to 7 years of age. Eleven percent of 24- to 27-week gestation infants have cerebral palsy. It appears that the outcome of these infants improves markedly once they reach 26 weeks' gestation. Therefore, it is important to delay delivery of these patients until 26 weeks' gestation if possible.

The problems of micropremies are similar to those of larger babies but worse. Because they are so immature, micropremies have no true alveoli and the distance between their capillaries and their gas exchange units is larger. Therefore, gas transfer is difficult and is made worse by interstitial edema. Micropremies have more difficulty maintaining their body temperature, because of their high surface/volume ratio. They have thin, fragile skin that increases fluid loss. Taking tape or monitors off of their skin often removes the skin and leaves large weeping areas. These infants often require very high volumes of fluid (often > 200 ml/kg/day) to maintain hydration. Failure to administer sufficient fluid to them causes dehydration and hypotension. The fluid should contain sufficient glucose

to maintain the blood glucose concentration between 40 and 100 mg/dl. What the normal arterial blood pressure is for infants of 24 to 26 weeks' gestation is debatable, but it is clear that the blood pressures measured by noninvasive means often give pressures that are too high (Table 14–11). Consequently, micropremies may be hypotensive despite having noninvasive blood pressures that would be considered normal (i.e., > 32 mm Hg). Determination of normal hydration is often difficult in these patients. They have little or no subcutaneous tissue, their skin is paper thin, and their pulses are often difficult to feel. Their fontanels are, however, normal and the skin over the fontanels are normally even with the skin of the outer table of the skull. Their urine output is usually greater than 1 ml/kg/h and the specific gravity is usually 1.005 or less.

The anesthesia requirement of infants of these gestational ages is unknown. However, from previous data it appears that the MAC for halothane is less than 0.55. We usually use narcotics to provide anesthesia for these infants because their arterial pressures are more stable than with halothane (Table 14–12). They are already mechanically ventilated preoperatively and will continue to be so postoperatively. Muscle paralysis with pancuronium 0.1 mg/kg and anesthesia with fentanyl 10 to 50 μg/kg usually provides adequate anesthesia for any surgery that is required. Care must be taken to provide adequate anesthesia to avoid inducing stress responses[85] and prevent intracranial hemorrhage. Although we have shown that even small premature infants have cerebrovascular autoregulation, it is fragile and easily disrupted, which increases the likelihood of intracranial hemorrhage and central nervous system injury.

Fluid requirements for micropremies during surgery may be very high. Failure to provide the correct amount of fluid will lead to hypotension and/or shock. However, it must be remembered that the blood volume of these infants is approximately 100 ml/kg. Therefore, the blood volume of a 500-g infant is 50 ml total. A loss of 5 ml of blood is equal to 10 percent of the blood volume. Ten milliliters of fluid per kilogram is 5 ml. All fluid should be administered via pumps that can be adjusted to infuse the correct amount of fluid per hour.

Where should this surgery be done? Should it be done in the operating room or in the NICU? Many institutions have chosen to perform the surgery in the NICU. It is easier to take nurses, doctors, and technicians to the intensive care nursery than it is to take patients to the operating room. There is no evidence that performing surgery in the intensive care unit is associated with more infections than performing surgery in the operating room. By operating

TABLE 14–10
NEUROLOGIC AND DEVELOPMENTAL OUTCOME OF MICROPREMIES*†

	24 Weeks	25 Weeks	26 Weeks
No. of infants followed	18	30	38
Neurologically normal	12 (67%)	22 (73%)	34 (89%)
Neurologically suspicious	4 (22%)	2 (7%)	0
Cerebral palsy	2 (11%)	6 (20%)	4 (11%)
Normal cognitive development	5 (28%)	14 (47%)	27 (71%)
Borderline cognitive development	6 (33%)	7 (23%)	7 (18%)
Deficient cognitive development	7 (39%)	9 (30%)	4 (11%)

* Data are presented as *n* (%).
† Kruskal-Wallis $\chi^2 = 10.6542$, $p = 0.005$ for cognitive outcome and gestational age. From Piecuch RE, Leonard CH, Cooper BA, et al: Outcome of infants born at 24-26 weeks' gestation: II. Neurodevelopmental outcome. Obstet Gynecol 90:809, 1997.

TABLE 14–11
ARTERIAL BLOOD PRESSURES DETERMINED NONINVASIVELY AND FROM AN INDWELLING ARTERIAL CATHETER: COMPARISON OF CUFF AND LINE PRESSURES

Method	N	MAP	Systolic/diastolic
Cuff	15	32 ± 5	46 ± 5/22 ± 3
Line	15	26 ± 6	38 ± 4/15 ± 3

TABLE 14-12
VITAL SIGNS DURING FENTANYL AND HALOTHANE ANESTHESIA (23–30 WK GESTATION)

	Halothane				Fentanyl		
	HR	*MAP*	*CVP*		*HR*	*MAP*	*CVP*
Awake	148 ± 17	31 ± 3	4 ± 1	Awake	152 ± 17	31 ± 3	4 ± 1
0.5 MAC	138 ± 26	28 ± 4	5 ± 1	10 μg/kg	148 ± 26	30 ± 4	4 ± 1
1.0	130 ± 28	27 ± 3	5 ± 2	30 μg/kg	147 ± 13	30 ± 3	3 ± 1

in the intensive care nursery, there is no transport of the patient, no disconnecting and reconnecting of monitors, and no need to remove the patient from the mechanical ventilation he or she is receiving. Since it is not possible to provide inhaled anesthesia via neonatal ventilators, it is usually necessary to induce and maintain anesthesia with intravenous agents. If the neonate is taken to the operating room, either a neonatal ventilator must be set up and the neonate must be hand-ventilated to and from the operating room or the lungs of the baby must be ventilated continuously by hand in the operating room. If the baby is on high-frequency ventilation, it may be difficult to reproduce this type of ventilation during the transport.

COMMON SURGICAL PROBLEMS

The common surgical problems that occur in preterm infants are described elsewhere in this book. Patent ductus arteriosus is covered in Chapter 18, thoracotomy for pulmonary resection in Chapter 17, hydrocephalus in Chapter 16, and necrotizing enterocolitis and inguinal hernia in Chapter 20. The following is a case study that illustrates many of the points discussed above.

Case Study

The infant was 5 days old at the time we were asked to see him. He was born after 29 weeks' gestation and weighed 980 g at birth. On the day of surgery his weight was 840 g. He was severely asphyxiated at birth and required immediate tracheal intubation and assisted ventilation. His initial blood gas values were pH 7.00, $Paco_2$ 63 mm Hg, and Pao_2 43 mm Hg despite ventilation with 100 percent oxygen. His mean arterial blood pressure was 16 mm Hg at 5 minutes of age. Ventilation was continued, and he was given 10 ml of whole blood over 5 minutes, which brought his arterial blood pressure to a mean of 28 mm Hg. His blood gases improved after the transfusion so that by 25 minutes of age the Pao_2 was 165 mm Hg, the $Paco_2$ 33 mm Hg, and the pH 7.34. He was transferred to the NICU after the Pao_2 had been reduced to 63 mm Hg by progressively decreasing the Fio_2 to 0.67. A chest radiograph was classic for RDS.

During the next 4 days, the respiratory distress decreased and the NICU staff was able to reduce the level of assisted ventilation. On day 1 he received 5 percent dextrose in water 50 ml/kg and electrolytes. This was increased to 70 ml/kg/day thereafter. He was covered with SaranWrap to reduce evaporative heat loss and was started on ampicillin and gentamicin (Garamycin) shortly after birth because it was uncertain if sepsis was present. When the blood, urine, and CSF cultures were negative on day 3, the antibiotics were discontinued. The initial hemoglobin value was 12.5 g/dl. Because of blood sampling it decreased to 9.5 g/dl. He was transfused to increase it to 11.2 g/dl on the third day after birth.

On day 5, the infant developed abdominal distention, vomiting, and bloody stools after two attempts at feeding with breast milk. Whereas his respiratory distress had been improving, it now worsened. His ventilator rate and pressure increased. A radiograph of the abdomen showed free air in the peritoneal cavity and a diagnosis of necrotizing enterocolitis was made. At this point, he was scheduled for surgery.

A review of the records and his physical examination demonstrated the following.

Hydration

His skin was pale and mottled and failed to return to its resting position for 8 seconds after being tented up. The fontanel was sunken below the inner table of his skull. It took more than 6 seconds for the skin of his fingers and toes to fill with blood after they were blanched. His extremities were cold from the groins and axillas outward. There were no pulses in his feet or wrists and his groin pulses were markedly diminished. The pulse rate was 150 beats per minute (bpm) and the arterial pressure 40/15 mm Hg, with a mean pressure of 23 mm Hg. There had been no urine output for 6 hours and only 2 ml during the 4 hours previous to that. The specific gravity of his last urine sample was 1.028.

Chest Findings

He had bilateral rales that did not clear when the ETT was suctioned. Air entry into the upper lobes of the lungs was good but was decreased in the bases. An ETT was in place and fixed securely. The Pao_2 was 72 mm Hg, the $Paco_2$ 30 mm Hg, and the pH 7.21. His base deficit was −15 mEq/L. He was ventilated 20 times per minute with pressures of 30/5 cm H_2O.

Cardiovascular Findings

His heart rate was normal (150 bpm) and there was no murmur or gallop. The point of maximal impulse was in the fourth interspace anteriorly. His pulses were as above.

Abdominal Findings

His abdomen was grossly distended, and loops of bowel were visible through the anterior abdominal wall, which was edematous, warm, and tender. The bowel sounds were absent. The liver was not palpable but could be percussed 1 cm below the right costal margin.

Laboratory Data

His WBC count was 29,300/mm³ with a shift to the left. Fifteen percent of these cells were bands. His hemoglobin was 14.5 g/dl. Electrolytes showed a sodium concentration of 147 mEq/L, potassium concentration of 5.3 mEq/L, chloride concentration of 120 mEq/L, and bicarbonate concentration of 17 mEq/L. His serum calcium concentration was 6.3 mg/dl, and the total protein concentration was 4.5 mg/dl.

Discussions with the nurses indicated that the infant became severely cyanotic and his transcutaneous oxygen tension fell abruptly to 30 to 40 mm Hg when the ETT was disconnected for tracheal suctioning. They also pointed out that his body temperature was labile and that he required increasing amounts of exogenous heat to maintain his body temperature in the normal range.

Preoperative Preparation

On the basis of the above information, it was clear that the infant was severely intravascularly volume-depleted, although his body weight had not changed over the past 12 hours. His peripheral perfusion and arterial blood pressure were decreased. The lack of urine output for 6 hours indicated not only that the intravascular volume was decreased but also that he had more than an 80 percent chance of becoming hypotensive with the induction of anesthesia. The rise in his hemoglobin concentration also indicated intravascular volume depletion. A central venous line was inserted with local anesthesia and was connected to a strain gauge. His CVP was found to be 0 cm H₂O. Lactated Ringer's solution 10 ml/kg was infused over 15 minutes, which increased his CVP to 2 cm H₂O. Additional lactated Ringer's solution 10 ml/kg raised the CVP to 5 cm H₂O. With this increase, the peripheral perfusion improved and the mean arterial pressure rose to 32 mm Hg. His urine output increased to 2 ml/kg/h, and the specific gravity was 1.006. The amount of mechanical ventilation was decreased because the PaO₂ rose to 123 mm Hg and the PaCO₂ decreased to 18 mm Hg. His base deficit rose to −15 without bicarbonate infusion. His blood glucose was now 128 mg/dl. We infused calcium gluconate 150 mg/kg because of the hypocalcemia. Repeat determination of electrolytes showed a calcium concentration of 8.1 mg/dl, sodium concentration of 140 mEq/L, potassium concentration of 4.5 mEq/L, and chloride concentration of 115 mEq/L.

After 90 minutes of preparation, the patient was ready for surgery. He was transported to the operating room while being ventilated by hand at the same ventilatory pressures, rates, and inspired oxygen concentration used in the nursery. The operating room had been previously prepared and was 37°C. His temperature was maintained during transport to the operating room with warmed blankets, SaranWrap, and a cap. The arterial line was always visible to the anesthesiologist. His arterial blood pressure and ECG were monitored with a battery-powered monitor during transport.

Surgery

The patient was anesthetized and operated on in his intensive care bed. Anesthesia was induced with fentanyl 20 µg/kg, and he was paralyzed with pancuronium. Surgery began within 5 minutes of the patient's arrival in the operating room. The inspired oxygen was maintained at a level that kept the PaO₂ within normal limits (50 to 70 mm Hg, SaO₂ 91 to 95 percent) by using air as the carrier gas and adding oxygen as needed. Oxygenation was measured continuously with a transcutaneous oxygen monitor. Blood gases and pH were measured intermittently, as was the serum glucose (Dextrostix). The calcium concentration was determined once during the 2-hour procedure and was found to be 6.9 mg/dl. Calcium gluconate 200 mg was administered slowly through the central venous line. The blood loss was 15 ml, which was replaced with packed RBCs, bringing the hemoglobin to 15 g/dl. He received 5 percent dextrose in lactated Ringer's solution 4 ml/h and lactated Ringer's solution without glucose 6 ml/h, which maintained the blood glucose concentration and the arterial and central venous pressures within normal limits. The bowel was resected and an end-to-end anastomosis performed in addition to a diverting colostomy. Body temperature was maintained within normal limits by wrapping the extremities with sheet wadding, covering his head with a cap, warming and humidifying the inspired gases to 37°C, and warming the infused fluids. At the end of the procedure, we continued to control his ventilation during transport to the NICU. Again, he was covered with warm blankets and SaranWrap. In the nursery, his ventilation and paralysis were continued. Once we were sure that the vital signs and ventilation were adequate, his care was transferred to the NICU staff.

His condition continued to improve over the next week, and he was weaned from mechanical ventilation and fed intravascularly through the central venous line. He was discharged from the hospital at 2 months of age neurologically intact and eating well. At 4 months of age, his colostomy was closed and he has done well since.

This case illustrates how severely dehydrated such patients can be and how well they respond to fluid replacement. It also shows how stable they can become once the deficits are replaced.

REFERENCES

1. Usher RH, Allen AC, McLean FH: Risk of respiratory distress syndrome related to gestational age, route of delivery and maternal diabetes. Am J Obstet Gynecol 111:826, 1971.
2. Bland RD, McMillan DD, Bressack MA, Dong L: Clearance of liquid from lungs of newborn rabbits. J Appl Physiol 49:171, 1980.
3. Karlberg P: The adaptive changes in the immediate postnatal period with particular reference to respiration. J Pediatr 56:585, 1960.
4. Usher RH: The special problems of the premature infant. In Avery GB (ed): Neonatology. Philadelphia, JB Lippincott, 1981.

5. Lou HC, Lassen NA, Friis HB: Low cerebral blood flow in hypotensive perinatal distress. Acta Neurol Scand 56:343, 1977.

6. Lou HC, Lassen NA, Friis HB: Impaired autoregulation of cerebral blood flow in the distressed newborn infant. J Pediatr 94:118, 1979.

7. Gregory GA: Resuscitation of the newborn. Anesthesiology 43:225, 1975.

8. Lou HC, Lassen NA, Friis HB: Decreased cerebral blood flow after administration of sodium bicarbonate in the distressed newborn infant. Acta Neurol Scand 57:239, 1978.

9. Lubchenco LD, Horner FA, Reed LH, et al: Sequelae of premature birth: evaluation of premature infants of low birth weights at ten years of age. Am J Dis Child 106:101, 1963.

10. Meyers RE: Focal patterns of perinatal brain damage and their conditions of occurrence in primates. Adv Neurol 10:2, 1975.

11. LeBlanc MH, Parker CC, Vig V, et al: Fructose-1,6-bisphosphate does not ameliorate hypoxic ischemic injury to the central nervous system in the newborn pig. Crit Care Med 20:1309, 1992.

12. Sheldon RA, Partridge JC, Ferriero DM: Postischemic hyperglycemia is not protective to the neonatal rat brain. Pediatr Res 32:489, 1992.

13. Hazan J, Maag U, Chessex P: Association between hypothermia and mortality rate of premature infants—revisited. Am J Obstet Gynecol 164:111, 1991.

14. Hey EN: The relation between environmental temperature and oxygen consumption in the newborn baby. J Physiol (Lond) 200:589, 1965.

15. Bach V, Telliez F, Krim G, Libert JP: Body temperature regulation in the newborn infant: interaction with sleep and clinical implications. Neurophysiol Clin 26:379, 1996.

16. Day R: Respiratory metabolism in infancy and childhood. XXVII. Regulation of body temperature of premature infants. Am J Dis Child 65:376, 1943.

17. Hey EN, Koty G: The range of thermal insulation in the tissues of the newborn baby. J Physiol (Lond) 207:667, 1970.

18. Hey EN, Koty G: Evaporative water loss in the newborn baby. J Physiol (Lond) 200:605, 1969.

19. Bruck K: Temperature regulation in the newborn infant. Biol Neonate 3:65, 1961.

20. Silverman WA, Sinclair JC: Temperature regulation in the newborn infant. N Engl J Med 279:146, 1966.

21. Hardman MJ, Hey EN, Hull D: Energy sources of thermogenesis in the newborn rabbit. J Physiol (Lond) 201:84P, 1969.

22. Baumgart S, Engle WD, Fox WW, Polen RA: Radiant warmer power and body size as determinants of insensible water loss in the critically ill neonate. Pediatr Res 15:1495, 1981.

23. Hurgoiu V: Thermal regulation in preterm infants. Early Hum Dev 28:1, 1992.

24. D' Alesssio JG, Ramanathan J: Effects of maternal anesthesia in the neonate. Semin Perinatol 22:350, 1998.

25. Okada Y, Powis M, McEwan A, Peirro A: Fentanyl analgesia increases the incidence of postoperative hypothermia in neonates. Pediatr Surg Int 13:508, 1998.

26. Jobe A, Ikegami M: Surfactant for the treatment of respiratory distress syndrome. Ann Rev Respir Dev 136:1256, 1987.

27. Phibbs RH, Ballard RA, Clements JA, et al: Initial clinical trial of EXOSURF, a protein-free synthetic surfactant, for the prophylaxis and early treatment of hyaline membrane disease. Pediatrics 88:1, 1991.

28. Rigatto H, Brady JP: Periodic breathing and apnea in preterm infants. 1. Evidence of hypoventilation possibly due to central respiratory depression. Pediatrics 50:202, 1972.

29. Rigatto H, Brady JP: Periodic breathing and apnea in preterm infants. II. Hypoxia as a primary event. Pediatrics 50:219, 1972.

30. Miller MJ, Martin RJ: Apnea of prematurity. Clin Perinatol 19:789, 1992.

31. Bjorklund LJ, Ingimarsson J, Curstedt T, et al: Manual ventilation with a few large breaths at birth compromises the therapeutic effect of subsequent surfactant replacement in immature lambs. Pediatr Res 42:348, 1997.

32. Clyman RI: Patent ductus arteriosus: a physiologic basis for current treatment practices. In Hanson TN, McIntosh N (eds): Current Topics in Neonatology. 4th ed. Philadelphia, WB Saunders Company, 2000.

33. Lim MK, Hanretty K, Houston AB, et al: Intermittent ductal patency in healthy newborn infants: demonstration by colour Doppler flow mapping. Arch Dis Child 67:1218, 1992.

34. Kitterman JA, Edmunds LH Jr, Gregory GA, et al: Patent ductus arteriosus in premature infants: incidence, relation to pulmonary disease and management. N Engl J Med 287:473, 1972.

35. Siassi B, Blanco C, Cabal LA, Corn AG: Incidence and clinical features of patent ductus arteriosus in low birth weight infants: a perspective analysis of 150 consecutively born infants. Pediatrics 57:347, 1976.

36. McGrath RC, McGuinness GA, Way GC, et al: The silent ductus arteriosus. J Pediatr 93:110, 1978.

37. Wolfgang AK, Radtke MD: Current therapy of the patent ductus arteriosus. Curr Opin Cardiol 13:59, 1998.

38. Stevenson JG: Fluid administration in the association of patent ductus arteriosus complicating respiratory distress syndrome. J Pediatr 90:257, 1977.

39. Heymann MA, Rudolph AM, Silverman NH: Closure of the ductus arteriosus in premature infants by inhibition of prostaglandin synthesis. N Engl J Med 295:530, 1976.

40. Merritt TA, DiSessa TG, Feldman BH, et al: Closure of the patent ductus arteriosus with ligation and indomethacin: a consecutive experience. J Pediatr 93:639, 1978.

41. Berman W Jr, Dubynsky O, Whitman V, et al: Digoxin therapy in low birth weight infants with patent ductus arteriosus. J Pediatr 93:652, 1978.

42. Burke RP, Jacobs JP, Cheng W, et al: Video-assisted thoracoscopic surgery for patent ductus arteriosus in low birth weight neonates and infants. Pediatrics 104:227, 1999.

43. Kitterman JA: Effects of intestinal ischemia in necrotizing enterocolitis in the newborn infant. In Moore TD (ed): Report of the Sixty-Eighth Ross Conference on Pediatric Research. Columbus, OH, Ross Laboratories, 1975, p 38.

44. Spector SA, Ticknor W, Grossman M: Study of the usefulness of clinical and hematologic findings in the diagnosis of neonatal bacterial infections. Clin Pediatr 20:285, 1981.

45. Avery GB (ed): Neonatology. 4th ed. Philadelphia, JB Lippincott, 1994.

46. Albanese CT, Rowe MI: Necrotizing enterocolitis. Semin Pediatr Surg 4:200, 1995.

47. Snyder CL, Gittes GK, Murphy JP, et al: Survival after necrotizing enterocolitis in infants weighing less than 1,000 g: 25 years' experience at a single institution. J Pediatr Surg 32:434, 1997.

48. Kabeer A, Gunnlaugsson S, Coren C: Neonatal necrotizing enterocolitis. A 12-year review at a county hospital. Dis Colon Rectum 38:866, 1995.

49. Phibbs RH, Shannon KM, Mentzer WC: Potential for treatment of anemia of prematurity with recombinant human erythropoietin: preliminary results. Acta Haematol 1:28, 1992.

50. Nelson N, Finnstrom O, Larsson L: Plasma ionized calcium, phosphate and magnesium in preterm and small for gestational age infants. Acta Paediatr Scand 78:351, 1989.

51. LeBlanc MH, Huang MH, Patel D, et al: Glucose affects severity of hypoxic ischemic brain injury in piglets. Pediatr Res 33:2212, 1993.

52. Sheldon RA, Partridge JC, Ferriero DM: Postischemic hyperglycemia is not protective to the neonatal rat brain. Pediatr Res 32:489, 1992.

53. Watchko JF, Oski FA: Kernicterus in preterm newborns: past, present and future. Pediatrics 90:707, 1992.

54. Gourley GR: Bilirubin metabolism and kernicterus. Adv Pediatr 44:173, 1997.

55. Gartner LM, Snyder RN, Choban S, et al: Kernicterus: high incidence in premature infants with low serum bilirubin concentrations. Pediatrics 45:906, 1970.

56. Palmer EA, Flynn JT, Hardy RJ, et al: Incidence and early course of retinopathy of prematurity. Ophthalmology 98:1628, 1991.

57. Purohit DM, Ellison RC, Zierler S, et al: Risks of retrolental fibroplasia: experience with 3,025 premature infants. Pediatrics 76:339, 1985.

58. Lucey JF, Dongman B: A re-examination of the role of oxygen in retrolental fibroplasia. Pediatrics 73:82, 1984.

59. Ashton N: Oxygen and the growth and development of retinal vessels. Am J Ophthalamol 62:412, 1966.

60. Avery GB, Glass P: Retinopathy of prematurity: what causes it? Clin Perinatol 15:917, 1988.

61. Phelps DL: Retinopathy of prematurity. Pediatr Clin North Am 40:705, 1993.

62. Kretzer FL, Mehta RS, Brown ES, Mintz HH: The pathogenesis of retinopathy of prematurity as it relates to surgical treatment. Doc Ophthalmol 74:205, 1990.

63. Muller DP: Vitamin E therapy in retinopathy of prematurity. Eye 6:221, 1992.
64. Johnson L, Quinn GE, Abbasi S, et al: Effect of sustained pharmacologic vitamin E levels on incidence and severity of retinopathy of prematurity: a controlled clinical trial. J Pediatr 114:827, 1989.
65. Phelps DL, Rosenbaum AL, Isenberg SL, et al: Tocopherol efficacy and safety for preventing retinopathy of prematurity: a randomized, controlled, double-masked trial. Pediatrics 79:489, 1987.
66. Finer NN, Peters KL, Hayek Z, Merel CL: Vitamin E and necrotizing enterocolitis. Pediatrics 73:387, 1984.
67. Johnson L, Bowen FW, Abbasi S, et al: Relationship of prolonged pharmacological serum levels of vitamin E to incidence of sepsis and necrotizing enterocolitis in infants with birth weight 1,500 gram or less. Pediatrics 75:619, 1985.
68. The Committee for the Classification of Retinopathy of Prematurity: an international classification of retinopathy of prematurity. Arch Ophthalmol 102:1130, 1984.
69. Hunter DG, Mukai S: Retinopathy of prematurity: pathogenesis, diagnosis, and treatment. Int Ophthalmol Clin 32:163, 1992.
70. Palmer EA: Results of U.S. randomized clinical trial of cryotherapy for ROP (CRYO-ROP). Doc Ophthalmol 74:245, 1990.
71. Kingham JD: Acute retrolental fibroplasia. Arch Ophthalmol 95:38, 1977.
72. Wasunna A, Whitelaw AGL: Pulse oximetry in preterm infants. Arch Dis Child 62:957, 1987.
73. Pryds O, Greisen G, Skov LL, Friis HB: Carbon dioxide-related changes in cerebral blood volume and cerebral blood flow in mechanically ventilated preterm neonates: comparison of near infrared spectrophotometry and ^{133}Xenon clearance. Pediatr Res 27:445, 1990.
74. Lou HC, Lassen NA, Friis-Hansen B: Is arterial hypertension crucial for the development of cerebral haemorrhage in premature infants. Lancet 1:1215, 1979.
75. Perkin RM, Levin DL, Clark R: Serum salicylate levels and right-to-left ductus shunts in newborn infants with persistent pulmonary hypertension. J Pediatr 96:721, 1980.
76. Peabody JL, Gregory GA, Willis MM, et al: Failure of conventional monitoring to detect apnea resulting from hypoxemia. Birth Defects 15:275, 1979.
77. Pape KE, Armstrong DL, Fitzhardinge PM: Central nervous system pathology associated with mask ventilation in very low birth weight infants: a new etiology—intracerebellar hemorrhage. Pediatrics 58:473, 1976.
78. Gregory GA: Respiratory care of the child. Crit Care Med 8:582, 1980.
79. Wilkinson AR, Phibbs RH, Gregory GA: Continuous in vivo oxygen saturation in newborn infants with pulmonary disease: a new fiberoptic catheter oximeter. Crit Care Med 7:232, 1979.
80. Graff TD, Benson DW: Systematic and pulmonary water changes with inhaled humid atmospheres: clinical applications. Anesthesiology 30:1, 1969.
81. Wu PY, Hodgman JE: Insensible water loss in preterm infants: changes with postnatal development and non-ionizing radiant energy. Pediatrics 54:704, 1974.
82. Sola A, Gregory GA: Colloid oncotic pressure of normal newborns and preterm infants. Crit Care Med 9:568, 1981.
83. Bhat R, Javed S, Malais L, Vidyasagar D: Critical care problems in neonates: colloid osmotic pressure in healthy and sick neonates. Crit Care Med 9:563, 1981.
84. Hathaway WE: The bleeding newborn. Semin Hematol 12:175, 1975.
85. Anand KJS, Sippell WG, Aynsley-Green A: Randomized trial of fentanyl anaesthesia in preterm babies undergoing surgery: effects on the stress response. Lancet 1:243, 1987.
86. Robinson SR, Gregory GA: Fentanyl-air oxygen anesthesia for ligation of patent ductus arteriosus in preterm infants. Anesth Analg 60:504, 1981.
87. Gregory GA: The baroresponses of preterm infants during halothane anesthesia. Can Anaesth Soc J 29:105, 1982.
88. LeDez KM, Lerman J: The minimum alveolar concentration (MAC) of isoflurane in neonates. Anesthesiology 67:301, 1987.
89. Nicodemus HF, Nassiri-Rahimi C, Bachman L, Smith TC: Median effective dose of halothane in adults and children. Anesthesiology 31:344, 1969.
90. Friesen RH, Henry DB: Cardiovascular changes in preterm neonates receiving isoflurane, halothane, fentanyl, and ketamine. Anesthesiology 64:238, 1986.
91. Duncan P, Gregory GA, Wade J: The effect of nitrous oxide on the baroreceptor response of newborn and adult rabbits. Can Anaesth Soc J 28:339, 1981.
92. Murat I, Levron J-C, Berg A, Saint-Maurice C: Effect of fentanyl on baroreceptor reflex control of heart rate in newborn infants. Anesthesiology 68:717, 1988.
93. Vidyasagar D, Raju TNK, Chiang J: Clinical significance of monitoring anterior fontanel pressure in sick neonates and children. Pediatrics 62:996, 1978.
94. Lerman J, Robinson S, Willis MM, Gregory GA: Anesthetic requirements for halothane in young children 0–1 month and 1–6 months of age. Anesthesiology 59:421, 1983.
95. Gregory GA, Eger EIF II, Munson E: The relationship between age and anesthetic requirement in man. Anesthesiology 30:488, 1969.
96. Buckley NM, Gootman PM, Reddy GD: Age-dependent cardiovascular effects of afferent stimulation of neonatal pigs. Biol Neonate 30:268, 1976.
97. Koehntop DE, Rodman JH, Brundage DM, et al: Pharmacokinetics of fentanyl in neonates. Anesth Analg 65:227, 1986.
98. Spears RJ, Yeh A, Fisher DM, Zwass MS: The "educated hand." Can anesthesiologists assess changes in neonatal pulmonary compliance manually? Anesthesiology 75:693, 1991.
99. Inkster JS: The T-piece technique in anaesthesia: an investigation into the inspired gas concentrations. Br J Anaesth 28:512, 1956.
100. Gothgen I, Jacobsen E: Transcutaneous oxygen tension measurements. II. The influence of halothane and hypotension. Acta Anaesth Scand Suppl 67:71, 1978.
101. Versmold HT, Kitterman JA, Phibbs RH, et al: Aortic blood pressure during the first 12 hours of life in infants with birth weight 610–4200 grams. Pediatrics 67:607, 1981.
102. Steward DJ: Preterm infants are more prone to complications following minor surgery than are term infants. Anesthesiology 56:304, 1982.
103. Liu LMP, Cote CJ, Goudsouzian NG, et al: Life-threatening apnea in infants recovering from anesthesia. Anesthesiology 59:506, 1983.
104. Welborn LG, Ramirez N, Oh TH, et al: Postanesthetic apnea and periodic breathing in infants. Anesthesiology 65:658, 1986.
105. Welborn LG, Greenspun JC: Anesthesia and apnea. Perioperative considerations in the former preterm infant. Pediatr Clin North Am 41:181, 1994.
106. Sims C, Johnson CM: Postoperative apnea in infants. Anaesth Intensive Care 22:40, 1994.
107. Poets CF, Samuels MP, Southall DP: Epidemiology and pathophysiology of apnoea of prematurity. Biol Neonate 65:211, 1994.
108. Calhoun LK: Pharmacologic management of apnea of prematurity. J Perinat Neonatal Nurs 9:56, 1996.
109. Wear R, Robinson S, Gregory GA: The effect of halothane on the baroresponse of adult and baby rabbits. Anesthesiology 56:188, 1982.
110. Henderson-Smart D, Pettigrew AG, Campbell DJ: Clinical apnea and brain stem neural function in preterm infants. N Engl J Med 308:353, 1983.
111. Allen GS, Cox CS, White N, et al: Postoperative respiratory complications in ex-premature infants after inguinal herniorrhaphy. J Pediatr Surg 33:1095, 1998.
112. Melone JH, Schwartz MZ, Tyson KR, et al: Outpatient inguinal herniorrhaphy in premature infants: is it safe? J Pediatr Surg 27:203, 1992.
113. Welborn LG, Hannallah RS, Luban NL, et al: Anemia and postoperative apnea in former preterm infants. Anesthesiology 74:1003, 1991.
114. Welborn LG, Rice LJ, Hannallah RS, et al: Postoperative apnea in former preterm infants: prospective comparison of spinal and general anesthesia. Anesthesiology 72:838, 1990.
115. Veverka TJ, Henry DN, Milroy MJ, et al: Spinal anesthesia reduces the hazard of apnea in high-risk infants. Am J Surg 57:531, 1991.
116. Cox RG, Goresky GV: Life-threatening apnea following spinal anesthesia in former premature infants. Anesthesiology 73:345, 1990.
117. Desparmet JF: Total spinal anesthesia after caudal anesthesia in an infant. Anesth Analg 70:665, 1990.
118. Kunst G, Linderkamp O, Holle R, et al: The proportion of high risk preterm infants with postoperative apnea and bradycardia is the same after general and spinal anesthesia. Can J Anaesth 46:94, 1999.
119. Krane EJ, Haberkern CM, Jacobson LE: Postoperative apnea, brady-

cardia and oxygen desaturation in formerly premature infants: prospective comparison of spinal and general anesthesia. Anesth Analg 80:7, 1995.

120. Tashiro C, Matsui Y, Nakano S, et al: Respiratory outcome in extremely premature infants following ketamine anaesthesia. Can J Anaesth 38:287, 1991.

121. Kurth CD, LeBard SE: Association of postoperative apnea, airway obstruction, and hypoxemia in former premature infants. Anesthesiology 75:22, 1991.

122. Welborn LG, De Soto H, Hannallah RS, et al: The use of caffeine in the control of postanesthetic apnea in former premature infants. Anesthesiology 68:796, 1988.

123. Kilpatrick SJ, Schluetter MA, Piecuch R, et al: Outcome of infants born at 24–26 weeks' gestation: I. survival and cost. Obstet Gynecol 90:803, 1997.

124. Piecuch RE, Leonard CH, Cooper BA, et al: Outcome of infants born at 24–26 weeks' gestation: II. neurodevelopmental outcome. Obstet Gynecol 90:809, 1997.

15

Anesthesia for the Expremature Infant

LAURA SIEDMAN

◆   ◆   ◆

The expremature child is a relatively recent addition to the already diverse population of patients cared for by pediatric anesthesiologists. Over the past three decades, greater numbers of premature babies of decreasing gestational age and birth weight have survived because of advances in neonatal intensive care and obstetrics. The use of exogenous surfactant and high-frequency ventilation for the treatment of respiratory distress syndrome has substantially reduced the high morbidity and mortality caused by lung immaturity in this population.[1, 2] The increased survival of premature neonates has produced a population of babies who are susceptible to a plethora of unique diseases and a host of potential anesthetic challenges.

Prematurity is defined as a gestational age less than 37 weeks from the last menstrual period. "Premies" may be further divided into borderline prematurity (36 to 37 weeks' gestation), moderate prematurity (31 to 36 weeks' gestation), and severe prematurity (24 to 30 weeks' gestation). Although borderline premies and moderate premies may suffer from temperature instability, feeding difficulties, and respiratory distress syndrome, these problems are generally short-lived and relatively mild in these 1,500-to 2,500-g babies. Severely premature infants weighing between 500 and 1,500 g, however, constitute a medically fragile population with numerous and often life–threatening physiologic derangements of multiple organ systems. Some of these include respiratory distress syndrome (RDS) with resultant difficulties in oxygenation and

ventilation, apnea and bradycardia, intraventricular hemorrhage (IVH), necrotizing enterocolitis (NEC), and congestive heart failure secondary to a patent ductus arteriosus (PDA) and chronic lung disease (CLD). These and other conditions often require these tiny babies to undergo early surgical intervention (e.g., PDA ligation, bowel resection, ventriculoperitoneal [VP] shunt placement). As these babies mature, they often require anesthesia for a host of operations and procedures (e.g., herniorrhaphy, stoma closure, VP shunt revision, magnetic resonance imaging). These procedures are performed in babies who are still "at risk" because of chronic lung disease, a propensity for apnea, and chronic anemia. Although these babies are generally bigger and more medically stable than the acutely ill premature neonates, they remain a complicated and often challenging subset of pediatric patients. This chapter focuses on that subset of patients who have survived the early challenges of extreme prematurity and are greater than 38 weeks' postconceptual age (PCA), a population known as the formerly premature or "expremie."

OUTCOME OF PREMATURE INFANTS

Many expremies suffer from chronic medical problems that extend well into childhood and adulthood. A series of outcome studies of premature infants born at 24 to 26 weeks' gestation shows that the severity of disabilities in later life correlates with the degree of prematurity.[3, 4] Many of these deficits have anesthetic implications, both physical and psychological (Table 15–1). Special attention must be paid to the physical and developmental limitations of these children. Psychological preparation and anesthesia induction techniques, including premedication, must be tailored to the neurodevelopmental stage of the child rather than to the chronologic age of the expremie.

Pulmonary Disease in the Expremie

Bronchopulmonary Dysplasia

Premature infants are at risk for RDS, which is also called hyaline membrane disease. Respiratory distress syndrome consists of a constellation of pulmonary changes that result from the increase in alveolar surface tension caused by a lack of surfactant. This lack of surfactant leads to alveolar collapse, a reduction in functional residual capacity (FRC), intrapulmonary shunting, and hyaline membrane formation. The highly compliant chest wall of the premature infant offers little resistance against the elastic recoil of the lungs; therefore, at the end of expiration, small airways collapse and lung volume approaches residual volume, further contributing to atelectasis. Atelectasis, hyaline membrane formation, and interstitial edema combine to reduce pulmonary compliance and necessitate the use of supplemental oxygen and positive pressure ventilation. This constellation of intrapulmonary shunting from atelectasis, plus an increase in physiologic dead space and an increased work of breathing, eventually give rise to insufficient alveolar ventilation and hypercarbia.

The severity of RDS has been reduced in the last few decades through maternal steroid administration and routine administration of exogenous surfactant to neonates of less than 28 weeks' gestation. More sophisticated ventilator technology, including high-frequency ventilation and an increased awareness of the long-term effects of hyperoxia and barotrauma on the premature lung, has also improved pulmonary outcome. The incidence and severity of RDS is inversely proportional to gestational age, although about 5 percent of infants with RDS are full-term infants.

Severe RDS requiring prolonged exposure to high concentrations of inspired oxygen and barotrauma from positive-pressure ventilation may give rise to pulmonary interstitial emphysema, a bullous disease of the lung that may progress to pneumomediastinum and/or pneumothorax. Chronic lung disease may then ensue. Bronchopulmonary dysplasia (BPD) is commonly defined as the need for supplemental oxygen beyond 30 days of life. BPD is a combination of pulmonary parenchymal and interstitial changes resulting from the effects of oxygen therapy and positive-pressure ventilation on the premature lung. It includes interstitial fibrosis, lobar emphysema, and components of reactive airway disease and may render the baby oxygen, steroid, or ventilator dependent. With progressive disease, BPD may lead to pulmonary hypertension and right heart failure. The treatment of BPD is supportive. The goals of therapy are to minimize the inspired oxygen concentration (Fio_2) and mean airway pressure, reduce the amount of lung water with diuretics, and to support cardiac contractility with inotropic agents (e.g., digoxin) when needed. For those infants who survive their BPD, the long-term sequelae include chronic reactive airways disease, structural and functional (i.e., tracheomalacia) abnormalities of the trachea from prolonged intubation or tracheostomy, and failure to thrive because of the tremendous metabolic cost of the increased work of breathing.

Though most apparent chronic lung disease subsides by the age of 2 years, infants with moderate to severe BPD continue to have moderately decreased vital capacity until age 3, and lower airway obstruction may persist well beyond age 3. FRC and forced vital capacity (FVC) tend to normalize during early childhood as alveolar formation and lung volume growth proceed. Residual volume (RV), however, tends to remain elevated because of air trapping well into later childhood.[5] The pattern of obstruction seems to be different from that of asthmatics. The airway hyperreactivity associated with BPD occurs primarily in small, peripheral airways, whereas the hyperreactivity associated with asthma occurs in the larger central airways.[6] Pulmonary reserve in patients with BPD may be limited. Consequently, careful consideration must be given to the potential consequences of anesthetizing expremies who have had recent upper respiratory infections, even when these children are much older.

Apnea and Control of Respiration

One impediment to discharge from the neonatal intensive care unit for many premature babies is the persistence of apnea and bradycardia. Some expremies go home with continuous cardiorespiratory monitoring and instructions to parents for neonatal resuscitation. Central stimulants such as theophylline and caffeine are often used to reduce the frequency and severity of apnea of prematurity. During the preoperative consultation, information must be sought about the occurrence of apnea because the presence of ongoing apnea alerts the anesthesiologist to the possibility

	24 Weeks	25 Weeks	26 Weeks
T A B L E 1 5 – 1 **OUTCOME OF PREMATURITY**			
Survival*	43%	74%	83%
No. of infants followed	18	30	38
Chronic lung disease	6 (33%)	5 (17%)	3 (8%)
IVH ≥ grade 3	2 (11%)	7 (23%)	4 (10%)
Neurologic			
Normal	12 (67%)	22 (73%)	34 (89%)
Suspicious	4 (22%)	2 (7%)	0
Cerebral palsy	2 (11%)	6 (20%)	4 (11%)
Cognitive development			
Normal	5 (28%)	14 (47%)	27 (71%)
Borderline	6 (33%)	7 (23%)	7 (18%)
Deficient	7 (39%)	9 (30%)	4 (11%)

* Of 138 nonanomalous newborns between 1990–1994 including stillbirths and nonresuscitated infants.
Adapted from Piecuch RE, Leonard CH, Cooper BA, et al: Outcome of infants born at 24-26 weeks' gestation: II. Neurodevelopmental outcome. Obstet Gynecol 90:809, 1997.

that the baby may develop postoperative apnea and require mechanical ventilation.

Central apnea of infancy is defined as the cessation of breathing for greater than 15 seconds, or less if it is associated with bradycardia, cyanosis, or pallor.[7, 8] Whereas apnea is rare in full-term neonates, up to 55 percent of preterm infants are affected.[8] The incidence of apnea of prematurity is inversely related to gestational age.

Control of respiration occurs via two sets of chemoreceptors, central (medullary) and peripheral (aortic and carotid bodies). The central chemoreceptors respond to changes in hydrogen ion concentration in the cerebrospinal fluid (CSF). Since CO_2 readily crosses the blood-brain barrier, respiratory acidosis stimulates the central chemoreceptors. In adults, the resultant increase in minute ventilation is linear. Each 1 mm Hg rise in $Paco_2$ causes a 2- to 3-L/min increase in minute ventilation up to a $Paco_2$ of 9 to 10 percent (68 to 76 mm Hg), where it begins to decrease.[9] Neonates also increase minute ventilation in response to an increase in $Paco_2$, but to a lesser extent. They are capable of increasing their minute ventilation three to four times baseline, whereas older children can increase it 10- to 20-fold. The slope of the CO_2 response curve increases with both gestational and postnatal age, but is independent of postconceptual age. Full-term infants have a much more robust response to increases in $Paco_2$ than premature infants during the first days of life. By the end of 1 month of age, the response to CO_2 in infants approaches that of an adult.[10]

Peripheral chemoreceptors are primarily responsible for an increase in ventilation in response to hypoxemia. The premature neonate's response to hypoxemia is even more profoundly affected than is its response to CO_2. Carotid body receptors remain relatively insensitive for the first few days of life because they are "set" for an in utero Pao_2 of 25 mm Hg. The sensitivity to Pao_2 increases to about 50 mm Hg at a few hours of life and to 70 mm Hg at a few days of life. Thus the relative hyperoxemia in the early postnatal period reduces responsiveness of the carotid bodies. Moderate to severe hypoxemia significantly increases ventilation in all patient populations, except newborns, and in particular premature newborn infants. Neonates show a biphasic response to hypoxemia. There is an initial short period of hyperventilation that is followed by sustained hypoventilation or apnea.[11] Sustained hyperventilation occurs by 3 weeks of age in full-term infants, much like that of adults. Premature infants, however, may have an initial increase in ventilation from the effect of peripheral chemoreceptors, but the central receptors remain depressed for longer periods of time, which contributes to subsequent hypoventilation or apnea.

Mechanoreceptors, located in the upper airway, lungs, and chest also play a role in the ventilatory response to stimuli. Pulmonary stretch receptors in the smooth muscle of the airway are activated during lung inflation to inhibit inspiratory activity. This so-called Hering-Breuer reflex is increased in premature infants.[12] Irritant receptors present on the surface of the airway epithelium respond to histamine, prostaglandins, irritant gases, and inhalation anesthetics and result in sneezing, coughing, or bronchoconstriction. Activation of laryngeal afferent nerves may cause coughing, apnea, or alterations in respiratory pattern. As infants mature, the central response to inhibitory input decreases and the response to stimulatory input increases, which modulates the frequency and intensity of the intrinsic respiratory rhythm. Some stimuli, such as small amounts of fluid in the hypopharynx (as may occur with gastroesophageal reflux) are potent inhibitors of breathing in preterm babies. Superior laryngeal nerve stimulation causes reflex inhibition of ventilation. Proprioceptors in the chest wall may inhibit the intercostophrenic pathway and cause airway obstruction and apnea.[13] Other factors that play a role in apnea of prematurity are hypothermia, hypoglycemia, anemia, and sepsis.

Henderson-Smart et al. demonstrated that auditory brainstem conduction time increases as gestational age decreases. The increase in conduction time correlated with an increase in frequency of apneic episodes; consequently, they concluded that apnea is probably related to immature brain stem function.[14]

Another factor implicated in the etiology of apnea of prematurity is the relative lack of type 1 muscle fibers in the premature baby's diaphragm. Up until 30 weeks' gestation, the diaphragm has about 10 percent type 1 fibers, the high oxidative fibers that are resistant to fatigue. Full-term babies have about 25 percent type 1 fibers and adults about 55 percent. The number of type 1 fibers in the intercostal muscles also increase with gestational and postnatal age, from 19 percent at less than 37 weeks' PCA to 46 percent at term and 65 percent after 48 weeks' PCA. This lack of type 1 fibers may predispose premature babies to fatigue and apnea, particularly during periods of stress. Conditions such as atelectasis or pain, which cause tachypnea, may contribute to the fatigue of these muscles in the postoperative period.[15, 16]

Gastrointestinal Disease

NEC is an intestinal disease found nearly exclusively in premature infants. It has a multifactorial etiology including gut ischemia, bacterial translocation across an immature gut wall, and a susceptible host. The occurrence of NEC typically coincides with the onset of enteral feeding. The usual age of onset for NEC is between 10 days and 2 weeks of life. The initial signs of NEC include abdominal distention, gastric residuals of previous feeds, occult blood in the stool, and periumbilical discoloration. A sepsis-like picture then ensues, which includes instability of temperature and blood glucose levels, reduced white blood cell count, and evidence of disseminated intravascular coagulation. There is evidence of pneumatosis intestinalis on abdominal radiograph. Broad-spectrum antibiotics and discontinuation of enteral feeding are the mainstay of therapy at this stage. However, if there is evidence of portal air or bowel perforation and free air on an abdominal radiograph, surgical intervention is required. The entire bowel may be involved or only a small segment of bowel may be affected. Bowel resection and stoma creation is the usual operation performed and requires that the infant return to the operating room at a later date to close the stoma or to resect the stricture. Strictures that result from bowel obstructions may follow NEC after medical treatment or they may occur when marginally viable bowel is left at the time of the initial operation. Extensive bowel resection, especially that which involves the ileocecal valve, may leave the child with short gut syndrome and unable to absorb sufficient calories and nutrients to meet requirements for growth. These patients may present for the insertion of indwelling central venous access catheters to allow the administration of total parenteral nutrition (TPN). Hepatic dysfunction from chronic TPN may complicate the anesthetic management in this subset of expremies because of the presence of a coagulopathy or ascites.

Even in the absence of severe intestinal disease, expremies typically remain small for age until they are 18 to 24 months of age, when they catch up to former full-term babies. Frequently, however, premature infants fail to thrive because they do not receive sufficient calories to compensate for the increased work associated with residual lung disease, or they have inadequate oral intake because of feeding difficulties including oral aversion, malabsorption, gastroesophageal reflux disease (GERD), and neurologic disease. This may necessitate the insertion of a gastrostomy tube, or if GERD is problematic, an antireflux operation (fundoplication) may be required.

Neurologic Disease

Intraventricular hemorrhage (IVH) is common in premature infants and is graded from 1 through 4 depending on the severity of the hemorrhage. A grade 1 IVH occurs in the germinal matrix of the subependymal areas of the brain. A grade 2 hemorrhage extends into the ventricle but causes no hydrocephalus. A grade 3 hemorrhage extends into the ventricles and is associated with hydrocephalus. A grade 4 IVH includes intraparenchymal bleeding plus blood in the ventricles and hydrocephalus. A grade 4 hemorrhage portends an adverse neurologic outcome. The obstructive hydrocephalus associated with grades 3 and 4 IVH usually requires lifelong CSF shunting. Expremies with shunt malfunctions or obstructions may present at any age for shunt revisions. The presence of increased intracranial pressure secondary to shunt obstruction must be addressed both preoperatively and intraoperatively. All patients with a VP shunt should receive prophylactic antibiotics intraoperatively.

The neurodevelopmental sequelae of prematurity are difficult to delineate. Cerebral palsy (CP) may occur in as many as 20 to 25 percent of very premature infants and may be limited to heelcord spasticity that is amenable to surgical correction, or the child may have severe motor and cognitive deficits.[3] These patients often present formidable problems with regard to positioning because of contractures of major joints. Consequently, care must be taken to prevent injuring the extremities by hyperextending them during the placement of intravenous lines or during positioning. Careful padding of bony prominences must be done to prevent ulcerations of the skin in these frequently cachectic patients. Patients with cerebral palsy may have severe scoliosis that may cause restrictive lung disease and compound the obstructive lung disease associated with prematurity.

Retinopathy of prematurity (ROP) may occur as a consequence of severe prematurity. The need for an increased inspired oxygen concentration, can elevate PaO_2 and retinal artery oxygen concentrations above normal, a factor long associated with the etiology of ROP. Otherwise normal low-birth-weight infants have a mean PaO_2 of 60 ± 8 mm Hg at 3 hours of age when breathing room air. This increases to 78 ± 16 mm Hg at 3 days and remains there for the first month of life. This is a hyperoxic state. The normal fetus of the same gestational age should have a PaO_2 of 30 to 40 mm Hg in utero. Consequently, premature infants may develop ROP at these relatively low PaO_2 levels. The retinal vasculature at the periphery of the temporal side of the retina is at risk for injury from oxygen until about 44 weeks' PCA.[17] ROP may necessitate laser therapy or vitrectomy in the expremie and in severe cases may lead to profound visual impairment or blindness.

Inguinal Hernia

Approximately 30 percent of premature neonates have inguinal hernias. Only 3 to 5 percent of full-term newborns have inguinal hernias.[18] Twenty percent of inguinal hernias are bilateral in premature infants. The repair of these hernias may be very difficult because the sac is friable and the hernias are often very large. The timing of repair is variable. If the hernia is very large and the baby is being mechanically ventilated, repair is often performed before tracheal extubation, since reduction of the hernia and the anesthetic often provide a temporary need for increased ventilation. Alternatively, inguinal hernias may be repaired shortly before discharge from the hospital to allow the neonate to be monitored in the neonatal intensive care unit for postoperative apnea. Still other infants are readmitted from home shortly after discharge for the repair of their hernias. The benefits of performing "elective" herniorrhaphy to prevent incarceration of the hernia must be weighed against the risks of apnea and general or regional anesthesia. Each expremie's chronic physiologic status must be evaluated and taken into account before anesthesia and herniorrhaphy are undertaken.

ANESTHETIC MANAGEMENT OF THE EXPREMIE

The Patient with Chronic Lung Disease

When providing general anesthesia for infants with BPD, it is important to know the baseline oxygen saturation, the current inspired oxygen concentration, whether the child has bullous lung disease, and the current drug therapy. The FIO_2 should be adjusted to maintain the oxygen saturation at baseline levels. Depending on the infant's age at operation, the oxygen saturation may be kept as low as 88 to 92 percent in an attempt to prevent further lung damage and further retinal injury. Severe lung disease and bullous disease preclude the use of nitrous oxide (N_2O) because the use of N_2O may cause a pneumothorax if N_2O diffuses into and expands and ruptures the blebs. Chronic diuretic therapy, particularly furosemide, is commonly used in this patient population and may deplete the intravascular volume, cause hypokalemia and hypochloremia, and induce a contraction alkalosis. Despite the contracted blood volume, fluid administration should be judicious to avoid increasing interstitial pulmonary edema. β-Agonists and steroids are often used to minimize the reactive and inflammatory components of the disease. These drugs should be continued or augmented up until the time of surgery, and steroids may have to be supplemented to compensate for the suppressed adrenal production of steroids that is caused by chronic steroid administration.

The anesthesiologist must be aware that infants with BPD and prolonged tracheal intubation may have wheezing or stridor caused by tracheo- or bronchomalacia and/or increased airway reactivity. Airway obstruction secondary to tracheomalacia may be exacerbated by increased or turbulent airflow as occurs during crying or pain.[19] Analgesics and changes in patient position, particularly to the prone position, may ameliorate symptoms in the postoperative period.

Prolonged tracheal intubation of premature infants may cause laryngeal injuries or subglottic stenosis. Consequently, it may be necessary to use endotracheal tubes (ETTs) smaller than appropriate for age-matched full-term infants. Diligence must be exercised in checking for an air leak after tracheal intubation to avoid causing edema in the already narrowed trachea. A leak of gas from around the ETT at inspiratory pressures of less than 20 cm H_2O is ideal. Laryngeal mask airways (LMA) have been used for the second stage of the open-sky vitrectomy for the treatment of ROP in expremies with BPD. Although patients for whom the LMA was used had a higher respiratory rate and end-tidal CO_2, heart rate, and blood pressure, the incidence of postoperative pulmonary complications (including coughing and oxygen desaturation) were lower than in intubated patients. No episodes of oxygen desaturation occurred in either the group with LMAs or the intubated group.[20] This suggests that it may be acceptable and prudent to use LMAs in expremies for short surgical procedures, particularly when coughing or bucking may be deleterious (e.g., eye surgery or in patients who have subglottic stenosis).

Anemia in the Expremie

Healthy full-term neonates have higher hematocrits (50 to 55 percent) than older children and adults. Within the first week of life, the hemoglobin concentration begins to decrease. Erythropoiesis abruptly declines as the postnatal oxygen saturation increases. Erythropoietin concentrations decrease and red blood cells (RBCs) containing fetal hemoglobin decrease because of their diminished life span. The increase in blood volume that accompanies the large weight gain characteristic of the first few months of extrauterine life leads to an apparent decrease in hematocrit.[21] This "physiologic nadir" usually occurs at 2 to 3 months of life.

The premature infant undergoes similar changes in hematocrit, but in an exaggerated fashion. The hemoglobin concentration is often as low as 7 to 9 g/dl by 6 weeks of age. However, this nadir frequently occurs at an even earlier age because of frequent phlebotomy. As fetal hemoglobin is replaced by adult hemoglobin, the affinity of the hemoglobin for oxygen is reduced (P_{50} of 19 mm Hg in the newborn vs. 30 mm Hg in the infant vs. 27 mm Hg in the adult).[22] Therefore, neonates, particularly premature

neonates, have a very high affinity of hemoglobin for oxygen because of the reduced P_{50}. Consequently, with the same hematocrit less oxygen is delivered to the tissues. When premature infants are transfused with hemoglobin A, oxygen delivery to the tissues is facilitated. Frequent blood sampling, combined with nutritional deficiencies of iron and folic acid caused by poor feeding or NEC, exaggerate the speed and depth of the decline in hemoglobin. A deficiency of vitamin E stores (vitamin E is necessary for RBC membrane stabilization) contributes to the shortened life span of the premature infant's RBCs. Even at several months of age, expremies may remain anemic because of poor nutrition and delayed hematopoiesis that is induced by earlier transfusion. It was traditionally, and arbitrarily, thought that elective surgery should not take place when the hemoglobin concentration was less than 10 g/dl. However, it is clear that several factors, including the tissue availability of the oxygen bound to hemoglobin (based on the age-dependent P_{50} and prior transfusions) and any additional oxygen requirements caused by lung disease, must be considered. Preoperative and intraoperative transfusion must, therefore, be based on the preoperative hematocrit, the type of operation the child is undergoing, and any ongoing physiologic derangements (e.g., BPD and apnea).

General Anesthesia

Preoperative evaluation of expremature infants should include a detailed history of the neonatal course. Specific attention should be paid to the severity of lung disease, duration of tracheal intubation, need for and duration of mechanical ventilation, and supplemental oxygen requirements. The presence of apnea of prematurity should be sought. It should be determined whether respiratory stimulants, including caffeine or theophylline, were used or are currently being used. Use of an apnea monitor on discharge from the hospital should be determined. If the child is having apnea at home, the likelihood of postoperative apnea is increased. Other medical problems of a chronic nature including hydrocephalus, cerebral palsy, and failure to thrive need to be addressed. Current medications, including supplemental nasal cannula oxygen, bronchodilators, and the use of diuretics, should be elicited, as should a history of drug allergies. A history of a recent upper respiratory infection, particularly respiratory syncytial virus (RSV), should be determined because of the additional airway reactivity it may impart. A history of gastroesophageal reflux should be specifically sought, since it is common in this patient population and may require precautions to prevent aspiration of gastric contents during the induction of general anesthesia. Prior anesthetic history should be determined and, when possible, the anesthetic record should be reviewed to determine the size of ETT used and whether there was an air leak around the ETT with positive-pressure ventilation. Parents should be questioned to determine if the child required postoperative mechanical ventilation after previous surgery. The NPO (nothing by mouth) status should be determined. At the University of California at San Francisco, babies less than 6 months are required to be NPO for formula for 4 hours or more, breast milk for 3 hours or more, and clear liquids for 2 hours or more. At greater than 6 months of age, the patient should be NPO for solids, including formula for 6 hours or more, breast milk for 4 hours, and clear liquids for 2 hours.

Premedication should be considered for expremies requiring surgery and anesthesia when the infant is greater than about 9 months of age. This is the time when infants begin to develop separation anxiety and apnea is less likely. Those infants with severe neurologic impairment may suffer exaggerated respiratory depression from routine doses of sedatives and probably should not receive premedication. The presence of a parent during the induction of anesthesia is often helpful for patients who do not receive premedication.

Inhalation versus intravenous induction of general anesthesia usually is decided by whether the patient has an intravenous catheter in place and whether there is a risk for pulmonary aspiration from either GERD or increased intra-abdominal pressure. For elective outpatient procedures, inhalation induction of anesthesia is common because intravenous access may be difficult after a long neonatal intensive care unit (NICU) stay. The size of the ETT chosen should be based on age and whether the child required prolonged tracheal intubation (>1 month) in the neonatal intensive care nursery. If he or she had a prolonged period of tracheal intubation, the endotracheal tube used should have an internal diameter that is 0.5 mm smaller than the tube usually chosen for a child of this age. Uncuffed endotracheal tubes provide a larger lumen with smaller outer diameter and therefore afford lower total airway resistance and improved suctioning capability. The anesthesiologist should ensure that there is an adequate air leak around the ETT during positive-pressure ventilation to prevent an excessively tight tube from contributing to postoperative tracheal edema and airway obstruction.

Particular intraoperative concerns for the expremie include maintenance of normal body temperature, judicious use of intravenous fluids, positioning to avoid injuries to contracted joints, and effective humidification of inhaled gases to promote effective pulmonary toilet and to help maintain a normal body temperature.

Until expremies attain normal weight for age (typically at 2 years of age), they have large surface area/volume ratios and lose body heat easily through their skin. For babies less than 6 months of age, the operating room should be prewarmed to prevent radiant heat loss during preparation and before the patient is covered with drapes. A warming mattress, a heated and humidified breathing circuit, and warmed intravenous and irrigation fluids further help prevent heat loss. A reduction of body temperature contributes to an increase in expenditure of metabolic energy postoperatively and may contribute to apnea in babies less than 60 weeks' PCA.

Intravenous access may be difficult, particularly during the first year of life, because the child may have had multiple percutaneous and cutdown intravenous catheters in the neonatal period. Saphenous, external jugular, and scalp veins often yield the greatest success when it is impossible to place a hand or foot intravenous (IV) cannula. Intravenous fluids should consist primarily of a balanced salt solution (such as lactated Ringer's solution) for replacement of intraoperative fluid losses. Maintenance fluids need not contain dextrose routinely, but should be used for patients receiving continuous infusions via total parenteral nutrition (TPN) or those with documented hypoglycemia. Reducing the rate of TPN by one third to one half will avoid the anesthesia- and surgery-induced hyperglycemia. Both hypoglycemia and hyperglycemia may contribute to brain injury if hypoxemia or a cardiac arrest occur. For the smallest expremies (those <3 months of age) who have inadequate glycogen stores, the routine administration of a 5 to 10 percent dextrose solution at maintenance rates usually will maintain normal blood glucose concentrations. Maintenance fluid rate can be calculated as 4 ml/kg/h for the first 10 kg of body weight plus 2 ml/kg for the next 10 kg body weight plus 1 ml/kg for each kilogram thereafter. However, it is important to measure glucose concentrations during surgery with Dextrostix or a glucometer to ensure that the glucose concentration is normal.

Positioning of the patient must be done in a way that prevents hyperextension of contracted joints. The extremities should be placed in their natural position and the areas that come in contact with hard surfaces padded. Bony prominences that have little overlying fat (including heels and elbow) must be padded well to prevent pressure ulcers. Placing a roll under the infant's upper back will align the airway of infants with large heads relative to their chest size.

Regional Anesthesia

Since 1909, there have been reports of spinal anesthesia for infants and children. However, until recently this technique was only rarely used in the United States. With the emergence of a large population of expremies at risk for postoperative apnea and oxygen desaturation, a resurgence of interest in regional anesthesia has occurred. This is primarily because there is less postoperative apnea when spinal anesthesia is used without added depressant drugs compared with general anesthesia.[23–27] The incidence of postoperative apnea following general anesthesia has been reported to be 11 to 37 percent, whereas the risk of postoperative apnea following spinal anesthesia without sedative supplementation is close to 0 percent.[23, 26–28] The risk of apnea, oxygen desaturation, and bradycardia is not completely abolished by the use of regional anesthesia because there is the occasional need to supplement regional anesthesia with IV or inhaled agents. However, the frequency of apnea, hemoglobin oxygen desaturation, and bradycardia is greater following general anesthesia.[23, 25]

Subarachnoid block, one-shot caudal epidural block, and continuous intrathecal and epidural blockade have been used successfully for lower abdominal, perineal, and lower extremity operations in expremies. Inguinal herniorrhaphy is the most common surgical indication for regional anesthesia in expremies. Herniorrhaphy should not be deferred for very long in this patient population because the incidence of bowel incarceration is high.

Spinal anesthesia can be accomplished with the infant either in the sitting or lateral decubitus position. Care should be taken to extend the head to avoid airway obstruction. Many different needles have been used to access the intrathecal space, ranging from 22- to 25-gauge, 3- to 4-cm nonstyletted needles to 22- to 25-gauge styletted Quincke needles. Tetracaine 1 percent that is mixed with an equal volume of 10 percent dextrose to create a hyperbaric solution, plus a wash of epinephrine (or approximately 0.02 ml of 1:1,000 solution) in a dose between 0.2 and 1.0 mg/kg, is the most common local anesthetic for this use. The smaller doses often require inhalation or intravenous supplementation because the duration of blockade is inadequate. The main limitation of a subarachnoid block is the limited duration of action of local anesthetics, even when relatively large doses per kilogram of body weight are administered. The duration of action is up to 80 percent shorter in the youngest children compared with adults. The maximum duration of spinal anesthesia is about 90 minutes, even when long-acting local anesthetics are administered in relatively large doses. The addition of epinephrine prolongs the blockade by approximately 30 percent.[29] The duration of the herniorrhaphy may be prolonged because hernias in the expremie are often quite large and are complicated by the small size of critical structures adjacent to the hernia sac, particularly the vas deferens in males. Nitrous oxide alone or in combination with halothane or sevoflurane administered by face mask has been used to supplement spinal blockade. This may become necessary when either the operation outlasts the block or when traction on the spermatic cord or manipulation of the peritoneum or bowel causes discomfort despite a functioning block. A patient that is crying may bear down and eviscerate bowel even when there is a functioning block. When this occurs, it is difficult or impossible to repair the hernia. Intravenous sedation with a myriad of depressant medications, including midazolam and ketamine, has been used for this purpose as well. Ketamine theoretically maintains spontaneous respiration better than other sedative/hypnotic drugs. However, there is controversy whether ketamine administration is associated with an increase in postoperative apnea. Veverka et al. found no increase in the incidence of postoperative apnea following ketamine supplementation of spinal anesthesia.[28] However, Welborn et al.[23] and Gallagher et al.[30] found that the use of ketamine supplementation increases the risk of postoperative apnea. In the study by Welborn et al., no patients in the spinal anesthetic alone group experienced postoperative apnea, but eight of nine patients who received ketamine supplementation developed postoperative apnea. This incidence of apnea is greater than that in the group receiving general anesthesia.[23] Supplementation with other intravenous drugs, including benzodiazepines and opiates, although not specifically studied, can be expected to contribute to respiratory depression and should therefore increase one's vigilance with postoperative monitoring.

Hemodynamic stability following a spinal block, despite wide variations in intrathecal dose, is the norm.[24, 29, 31] Dohi et al. found little or no decrease in systolic blood pressure following the onset of spinal block in children less than 5 years of age ($n = 23$), whereas children and adults over 5 years of age had decreases in blood pressure of at least 20 percent ($n = 54$). The levels of sensory block were similar in both groups.[29] This has prompted many anesthe-

siologists to establish intravenous access following the onset of sensory loss in the lower extremities to avoid the discomfort associated with inserting an IV cannula, particularly in expremies who often pose a formidable challenge for IV cannulation. The spinal block often dilates vessels in the lower extremities and makes inserting cannula easier.

The short duration of action of intrathecal drugs in this youngest population has prompted interest in continuous regional anesthesia techniques so that the duration of anesthesia may be extended while drug toxicity is minimized. Continuous spinal anesthesia is often accomplished using bupivacaine in 10 percent dextrose as a 0.5 percent solution and administering 0.3 mg/kg hourly to maintain a T2–T4 sensory level. The block may be performed using a 24-gauge epidural catheter that is inserted into the subarachnoid space through a 20-gauge, 2-inch Crawford needle. Continuous spinal techniques have the advantage of providing adequate anesthesia with smaller total doses of local anesthetics. However, concerns regarding direct neurotoxicity of local anesthetics and specific concerns regarding the cauda equina syndrome in adults following continuous spinal anesthetics using microcatheters raise concern about the safety of this technique.

Continuous caudal anesthesia is often used because pediatric anesthesiologists are familiar and facile with performing this common block in pediatric patients. The ability to thread catheters so that the tip of the catheter is in closer proximity to the dermatome of the operative field may allow less local anesthetic to be used. This is especially important because of the relatively high volume of local anesthetic required to perform a successful caudal anesthetic. While the ability to provide "top-up" doses is advantageous, long-acting local anesthetics like bupivacaine (mean elimination half-life of 7.7 hours) may cause toxic blood levels if frequent intermittent doses of the drug are given in addition to the large initial dose of anesthetic required for caudal anesthesia.[32, 33] The use of 3 percent 2-chloroprocaine has utility for this purpose because its serum half-life is less than 60 seconds. Therefore, the likelihood of systemic toxicity is very low.

Caudal epidural anesthesia may be accomplished through an indwelling intravenous catheter that is connected to a T-piece and is affixed to the skin or via an indwelling epidural catheter that is placed through an IV catheter in the caudal space and then threaded to 5 to 8 cm from the skin. In two separate studies, the cumulative dose of 3 percent 2-chloroprocaine administered over a mean of 95 minutes was 2.8 ml/kg/h. The initial loading dose was 30 mg/kg (1 ml/kg), which was followed by incremental doses of 0.3 ml/kg to achieve a T2–T4 sensory level. The initial dose was immediately followed by an infusion of 1 ml/kg/h. Even with these large total doses of 3 percent 2-chloroprocaine, the plasma concentration was undetectable in four of the five infants studied by Henderson et al. and was 0.5 μg/ml in the fifth patient, even though this population has low serum cholinesterase levels.[34] Surgical conditions are reportedly good to excellent with continuous epidural anesthesia without systemic sedatives.[34-36]

Successful regional anesthesia techniques offer many advantages in this high-risk population. Aside from the obvious advantages of reducing the incidence of postoperative complications, particularly apnea and the need for postoperative tracheal intubation and mechanical ventilation, early discharge from the hospital may reduce the number of infants who acquire nosocomial infections. The cost of care for these babies could be dramatically reduced by avoiding postoperative admission, particularly if the cost of prolonged tracheal intubation and mechanical ventilation in an intensive care unit is avoided.[26, 28]

POSTOPERATIVE APNEA

Incidence and Risk Factors

Expremies may experience cardiopulmonary compromise in the perioperative period of which apnea, bradycardia, and cyanosis are the most common.[37] The incidence of apnea following general anesthesia is reported to be 11 to 37 percent.[23, 25, 37, 38] Anecdotal reports appeared in the 1970s describing fatal postoperative apnea in former premature babies. In 1982, Steward reported a higher incidence of respiratory complications, especially apnea in expremies (33 percent) compared with full-term infants (0 percent) receiving general anesthesia for herniorrhaphy.[39] Since that time, several investigators have attempted to quantify the incidence and identify indicators that put particular expremies at increased risk. There is clear correlation between younger postconceptual age and a weaker but significant association with gestational age on the incidence of postoperative apnea. The presence of anemia (hematocrit <30 percent) is the only other independent risk factor for postoperative apnea. In a prospective study of 24 expremies, Welborn et al. found an 80 percent incidence of postoperative apnea in anemic compared with 21 percent in age-matched nonanemic expremies.[40]

Because of the small number of patients in this category at any one institution, results of studies that attempt to determine risk factors for postoperative apnea must be interpreted with caution. In the combined analysis of 255 patients from eight studies at four institutions, multiple variables were evaluated to determine their impact on the rate of postanesthetic apnea by Coté et al. Postconceptual age, gestational age, and the continued use of a home monitor were found to be independently related to the probability of apnea. The presence of anemia (hematocrit <30 percent) had only a weak correlation. It appears from this study that the probability of apnea does not decline with postconceptual and gestational age in anemic infants as it does for infants with hematocrits greater than or equal to 30 percent. Anemia appears to be a significant risk factor, particularly for the older infants (>43 weeks' PCA) whose risk might otherwise be low, whereas anemia is less of a factor in the younger infants where postconceptual age and gestational age override its impact on the incidence of postoperative apnea. A history of neonatal apnea, NEC, RDS, BPD, or the use of opioids or nondepolarizing muscle relaxants bore no significant relationship to the incidence of postoperative apnea. In this combined analysis of data from several institutions, postconceptual age was the most significant factor in the development of postoperative apnea, followed by gestational age. The use

of a home monitor was found not significant by itself when the investigator controlled for PCA. When postconceptual and gestational age were controlled, birth weight was related to the probability of apnea. Small-for-gestational-age babies had a less than expected rate of postoperative apnea when compared to appropriate-for-gestational-age and large-for-gestational-age babies.[41]

Kurth reported that, although most apnea is central in origin, nearly one third of apnea is associated with upper airway obstruction, so-called mixed apnea. Nasal airflow, pneumocardiography, and pulse oximetry were evaluated in 74 expremies (<37 weeks' gestation, <50 weeks PCA) for 2 hours following recovery from inhalation anesthesia looking for central, obstructive, or mixed apnea. Postoperative apnea occurred in 23 infants who were 31 to 48 weeks postconceptual age. Arterial hemoglobin desaturation was significantly more frequent following mixed apnea than central apnea alone.[42]

Caffeine/Theophylline Use

Since the discovery that aminophylline decreases the frequency of apneic episodes in newborns,[43] xanthine derivatives such as theophylline and caffeine have been widely used to treat apnea of prematurity. Theophylline undergoes marked demethylation and oxidation in adults. Infants, however, tend to methylate theophylline to produce caffeine. Although both possess respiratory stimulant effects, caffeine has a greater therapeutic index, a longer half-life, a more stable plasma concentration, and fewer cardiac side effects, making it easier to administer and monitor the drug. Preparation of the drug requires special attention, because the caffeine base is only slightly soluble in water. Caffeine citrate is available in powder form and may be prepared by a hospital pharmacist to make it suitable for intravenous use. Twenty milligrams of caffeine citrate is equivalent to 10 mg of caffeine base. Optimal response to the drug is achieved with plasma levels between 8 and 20 mg/L, but an effect can be demonstrated with levels as low as 3 to 5 mg/L.[44] Administering 5 mg/kg of caffeine base results in plasma caffeine concentrations of 5 to 8.6 mg/L, and these plasma concentrations of caffeine have reduced prolonged apnea but have not eradicated all ventilatory dysfunction.[45, 46] Because the plasma concentrations of caffeine in these studies fell below therapeutic level (5 to 8.6 mg/L vs. 8 to 20 mg/L), a randomized, double-blind study using 10 mg/kg was undertaken by Welborn et al. and this achieved plasma levels of 15 to 19 mg/L. None of the patients in this study who received caffeine developed adverse airway events, including prolonged apnea, periodic breathing, bradycardia, or oxygen desaturation to less than 90 percent. Eighty-one percent of the control patients (13 infants) developed prolonged apnea 4 to 6 hours postoperatively (Tables 15–2 through 15–5).

In newborns, the half-lives of xanthine derivatives are much longer than they are in adults. In adults, the half-life of caffeine is approximately 6 hours, and the half-life of theophylline is approximately 9 hours. In neonates, caffeine's half-life is between 37 and 231 hours and theophylline's half-life is between 12 and 64 hours. The half-life

TABLE 15-2
PERIOPERATIVE DATA OF STUDY PATIENTS: CAFFEINE BASE 5 mg/kg

	Group 1: Caffeine (*n* = 9)	Group 2: Controls (*n* = 11)
Gestational age (wk)		
Mean ± SD	29.8 ± 3	31.6 ± 3
Range	25–35	26–36
Conceptual age (wk)		
Mean ± SD	40.6 ± 2	40.6 ± 2
Range	38–44	35–44
History of preoperative apnea	8 (89%)*	5 (45%)

* *p* < 0.001, Fisher's exact test.
From Welborn LG, De Soto H, Hannallah RS, et al: The use of caffeine in the control of postanesthetic apnea in former premature infants. Anesthesiology 68:796, 1988, with permission.

TABLE 15-4
PERIOPERATIVE DATA OF STUDY PATIENTS CAFFEINE BASE 10 mg/kg (*n* = 32)

	Group 1: Caffeine (*n* = 16)	Group 2: Controls (*n* = 16)
Gestational age (wk)		
Mean ± SD	30.0	30.4
Range	24–35	25–36
Conceptual age (wk)		
Mean ± SD	40.9	40.5
Range	37–44	37–44
History of preoperative apnea	10 (63%)	8 (50%)

From Welborn LG, Hannallah RS, Fink R, et al: High-dose caffeine suppresses postoperative apnea in former preterm infants. Anesthesiology 71:347, 1989 with permission.

of caffeine approaches that of the adult by about 4 months of age.[44]

Same-Day Discharge Criteria

With the increasing expremie population and the ever-increasing pressure to admit and discharge patients on the same day as surgery occurs, it is critical that guidelines and common sense prevail when deciding when an expremie should be admitted to the hospital postoperatively. Recommendations for routine postoperative admission vary widely, from 44 to 60 weeks' PCA, following minor surgery. It is imperative that each expremie be considered on a case-by-case basis, giving consideration to factors including PCA, gestational age, persistence of apnea requiring home monitor or supplemental O_2, hemoglobin concentration, and the nature of the surgical procedure. Many investigators have attempted to determine the risk of postoperative apnea in expremies by various monitoring techniques, including pneumocardiograms, impedance pneumography, nasal thermistry, pulse oximetry, and electrocardiography.

Many prospective studies have attempted to define the group at highest risk for postoperative apnea. In 1983, Liu et al. studied 41 prematurely born infants under 12 months of age who were undergoing a variety of surgical and radiologic procedures. Apnea was defined as the cessation of breathing for longer than 20 seconds, or shorter if associated with bradycardia, cyanosis, or pallor. Postoperatively, 18 of these infants required postoperative mechanical ventilation; 10 of them did so because of preoperative mechanical ventilation or surgical indications. Seven required tracheal intubation secondary to postoperative apnea, all of whom had a history of apnea but did not require tracheal intubation just prior to surgery. All infants requiring postoperative mechanical ventilation were less than 41 weeks' PCA. Those who did not require postoperative mechanical ventilation were greater than 46 weeks' PCA. This led to the recommendation that all infants less than 46 weeks' PCA be admitted to the hospital and closely monitored for 24 hours postoperatively.[37]

TABLE 15-3
INCIDENCE OF POSTOPERATIVE APNEA AND PERIODIC BREATHING: CAFFEINE BASE 5 mg/kg

	Group 1: Caffeine (*n* = 9)	Group 2: Controls (*n* = 11)
Postoperative prolonged apnea with bradycardia	None	8 (73%)*
Postoperative PB > 1%	None	2 (18%)
Postoperative apnea < 15 s	8 (89%)	1 (9%)
Postoperative intubation or ventilation	None	None
Postoperative caffeine level (mg/L, range)	5–8.6	0

* *p* < 0.002, Fisher's exact test.
From Welborn LG, De Soto H, Hannallah RS, et al: The use of caffeine in the control of postanesthetic apnea in former premature infants. Anesthesiology 68:796, 1988, with permission.

TABLE 15-5
INCIDENCE OF POSTOPERATIVE APNEA AND PERIODIC BREATHING AND DESATURATION: CAFFEINE BASE 10 mg/kg

	Group 1: Caffeine (*n* = 16)	Group 2: Controls (*n* = 16)
Postoperative prolonged apnea with bradycardia	None	13 (81%)*
Postoperative PB > 1%	None	4 (25%)
Postoperative desaturation <90%	None	8 (50%)*
Postoperative intubation or ventilation	None	None
Postoperative caffeine level (mg/L, range)	15–19	0

* *p* < 0.05, Fisher's exact test.
From Welborn LG, Hannallah RS, Fink R, et al: High-dose caffeine suppresses postoperative apnea in former preterm infants. Anesthesiology 71:347, 1989, with permission.

In 1986, Welborn et al. studied 86 infants less than 12 months postnatal age undergoing inguinal herniorrhaphy. Two groups of infants, one with 38 infants with a birth weight of 2,500 or less (22 ≤44 weeks and 16 >44 weeks) and/or less than or equal to 37 weeks of gestation and a second with 48 infants greater than 37 weeks (7 ≤44 weeks and 41 >44 weeks), were delineated. All infants were free of cardiac, neurologic, endocrine, and metabolic disease. Infants were monitored by chest wall impedance pneumography so that apnea (absence of chest wall motion) would be immediately detected. The electrocardiogram was detected and amplified and was used to measure heart rate. Prolonged apnea was defined as a respiratory pause 15 seconds or longer; apnea was defined as a respiratory pause less than 15 seconds; periodic breathing (PB) was defined as three or more periods of apnea of 3 to 15 seconds separated by less than 20 seconds of normal respiration. The significance of PB was interpreted by determining its duration relative to the total sleep time to achieve a PB percentage. Periodic breathing percentage less than 0.5 percent was considered normal. Bradycardia was defined as a heart rate of less than 100 bpm for at least 5 seconds in neonates less than 1 month of age, less than 90 bpm in infants 1 to 3 months of age, and less than 80 bpm in infants 3 months of age or older. The incidence of prolonged apnea and/or PB in expremies less than or equal to 44 weeks' PCA versus those greater than 44 weeks was tested for statistical significance. None of the full-term infants had a history of apnea and none developed prolonged apnea or PB. Twelve of the 16 expremies greater than 44 weeks had a history of apnea, but none showed perioperative prolonged apnea or PB and subsequently none required postoperative intubation or ventilation. Eighteen of the 22 expremies less than or equal to 44 weeks had a history of apnea, but none showed preoperative prolonged apnea or PB. Postoperatively, there were no episodes of prolonged apnea; PB was noted in 14. These 14 (63.6 percent) had postoperative PB greater than 0.5 percent without bradycardia. Two of these patients showed PB as late as 5 hours postoperatively, but none required endotracheal intubation. Based on this study, it was concluded that premature infants less than 44 weeks' PCA are at high risk for postoperative ventilatory dysfunction, and it is therefore recommended that nonessential surgery be delayed.[48] Though the significance is not clear, there is a gradual reduction in ventilation and oxygenation during periodic breathing. This may eventually result in prolonged apnea.[49] An increase in periodic breathing has been noted in babies with near-miss sudden infant death syndrome.[50] Their recommendations are therefore that when surgery is deemed necessary, infants less than 44 weeks' PCA should be admitted to a hospital and monitored for at least 12 hours postoperatively.

Kurth et al., in 1987, published a series of 47 expremies less than 60 weeks' PCA undergoing a variety of surgical procedures. Each infant was monitored before and after inhalation anesthesia by pneumocardiogram. Eighteen (37 percent) had prolonged apnea (>15 seconds) postoperatively. Seven (14 percent) had short apnea (6 to 15 seconds). The first apneic event occurred within 2 hours of anesthesia in 72 percent of patients, and the remaining 28 percent had their initial episode as late as 12 hours postoperatively. In this series, it was concluded that the risk of apnea was proportional to young postconceptual age and a history of NEC. The postoperative elapsed time to the last long apnea was inversely proportional to PCA. It was also found that the preoperative pneumocardiogram was not a reliable predictor of postoperative apnea.[51]

In 1991, Malviya et al. published a study of 91 infants less than 60 weeks' PCA undergoing general anesthesia; 38 procedures in 35 infants less than 44 weeks' PCA. Ten procedures (26.3 percent) in nine infants resulted in postoperative apnea, eight of which were not self-limited; four required manual stimulation and four required supplemental ventilation by face mask. Apnea occurred after 2 of the 63 procedures in infants greater than or equal to 44 weeks, both episodes in the same patient with neurologic deficits. Seven infants had episodes of bradycardia, defined as a decrease in heart rate greater than 40 bpm below the resting heart rate. All lasted less than 5 seconds and were self-limited, with a minimum heart rate of 79 bpm, without the occurrence of apnea or cyanosis. All episodes began within 12 hours of surgery. It was concluded that the "maximum long-run risk of postanesthetic apnea in preterm infants older than 44 weeks' PCA is 5 percent with 95 percent confidence." The incidence of apnea in infants undergoing procedures appropriate for an inpatient setting did not differ from that of patients undergoing operations appropriate for an outpatient setting.[52] Therefore, the type of surgery was not predictive of the incidence of postoperative apnea.

It is difficult to draw conclusions based on these studies because they each used different modalities to detect apnea, some of the studies controlled for associated medical conditions whereas others did not; and some looked solely at herniorrhaphy whereas others included all types of surgery, including laparotomy and neurosurgery.

In an attempt to attain greater statistical power and thereby make recommendations regarding the postoperative disposition of expremies undergoing minor surgery, a combined analysis of eight prospective studies was done by Coté et al. They compiled the original data from the aforementioned authors. This allowed them to analyze the results of 255 patients. They concluded that the incidence of apnea in a baby born at 32 weeks does not decrease to less than 1 percent until a PCA of 54 to 56 weeks.[41] Even this larger sample size may not be sufficient. It has been argued that a sample size of at least 300 patients would be required to ensure a 95 percent probability that the incidence of apnea does not exceed 1 percent in a particular group.[53, 54]

Recommendations for same-day discharge in this group of patients therefore remain controversial. In an editorial by Gregory and Steward, it was recommended to:

1. Delay nonessential surgery for preterm infants until they were beyond 44 weeks' PCA.
2. Where such surgery cannot be delayed, the patient should be admitted to the hospital and monitored with an apnea monitor for at least 18 hours postoperatively. The hospital must be able to mechanically ventilate infants postoperatively.
3. Pediatric surgeons must reexamine the indications for surgery in the preterm infant and define those

conditions that safely can be managed nonoperatively until the patient is older and more mature.[12]

REFERENCES

1. Jobe A, Ikegami M: Surfactant for the treatment of respiratory distress syndrome. Am Rev Respir Dis 136:1256, 1987.
2. Phibbs RH, Ballard RA, Clements JA, et al: Initial clinical trial of EXOSURF, a protein-free synthetic surfactant, for the prophylaxis and early treatment of hyaline membrane disease. Pediatrics 88:1, 1991.
3. Piecuch RE, Leonard CH, Cooper BA, et al: Outcome of infants born at 24-26 weeks' gestation: II. Neurodevelopmental outcome. Obstet Gynecol 90:809, 1997.
4. Kilpatrick SJ, Schlueter MA, Piecuch R, et al: Outcome of infants born at 24-26 weeks' gestation: I. Survival and cost. Obstet Gynecol 90:803, 1997.
5. Mallory GB Jr, Chaney H, Mutich RL, Motoyama EK: Longitudinal changes in lung function during the first three years of premature infants with moderate to severe bronchopulmonary dysplasia. Pediatr Pulmonol 11:8, 1991.
6. Loke J, Ganeshananthan M, Palm CR, Motoyama EK: Site of airway obstruction in asymptomatic asthmatic children. Lung 159:35, 1981.
7. Brooks JG: Apnea of infancy and sudden infant death syndrome. Am J Dis Child 136:1012, 1982.
8. Glotzbach SF, Tansey PA, Baldwin RB, Ariagno RL: Periodic breathing in preterm infants: influence of bronchopulmonary dysplasia and theophylline. Pediatr Pulmonol 7:78, 1989.
9. Dripps RD, Comroe JH Jr: The respiratory and circulatory response of normal man to inhalation of 7.6 and 10.4 percent CO_2 with a comparison of the maximal ventilation produced by severe muscle exercise, inhalation of CO_2 and maximum voluntary hyperventilation. Am J Physiol 149:43, 1947.
10. Rigatto H, Brady JP, de la Torre Verduzco R: Chemoreceptor reflexes in preterm infants: II. The effect of gestational and postnatal age on the ventilatory response to inhaled carbon dioxide. Pediatrics 55:614, 1975.
11. Rigatto H, Brady JP, de la Torre Verduzco R: Chemoreceptor reflexes in preterm infants: I. The effect of gestational and postnatal age on the ventilatory response to inhalation of 100% and 15% oxygen. Pediatrics 55:604, 1975
12. Rigatto H, de la Torre Verduzco R, Gates DB: Effects of O_2 on the ventilatory response to CO2 in preterm infants. J Appl Physiol 39:896, 1975.
13. Knill R, Bryan AC: An intercostal-phrenic inhibitory reflex in human newborn infants. J Appl Physiol 40:352, 1976.
14. Henderson-Smart DJ, Pettigrew AG, Campbell DJ: Clinical apnea and brain-stem neural function in preterm infants. N Engl J Med 308:353, 1983.
15. Gregory GA, Steward DJ: Life-threatening perioperative apnea in the ex-"premie" [editorial]. Anesthesiology 59:495, 1983.
16. Muller NL, Bryan AC: Chest wall mechanics and respiratory muscles in infants. Pediatr Clin North Am 26:503, 1979.
17. Betts EK, Downes JJ, Schaffer DB, Johns R: Retrolental fibroplasia and oxygen administration during general anesthesia. Anesthesiology 47:518, 1977.
18. Holl J: Anesthesia for abdominal surgery. In Gregory GA (ed): Pediatric Anesthesia. New York, Churchill Livingstone, 1994, p 561.
19. McCubbin M, Frey EE, Wagener JS, et al: Large airway collapse in bronchopulmonary dysplasia. J Pediatr 114:304, 1989.
20. Ferrari LR, Goudsouzian NG: The use of the laryngeal mask airway in children with bronchopulmonary dysplasia. Anesth Analg 81:310, 1995.
21. Pearson HA: Diseases of the blood. In Nelson WE (ed): Textbook of Pediatrics. Philadelphia, WB Saunders Company, 1987, p 1038.
22. Motoyama EK: Respiratory physiology in infants and children. In Motoyama EK, Davis PJ (eds): Anesthesia for Infants and Children. St Louis, Mosby-Year Book, 1996, p 46.
23. Welborn LG, Rice LJ, Hannallah RS, et al: Postoperative apnea in former preterm infants: prospective comparison of spinal and general anesthesia. Anesthesiology 72:838, 1990.
24. Harnik EV, Hoy GR, Potolicchio S, et al: Spinal anesthesia in premature infants recovering from respiratory distress syndrome. Anesthesiology 64:95, 1986.
25. Krane EJ, Haberkern CM, Jacobson LE: Postoperative apnea, bradycardia, and oxygen desaturation in formerly premature infants: prospective comparison of spinal and general anesthesia. Anesth Analg 80:7, 1995.
26. Sartorelli KH, Abajian JC, Kreutz JM, Vane DW: Improved outcome utilizing spinal anesthesia in high-risk infants. J Pediatr Surg 27:1022, 1992.
27. Krane EJH, Haberkern CM, Jacobson LE: Postoperative apnea, bradycardia, and oxygen desaturation in formerly premature infants: prospective comparison of spinal and general anesthesia. Anesth Analg 80:7, 1995.
28. Veverka TJ, Henry DN, Milroy MJ, et al: Spinal anesthesia reduces the hazard of apnea in high-risk infants. Am Surg 57:531, 1991.
29. Dohi S, Naito H, Takahashi T: Age-related changes in blood pressure and duration of motor block in spinal anesthesia. Anesthesiology 50:319, 1979.
30. Gallagher TM, Crean PM: Spinal anaesthesia in infants born prematurely. Anaesthesia 44:434, 1989.
31. Abajian JC, Mellish RW, Browne AF, et al: Spinal anesthesia for surgery in the high-risk infant. Anesth Analg 63:359, 1984.
32. Mazoit JX, Denson DD, Samii K: Pharmacokinetics of bupivacaine following caudal anesthesia in infants. Anesthesiology 68:387, 1988.
33. Berde CB: Convulsions associated with pediatric regional anesthesia [editorial; comment]. Anesth Analg 75:164, 1992.
34. Henderson K, Sethna NF, Berde CB: Continuous caudal anesthesia for inguinal hernia repair in former preterm infants. J Clin Anesth 5:129, 1993.
35. Tobias JD, Lowe S, O'Dell N, et al: Continuous regional anaesthesia in infants. Can J Anaesth 40:1065, 1993.
36. Peutrell JM, Hughes DG: Epidural anaesthesia through caudal catheters for inguinal herniotomies in awake ex-premature babies. Anaesthesia 48:128, 1993.
37. Liu LM, Cote CJ, Goudsouzian NG, et al: Life-threatening apnea in infants recovering from anesthesia. Anesthesiology 59:506, 1983.
38. Welborn LG, Hannallah RS, Luban NL, et al: Anemia and postoperative apnea in former preterm infants. Anesthesiology 74:1003, 1991.
39. Steward DJ: Preterm infants are more prone to complications following minor surgery than are term infants. Anesthesiology 56:304, 1982.
40. Welborn LG, Hannallah RS, Higgins T, et al: Postoperative apnoea in former preterm infants: does anaemia increase the risk? Can J Anaesth 37:S92, 1990.
41. Coté CJ, Zaslavsky A, Downes JJ, et al: Postoperative apnea in former preterm infants after inguinal herniorrhaphy. A combined analysis. Anesthesiology 82:809, 1995.
42. Kurth CD, LeBard SE: Association of postoperative apnea, airway obstruction, and hypoxemia in former premature infants. Anesthesiology 75:22, 1991.
43. Kuzemko JA, Paala J: Apnoeic attacks in the newborn treated with aminophylline. Arch Dis Child 48:404, 1973.
44. Aranda JV, Cook CE, Gorman W, et al: Pharmacokinetic profile of caffeine in the premature newborn infant with apnea. J Pediatr 94:663, 1979.
45. Welborn LG, de Soto H, Hannallah RS, et al: The use of caffeine in the control of post-anesthetic apnea in former premature infants. Anesthesiology 68:796, 1988.
46. Turmen T, Davis J, Aranda JV: Relationship of dose and plasma concentrations of caffeine and ventilation in neonatal apnea. Semin Perinatol 5:326, 1981.
47. Welborn LG, Hannallah RS, Fink R, et al: High-dose caffeine suppresses postoperative apnea in former preterm infants. Anesthesiology 71:347, 1989.
48. Welborn LG, Ramirez N, Oh TH, et al: Postanesthetic apnea and periodic breathing in infants. Anesthesiology 65:658, 1986.
49. Rigatto H, Brady JP: Periodic breathing and apnea in preterm infants. I. Evidence for hypoventilation possibly due to central respiratory depression. Pediatrics 50:202, 1972.
50. Kelly DH, Shannon DC: Periodic breathing in infants with near-miss sudden infant death syndrome. Pediatrics 63:355, 1979.
51. Kurth CD, Spitzer AR, Broennle AM, Downes JJ: Postoperative apnea in preterm infants. Anesthesiology 66:483, 1987.
52. Malviya S, Swartz J, Lerman J: Are all preterm infants younger than 60 weeks postconceptual age at risk for postanesthetic apnea? Anesthesiology 78:1076, 1993.
53. Fisher DM: When is the ex-premature infant no longer at risk for apnea? [editorial; comment]. Anesthesiology 82:807, 1995.
54. Hanley JA, Lippman-Hand A: If nothing goes wrong, is everything all right? Interpreting zero numerators. JAMA 249:1743, 1983.

16

Anesthesia for Neurosurgical Procedures

BRUNO BISSONNETTE
PARVINE SADEGHI

♦   ♦   ♦

The child is not merely a small adult. At birth, central nervous system (CNS) development is incomplete and will not be mature until the end of the first year of life. Because of this delay in the maturation, several specific pathophysiologic and psychological differences ensue.

Anesthesia for neurosurgery presents an interesting challenge to the anesthesiologist. Although one has little control over the patient's primary lesion, the selection of anesthetic technique and the recognition of perioperative events and changes may profoundly reduce or prevent significant morbidity. Current neuroanesthetic practice is based on the understanding of cerebral physiology and how it can be manipulated in the presence of intracranial pathology. The pediatric neuroanesthesiologist also must contend with the physiologic differences in developing children. In addition to the common problems of administering anesthesia to the general pediatric population, special consideration must be given to the effects of anesthesia on the CNS of children with neurologic diseases. This chapter reviews the basic concepts necessary for clinical management and understanding of anesthetic problems in neurosurgical patients. A section on anesthetic management of specific neurosurgical conditions addresses the particular problems encountered by the pediatric neuroanesthesiologist.

THE CENTRAL NERVOUS SYSTEM: BASIC CONCEPTS

The practice of anesthesia for pediatric neurosurgery requires some knowledge of neuroembryology and development, neuroanatomy, and neurophysiology.

Neuroembryology and Development

The CNS is the system first to begin and probably last to complete its development in human maturation. To understand the various disorders encountered in pediatric neurologic practice, the time sequences for the major events in CNS development are important. The nature of several neurologic dysfunctions or disorders will be related to a specific developmental stage of the CNS. Central nervous system development begins from a relatively simple single layer of cells and progresses to a very complex, multilayered central structure that eventually connects it with every part of the body. The processes by which the CNS develops follow three steps: (1) neurulation, (2) canalization, and (3) retrogressive differentiation.

Early Stage of Neurulation in Humans

The process by which the neural tube initially folds is called neurulation. This occurs very early in embryonic

381

development and it is vitally important. Although this process has been well studied, many of its mechanisms remain unclear. Several factors have been identified as possible determinants involved in the process of neurulation.[1]

Neural tube differentiation is part of a long process of neurologic development, which occurs in the first 56 to 60 days after fertilization of the ovum.[2-5] Table 16–1 indicates the stages of development. The nervous system does not appear until stage 6 (i.e., during the second week of gestation). Primary orientation of the embryo arises when the primitive streak and Hensen's node are present. Shortly thereafter (stage 7), the notochord is found extending rostrally from Hensen's node. Over the next 2 days, when there are six or seven somites, fusion of the neural folds occurs (stage 10). Initial site fusion occurs at the level of the third or fourth somite, which correlates with the future rhombencephalon (hindbrain) region.[6] By early stage 11, the embryo possesses fused neural folds to the level of the colliculi rostrally. The primordia of the thalamus and corpus striatum distort the terminal hole and may be involved in its closure. At this time, the only contact between the neuroectoderm and the amniotic cavity is through the posterior neuropore.

Later Development of the Neural Tube

Cerebral Cortex and Cerebellum

After closure of the anterior neuropore in stage 11, there is an interval before the first indication of differentiation of the telencephalon (forebrain). In stage 15, bilateral cerebral vesicles appear, and their connections with the existing neural tube later become the foramina of Monro. The midline lamina terminalis forms a keel to these enlarging structures. By stage 17, areas that become frontal and parietal lobes are identifiable. Primordia of the occipital lobe are present at stage 19, and the temporal pole appears at stage 23 (Fig. 16–1).

At this early stage, these poles bear no resemblance to their final form. The main differentiation of the cerebral cortex takes place throughout the gestational period but mainly during the third trimester.[7] The external surfaces of the developing brain provide information about gestational age. Fissures and sulci develop. A majority of the cortical surface becomes buried as the gyri are formed. The primordium of cortical gray matter is formed when a layer of neuroblasts, derived mainly from pyramidal cells, migrates into the marginal zone during stage 22. The progressive formation of upper and lower fibers divides the

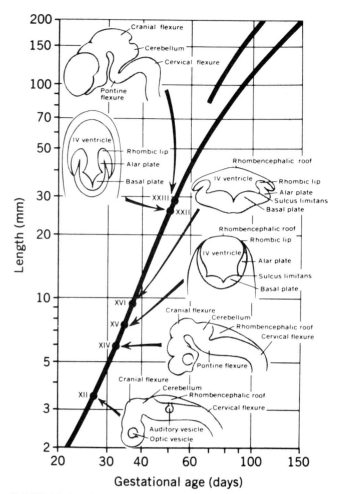

FIGURE 16–1. Schematic representation of early development of the human cerebellum as correlated with developmental stage (Roman numerals), gestational age, and crown-rump length. (From Lemire R, Loeser J, Leedh R, Alvord E: Normal and Abnormal Development of the Normal Nervous System. New York, Harper & Row, 1975, with permission.)

caudate nucleus from the putamen and the globus pallidus at stage 23.

The deep cerebral nuclei, which are derived from the diencephalon (midbrain), appear at different stages. The thalamic structure begins to appear at stage 15, with a separate lateral part becoming identifiable later. The anlage of the cerebellum are found when the pontine and cervical flexures begin to form during stage 13. Interestingly, most of the early development of the cerebellum takes place about 1 month after the embryonic period begins, even though the paired cerebellar primordia have not acquired a recognizable pattern. Development of the cerebral cortex and the white matter is relatively primitive by the time of transition from embryo to fetus. This supports the concept that the brain grows mainly during the later phases of gestation and will be continued postnatally.

Canalization and Retrogressive Differentiation

The process of neural tube formation that occurs caudal to the neural tube formed by neurulation is called *canalization* and involves development of the lower lumbar, sacral,

---

T A B L E   1 6 – 1
PHASES AND STAGES OF NEURAL DEVELOPMENT DURING GESTATION

Phase	Stages	Age (Days)	Outcome
Neurulation	7	16–28	Brain, spinal cord through L2–L4
Canalization	13–20	30–52	Sacral, coccygeal segments
Retrogressive differentiation	18–Birth	46–Birth	Filum terminale

and coccygeal segments. Cells proliferate in the neural tube wall in this region. This "secondary" phase of caudal neural tube development and the development of the associated vertebrae produce an excess number of segments. Formation of the filum terminale and the cauda equina is the result of *retrogressive differentiation.*[8] It consists of a degenerative process in which the excess segments formed by canalization are remodeled. It eventually brings the conus medullaris to its adult level opposite L1–L2.

Development defects of the CNS are referred to as *neural tube defects.* Neurulation defects fall into three general categories: (1) those involving the brain and spinal cord, (2) those involving the brain alone, and (3) those involving the spinal cord alone. For example, in early development, failure of both the brain and the spinal column to undergo proper neurulation results in total dysrhaphism (or craniorachischis). If the brain alone fails to close, anencephaly occurs.

In the later stages of development, many brain malformations can occur that have clinical relevance for the pediatric anesthesiologist. *Microencephaly* is characterized by a small brain enclosed in a small skull. It is seldom a neurosurgical problem in itself, but craniosysnostosis and encephalocele must be considered in the differential diagnosis. *Congenital hydrocephaly,* an increase in the amount of cerebrospinal fluid in the cranial cavity, is a common complication. Cortical malformations are most often the result of neuronal migration and can also be visible on the surface.

Schizencephaly (clefts in the cerebral wall), *pachygyri* (sparse, broad gyri), and *polymicrogyria* are anomalies strongly associated with migrational abnormalities. *Lissencephaly,* or smooth brain, is a severe anomaly that may be produced by either migrational anomalies or earlier disruptions in neurogenesis. *Agenesis of the corpus callosum,* which is not believed to be a migrational anomaly, is, however, often associated with such anomalies, and may be complete or partial. Caudally defective neurulation results in *myelocele* if the lesion is flat or *meningomyelocele* if there is an enlarged subarachnoid space dorsal to the dysplastic cord. The correlation of these anatomic locations with the probable stages in which they arise is shown in Table 16–1.

The Ventricular System and Cerebrospinal Fluid Pathway

When closure of the posterior neuropore occurs in stage 12, the ventricular system is closed and consists of that within the prosencephalon, diencephalon, mesencephalon, rhombencephalon (metencephalon, myelencephalon), and central canal of the spinal cord. During stage 14 the rhombencephalic roof becomes thinner, and in stage 15 evaginations of the cerebral hemispheres develop. This demarcates the anlage of the lateral ventricles, the third ventricle, and the foramen of Monro. By stage 20 the cerebral hemispheres have overlapped the diencephalon. At this stage the lateral ventricles are the largest of the ventricular system. At about this stage a perforation of the roof of the fourth ventricle occurs, creating the foramen of Magendie.[9] The foramina of Luschka form

about 10 to 11 weeks later. Within the cranium the aqueduct of Sylvius narrows as the tectum and tegmentum enlarge. The actual volume within the lateral, third, and fourth ventricles becomes somewhat reduced as the choroid plexuses differentiate and the brain substance increases. The central canal of the spinal cord is normally obliterated after birth by the cellular proliferation of the spinal cord. Therefore, the ventricular system terminates at the obex in the caudal floor of the fourth ventricle. The disturbed embryology of the caudal cerebellum in the spina bifida–Arnold-Chiari malformation complex frequently alters this normal course of events. It causes the central canal to remain enlarged and patent to the point of causing symptomatic hydrosyringomyelia.

Cerebral Vascular Development

There are five periods in the development of the cerebral vasculature.[10] The first period corresponds to stage 8 or 9, in which there are neither arteries nor veins. The primordial endothelium-lined channels then form a plexiform network, which eventually, during the second period (stages 10 to 13), differentiates into arteries and veins. This provides the initial circulation to the head. Direct connections with the primitive aortic system supply the arterial side, and the venous drainage joins the jugular system. At stage 19, corresponding to the fourth period and leading into fetal life, there is separation of the arterial and venous systems. The final period extends beyond birth and consists of late histologic changes in vascular walls, transforming then into the adult form. It is believed that most vascular malformations occur before the embryo attains a length of 40 mm (i.e., before the arterial walls thicken). This is a structural defect in the formation of the primitive arteriolar-capillary network.[11]

Neuroanatomy

The CNS is unique in its vulnerability to trauma, hypoxia, ischemia, and other pathophysiologic phenomena. The management of these events by up-to-date techniques in cerebral protection, resuscitation, and monitoring is as important as the provision of excellent anesthesia in the operating room. For this reason a knowledge of normal CNS anatomy and physiology is essential for the neuroanesthesiologist.

Central Nervous System

The craniospinal compartment is limited by the calvaria and the vertebral column. It is a single continuous space well developed to protect the vulnerable neural tissue of the brain and the spinal cord. However, the compliance of the system is low because of a lack of distensibility within the subdural space. The contents of this space include the brain parenchyma (neurons, glial tissue, and the interstitial fluid), cerebrospinal fluid (10 percent), and cerebral blood volume (10 percent). An increase in volume of any of these compartments caused by, for example, tumor growth, hydrocephalus, or hemorrhage will result in compression of vital tissue and displacement of adjacent structures. The change in volume produces a rapid rise in intracranial pressure (ICP).

At birth the brain weighs about 335 g and accounts for 10 to 15 percent of total body weight. During the first year of life the brain grows rapidly. It doubles in weight within 6 months and at 1 year weighs 900 g. At the end of the second year it weighs 1,000 g. It reaches adult weight by about 12 years of age (1,200 to 1,400 g). The weight ratio of the CNS to the total body in adulthood is about 2 percent.[12] The calvaria at birth consists of ossified plates, which cover the dura mater and are separated by fibrous sutures and the fontanelles (Fig. 16–2). Two fontanelles are identifiable at birth. The posterior fontanelle closes during the second or third postnatal month, and the anterior fontanelle usually closes at 10 to 16 months.[12] The fontanelles do not totally ossify until the teenage years.[12] However, even before closure of the fibrous fontanelle, the ability to accommodate to an acute increase in ICP is limited, if not nonexistent. The distensibility of the dura mater and the osteofibrous cranium resembles that of a leather bag and offers a high resistance to an acute rise in pressure. Slow pressure rises can, to a certain point, be accommodated by expansion of the fontanelle and separation of the suture lines.[13] Palpation or application of a skin transducer on the fontanelles can be used clinically to assess ICP.[14] The intracranial space is separated into two major compartments by a layer of dura called the tentorium cerebelli.

The Supratentorial Compartment

The supratentorial compartment is the largest compartment of the craniospinal space. Its size is determined by

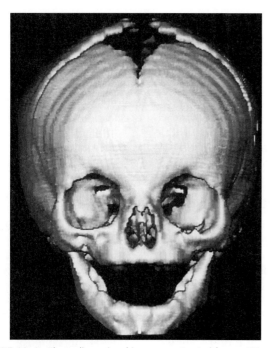

FIGURE 16–2. Three-dimensional image constructed from a CT scan of a 10-month-old infant, showing craniofacial contours. The small size of the face relative to the cranium is evident. The open anterior fontanelle is easily seen, as are the coronal and the metopic sutures.

the calvaria and the tentorium cerebelli (Fig. 16–3). The two hemispheres are separated by the falx cerebri. Each hemisphere consists of three lobes (frontal, temporal, and parieto-occipital), each of which has several complex and specialized functions. Lesions of the temporal and parieto-occipital lobes have more serious clinical consequences than lesions in the frontal lobe.

The diencephalon forms the central part of the supratentorial compartment and is the rostral end of the brain stem. It consists of the thalamus, hypothalamus, epithalamus, and subthalamus, and it surrounds the third ventricle. It is vulnerable to involvement by neoplasms and ischemia. The impairment of blood supply is often because of compression by the hemispheric masses.

In neuroanesthesia, intracranial procedures are described as supratentorial or infratentorial. The supratentorial compartment includes the anterior and the middle cranial fossae. The anterior cranial fossa is occupied by the inferior part and anterior extremities of the frontal lobe. The tentorium is a tent-shaped dural septum, which forms a roof over the posterior cranial fossa separating the supratentorial compartment and the cerebellum. Between the anteromedial parts of the right and left leaves of the tentorium is an oval opening called the tentorial incisura (notch). It allows the brain stem to pass from the middle cranial fossa to the posterior cranial fossa (Fig. 16–3).

Clinically, if a severe primary injury to the brain results in marked hemorrhage or edema, both the inferior edge of the falx cerebri (a large sickle-shaped vertical formation of dura in the longitudinal fissure between the two cerebral hemispheres) and the tentoria incisura become important sites of secondary injury. This injury is caused by a differential pressure across the tentorial incisura that leads to herniation of the brain stem and other vital structures. It can also lead to cerebral ischemia if it occludes the anterior cerebral artery. If the pressure increases even more, the diencephalic brain stem, cerebral peduncles, oculomotor nerve, and the posterior communicating artery will herniate through the tentoria incisura. Because the medial aspect of the temporal lobe is in the medial cranial fossa on either side of the tentoria incisura, the uncus will herniate and cause contralateral hemiplegia, posturing problems, and an ipsilateral, large, irregular, poorly reactive pupil.

The Infratentorial Compartment

The posterior cranial fossa is the largest and deepest of all three cranial fossae. It contains the cerebellum, the pons, and the medulla oblongata. The skull covering the posterior fossa is formed largely by the inferior and anterior parts of the occipital bone.

The clinical consequences of injury or disease in the posterior cranial fossa may be devastating owing to physical compression of many vital structures, including the reticular system, cardiac and respiratory centers, and cranial nerves. The cerebellum occupies most of the posterior cranial fossa and is mainly concerned with motor functions that regulate posture, muscle tone, and coordination. Midline or bilateral lesions on the cerebellum may cause unsteady gait, hypotonia, and tremor.

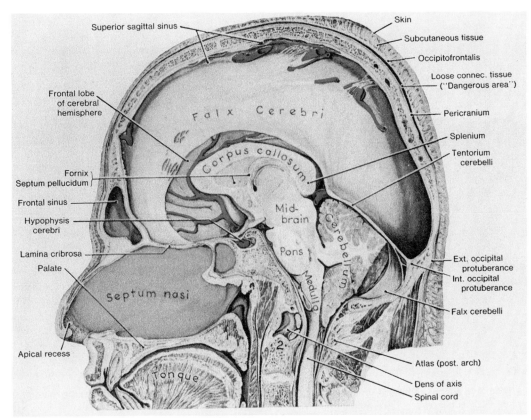

FIGURE 16–3. A median section of the head, showing supratentorial and posterior fossa structures. (Modified from Moore KL: Clinically Oriented Anatomy. Baltimore, Williams & Wilkins, 1985, with permission.)

From a clinical standpoint, the cerebellar tonsils (posteroinferior prolongations of cerebellar tissues) are of considerable importance. Pressure produced by posterior cranial fossa pathology causes herniation of the cerebellar tonsils, mainly the vermis, through the foramen magnum and results in a syndrome called the "pressure cone" phenomenon, which is commonly fatal. The neuroanesthesiologist should keep in mind that identification of increasing posterior cranial fossa pressure, which can eventually lead to herniation, may be relatively subtle and requires a high index of suspicion for its diagnosis.

The Spinal Canal Compartment

The spinal cord, which represents a significant proportion of CNS volume, lies in the vertebral canal. It is a cylindrical structure that is slightly flattened anteriorly and posteriorly where the vascularization predominates. The spinal cord is a continuation of the medulla, the inferior part of the brain stem. The spinal cord in adults is usually 42 to 45 cm long and ends opposite to the intervertebral disk between L1 and L2, but it may terminate anywhere between T12 and L3 (Fig. 16–4). At birth, after retrogressive differentiation is accomplished, the spinal cord ends at the intervertebral space of L3 (Fig. 16–4C). The end of the spinal cord reaches the adult level at 8 years of age (Fig. 16–4D). The intradural space is much longer than the spinal cord and ends at S2 (Fig. 16–4D). The spinal cord occupies approximately two thirds of the entire vertebral space. The total space is occupied by the cerebrospi-

nal fluid (CSF). The L2–S2 segments, therefore, consist of a reservoir of CSF, which may provide a relief mechanism during increases in ICP. It must be remembered that the spinal compartment is larger than the posterior cranial fossa and that the greater compliance of the spinal compartment, associated with the slight distensibility of the spinal dura mater and the compressibility of the venous plexuses, sets the stage for transforaminal tonsil herniation. Consequently, acute decompression of the spinal compartment by lumbar puncture may readily precipitate such herniation.

Vascular Anatomy

The brain is supplied by an extensive system of branches from two pairs of vessels, the internal carotid and the vertebral arteries. Each contributes to the circulus arteriosus cerebri (circle of Willis), which is formed by the posterior cerebral artery, the posterior communicating artery, the internal carotid siphon, the anterior cerebral artery, and the anterior communicating artery. Although this structure seems to be designed to prevent cerebral infarction in the event of occlusion of one of these vessels, in most cases insufficient blood is supplied by these collateral routes to do so. Twenty-eight percent of individuals lack at least one anastomotic component of the circle of Willis, with the anterior communicating artery being the most frequently absent.

Venous drainage of the brain is achieved mainly by the venous sinuses of the dura mater. These sinuses and

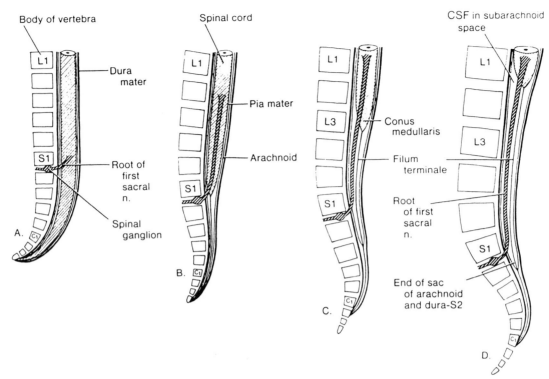

FIGURE 16–4. The position of the inferior end of the spinal cord in relation to the vertebral column and meninges at various stages of development: 8 weeks (*A*), 24 weeks (*B*), newborn (*C*), and 8-year-old child and adult (*D*). (From Moore KL: Clinically Oriented Anatomy. Baltimore, Williams & Wilkins, 1985, with permission.)

lacunae are venous channels located between the dura mater and the periosteum lining the cranium. The venous sinuses are lined with endothelium that is continuous with that of the cerebral veins. These sinuses have no valves and no muscle in their walls. Although the brain itself is insensitive to pain, the cerebral dura mater has nociceptive responses, especially around the venous sinuses of the dura. Several sinuses form the venous drainage system. The *superior sagittal sinus,* which travels in the midline, may be lacerated during surgical correction of a craniosynostosis or during a morcellation craniectomy. In about 60 percent of cases, the superior sagittal sinus ends by becoming the *right transverse sinus.* The transverse sinus runs above the tentorium cerebelli to the *sigmoid sinus.* The sigmoid sinus is so named because of its S-shaped course in the posterior cranial fossa. It eventually enters the superior bulbs of the internal jugular veins. All the venous sinuses of the dura mater deliver their blood to the sigmoid sinuses and then to the internal jugular vein, except the inferior petrosal sinuses, which enter the jugular veins directly. Finally, the *occipital sinus,* which is the smallest, lies along the foramen magnum and communicates with the internal vertebral plexus. The large and short *cavernous sinuses* surround the sella turcica. They join the inferior petrosal sinuses, which drain into the transverse sinus.

Spinal Cord Vascular Anatomy

The spinal cord vascular anatomy comprises separate anterior and posterior circulations that arise from the vertebral arteries and are supplemented by intercostal and lum-

bar vessels from the descending aorta (Fig. 16–5). The ventral two thirds of the spinal cord, which includes the corticospinal tracts and motor neurons, is supplied by a single anterior spinal artery. The dorsal one third of spinal cord parenchyma, which transmits proprioception and light touch, is supplied by paired posterior spinal arteries that actually form a plexus-like arrangement on the surface of the cord.[15] There is essentially no collateral flow between the anterior and the posterior circulations.

The anterior spinal artery is of great clinical importance because it supplies motor neurons and tracts. Some of its branches run circumferentially on the ventrolateral surface of the spinal cord to supply white matter tracts; sulcal branches penetrate the cord parenchyma and divide in the ventral gray matter. The anterior spinal artery is of uneven caliber and not functionally continuous throughout its length. The blood flow to the ventral spinal cord in some patients may be heavily dependent on collateral flow through radicular arteries arising from the aorta. These radicular vessels are unpaired and typically arise from intercostal or lumbar arteries on the left side of the aorta. Only six to eight of the 62 radicular vessels present during development persist into adult life, and 45 percent of the population have fewer than five (generally one or two cervical, two or three thoracic, and one or two lumbar). The large distance between these radicular vessels leaves watershed areas at the upper thoracic and lumbar levels; consequently, the spinal cord in these areas is particularly vulnerable to ischemia. For this reason, the great radicular artery of Adamkiewicz, which arises from the aorta between the T8 and L3 nerve roots and supplements

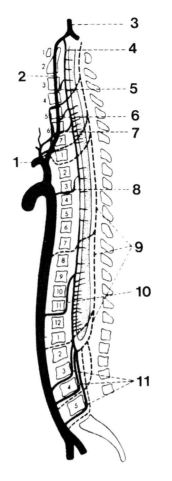

① subclavian artery
② vertebral artery
③ basilar artery
④ anterior spinal artery
⑤ ventral radicular artery $(C_3\text{-}C_4)$
⑥ ventral radicular artery $(C_5\text{-}C_6)$
⑦ ventral radicular artery $(C_7\text{-}C_8)$
⑧ ventral radicular artery $(T_3\text{-}T_4)$
⑨ posterior spinal artery
   dorsal radicular artery
⑩ great ventral radicular artery
   (Adamkiewicz's artery, $T_{11}\text{-}T_{12}$)
⑪ lumbosacral artery

FIGURE 16–5. Blood supply to the spinal cord. (From Goto T, Crosby B: Anesthesia and the spinal cord. *In* Bissonnette B (ed): Cerebral Protection, Resuscitation and Monitoring: A Look into the Future of Neuroanesthesia. Anesthesiology Clinics of North America. Vol 10. Philadelphia, WB Saunders Company, 1992, p 493, with permission.)

flow to the ventral portion of the distal thoracic spinal cord and lumbar enlargement, is a particularly important collateral vessel. It provides up to 50 percent of the entire spinal cord blood flow and may be injured during aortic or spinal surgery or after spinal trauma.

The venous outflow of the spinal cord is divided into two systems called the *vertebral venous plexuses*.[16] These internal and external plexuses communicate with each other and with the segmental systemic veins and the portal system.

The *internal plexus* consists of thin-walled, valveless veins in a basketwork pattern, which surround the dura mater of the spinal cord and the posterior longitudinal ligament. This plexus communicates through the foramen magnum with the occipital and basilar sinuses. At each spinal segment the plexus receives veins from the spinal cord and a basivertebral vein from the body of the vertebra. The plexus, in turn, is drained by intervertebral veins, which pass through the intervertebral and sacral foramina to the vertebral, intercostal, lumbar, and lateral sacral veins.

The *external plexus* is formed by the veins coming from each vertebral body, which join to form the anterior vertebral plexus. Veins passing through the ligamenta flava form the posterior vertebral plexus.

Neurophysiology

To understand the effect of anesthetic agents on the CNS and how these anesthetic actions may affect the outcome of neuroanesthesia, it is necessary to understand the basic principles of neurophysiology. This section reviews the physiology of the energetics of cerebral metabolism, cerebral blood flow, CSF dynamics, and spinal cord blood flow.

Energetics of Cerebral Metabolism

An analysis of the structure, physiology, and function of the human brain represents one of the most complex of all biologic problems. A major aspect of this complexity is the myriad of synaptic connections, voltage- and ligand-gated channels, and intracellular second-messenger systems that mediate interneuronal communications.[17] The energy required to maintain and regulate these systems is considerable. After 7 years of age the brain weighs a mere 2 percent of the total body weight but consumes more than 20 percent of the entire adenosine triphosphate (ATP) produced in the body. Under normal conditions, the main substance used for energy production in the brain is glucose.[18] In the presence of oxygen, glucose is the primary source of metabolic fuel to generate high-energy intermediates from the Krebs cycle. ATP is generated from adenosine diphosphate (ADP) and inorganic phosphate and the reduced form of nicotinamide-adenine dinucleotide (NAD) methemoglobin reductase (NADH) is produced from the oxidized form of NAD (NAD^+).

Glucose depletion rapidly leads to coma and eventually to brain death. The brain stores minuscule amounts of glucose and glycogen; muscle stores 10 times and the liver tissue 100 times as much glycogen per unit of mass as the brain. The glycogen content of the brain is sufficient to provide less than 3 minutes of normal ATP consumption. Therefore, the brain is entirely dependent on blood circulation for the 120 g of glucose it requires each day. Neonatal mammals have much greater brain glycogen stores, which may explain why they are more resistant to oxygen deprivation. The overall metabolic rate for the brains of children (mean age, 6 years) is markedly higher than in adults for both oxygen (5.8 vs. 3.5 ml O_2/min/100 g of brain tissue) and for glucose (6.8 vs. 5.5 mg glucose/min/100 g).[18]

In the absence of oxygen, glycogen is broken down, and the resultant glucose is used in the anaerobic glycolysis pathway to form ATP and NAD^+. This energy production is accompanied by the generation of hydrogen ions, which decrease intracellular pH and eventually alter conductivity and viability. When the oxygen supply to neurons is reduced to a minimum, survival mechanisms are triggered that reduce and/or slow the fall in ATP concentration until reestablishment of cerebral perfusion and substrate intake occurs. These include (1) the utilization of phosphate phosphocreatinine stores (a high-energy phosphate that can donate its energy passively to maintain ATP), (2) the production of ATP at low levels by anaerobic glycolysis, and (3) a rapid cessation of spontaneous electrophysiologic activity, reducing the energy demand by 60 percent.[19]

Cerebral Blood Flow and Cerebral Blood Volume

Cerebral blood flow is readily altered by the anesthesiologist and, to the extent that cerebral blood flow is related to cerebral blood volume, decreasing cerebral blood flow reduces ICP. Although intracranial pathology may alter or even reverse this relationship, it is, for the most part, the clinician's most useful tool in controlling ICP. Global cerebral blood flow in children between the ages of 3 and 12 years is higher than in adults and is around 100 ml/100 g of brain tissue per minute.[20, 21] Infants and small children between the ages of 6 and 40 months have a cerebral blood flow of about 90 ml/100 g/min.[22] Values for cerebral blood flow in premature and newborn infants are only 40 to 42 ml/100 g/min.[23, 24] The cerebral blood flow in gray matter is higher than that in white matter, and areas of predominant brain activity in children shift as they develop.[25] Regional areas in the brain that exhibit high levels of metabolic activity have higher levels of blood flow. As the cerebral metabolic rate of oxygen consumption ($CMRO_2$) increases or decreases, cerebral vasoconstriction or vasodilation occurs and alters cerebral blood flow to meet the current demand for oxygen. This phenomenon is known as autoregulation, and experimental evidence suggests that changes in local adenosine concentration that occur in response to changes in lactate levels are responsible for this vasoactivity. As $CMRO_2$ rises, as in fever or during seizure activity, cerebral blood flow and blood volume increase. ICP will potentially increase. Conversely, hypothermia and anesthetic agents that decrease $CMRO_2$ reduce cerebral blood flow. During mild to moderate hypothermia, $CMRO_2$ and cerebral blood flow initialy decrease on the order of 7 percent per degree centigrade.[26]

The global $CMRO_2$ of children 3 to 12 years old is 5.2 ml O_2/100 g of brain mass per minute, which is substantially greater than that of adults.[20-26] The $CMRO_2$ in anesthetized newborns and infants is 2.3 ml O_2/100 g of brain mass per minute.[21] The above discussion has looked at changes in cerebral blood flow from the demand side, yet important relationships exist on the supply side as well. Cerebral blood flow will autoregulate to maintain constant O_2 delivery over a wide range of perfusion pressures. Adults maintain a constant cerebral blood flow over a range of mean arterial pressures (MAP) between 60 and 150 mm Hg.[27] The autoregulatory thresholds for infants and children are not well known. Studies in neonatal animals suggest that the lower limit for autoregulation may be around 40 mm Hg and the upper limit at 90 mm Hg.[28, 29] Although it is not possible to calculate the effect of hypotension or hypertension on cerebral blood flow, it seems reasonable to assume that neonates with MAPs below 60 mm Hg autoregulate cerebral blood flow. Induced hypotension in infants seems to be well tolerated.[30]

Evidence suggests that neonates in severe distress have altered autoregulation.[31] Above and below the limits for autoregulation, cerebral blood flow changes passively with arterial blood pressure. Arterial blood pressure alone is an insufficient measure of cerebral perfusion. Cerebral perfusion pressure (CPP) is also important. CPP is the MAP minus the central venous pressure (CVP) or, in the case of the intact cranium, is MAP minus ICP when ICP exceds CVP. Again, on the supply side, anemia, hemodilution, and drugs that alter the rheologic properties of blood increase O_2 delivery by decreasing viscosity. Adenosine concentrations decrease, venoconstriction occurs, and cerebral blood volume decreases despite constant cerebral blood flow; this concept is known as *blood viscosity autoregulation*. Autoregulation is impaired or abolished by hypoxia,[32] vasodilators, and high concentrations of volatile anesthetics. However, as in adults, hyperventilation has been reported to restore autoregulation in the neonate.[33] Intracranial pathology owing to trauma, areas of inflammation surrounding tumors, abscesses, or sites of focal ischemia leads to altered autoregulation.[34] Autoregulation is easily impaired or lost in the newborn, and its loss may lead to intraventricular hemorrhage, CNS damage, or death.[35]

Cerebrovascular reactivity to hypocarbia is the anesthesiologist's most useful means of reducing cerebral blood flow. In adults, the cerebral blood flow varies linearly with a $Paco_2$ between 20 and 80 mm Hg. A 1-mm Hg fall in $Paco_2$ results in a 4 percent decrease in cerebral blood flow. As $Paco_2$ falls, cerebrospinal fluid pH rises and periarteriolar changes in pH are reflected in vasoconstriction. Chronic hyperventilation causes slow movement of bicarbonate ions out of the CSF and normalization of CSF pH and cerebral blood flow within 24 hours.[26] Sudden increases in $Paco_2$ after hyperventilation can result in cerebral vasodilation and increased ICP. Experimental evidence suggests that the immature brain is relatively unresponsive to small changes in $Paco_2$. However, a study in anesthetized infants and children (using transcranial Doppler sonography) has demonstrated that cerebral blood flow velocity changes logarithmically and directly with end-tidal carbon dioxide ($Petco_2$).[36] This study suggests that the vasodilatory effect of CO_2 on the cerebral vasculature may occur at much lower $Paco_2s$ than in adults. The cerebral vascular response to hypoxia is not well studied in children. Adults show no change in cerebral blood flow until Pao_2 falls below 50 mm Hg, after which cerebral blood flow increases exponentially.

Cerebrospinal Fluid

Fifty to 80 percent of the CSF is produced by the choroid plexuses lining the ventricular system. Extrachoroidal sites of production are not well identified, but it was suggested that the brain's ependymal surface and the brain parenchyma are possible sites of production.[37] Under normal circumstances, CSF production and absorption exist in equilibrium. The mean CSF production rate in children is 0.35 ml/min.[38] The composition of CSF differs from that of plasma, suggesting that it is the product of active secretion via an Na^+/K^+-dependent adenosine triphosphatase (ATPase) pump. Cerebrospinal fluid from the ventricular system exits from the fourth ventricle through the foramina of Magendie and Luschka into the subarachnoid space surrounding the brain and spinal cord. The main absorption of CSF is thought to occur in the arachnoid villi that project into the veins and sinuses of the brain. The exact mechanism of resorption is unknown, and both passive and active transport mechanisms have been proposed. Even the choroid plexus itself has been suggested as a possible site of absorption.[39] Under normal conditions, the ICP is much more dependent on cerebral blood flow and cerebral blood volume than on CSF production. Reduction of CSF production by one third reduces ICP by only 1.1 mm Hg.[40] It is therefore not surprising that drugs such as acetazolamide, which reduce CSF production, have minimal effects on ICP, and these effects become significant only in patients whose intracranial compliance curves lie to the right. In this group of patients, anesthetic agents that increase CSF production or decrease CSF absorption should be avoided.

Intracranial Pressure

Uncontrolled increases in ICP constitute one of the most deleterious pathophysiologic derangements faced by the anesthesiologist. In general, the cranium can be viewed as a closed space occupied by brain mass (70 percent), extracellular fluid (10 percent), blood volume (10 percent), and CSF (10 percent). Increases in the volume of any one of these must be offset by a reduction in the others to maintain an overall constant volume. The brain mass itself is relatively incompressible, and changes in CSF volume serve as the primary buffer against increases in the other volumes. When increases in intracranial volume can no longer be offset, ICP increases. ICP has been measured in neonates and infants.[41, 42] Normal ICP in adults is between 8 and 18 mm Hg, and that of children usually is 2 to 4 mm Hg. Newborns normally have a positive ICP on the day of birth but exhibit subatmospheric ICP in early life.[41] Newborn babies usually lose salt and water during the first few days after birth, and the brain contributes to this loss by reducing the intracerbral volume, which is reflected in less head growth during this period.[41] As pre-

viously stated, it is postulated that negative ICP promotes intraventricular hemorrhage, especially in premature infants.

Although the cranium is most easily viewed as a rigid space, the pediatric patient with open fontanelles or sutures may be able to compensate for a slow increase in intracranial volume by expansion of the skull. Sutures that are bridged by fibrous connective tissue are relatively difficult to separate and cannot compensate for acute increases in intracranial volume. In the older child, as in the adult, the skull is a rigid, nonexpandable container in which the pressure depends on the total volume of brain substance, interstitial fluid, CSF, and blood. A patient may have normal ICP yet be at a noncompliant point on the curve. If so, a small change in volume will result in a large and potentially dangerous increase in ICP. This is, of course, an idealized relationship, and there is evidence suggesting that the intracranial compliance curve is a smooth logarithmic curve, accounted for by the buffering of intracranial mass by the compliance of cerebral blood vessels and a pressure-driven increase in CSF absorption.[43–45] A review of the pressure–volume intracranial compliance curve demonstrates that with initial volume changes in one compartment, compensation is possible allowing only a small change in pressure.[46] The pressure–volume index (PVI) is an assessment of this compliance such that

$$PVI = \Delta V/\log_{10}(P_p/P_o),$$

where ΔV is the volume of the fluid bolus, P_p is the peak ICP after bolus injection, and P_o is the baseline ICP. In normal adults, about 25 ml is required to raise baseline ICP by a factor of 10, whereas in infants the normal PVI is 10 ml, because PVI is proportional to the neural axis volume.[47] Therefore, the ICP in infants and children rises much faster than it does in adults, which explains why a child can progress from neurologically well to moribund in 30 minutes.

Intervention by the anesthesiologist is based on the ability to shift the patient's intracranial compliance curve to the right, to change the slope of the patient's curve, or to move to the left along his own curve.

Spinal Cord Blood Flow

The use of Doppler flowmetry has simplified certain methodologic problems that researchers and clinicians have encountered in measuring spinal cord blood flow. Until recently, nearly all available data concerning spinal cord circulation physiology was obtained in animals. Within the limits of the Doppler technology and the determination of flow velocities, it is interesting to see that the rate of flow inferred with these measurements correlates well with those determined in cats.[48] Animal data suggest that the spinal cord blood flow is controlled by the same factors and operates according to the same general physiologic principles as the brain.[49, 50] It is known, however, that spinal cord blood flow is lower because absolute spinal cord metabolism is lower than that of the brain. The blood flow to spinal gray matter is about 50 percent that of the cerebral cortex and the flow to the white matter is lower still, which is approximately one third of the rate of the spinal gray matter.[51] The metabolic rate in the spinal cord is proportionally lower, so the ratio of supply to demand is probably similar to that of brain.

Regulation of Spinal Cord Blood Flow

The concept of spinal cord perfusion pressure (SCPP) (SCPP equals mean arterial pressure minus extrinsic pressure on the cord) is clinically useful because it describes factors that affect the adequacy of spinal perfusion.[52] Pressures exerted by local extrinsic mechanical compression,[53] such as tumor, hematoma, spinal venous congestion, and increased intraspinal fluid pressure, can be important determinants of the SCPP. Because spinal blood flow is maintained constant by vasodilation or vasoconstriction of the cord's vasculature to accommodate changes in mean arterial blood pressure,[49, 50] this suggests that blood pressure is not a determining factor in spinal cord perfusion. The limits of spinal cord blood flow autoregulation are inconsistent in the literature, and a range of 60 to 150 mm Hg is often cited. However, a lower limit of 45 mm Hg[54] and an upper limit of 180 mm Hg[55] have been suggested. Several conditions affect this autoregulatory mechanism: (1) blood pressure exceeding these limits, (2) severe hypoxia,[56] (3) hypercapnia,[56] and (4) trauma that abolishes vascular reactivity.[55] Epidural anesthesia may affect the spinal fluid pressure. Administration of 10 ml of solution into the epidural space increases CSF pressure,[57] but this effect is transient and probably has little significance for the SCPP. Much like the cerebral circulation, the spinal cord vasculature is very reactive to changes in oxygenation and CO_2 concentrations. Like the cerebral vasculature, the spinal cord does not respond to changes in Pa_{O_2} until the Pa_{O_2} decreases below about 60 mm Hg, after which the spinal cord blood flow increases sharply.[56] Many investigators have suggested that spinal cord blood flow is linear between a Pa_{CO_2} of 20 and 80 mm Hg, with an absolute change in spinal cord blood flow of about 0.5 to 1 ml/100 g/min/mm Hg change in Pa_{CO_2}.[51] The cerebral circulation changes approximately 1 to 2 ml/100 g/min/mm Hg change in Pa_{CO_2}.[58] This difference probably reflects baseline differences in the absolute rate of spinal blood flow and cerebral blood flow rather than differences in the sensitivities of the two vascular systems to CO_2.

NEUROPHARMACOLOGY

General Principles

Evidence from animals suggests that the lethal dose in 50 percent of the animals (LD_{50}) for many medications is significantly lower in the neonatal and infancy periods than in adults.[59] The sensitivity of the human newborn to most of the sedatives, hypnotics, and narcotics is increased, probably owing to increased brain immaturity (incomplete myelination and blood-brain barrier) and to increased permeability for some medications (i.e., the lipid-soluble drugs used in anesthesia).[60] In addition, the effect of volatile anesthetic agents is influenced by the age of the patient. The minimal alveolar concentration in the neonate (0 to 31 days) is much lower than in infants aged 30 to 180 days.[61] Although there is an increase in anesthetic requirements in infancy, it must be emphasized that there is a smaller margin of safety between adequate anesthesia and severe cardiopulmonary depression in the infant and child compared with the adult.[62] Therefore, dosages must be appropriately calculated and therapeutic effects must be monitored to avoid inadvertent adverse clinical consequences and prolonged effects.

Inhalational Anesthetic Agents

All currently used inhalational anesthetic agents have variable degrees of cerebrovascular effects.

Nitrous Oxide

The effect of nitrous oxide on cerebral circulation remains controversial. The reported variability of its effects on cerebral blood flow and ICP is probably because of differences in experimental species and background anesthesia. Subanesthetic doses of nitrous oxide 60 to 70 percent cause excitement, cerebral metabolic stimulation, and increased cerebral blood flow.[63–65] Because nitrous oxide is not an adequate anesthetic in the absence of other inhalational or intravenous (IV) anesthetics, studies reporting an increase in cerebral blood flow with nitrous oxide were accomplished in the presence of such medications. A study in infants and children showed that 70 percent nitrous oxide in oxygen with fentanyl–diazepam–caudal epidural anesthesia increased cerebral blood flow significantly compared with an air/O_2 mixture.[66] This increase in cerebral blood flow was not associated with significant changes in MAP, heart rate, or cerebrovascular resistance. It was suggested that nitrous oxide has a direct effect on cerebral mitochondrial metabolic activity. In animals, $CMRO_2$ increased without alterations in arterial blood pressure and heart rate.[64] It was hypothesized that nitrous oxide has direct effects on cerebral metabolism.[64] Clinically, nitrous oxide increases cerebral blood flow and ICP in adults and children.[66, 67] Barbiturates and hypocapnia in combination may prevent these increases. Given individually, barbiturates, benzodiazepines, and morphine can reduce the effect of nitrous oxide on cerebral blood flow.[68, 69] In contrast, volatile agents can further increase cerebral blood flow.[70] Although nitrous oxide is commonly used in neuroanesthesia, it may be prudent to discontinue its administration if the brain is tight. Furthermore, because of its ability to increase $CMRO_2$, it would be unwise to continue nitrous oxide administration when cerebral perfusion is reduced.

Halothane

Halothane is a cerebral vasodilator that decreases cerebrovascular resistance and increases cerebral blood flow in a dose-dependent fashion.[71, 72] In pediatric neuroanesthesia, halothane remains an excellent anesthetic agent and is thus widely used in combination with hyperventilation. Halothane is a potent vasodilator whose effects are maximal at 1 MAC. In animals, no additional vasodilation was caused by increasing the level of CO_2 when 0.5 MAC or

1 MAC halothane was administered.[73] In children with normocapnia, cerebral blood flow velocity (Doppler) changed between 0.5 MAC and 1 MAC but failed to increase further at 1.5 MAC (B. Bissonnette, unpublished data). Despite decreasing the halothane concentration from 1.5 MAC to 0.2 MAC, cerebral blood flow velocity remained increased for approximately 30 to 45 minutes (B. Bissonnette, unpublished data). This was thought to be because of a hysteresis phenomenon in the cerebral vasculature and may be important in patients with raised ICP. Halothane decreases cerebrovascular resistance, increases cerebral blood flow, and increases ICP in animals.[74] Many human studies have reported similar findings.[75, 76] Another study in children showed that the cerebrovascular reactivity to carbon dioxide during halothane anesthesia (0.5 or 1 MAC) was preserved, but that the vasoconstrictive effect of 20 mm Hg of carbon dioxide was not as strong at 1 MAC halothane as at 0.5 MAC halothane.[77] Therefore, if ICP is not being monitored, halothane should be avoided in patients known to have reduced intracerebral compliance until after the dura has been opened and halothane effects on the brain can be directly observed.

Isoflurane

Isoflurane is the most popular of the volatile anesthetics for neuroanesthesia. Its popularity is based on the fact that isoflurane affects cerebral blood flow less than halothane at equivalent MAC doses and on the belief that isoflurane may provide cerebral protection.[78, 79] Cerebral autoregulation is less affected by isoflurane than by halothane.[72] Also, isoflurane does not change CSF production and resorption as does enflurane.[80] Studies in children suggest that isoflurane has minimal effects on the cerebrovascular reactivity to CO_2.[81] During normocapnia, varying the concentration of isoflurane between 0.5 MAC and 1.5 MAC did not change cerebral blood flow velocity. Furthermore, there were no time–response effects of 1 MAC isoflurane on cerebral blood flow velocity in anesthetized children during 90 minutes.[82] Similar results were found by other investigators.[83, 84] However, despite their dissimilar effects on cerebral blood flow, isoflurane and halothane increase ICP equally in an animal model of brain injury,[85, 86] probably because both agents increase cerebral blood volume to a similar degree.[87]

Enflurane

Enflurane increases cerebral blood flow by a maximum of 8 to 37 percent, depending on the concentration used. This increase is less than that with halothane.[88, 89] Enflurane and halothane reduce $CMRO_2$ to a similar degree.[89] Enflurane in high concentration disrupts cerebrovascular autoregulation but does not affect cerebrovascular reactivity to CO_2. There are no data describing the effects of enflurane in pediatric anesthesia. Two effects of enflurane make it less suitable for neuroanesthesia. First, it increases the rate of CSF production[90] and decreases its reabsorption; the latter effect is greater than that observed with halothane.[91] Second, and by far the most important disadvantage of enflurane, is its ability to induce seizure-like electro-

encephalographic (EEG) activity (high-voltage spike waves with burst suppression [2 MAC]).[89–93]

Sevoflurane

Sevoflurane offers the advantages of rapid onset and titrability for close hemodynamic control, as well as rapid emergence for postoperative neurologic assessment.[94] Sevoflurane is similar to isoflurane with regard to its effects on $CMRO_2$ and ICP in adult neurosurgical patients.[95] It has been suggested that isoflurane may have a greater capacity to preserve global cerebral blood flow relative to $CMRO_2$ than halothane and sevoflurane.[96] Interestingly, another adult study found a better preservation of dynamic cerebral autoregulation during sevoflurane than isoflurane anesthesia.[97] In children, changes in arterial blood pressure and in cerebral blood flow velocity were studied during induction of anesthesia with sevoflurane or halothane with nitrous oxide in oxygen. Sevoflurane produced similar cerebrovasvular effects to those of halothane.[98] In pediatric patients with and without a history of epilepsy, tonicoclonic as well as clinically silent electrical seizures have been reported upon induction and during maintenance of anesthesia with sevoflurane.[99–101]

Desflurane

Desflurane increases cerebral blood flow and ICP, but decreases $CMRO_2$ in animals.[102, 103] One MAC desflurane has been shown to increase ICP significantly in neurosurgical patients with supratentorial mass lesions, despite the induction of hypocapnia. This was in contrast with one MAC isoflurane which did not increase ICP in the same group of patients.[104] There are no available data on the effects of desflurane on the cerebral circulation of children.

Intravenous Anesthetics

Barbiturates

Barbiturates decrease cerebral blood flow and $CMRO_2$ in a dose-dependent manner[105, 106] and reduce ICP. A major problem with barbiturates is that they can significantly reduce myocardial contractility, systemic arterial blood pressure, and CPP. In nonclinical doses (10 to 55 mg/kg), thiopental produces an isoelectric EEG and decreases the $CMRO_2$ by 50 percent.[106] Barbiturates can prevent an increase in ICP during laryngoscopy and tracheal intubation owing to their ability to decrease cerebral blood flow.[107] Cerebral autoregulation and cerebrovascular reactivity to CO_2 are preserved with barbiturates. Production and reabsorption of CSF is not altered.[108] Barbiturates are also effective in controlling epileptiform activity, except methohexital, which may activate seizure foci in patients with temporal lobe epilepsy.[109]

Etomidate

Etomidate reduces cerebral blood flow (34 percent) and $CMRO_2$ (45 percent).[110] Etomidate directly vasoconstricts the cerebral vasculature, even before the metabolism is suppressed.[111] Cerebrovascular reactivity to CO_2 is maintained.[110] Its advantage over barbiturates is that it does not produce cardiovascular depression. However, two disadvantages to its use are suppression of the adreno-cortical response to stress[112] and its ability to trigger my-oclonic activity, especially after prolonged infusion.[113]

Droperidol

Droperidol is a cerebral vasoconstrictor that reduces cere-bral blood flow (40 percent in dogs) without changing $CMRO_2$.[114] Failure to lower $CMRO_2$, despite reduced cere-bral blood flow, could be undesirable in patients with cerebral vascular disease or increased ICP. The combina-tion of fentanyl and droperidol has little effect on cerebral blood flow.[115]

Propofol

Propofol is a rapidly acting agent that reduces cerebral blood flow and $CMRO_2$.[116] It can reduce ICP, but its ability to reduce MAP may jeopardize CPP.[117] Propofol sedation is now widely used during awake craniotomy for sei-zures.[118] In epileptic patients, propofol at low doses causes activation of the electrocorticogram, whereas at higher doses, it is an anticonvulsant through its ability to induce burst suppression.[119]

Benzodiazepines

Benzodiazepines have been reported to decrease cerebral blood flow by a 25 percent decrease in $CMRO_2$.[120, 121] Benzo-diazepines can reduce ICP. Flumazenil is a benzodiaze-pine antagonist that reverses the beneficial effects of ben-zodiazepines on cerebral blood flow,[122] $CMRO_2$, and ICP.[123] Consequently, Flumazenil may have detrimental effects in patients with high ICP or abnormal intracranial elastance.

Opioid Anesthetics

The opioid agents have little or no effect on cerebral blood flow, $CMRO_2$, and ICP.[124] However, if patients are experiencing pain, opioids cause a modest reduction in these variables through indirect effects on the sympathetic nervous system.[125] Fentanyl combined with nitrous oxide decreases cerebral blood flow and $CMRO_2$ by 47 percent and 18 percent, respectively.[89] Cerebrovascular reactivity to CO_2 and cerebral autoregulation are preserved with narcotics. Finally, fentanyl has no effects on CSF produc-tion, but it reduces CSF reabsorption by at least 50 per-cent.[126, 127] In head trauma patients, both fentanyl and sufen-tanil, when given as an intravenous bolus, significantly increase ICP.[128, 129] Fentanyl has no effects on the cerebral circulation of neonatal animals, but alfentanil increases CSF pressure in patients with brain tumors.[130] This effect was less than that observed with sufentanil but greater than that observed with fentanyl. Alfentanil has the great-est effect on MAP and CPP.[131] Some studies reported a decrease in cerebral blood flow and $CMRO_2$,[132] whereas others suggested an increase in cerebral blood flow and ICP.[133] Remifentanil with its ultrashort elimination half-life, offers the advantage of not delaying postoperative neuro-logic assessment. Equipotent loading infusions of remifen-

tanil or fentanyl, followed by titration to hemodynamic effects, were studied in patients undergoing supratentorial tumor surgery with isoflurane and 2:1 nitrous–oxygen. Re-mifentanil and fentanyl had similar effects on absolute cerebral blood flow and cerebrovascular carbon diox-ide reactivity.[134]

Ketamine

Ketamine is a potent cerebral vasodilator capable of in-creasing cerebral blood flow by 60 percent in normocap-nic humans.[135] It has negligible effects on the $CMRO_2$. Pa-tients with increased ICP have had their condition deteriorate after ketamine administration.[136] Although it is suggested that ketamine may have some cerebral protec-tive effects, and even potentially decrease intracranial pressure in traumatic brain injury patients during propofol sedation, its use remains controversial in neuroanes-thesia.[137]

Muscle Relaxants

Muscle relaxants have little effect on cerebral circulation.

Succinylcholine

Succinylcholine produces an initial fall followed by a rise in ICP, especially in patients with decreased intracranial compliance resulting from increased cerebral blood flow.[138, 139] The increase in ICP is probably related to cere-bral stimulation caused by increases in afferent muscle spindle activity.[140] The increase in ICP and cerebral blood flow with succinylcholine is reduced by prior adminis-tration of deep general anesthesia or by precurariza-tion.[141, 142] However, the benefits to pediatric patients with increased ICP from rapid control of the airway and hy-perventilation offset the slight increase in ICP caused by succinylcholine. It is important to remember that life-threatening hyperkalemia may occur after administration of succinylcholine to patients with closed head injury even though they do not have motor deficits,[143] severe cerebral hypoxia,[144] subarachnoid hemorrhage,[145] cerebrovascular accident with loss of brain substance,[146] and paraplegia.[147]

Rocuronium and Rapacuronium

Rocuronium offers a perfect substitute to succinylcholine for rapid control of the airway when rapid restoration of spontaneous respiration is not anticipated.[148, 149] Rapacuro-nium, a short-acting nondepolarizing muscle relaxant, is currently being investigated in the pediatric population. When given intravenously, its rapid onset and short dura-tion of action rival that of succinylcholine.[150]

Pancuronium, Atracurium, Cis-Atracurium, and Mivacurium

Pancuronium and atracurium have no effect on cerebral blood volume, ICP, or $CMRO_2$ in the presence of halo-thane.[151] Large doses of d-tubocurarine, atracurium, meto-curine, or mivacurium may release histamine and cause transient cerebrovascular dilatation, which could account for a slight increase in ICP. However, a slight decrease in MAP may offset any change in intracerebral blood volume.[152] Cis-atracurium does not release histamine, which should offer greater cardiovascular stability.[153]

Vecuronium

Vecuronium is known for its cardiovascular stability and its relatively short duration of action. In patients with reduced intracranial compliance, vecuronium slightly decreased ICP, probably because there was a concomitant decrease in CVP.[154]

PATHOPHYSIOLOGY OF INTRACRANIAL PRESSURE

Limiting blood supply to the brain usually results in ischemia and neuronal damage. The brain is the organ most sensitive to ischemic damage.[19] To understand how to protect the brain against hypoxic-ischemic damage, it is essential for the anesthesiologist to appreciate the pathophysiologic mechanisms associated with this insult.

The central event that precipitates cell damage is reduced production of energy (ATP), decreased activity of the ATP-dependent ion pumps, increased intracellular concentrations of sodium and calcium, and decreased intracellular concentrations of potassium. These ion changes cause the neurons to depolarize and to release excitatory amino acids such as glutamate and aspartate. The increase in glutamate increases neuronal depolarization and calcium entry through the N-methyl-D-aspartate (NMDA) receptor channel. The high intracellular calcium concentrations increase the activity of proteases and phospholipases and activate the Haber-Weiss reaction. The increased phospholipase activity causes free radical production and lipid peroxidation, which leads to release of free fatty acids and membrane destruction. Although the mechanisms of neuronal damage are similar in global and focal ischemia, there are important distinctions between the two. In focal ischemia, three anatomohistologic factors are identifiable. First, the region affected has no blood flow and responds in the same way as globally ischemic tissue. Second, a transitional zone called the *penumbra* receives collateral blood flow. Although this area is salvageable, it remains vulnerable to ischemia and dependent on the reestablishment of perfusion. Third, the region surrounding the penumbra is well perfused and normal.

Brain trauma may cause permanent neuronal damage. The mechanism of this damage can be either brain herniation or severing of blood vessels in brain tissue, both of which lead to ischemia. In these circumstances, it is important to prevent the ischemia caused by release of vasoconstrictive substances during reperfusion. Calcium influx after trauma has been implicated as the trigger for this damage.[155]

Trauma-induced hemorrhage may increase ICP by changing intracranial blood volume and decreasing CPP. The extravasated blood can cause additional damage by increasing the release of free radicals after release of iron from hemoglobin.

These pathophysiologic events associated with brain damage may be ameliorated by vigorous treatment, including maintaining ATP levels (either by increasing substrate use or reducing the metabolic rate), blocking the ionic flux across the cell membrane, limiting free radical production or increasing the efficiency of scavenging mechanisms, and avoiding the production of acidic metabolites (such as glutamate and asparate) that favor neuronal depolarization and destruction. Most importantly, cerebral blood flow and oxygen delivery to the tissues must be maintained.

Hydrocephalus

Hydrocephalus is characterized by an increased volume of CSF within the ventricular system and, with few exceptions, is caused by obstruction of CSF circulation or reduced reabsorption. The obstruction may lie within the ventricles themselves, within the subarachnoid space, or at sites of CSF egress or absorption. Patients with obstructive hydrocephalus and blocked access to the arachnoid villi appear to have alternative sites of CSF absorption. There is evidence of some lymphatic-type drainage and of transependymal absorption of CSF.[156] Many classifications of hydrocephalus have been proposed. Increased ICP may occur without hydrocephalus, and vice versa.

In the newborn period, and especially in premature infants, hydrocephalus is usually secondary to intraventricular hemorrhage, aqueductal stenosis, or an Arnold-Chiari malformation. Bleeding into the subependymal germinal matrix may extend into the ventricle and block CSF flow.[157] An obliterative arachnoiditis also may obstruct CSF flow, even after the blood is resorbed. In the neonate, hydrocephalus may exist despite normal ICP. Any increase in CSF volume is compensated for by a decrease in brain mass until the compliance limit of immature brain tissue is reached. Arnold-Chiari malformations are common and consist of an array of abnormalities, mainly in the posterior fossa and cervical region. The brain stem is displaced downward and, together with an abnormal vermis, extends below the foramen magnum and into the cervical canal. The fourth ventricle becomes compressed and its foramina become obstructed. The cranial nerves may be stretched or entrapped secondary to downward displacement of the brain stem, which causes a variety of bulbar symptoms. Hydrocephalus is present in about 90 percent of cases. Other diseases of childhood characterized by hydrocephalus include the mucopolysaccharidoses (which obliterate the subarachnoid space) and achondroplastic disorders (which alter occipital bone growth and impede venous outflow).[158, 159] Similarly, any condition that causes significant cranial deformity can lead to hydrocephalus. In childhood, brain tumors are the most common cause of hydrocephalus.

Brain Tumors

Half of all childhood brain tumors arise in the posterior fossa, with a predisposition for midline structures, and are frequently associated with obstructive hydrocephalus, headache, and vomiting.[160] Medulloblastomas (composing 15 to 20 percent of CNS tumors in children) are usually found growing adjacent to or within the fourth ventricle. Ependymomas also are found most frequently in the fourth ventricle. A posterior fossa tumor should be suspected in all children who present with increased ICP or cranial nerve symptoms. Choroid plexus papillomas are the only known pathologic cause of CSF overproduction and hydrocephalus.

Brain tumors are expanding, space-occupying lesions, which lead eventually to increased ICP and to a reduction in CPP. Nonautoregulated vessels associated with these tumors contribute to peritumoral vasogenic edema, which further elevates ICP. Ultimately, nontreated brain masses lead to brain stem herniation and death.

Before surgical excision of CNS tumors, administration of dexamethasone will reduce the vasogenic edema surrounding the tumor. Brain bulk can be reduced by dehydration with mannitol, hypertonic saline, and furosemide. Furosemide also may secondarily decrease ICP by reducing CSF production and by reducing CVP by peripheral venodilation. The administration of osmotically active agents will be discussed below.

Complications of Elevated Intracranial Pressure

It is usual to consider the cranial space as a closed box. However, the cranial space is divided into distinct spaces, with the cerebral hemispheres divided by the falx cerebri and the elements of the posterior fossa separated from the hemispheres by the tentorium cerebelli. Shifts of intracranial contents occur when asymmetric increases in pressure create gradients across the falx, the tentorium, and the foramen magnum. Tentorial herniation (the uncal syndrome) results in typical eye and motor signs as the diencephalon moves backward through the tentorial notch. Compression of the superior colliculus causes vertical gaze palsy (sunset sign). When a mass effect occurs within one compartment, extrusion of brain from one compartment to another occurs when the limits of compensation or buffering have been exceeded. As a mass expands in one hemisphere, one anterior cerebral artery may be compressed as brain tissue gains access into the opposite hemisphere under the falx cerebri. The resulting ischemia produces further edema and swelling. Herniation at this level often disrupts cortical pathways to the contralateral limbs and the bladder sphincter. Compression of the posterior cerebral artery against the tentorium results in hemianopsia. Calcarine infarction may arise from bilateral compression of the basal arteries and lead to irreversible blindness. Protrusion of the parahippocampal gyrus (uncus) of the temporal lobe beneath the tentorium cerebelli and through the tentorial hiatus cause signs of brain stem compression: progressive obtunding of reflexes, ipsilateral pupillary dilation, contralateral hemiparesis and, if uncontrolled, cardiorespiratory arrest. Midbrain compression in children is associated with hypertonic extension of the upper arms and legs (dog-paddling arms and cycling legs), opisthotonos, decerebrate rigidity, decorticate posturing, and hypotonia. Further compression of the midbrain results in coma, hypertension, bradycardia, tachypnea, and periodic respirations.[161] As pressure on the medullary respiratory center increases, bradypnea is replaced by apnea.

Distortion of posterior fossa contents by a mass effect may obstruct the flow of CSF and lead to obstructive hydrocephalus. Even without herniation, increases in ICP result in global or regional cerebral ischemia. As ICP approaches MAP, cerebral perfusion pressure falls below critical levels. This causes tissue hypoxia, cell injury or death, swelling from increased brain edema from fluid shifts in response to disturbed electrolyte balance, and a vicious cycle of increasing brain volume and ICP. Herniation of brain from the posterior fossa usually includes the cerebellar tonsils and vermis, which protrude through the foramen magnum. This protrusion causes compression of the medullary cardiorespiratory centers. Loss of upward gaze (sunset sign), projectile vomiting, miotic fixed pupils, and central hyperventilation are suggestive of increased pressure in the posterior fossa. Failure of vocal cord abduction may result in inspiratory stridor. Gross displacement of the brain (the final manifestation of severe posterior fossa hypertension) compresses the vascular supply to the medulla as it protrudes through the foramen magnum. This results in Cushing's triad (tachypnea, hypertension, and bradycardia) and eventually leads to apnea and death.[162]

GENERAL ANESTHETIC CONSIDERATIONS

The following sections discuss the anesthetic management of pediatric neurosurgical procedures. Topics common to most procedures are reviewed first, followed by discussion of specific considerations and surgical procedures.

Preoperative Assessment of the Neurosurgical Patient

In recent years, increased understanding of cerebral pathophysiology and improved diagnostic imaging techniques have improved the preoperative assessment of neurosurgical patients. However, the cornerstone of assessment of cerebral function is still the history and physical examination. The preoperative anesthetic work-up of the neurosurgical patient includes an assessment of ICP, assessment of the function of vital respiratory and cardiovascular centers that can be affected by neuropathologic processes, either in the brain stem or in the spinal cord, and assessment of the specific disturbances in neurologic function.[163]

Of primary importance is the preoperative recognition of intracranial hypertension and major neurologic deficits. The history and physical findings of intracranial hypertension differ somewhat according to the age group. In general, the clinical presentation of patients with intracranial hypertension varies with the duration of increased ICP. Sudden massive increases in ICP often cause coma. In a less acute case, however, there may be a history of headache on awakening, suggestive of vasodilation caused by sleep-induced hypercapnia and reduced intracranial compliance. Vomiting is a common sign. Neonates and infants often present with a history of increased irritability, poor feeding, or lethargy. A bulging anterior fontanelle, dilated scalp veins, cranial enlargement or deformity, and lower extremity motor deficits are also common signs of increased ICP in this age group.[164] Increased ICP in children is frequently caused by a tumor. As ICP reaches critical levels, vomiting, decreased level of consciousness, and evidence of herniation may develop. Other symptoms include diplopia caused by oculomotor or gaze palsies (sunset sign), dysphonia, dysphagia, and/or gait disturbances. Injury to the third cranial nerve may result in ptosis. Injury to the sixth cranial nerve produces a strabismus caused by loss of abduction. Nausea and vomiting usually occur, and older children complain of morning headache. Papilledema and absent venous pulsation of the retinal vessels may be seen on funduscopy.[47, 161–164]

Neurogenic pulmonary edema is a syndrome that includes acute hypoxia, pulmonary congestion, pink, frothy, protein-rich pulmonary edema, and radiologic evidence of pulmonary infiltrates.[165, 166] It is associated with a variety of intracranial pathologic occurrences, including hemorrhage,[167] head trauma,[168] and seizures.[169] The mechanisms responsible for activating the sympathetic nervous system and the vagal centers, which leads to pulmonary edema, are related to ischemia of the medulla and distortion of the brain stem.[170] Cranial nerve function and the patient's ability to protect the airway must be evaluated. During the preoperative assessment, the possibility of spinal cord dysfunction must be determined. Neurologic dysfunction arising from cervical spinal cord injury may affect the respiratory and cardiovascular centers (see below).

Laboratory tests may yield evidence of syndrome of inappropriate antidiuretic hormone (SIADH) and of electrolyte abnormalities or volume contraction from protracted vomiting. Diabetes insipidus may result in hypernatremia.[171] Disturbances in metabolism, such as hypo- or hyperglycemia, may be present. The preoperative history and chart review may reveal that the patient is receiving steroids to reduce tumor edema. If so, steroids will be required during surgery. Neurosurgical patients may be receiving anticonvulsant medication either to treat seizures or to prevent them. These drugs may have profound effects on the metabolism of other drugs (e.g., barbiturates, narcotics). Patients with suprasellar tumors, such as craniopharyngioma, frequently have pituitary dysfunction and should have a complete endocrine evaluation before surgery.

Skull radiographs, ultrasonography, computed tomographic (CT) scan, and magnetic resonance imaging (MRI) aid in the assessment of intracranial hypertension. Skull radiographs may show the "beaten copper sign" (Fig. 16–6) and widening of the sagittal sutures in response to chronic increased ICP and universal suture stenosis. In infants and young children, the width of the cranial sutures should not exceed 2 mm, and they should not have bridges or closures.[172] Ultrasonography of the brain is useful in premature infants and neonates because it is relatively inexpensive, does not require sedation, and can be performed at the bedside through the fontanelle. The real-time sector scanner can visualize virtually all parts of the brain.[173] Development of CT scan and MRI has revolutionized the investigation of brain disease.

Premedication

The routine use of sedation in pediatric neurosurgical patients is best avoided. If sedatives and narcotics are

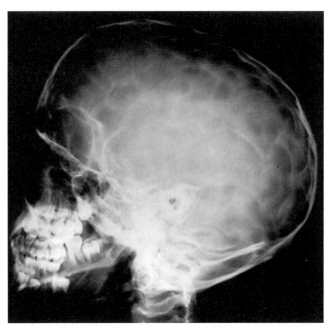

FIGURE 16–6. Plain film of the skull in lateral projection, showing extensive "beaten copper" or "thumb printing," which is the result of sustained increased ICP caused by universal suture stenosis.

given, the patient must be closely monitored because the drugs may precipitate respiratory depression, hypercarbia, loss of airway integrity, and increased ICP.

Exceptions to this rule include patients with intracranial vascular lesions (with no increase in ICP) who may benefit from sedation to reduce the likelihood of precipitating a preoperative hemorrhage. Sedation can be accomplished in small children with pentobarbital 4 mg/kg or chloral hydrate 50 mg/kg administered orally or rectally 1 hour before surgery. Emotional preparation is essential and is accomplished by the anesthesiologist and the parents working together. In older children, a simple explanation of what to expect before induction of anesthesia will reduce the element of surprise and the incidence of hemodynamic responses in a threatening environment.

Patient Positioning

Planning of a successful anesthetic includes the preparation of the operating table with proper equipment to protect the patient after positioning. The anesthesiologist's preoperative visit should provide information on patient positioning during surgery.

Although patient positioning varies according to the neurosurgical procedure, the general principles remain the same. The eyes must be securely taped closed and, if the patient is prone, the face and other vulnerable areas must be padded to prevent localized pressure. Since ventilation may be compromised by incorrect positioning, it is mandatory to ensure that chest excursion remains adequate, especially when the patient is prone. This can be achieved by using suitable bolsters or a frame that allows the abdomen to be pendulous and facilitates respiratory movement during intermittent positive-pressure ventilation. The endotracheal tube (ETT) should be taped securely in place; in the prone position, secretions may loosen the tape. A 10-degree head-up position is usually advisable to improve cerebral venous return and reduce venous congestion. Rotation of the head to one side may kink the jugular veins and reduce venous return. This kinking can be avoided by rotating the trunk to maintain the axial position. During any surgical procedure, it is important for the anesthesiologist to be able to inspect the ETT and circuit connection and to have access to the tube for possible endotracheal suctioning. In addition, it is desirable to have a body part, such as a hand or foot, visible during surgery so that peripheral perfusion and color can be readily assessed.

Monitoring

Basic monitoring consists of a precordial/esophageal stethoscope, electrocardiography (ECG), a noninvasive blood pressure measuring device, a temperature probe, a pulse oximeter, and capnometry. In addition, a radial pulse Doppler allows continuous monitoring of peripheral perfusion on a beat-to-beat basis and provides a noninvasive measurement of blood pressure. The Doppler device is especially useful in neonatal anesthesia. A peripheral nerve stimulator for monitoring neuromuscular blockade is desirable. A urinary catheter is required for long surgical procedures and is mandatory if osmotic diuretics are administered.

Induction of Anesthesia: General Principles

Anesthesia for pediatric neurosurgical procedures often presents a challenge to the anesthesiologist. The anesthetic technique chosen and recognition of perioperative events may have profound effects on morbidity. Pediatric patients range from premature neonates to 16-year-old young adults. Knowledge of normal physiology in these differing age groups is essential. Neonatal anesthesia differs from that in the older child and adult, particularly with regard to the respiratory system, the cardiovascular system, and thermoregulation.

Anesthesia for patients with elevated ICP is fraught with danger. After induction of anesthesia, rapid tracheal intubation and hyperventilation will lower the ICP. The systemic hypertension associated with laryngoscopy may be avoided by giving IV lidocaine at induction of anesthesia. However, it is important to limit the bolus dose of lidocaine in infants and small children, since severe cardiovascular depression can occur.[174] The authors recommend that the dose of lidocaine should be limited to 0.5 mg/kg. Rapid-sequence induction of anesthesia can be achieved using thiopental and atropine. The use of carefully applied cricoid pressure and manual hyperventilation is recommended unless the patient has evidence of unstable cervical spine. With appropriate cricoid pressure, manual ventilation can be performed without distention of the stomach, which will prevent the transient increase in cerebral blood volume and intracranial pressure.[175] Cricoid pressure reduces the likelihood of aspirating gastric contents; delayed gastric emptying is often associated with increased ICP. Muscle relaxation to facilitate tracheal intubation can be provided with succinylcholine or rocuro-

nium. The rapid rate at which succinylcholine produces satisfactory intubation conditions outweighs the small increase in ICP that it causes.[141] Consequently, succinylcholine is routinely used in pediatric neuroanesthesia. Rocuronium 1.0 to 1.2 mg/kg produces intubation conditions comparable to succinylcholine.[148] In patients without ready IV access, anesthesia can be induced via a small butterfly needle, which can be inserted with minimal patient stress or hemodynamic fluctuation. Failing this, it is probably less injurious to children with raised ICP to perform a skillful inhalation induction of anesthesia than it is to subject them to a difficult IV placement. Anesthesia is best maintained with nitrous oxide in oxygen, isoflurane, and a suitable muscle relaxant. It is important to remember that sevoflurane should be used with caution, especially when high concentrations are given to children known to have seizure activity.[99–101] Intermittent positive-pressure mechanical ventilation is provided. Hypoventilation and hypercarbia are best avoided. An IV narcotic can be used in children. Deep levels of anesthesia are not needed and are contraindicated.

Fluid Management and Intracranial Pressure Control

Fluid Management

Fluid administration to neurosurgical patients depends on the pathology or brain insult being treated. A frequent result of these insults is the development of brain edema, with a resultant increase in ICP. It is essential for the neuroanesthesiologist to understand the principles of fluid movement in the injured brain to administer the proper fluid regimen.

Edema formation occurs when there is inequality of net movement of fluid between the intra- and extracellular compartments. Edema is the result of pressure gradients between the hydrostatic, osmotic, colloid oncotic pressures, and the properties of the barrier that separate them. The blood-brain barrier is composed of capillary endothelial cells, which are connected in continuous fashion by tight junctions. This system forms a barrier that excludes polar hydrophilic molecules. The endothelium of the brain differs from that of the rest of the body. In most noncentral neural tissue, the tight junction between endothelial cells is 65 Å (angstroms), whereas it is 7 Å in the CNS. In the brain, the size of these junctions is sufficiently small to prevent sodium from traversing them freely. Essential molecules, such as glucose and amino acids, cross the blood-brain barrier by energy-mediated transport systems. Only water freely communicates with both sides of the membrane. This passive movement of water is regulated by oncotic, osmotic, and hydrostatic pressure changes across the barrier. The colloid oncotic pressure is a relatively weak driving force, although in very low concentration, it can aggravate brain edema after mechanical head injury.[176] A reduction of 50 percent of the colloid oncotic pressure (normal, 20 mm Hg) results in a pressure gradient across the membrane, which is less than that caused by a transcapillary osmolarity difference of 1 mOsm/L. A reduction in the colloid oncotic pressure of the brain does not have the same impact as that observed in the bowel.

This is because the brain's extracellular space is poorly compliant, because of its network of glial cells, and discourages edema formation, even in the presence of a severe colloid oncotic pressure gradient. Administration of lactated Ringer's solution alone will lead eventually to hemodilution and reduced plasma osmolarity (osmolarity, 273 mOsm/L^{-1}), which would encourage cerebral edema.[177]

The choice of fluid must be dictated by the neuropathologic process involved. It should maintain an isovolemic, iso-osmolar, and relatively iso-oncotic intravascular volume. For example, a patient with increased ICP and/or a brain mass requires a fluid regimen that balances adequate intravascular volume against efforts to dehydrate the brain mass. In a patient undergoing insertion of a ventricular shunt and/or repair of myelomeningocele, fluid management should replace third-space losses.

An osmolar gradient can be maintained only in areas where the blood-brain barrier is intact. Under normal circumstances, osmotic diuretics and plasma expanders, such as albumin, are excluded. Unfortunately, areas that might benefit the most from dehydration therapy, such as tumor edema, exhibit blood-brain barrier incompetence. Agents of high osmolality move into these tissues and increase the edema.[178]

Efforts to dehydrate the brain are complicated by the need to maintain adequate circulating blood volume. In many neurosurgical procedures, a substantial portion of the blood loss is onto the drapes and is difficult to measure. Furthermore, the use of large amounts of irrigation solution makes it impossible to assess blood loss accurately. The initial phase of any neurosurgical procedure produces blood loss, especially scalp incisions. Infiltration of the scalp with bupivacaine 0.125 percent with 1:200,000 epinephrine reduces blood loss and reduces hemodynamic responses (increased heart rate and blood pressure) during incision.[179] In all cases, bupivacaine blood levels were within the therapeutic range. Resection of a vascular malformation may require massive volume replacement. Placing large-bore lines and having available sufficient blood products are part of appropriate planning for anesthesia and surgery. Urine output in the face of aggressive diuresis is a misleading indicator of adequate volume replacement. In this instance, CVP monitoring is very useful.

There is no perfect protocol for fluid replacement in neurosurgical patients with increased ICP. However, maintenance of cerebral perfusion should represent the optimal goal of fluid therapy. Most anesthesiologists start osmotic diuretic therapy at the beginning of anesthesia and measure the resulting urine output. As surgery and blood loss progress, volume replacement usually consists of a mixture of crystalloid and colloid solutions to maintain an isovolemic, iso-osmolar, and iso-oncotic intravascular volume. After an initial 20 ml/kg of crystalloid solution, a mixture of normal saline with albumin 5 percent in a ratio of 3:1 can be given. A suitable alternative to albumin is the use of a synthetic colloid such as pentastarch.[180] In a rat model of brain injury, the group receiving normal saline had a significant increase of brain water content accompanied by a reduction of colloid osmotic pressure, when compared to the hetastarch and whole blood groups.[176] In another animal model of spinal cord ischemia, pentast-

arch reduced microvascular permeability, neuron membrane injury, and incidence of paraplegia when compared to normal saline and hetastarch.[181] As described earlier, the brain that has sustained a recent insult (primary lesion) is vulnerable to so-called secondary brain injury (penumbra area) either for a short period of mechanical compromise (retraction)[182, 183] or to a minor episode of hypotension, hypoxia or ischemia (hemodynamic instability).[184] Although rapid administration of normal saline (10 ml/kg) has little effect on cerebral blood volume and ICP, it may reinstitute hemodynamic stability.[185] Blood products should be administered only on the basis of hemodynamic instability and diminished oxygen-carrying capacity.

Dextrose-containing solutions are associated with a poorer neurologic outcome and are best avoided unless hypoglycemia has been confirmed.[186, 187] Stressed neonates have reduced glycogen stores, and patients from the intensive care unit may have high glucose loads in their parenteral nutrition. Abrupt cessation of high-dextrose solutions can precipitate an insulin-induced hypoglycemia. In these patients, blood glucose levels should be sampled frequently and normoglycemia maintained.

Diuretics to Reduce Intracranial Pressure

Hypertonic Saline

Some investigators have suggested that extracellular volume dehydration can be accomplished by raising serum osmolality with hypertonic saline (3 percent saline).[188] Hypertonic saline solution has been shown to be effective for volume resuscitation, while resulting in less cerebral edema and/or ICP elevation.[190] In children with severe head injury, fluid resuscitation with hypertonic saline (sodium 268 mmol/L, 598 mOsm/L) is superior to resuscitation with lactated Ringer's solution (sodium 131 mmol/L, 277 mOsm/L). Children who received hypertonic saline required less interventions to maintain their ICP below 15 mm Hg, received less fluid on day 1, had diminished mechanical ventilation requirements, and had a lower frequency of acute respiratory distress syndrome than children receiving lactated Ringer's solution. Despite the fact that children treated with hypertonic saline had a shorter intensive care unit (ICU) stay, the overall survival rate and duration of hospitalization were similar in both groups.[189] In another study of children after head trauma, 3 percent hypertonic saline significantly reduced ICP when compared with normal saline.[150]

Mannitol

Mannitol (20 percent solution) remains the most popular diuretic for reducing ICP and providing brain relaxation. Small doses, such as 0.25 to 0.5 g/kg, will raise osmolality by 10 mOsm and reduce cerebral edema and ICP.[190, 191] Mannitol's effects begin within 10 to 15 minutes of its administration and persist for at least 2 hours. Mannitol-induced vasodilation affects intracranial and extracranial vessels and transiently increases CBV and ICP while simultaneously reducing systemic blood pressure.[192] In particular, some children may show transient hemodynamic instability (during the first 1 to 2 minutes) after rapid administration of mannitol.[193] Therefore, the drug should be given at a rate not to exceed 0.5 g/kg over 20 to 30 minutes. The initial period of hypotension will be followed by increases in cardiac index, blood volume, and pulmonary capillary wedge pressure, all of which reach peak values 15 minutes after infusion.[194] The changes in intravascular volume last for about 30 minutes and then return to normal levels. Administration of furosemide before administering mannitol may increase venous capacitance, reduce transient increases in intravascular volume, and provide more effective dehydration. There is, however, a danger of producing profound dehydration and severe electrolyte imbalance.[195] Larger doses of mannitol produce a longer duration of action, but there is no scientific evidence that they reduce ICP further.[190] In the presence of cerebral ischemia, larger doses of mannitol 2 g/kg can be used.[196] This has been shown to increase cerebral blood flow[197] and cardiac output,[198] probably by reducing blood viscosity (rheology)[199] or by increasing intravascular volume. It has been suggested that with decreased viscosity, cerebral blood flow increases, causing autoregulatory vasoconstriction and therefore decreased cerebral blood volume. ICP decreases as a consequence of decreased cerebral blood volume.[200] Mannitol also has the ability to decrease brain tissue volume by decreasing brain tissue water content. Furthermore, mannitol significantly decreases the rate of CSF formation when administered at high-dose in animal studies.[201]

Loop Diuretics

The loop diuretics, such as furosemide and ethacrynic acid, may reduce brain edema by inducing a systemic diuresis, decreasing CSF production,[202] and improving cellular water transport.[203, 204] Although furosemide can reduce ICP without increasing cerebral blood volume or blood osmolality, it is not as effective as mannitol.[203] The initial dose of furosemide should be 0.6 to 1 mg/kg if administered alone or 0.3 to 0.4 mg/kg if administered with mannitol to children. It has been suggested that ethacrynic acid reduces secondary brain injury by decreasing glial swelling.[205] Raising serum osmolality above 320 mOsm may precipitate acute renal failure, water retention, and a falling serum osmolality. Periods of aggressive dehydration may be followed by rebound intracranial hypertension.

Corticosteroids

Corticosteroids are an important part of the therapeutic regimen in neurosurgical patients with raised ICP. They reduce edema around brain tumors, but hours or days may be required to produce an effect.[206] However, the administration of dexamethasone preoperatively or at the induction of anesthesia frequently improves the neurologic status before the ICP decreases. It has been suggested that this is in response to a partial restoration of blood-brain barrier function.[207]

Temperature Homeostasis

Although hypothermia reduces the cerebral metabolic rate for oxygen, it frequently delays drug clearance, slows reversal of muscle relaxants, decreases cardiac output, causes conduction abnormalities, attenuates hypoxic pulmonary vasoconstriction, alters platelet function, causes electrolyte abnormalities, and induces postoperative shivering.[208] The intraoperative vasoconstriction produced by hypothermia reverts to vasodilation and redistribution of body heat on rewarming, and the core temperature falls.[209]

Neonates and infants are at greatest risk of hypothermia because of their large surface area relative to body mass. Despite a warm operating room, body temperature falls immediately after induction of anesthesia owing to internal redistribution of body heat from the central compartment to the periphery.[210] As heat loss continues, young pediatric patients trigger nonshivering thermogenesis in an attempt to rewarm themselves. In the paralyzed and ventilated patient, body temperature and P_{ETCO_2} concentration may increase at constant minute ventilation.[211] This phenomenon may not be readily apparent owing to cold fluid administration. Temperature monitoring is essential, but the actual site of the probe placement is less important than probe reliability.[212] For this reason, we usually place the probe in the esophagus or rectum. During induction of anesthesia and during placement of IV lines and monitors, a large body surface area is exposed. During these procedures, premature infants and small infants should be placed under a radiant heat lamp. Extremities can be covered with plastic wrap or sheet wadding. Dry inspired gases should be warmed and moisturized with a heat exchanger.[212-214] Although the usefulness of warming blankets has been questioned, they appear to work well, provided they are positioned both above and below the patient. Blood warmers should always be used if substantial fluid replacement is required. Rewarming measures, such as a forced warm air system (Bair Hugger), can be used in the postoperative period.

Venous Air Embolism

Venous air embolism is one of the most serious complications of anesthesia and surgery. It may occur whenever the operative site is elevated above the heart, and the risk increases as the height difference increases. Classically, it is associated with posterior fossa surgery in the sitting position, but it is not confined to this procedure. It has been reported in infants and children during procedures involving the skull, such as morcellation of the cranial vault, craniectomy for craniosysnostosis, and spinal cord procedures.[215, 216] It has also occurred with the patient in the lateral position.[217] The incidence of venous air embolism has been reduced considerably by use of the prone position for posterior fossa surgery[218] and by use of mechanical ventilation.

Air entrainment occurs when a number of conditions are met, including (1) venous pressure at the operative site that is below atmospheric pressure, (2) a vein that is open to the atmosphere, and (3) a vein that is prevented from collapsing. It most commonly occurs during the first hour of surgery, and the most frequent sites of air entrainment are the cranial diploic veins, the emissary veins, and the intracranial venous sinuses, which are kept open by their dural attachment. Venous air embolism can also occur from veins in muscles and from the puncture site of the multipoint head-holder used in children over 3 years of age.[219, 220] Detection of venous air embolism depends entirely on the sensitivity of the monitors used. The reported incidence of air emboli varies widely.[221, 222] Using highly sensitive precordial Doppler, the reported incidence of air embolus is as high as 58 percent in adult patients undergoing posterior fossa surgery in a sitting position.[223] Less than half of the cases of detected emboli produce systemic hypotension.[224] In pediatric neurosurgery the incidence of detectable air emboli is about 33 percent,[225] but systemic complications occur in more than half of the cases. Although children are not more prone to air emboli than adults, they are more susceptible to them. For example, the incidence of air embolism during craniosysnostosis repair in supine infants may be as high as 67 percent.[216] This may explain why, without any obvious reason, some patients experience periods of hypotension. In addition, the increased right-sided pressure may cause air to pass from the right side of the heart to the left via an atrial septal defect,[226] causing paradoxical air embolus (PAE). Anatomically, some 27 percent of patients have a patent foramen ovale and are potentially at risk for embolization to the left heart. Air also may reach the systemic circulation without the presence of an intracardiac septal defect,[227] and may result in cerebral or myocardial infarction.

It is essential to take measures to avoid this potentially disastrous complication. Meticulous avoidance of a pressure gradient between the open tissue and the heart and the routine use of positive-pressure ventilation are mandatory. On detecting air entrainment, the anesthesiologist must (1) advise the neurosurgeon to discontinue surgery, flood the surgical field with fluid, and compress the jugular veins to prevent further ingress of air; (2) ventilate the lungs with 100 percent oxygen; (3) attempt to withdraw air through the central venous catheter; (4) treat any hemodynamic consequences; and (5) if hemodynamic instability persists, turn the patient into a left-side-down position. When venous air is detected during craniotomy in children, air can be successfully aspirated in veins 38 to 60 percent of the time.[225] IV fluids,[228] appropriate antiarrhythmic and inotropic agents, or vasopressors may be necessary and should be administered as needed. Nitrous oxide must be discontinued because it increases the size of the embolus severalfold, causing further physiologic compromise.[229] Some authors have proposed that a positive end-expiratory pressure (PEEP) of 10 cm H_2O might decrease the rate of air entry by increasing venous pressure, but 10 cm H_2O pressure is not adequate to do so.[230] It is possible that the use of PEEP may cause paradoxical air embolism. However, 8 cm H_2O pressure did not raise the right atrial pressure above left atrial pressure.[231]

SPECIFIC ANESTHETIC CONSIDERATIONS

Neuroradiology

Children and infants, unlike adults, frequently require general anesthesia or sedation for neuroradiologic diagnostic or interventional therapeutic procedures. Several special problems are related to the administration of anesthesia in this context. Among these is the delivery of care in a remote area away from skilled help, the limitations imposed by cumbersome equipment, the necessity to be at a distance from the patient during the procedure, and the occasional adverse effects of contrast agents. The principal indication for anesthesia in these circumstances is to provide total immobility for extended periods for young patients who cannot cooperate.

The most common procedures are CT scanning, cerebral angiography, lumbar myelography, radiation therapy, and MRI. Specific anesthetic considerations for these procedures depend on the patient's condition and the radiologic demands.

Skull Abnormalities

The most common skull anomalies in pediatric anesthesia are the craniosysnostoses (Fig. 16–7) and craniofacial dysmorphism (Fig. 16–8).

Craniosynostosis

Special considerations for patients with craniosynostosis include (1) increased ICP and (2) blood loss.

Children and infants undergoing craniectomy may have increased ICP, and induction of anesthesia should proceed as discussed before. The degree of blood loss is increased in patients with multiple suture synostoses and in those more than 6 months old with thicker bone tables. Most craniosynostosis surgery is performed between 2 and 6 months of age, a period that coincides with physiologic anemia. Transfusion may therefore be required to main-

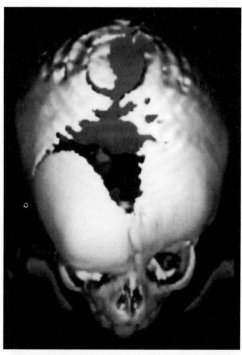

FIGURE 16–7. Three-dimensional CT scan image of a 6-month-old infant, showing the cranial vault contours. The asymmetric deformity of the skull is because of premature synostosis of the coronal and metopic sutures.

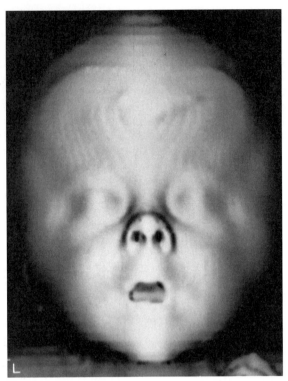

FIGURE 16–8. Three-dimensional CT scan image of an infant face, showing craniofacial contours of a patient with Crouzon syndrome.

tain an acceptable hemoglobin level. Simple suture craniectomy in the young child with normal ICP seldom requires arterial line placement. However, adequate IV access for fluid and blood replacement is essential. Children with elevated ICP and those undergoing extensive multiple suture procedures usually require arterial line placement.

Craniofacial Procedures

Special considerations for craniofacial procedures (see Chapter 24) include (1) difficult intubation, (2) blood loss, and (3) extubation and airway edema. Many craniofacial procedures require frontal bone advancement or reshaping, which involves intracranial surgery. Efforts to reduce brain bulk are often necessary. Occasionally a lumbar subarachnoid drain is placed for continuous cerebrospinal fluid drainage.

Tracheal Intubation

Patients undergoing craniofacial procedures present a multiplicity of tracheal intubation problems, from mandibular hypoplasia, or lack of neck or trachea mobility, to macroglossia and poor mouth opening. Few children can tolerate awake laryngoscopy or awake fiberoptic intubation. Therefore, anesthesia is usually induced by inhalation of halothane or isoflurane. After successful induction of anesthesia, direct laryngoscopy or fiberoptic-guided intubation of the trachea (possible with endotracheal tubes of 3 mm diameter and above) can usually be accomplished. In the older child or teenager, local anesthesia combined with neuroleptic drugs can be used. Help should always be available for difficult tracheal intu-

bations, as well as equipment for surgically securing the airway. After the ETT is placed, it should be wired to the mandible by the surgeon, and the eyes should be sewn closed. Mono-bloc procedures require intraoperative replacement of a nasal and tracheal tube.

Blood Loss

Craniofacial surgery often includes multiple suture craniectomies, dissection of large skin flaps, and facial bone repositioning, all of which result in copious blood loss.[232] Rapid blood transfusion may increase potassium acutely and lead to serious problems in very small children.[233, 234] Blood loss can be reduced by using a hypotensive anesthetic technique. At least two large-bore IV catheters, an arterial line, and a urinary catheter should be placed. Central line placement is often very helpful for determining adequacy of fluid replacement and for aspiration of intracardiac air should an air embolism occur. Patients in whom air embolism is likely require precordial Doppler monitoring.

Extubation and Airway Edema

Patients undergoing facial procedures below the orbits frequently have significantly edema of the upper airway. In our institution and many others, patients who have undergone extensive frontal craniotomies remain intubated, sedated, and ventilated, with subarachnoid drains in place, for 24 to 48 hours postoperatively in an effort to reduce CSF leakage through the dura before extubation. These patients should be fully awake and carefully suctioned to remove any clots and residual blood in the oropharynx before their tracheal tubes are removed.

Hydrocephalus

Hydrocephalus is a congenital or acquired pathologic condition with many variations, but it is always characterized by an increase in the amount of CSF that is now or has been under increased pressure (Fig. 16–9). It can occur at any age. It is caused by one of four basic disease processes: (1) congenital anomalies (e.g., Arnold-Chiari malformation), (2) neoplasms, (3) inflammatory conditions, and (4) overproduction of CSF (choroid plexus papillomas).

Ventricular Shunts

Three types of ventricular shunts are in current use: ventriculoperitoneal, ventriculo-atrial, and ventriculopleural. Each has its indications and anesthetic implications. Often, as the pediatric patient grows, the shunt must be revised. It must be replaced if it malfunctions or becomes infected. Placement or revision of shunts is common in both severely neurologically impaired children and in otherwise healthy patients. These children may present to the operating room multiple times and may request a specific anesthesia induction technique. Patients who present for CSF shunting procedures may exhibit a broad spectrum of symptoms and clinical signs, ranging from an apparently

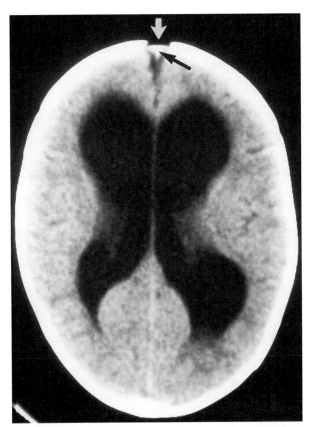

FIGURE 16–9. Axial CT scan image showing significant dilation of the lateral ventricle in hydrocephalus. The open anterior fontanelle is seen (*white arrow*) with the unprotected superior sagittal sinus lying within it (*black arrow*).

healthy child with minimal disability to a seriously ill, comatose patient for whom surgery is urgent.

Considerations

Preanesthetic assessment must include the following:

1. Level of consciousness. Patients presenting for primary shunting, shunt revision, or malfunction may exhibit severe elevations in ICP that require aggressive treatment.
2. Full stomach. Evidence of vomiting or delayed gastric emptying are indications to take precautions against aspiration of gastric contents (e.g., a rapid-sequence induction).
3. Coexisting pathology. Does the child have evidence of other significant organ system compromise, such as the child with cerebral palsy who frequently aspirates?
4. Age-related pathophysiology. Is the patient likely to have apnea, poor pulmonary compliance, or immature renal function?

Monitoring

Routine monitoring has been discussed earlier. Arterial line placement is usually reserved for the patient with uncontrolled ICP and hemodynamic instability.

Preinduction

A shunt scan helps to determine the site of malfunction. In some cases, the increased ICP caused by shunt malfunction can be reduced acutely by tapping the proximal reservoir. Infiltration of the skin with local anesthetic allows the tap to proceed with minimal trauma to the patient. The needle can be left in place to monitor ICP during induction. In the patient at risk for emesis during induction of anesthesia, placement of a nasogastric tube may precipitate coughing and bucking and increase ICP. Severely neurologically compromised children often have gastrostomy tubes, and opening these tubes before induction of anesthesia is recommended. However, this does not guarantee that the patient will not vomit and aspirate gastric contents.

Induction and Intubation

Many patients with hydrocephalus have undergone multiple surgical procedures. If there is no clinical evidence of elevated ICP, anesthesia can be induced by mask or with IV drugs; we usually allow children their preference. On the other hand, children with increased ICP and delayed gastric emptying usually have anesthesia induced with thiopentone, atropine, lidocaine, a narcotic, and a nondepolarizing muscle relaxant after preoxygenation. Cricoid pressure is applied and the patient is hyperventilated at low peak inspiratory pressures. Since laryngoscopy is a potent stimulus for increasing ICP, an oral tracheal tube is placed as smoothly as possible.

Maintenance

The considerations of maintenance of anesthesia are as follows:

1. Positioning
2. Ventilation
3. Anesthetic agents
4. Muscle relaxants
5. Fluid management
6. Maintenance of body temperature

Patients are placed in a supine position with the head turned, or in a slightly lateral position. Patients with increased ICP should be placed in a 30-degree head-up position with minimal neck rotation or flexion to improve cerebral venous drainage. Patients whose shunt tubing is placed posteriorly and those who are placed in a lateral position should have an axillary roll placed and all extremities padded.

After the airway is secured, patients with increased ICP are hyperventilated to a $Paco_2$ of 25 to 30 mm Hg. Patients with normal ICP are maintained at normocapnia. Spontaneous ventilation should be avoided in patients with ventriculopleural shunts to reduce the risk of pneumothorax and in those with ventriculoatrial shunts to avoid air embolism. Also, spontaneous ventilation should be avoided when the cranium is opened. Patients with poor pulmonary compliance and those at risk for apnea should be mechanically ventilated during anesthesia.

Anesthesia is usually maintained with nitrous oxide in oxygen, low concentrations of isoflurane or sevoflurane, and minimal narcotic supplementation. Although nitrous oxide increases cerebral blood flow in anesthetized pediatric patients,[66] increases in cerebral blood flow and $CMRO_2$ are effectively blunted by hyperventilation and pretreatment with thiopentone. As previously mentioned, halogenated anesthetics increase cerebral blood flow, cerebral blood volume, and ICP in a dose-dependent manner, with isoflurane having a less adverse effect than halothane. These agents are therefore either used in low concentrations in patients with elevated ICP or avoided entirely until the CSF is drained. Muscle relaxation is usually maintained with an intermediate-acting muscle relaxant if the procedure is expected to last a short time.

Ventricular shunt procedures usually are not associated with significant blood loss or third-space losses, and fluid management centers around replacement of intravascular volume associated with emesis or drug-induced diuresis.

The body temperature may decrease during shunt procedures, despite their relatively short duration. Exposure of a large body surface area and cold preparation solution, particularly for ventriculoperitoneal shunting, may cause infants to cool rapidly.

Emergence from Anesthesia

Anesthetic considerations for emergence from anesthesia are the following:

1. Elimination of anesthetics
2. Reversal of neuromuscular blockade
3. Delayed gastric emptying

Adequate time for elimination of the anesthetic agents and adequate reversal of neuromuscular blockade should be ensured before extubation of the trachea. Although it does not provide absolute insurance against regurgitation, the stomach should be suctioned before extubation of the trachea in patients suspected of having increased gastric contents. The patient should be fully awake and have an appropriate gag reflex to protect his airway against emesis. Many patients coming for shunt procedures are severely neurologically impaired and have poor airway control.

Postoperative Management

The anesthetic considerations for postoperative care are similar to those required for any general anesthetic. They include the following:

1. Oxygen and respiration
2. Maintenance of body temperature
3. Analgesia

As with any postsurgical patient, supplemental oxygen should be given and the respiratory pattern and adequacy assessed. Neurosurgical patients in general, and preterm infants who are less than 50 weeks' postconceptual age in particular, are likely to have abnormal respiratory patterns or apnea after surgery. Hypothermic patients should be rewarmed before extubation of the trachea.

Analgesics should be used judiciously in neurologically impaired patients. Infiltration of the skin with local anesthetic at the time of surgery substantially reduces the requirement for postoperative analgesia. Patients without preoperative neurologic impairment can be given routine postoperative narcotics.

Intracranial Tumors

Malignancy is second only to unintentional injury as a cause of death in children less than 15 years of age in the United States.[235] The second most common cancer of childhood (after leukemia) is CNS neoplasm, which accounts for 21 percent of all cancers in children.[236] The incidence of CNS tumors is 14 percent higher for males than females. The annual incidence rate for all CNS tumors is 27.6 per 1 million children younger than 15 years of age.[236] The mortality rate from pediatric brain cancer has declined over the past two decades, from 2 per 100,000 to less than 0.9 per 100,000 per year.[160] Despite this improvement, much remains to be accomplished, especially in children less than 2 to 3 years of age at the time of diagnosis.

From the anesthesiologist's point of view, intracranial brain tumors are divided according to the site of the tumor. The following section describes an anesthetic approach for supratentorial and posterior fossa craniotomies and for surgical excision of craniopharyngiomata.

Supratentorial Craniotomy

Supratentorial lesions account for about half of all pediatric brain neoplasms. For reasons related to embryogenesis, pediatric brain tumors often arise from midline structures, including the hypothalamus, epithalamus, and thalamus, and the basal ganglia (Fig. 16–10). These tumors tend to impinge on the ventricular system and cause obstructive hydrocephalus. Hemispheric masses are more common during the first year of life.[237] Their frequency in infants is approximately twice as high as in children (i.e., 37 percent compared with 16 to 24 percent).[238] The relative incidence of hemispheric tumors also increases after 8 to 10 years of age.[239]

Anesthetic Considerations

1. Increased intracranial pressure. The ICP should be estimated. The CT scan and MRI film should be reviewed.
2. Full stomach. Delayed gastric emptying occurs in the patient with raised ICP.
3. Electrolytes and fluid. Hydration state and electrolyte balance may be altered in the child with intracranial pathology and SIADH.
4. Age-related pathophysiology. Anesthetic considerations are identical to those discussed earlier.
5. Positioning. The head should be elevated not more than 10 degrees from level. It should be confirmed that venous return is not obstructed.

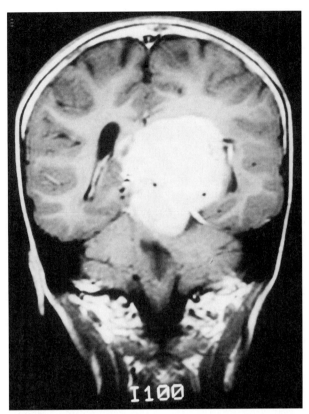

FIGURE 16–10. Midsagittal MRI scan demonstrating a midline glioma in a child. The rounded black spots within the tumor represent the basal cerebral arteries.

Monitoring

To the routine monitoring previously described, we add an arterial line for hemodynamic monitoring and blood sampling. In patients in whom we expect significant blood loss, hemodynamic instability, or air embolism, we insert a central venous catheter. A urinary catheter is inserted because of the duration of the surgical procedure and the use of osmotic diuretics.

Preinduction

Detection of preoperative elevation of ICP in patients undergoing craniotomy is essential. Most patients with large mass lesions, significant tumor edema, or obstruction to CSF outflow require an anesthetic approach that aims to reduce ICP. Some children undergo ventriculostomy placement before their definitive surgical procedure, as discussed earlier. Preoperative neurologic deficits should be detected and documented. Many patients with intracranial pathology present with SIADH. Such children have evidence of hyponatremia, low serum osmolality, high urine osmolality, and oliguria. Peripheral edema is rarely present. Preoperative treatment of SIADH usually includes fluid restriction.

Induction of Anesthesia and Tracheal Intubation

Unlike children with normal ICP, induction of anesthesia, followed by rapid securing of the airway and hyperventila-

tion are of paramount importance in patients with significantly elevated ICP. Induction of anesthesia generally proceeds as discussed in the section on hydrocephalus and includes IV thiopentone, lidocaine, a narcotic, and a nondepolarizing muscle relaxant. Cricoid pressure is applied and the patient hyperventilated with low peak inspiratory pressures to avoid inflation of the stomach. Laryngoscopy should proceed as smoothly as possible. Some anesthetists prefer nasotracheal intubation for patients in whom postoperative ventilation is expected or to better stabilize the ETTs of small infants.

Maintenance

The considerations for maintenance of anesthesia include the following:

1. Ventilation
2. Positioning
3. Anesthetic agents and muscle relaxants
4. Fluid management
5. Maintenance of body temperatures

Patients with increased ICP are generally ventilated to a $Paco_2$ of 25 to 30 mm Hg. Occasionally, lower levels of $Paco_2$ are required if the brain is very "tight" and there is uncontrollable intracranial hypertension. Caution must be exercised because extreme hyperventilation may decrease CPP sufficiently to induce cerebral ischemia or to shift blood flow from brain with low flow to areas of brain with impaired autoregulation and high flow. PEEP is generally avoided to facilitate cerebral venous drainage. PEEP may also decrease MAP, which should be considered in patients with decreased CPP. In patients with impaired oxygenation, small amounts of PEEP may correct hypoxia without obstructing venous return.

Pediatric patients are usually placed supine for supratentorial procedures, with the head elevated slightly to facilitate venous drainage. Extremities should be well padded and the eyes protected from injury. Care must be taken to avoid undue flexion, extension, or rotation of the neck.

Discussion of the specific pharmacology of each anesthetic agent is beyond the scope of this chapter. We use one of two techniques: neuroleptanalgesia or balanced inhalational anesthesia. The neurolept technique combines nitrous oxide, a synthetic short-acting narcotic (usually fentanyl citrate or remifentanil), a nondepolarizing muscle relaxant, and either a benzodiazepine or droperidol. With balanced anesthesia, sub-MAC concentrations of isoflurane are used with nitrous oxide, fentanyl, and a nondepolarizing muscle relaxant. Any nondepolarizing muscle relaxant is acceptable for neurosurgery, but pancuronium, because it is vagolytic and does not stimulate histamine release, which could increase ICP, is preferred in infants and small children.

Fluid management can be a problem. Patients with increased ICP are usually dehydrated after receiving mannitol. This increases the potential for hypovolemia and hypotension, especially when there is significant blood loss. CVP monitoring allows early detection of hypovolemia and volume expansion with colloid solutions such as 5 percent albumin or pentastarch. This synthetic colloid (average molecular weight of 260,000 Da) offers the advantage of reducing blood-brain barrier permeability and cerebral edema in animal models of temporary focal cerebral ischemia. In a study where pentastarch was compared to albumin, brain injury and vasogenic edema were substantially decreased in the pentastarch group. Reduction by pentastarch of transcytosis of serum proteins into brain parenchyma could be one of the mechanisms by which vasogenic edema is decreased.[180] Another study failed to show the same beneficial effect of pentastarch when compared with 0.9 percent saline in an animal model of transient global cerebral ischemia.[240] Both pentastarch and hetastarch can be used safely in children to a maximum dose of 25 and 20 ml/kg respectively (coagulopathies have been described with higher doses).[241] Simple craniotomy in patients without significantly increased ICP and in procedures with little blood loss frequently requires crystalloid replacement only.

Emergence

Anesthetic considerations for emergence include the following:

1. Elimination of anesthetic agents
2. Reversal of neuromuscular blockade
3. Delayed gastric emptying
4. Increased intracranial pressure

The decision to extubate the trachea at the end of the procedure is made on the basis of the success of the surgical intervention, smoothness of the intraoperative course, normalization of ICP, age of the patient, degree of residual neurologic deficit, and the presence of factors that affect respiration and airway protection. Patients with inadequate respiratory efforts retain CO_2 and their ICP may therefore be increased. Those without a gag reflex cannot protect their airway. Children who remain sedated and who hyperventilate during the postoperative period should be suspected of having increased ICP. Neonates with poor pulmonary compliance or an immature respiratory drive may require postoperative mechanical ventilation. Barring any of these complications, a child's trachea can be extubated after awakening and after reversal of the neuromuscular blockade and elimination of anesthetic agents.

Postoperative Management

Considerations for postoperative management after supratentorial craniotomy include the following:

1. Oxygen and respiration
2. Temperature homeostasis
3. Analgesia
4. Neurologic assessment
5. Hypertension
6. Seizures

As with any postsurgical patient, supplemental oxygen should be administered and the adequacy of respiration

assessed. Patients who require postoperative ventilation also require sedation and possibly muscle relaxation, to prevent agitation and increased ICP. Infiltration of local anesthetics into the wound intraoperatively or performance of a cervical superficial plexus block at the end of the procedure can reduce the requirement for postoperative analgesics. A balance between patient comfort and the ability to follow the patient's neurologic status must be sought. An obtunded patient must be investigated for increased ICP or other surgically correctible pathology, such as intracranial bleeding. Body temperature should be maintained at a normal level.

The most common cause of increased ICP after surgery is uncontrolled systemic hypertension. When postoperative pain control has been achieved, blood pressure can be controlled with vasodilators. β-Blocking medications have been used successfully, particularly labetolol, which normally does not cross the blood-brain barrier.

Seizures frequently occur during the immediate postoperative period. Therefore, many surgeons administer anticonvulsants before surgery and continue these drugs postoperatively. Phenobarbital is the most commonly used drug, and phenytoin or other medications are added if the seizures are refractory to treatment.

Craniopharyngioma

Special considerations for craniopharyngioma surgery include the following:

1. Positioning
2. Hypopituitarism
3. Diabetes insipidus (DI)
4. Altered insulin requirement
5. Hyperthermia
6. Seizures

Craniopharyngioma is a benign encapsulated tumor of the hypophysis cerebri (Fig. 16–11). Children with this tumor often present with symptoms of endocrine failure, visual disturbances, or hydrocephalus, as the tumor grows beyond the sella turcica and compresses the optic chiasm or other midline structures. The transsphenoidal approach to this tumor is rarely used in pediatric patients, and most resections are therefore performed through a frontal craniotomy. Anesthesia for craniopharyngioma and hypothalamic tumor surgery is similar to that for supratentorial craniotomy.

Preoperative evaluation of the child with craniopharyngioma focuses on determining the presence of hydrocephalus and on the types of endocrine dysfunction that could affect anesthetic management. Children may present with symptoms of hypothyroidism, growth hormone deficiency, adrenocorticotropic hormone (ACTH) deficiency, or DI. Hormone replacement, including thyroid hormone and corticosteroids, may be necessary pre- and postoperatively.

Diabetes insipidus is a complication of pituitary surgery and of head injury. It is caused by disruption of antidiuretic hormone (ADH)-secreting cells. It is rarely present preoperatively, but usually begins 4 to 6 hours after surgery, although it occasionally becomes evident intraoperatively.

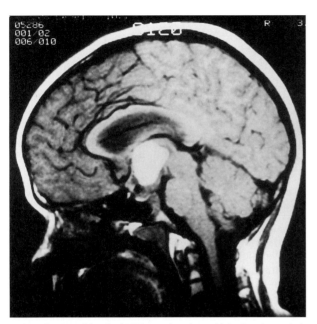

FIGURE 16–11. Midsagittal MRI scan showing, a high-signal mass lesion filling the suprasellar cistern (craniopharyngioma). The lesion extends from the pituitary fossa and herniates into the third ventricle.

Characteristically, patients produce a large quantity of dilute urine. Their serum osmolality increases, and their urine osmolality is low (<200 mOsm/L). The urine specific gravity is below 1.002. The patient becomes hypernatremic and hypovolemic. Treatment of DI requires careful determination of the patient's hourly urine output and administration of maintenance fluids plus 75 percent of the previous hour's urine output. The type of fluid to be administered is determined by the patient's serum electrolyte concentrations. Urine is low in sodium content and should be replaced with hypotonic solutions, such as 5 percent dextrose in water (D_5W) half-normal saline. Hyperglycemia and osmotic diuresis may occur if a large volume of D_5W is used. Vasopressin or one of its analogues, such as 1-deamino-8-D-arginine vasopressin (DDAVP), should be administered at an early stage of DI. When administered intraoperatively, aqueous DDAVP occasionally produces hypertension. Postoperatively, DDAVP 0.05 to 0.3 ml/kg is divided into two doses (5 to 30 mg/day) and given transnasally. If DDAVP is given IV, the dose is one tenth the intranasal dose, divided into two doses. DDAVP also can be administered by constant infusion at 0.5 U/kg. The rate must be adjusted to achieve the desired degree of antidiuresis.

Postoperative management should include administration of steroids, thyroid, mineralocorticoid, and sex hormone supplements. Insulin-dependent diabetics may have reduced insulin requirements after surgery. Therefore, the amount of glucose in their blood must be closely monitored and their insulin regimens altered as necessary.[242]

Other problems that arise postoperatively include seizures and hyperthermia. Surgical exposure often requires significant retraction of the frontal lobes. Consequently, anticonvulsant prophylaxis may be necessary intraoperatively and should be continued postoperatively. Injury to the hypothalamic thermoregulatory mechanisms may re-

sult in hyperthermia. Efforts should be made to maintain normothermia and reduce the risk of hypermetabolic cell injury.

Posterior Fossa Surgery

Posterior fossa tumors (Fig. 16–12) are more frequent in children than in adults and account for about half of all pediatric brain tumors.[243] The four most common tumors are medulloblastoma (30 percent), cerebellar astrocytoma (30 percent), brain stem glioma (30 percent), and ependymoma (7 percent). The remaining 3 percent include acoustic neuroma (Fig. 16–13), meningioma, ganglioglioma, and other much rarer tumors. Cerebellar astrocytomas have no sex predilection, but medulloblastoma occurs more frequently in males.[244] Hydrocephalus occurs in 90 percent of children with medulloblastoma and in virtually all children with cerebellar astrocytoma (Fig. 16–12).[245]

The most frequent surgical procedure, other than for tumors, is decompression for Arnold-Chiari malformation with obex occlusion (Fig. 16–14A,B). The Arnold-Chiari malformation is a complex developmental anomaly that characteristically presents with downward displacement of the inferior cerebellar vermis into the upper cervical spinal canal and elongation of the medulla oblongata and the fourth ventricle. Preoperatively, the anesthesiologist should pay particular attention to the neurologic symptoms, such as cerebellar dysfunction, upper airway obstruction (inspiratory stridor), cardiovascular instability, and increased intracranial pressure.

Anesthetic Considerations

1. Age-related pathophysiology.
2. Intracranial pressure. Symptomatic hydrocephalus may require placement of an external ventricular

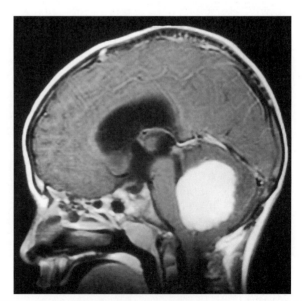

FIGURE 16–12. Midsagittal MRI scan showing a large fourth ventricle tumor. The tumor obstructs the aqueduct of Sylvius, resulting in hydrocephalus. The mass effect bulges the tentorium upward, compresses the pons against the clivus, and herniates the cerebellar tonsils through the foramen magnum.

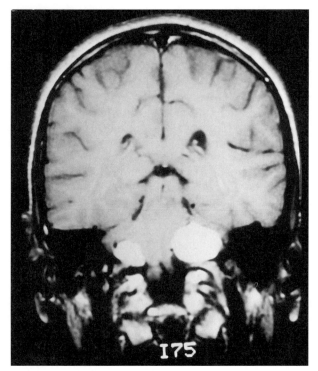

FIGURE 16–13. Coronal MRI scan through the brain stem and cerebellar pontine, showing large, round bilateral acoustic neuromas in a patient with neurofibromatosis.

drain (EVD) after induction of anesthesia. Maintenance of cerebral perfusion is essential. Mannitol, furosemide, and corticosteroids may be required.

3. Full stomach. Pathology in the posterior fossa decreases gastric emptying in children and makes them prone to regurgitation and aspiration of gastric contents with induction of anesthesia.

4. Associated preexisting problems. Cardiovascular: some patients may be hypertensive in response to brain stem compression; pulmonary: recurrent aspiration pneumonia is a common occurrence; nervous system: central sleep apnea occurs and may persist postoperatively.

5. Air embolism. See above.

6. Airway management. Arnold-Chiari malformation or brain stem compression may cause upper airway dysfunction and inspiratory stridor.

7. Fluid and electrolytes. Preoperative attempts to reduce ICP may cause electrolyte imbalance and contraction of the intravascular volume.

8. Premedication. See above.

Preoperative Evaluation and Induction of Anesthesia

Preoperative assessment of these patients is similar to that described previously.

During the induction of anesthesia, attempts must be made to preserve CPP, to avoid ICP elevations, and to provide an appropriate depth of anesthesia. The choice of anesthetic is not as crucial as the manner in which it

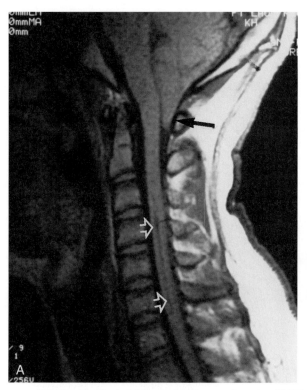
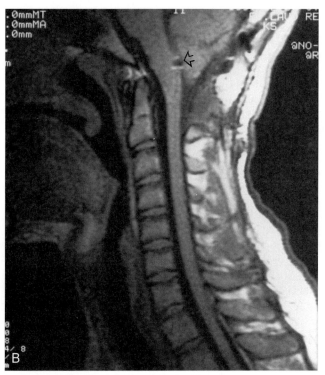

FIGURE 16–14. *A,* Midsagittal MRI scan of an Arnold-Chiari malformation type I, showing the cerebellar vermis extending through the foramen magnum (*black arrow*) and the association of cervicospinal syringomyelia (*open white arrows*). *B,* Posterior fossa decompression with occlusion of the obex with fat (*open black arrow*). The cervicospinal syrinx has disappeared.

is administered. A combination of thiopental, atropine, and a nondepolarizing muscle relaxant associated with a narcotic, such as fentanyl or remifentanil, is common. Succinylcholine can be used safely[246] unless the patient shows signs of severe increased ICP with hemodynamic instability. Rocuronium is the perfect alternative for a rapid-sequence induction in these patients. To minimize the possibility of kinking and obstructing the ETT during positioning, a reinforced armored orotracheal tube can be used. Many neuroanesthesiologists, however, prefer to use a nasotracheal tube for better stability and fixation. Use of an oral tracheal tube with a soft bite block reduces epistaxis and avoids possible nasal mucosal injury and infection.

Maintenance of Anesthesia

As with induction of anesthesia, no single anesthetic technique has been shown to be superior,[247] and the maintenance regimen must be tailored to the needs of the patient and the requirement of the surgical procedure. After skin preparation, local anesthetic (bupivacaine 0.125 percent with epinephrine 1:200,000) should be infiltrated along the incision line,[179] and anesthesia depth should be increased with fentanyl/remifentanil, and/or isoflurane. The aim is to provide a "slack brain," which will reduce the amount of pressure caused by retractors and allow adequate cerebral perfusion. Muscle paralysis is provided by a nondepolarizing muscle relaxant, and the ICP is reduced by mannitol and furosemide. The intermittent positive-pressure ventilation is adjusted to maintain the Paco$_2$ between 25 and 28 mm Hg.

Patient Positioning

Three common patient positions are used for posterior fossa tumor operations. The prone position is used in 55 percent of cases, the sitting position in 30 percent, and the lateral position in 15 percent.[245] At our institution, all surgical procedures in the posterior cranial fossa or the upper cervical spine are performed in the prone position (Fig. 16–15)[248] with the patient lying on a U-bolster or a Relton frame.[249] It is the anesthesiologist's responsibility to ensure that during positioning the ETT is not advanced into or withdrawn from the trachea, that ventilation is adequate, that pressure points are well padded, and that the neck is not flexed enough to occlude jugular venous drainage. The method of head fixation depends on the age of the patient, the skull thickness, and the surgeon's needs. Horseshoe head rests are useful, but the patient's face must be padded carefully and the eyes must be free of compression. After 3 years of age, the multipin headholder is preferable. Infiltration of the pin sites with local anesthetic reduces nociceptive responses.

Monitoring

Monitoring for posterior fossa surgery is basically the same as for supratentorial craniotomy, with one important exception. The precordial Doppler should be used to detect air embolism (see above). Occasionally, sensory-evoked

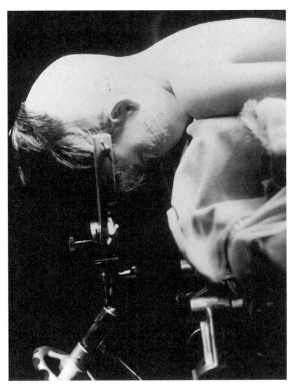

FIGURE 16–15. Prone position in a 3-year-old child undergoing posterior fossa surgery. The anesthesiologist must (1) give special attention to ventilation (U-bolsters or frame), (2) pad pressure points, (3) prevent flexion of the head to avoid occluding the jugular veins, and (4) prevent kinking of the endotracheal tube.

potentials should be obtained during resection of intramedullary or brain stem tumors.

Emergence and Recovery from Anesthesia

Prompt awakening is mandatory, but it is important to keep the patient hemodynamically stable and unstimulated during tracheal extubation. The pathologic process often dictates the appropriate postoperative airway management (e.g., postoperative tracheal intubation is essential after resection of intramedullary tumor). When early tracheal extubation is appropriate, intraoperative administration of narcotics plus lidocaine 0.5 to 1 mg/kg to infants and children will allow emergence from anesthesia without coughing and straining, which might otherwise lead to a hypertensive episode and intracerebral bleeding. Postoperative pain can usually be managed with morphine 0.05 to 0.2 mg/kg, with or without acetaminophen. Avoidance of medications that affect the sensorium or the pupils is important.

Cerebrovascular Anomalies

Arteriovenous malformations (AVMs) are congenital or acquired lesions that constitute an important anesthetic challenge, mainly in infants and children.[250] Congenital AVMs and arterial aneurysms arise from abnormal development of the arteriolar-capillary network that connects the arterial and venous systems. These vascular malformations consist of large arterial feeding vessels that lead to dilated communicating vessels and finally to veins, which are easily identifiable because they carry arterialized blood. Flow of blood through the low-resistance arteriocapillary circuit results in progressive distention and dilation of the entire venous system of the brain and cranium. Several specific vascular anomalies occur in pediatric patients, including those involving the posterior cerebral artery and the great vein of Galen[251] (Fig. 16–16). These anomalies often present in the neonatal period with congestive heart failure (CHF). Saccular dilation of the vein of Galen may be associated with hydrocephalus because the aqueduct of Sylvius is obstructed. Although Moyamoya disease is not really an AVM, similar anesthetic considerations apply. Moyamoya disease is a chronic occlusive cerebrovascular disease of the basal cerebral arteries that leads to severe dilation of perforating arteries at the base of the brain to form the so-called Moyamoya vessel.

Most AVMs go undetected until the fourth or fifth decade of life. Only 18 percent of them are present before 15 years of age. Cerebral injury may ensue because of one or more causes: (1) hemorrhage with thrombosis and infarction, (2) compression of adjacent neural structures, (3) parenchymal ischemia caused by "steal" of blood flow to the low-resistance network, (4) CHF and hypoperfusion, and (5) surgical disruption or diversion of the blood flow. Patients with AVMs may undergo radiologically controlled embolization of the arterial blood supply or stereotactic radiosurgery as definitive or adjunctive therapy. Surgical clipping of feeding vessels may be performed as a single or a staged procedure.

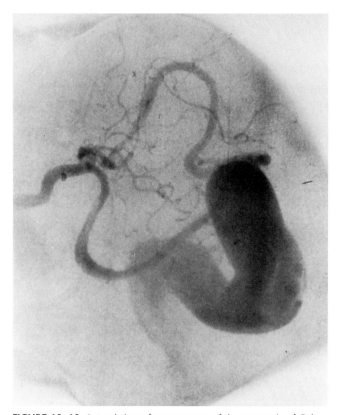

FIGURE 16–16. Lateral view of an aneurysm of the great vein of Galen. The main arterial contribution is from the anterior cerebral artery. The dilated vein of Galen empties directly into an enlarged straight sinus.

Anesthetic Considerations

Considerations for patients undergoing AVM resection include the following:

1. Preexisting pathophysiology. Does the patient present with increased ICP or CHF? Does the patient have associated congenital defects?
2. Age-related pathophysiology. Will organ system immaturity impact on the anesthetic technique?
3. Blood loss. The possibility of massive blood loss is real. Appropriate precautions must be taken.
4. Ventilation pattern. Hyperventilation is indicated for patients with vascular anomalies, but is contraindicated for patients with Moyamoya disease.

Monitoring

Routine monitoring is as described above. Patients undergoing AVM resection should have at least two large-bore IV catheters inserted, and the catheters should be connected to blood pumps before surgery begins. IV solutions should be warmed throughout anesthesia and surgery. Arterial line placement is essential. CVP monitoring should always be utilized for all but the smallest AVMs. Urinary catheter placement is mandatory after induction of anesthesia.

Preinduction

Symptoms vary with the age at which the disease presents.[250] Older children most commonly present with evidence of subarachnoid hemorrhage (SAH) or intraventricular hemorrhage (IVH). More than 70 percent of pediatric patients who present with spontaneous SAH have an AVM as the etiology. Seizure is the presenting symptom in approximately 25 percent of patients. The neonatal presentation of cerebral arteriovenous malformation is often associated with CHF.

The low-resistance pathway of the AVM results in volume overload and heart failure. CHF rarely presents in utero because the ductus arteriosus may provide a pressure release for the right ventricle by enabling it to pump blood into the low-resistance placental circulation. After birth, the demand for increased cardiac output and the increased pulmonary blood flow associated with decreased pulmonary vascular resistance may precipitate left ventricular failure. The low resistance of the cerebral AVM results in a low systemic diastolic pressure. This is combined with an increased left ventricular end-diastolic pressure because of ventricular failure. Coronary perfusion pressure is reduced, and myocardial ischemia ensues.[252] Right-to-left ductal shunting may occur and may divert a majority of descending aortic blood flow to the cerebral circulation. Therefore, cardiac failure in these infants is secondary to both pressure and volume overload, and they present with a picture similar to that of persistent fetal circulation.[250, 253, 254] Physical examination shows signs of left and/or right heart failure, such as tachypnea, tachycardia, cyanosis, pulmonary edema, hepatomegaly, and ECG changes. Laboratory studies may provide evidence of severe electrolyte imbalances caused by aggressive diuretic therapy. Neonates in severe CHF are treated with digoxin and may well require tracheal intubation, mechanical ventilation, and continuous IV inotropic support. Patients without evidence of CHF can be premedicated to reduce agitation and hypertension before induction of anesthesia.

Induction of Anesthesia and Tracheal Intubation

Prevention of hypertension during laryngoscopy is a major goal of induction of anesthesia in children with AVM if they do not have CHF. Inhalation or IV induction of anesthesia can be performed if there is no evidence of increased ICP. Incremental doses of pentothal and narcotic are given, along with lidocaine, before laryngoscopy. Use of a nondepolarizing muscle relaxant is recommended. Neonates who have CHF must have adequate IV access before induction of anesthesia. Extreme caution must be observed, as many anesthetic agents used for anesthesia induction, including lidocaine, are myocardial depressants and may precipitate cardiovascular collapse in infants and small children.[174] Oral or nasal tracheal intubation can proceed once the patient is adequately anesthetized.

Maintenance of Anesthesia

Considerations for maintenance of anesthesia include the following:

1. Positioning
2. Ventilation
3. Anesthetic agents
4. Blood loss and fluid management
5. Temperature maintenance

Positioning for surgery depends on the site of the AVM. AVMs most commonly receive their blood supply from the distribution of the middle meningeal artery and are approached by supratentorial craniotomy.

All patients are mechanically ventilated for control of $Paco_2$. Patients with hydrocephalus may require hyperventilation to reduce pressure. We usually maintain normocarbia in children undergoing resection of an AVM because we assume that hypocarbia will decrease cerebral blood flow in normal vessels and shunt additional blood to low-resistance, malformed vessels. This could cause cerebral ischemia and increase bleeding from the AVM.

The agents selected for maintenance of anesthesia are similar to those used for any intracranial procedure. In the absence of CHF, controlled hypotension can be employed when the AVM is ligated (see Chapter 13). An infusion of phentolamine has proven to be particularly useful, easily titratable, and to have predictable effects. Neonates with CHF are usually receiving inotropic support and cannot tolerate hypotensive anesthesia. Vasoactive drugs should be infused via central lines if possible. Temporary clipping has reduced the need for controlled hypotension.

Fluid management in these patients is often difficult and challenging. Neonates may not tolerate large volumes of fluid at all, and children with reduced intravascular volume after attempts at brain dehydration undergo rapid circulatory collapse after brisk intraoperative bleeding.

Maintaining a normal body temperature can be quite difficult in these children, especially if massive transfusions are required.[255] Allowing the patient's core temperature to decrease to 34°C may reduce the cerebral metabolic rate and ensure a certain degree of cerebral protection, without increasing postoperative complications.[256-258]

Emergence from Anesthesia

Considerations for emergence from anesthesia include the following:

1. Elimination of anesthetic agents
2. Reversal of neuromuscular blockade
3. Assessment of airway patency and respiration

Patients without a history of CHF can be extubated at the end of surgery. Patients with a likelihood of significant neurologic deficit or who have had extensive resection of brain, extensive brain retraction, cerebral edema, or CHF should remain sedated and intubated after surgery.

Postoperative Management

The basic anesthetic considerations for postoperative care of these patients includes consideration of the following:

1. Cerebral edema
2. Congestive heart failure
3. Hypertension
4. Vasospasm

Cerebral edema, which can be caused by the lesion itself or by the surgical procedure, may require mechanical ventilatory support and treatment with pharmaceutical adjuncts. Transfer to the ICU is indicated. It is usual for patients with large AVMs not to return to full consciousness for several days after surgical removal of the malformation. During this period, close neurologic observation is required.

Although obliteration of an AVM reduces right-to-left shunting of blood, patients with preoperative CHF usually remain in a precarious medical state for several days and require close observation and treatment in an ICU. The necessity to maintain adequate CPP and the need to reduce cardiac overload at the same time makes management of these patients difficult. Analgesics and antihypertensive drugs may be required to prevent sudden increases in arterial blood pressure, which could precipitate rebleeding.

Vasospasm is not a common postoperative complication of cerebrovascular surgery but must be considered if the patient's neurologic status deteriorates. The pathogenesis of vasospasm is poorly understood, and early diagnosis is crucial. Transcranial Doppler sonography allows detection of changes in cerebral blood flow and is useful in the diagnosis of this complication. Treatment of vasospasm is limited, but calcium blockers such as nimodipine have been used with certain success.[259] Endothelins are potent vasoconstrictors released following CNS insults such as subarachnoid hemorrhage, or head injury. Endothelin antagonist compounds prevent vasospasms in animal models of brain injury and show some promise.[260]

Surgery for Epilepsy

Specific anesthetic considerations for a surgical procedure for the relief of epilepsy include

1. The awake patient
2. Analgesia
3. Airway maintenance

Excision of a seizure focus requires a cooperative, sedated patient to identify the precise surgical site by cortical electroencephalography (ECoG) (Fig. 16–17). Neuroleptanalgesia is the technique of choice,[118] and anesthesia is induced with droperidol and fentanyl. The analgesic state is maintained with enough fentanyl citrate to keep the respiratory rate between 8 and 16 breaths/min. Additional doses of droperidol are avoided so that the patient's ability to cooperate in identification of the speech and motor areas is not impaired. Nitrous oxide/O_2 by face mask or soft nasopharyngeal cannula can be used to supplement IV analgesia until cortical mapping is performed. Use of a nasopharyngeal cannula makes PETCO$_2$ measurement possible and fresh gas administration more efficient.

Arterial and central line placement and placement of the multipin head-holder before skin incision[179] are accomplished after local anesthetic infiltration. We have found this technique acceptable for children above 4 years of age. Younger pediatric patients are usually unable to cooperate and require tracheal intubation and general anesthesia. The limitations of a neuroleptanalgesia technique include (1) restlessness in children, who must remain motionless and in an uncomfortable position for a long period of time; (2) breakthrough pain; and (3) poor cooperation in psychologically disturbed children. Propofol sedation represents an effective alternative to neuroleptanalgesia.[118] Propofol can either be entirely administered by the anesthesiologist along with fentanyl or remifentanil, or it can be dispensed, in older children as patient-controlled propofol sedation (PCS).[261, 262] The higher frequency background ECoG activity associated with propofol sedation does not interfere with ECoG interpretation, provided propofol administration is suspended at least 15 minutes before recording.[261] In an adult study of awake craniotomy for seizures, the frequency of intraoperative seizure was higher among the neurolept (droperidol/fentanyl) patients than in the propofol group.[263]

Electrical currents generated by seizure activity produce magnetic fields that can be measured by magnetoencephalography (MEG), a new noninvasive imaging technique. MEG signal is not affected by cranium and soft tissue and provides three-dimensional localization of epileptic spike sources. Its combination with EEG has substantially improved the accuracy of cortical epileptic loci mapping.[264–266] Children immobilized within the MRI machine often have difficulty remaining motionless, and they may also be going through an interictal period with limited seizure activity. In order to increase the number of epileptiform discharges during the EEG/MEG recording sessions, methohexital (1 to 1.5 mg/kg) becomes a helpful diagnostic medication when administered only by an anesthesiologist using proper monitoring.[265] A recent study in adults reported that the use of clonidine premedication followed by methohexital anesthesia could further increase focal epileptiform discharges.[267]

Image Guidance Technology

The combination of new image guidance technologies allows better surgical planning and positioning of bone flaps, as well as optimal delineation and resection of cerebral lesions. Functional magnetic resonance imaging (fMRI), frameless stereotaxy, direct cortical mapping (Fig. 16–17), and ISG wand all contribute to the reduction of neurologic morbidity in children.

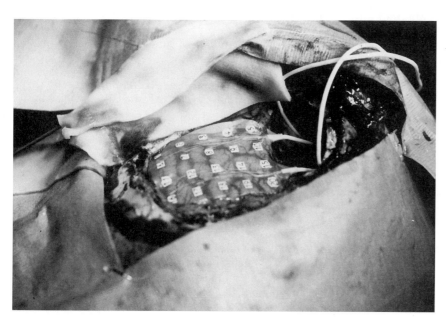

FIGURE 16–17. Cortical electrode application on the surface of the brain to detect epileptic foci.

Functional MRI uses blood-oxygenation-level-dependent (BOLD) contrast imaging where activity-related increases in regional blood flow result in augmentation of oxygen delivery to areas of activated brain tissues and fall in concentration of deoxyhemoglobin (Fig. 16–18). These images are detectable by increases in T2 and T2* signals and, when combined with standard MRI images, can correlate areas of functional cerebral cortex to pathologic areas such as arteriovenous malformations, tumors, and intracranial cysts.[268, 269] Only a cooperative child can execute the tasks required for fMRI and parental presence into the scanning room is often the key to a successful procedure.[268]

Frameless stereotaxy, which allows accurate localization of specific brain areas and lesions, can be done intraoperatively. This technique relates fixed points on the face and skull to regions of interest previously seen on CT scan or MRI three-dimensional reconstructions.[268]

The ISG wand is a three-dimensional intraoperative navigation system, guiding the neurosurgeon to the lesion to be resected through an optimal trajectory. Coupling information from the ISG wand to fMRI and, when possible, to direct cortical stimulation of language or motor areas, allows optimization of surgical resection with preservation of adjacent task-activated cortex.[268, 270, 271]

Specific anesthetic considerations for a surgical procedure involving these new imaging technologies include

1. The awake patient
2. Analgesia
3. Airway maintenance

These procedures can be performed in a cooperative patient with infiltration of local anesthetic under neuroleptanalgesia or with propofol/opioids (fentanyl or remifentanil).[179, 262, 268] Younger children or anxious patients unable to cooperate require general anesthesia. Should propofol be used, the infusion would have to be stopped at least 15 minutes prior to ECoG recording.[261, 268] Nitrous oxide, in concentrations up to 70 percent, has no significant effect on spike rate and can be used during epilepsy surgery with ECoG.[272]

Myelodysplasia

Hydrocephalus is accompanied by abnormalities in the spinal column and spinal cord in 70 percent of infants.[273] Myelodysplasia is an abnormality in fusion of the embryologic neural groove during the first month of gestation. Failure of neural tube closure results in a sac-like herniation of meninges (meningocele) or a herniation of neural elements (myelomeningocele). The spinal cord is often tethered caudally by the sacral roots, causing orthopedic or urologic symptoms in later childhood if the tethered cord is not surgically corrected (Fig. 16–19).

Myelomeningoceles most commonly occur in the lumbosacral region, but they can occur at any level in the neuraxis. Most children with meningomyelocele have an

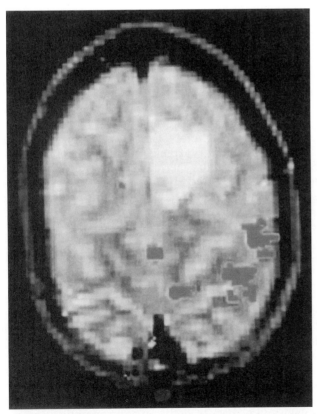

FIGURE 16–18. fMRI mapping of a 3-year-old female. The gray pixels represent activated cortex during the performance of a sensorimotor task with the right hand.

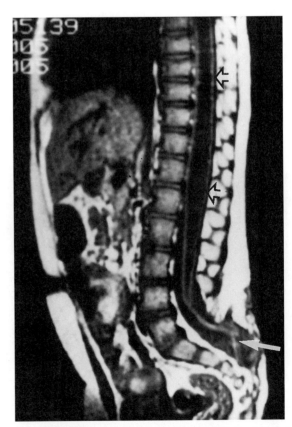

FIGURE 16–19. Midsagittal CT scan of the lumbosacral spine, demonstrating a myelomeningocele. The spinal cord is tethered at the site of the meningocele (*white arrow*). A large syrinx is seen running the length of the spinal cord (*open black arrows*).

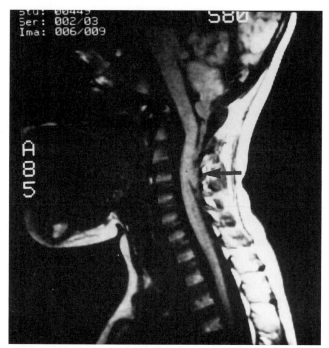

FIGURE 16–20. Midsagittal MRI scan demonstrating an Arnold-Chiari malformation type II. The cerebellar tonsils can be seen as low as the fifth cervical vertebral body within the cervical spinal canal (*arrow*).

associated Arnold-Chiari type II malformation (Fig. 16–20) and hydrocephaly. An encephalocele is most frequently found in the occipital/suboccipital areas or nasally (Fig. 16–21). Anencephaly results from a defect in anterior closure of the neural groove.

Myelodysplasia causes exposure of CNS tissue (see Fig. 16–22) and places the patient at risk for infection and death. The incidence of infection increases the longer the lesion remains unrepaired but occurs in less than 7 percent of patients if the defect is repaired within 48 hours of birth. Furthermore, delay in closure of the defect increases the

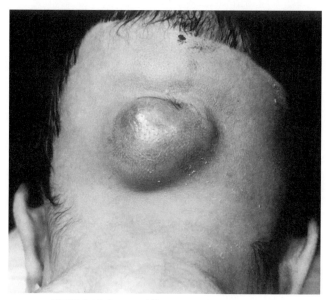

FIGURE 16–21. A midline occipital encephalocele.

likelihood of progressive neural damage and decreased motor function.[273] For these reasons, myelodysplasia is regarded as a surgical emergency, and most neonates present for surgery in the first 24 hours of life.

Anesthetic Considerations

1. Coexisting disease. Additional pathology may accompany myelodysplasia (Arnold-Chiari, hydrocephalus).
2. Age-related pathophysiology.
3. Airway management. Encephaloceles may be associated with difficulty in control of the airway.
4. Positioning. Protection of the neuroplaque.
5. Volume status. High third-space losses from the skin defect.
6. Potential for hypothermia. Exposure of large body surface area and loss of third-space fluid.

Monitoring

Routine monitoring is necessary. Blood loss can be insidious, especially if the sac is large and significant undermining of skin, relaxing incisions, or skin grafting is required for closure of the defect. Blood transfusion may be necessary. Patients with encephaloceles who must undergo craniotomy for repair should have an arterial line placed for blood pressure and hemoglobin measurement. A central venous line may be indicated for repair of a nasal encephalocele when the repair is done in a semisitting position.

Preinduction of Anesthesia

Infants presenting for repair of meningomyeloceles rarely exhibit increased ICP. The majority of myelodysplastic patients have an associated Arnold-Chiari malformation, and most have hydrocephalus, which usually requires ventricular shunt placement. Preoperative assessment of these children reveals a variety of neurologic deficits, depending on the level of the lesion. Seventy-five percent of all lesions occur in the lumbosacral region. Lesions above the level of T4 usually result in paraplegia, whereas lesions below S1 allow ambulation. The legs are severely affected by lesions between L4 and S1.[273] Before induction of anesthesia, the patient's volume status should be assessed. These patients have the potential for large third-space losses from the exposed myelomeningocele.

Induction of Anesthesia and Tracheal Intubation

Anesthesia for patients with lumbosacral or thoracic myelomeningoceles can be induced either in the left lateral position or supine with the sac protected by a cushioned ring. Anesthesia can be induced in a majority of patients with thiopentone, atropine, and a muscle relaxant. Either a nondepolarizing muscle relaxant or succinylcholine can be used safely.[274] Patients with nasal encephalocele commonly have airway obstruction, and it may be difficult to obtain a good mask fit. Sedation and fiberoptic technique might be useful to facilitate tracheal intubation in these patients.

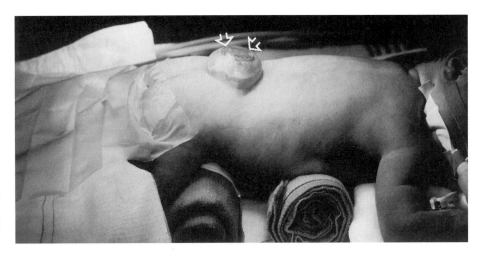

FIGURE 16–22. Newborn infant in the prone position undergoing closure of a myelomeningocele. The central darker region represents the neuroplaque (unprotected neural tissue) (*arrows*).

Maintenance of Anesthesia

The anesthetic considerations for maintenance of anesthesia are as follows:

1. Positioning of the patient
2. Ventilation of the lungs
3. Anesthetic agents
4. Muscle relaxants
5. Fluid management
6. Maintenance of body temperature

After tracheal intubation the patient is turned to the prone position. Injury to the exposed neural tissue must be prevented. Chest and hip rolls are placed to ensure that the abdomen is free, to facilitate ventilation, and to reduce intra-abdominal pressure and decrease bleeding from the epidural plexus. Since most of these children have an Arnold-Chiari malformation, excessive rotation of the neck should be avoided. The extremities should lie in a relaxed position and be well padded.

The lungs are mechanically ventilated. Barotrauma in the immature lung must be prevented. Premature infants (especially those <32 weeks' gestation) are at increased risk for retinopathy of prematurity[275] and lung injury from prolonged exposure to high oxygen concentrations[276] (see Chapter 14).

Anesthesia can be maintained with a variety of agents, but higher dose narcotics and ketamine may cause postoperative apnea. Muscle relaxants are contraindicated during maintenance of anesthesia because nerve stimulation is often required to identify neural structures.

The large area of exposed tissue and the liberal use of cold surgical preparation solutions increase the risk of hypothermia in these patients. Care must be taken to prevent drying or thermal injury to the exposed neural tissue by radiant heat lamps.

Emergence

Anesthetic considerations for emergence include the following:

1. Elimination of anesthetic agents
2. Reversal of neuromuscular blockade
3. Assessment of airway patency

Neonates at risk for apnea after anesthesia, patients with severe central neurologic deficits, and those undergoing craniotomy for encephalocele repair should be extubated fully awake. Patients with nasal encephalocele repairs may have residual airway obstruction or blood in the oropharynx, and may require postoperative tracheal intubation.

Postoperative Management

Basic anesthetic considerations for the postoperative period have been discussed above.

Spinal Cord Surgery

Common diseases of the spinal cord that require surgery include herniated disks, spondylosis, syringomyelia, primary or metastatic tumors, hematomas or abscesses, and trauma. In all cases, compression of the spinal cord may produce ischemia,[277] interstitial edema, and venous congestion,[278] and may interfere with nerve transmission.[53] Maintaining spinal cord perfusion pressure and reducing spinal cord compression are crucial.

Despite apparently optimal surgical and anesthetic management, devastating neurologic complications still occur with spinal surgery. Intraoperative monitoring of spinal cord function includes (1) the wake-up test, (2) somatosensory-evoked potentials (SSEP), and (3) motor-evoked potentials (MEP).[279] The wake-up test remains the traditional method for assessing spinal cord well-being during corrective procedures on the spinal column. Its main advantage is that it assesses anterior spinal cord (i.e., motor) function, but it does so only at one time. Evoked potential monitors (e.g., SSEP monitoring) generate an electrical potential by stimulation of peripheral nerves (e.g., the median nerve at the wrist or the posterior tibial nerve at the ankle). If nerve transmission in intact, a signal is recorded from the scalp or at various sites along the neural pathway. The electrical signals arise from axonal action potentials and graded postsynaptic potentials as the impulse is propagated from the periphery to the brain. The technique measures only the response of the sensory nervous system. This limitation can be overcome by use of MEPs, in which the motor cortex is stimulated by a transcranial electric current or a pulsed magnetic field generated by a coil placed over the scalp.[280]

Head Injury

Unintentional injury is the leading cause of death among children in the United States.[235] Head injury is a major cause of morbidity and mortality in these children and remains the most frequent cause of pediatric trauma hospitalization.[281] Brain injury is also the leading cause of death from child abuse[282] and it can be difficult to diagnose in young children.[283] The overall mortality rate for children sustaining severe head injury (Glasgow Coma Scale [GCS] score <8) is 36.5 percent in the United States.[284] The presence of skull fracture on radiographs appears to be a poor predictor of intracranial morbidity. However, skull radiography remains indicated when there is suspicion of depressed fracture (Fig. 16–23) or penetrating injury. It is also recommended in patients suspected of nonaccidental injury, especially those younger than 2 years of age.[285] Clinical neurologic abnormalities are the major indication of intracranial injury. Children with such symptoms should undergo a brain CT scan, which is the most readily available "gold standard" for detection of intracranial injury.[285, 286]

Head injury causes several different pathophysiologic events, including intracranial hematomas (epidural, subdural, intracerebral, and brain contusion), brain edema, and systemic effects. Adults suffer more hematomas than children, and children ahve diffuse cerebral edema more frequently.[287]

Epidural Hematoma

This lesion is frequently caused by laceration of a middle meningeal artery during a deceleration injury. Children do not necessarily have an overlying skull fracture (Fig. 16–24). Epidural hematomas constitute 25 percent of all intracranial hematomas in pediatric patients and are a true neurosurgical emergency. In adults, there is a lucid interval between the initial loss of consciousness and later neurologic deterioration. Children often do not have the initial alteration in the state of consciousness observed in adults. The child who is old enough to talk complains of an increasing headache and then becomes confused or lethargic. Rapid development of hemiparesis, posturing, and pupillary dilation occurs frequently and may confuse the diagnosis. Rapid expansion of the hematoma causes herniation of the temporal lobe downward through the tentoria incisura. Anisocoria is an early sign. Herniation eventually leads to rostrocaudal deterioration and is associated with bradycardia, slowed and irregular breathing, and widened pulse pressure (Cushing triad). The relationship between the degree of brain shift and the level of consciousness has been confirmed, however, the role of uncal herniation in the syndrome has been questioned.[288]

Subdural Hematoma

Subdural hematomas are associated with parenchymal contusion, blood vessel laceration, and cortical damage. The mass effect of the contused and edematous brain may

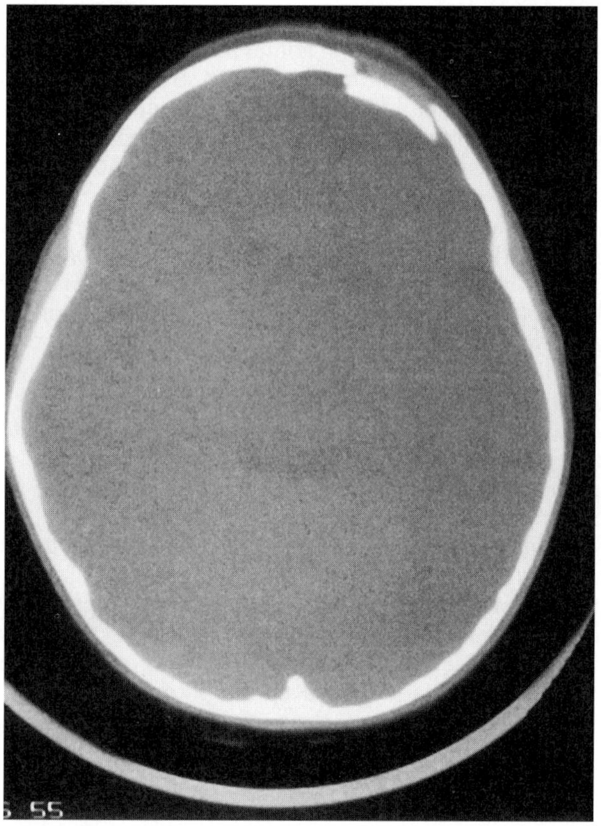

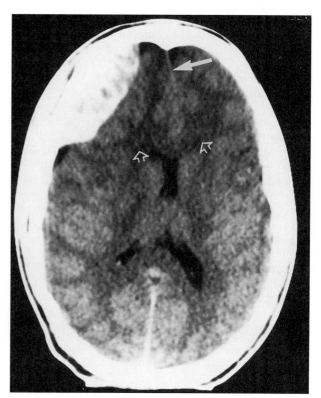

FIGURE 16–23. Axial CT scan showing a depressed skull fracture in the left frontal region.

FIGURE 16–24. Axial CT scan showing a large, rounded high-density collection in the right frontal region, indicating the presence of an acute epidural hematoma. There is a significant shift of the midline structures (*white arrow*) from the expanding mass and the associated cerebral edema in the subfrontal lobe (*open white arrows*).

prompt surgical removal of the hematoma if the brain region involved is not functionally important. Studies using positron emission tomography have demonstrated that cerebral metabolism and blood flow are reduced by 50 percent with brain contusion.[289] Severe edema and elevated ICP often lead to persistent neurologic deficits.

Intracerebral Hematoma

Intracerebral hematomas are rare but carry a poor prognosis. Surgery is usually avoided for fear of damaging viable brain tissue.

Anesthetic Considerations

The anesthetic considerations are as follows:

1. Resuscitation and stabilization. Airway, breathing, and circulation are essential components of the initial clinical assessment. Traumatized patients often have a variety of physiologic disturbances, including acid–base and electrolyte imbalances and abnormalities of glucose homeostasis and body temperature control.
2. Neurologic status. The GCS provides a means of detecting changes in the patient's condition. Symptoms of raised ICP must be evaluated.
3. Associated injuries. Pediatric trauma often occurs from high-velocity energy transfer, which leads to injuries to the neck, chest, and abdominal organs.
4. Full stomach. Vomiting leads to pulmonary aspiration and respiratory complications.
5. Age-related pathophysiology.

Monitoring

Arterial catheter and central venous line placement are indicated. A urinary catheter should be inserted unless contraindicated by an associated bladder neck injury. Central body temperature should be monitored at all times.

Preinduction of Anesthesia

A CT scan is the procedure of choice for evaluation of head injury during the first 72 hours after the accident. Management of an elevated ICP is essential to provide a safe anesthetic. Adequate hemodynamic resuscitation and stabilization must be achieved to maintain a normal CPP and brain tissue oxygenation.

Induction and Intubation

Providing a patent airway is an essential part of the management of patients with head injury. Although the airway of an unconscious patient may not be compromised by the injury, tracheal intubation will protect the lungs against aspiration of stomach contents or secretions and allow ventilatory support of patients with increased ICP. The association of head injury and neck injury occurs so often in infants and children that tracheal intubation must be accomplished with minimal manipulation of the neck.

The neck should be stabilized by an assistant who applies axial traction. Since a cervical spine fracture is always considered present until proven otherwise in patients with head injury, use of the Sellick maneuver is contraindicated. Patients should be hemodynamically stable before anesthesia is induced. After airway injury has been ruled out, anesthesia should be induced rapidly with atropine, thiopentone or propofol, lidocaine, and either succinylcholine or a nondepolarizing muscle relaxant such as rocuronium. Although it has been suggested that the use of ketamine with propofol might reduce ICP,[137] the authors believe that its use in head injury patients remains controversial. If the patient is suspected to have a difficult airway, a two-person technique or a fiberoptic intubation may be required. Depending on the age of the patient, the use of a volatile anesthetic and assisted ventilation or the use of neuroleptanesthesia with topicalization of the larynx is recommended.

Maintenance of Anesthesia

Anesthetic considerations for maintenance of anesthesia are similar to those previously described for supratentorial surgery. Evacuation of an intracranial hematoma usually requires a craniotomy, which can commonly be done without opening the dura mater. Evacuation of a large hematoma may suddenly decrease ICP and allow upward movement of the brain stem through the tentoria incisura. This may result in transient hemodynamic instability and cardiac arrhythmias.

Emergence and Postoperative Management

Patients with severe head injury remain intubated after surgery to provide ventilatory support and to control elevated ICP. Transfer to an ICU is indicated for continued care.

Cervical Spinal Cord Injury

Isolated cervical spine injury is uncommon in the pediatric population. However, all children with severe head injury should be treated as though they have a cervical spine injury until proven otherwise. Injury to the high cervical cord is usually caused by high-velocity injuries to the cranium (Fig. 16–25). Children with cord injury or disruption of the cord often present without respiratory efforts, often in cardiac arrest or with profound hypotension. They frequently die from hypoxic/ischemic encephalopathy and may have serious traumatic brain injury.[290] In this study, all patients with absent vital signs had high cervical cord luxation on a lateral view radiograph of the neck. Physicians caring for such patients might think that the hypotension is related to blood loss from intra-abdominal, pelvic, or thoracic injury, or even from devastating cerebral injury and loss of brain stem function.

Anesthetic Considerations and Management

Some cervical spine injury victims have signs of brain shift and elevated ICP. The anesthetic considerations for these patients include the following:

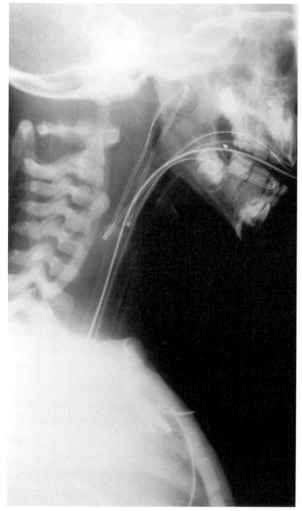

FIGURE 16–25. Lateral view of the cervical spine, showing craniocervical dislocation in a 3-year-old child.

1. Resuscitation and stabilization of cardiopulmonary function
2. Decreasing ICP and improving cerebral perfusion
3. Stabilization of the cervical spine
4. Correction of metabolic disturbances
5. Treatment of ARDS
6. Identification of the central rostrocaudal deterioration and uncal herniation
7. Consider the use of colloids such as pentastarch as part of the intravenous fluid resuscitation[180, 181]
8. Monitoring arterial pressure, CVP, and urine output
9. Correcting the coagulopathy often caused by brain tissue thromboplastin release
10. Treatment of DI (see craniopharyngioma)
11. Treatment of SIADH
12. Controlling the hyperglycemia that frequently occurs in head-injured patients, which is thought to be a good indicator of the severity of the injury and a predictor of outcome.[291] It is advisable to prevent the increase in glucose associated with head injury.[292]

CEREBRAL PROTECTION, RESUSCITATION, AND OUTCOME

An extensive discussion of these topics is beyond the scope of this chapter, and readers are referred to previously published reviews.[293–295] General principles are presented for completeness.

Cerebral Protection

After ischemic injury the CNS has limited regenerative ability. *Brain protection* has been defined as the "prevention or amelioration of neuronal damage evidenced by abnormalities in cerebral metabolism, histopathology, or neurologic function occurring after an hypoxic or ischemic event"[296] (i.e., treatment that is instituted before and often sustained throughout the insult). *Brain resuscitation* refers to the treatment of the secondary brain injury or simply to therapy given after the primary insult.[297] The secondary consequences of ischemia are those that occur after the cerebral circulation is restored and are usually termed postischemic injury or reperfusion injury. Cell vulnerability differs, depending on the type of neuron. For example, the limbic system, especially the pyramidal cells of the CA_1 layer of the hippocampus; Purkinje cells of the cerebellum; and layers 3, 4, and 6 of the cortex, are extremely vulnerable to ischemia; spinal cord cells, on the other hand, seem to tolerate a longer period of oxygen deprivation before they are injured.[297]

Cerebral protection either increases oxygen delivery, reduces its demands, or ameliorates the pathologic process by free radical scavenging or by reducing the effects of excitatory amino acids (glutamate, aspartate) and ionic fluxes. The difficulty with cerebral protection is that these strategies must be instituted before the onset of ischemia. With complete global ischemia, the brain tolerates 4 but maybe up to 6 minutes of oxygen deprivation. The goal of cerebral protection is to delay the onset of irreversible CNS damage. There are no proven methods of cerebral protection except for mild hypothermia.[298–300] Therefore, maintaining adequate cerebral perfusion and oxygen delivery and avoiding hyperglycemia are, at this time, the only means we have to reduce CNS injury.

Cerebral Resuscitation

Intracellular events that occur during ischemia or after restoration of circulation and oxygenation contribute to the ultimate neurologic damage. Ischemia depolarizes neurons and allows ionic fluxes (Na^+ and Ca^{2+}) into the cells, probably owing to release of glutamate and aspartate and activation of the NMDA and α-amino-3-hydroxy-5-methyl-4-isoxazolepropionic acid (AMPA) receptors.[301] Depletion of ATP stores leads to the energy-dependent ion pump's failure to eject Na^+ and Ca^{2+} from the cells. This leads to formation of prostaglandins, oxygen free radicals, to mitochondrial respiratory chain paralysis, to acidosis, and finally to membrane destruction.

Cerebral Outcome

Premature but also term infants with refractory hypoxemic respiratory failure are often treated with inhaled nitric oxide (INO). Despite significant improvements in systemic oxygenation with INO, the question of higher frequency of intraventricular hemorrhage as well as poor neurodevelopmental outcome has been raised.[302] Production of cytotoxic oxidants, brain mitochondrial damage during perinatal asphyxia, as well as inhibition of platelet function have been described as part of nitric oxide–mediated processes.[303-305] The future of cerebral well-being depends on our level of understanding of the pathophysiology of hypoxic-ischemic injury and our broad-based medical and pharmacologic knowledge. Future therapy depends on development of a better understanding of the molecular and cellular processes that cause CNS injury and the development of specific treatments to salvage or protect injured tissue.[303, 306] Ultimately, the goal is to provide effective therapeutic measures that reverse the cascade of cellular events leading to injury.

REFERENCES

1. Karfunkel P: The mechanisms of neural tube formation. Int Rev Cytol 38:245, 1974.
2. Streeter G: Developmental horizons in humans embryos. Description of age group XIII, embryos about 4 or 5 millimeters long and age group XIV, period of indentation of the lens vesicle. Contrib Embryol 31:211, 1942.
3. Streeter G: Developmental horizons in human embryos. Description of age group XV, XVI, XVII and XVIII, being the third issue of a survey on the Carnegie collection. Contrib Embryol 32:133, 1948.
4. Streeter G: Developmental horizons in human embryos (fourth issue). A review of the histogenesis of bone and cartilage. Contrib Embryol 33:149, 1949.
5. Streeter G: Developmental horizons in human embryos. Description of age groups XIX, XX, XXi, XXII, XXIII, being the fifth issue of a survey of the Carnegie collection. Contrib Embryol 34:165, 1951.
6. Heuser C, Corner G: Development horizons in human embryos. Description of age group X, 4 to 12 somites. Contrib Embryol 36:29, 1975.
7. Lemire R, Loeser J, Leedh R, Alvord E: Normal and Abnormal Development of the Normal Nervous System. New York, Harper & Row, 1975.
8. Streeter G: Factors involved in the formation of the filum terminale. Am J Anat 25:1, 1919.
9. Brocklehurst G: The development of the human cerebrospinal fluid pathway with particular reference to the roof of the fourth ventricle. J Anat 105:467, 1969.
10. Streeter G: The development of the human cerebrospinal fluid pathway with particular references to the roof of the fourth ventricle. J Anat 105:467, 1918.
11. Padget D: The cranial venous system in man in reference to development, adult configuration and relation to the arteries. Am J Anat 98:307, 1956.
12. Milhorat T: Circulation of the cerebrospinal fluid. In McLaurin R, Schut L, Venes J, Epstein F (eds): Pediatric Neurosurgery of the Developing Nervous System. Philadelphia, WB Saunders Company, 1989, p 170.
13. Loefgren J, Zwetnow NN: Cranial and spinal components of the cerebrospinal fluid pressure-volume curve. Acta Neurol Scand 49:575, 1973.
14. Hill A, Volpe J: Measurement of intracranial pressure using the Ladd intracranial pressure monitor. J Paediatr 98:974, 1984.
15. Ross RT: Spinal cord infarction in disease and surgery of the aorta. Can J Neurol Sci 12:289, 1985.
16. Batson O: The vertebral vein system. AJR Am J Roentgenol 78:195, 1957.
17. Bickler P: Energetics of cerebral metabolism and ion transport. In Bissonnette B (ed): Cerebral Protection, Resuscitation and Monitoring: A Look into the Future of Neuroanesthesia. Anesthesiology Clinics of North America. Vol 10. Philadelphia, WB Saunders Company, 1992, p 563.
18. Sokoloff L: Circulation and energy metabolism of the brain. In Siegel G, Agranoff B, Albers R, Molinoff P (eds): Basic Neurochemistry: Molecular, Cellular and Medical Aspects. New York, Raven Press, 1989, p 565.
19. Siesjo BK: Cell damage in the brain: a speculative synthesis. J Cereb Blood Flow Metab 1:155, 1981.
20. Kennedy C, Sokoloff L: An adaptation of nitrous oxide method to the study of the circulation in children: normal values for cerebral blood flow and cerebral metabolic rate in childhood. J Clin Invest 36:1130, 1957.
21. Settergren G, Lindblad BS, Persson B: Cerebral blood flow and exchange of oxygen, glucose ketone bodies, lactate, pyruvate and amino acids in anesthetized children. Acta Paediatr Scand 69:457, 1980.
22. Mehta S, Kalsi HK, Nain CK, Menkes JH: Energy metabolism of brain in human protein-calorie malnutrition. Pediatr Res 11:290, 1977.
23. Younkin DP, Reivich M, Jaggi J, et al: Noninvasive method of estimating human newborn regional cerebral blood flow. J Cereb Blood Flow Metab 2:415, 1982.
24. Cross KW, Dear PR, Hathorn MK, et al: An estimation of intracranial blood flow in the new-born infant. J Physiol (Lond) 289:329, 1979.
25. Ogawa A, Sakurai Y, Kayama T, Yoshimoto T: Regional cerebral blood flow with age: changes in rCBF in childhood. Neurol Res 11:173, 1989.
26. Rosomoff H, Holaday D: Cerebral blood flow and cerebral oxygen consumption during hypothermia. Am J Physiol 179:85, 1954.
27. Lassen NA, Christensen MS: Physiology of cerebral blood flow. Br J Anaesth 48:719, 1976.
28. Hernandez MJ, Brennan RW, Bowman GS: Autoregulation of cerebral blood flow in the newborn dog. Brain Res 184:199, 1980.
29. Purves MJ, James IM: Observations on the control of cerebral blood flow in the sheep fetus and newborn lamb. Circ Res 25:651, 1969.
30. McLeod ME, Creighton RE, Humphreys RP: Anaesthesia for cerebral arteriovenous malformations in children. Can Anaesth Soc J 29:299, 1982.
31. Muizelaar JP, Wei EP, Kontos HA, Becker DP: Cerebral blood flow is regulated by changes in blood pressure and in blood viscosity alone. Stroke 17:44, 1986.
32. Tweed A, Cote J, Lou H, et al: Impairment of cerebral blood flow autoregulation in the newborn lamb by hypoxia. Pediatr Res 20:516, 1986.
33. Gregory G, Ong B, Tweed A: Hyperventilation restores autoregulation in the cerebral circulation in the neonate. Anesthesiology 59:427, 1983.
34. Lassen NA: Control of cerebral circulation in health and disease. Circ Res 34:749, 1974.
35. Lou HC, Lassen NA, Friis HB: Impaired autoregulation of cerebral blood flow in the distressed newborn infant. J Pediatr 94:118, 1979.
36. Pilato MA, Bissonnette B, Lerman J: Transcranial Doppler: response of cerebral blood-flow velocity to carbon dioxide in anaesthetized children. Can J Anaesth 38:37, 1991.
37. Pollay M: Formation of cerebrospinal fluid. Relation of studies of isolated choroid plexus to the standing gradient hypothesis. J Neurosurg 42:665, 1975.
38. Ruben RC, Henderson ES, Ommaya AK, et al: The production of cerebrospinal fluid in man and its modification by acetazolamide. J Neurosurg 25:430, 1966.
39. Milhorat TH, Hammock MK, Fenstermacher JD, Levin VA: Cerebrospinal fluid production by the choroid plexus and brain. Science 173:330, 1971.
40. Cutler RW, Page L, Galicich J, Watters GV: Formation and absorption of cerebrospinal fluid in man. Brain 91:707, 1968.
41. Welch K: The intracranial pressure in infants. J Neurosurg 52:693, 1980.
42. Raju TN, Vidyasagar D, Papazafiratou C: Intracranial pressure monitoring in the neonatal ICU. Crit Care Med 8:575, 1980.
43. Kosteljanetz M: Pressure-volume conditions in patients with subarachnoid and/or intraventricular hemorrhage. J Neurosurg 63:398, 1985.
44. Chopp M, Portnoy HD, Branch C: Hydraulic model of the cerebrovascular bed: an aid to understanding the volume-pressure test. Neurosurgery 13:5, 1983.
45. Marmarou A, Maset AL, Ward JD, et al: Contribution of CSF and vascular factors to elevation of ICP in severely head-injured patients. J Neurosurg 66:883, 1987.

46. Shapiro HM: Intracranial hypertension: therpeutic and anesthetic considerations [review]. Anesthesiology 43:445, 1975.
47. Shapiro K, Marmarou A: Mechanism of intracranial hypertension in children. In McLaurin R, Venes J, Schut L, Epstein F (eds): Pediatric Neurosurgery. Philadelphia, WB Saunders Company, 1989, p 338.
48. Lindberg PJ, O'Neill JT, Paakkari IA, et al: Validation of laser-Doppler flowmetry in measurement of spinal cord blood flow. Am J Physiol 257:H264, 1989.
49. Hickey R, Albin MS, Bunegin L, Gelineau J: Autoregulation of spinal cord blood flow: is the cord a microcosm of the brain? Stroke 17:1183, 1986.
50. Marcus ML, Heistad DD, Ehrhardt JC, Abboud FM: Regulation of total and regional spinal cord blood flow. Circ Res 41:128, 1977.
51. Sandler AN, Tator CH: Review of the effect of spinal cord trauma on the vessels and blood flow in the spinal cord. J Neurosurg 45:638, 1976.
52. Goto T, Crosby G: Anesthesia and the spinal cord. In Bissonnette B (ed): Cerebral Protection, Resuscitation and Monitoring: A Look into the Future of Neuroanesthesia. Anesthesiology Clinics of North America. Vol 10. Philadelphia, WB Saunders Company, 1992, p 493.
53. Griffiths IR, Trench JG, Crawford RA: Spinal cord blood flow and conduction during experimental cord compression in normotensive and hypotensive dogs. J Neurosurg 50:353, 1979.
54. Rubinstein A, Arbit E: Spinal cord blood flow in the rat under normal physiological conditions. Neurosurgery 27:882, 1990.
55. Guha A, Tator CH, Rochon J: Spinal cord blood flow and systemic blood pressure after experimental spinal cord injury in rats. Stroke 20:372, 1989.
56. Griffiths IR: Spinal cord blood flow in dogs. 2. The effect of the blood gases. J Neurol Neurosurg Psychiatry 36:42, 1973.
57. Usubiaga JE, Usubiaga LE, Brea LM, Goyena R: Effect of saline injections on epidural and subarachnoid space pressures and relation to postspinal anesthesia headache. Anesth Analg 46:293, 1967.
58. Lassen N: Cerebral and spinal cord blood flow. In Cottrell J (ed): Anesthesia and Neurosurgery. St Louis, CV Mosby, 1986, p 1.
59. Goldenthal EI: A compilation of LD50 values in newborn and adult animals. Toxicol Appl Pharmacol 18:185, 1971.
60. Kupferberg H, Way E: Pharmacologic basis for the increased sensitivity of the newborn rat to morphine. J Pharmacol Exp Ther 141:105, 1963.
61. Lerman J, Robinson S, Willis MM, Gregory GA: Anesthetic requirements for halothane in young children 0-1 month and 1-6 months of age. Anesthesiology 59:421, 1983.
62. Cook DR, Brandom BW, Shiu G, Wolfson B: The inspired median effective dose, brain concentration at anesthesia, and cardiovascular index for halothane in young rats. Anesth Analg 60:182, 1981.
63. Sakabe T, Kuramoto T, Inoue S, Takeshita H: Cerebral effects of nitrous oxide in the dog. Anesthesiology 48:195, 1978.
64. Pelligrino DA, Miletich DJ, Hoffman WE, Albrecht RF: Nitrous oxide markedly increases cerebral cortical metabolic rate and blood flow in the goat. Anesthesiology 60:405, 1984.
65. Theye RA, Michenfelder JD: The effect of nitrous oxide on canine cerebral metabolism. Anesthesiology 29:1119, 1968.
66. Leon JE, Bissonnette B: Transcranial Doppler sonography: nitrous oxide and cerebral blood flow velocity in children [published erratum appears in Can J Anaesth 39(4):409, 1992]. Can J Anaesth 38:974, 1991.
67. Moss E, McDowall DG: I.c.p. increases with 50% nitrous oxide in oxygen in severe head injuries during controlled ventilation. Br J Anaesth 51:757, 1979.
68. Hoffman WE, Miletich DJ, Albrecht RF: The effects of midazolam on cerebral blood flow and oxygen consumption and its interaction with nitrous oxide. Anesth Analg 65:729, 1986.
69. Phirman JR, Shapiro HM: Modification of nitrous oxide-induced intracranial hypertension by prior induction of anesthesia. Anesthesiology 46:150, 1977.
70. Sakabe T, Kuramoto T, Kumagae S, Takeshita H: Cerebral responses to the addition of nitrous oxide to halothane in man. Br J Anaesth 48:957, 1976.
71. Albrecht RF, Miletich DJ, Rosenberg R, Zahed B: Cerebral blood flow and metabolic changes from induction to onset of anesthesia with halothane or pentobarbital. Anesthesiology 47:252, 1977.
72. Todd MM, Drummond JC: A comparison of the cerebrovascular and metabolic effects of halothane and isoflurane in the cat. Anesthesiology 60:276, 1984.
73. Manohar M, Goetz TE: Cerebral, renal, adrenal, intestinal, and pancreatic circulation in conscious ponies and during 1.0, 1.5, and 2.0 minimal alveolar concentrations of halothane-O2 anesthesia. Am J Vet Res 46:2492, 1985.
74. Madsen JB, Cold GE, Hansen ES, Bardrum B: Cerebral blood flow, cerebral metabolic rate of oxygen and relative CO2-reactivity during craniotomy for supratentorial cerebral tumours in halothane anaesthesia. A dose-response study. Acta Anaesthesiol Scand 31:454, 1987.
75. Christensen MS, Hoedt RK, Lassen NA: Cerebral vasodilatation by halothane anaesthesia in man and its potentiation by hypotension and hypercapnia. Br J Anaesth 39:927, 1967.
76. Adams RW, Gronert GA, Sundt TJ, Michenfelder JD: Halothane, hypocapnia, and cerebrospinal fluid pressure in neurosurgery. Anesthesiology 37:510, 1972.
77. Leon JE, Bissonnette B: Cerebrovascular responses to carbon dioxide in children anaesthetized with halothane and isoflurane. Can J Anaesth 38:817, 1991.
78. Drummond JC, Todd MM: The response of the feline cerebral circulation to PaCO2 during anesthesia with isoflurane and halothane and during sedation with nitrous oxide. Anesthesiology 62:268, 1985.
79. Newberg LA, Michenfelder JD: Cerebral protection by isoflurane during hypoxemia or ischemia. Anesthesiology 59:29, 1983.
80. Artru AA: Effects of enflurane and isoflurane on resistance to reabsorption of cerebrospinal fluid in dogs. Anesthesiology 61:529, 1984.
81. Leon JE, Bissonnette B: Cerebrovascular responses to carbon dioxide in children anaesthetized with halothane and isoflurane. Can J Anaesth 38:817, 1991.
82. Bissonnette B, Leon JE: Cerebrovascular stability during isoflurane anaesthesia in children. Can J Anaesth 39:128, 1992.
83. Algotsson L, Messeter K, Nordstrom CH, Ryding E: Cerebral blood flow and oxygen consumption during isoflurane and halothane anesthesia in man. Acta Anaesthesiol Scand 32:15, 1988.
84. Eintrei C, Leszniewski W, Carlsson C: Local application of 133Xenon for measurement of regional cerebral blood flow (rCBF) during halothane, enflurane, and isoflurane anesthesia in humans. Anesthesiology 63:391, 1985.
85. Archer DP, Labrecque P, Tyler JL, et al: Cerebral blood volume is increased in dogs during administration of nitrous oxide or isoflurane. Anesthesiology 67:642, 1987.
86. Scheller MS, Todd MM, Drummond JC, Zornow MH: The intracranial pressure effects of isoflurane and halothane administered following cryogenic brain injury in rabbits. Anesthesiology 67:507, 1987.
87. Artru AA: Relationship between cerebral blood volume and CSF pressure during anesthesia with isoflurane or fentanyl in dogs. Anesthesiology 60:575, 1984.
88. Sakabe T, Maekawa T, Fujii S, et al: Cerebral circulation and metabolism during enflurane anesthesia in humans. Anesthesiology 59:532, 1983.
89. Michenfelder JD, Cucciara RF: Canine cerebral oxygen consumption during enflurane anesthesia and its modification during induced seizures. Anesthesiology 40:575, 1974.
90. Artru AA, Nugent M, Michenfelder JD: Enflurane causes a prolonged and reversible increase in the rate of CSF production in the dog. Anesthesiology 57:255, 1982.
91. Artru AA: Effects of halothane and fentanyl anesthesia on resistance to reabsorption of CSF. J Neurosurg 60:252, 1984.
92. Artru AA: Relationship between cerebral blood volume and CSF pressure during anesthesia with halothane or enflurane in dogs. Anesthesiology 58:533, 1983.
93. Lebowitz MH, Blitt CD, Dillon JB: Enflurane-induced central nervous system excitation and its relation to carbon dioxide tension. Anesth Analg 51:355, 1972.
94. Hormann C, Kolbitsch C, Benzer A: The role of sevoflurane in neuroanesthesia practice. Acta Anaesthesiol Scand Suppl 111: 148, 1997.
95. Artru AA, Lam AM, Johnson JO, Sperry RJ: Intracranial pressure, middle cerebral artery flow velocity, and plasma inorganic fluoride concentrations in neurosurgical patients receiving sevoflurane or isoflurane. Anesth Analg 85:587, 1997.
96. Kuroda Y, Murakami M, Tsuruta J, et al: Preservation of the ration of cerebral blood flow/metabolic rate for oxygen during prolonged anesthesia with isoflurane, sevoflurane, and halothane in humans. Anesthesiology 84:555, 1996.
97. Summors AC, Gupta AK, Matta BF: Dynamic cerebral autoregulation during sevoflurane anesthesia: a comparison with isoflurane. Anesth Analg 88:341, 1999.

98. Berkowitz RA, Hoffman WE, Cunningham F, McDonald T: Changes in cerebral blood flow velocity in children during sevoflurane and halothane anesthesia. J Neurosurg Anesthesiol 8:194, 1996.

99. Komatsu H, Taie S, Endo S, et al: Electrical seizures during sevoflurane anesthesia in two pediatric patients with epilepsy. Anesthesiology 81:1535, 1994.

100. Woodforth IJ, Hicks RG, Crawford MR, et al: Electroencephalographic evidence of seizure activity under deep sevoflurane anesthesia in a nonepileptic patient. Anesthesiology 87:1579, 1997.

101. Bosenberg AT: Convulsions and sevoflurane. Paediatr Anaesth 7:477, 1997.

102. Lutz LJ, Milde JH, Milde LN: The cerebral functional, metabolic, and hemodynamic effects of desflurane in dogs. Anesthesiology 73:125, 1990.

103. Artru AA: Intracranial volume/pressure relationship during desflurane anesthesia in dogs: comparison with isoflurane and thiopental/halothane. Anesth Analg 79:751, 1994.

104. Muzzi DA, Losasso TJ, Dietz NM, et al: The effect of desflurane and isoflurane on cerebrospinal fluid pressure in humans with supratentorial mass lesions. Anesthesiology 76:720, 1992.

105. Pierce E, Lambertson C, Deutsch S: Cerebral circulation and metabolism during thiopental anesthesia and hyperventilation in man. J Clin Invest 41:1664, 1962.

106. Michenfelder JD: The interdependency of cerebral functional and metabolic effects following massive doses of thiopental in the dog. Anesthesiology 41:231, 1974.

107. Shapiro HM, Galindo A, Wyte SR, Harris AB: Rapid intraoperative reduction of intracranial pressure with thiopentone. Br J Anaesth 45:1057, 1973.

108. Mann J, Mann E, Cookson S: Differential effects of pentobarbital, ketamine hydrochloride and enflurane anesthesia on cerebrospinal fluid formation rate and outflow resistance in the rat. Neurosurgery 2:482, 1979.

109. Rockoff MA, Goudsouzian NG: Seizures induced by methohexital. Anesthesiology 54:333, 1981.

110. Renou AM, Vernhiet J, Macrez P, et al: Cerebral blood flow and metabolism during etomidate anaesthesia in man. Br J Anaesth 50:1047, 1978.

111. Milde LN, Milde JH, Michenfelder JD: Cerebral functional, metabolic, and hemodynamic effects of etomidate in dogs. Anesthesiology 63:371, 1985.

112. Fragen RJ, Shanks CA, Molteni A, Avram MJ: Effects of etomidate on hormonal responses to surgical stress. Anesthesiology 61:652, 1984.

113. Laughlin TP, Newberg LA: Prolonged myoclonus after etomidate anesthesia. Anesth Analg 64:80, 1985.

114. Michenfelder JD, Theye RA: Effects of fentanyl, droperidol, and innovar on canine cerebral metabolism and blood flow. Br J Anaesth 43:630, 1971.

115. Sari A, Okuda Y, Takeshita H: The effects of thalamonal on cerebral circulation and oxygen consumption in man. Br J Anaesth 44:330, 1972.

116. Van Hemelrijck J, Fitch W, Mattheussen M, et al: Effect of propofol on cerebral circulation and autoregulation in the baboon. Anesth Analg 71:49, 1990.

117. Pinaud M, Lelausque JN, Chetanneau A, et al: Effects of propofol on cerebral hemodynamics and metabolism in patients with brain trauma. Anesthesiology 73:404, 1990.

118. Bissonnette B, Swan H, Ravussin P, Un V: Neuroleptanesthesia: current status. Can J Anaesth 46:154, 1999.

119. Smith M, Smith SJ, Scott CA, Harkness WF: Activation of the electrocorticogram by propofol during surgery for epilepsy. Br J Anaesth 76:499, 1996.

120. Forster A, Juge O, Morel D: Effects of midazolam on cerebral hemodynamics and cerebral vasomotor responsiveness to carbon dioxide. J Cereb Blood Flow Metab 3:246, 1983.

121. Nugent M, Artru AA, Michenfelder JD: Cerebral metabolic, vascular and protective effects of midazolam maleate: comparison to diazepam. Anesthesiology 56:172, 1982.

122. Forster A, Juge O, Louis M, Nahory A: Effects of a specific benzodiazepine antagonist (RO 15-1788) on cerebral blood flow. Anesth Analg 66:309, 1987.

123. Fleischer JE, Milde JH, Moyer TP, Michenfelder JD: Cerebral effects of high-dose midazolam and subsequent reversal with Ro 15-1788 in dogs. Anesthesiology 68:234, 1988.

124. Jobes DR, Kennell EM, Bush GL, et al: Cerebral blood flow and metabolism during morphine–nitrous oxide anesthesia in man. Anesthesiology 47:16, 1977.

125. Drummond J, Shapiro H: Cerebral physiology. In Miller R (ed): Anesthesia. New York, Churchill Livingstone, 1990, p 621.

126. Artru AA: Effects of halothane and fentanyl on the rate of CSF production in dogs. Anesth Analg 62:581, 1983.

127. Yaster M, Koehler RC, Traystman RJ: Effects of fentanyl on peripheral and cerebral hemodynamics in neonatal lambs. Anesthesiology 66:524, 1987.

128. Albanese J, Durbec O, Viviand X, et al: Sufentanil increases intracranial pressure in patients with head trauma. Anesthesiology 79:493, 1993.

129. Sperry RJ, Bailey PL, Reichman MV, et al: Fentanyl and sufentanil increase intracranial pressure in head trauma patient. Anesthesiology 77:416, 1992.

130. Jung R, Free K, Shah N, et al: Cerebrospinal fluid pressure in anesthetized patients with brain tumors: impact of fentanyl vs. alfentanil. J Neurosurg Anesthesiol 1:136, 1989.

131. Marx W, Shah N, Long C, et al: Sufentanil, alfentanil and fentanyl: impact on cerebrospinal fluid pressure in patients with brain tumors. J Neurosurg Anesthesiol 1:3, 1989.

132. Young WL, Prohovnik I, Correll JW, et al: A comparison of the cerebral hemodynamic effects of sufentanil and isoflurane in humans undergoing carotid endarterectomy. Anesthesiology 71:863, 1989.

133. Milde LN, Milde JH, Gallagher WJ: Effects of sufentanil on cerebral circulation and metabolism in dogs. Anesth Analg 70:138, 1990.

134. Ostapkovich ND, Baker KZ, Fogarty MP, et al: Cerebral blood flow and CO2 reactivity is similar during remifentanil/N2O fentanyl/N2O anesthesia. Anesthesiology 89:358, 1998.

135. Takeshita H, Okuda Y, Sari A: The effects of ketamine on cerebral circulation and metabolism in man. Anesthesiology 36:69, 1972.

136. Shapiro H, Wyte S, Harris A: Ketamine anaesthesia in patients with intracranial pathology. Br J Anaesth 44:1200, 1972.

137. Albanese J, Arnaud S, Rey M, et al: Ketamine decreases intracranial pressure and electroencephalographic activity in traumatic brain injury patients during propofol sedation. Anesthesiology 87:1328, 1997.

138. Ducey JP, Deppe SA, Foley KT: A comparison of the effects of suxamethonium, atracurium and vecuronium on intracranial haemodynamics in swine. Anaesth Intensive Care 17:448, 1989.

139. Cottrell JE, Hartung J, Giffin JP, Shwiry B: Intracranial and hemodynamic changes after succinylcholine administration in cats. Anesth Analg 62:1006, 1983.

140. Lanier WL, Milde JH, Michenfelder JD: Cerebral stimulation following succinylcholine in dogs. Anesthesiology 64:551, 1986.

141. Millar C, Bissonnette B: Awake intubation increases intracranial pressure without affecting cerebral blood flow velocity in infants. Can J Anaesth 41:281, 1994.

142. Minton MD, Grosslight K, Stirt JA, Bedford RF: Increases in intracranial pressure from succinylcholine: prevention by prior nondepolarizing blockade. Anesthesiology 65:165, 1986.

143. Frankville DD, Drummond JC: Hyperkalemia after succinylcholine administration in a patient with closed head injury without paresis. Anesthesiology 67:264, 1987.

144. Tong TK: Succinylcholine-induced hyperkalemia in near-drowning. Anesthesiology 66:720, 1987.

145. Iwatsuki N, Kuroda N, Amaha K, Iwatsuki K: Succinylcholine-induced hyperkalemia in patients with ruptured cerebral aneurysms. Anesthesiology 53:64, 1980.

146. Cooperman LH: Succinylcholine-induced hyperkalemia in neuromuscular disease. JAMA 213:1867, 1970.

147. John DA, Tobey RE, Homer LD, Rice CL: Onset of succinylcholine-induced hyperkalemia following denervation. Anesthesiology 45:294, 1976.

148. Mazurek AJ, Rae B, Hann S, et al: Rocuronium versus succinylcholine: are they equally effective during rapid-sequence induction of anesthesia? Anesth Analg 87:1259, 1998.

149. Stoddart PA, Mather SJ: Onset of neuromuscular blockade and intubating conditions one minute after the administration of rocuronium in children. Paediatr Anaesth 8:37, 1998.

150. Fisher D: Neuromuscular blocking agents in paediatric anaesthesia. Br J Anaesth 83:58, 1999.

151. Lanier WL, Milde JH, Michenfelder JD: The cerebral effects of pancuronium and atracurium in halothane-anesthetized dogs. Anesthesiology 63:589, 1985.

152. Vesely R, Hoffman WE, Gil KS, et al: The cerebrovascular effects of curare and histamine in the rat. Anesthesiology 66:519, 1987.

153. Lien CA, Belmont MR, Abalos A, et al: The cardiovascular effects and histamine-releasing properties of 51W89 in patients receiving nitrous oxide/opioid/barbiturate anesthesia. Anesthesiology 82:1131, 1995.

154. Rosa G, Sanfilippo M, Vilardi V, et al: Effects of vecuronium bromide on intracranial pressure and cerebral perfusion pressure. A preliminary report. Br J Anaesth 58:437, 1986.

155. Young W, Koreh I: Potassium and calcium changes injured spinal cords. Brain Res 365:42, 1986.

156. Casley-Smith J, Foldi BE, Foldi M: The prelymphatic pathways of the brain as revealed by cervical lymphatic obstruction and the passage of particles. Br J Exp Pathol 57:179, 1976.

157. Chaplin ER, Goldstein GW, Myerberg DZ, et al: Posthemorrhagic hydrocephalus in the preterm infant. Pediatrics 65:901, 1980.

158. Friedman WA, Mickle JP: Hydrocephalus in achondroplasia: a possible mechanism. Neurosurgery 7:150, 1980.

159. Pierre-Kahn A, Hirsch JF, Renier D, et al: Hydrocephalus and achondroplasia. A study of 25 observations. Childs Brain 7:205, 1980.

160. Valentino TL, Conway EJ, Shiminski MT, Siffert J: Pediatric brain tumors. Pediatr Ann 26:579, 1997.

161. Brown J: The pathological effects of raised intracranial pressure. Clin Dev Med 38:113, 1991.

162. Cushing H: Some experimental and clinical observations concerning the states of increased intracranial pressure. Am J Med Sci 124:375, 1902.

163. Brown K: Preoperative assessment of neurologic function in the neurosurgical patient. In Bissonnette B (ed): Cerebral protection, Resuscitation and Monitoring: A Look into the Future of Neuroanesthesia. Anesthesiology Clinics of North America. Vol 10. Philadelphia, WB Saunders Company, 1992, p 645.

164. Gascon G, Leech R: Medical evaluation. In Leech R, Brunback R (eds): Hydrocephalus: Current Clinical Concepts. St Louis, CV Mosby, 1991, p 105.

165. Bekemeyer WB, Pinstein ML: Neurogenic pulmonary edema: new concepts of an old disorder. South Med J 82:380, 1989.

166. Milley JR, Nugent SK, Rogers MC: Neurogenic pulmonary edema in childhood. J Pediatr 94:706, 1979.

167. Carlson RW, Schaeffer RJ, Michaels SG, Weil MH: Pulmonary edema following intracranial hemorrhage. Chest 75:731, 1979.

168. Baigelman W, O'Brien JC: Pulmonary effects of head trauma. Neurosurgery 9:729, 1981.

169. Terrence CF, Rao GR, Perper JA: Neurogenic pulmonary edema in unexpected, unexplained death of epileptic patients. Ann Neurol 9:458, 1981.

170. Malik AB: Mechanisms of neurogenic pulmonary edema. Circ Res 57:1, 1985.

171. Shucart WA, Jackson I: Management of diabetes insipidus in neurosurgical patients. J Neurosurg 44:65, 1976.

172. Hodges FI: Pathology of the skull. In Tavaras J (ed): Radiology Diagnosis—Imaging—Intervention: Neuroradiology and Radiology of the Head and Neck. Philadelphia, JB Lippincott, 1989, p 123.

173. Grant E, Richardson J: Infant and neonatal neurosonography technique and normal anatomy. In Tavaras J (ed): Radiology Diagnosis—Imaging—Intervention: Neuroradiology and Radiology of the Head and Neck. Philadelphia, JB Lippincott, 1989, p 453.

174. Garner L, Stirt JA, Finholt DA: Heart block after intravenous lidocaine in an infant. Can Anaesth Soc J 32:425, 1985.

175. Moynihan RJ, Brock UJ, Archer JH, et al: The effect of cricoid pressure on preventing gastric insufflation in infants and children. Anesthesiology 78:652, 1993.

176. Drummond JC, Patel PM, Cole DJ, Kelly PJ: The effect of the reduction of colloid oncotic pressure, with and without reduction of osmolality, on post-traumatic cerebral edema. Anesthesiology 88:993, 1998.

177. Korosue K, Heros RC, Ogilvy CS, et al: Comparison of crystalloids and colloids for hemodilution in a model of focal cerebral ischemia. J Neurosurg 73:576, 1990.

178. Kaieda R, Todd MM, Cook LN, Warner DS: Acute effects of changing plasma osmolality and colloid oncotic pressure on the formation of brain edema after cryogenic injury. Neurosurgery 24:671, 1989.

179. Hartley E, Bissonnette B, St-Louis P, et al: Scalp infiltration with bupivacaine in paediatric brain surgery. Can J Anaesth 73:29, 1991.

180. Schell RM, Cole DJ, Schultz RL, Osborne TN: Temporary cerebral ischemia. Effects of pentastarch or albumin on reperfusion injury. Anesthesiology 77:86, 1992.

181. Wisselink W, Patetsios P, Panetta TF, et al: Medium molecular weight pentastarch reduces reperfusion injury by decreasing capillary leak in an animal model of spinal cord ischemia. J Vasc Surg 27:109, 1998.

182. Ishige N, Pitts LH, Berry I, et al: The effect of hypoxia on traumatic head injury in rats: alterations in neurologic function, brain edema, and cerebral blood flow. J Cereb Blood Flow Metab 7:759, 1987.

183. Albin MS, Bunegin L, Dujovny M, et al: Brain retraction pressure during intracranial procedures. Surg Forum 26:499, 1975.

184. Araki T, Kato H, Kogure K: Neuronal damage and calcium accumulation following repeated brief cerebral ischemia in the gerbil. Brain Res 528:114, 1990.

185. Ravussin P, Archer DP, Meyer E, et al: The effects of rapid infusions of saline and mannitol on cerebral blood volume and intracranial pressure in dogs. Can Anaesth Soc J 32:506, 1985.

186. Lanier WL, Stangland KJ, Scheithauer BW: The effects of dextrose infusion and head position on neurologic outcome after complete cerebral ischemia in primates: examination of a model. Anesthesiology 66:39, 1987.

187. Pulsinelli WA, Levy DE, Sigsbee B, et al: Increased damage after ischemic stroke in patients with hyperglycemia with or without established diabetes mellitus. Am J Med 74:540, 1983.

188. Smerling A: Hypertonic saline in head trauma: a new recipe for drying and salting. J Neurosurg Anesthesiol 4:1, 1992.

189. Simma B, Burger R, Falk M, et al: A prospective, randomized, and controlled study of fluid management in children with severe head injury: lactated Ringer's solution versus hypertonic saline. Crit Care Med 26:1265, 1998.

190. Marshall LF, Smith RW, Rauscher LA, Shapiro HM: Mannitol dose requirements in brain-injured patients. J Neurosurg 48:169, 1978.

191. Nath F, Galbraith S: The effect of mannitol on cerebral white matter water content. J Neurosurg 65:41, 1986.

192. Ravussin P, Abou MM, Archer D, et al: Changes in CSF pressure after mannitol in patients with and without elevated CSF pressure [published erratum appears in J Neurosurg 70(4):662, 1989]. J Neurosurg 69:869, 1988.

193. Cote CJ, Greenhow DE, Marshall BE: The hypotensive response to rapid intravenous administration of hypertonic solutions in man and in the rabbit. Anesthesiology 50:30, 1979.

194. Rudehill A, Lagerkranser M, Lindquist C, Gordon E: Effects of mannitol on blood volume and central hemodynamics in patients undergoing cerebral aneurysm surgery. Anesth Analg 62:875, 1983.

195. Schettini A, Stahurski B, Young HF: Osmotic and osmotic-loop diuresis in brain surgery. Effects on plasma and CSF electrolytes and ion excretion. J Neurosurg 56:679, 1982.

196. Suzuki J, Takahashi A, Yoshimoto T, Seki H: Use of balloon occlusion and substances to protect ischemic brain during resection of posterior fossa AVM. Case report. J Neurosurg 63:626, 1985.

197. Jafar JJ, Johns LM, Mullan SF: The effect of mannitol on cerebral blood flow. J Neurosurg 64:754, 1986.

198. Warren SE, Blantz RC: Mannitol. Arch Intern Med 141:493, 1981.

199. Muizelaar JP, Wei EP, Kontos HA, Becker DP: Mannitol causes compensatory cerebral vasoconstriction and vasodilation in response to blood viscosity changes. J Neurosurg 59:822, 1983.

200. Muizelaar JP, Lutz HD, Becker DP: Effect of mannitol on ICP and CBF and correlation with pressure autoregulation in severely head-injured patients. J Neurosurg 61:700, 1984.

201. Donato T, Shapira Y, Artru A, Powers K: Effect of mannitol on cerebrospinal fluid dynamics and brain tissue edema. Anesth Analg 78:58, 1994.

202. Pollay M, Fullenwider C, Roberts PA, Stevens FA: Effect of mannitol and furosemide on blood-brain osmotic gradient and intracranial pressure. J Neurosurg 59:945, 1983.

203. Cottrell JE, Robustelli A, Post K, Turndorf H: Furosemide- and mannitol-induced changes in intracranial pressure and serum osmolality and electrolytes. Anesthesiology 47:28, 1977.

204. Clasen RA, Pandolfi S, Casey DJ: Furosemide and pentobarbital in cryogenic cerebral injury and edema. Neurology 24:642, 1974.

205. Bourke R, Kimmelberg H, Daze M, et al: Studies on the formation of astroglial swelling and its inhibition by clinically usefull agents.

In Popp A, Bourke R, Nelson L (eds): Neural Trauma. New York, Raven Press, 1979, p 95.

206. Galicich J, French L: Use of dexamethasone in the treatment of brain tumors and brain surgery. Am Proc 12:169, 1961.

207. Bouzarth WF, Shenkin HA: Possible mechanisms of action of dexamethasone in brain injury. J Trauma 14:134, 1974.

208. Bissonnette B, Davis P: Thermal regulation—physiology and perioperative management in infants and children. *In* Motoyama E, Davis P (eds): Smith's Anesthesia for Infants and Children. St Louis, Mosby-Year Book, 1996, p 5.1.

209. Davis A, Bissonnette B: Thermal regulation and mild intraoperative hypothermia. Curr Opin Anesthesiol 12:303, 1999.

210. Bissonnette B, Sessler DI: Thermoregulatory thresholds for vasoconstriction in pediatric patients anesthetized with halothane or halothane and caudal bupivacaine. Anesthesiology 76:387, 1992.

211. Bissonnette B, Sessler DI: The thermoregulatory threshold in infants and children anesthetized with isoflurane and caudal bupivacaine. Anesthesiology 73:1114, 1990.

212. Bissonnette B: Temperature monitoring in pediatric anesthesia. Int Anesthesiol Clin 30:63, 1992.

213. Bissonnette B, Sessler DI: Passive or active inspired gas humidification increases thermal steady-state temperatures in anesthetized infants. Anesth Analg 69:783, 1989.

214. Bissonnette B, Sessler DI, LaFlamme P: Passive and active inspired gas humidification in infants and children. Anesthesiology 71:350, 1989.

215. Harris MM, Strafford MA, Rowe RW, et al: Venous air embolism and cardiac arrest during craniectomy in a supine infant. Anesthesiology 65:547, 1986.

216. Harris MM, Yemen TA, Davidson A, et al: Venous embolism during craniectomy in supine infants. Anesthesiology 67:816, 1987.

217. Joseph M, Leopold G, Carillo J: Venous air embolism during repair of craniosynostosis in the lateral position. Anesth Rev 12:46, 1985.

218. Meridy HW, Creighton RE, Humphreys RP: Complications during neurosurgery in the prone position in children. Can Anaesth Soc J 21:445, 1974.

219. Cabezudo JM, Gilsanz F, Vaquero J, et al: Air embolism from wounds from a pin-type head-holder as a complication of posterior fossa surgery in the sitting position. Case report. J Neurosurg 55:147, 1981.

220. Wilkins RH, Albin MS: An unusual entrance site of venous air embolism during operations in the sitting position. Surg Neurol 7:71, 1977.

221. Michenfelder J, Terry H, Daw E: Air embolism during neurosurgery. Anesth Analg 45:390, 1976.

222. Marshall WK, Bedford RF: Use of a pulmonary-artery catheter for detection and treatment of venous air embolism: a prospective study in man. Anesthesiology 52:131, 1980.

223. Black S, Ockert DB, Oliver WJ, Cucchiara RF: Outcome following posterior fossa craniectomy in patients in the sitting or horizontal positions. Anesthesiology 69:49, 1988.

224. Michenfelder JD, Miller RH, Gronert GA: Evaluation of an ultrasonic device (Doppler) for the diagnosis of venous air embolism. Anesthesiology 36:164, 1972.

225. Cucchiara RF, Bowers B: Air embolism in children undergoing suboccipital craniotomy. Anesthesiology 57:338, 1982.

226. Gronert GA, Messick JJ, Cucchiara RF, Michenfelder JD: Paradoxical air embolism from a patent foramen ovale. Anesthesiology 50:548, 1979.

227. Marquez J, Sladen A, Gendell H, et al: Paradoxical cerebral air embolism without an intracardiac septal defect. Case report. J Neurosurg 55:997, 1981.

228. Colohan AR, Perkins NA, Bedford RF, Jane JA: Intravenous fluid loading as prophylaxis for paradoxical air embolism. J Neurosurg 62:839, 1985.

229. Munson ES: Effect of nitrous oxide on the pulmonary circulation during venous air embolism. Anesth Analg 50:785, 1971.

230. Bedford R: Perioperative venous air embolism. Semin Anesth 6:163, 1987.

231. Pearl RG, Larson CJ: Hemodynamic effects of positive end-expiratory pressure during continuous venous air embolism in the dog. Anesthesiology 64:724, 1986.

232. Davies D, Munro I: The anesthetic management and intraoperative care of patient undergoing major facial osteotomies. Plast Reconstr Surg 55:50, 1975.

233. Brown KA, Bissonnette B, McIntyre B: Hyperkalaemia during rapid blood transfusion and hypovolaemic cardiac arrest in children. Can J Anaesth 37:747, 1990.

234. Brown KA, Bissonnette B, MacDonald M, Poon AO: Hyperkalaemia during massive blood transfusion in paediatric craniofacial surgery. Can J Anaesth 37:747, 1990.

235. Guyer B, MacDorman MF, Martin JA, et al: Annual summary of vital statistics—1997. Pediatrics 102:1333, 1998.

236. Gurney JG, Severson RK, Davis S, Robison LL: Incidence of cancer in children in the United States. Sex-, race-, and 1-year age-specific rates by histologic type. Cancer 75:2186, 1995.

237. Farwell JR, Dohrmann GJ, Flannery JT: Central nervous system tumors in children. Cancer 40:3123, 1977.

238. Farwell JR, Dohrmann GJ, Flannery JT: Intracranial neoplasms in infants. Arch Neurol 35:533, 1978.

239. Childhood Brain Tumor Consortium: A study of childhood brain tumors based on surgical biopsies from ten North American institutions: sample description. J Neurooncol 6:9, 1988.

240. Goulin GD, Duthie SE, Zornow MH, et al: Global cerebral ischemia: effects of pentastarch after reperfusion. Anesth Analg 79:1036, 1994.

241. Cully MD, Larson CJ, Silverberg GD: Hetastarch coagulopathy in a neurosurgical patient. Anesthesiology 66:706, 1987.

242. Ravin MB, Feinberg G: Anesthetic management of hypophysectomy. N Y State J Med 68:776, 1968.

243. Bruno L, Schut L, Bruce D: Survey of pediatric brain tumors. *In* Pediatric Neurosurgery. New York, Grune & Stratton, 1992, p 361.

244. Chatty EM, Earle KM: Medulloblastoma. A report of 201 cases with emphasis on the relationship of histologic variants to survival. Cancer 28:977, 1971.

245. Albright AL, Wisoff JH, Zeltzer PM, et al: Current neurosurgical treatment of medulloblastomas in children. A report from the Children's Cancer Study Group. Pediatr Neurosci 15:276, 1989.

246. Stirt JA, Grosslight KR, Bedford RF, Vollmer D: "Defasciculation" with metocurine prevents succinylcholine-induced increases in intracranial pressure. Anesthesiology 67:50, 1987.

247. Todd MM, Warner DS, Sokoll MD, et al: A prospective, comparative trial of three anesthetics for elective supratentorial craniotomy. Propofol/fentanyl, isoflurane/nitrous oxide, and fentanyl/nitrous oxide. Anesthesiology 78:1005, 1993.

248. Humphreys RP, Creighton RE, Hendrick EB, Hoffman HJ: Advantages of the prone position for neurosurgical procedures on the upper cervical spine and posterior cranial fossa in children. Childs Brain 1:325, 1975.

249. Relton JE, Hall JE: An operation frame for spinal fusion. A new apparatus designed to reduce haemorrhage during operation. J Bone Joint Surg Br 49:327, 1967.

250. Millar C, Bissonnette B, Humphreys RP: Cerebral arteriovenous malformations in children. Can J Anaesth 41:321, 1994.

251. McLeod ME, Creighton RE, Humphreys RP: Anaesthetic management of arteriovenous malformations of the vein of Galen. Can Anaesth Soc J 29:307, 1982.

252. Jedeikin R, Rowe RD, Freedom RM, et al: Cerebral arteriovenous malformation in neonates. The role of myocardial ischemia. Pediatr Cardiol 4:29, 1983.

253. Cumming GR: Circulation in neonates with intracranial arteriovenous fistula and cardiac failure. Am J Cardiol 45:1019, 1980.

254. Levy AM, Hanson JS, Tabakin BS: Congestive heart failure in the newborn infant in the absence of primary cardiac disease. Am J Cardiol 26:409, 1970.

255. Bissonnette B: Temperature monitoring in pediatric anesthesia. *In* Pullerits J, Holtzman R (eds): Anesthesia Equipment for Infants and Children. Boston, Little, Brown, 1992, p 63.

256. Busto R, Dietrich WD, Globus MY, Ginsberg MD: The importance of brain temperature in cerebral ischemic injury. Stroke 20:1113, 1989.

257. Busto R, Globus MY, Dietrich WD, et al: Effect of mild hypothermia on ischemia-induced release of neurotransmitters and free fatty acids in rat brain. Stroke 20:904, 1989.

258. Bissonnette B, Sessler DI: Mild hypothermia does not impair postanesthetic recovery in infants and children. Anesth Analg 76:168, 1993.

259. Barker FN, Ogilvy CS: Efficacy of prophylactic nimodipine for delayed ischemic deficit after subarachnoid hemorrhage: a metaanalysis. J Neurosurg 84:405, 1996.

260. Hino A, Weir BK, Macdonald RL, et al: Prospective, randomized, double-blind trial of BQ-123 and bosentan for prevention of vasospasm following subarachnoid hemorrhage in monkeys. J Neurosurg 83:503, 1995.

261. Herrick IA, Craen RA, Gelb AW, et al: Propofol sedation during awake craniotomy for seizures: electrocorticographic and epileptogenic effects. Anesth Analg 84:1280, 1997.

262. Johnson KB, Egan TD: Remifentanil and propofol combination for awake craniotomy: case report with pharmacokinetic simulations [published erratum appears in J Neurosurg Anesthesiol 10(2):69, 1998]. J Neurosurg Anesthesiol 10:25, 1998.

263. Herrick IA, Craen RA, Gelb AW, et al: Propofol sedation during awake craniotomy for seizures: patient-controlled administration versus neurolept analgesia. Anesth Analg 84:1285, 1997.

264. Ebersole JS: New applications of EEG/MEG in epilepsy evaluation. Epilepsy Res Suppl 11:227, 1996.

265. Diekmann V, Becker W, Jürgens R, et al: Localisation of epileptic foci with electric, magnetic and combined electromagnetic models. Electroencephalogr Clin Neurophysiol 106:297, 1998.

266. Ko DY, Kufta C, Scaffidi D, Sato S: Source localization determined by magnetoencephalography and electroencephalography in temporal lobe epilepsy: comparison with electrocorticography: technical case report. Neurosurgery 42:414, 1998.

267. Kirchberger K, Schmitt H, Hummel C, et al: Clonidine- and methohexital-induced epileptiform discharges detected by magnetoencephalography (MEG) in patients with localization-related epilepsies. Epilepsia 39:1104, 1998.

268. Stapleton SR, Kiriakopoulos E, Mikulis D, et al: Combined utility of functional MRI, cortical mapping, and frameless stereotaxy in the resection of lesions in eloquent areas of brain in children. Pediatr Neurosurg 26:68, 1997.

269. Atlas SW, Howard RD, Maldjian J, et al: Functional magnetic resonance imaging of regional brain activity in patients with intracerebral gliomas: findings and implications for clinical management. Neurosurgery 38:329, 1996.

270. Sipos EP, Tebo SA, Zinreich SJ, et al: In vivo accuracy testing and clinical experience with the ISG Viewing Wand. Neurosurgery 39:194, 1996.

271. Arginteanu M, Abbott R, Frempong A: ISG viewing wand-guided endoscopic catheter placement for treatment of posterior fossa CSF collections. Pediatr Neurosurg 27:319, 1997.

272. Hosain S, Nagarajan L, Fraser R, et al: Effects of nitrous oxide on electrocorticography during epilepsy surgery. Electroencephalogr Clin Neurophysiol 102:340, 1997.

273. Leech R: Myelodysplasia, Arnold-Chiari malformation and hydrocephalus. In Leech R, Brumbaric R (eds): Hydrocephalus: Current Clinical Concepts. St Louis, Mosby-Year Book, 1991, p 129.

274. Dierdorf SF, McNiece WL, Rao CC, et al: Failure of succinylcholine to alter plasma potassium in children with myelomeningocoele. Anesthesiology 64:272, 1986.

275. Flynn J: Retinopathy of prematurity. In Martyn L (ed): Pediatric Ophthalmology. Philadelphia, WB Saunders Company, 1987, p 1487.

276. Bryan MH, Hardie MJ, Reilly BJ, Swyer PR: Pulmonary function studies during the first year of life in infants recovering from the respiratory distress syndrome. Pediatrics 52:169, 1973.

277. Sandler AN, Tator CH: Effect of acute spinal cord compression injury on regional spinal cord blood flow in primates. J Neurosurg 45:660, 1976.

278. Kato A, Ushio Y, Hayakawa T, et al: Circulatory disturbance of the spinal cord with epidural neoplasm in rats. J Neurosurg 63:260, 1985.

279. Lam A: Do evoked potentials have any value in anesthesia? In Bissonnette B (ed): Cerebral Protection, Resuscitation and Monitoring: A Look into the Future of Neuroanesthesia. Anesthesiology Clinics of North America. Vol 10. Philadelphia, WB Saunders Company, 1992, p 657.

280. Maertens de Noordhout A, Remacle JM, Pepin JL, et al: Magnetic stimulation of the motor cortex in cervical spondylosis. Neurology 41:75, 1991.

281. Lavelle JM, Shaw KN: Evaluation of head injury in a pediatric emergency department: pretrauma and posttrauma system. Arch Pediatr Adolesc Med 152:1220, 1998.

282. Levitt C, Smith W, Alexander R: Abusive head trauma. In Reece R (ed): Child Abuse: Medical Diagnosis and Management. Philadelphia, Lea & Febiger, 1994, p 1.

283. Jenny C, Hymel KP, Ritzen A, et al: Analysis of missed cases of abusive head trauma. JAMA 281:621, 1999.

284. Johnson DL, Krishnamurthy S: Severe pediatric head injury: myth, magic, and actual fact [review]. Pediatr Neurosurg 28:167, 1998.

285. Lloyd DA, Carty H, Patterson M, et al: Predictive value of skull radiography for intracranial injury in children with blunt head injury. Lancet 349:821, 1997.

286. Carty H, Lloyd D: Commentary: head injury in children. Who needs a skull x-ray? Pediatr Radiol 28:815, 1998.

287. Bruce DA, Alavi A, Bilaniuk L, et al: Diffuse cerebral swelling following head injuries in children: the syndrome of "malignant brain edema". J Neurosurg 54:170, 1981.

288. Ross DA, Olsen WL, Ross AM, et al: Brain shift, level of consciousness, and restoration of consciousness in patients with acute intracranial hematoma. J Neurosurg 71:498, 1989.

289. Langfitt TW, Obrist WD, Alavi A, et al: Computerized tomography, magnetic resonance imaging, and positron emission tomography in the study of brain trauma. Preliminary observations. J Neurosurg 64:760, 1986.

290. Bohn D, Armstrong D, Becker L, Humphreys R: Cervical spine injuries in children. J Trauma 30:463, 1990.

291. Young B, Ott L, Dempsey R, et al: Relationship between admission hyperglycemia and neurologic outcome of severely brain-injured patients. Ann Surg 210:466, 1989.

292. Pulsinelli WA, Waldman S, Rawlinson D, Plum F: Moderate hyperglycemia augments ischemic brain damage: a neuropathologic study in the rat. Neurology 32:1239, 1982.

293. Schell R, Cole D: Cerebral protection and neuroanesthesia. In Bissonnette B (ed): Cerebral Protection, Resuscitation and Monitoring: A Look into the Future of Neuroanesthesia. Anesthesiology Clinics of North America. Vol 10. Philadelphia, WB Saunders Company, 1992, p 453.

294. Milde Newberg L: Cerebral resuscitation, is it possible? In Bissonnette B (ed): Cerebral Protection, Resuscitation and Monitoring: A Look into the Future of Neuroanesthesia. Anesthesiology Clinics of North America. Vol 10. Philadelphia, WB Saunders Company, 1992, p 575.

295. Skippen P: Cardiopulmonary resuscitation and cerebral outcome: Is there any hope? In Bissonnette B (ed): Cerebral Protection, Resuscitation and Monitoring: A Look into the Future of Neuroanesthesia. Anesthesiology Clinics of North America. Vol 10. Philadelphia, WB Saunders Company, 1992, p 619.

296. Messick J, Milde L: Brain protection. Adv Anesth 4:47, 1987.

297. Hossmann KA: Post-ischemic resuscitation of the brain: selective vulnerability versus global resistance. Prog Brain Res 63:3, 1985.

298. Sano T, Drummond JC, Patel PM, et al: A comparison of the cerebral protective effects of isoflurane and mild hypothermia in a model of incomplete forebrain ischemia in the rat. Anesthesiology 76:221, 1992.

299. Matsumoto M, Iida Y, Sakabe T, et al: Mild and moderate hypothermia provide better protection than a burst-suppression dose of thiopental against ischemic spinal cord injury in rabbits. Anesthesiology 86:1120, 1997.

300. Nakashima K, Todd MM, Warner DS: The relation between cerebral metabolic rate and ischemic depolarization. A comparison of the effects of hypothermia, pentobarbital, and isoflurane. Anesthesiology 82:1199, 1995.

301. Kawai F, Sterling P: AMPA receptor activates a G-protein that suppresses a cGMP-gated current. J Neurosci 19:2954, 1999.

302. Cheung PY, Peliowski A, Robertson CM: The outcome of very low birth weight neonates ($</= 1500$ g) rescued by inhaled nitric oxide: neurodevelopment in early childhood. J Pediatr 133:735, 1998.

303. Beckman JS: The double-edged role of nitric oxide in brain function and superoxide-mediated injury. J Dev Physiol 15:53, 1991.

304. Bolanos JP, Almeida A, Medina JM: Nitric oxide mediates brain mitochondrial damage during perinatal anoxia. Brain Res 787:117, 1998.

305. Cheung PY, Salas E, Etches PC, et al: Inhaled nitric oxide and inhibition of platelet aggregation in critically ill neonates [letter]. Lancet 351:1181, 1998.

306. Young W: Neuroanesthesia: a look into the future. In Bissonnette B (ed): Cerebral Protection, Resuscitation and Monitoring: A Look into the Future of Neuroanesthesia. Anesthesiology Clinics of North America. Vol 10. Philadelphia, WB Saunders Company, 1992, p 727.

17

Anesthesia for Thoracic Surgery

GEORGE ULMA
JEREMY M. GEIDUSCHEK
A. ANDREW ZIMMERMAN
JEFFREY P. MORRAY

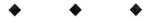

Thoracic surgery in the pediatric patient may be performed for a wide variety of congenital, neoplastic, traumatic, and infectious processes. This chapter discusses relevant pulmonary anatomy and physiology, then addresses the clinical approach to the child who presents for thoracic surgery, including preoperative preparation and intraoperative management. The approach to anesthetic management of specific surgical lesions follows, and the chapter concludes by discussing the management of children with chronic respiratory disease.

EMBRYOLOGY OF THE LUNG

Airways and Alveoli

Lung development begins in the fourth week of fetal life as lung buds divide first into main-stem bronchi and then into lobar and subsegmental airways. By 16 weeks' gestation the number of airway generations is similar to that in the adult[1, 2] and alveolar development begins. Terminal airways remodel to form clusters of large saccules, which ultimately become true alveoli.[3] Surfactant-producing type II cells first appear at approximately 24 weeks of fetal life.[4]

Postnatally, the number of alveoli rapidly increases during the first 8 years of life.[5–7] Once this multiplication is complete, further lung growth occurs, principally by an increase in alveolar size. Postnatal increase in airway caliber occurs in a nonuniform manner, with peripheral airway growth delayed compared with that of central airways. Most of the increase in peripheral airway caliber occurs after 8 years of age.[8]

Pulmonary Circulation

Development of the pulmonary circulation parallels airway development. An adult pattern of arterial branching is present by 20 weeks' gestation.[9] From later fetal life until approximately 3 years after birth, the development of new arteries follows the pattern of terminal airway branching and alveolar development. Supernumerary arteries, which directly supply alveoli, continue to grow as the number of alveoli increases.[10]

The vascular microanatomy changes during fetal and postnatal life. In the adult, muscular arteries are present all the way to the pleural surface, whereas at birth, smooth muscle extends only to the level of the terminal bronchioles.[5] However, in the newborn, arteries that are muscularized are thicker-walled than similar-sized arteries in the adult, a feature that is important for determining pulmonary flow during fetal life.[11] During the first years of life this smooth muscle thins to adult levels and extends distally toward the periphery of the acinus (Fig. 17–1).

THE TRANSITIONAL CIRCULATION

The transition from intrauterine to extrauterine life requires a number of dynamic cardiopulmonary events. The vascular system of the fetus is characterized by high pulmonary vascular resistance (PVR) and low systemic vascular resistance (SVR), partly the result of the low-resistance placental circulation. This differential in systemic and pulmonary resistance causes blood to bypass the lungs in favor of right-to-left shunts through the foramen ovale and the ductus arteriosus.[12] At birth, with placental separation, SVR increases. A concomitant decrease in PVR is mediated through a number of only partially understood mechanisms (Fig. 17–2). Inflation of the lungs mechanically decreases PVR.[13] The abrupt increase in Pa_{O_2} and the decrease in Pa_{CO_2} decrease pulmonary vascular smooth muscle tone. In addition, circulating mediators such as endothelium-derived relaxant factor (EDRF) and prostaglandins play an active role.[14–17]

At the same time, the foramen ovale and the ductus arteriosus close. The foramen ovale is functionally closed as left atrial pressure increases. The ductus arteriosus constricts in response to changes in Pa_{O_2}, Pa_{CO_2}, and pH, as well as to circulating factors.

This transition from fetal to extrauterine life is dynamic and can reverse during the immediate postnatal period to a fetal-like circulation characterized by increased PVR

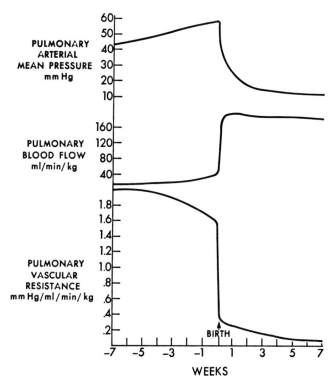

FIGURE 17–2. Changes in pulmonary arterial pressure, pulmonary blood flow, and calculated pulmonary vascular resistance during the 7 weeks preceding birth, at birth, and during the 7 weeks postnatally. The prenatal data were derived from lambs and the postnatal data from other species. (From Rudolph AM: Congenital Diseases of the Heart. Chicago, Year Book Medical Publishers, 1974, with permission.)

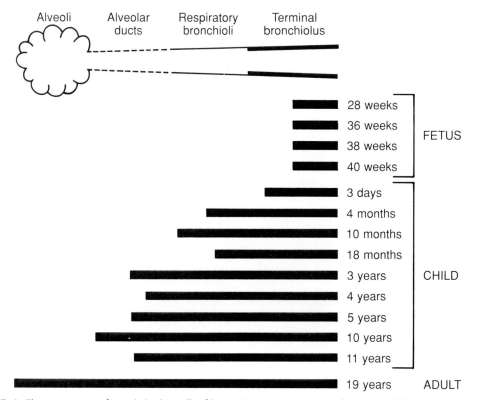

FIGURE 17–1. The appearance of muscle in the walls of intra-acinar arteries. No muscle is seen within the acinus in the fetus, but with age muscle extends gradually within the acinus. However, even at 11 years, extension of muscle is not as great as in the adult.

and extreme hypoxemia secondary to right-to-left shunting of blood. PVR can be elevated in the postnatal period by hypoxemia, acidosis, pneumonia, and hypothermia. This clinical state has been termed persistent fetal circulation (PFC) or persistent pulmonary hypertension of the newborn (PPHN).[18, 19] Sustained increases in pulmonary artery resistance and pressure can result in right ventricular hypertrophy and dilation (cor pulmonale).

THE PEDIATRIC LUNG

Compliance

The pediatric lung is less compliant than the adult lung because of differences in alveolar architecture, elastin, and surfactant. Alveolar anatomy has the greatest impact during the postnatal period when alveoli are small and many airspaces are in the prealveolar or saccular stage with thickened walls.[20]

The amount of elastin in the alveoli and airways determines the elasticity of the lung. Less elastin results in less elastic recoil and more likely collapse of airways and alveoli. When there is little elastin, airways collapse before the end-exhalation and at a closing volume that is larger than the functional residual capacity (FRC), producing a right-to-left intrapulmonary shunt (Fig. 17–3). At birth, elastin extends only to the level of the terminal bronchus.[21] The amount of elastin increases over the first 18 years of age and then gradually decreases over the next five decades.[22] Consequently, lung compliance peaks during late adolescence and is relatively low in the very young and the very old.

Finally, either immaturity of or damage to the surfactant system results in a decrease in compliance. Hyaline membrane disease or infant respiratory distress syndrome (IRDS) occurs in premature infants with inadequate surfactant production and is characterized by respiratory failure secondary to poor lung compliance and alveolar collapse.

Airway Resistance

Airway resistance is greater in children than in adults. Although the adult number of airway generations is present by 16 weeks' gestation, the airway caliber is smaller than that of the adult. Poiseuille's law holds that resistance is inversely proportional to the fourth power of the radius (of the airway) during laminar flow:

$$Resistance = 8Ln/\pi r^4$$

where L = length and n = flow constant. Hence, the smaller the airway, the more resistance to flow through that airway. The distribution of resistance is not uniform and changes with age. Hogg et al.[8] demonstrated that whereas the conductance (conductance = 1/resistance) of the large, central airways remains relatively constant, the conductance of the smaller peripheral airways is low in young children and dramatically increases after the age of 5 years (Fig. 17–4). The increased airway resistance in the younger child results in increased work of breathing and increased vulnerability to diseases affecting the small airways.

The Chest Wall

The configuration of the child's chest differs from that of the adult. The child's chest is box-like, with ribs positioned

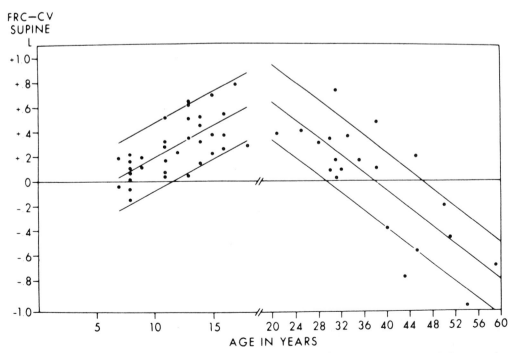

FIGURE 17–3. Functional residual capacity minus closing volume as a function of age. Negative values imply that some dependent units are closed throughout all or part of the tidal volume.

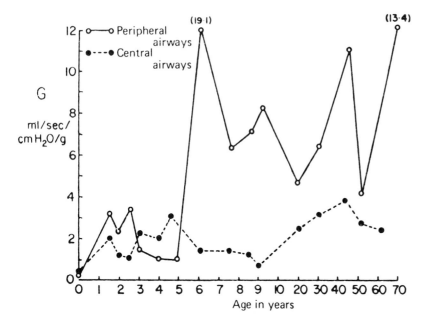

FIGURE 17-4. Central and peripheral conductance per gram of lung tissue as a function of age. Central conductance is almost constant with growth, but there is a sharp rise in peripheral conductance at about the age of 5 years. (From Hogg JC, Williams J, Richardson B, et al: Age as a factor in the distribution of lower airway conductance and in the pathologic anatomy of obstructive lung disease. N Engl J Med 282:1283, 1970, with permission.)

at nearly right angles to the vertebral column. The adult's chest is flattened dorsoventrally and has ribs that slant in a caudal direction[23] (Fig. 17-5). The shape of the adult chest is mechanically more efficient, in that intrathoracic volume can be increased by raising the ribs into a horizontal position.[24]

The chest wall of the child is very compliant. The child's ribs are cartilaginous rather than bony. Because the chest wall is so compliant, negative intrapleural pressure in the presence of high airway resistance or low lung compliance can result in chest wall collapse with little air entry. Therefore, the neonate's chest can behave much like a "flail" chest.

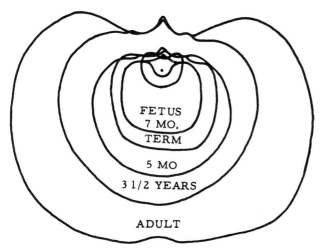

FIGURE 17-5. Superimposed outlines of thoracic skeletal contours at various ages to illustrate the transition from the rounded thorax of the fetus to the dorsoventrally flattened thorax of the adult. (From Krahl VE: Anatomy of the mammalian lung. In Fenn WO, Rahn H [eds]: Handbook of Physiology. Section 3: Respiration. Vol 1. Washington, DC, American Physiological Society, 1964, p 472, with permission.)

Physiology of the Lateral Decubitus Position

Because most thoracic surgical procedures are done in the lateral decubitus position (LDP), an understanding of the factors that influence the distribution of ventilation and perfusion in the LDP is important.

LDP, Awake, Closed Chest

Because gravity causes a vertical gradient for pulmonary blood flow in the LDP and in the upright position, blood flow to the dependent lung is much greater than blood flow to the nondependent lung (Fig. 17-6). Gravity also causes a vertical gradient in pleural pressure, resulting in the most positive pleural pressure in the dependent lung. This places the dependent lung on a more favorable position on the compliance curve (Fig. 17-7). In addition, the abdominal contents exert more pressure on the dependent versus the nondependent diaphragm, resulting in doming and more efficient contraction during spontaneous ventilation.[25] For these reasons, ventilation is also preferentially distributed to the dependent lung, and ventilation-perfusion ratios ($\dot{V}/\dot{Q}$) are not significantly altered when the awake subject assumes the LDP.

LDP, Anesthetized, Closed Chest

The induction of anesthesia does not produce any qualitative change in the distribution of pulmonary blood flow but does alter the distribution of ventilation. There is a loss of FRC in both lungs, perhaps to a greater extent in the lower lung because of the weight of the mediastinum and abdominal contents. The loss of FRC usually results in a change in compliance, as illustrated in Figure 17-7. The nondependent lung moves from the flat, noncompliant portion to the steep, compliant portion of the pressure-volume curve, whereas the dependent lung moves from

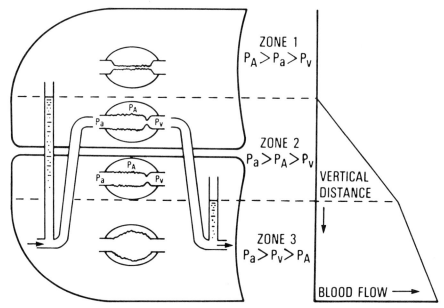

FIGURE 17-6. The effect of gravity on distribution of pulmonary blood flow in the lateral decubitus position. Pulmonary blood flow increases with lung dependency and is greatest in the most dependent zone 3, where both arterial (Pa) and venous (Pv) pressure exceed alveolar pressure (PA), and the amount of flow depends on the Pa–Pv gradient. (From Benumof JL, Alfery DD: Anesthesia for thoracic surgery. *In* Miller RD [ed]: Anesthesia. 3rd ed. New York, Churchill Livingstone, 1990, p 1517, with permission.)

the steep, compliant portion to the flat, noncompliant portion. This shifts ventilation away from the dependent lung to the upper, nondependent lung.[26, 27] If the patient is given muscle relaxants and mechanical ventilation, the mechanical advantage of the dependent diaphragm is also eliminated, which also favors redistribution of ventilation away from the lower lung. Therefore, $\dot{V}/\dot{Q}$ matching is disturbed and a decreased Pa_{O_2} frequently results. The application of PEEP to both lungs usually restores the preponderance of ventilation to the lower lung and improves $\dot{V}/\dot{Q}$ matching,[28] presumably by reverting each lung toward its preanesthesia position on the pressure–volume curve.[29]

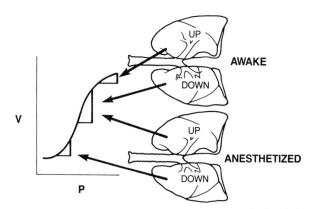

FIGURE 17-7. In the lateral decubitus position (LDP) with closed chest, the induction of anesthesia results in a change in position on the volume (V) versus pressure (P) curve for both the dependent and nondependent lungs. The nondependent lung moves from the upper, flat portion, to the steep, more favorable portion of the curve, whereas the dependent lung moves from the steep portion to the flat lower portion. (Adapted from Benumof JL, Alfery DD: Anesthesia for thoracic surgery. *In* Miller RD [ed]: Anesthesia. 2nd ed. New York, Churchill Livingstone, 1986, p 1371, with permission.)

LDP, Anesthetized, Open Chest

Opening the chest cavity exacerbates the $\dot{V}/\dot{Q}$ mismatch seen in the LDP in the anesthetized, closed-chest state. The qualitative distribution of pulmonary blood flow is not affected but the distribution of ventilation is altered. Positive-pressure ventilation becomes mandatory; because the chest wall and pleura are open, total compliance of the upper lung is reduced to that of the lung parenchyma alone. If muscle relaxants are added, any restrictive effect of the diaphragm is also eliminated and the diaphragm is displaced preferentially in the nondependent area, where the weight of the abdominal contents is the least.[25] The lower lung remains compressed by the chest wall, mediastinum, and abdominal contents. Thus, the upper lung is overventilated and underperfused, whereas the lower lung is underventilated and overperfused.[26]

A logical solution to the $\dot{V}/\dot{Q}$ mismatch induced by the LDP, anesthetized, open-chest situation would be selective application of positive end-expiratory pressure (PEEP) to the dependent lung via a double-lumen endotracheal tube (ETT). This has been done successfully in adults but is not practical in children because appropriately sized double-lumen tubes are not manufactured. A less physiologic, although more practical solution to the problem, is often provided by the surgeon, whose retraction of the nondependent lung redistributes ventilation to the dependent, better-perfused lung.

The factors that influence distribution of ventilation and perfusion are also important during the postoperative period when a decision is made about the position in which to nurse the patient to achieve optimal gas exchange. In adults with unilateral lung disease, gas exchange is optimal when the good lung is dependent.[27, 28] Data have been published suggesting that infants, both those breathing spontaneously and those receiving positive-pressure ventilation, distribute more ventilation to the nondependent lung.[30, 31] Infants with unilateral lung disease have been oxygenated when the good lung is nondependent, a finding opposite to that in adults. Ventilation may be distributed differently in infants and adults because the more unstable rib cage in infants cannot fully support the underlying lung. This results in a lower FRC close to residual volume, making airway closure likely to occur in the dependent lung, even during tidal breathing, and thereby redistributing ventilation to the nondependent lung. It is not known at what age the adult pattern appears. It is suggested that during the postoperative period the child with unilateral lung disease should be nursed in both lateral decubitus positions, as well as supine, to determine the position of optimal gas exchange.

CONTROL OF BREATHING

Ventilation is adjusted to minimize variations in arterial $Paco_2$, Pao_2, and pH despite major changes in metabolic demand (exercise) or oxygen availability (high altitude). The rate and depth of breathing are also controlled to minimize the energy expended to overcome the elastic, resistive, and inertial forces associated with respiration.[32]

Two systems are involved in the regulatory process: (1) the neural system, which is responsible for maintaining the coordinated, rhythmic respiratory cycle and regulating the depth of respiration; and (2) a chemical system (also, in part, neurally mediated) that regulates minute ventilation and maintains normal blood gas tensions.

Neural Control

Four centers in the brain are responsible for respiratory control: the apneustic and pneumotaxic centers are located in the pons, and the inspiratory and expiratory centers are located in the medulla. The medullary centers receive information from proprioceptors in the lung and the intercostal muscles, which provide mechanical feedback. The Hering-Breuer reflex is the best described mechanical feedback pathway: with inspiration and inflation of the lungs, inhibitory feedback is sent to the inspiratory center via the vagus nerve. This peripheral control modulates central medullary activity. In addition, the respiratory control areas are influenced by the hypothalamus and the cerebral cortex.[33] Tachypnea associated with fever is thought to be controlled by the hypothalamus, and conscious control of respiration (anxiety-hyperventilation syndrome) is controlled by the cerebral cortex. The medullary reticular activating system also may affect respiration. It has been postulated that this area mediates the initiation of spontaneous ventilation in the neonate.

Chemical Control

Chemical control of alveolar ventilation is mediated by central chemoreceptors and chromaffin tissue positioned along the great vessels (carotid and aortic bodies). The central chemoreceptor, thought to be located in the medulla, responds to changes in cerebrospinal fluid pH or $Paco_2$. Direct stimulation by increased $Paco_2$ or hydrogen

ion concentration increases ventilation, whereas a decrease in $Paco_2$ or hydrogen ion concentration decreases ventilation.[34]

The two principal peripheral chemoreceptors are the carotid bodies, located at the division of the common carotid artery into its external and internal branches, and the aortic bodies, which lie between the ascending aorta and the pulmonary artery. Afferent impulses are mediated by the glossopharyngeal and recurrent laryngeal nerves. The peripheral receptors have resting tone and respond primarily to changes in arterial oxygen tension. An increase in arterial oxygen tension (not oxygen content) inhibits respiration, whereas a decrease in Pao_2 to less than 50 mm Hg causes a significant rise in ventilation. Changes in arterial pH stimulate the peripheral chemoreceptors to a lesser degree than hypoxia, but the effect of changes in $Paco_2$ or pH is greater during hypoxia, suggesting a synergistic effect.

Respiratory control in the neonate may be somewhat different from that in the child or adult. In response to hypoxia, ventilation in the neonate initially increases, then decreases. This "biphasic" response is more exaggerated in the preterm neonate and disappears in the full-term infant after several weeks. Irregular respiration, known as periodic breathing, which is seen most commonly in infants, particularly premature infants, suggests incomplete development of the medullary respiratory centers.[35]

ANESTHETIC MANAGEMENT: GENERAL CONSIDERATIONS

Preoperative Management

History

Preoperative assessment of the child who presents for a thoracic surgical procedure focuses on the nature and degree of cardiopulmonary compromise. The history must include inquiries about exercise intolerance, cyanosis, respiratory tract infections, and symptoms of respiratory distress, such as cough, tachypnea, dyspnea, chest wall retractions, and nasal flaring. Generalized complaints may accompany such symptoms, including weight loss, fatigue, and anorexia.

Physical Examination

The physical examination also focuses on the cardiopulmonary system, but begins with a general assessment of the patient. The upper airway is examined to assess potential difficulty in airway management. The heart is examined for murmurs, gallops, or rubs. The chest is auscultated for rales, rhonchi, or wheezes. The presence of active bronchospasm has particular significance, since further preoperative evaluation and therapy may be necessary and intraoperative anesthetic techniques may require alterations to prevent exacerbation of bronchospasm.

Laboratory Evaluation

Because of economic concerns, it is becoming increasingly common for the otherwise healthy child to undergo minor surgery without any preoperative laboratory tests. The decision to perform a preoperative laboratory test is driven by the severity of the child's underlying disease and the nature of the surgery planned. The hematocrit may indicate polycythemia as a reflection of chronic hemoglobin desaturation or anemia of chronic disease. In addition, the hematocrit is used to estimate the degree of surgical blood loss that can occur before transfusion is necessary. The white blood cell (WBC) count and differential may indicate the presence of active pulmonary infection, although the sensitivity and specificity of both tests are low. In the presence of pulmonary infection, a sputum sample, if obtainable, is sent for Gram's stain, culture, and sensitivity to guide antibiotic therapy.

Anteroposterior (AP) and lateral chest radiographs are obtained in most patients scheduled for thoracic surgery. These must be viewed carefully, looking in particular for findings that may influence anesthetic management (Table 17–1). Computed tomographic (CT) scans or magnetic resonance imaging (MRI), if available, should also be reviewed for any additional information concerning intrathoracic anatomy. Rapid three-dimensional reconstruction by ultrafast chest CT can be performed in minutes and may offer an alternative to MRI for children at risk for respiratory complications with sedation or anesthesia.[36]

Arterial blood gas analysis is obtained in patients with significant signs and symptoms of respiratory compromise. Patients who are hypoxic and hypercarbic while breathing room air are at increased risk for intraoperative problems and postoperative ventilatory failure.

Pulmonary function testing has been widely used in adults with pulmonary dysfunction who are scheduled for thoracic or abdominal surgery. The results of such tests are generally used to estimate intra- or postoperative risk. The role of routine pulmonary function testing in children has not been established, though awareness of reduction in lung volumes may help guide management during postoperative separation from the ventilator.[37] Pulmonary function testing may also be useful in the presence of airway obstruction (see sections "Anterior Mediastinal Mass" and "Asthma"). Pulmonary function standards are available for children,[38] although patient cooperation is not feasible until the age of 5 or 6 years.

T A B L E   1 7 – 1
SIGNIFICANT FINDINGS ON CHEST RADIOGRAPH THAT MIGHT INFLUENCE THE COURSE OF ANESTHESIA

Radiographic Finding	Potential Anesthetic Problem
Tracheal deviation or compression	Difficulty with intubation or ventilation
Intraparenchymal infiltrate, pleural effusion	Decreased lung compliance
	Increased $\dot{V}/\dot{Q}$ mismatch
	Increased transpulmonary shunt with poor systemic oxygenation
Cardiac enlargement	Cardiac depression from anesthetics, possible tamponade
Air–fluid levels (abscess)	Rupture of abscess with soiling of healthy lung

---

T A B L E   1 7 – 2
PREPARATION OF THE CHILD FOR THORACIC SURGERY

Achieve positive caloric balance with sustained weight gain

Treat infection
  Select antibiotic on basis of Gram's stain, culture, and sensitivity of tracheal secretions, if possible
  Attempt to mobilize secretions with chest percussion and postural drainage
  Teach deep breathing, coughing exercises, and incentive spirometry if possible

Treat bronchospasm (see section on asthma)
  β_2-Adrenergic agents
  Methylxanthines (e.g., aminophylline)
  Steroids
  Cromolyn sodium

Increased inspired oxygen concentration, if necessary

Treat cor pulmonale, if present
  Supplemental oxygen
  Diuretics
  Digitalis

Preoperative Preparation

Adult patients with pulmonary dysfunction appear to have fewer postoperative pulmonary complications when preoperative pulmonary therapy is performed.[39] Similar data do not exist for children, although it makes intuitive sense that fewer intra- and postoperative problems would occur after preoperative treatment of the reversible components of respiratory disease. Preoperative treatments that should be considered are summarized in Table 17–2.

The approach to the patient with cor pulmonale includes the preoperative use of oxygen to reverse the pulmonary vasoconstriction and subsequent right ventricular strain that results from chronic hypoxemia. Diuretics are used to decrease the excess lung water commonly seen in cor pulmonale. Digitalis can be used for patients in overt congestive heart failure (CHF) or for patients who have supraventricular dysrhythmias with a rapid ventricular response.[40] Serum potassium levels must be monitored closely and supplemented if low, to avoid digitalis toxicity. Digitalis should probably be withheld on the day of surgery to lessen the risk of digitalis toxicity.

The patient and family must be prepared emotionally for the impending procedure. Pertinent preoperative procedures should be explained in as benign a way as possible. The patient's postoperative experience (intravenous [IV] lines, monitoring devices, ETTs, and chest tubes) is explained, not so explicitly as to frighten the child but simply and gently to help allay the fear of the unknown. The needs of the parents must also be considered. Although an exhaustive description of possible complications is not indicated, discussion of the most likely complications in the high-risk patient is appropriate, usually in the child's absence. Finally, both the parents and the child should be given ample opportunity to ask questions about the impending procedure. Adequate psychological preparation of the child can significantly reduce the emotional trauma associated with impending surgery.

Premedication

Children who are hypoxemic (Pa_{O_2} <60 mm Hg) on room air, who are hypercarbic (Pa_{CO_2} >50 mm Hg), or who have compromised airways are given no premedication that might depress respiratory drive or result in airway obstruction. For children without these difficulties there is no general agreement as to the optimal regimen. The choice of drugs is individualized to the psychological needs of the patient, based on clinical experience. Anticholinergic agents, if needed to dry secretions or block vagal effects, can be given intravenously at the time of induction.

Intraoperative Management

Monitoring

Anesthesia for thoracotomy requires monitoring of the electrocardiogram (ECG), blood pressure, temperature, heart and breath sounds, inspired oxygen concentration, airway pressure, and oxygen saturation. A nerve stimulator is used when muscle relaxants are employed. Continual end-tidal carbon dioxide (Pet_{CO_2}) measurement is now included in the American Society of Anesthesiologists Standards for Basic Anesthesia Monitoring.[41] In infants with small tidal volumes and rapid respiratory rates, true end-tidal sampling is difficult and expired CO_2 values may be falsely low. When sampling is performed from the distal end of the ETT, the value obtained is more likely to approximate the Pa_{CO_2}.[42] The gradient between arterial and alveolar carbon dioxide is also increased in the presence of increased dead space ventilation or other abnormalities of matching between ventilation and perfusion.[43] Despite these limitations, end-tidal carbon dioxide measurement is useful as a reflection of the Pa_{CO_2} and alveolar ventilation and also as a means of detecting complications such as esophageal intubation, inadvertent extubation, or ETT obstruction.

Hypothermia is a significant risk in the premature or newborn child but may occur in any child undergoing thoracotomy because of evaporative and radiant heat loss. Core temperature is monitored with an esophageal or rectal probe in all patients. In the infant, core temperature is supported with a radiant warmer, a heating blanket, increased environmental temperature, warmed IV solutions, and warmed, humidified inspired gases.

For patients with preoperative cardiopulmonary disease and for those scheduled for invasive intrathoracic surgery, the use of intra-arterial and central venous pressure (CVP) monitoring should be considered. Direct arterial cannulation permits beat-to-beat blood pressure monitoring and frequent blood gas analysis. Central venous cannulation allows rapid administration of fluids and blood products to maintain or restore intravascular volume; it also allows administration of drugs that are potentially sclerosing (e.g., $CaCl_2$) or vasoconstricting (e.g., high-dose dopamine) when given through a peripheral vein. In addition, measurement of CVP permits assessment of circulating blood volume and right ventricular function.

Anesthetic Agents

Although a variety of anesthetic agents can be chosen for use in thoracic procedures, the halogenated agents are most frequently used for the following reasons:

1. They can be delivered with high concentrations of inspired oxygen. Although "balanced" techniques that include nitrous oxide can be used, the concomitant reduction in inspired oxygen concentration increases the chance of intraoperative hypoxemia.
2. They obtund airway reflexes, and thereby lessen the risk of bronchoconstriction (see the section "Asthma").
3. They are relatively insoluble and therefore are eliminated quickly, allowing rapid emergence and perhaps a diminished risk of hypoventilation during the postoperative period.

Opioids can be used as adjuncts to the halogenated agents. Fentanyl 2 to 3 $\mu g/kg$ or morphine sulfate 0.1 mg/kg IV decreases the intraoperative requirements for potent vapors. However, delayed awakening and prolonged respiratory depression may be seen after opioid administration, particularly in neonates, in whom opioid clearance is decreased compared with older children.[44] The use of ultra–short-acting agents such as remifentanil should be considered in patients in whom prolonged opioid clearance would be problematic.

Muscle relaxants are useful adjuncts in the maintenance of anesthesia; they may facilitate rib spreading and surgical exposure. More importantly, they reduce the requirement for halogenated agents, thereby decreasing both the total amount of anesthetic drug given and the emergence time.

A potential disadvantage of the halogenated agents is their tendency to block hypoxic pulmonary vasoconstriction (HPV). Normally, poorly ventilated areas of lung (e.g., areas of atelectasis) have a parallel reduction in blood flow as HPV redirects blood flow away from hypoxic lung to well-ventilated areas. This autoregulatory mechanism reduces intrapulmonary shunting and maintains Pa_{O_2}. Because of the need for surgical exposure in many thoracic procedures, atelectasis and other causes of ventilation abnormalities are common. Anesthetic agents that maintain HPV would be advantageous; agents that block HPV would be undesirable. All injectable anesthetics studied to date have had no effect on HPV.[45–50] Of the inhaled anesthetics, halothane has been the most extensively studied.[48, 57, 58] The results of these studies have been species and experimental model dependent. In the in vitro and in isolated in vivo models,[42–47] halothane inhibited HPV; in intact in vivo[48–50] models and in human studies,[59] halothane caused either no change or only a slight decrease in HPV.

The other inhaled anesthetics in common clinical use have been less extensively studied. Isoflurane has been shown to inhibit HPV in isolated perfused lungs.[52] However, in intact in vivo preparations[48, 58, 60] and in adult human[61, 62] the effect of isoflurane on HPV has been much less pronounced. In vivo experiments are complicated by the effects of the anesthetic agent on other variables that influence HPV. For example, mixed venous oxygen tension is a primary determinant of HPV, especially in the setting of low alveolar P_{O_2}.[63] Isoflurane reduces cardiac output and therefore mixed venous oxygen tension, resulting in HPV stimulation; this might negate the direct HPV-inhibiting effect of the agent.[64]

In vitro studies of enflurane's effect on HPV have revealed a dose-related HPV depression of 60 to 100 percent.[51, 52, 65] Nitrous oxide seems to cause a more modest HPV inhibition of 10 to 40 percent in the intact in vivo dog model.[48, 58, 66]

Therefore, although the inhalation agents seem to inhibit HPV to a variable and often dose-related degree, the effect in vivo appears to be diminished by other hemodynamic effects that stimulate HPV. Because of their multiple advantages and in spite of this potential disadvantage, the inhalation agents remain the agents of choice during thoracic surgery in childhood.

One-Lung Anesthesia

One-lung anesthesia with double-lumen ETTs is widely practiced in adult patients to (1) prevent spread of blood or purulent secretions into the trachea and dependent lung, (2) ventilate only the uninvolved lung in the presence of a large bronchopleural cutaneous fistula, (3) perform unilateral bronchopulmonary lavage for pulmonary alveolar proteinosis, and (4) improve surgical exposure during an intrathoracic procedure, including video-assisted thoracoscopic surgery.[67] A complete discussion of the use of double-lumen ETTs is available elsewhere.[68]

The indications for single-lung ventilation in children do not differ from those in adults. Video-assisted thoracoscopic surgery is increasing in frequency in most pediatric centers and is discussed elsewhere in this chapter. As shown in Table 17–3, the smallest double-lumen tube, 28-Fr, has an outside diameter of 9.8 mm, comparable to a 7.0 mm ETT; this tube can generally not be used in children younger than 8 to 9 years of age. However, lung separation can still be achieved with alternative techniques, described below.

Selective Endobronchial Intubation

An endotracheal tube can be advanced blindly into either bronchus. The right side is favored because of the angles of the main-stem bronchi and because of the left-facing bevel of the tube.[69] Intubation of the left main-stem bronchus can be achieved by turning the bevel of the ETT to the right. This enables the tip of the tube to advance down the left side of the trachea into the left main-stem

TABLE 17 – 3
INNER AND OUTER DIAMETER OF STANDARD DOUBLE-LUMEN ENDOBRONCHIAL TUBES AND THE UNIVENT TUBE

	Inner Diameter (mm)	Outer Diameter (mm)
Double-lumen tube*		
28 Fr	4.5	9.8
35 Fr	6.0	12.1
37 Fr	6.5	13.2
Univent Tube†		
3.5 mm	3.5	7.5
4.5 mm	4.5	8.5
6.0 mm	6.0	10.0
6.5 mm	6.5	10.5
7.0 mm	7.0	11.0

* Sheridan Catheter Corporation, Argyle, NY.
† Fuji Systems Corporation, Tokyo, Japan.

TABLE 17 – 4
BRONCHOSCOPE SPECIFICATIONS WITH ETT AND DOUBLE-LINE EBT COMPATIBILITIES*

Model #	OD mm	Smallest ETT (ID mm)	Smallest EBT
LF-P	2.2	2.5	—
BF-3C30	3.6	4.5	28 Fr
LF-2	4.0	5.0	35 Fr
BF-P20D	5.0	6.0	35 Fr

ETT, endotracheal tube; EBT, endobronchial tube; OD, outside diameter; ID, inside diameter.
* Olympus, Surgical Endoscopy Division, Tokyo, Japan.

bronchus.[69] Correct endobronchial tube position can also be accomplished or confirmed using the flexible fiberoptic bronchoscope.[70] A variety of bronchoscopes are available that permit use of endotracheal tubes as small as 2.5 mm inside diameter (ID) (see Table 17–4). Direct guidance by the surgeon is also possible when the carina is exposed during surgery.

Bronchial Blockade

Lung separation can also be achieved with an ETT and a bronchial blocker, usually a Fogarty embolectomy catheter. Bronchial blockade has been described in children using a 4- (for 2 years and under) or 5-Fr (for over 2 years) Fogarty catheter,[71] a Foley catheter, or a balloon-tipped wedge pressure catheter.[72] The trachea is intubated with an ETT appropriate for the age and size of the patient. The Fogarty catheter is passed alongside the ETT and an appropriately sized (Table 17–4) fiberoptic bronchoscope is passed through a self-sealing diaphragm in the elbow connector to the end of the ETT (Fig. 17–8). The Fogarty catheter is visualized and manipulated into the desired bronchus under direct vision. Proper placement of the bronchial blocker is confirmed by fiberoptic bronchoscopic examination and by loss of breath sounds over the ipsilateral chest when the blocker is inflated. Using a catheter with an end hole allows the lung to deflate, and also allows suctioning or the delivery of continuous positive airway pressure (CPAP) or oxygen as desired.

The Univent tube (Fuji Systems Corporation, Tokyo, Japan) is an alternative to balloon-tipped catheters for bronchial blockade.[73] This device is a conventional ETT with an additional smaller lumen that contains a movable blocker tube with an inflatable balloon at the distal tip (Fig. 17–9). A range of sizes is now available, including a 3.5-mm tube, which has an outer diameter equivalent to a 5.5-mm-ID tube (7.5 to 8.0 mm) (Table 17–3).

Alternatively, the Fogarty catheter can be placed under direct vision with a rigid bronchoscope.[71, 74] Blind passage of the catheter[75] and passage under fluoroscopic guidance[76] have also been described; neither of these latter techniques offers the same degree of control as placement with fiberoptic or rigid bronchoscopy.

The blocker is taped securely to prevent dislodgment. Care must be taken to ensure that the bronchial blocker is not pulled back into the main-stem trachea, which would risk tracheal obstruction or contamination of the

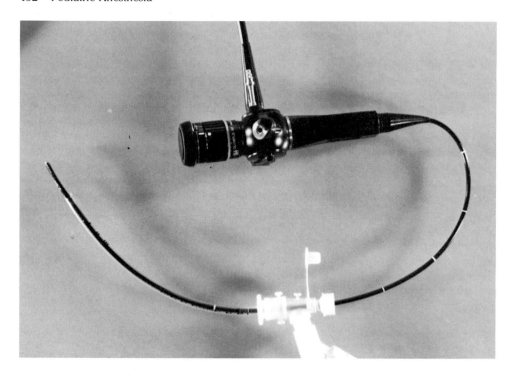

FIGURE 17–8. A 3.7-mm fiberoptic bronchoscope (Olympus BF3C) can be used to guide endotracheal or endobronchial intubation with tubes of 4.5 mm or greater (ID). A self-sealing adaptor (Portex 625207, Wilmington, MA) allows continuous ventilation through an anesthesia circuit.

dependent lung. Continuous monitoring of compliance and breath sounds is mandatory when bronchial blockade is employed.

During one-lung ventilation, any blood that flows through the nonventilated, nondependent lung contributes to a right-to-left transpulmonary shunt and decreased Pao_2. The amount of perfusion to the atelectatic lung is influenced by the degree of surgical compression and by the integrity of HPV. HPV, in turn, is influenced by a number of factors (Table 17–5), many of which are under direct control of the anesthesiologist. Hypocapnia is avoided, since HPV may be inhibited.[77] The use of excessive airway pressures may increase pulmonary vascular resistance in the dependent lung and increase flow through the nondependent lung.[78, 79] Therefore, a tidal volume (10 to 12 ml/kg) and respiratory rate are selected to produce normocapnia at the lowest possible airway pressures. CO_2 elimination is usually not a problem in one-

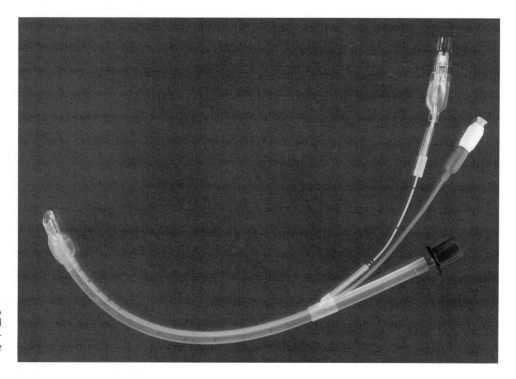

FIGURE 17–9. The Univent Tube: A conventional ETT with an additional smaller lumen that contains a movable blocker tube with an inflatable balloon at the distal tip.

T A B L E   1 7 – 5
FACTORS THAT INFLUENCE HYPOXIC PULMONARY VASOCONSTRICTION

Factor	Effect on HPV (Inhibition ↓; Stimulation ↑; → No Effect)	Mechanism
Increased pulmonary artery pressure		Elevated pulmonary artery pressure overcomes
Volume overload[79]	↓	vasoconstriction
PEEP/increased airway pressure[78, 79, 359]	↓	Increased alveolar pressure compresses intra-alveolar vessels, raising pulmonary vascular resistance and pressure
Vasoconstrictive drugs	↓	Direct vasoconstrictive effect
Decreased pulmonary artery pressure	↓	Conversion of ventilated lung to zone 1, thereby compressing intra-alveolar vessels and redirecting flow to hypoxic lung
Hypocapnia[77]	↓	Direct effect (may be accentuated by increased airway pressures)
Hypercapnia[77]	↑	Direct effect
Vasodilator drugs		
Nitroglycerin[360]	↓	Direct effect
Nitroprusside	↓	Direct effect
Calcium antagonist[361, 362]	↓	Direct effect
β_2-Agonists[363]	↓	Direct effect
Hydralazine	→	
Anesthetic agents (see previous section)		
Hypothermia[364]	↓	Direct effect
Hyperthermia[364]	↑	Direct effect
Increasing FiO_2[80, 81, 365]	↓	Direct effect vs. reabsorption atelectasis in low $\dot{V}/\dot{Q}$ areas
Atelectasis[366–368]	↑	Alveolar hypoxia[366]; some mechanical effect on blood vessels[368]
Elevated Pv_{O_2}[369]	↓	Back-diffusion of O_2 into alveolar or interstitial spaces
Decreased Pv_{O_2}[370]	↓	Decrease in alveolar O_2 tension produces vasoconstriction in normoxic lung

HPV, hypoxic pulmonary vasoconstriction; PEEP, positive end-expiratory pressure.

lung anesthesia, since overventilated alveoli can eliminate an excessive amount of CO_2. The selection of anesthetic agents has been previously discussed. A high inspired oxygen concentration is used; in most instances, the potential benefits of high FiO_2 (increased alveolar oxygen tension, vasodilation in the dependent lung) outweigh the potential disadvantage of absorption atelectasis caused by high inspired oxygen concentration to low $\dot{V}/\dot{Q}$ areas in the dependent lung.[80, 81] Continuous monitoring of hemoglobin saturation with pulse oximetry is mandatory during one-lung anesthesia, supplemented with arterial blood gas analysis. If hypoxia is present in spite of the above measures, 2- to 3-cm H_2O increments of PEEP can be applied to the dependent lung, keeping in mind the potential hazards as well as the benefits of this therapy. If hypoxia persists, the pulmonary artery of the diseased lung is clamped as soon as possible to decrease venous admixture.

Postoperative Management

The decision whether to extubate the trachea at the conclusion of the procedure is based on the nature of the patient's underlying condition, the extent of the surgery, the integrity of gas exchange, and the expected postoperative course. Before extubation, the patient must be awake, able to cough and maintain an adequate airway, and able to sustain adequate oxygenation and ventilation in 50

percent oxygen or less. If this is not possible, the trachea should be left intubated and the patient should be transferred to intensive care for further management (see Chapter 29).

Regional Techniques

Although regional anesthesia is the subject of another chapter, several regional techniques deserve emphasis in a discussion of anesthesia for thoracic surgery. Regional techniques may confer specific advantages during and after thoracic surgery compared with use of systemic agents. Adult patients receiving regional techniques have improved postoperative pulmonary function compared with patients receiving general anesthesia.[82] In Ballantyne's meta-analysis, the use of epidural opioids decreased the incidence of atelectasis and pulmonary infections compared with systemic opioids. The use of epidural local anesthetics was associated with a decreased incidence of pulmonary infections and overall pulmonary complications, compared with systemic opioids. Earlier ambulation and shortened convalescent times have been demonstrated in adults receiving epidural analgesia compared with those receiving systemic morphine.[83] Intercostal nerve blocks may improve pulmonary outcome measures, including the incidence of atelectasis and overall pulmonary complications.[82] In adults, significant improvements following intercostal blocks have been shown in Pa_{O_2},

Pa_{CO_2}, vital capacity, forced expiratory flow rates, and patient comfort.[84, 85] However, not all authors have demonstrated beneficial effects.[86] Using small amounts of bupivacaine 0.25 to 0.5 percent, dermatome-level analgesia can be achieved that lasts 4 to 8 hours. The most common complication is pneumothorax, though Moore reported an incidence of only 0.073 percent in over 10,000 cases.[87] Because the intercostal space is highly vascular, rapid rates of anesthetic absorption are seen, with the associated risk of local anesthetic toxicity.[88, 89] The block may need to be repeated after several hours, which may not be possible on a child that is not heavily sedated or anesthetized. The duration of the block can be extended to over 30 hours with the addition of low-molecular-weight dextran.[84] Placement of a catheter in the intercostal space by the surgeon prior to closure of the incision allows a constant infusion of local anesthetic in the postoperative period.[90] This technique has not been subjected to controlled trials; in addition, serum levels of local anesthetic have not been assessed.

Intrapleural analgesia (IPA) involves injection of local anesthetics through a catheter into the intrapleural space, usually placed under direct vision by the surgeon.[91] Applications of this technique have been reported for coarctation repair and anterior spinal fusion,[92] pectus excavatum repair, multiple trauma,[93] and nonthoracic procedures, such as Nissen fundoplication or splenectomy.[94] It has even been used in newborns after tracheoesophageal fistula repair.[95] The technique tends to be more efficacious in younger patients; patients older than 10 years often require supplemental analgesics.[96]

Intrapleural catheters are easy to place and have few associated risks; unlike epidural catheters, intrapleural catheters are not contraindicated in the presence of coagulation defects. A limited amount of sympathectomy is produced, given the unilateral nature of the block. On the other hand, high plasma levels of local anesthetic may occur, particularly in the presence of an inflammatory response. In adults, a continuous infusion of extrapleural bupivicaine resulted in a steady increase in total serum bupivicaine concentration, with no elevation in free serum bupivicaine.[97] Seizures have been reported after IPA.[98] One study of intrapleural bupivicaine for postthoracotomy patients as young as 6 months utilized an initial loading dose of 0.625 mg/kg followed by a continuous infusion starting at 1.25 mg/kg/h, and reduced to 0.75 mg/kg/h.[99] Although toxicity was not reported, serum levels of bupivicaine were not reported. Maximum rates of 0.4 mg/kg/h for older children and 0.2 mg/h for neonates have been recommended to avoid toxicity.[100] Some authors have reported inadequate analgesia using intrapleural techniques.[101, 102] Other possible complications include injury to the intercostal vasculature, catheter breakage, infection, and phrenic nerve blockade.

Epidural analgesia can provide effective postoperative pain control after thoracic surgery. Low doses of local anesthetics can be used, with less risk of local anesthetic toxicity compared with intercostal blocks or IPA. Placement near the dermatomal levels in question allows the safest and most effective application of local anesthetics. Thoracic catheter placement can be achieved via the caudal space with cephalad threading of a styleted catheter.[103, 104] If a lumbar or caudal epidural is the only option, thoracic analgesia can be effective with the use of hydrophilic opiate preparations, such as morphine.[105–107]

Although placement of epidural catheters is associated with a risk of neurologic injury, the risk is low in experienced hands.[108–110] Placement of epidural catheters is contraindicated in the presence of coagulopathy, because of the risk of epidural hematoma. Some authors consider placement of epidural catheters safe for patients undergoing cardiopulmonary bypass if the catheter placement is uncomplicated and completed at least 1 hour prior to anticoagulation.[111, 112]

ANESTHESIA FOR SPECIFIC LESIONS

Congenital Diaphragmatic Hernia

Congenital diaphragmatic hernias (CDHs) occur in approximately 1 in 5, 000 births. Although the clinical presentation and pathology were first described in 1804, operative repair was considered impossible until 1940, when Ladd and Gross[113] published the first large series with long-term survivors. Despite improvements in diagnosis and clinical management of these patients, mortality remains high as a result of lung hypoplasia and associated defects.

Classification

CDHs are classified by the site of the diaphragmatic herniation (Fig. 17–10). Eighty percent are posterolateral defects (Bochdalek), with left-sided lesions occurring five times more often than right-sided lesions. The Bochdalek hernias are the largest and are associated with the greatest degree of pulmonary hypoplasia. Two percent of hernias occur at the anterior foramen of Morgagni and are relatively small. The remainder are herniations through the esophageal hiatus.

Included in the differential diagnosis of CDH is eventration of the diaphragm, which results from a lack of development of the muscular component of the diaphragm, leaving only a compliant pleuroperitoneal membrane. Clinical presentations of eventration vary from asymptomatic to profound respiratory compromise.

Embryology

Two alternate primary defects causing CDH have been proposed: (1) abnormal lung growth with secondary abnormal diaphragmatic development or (2) a primary diaphragm defect with secondary pulmonary hypoplasia resulting from compression by eviscerated bowel.[114, 115] The predominance of left-sided Bochdalek hernias is supported by the latter hypothesis. A common pleuroperitoneal cavity exists during the first month of fetal life. Between 4 and 9 weeks' gestation the pleuroperitoneal membrane forms, creating separate pleural and peritoneal cavities. The posterolateral section is the last portion of this membrane to form, with the left side closing after the right. The developing gut returns from the yolk sac to the peritoneum at 9 weeks' gestation: if the gut returns before pleuroperitoneal closure is complete, the stomach, spleen, liver, and the small and large bowel can migrate into the chest cavity.

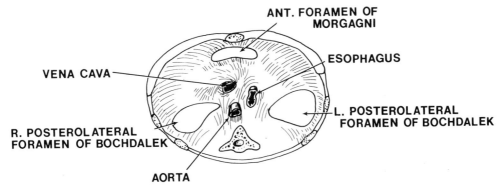

FIGURE 17–10. Inferior surface of the diaphragm, showing potential sites of herniation of abdominal contents with congenital diaphragmatic hernia.

Anatomic Defects of the Lung

Abdominal contents that migrate into the chest become a space-occupying mass that affects the normal development of the lung. The degree of lung abnormality is determined both by the time of the migration and the amount of abdominal contents in the chest. Although the ipsilateral lung is the most profoundly affected, both lungs are abnormal. In severe cases (early migration of large-volume abdominal contents), both lungs are usually small, and bronchial and bronchiolar development arrest occurs at 11 to 13 weeks' gestation.[116] The total number of airway generations can be decreased by 50 percent. Alveolar maturation continues around the existing airways, but with fewer airways there are fewer alveoli.[117]

The pulmonary artery is diminished in size, usually in proportion to the size of the lung. Arterial branching is also decreased. Infants who have a CDH have a normal ratio of alveoli to capillaries, but because of the decreased number of alveoli the total vascular cross-sectional area is decreased.[118, 119] This can contribute to pulmonary hypertension. In addition, the existing arteries may have precocious distal growth of smooth muscle, which also contributes to pulmonary hypertension.[120, 121]

Pathophysiology

The primary cause of death in CDH is progressive hypoxemia and acidosis. Although the causes of hypoxia and acidosis are multifactorial, elevated PVR and PPHN are the final common pathway. The increased PVR in CDH patients results from pulmonary hypoplasia (decreased vascular cross-sectional area), the presence of inappropriately muscularized pulmonary arteries, and/or from active vasoconstriction of normal pulmonary arteries.[120, 121] Therefore, pulmonary hypertension in the CDH infant is caused by a combination of irreversible (hypoplasia, dysplastic arteries) and reversible (constriction of relatively normal arteries) factors. It would be helpful to differentiate how much of the hypertension was caused by reversible factors, but at present there are no clinical parameters that adequately address this question.

The effect of lung compression (by intrathoracic abdominal contents on respiratory function) is controversial. Most clinicians agree that the herniated contents do not cause respiratory failure unless there is massive gaseous distention of the stomach and intestine.[122] It must also be

noted that pneumothorax is a common and significant complication of mechanical ventilation in the hypoplastic lung. Pneumothorax is most clinically significant when it occurs on the contralateral side.[123]

Clinical Presentation and Diagnosis

The diagnosis of CDH can be made either pre- or postnatally. Prenatal diagnosis is made with ultrasonography. Findings correlated with poor prognosis include the presence of polyhydramnios, stomach placement above the diaphragm, and diagnosis made before 20 weeks' gestation. The increase in the use of routine ultrasound has made the prenatal diagnosis of CDH a common event.[124, 125]

This diagnosis should be considered in any child who presents with respiratory compromise during the immediate postnatal period. These children usually have a scaphoid abdomen with a barrel-shaped chest, reflecting the presence of abdominal contents in the thorax. Because the mediastinum is shifted into the contralateral chest, the cardiac sounds and impulse are also shifted. The presence of bowel sounds in the chest is an uncommon finding.

A chest radiograph usually shows intestinal loops and possibly stomach, spleen, or liver in the thorax (Fig. 17–11). The ipsilateral lung is usually compressed into the mediastinum, which, in turn, is shifted into the contralateral hemithorax.

Timing of the clinical diagnosis often correlates with prognosis, because the time of onset of symptoms reflects the degree of lung hypoplasia, the size of the defect, and the effective size of the space-occupying mass. Children who present with respiratory failure in the first 6 hours of life are considered at high risk; those who present in the first hour of life have the highest mortality. Children who are diagnosed later than 6 hours of life enjoy excellent outcomes.[126, 127] CDH can present in adolescents and adults; these cases generally have small defects and relatively normal lungs.

Initial Care

The presence and severity of associated congenital anomalies should be determined, since some of these may influence outcome[128] (Table 17–6). The philosophy of initial care for the CDH patient has changed. In the past, the hernia was repaired as an emergency, in the belief that the herniated contents caused lung collapse and respiratory

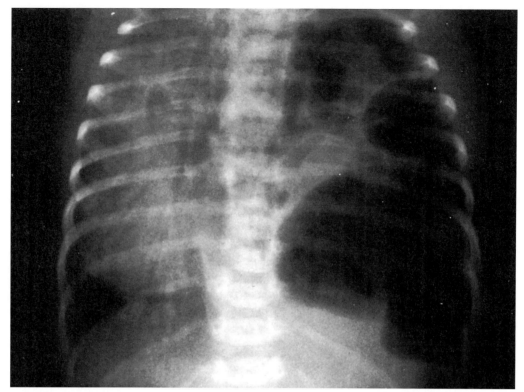

FIGURE 17–11. Preoperative chest radiograph of child with left-sided congenital diaphragmatic hernia, showing intestinal loops in the left hemithorax, compression of the left lung, and shift of the mediastinal contents to the right.

failure. As a result, many patients were rushed to the operating room without taking time for medical stabilization.[129] Now, it is common to delay surgery and concentrate on medical stabilization. This new approach reflects the belief that lung compression is not the primary problem. In addition, surgery does not cure the respiratory failure, and may worsen respiratory mechanics.[130] The goal is to schedule semielective surgery when the neonate is medically stable. The optimal length of delay is unknown; delays of hours to many days are being evaluated.[122, 131] Improved survival has been reported during an era of delayed surgery with or without extracorporeal membrane oxygenation (ECMO) support compared with historical control data.[132]

T A B L E 1 7 – 6
CONGENITAL ANOMALIES ASSOCIATED WITH CONGENITAL DIAPHRAGMATIC HERNIA

Anomaly	Incidence in Newborns with CDH (%)
Central nervous system (spina bifida, hydrocephalus, anencephaly)	28
Gastrointestinal (malrotation, atresia)	20
Genitourinary (hypospadius)	15
Cardiovascular (ASD, VSD, coarctation, tetralogy of Fallot)	23[128]

CDH, congenital diaphragmatic hernia; ASD, atrial septal defect; VSD, ventricular septal defect.
From David TJ, Illingworth CA: Diaphragmatic hernia in the southwest of England. J Med Genet 13:253, 1976, with permission.

Initial care is determined by the child's degree of illness. Physiologic perturbations known to precipitate PPHN are avoided. Efforts should be made to maintain normoxia, normo- or hypocarbia, and a normal or high pH. In minimally affected children this may require only an isolette with increased ambient oxygen. In the more compromised child, endotracheal intubation, sedation, paralysis, positive-pressure ventilation (PPV), and even ECMO may be required.[133–135]

It is also important to avoid gaseous distention of the stomach and intestine; therefore, early placement of a nasogastric tube is mandatory. In addition, any ventilatory assistance that may cause gastric distention should be avoided, such as nasal CPAP or prolonged mask ventilation.

If PPHN is a problem, a number of strategies can be used to improve pulmonary blood flow by causing active pulmonary vasodilation. Hyperoxia and alkalosis with hypocarbia are used, although elevated inspired oxygen concentrations and airway pressure may cause secondary lung damage.[130]

The most consistently successful therapeutic modality is the alkalosis achieved with hyperventilation.[137, 138] Often, a threshold effect is observed, such that PaO_2 does not rise until pH reaches 7.55 to 7.6.[138]

A number of pharmacologic pulmonary vasodilators have been tried, including morphine,[139] prednisolone,[139] chlorpromazine,[139] tolazoline,[138–140, 142] bradykinin, acetylcholine,[141] and prostaglandin E[143] and D_2.[144] Inhaled nitric oxide (NO), an EDRF, may provide selective pulmonary vasodilation in some patients. Clinical studies are limited but have shown excellent improvement in oxygenation in neonates with persistent pulmonary hypertension exposed to 20 to 80 ppm NO.[145, 146] Inhaled NO is unique in that it is a selective pulmonary vasodilator; it is inactivated immediately on exposure to hemoglobin and therefore has no effect on systemic circulation.[147]

Another important aspect of care is attention to the systemic circulation and myocardial function. Systemic hypotension and hypoxia may result in cardiac failure. Close monitoring of intravascular volume and the need for inotropes and vasoactive drugs is mandatory.

All infants with CDH and respiratory distress require invasive monitoring. Peripheral venous access is best done in the upper extremities because reduction of the hernia may increase intra-abdominal pressure and partially obstruct the inferior vena cava. Central venous access should be attempted via the umbilical or femoral vein. Neck veins should be avoided in case ECMO is required. Cannulation of the right radial artery is preferable so that preductal blood can be sampled. In severely compromised children, both pre- and postductal catheters are placed. Pre- and postductal oximetry (above and below the nipple line) is routine in these patients.

Intraoperative Care

Positioning of the patient is at the discretion of the surgeon, although the supine position is usually chosen, with the affected side slightly elevated. Most surgeons prefer a transabdominal approach, since this facilitates both correction of intestinal malrotation and return of the abdominal organs to the peritoneal cavity. Small defects are closed primarily by suturing together the existing diaphragmatic tissue. If little or no tissue is present, an artificial diaphragm is constructed. These are akinetic membranes that will not participate in the mechanics of gas movement, an issue that may later become a problem during weaning from mechanical ventilation. In most cases, the abdominal cavity is closed primarily, but if the abdomen is too small to accommodate the returned contents, a Silastic pouch is created to house the abdominal contents without excessive increase in the intra-abdominal pressure.[148]

Mechanical ventilation during surgery should maintain normoxia or hyperoxia and normo- or hypocarbia, using minimal airway pressure (<20 to 30 cm H_2O) and relatively rapid rates (60 to 120 breaths/min). The use of a ventilator from the intensive care unit (ICU) should be considered if these settings cannot be achieved with the operating room ventilator. Pulmonary mechanics change during surgery; compliance may actually decrease.[149] Therefore, hand ventilation with close attention to the progress of the surgery is mandatory. Any sudden deterioration in lung compliance or in oxygenation or blood pressure suggests a pneumothorax. The equipment necessary for chest tube insertion should be immediately available. Some authors have recommended the prophylactic insertion of a contralateral chest tube before surgery.[123, 149]

To avoid any triggers for the development of pulmonary vasoconstriction, Pa_{O_2} above 80 mm Hg, Pa_{CO_2} of 25 to 30 mm Hg, and a normal or elevated pH are maintained. Continuous monitoring of pre- and postductal oxygen saturations allows early recognition of right-to-left shunting. Arterial blood gases should be monitored frequently. Any metabolic acidosis should be appropriately treated with an infusion of sodium bicarbonate. Blood loss during the procedure is usually minor, but any significant loss should be replaced.

Hypothermia is known to increase oxygen consumption, which may exacerbate systemic desaturation. The room temperature is maintained at 80°F. A warming blanket, radiant warmer, blood warmer, and humidifier are employed.

The choice of anesthetic agent depends on the cardiovascular stability of the child. Inhaled halogenated anesthetics, even in low concentration, may cause significant hypotension. Opioids such as fentanyl or sufentanil are usually well tolerated. In either case, muscle relaxants are useful adjuncts. Nitrous oxide should be avoided because it may distend gas-filled intestinal loops. Preoperatively, this could increase respiratory compromise; intraoperatively, it could make abdominal closure more difficult.

At the conclusion of surgery, the child is carefully returned to the ICU for continued monitoring and care.

Postoperative Care

Once the infant's condition has been stabilized in the ICU, the need for continued respiratory assistance must be assessed. Factors involved in this assessment include the preoperative status of the baby, the size of the defect in the diaphragm, the tension of the abdominal wall, the presence of associated congenital defects, and the degree of pulmonary hypoplasia, as judged by the alveolar–arterial oxygen gradient ([A–a]D_{O_2}).[126, 150] In infants with mild pulmonary disease, controlled ventilation is continued for 2 to 12 hours.

Infants with severe lung disease ([A–a]D_{O_2} > 400 mm Hg) and those who demonstrate cardiopulmonary deterioration at any time during the postoperative period require continued mechanical ventilation. Persistent hypoxemia while on high F_{IO_2} suggests PPHN with right-to-left shunting of desaturated blood at preductal or ductal levels. Hypoxemia can be triggered by minimal changes in inspired oxygen concentration or by hypoxemia, acidosis, or sudden changes in pulmonary blood volume. Metabolic acidosis is treated with intravascular volume expansion (when appropriate) and infusion of sodium bicarbonate. Endotracheal suctioning is minimized to avoid even transient changes in F_{IO_2} or Pa_{O_2}. Hyperventilation is induced to achieve and maintain a respiratory alkalosis. A variety of pulmonary vasodilators have been tried, as previously mentioned, although none other than NO offers the promise of a more selective effect.

Delivery of adequate nutrition is an integral part of the postoperative care of these infants. If enteral feedings are not possible after the first postoperative week, IV alimentation is begun with high-concentration glucose, amino acids, lipids, trace minerals, and vitamins. If IV alimentation is necessary only for a few days, peripheral intravenous alimentation may be sufficient. For longer periods, central venous alimentation is indicated.

Extracorporeal Membrane Oxygenation

Infants who have severe pulmonary hypertension, hypoxemia, and/or hypercarbia, despite maximal conventional management, are routinely offered ECMO.[151] ECMO has been used to support infants with PPHN since the mid-1980s. The survival by specific entry diagnosis varies widely: infants with meconium aspiration have a survival of 92 percent, whereas infants with CDH have a survival of only 60 percent.[152]

ECMO, a form of partial cardiopulmonary bypass, is usually venoarterial (VA) (Fig. 17–12). In VA ECMO, a large cannula (12- to 14-Fr) is placed in the right jugular vein. Blood is allowed to passively flow by gravity into the ECMO circuit, where it is pumped with an occlusive blood pump into the membrane oxygenator, where oxygen is added and CO_2 is eliminated. From the oxygenator, blood passes through a heat exchanger and is returned to the child via a catheter placed through the right common carotid artery into the ascending aorta. In VA bypass, the ECMO circuit assumes not only the function of the lungs but also a portion of the function of the heart. In venovenous (VV) ECMO, blood is both removed from and returned to the venous system. Most VV ECMO is performed through a double-lumen catheter placed in the right atrium via the right internal jugular vein. This catheter allows continuous drainage via the proximal port and return through the distal port. VV ECMO is effective if myocardial function is normal, but in many of these neonates it is not normal. In both VA and VV ECMO, the priming volume of the circuit is 500 to 600 ml. During ECMO, the patient and the circuit are heparinized to an activated clotting time (ACT) of 200 to 240 seconds. A pump flow of approximately 100 ml/kg/min is required to maintain adequate gas exchange. During VA ECMO, the child's lungs are ventilated with minimal settings (room air, respirator rate of 4 to 20 breaths/min), and peak inspiratory pressures of 20 cm H_2O. Because VV ECMO is less efficient than VA ECMO for supporting gas exchange, more aggressive ventilator support is required.[153, 154]

Regardless of which type of ECMO is employed, it is important to recognize that ECMO does not cure lung disease but merely supports the child long enough for the pulmonary problem to resolve, either spontaneously or in response to other therapy. The duration of ECMO support for infants with CDH averages 7 to 10 days.[154]

A number of risks and potential morbidity are associated with ECMO. Bleeding is the biggest problem; factors that predispose to this complication include the use of heparin and the consumption and inactivation of platelets in the circuit. Although bleeding can occur anywhere, central nervous system (CNS) hemorrhage is the most worrisome. The risk of CNS bleeding is increased by the disruption of normal intracranial blood flow by placement of cannulae in the central venous and arterial system, embolization of particulate matter or gas, and the propensity of neonates to develop intracranial hemorrhage.[155, 156] Long-term follow-up of ECMO survivors has been encouraging, with many children enjoying normal physical and mental development. However, 5 to 15 percent of children supported with ECMO reportedly have evidence of intracranial pathology, ranging from minor to severe handicaps.[157, 158]

The limits and complications of ECMO strongly influence the inclusion and exclusion criteria for the selection

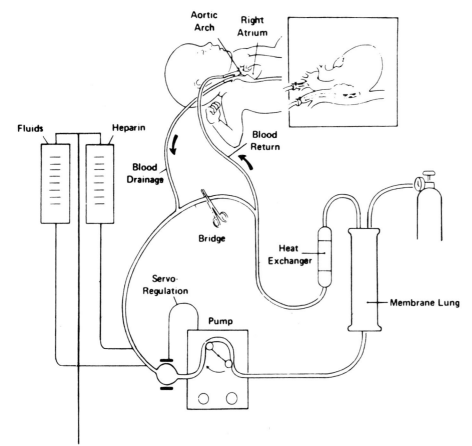

FIGURE 17–12. The ECMO circuit employs gravity venous drainage to a servo-regulated pump, a heat exchanger, and an oxygenator. (From Bartlett RH, Roloff DW, Cornell RG, et al: Extracorporeal circulation in neonatal respiratory failure: a prospective randomized study. Pediatrics 76:479, 1985, with permission.)

of ECMO candidates. The entry criteria include a gestational age of 34 weeks or greater, the presence of a reversible disease process, a minimal weight (usually 2 kg), and a predicted mortality of at least 80 percent. Exclusion criteria include the presence of a grade II or greater intracranial hemorrhage or the presence of another life-threatening congenital anomaly.[151]

The most difficult criterion to define is predicated mortality; most ECMO centers use some measurement of oxygenation to predict mortality. The oxygenation index (OI) is the most common of these:

$$OI = F_{IO_2} \times \frac{\text{Mean airway pressure} \times 100}{Pa_{O_2}}$$

Values in excess of 40 to 50 are thought to identify infants with a predicted mortality greater than 80 percent.[151]

Whereas ECMO is presently considered the standard of care for neonates with PPHN, the child with CDH must be considered separately. The most important entry criterion for ECMO support is the presence of reversible disease, and CDH includes both reversible and irreversible components. Because there are no clinical markers to adequately differentiate the relative effect of irreversible factors, ECMO is frequently offered to all CDH infants who fail conventional support. Hence, a number of infants are placed on ECMO without known reversible disease. This probably explains why infants with CDH have a lower survival rate than other infants with PPHN after ECMO support and why some infants require prolonged mechanical ventilation after ECMO.

ECMO support can be started either pre- or postoperatively. The anesthesiologist must have a working knowledge of ECMO to care for those patients who have surgery while on ECMO support.[159] In some institutions, the child is moved to the operating room for repair; this requires that the ECMO circuit have a battery pack. Even when all goes well, transport of the child on ECMO is time consuming and exposes the child to numerous risks. Some ECMO centers bring the necessary operating room equipment to the ICU and perform surgery at the bedside without moving the child. Hence, the anesthesiologist must be flexible regarding the site of the anesthetic.

Children on ECMO are lightly sedated and usually do not require muscle relaxants. For surgery, an opioid-relaxant technique is usually used. Because the lungs do not participate in significant gas exchange, the use of any inhalational drug is virtually impossible unless the inhaled anesthetic is added directly to the ECMO circuit. Drugs can be given directly to the child or through the ECMO circuit itself. The anesthesiologist must work in concert with the ECMO physicians, nurses, and technicians. Because the child on ECMO is heparinized, hemostasis is not normal. In an attempt to minimize intraoperative bleeding, the ACTs are kept at 180 to 200 seconds and the platelet count is maintained over 150,000/mm³.[134] The use of aminocaproic acid has been advocated to reduce hemorrhagic complications.[160]

ECMO support is continued until the native lungs can support gas exchange with minimal ventilator settings. Most institutions limit the duration of ECMO to 14 to 21 days, because the likelihood of successful weaning of the

child from ECMO after that time is negligible. The outcome of CDH infants after ECMO varies. Although some infants may be weaned from conventional mechanical support within a few days, others require prolonged weaning, which can last for months. Others cannot survive without ECMO and die as soon as bypass is discontinued.[161]

Mortality Rate

Mortality in infants with CDH is variously reported as 30 to 60 percent.[162] Reported mortality rates may be conservative, since aborted and stillborn fetuses are not reliably included in survey data and not all neonatal deaths are investigated by radiography or by autopsy. Factors that affect mortality are shown in Table 17–7. Inhaled NO has not been shown to decrease the need for ECMO or reduce the overall mortality rate.[163] The impact of ECMO on survival rate remains controversial. Survival is highest in children with adequate lung volumes in whom ECMO is not necessary.[164] For those patients sick enough to warrant ECMO, several centers have reported improved survival associated with the use of ECMO,[164, 165] though the incidence of neurologic sequelae may be increased.[166] Not all centers have seen improved survival.[167] Even centers reporting improved outcomes with the use of ECMO have overall mortality rates of 30 to 40 percent, suggesting that the problem is far from being solved.

Long-Term Follow-up

Pulmonary outcomes of children who survive CDH are usually good. A small percentage have intermittent episodes of wheezing.[168, 169] Chest radiographs are usually normal, with the exception of decreased vascular markings on the affected side. Likewise, lung scans show a consistent decrease in perfusion on the affected side. Measurements of lung volumes are generally normal, suggesting either that alveolar number has increased to the normal range postoperatively or that existing alveoli have enlarged to become emphysematous.[170] Studies of airway resistance have been conflicting, with some studies demonstrating normal values[169, 171] and others indicating minor degrees of airway obstruction during forced expiration.[168, 172]

TABLE 17–7
FACTORS AFFECTING MORTALITY FROM CDH

Pulmonary hypoplasia
Associated malformations
  CNS
  Cardiovascular

Inadequate preoperative management
  Hypothermia
  Acidosis
  Shock
  Tension pneumothorax

Ineffective postoperative care
  Tension pneumothorax

Hemorrhage
  Excessive suction on chest tube
  Inferior vena cava compression
  Persistent fetal circulation (PFC)

Long-term neurologic complications have been reported. One study has reported a 10 percent incidence of developmental delay, presumably secondary to hypoxia during the neonatal period.[171] Children who received ECMO as part of their early management appear to be at increased risk for developmental delays.[166]

Esophageal Atresia and Tracheoesophageal Fistula

History

The history of treatment of congenital esophageal atresia (EA) and tracheoesophageal fistula (TEF) illustrates the remarkable progress that has been made in pediatric anesthesia and surgery over the last four decades. Although EA with TEF was accurately described by Thomas Gibson in 1697, no infant with this lesion survived until 1939, when Dr. Logan Leven performed the first successful staged operative repair. The first primary repair of EA with TEF was reported in 1943. Since that time there have been progressive improvements in perioperative care, all of which have reduced mortality figures. Prematurity and severe associated congenital anomalies continue to contribute to mortality of TEF; in the absence of these factors, survival currently approaches 100 percent.[173, 174]

Incidence

The incidence of EA and TEF is 1 in 3,000 births,[175] with no particular preponderance of sex or race. Mean birth weight is low compared with that of the general population.[177] Risk of recurrence among siblings is approximately 0.5 percent.[176]

Embryology

Development of the respiratory system begins at 3 weeks of gestational age with the appearance of a diverticulum from the ventral wall of the foregut, which becomes separated from the foregut by the esophagotracheal septum. Thereafter, under normal circumstances, the developing trachea and lungs remain in contact with the gut only at the level of the laryngeal aditus. The normal laryngotracheal tube grows faster than the esophagus; if the separation of the esophagus and trachea is slightly delayed, the rapidly growing trachea separates the proximal and distal esophagus, resulting in the typical combination of EA and distal TEF.[177] In some cases, vascular anomalies, such as an anomalous right subclavian artery or a persistent right descending aorta, may cause localized pressure, accounting for the loss of esophageal continuity. However it occurs, TEF is the result of an error in separation of the trachea from the floor of the foregut in the fourth or fifth week of intrauterine life. The resulting defect is likely to be associated with anomalies of other body parts developing at about the same time.[178]

Classification

The most common classification of this anomaly is that of Gross,[179] who described types A through F (Fig. 17–13).[179] In 1976, Kluth[180] published 97 different anatomic types and subtypes of congenital esophageal anomalies. Hence, an anatomic description of the lesion is more appropriate than the use of letters and numbers. Esophageal atresia with distal fistula is by far the most common of these, occurring in 80 to 90 percent of cases. Seven to 9 percent have EA without TEF. The other types are less common.

Associated Anomalies

The incidence of other anomalies in infants with EA and TEF is 30 to 50 percent.[176] The incidence of associated anomalies by organ system is shown in Table 17–8. The cardiovascular anomalies seen, in approximate order of occurrence, are ventricular septal defect, patent ductus arteriosus, tetralogy of Fallot, atrial septal defect, and coarctation of the aorta.[176, 181] The musculoskeletal anomalies include vertebral malformation, radial aplasia, polydactyly, wrist anomalies, and knee malformations.[176] The associated gastrointestinal anomalies include imperforate anus, midgut malrotation, duodenal atresia, pyloric stenosis, Meckel's diverticulum, and ectopic or annular pancreas.[182] Genitourinary anomalies include renal lobulation or malposition, renal agenesis, hydronephrosis, ureteral abnormalities, and hypospadius.[182] The most common craniofacial abnormality is cleft lip and/or palate.

Particular combinations of anomalies have been described. The VATER association, first described in 1972,[178] consists of *v*ertebral defect, *a*nal defect, and *t*racheal

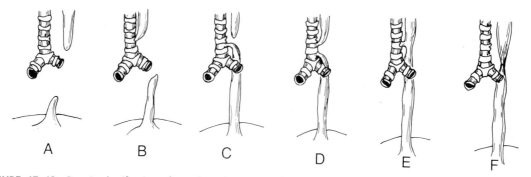

FIGURE 17–13. Gross's classification of esophageal atresia without fistula (*A*), esophageal atresia with proximal fistula (*B*), esophageal atresia with distal fistula (*C*), esophageal atresia with proximal and distal fistula (*D*), tracheoesophageal fistula without atresia (*E*), and esophageal stenosis (*F*).

TABLE 17 – 8
ANOMALIES ASSOCIATED WITH ESOPHAGEAL ATRESIA AND TRACHEOESOPHAGEAL FISTULA BY ORGAN SYSTEM

Anomaly	Incidence(%)
Cardiovascular	35
Musculoskeletal	30
Gastrointestinal	20
Genitourinary	10
Craniofacial	4

esophageal fistula with *e*sophageal atresia and *r*adial anomalies. The *v* can also indicate *v*entricular septal defect, whereas the *r* may indicate *r*enal anomalies.

Clinical Presentation

Atresia of the esophagus may be suspected before delivery if polyhydramnios is present. The diagnosis may be made at the time of delivery, when a tube cannot be passed into the infant's stomach, but is usually delayed until the first feeding, when coughing, choking, and cyanosis occur. In the presence of a fistula between the trachea and lower esophagus, the abdomen is tympanitic; occasionally, it becomes so distended that it interferes with the infant's breathing. The diagnosis is confirmed by passing a radiopaque catheter into the proximal esophageal segment. If the catheter passes into the stomach, atresia is obviously not present. If the catheter stops abruptly at a distance of 10 ± 1 cm from the gum line, the diagnosis is virtually ensured. Posteroanterior and lateral chest films are taken to determine the position of the tip of the esophagus (Fig. 17–14).

Although the injection of a small amount of contrast can outline the proximal esophageal segment and identify a proximal TEF, radiopaque material may be aspirated, resulting in respiratory problems that range in severity from a barium plug in a bronchus to chemical pneumonitis. An increased mortality from respiratory complications has been demonstrated in patients who have undergone contrast studies.[183]

Radiographic studies should include the entire abdomen, so that presence or absence of air in the stomach and intestines can be determined. When the upper esophagus is atretic, air in the stomach is pathognomonic of a fistula between trachea and lower esophagus. Absence of air in the gastrointestinal tract usually indicates the presence of EA without TEF.

TEF without atresia usually presents later in infancy but may not present until adolescence or adulthood. The signs and symptoms include choking during feedings, abdominal distention, and recurrent pneumonitis. The diagnosis is usually determined by bronchoscopy or contrast studies, although the lesion may be difficult to demonstrate and surgical exploration is sometimes necessary without prior demonstration of the fistula. The lesion has also been diagnosed by measuring elevated intragastric oxygen concentrations during ventilation with 100 percent oxygen.[184]

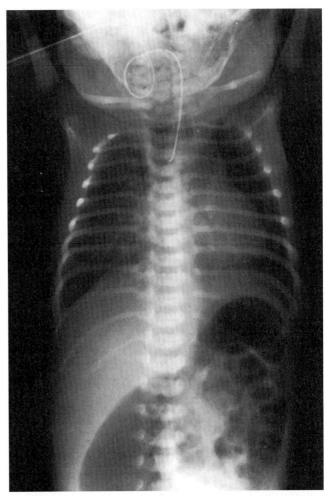

FIGURE 17–14. Preoperative chest radiograph of child with distal tracheoesophageal fistula. Proximal esophageal segment is dilated with air. The presence of intestinal air implies a distal tracheoesophageal fistula. Colonic dilation was caused by an associated anal atresia.

The diagnosis should be considered in any patient who develops gastric distention during tracheal intubation and PPV.

Preoperative Management

Pulmonary complications in the preoperative period contribute to infant morbidity and mortality; one of the primary goals of preoperative management is prevention of such complications until surgery can be performed. Oral feeds are discontinued and the baby is kept in a semi-upright position to minimize regurgitation of gastric juice through the fistula. The proximal esophageal segment is suctioned continuously to prevent aspiration of nasopharyngeal secretions.

Severity of pulmonary disease is evaluated with clinical examination, chest radiography, and arterial blood gases. Because repeated blood gas determinations are required before, during, and after surgery, an arterial catheter greatly facilitates care. Pneumonitis and atelectasis are common findings, particularly in the right upper lobe. Hypoxemia is treated with humidified oxygen and metabolic acidosis with sodium bicarbonate. In cases of refractory hypoxemia or respiratory failure, intubation of the trachea and mechanical ventilation may be necessary. Infants should be maintained in a thermally neutral environment (30° to 40°C), as hypothermia has been associated with a high mortality rate.[173]

For premature infants, associated IRDS, hypoglycemia, hypocalcemia, and hyperbilirubinemia must be evaluated and treated.[185] In infants with extreme prematurity or severe lung disease, a gastrostomy is performed under local anesthesia and the thoracotomy is postponed until respiratory function has improved.[186, 187] Templeton et al.[188] have argued that the presence of severe RDS with noncompliant lungs represents an indication for early thoracotomy and ligation of the fistula.

Associated anomalies also affect survival and should be looked for with chest and abdominal radiographs. Gas in the small bowel rules out duodenal atresia, and gas in the rectum may help in assessing coincidental anal atresia (Fig. 17–14). The heart and lungs are examined closely for evidence of congenital heart disease; an echocardiogram and/or cardiac catheterization may be indicated if a problem is suspected. Vertebral or other skeletal anomalies may be seen on chest or abdominal films. The abdomen is examined to screen for renal anomalies, and a urine collection bag is applied to document adequate urine output. If problems are suspected, abdominal ultrasound is indicated. Limb anomalies can be examined later, since they are not of vital importance.

Reliable venous access is established with a plastic catheter in a peripheral vein. Central venous cannulation is generally not necessary. Fluid and electrolyte status is evaluated and abnormalities are corrected, although fluid and electrolyte depletion is unusual with this lesion. Blood typing and crossmatch are performed for whole blood or packed red blood cells (RBCs).

Anesthetic Management

The operating room and anesthesia equipment are thoroughly prepared and the room is warmed to 27°C. Routine monitors include ECG, blood pressure cuff, temperature probe, and pulse oximeter. Special care is taken to place a precordial stethoscope securely in the left axilla, since this device is essential for detecting intraoperative airway obstruction.

Awake tracheal intubation can be performed, though this may be difficult and traumatic in a vigorous child. Alternatively, an inhalation or intravenous induction can be done. Some practitioners prefer to intubate the trachea without muscle relaxants, and allow the child to ventilate spontaneously. Others provide muscle relaxation prior to intubation.[189] The ETT is positioned to avoid gaseous distention of the stomach, a complication that can impede ventilatory efforts and venous return and may lead to cardiopulmonary arrest or gastric rupture.[190, 191] Because the fistula is usually located just proximal to the carina on the posterior aspect of the trachea (Fig. 17–15), the endotracheal tube is advanced gently into the right mainstem bronchus and then withdrawn slowly to a position just above the carina, where breath sounds can be heard equally on both sides.[192] Rotating the tube so that the bevel faces posteriorly may prevent intubation and ventilation

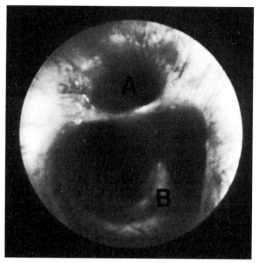

FIGURE 17–15. Endoscopic view of the main-stem bronchus in patient with esophageal atresia with distal fistula. The fistula (*A*) arises just above the level of the carina (*B*).

of the fistula itself. Observation of P_{ETCO_2} and oxygen saturation, as well as auscultation of the stomach and chest, are essential to achieve proper ETT placement. Some practitioners perform rigid[193] or fiberoptic[189] bronchoscopy routinely; this allows exact localization of the fistula and placement of the endotracheal tube distal to the fistula. If the fistula is large or located close to the carina, a Fogarty catheter can be placed and manipulated into the fistula under visual guidance for balloon occlusion. The ETT is taped securely to the face, well clear of the nasoesophageal tube, which often requires intraoperative manipulation to identify the proximal pouch for the surgeon.

Placement of a gastrostomy may only provide a low-pressure escape route for fresh gas under positive pressure (particularly in the presence of low lung compliance), thereby increasing flow through the fistula and decreasing pulmonary ventilation. Several strategies have been attempted under these circumstances. Filston et al.[194] described placement of a Fogarty balloon catheter through a bronchoscope into the fistula and inflating the balloon to occlude the fistula. Alternatively, Karl[195] described the insertion of the Fogarty catheter retrograde through the gastrostomy into the distal esophagus under fluoroscopic control for the same purpose. This technique may present lower risk than bronchoscopy in the child with noncompliant lungs.

After induction of anesthesia, the patient is turned to the left LDP for a right thoracotomy, ligation of the fistula, and primary esophageal anastomosis. If the patient has a right aortic arch, a left thoracotomy is necessary. Anesthesia is maintained with a nondepolarizing muscle relaxant and either inhaled or IV agents in amounts that do not cause significant cardiovascular depression. In premature infants at risk for retinopathy of prematurity, an F_{IO_2} that results in a Pa_{O_2} no higher than 90 to 100 mm Hg is selected.

Suction apparatus, gloves, and catheters should be available for sterile tracheal suctioning, because accumulation of secretions or blood can cause complete airway occlusion. Airway obstruction also may result from surgical manipulation of the trachea; the surgeon must be informed when this occurs. Occasionally, the ETT becomes occluded by a clot that cannot be removed by suctioning. This life-threatening situation necessitates immediate replacement of the tube, a difficult procedure given the position of the child.

Temperature is maintained with a warming mattress and with delivery of warmed humidified gases through the anesthesia circuit. Transfused blood should be warmed to approximately 37°C before administration.

IV fluids consisting of 5 percent dextrose and saline are administered to provide maintenance fluids (4 ml/kg/h), and intraoperatively estimated evaporative and third-space losses (6 to 8 ml/kg/h) are replaced with crystalloid. Blood lost in the suction bottle and in sponges is quantitated. Urine output, heart rate, blood pressure, serial hematocrits, and sodium and glucose concentrations are useful to follow the adequacy of fluid therapy and to determine the need for blood replacement.

Postoperative Care

The postoperative management of infants with EA and TEF is determined by the severity of pulmonary dysfunction, the presence of associated anomalies, and prematurity. In vigorous, otherwise healthy term infants, extubation can usually be accomplished postoperatively without difficulty. These infants are then placed in sufficient humidified oxygen to maintain a PaO_2 of 60 to 80 mm Hg. The most frequent complication in the early postoperative period is pneumonitis or atelectasis resulting from retained secretions in the tracheobronchial tree. Nasopharyngeal and oropharyngeal suctioning is done as needed, using a catheter that is marked to prevent insertion into the esophagus as far as the anastomosis. If atelectasis occurs, tracheal suction and manual hyperventilation are performed through an ETT, which is inserted for the procedure and then removed. Excessive neck extension is avoided because it puts the esophageal anastomosis under tension.

Infants who are likely to develop respiratory failure are returned to the ICU with an endotracheal tube in place. Respiration is supported with intermittent mandatory ventilation (IMV), supplemental oxygen, and PEEP. Manual percussion and vibration of the chest are often delayed until the third postoperative day to facilitate healing of the anastomosis. Weaning and discontinuation of ventilatory support can occur once the infant demonstrates adequate gas exchange and mechanics of breathing.

Tracheomalacia is commonly associated with the tracheoesophageal fistula and may result in life-threatening cyanotic and apneic spells during the postoperative period.[196] Tracheostomy may be necessary if the patient is unable to maintain a patent airway without an ETT. Tracheopexy has been recommended as an alternate approach to this problem.[196]

Outcome of Survivors

Most survivors of EA and TEF are asymptomatic 15 to 20 years after its repair. Nonetheless, the young child who has had EA and TEF repair is at risk for problems with dysphagia and recurrent respiratory infections. Children in the first year after repair are likely to have some degree of esophageal stricture,[197] which may require dilation. The esophagus may even become totally obstructed by food, necessitating esophagoscopy. Strictures seem to be less severe as the child grows; by the second to third decade, more than 90 percent of patients are either asymptomatic or have only mild dysphagia. However, almost all have demonstrable abnormalities in esophageal motility, which probably accounts for many of the cases of mild to moderate dysphagia.[198]

Abnormal esophageal motility also predisposes the child to recurrent aspiration of food and milk, which has been implicated in the etiology of recurrent pneumonia, asthma, bronchitis, and pulmonary fibrosis. These factors probably account for the increased incidence of recurrent upper and lower respiratory infection in survivors, which varies from 33 to 75 percent.[198, 199] In addition, the finding of squamous epithelium extending from the trachea to the peripheral bronchi in children dying with EA and TEF[200] suggests that the mucociliary clearance in these patients is impaired. Studies of lung function and bronchial reactivity in survivors 7 to 18 years after repair have shown an increased incidence of obstructive and restrictive lung disease, as well as sensitivity to methacholine.[201] It has been postulated that recurrent aspiration and infection damages bronchial walls and leads to airway obstruction and sensitivity. After correction of EA and TEF, a regimen of thickened feedings and upright positioning after feedings might reduce the incidence of further aspiration during the early postoperative period.

Laryngotracheoesophageal Cleft

Laryngotracheoesophageal cleft is a rare midline defect of variable length between the posterior larynx, posterior trachea, and the anterior wall of the esophagus (Fig. 17–16). The defect results from failure of caudal-rostral advancement of the mesenchymal tracheoesophageal septum and lack of dorsal fusion of the cricoid cartilages.[202] Patients may present with increased oral secretions (be-

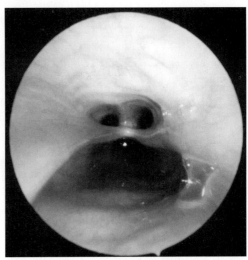

FIGURE 17–16. Tracheoesophageal lumen in an infant with a complete tracheoesophageal cleft. The carina and main-stem bronchi are clearly seen below the cleft.

cause of a swallowing defect); aphonia or a hoarse cry; and coughing, choking, or cyanosis associated with feeding. Diagnosis is often difficult and usually requires direct laryngoscopy and bronchoscopy.

The extent of the defect determines the surgical approach to repair. Clefts involving the larynx above the cricoid ring can be repaired endoscopically, and defects through the ring can be repaired using a cervical and/or thoracic approach.[203, 204] Defects extending into the trachea and to the carina are the most severe. These patients usually suffer from recurrent aspiration pneumonias and are difficult to prepare for surgery. There are very few reported survivors with a defect extending to the carina or beyond.[205–210]

The major concern with anesthetic management is stabilization of the airway. Endotracheal intubation does not guarantee a safe airway. Positioning of the patient and manipulation of the trachea and esophagus during surgery can cause the ETT to slip into the common tracheoesophagus. The use of PPV or assisted ventilation may force gas into the stomach, making ventilation progressively more difficult and increasing the risk for aspiration. One way to prevent gastric distention is to pass a No. 10 Foley catheter into the stomach, inflate the balloon, and retract the balloon into the gastroesophageal junction.[208] The trachea is repaired around the ETT, while the esophagus is repaired around the Foley catheter. Use of a bifurcated ETT with each lumen entering a main-stem bronchus has been reported.[205, 206]

Use of an ETT interferes with access to the defect when an anterior cervical surgical approach is used. In this situa-tion, the use of cardiopulmonary bypass or ECMO to facilitate repair has been reported.[204, 211]

Congenital Lobar Emphysema

Congenital lobar emphysema (CLE) is a pathologic accumulation of air in one lobe of the lung, usually an upper lobe or the right middle lobe.[212] The etiology of this condition is unknown in more than half of the reported cases. In cases with a defined etiology, extrinsic or intrinsic bronchial obstruction is most commonly cited. Intrinsic obstruction may result from cartilage deficiency, bronchial stenosis, or redundant bronchial mucosa. Abnormal vessels or enlarged lymph nodes are usually responsible for extrinsic bronchial compression.

The clinical presentation of CLE is variable. The usual age at presentation ranges from birth to 6 months. Age of onset and severity of symptoms relate to the degree of cardiopulmonary compromise caused by air accumulation under tension. Symptoms include dyspnea, cyanosis, wheezing, grunting, and coughing.

Physical examination is usually remarkable for tachypnea, intercostal retractions, nasal flaring, labored breathing, and expiratory wheezing. The involved hemithorax may be prominent but with decreased breath sounds.

Radiographic findings include unilateral radiolucency caused by lobar distention, mediastinal shift away from the affected side, atelectasis of unaffected lobes, and a flattened diaphragm (Fig. 17–17). The presence of bronchovascular markings may help to differentiate CLE from congenital lung cysts. The chest radiograph also helps to

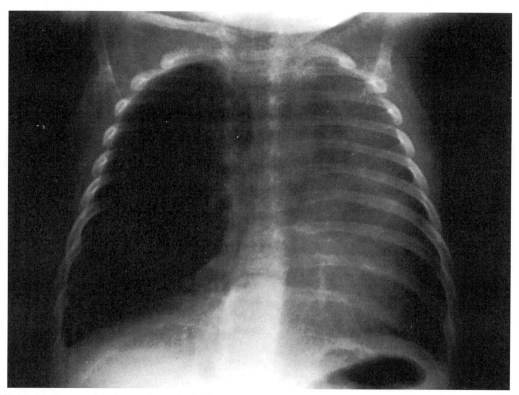

FIGURE 17–17. Preoperative chest radiograph of infant with congenital lobar emphysema, showing overdistention of the right hemithorax, flattening of the right hemidiaphragm, and shift of mediastinal contents to the left.

rule out other possible diagnoses, including pneumothorax, foreign body aspiration, and diaphragmatic hernia.[213]

The course of CLE is usually progressive, and lobectomy is the treatment of choice. Conservative therapy such as needle aspiration, tube thoracostomy, and administration of antibiotics and oxygen has been associated with a 50 to 75 percent mortality rate, whereas operative mortality is 3 to 7 percent. Infants who survive without operation develop persistent emphysema, but those that survive operation have minimal respiratory function differences from normal individuals.[212, 214, 215] Infants who have undergone lobectomy compensate with new alveolar development, whereas adults develop overdistention of the remaining lung.

Anesthetic Management

Emergency lobectomy is occasionally required because of severe cardiorespiratory failure. Whenever possible, a complete preoperative evaluation should be performed to rule out coexisting congenital anomalies. There is an increased incidence of ventricular septal defect and patent ductus arteriosus in patients with CLE.[216, 217] An IV catheter should be placed and anesthesia induced using oxygen and a volatile agent. Nitrous oxide is avoided initially, as it may expand the emphysematous segment, causing lung compression and mediastinal shift. Most practitioners favor tracheal intubation without muscle relaxants, and allow spontaneous ventilation, at least until the involved lobe is delivered through the incision. Because higher levels of inhaled anesthetic agents are required with this technique, hypotension is possible. For this reason, some authors intubate the contralateral bronchus, and use PPV, facilitated by the use of muscle relaxants.[218] Placement of an arterial catheter allows the anesthesiologist to draw serial blood gases and to monitor beat-to-beat blood pressure changes during surgical manipulations.

Once the lobectomy is completed, nitrous oxide can be added. After completion of surgery, most infants tolerate spontaneous ventilation and tracheal extubation. In most institutions these patients receive their postoperative care in an ICU where continuous ECG, respiratory monitoring, and pulse oximetry are available.

Anterior Mediastinal Mass

The anterior mediastinum contains the thymus and lymph nodes, and it occasionally contains the parathyroid glands or extensions of the thyroid glands. The most common anterior mediastinal masses in children are teratomas, masses of thymic origin, lymphomas, and angiomatous tumors. Roughly 40 percent of anterior mediastinal masses are either Hodgkin's or non-Hodgkin's lymphoma.[219] Appropriate treatment may include surgical resection, chemotherapy, and/or radiation therapy, depending on the histologic diagnosis. Therefore, children with anterior mediastinal masses may be scheduled to receive an anesthetic for tumor biopsy or resection.

The tumor may surround the large airways, the heart, and the great vessels, resulting in three types of intrathoracic compromise: compression of the tracheobronchial tree, compression of the pulmonary artery, and superior vena cava syndrome. As documented in a series of case reports,[219–226] children with anterior mediastinal masses may demonstrate severe cardiopulmonary compromise on induction of anesthesia, including cardiac arrest and death.

A recurrent theme in the reported cardiac arrests caused by airway obstruction has been loss of airway patency concomitant with loss of spontaneous ventilation, either with induction of anesthesia or administration of muscle relaxants. Some patients are in such precarious condition that even a change from the sitting to the supine position results in deterioration of their condition. This implies that critical airway diameter, previously maintained by the upright position and transpleural pressure gradients, is lost with change in body position or loss of negative intrapleural pressure. Anesthesia in the supine patient also leads to a decrease in chest wall dimensions, a cephalad displacement of the dome of the diaphragm, and a reduction in thoracic volume, thereby limiting the space available for the trachea. Application of positive airway pressure may not overcome extrinsic airway compression, as pressure is dissipated at the proximal end of the obstruction. The obstruction may be resolved with endotracheal intubation, although insertion of the tube down to or below the level of the carina may be required. However, rigid bronchoscopy is sometimes necessary to relieve the obstruction. Todres et al.[222] reported a case of severe airway obstruction that required selective intubation of each main-stem bronchus, the left side through a tracheostomy and the right side through a cuffed oral ETT positioned just below the tracheostomy stoma. Similarly, John and Narong[221] reported successful resolution of airway obstruction with the passage of two small-diameter, uncut ETTs through the larynx into each main-stem bronchus, thereby bypassing the area of obstruction. One of the authors (J.P.M.) has cared for a child who required emergency sternotomy to achieve adequate ventilation after induction of anesthesia led to complete airway obstruction.

A critical reduction in preload during induction of anesthesia may be responsible for some of the cardiac arrests. Alternatively, a change in body position may cause the tumor to compress right ventricular outflow. Such a phenomenon has been demonstrated in a canine model of anterior mediastinal mass, resulting in right ventricular enlargement and a decrease in left ventricular output because the interventricular septum impinged on left ventricular volume.[227]

Preoperative Evaluation

Identification of the patient at risk depends on a thorough history, physical examination, and laboratory evaluation (Table 17–9). Particularly ominous is the child with signs and symptoms of marked airway obstruction who refuses to lie down. Even asymptomatic patients with mediastinal masses have the potential to develop catastrophic airway obstruction. AP and lateral chest radiographs can be helpful in assessing airway compression (Fig. 17–18). Even better anatomic definition can be obtained with a CT scan of the chest (Fig. 17–19) and a cardiac echocardiogram. The CT scan is particularly helpful in planning strategy

T A B L E   1 7 – 9
EVALUATION OF PATIENTS WITH AN ANTERIOR MEDIASTINAL MASS

Diagnosis	History	Physical Examination	Other
Airway radiograph compromise	Cyanosis Cough Wheezing Dyspnea Refusal to lie down	Decreased breath sounds Wheezing Cyanosis Retractions	AP + lateral chest CT scan Flow-volume loop Fiberoptic endoscopy
Cardiovascular compromise	Syncope Dizziness Sudden pallor Facial swelling Exacerbation with Valsalva maneuver	Jugular distention Head/neck swelling Postural blood pressure changes Increased pulsus paradoxus Papilledema	Echocardiogram CT scan

AP, anteroposterior; CT, computed tomographic.

for airway management.[228] Special consideration must be made in all patients where there is compression of the trachea or major vascular structures. The induction of anesthesia in this subset of patients can lead to airway and cardiovascular collapse.[229] The flow volume loop (Fig. 17–20) can be useful in assessing degree of airway obstruction in the upright and supine position in the patient who is old enough to cooperate (>5 years).[226]

Anesthetic Management

A systematic approach to the patient with an anterior mediastinal mass is presented in Figure 17–21. In patients with enlarged cervical nodes, biopsy should be performed under local anesthesia, whether or not symptoms are present. When no cervical nodes are present, a mediastinal biopsy may be required. The symptomatic patient is assumed to be a poor anesthetic risk. If possible, empiric therapy should be initiated, including 24 hours of corticosteroids or mediastinal irradiation.[219, 226] If there is concern that prior treatment may preclude tissue diagnosis, treatment can be limited to radiation with a portion of the tumor excluded from the field.[229]

Once the decision has been made to proceed with a general anesthetic for biopsy or for tumor resection, careful preparation is necessary. Awake fiberoptic bron-

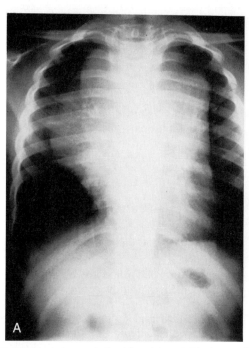
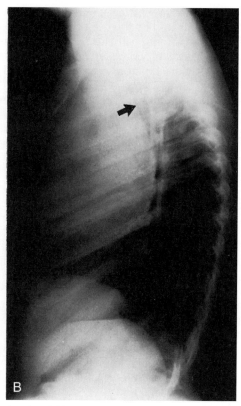

FIGURE 17–18. Anteroposterior (*A*) and lateral (*B*) chest radiographs of a child with an anterior mediastinal mass. The child was stridorous and refused to lie down because of increased respiratory distress. Note that the caliber of the airway appears normal on the AP view (*A*), but that the airway is posteriorly displaced and narrowed on the lateral view (*B, arrow*).

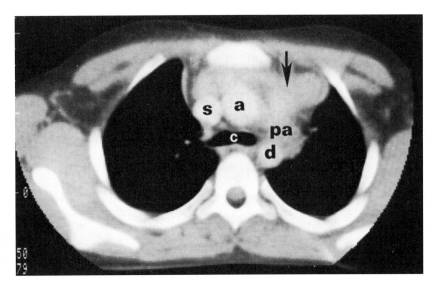

FIGURE 17–19. CT scan of the chest in a patient with an anterior mediastinal lymphoma (*arrow*). The proximity of the tumor to the ascending (*a*) and descending (*d*) aorta, left pulmonary artery (*pa*), superior vena cava (*s*), and trachea at the carinal level (*c*) is well shown.

choscopy under local anesthesia can provide useful information about the location and dynamic nature of tracheobronchial compression. The bronchoscope can also facilitate and confirm correct placement of the ETT before induction of anesthesia.[231] If fiberoptic bronchoscopy is not possible, induction of anesthesia is performed with oxygen and halothane or sevoflurane, with the patient breathing spontaneously in the semi-Fowler's position. Intubation of the trachea is performed without the aid of muscle relaxants; the ETT is positioned as determined during the preoperative evaluation, and both sides of the chest are carefully auscultated.

If the airway becomes obstructed, positive pressure can be applied, although frequently this does not relieve the obstruction. The lateral and/or prone position may help to relieve the obstruction. If not, a rigid bronchoscope, set up before induction of anesthesia, should be inserted beyond the obstruction, at which point ventilation and oxygenation of the lungs should improve. If obstruction is unabated, two alternatives remain: median sternotomy

and femorofemoral bypass. Regardless of the option chosen, the necessary equipment must be available at the time anesthesia is induced. The key to successful management of these difficult patients is careful planning and preparation, with a back-up plan readily available for each step.

At the end of the procedure the trachea is extubated with the patient awake and breathing spontaneously. The equipment required to reinsert the endotracheal tube must be readily available in case airway obstruction occurs after tracheal extubation.

Pectus Excavatum

Pectus excavatum is a concave depression of the lower sternum that generally presents at birth and often is progressive (Fig. 17–22). Although the etiology is unknown, the condition frequently is familial, is particularly common in Marfan syndrome, and may occur in patients with congenital heart disease.[231]

Most patients are asymptomatic, although some complain of exercise intolerance, occasionally to a degree that is a sufficient indication for surgery. Although early studies of cardiac and pulmonary function revealed no abnormalities,[232, 233] studies using more sophisticated techniques have shown mild decreases in forced expiratory flow and lung volumes.[231, 234] A decrease in cardiac output resulting from limitation of diastolic filling has been demonstrated during exercise and with changing from the supine to sitting position.[235, 236] Encroachment by the depressed sternum can also cause leftward displacement of the heart, a functional systolic murmur, right axis deviation on ECG, and atrial and ventricular arrhythmias.[231] Several studies have demonstrated that pulmonary function does not improve after repair. Whether improvement in exercise tolerance follows surgical repair remains controversial.[235, 237–240] In addition to physiologic considerations, indications for surgery include severe cosmetic or postural defects. Predictive indices of progression are difficult to identify. Pectus excavatum presenting in infancy may improve by the age of 3 years and therefore may not require surgery.[241]

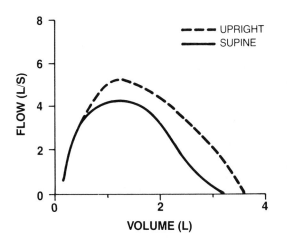

FIGURE 17–20. Flow–volume loop in patient with an anterior mediastinal mass in upright and supine positions. Reduction in expiratory flow rate is seen in both positions. In the supine position, the expiratory flow rate has a lower peak and a plateau, indicating intrathoracic airway obstruction.

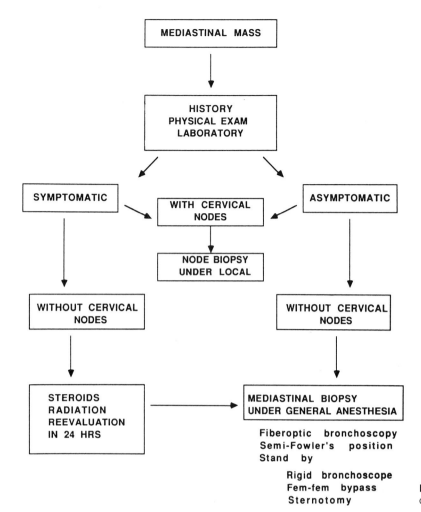

FIGURE 17–21. Decision tree in the management of the child with anterior mediastinal mass.

Otherwise, operative repair is generally advised for any child with a marked or progressive deformity.

Preoperative assessment includes a thorough history and physical examination to elicit evidence of cardiopulmonary compromise. Laboratory assessment, including chest radiograph, ECG, pulmonary function studies, and arterial blood gases should be obtained only when the initial evaluation indicates significant cardiopulmonary disease.

The surgical technique most commonly used involves an extrapleural, subperichondral resection of the depressed rib cartilage and a sternal osteotomy. Metallic struts or wires can be placed to support the sternum during the early postoperative period.[242] Although blood replacement is usually not necessary, 1 unit of whole blood or packed RBCs should be available. General endotracheal anesthesia with controlled ventilation is employed. If nitrous oxide is used, the anesthesiologist should be aware that the pleura may be punctured during the procedure and that nitrous oxide may enlarge a pneumothorax. Placement of an epidural catheter allows intraoperative supplementation with local anesthetics and postoperative pain management with epidural opioids. An arterial catheter is not indicated unless dictated by significant preoperative cardiopulmonary disease.

At the conclusion of surgery, the tracheas of most patients can be extubated unless significant cardiopulmonary compromise is present. A chest radiograph should be obtained in the recovery room to rule out pneumothorax or lobar atelectasis. Supplemental oxygen should be administered on the basis of pulse oximetry readings.

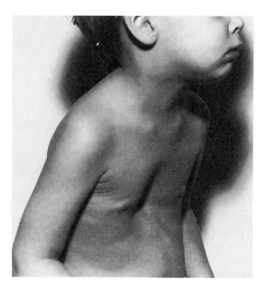

FIGURE 17–22. Child with pectus excavatum.

Pectus Carinatum

Pectus carinatum, a convex defect of the sternum, is much less common than pectus excavatum. Although the cosmetic deformity is the usual presenting complaint, a few children have exertional dyspnea and cardiac arrhythmias. No studies have been done to document the presence of cardiac or pulmonary compromise in these patients. Anesthetic management is similar to that for pectus excavatum.

RIGID BRONCHOSCOPY

Direct examination of the airway is often indicated for diagnosis of upper and lower airway lesions, for removal of aspirated foreign bodies, for obtaining microbiologic specimens for laboratory diagnosis, and for treatment of refractory lobar atelectasis. Anesthesia for bronchoscopy is a challenge for the anesthesiologist, who must share access to the airway with the bronchoscopist and must, to the extent possible, prevent hypoventilation, hypoxia, and inadequate depth of anesthesia, which can lead to coughing, movement, and secondary trauma to the airway.

Indications

Retrospective reviews[243–245] have shown that the indications for bronchoscopy in children fall into two broad groups. The first group consists of children with symptoms of airway obstruction, most commonly dyspnea associated with stridor on inspiration. Table 17–10 shows that children who fall into this group tend to be younger and to have a greater incidence of congenital malformations of the airway.

The second group consists of children with lower airway disease. This group, about twice as common as the former, comprises older children with acquired (rather than congenital) abnormalities, most commonly recurrent pneumonia, foreign body aspiration, bronchiectasis, or suspected tuberculosis.[244] Therefore, children undergoing rigid bronchoscopy are often physiologically abnormal and have some combination of airway obstruction and ventilation and perfusion abnormalities.

Anesthetic Management

Equipment

Of the several techniques for providing fresh gas and anesthetic gas flow to the lungs during rigid bronchoscopy, the use of a bronchoscope with a side-arm for delivery of anesthetic gases has become the most popular. Anesthetic management of patients for bronchoscopy has improved significantly since the introduction of bronchoscopes with miniature lens systems, improved illumination, and a standard 15-mm connector for the anesthesia circuit (Fig. 17–23).[246] Because this is a closed system, controlled ventilation is possible, even during examination by the bronchoscopist, except when a 2.5-mm scope is used. When the latter is used, the lens and light carrier must be removed periodically, and the proximal end of the bronchoscope must be occluded to allow ventilation by the lungs. Usually, the surgeons can continue to examine the airways if the SaO_2 is greater than 95 percent.

In 1967, Sanders[247] described a system in which oxygen at hospital pipeline pressure (50 to 60 psi) was intermittently directed down the bronchoscope. Because of the Venturi effect, room air was entrained in the process, often resulting in a progressive decrease in arterial oxygen tension. Improvements in the apparatus that limit air entrainment have since been made.[248, 249] The ability to provide high arterial oxygen tensions and hypocarbic CO_2 tensions with this apparatus has been claimed[250] but not extensively studied in children. With the Sanders device, peak infla-

Modified from Wiseman NE, Sanchez I, Powell RE: Rigid bronchoscopy in the pediatric age group; diagnostic effectiveness. J Pediatr Surg 27:1294, 1992, with permission.

T A B L E   1 7 – 1 0
DIAGNOSIS AND AGE OF CHILDREN UNDERGOING BRONCHOSCOPY FOR AIRWAY OBSTRUCTION

Diagnosis	No. of Patients		
	<1 yr	1–3 yr	>3 yr
Laryngomalacia	7		
Tracheomalacia	11	4	3
Bronchomalacia	3		
Vocal cord paralysis	3		
Subglottic stenosis	6	8	7
Vascular ring	3	2	
Papillomatosis			3
Hemangioma, cysts	13	1	
Infection (tracheitis, epiglottitis)	5	4	4
Normal findings	4	1	1
Total	55	20	18

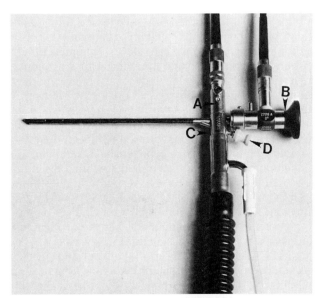

FIGURE 17–23. Rigid bronchoscope that includes a proximal light prism (*A*), miniature lens system (*B*), 15-mm connector for anesthesia circuit (*C*), and channel for suction or biopsy forceps (*D*).

tion pressures and flow rates are influenced by the driving pressure, diameter and shape of the bronchoscope, diameter and length of the injector, and angle from the axial line of the bronchoscope.[251, 252] Because of the smaller diameter, pediatric bronchoscopes tend to have lower flow rates and higher inflation pressures than adult bronchoscopes.

Miyasaka et al.[252] demonstrated that conventional tidal volumes (6 to 16 ml/kg) could be obtained with driving pressures of 20 to 40 psi, although there were differences in the properties of each bronchoscope evaluated that influenced the resultant tidal volumes and inflation pressures. Excessive inflation pressures may occur with some systems,[253] as may inadequate tidal volumes in patients with abnormally low pulmonary compliance.[249] Jet ventilation must be individualized to the needs of each patient on a case-by-case basis.

Monitors routinely used include ECG, an automated blood pressure device, a monitor for body temperature, a peripheral nerve stimulator (if neuromuscular relaxants are used), a precordial stethoscope for auscultating respirations and monitoring heart tones, and a pulse oximeter for continuous determination of arterial hemoglobin-oxygen saturation. Because the rise and fall of the child's chest must be observed, the thorax should be left uncovered throughout the procedure. The anesthesiologist should have available an atomizer for administering topical local anesthetic to the airway and an assortment of sizes of uncut ETTs.

Anesthetic Management

Atropine 0.02 mg/kg can be administered intravenously at the time of induction of anesthesia for its effects on secretions and vagal tone. Anesthesia is usually induced with an IV induction agent (e.g., sodium thiopental, ketamine, or propofol), by rectal induction agents (e.g., methohexital) or, most commonly, by inhalation of halothane or sevoflurane. When there is a suspicion of a high-grade obstruction of the upper airway, induction of anesthesia by inhalation of halothane or sevoflurane and maintenance of spontaneous respiration is generally felt to be safer than administering fixed agents. Examples of such obstructions would include the child with epiglottitis, a laryngeal or tracheal foreign body, or an anterior mediastinal mass causing compression of the thoracic airway. In the presence of normal oxygenation, nitrous oxide can be used at the time of anesthetic induction, but is contraindicated during maintenance of anesthesia to minimize the possibility of intraoperative hypoxemia. The maintenance concentration of inhaled agent is determined by the patient's cardiovascular status and response to anesthesia.

An intravenous infusion of propofol (100 to 200 μg/kg/min) can be used as an adjunctive or primary agent; a continuous intravenous anesthetic has the advantage of a constant level of anesthesia despite changes in alveolar ventilation. The combination of alfentanil and propofol has been compared to propofol alone for bronchoscopy in adults.[254] An intravenous bolus of 10 μg/kg of alfentanil reduced the required induction dose of propofol from 2.2 mg/kg to 1.7 mg/kg. The incidence of hypotension was higher in the patients receiving alfentanil. Alfentanil and propofol can be combined as a single infusion (20 μg alfentanil per 1 ml [10 mg] of propofol) and infused at the standard rate for propofol without causing significant hypotension.

When the patient has been anesthetized, the larynx, vocal cords, and tracheal mucosa can be sprayed with 4 percent lidocaine, thus reducing the anesthetic requirement. Amitai et al.[255] studied the safety of topical lidocaine 3.2 to 8.5 mg/kg in children undergoing fiberoptic bronchoscopy. They found that peak serum lidocaine concentrations were 1 to 3.5 μg/ml, well below the toxic serum level. They concluded that lidocaine doses of up to 7 mg/kg were safe, provided that the dose is administered slowly (over 15 minutes) and that doses up to 8.5 mg/kg could be administered over longer periods. After the topical anesthesia is applied and after another brief period of assisted ventilation, the patient can then be turned over to the bronchoscopist, who inserts the bronchoscope after visualizing the larynx with a laryngoscope with a straight blade. Spontaneous ventilation through, and possibly around, the bronchoscope is usually well tolerated and may be preferred so that the bronchoscopist can evaluate vocal cord movement and the effects of any dynamic intrathoracic obstruction. Muscle relaxation, if desired, can be achieved by any one of a number of conventional techniques, including succinylcholine by bolus and continuous infusion, or nondepolarizing relaxants. Of the latter, shorter acting agents (e.g., mivacurium or atracurium) may be preferred to avoid excessive neuromuscular blockade at the end of a brief bronchoscopy. Muscle relaxation necessitates controlled ventilation but also allows delivery of less anesthesia, prevents coughing, and facilitates removal of foreign bodies through the vocal cords.[256]

Throughout the procedure, adequacy of ventilation is monitored by chest auscultation with the precordial stethoscope and by inspection of chest wall excursion. Capnometry is generally of little use during bronchoscopy if a T-piece breathing circuit is used, because of contamination of exhaled gas by high fresh gas flows. During PPV, gas leaks around the bronchoscope can usually be remedied by gentle compression of the thyroid cartilage between the thumb and forefinger. Constant communication with the endoscopist is vital, as manipulations of the bronchoscope may cause ineffective ventilation. It may be necessary, for example, to instruct the bronchoscopist to remove the telescope from the bronchoscope and occlude the end of the scope a finger to more effectively ventilate the lungs, or to cease suctioning, which is known to produce hypoxemia if prolonged.[257]

Complications

The most common complications of bronchoscopy in children are cardiac arrhythmias, which are the consequence of light anesthesia, hypoventilation, and possibly increased vagal tone and hypoxemia. Cardiac arrhythmias are usually ventricular in origin and include premature ventricular contractions, bigeminy, and (rarely) ventricular tachycardia. Ventricular arrhythmias usually resolve with manual hyperventilation of the lungs, provision of adequate oxygenation, and deepening of the anesthetic.

If these measures are unsuccessful, lidocaine 1 mg/kg given IV usually controls cardiac irritability.

Bronchospasm may occur in children with a known or unknown history of reactive airway disease, usually as a consequence of bronchial or carinal stimulation during light anesthesia. Treatment consists of deepening the anesthesia and administrating bronchodilators and topical anesthetics (see below).

Mechanical complications occur less frequently. Foreign bodies of organic origin (particularly nuts and seeds, as well as pieces of hard fruits or vegetables) often induce an intense inflammatory response in adjacent mucosa. Such organic material is subjected to enzymatic effects that may make them too friable to remove in one piece if they have been in situ for more than a few hours. Impaction and fragmentation of such a foreign body may occur during attempts to retrieve it, especially when PPV is utilized. PPV, by increasing intrathoracic pressure, may also reduce the caliber of the bronchus containing the foreign body. Administration of a bronchodilator, such as terbutaline 5 to 10 μg/kg intramuscularly or subcutaneously to a maximal dose of 0.4 mg, may provide enough airway dilation to allow successful foreign body removal. Pneumothorax may occur,[258] particularly with PPV in the setting of a necrotizing bronchopneumonia or when a foreign body causes a ball-valve obstruction of a bronchus.

On completion of the examination, the bronchoscope is removed from the trachea and the anesthesiologist institutes bag-and-mask ventilation of the lungs with 100 percent oxygen. The trachea is intubated as needed to provide pulmonary toilet, to protect the airway from aspiration of gastric contents (in the child who was not adequately fasted before bronchoscopy), or to manage pulmonary insufficiency.

Postoperative Care

After bronchoscopy, the child is observed in an anesthesia recovery area for stridor, respiratory distress, or other signs suggestive of subglottic edema. A chest radiograph should be obtained to rule out new pulmonary parenchymal abnormalities or pneumothorax. Subglottic edema, if present, usually responds to humidified oxygen, racemic epinephrine, and steroids (e.g., dexamethasone 0.3 to 0.5 mg/kg),[259] although the latter's effect requires several hours.

THORACOSCOPIC SURGERY

Thoracoscopy was first described in 1910 by Jacobeus, when he used a cystoscope via a rigid trocar to lyse pleural adhesions in a patient with tuberculosis.[260] Although the first use of thoracoscopy in children was reported by Rodgers in 1976,[261, 262] in the 1990s more advanced diagnostic and therapeutic procedures have been performed in children.[263-267] Initially limited to small biopsies, diagnostic evaluations, and pleural debridement of empyemas,[268-270] indications for thoracoscopy have expanded to include extensive pulmonary resections, bullous disease, metastatic lesions,[271, 272] mediastinal masses,[273] and congenital vascular malformations, such as patent ductus arteriosus and vascular rings.[274-277] In patients who have scoliosis, thoracoscopy has been used to facilitate anterior thoracic spinal fusions.[278, 279]

Preoperative Evaluation

When developing an anesthetic plan for children undergoing thoracoscopic surgery, both the patient's underlying physiologic condition as well as the alterations imposed by the surgical procedure must be considered. All thoracoscopic procedures require one-lung ventilation and collapse of the ipsilateral lung to facilitate surgical exposure. In patients with marginal lung function, pulmonary function studies may assist in determining whether one-lung ventilation will be tolerated.

Anesthetic Management

All pediatric patients undergoing thoracoscopy require general anesthesia.[280, 281] The local anesthesia and interpleural techniques have been described in adults are impractical for children.[282] Induction of anesthesia can be accomplished with either an intravenous or inhalational technique. Although blood loss is generally minimal, large-bore venous access should be established. Central venous monitoring is not necessary in patients with normal cardiovascular function. If a central venous catheter is inserted, placement of the catheter on the side of the surgery minimizes the risk of bilateral pneumothoracies.

Surgical exposure during thoracoscopic procedures is improved with techniques for achieving one lung ventilation. Techniques for achieving one-lung ventilation are described on p 431.

Complications

Hypoxia during one-lung ventilation is a common problem. Etiologies include tube malposition, inadequate ventilation of the dependant lung, shunting of blood in the unventilated lung, and underlying lung disease. Pa_{O_2} can often be improved by increasing the inspired oxygen concentration or adding PEEP to the ventilated lung. The application of CPAP to the operative side may improve oxygenation, but may also reduce surgical exposure.

Progressive hyperthermia has been reported during thoracoscopic procedures in children, secondary to local heat production by the endoscope.[283] Hyperthermia is more common in infants less than 5 kg or during procedures lasting more than 200 minutes. Other reported complications are inadvertent esophageal injury and tension pneumothorax.[284] Although CO_2 embolization is theoretically possible during thoracoscopic procedures, there are no reports of this in children.

ANESTHESIA FOR PATIENTS WITH CHRONIC LUNG DISEASE

Asthma

It is common in the practice of pediatric anesthesia to deal with children who have a history of asthma or who develop bronchospasm intraoperatively. A discussion of

T A B L E   1 7 - 1 1
ASTHMA: PRECIPITATING FACTORS

Respiratory infection

Allergic reaction to inhaled antigen

Mechanical stimulation: coughing, exercise, cold air inhalation

Occupational or environmental exposure to irritant

Emotional stress

Idiosyncratic reaction to nonsteroidal anti-inflammatory drug (e.g., aspirin)

the pathophysiology of this process will be followed by recommendations for management.

Pathophysiology

Asthma includes a variety of bronchospastic diseases that have in common airway hyperreactivity in response to physical, chemical, or immunologic stimulation (Table 17–11). Asthma can be classified as intrinsic or extrinsic. Intrinsic asthma, most common in adults, is associated with a negative allergic history and skin tests, and low immunoglobulin E (IgE) levels. Extrinsic asthma, most common in childhood, is caused by the patient's immunologic response to an allergen. Such exposure stimulates the production of IgE, which becomes fixed to mast cells, either in the tissues or circulating in blood. On repeated exposure, the same antigen reacts with receptors on two IgE molecules, triggering release of mediators from mast cells. The responsiveness of the airway to the effect of these mediators is largely determined by background adrenergic and cholinergic input and by the presence of inflammation (Fig. 17–24). β-Adrenergic input, via regulation of cyclic adenosine monophosphate (cAMP) in airway smooth muscle cells, produces bronchodilation and pulmonary vasodilation. Therapeutically, cAMP levels can be increased with β-agonists that stimulate its formation or with phosphodiesterase inhibitors (e.g., xanthines) that block its breakdown.[285]

Cholinergic input to the smooth muscle cell occurs via acetylcholine stimulation and results in bronchoconstric-tion and mucous gland constriction. Acetylcholine production is regulated, in turn, by the intracellular concentration of cyclic guanosine monophosphate (cGMP). Anticholinergic drugs such as atropine inhibit acetylcholine stimulation, usually resulting in dilation of proximal airways.[286] Thus, the addition of an anticholinergic drug to β-agonist therapy may augment bronchodilation, since β-agonists affect more distal airways.[286]

Inflammation may cause bronchospasm by stimulating mediator release and by lowering the threshold of airway reactivity. Therefore, wheezing is frequently triggered by respiratory infections. Increased bronchomotor response to a viral challenge can be demonstrated for up to 8 weeks after a viral respiratory infection.

Histamine acts at H_1 receptors to produce smooth muscle contraction. Stimulation of H_2 receptors may provide negative feedback or modulation of H_1-induced bronchoconstriction. Thus, H_2-receptor antagonists, such as cimetidine, may provoke or exacerbate bronchoconstriction.

Lung tissue synthesizes a variety of prostaglandin-like substances, which play a role of undetermined importance in inflammatory mediation and regulation of bronchomotor tone. Prostaglandins F and D are bronchoconstrictors, whereas type E prostaglandins are bronchodilators. Disturbance of prostaglandin balance may play a role in aspirin-induced asthma.

Pulmonary Mechanics and Gas Exchange

Bronchospasm, intraluminal secretions, and an inflammatory response of the walls of the airway result in obstruction to airflow in both large and small airways, although peripheral airway obstruction seems to predominate in severe asthma.[287] Increased resistance to expiratory flow results in increased residual volume (RV), FRC, and total lung volume (TLV), whereas vital capacity (VC), expiratory reserve volume (ERV), and inspiratory capacity (IC) are reduced.[288, 289]

Dynamic pulmonary compliance decreases in asthma as a result of overinflation,[289] as shown in Figure 17–25. Decreased compliance and increased airway resistance result in increased work of breathing, with recruitment of accessory muscles of respiration. Alveolar overinflation

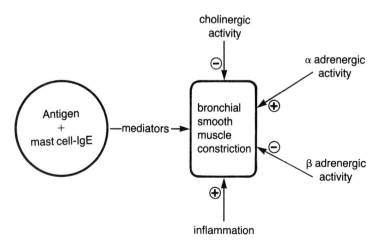

FIGURE 17–24. Mediators released from IgE-coated mast cells are the primary effectors of bronchial smooth muscle constriction. The responsiveness of smooth muscle to mediators is influenced by other factors, as shown. +, bronchoconstriction; −, bronchodilation.

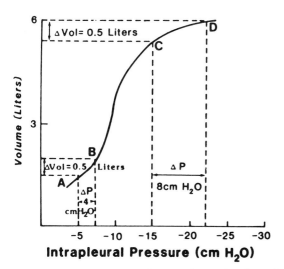

FIGURE 17–25. Compliance curve showing change in volume (ΔVol) for change in intrapleural pressure (ΔP). In the normal subject (*AB*), a ΔP of 4 cm H_2O and a peak airway pressure of 7 cm H_2O generate a volume of 500 ml. In the asthmatic child with hyperinflated lung (*CD*), a ΔP of 8 cm H_2O and a peak pressure of 22 cm H_2O are required to produce the same volume change. (From Kingston HGG, Hirshman CA: Perioperative management of the patient with asthma. Anesth Analg 63:844, 1984, with permission.)

causes constriction of intra-alveolar vessels, with a resultant increase in dead space fraction (V_D/V_T).[288] Therefore, minute ventilation must increase to maintain eucapnia; respiratory failure may ensue if excessive work of breathing precludes maintenance of a high minute ventilation.

Hypoxia also is seen frequently in asthma and results from $\dot{V}/\dot{Q}$ mismatch and shunting of blood through areas of lung made atelectatic by intraluminal secretions. Therefore, oxygen delivery to tissues may be compromised in the face of elevated oxygen demands.

Preoperative Assessment

It has long been recognized that intraoperative morbidity and mortality are higher in asthmatic than in nonasthmatic patients.[290] Preoperative evaluation often provides clues as to how a patient might respond to general anesthesia and what therapies might be effective if bronchospasm occurs.

History

A complete history includes questions concerning the following:

1. Current medications, including all bronchodilators and steroids.
2. Previous response to anesthesia.
3. Recent upper respiratory infections (URIs) or episodes of wheezing. Ideally, 4 to 6 weeks should elapse after a URI or an episode of bronchospasm because of the risk of exacerbation. This is not always feasible, and frequently a more flexible approach must be adopted.

4. Number of emergency room visits or hospitalization in the past year.
5. The patient's own assessment of current status compared with baseline.

Physical Examination

A patient's general appearance often reflects the degree of bronchospasm (e.g., agitation, obvious respiratory distress, or somnolence). During bronchospasm, the respiratory rate is usually elevated and the expiratory phase prolonged. On chest auscultation, wheezing is most often audible during expiration. In the severely distressed patient, absence of significant wheezing can be ominous, reflecting little air movement. Severe bronchospasm also may produce chest hyperinflation, cyanosis, intercostal retractions, and use of accessory muscles. A pulsus paradoxus of greater than 20 mm Hg is often seen but may be absent even in patients with an FEV_1 of less than 1 L.[291] Physical examination should include a search for nasal polyps, the presence of which would contraindicate nasal intubation.

Pulmonary Function Testing

Preoperative spirometry may be useful for documenting the extent of obstructive airway disease and, more importantly, the potential for reversal with bronchodilators. The degree of airway constriction is most often quantitated with a measurement of forced expired volume over time. With the resulting spirogram (Fig. 17–26), one can calculate the total amount of volume forcibly expired after a maximal breath (forced vital capacity [FVC]) and the volume forcibly expired in one second (FEV_1). Both the FVC and the FEV_1 are reduced during an asthma attack; however, both are subject to inaccuracy because of poor patient cooperation. In addition, the FEV_1 is sensitive to proximal but not to distal airway obstruction.[292] However, the maximal midexpiratory flow rate ($FEF_{25-75\%}$) can also be calculated from the spirogram and is a better indicator of distal airway obstruction.[293] The $FEF_{25-75\%}$, obtained by identifying the points at which 25 and 75 percent of the FVC have been expelled, is independent of patient effort. Comparing such parameters of pulmonary function against predicted values allows a classification of clinical impairment (Table 17–12).[294]

Airway obstruction can also be quantitated by plotting flow versus lung volume (flow–volume curve; Fig. 17–27). The flow–volume loop is a sensitive indicator of small airway disease and can provide useful information independent of patient effort.

Improvement in such pulmonary function parameters after a trial of bronchodilators in a child with acute bronchospasm implies a reversible component and suggests that adjustments in bronchodilator therapy before elective surgery may be beneficial. Elective surgery should be postponed until the patient's status is optimal.

Other Laboratory Tests

Baseline arterial blood gas analysis is indicated in the asthmatic patient with severe impairment of pulmonary

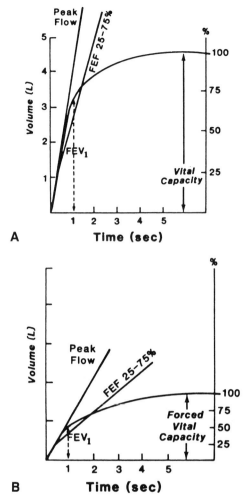

FIGURE 17–26. Spirograms in nonasthmatic patient (*A*) and asthmatic patient (*B*) demonstrating reductions in FVC, FEF$_{25-75\%}$, FEV$_1$ and peak flow associated with bronchospasm. (From Kingston HGG, Hirshman CA: Perioperative management of the patient with asthma. Anesth Analg 63:844, 1984, with permission.)

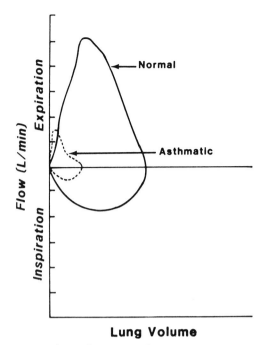

FIGURE 17–27. Flow–volume curves from normal and asthmatic subjects, showing decreased lung volume and inspiratory and expiratory flows in the asthmatic patient. (From Kingston HGG, Hirshman CA: Perioperative management of the patient with asthma. Anesth Analg 63:844, 1984, with permission.)

T A B L E 1 7 – 1 2		
CLINICAL CLASSIFICATION OF IMPAIRMENT OF PULMONARY FUNCTION IN ASTHMA		
	FVC, FEV$_1$ (% of Predicted)	FEF$_{25-75\%}$ (% of Predicted)
Normal	>80	>75
Mild	65–80	60–75
Moderate	56–64	45–59
Severe	35–55	30–44
Very severe	<35	<30

From Kingston HGG, Hirshman CA: Perioperative management of the Patient with asthma. Anesth Analg 63:844, 1984, with permission.

function, in whom hypercarbia and hypoxia may be seen. Chest radiographs usually show only lung hyperinflation and peribronchial thickening, which do not demand alterations in therapy.[295] However, complicating factors, such as pneumonia or pulmonary edema, also may be revealed.

Specific Medications

Anti-inflammatory Drugs

Corticosteroids. Corticosteroids are now heavily relied on in the treatment of chronic asthma and are also useful in the treatment of acute asthma. Their mechanism of action is not well understood.[296] The preparation used most frequently is hydrocortisone 1 to 3 mg/kg intravenously. The onset of action is 1 to 2 hours after administration. Methylprednisolone 1 to 2 mg/kg is an alternate choice, with less mineralocorticoid effect. Improvement in oxygenation and peak flow rates has been demonstrated after corticosteroid administration.[297]

Cromolyn. Cromolyn prevents release of mediators from mast cells and is frequently given in aerosol form for treatment of chronic asthma. It is relatively free of side effects and has no known interactions with drugs used in anesthesia. Therefore, it can be given until the time of induction of anesthesia.[298]

Bronchodilators

Sympathomimetics. For mild to moderate asthma attacks, β-agonists such as terbutaline are preferred to agents with both β_1 and β_2 properties (e.g., isoproterenol) because of the latter's propensity to cause tachycardia and arrhythmias. Terbutaline can be given either by jet nebulizer (0.1 percent solution, 3 ml over 10 minutes) or by subcutaneous injection of 5 to 10 μg/kg. For patients with severe asthma associated with respiratory failure, IV isoproterenol[299] or terbutaline can be used. This should be done in an ICU with continuous ECG and arterial pressure monitoring, as arrhythmias and marked tachycardia may result.

Xanthine Derivatives. The xanthine derivative aminophylline is commonly used in the management of bronchospasm. For children without prior aminophylline therapy, an IV loading dose of 5 to 7 mg/kg is given over 20 to 30 minutes. When previous doses of theophylline have been given, a serum level is obtained and the dose is adjusted to achieve a serum drug level of 10 to 20 μg/ml. A bolus of 1 mg/kg usually raises the serum level by 2 μg/ml.[300] Maintenance aminophylline can be given either by bolus administration every 4 hours or by a continuous infusion of 0.6 to 1 mg/kg/h. Serum levels higher than 10 to 20 μg/ml are associated with tachyarrhythmias, hypotension, and seizures.

Anticholinergics. Anticholinergics are less effective bronchodilators than the β-adrenergic agonists or the xanthines, and should be viewed as adjunctive agents. They produce bronchodilation by inhibiting cholinergic activation of airway smooth muscle.[301] Atropine 1 to 5 mg can be dissolved in saline and administered in a hand-held nebulizer. As a tertiary ammonium compound, it is rapidly absorbed and distributed throughout the body, which may result in undesirable cardiovascular and CNS side effects. Ipratropium bromide, a quaternary ammonium compound, is poorly absorbed when inhaled and can be viewed as a topical form of atropine. It has recently been released for clinical use in a metered dose inhaler. The optimal dose is 50 to 125 μg.[302]

Anesthetic Management

In adults with a documented history of asthma, the incidence of intraoperative bronchospasm is only 1 to 2 percent.[303] Patient characteristics associated with complications included the recent use of antiasthma drugs, recent asthma symptoms, and recent therapy in a medical facility for asthma.

Premedication

No controlled investigation of premedication for asthmatic patients has been reported. In theory, opioids in doses sufficient to depress respiration should be avoided. The risk of inspissation of bronchial secretions by anticholinergic medications, such as atropine, is probably outweighed by the potential benefit of inhibition of parasympathetic-induced bronchoconstriction. Atropine in combination with either meperidine or a barbiturate has been used without apparent risk of bronchospasm.[304]

The role of histamine release in precipitation of bronchospasm is unclear. Although histamine produces bronchoconstriction, antihistamines have not been effective in reversing bronchospasm. Because H_2 receptors are thought to be responsible for inhibitory feedback control of mediator release,[305] H_2-receptor antagonists, such as cimetidine, should probably be avoided.

Patients who have been on chronic steroid therapy within 6 months of surgery are at risk for adrenal suppression and should receive steroid coverage. Hydrocortisone 1 to 2 mg/kg every 6 to 12 hours is initiated 1 day before surgery and is continued for at least 2 days postoperatively.

Choice of Anesthetic Technique

Regional anesthesia should be considered for extremity procedures in children old enough to accept and tolerate the procedure. In adults with chronic bronchitis or chronic obstructive pulmonary disease, regional anesthesia is safer than general anesthesia.[306] However, bronchospasm certainly can occur during regional anesthesia. In the series of Shnider and Papper,[304] 1.9 percent of asthmatic patients undergoing regional anesthesia developed active wheezing during surgery. Bronchospasm has also been reported in an asthmatic patient after interscalene block of the brachial plexus.[307] This may result from block of the upper thoracic portion of the sympathetic chain, with a relative excess of parasympathetic activity resulting in bronchoconstriction.

When regional anesthesia is inappropriate, general anesthesia is used. Probably the most important cause of bronchospasm during general anesthesia is tracheal intubation.[304] For this reason, tracheal intubation is avoided when possible and, when necessary, is performed only after airway reflexes have been thoroughly depressed with both general and local anesthetic agents. Lidocaine prevents reflex-induced bronchospasm[308] and can be given intravenously 1 to 2 mg/kg, since intratracheal administration has a longer onset of action and may precipitate bronchospasm.[309] Lidocaine 1 to 3 mg/kg/h by infusion may also be a useful adjunct in patients whose airways require more anesthesia than their cardiovascular systems can tolerate.

Induction of anesthesia with thiopental has been reported to produce bronchospasm, although its cause is more likely to be instrumentation of the airway under light planes of anesthesia than a direct effect of the drug. In practice, thiopental has been used frequently for successful induction of anesthesia for asthmatic patients.[304] For patients who demonstrate active bronchospasm at the time anesthesia is induced, ketamine 1 to 2 mg/kg intravenously is probably the drug of choice,[310] since it increases circulating concentrations of epinephrine[311] and directly dilates tracheal smooth muscle.[312] Ketamine's protective effect against antigen-induced bronchospasm is precluded by β-adrenergic blockade. Ketamine decreases airway resistance in patients with active bronchospasm[313] and can eliminate bronchospasm during anesthesia.[310,314] Ketamine also improved bronchospasm in children in respiratory failure that is refractory to conventional asthma therapy.[315]

Propofol appears to be a safe anesthetic in asthmatic patients. In adults, propofol has been shown to provide more protection against tracheal intubation–induced bronchoconstriction than an induction dose of thiopental.[316] However, there is insufficient evidence to distinguish the beneficial effects of propofol related to depth of anesthesia and a specific effect of this agent on bronchial tone.

Potent inhalational anesthetics may prevent development of bronchospasm by blocking airway reflexes, by directly relaxing airway smooth muscle, or by inhibiting mediator release.[317] The choice of inhalational agent is hindered by the lack of controlled studies. Nonetheless, halothane has been proposed to be the drug of choice for maintaining anesthesia, since it is associated with the lowest incidence of bronchospasm.[290, 305] Halothane has been associated with an increase in bronchial caliber and pulmonary compliance,[318] a decrease in pulmonary resistance, and improved gas exchange during asthma attacks.[319] Halothane has even been used in the ICU for treatment of status asthmaticus refractory to other forms of therapy.[320, 321] However, halothane may be associated with cardiac arrhythmias, especially when given in combination with agents that also increase myocardial irritability, such as isoproterenol and aminophylline. If significant arrhythmias arise during halothane administration, increasing minute volume and the depth of anesthesia usually resolves the problem. If not, another agent should be chosen for maintaining anesthesia. Halothane and isoflurane appear to be equally effective in preventing[322] and reversing[323] bronchoconstriction, and isoflurane does not sensitize the myocardium to catecholamines. In the presence of toxic aminophylline levels, halothane is particularly likely to produce ventricular dysrhythmias.[324, 325] In this situation, isoflurane[326] or sevoflurane would be preferred over halothane.

Sevoflurane relaxes bronchial smooth muscle, though perhaps less effectively than does halothane.[327] In a clinical trial comparing sevoflurane and halothane for pediatric day surgery patients, respiratory events, including bronchospasm, were more common during induction with sevoflurane than with halothane.[328] However, sevoflurane has been used safely in patients with asthma.[329]

No clear advantage has been shown in the choice of neuromuscular blocking agents. Pancuronium has been used frequently in asthmatic patients without adverse effects.[330, 331] Succinylcholine, although frequently used without difficulty, increases parasympathetic tone and has been associated with bronchospasm by a cholinergic mechanism,[332] but this can be prevented and reversed with an appropriate dose of atropine.

If wheezing develops during the course of anesthesia, bronchospasm is the mostly likely cause, although other causes of wheezing (i.e., pneumothorax, bronchial intubation, pulmonary edema, or partial ETT obstruction) must be ruled out. Once bronchospasm is assumed to be present, 100 percent oxygen and an increased concentration of inhalation agent are delivered. If increasing anesthetic depth does not resolve the bronchospasm, the β-agonists (e.g., terbutaline, albuterol) are the drugs of choice, usually given in nebulized form. Terbutaline can also be given subcutaneously 5 to 10 μg/kg. This mode of administration is particularly useful for the severely bronchospastic patient in whom a nebulized drug may not be effective. Steroids are also appropriate, although their slow onset of action limits their utility in an episode of acute bronchospasm. The anticholinergics should be viewed as useful adjuncts. The xanthines should be used with caution,

given their propensity to cause arrhythmias, particularly during halothane anesthesia.

A slow, smooth emergence from anesthesia minimizes the risk of bronchospasm. Therefore, unless contraindicated by other considerations, the trachea is extubated while the patient is still deeply anesthetized and is taken to the recovery room for postoperative observation and care.

If a deep extubation is contraindicated, the patient is left intubated, although the presence of the ETT may stimulate bronchospasm as airway reflexes return. A slow emergence from anesthesia achieved by the use of IV opioids may improve the patient's tolerance of the ETT and decrease the incidence and severity of bronchospasm.

Cystic Fibrosis

Cystic fibrosis (CF) is the most common cause of progressive chronic respiratory disease in childhood and accounts for a large proportion of pediatric deaths caused by respiratory failure. The incidence of this autosomal recessive disease is approximately 1 in 2,000.[333] In the last 15 years, the gene responsible for CF has been located on chromosome 7.[334, 335] Several mutations in the gene have been identified causing altered chloride transport in epithelium, presumably the cause of abnormal exocrine secretions in patients with CF.[336–338] The result is altered electrolyte content and viscid mucus production leading to exocrine gland duct obstruction common to all CF patients.

Although several organ systems become involved, it is the pulmonary pathology that limits life expectancy and is of most concern to the anesthesiologist. As shown in Figure 17–28, the combination of viscous tracheobronchial secretions and defective mucociliary transport results in obstruction, chronic infection, and tissue destruction. Bronchiectasis, fibrosis, and airway obstruction lead to progressive respiratory insufficiency, eventually resulting in death.

Pulmonary function abnormalities include increased airway resistance, gas trapping, increased FRC, and a decrease in the FEV_1 and vital capacity. Pulmonary fibrosis and intraluminal secretions cause areas of low $\dot{V}/\dot{Q}$ ratios, resulting in lowered Pao_2. $Paco_2$ is usually low or normal; the presence of an elevated $Paco_2$ usually indicates advanced disease. Such patients may rely entirely on hypoxic respiratory drive; when oxygen must be given, assisted or control ventilation may be required. Many patients with

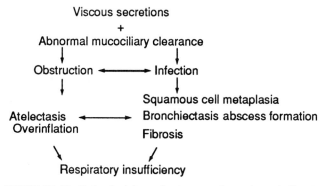

FIGURE 17–28. Pathophysiology of pulmonary disease in cystic fibrosis.

CF have bronchial hyperactivity, requiring bronchodilator therapy.[339] In addition to reducing airway resistance, bronchodilators may enhance clearance of mucus by stimulating ciliary movement.[340] Nebulized recombinant human DNAase may also improve lung function; DNA is a major component of viscid pulmonary secretions, and DNA breakdown improves secretion clearance.[341]

The pulmonary disease, in particular the chronic hypoxemia, leads to cor pulmonale, with cardiomegaly, hepatomegaly, fluid retention, and hypoalbuminemia. Liver dysfunction, in turn, leads to low levels of plasma cholinesterase and of clotting factors II, VII, IX, and X.[342]

The time course of pulmonary deterioration has been greatly prolonged in the last 30 years by improved care, although it is unclear which aspects of care have been most important. Antibiotics are often used to treat chronic pulmonary infection, thereby decreasing both the inflammation within the lung and perhaps the viscosity of sputum. Clinical improvement commonly follows the use of antibiotics, although complete eradication of organisms (frequently *Pseudomonas*) rarely occurs and, when achieved, is transient. Nebulized tobramycin may improve control of pulmonary infection.[343] Chest physiotherapy, including coughing, vibration, and postural drainage, is advocated to enhance removal of airway secretions. Humidified oxygen therapy is provided for patients with severe lung disease to prevent the complications of chronic hypoxemia, including cor pulmonale.[344] Adequate nutrition, supplemented with pancreatic enzymes and fat-soluble vitamins, may retard progression of pulmonary disease. The use of bronchodilators is controversial, although terbutaline may enhance mucociliary clearance by directly stimulating ciliary movement.[340]

Anesthetic Management

The most common surgical procedures performed on patients with cystic fibrosis include nasal polypectomy, vascular access, bronchoscopy, pleural stripping, and (in the neonate) laparotomy for meconium ileus.[345] For patients with cor pulmonale or end-stage pulmonary disease, heart–lung or lung transplantation is also performed.[346] Preoperative evaluation of patients with CF is important in minimizing postanesthetic morbidity; an attempt should be made to quantitate the severity of pulmonary disease. The degree of exercise intolerance and quantity of sputum production are important historical features. Signs of respiratory distress, respiratory rate, cardiomegaly or a loud second heart sound, quality of breath sounds, liver enlargement, and peripheral edema or cyanosis constitute evidence of cardiopulmonary compromise. If cor pulmonale is suspected a preoperative ECG and echocardiogram should be obtained. If a nasal intubation is planned, the turbinates are examined for polyps. Pulmonary function tests can quantitate pulmonary compromise in patients old enough to cooperate, although they do not necessarily predict postoperative complications. Hypoxemia or hypercarbia may be seen on arterial blood gas analysis in patients with significant respiratory disease. Liver function tests are useful in screening patients for hepatic involvement.

Every attempt is made to improve the pulmonary status preoperatively. A regular program of chest physiotherapy is begun, including chest percussion and postural drainage. Sputum samples are sent for culture and sensitivity, and the patient receives an aminoglycoside and a synthetic penicillin until culture results are available. The patient is well hydrated to prevent further inspissation of secretions. Patients not on oral vitamin K supplements are given parenteral vitamin K.

Premedication with a benzodiazepine or a barbiturate is designed to relieve anxiety. Atropine is also generally avoided because it may inhibit clearance of secretions, although atropine administration has not been associated with an increase in pulmonary complications.

Regional anesthesia may be useful for extremity procedures, although high-level spinal or epidural anesthesia depresses the ability to cough and should be avoided. Coagulopathy should be ruled out before regional conduction anesthesia is performed. If a general anesthetic is required, halothane is useful because it allows rapid induction of an emergence from anesthesia, is potent enough to allow administration of high-concentration oxygen, and is bronchodilating. In older patients with severe lung disease, inhalation induction or anesthesia may be slowed because of marked $\dot{V}/\dot{Q}$ mismatching.

In most patients with cystic fibrosis who receive a general anesthetic, the trachea is intubated to facilitate airway control and to permit suctioning of secretions. Most complications reported are caused by difficulties with secretions, airway irritability, and oxygenation.[347] A cuffed ETT is used for patients with severe lung disease because poor chest compliance necessitates high airway pressures for adequate ventilation. Ventilation generally is assisted or controlled to prevent intraoperative loss of lung volume and subsequent atelectasis. All delivered gases are humidified, and IV hydration is maintained to facilitate clearance of secretions. Tracheal suctioning is performed during the procedure as necessary. All cystic fibrosis patients are at risk for rupture of emphysematous bullae, resulting in pneumothorax.

At the conclusion of surgery, the patient is allowed to awaken with the ETT in place. Adequate reversal of neuromuscular blocking agents is confirmed with a nerve stimulator and the trachea is extubated after thorough suctioning and demonstration of adequate gas exchange.

During the postoperative period, the patient with cystic fibrosis is at risk for respiratory failure and arrest, pneumothorax, pneumonia, atelectasis, and airway obstruction. Reductions in flow rates and lung volumes have been documented in patients with cystic fibrosis after general anesthesia. For high-risk patients, an ICU should be considered for close observation, continued IV hydration, airway humidification, chest physiotherapy, and antibiotics. Postoperative analgesia, if desired, can be provided with low-dose narcotics or with intercostal nerve blocks or epidural opioids.

Bronchopulmonary Dysplasia
Definition

The advances of the past three decades in extending the limits of viability after premature birth to smaller and smaller infants has created a new population of infants and children. The lungs of the survivors of high-technology neonatal intensive care units (NICUs) frequently bear the residual effects of hyaline membrane disease and its treatments, oxygen, and positive airway pressure. The deleterious effects of these life-saving therapies result in a variable constellation of parenchymal abnormalities termed bronchopulmonary dysplasia (BPD). These abnormalities include pulmonary fibrosis, acquired lobar emphysema, tracheo- and bronchomalacia, reactive airway disease, and chronic inflammatory bronchitis. BPD has a wide spectrum of manifestations, from the child whose only abnormality may be radiologic to the severely impaired steroid-dependent infant with chronic respiratory insufficiency, ventilator dependency, cor pulmonale, and growth failure.

Common surgical procedures performed for graduates of NICUs are often directly related to the effects of prematurity or its therapy, such as hydrocephalus, tracheal stenosis, tracheomalacia, acquired lobar emphysema, patent ductus arteriosus, malabsorption requiring total parenteral nutrition, or inguinale hernia, to name a few.[348] Lung transplantation has even been suggested as therapy for some children with severe BPD.[349] Gastroesophageal reflux associated with pulmonary disease may require surgical treatment if medical management fails.[350]

Anesthetic Management

During the preoperative evaluation, the anesthesiologist should evaluate the degree of pulmonary impairment, as manifested by the requirement for oxygen and positive airway pressure. Children with BPD are usually treated with supplemental oxygen, especially during sleep, to minimize secondary pulmonary vascular changes that occur with intermittent hypoxia. Moderate and severe BPD are often associated with CO_2 retention, which produces a compensatory metabolic alkalosis, hypochloremia, and hypokalemia. These electrolyte abnormalities are accentuated by the use of loop diuretics.

The presence of cor pulmonale and pulmonary hypertension is suggested by accentuation of the pulmonic component of the second heart sound; by hepatomegaly; and by right axis deviation, right ventricular hypertrophy, and right atrial enlargement on ECG. Echocardiography may be helpful in confirming the presence of right-sided cardiac dilation. Patients with over right ventricular failure may benefit preoperatively from digitalis and diuretics.

Preoperative evaluation also should focus on other systems secondarily affected by the abnormalities of the lungs and heart. Chronically mechanically ventilated infants who have been chronically exposed to sedatives or opioids may exhibit remarkable tolerance to opioids and benzodiazepines. Growth failure and chronic malnutrition, with secondary hypoproteinemia, may affect the pharmacology of anesthetic drugs (see Chapter 3). Poorly controlled cor pulmonale, with passive hepatic congestion, may also impair hepatic clearance of drugs. Prolonged diuretic therapy may cause calcium wasting, nephrocalcinosis, and impaired renal function. Infants treated with long-term corticosteroids should be considered as having adrenal insufficiency and should be treated with pharmacologic "stress" doses of steroids in the perioperative period. Infants with a history of intraventricular hemorrhage may be at risk for seizure disorders. Finally, the risk of apnea in the former premature infant has been well established (see Chapter 15), and should influence the decision regarding ambulatory surgery for the less severely affected child with BPD.[351–354]

Intraoperative management of the child with BPD depends entirely on the severity of the underlying pulmonary disease and on the nature of the surgery being performed. Many infants with BPD have borderline right ventricular function and tolerate overhydration poorly. Therefore, careful attention should be paid to the quantity of IV fluid and to the sodium load administered. $\dot{V}/\dot{Q}$ inequality may be worsened by PPV, by directing ventilation preferentially to emphysematous segments of lung to the exclusion of more physiologically normal lung. Instrumentation of the trachea under inadequate anesthesia may promote bronchospasm and increase the quantity of mucous secretions in the airway.

Several centers have expressed enthusiasm for regional anesthetic techniques in lieu of general anesthesia, in the hope that the former would be associated with a lower incidence or severity of postoperative apnea.[354–358] Currently, the published experience with spinal anesthesia remains too small for definitive conclusions regarding the reduction of postoperative apnea. However, intuitively one would expect that a well-conducted regional anesthetic might successfully avoid many of the cardiorespiratory complications associated with general anesthesia. This must be balanced against the relative loss of control of the airway with regional anesthesia, as well as the inability to titrate spinal anesthesia. Without the benefit of randomized controlled studies to compare these anesthetic techniques in this patient population, the putative risks and benefits of each technique must be weighed on a case-by-case basis.

REFERENCES

1. Well LJ, Boyden EA: The development of bronchopulmonary segments in human embryos of horizons XVII to XIX. Am J Anat 95:153, 1954.
2. Bucher U, Reid L: Development of the intrasegmental bronchial tree: the pattern of branching and development of cartilage at various stages of intrauterine life. Thorax 16:207, 1961.
3. Loosli CG, Potter EL: Pre- and post-natal development of the respiratory portion of the human lung. Am Rev Respir Dis 80:5, 1959.
4. Campiche M: Les inclusions lamellaires des cellules alvéolaires, dans le poumon duration: relations entre l'ultrastructure et la fixation. J Ultrastruct Res 3:302, 1960.
5. Davies GM, Reid L: Growth of the alveoli and pulmonary arteries in childhood. Thorax 25:669, 1970.
6. Hislop AA, Wigglesworth JS, Desai R: Alveolar development in the human fetus and infant. Early Hum Dev 13:1, 1986.
7. Langston C, Kida K, Reed M, Thurlbeck WM: Human lung growth in late gestation and in the neonate. Am Rev Respir Dis 129:607, 1984.
8. Hogg JC, Williams J, Richardson B, et al: Age as a factor in the distribution of lower airway conductance and in the pathologic anatomy of obstructive lung disease. N Engl J Med 282:1283, 1970.
9. Elliott FW, Reid L: Some unfamiliar facts about the pulmonary artery and its branching pattern. Clin Radiol 16:193, 1965.
10. Hislop A, Reid L: Intrapulmonary arterial development during childhood: branching pattern and structure. Thorax 28:129, 1973.

11. Hislop A, Reid L: Intrapulmonary arterial development during fetal life—branching pattern and structure. J Anat 113:35, 1972.
12. Lyrene RK, Philips JB: Control of pulmonary vascular resistance in the fetus and newborn. Clin Perinatol 11:551, 1984.
13. Enhorning G, Adams FH, Norman A: Effect of lung expansion on the fetal lamb circulation. Acta Pediatr Scand 55:441, 1966.
14. Rudolph AM: The changes in the circulation after birth: their importance in congenital heart disease. Circulation 41:343, 1970.
15. Oh W, Lind J, Gessner JH: The circulatory and respiratory adaptations to early and late cord clamping in new born infants. Acta Paediatr Scand 55:17, 1966.
16. Gessner I, Krovetz LJ, Benson RW, et al: Hemodynamic adaptations in the newborn infant. Pediatrics 36:752, 1965.
17. Luscher TF: Endothelium derived nitric oxide: the endogenous nitro-vasodilator in the human cardiovascular system. Eur Heart J 12(Suppl E):2, 1991.
18. Haworth SG, Reid LR: Persistent fetal circulation—newly recognized structural features. J Pediatr 88:614, 1976.
19. Gersony WM, Duc CV, Sinclair JD: "PFC" syndrome (persistence of the fetal circulation). Circulation 40(Suppl III):87, 1969.
20. Hislop A, Reid L: Development of the acinus in the human lung. Thorax 29:90, 1974.
21. Pierce J, Hobcott J: Studies on the collagen and elastin content of the human lung. J Clin Invest 39:8, 1960.
22. Mansell A, Bryan C, Levison H: Airway closure in children. J Appl Physiol 33:711, 1972.
23. Krahl VE: Anatomy of the mammalian lung. In Fenn WO, Rahn H (eds): Handbook of Physiology. Section 3: Respiration. Vol 1. Washington, DC, American Physiological Society, 1964, p 472.
24. Jordanoglou J: Vector analysis of rib movement. Respir Physiol 10:109, 1970.
25. Froese AR, Bryan CA: Effects of anesthesia and paralysis on diaphragmatic mechanics in man. Anesthesiology 41:242, 1974.
26. Wulff EK, Aulin I: The regional lung function in the lateral decubitus position during anesthesia and operation. Acta Anaesthesiol Scand 16:195, 1972.
27. Zack MR, Pontoppidan H, Kazemi H: The effect of lateral positions on gas exchange in pulmonary disease: a prospective evaluation. Am Rev Respir Dis 110:49, 1974.
28. Remolina C, Khan AU, Santiago TV, et al: Positional hypoxemia in unilateral lung disease. N Engl J Med 304:523, 1981.
29. Rheder K, Wenthe PM, Sessler AD: Function of each lung during mechanical ventilation with SEEP and with PEEP in man anesthetized with thiopental-meperidine. Anesthesiology 39:597, 1973.
30. Heaf DP, Hehns P, Gordon I, et al: Postural effects of gas exchange in infants. N Engl J Med 308:1505, 1983.
31. Davies H, Kitchman R, Gordon I, et al: Regional ventilation in infancy. N Engl J Med 313:1626, 1985.
32. Cherniak NS, Longobardo GS: Oxygen and carbon dioxide gas stores of the body. Physiol Rev 50:196, 1970.
33. Cummingham DJC: The control system regulating breathing in man. Q Rev Biophys 6:433, 1974.
34. Leusen I: Regulation of cerebrospinal fluid composition with reference to breathing. Physiol Rev 52:1, 1972.
35. Rigatto H, Brady JP: Periodic breathing and apnea in the preterm infant. I. Evidence for hypoventilation possibly due to central depression. Pediatrics 50:202, 1971.
36. Newman R, Cleveland DC: Three dimensional reconstruction of ultrafast chest CT for diagnosis and operative planning in a child with right pneumonectomy syndrome. Chest 106:973, 1994.
37. Motoyama EK, Glazener CH: Hypoxemia after general anesthesia in children. Anesth Analg 65:267, 1986.
38. Polgar G, Promadhat V: Pulmonary Function Testing in Children: Techniques and Standards. Philadelphia, WB Saunders Company, 1971.
39. Gracey DR, Divertie MB, Didier EP: Preoperative pulmonary preparation of patients with chronic obstructive pulmonary disease. Chest 76:123, 1979.
40. Deutsch S, Dalen JE: Indications for prophylactic digitalization. Anesthesiology 30:648, 1969.
41. American Society of Anesthesiologists House of Delegates Standards of Basic Anesthetic Monitoring, October 21, 1998.
42. Badgwell TM, Heavner JE, May WS, et al: End-tidal P_{CO_2} monitoring in infants and children ventilated with either a partial rebreathing or a non-rebreathing circuit. Anesthesiology 66:405, 1987.
43. Raemer DB, Francis D, Philip JH, et al: Variation in P_{CO_2} between arterial blood and peak expired gas during anesthesia. Anesth Analg 62:1065, 1983.
44. Lynn AM, Slattery JT: Morphine pharmacokinetics in early infancy. Anesthesiology 66:136, 1987.
45. Weinrich Al, Silvay G, Lumb PD: Continuous ketamine infusion for one lung anesthesia. Can Anaesth Soc J 27:485, 1980.
46. Bjertnaes LJ, Hauge A, Torgrinsen T: The pulmonary vasoconstriction response to hypoxia. The hypoxia-sensitive site studied with a volatile inhibitor. Acta Physiol Scand 109:447, 1980.
47. Lumb PD, Silvay G, Weinreich A, et al: A comparison of the effects of continuous ketamine infusion and halothane on oxygenation during one lung anesthesia in dogs. Can Anaesth Soc J 26:394, 1979.
48. Benumof JL, Wahrenbrock EA: Local effects of anesthetics on regional hypoxic pulmonary vasoconstriction. Anesthesiology 43:525, 1975.
49. Bjertnaes L, Hauge A, Kriz M: Hypoxia induced pulmonary vasoconstriction: effects of fentanyl following different routes of administration. Acta Anaesthesiol Scand 24:53, 1980.
50. Gibbs JM, Johnson H: Lack of effect of morphine and buprenorphine on hypoxic pulmonary vasoconstriction in the isolated perfused cat lung and the perfused lobe of the dog lung. Br J Anaesth 50:1197, 1978.
51. Bjertnaes LJ, Mundal R, Hauge A, et al: Vascular resistance in atelectatic lungs. Effect of inhalation anesthetics. Acta Anaesthesiol Scand 24:109, 1980.
52. Marshall C, Lindgren L, Marshall RE: The effect of inhalation anesthetics on HPV [abstract]. Anesthesiology 59:A527, 1983.
53. Sykes MK, Davies DM, Chakrabarti MK, et al: The effects of halothane, trichlorethylene and ether on the hypoxic pressor response and pulmonary vascular resistance in the isolated, perfused lung. Br J Anaesth 45:655, 1973.
54. Gibbs JM, Sykes MK, Tart AR: Effects of halothane and hydrogen ion concentration on the alteration of pulmonary vascular resistance induced by graded alveolar hypoxia in the isolated perfused cat lung. Anaesth Intensive Care 2:231, 1974.
55. Loh L, Sykes MK, Chakrabarti MK: The effects of halothane and ether on the pulmonary circulation in the isolated perfused cat lung. Br J Anaesth 49:309, 1977.
56. Babjak AF, Forrest JB: Effects of halothane on the pulmonary vascular response to hypoxia in dogs. Can Anaesth Soc J 26:6, 1979.
57. Sykes MK, Gibbs JM, Loh L, et al: Preservation of the pulmonary vasoconstrictor response to alveolar hypoxia during the administration of halothane to dogs. Br J Anaesth 50:1185, 1978.
58. Mathers J, Benumof JL, Wahrenbrock EA: General anesthetics and regional hypoxic pulmonary vasoconstriction. Anesthesiology 46:111, 1977.
59. Bjertnaes LJ: Hypoxia induced pulmonary vasoconstriction in man: inhibition due to diethyl ether and halothane anesthesia. Acta Anaesthesiol Scand 22:570, 1978.
60. Saidman LJ, Troudsale FR: Isoflurane does not inhibit hypoxic pulmonary vasoconstriction. Anesthesiology 57:A472, 1982.
61. Rogers SN, Benumof JL: Halothane and isoflurane do not decrease PaO_2 during one lung ventilation in intravenously anesthetized patients. Anesth Analg 64:946, 1985.
62. Augustine SD, Benumof JL: Halothane and isoflurane do not impair arterial oxygenation during one lung ventilation in patients undergoing thoracotomy. Anesthesiology 61:A484, 1984.
63. Marshall C, Marshall BE: Site and sensitivity for stimulation of hypoxic pulmonary vasoconstriction. J Appl Physiol 55:711, 1983.
64. Domino KB, Borowec L, Alexander CM, et al: Influence of isoflurane on hypoxic pulmonary vasoconstriction in dogs. Anesthesiology 64:423, 1986.
65. Bjertnaes LJ, Mundal R: The pulmonary vasoconstrictor response to hypoxia during enflurane anesthesia. Acta Anaesthesiol Scand 24:252, 1980.
66. Sykes MK, Hurtig JR, Tait AR, et al: Reduction of hypoxic pulmonary constriction in the dog during administration of nitrous oxide. Br J Anaesth 49:301, 1977.
67. Hasnain JU, Krasna MJ, Barker SJ, et al: Anesthetic considerations for thoracoscopic procedures. J Cardiothorac Vasc Anesth 6:624, 1992.
68. Benumof JL: Separation of the two lungs (double-lumen tube intubation). In Benumof JL (ed): Anesthesia for Thoracic Surgery. Philadelphia, WB Saunders Company, 1987, p 223.

69. Bloch EC: Tracheo-bronchial angles in infants and children. Anesthesiology 65:236, 1986.
70. Watson CR, Rowe EA, Rurk W: One-lung anesthesia for pediatric surgery: a new use for the fiberoptic bronchoscope. Anesthesiology 56:314, 1982.
71. Vale R: Selective bronchial blocking in a small child. Br J Anaesth 41:453, 1969.
72. Hammer GB, Manos SJ, Smith BM, et al: Single lung ventilation in pediatric patients. Anesthesiology 84:1503, 1996.
73. Inoue H, Shohtsua A, Ogawa J, et al: Endotracheal tube with movable blocker to prevent aspiration of intratracheal bleeding. Ann Thorac Surg 37:497, 1984.
74. Rao CC, Krishna G, Grosfeld JL, Weber TR: One lung pediatric anaesthesia. Anesth Analg 60:450, 1981.
75. Hogg CE, Lorhan PH: Pediatric bronchial blocking. Anesthesiology 33:560, 1970.
76. Cay DL, Csenderits LE, Lines V, et al: Selective bronchial blocking in children. Anaesth Intensive Care 3:117, 1975.
77. Benumof JL, Mathers JM, Wahrenbrock EA: Cyclic hypoxic pulmonary vasoconstriction induced by concomitant carbon dioxide changes. J Appl Physiol 41:466, 1976.
78. Benumof JL, Rogers SN, Moyce PR, et al: Hypoxic pulmonary vasoconstriction and whole lung PEEP in the dog. Anesthesiology 51:503, 1979.
79. Katz JA, Laverue RG, Fairley HB, et al: Pulmonary oxygen exchange during endobronchial anesthesia: effects of tidal volume and PEEP. Anesthesiology 56:164, 1982.
80. Johansen I, Benumof JL: Flow distribution in abnormal lung as a function of FIO2. Anesthesiology 51:369, 1979.
81. Dansker DR, Wagner PD, West JB: Instability of lung units with low $\dot{V}/\dot{Q}$ ratios during O2 breathing. J Appl Physiol 38:886, 1975.
82. Ballantyne JC, Carr DB, deFerranti S, et al: The comparative effects of postoperative analgesic therapies on pulmonary outcome: cumulative meta-analyses of randomized, controlled trials. Anesth Analg 86:598, 1998.
83. Pflug AE, Murphy TM, Butler SH, Tucker, GT: The effects of postoperative peridural analgesia on pulmonary therapy and pulmonary complications. Anesthesiology 41:8, 1974.
84. Kaplan JA, Miller ED, Gallagher EG: Postoperative analgesia for thoracotomy patients. Anesth Analg 54:773, 1974.
85. Bridenbaugh PO, DuPen S, Moore DC, et al: Postoperative intercostal nerve block analgesia versus narcotic analgesia. Anesth Analg 52:81, 1973.
86. Galway JE, Caves PK, Dundee JW: Effect of intercostal nerve blockade during operation on lung function and the relief of pain following thoracotomy. Br J Anaesth 47:730, 1975.
87. Moore DC: Intercostal nerve block for postoperative somatic pain following surgery of thorax and upper abdomen. Br J Anaesth 47:284, 1975.
88. Braid DP, Scott DD: The systemic absorption of local anesthetic drugs. Br J Anaesth 37:934, 1965.
89. Moore DC, Bush WH, Scurlock JE: Intercostal nerve block: a roentgenographic anatomic study of technique and absorption in humans. Anesth Analg 59:815, 1980.
90. Downs CS, Cooper MG: Continuous extrapleural intercostal nerve block for post thoracotomy analgesia in children. Anaesth Intensive Care 25:390, 1997.
91. Swinhoe CF, Pereira NH: Intrapleural analgesia in a child with a mediastinal tumor. Can J Anaesth 41:427, 1994.
92. McIlvaine WB, Knox RF, Fennesse PV, Goldstein M: Continuous infusion of bupivacaine via intrapleural catheter for analgesia after thoracotomy in children. Anesthesiology 69:261, 1988.
93. Queen JS, Kahana MD, Difazia CA, et al: An evaluation of interpleural analgesia with etidocaine in children. Anesth Analg 68:S228, 1989.
94. McIlvaine WB, Chang JHT, Jones M: The effective use of intrapleural bupivacaine for analgesia after thoracic and subcostal incisions in children. J Pediatr Surg 23:1184, 1988.
95. Holland R, Anderson B, Watson T, McCall E: Introduction of continuous regional anesthetic techniques for postoperative paediatric patients: one year's experience from two hospitals. N Z Med J 107:80, 1994.
96. Tobias JD, Marin LD, Oakes L, et al: Postoperative analgesia following thoracotomy in children: intrapleural catheters. J Pediatr Surg 28:1466, 1993.
97. Dauphin A, Gupta RN, Young JE: Serum bupivicaine concentrations during continuous extrapleural infusion. Can J Anaesth 44:367, 1997.
98. Agarwal R, Gutlove DP, Lockhart CH: Seizures occurring in pediatric patients receiving continuous infusion of bupivacaine. Anesth Analg 75:284, 1992.
99. Semsroth M, Plattner O, Horcher E: Effective pain relief with continuous intrapleural bupivicaine after thoracotomy in infants and children. Paediatr Anaesth 6:303, 1996.
100. Berde CB: Convulsions associated with pediatric regional anesthesia. Anesth Analg 75:284, 1992.
101. Riegleer FX: IPA: unreliable benefit after thoracotomy—epidural is a better choice. J Cardiothorac Vasc Anesth 10:429, 1996.
102. Schneider RF, Villamena PC, Harvey J, et al: Lack of efficacy of intrapleural bupivacaine for postoperative analgesia following thoracotomy. Chest 103:414, 1993.
103. Bosenberg A, Bland B, Schulte-Steinberg O, Downing J: Thoracic epidural anesthesia via caudal route in infants. Anesthesiology 69:265, 1988.
104. Gunter J, Eng C: Thoracic epidural anesthesia via the caudal approach in children. Anesthesiology 76:935, 1992.
105. Rosen K, Rosen D, Bank E: Caudal morphine for postoperative pain control in children undergoing cardiac surgery. Anesthesiology 67:A510, 1987.
106. Haberkern C, Lynn A, Geiduschek J, Jacobson L: Epidural and intravenous bolus morphine for postoperative analgesia in infants. Can J Anaesth 43:1203, 1996.
107. Krane E, Tyler D, Jacobson L: The dose response of caudal morphine in children. Anesthesiology 71:48, 1989.
108. Murrell D, Gibson P, Cohen R: Continuous epidural analgesia in newborn infants undergoing major surgery. J Pediatr Surg 28:548, 1993.
109. Flandin-Blety C, Barrier G: Accidents following extradural analgesia in children. The results of a retrospective study. Paediatr Anaesth 5:41, 1995.
110. Giufre E, Dalens B, Gombert A: Epidemiology and morbidity of regional anesthesia in children: a one-year prospective survey of the French language society of pediatric anesthesiologists. Anesth Analg 83:904, 1996.
111. Vandermeulen EP, Van Aken H, Vermylen J: Anticoagulants and spinal-epidural anesthesia. Anesth Analg 79:1165, 1994.
112. Rao T, El-Etr A: Anticoagulation following placement of epidural and subarachnoid catheters: an evaluation of neurologic sequelae. Anesthesiology 55:618, 1981.
113. Ladd WE, Gross RE: Congenital diaphragmatic hernia. N Engl J Med 223:917, 1940.
114. Iriani I: Experimental study on embryogenesis of congenital diaphragmatic hernia. Anat Embryol 169:133, 1984.
115. deLorimer AA, Tierney DF, Parker HR: Hypoplastic lungs in fetal lambs with surgically produced congenital diaphragmatic hernia. Surgery 62:12, 1967.
116. Kitagawa N, Hislop A, Boyden EA, Reid L: Lung hypoplasia in congenital diaphragmatic hernia. A quantitative study of airway, artery, and alveolar development. Br J Surg 58:342, 1971.
117. Areechon W, Reid L: Hypoplasia of lung with congenital diaphragmatic hernia. BMJ 1:230, 1963.
118. Reale FR, Esterly JR: Pulmonary hypoplasia: a morphometric study of the lungs of infants with diaphragmatic hernia, anencephaly and renal malformations. Pediatrics 51:91, 1973.
119. Bohn D, Tamura M, Perrin D, et al: Ventilatory predictors of pulmonary hypoplasia in congenital diaphragmatic hernia, confirmed by morphologic assessment. J Pediatr 11:423, 1987.
120. Levin DL: Morphologic analysis of pulmonary vascular bed in congenital left-sided diaphragmatic hernia. J Pediatr 92:805, 1978.
121. Naeye RL, Shochat SJ, Whitman V, Naisels NJ: Unsuspected pulmonary vascular abnormalities associated with diaphragmatic hernia. Pediatrics 58:902, 1976.
122. West WW, Bengston K, Rescorla FJ, et al: Delayed surgical repair and ECMO improves survival in congenital diaphragmatic hernia. Ann Surg 216:454, 1992.
123. Bray RJ: Congenital diaphragmatic hernia. Anaesthesia 34:567, 1979.
124. Adzick NS, Harrison MR, Glick PL, et al: Diaphragmatic hernia in the fetus: prenatal diagnosis and outcome in 94 cases. J Pediatr Surg 20:357, 1985.
125. Adzick NS, Vacanti JP, Lillehei CW, et al: Fetal diaphragmatic hernia: ultrasound diagnosis and clinical outcome in 38 cases. J Pediatr Surg 24:654, 1989.

126. Raphaely RC, Downes JJ: Congenital diaphragmatic hernia: prediction of survival. J Pediatr Surg 8:815, 1973.
127. Wilson JM, Lund DP, Lillehei CW, Vacanti JP: Congenital diaphragmatic hernia: predictors of severity in the ECMO era. J Pediatr Surg 26:1028, 1991.
128. Greenwood RD, Rosental A, Nadas AS: Cardiovascular abnormalities associated with congenital diaphragmatic hernia. Pediatrics 57:92, 1976.
129. Rowe MI, Uribe FL: Diaphragmatic hernia in the newborn infant: blood gas and pH considerations. Surgery 70:758, 1971.
130. Sakai H, Tamura M, Hosokawa Y, et al: Effect of surgical repair on respiratory mechanics in congenital diaphragmatic hernia. J Pediatr 111:432, 1987.
131. Hazebroek FWJ, Tibboel D, Bos AP, et al: Congenital diaphragmatic hernia: impact of preoperative stabilization. A prospective pilot study in 13 patients. J Pediatr Surg 23:1139, 1988.
132. Reyes C, Chang LK, Waffarn F, et al: Delayed repair of congenital diaphragmatic hernia with early high-frequency oscillatory ventilation during preoperative stabilization. J Pediatr Surg 33:1010, 1998.
133. German JC, Gazzaniga AB, Amile R, et al: Management of pulmonary insufficiency in diaphragmatic hernia using extracorporeal circulation with a membrane oxygenator (EMCO). J Pediatr Surg 12:905, 1977.
134. Truog RD, Schena JA, Hershenson MB, et al: Repair of congenital diaphragmatic hernia during extracorporeal membrane oxygenation. Anesthesiology 72:750, 1990.
135. Connors RH, Tracy T, Baily PV, et al: Congenital diaphragmatic hernia repair on ECMO. J Pediatr Surg 25:1043, 1990.
136. Wung JT, James LS, Kilchevsky E, James E: Management of infants with severe respiratory failure and persistence of fetal circulation without hyperventilation. Pediatrics 76:488, 1985.
137. Peckham GJ, Fox WW: Physiologic factors affecting pulmonary artery pressure in infants with persistent pulmonary hypertension. J Pediatr 93:1005, 1978.
138. Drummand WH, Gregory GA, Heymann MA, Phibbs RA: The independent effects of hyperventilation, tolaxoline, and dopamine on infants with persistent pulmonary hypertension. J Pediatr 98:603, 1981.
139. Dibbins AW, Wiener ES: Mortality from neonatal diaphragmatic hernia. J Pediatr Surg 9:653, 1974.
140. Goetzman BW, Sunshine P, Johnson JD, et al: Neonatal hypoxic and pulmonary vasospasm: response to tolazoline. J Pediatr 89:617, 1976.
141. Collins D, Pomerance JJ, Travis KW, et al: New approach to congenital posterolateral diaphragmatic hernia. J Pediatr Surg 12:149, 1977.
142. Maisels NJ, Shochat SJ, Friedman A, et al: Pulmonary vascular resistance in diaphragmatic hernia: response to tolazoline [abstract]. Pediatr Res 10:427, 1976.
143. Graham TP Jr, Atwood GF, Boucek RJ: Pharmacological dilatation of the ductus arteriosus with prostaglandin E1 in infants with congenital heart disease. South Med J 71:1238, 1978.
144. Soifer SJ, Morris FC III, Heymann MA: Prostaglandin D2 reverses induced pulmonary hypertension in the newborn lamb. J Pediatr 100:33, 1984.
145. Roberts JD, Polaner DM, Lang P, Zapol WM: Inhaled nitric oxide in persistent pulmonary hypertension of the newborn. Lancet 340:818, 1992.
146. Kinsella JP, Neish SR, Shaffer E, Abman SH: Low-dose inhalational nitric oxide in persistent pulmonary hypertension of the newborn. Lancet 340:819, 1992.
147. Frostell C, Fratacci MD, Wain JC, et al: Inhaled nitric oxide: a selective pulmonary vasodilator reversing hypoxic pulmonary vasoconstriction. Circulation 83:2038, 1991.
148. Lister J: Recent advances in the surgery of the diaphragm of the newborn. Prog Pediatr Surg 2:29, 1971.
149. Ehrlich FE, Salzberg AM: Pathophysiology and management of congenital posterolateral diaphragmatic hernias. Am Surgeon 44:26, 1978.
150. Boix-Ochoa J, Pegeuro G, Seijo G, et al: Acid-base balance and blood gases in prognosis and therapy of congenital diaphragmatic hernia. J Pediatr Surg 9:49, 1974.
151. Stolar CJ, Snedecor SS, Bartlett RH: Extracorporeal membrane oxygenation and neonatal respiratory failure: experience from the Extracorporeal Life Support Organization. J Pediatr Surg 26:563, 1991.

152. Extracorporeal Life Support Organization (ELSO) Registry, Ann Arbor, MI, September, 1993.
153. Barlett RH, Andrews AF, Toomasian JM, et al: Extracorporeal membrane oxygenation for newborn respiratory failure: forty-five cases. Surgery 92:425, 1982.
154. Andres AF, Zwischenberger JB, Cilley RE, Drake KL: Veno-venous extracorporeal membrane oxygenation (ECMO) using a double-lumen catheter. Artif Organs 33:429, 1987.
155. Levy FH, O'Rourke PP, Crone RK: Extracorporeal membrane oxygenation, review article. Anaesth Analg 75:1053, 1992.
156. Bartlett RH, Gazzaniga AB, Toomasian J, et al: Extracorporeal membrane oxygenation (ECMO) in neonatal respiratory failure: 100 cases. Ann Surg 204:236, 1986.
157. Glass P, Miller M, Short B: Morbidity for survivors of extracorporeal membrane oxygenation: neurodevelopment outcome at 1 year of age. Pediatrics 83:72, 1989.
158. Hofkosh D, Thompson AE, Nozza RJ, et al: Ten years of extracorporeal membrane oxygenation: neurodevelopmental outcome. Pediatrics 87:549, 1991.
159. Coleman DM, Geiduschek JM: Use of extracorporeal membrane oxygenation for the treatment of persistent pulmonary hypertension: an anesthesiologist's perspective. In Eisencraft JB (ed): Progress in Anesthesiology. Vol XI. San Antonio, TX, Dannemiller Memorial Education Foundation, 1997, p 323.
160. Wilson JM, Bower LK, Fackler, et al: Aminocaproic acid decreases the incidence of intracranial hemorrhage and other hemorrhagic complications of ECMO. J Pediatr Surg 28:536, 1993.
161. O'Rourke PP, Lillehei CW, Crone RK, Vacanti JP: The effect of extracorporeal membrane oxygenation (ECMO) on the survival of neonates with high-risk congenital diaphragmatic hernia: 45 cases from a single institution. J Pediatr Surg 26:147, 1991.
162. Clark RH, Hardin WD, Hirsch RB, et al: Current surgical management of congenital diaphragmatic hernia: a report from the Congenital Diaphragmatic Hernia Study Group. J Pediatr Surg 33:1004, 1998.
163. Anonymous: Inhaled nitric oxide and hypoxic respiratory failure in infants with congenital diaphragmatic hernia. The Neonatal Inhaled Nitric Oxide Study Group (NINOS). Pediatrics 99:838, 1997.
164. Ssemakula N, Stewart DL, Goldsmith LJ, et al: Survival of patients with congenital diaphragmatic hernia during the ECMO era: an 11 year experience. J Pediatr Surg 32:1683, 1997.
165. Weber TR, Kountzman B, Dillon PA, Silen ML: Improved survival in congenital diaphragmatic hernia with evolving therapeutic strategies. Arch Surg 133:498, 1998.
166. McGahren ED, Mallik K, Rogers BM: Neurologic outcome is diminished in survivors of congenital diaphragmatic hernia requiring extracorporeal oxygenation. J Pediatr Surg 32:1216, 1997.
167. Keshen TH, Gursoy M, Shew SB, et al: Does extracorporal membrane oxygenation benefit neonates with congenital diaphragmatic hernia? Application of a predictive equation. J Pediatr Surg 32:818, 1997.
168. Kerr AA: Lung function in children after repair of congenital diaphragmatic hernia. Arch Dis Child 52:902, 1977.
169. Landau LI, Phelan PD, Gillam GL, et al: Respiratory function after repair of congenital diaphragmatic hernia. Arch Dis Child 52:282, 1977.
170. Wohl MEB, Griscom NT, Strieder DJ, et al: The lung following repair of congenital diaphragmatic hernia. J Pediatr 90:405, 1977.
171. Reid IS, Hutcherson RJ: Long term follow-up of patients with congenital diaphragmatic hernia. J Pediatr Surg 11:939, 1976.
172. Chatrath RR, El Shafie M, Jones RS: Fate of hypoplastic lungs after repair of congenital diaphragmatic hernia. Arch Dis Child 46:633, 1971.
173. Koop CE, Schnaufer L, Broennle AM: Esophageal atresia and tracheoesophageal fistula: supportive measures that affect survival. Pediatrics 54:558, 1974.
174. Calverley RK, Johnston AE: The anesthetic management of tracheoesophageal fistula: a review of ten years' experience. Can Anaesth Soc J 129:270, 1972.
175. Humphreys GH, Hogg BM, Ferrer J: Congenital atresia of the esophagus. J Thorac Surg 32:332, 1956.
176. Chen H, Goei GS, Hertzler JH: Family studies on congenital esophageal atresia with or without tracheoesophageal fistula. Birth Defects 15:117, 1979.
177. Gruenwald P: A case of atresia of the esophagus combined with tracheoesophageal fistula in a 9 mm human embryo, and its embryologic explanation. Anat Rec 78:293, 1940.

178. Quan L, Smith DW: The VATER association: vertebral defects, anal atresia, tracheoesophageal fistula with esophageal atresia, radial dysplasia. Birth Defects 8:75, 1972.

179. Gross RE: The Surgery of Infancy and Childhood. Philadelphia, WB Saunders Company, 1953.

180. Kluth D: Atlas of esophageal atresia. J Pediatr Surg 11:901, 1976.

181. Greenwood RD, Rosenthal A: Cardiovascular malformations associated with tracheoesophageal fistula and esophageal atresia. Pediatrics 57:87, 1976.

182. Andrassy RJ, Mahour GH: Gastrointestinal anomalies associated with esophageal atresia or tracheoesophageal fistula. Arch Surg 114:1125, 1979.

183. Koop CE: Recent advances in the surgery of esophageal atresia. Prog Pediatr Surg 2:41, 1971.

184. Korones SB, Evans LJ: Measurement of intragastric oxygen concentration for the diagnosis of H-type tracheoesophageal fistula. Pediatrics 60:450, 1977.

185. Cozzi F, Wilkinson AW: Low birth weight babies with esophageal atresia or tracheoesophageal fistula. Arch Dis Child 50:791, 1975.

186. Grosfeld JL, Ballantine TV: Esophageal atresia and tracheoesophageal fistula: effect of delayed thoracotomy on survival. Surgery 84:394, 1978.

187. Holder TN, McDonald VG, Woolley MW: The premature or critically ill infant with esophageal atresia: increased success with a staged approach. J Thorac Cardiovasc Surg 44:344, 1962.

188. Templeton JN, Templeton JJ, Schnaufer L, et al: Management of esophageal atresia and tracheoesophageal fistula in the neonate with severe respiratory distress syndrome. J Pediatr Surg 20:394, 1985.

189. Andropoulos DB, Rowe RW, Betts JM: Anaesthetic and surgical airway management during tracheo-oesophageal fistual repair. Paediatr Anaesth 8:313, 1998.

190. Baraka A, Slim N: Cardiac arrest during IPPV in a newborn with tracheoesophageal fistula. Anesthesiology 32:564, 1970.

191. Jones TB, Kirchner SG, Lee FA, Heller RM: Stomach rupture associated with esophageal atresia, tracheoesophageal fistula, and ventilatory assistance. Am J Radiol 134:675, 1980.

192. Salem MR, Wong AY, Lin YH, et al: Prevention of gastric distension during anesthesia for newborns with tracheoesophageal fistulas. Anesthesiology 38:82, 1973.

193. Reeves ST, Burt N, Smith CD: Is it time to reevaluate the airway management of tracheoesophageal fistual? Anesth Analg 81:866, 1995.

194. Filston HC, Chitwood WR Jr, Schkolne B, et al: The Fogarty balloon catheter as an aid to management of the infant with esophageal atresia and tracheoesophageal fistula complicated by severe RDS or pneumonia. J Pediatr Surg 17:149, 1982.

195. Karl HW: Control of life-threatening air leak after gastrostomy in an infant with respiratory distress syndrome and tracheoesophageal fistula. Anesthesiology 62:671, 1985.

196. Conroy PT, Bennett NR: Management of tracheomalacia in association with congenital tracheo-esophageal fistula. Br J Anaesth 59:1313, 1987.

197. Desjardins JG, Stephens CA, Moes CAF: Results of surgical treatment of congenital tracheoesophageal fistula with a note on cinefluorographic findings. Am Surg 160:141, 1964.

198. Laks H, Wilkinson RH, Schuster SR: Long term results following correction of esophageal atresia with tracheoesophageal fistula: a clinical and cinefluorographic study. J Pediatr Surg 7:591, 1972.

199. Dudley NE, Phelan PD: Respiratory complications in long term survivors of oesophageal atresia. Arch Dis Child 51:279, 1976.

200. Emery JL, Haddadin AJ: Squamous epithelium in respiratory tract of children with tracheoesophageal fistula. Arch Dis Child 46:236, 1971.

201. Milligan DWA, Levison H: Lung function in children following repair of tracheoesophageal fistula. J Pediatr 95:24, 1979.

202. Blumberg JB, Stevenson JK, Lemire RJ, Boyden EA: Laryngotracheoesophageal cleft, the embryologic implications: review of the literature. Surgery 57:559, 1965.

203. Benjamin B, Inglis A: Minor congenital laryngeal clefts: diagnosis and classification. Ann Otol Rhinol Laryngol 98:417, 1989.

204. Evans KL, Courtney-Harris R, Baily CM, et al: Management of posterior laryngeal and laryngotracheoesophageal clefts. Arch Otolaryngol Head Neck Surg 121:1380, 1995.

205. Donahoe PK, Gee PE: Complete laryngotracheoesophageal cleft: management and repair. J Pediatr Surg 19:143, 1984.

206. Ogawa T, Yamataka A, Miyanon T, et al: Treatment of laryngotracheoesophageal cleft. J Pediatr Surg 24:341, 1989.

207. Ryan DP, Muehrcke DD, Doody DP, et al: Laryngotracheoesophageal cleft (type IV): management and repair of lesions beyond the carina. J Pediatr Surg 26:962, 1991.

208. Ruder CV, Glaser LC: Anesthetic management of laryngotracheoesophageal cleft. Anesthesiology 47:65, 1977.

209. Pinlong E, Lesage V, Robert M, et al: Type III-IV laryngotracheoesophageal cleft: report of a successfully treated case. Int J Pediatr Otorhinolaryngol 36:253, 1996.

210. Carr MM, Clark KD, Webber E, Giacomartonio M: Congenital laryngotracheoesophageal cleft. J Otolaryngol 28:112, 1999.

211. Geiduschek JM, Inglis AF, O'Rourke PP, et al: Repair of a laryngotracheoesophageal cleft in an infant by means of extracorporeal membrane oxygenation. Ann Otol Rhino Laryngol 132:827, 1993.

212. Raynor AC, Capp NP, Sealy WC: Lobar emphysema of infancy. Ann Thorac Surg 4:374, 1967.

213. Cambell DP, Raffensperger JG: Congenital cystic disease of the lung masquerading as diaphragmatic hernia. J Thorac Cardiovasc Surg 64:592, 1972.

214. Murray GF: Congenital lobar emphysema. Surg Gynecol Obstet 124:611, 1967.

215. De Muth GR, Sloan H: Congenital lobar emphysema: long term effects and sequelae in treated cases. Surgery 59:601, 1966.

216. Pierce WS, DeParedes CG, Friedman S, et al: Concomitant congenital heart disease and lobar emphysema in infants: incidence, diagnosis and operative management. Ann Surg 172:951, 1970.

217. Jones JC, Almond CH, Snyder HN, et al: Lobar emphysema and congenital heart disease in infancy. J Thorac Cardiovasc Surg 49:1, 1965.

218. Gupta R, Singhal SK, Rattan KN, et al: Management of congenital lobal emphysema with endobronchial intubation and controlled ventilation. Anesth Analg 86:71, 1998.

219. Halpern SH, Chatten J, Meadows AT, et al: Anterior mediastinal masses: anesthesia hazards and other problems. J Pediatr 102:407, 1983.

220. Bittar D: Case history number 84: respiratory obstruction associated with induction of general anesthesia in a patient with mediastinal Hodgkin's disease. Anesth Analg 54:399, 1975.

221. John RE, Narang VPS: A boy with an anterior mediastinal mass. Anaesthesia 43:864, 1988.

222. Todres ID, Reppert SM, Walker PF, Grillo HC: Management of critical airway obstruction in a child with a mediastinal tumor. Anesthesiology 45:100, 1976.

223. Keon TP: Death on induction of anesthesia for cervical node biopsy. Anesthesiology 55:471, 1981.

224. Bray RJ, Fernandez FJ: Mediastinal tumour causing airway obstruction in anaesthetised children. Anaesthesia 37:571, 1982.

225. Levin H, Bursztein S, Heifetz M: Cardiac arrest in a child with an anterior mediastinal mass. Anesth Analg 64:1129, 1985.

226. Neuman GG, Weingarten AE, Abramowitz RM, et al: The anesthetic management of the patient with an anterior mediastinal mass. Anesthesiology 60:14, 1984.

227. Johnson C, Hurst D, Cujec B, Mayers I: Cardiopulmonary effects of an anterior mediastinal mass in dogs anesthetized with halothane. Anesthesiology 74:725, 1991.

228. Shamberger RC, Holzman RS, Griscom NT, et al: CT quantitation of tracheal cross-sectional area as a guide to the surgical and anesthetic management of children with anterior mediastinal masses. J Pediatr Surg 26:138, 1991.

229. Pullerits J, Holzman R: Anaesthesia for patients with mediastinal masses. Can J Anaesth 36:681, 1989.

230. Mackie AM, Watson CB: Anaesthesia and mediastinal masses. A case report and review of the literature. Anaesthesia 39:899, 1984.

231. Ravitch MN: Disorders of the sternum and the thoracic wall. In Sabiston DC, Spencer FC (eds): Surgery of the Chest. Philadelphia, WB Saunders Company, 1976, p 411.

232. Polgar G, Koop CE: Pulmonary function in pectus excavatum. Pediatrics 32:209, 1963.

233. Reusch CS: Hemodynamic studies in pectus excavatum. Circulation 24:1143, 1961.

234. Quigley PM, Haller JA, Jelus KL, et al: Cardiorespiratory function before and after corrective surgery in pectus excavatum. J Pediatr 128:638, 1996.

235. Beiser GD, Epstein SE, Stampfer M, et al: Impairment of cardiac function in patients with pectus excavatum with improvement after operative correction. N Engl J Med 287:267, 1972.
236. Berregard S: Postural circulatory changes at rest and during exercise in patients with funnel chest, with special reference to factors affecting the stroke volume. Acta Med Scand 171:695, 1962.
237. Derveaux L, Ivanoff I, Rochette F, Demedts M: Mechanism of pulmonary function changes after correction for funnel chest. Eur Resp J 1:823, 1988.
238. Kaguraoka H, Ohnuki T, Iutaoka T, et al: Degree of severity of pectus excavatum and pulmonary function in preoperative and postoperative periods. J Thorac Cardiovasc Surg 104:1483, 1992.
239. Wynn SR, Driscoll DJ, Ostrom NK, et al: Exercise cardiorespiratory function in adolescents with pectus excavatum. J Thorac Cardiovasc Surg 99:41, 1990.
240. Morshuis W, Folgering H, Barents J, et al: Pulmonary function before surgery for pectus excavatum and at long-term followup. Chest 105:1646, 1994.
241. Humphreys GH, Jaretzki A: Pectus excavatum: late results with and without repair. J Thorac Cardiovasc Surg 80:686, 1980.
242. Shamberger RC, Welch KJ: Surgical repair of pectus excavatum. J Pediatr Surg 23:615, 1988.
243. Wiseman NE, Sanchez I, Powell RE: Rigid bronchoscopy in the pediatric age group: diagnostic effectiveness. J Pediatr Surg 27:1294, 1992.
244. Puhakka H, Kero P, Erkinjuntti M: Pediatric bronchoscopy during a 17-year period. Int J Pediatr Otorhinolaryngol 13:171, 1987.
245. Puhakka H, Kero P, Valli P, et al: Pediatric bronchoscopy: a report of methodology and results. Clin Pediatr 28:253, 1989.
246. Gans SL, Berci G: Advances in endoscopy of infants and children. J Pediatr Surg 6:199, 1971.
247. Sanders RD: Two ventilating attachments for bronchoscopy. Del Med J 39:170, 1967.
248. Carden E, Trapp WG, Oulton J: A new and simple method of ventilating patients for bronchoscopy. Anesthesiology 33:454, 1970.
249. Komersaroff D, Mekie B: "The bronchoflator": a new technique for bronchoscopy under general anesthesia. Br J Anaesth 44:1057, 1972.
250. Carden E: Recent improvements in techniques for general anesthesia for bronchoscopy. Chest 73:697, 1978.
251. Sloan IA, McLeod ME: Evaluation of the jet injector in paediatric fibreoptic bronchoscopes. Can Anaesth Soc J 32:79, 1985.
252. Miyasaka K, Sloan IA, Froese AB: An evaluation of the jet injector (Sanders) technique for bronchoscopy in paediatric patients. Can Anaesth Soc J 27:117, 1980.
253. Ostfeld E, Ovadia L: Bilateral tension pneumothorax during pediatric bronchoscopy (high frequency jet injection ventilation). Int J Pediatr Otorhinolaryngol 7:301, 1984.
254. Kestin IG, Chapman JM, Coates MB: Alfentanil used to supplement propofol infusions for oesophagoscopy and bronchoscopy. Anaesthesia 44:994, 1989.
255. Amitai Y, Zylber KE, Avital A, et al: Serum lidocaine concentrations in children during bronchoscopy with topical anesthesia. Chest 98:1370, 1990.
256. Baraka A: Bronchoscopic removal of inhaled foreign bodies in children. Br J Anaesth 46:124, 1974.
257. Boutious A: Arterial blood oxygenation during and after tracheal suctioning in the apneic patient. Anesthesiology 32:114, 1970.
258. Gallagher MJ, Muller BJ: Tension pneumothorax during pediatric bronchoscopy. Anesthesiology 55:685, 1981.
259. Maze A, Block E: Stridor in pediatric patients. Anesthesiology 50:132, 1979.
260. Jacobeus H: The practical importance of thoracoscopy in surgery of the chest. Surg Gynecol Obstet 4:289, 1921.
261. Rodgers BM, Talbert JL: Thoracoscopy for diagnosis of intrathoracic lesions in children. J Pediatr Surg 11:703, 1976.
262. Rodgers BM, Moazam F, Talbert JL: Thoracoscopy in children. Ann Surg 189:176, 1979.
263. Rodgers BM: Pediatric thoracoscopy: where have we come and what have we learned? Ann Thorac Surg 56:704, 1993.
264. Rodgers BM: Thoracoscopic procedures in children. Semin Pediatr Surg 2:182, 1993.
265. Rothenberg SS: Thoracoscopy in infants and children. Semin Pediatr Surg 3:277, 1994.
266. Rothenberg SS, Chang JH: Thoracoscopic decortication in infants and children. Surg Endosc 11:93, 1997.
267. Rothenberg SS: Thoracoscopy in infants and children. Semin Pediatr Surg 7:194, 1998.
268. Kern JA, Rodgers BM: Thoracoscopy in the management of empyema in children. J Pediatr Surg 28:1128, 1993.
269. Kern JA, Daniel TM, Tribble CG, et al: Thoracoscopic diagnosis and treatment of mediastinal masses. Ann Thorac Surg 56:92, 1993.
270. Ryckman FC, Rodgers BM: Thoracoscopy for intrathoracic neoplasia in children. J Pediatr Surg 17:521, 1982.
271. Rothenberg SS: The safety and efficacy of thoracoscopic lung biopsy for diagnosis and treatment in infants and children. J Pediatr Surg 31:100, 1996.
272. Hazelrigg SR, Landreneau RJ, Mack MJ, Acuff TE: Thoracoscopic resection of mediastinal cysts. Ann Thorac Surg 56:659, 1993.
273. Mack MJ: Thoracoscopy and its role in mediastinal disease and sympathectomy. Semin Thorac Cardiovasc Surg 5:332, 1993.
274. Laborde F: Video-assisted thoracoscopic surgical interruption: the technique of choice for patent ductus arteriosus. Routine experience in 230 pediatric cases. J Thorac Cardiovasc Surg 110:1681, 1995.
275. Rothenberg SS: Transcatheter versus surgical closure of patent ductus arteriosus [letter; comment]. N Engl J Med 330:1014, 1994.
276. Burke RP, Wernovsky G, van der Velde M: Video-assisted thoracoscopic surgery for congenital heart disease. J Thorac Cardiovasc Surg 109:499, 1995.
277. Burke RP, Rosenfeld HM, Wernovsky G, Jonas RA: Video-assisted thoracoscopic vascular ring division in infants and children. J Am Coll Cardiol 25:943, 1995.
278. Mack M: Video-assisted thoracic surgery for the anterior approach to the thoracic spine. Ann Thorac Surg 59:1100, 1995.
279. Rothenberg S, Erickson M, Eilert R, et al: Thoracoscopic anterior spinal procedures in children. J Pediatr Surg 33:1168, 1998.
280. Tobias JD: Anaesthetic implications of thoracoscopic surgery in children. Paediatr Anaesth 9:103, 1999.
281. Rowe R, Andropoulos D, Heard M, et al: Anesthetic management of pediatric patients undergoing thoracoscopy. J Cardiothorac Vasc Anesth 8:563, 1994.
282. Morton JR, Guinn GA: Mediastinoscopy using local anesthesia. Am J Surg 122:696, 1971.
283. Sugi K, Katoh T, Gohra H, et al: Progressive hyperthermia during thoracoscopic procedures in infants and children. Paediatr Anaesth 8:211, 1998.
284. Chen MK, Schropp KP, Lobe TE: Complications of minimal-access surgery in children. J Pediatr Surg 31:1161, 1996.
285. Webb-Johnson DC, Andrews JL: Bronchodilator therapy (part 1). N Engl J Med 297:476, 1977.
286. Ingram RH, McFadden ER: Localization and mechanisms of airway responses. N Engl J Med 297:596, 1977.
287. Fairshter RD, Wilson AF: Relationship between site of airflow limitation and localization of the bronchodilator response in asthma. Am Rev Respir Dis 122:27, 1980.
288. Woolcock AJ, Read J: Lung volumes in exacerbations of asthma. Am J Med 41:259, 1966.
289. Cade JF, Woolcock AJ, Rebuck AS, Pain MCF: Lung mechanics during provocation of asthma. Clin Sci 40:381, 1971.
290. Gold MI, Helrich M: A study of the complications related to anesthesia in asthmatic patients. Anesth Analg 42:283, 1963.
291. McFadden ER, Kiser R, de Groot WJ: Acute bronchial asthma: relations between clinical and physiological manifestations. N Engl J Med 288:221, 1973.
292. Berman NA: New tests of pulmonary function: physiological basis and interpretation. Anesthesiology 44:220, 1976.
293. McFadden ER Jr, Linden DA: A reduction in maximum mid-expiratory flow rate. A spirographic manifestation of small airway disease. Am J Med 52:725, 1972.
294. Kingston HGG, Hirshman CA: Perioperative management of the patient with asthma. Anesth Analg 63:844, 1984.
295. Gershel JC, Goldman HS, Stein REK, et al: The usefulness of chest radiographs in first asthma attacks. N Engl J Med 309:336, 1983.
296. Pauwels R: Mode of action of corticosteroids in asthma and rhinitis. Clin Allergy 16:281, 1986.
297. Pierson WE, Bierman CW, Kelley VC: A double-blind trial of corticosteroid therapy in status asthmaticus. Pediatrics 54:282, 1974.
298. Bernstein IL, Johnson JL, Tse CST: Therapy with cromolyn sodium. Ann Intern Med 89:228, 1978.

299. Downes JJ, Heiser MS: Status asthmaticus in children. *In* Gregory GA (ed): Respiratory Failure in the Child. New York, Churchill Livingstone, 1981, p 107.
300. Mitenko PA, Ogilvie RI: Rational intravenous doses of theophylline. N Engl J Med 289:600, 1973.
301. Gross NJ: Ipratropium bromide. N Engl J Med 319:486, 1988.
302. Davis A, Vickerson F, Worsley G, et al: Determination of dose-response relationship for nebulized ipratropium in asthmatic children. J Pediatr 105:1002, 1984.
303. Warner DO, Warner MA, Barnes RD: Perioperative respiratory complications in patients with asthma. Anesthesiology 85:455, 1996.
304. Shnider SN, Papper EN: Anesthesia for the asthmatic patient. Anesthesiology 22:886, 1962.
305. Lichtenstein LM, Gillespie E: Inhibition of histamine release controlled by H2 receptor. Nature 244:287, 1973.
306. Tarhan S, Moffitt EA, Sessler AD, et al: Risk of anesthesia and surgery in patients with chronic bronchitis and chronic obstructive pulmonary disease. Surgery 74:720, 1973.
307. Lim EK: Interscalene brachial plexus block in the asthmatic patient [correspondence]. Anaesthesia 34:370, 1979.
308. Downes H, Gerber N, Hirshman CA: IV lignocaine in reflex and allergic bronchoconstriction. Br J Anaesth 52:873, 1980.
309. Downes H, Hirshman CA: Lidocaine aerosols do not prevent allergic bronchoconstriction. Anesth Analg 60:28, 1981.
310. Corssen G, Gutierrez J, Reves JG, Huber FC: Ketamine in the anesthetic management of asthmatic patients. Anesth Analg 51:588, 1972.
311. Takki S, Nikki P, Jaattela A, Tammisto T: Ketamine and plasma catecholamines. Br J Anaesth 44:1318, 1972.
312. Lundy PM, Gowdey CW, Calhoun EH: Tracheal smooth muscle relaxant effect of ketamine. Br J Anaesth 46:333, 1974.
313. Huber FC, Reves JG, Gutierrez J, Corssen G: Ketamine: its effect on airway resistance in man. South Med J 65:1176, 1972.
314. Betts EK, Parkin CE: Use of ketamine in an asthmatic child. Anesth Analg 50:420, 1971.
315. Rock MJ, de la Rocha SR, L'Hommedieu CS, et al: Use of ketamine in asthmatic children to treat respiratory failure refractory to conventional therapy. Crit Care Med 14:514, 1986.
316. Wu RS, Wu KC, Sum DC, Bishop MJ: Comparative effects of thiopentone and propofol on respiratory resistance after tracheal intubation. Br J Anaesth 77:735, 1996.
317. Hirshman CA, Bergman NA: Factors influencing intrapulmonary airway calibre during anaesthesia. Br J Anaesth 65:30, 1990.
318. Colgan FJ: Performance of lungs and bronchi during inhalation anesthesia. Anesthesiology 26:778, 1965.
319. Gold MI, Han YH, Helrich M: Pulmonary mechanics and blood gas tensions during anesthesia in asthmatics. Anesthesiology 27:216, 1966.
320. O'Rourke PP, Crone RK: Halothane in status asthmaticus. Crit Care Med 10:341, 1982.
321. Rosseel P, Lauwers LF, Bante L: Halothane treatment in life-threatening asthma. Intensive Care Med 11:241, 1985.
322. Hirshman CA, Bergman NA: Halothane and enflurane protect against bronchospasm in an asthma dog model. Anesth Analg 57:629, 1978.
323. Hirshman CA, Edelstein G, Peetz S, et al: Mechanism of action of inhalational anesthesia on airways. Anesthesiology 56:107, 1982.
324. Roizen NF, Stevens WC: Multiform ventricular tachycardia due to the interaction of aminophylline and halothane. Anesth Analg 57:738, 1978.
325. Stirt JA, Berger JM, Ricker SM, Sullivan SF: Arrhythmogenic effect of aminophylline during halothane anesthesia in experimental animals. Anesth Analg 59:410, 1980.
326. Stirt JA, Berger JM, Sullivan SF: Lack of arrhythmogenicity of isoflurane following administration of aminophylline in dogs. Anesth Analg 62:548, 1983.
327. Katoh T, Ikeda K: Effect of sevoflurane on bronchoconstriction caused by histamine or acetylcholine [abstract]. Anesthesiology 75:A973, 1991.
328. Walker SM, Haugen RD, Richards A: A comparison of sevoflurane with halothane for paediatric day case surgery. Anaesth Intensive Care 25:643, 1997.
329. Fujibayashi T, Mizogami M, Niwa M, et al: About the merits of use of laryngeal mask airway and sevoflurane in five cases of bronchial asthma. Hiroshima J Anesth 27:383, 1991.

330. Narra A, Cardan E, Leitersdorfer T: Pancuronium bromide. Its use in asthmatics and patients with liver disease. Anaesthesia 27:154, 1972.
331. Levin N, Dillon JB: Status asthmaticus and pancuronium bromide. JAMA 222:1265, 1972.
332. Miller MM, Fish JE, Patterson R: Methacholine and physostigmine airway reactivity in asthmatic and nonasthmatic subjects. J Allergy Clin Immunol 60:116, 1977.
333. Doershuk CF, Reyes AL, Regan AG, Matthews LW: Anesthesia and surgery in cystic fibrosis. Anesth Analg 51:413, 1972.
334. Knowlton RG, Cohen-Haguenauer O, Van Cong N, et al: A polymorphic DNA marker linked to cystic fibrosis is located on chromosome 7. Nature 318:380, 1985.
335. White R, Woodward S, Seppart M, et al: A closely linked genetic marker for cystic fibrosis. Nature 318:382, 1985.
336. McPherson MA, Goodchild MC: The biochemical defect in cystic fibrosis. Clinical Science 74:337, 1988.
337. Lemma WK, Feldman GL, Kerem B, et al: Mutation analysis for heterozygote detection and the prenatal diagnosis of cystic fibrosis. N Engl J Med 322:291, 1990.
338. Dean M, White MB, Amos J, et al: Multiple mutations in highly conserved residues are found in mildly affected cystic fibrosis patients. Cell 61:863, 1990.
339. Mitchell I, Corey M, Woenne R, et al: Bronchial hyperactivity in cystic fibrosis and asthma. J Pediatr 93:747, 1978.
340. Wood RE, Wanner A, Hirsch J, Farrell PM: Tracheal mucociliary transport in patients with cystic fibrosis and its stimulation by terbutaline. Am Rev Respir Dis 111:733, 1975.
341. Johnson CA, Butler SM, Konstar MW, et al: Estimating effectiveness in an observational study: a case study of dornase in cystic fibrosis. J Pediatr 134:734, 1999.
342. Komp DM, Selden RF: Coagulation abnormalities in cystic fibrosis. Chest 58:501, 1970.
343. Ramsey BW, Pepe MS, Quan JM, et al: Intermittent administration of inhaled tobramycin in patients with cystic fibrosis. N Engl J Med 340:23, 1999.
344. Goldring RM, Fishman AP, Turino GM, et al: Pulmonary hypertension and cor pulmonale in cystic fibrosis of the pancreas. J Pediatr 65:501, 1964.
345. Olsen MM, Ganderer MWL, Girz MK, Izant RJ: Surgery in patients with cystic fibrosis. J Pediatr Surg 22:613, 1987.
346. Mauer JT, Chaparro C: Lung transplantation in cystic fibrosis. Curr Opin Pulm Med 1:465, 1995.
347. Lamberty JM, Rubin BK: The management of anaesthesia for patients with cystic fibrosis. Anaesthesia 40:448, 1985.
348. Greenholz SK, Hall RJ, Lilly JR, Shikes RH: Surgical implications of bronchopulmonary dysplasia. J Pediatr Surg 22:1132, 1987.
349. Kaiser LR, Cooper JK: The current status of lung transplantation. Adv Surg 25:259, 1992.
350. Giuffre RM, Rubin S, Mitchell I: Antireflux surgery in infants with bronchopulmonary dysplasia. Am J Dis Child 141:648, 1987.
351. Kurth CD, Spitzer AR, Broennle AM, Downes JJ: Postoperative apnea in preterm infants. Anesthesiology 66:483, 1987.
352. Liu LMP, Coté CJ, Goudsouzian NG, et al: Life-threatening apnea in infants recovering from anesthesia. Anesthesiology 59:506, 1983.
353. Melone JH, Schwartz MZ, Tyson KR, et al: Outpatient inguinal herniorrhaphy in premature infants: is it safe? J Pediatr Surg 27:203, 1992.
354. Mayhew JK, Bourke DL, Guinee WS: Evaluation of the premature infant at risk for postoperative complications. Can J Anaesth 34:627, 1987.
355. Webster AC, McKishnie JD, Kenyon CF, Marshall DG: Spinal anaesthesia for inguinal hernia repair in high-risk neonates. Can J Anaesth 38:281, 1991.
356. Harnik EV, Gregory RH, Potolicchio S, et al: Spinal anesthesia in premature infants recovering from respiratory distress syndrome. Anesthesiology 64:95, 1986.
357. Welborn LG, Rice LJ, Hannallah RS, et al: Postoperative apnea in former premature infants: prospective comparison of spinal and general anesthesia. Anesthesiology 72:838, 1990.
358. Krane EJ, Haberkern CM, Jacobson LE: A comparison of spinal and general anesthesia in the former premature infant. Anesthesiology 75:A912, 1991.
359. Kanarck DJ, Shannon DL: Adverse effect of positive end-expiratory pressure on pulmonary perfusion and arterial oxygenation. Am Rev Respir Dis 112:457, 1975.

360. Benumof JL: Hypoxic pulmonary vasoconstriction and sodium nitroprusside infusion [editorial]. Anesthesiology 50:481, 1979.

361. Bishop MJ, Cheney FW: Minoxidil and nifedipine inhibit hypoxic pulmonary vasoconstriction. J Cardiovasc Pharmacol 5:184, 1983.

362. Tucker A, McMurty IF, Grover RF, et al: Alteration of hypoxic pulmonary vasoconstriction by verapamil in intact dogs. Proc Soc Exp Biol Med 151:611, 1976.

363. Conover WB, Benumof JL, Key TC: Ritodrine inhibition of hypoxic pulmonary vasoconstriction. Am J Obstet Gyneol 146:652, 1983.

364. Beumof JL, Wahrenberg EA: Dependency of hypoxic pulmonary vasoconstriction on temperature. J Appl Physiol 42:56, 1977.

365. Suter PM, Fairley HB, Schlobohm RM: Shunt, lung volume, and perfusion during short periods of ventilation with oxygen. Anesthesiology 43:617, 1975.

366. Benumof JL: Mechanism of decreased blood flow to atelectatic lung. J Appl Physiol 46:1047, 1978.

367. Pirlo AF, Benumof JL, Trousdale FR: Atelectatic lung lobe blood flow. Open vs. closed chest, positive pressure vs. spontaneous ventilation. J Appl Physiol 50:1022, 1981.

368. Glasser SA, Domino KB, Lindgren L, et al: Pulmonary artery pressure and flow during atelectasis [abstract]. Anesthesiology 57:A504, 1982.

369. Domino KB, Glasser SA, Wetstein L, et al: Infuence of PvO_2 on blood flow to atelectatic lung [abstract]. Anesthesiology 57:A471, 1982.

370. Benumof JL, Pirlo AF, Trousdale FR: Inhibition of hypoxic pulmonary vasoconstriction by decreased PvO_2: a new indirect mechanism. J Appl Physiol 51:871, 1981.

18

Anesthesia for Congenital Heart Disease

PETER C. LAUSSEN
DAVID L. WESSEL

◆　◆　◆

Among the causes of infant mortality in the United States, congenital anomalies account for the largest diagnostic category.[1] Structural heart disease leads the list of congenital malformations. Over 4 million children are born each year in the United States, and nearly 40,000 of these have some form of congenital heart disease (CHD). Approximately half of these children appear for therapeutic intervention within the first year of life, and the vast majority of them require care by an anesthesiologist.

Initial reports of anesthetic mortality ranging from 3 to 10 percent in operations for CHD indicated a significant risk of anesthesia in this patient population.[2, 3] However, the principles and techniques of pediatric anesthesia presented in this volume allow one to anesthetize CHD patients with minimal anesthetic mortality and morbidity.[4] This low anesthetic risk is predicated not only on adherence to these principles but also on an understanding of the pathophysiologic circumstance of each patient and the nature of the planned surgical procedure. Implicit in all surgical procedures are potential complications that anesthesiologists, by virtue of their primary role in monitoring and maintaining vital functions, are able to identify and treat. For cardiac surgery, knowledge of specific problems related to each type of cardiac repair helps to identify complications during the postbypass and postoperative periods, as well as later complications that affect subsequent anesthesia for noncardiac procedures. The diagnostic information now available intraoperatively, in the form of intracardiac pressures and oxygen saturations plus echocardiographic diagnoses, provides the pediatric cardiac anesthesiologist with the opportunity and responsibility to assess the adequacy of surgical intervention and its impact on hemodynamics.

This chapter describes general principles relevant to anesthesia for children with CHD; it does not present "recipes" for individual cardiac defects. The pathophysiology is presented as it relates to principles of management, patient assessment, selection and application of an anesthetic regimen, and specific cardiac lesions and procedures. Knowledge of these principles should permit safe administration of anesthesia to children with CHD undergoing both cardiac and noncardiac operations. Optimal management will occur when the anesthesiologist regularly becomes involved in the care of these patients and has special insight and rapport with the entire cardiovascular staff, such that care is provided by a cohesive team in a smooth continuum from the preoperative preparation and diagnosis through the postoperative discharge.

MYOCARDIAL FUNCTION AND FAILURE

Congestive Heart Failure

Determinants of myocardial performance, well described for the adult heart, are usually valid for children with CHD provided that special consideration is given to the immature myocardium. Factors that influence ventricular performance include the force that distends the ventricular muscle to its precontraction length (preload), the load or impedance that is faced by the contracting heart (afterload), and the contractile state of the muscle that is influenced not by preload or afterload but rather by the degree of activation and rapidity of cross-bridge formation within the myocyte (contractility). When considered along with heart rate, these factors describe overall ventricular performance, which is manifest by the adequacy of systemic perfusion (Fig. 18–1). The measure of performance is commonly associated with cardiac output but must be more broadly interpreted in terms of the adequacy of oxygen and nutrient delivery in fulfilling the needs of growth and development of the child. Congestive heart failure (CHF) occurs in children with CHD, as in adults, when cardiac performance is depressed and high preload requirements are expressed as the typical congestive symptoms of dyspnea with pulmonary edema (from elevated left heart preload) or peripheral edema (elevated right heart preload). However, CHF symptoms typically appear in CHD when there may be increased ventricular output and only moderately elevated preload. Therefore, comparable terminology may describe similar symptoms in patients with congenital versus acquired heart disease, but the pathophysiologic basis for similar clinical symptoms may be strikingly different. The term "congestive heart failure" in the dyspneic adult with ischemic heart disease and left ventricular dysfunctions has entirely different pathophysiologic connotations from the description of "congestive heart failure" in a 3-month-old patient with a hyperdynamic left ventricle and a large left-to-right shunt through a ventricular septal defect. When there is a large ventricular septal defect, and the majority of left ventricular output recirculates to the lungs without benefit to the systemic circulation, the pulmonary circulation is overcome with high flow and pressure. This flow and pressure is communicated from the left ventricle and provides hydrostatic forces that promote increased lung water and an excessive volume of return to the left heart (increased preload). This results in the typical findings of tachypnea, wheezing, diaphoresis, tachycardia, cardiomegaly, and failure to thrive, referred to as congestive heart failure. In this instance CHF is notably different in etiology and physiology from the adult with ischemic heart disease who has high left atrial pressures and poor left ventricular function and ejection.

Low Cardiac Output States

Although many causes of morbidity and mortality after cardiopulmonary bypass (CPB) are attributable to residual or undiagnosed structural lesions (supporting the notion of aggressive diagnostic intervention), low cardiac output states do occur.[5, 6] In neonates studied after an arterial switch operation, the cardiac index fell to less than 2 L/min/m^2 in a quarter of the patients during the first postoperative night, while pulmonary and systemic vascular resistance rose.[6] The addition of afterload reduction and inotropic support can oppose this trend.[7]

After CPB, the factors that influence cardiac output, preload, afterload, myocardial contractility, heart rate, and rhythm must be assessed and manipulated. Volume therapy (increased preload), followed by appropriate use of inotropic and afterload-reducing agents, is commonly necessary.[8] Atrial pressure and the ventricular response to changes in atrial pressure must be evaluated. Ventricular response is judged by observing systemic arterial pressure and waveform, heart rate, skin color and peripheral extremity temperature, peripheral pulse magnitude, urine flow, core body temperature, and acid–base balance.

For more refractory but potentially reversible ventricular dysfunction, ventricular assist devices may be useful when gas exchange appears satisfactory.[9] While this technique offers potential advantages for selected patients over extracorporeal membrane oxygenation (ECMO), ECMO is indicated when pulmonary function is also significantly impaired.[10, 11] It also is a more reliable therapy for

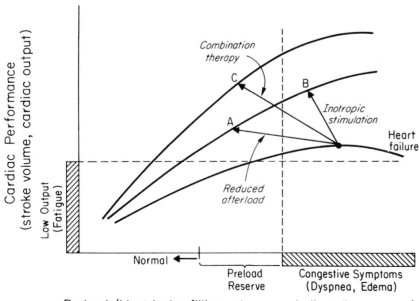

FIGURE 18–1. Vasodilating agents move the cardiac performance curve along line A to reduce afterload; there is a concomitant reduction in filling pressure (preload). Inotropic stimulation shifts the performance curve upward toward B. Maximal benefit is gained by combination therapy whereby vasodilators reduce symptoms associated with high filling pressures (congestive heart failure). Cardiac output is maintained by reducing afterload and enhanced by inotropic stimulation. (From Friedman WF, George BL: Treatment of congestive heart failure by altering loading conditions of the heart. J Pediatr 106:697, 1985, with permission.)

biventricular dysfunction. In our experience, which is similar to that of many other centers, mechanical support is necessary in less than 3 percent of all patients who undergo CPB.[12]

Selected children with low cardiac output may benefit from strategies that allow right-to-left shunting at the atrial level when there is postoperative right ventricular dysfunction. A typical example is early repair of tetralogy of Fallot, when the moderately hypertrophied, noncompliant right ventricle has undergone a ventriculotomy and may be further compromised by an increased volume load from pulmonary regurgitation secondary to a transannular patch on the right ventricular outflow tract. In these children it is very useful to leave the foramen ovale patent to permit right-to-left shunting of blood, thus preserving cardiac output and oxygen delivery despite the attendant transient cyanosis. If the foramen is not patent or is surgically closed, right ventricular dysfunction can lead to reduced left ventricular filling, low cardiac output and, ultimately, to left ventricular dysfunction. In infants and neonates with repaired truncus arteriosus, the same concerns apply and may even be exaggerated if right ventricular afterload is elevated because of pulmonary artery hypertension.[13] This concept has been extended to older patients with single-ventricle physiology who are at high risk after Fontan operations. If an atrial septal communication or fenestration is not repaired at the time of the Fontan procedure, the resulting right-to-left shunt helps preserve cardiac output. Children treated this way have fewer postoperative complications.[13] It is better to shunt blood right to left, and accept some decrement in oxygen saturation while maintaining ventricular filling and cardiac output, than it is to have a high oxygen saturation and low blood pressure and cardiac output.

Pharmacologic Support

Inotropic Agents

Failure to improve cardiac output after volume adjustments requires the additional use of an inotropic drug.[8, 14–17] Tables 18–1 and 18–2 list commonly used vasoactive drugs and their actions. Many clinicians prefer to use dopamine first in doses of 3 to 10 μg/kg/min. One rarely uses more than 15 μg/kg/min because of the known vasoconstrictor and chronotropic properties of dopamine at very high doses. However, extreme biologic variability in pharmacokinetics and pharmacodynamics defies placing narrow limits on recommended dosages. Dobutamine's chronotropic and vasodilatory advantages recognized in adults with coronary artery disease have not always proven equally efficacious in clinical studies in children. In fact, dobutamine has fewer, or no, dopaminergic advantages for the kidney. This may be an especially important limitation in infants with excess total body water and interstitial edema. The significant chronotropic effect and increased oxygen consumption induced by isoproterenol have increasingly limited its use in neonates and infants. Epinephrine is occasionally useful for short-term therapy when high systemic pressures are sought, provided that the temporary increase in peripheral vascular resistance is tolerated. High doses of epinephrine are occasionally neces-

sary to increase pulmonary blood flow across significantly narrowed systemic-to-pulmonary artery shunts when oxygen saturations are low and falling. Arginine vasopressin has been advocated for states of refractory vasodilation associated with low circulating vasopressin levels as occurs rarely after CPB in children.[18]

In the past, the side effects of inotropic support of the heart with catecholamines seemed a lesser concern in children than in adults with an ischemic, noncompliant heart. Tachycardia, an increased end-diastolic pressure and afterload, or increased myocardial oxygen consumption, in spite of their undesirable side effects, were tolerated by most children in need of inotropic support after CPB. However, with increasing perioperative experience in neonates and young infants, the adverse effects of vasoactive drugs have become more evident. The less compliant neonatal myocardium, like the ischemic adult heart, may raise its end-diastolic pressure during infusion of higher doses of dopamine or may develop even more extreme noncompliance. Actual myocardial necrosis has been identified in neonatal animal models after CPB following infusion of high doses of epinephrine.[19, 20] Although these agents do increase the cardiac output, the concomitant increase in ventricular filling pressure is less well tolerated by the immature myocardium than it is by the myocardium of older children (Fig. 18–2). Many of the complex corrective procedures performed in neonates and small infants are accompanied by transient postoperative arrhythmias that are either induced or exacerbated by catecholamines. These arrhythmias can have profound adverse effects on the patient's recovery after surgery. Diastolic function is crucial in older patients with single ventricles and can be adversely affected by catecholamines. Nevertheless, the predictable and often significant decrease in cardiac output documented by many investigators after CPB in infants and older children continues to justify the practice of judiciously using inotropic agents to support the heart and circulation while weaning these children from CPB and during the immediate postoperative period.[14]

Amrinone and milrinone have emerged as important inotropic agents for use in children after open heart surgery. These drugs are nonglycosidic, noncatecholamine inotropic agents with additional vasodilatory and lusitropic properties. They have been used extensively in adults for treatment of chronic CHF, and more recently introduced to pediatric practice.[21–23] These drugs exert their principal effects by inhibiting phosphodiesterase, the enzyme that metabolizes cyclic adenosine monophosphate (cAMP). By increasing intracellular cAMP, calcium transport into the cell is favored, and the increased intracellular calcium stores enhance the contractile state of the myocyte. In addition, the reuptake of calcium is a cAMP-dependent process, and these agents may, therefore, enhance diastolic relaxation of the myocardium by increasing the rate of calcium reuptake after systole (lusitropy). The drug also appears to work synergistically with low doses of β-agonists and has fewer side effects than other catecholamine vasodilators, such as isoproterenol. While the use of amrinone, beginning in the operating room, has become more commonplace in many cardiovascular centers,[17, 24] the half-life of 2 to 4 hours rather than

T A B L E   1 8 – 1
SUMMARY OF SELECTED VASOACTIVE AGENTS: NONCATECHOLAMINES

Agent	Doses (IV)	Peripheral Vascular Effect	Cardiac Effect	Conduction System Effect
Digoxin (total digitalizing dose)	20 μg/kg premature 30 μg/kg neonate (0–1 mo) 40 μg/kg infant (<2 yr) 30 μg/kg child (2–5 yr) 20 μg/kg child (>5 yr)	Increases peripheral vascular resistance 1–2+; acts directly on vascular smooth muscle	Inotropic effect 3–4+; acts directly on myocardium	Slows sinus node slightly; decreases AV conduction more
Calcium chloride	10–20 mg/kg/dose (slowly)	Variable; age dependent; vasoconstrictor	Inotropic effect 3+; depends on ionized Ca^{2+}	Slows sinus node; decreases AV conduction
Gluconate	50–100 mg/kg/dose (slowly)			
Nitroprusside	0.5–5 μg/kg/min	Donates nitric oxide group to relax smooth muscle and dilate pulmonary and systemic vessels	Indirectly increases cardiac output by decreasing afterload	Reflex tachycardia
Nitroglycerin	0.5–10 μg/kg/min	Primarily venodilator; as a nitric oxide donor may cause pulmonary vasodilation, and enhance coronary vasoreactivity after aortic cross-clamping	Decreases preload, may decrease afterload; reduces myocardial work related to change in wall stress	Minimal
Amrinone	1–3 mg/kg loading dose 5–20 μg/kg/min maintenance	Systemic and pulmonary vasodilator; thrombocytopenia	Diastolic relaxation (lusitropy)	Minimal tachycardia
Milrinone	50 μg/kg loading dose 0.25–1.0 μg/kg/min maintenance	As above Shorter half-life	As above	As above
Vasopressin	0.003–0.002 U/kg/min	Potent vasoconstrictor	No direct effect	None known

T A B L E   1 8 – 2
SUMMARY OF SELECTED VASOACTIVE AGENTS: CATECHOLAMINES

Agent	Dose Range	Peripheral Vascular Effect			Cardiac Effect		Comment
		Alpha	Beta₂	Delta	Beta₁	Beta₂	
Phenylephrine	0.1–0.5 μg/kg/min	4+	0	0	0	0	Increases systemic resistance, no inotropy; may cause renal ischemia; useful for treatment of TOF spells
Isoproterenol	0.05–0.5 μg/kg/min	0	4+	0	4+	4+	Strong inotropic and chronotropic agent; peripheral vasodilator; reduces preload; pulmonary vasodilator. Limited by tachycardia and oxygen consumption
Norepinephrine	0.1–0.5 μg/kg/min	4+	0	0	2+	0	Increases systemic resistance; moderately inotropic; may cause renal ischemia
Epinephrine	0.03–0.1 μg/kg/min 0.2–0.5 μg/kg/min	2+ 4+	1–2+ 0	0 0	2–3+ 4+	2+ 3+	Beta₂ effect with lower doses; best for blood pressure in anaphylaxis and drug toxicity
Dopamine	2–4 μg/kg/min 4–8 μg/kg/min >10 μg/kg/min	0 0 2–4+	0 2+ 0	2+ 2+ 0	0 1–2+ 1–2+	0 1+ 2+	Splanchnic and renal vasodilator; may be used with isoproterenol; increasing doses produce increasing alpha effect
Dobutamine	2–10 μg/kg/min	1+	2+	0	3–4+	1–2+	Less chronotropy and arrhythmias at lower doses; effects vary with dose similar to dopamine; chronotropic advantage compared with dopamine may not be apparent in neonates

TOF, Tetralogy of Fallot.

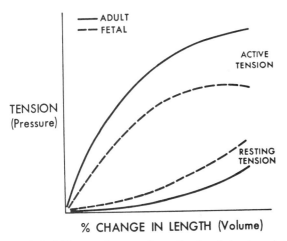

FIGURE 18–2. Differences between the resting length-tension relationship of the adult and the fetal myocardium. Note that the adult myocardium develops greater active tension than does that of the fetus. (From Rudolph AM: Congenital Diseases of the Heart. Chicago, Year Book Medical Publishers, 1974, p 79, with permission.)

minutes, and its potential toxicity in the face of hepatic and renal failure, have discouraged some from using this drug more frequently. Milrinone has the advantage of a shorter half-life and may, therefore, be more titratable when there is hemodynamic instability.[25, 26] This drug also may be associated with a lower incidence of thrombocytopenia and its use is preferable when longer term use of a phosphodiesterase inhibitor is indicated.

Afterload-Reducing Agents

When systemic blood pressure is elevated and cardiac output appears normal, a primary vasodilator is indicated to normalize blood pressure and to decrease the afterload on the left ventricle. Although nitroprusside has no known direct inotropic effects, this potent vasodilator has the advantage of being readily titratable and of possessing a short biologic half-life. Use of nitroglycerin avoids the toxic metabolites, cyanide and thiocyanate, associated with the use of nitroprusside (especially when there is hepatic and renal insufficiency), but the potency of nitroglycerin as a vasodilator is less than that of nitroprusside. Inhibitors of angiotensin-converting enzyme have proven to be important adjuvants to chronic anticongestive therapy in pediatric patients. Intravenous forms are available and may be useful in treatment of systemic hypertension immediately after repair of a coarctation of the aorta or when afterload reduction with these inhibitors would benefit patients unable to take oral medications.[27]

Pulmonary Vasodilators

Children with many forms of CHD are prone to develop perioperative elevations of pulmonary vascular resistance (PVR).[28, 29] Increases in PVR may complicate the postoperative course when transient myocardial dysfunction requires optimal control of right ventricular afterload.[30–33] Success with vasodilators for treatment of pulmonary hypertension has had mixed results because the systemic vasodilating effects of these drugs often predominate and

limit their effectiveness. Tolazine, prostaglandin E_1 (PGE_1), and prostacyclin have all been suggested as useful pharmacologic treatments for this condition.[34–37] Several factors peculiar to CPB may raise PVR: microemboli, pulmonary leukosequestration, excess thromboxane production, atelectasis, hypoxic pulmonary vasoconstriction, and adrenergic events have all been suggested to play a role in postoperative pulmonary hypertension.[32, 38] Postoperative pulmonary vascular reactivity has been related not only to the presence of preoperative pulmonary hypertension and left-to-right shunts,[28, 31, 39] but also to the duration of total CPB.[40, 41] Treatment of postoperative pulmonary hypertensive crises has been partially addressed by surgery at earlier ages, pharmacologic intervention, and other postoperative management strategies. However, recent developments in vascular biology have offered new insights into the possible causes and correction of post-CPB pulmonary hypertension.

Nitric oxide (NO) is formed by the endothelium from L-arginine and molecular oxygen in a reaction catalyzed by NO synthase. NO then diffuses to the adjacent vascular smooth muscle cells where it induces vasodilation through a cyclic guanosine monophosphate–dependent pathway.[42–46] Since NO exists as a gas, it can be delivered by inhalation to the alveoli and then to the blood vessels that lie in close proximity to ventilated lung. Because of its rapid inactivation by hemoglobin, inhaled NO may achieve selective pulmonary vasodilation when pulmonary vasoconstriction exists. NO has advantages over intravenously administered vasodilators that cause systemic hypotension and increase intrapulmonary shunting. Inhaled NO lowers pulmonary artery pressure in a number of diseases without the unwanted effect of systemic hypotension. This is especially dramatic in children with cardiovascular disorders and postoperative patients with pulmonary hypertensive crises.

Pulmonary vascular endothelial dysfunction may be a contributing factor in post-CPB pulmonary hypertension. Structural damage to the pulmonary endothelium is demonstrable after CPB, and the degree of pulmonary hypertension is correlated with the extent of endothelial damage after CPB.[40, 41] The decreased pulmonary blood flow on CPB may result in postoperative impairment of endothelial function and inability to release nitric oxide. Transient pulmonary vascular endothelial cell dysfunction has been demonstrated in neonates and older children by documenting the transient loss of endothelium-dependent vasodilation immediately after cardiopulmonary bypass[47] (Fig. 18–3). NO production, as measured by exhaled NO, is reduced postoperatively.[48] This and other evidence provides a theoretical basis for administering NO after surgery.

Therapeutic uses of inhaled NO in children with congenital heart disease abound. For example, newborns with total anomalous pulmonary venous connection (TAPVC) frequently have obstruction of the pulmonary venous pathway as it connects anomalously to the systemic venous circulation. When pulmonary venous return is obstructed preoperatively, pulmonary hypertension is severe and demands urgent surgical relief. Increased neonatal pulmonary vasoreactivity, endothelial injury induced by cardiopulmonary bypass, and intrauterine anatomic changes in the pulmonary vascular bed in this disease[49] contribute to

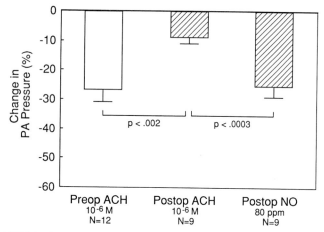

FIGURE 18–3. Percentage change in pulmonary artery (PA) pressure with 10^{-6} M dose of acetylcholine (ACh) in preoperative (Preop) patients and postoperative (Postop) patients. The vasodilating response to acetylcholine is attenuated in postoperative patients, but the capacity for vasodilation, as indicated by the response to inhaled nitric oxide (NO), is retained. (Modified from Wessel DL, Adatia I, Gaglia TM, et al: Use of inhaled nitric oxide and acetylcholine in the evaluation of pulmonary hypertension and endothelial function after cardiopulmonary bypass. Circulation 88:2128, 1993, with permission.)

postoperative pulmonary hypertension. In one study, 20 infants presenting with isolated TAPVC were monitored for pulmonary hypertension. A mean percentage decrease of 42 percent in pulmonary vascular resistance and 32 percent in mean pulmonary artery pressure was demonstrated with 80 ppm of NO. There was no significant change in heart rate, systemic blood pressure, or vascular resistance.[50]

Inhaled NO can also be used diagnostically in neonates with right ventricular hypertension after cardiac surgery to determine which infants have reversible vasoconstriction. Failure of the postoperative newborn with pulmonary hypertension to respond to NO successfully discriminated anatomic obstruction to pulmonary blood flow from pulmonary vasoconstriction.[51] Failure of the postoperative newborn to respond to NO should be regarded as strong evidence of anatomic and possibly surgically remediable obstruction.

Patients with TAPVC, congenital mitral stenosis, and other disorders that cause pulmonary venous hypertension appear to be among the most responsive to NO. These infants are born with significantly increased amounts of smooth muscle in their pulmonary veins. Histologic evidence of muscularized pulmonary veins, as well as pulmonary arteries, suggest the presence of vascular tone and capacity for change in resistance at both the arterial and venous sites. The increased responsiveness seen in younger patients with pulmonary venous hypertension to NO may result from pulmonary vasorelaxation of both pre- and postcapillary vessels.

Successful use of inhaled NO in a variety of congenital heart defects following cardiac surgery has been reported by several groups.[52-56] It may be especially helpful when administered during a pulmonary hypertensive crisis. Descriptions of use after Fontan procedures[57] and following ventricular septal defect (VSD) repair have been described along with a variety of other anatomic lesions.

Very young infants who are excessively cyanotic after a bidirectional Glenn anastomosis do not generally improve their oxygen saturation in response to inhaled NO.

Some studies suggest that there is a correlation between the response to NO and the extent of preoperative pulmonary hypertension.[58, 59] However, as pulmonary vascular obstructive disease progresses in the unrepaired patient, the pulmonary vasculature becomes less responsive acutely to NO as well as other vasodilators.

Reports have shown dramatic improvement in the oxygenation of children who have pneumonia that is caused by the respiratory syncytial virus, group B streptococcus, and other organisms.[60, 61] This is presumably attributable to improved ventilation–perfusion matching. In animal models of endotoxemia, inhaled NO improved pulmonary hypertension, pulmonary edema, and oxygenation.[62] Overwhelming pneumonia is a devastating complication of heart disease that may be exacerbated by cardiopulmonary bypass. Mild infectious pneumonitis or bronchiolitis in the young preoperative infant can turn to life-threatening respiratory failure during postoperative recovery from surgery. As an inhaled vasodilator, NO therapy addresses both aspects of the disease: pulmonary hypertension and hypoxia. Inhaled NO, by virtue of its antioxidant effects, inhibition of unwanted platelet aggregation, and suppression of deleterious inflammatory responses during reperfusion injury, may even have a role in routine prophylactic use for all patients at risk of postbypass respiratory complications. The use of NO in adults with acute respiratory distress syndrome has been shown to improve oxygenation, but improvement in meaningful clinical end points has been difficult to prove in this heterogeneous population. However, use of NO in patients with transient graft dysfunction after lung transplantation is now well described.

When administered chronically, other actions of inhaled NO may further increase its therapeutic potential, even in Eisenmenger's disease and other advanced forms of primary pulmonary hypertension or pulmonary vascular hypoplasia. Inhaled NO attenuates proliferation of vascular smooth muscle, inhibits platelet aggregation, provides cytoprotection of donor organs, ameliorates harmful aspects of ischemia-reperfusion injury, and improves the oxygen-carrying capacity of sickle hemoglobin. Chronic inhalation of NO also may promote angiogenesis in the immature lung. Although outpatient use of inhaled NO has been reported in a small number of adults,[63] its use in younger patients with heart disease is largely unstudied.[64] It also reduces hypoxic remodeling in the rat lung,[65] suggesting that it might have a salutary effect on scarring or pathologic remodeling in the human lung. The antioxidant and antiproliferative effects of NO combined with its antihypertensive action might provide a theoretical basis for prolonged treatment of primary pulmonary hypertension. This might be particularly applicable to infants, who by virtue of their young age, have substantial capacity for smooth muscle regression, alveolar growth, and angiogenesis. Apparent reversal of presumed fatal forms of primary pulmonary hypertension in infancy has been seen with prolonged administration of NO (inhibition of smooth muscle growth) and heparin (angiogenesis).[66]

At the relatively low levels of NO used therapeutically (1 to 80 ppm), the metabolic fate of inhaled NO is an accumulation of nitrate and nitrite in plasma and a small increase in methemoglobin; there is little detectable nitrosylhemoglobin present.[67] Possible toxicities of inhaled NO include methemoglobinemia due to the intravascular binding to hemoglobin,[68] cytotoxic effects in the lung due to either free radical formation, development of excess nitrogen dioxide, peroxynitirite production, or injury to the pulmonary surfactant system.[69] Carcinogenic potential and teratogenic potential of inhaled NO exist, as well as effects on glutathione metabolism, unknown effects on immature or immunocompromised lung, potential interaction with other heme-containing proteins, and effects on platelet function and hemostasis.

Caution must be exercised when administering NO to patients with severe left ventricular dysfunction and pulmonary hypertension. In adults with ischemic cardiomyopathy, sudden pulmonary vasodilation may occasionally unload the right ventricle sufficiently to increase pulmonary blood flow and harmfully augment preload of a compromised left ventricle.[70, 71] The attendant rise in left atrial pressure may produce pulmonary edema.[72] This increase in left atrial pressure is not likely to arise from any negative inotropic effect of NO[73] and may be ameliorated by vasodilators or diuretics. Anesthesiologists should be cognizant of this potential adverse effect during acute testing of unstable patients during cardiac catheterization, even though it has not been reported to occur in children with congenital heart disease.

Abrupt withdrawal effects of NO or even rebound pulmonary hypertension are important issues. Appreciation of the transient characteristics of withdrawal of NO may facilitate weaning from NO and has important implications for patients with persistent pulmonary hypertensive disorders when interruption of NO is necessary.[50, 74] If the underlying pulmonary hypertensive process has not resolved, then the tendency for an abrupt increase in pulmonary artery pressure may be hazardous when NO therapy is withdrawn or interrupted.[75, 76] If withdrawal of NO is necessary before resolution of the pathologic process, hemodynamic instability may be expected. If labile pulmonary hypertension is stabilized with NO prior to transfer to a specialized center, NO should be administered during transport of the patient. Recent work suggests that the withdrawal response to inhaled NO can be attenuated by pretreatment with the type V phosphodiesterase inhibitor, sildenafil (Viagra).[77]

Diastolic Function

Occasionally there is an alteration of ventricular relaxation, an active energy-dependent process, which reduces ventricular compliance. This is particularly problematic when patients with a hypertrophied ventricle are undergoing surgical repair (e.g., tetralogy of Fallot) and following CPB in some neonates when myocardial edema may significantly restrict diastolic function (i.e., "restrictive physiology"). The ventricular cavity size is small and the stroke volume is decreased. β-Adrenergic antagonists and calcium channel blockers add little to the treatment of this condition. In fact, hypotension or myocardial depression produced by these agents frequently outweighs any gain from slowing the heart rate. Calcium channel blockers are relatively contraindicated in neonates and small infants because of their dependence on transsarcolemal flux of calcium to both initiate and sustain myocardial contraction (see below).

A gradual increase in intravascular volume to augment ventricular capacity, in addition to the use of low doses of inotropic agents, has proven to provide modest benefit in patients with diastolic dysfunction. Tachycardia must be avoided to optimize diastolic filling time and to decrease myocardial oxygen demands. If low cardiac output continues despite the above-outlined treatment, therapy with vasodilators can be attempted to alter systolic wall tension (afterload) and thus decrease the impediment to ventricular ejection. Intuitively, one may hesitate to use vasodilators in the presence of marginal systemic arterial blood pressure because blood pressure is the product of cardiac output and systemic vascular resistance (SVR). But a decrease in SVR could increase flow with no undesirable changes in arterial pressure.[8] Because the capacity of the vascular bed increases after vasodilation, simultaneous volume replacement is indicated. Amrinone, milrinone, or enoximone are useful under these circumstances, since these agents are noncatecholamine so-called inodilators with vasodilating and lusitropic (improved diastolic state) properties, in contrast to other inotropic agents.[78–83]

THE NEONATE WITH CHD

Anesthetic Considerations for Surgical Repair

The disappointing cumulative morbidity and mortality of palliative operations, compared with those of reparative procedures, have become apparent over the past 10 to 20 years. Primary reparative surgery for CHD has had a significant impact on both the mortality due to the underlying defect and the secondary effects of the CHD on development of other organ systems. Nowhere has this impact been more dramatic than among neonates.[84]

Expanding the scope of reparative operations to the neonate has altered the demographic makeup of cardiac patients scheduled for operations and has created new challenges for anesthesiologists. The proportion of children undergoing cardiac surgery at Children's Hospital in Boston in the first year of life now exceeds 50 percent. Consequently, anesthesiologists must now be familiar not only with the pathophysiologic mechanisms of complex congenital heart disease but also with the special physiologic considerations specific to the neonate, especially concerning their response to anesthesia and surgery.

Care of the critically ill neonate requires an appreciation of the special structural and functional features of immature organs. The neonate appears to respond more quickly and extremely to physiologically stressful circumstances; this may be expressed in terms of rapid changes in, for example, pH, lactic acid, glucose, and temperature.[85] Neonates and infants have limited physiologic reserve. The mechanical disadvantage of an increased chest wall compliance and reliance on the diaphragm as the main muscle of respiration limits their capacity for ventilation. The diaphragm and intercostal muscles have fewer type I muscle fibers (i.e., slow-contracting, high-oxidative fibers for sustained activity), and this contributes to early fatigue when the work of breathing is increased. The neonate has a reduced functional residual capacity (FRC) secondary to their increased chest wall compliance (FRC being determined by the balance between chest wall and lung compliance). Closing capacity is also increased in newborns, which reduces oxygen reserve. This plus the increased basal metabolic rate and an oxygen consumption two to three times that of adults, put neonates and infants at risk for hypoxemia. When the work of breathing increases (e.g., with parenchymal lung disease, airway obstruction, cardiac failure or increased pulmonary blood flow), a larger proportion of total energy expenditure is required to maintain adequate ventilation. In addition, the neonate has diminished nutrient reserves in terms of fat and carbohydrate, which must be factored into the care of these infants. Infants with CHF therefore fatigue readily and fail to thrive.

Cardiorespiratory interactions are significant in neonates and infants. Ventricular interdependence means that a relative increase in right ventricle (RV) end-diastolic volume and pressure results in a leftward shift of the ventricular septum and diminished diastolic compliance of the left ventricle (LV). Therefore, a volume load from an intracardiac shunt or valve regurgitation, and a pressure load from ventricular outflow obstruction or increased vascular resistance, may cause biventricular dysfunction.

The myocardium in the neonate is immature; only 30 percent of the myocardial mass comprises contractile tissue versus 60 percent in mature myocardium. In addition, neonates have a lower velocity of shortening, a diminished length–tension relationship, and a reduced ability to respond to afterload stress.[86-90] The stroke volume is relatively fixed and cardiac output is heart rate dependent. The cytoplasmic reticulum and T-tubular system are underdeveloped, and the neonatal heart is dependent on the transsarcolemmal flux of extracellular calcium that both initiates and sustains contraction.

Immaturity of the liver and kidney may be associated with reduced protein synthesis and glomerular filtration, reducing drug metabolism and synthetic function. These problems may be compounded by the normally increased total body water of the neonate and by the propensity of the neonatal capillary system to leak fluid out of the intravascular space.[91] This is especially pronounced in the neonatal lung where the pulmonary vascular bed is almost fully recruited at rest, and the ability to recruit the additional lymphatic flow required to handle the increased mean capillary pressures associated with increases in pulmonary blood flow are unavailable.[92]

The neonate is infamous for maintaining blood pressure and luring the practitioner into a sense of security when, in fact, there exists a state of impending shock. Systemic blood pressure is not always a reliable indicator of the adequacy of preload or satisfactory oxygen delivery. The potential for sustained or labile increases in pulmonary vascular resistance is well known in neonates, especially those with CHD, and concern over evoking pulmonary hypertensive crisis has deterred some practitioners from

pursuing a reparative approach in neonates. Finally, the stress responses demonstrated in response to CPB (see below) must be considered in the overall approach to the postoperative management of these patients.[93, 94]

These factors do not preclude intervention in the case of neonates but merely dictate that extraordinary vigilance be applied to the care of these children and that management plans must take into account the immature physiology of these patients. Caring for the neonate therefore demands close monitoring of *more* physiologic variables, not fewer, and requires rapid analysis of events with appropriate and timely intervention.[84]

Whereas the neonate may be more labile to changes in intravascular pressures, PVR, and cardiac output than the older child, there is ample evidence that this age group is more resilient in its response to metabolic or ischemic injury. In fact, the neonate may be particularly capable of coping with some forms of stress. Tolerance of hypoxia in the neonate is characteristic of many species,[95] and the plasticity of the neurologic system in the neonate is well known. Neonates with obstructive left heart lesions often present with profound metabolic acidosis but can be effectively resuscitated without persistent organ system impairment or sequelae as the rule rather than the exception. The pliability and mobility of vascular structures in the neonate improve the technical aspects of surgery. Reparative operations in neonates take best advantage of normal postnatal changes, allowing more normal growth and development in crucial areas, such as myocardial muscle, pulmonary parenchyma, and coronary and pulmonary angiogenesis. Neonatal repair may obviate irreversible secondary organ damage arising from unrepaired or palliative approaches. Postoperative pulmonary hypertensive events are more common in the infant who has been exposed to weeks or months of high pulmonary pressure and flow.[13, 30] These events especially are more common for such lesions as truncus arteriosus, complete atrioventricular canal defects, and transposition of the great arteries with ventricular septal defects. Finally, cognitive and psychomotor abnormalities associated with months of hypoxemia or abnormal hemodynamics may be diminished or eliminated by early repair of cyanotic congenital heart lesions.

Although the technical aspects of CPB in small neonates seem formidable, surgical advances now allow routine corrective repair of complex heart disease in neonates weighing less than 2,000 g. In our experience, neither gestational age nor patient size precludes successful complete repair of lesions such as tetralogy of Fallot, truncus arteriosus, and transposition of the great arteries; survival for corrective surgery in neonates weighing less than 2,000 g now approaches 90 percent.[96, 97]

Hemodynamic Responses to Perioperative Pain and Stress

Neonates and infants are able to generate a significant metabolic and hormonal response to stress. In newborns without cardiac disease, adverse cardiorespiratory effects of the stress of awake intubation include bradycardia, hypoxia, lability in systemic blood pressure, and increased intracranial pressure. Similarly, the infant or neonate with cardiac disease may respond to stressful perioperative stimuli with altered hemodynamics and stress hormone levels.[98, 99] As a result, we do not recommend awake tracheal intubation of patients with cardiac disease, unless there is a dire emergency. Patients with CHD who are recovering from surgery are especially sensitive to stressful interventions; they have marginal organ system reserve and insufficient compensatory mechanisms to respond adequately. Extending anesthesia into the immediate postoperative period may blunt the adverse hemodynamic lability and hormonal stress response and improve outcome without complicating or extending postoperative care.

The postoperative myocardium previously exposed to the effects of cardiopulmonary bypass, the sequelae of deep hypothermia, or myocardial ischemic and hypoxic-ischemic reperfusion injury may not be capable of increasing stroke volume during a bradycardic episode or of maintaining cardiac output during an acute increase in afterload after surgical procedures. This is especially true when myocardial performance has been impaired by ventriculotomy, as is often required for repair of a variety of CHDs.

Neonates and infants are capable of generating an impressive rise in stress hormone levels in response to cardiopulmonary bypass.[93, 100] Infants who have a healthy heart and normal cardiovascular reserve may produce tachycardia, hypertension, and a transient decrease in arterial Po_2 to a painful or stressful stimulus.[98, 101] However, in a postoperative cardiac patient the tachycardia may evolve into a hemodynamically compromising tachyarrhythmia, and the hypertension may represent a critical and intolerable increase in ventricular afterload. Hypoxia may be profound and prolonged if the child has cyanotic heart disease or if there is an opportunity for right-to-left shunting during periods of agitation that result in increased intrathoracic pressure and right ventricular afterload.

Wakefulness, agitation, and stress responses may increase the work of breathing, exacerbate asynchrony between patient and ventilator, and allow an increase in a $Paco_2$ in mechanically ventilated children. The associated decrease in pH significantly raises pulmonary vascular resistance in children after cardiopulmonary bypass. Endotracheal suctioning causes sympathetic stimulation and marked elevation of pulmonary vascular resistance, which can be attenuated by pretreatment with high doses of narcotics,[102] or instillation of 1 percent lidocaine through the endotracheal tube.

This sensitivity to stimuli and the lability in hemodynamic response may be expressed as sudden death during the first postoperative night following apparently successful and uncomplicated surgery for congenital heart disease. This appears to be especially true for patients with labile pulmonary artery hypertension and for those who undergo palliative surgery for a single ventricle, in whom the balance between systemic and pulmonary vascular resistance plays an important role in hemodynamic stability.

These observations have motivated some to extend anesthesia through the first postoperative night in selected patients, using high-dose continuous infusions of fentanyl (10 to 15 μg/kg/h) after intraoperative anesthetic doses (50 to 100 μg/kg).[94] This philosophy has been applied to patients with unstable hemodynamics and pulmonary artery hypertension, and to high-risk neonates after CPB. The objective is to minimize hemodynamic lability in patients who may be unstable during the first postoperative night when their cardiac output reaches its nadir and their myocardial reserve is diminished. Precise control of Pco_2/pH and, hence, pulmonary vascular resistance is more easily achieved in a paralyzed and anesthetized patient. This approach to patient care requires close monitoring of intracardiac, pulmonary, and systemic artery pressure.

Another example where extending anesthesia into the postoperative period is important is in patients with an open sternum. Pericardial and sternal closure following cardiac surgery restricts cardiac function and may interfere with efficient mechanical ventilation. Leaving the chest open is particularly important for neonates and infants in whom considerable capillary leak and edema may develop following CPB, and in whom cardiopulmonary interactions have a significant impact on immediate postoperative recovery. In the operating room, mediastinal edema, unstable hemodynamic conditions, and bleeding are indications for delayed sternal closure. Sternal closure also may be considered semielectively for patients in whom hemodynamic or respiratory instability may be anticipated in the immediate postoperative period (e.g., following a Norwood procedure for hypoplastic left heart syndrome [HLHS]). Urgent reopening of the sternum in the intensive care unit (ICU) after surgery is associated with higher mortality than occurs when the sternum is left open in the operating room; successful sternal closure can be achieved for most patients by postoperative day 4; and the risk for surgical site infection is low.[103]

Critics of continuing the use of high-dose opioids into the postoperative period have argued that the use of any anesthetic depresses myocardial function and that blunting the endogenous sympathetic response to stimuli lowers vascular tone and invites an increase in the use of inotropic agents. They argue that controlled ventilation may be hazardous, as inadvertent extubation or other compromise of the airway will leave the patient unable to make spontaneous compensatory effort. However, two significant prospective studies support the notion that high-dose narcotic anesthesia for *selected* patients during the first postoperative night can be accomplished without additional morbidity and may prove advantageous over conventional analgesic regimens. In a randomized trial of neonates undergoing congenital heart surgery with either morphine/halothane or a high-dose synthetic narcotic for anesthesia and continued infusion of high-dose fentanyl through the first postoperative day, the authors demonstrated that the high-dose synthetic narcotic anesthesia group had lower levels of stress hormones, a decreased incidence of metabolic acidosis, fewer instances of hypotension, and a shorter ICU stay than the group that received morphine.[94]

Neurologic outcome following arterial switch operations in neonates with transposition of the great arteries was determined following detailed evaluation of hemodynamic changes and neurologic outcome in patients prospectively monitored in the operating room and ICU.[104] One hundred seventy-three patients were anesthetized with a high-dose synthetic narcotic (fentanyl 100 μg/kg [total dose]) for an arterial switch operation. The anesthesia was continued with fentanyl 10 to 15 μg/kg/h for the first postoperative night in the ICU. Patients who were hemodynamically unstable or in whom the chest could not be closed in the operating room were continued on the infusion of fentanyl for longer periods. There were no deaths during the first 72 postoperative hours and there was only 1 ICU death in 173 patients. This low mortality was achieved despite a low cardiac index (< 2 L/min/m^2) in 24 percent of patients and sufficient hemodynamic instability to delay sternal closure or dictate opening of the sternum in 18 patients. These results support the potential value of analgesia or extended anesthesia for selected patients.

Currently, we continue high-dose opioid infusions in the immediate postoperative period in patients who have limited systolic and diastolic function, or who have labile pulmonary hypertension. Specific circumstances include neonates following stage I palliation for hypoplastic left heart syndrome or similar single-ventricle physiology, and neonates following right ventricular outflow tract reconstruction, such as repair of tetralogy of Fallot and truncus arteriosus.

Early Extubation

For most patients undergoing congenital cardiac surgery, postoperative recovery is uncomplicated. This largely reflects the improvements in preoperative diagnosis and stabilization, surgical techniques and, in particular, cardiopulmonary bypass management, over the past decade. Indeed, the low mortality that is now evident after most congenital cardiac procedures means that this is no longer a significant outcome variable when comparing results of surgical techniques or changes in management practices. Postoperative morbidity is low, and it is difficult to evaluate or compare between institutions because of variable management practices. With the evolving changes in the economics of health care delivery, cost-effective management has become an important outcome variable. Many institutions have developed clinical practice guidelines to provide efficient and safe care for patients after cardiac surgery. Usually included within these practices are guidelines for early tracheal extubation protocols and early discharge from hospital. This clearly impacts on the anesthesia technique used. It is not necessary to use high-dose opioid anesthesia for all patients, nor is it necessary to continue the use of these drugs into the postoperative period.

Recovery following cardiac surgery and duration of mechanical ventilation depend upon numerous factors, including the patient's preoperative clinical condition, type and duration of surgical repair, hemodynamic stability, and complications such as postoperative bleeding and dysrhythmias. For the majority of patients with stable preoperative hemodynamics undergoing uncomplicated surgical repair, prolonged postoperative mechanical ventilation in the ICU is not necessary. Once hemodynamically stable, normothermic, and when hemostasis has been established following surgery, patients can be rapidly weaned from mechanical ventilation and the trachea can

be extubated. Examples include infants and older children undergoing uncomplicated atrial septal defect (ASD) and VSD repair, RV outflow tract reconstruction and conduit replacement, and following LV outflow tract reconstruction, such as aortic valve repair or replacement. Low-dose opioid techniques are used to maintain anesthesia, and following repair of lesions such as an ASD, tracheal extubation is possible in the operating room.[105] A similar approach for early tracheal extubation is applicable to patients following a cavopulmonary anastomosis when early resumption of spontaneous ventilation is preferable because of the potential deleterious effects of positive pressure ventilation on preload and pulmonary blood flow.

Patients undergoing early tracheal extubation can be managed with intermittent doses of opioids. This ensures adequate analgesia without the occurrence of respiratory depression. Sedation with benzodiazepines may be indicated for restlessness or agitation as patients emerge from anesthesia; this will prevent dislodgment of transthoracic catheters and chest drains.

A mild respiratory acidosis is common following tracheal extubation in the operating room or soon after transfer to the ICU, although the acidosis usually resolves within the first 6 hours or so after surgery.[105] Hypertension and tachycardia are common during emergence from anesthesia and sedation, which may increase the risk for bleeding from operative suture lines; antihypertensive agents may be necessary. Warming blankets should be used to prevent hypothermia and shivering in those patients who are extubated early. The patient must be closely observed for possible airway obstruction.

PATHOPHYSIOLOGY OF CHD

Principles of Management

The pathophysiologic consequences of CHD are derived primarily from anatomic circumstances that produce abnormalities of flow: outflow obstruction, regurgitant lesions, shunt lesions, and common mixing lesions. Typically, in more complex disease, shunts and obstructions may occur in combination. The pathophysiology of the most common purely obstructive lesions occurring outside the neonatal period are comparable to adult disease (e.g., aortic and mitral valve stenosis) and are not extensively reviewed here. Regurgitant lesions rarely exist as pure primary congenital defects except in Ebstein's malformation of the tricuspid valve, in which a regurgitant volume flows back through the tricuspid valve and is directed across the patent foramen ovale to produce cyanosis and various degrees of heart failure. However, as a complicating feature of other CHDs, regurgitant lesions produce a volume-overload circulation with progressive ventricular dilation and failure. This is seen most commonly when regurgitation is associated with atrioventricular canal defects, semilunar valve incompetence (as seen in tetralogy of Fallot with absent pulmonary valve), in truncal valve regurgitation in truncus arteriosus, or after interventions for aortic stenosis. Much of the remaining pathophysiology of congenital heart disease can be best understood by characterizing lesions with regard to the nature and magnitude of the shunt and the interaction of these shunts with obstructive lesions. Understanding the interactions of the various types of shunts and obstructions simplifies the bewildering variety of congenital heart lesions.

Many congenital heart lesions give rise to some degree of mixing of pulmonary and systemic venous blood, and they alter pulmonary blood flow. Varying degrees of hypoxemia may occur. These pathophysiologic mechanisms alter the volume and pressure load of the heart, as well as cardiovascular development. Although such acquired developmental abnormalities may be adaptive, they also can compound further the effects of the original congenital heart defect. The resultant cardiac and pulmonary vascular structural abnormalities may become as important as the original heart defects when the pathophysiology is determined (e.g., severe left ventricular hypertrophy, seen with coarctation of the aorta, and right ventricular hypertrophy with progressive outflow obstruction, seen with tetralogy of Fallot). However, the intracardiac shunting and alterations in pulmonary blood flow constitute the major, unique problems encountered with CHD. These problems complicate the task of administering adequate anesthesia while still maintaining normal cardiac output and oxygen transport.

Shunt Lesions

Central cardiac shunts are defined as direct communications across normally intact anatomic structures that divide the systemic and pulmonary circulations. Central shunts may occur alone as simple shunts (e.g., a VSD), or with complicating obstructive lesions in complex shunts such as tetralogy of Fallot. The direction and magnitude of shunts are variable, both within each cardiac cycle and over longer periods of cardiovascular development.[106] Shunts also change with anesthesia and with operative manipulation of the heart, great vessels and lungs, potentially destabilizing the circulation.

Control of Shunting

The hemodynamics in intracardiac shunts are complex and depend on many factors that determine shunt magnitude and direction (Fig. 18–4). Complete description of the dynamics of a particular shunt requires more data than are usually clinically available.[107] The determinants of shunting may change considerably during anesthesia and operative manipulations without being readily measurable. Nevertheless, the concepts of control of central shunting outlined below are useful during the perioperative period when it must be decided which shunts are hemodynamically significant and which are subject to intraoperative change.

Shunt orifice and outflow resistance are the most important determinants of shunting, particularly in ventricular and great vessel shunts. Ventricular compliance also may be important, but primarily as it relates to atrial level shunts. To simplify this discussion, ventricular compliance as a determinant of shunting is not further considered.

Simple Shunts

With simple shunts (those without associated obstructive lesions), outflow resistance is equivalent to PVR on the right and SVR on the left (Fig. 18–5). The effects of shunt orifice and vascular resistances on simple shunts are outlined in Table 18–3. Although restrictive shunts are relatively fixed in magnitude by the small shunt orifice, shunt direction and magnitude become more dependent on the ratio of outflow resistances (i.e., the relative resistances of the pulmonary and systemic vascular beds [PVR/SVR]), as the communication becomes larger and nonrestrictive (equal to or exceeding the aortic valve area).[108]

When the communication becomes large enough, the two structures effectively become a common chamber and complete mixing occurs. With complete mixing in a common chamber and no outflow obstruction, the amount of pulmonary and systemic blood flow depend on PVR/SVR. Because normal PVR is often much less than SVR (as little as 5 percent of SVR in older children and adults), pulmonary blood flows can become large with a nonrestrictive simple shunt, even during the neonatal period.

Although a number of factors affect PVR/SVR, some are relatively fixed, whereas others are variable and dynamic. Simple shunting can change intraoperatively as dynamic factors change. Thus, shunting may be manipulated to variable degrees depending on the size of the communication and the ability to manipulate the dynamic portions of the relative vascular resistance. When shunt orifices are large and nonrestrictive, simple shunts are more subject to some manipulation.

Complex Shunt Lesions

With complex shunts (Fig. 18–6), a fixed outflow obstruction is present at the ventricular outflow, subvalvular, valvular, or supravalvular level, or in major vessels such as the pulmonary artery or aorta. The fixed resistance offered by the obstruction is added to the outflow resistance of the downstream vascular bed, which increases shunting to the opposite side of the circulation. When the fixed resistance is high, the resultant shunting away from the obstructed side is substantially fixed by the high resistance. Therefore, only a portion of a complex shunt is related to the relative resistances in the distal pulmonary and systemic vascular beds, and shunting through any communication is less dependent on PVR/SVR. As the outflow obstruction increases, changes in PVR or SVR become less important for determining flow. This is particularly true for the right side of the circulation, where normal PVR is low compared with the resistance offered by most right-sided obstructive lesions. For example, in tetralogy of Fallot with severe pulmonic stenosis, a component of the right-to-left shunting across the VSD is fixed by the pulmonary valve stenosis. An additional variable component of shunting may be due to variations in PVR or, more commonly, dynamic infundibular obstruction in the right ventricular outflow tract. Dynamic changes in variable portions of the total right-sided outflow obstruction may increase or decrease the total amount of right-to-left shunting, thereby increasing or decreasing cyanosis. Right-to-left shunting in the baseline state, when the dynamic obstructive components are minimal, is determined largely by the fixed pulmonary stenosis. These statements presume a constant SVR and cardiac output; large changes

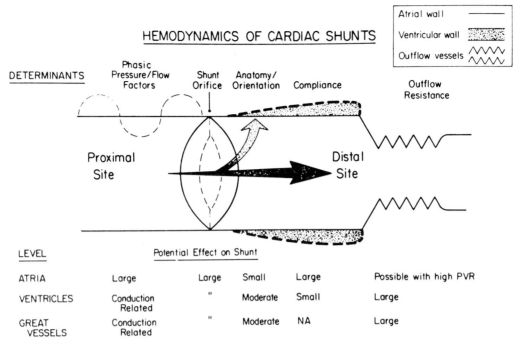

HEMODYNAMICS OF CARDIAC SHUNTS

LEVEL	Potential Effect on Shunt				
ATRIA	Large	Large	Small	Large	Possible with high PVR
VENTRICLES	Conduction Related	"	Moderate	Small	Large
GREAT VESSELS	Conduction Related	"	Moderate	NA	Large

FIGURE 18–4. Effects of the many determinants on central cardiac shunting at various levels. PVR, pulmonary vascular resistance. (From Berman W: Cardiovascular Shunts: Phylogenetic, Ontogenetic, and Clinical Aspects. New York, Raven Press, 1985, p 399, with permission.)

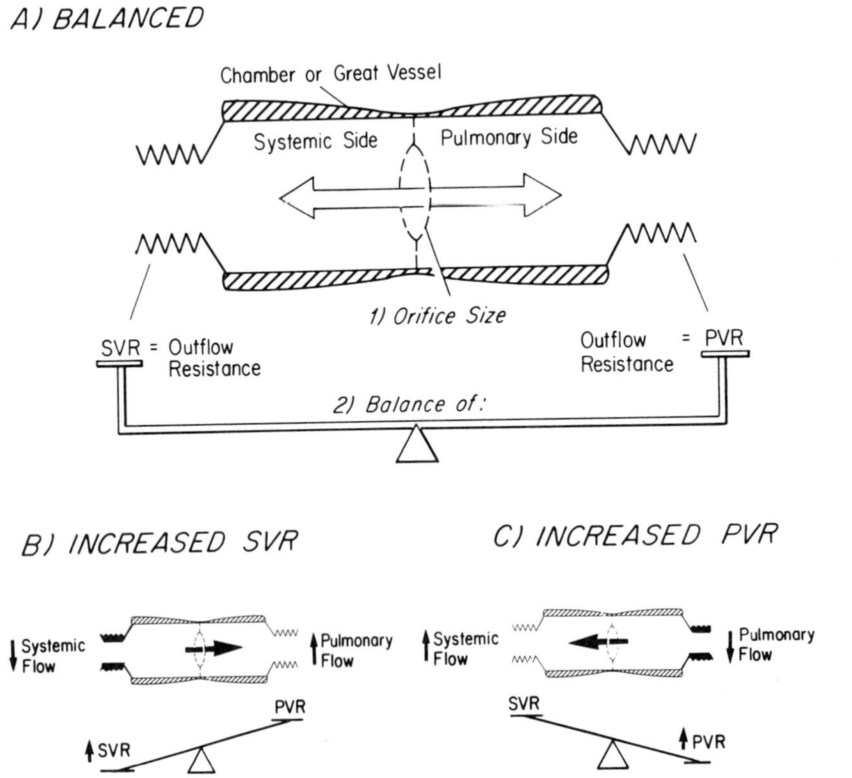

FIGURE 18–5. Determinants of the magnitude and direction of simple central shunts. *A*, Balanced PVR/SVR. *B*, Increased pulmonary flow with increased SVR. *C*, Increased systemic flow with increased PVR. (*1*) Orifice size generally fixed, is important for determining the magnitude of shunting and the pressure gradient across a shunt. (*2*) Balance of pulmonary vascular resistance (PVR) and systemic vascular resistance (SVR) is dynamic and determines the direction of shunt and variations in magnitude around the limits fixed by the orifice size. (From Hickey PR, Wessel DL: Anesthesia for treatment of congenital heart disease. *In* Kaplan JA [ed]: Cardiac Anesthesia. Orlando, FL, Grune & Stratton, 1987, with permission.)

TABLE 18-3
SIMPLE SHUNTS (NO OBSTRUCTIVE LESIONS)

Restrictive Shunts (Small Communications)	Nonrestrictive Shunts (Large Communications)	Common Chambers (Complete Mixing)
Large pressure gradient	Small pressure gradient	No pressure gradient
Direction and magnitude more *independent* of PVR/SVR	Direction and magnitude more dependent on PVR/SVR	Bidirectional shunting
Less subject to control	More subject to control	Net $\dot{Q}p/\dot{Q}s$ totally depends on PVR/SVR
Examples: small VSD, small PDA, Blalock shunts, small ASD	*Examples:* large VSD, large PDA, large Aortopulmonary shunts	*Examples:* single ventricle, truncus arteriosus, single atrium

PVR, pulmonary vascular resistance; SVR, systemic vascular resistance; $\dot{Q}p$, pulmonary blood flow; $\dot{Q}s$, systemic blood flow; PDA, patent ductus arteriosus; VSD, ventricular septal defect.

in SVR, of course, change shunting by altering the other side of the balance (Fig. 18–6). Characteristics and examples of complex shunts are listed in Table 18–4.

Complete Obstruction and Shunts

When obstruction to central outflow of blood becomes complete, as in tricuspid atresia, pulmonary atresia, or aortic atresia, shunting across communications proximal to the obstruction becomes total and obligatory. This type of shunting must be associated with another downstream shunt, which provides flow to the obstructed side of the circulation. This associated shunt is exemplified by a patent ductus arteriosus, which provides pulmonary blood flow with pulmonary valvular atresia or provides systemic blood flow with aortic valvular atresia. The downstream shunting is variably dependent on PVR/SVR, depending on the restrictive nature of the shunt orifice.

Manipulation of Pulmonary and Systemic Resistance

Manipulation of PVR/SVR allows some measure of control over shunting, depending on the specific pathophysiology.

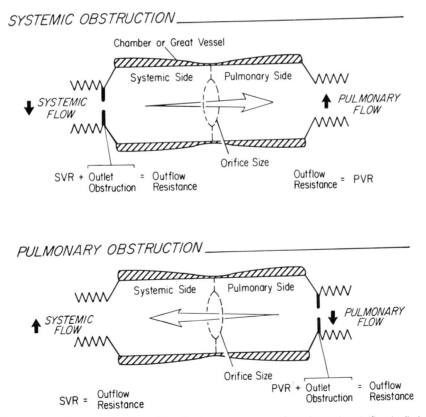

FIGURE 18–6. Determinants of complex shunting with systemic or pulmonary outflow obstruction. Orifice size limits the magnitude of the shunt. Outflow resistances are balanced by outlet obstruction on either side of the circulation and by the systemic vascular resistance (SVR) or pulmonary vascular resistance (PVR). Addition of outlet obstruction increases flow on the opposite side and decreases flow on the same side. (From Hickey PR, Wessel DL: Anesthesia for treatment of congenital heart disease. *In* Kaplan JA [ed]: Cardiac Anesthesia. Orlando, FL, Grune & Stratton, 1987, with permission.)

TABLE 18–4
COMPLEX SHUNTS (SHUNT AND OBSTRUCTIVE LESION)

Partial Outflow Obstruction	Total Outflow Obstruction
Shunt magnitude and direction largely fixed by obstructions	Shunt magnitude and direction totally fixed
Shunt depends less on PVR/SVR	All flow goes through shunt
Orifice and obstruction determine pressure gradient	Pressure gradient depends on orifice
Examples: tetralogy of Fallot, VSD and pulmonic stenosis, VSD with coarctation	*Examples:* tricuspid atresia, mitral atresia, pulmonary atresia, aortic atresia

PVR, pulmonary vascular resistance; SVR, systemic vascular resistance.

PVR is particularly important because of the frequency of disturbances of pulmonary blood flow and right-sided defects in CHD. Usually, PVR is decreased to improve pulmonary blood flow and right heart function, but with some lesions pulmonary flow may be excessively high at the expense of systemic blood flow and require increases in PVR. Some intraoperative manipulations may increase PVR, a common problem because of the increased reactivity and resistance of the abnormal pulmonary vasculature often found with CHD. These manipulations include sympathetic stimulation, encroachments on lung volumes that produce atelectasis (surgical retraction, pleural and peritoneal collections, abdominal packing), CPB, alveolar hypoxia, and hypoventilation. Ventilation is important because it is subject to control by the anesthesiologist and is crucial for determining PVR via airway pressure, lung volumes, $Paco_2$, pH, and Fio_2.

Ventilatory Control of PVR

The PVR can be controlled independently of the SVR by manipulating various aspects of ventilation (Table 18–5), whereas specific or selective pharmacologic control of PVR is difficult unless the pulmonary vascular bed is responsive to nitric oxide (see above). Even with selective infusions of rapidly metabolized vasoactive drugs into the pulmonary circulation, systemic drug concentrations and systemic hemodynamic effects can be appreciable.[109] In contrast, high levels of inspired oxygen, especially 100

TABLE 18–5
MANIPULATIONS ALTERING PULMONARY VASCULAR RESISTANCE

Increased PVR	Decreased PVR
Hypoxia	Oxygen
Hypercarbia	Hypocarbia
Acidosis	Alkalosis
Hyperinflation	Normal FRC
Atelectasis	Blocking sympathetic stimulation
High hematocrit	Low hematocrit
Surgical constriction	

PVR, pulmonary vascular resistance; FRC, functional residual capacity.

percent O_2, decrease elevated PVR in infants without changing (or slightly increasing) SVR, whereas inspired oxygen concentrations of 21 percent or less increase PVR.[97, 98, 110, 111] The effectiveness of oxygen (i.e., hyperoxia) as a pulmonary vasodilator after CPB, however, is unclear.[112] Hypoventilation, with associated acidosis and hypercapnia, also increases PVR (Fig. 18–7).[111] In contrast, hyperventilation to a pH of more than 7.5 reliably decreases PVR in infants with dynamically vasoconstricted small vessels.[113, 114] This maneuver increases pulmonary blood flow and decreases right-to-left shunting in neonates, increasing the Pao_2.[35, 115] Although prolonged hyperventilation to decrease PVR may in theory cause problems from decreased cerebral blood flow, clinical experimental studies in hyperventilated infants show little evidence of cerebral damage.[116–118]

The pattern of ventilation and use of positive end-expiratory pressure (PEEP) also can alter PVR. PVR is lowest at normal FRC. At low lung volumes (collapsed alveoli), PVR increases.[119] If atelectasis and pulmonary edema are corrected by PEEP, the PVR may in fact decrease. High levels of PEEP, however, may increase PVR, primarily by hyperinflating the alveoli. Different patterns of ventilation may further reduce PVR by stimulating production of prostacyclin in the pulmonary vasculature.[120, 121]

Anesthetics and PVR

The effects of anesthetic agents on PVR for the most part are minimal, although this depends to some extent on the underlying cause of the increase in PVR. Ketamine and nitrous oxide reportedly increase PVR in adults, particularly in patients with mitral stenosis, but do not affect the PVR of infants with normal or elevated PVR when ventilation and Fio_2 are held constant.[122–124] However, some workers have observed a rise in PVR when ketamine is given to sedated children spontaneously breathing room air during cardiac catheterization.[125] Stress responses in

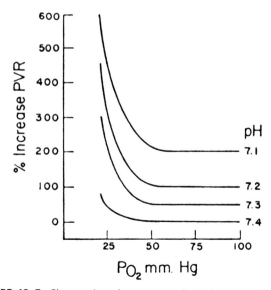

FIGURE 18–7. Changes in pulmonary vascular resistance (PVR) with changes in Pao₂ and arterial pH. (From Rudolph AM, Yuan S: Response to the pulmonary circulation to hypoxia and H+ ion changes. J Clin Invest 45:399, 1966, with permission.)

the pulmonary circulation of patients with CHD are of primary concern in some patients during the perioperative period. Large doses of synthetic opioids (e.g., fentanyl) attenuate pulmonary vascular responses to noxious stimuli, such as endotracheal suctioning, in infants, but they do not change the baseline PVR.[126, 127] Reactive hypertensive responses in the pulmonary bed are partially mediated by the sympathoadrenal axis and therefore are attenuated by an adequate depth of anesthesia, usually without changing the baseline PVR.

Manipulation of SVR

When deleterious intracardiac shunting cannot be controlled by manipulating PVR, it may be necessary to change SVR. In the presence of a complex shunt with *fixed* pulmonary outflow obstruction and right-to-left shunting (e.g., tetralogy of Fallot), an increase in SVR decreases the right-to-left shunting and increases arterial oxygen saturations.[128] Dynamic increases in infundibular outflow obstruction with tetralogy of Fallot that acutely increase baseline right-to-left shunting and hypercyanotic spells can be treated with intravenous (IV) pressor agents, which are shunted right-to-left directly into the systemic circulation, thus increasing SVR and decreasing right-to-left shunting. In the presence of a severely restrictive aortopulmonary shunt (e.g., Blalock-Taussig, Waterston) or when coronary perfusion is compromised, increases in systemic arterial pressure with pressor agents may increase pulmonary and coronary blood flow. Use of phenylephrine, norepinephrine, or other ∝-agonists to maintain high systemic perfusion pressure may be beneficial under these circumstances.[128] Alternatively, proximal aortic (or left ventricular) pressure can occasionally be increased by partially occluding the aorta with a clamp to increase SVR.

Pulmonary Circulation

Alterations in pulmonary blood flow caused by central shunting in patients with CHD may produce several problems: pulmonary vascular obstructive disease, arterial desaturation, or an increased volume load on the heart. These alterations are variable because of the changes in PVR that occur during development (Fig. 18–8). Because of these changes, associated problems may appear at different times during development. Dramatic alterations in pulmonary blood flow are seen during the neonatal period at the time of transition to adult-type circulation.

Transitional Circulation

The transitional circulation of normal neonates can be viewed as a transient form of CHD. Shunting occurs in either direction through the ductus arteriosus and the foramen ovale until these structures functionally, and later anatomically, close. Initially, high PVR promotes right-to-left shunting through the ductus arteriosus and foramen ovale, which causes hypoxemia (Figs. 18–8 and 18–9). Later, as PVR decreases, shunting through the ductus reverses and becomes left-to-right until the ductus closes anatomically (Figs. 18–8 and 18–9). When undergoing major noncardiac surgery, neonates may revert to this

transitional circulation despite previous *functional* closure of the ductus arteriosus and foramen ovale. The anesthetic plan should anticipate this possibility, and all neonates should be considered to have potential for intracardiac shunting. Intraoperatively, hypoxia, acidosis, hypercapnia, hypothermia, sepsis, and prolonged stress favor return to the transitional circulation pattern. This pattern occurs because the degree of hypoxic pulmonary vasoconstriction is much greater in normal newborns than in adults. The resulting high pulmonary artery pressures may exceed aortic pressures and produce intermittent or continuous right-to-left shunting through a patent ductus arteriosus or foramen ovale.[129] Once the period of perioperative stress is over, normal developmental changes modify and functionally eliminate the ductus arteriosus, foramen ovale, and high PVR.

In children with forms of CHD that are "ductus-dependent," the transitional circulation serves a palliative role by providing either adequate pulmonary or systemic flow until intervention can establish more normal patterns of flow. In these patients, the transitional circulation is actively supported with PGE₁ (see below).

Pulmonary Vascular Obstructive Disease

In the presence of a nonrestricted simple shunt (e.g., a large VSD), blood flow into the lungs increases as PVR decreases (Fig. 18–8). However, the pulmonary artery pressure and volume overload resulting from such shunts may, over time, alter pulmonary vascular development and cause pulmonary vascular obstructive disease (Figs. 18–8 and 18–10).[29, 130, 131] This occurs with large VSDs, an atrioventricular canal, transposition of the great arteries, truncus arteriosus, and a large patent ductus arteriosus. In lesions such as atrial septal defects (ASDs), where only flow is increased and pulmonary artery pressures are initially normal, pulmonary vascular disease takes decades to develop.[132] In contrast, pulmonary vascular disease can occur even during the first year of life in patients with an atrioventricular canal or in the first weeks of life in those with transposition of the great arteries and VSD.[133] A progressive increase in PVR may lead to chronic right-to-left shunting and right ventricular failure.

Intraoperatively, the more muscular and less well-arborized pulmonary arterial tree of patients with pulmonary vascular obstructive disease is capable of additional increases in PVR in response to surgical stimuli and stress. Right-to-left shunting may appear or dramatically increase during this time. Minimizing the reactive component of PVR without lowering SVR is often critical in anesthetic management.

Decreased flow in the pulmonary circulation during development also can lead to early significant abnormalities in the pulmonary arterial tree, including hypoplasia in some areas and excessive flow producing vascular obstructive disease in other regions.[28] This is especially true in patients with tetralogy of Fallot and pulmonary atresia, in whom the pulmonary artery anatomy must be addressed early in life.

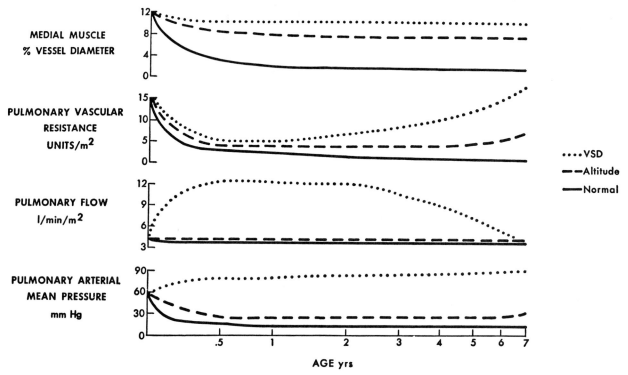

FIGURE 18–8. Normal and abnormal developmental changes in the pulmonary arterial tree during the first years of life. Pulmonary vascular resistance, arterial smooth muscle (%), and pressure normally decrease during the first year of life. A large, nonrestrictive VSD with a large left-to-right shunt results in an immediate increase in flow and a later increase in vascular resistance. (From Rudolph AM: Congenital Diseases of the Heart. Chicago, Year Book Medical Publishers, 1974, p 79, with permission.)

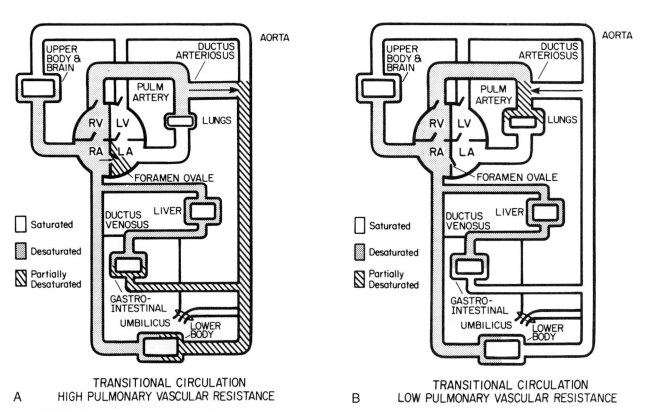

FIGURE 18–9. Central shunting and blood saturations that occur normally in the transitional circulation during the first few hours and days after birth. During the first few hours *A*, the foramen oval is widely patent and pulmonary vascular resistance is high, leading to right-to-left shunting. *B*, A second, later stage of transitional circulation when pulmonary vascular resistance decreases and the ductus arteriosus remains patent, resulting in left-to-right shunting. The foramen ovale is functionally closed. (From Hickey PR, Crone RK: Cardiovascular physiology and pharmacology in children. *In* Ryan J, Todres D, Cote C, Goudsouzian N [eds]: A Practice of Anesthesia for Infants and Children. Orlando, FL, Grune & Stratton, 1986, p 175, with permission.)

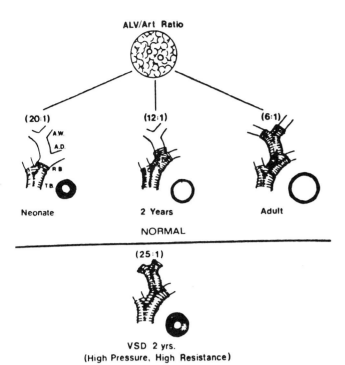

FIGURE 18–10. Developmental changes in the peripheral pulmonary arterial tree in normal infants and in those with a VSD and a large left-to-right shunt. The alveolar/arteriolar (ALV/art) ratio decreases with age because of extensive arborization of the arterial tree as the arteriolar lumen increases and the muscle layer thins and spreads distally. Pulmonary hypertension and high flow of blood from a left-to-right shunt in a patient with a VSD cause pulmonary vascular obstructive disease as evidenced by a decreased number of pulmonary arterioles (ALV/art of 25:1), a decrease in vessel lumen, an increase in muscle thickness, and a more distal spread of muscle. Letters indicate arterioles from the level of the terminal bronchiolus (T.B.) to the alveolar wall (A.W.). RB, respiratory bronchiolus; AD, alveolar duct. (From Rabinovitch MB, Hawroth SG, Castaneda AR: Lung biopsy in congenital heart disease: a morphometric approach to pulmonary vascular disease. Circulation 58:1107, 1978, with permission.)

Arterial Desaturation

Systemic arterial desaturation in CHD frequently results from shunting of systemic venous blood into the systemic arterial circulation rather than from pulmonary parenchymal problems. If pulmonary parenchymal disease is also present, it is even more difficult to achieve adequate arterial oxygenation. Shunt-related arterial desaturation can occur whether pulmonary blood flow is greater than, equal to, or less than systemic flow. The effects of alterations in pulmonary blood flow on arterial oxygenation in the presence of various shunts are listed in Table 18–6. It is important to realize that an F_{IO_2} of more than 0.21 has little effect on arterial oxygen tension in the presence of a large right-to-left shunt, but it has more effect as the shunt becomes smaller (Fig. 18–11). This statement presumes no pulmonary parenchymal disease and fully saturated pulmonary venous blood.

Many poorly understood adaptations occur in patients with severe hypoxemia to allow reasonable levels of oxygen transport and consumption, including polycythemia, increases in 2,3-diphosphoglycerate (2,3-DPG) concentrations, vasodilation with increased blood volume, neovascularization, and alveolar hyperventilation with chronic

T A B L E   18 – 6
EFFECTS OF CENTRAL SHUNTING AND PULMONARY BLOOD FLOW ON OXYGENATION

Pulmonary Blood Flow ($\dot{Q}p$)	L→R Shunt Only	L→R + R→L (mixing)	R→L Shunt Only
$\dot{Q}p > \dot{Q}s$	Normoxemia	Hypoxemia*	—
$\dot{Q}p = \dot{Q}s$	—	Hypoxemia	—
$\dot{Q}p < \dot{Q}s$	—	Hypoxemia (severe)	Hypoxemia (severe)

$\dot{Q}p$, pulmonary blood flow; $\dot{Q}s$, systemic blood flow; —, does not occur.
* Normoxemia when $\dot{Q}p/\dot{Q}s \geq 7$–10.

respiratory alkalosis.[134] These and other poorly defined adaptive mechanisms maintain near-normal levels of mitochondrial oxygen utilization at rest without increased lactate production. Elevated cardiac output and substantial shifts in the oxyhemoglobin dissociation curve are not essential adaptations for patients with severe hypoxemia.[135]

The adaptations, however, may be associated with adverse physiologic effects. Polycythemia increases blood viscosity, vascular resistance, and therefore ventricular afterload, especially in the pulmonary circulation.[136, 137] As increasing viscosity elevates afterload, it decreases cardiac output, which opposes the benefit of polycythemia to oxygen-carrying capacity. The net reduction in oxygen transport is maladaptive and occurs when the hematocrit

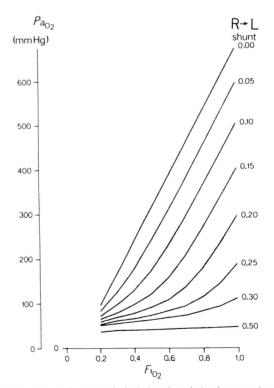

FIGURE 18–11. Isoshunt graph depicting the relation between inspired F_{IO_2} and arterial Pa_{O_2} with different amounts of right-to-left shunting. It assumes normal values of pH, Pa_{CO_2}, pulmonary venous saturation, and mixed venous saturation. (Adapted from Lawler PGP, Nunn JF: A reassessment of the validity of the isoshunt graph. Br J Anaesth 56:1325, 1984, with permission.)

exceeds 60 percent. Such high hematocrits are associated with an appreciable incidence of cerebral and renal thrombosis, which increases with dehydration. This situation makes pre- and postoperative hydration crucial in these patients.[138] Also associated with polycythemia are poorly defined coagulopathies, which generally improve, along with the risk of thrombosis, when the hematocrit is lowered.[139] Such coagulopathies are due in part to decreased fibrinogen and platelets, both of which correlate with the degree of hypoxemia in older patients.[140–142] An adequate supply of blood products is necessary for surgical operations because major bleeding may occur. Because of these problems, preoperative erythropheresis should be considered in patients with hematocrits of more than 70 percent.

Hypoxemia also occurs in situations other than those with a pure right-to-left shunt with decreased pulmonary blood flow. If systemic and pulmonary venous blood mix in a vascular chamber, arterial desaturation occurs, even though pulmonary blood flow may be normal or increased (Table 18–6). Mixing can occur at any anatomic level: right atrium (e.g., total anomalous pulmonary venous connection), left atrium (e.g., tricuspid atresia), ventricle (e.g., single ventricle), or great vessel (e.g., truncus arteriosus). When mixing is complete and pulmonary blood flow is normal or increased, hypoxemia is mild. When mixing is incomplete, hypoxemia may be severe, as occurs with the parallel circulation occurring in patients with transposition of the great arteries.

Increased Pulmonary Blood Flow

When pulmonary flow is greater than systemic flow ($\dot{Q}p/\dot{Q}s > 1$), a volume load is imposed on the heart. With pure left-to-right shunts, the additional pulmonary flow does not increase arterial oxygen content. This increased load decreases not only cardiovascular reserve but also pulmonary reserve, because the work of breathing is increased owing to decreased pulmonary compliance and increased airway resistance.[143] These changes in pulmonary function are due to increased lung water, compression of bronchi by distended pulmonary vessels, and general pulmonary vascular congestion. When left-to-right shunts are closed (e.g., ligation of a patent ductus arteriosus), lung compliance improves immediately.[144]

PREOPERATIVE ASSESSMENT AND PREPARATION

Successful anesthetic management of patients with CHD is based on complete, accurate preoperative assessment and adequate preoperative patient preparation. The clinical and laboratory information routinely available preoperatively (Table 18–7) should be frequently reassessed and integrated with information from continuous monitoring during surgery and the immediate recovery phase. The anesthesiologist must be cognizant of the physical and laboratory findings that are of particular importance for CHD. Involvement of the anesthesiologist in the preoperative preparation and early postoperative management pro-

TABLE 18–7
CLINICAL AND LABORATORY PREOPERATIVE ASSESSMENT

History and physical examination
Chest radiograph
Electrocardiogram
Complete blood count, blood urea nitrogen, creatinine, electrolytes
Calcium and glucose in newborns and critically ill children
Two-dimensional echocardiogram and Doppler flow study
Cardiac catheterization

vides a perspective on the pathophysiology that improves perioperative care.

Physical Examination and Laboratory Data

A complete history and physical examination are required; attention should be directed to the extent of cardiopulmonary impairment, airway abnormalities, and associated extracardiac congenital anomalies.[145, 146] Upper and lower airway problems in patients with Down syndrome, calcium and immunologic deficiencies in patients with aortic arch abnormalities, and renal abnormalities in patients with esophageal atresia and CHD are a few of the associated congenital abnormalities with which the anesthesiologist should be familiar. Intercurrent pulmonary infection is common in chronically overcirculated lungs. The presence, degree, and duration of hypoxemia are important details which, in the absence of iron deficiency, are reflected in the hematocrit. The nadir of physiologic anemia during infancy may contribute to left-to-right shunting by decreasing the relative PVR.[136]

Chest radiography shows heart size, pulmonary vascular congestion, airway compression, and areas of consolidation or atelectasis. The electrocardiogram (ECG) may reveal rhythm disturbances and demonstrate ventricular strain patterns (ST segment and T-wave changes) characteristic of unphysiologic pressure or volume burdens on the ventricles. Electrolyte abnormalities caused by congestive heart failure and forced diuresis also must be evaluated preoperatively. Severe hypochloremic metabolic alkalosis may occur in some patients. It is important to discontinue digoxin preoperatively and to avoid hyperventilation and administration of calcium to these patients during the induction of anesthesia. The alkalotic hypokalemic, hypercalcemic, hypotensive, dilated, digoxin-bound myocardium fibrillates with ease.

Echocardiographic and Doppler Assessment

Advances in echocardiographic imaging have had an enormous impact on the diagnosis of CHD.[147] Accurate anatomic diagnosis is now routine in children without the need for cardiac catheterization. Echocardiography is the preferred imaging modality for assessment of intracardiac anatomic features in young children. However, the anesthesiologist should be aware of the current limitations of echocardiographic and Doppler techniques so that alternative diagnoses can be considered when intraoperative or postoperative findings are inconsistent with the working echocardiographic diagnosis.

Skilled echocardiographers accurately interpret the alignment of cardiac chambers and great vessels but cannot always visualize an ASD or VSD, although color flow mapping techniques have vastly improved diagnostic capabilities. An ASD can be indirectly inferred from right ventricular volume overload and interventricular septal shift. Distal pulmonary artery architecture and conduits between a ventricle and a great artery are poorly imaged by echocardiography, and pressure gradients in these areas are not always measurable with Doppler techniques. Quantification of atrioventricular valve regurgitation may be subjective and nonquantitative. An inadequate window for imaging in the obese patient, the older child, and some postoperative patients limits accuracy of echocardiographic diagnoses. Although real-time three-dimensional imaging is currently not readily available, techniques for three-dimensional echocardiography are available and may improve diagnostic capabilities, such as defining the mechanism of valve regurgitation.

Doppler measurements add greatly to noninvasive diagnostic capabilities. Measurements of pressure gradients across semilunar valves and other obstructions are frequently accurate but may not always correlate with peak systolic ejection gradients measured at catheterization. As good as echocardiographic diagnosis of anatomic defects and Doppler measurements of pressure gradients and valve function have become, the standard for assessment of physiology when other clinical information is ambiguous or contradictory remains cardiac catheterization.

Cardiac Catheterization

When echocardiographic analysis with Doppler measurements and color flow mapping is complete and unambiguous, preoperative assessment may no longer require cardiac catheterization. Catheterization is not typically performed before infant or neonatal operations for ventricular septal defects, complete atrioventricular canal defects, tetralogy of Fallot, interrupted aortic arch, hypoplastic left heart syndrome, or coarction of the aorta. However, in older patients with complex anatomy, such as a single ventricle, physiologic data from catheterization may be essential. This technique allows description of the direction, magnitude, and approximate location of intracardiac shunts. Intracardiac and intravascular pressures are measured to determine the presence of obstructions and whether shunt orifices are restrictive or nonrestrictive. Pressure gradients across sites of obstruction must be considered in light of simultaneous blood flow; a small pressure gradient measured at a time of low cardiac output is misleading.

Normal intracardiac pressure and saturation values in children are shown in Figure 18–12. Normally, there is no significant change in oxygen saturation from vena cava to pulmonary artery. In the child with CHD, the superior vena cava gives the best indication of true mixed venous oxygen saturation; a 5 percent or greater step-up in saturation downstream suggests the presence of a left-to-right shunt.[148] It would occur at the level of the right atrium

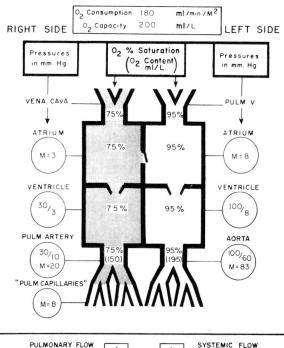

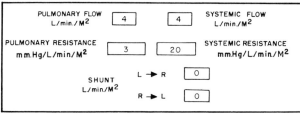

FIGURE 18–12. Cardiac catheterization findings in a normal child. Numbers in chambers are oxygen saturation (percent), and numbers in parentheses are oxygen content. Pressures in chambers are shown in circles. Note "probe-patent" foramen ovale. (From Nadas AS, Fyler DC: Pediatric Cardiology. Philadelphia, WB Saunders Company, 1972, with permission.)

with an ASD, in the right ventricle with a VSD, and in the pulmonary artery with a patent ductus arteriosus. The magnitude of the left-to-right shunt can be calculated from the Fick equation. The oxygen consumption of the patient is measured (assumed values are unreliable), as are the saturation values, but subsequent flow and resistance calculations can be in error. The frequently used term $\dot{Q}p/\dot{Q}s$ (pulmonary to systemic blood flow ratio) can be derived simply from the measured oxygen saturation values.

The patient whose aortic blood is fully saturated can be safely assumed to have no significant right-to-left shunting. However, when a right-to-left shunt is present, aortic blood is hypoxemic. Blood samples should also be obtained from the pulmonary veins, left atrium, and left ventricle for oxygen saturation determination and ascertainment of the source of desaturated blood. Pulmonary venous desaturation implies a pulmonary source of venous admixture (e.g., pneumonia, atelectasis, or other pulmonary disease). Intrapulmonary shunting may substantially alter the anesthetic plan and the postoperative ventilatory requirements of the patient.

In the presence of a left-to-right shunt and elevated PVR, pressure and saturation measurements are often repeated with the patient breathing 100 percent oxygen to assess both the reactivity of the pulmonary vascular bed and any contribution of ventilation–perfusion abnormalities to hypoxemia. If breathing 100 percent oxygen increases pulmonary blood flow and dramatically increases $\dot{Q}p/\dot{Q}s$ (with a decrease in PVR), potentially reversible processes such as hypoxic pulmonary vasoconstriction are probably contributing to the elevated PVR. The patient with a high, unresponsive PVR and a small left-to-right shunt, despite a large shunt orifice, may have extensive pulmonary vascular damage from irreversible obstructive pulmonary vascular disease. If so, surgical repair is usually contraindicated if the child is beyond 1 year of age.[149]

During cardiac catheterization, anatomic abnormalities are identified angiographically. Special angled views provide specific information about the location and extent of congenital defects.[150, 151] Ventricular function is assessed angiographically and physiologically (e.g., by pressure measurements). The calculated size of a cardiac chamber may have an important bearing on its ability to support the circulation of a child with hypoplastic ventricles.

Magnetic Resonance Imaging and Angiography

Magnetic resonance imaging and angiography (MRI/A) has emerged as an important diagnostic modality in the evaluation of the cardiovascular system following the development of ECG-gated MRI. Image acquisition is triggered to the patient's ECG to counter motion artifacts and to acquire cine sequences that allow imaging of cardiac structures and visualization of blood flow throughout the cardiac cycle. In addition to providing excellent anatomical and three-dimensional images, particularly of the pulmonary veins and thoracic aorta, it is also possible with magnetic resonance angiography (MRA) to qualitatively assess valve and ventricular function, and to quantify flow, ventricular volume, mass, and ejection fraction.[152, 153] While ferromagnetic implants near the region of interest might produce an artifact, sternal wires and vascular clips produce relatively minor disturbances and therefore MRI can be performed in patients who have undergone previous cardiac surgery. Contraindications to MRI/A include patients with pacemakers, recently implanted endovascular or intracardiac implants, and aneurysm clips on vessels that will be exposed directly to the magnetic field.

The claustrophobic small bore of the MRI machine and noise during imaging means that sedation is necessary for most children undergoing cardiac MRI/A. To allow three-dimensional MRA and gradient echo sequences for images of blood flow, breath-hold is necessary during image acquisition, and therefore general anesthesia is frequently required for neonates, infants, and young children. As for procedures in the catheterization laboratory, the environment for magnetic resonance imaging is often a difficult one in which to administer general anesthesia, and hemodynamic monitoring may be limited (see Chapter 28).

Assessment of Patient Status and Predominant Pathophysiology

Frequently, congenital heart defects are complex, and can be difficult to categorize or conceptualize. Rather than trying to determine the management for each individual

anatomic defect, a physiologic approach can be taken. The following questions should be asked:

1. How does the systemic venous return reach the systemic arterial circulation to maintain cardiac output? What intracardiac mixing, shunting, or outflow obstruction exists?
2. Is the circulation in series or parallel? Are the defects amenable to a two-ventricle or single-ventricle repair?
3. Is pulmonary blood flow increased or decreased?
4. Is there a volume load or pressure load on the ventricles?

Appropriate organization of preoperative patient data; preparation of the patient; and decisions about monitoring, anesthetic agents, and postoperative care are best accomplished by focusing on a few major pathophysiologic problems, beginning with whether the patient is cyanotic or in CHF (or both). Most pathophysiologic mechanisms in the patient's disease that are pertinent to the anesthetic plan and to optimal preparation of the patient will focus on one of the following major problems: severe hypoxemia, excessive pulmonary blood flow, CHF, obstruction of blood flow from the left heart, and poor ventricular function. Although some patients with CHD present with only one problem, many have multiple interrelated problems.

Severe Hypoxemia

Many of the cyanotic forms of CHD present with severe hypoxemia ($PaO_2 < 50$ mm Hg) during the first few days of life, but without respiratory distress. Infusion of PGE_1 in patients with decreased pulmonary blood flow maintains or reestablishes pulmonary flow through the ductus arteriosus. This also may improve mixing of venous and arterial blood at the atrial level in patients with transposition of the great arteries.[154] Consequently, neonates rarely require surgery while they are severely hypoxemic. During preoperative preparation with PGE_1, neurologic examination, as well as blood chemistry analysis of renal, hepatic, and hematologic function, is necessary to assess the effects of severe hypoxemia during or after birth on end-organ dysfunction.

Cyanotic patients who present for surgery after infancy require adequate pre- and postoperative hydration to prevent the thrombotic problems caused by their high hematocrits. Adequate quantities of blood products for treatment of the coagulopathies also are needed, as outlined above. Premedication must be given cautiously to avoid causing hypoventilation in these patients.

PGE_1 dilates the ductus arteriosus of the neonate with life-threatening ductus-dependent cardiac lesions and improves the patient's condition before surgery. PGE_1 can reopen a functionally closed ductus arteriosus for several days after birth, or it can maintain patency of the ductus arteriosus for several months postnatally.[154, 155] The common side effects of PGE_1 infusion—apnea, hypotension, fever, central nervous system (CNS) excitation—are easily managed in the neonate when normal therapeutic doses of the drug (0.02 to 0.1 μg/kg/min) are used.[156] However,

PGE_1 is a potent vasodilator, so intravascular volume frequently requires augmentation. Patients with intermittent apnea resulting from administration of PGE_1 may require mechanical ventilation preoperatively.

PGE_1 usually improves the arterial oxygenation of hypoxemic neonates who have poor pulmonary perfusion that is caused by obstructed pulmonary flow (critical pulmonic stenosis or pulmonary atresia). By providing pulmonary blood flow from the aorta via the ductus arteriosus, an infusion of PGE_1 improves oxygenation and stabilizes the condition of neonates with these lesions. The improved oxygenation reverses the lactic acidosis that may have developed during episodes of severe hypoxia. PGE_1 administration for 24 hours usually markedly improves the condition of a severely hypoxemic neonate with restricted pulmonary blood flow.[157]

Excessive Pulmonary Blood Flow

Excessive pulmonary blood flow is frequently the primary problem of patients with CHD. The anesthesiologist must carefully evaluate the hemodynamic and respiratory impact of left-to-right shunts (see above). Children with left-to-right shunts may have a chronic low-grade pulmonary infection and congestion that cannot be eliminated despite optimal preoperative preparation. If so, surgery should not be postponed further. Respiratory syncytial virus infections are particularly prevalent in this population, but improvements in intensive care have markedly improved outcome of patients with this and other viral pneumonias.[158]

Aside from the respiratory impairment caused by increased pulmonary blood flow, the left heart must dilate to accept pulmonary venous return that is several times normal. If the body requires more systemic blood flow, the heart responds inefficiently. Most of the increment in cardiac output is recirculated to the lungs. Eventually, symptoms of CHF appear.

Children with failing hearts increase endogenous catecholamine production and redistribute cardiac output to favored organs by their increased heart rate and decreased extremity perfusion.[159] In the most severe cases, the evaluation reveals a child whose body weight is below the third percentile for age and who is tachypneic, tachycardic, and dusky in room air. The child may have intercostal and substernal retractions and skin that is cool to the touch. Capillary refill may be prolonged. Expiratory wheezes are usually audible (Table 18–8). Medical management with digoxin and diuretics may improve the patient's condition, but the diuretics may induce a profound hypochloremic alkalosis and potassium depletion.

These clinical signs and symptoms suggest that profound pathophysiologic alterations have occurred. This information, combined with the anatomic description from the two-dimensional echocardiogram and the physiologic data from cardiac catheterization, permit accurate assessment of the severity of the illness and formulation of an anesthetic plan. For example, it may be prudent to minimize premedication, begin an IV infusion while the patient is awake, induce anesthesia with an IV narcotic while the patient breathes oxygen, and be prepared to support the circulation immediately with inotropic and

TABLE 18–8
SYMPTOMS AND SIGNS OF CARDIAC FAILURE IN A NEONATE AND INFANT

Failure to thrive
   Poor feeding
   Diaphoresis

Increased respiratory work
   Tachypnea
   Wheezing
   Grunting
   Flaring of ala nasi
   Chest wall retraction

Altered cardiac output
   Tachycardia
   Gallop rhythm
   Cardiomegaly
   Poor extremity perfusion
   Hepatomegaly

pressor drugs when necessary in the sickest patients with respiratory compromise and minimal cardiac reserve. Alternatively, the physical examination may indicate that the patient is only mildly symptomatic and should tolerate a standard premedication and sevoflurane or halothane/nitrous oxide inhalation induction of anesthesia for an elective operation.

Obstruction of Left Heart Outflow

Patients who require surgery to relieve obstruction of outflow of blood from the left heart are among the most critically ill children for whom the anesthesiologist must care. These lesions include interruption of the aortic arch, coarctation of the aorta, aortic stenosis, and mitral stenosis or atresia that occurs as part of the hypoplastic left heart syndrome. These neonates present with inadequate systemic perfusion and profound metabolic acidosis. The initial pH may be less than 7.0 despite a $PaCO_2$ of less than 20 mm Hg. Systemic blood flow is largely or completely dependent on blood flow into the aorta from the ductus arteriosus.

Closure of the ductus arteriosus in the neonate who has any of these problems causes dramatic worsening of the patient's condition. The patient becomes critically ill or even moribund and requires PGE_1 infusion (see above) for survival. PGE_1 allows blood flow into the aorta from the pulmonary artery because it maintains the patency of the ductus arteriosus.[157, 160, 161] In neonates with acidosis, metabolic derangements, and renal failure due to inadequate systemic perfusion, PGE_1 infusion improves perfusion and metabolism, and surgery can be deferred until the patient's condition improves. Ventilatory and inotropic support and correction of metabolic acidosis, along with calcium, glucose, and electrolyte abnormalities, are often indicated preoperatively. The stabilization period also allows assessment of the magnitude of end-organ dysfunction caused by the preceding period of inadequate systemic perfusion. Adequacy of resuscitation, rather than severity of illness at presentation, appears to influence postoperative outcome.[162]

Ventricular Dysfunction

Older patients with CHD and poor ventricular function due to chronic ventricular volume overload (aortic or mitral valve regurgitation or longstanding pulmonary-to-systemic arterial shunts) present a different problem. Although patients with large shunts may have complete mixing of systemic and venous blood and only mild to moderate hypoxemia as a result of their excessive pulmonary blood flow, the price paid for near-normal arterial oxygen saturation is chronic ventricular dilation and dysfunction as well as pulmonary vascular obstructive disease. Consequently, narrowing of the shunt or a staged approach to single-ventricle repair may be indicated before any other elective surgery can be undertaken.

Assessment should include an estimation of the patient's functional limitation as an indicator of myocardial performance and reserve, quantification of the degree of hypoxia and the amount of pulmonary blood flow, and evaluation of PVR. For patients with an increased $\dot{Q}p/\dot{Q}s$, during induction of anesthesia, systemic blood flow should be optimized without further augmenting pulmonary flow. However, during maintenance and emergence from anesthesia, retraction of the lung, changes in position, and abdominal distention may increase the hypoxemia and compromise the function of a dilated, poorly contractile ventricle. If this sequence occurs during surgery, the anesthetic management must be altered to improve pulmonary blood flow.

In addition, systolic function of the ventricle may be impaired by intrinsic myopathic abnormalities related to drug toxicity (e.g., Adriamycin), inborn enzyme deficiencies, or acquired inflammatory or infectious disease. Patients with such dilated cardiomyopathies require optimization of ventricular performance with emphasis on inotropic support and afterload reduction.

MONITORING FOR CONGENITAL HEART OPERATIONS

Preoperative assessment of the patient includes determining the appropriate monitors for the particular patient and the risks and benefits of the monitoring. The information from the monitoring devices must be interpreted in light of preoperative data, events in the surgical field, and the appearance of the patient. When the chest is open, direct observation of the heart's contractile state and performance and the adequacy of lung inflation and deflation are important sources of information.

Standard Monitoring

In addition to the standard monitoring employed for any pediatric patient undergoing anesthesia, a pulse oximeter must be used, particularly for patients with potential for right-to-left shunting and hypoxemia. Pulse oximetry is a sensitive, on-line monitor of intraoperative circulatory homeostasis, and reflects adequacy of gas exchange, cardiac output, pulmonary blood flow, and intracardiac shunting. Although its accuracy at the low oxygen saturations commonly seen in children with CHD is diminished,

pulse oximetry provides valuable information in the care of these patients.[163, 164] Continuous intra-arterial oximetry or blood gas determination also is possible.[165] In addition to a standard lead II, simultaneous monitoring of a V lead is recommended in children with any type of left ventricular outflow obstruction or coronary artery anomaly. Monitoring of at least two leads is recommended for all patients undergoing cardiac surgery.

Direct arterial pressure monitoring yields important beat-to-beat information in cardiac patients, but because arterial catheters are not without risk, especially in infants, they are not always indicated for less complex procedures and less symptomatic patients.[166] In general, radial arterial lines are preferred, but previous Blalock-Taussig shunts or repairs of aortic coarctation make ipsilateral radial arterial pressure monitoring inaccurate. Although femoral arterial lines are an excellent alternative to radial artery lines in older children, they may be associated with a high complication rate in neonates.[167] Caution is required in flushing radial artery catheters because volumes as small as 0.3 ml force microbubbles and small thrombi retrogradely into the carotid arteries.[168] Peripheral arterial lines, particularly those in the foot, may not accurately reflect the central aortic pressure of hypothermic children, especially during CPB and deep hypothermia.

End-tidal CO_2 (P_{ETCO_2}) monitoring should be used for all intubated patients. Besides providing valuable information regarding correct placement of the endotracheal tube following tracheal intubation, loss of the P_{ETCO_2} tracing may provide early warning that the endotracheal tube has been dislodged inadvertently by the cardiac surgeon during the procedure. If intraoperative transeophageal echocardiography (TEE) is used, placement or removal of the TEE probe may dislodge the endotracheal tube. Anterior flexion of the TEE probe may also compress the left or right mainstem bronchi, often manifesting itself as hyperinflation of one lung or a sudden increase in P_{ETCO_2}.[169]

The amount of pulmonary blood flow also has a significant impact on P_{ETCO_2}. Patients with an increased $\dot{Q}p/\dot{Q}s$ (>2:1) may have congested lung fields and pulmonary edema; total lung compliance is decreased and airway resistance is increased. Extrinsic compression of larger airways by a dilated pulmonary artery or dilated left atrium may cause lobar collapse. The lung fields may appear hyperinflated on chest x-ray because the distal airway is compressed by dilated pulmonary vessels within the lung. All these factors may significantly alter ventilation–perfusion matching in the lung.[170] The gradient between the P_{ETCO_2} and Pa_{CO_2} may, therefore, be significantly increased. It is essential that this relationship be established soon after tracheal intubation when arterial access has been established. Aggressively hyperventilating a patient to a normal or low P_{ETCO_2} may result in a very low Pa_{CO_2} and a significant respiratory alkalosis. The alkalosis will increase pulmonary blood flow, increase lung congestion, and increase volume load to the systemic ventricle by decreasing PVR. The alkalosis also may decrease cerebral blood flow, which is detrimental prior to deep hypothermic cardiopulmonary bypass and circulatory arrest. A sudden decrease in pulmonary blood flow, as occurs with a decrease in cardiac output, an increase in right-to-left intracardiac shunt, air embolism, or surgical restriction of pulmonary blood flow (e.g., from a vessel loop) will cause a sudden reduction in P_{ETCO_2}.

For operations involving CPB, temperature is monitored at a number of sites, including the rectum, esophagus, and tympanic membrane, to demonstrate how different regions of the body cool and rewarm. A nasopharyngeal thermistor can estimate brain temperature and is essential for procedures involving deep hypothermic circulatory arrest because brain temperature may differ substantially from core or rectal temperature. Large discrepancies between rectal, core, and tympanic temperatures may reflect inadequate arterial perfusion or inadequate venous drainage of the head or lower body during CPB. For noncardiac surgery, a single site for measuring core temperature is usually adequate.

Intracardiac Pressure Measurement

Transthoracic or transvenous measurement of atrial and pulmonary arterial pressures provides important physiologic data intraoperatively and during recovery from surgery. Placement of a percutaneous central venous line is not necessary for all patients. Central venous lines are indicated in situations where large blood loss may be anticipated, and when inotrope support is necessary prior to cardipulmonary bypass. Measurement of the superior vena cava (SVC) O_2 saturation and the (arterial–SVC) O_2 saturation difference (Sao_2–Svo_2, normally < 20 to 30 percent) may provide information about the adequacy of the cardiac output. During surgery and bypass, the central venous pressure may be a useful monitor for adequate cerebral venous drainage after placement of the SVC venous cannula. Postoperative complications of transvenous central lines include venous thrombus and infection, particularly in neonates and infants, which may cause SVC syndrome and persistent pleural effusions, and may significantly affect the success of later surgical procedures in patients undergoing staged repairs. The central venous line should, therefore, be removed as soon as possible after surgery.

Transthoracic atrial lines, placed by the surgeon prior to discontinuing cardiopulmonary bypass, can be used for volume replacement and drug infusions, and can generally remain for a longer period of time after surgery.[171] Left atrial pressure measurement gives useful information about the adequacy of circulating blood volume and the adequacy of ventricular and atrioventricular valve function. Oxygen saturation data and pressure recording from pulmonary arterial and atrial catheters provides reliable clues about the presence of residual shunts. Changes in pressure recorded when the pulmonary artery catheter is pulled back from the pulmonary artery to the right ventricle provide useful information about the adequacy of the right ventricular outflow tract repair.[172] Transcutaneous pulmonary artery balloon catheters may be difficult to place, and measurement of the thermodilution cardiac output is inaccurate in patients with intracardiac shunting.

Intraoperative Echocardiography

Intraoperative echocardiography has an established role in intraoperative monitoring of patients undergoing repair of CHD.[173–175] The development of smaller probes has allowed transesophageal monitoring to replace epicardial echocardiographic imaging in neonates, and such monitoring is routinely performed in some centers. Placement of a transesophageal probe after the induction of anesthesia affords anesthesiologists the opportunity to reevaluate the anatomy of the heart and great vessels before surgical intervention, and it allows the surgeons to determine the adequacy of surgical repair as soon as the patient is weaned from CPB. The effects of the probe on the airway and on unstable hemodynamics must be carefully evaluated before and after CPB to detect complications caused by this form of monitoring.

PRINCIPLES OF ANESTHETIC MANAGEMENT

The diversity of CHD lesions and the variations of severity and pathophysiology of each lesion mandate individualized anesthetic management based on the known effects of anesthetics and other drugs in patients with CHD. Once the critical aspects of the patient's pathophysiology are understood, the anesthetic management plan is formulated, including plans for the surgery, plans for dealing with anticipated problems and complications, and plans for pre- and postoperative care.

General Care of Patients with CHD

The patient's condition should be optimal within the limits set by the lesion. Cardiac medications such as antiarrhythmic drugs should be continued preoperatively and anesthetic plans adjusted accordingly. The general preparation for each major pathophysiologic problem is outlined above.

Systemic air emboli are a constant threat in children with CHD, regardless of their usual shunting pattern, because of the dynamic nature of shunts during anesthesia and surgery. Air traps are advisable for all IV lines but are not a substitute for meticulous attention and constant vigilance and purging of air bubbles. Direct shunting of micro- and macrobubbles of air into the systemic circulation from multiple IV lines is always possible. Even when shunting patterns are nominally left-to-right, transient right-to-left shunts may occur during some portions of the cardiac cycle or during straining or coughing in patients with open communications between the left and right sides of the heart when normal transatrial pressure gradients are transiently reversed.[176] Right-to-left shunting may occur, even across functionally "closed" communications. A "probe-patent" foramen ovale is common in children, regardless of whether or not they have CHD, and transient right-to-left shunting through the foramen ovale has been documented in a normal child during emergence from anesthesia.[177]

Prevention of bacterial endocarditis is an important consideration in patients with CHD undergoing noncardiac surgery.[178] The majority of patients with CHD in whom antibiotic prophylaxis is not recommended are those with isolated secundum ASD (unrepaired), an isolated secundum atrial defect repaired without a prosthetic patch, and a previously ligated patent ductus arteriosus. Details of recommendations for antibiotic prophylaxis for all other patients with repaired or unrepaired CHD are given in the references.[179, 180]

The immediate preoperative period is an anxious time for patients and parents. Many patients may have undergone prior surgery or investigational procedures and separation from parents may be difficult. Because many patients are now admitted on the day of surgery, adequate preparation for surgery in the preoperative clinic with a thorough explanation of the planned procedure and conduct of anesthesia, including a plan for induction of anesthesia, is essential. Clear fluids can be ingested up to 2 hours preoperatively, and an extended period of fasting should be avoided where possible, particularly in cyanotic patients.

Given the many types of pathophysiology in CHD patients, no single premedication regimen is recommended. Ideally, one wants a sedated, quiet patient who has adequate ventilation and circulation. Oral midazolam 0.5 to 0.75 mg/kg, is often an effective anxiolytic, and although this drug may not produce hypnosis, it will enable separation from parents. An intramuscular premedication with ketamine 4 to 5 mg/kg, glycopyrolate 10 to 20 μg/kg, and midazolam 0.1 mg/kg is effective for young children who will not separate from their parents in the preoperative holding area, or who have limited hemodynamic reserve and are unsuited for an inhalation induction of anesthesia. However, the effects of premedication on the often fragile circulatory and ventilatory status of these patients must be appreciated, especially as cyanotic patients have decreased hypoxic drive.[181]

Induction of Anesthesia

Because of the potential for rapid and dramatic hemodynamic changes in young patients with CHD, especially infants, complete preparation of anesthetic and monitoring equipment and required drugs is essential. Adequate assistance should be immediately available during the induction of anesthesia in case problems develop.

The choice of induction technique is influenced by the response to premedication, the parent–child–anesthesiologist relationship, and the anesthetic management plan. In older, nonhypoxemic patients who have minimal compromise of their cardiac reserve, the choice of induction techniques is large. Inhalation, intravenous, intramuscular, or rectal induction of anesthesia can be accomplished with a variety of drugs with reasonable degrees of safety if individual pathophysiologic limitations are understood. For younger, sicker, and less cooperative patients, the choices diminish.

In children with good IV access, quick insertion of a small-bore IV needle for induction of anesthesia can be virtually painless. Preoperative use of EMLA cream may facilitate IV placement. Cooperative children with an adequate cardiac reserve and difficult IV access or a morbid fear of needles can have anesthesia induced cautiously with inhaled anesthetics, even if the patients are cyanotic. An IV catheter can then be inserted to facilitate administration of muscle relaxants; these drugs facilitate tracheal intubation and avoid the risk of deep levels of inhalational anesthesia for tracheal intubation in patients whose circulatory systems may have little reserve.

Intravenous induction of anesthesia should be used for all patients with severely limited hemodynamic reserve, particularly those with severe ventricular failure or pulmonary hypertension. In situations where hemodynamic instability during induction of anesthesia is likely, administering an inotrope agent such as dobutamine or dopamine prior to induction should be considered. While the stress of placing an IV may be considerable for some patients, particularly those with difficult IV access, this is preferable to the potential myocardial depression that may occur during an inhalation induction of anesthesia with sevoflurane or halothane.

Fentanyl 15 to 25 μg/kg, in combination with pancuronium 0.2 mg/kg, provides hemodynamic stability and prompt airway control, and attenuates the stress-induced increase in PVR associated with tracheal intubation. Ketamine 1 to 3 mg/kg IV is safe and reliable, provided there is hemodynamic stability and minimal increases in PVR. It is particularly useful in patients with severe CHF and ventricular outflow obstructions. Atropine 20 μg/kg or glycopyrrolate 10 μg/kg are traditionally given concurrently due to increased secretions. If IV access is difficult and stressful in infants, a combination 4 mg/kg ketamine, glycopyrrolate 10 μg/kg, and suxamethonium 2 mg/kg intramuscularly allows prompt induction of anesthesia and control of the airway.

Barbiturates and propofol can be used in patients with normal ventricular function. Titrated doses of these drugs are suitable for short procedures such as cardioversion or TEE. Midazolam 0.1 to 0.2 mg/kg is also a useful adjunct during induction of anesthesia with narcotics but may cause hypotension in patients who are dependent on a high sympathetic drive.

An inhalation induction of anesthesia with sevoflurane is suitable for most infants and children, provided they have stable ventricular function and adequate hemodynamic reserve. This emphasizes the importance of preoperative evaluation when planning the anesthesia induction technique. Inhalational induction of anesthesia can be used safely in patients with cyanotic heart disease, although uptake of the inhaled agent may be slower due to the right-to-left shunt.[182] Oxygen saturations will generally increase, provided cardiac output is maintained and airway obstruction is avoided.

For many younger children, the presence of a parent during inhalation induction may be preferable for both the patient and parent. This is commonly done for normal children undergoing induction of anesthesia for noncardiac surgery; however, careful preoperative preparation and explanation is necessary before this is undertaken in the cardiac operating room.

Maintenance of Anesthesia

Anesthesia maintenance techniques depend on the patient's preoperative cardiorespiratory status and the pathophysiology of the underlying cardiac defect, the surgical procedure, the conduct of CPB, potential postoperative surgical problems, and the anticipated postoperative management. Once induction of anesthesia and control of the airway are accomplished and monitoring is adequate, anesthesia can be maintained with inhaled anesthetics or additional intravenous drugs as dictated by the response of each patient, intraoperative events, and postoperative plans.

Stress responses to pain and other noxious stimuli are profound in even the youngest neonates, regardless of postconceptual age.[98, 101, 183] These hormonal and metabolic stress responses can be deleterious,[93] particularly in patients with marginal hemodynamic reserve. Intraoperative deterioration of the patient's condition is not always clear, but changes in shunting, surgical manipulation of the heart, lungs, or great vessels, and depression of the myocardium by anesthetics are common causes of the deterioration. Decreases in arterial oxygenation or in systemic blood flow and pressure frequently are due to alterations in intracardiac shunting. When circulating blood volume is adequate and anesthesia-related myocardial depression is unlikely, these problems are corrected by appropriately manipulating PVR and SVR. If PVR cannot be altered or is not part of the problem, vasopressor and inotropic drugs are used where indicated to increase SVR and cardiac function.

CHOICE OF ANESTHETIC AGENTS

Inhaled Anesthetics

Use of inhaled anesthetics in children with intracardiac shunting is complicated by differences in uptake and distribution of these agents. A complex computer model suggested that induction of anesthesia is slowed by the presence of central right-to-left shunts, slowed less by mixed shunts, and changed little by pure left-to-right shunts; the changes are proportional to the size of the shunt.[182] These theoretical effects assume a constant cardiac output and are most marked for insoluble gases (e.g., nitrous oxide). Induction of anesthesia with more soluble gases (e.g., halothane) is less affected (Fig. 18–13). Similar studies

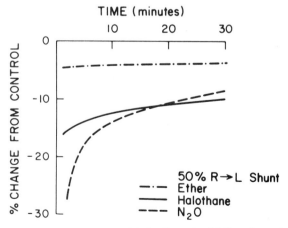

FIGURE 18–13. Computer modeled effect of solubility of anesthetic gases on delay of uptake (arterial/inspired gases concentration ratio) in children caused by a 50 percent right-to-left shunt. Ether is most soluble and thus least affected; nitrous oxide is least soluble. (From Tanner GE, Angers DG, Barash PG: Effect of left-to-right, mixed left-to-right, and right-to-left shunts on inhalational anesthetic induction in children. Anesth Analg 64:101, 1985, with permission.)

comparing the speed of induction with sevoflurane to other potent inhalation agents has not been performed; however, because it is less soluble than halothane, induction of anesthesia with sevoflurane should be expected to be slower in patients with a right-to-left shunt. In children with left-to-right shunts, the speed of inhalation induction is little altered clinically.[184] Data from animals with right-to-left shunts confirm that induction of anesthesia is slowed; data from children with right-to-left shunts are not available.[185] Inhalation induction often seems slower in children with pure right-to-left shunts, but this effect is not marked, probably because multiple other variables are affecting uptake. The potentially slow induction of anesthesia in children with pure right-to-left shunts should be remembered when one must rapidly increase the concentration of potent inhaled anesthetics in these patients.

Potent Inhaled Anesthetics

The volatile agents most commonly used during pediatric anesthesia are halothane, isoflurane, and sevoflurane. All three can be used safely to maintain anesthesia in children with cardiac disease, although this depends to some extent on the child's cardiac anomaly and related pathophysiology. Cyanotic children with reasonable functional cardiac reserve can have anesthesia induced with sevoflurane or halothane and oxygen (even 70 percent nitrous oxide does not significantly decrease arterial oxygen saturation).[186–188] Nevertheless, it is important for the anesthesiologist to have an understanding of the potential effects of these anesthetics in young children with CHD.

Increased sensitivity of the immature cardiovascular system and decreased cardiovascular reserves are more serious problems with potent inhaled anesthetics. Use of these agents may considerably reduce the margin of safety in infants and younger children with severe CHD. Volatile anesthetics depress myocardial function primarily by limiting calcium availability within the myocyte (i.e. by reducing transsarcolemmal and sarcoplasmic reticulum calcium flux). The net result is depletion of intracellular calcium stores, and given the immaturity of the neonatal and infant myocardium, the potential for systolic dysfunction in these patients may be increased when volatile agents are used. In addition, diastolic ventricular function may be also impaired because of limited reuptake of calcium into the immature sarcoplasmic reticulum, and dependence upon transsarcolemmal sodium–calcium exchange.[90] Therefore, it is not surprising that numerous studies have shown that the immature cardiovascular system of normal infants does not tolerate halothane and isoflurane well; up to 50 percent of infants with *normal cardiovascular systems* develop substantial hypotension and bradycardia during induction of anesthesia with these agents unless the cardiovascular system is supported.[189, 190] The ventricular function of normal infants declines when anesthesia is induced with halothane or isoflurane; stroke volume and ejection fraction decrease by as much as 38 percent.[190] Somewhat less myocardial depression occurs with halothane in older children.[191]

A problem interpreting these clinical studies in pediatric patients, however, is the variability in response as the myocardium matures (fully mature by 2 years of age), and differences in techniques and inability to use load-independent measures of contractility. Furthermore, no prospective studies have been undertaken in children with specific congenital cardiac lesions. In vitro, halothane depresses contractility more than isoflurane, secondary to a more substantial decrease in peak intracellular calcium concentration.[192] However, using echocardiographic derived indices of cardiac function in a group of neonates and infants, Murray et al. were unable to demonstrate a difference in myocardial depression between isoflurane and halothane in equipotent concentrations.[193]

Halothane and isoflurane have been reported to prolong atrioventricular (AV) conduction time in vitro and depress baroreflex control of heart rate. This effect is greater with halothane and more prominent in infants compared to older patients, which may reflect a direct inhibition of the slow inward calcium current upon which AV node depolarization depends. However, in recent clinical studies of older children undergoing radiofrequency catheter ablation, 1.0 MAC of halothane, isoflurane, and sevoflurane did not cause intracardiac conduction delay.[194, 195]

Halothane has been used successfully during pediatric cardiac anesthesia for many years, both as an induction agent and to maintain anesthesia. Although mildly pungent, it is generally well tolerated by children during induction of anesthesia, although airway reflexes are heightened compared to sevoflurane, and the incidence of laryngospasm during induction is therefore increased. Because of the significant cardiorespiratory interactions for many congenital cardiac defects, any airway compromise may significantly reduce cardiac output. Therefore, halothane must be used with caution during induction of anesthesia, and for most patients, sevoflurane may be preferable.

The potential for significant myocardial depression and bradycardia during induction of anesthesia are important considerations for avoiding halothane in children with limited hemodynamic reserve. Halothane sensitizes the myocardium to endogenous and exogenous catecholamines, which may cause ventricular tachycardia, particularly in lightly anesthetized or stressed patients, and those with ventricular hypertrophy. Halothane also can abolish or alter normal sinus rhythm. Because ventricular function is dependent on normal sinus rhythm in hearts with compromised function, loss of sinus rhythm in patients with CHD may be especially detrimental. This condition applies to right and left ventricular function in cases where right ventricular dysfunction might be expected to become a problem (e.g., tetralogy of Fallot) (Fig. 18–14).[196] Although greater reductive metabolism of halothane has been demonstrated in patients with cyanotic CHD, no increase in postoperative hepatic and renal dysfunction has been documented; "halothane hepatitis" has not been a problem in cyanotic children.[197]

The negative inotropic properties of halothane are sometimes advantageous in patients who have dynamic right ventricular outflow tract obstruction, such as in forms of tetralogy of Fallot. In the circumstance of an increased right-to-left shunt during a "spell," deepening the anesthetic and relaxation of the infundibular muscle with halothane may enhance antegrade pulmonary blood flow and increase the arterial oxygen saturation.

Other than being a cheaper inhalation agent, on balance there appears little indication for the continued use of halothane in children with cardiac disease in view of its potential for myocardial irritability. Isoflurane causes less direct myocardial depression, is less soluble and therefore has a faster uptake and emergence, has no effect on intracardiac conduction, and has much less sensitization of the myocardium to catecholamines compared to halothane. Isoflurane may be an unwise choice for the induction of anesthesia in cyanotic children with decreased oxygen reserves because of the increased incidence of airway problems with this drug.[190] On the other hand, it is a very useful agent to maintain anesthesia throughout cardiac surgery and bypass. It may be used as a sole agent for patients in whom extubation in the immediate postoperative period is planned. Because of peripheral vasodilating properties, isoflurane is a useful adjunct during high-dose opioid anesthesia, particularly if the patient is hypertensive. During cardiopulmonary bypass, isoflurane 0.5 to 1.0 percent can be delivered into the fresh gas flow of the bypass circuit and titrated to the desired hemodynamic response.

Sevoflurane is a popular agent for induction of anesthesia in children, and can be safely used for most patients with congenital heart disease and a stable hemodynamic status. Its low solubility contributes to faster onset of action and subsequent emergence from anesthesia. As with isoflurane, it causes less myocardial depression and has a low risk for arrhythmias in children compared to halothane.[198–200] However, because of cost and rapid emergence from anesthesia, there appears little advantage to continue the use of sevoflurane during maintenance of anesthesia.

Desflurane is the least soluble and least metabolized of the volatile anesthetics. It is very pungent and therefore not indicated for induction of anesthesia, but it is used to maintain anesthesia because it provides rapid emergence from anesthesia. It is expensive and requires a special vaporizer because of it low boiling point and high vapor pressure (664 mm Hg). Desflurane has hemodynamic and physiologic effects similar to isoflurane, although at higher concentrations (>6 percent inspired) desflurane has been reported to cause tachycardia and hypertension secondary to sympathetic stimulation. Overall, there is little indication for the use of desflurane to maintain anesthesia during cardiac surgery. However, it may be a useful anesthetic for patients with congenital heart disease undergoing noncardiac surgery.[201]

Nitrous Oxide

The use of nitrous oxide in children with CHD and shunts is controversial because of its potential for enlarging systemic air emboli and for increasing PVR. Nitrous oxide may expand intravascular air emboli and exaggerate the effects of other anesthetics on the circulation, even without systemic air embolization.[202] However, neither has been demonstrated to be a clinical problem in patients with CHD.

Nitrous oxide has been reported to decrease cardiac output, systemic arterial pressure, and heart rate in adults, and it increases PVR, especially when the preexisting PVR

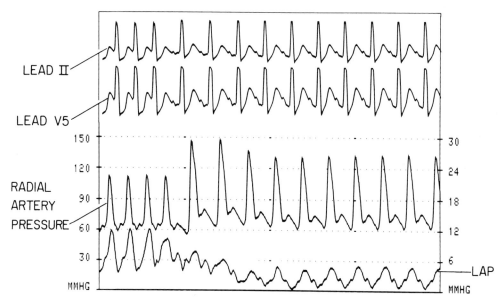

FIGURE 18–14. Improvement in hemodynamics with onset of sinus rhythm secondary to discontinuing halothane in a 2-year-old child after tetralogy of Fallot repair. Adding and deleting halothane to the inspired gas mixture resulted in nodal rhythm and then spontaneous conversion to sinus rhythm on several occasions when halothane was discontinued. (From Hickey PR, Wessel DL: Anesthesia for treatment of congenital heart disease. *In* Kaplan JA [ed]: Cardiac Anesthesia. Orlando, FL, Grune & Stratton, 1987, with permission.)

is elevated.[203, 205] The latter would be detrimental to children with right-to-left shunts, pulmonary hypertension, and decreased pulmonary flow. However, Hickey et al. reported no increase in pulmonary artery pressure or PVR in infants given 50 percent nitrous oxide, regardless of preexisting PVR.[206] Mild but significant decreases in cardiac output, systemic arterial pressure, and heart rate were seen in these infants. Furthermore, inhalation induction of anesthesia with 70 percent nitrous oxide and halothane did not decrease the arterial oxygen saturation of cyanotic children, suggesting that pulmonary blood flow is not decreased and that PVR is not substantially increased by nitrous oxide.[186, 187] Although the administration of nitrous oxide prevents the use of 100 percent oxygen, the arterial oxygen saturation of cyanotic children may not decrease because changes in FIO$_2$ have little effect on the arterial oxygenation of these patients (Fig. 18–11).[207] Arterial desaturation that is caused by pulmonary disease is, however, probably a contraindication to the use of nitrous oxide.

Intravenous Anesthetics

Some intravenous anesthetics provide a larger margin of safety for induction of anesthesia in the immature and compromised cardiovascular system of neonates and infants with severe cardiac disease. However, very high, transient arterial, cardiac, and brain concentrations of IV agents can occur when normal IV doses of drugs are given as a rapid infusion in children with known right-to-left shunts because mixing, uptake, and metabolism in the pulmonary circulation are bypassed. In dogs with right-to-left shunts, a 1 mg/kg bolus of IV lidocaine resulted in arterial drug concentrations above those reported to cause irreversible myocardial toxicity.[208] Routinely administered bolus doses of lidocaine used for dysrhythmias or intuba-

tion, or other drugs such as barbiturates, β-blockers, or calcium channel blockers, may be potentially toxic to children with substantial right-to-left shunts.

Ketamine

When IV access or lack of patient cooperation is a problem, intramuscular ketamine (3 to 5 mg/kg) is well tolerated in sick infants and children with cyanosis or congestive heart failure.[209, 210] Because of the potential effects of ketamine on airways, ventilation, and secretions, it should be given in combination with an antisialagogue (e.g., atropine or glycopyrrolate) while the airway and ventilation are carefully maintained, especially in children with decreased oxygen reserves.[211, 212] Ketamine can be mixed with atropine and succinylcholine in the same syringe, the final volume being relatively small, and injection of this mixture allows rapid control of the airway. Small IV doses of ketamine (1 to 3 mg/kg) are effective for supplemental sedation in uncooperative or apprehensive children who are unwilling to leave their parents. Excessive secretions, airway problems, and apnea do not occur with these doses as they occasionally do with larger intramuscular (IM) doses and frequently do with IV doses of ketamine.

Although increased PVR is reported with ketamine in adults, 2 mg/kg IV in premedicated infants and young children usually does not increase pulmonary artery pressure or PVR, even when the baseline PVR is elevated.[124, 213] However, reports are not consistent in this regard.[125] If hypoventilation or apnea occurs after an IV dose of ketamine, undesirable increases in PVR can occur because of the associated changes in PaO$_2$ and PaCO$_2$.[213] Little change in cardiac output, heart rate, or arterial pressure is seen after IV ketamine in infants and small children with CHD.[124, 213] Despite reports of ketamine having a negative inotropic effect on isolated heart muscle of animals at very high doses, the ejection fraction of children with CHD is well preserved after ketamine. Furthermore, arterial saturation for the most part is improved when ketamine is used to induce anesthesia in cyanotic patients. Clinical experience with ketamine as the induction agent has been excellent for sick infants and children with most forms of heart disease, including those with limited pulmonary blood flow and cyanosis. Ketamine also is useful for sedation and for anesthesia for cardiac catheterization of children with CHD,[212, 214] although the recovery time is delayed compared with drugs such as propofol.[215]

Narcotic Anesthesia

High-dose narcotic anesthesia provides excellent cardiovascular stability in children with CHD. Morphine (1 mg/kg or more) given slowly over a prolonged period provides reasonable cardiovascular stability in children; however, as in adults, histamine release can occur and cause hypotension. The more potent synthetic opioids, fentanyl (25 to 75 μg/kg) and sufentanil (5 to 15 μg/kg), given more slowly, provide better stability of the cardiovascular system on induction of anesthesia when used with pancuronium in very sick infants with CHD.[216–220] Because of its effect on the sympathetic nervous system and duration of action, pancuronium remains the muscle relaxant of choice for use with high-dose synthetic opioids. Shorter acting muscle relaxants such as cis-atracurium have a relatively benign hemodynamic profile, but should be administered as a continuous infusion during cardiac surgery because of their short duration of action. The doses of synthetic opioids required to blunt the systemic and pulmonary stress responses in younger and sicker children are generally well tolerated.[101, 126, 127] Changes in pulmonary and systemic hemodynamics are insignificant in infants following a bolus of fentanyl 15 to 25 μg/kg, but mild hypotension and bradycardia have been reported with the shorter acting synthetic narcotic alfentanil.[213, 221] Used with 100 percent oxygen, these high-dose narcotics are safe and result in increased arterial oxygenation in cyanotic children.[213, 217] Fentanyl doses as low as 10 μg/kg may be sufficient for effective baseline anesthesia in neonates, but larger doses are necessary for prolonged anesthesia.[222–224] A bolus dose of 10 to 15 μg/kg effectively ameliorates the hemodynamic response to tracheal intubation in neonates.[222] For complete suppression of hemodynamic responses to intense stimulation of more vigorous children, supplementation of high-dose narcotics with small amounts of inhaled anesthetic may be necessary. Although low doses of fentanyl 2 to 5 μg/kg facilitate mechanical ventilation and decrease total lung compliance in an awake child, high-dose narcotics produce chest wall rigidity in adults and neonates.[225] A muscle relaxant is required with rapid infusion of high-dose synthetic narcotics.

The high-dose narcotic technique is most suitable for sick infants and older children in whom postoperative mechanical ventilation is planned. This technique provides hemodynamic stability, although it does not guarantee suppression of the endocrine response to surgical stimulation. Neonates and infants undergoing deep hypothermic CPB surgery are able to generate a significant stress response.[94] Wood et al. reported a 17-fold increase in epinephrine and 10-fold increase in norepinephrine concentrations in infants after 1 hour of circulatory arrest at 18°C.[226] Nevertheless, the reported magnitude of the stress response after cardiac surgery is variable, and influenced by patient age, type of anesthesia, level of hypothermia, and the duration of CPB and circulatory arrest.[227]

It has been previously demonstrated from Children's Hospital, Boston, that sufentanil anesthesia (total dose, 30 μg/kg), compared to anesthesia consisting of primarily halothane and morphine, was associated with less stress hormone release and improved outcome after neonatal cardiac surgery.[94] In our current practice, fentanyl is more commonly used, with a usual dosing strategy of 50 μg/kg administered prior to CPB, a further 25 μg/kg at the onset of rewarming on CPB, and a further 25 μg/kg after bypass depending on hemodynamic stability. In a recent study of stress hormone release during infant cardiac surgery and deep hypothermic cardiopulmonary bypass using this fentanyl dosing regimen, the endocrine response was not obtunded, yet there were no adverse outcomes. In addition, no specific relationship between opioid dose, plasma fentanyl level, and hormone or metabolic stress response was established.[100] Considering the advances in surgical techniques, conduct of CPB, and perioperative management over the past decade that have lead to a significant improvement in patient outcome, a strategy of high-dose opioid anesthesia to blunt the stress response may be less critical.

Additional doses or a continuous infusion of potent narcotics may be necessary for surgery involving cardiopulmonary bypass because narcotic concentrations decrease markedly during CPB.[228] Drug pharmacokinetics may be substantially altered by hypothermia, hemodilution, reduced protein binding, binding of drugs to the bypass circuit and oxygenator membrane, sequestration of drugs within the pulmonary vascular bed, and reduced hepatic and renal clearance. Drug pharmacodynamics may be altered by CPB variables such as flow rate, perfusion pressure, and the use of vasoactive drugs. Cardiac anesthesia with cardiopulmonary bypass is associated with an increased risk of awareness.[229, 230] Although these studies have been performed in adults, there is no reason to suspect that infants and children do not have the same potential risk. Monitoring the adequacy of anesthetic depth during CPB is difficult but possible. Indices frequently monitored include changes in autonomic responses such as an increase in perfusion pressure for a given flow rate, tearing and diaphoresis, and metabolic responses such as a decrease in mixed venous oxygen saturation and an increase in lactate concentrations.

Remifentanil is a new synthetic ultra-short acting opioid, rapidly metabolized by nonspecific tissue esterases.[231] It is unique among the currently available opioids because of its extremely short context-sensitive half-life (3 to 5 minutes), which is largely independent of the duration of infusion. Remifentanil may cause significant respiratory depression and is usually administered to patients who are mechanically ventilated. It may be useful for patients with limited cardiorespiratory reserve undergoing procedures such as cardiac catheterization or pacemaker placement because intense analgesia is provided without significant hemodynamic complications. It may also be used to maintain anesthesia during mild hypothermic CPB for patients who are extubated immediately after surgery in the operating room, such as after atrial septal defect repair.[232] Patients usually emerge quickly once the infusion has been stopped. Opioid side effects are reduced because of the short duration of action of this drug.

Other Intravenous Agents

The benzodiazepine derivatives (e.g., midazolam or diazepam) can be useful when titrated in small doses (0.05 to 0.1 mg/kg), especially in older patients with CHD. Lack of pain on injection and lack of vascular damage make the water-soluble midazolam a more useful benzodiazepine than diazepam, particularly because it has a shorter duration of action. Benzodiazepines are commonly used to ensure adequate hypnosis during opioid-based anesthesia, but may also improve hemodynamic stability. In a study of children with acyanotic heart disease undergoing cardiac surgery, the addition of diazepam to fentanyl-based anesthesia (75 μg/kg) resulted in a more stable hemodynamic profile without an increase in epinephrine levels when compared to an isoflurane based anesthetic.[233] In a study of younger children undergoing correction of tetralogy of Fallot, the combined use of sufentanil and flunitrazepam provided a more stable hemodynamic profile and catecholamine response compared to a sufentanil-based technique alone.[234]

Published studies of the effects of other IV agents are sparse in small children with CHD. Incremental doses of thiopental (2 to 5 mg/kg) and propofol (1 to 3 mg/kg) are suitable for induction of anesthesia in small children who have stable hemodynamics. In the older age group, thiopental does not reduce the arterial oxygenation of cyanotic patients.[188] Rectal barbiturates, notably methohexital, may be acceptable agents for the induction of anesthesia in an otherwise uncooperative child with less severe CHD and good cardiac reserve, but absorption of the drug is variable and myocardial depression is possible. These agents cause venodilation and must be used with caution in patients who have undergone a previous cavopulmonary connection. The resting venous tone may be increased in this patient group, and the fall in preload could result in significant hypotension during induction of anesthesia.

Etomidate is an anesthetic induction agent with the advantage of minimal cardiovascular and respiratory depression. An intravenous dose of 0.3 mg/kg induces a rapid loss of consciousness with a duration of action of 3 to 5 minutes. It may cause pain on injection and is associated with spontaneous movements, hiccuping, and myoclonus. Etomidate may be used as an alternative to the synthetic opioids for induction of anesthesia in patients with limited myocardial reserve. It is not approved for continuous infusion because of depression to adrenal steroidogenesis.[235]

Muscle Relaxants

Dosage requirements for pancuronium are unchanged in children with CHD and intracardiac shunts; this agent produces virtually no heart rate or blood pressure changes when given slowly to such patients.[236] However, a bolus dose of pancuronium can produce tachycardia and hypertension in children through its sympathomimetic effect, which is sometimes desirable to support the cardiac output of infants with relatively fixed stroke volumes.[237] If tachycardia is undesirable, metocurine (Metubine), which causes minimal change in heart rate, blood pressure, and cardiac rhythm in small children (even at doses of 0.5 mg/kg), is often appropriate.[238] For patients in whom a short-acting, nondepolarizing muscle relaxant is desirable, atracurium, cis-atracurium, and vecuronium have few cardiovascular side effects in children when given in low doses.[239-241]

If succinylcholine is given to children with CHD, atropine also should be given to avoid associated bradycardia or sinus arrest. Although not reported as a clinical problem in normal children, simultaneous use of the potent narcotics and succinylcholine without atropine should be avoided in children with compromised cardiovascular function because of the potential for severe bradycardia with this combination of drugs.

Rocuronium is an aminosteroid, nondepolarizing muscle relaxant with fast onset and intermediate duration of action. Time to complete neuromuscular blockade for an intubating dose of 0.6 mg/kg ranges from 30 to 180 seconds, although adequate intubating conditions are usually achieved within 60 seconds. It is, therefore, a suitable alternative to the use of succinylcholine during rapid-sequence induction of anesthesia.[241] The duration of action averages 25 minutes, although recovery from paralysis is slower in infants. It is a safe drug to administer to patients with limited hemodynamic reserve and does not cause histamine release.

ANESTHESIA FOR CARDIAC SURGERY

Communication between the anesthesia and surgical teams is of utmost importance during surgery for CHD. The manipulations of each team influence the other, and close coordination of activities is necessary for optimal patient care. Specific problems occurring with total repair or palliation of specific congenital cardiac lesions are covered later in the chapter. General problems that occur with various types of closed and open cardiac surgical procedures are considered here.

Anesthetic Management of Closed Cardiac Procedures

Patent ductus arteriosus, coarctation of the aorta, and repair of vascular rings are the only congenital cardiac anomalies *corrected* with closed procedures. Closed palliative procedures including systemic-to-pulmonary shunts, pulmonary artery banding, and procedures to improve interatrial mixing (Blalock-Hanlon atrial septectomy) are performed infrequently, as the trend to definitively correct the CHD early continues. Anesthesia for closed palliative procedures is in some ways more demanding, because CPB is not available if the patient's hemodynamic status deteriorates. Therefore, monitoring requirements are stringent, and venous and arterial access are usually mandatory. Pulse oximetry is invaluable in these cases to evaluate the infant's condition and to assess the effectiveness of the closed surgical procedure.

Acid–base and electrolyte balance are meticulously maintained at normal levels throughout closed procedures. When these procedures are done via a thoracotomy, the operative field is rarely visible to the anesthesiologist, and marked deterioration of cardiopulmonary function may result from surgical manipulations. Any deterioration in the infant's condition should be immediately communicated to the surgeon, who has a view of the surgical field and knows what is being done there. Some compromise of ventilation and pulmonary blood flow inevitably occurs during these procedures, occasionally with severe decreases in arterial oxygen saturations.

Mechanical Ventilation

Altered lung mechanics and ventilation–perfusion abnormalities are common problems in the immediate postoperative period.[170, 242, 243] Besides preoperative problems due to increased $\dot{Q}p/\dot{Q}s$, additional considerations include the surgical incision and lung retraction, increased lung water following CPB, possible pulmonary reperfusion injury, surfactant depletion and restrictive defects from atelectasis, and pleural effusions.

In general, neonates and infants with their limited physiologic reserve should not be weaned from mechanical ventilation until hemodynamically stable and factors contributing to an increase in intrapulmonary shunt and altered respiratory mechanics have improved.

Volume-Limited Ventilation

A traditional approach to mechanical ventilation in children with congenital heart disease has been the use of a volume-limited, time-cycled mode, with large tidal volumes of 15 to 20 ml/kg and no PEEP. This approach was developed in the early years of congenital heart surgery when older generations of ventilators existed and the monitoring of ventilation was frequently less than ideal. While the peak inspiratory and mean airway pressure are usually increased using large tidal volumes in this mode, changes in compliance and resistance can be readily detected. If there is a sudden change in pulmonary mechanics from atelectasis, pneumothorax, or endotracheal tube obstruction, the peak inspiratory pressure alarm limit is reached as the ventilator tries to deliver the preset tidal volume.

However, for neonates and infants, the compressible volume of the ventilator circuit (1 to 1.5 ml/cm H_2O peak inspiratory pressure) means that the delivered tidal volume is less than the preset volume. For older patients receiving larger tidal breaths, the volume lost by compression of gas in the circuit is minimal and rarely impacts on their tidal ventilation. However, for neonates and infants, this compressible volume may be a considerable portion of their tidal ventilation. Furthermore, any leak around the endotracheal tube means a proportion of the delivered tidal volume also may be lost. Inspiratory and expiratory times also need to be closely observed to prevent excessive auto-PEEP. Variable time constants (i.e. compliance

× resistance), within regions of the lung are common in children with defects associated with high pulmonary blood flow, as well as following CPB. Using a volume-limited, time-cycled mode, those areas of lung with an increased time constant may be preferentially ventilated and overdistended, contributing to ventilation–perfusion mismatch and potential lung injury.

Pressure-Limited Ventilation

A pressure-limited, time-cycled mode of ventilation is often appropriate in children less than 10 kg, particularly those with significant alteration in lung compliance and airway resistance. A decelerating flow pattern is used when a breath is delivered to the patient until a preset peak inspiratory pressure is achieved. The delivered tidal volume will vary according to the compliance and resistance of the lung, and therefore from breath to breath. Both the peak inspiratory pressure and the inspiratory time can be manipulated to increase or decrease the delivered tidal volume. A square-wave pressure waveform is generated by changing the inspiratory time, which also will alter the mean airway pressure. In general, it is preferable to set a minute ventilation using the lowest possible mean airway pressure. In-line monitoring that enables breath-to-breath assessment of tidal volume and mean airway pressure is essential, with appropriate alarm limits set to detect acute changes in compliance and resistance.

Cardiorespiratory Interactions

Cardiorespiratory interactions vary significantly between patients, and it is not possible to provide specific ventilation strategies or protocols that will cover all patients. Rather, the mode of ventilation must be matched to the hemodynamic status of each patient to achieve the appropriate cardiac output and gas exchange. Frequent modifications to the mode and pattern of ventilation may be necessary during recovery after surgery, with attention paid to changes in lung volume and airway pressure.

Lung Volume

Changes in lung volume have a major effect on PVR, which is lowest at FRC. Both hypo- and hyperinflation may result in a significant increase in PVR. At low tidal volumes, alveolar collapse occurs because of reduced interstitial traction on alveolar septae. In addition, radial traction on extra-alveolar vessels such as the branch pulmonary arteries is reduced, which reduces the cross-sectional diameter of the vessels. Conversely, hyperinflation of the lung may stretch the alveolar septae and compress extra-alveolar vessels.

An increase in PVR increases the afterload or wall stress on the RV, potentially compromising RV function and contributing to decreased LV compliance secondary to interventricular septal shift. In addition to low cardiac output, signs of RV dysfunction, including tricuspid regurgitation, hepatomegaly, ascites, and pleural effusions, may be observed.

Intrathoracic Pressure

An increase in mean intrathoracic pressure during positive-pressure ventilation decreases preload to both pulmonary and systemic ventricles, but it has opposite effects on afterload to each ventricle.[244, 245]

Right Ventricle

The reduction in RV preload that occurs with positive-pressure ventilation may reduce cardiac output. Normally, the RV diastolic compliance is extremely high and the pulmonary circulation is able to accommodate changes in flow without a large change in pressure. An increase in mean intrathoracic pressure increases the afterload on the RV from direct compression of extra-alveolar and alveolar pulmonary vessels.

Patients with normal RV compliance, and without residual volume load or pressure load on the ventricle following surgery, usually show little change in RV function from the alteration in preload and afterload that occurs with positive-pressure ventilation. However, these effects can be magnified in patients with restrictive RV physiology, in particular neonates who have required a right ventriculotomy for repair of tetralogy of Fallot (TOF), pulmonary atresia, or truncus arteriosus. Whereas systolic RV function may be preserved, diastolic dysfunction is common, with increased RV end-diastolic pressure and impaired RV filling.

The potential deleterious effects of mechanical ventilation on RV function are important to emphasize. The aim should be to ventilate with a mode that enables the lowest possible mean airway pressure, while maintaining lung volume. The use of a low peak inspiratory pressure, short inspiratory time, increased intermittent mandatory ventilation (IMV) rate, and low levels of PEEP has been recommended as one ventilation strategy in patients with restrictive RV physiology. The smaller tidal volumes (6 to 8 ml/kg) used during this pattern of ventilation may reduce lung volume and FRC, thereby increasing PVR and afterload on the RV. An alternative strategy is to use tidal volumes of 12 to 15 ml/kg, with a longer inspiratory time of 0.8 to 1.0 second, an increased peak inspiratory pressure of around 30 cm H_2O, low PEEP (i.e., wide ΔP), and slow IMV rate of 12 to 15 breaths/min. For the same mean airway pressure, RV filling is maintained and RV output is augmented by maintaining lung volume and reduced RV afterload.

Left Ventricle

Left ventricular preload also is affected by changes in lung volume. Pulmonary blood flow, and therefore preload to the systemic ventricle, may be reduced by an increase or decrease in lung volume caused by alteration in radial traction on alveoli and extra-alveolar vessels.

The systemic arteries are under higher pressure and are not exposed to the effects of radial traction during inflation or deflation of the lungs. Therefore, changes in lung volume will affect LV preload, but the effect on afterload is dependent on changes in intrathoracic pressure alone rather than changes in lung volume.

In contrast to the RV, a major effect of positive-pressure ventilation on the LV is a reduction in afterload. Using Laplace's law, wall stress is directly proportional to the transmural LV pressure and the radius of curvature of the LV. The transmural pressure across the LV is the difference between the intracavity LV pressure and surrounding intrathoracic pressure. Assuming a constant arterial pressure and ventricular dimension, an increase in intrathoracic pressure, as occurs during positive-pressure ventilation, will reduce the transmural gradient and the wall stress on the LV. Therefore, positive-pressure ventilation and PEEP can have significant beneficial effects in patients with left ventricular failure.

Patients with LV dysfunction and increased end-diastolic volume and pressure can have impaired pulmonary mechanics secondary to increased lung water, decreased lung compliance, and increased airway resistance. The work of breathing is increased and neonates can fatigue early because of limited respiratory reserve. A significant proportion of total body oxygen consumption is directed at the increased work of breathing in neonates and infants with LV dysfunction, contributing to poor feeding and failure to thrive. Therefore, positive-pressure ventilation has an additional benefit in patients with significant volume overload and systemic ventricular dysfunction by reducing the work of breathing and oxygen demand.

Lung Injury

It is important to appreciate that mechanical ventilation may result in significant lung injury, particularly when high tidal volumes are used.[246] Large, rapid changes in tidal volumes may lead to shear stress on the alveolar septae and subsequent alveolar capillary disruption. The same mechanisms that result in air leak also may result in disruption of the microcirculation, causing an increase in total lung water, an increase in airway resistance, and a reduction in lung compliance.

Lung disease usually is not homogenous, with regions of the lung having different time constants (i.e., "fast" alveoli and "slow" alveoli). When using a volume-limited ventilation strategy, the more compliant alveoli will distend in preference to regions of lung that are collapsed or have slow time constants, thereby resulting in regional alveolar overdistention and trauma. This may be less evident when using pressure-limited ventilation, as the more compliant or faster alveoli will distend to the preset pressure limit and then, depending on the inspiratory time, regions of lung with reduced time constants will gradually distend and be recruited.

Although a relatively large tidal volume of 12 to 15 ml/kg is beneficial to maintain lung volume at lower PVR for many patients after congenital heart surgery, lung injury may occur if a high-volume strategy is continued for a prolonged period (i.e., volutrauma). Using a pressure-limited mode of ventilation will enable the use of a relatively constant tidal volume without a wide swing in peak inspiratory pressure or regional alveolar overdistention. It is essential to continually reevaluate the mode of ventilation and modify it according to hemodynamic responses. Fortunately, most patients undergoing congenital cardiac surgery do not have parenchymal lung disease; and changes in pulmonary mechanics, such as those due to changes in lung water, are generally resolved following complete surgical repair and diuresis after CPB. Further-more, the common use of ultrafiltration techniques during and after CPB also has been associated with improved postoperative pulmonary function. Therefore, the need for sustained postoperative higher lung volume ventilation strategies is reduced.[247]

PEEP

The use of PEEP in patients with congenital heart disease has been controversial. It was initially perceived not to have a significant effect in terms of improving gas exchange, and there was concern that the increased airway pressure could have a detrimental effect on hemodynamics and contribute to lung injury and air leak.

Nevertheless, PEEP increases FRC, which enables lung recruitment and redistribution of lung water from alveolar septal regions to the more compliant perihilar regions. Both of these effects will improve gas exchange and reduce PVR. However, excessive levels of PEEP may be detrimental by increasing afterload on the RV. Usually 3 to 5 cm H_2O of PEEP will help maintain FRC and redistribute lung water without causing hemodynamic compromise.

Management of Cardiopulmonary Bypass

The advantages of a primary corrective operation over a staged approach that uses an initial palliative procedure have been addressed above and elsewhere.[84] Inasmuch as reparative procedures usually entail CPB techniques, the care of these patients must incorporate technical knowledge of CPB issues and take into account the effects of CPB on the function of multiple organ systems. An important component of the improvement in early outcome after congenital heart surgery has been the advances in cardiovascular support, especially cardiopulmonary bypass techniques, myocardial protection, pharmacologic support, and mechanical support. It is well recognized that the exposure of blood elements to the nonepithelialized cardiopulmonary bypass circuit, along with ischemic-reperfusion injury, induces a systemic inflammatory response (Fig. 18–15). The effects of the interactions of blood components with the extracorporeal circuit is magnified in children because of the large bypass circuit surface area and priming volume relative to patient blood volume. Humoral responses include activation of complement, kallikrein, eicosanoid, and fibrinolytic cascades; cellular responses include platelet activation and an inflammatory response with an adhesion molecule cascade that stimulates neutrophil activation and release of proteolytic and vasoactive substances.[248, 249]

The clinical consequences of activating these pathways include increased interstitial fluid, generalized capillary leak, and potential multiorgan dysfunction. Total lung water is increased and there is an associated decrease in lung compliance and increase in the alveolar to arterial O_2 ($[A–a]O_2$) gradient. Myocardial edema results in impaired ventricular systolic and diastolic function. A secondary decrease in cardiac output of 20 to 30 percent is common in neonates in the first 6 to 12 hours after surgery, contribut-

ing to decreased renal function and oliguria.[250] It may be necessary to delay sternal closure due to mediastinal edema and the associated cardiorespiratory compromise that occurs when closure is attempted. Ascites, hepatic congestion, and bowel edema may affect mechanical ventilation, cause a prolonged ileus, and delay feeding. A coagulopathy after CPB may contribute to delayed hemostasis.

Numerous strategies have evolved over recent years to limit the effect of the endothelial injury that results from the systemic inflammatory response. Of these, the most important strategy is limiting the time spent on bypass and limiting the use of deep hypothermic circulatory arrest (DHCA). This is clearly dependent, however, on surgical expertise and experience, and in certain situations DHCA is necessary to effect surgical repair. Hypothermia, steroids, and aprotinin (a serine protease inhibitor) are important prebypass measures to limit activation of the inflammatory response. Attenuating the stress response, the use of antioxidants such as mannitol, altering pump-prime composition to maintain oncotic pressure, and ultrafiltration during rewarming or immediately after bypass also are used to limit the clinical consequences of the inflammatory response.

There are no specific guidelines that delineate which techniques are preferable, and opinions about this matter vary considerably between institutions. However, hemofiltration is commonly used to hemoconcentrate and to possibly remove inflammatory mediators such as complement, endotoxin, and cytokines.[52, 251, 252] Early clinical experience reported improved systolic and diastolic pressures during hemofiltration. Improved pulmonary function also has been noted with reduction in pulmonary vascular resistance and total lung water.[253, 254] The duration of postoperative mechanical ventilation and cardiac intensive care unit (CICU) and hospital stay also have been reduced.[247, 251] Hemofiltration techniques include modified ultrafiltration (MUF) in which the patient's blood volume is filtered after completion of bypass; conventional hemofiltration in which both the patient and circuit blood are filtered during rewarming on bypass; and zero-balance ultrafiltration in which high-volume ultrafiltration essentially washes the patient and circuit blood during the rewarming process.[252]

Although these techniques are useful to hemoconcentrate and remove total body water immediately after cardiopulmonary bypass, they do not prevent the inflammatory response. Although this response is perhaps modified by these techniques, this response is nevertheless idiosyncratic. Despite all the above maneuvers, some neonates and infants will still manifest significant clinical signs and delayed postoperative recovery.[255] The development of drugs that will prevent the adhesion molecule–endothelial interaction, which is pivotal in the inflammatory response, continues to be pursued in both laboratory and clinical studies. To date, however, no one specific drug or treatment has proven beneficial. This highlights the multifactorial nature of the inflammatory response and that attention must be paid to multiple functions.

Special circumstances exist during management of CPB in patients with CHD that may not apply to adults undergoing correction of acquired heart disease. Venous cannula-

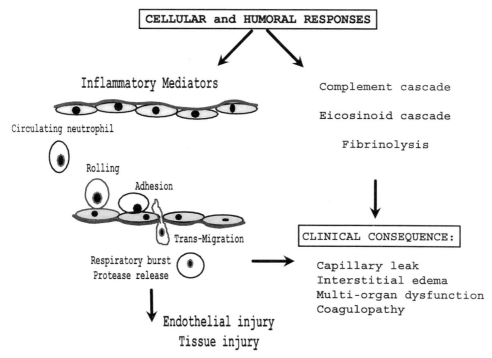

FIGURE 18–15. Cellular and humoral response to cardiopulmonary bypass.

tion in neonates and infants may be single or multiple, depending on the anatomy and the bypass technique. Obstruction of venous return is often due to the small vessel size and will increase venous pressures, thereby decreasing perfusion pressure to the cerebral and splanchnic circulations. A decrease in venous return to the bypass circuit, abdominal distention, and head suffusion all indicate problems with venous cannulation. Elevated SVC pressures will reduce cerebral blood flow, increase the risk of cerebral edema, and reduce the rate of cerebral cooling. Systemic-to-pulmonary shunts and collateral vessels must be controlled when going onto bypass to prevent excessive pulmonary flow and increased blood return to the heart, myocardial distention, systemic hypoperfusion, and uneven cooling or rewarming. Most importantly, a high perfusion rate at the pump head does not ensure an equally high systemic flow unless all sources of potential aortopulmonary shunts (e.g., Blalock-Taussig), patent ductus arteriosus, or native aortopulmonary collaterals are occluded. If these shunts are not occluded, other indices of the adequacy of the flow should be followed.

There are two broad bypass management strategies:

1. *Deep hypothermia (< 18°C) with low/intermittent flow or circulatory arrest:* DHCA provides optimal operating conditions for intracardiac repairs with an empty, relaxed heart, and reduces the duration on bypass and exposure of circulating blood to foreign surfaces. Prolonged ischemia to the brain is a major disadvantage and is both time and temperature dependent.[256] Low-flow deep hypothermic bypass is associated with improved neurologic protection. Flow rates between 30 and 50 ml/kg/min are often referred to as "low flow," but the optimal flow rates during low-flow bypass are not firmly established. Flows as low as 10 ml/kg have been used in animal studies evaluating low-flow bypass, with maintenance of cerebral phosphocreatine, adenosine triphosphate (ATP), and intracellular pH at or above baseline both during bypass and reperfusion.[257–259]

2. *Moderate hypothermia with normal or increased pump flow:* Bicaval cannulation is generally used, and the risk of cerebral ischemia is reduced. However, CPB is prolonged and operative conditions may not be ideal. Pump flow rates are generally higher in neonates and infants, reflecting the increased metabolic rate. During bypass, there is no one measure or index that ensures adequate perfusion. Generally, flow rates of 100 to 150 ml/kg/min, or indexed flows to 2.2 to 2.5 L/min/m², should provide adequate flow at normothermia. Pump perfusion in young patients is regulated primarily by flow rate, so that perfusion pressures of 30 mm Hg or less are common in these patients when hemodilution has decreased SVR (low viscosity). A venous oxygen saturation of greater than 75 percent, even differential temperature cooling, and low lactate levels suggest adequate perfusion.[260] However, these values may be misleading in patients with poor venous drainage, severe hemodilution, malposition of the aortic cannula, or in the presence of a large left-to-right shunt. On-line continuous monitoring of blood gases and oxygen saturation of hemoglobin is important to identify trends in oxygen extraction. These measures only provide global indices of perfusion, and monitoring regional perfusion would be ideal. Although cerebral perfusion can be monitored using transcranial sonography, near-infrared spectroscopy, and the electroencephalogram (EEG), to date there are no monitors available

for routine clinical use to monitor perfusion of other vascular beds.

Because of the large body surface area/mass ratio in neonates and infants, a 2° to 3°C reduction in core temperature is common prior to cardiopulmonary bypass following induction of anesthesia. The use of cooling/warming blankets, low ambient temperature, and reduced overhead operating light intensity helps maintain a low temperature during bypass and minimizes radiant heating of the myocardium. Surface cooling is aided by placement of ice bags on and around the head and will assist with brain cooling.

Neurologic injury is an inherent risk for any patient undergoing cardiac surgery and cardiopulmonary bypass. This has been particularly the case in neonates and infants where DHCA or low-flow techniques have been commonly used. Early in the development of cardiopulmonary bypass strategies, postoperative seizures were a relatively common occurrence. They were generally self-limiting and did not imply longer term seizure activity. However, it is now clear that seizures are a manifestation of ongoing neurologic injury. During seizures, excitatory neurotransmitters such as glutamate are released and produce neuronal injury by N-methyl-D-aspartate (NMDA) receptor-gated calcium channels.[261] Adverse neurologic sequelae are multifactorial after bypass and may be secondary to the duration of CPB,[262, 263] rate and depth of cooling,[264–266] perfusion flow rate,[267] duration of circulatory arrest, pH management on bypass,[268, 269] hematocrit[270, 271] and embolic events. Our current strategies to optimize cerebral protection during deep hypothermic bypass, with or without circulatory arrest, include a longer duration of cooling over 20 minutes, the use a pH-stat strategy of blood gas management during cooling (i.e., addition of CO_2 to the oxygenator), and a higher hematocrit (approximately 30 percent). The optimal hematocrit remains to be determined. While acting as an O_2 reservoir during DHCA or low-flow bypass, the hematocrit must not be too high because the increased hematocrit can be associated with an increase in viscosity when the temperatures decrease.

In many centers, the practice of using DHCA for periods beyond 30 to 40 minutes has decreased if the repair can be satisfactorily accomplished using low-flow techniques.[104, 256] Although there is no optimal "safe" duration of DHCA, the accepted limit has declined over recent years from approximately 60 minutes to about 40 minutes if the temperature is less than 20°C.[104] With improvements in neurologic protection over recent years, the incidence of overt injury (i.e., postoperative seizures) has declined substantially. Although long-term neurodevelopmental outcome after DHCA in children is still being clarified, this has nevertheless become an important outcome variable when evaluating neurologic protection strategies.[272]

Weaning from Cardiopulmonary Bypass

During the rewarming phase, air is vented from the heart before blood is injected into the systemic circulation. Arterial blood gases, electrolytes, and concentrations of anticoagulation are checked periodically during bypass, but especially during rewarming. Electrolytes, especially ionized calcium, are normalized before separation from cardiopulmonary bypass is attempted. Adequacy of corporal rewarming is judged by temperature recordings from multiple sites.

The need for vasopressor and inotropic support during weaning from cardiopulmonary bypass is determined by close observation of the heart during the rewarming phase. Rhythm problems, coronary perfusion problems, and the general state of myocardial contractility can be estimated by directly observing the heart during this period. Separation from cardiopulmonary bypass is accomplished in concert with the surgical team. Although monitoring of the appropriate intracardiac and intra-arterial pressures and waveforms may accurately indicate both left and right ventricular function, slavish adherence to the monitored values without visual confirmation of the adequacy of cardiac filling and performance can lead to many errors. The small size of the heart and the presence of unsuspected congenital defects sometimes make interpretation of intravascular pressures difficult. When rewarming is complete and cardiac function is judged adequate, weaning from the extracorporeal circulation is accomplished by slowly allowing the heart to fill and eject while ventilation is reestablished. Optimal ventricular filling pressures are estimated using filling pressures from preoperative catheterization data, the appearance of the heart, and the infusion of small increments of volume while watching filling and systemic arterial pressures. The direct measurement of oxygen saturations from chambers of the heart enables calculation of a residual intracardiac shunt immediately following surgery, and direct pressure measurements across systemic and pulmonary outflow tracts enables detection of residual significant obstruction across these tracts. Transesophageal echocardiography has become an important diagnostic method to evaluate ventricular function, as well as to assess atrioventricular and semilunar valve competence, outflow obstruction, and significant residual intracardiac shunting across the ventricular or atrial septums. If systemic arterial pressures or gas exchange are inadequate, CPB is reinstituted while the problem is analyzed and appropriate corrective measures are taken.

After discontinuing cardiopulmonary bypass, and despite full rewarming on bypass, mild hypothermia often develops in neonates and infants. Active measures to decrease radiant and evaporative losses are necessary because of the increased metabolic stress, pulmonary vasoreactivity, coagulopathy, and potential for dysrhythmias associated with hypothermia. However, hyperthermia also must be be actively avoided because of the associated increased metabolic rate and potential for ongoing neurologic injury, particularly when myocardial function may be depressed and cerebral autoregulation impaired.[273]

Hemostasis may be difficult to obtain if bypass has been prolonged and if there are extensive, high-pressure (often concealed) suture lines. Prompt management and meticulous control of surgical bleeding is essential to prevent the complications associated with a massive transfusion. Besides hemodilution of coagulation factors and platelets, complex surgery with long bypass times increases endothelial injury and exposure to the nonendothelialized surface of the pump circuit, thereby stimulating the intrinsic pathway, and platelet activation and aggregation. Preoperative factors, including chronic cyanosis in older patients, a low cardiac output (CO) with tissue hypoperfusion and disseminated intravascular coagulation (DIC), hepatic immaturity, and the use of platelet inhibitors such as PGE_1 in neonates and infants, also contribute to prolonged bleeding after bypass.[274, 275]

Chest Closure and Tamponade After Cardiac Operations

Chest closure is a time of particular instability after operations for CHD. The small infant's mediastinum makes compression of the heart and cardiac tamponade ever-present possibilities after chest closure, despite patent drainage tubes. The warning signs of tamponade are frequently not present in small children, even minutes before cardiovascular collapse from tamponade. Any significant deterioration in hemodynamics after chest closure should be first attributed to tamponade if ventilation and cardiac rhythm are adequate. Until the patient is safely transported to the intensive care unit and cardiovascular stability is ensured, continuous attention must be paid to the patient's hemodynamic status after chest closure.

ANESTHESIA FOR NONCARDIAC SURGERY

The approach to anesthesia for children with CHD outlined above is the same whether the proposed operation is cardiac or noncardiac. Because noncardiac surgeons may have less appreciation of the delicate homeostatic balance of the child's cardiac pathophysiology, it is particularly important during noncardiac surgery that the anesthesiologist understand the pathophysiology of the patient's problem(s). Furthermore, CPB is not immediately available for cardiovascular support if surgery and anesthesia overwhelm the patient's circulatory homeostasis. Because the anesthesiologist must understand and maintain the often fragile circulatory balance during surgery, surgical insults must be anticipated preoperatively and planned for. Familiarity with the child's pathophysiology and the planned noncardiac procedure should avoid major problems in anesthetic management. Evaluation, preoperative preparation, choice of monitors, induction, maintenance, emergence from anesthesia, and plans for postoperative care are predicated on this familiarity.

An important aspect of the care of children with CHD who are undergoing noncardiac surgery is a cardiology consultation to delineate the pathologic lesion and provide objective assessment of the patient's current hemodynamic status. Most cardiologists have an incomplete appreciation of the physiologic stresses that major noncardiac surgical procedures impose on the cardiopulmonary system. When major blood loss is anticipated; when intrusion into the airway, peritoneal, thoracic, or cranial cavity is necessary, or when a prolonged operative procedure is planned, a cardiology consult is often helpful *if* the cardiologist is informed about the anticipated perioperative stresses to homeostasis.

Status of the Disease

Children with CHD may present for noncardiac operations before cardiac surgical treatment, after palliation, or after "repair" of their CHD. Palliated patients still have a distinctly abnormal circulation, and the consequences of CHD (e.g., CHF, hypoxemia, polycythemia, pulmonary vascular disease) may be a problem. It is important to note that even patients whose heart disease has been surgically "corrected" can have significant residual problems. Arrhythmias, ventricular dysfunction, shunts, valvular stenosis or regurgitation, and pulmonary hypertension may remain or develop after surgical "repair" of the CHD. Surgical "corrections" may be classified as "anatomical," whereby the circulation is in series and the left ventricle is connected to the aorta, or "physiologic," where the circulation is also in series and the patient is no longer cyanosed; however they may function with the RV as the systemic ventricle or have undergone a single ventricle repair (Table 18–9).

ANESTHESIA FOR INTERVENTIONAL PROCEDURES

Cardiac Catheterization Laboratory

Adequate sedation and anesthesia during cardiac catheterization is essential to facilitate acquisition of meaningful hemodynamic data and to assist during interventional procedures. For the most part, hemodynamic or diagnostic catheterization procedures can be performed under sedation in all age groups.[276] For many interventional procedures, sedation may be appropriate; however, for procedures that are associated with significant hemodynamic compromise or are prolonged, general anesthesia is preferable. Whatever technique is used, it is essential that hemodynamic data be attained in conditions as close to normal as possible. When using sedation, full monitoring is essential to ensure that respiratory depression is avoided. During

T A B L E   1 8 – 9
A CLASSIFICATION FOR CONGENITAL CARDIAC SURGICAL REPAIRS

Type of Repair	Outcome

Anatomic
  LV = systemic ventricle
  RV = pulmonary ventricle
  Circulation in series
  Cyanosis corrected
	1. Simple reconstruction;
	   Structurally normal after repair
	   (e.g., ASD, VSD, PDA)
	   Late complications unlikely
	2. Complex reconstruction;
	   Baffle, conduit, outflow
	   reconstruction or AV valve
	   repair; late complications
	   likely

Physiologic
  Circulation in series
  Cyanosis corrected
	1. Two ventricles:
	   RV = systemic ventricle
	   LV = systemic ventricle (e.g.,
	   Senning or Mustard
	   procedure)
	2. Single ventricle:
	   Fontan procedure

RV, right ventricle; LV, left ventricle; ASD, atrial septal defect; VSD, ventricular septal defect; PDA, patent ductus arteriosus; AV, atrioventricular valve.

anesthesia, the effects of inspired oxygen concentration, mechanical ventilation, and hemodynamic side effects of various anesthesia agents must also be appreciated. Postprocedure monitoring, either in a recovery room or intensive care unit, is mandatory.

Cardiac catheterization laboratories are usually remote from the operating room, and are rarely configured to accommodate anesthetic personnel. Relative to patient size, the lateral and anteroposterior cameras used for imaging are in close proximity to the patient's head and neck, limiting access to the airway. An anesthetic machine and monitors around the patient will further confine the space in which the anesthesiologist may work and limit access to the patient. In addition, the environment is darkened to facilitate viewing of images. This may make monitoring with capnography and pulse oximetry difficult unless the monitors are well lit. The environment is also cooler because of computer and cine equipment, and children may become hypothermic from conductive and convective heat loss. In addition, frequent flushing of the catheters and sheaths to prevent clotting or air embolism may contribute to hypothermia and to fluid overload. Unnecessary exposure of the child must be avoided and convective warming blankets should be used when possible. Care must be taken when positioning a patient on the catheterization table because of the risk for pressure areas and nerve traction injury. In particular, brachial plexus injury may occur when patients have their arms positioned above their heads for a prolonged period of time to make room for the lateral cameras. To facilitate femoral vein and arterial access, the pelvis is commonly elevated from the catheterization table. This may displace abdominal contents cephalad, restricting diaphragm excursion, and increasing the risk for respiratory depression in a sedated, spontaneously breathing patient.

In addition to considerations related to the environment, there are a number of potential problems and complications that are inherent to any catheterization procedure, and some related to specific interventions (see below). The minimal monitoring available to all patients in the catheterization laboratory includes automated blood pressure, ECG, pulse oximetry, P_{ETCO_2}, and direct observation of the patient's airway and breathing.

Interventional Cardiology

Transcatheter treatment of CHD is replacing a number of conventional intraoperative surgical procedures.[277-279] This form of therapy has had a significant impact on the severity and complexity of illness seen in the operating room and in the interventional laboratory. Procedures that are routinely performed in the catheterization laboratory now include (1) balloon valvuloplasty of congenitally stenotic aortic, mitral, and pulmonary valves; (2) angioplasty for pulmonary arterial stenoses and postoperative aortic recoarctation, or angioplasty combined with transcatheter placement of endovascular stents for sustained relief of obstruction in arterial or subarterial (intracardiac) locations; (3) radiofrequency ablation of abnormal conduction pathways; and (4) embolization or device occlusion procedures of systemic-to-pulmonary arterial communications, venous channels, fistulae, muscular VSDs, ASDs, or

patent ductus arteriosus (PDA). Many procedures (e.g., PDA closure) are performed on an outpatient basis with the full participation of the anesthesiologist.[280]

Although many relatively uncomplicated procedures previously performed in the operating room are now performed in the catheterization laboratory, they have been replaced by surgical procedures for previously inoperable patients with more complex disease who have derived benefit from interventional catheterization techniques. These interventions have established an anatomic or physiologic circumstance that lends itself to intraoperative repair. Among the best examples are patients with tetralogy of Fallot and pulmonary atresia with hypoplastic pulmonary arteries who are deemed inoperable after an early palliative shunt has failed to provide any meaningful growth of pulmonary arteries. By establishing antegrade flow to the pulmonary artery early in life with a surgically placed homograft from right ventricle to pulmonary artery, the child can undergo serial balloon dilations of the pulmonary arteries with subsequent growth that allows eventual surgical correction with VSD closure. Among patients with single ventricles who have undergone a modified Fontan procedure, high-risk candidates can be assisted during the postoperative period by leaving a communication at the atrial level that allows right-to-left shunting, and hence cardiac output, to be maintained during transient postoperative elevation in pulmonary vascular resistance. This fenestration can subsequently be test-occluded in the catheterization laboratory and permanently occluded with a device if indicated.[281]

This collaborative approach to intervention and repair has offered improved results and new futures for patients with many types of serious congenital heart disease.[278] Therefore, the cardiac anesthesiologist is faced with more complex, previously inoperable patients in the operating room, and with more demand for presence in the catheterization laboratory, where the environment is rapidly evolving into a hybrid operating room in need of the skills and balance of the anesthesiologist.

Risks and Complications

Placement of catheters in and through the heart increases the risk for dysrhythmias, perforation of the myocardium, damage to valve leaflets and cordae, cerebral vascular accidents, and air embolism. The use of radiopaque contrast material may cause an acute allergic reaction (although this is rare in children when nonionic contrast media is used), pulmonary hypertension, and myocardial depression. Blood loss may be sudden and unexpected when large-bore catheters are used or vessels are ruptured. More insidious blood loss may occur over several hours in heparinized small children or neonates owing to bleeding around the catheter site or multiple aspirations and flushes of catheters. Transfusion requirements and appropriate vascular access should be continually assessed.

Arrhythmias, albeit transient, may be recurrent and fatal if not promptly treated. These include catheter-induced supraventricular tachyarrhythmias, ventricular tachycardia, ventricular fibrillation, and occasionally complete heart block requiring temporary transvenous pacing support. On most occasions, removal of the wire or catheter is sufficient for the arrhythmia to resolve, but when this does not happen, it is important that full resuscitation and cardioversion equipment be available. An algorithm for treating catheter-induced arrhythmias is shown in Figure 18–16.

Complications of various interventional procedures are related in part to the type of procedure, but all share the risks associated with percutaneous vascular access with large catheters that course through the heart and vessels. The specific problems that may occur during various interventional transcatheter procedures are listed in Table 18–10. Although the underlying cardiac status or American Society of Anesthesiologists (ASA) classification of the patient may increase their risk for adverse events during catheterization, in many circumstances complications are sudden, occurring without warning, and reflect the inherent risk for a specific procedure. Many complications are potentially life threatening, and successful treatment of complications depends on prompt action by anesthesiologists cooperating closely with the interventional cardiologists who are manipulating the catheters.

Inadvertent release or detachment of embolic and closure devices results in systemic and pulmonary arterial embolization. Embolization usually occurs immediately after placement, and devices can often be retrieved by use of a variety of retrieval catheters, but in a small minority of cases surgical removal of these devices is required. If the device is lodged in the heart or a great vessel, CPB may be required for its removal. Device embolization does not usually cause extreme hemodynamic instability or cardiovascular decompensation requiring emergency surgical removal, but an unscheduled surgical procedure is still required. Even after successful transcatheter retrieval, femoral artery and vein reconstruction during anesthesia is occasionally necessary when embolized devices or large dilation balloons are removed through these vessels. Deliberate embolization of aortopulmonary collaterals may decrease pulmonary blood flow excessively and cause severe hypoxemia. General anesthesia and muscle paraly-sis may be necessary to increase arterial oxygen saturation to acceptable levels by decreasing oxygen consumption while the operating room is being prepared.

Balloon Dilation of Pulmonary Arteries

Balloon dilation and stent placement of the pulmonary artery to relieve stenosis is a common procedure performed in the catheterization laboratory. Complications that occur during this procedure exemplify many of the potential problems that can occur during any catheterization. Pulmonary artery stenoses may be congenital or acquired. The lesions may be discrete, involving the main or branch pulmonary arteries, or the lesions may be multiple and involve distal segmental vessels. Some factors that determine whether dilation should be performed under sedation or general anesthesia include the extent of balloon dilation, anticipated complications, and the duration of the procedure.

Pulmonary artery disruption is signaled by hemoptysis or by the appearance of intravascular contrast medium in the pleural space or major lung fissures.[282] In the presence of substantial hemoptysis, immediate endotracheal intubation is indicated for airway control and ventilation. Hypertension and further airway stimulation are avoided. Addition of PEEP may be useful. Heparinization is reversed and blood for transfusion is made immediately available. Intrapulmonary hemorrhage is often self-limited, but hemothorax can be severe and may lead to hypotension and death. Transient unilateral or unilobar pulmonary edema also is seen with pulmonary artery dilation. Edema occurs following sudden large increases in pulmonary blood flow and distal pulmonary artery pressure following dilation in a previously underperfused pulmonary vascular bed. These two distinct entities, unilateral pulmonary edema and disruption of pulmonary artery integrity, can both occur abruptly, in isolation or together, during pulmonary artery dilation procedures, and both can cause the appearance in the airway of frank blood or blood-tinged

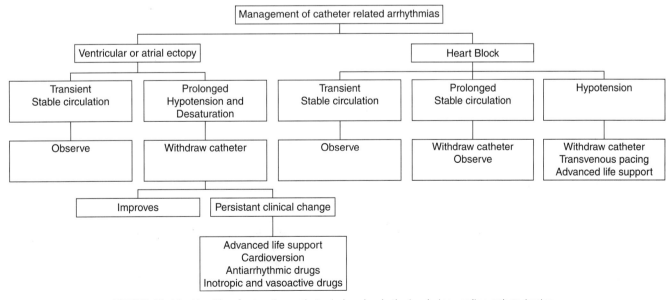

FIGURE 18–16. Algorithm for treating catheter-induced arrhythmias during cardiac catheterization.

TABLE 18-10
COMPLICATIONS IN THE CARDIAC CATHETERIZATION LABORATORY

Procedure	Representative Lesion	Complications
Diagnostic catheterization	Congenital heart disease	Blood loss requiring transfusion Air embolism Cerebral vascular accident Myocardial perforation and tamponade Femoral vessel occusion Arrhythmias; ventricular and supraventricular tachycardia, ventricular fibrillation, complete heart block
Coil embolization	Aortopulmonary collaterals Blalock–Taussig shunts Anomalous coronary arteries Hepatic hemangiomas	Fevers Excessive hypoxemia Systemic embolization Hepatic necrosis
Transcatheter device closure	Patent ductus arteriosus Atrial septal defect Ventricular septal defect Baffle leak	Air or device embolization Blood loss Interference with atrioventricular value function, ventricular arrhythmias, complete heart block
Balloon and stent dilations	Pulmonary artery stenosis	Pulmonary artery tear and bleeding
		Unilateral pulmonary edema False aneurysm Cardiac arrest (William's syndrome)
	Blalock–Taussig shunt	Pulmonary artery tear and bleeding Thrombosis Pulmonary edema
	Pulmonary valve stenosis	Pulmonary insufficiency
	Aortic valve stenosis	Aortic regurgitation Ventricular fibrillation (neonate)
	Mitral valve stenosis	Mitral insufficiency Pulmonary hypertension
	Coarctation of the aorta	Aortic dissection Hypertension
	Right ventricular conduit	False aneurysms Stent embolization
Atrial septotomy	Transposition of the great arteries, mitral stenosis (atresia), and restrictive atrial septum	Perforation of the heart and tamponade
Radiofrequency mapping and ablation	Anomalous conduction pathways	Complete heart block Supraventricular tachycardia Thromboembolus from long sheath and prolonged procedure
Myocardial biopsy	Cardiomyopathy or transplantation	Myocardial perforation Complete heart block

edema fluid in substantial quantities. Treatment of both entities starts with endotracheal intubation unless the symptoms are minimal.

The function of the right ventricle is critical. At the time of balloon dilation, cardiac output may decrease significantly, causing hypotension, bradycardia, arterial oxygen desaturation, and a decrease in PETCO$_2$. As the balloon is only inflated for a few seconds, the procedure is usually well tolerated and the circulation usually recovers spontaneously if the preload is maintained. Patients who have a hypertrophied, poorly compliant right ventricle and intraventricular pressures at systemic or suprasystemic levels may not tolerate the sudden increase in afterload associated with balloon dilation, even for a short period. In particular, myocardial ischemia and arrhythmias may occur, causing severe acute RV failure and loss of cardiac output. General anesthesia and controlled ventilation is recommended prior to the intervention in this at-risk group of patients.

Patients who have a dilated right ventricle that is caused by a longstanding volume load, such as chronic pulmonary regurgitation, also are at risk for arrhythmias and low output during catheter manipulations and interventions. On most occasions, the changes in rhythm are short lived and disappear once the catheters are withdrawn. Nevertheless, anesthesia and airway control is recommended if the circulation is compromised, and a defibrillator and transvenous pacing must be immediately available.

Potential movement at the time of critical balloon dilation or stent placement must be avoided. The dilation of pulmonary arteries is painful and will often cause patients to waken from sedation and move. In addition, dilation of the pulmonary arteries may induce coughing. This is usually not a problem for isolated pulmonary artery dilation; however, if the patient moves during stent placement, it is possible to obstruct lobar or segmental branch pulmonary arteries inadvertently by placing the stent in the wrong place. Therefore, it is essential the patient is immobile when the stent is placed. Additional sedation should be considered immediately prior to stent placement.

Balloon dilation of multiple peripheral pulmonary artery stenoses, such as occur in patients with Williams' syndrome, are often prolonged procedures and associated with significant hemodynamic changes. Endotracheal general anesthesia is usually required from the outset of the procedure. Besides right ventricular hypertension, an additional concern in this group of patients is the risk for pulmonary edema after dilation of the artery. This usually occurs immediately following balloon dilation of the vessel, but can be delayed for up to 24 hours. Endotracheal intubation and controlled ventilation are usually necessary until the edema resolves.

Occlusion Device Insertion

"Umbrella" or "clamshell" device closure of a PDA, ASDs, and VSDs are commonly performed in the cardiac catheterization laboratory. Placement of a device to close a PDA or ASD is usually associated with minimal hemodynamic disturbance and can be performed in most patients using sedation only.[280] General anesthesia may be necessary for airway protection if transesophageal echocardiography is used to guide device placement or if the procedure is prolonged and a procedural complication, such as device embolization, occurs.

In contrast to our experience with closure of PDAs or ASDs, transcatheter closure of a VSD with one of these devices is a long procedure and often is associated with profound hemodynamic instability and blood loss.[283] Intensive care management of the patient frequently is required following placement of the device. The indications for VSD device placement include closure of a residual or recurrent septal defect, preoperative closure of defects that may be difficult to reach surgically while on cardiopulmonary bypass, and closure of acquired defects, such as occur after myocardial infarction or trauma. Although the clinical condition of patients undergoing VSD device placement may vary considerably, the preoperative clinical condition or ASA status is not a predictor of hemodynamic disturbance during device placement.[283] Rather, it is the technique necessary for deploying the occlusion device that results in significant hemodynamic compromise and all patients are therefore susceptible.

Factors contributing to hemodynamic instability include blood loss; arrhythmias from catheter manipulation in the ventricles and across the septum; atrioventricular (AV) or aortic valve regurgitation after stenting open of valve leaflets by stiff-walled catheters; and device-related factors, such as malposition of the umbrella with impingement of the arms of the device on valve leaflets or dislodgment of the device from the ventricular septum.

The procedures are often prolonged. Because of the large sheath required to position the delivery pod and folded umbrella, and because of the need for frequent catheter changes through the sheath, considerable blood loss may occur (often concealed by drapes) and the risk for air embolism also is increased. Air embolization may be life threatening in patients with intracardiac shunts. When unoccupied by the device carrier system and collapsed device, the large delivery sheath represents a poten-

tial space for air accumulation and subsequent delivery of air into the heart. In addition, when the entry port of the large delivery sheath is open during removal and reinsertion of various catheters and devices, extreme inspiratory efforts may entrain air into the heart. Air delivered into the right atrium may be shunted across the ASD, even in the presence of nominal left-to-right shunting. Left atrial air embolization during these procedures can be seen with fluoroscopy; it produces ST-segment elevation and often produces hemodynamic changes as the air passes into the aorta. The resultant ST-segment changes, hypotension, arterial desaturation, and bradycardia generally respond to aspirating the air and sealing the entry port, along with administration of atropine, and the use of inotropic and pressor support to maintain coronary perfusion. Meticulous purging of air from the catheter system and sealing of open ports should minimize the incidence of air embolism. Use of controlled positive-pressure ventilation through an endotracheal tube in an anesthetized, paralyzed patient also may decrease the potential for transcatheter air entrainment during transcatheter closure of intracardiac defects.

Transcatheter Radiofrequency Ablation

Pediatric patients undergoing radiofrequency ablation of abnormal conduction pathways vary in age and diagnosis.[284] Ablation may be necessary in the newborn with persistent reentrant tachycardia or ectopic atrial tachycardia and cardiac failure. It is required in older children who have an ectopic focus and otherwise structurally normal heart. An increasing number of patients undergoing ablation of these pathways are those who have undergone previous surgical repair of congenital heart defects. Patients with persistent volume or pressure load on the right atrium and those who have required extensive incisions and suture lines within the right atrium, such as occurs with a Mustard, Senning, or Fontan procedure, may be at increased risk for supraventricular tachyarrhythmia (SVT), including atrial flutter and fibrillation. Ventricular tachyarrhythmias also may develop late following repair of certain congenital heart defects, such as RV outflow tract reconstruction for tetralogy of Fallot.

Radiofrequency catheter ablations (RFCAs) are usually prolonged procedures. It is difficult for children to lie still for some hours and, therefore, endotracheal general anesthesia is preferred. In addition, it is important patients remain immobile to avoid catheter movement at the time of ablation because sudden patient movement may result in a radiofrequency lesion being created at an incorrect site. For instance, if the focus is close to the AV node, inadvertent movement might displace the catheter and cause permanent AV conduction blockade. On occasions, holding the ventilation either in inspiration or expiration may be necessary to ensure adequate contact of the ablation catheter with the arrhythmic focus.

Although these procedures are long, for the most part they are hemodynamically well tolerated and blood loss is minimal. During mapping, the focus is stimulated and the tachyarrhythmia induced. This may result in hypotension. However, the hypotension usually is short lived and can be converted readily via intracardiac pacing. If hypotension is prolonged and intracardiac conversion unsuccessful, transthoracic cardioversion may be necessary. Therefore, a defibrillator should be immediately available.

Because anesthetic drugs have minimal effect on intrinsic conduction of impulses,[194, 195, 285] a range of techniques can be used to maintain general anesthesia during RFCA. Some tachyarrhythmias, such as ectopic atrial tachycardia, are catecholamine sensitive, and the abnormal conduction focus may be difficult to localize after the induction of anesthesia. For this reason, it is preferable to perform the procedure under light sedation or light general anesthesia in these patients.

Cardiac Tamponade

Acute myocardial perforation and cardiac tamponade occasionally occurs during interventional cardiac catheterization procedures. Prompt support of the circulation with volume infusions and pressor support, along with immediate catheter drainage of the pericardial space, are essential when this complication occurs. Hemopericardium following ventricular puncture usually is self-limited, because the muscular ventricle seals the perforation after the responsible wire or catheter is removed. However, laceration of the thin-walled atrium may require suture closure of the laceration in the operating room.

Other causes of cardiac tamponade occur in patients with CHD and treatment frequently requires the assistance of an anesthesiologist. Tamponade that occurs immediately after surgery is best handled by chest tube drainage or reopening the sternotomy. These patients usually are still anesthetized and mechanically ventilated so that new anesthetic considerations and choices are limited. However, some children develop pericardial effusions at other phases of their illness, owing to hydrostatic influences (e.g., patients with modified Fontan operations) or postpericardiotomy syndrome. Fluid in the pericardial space may accumulate under considerable pressure, and filling of the heart is impaired. If this problem is left unattended, the transmural pressure in the atria diminishes as the intraatrial pressures rise and diastolic collapse of the atria can be observed by echocardiography. The patients develop a narrow pulse pressure, pulsus paradoxus, tachycardia, respiratory distress, abdominal pain, decreased urine output, hyperkalemia, metabolic acidosis, and hypotension. There usually is a tremendous endogenous catecholamine response.

When the patient's hemodynamics are compromised, draining the pericardial fluid is imperative. If the fluid is accessible through a subxiphoid approach, percutaneous drainage of the fluid is preferred. This may be a formidable task in a frightened, combative child who has impending shock. Anesthetic principles guiding sedation for pericardial drainage should focus on maintaining or improving intravascular volume, vascular tone, and the contractile state of the ventricle. Anesthetic agents used for sedation that excessively decrease preload or afterload and transiently impair myocardial function may have disastrous consequences, especially when they are combined with muscle paralysis and positive-pressure ventilation. The latter further impairs ventricular filling. If a child demonstrates serious symptoms of cardiac tamponade and a large circumferential, percutaneously accessible pericardial effusion is identified echocardiographically, drainage of the fluid can occur after the child is sedated with a narcotic, benzodiazepine, or ketamine and the skin and subcutaneous tissues are anesthetized with local anesthetic. This approach usually is safer than doing a rapid-sequence induction of anesthesia, initiating positive-pressure ventilation, and draining the fluid surgically.

PATHOPHYSIOLOGY AND ANESTHETIC MANAGEMENT OF SPECIFIC LESIONS AND PROCEDURES

A unique feature of managing patients with congenital heart defects is the knowledge, expertise, and technical skills required to manage a heterogeneous population of patients with a wide variety of diagnoses and pathophysiology. The experience at Children's Hospital, Boston, over the past 5 years is shown in Figure 18–17. In addition, there has been a change in management philosophy over the past 20 years towards performing reparative operations on neonates and infants rather than performing an initial palliative procedure and doing the complete repair later.[84] The change in surgical practice and age at which procedures are undertaken at Children's Hospital, Boston, is shown in Figure 18–18. Emphasis now is on early surgical repair of congenital heart lesions. The aim in doing so is to promote normal growth and development and to limit the pathophysiologic consequences of congenital cardiac defects such as volume overload, pressure overload, and chronic hypoxemia. It is important to note, however, that an increasing number of older children and adults with congenital heart disease are presenting themselves for cardiac and noncardiac surgery. This includes patients undergoing a reparative operation, often some years following an initial palliative procedure, and patients who have had previous reparative surgery who subsequently require surgery because of residual or progressive defects, such as conduit stenosis.

Virtually all congenital cardiac defects are now amenable to either an anatomic or functional repair. However, these lesions are often "corrected" but not "cured." Palliative procedures are often necessary to control pulmonary blood flow prior to repair because of extreme lesion size, anatomic variations, or need for maturation of the child before repair can be accomplished. For example, a modified Fontan procedure is the definitive operation for many classes of complex CHD. However, the Fontan procedure requires low PVR and large pulmonary arteries, which are not characteristic of the neonate. Therefore, a shunt may be required to relieve hypoxemia and allow growth of the pulmonary arteries until the child is a few months older. Alternatively, if the pulmonary blood flow is excessive, a pulmonary band may be required to minimize the occurrence of CHF and to prevent *any* pulmonary vascular obstructive disease from developing until a Fontan repair can be done. Nevertheless palliative procedures have immediate complications and may seriously compromise subsequent complete surgical repair of the lesion.[286–294]

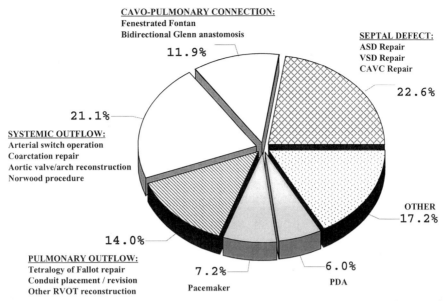

FIGURE 18–17. Spectrum of congenital cardiac surgical procedures performed at Children's Hospital, Boston, between 1995 and 1999. Abbreviations: ASD, atrial septal defect; VSD, ventricular septal defect; CAVC, complete atrioventricular canal; PDA, patent ductus arteriosus; RVOT, right ventricle outflow tract.

This section summarizes the basic pathophysiology of each lesion or procedure as a prelude to discussion of anesthetic management of the lesion. The discussion of anesthetic management before the repair applies equally well to noncardiac procedures in unrepaired patients and to patients undergoing repair of the CHD before CPD support is initiated. For some lesions, a separate discussion considers the anesthetic complications that occur after repair of the lesion. This heading, where appropriate, outlines specific complications and problems that may be encountered months or years after repair of the anomaly. Otherwise, this information is found at the end of the section on anesthetic management.

Surgical Shunts

Pathophysiology

When the anatomy or physiology includes severe obstruction of pulmonary blood flow and is unsuitable for immediate physiologic repair, a shunt is required. This situation is seen most commonly in patients who have tricuspid atresia with restricted pulmonary blood flow, pulmonary atresia, or a single ventricle and severe obstruction to pulmonary blood flow. The surgically created shunt provides sufficient pulmonary blood flow to maintain acceptable arterial oxygen saturation in a circumstance where oxygenated pulmonary venous blood mixes with systemic

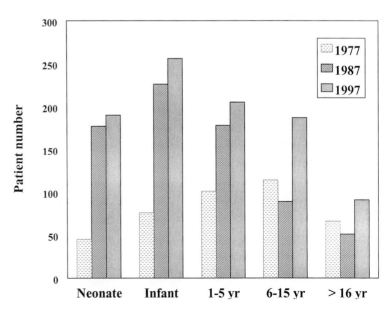

FIGURE 18–18. Changes in the age spectrum of patients undergoing congenital cardiac procedures at Children's Hospital, Boston, over the past 20 years.

venous blood. Optimally, the surgical shunt (a simple shunt) provides restrictive flow to the pulmonary circuit, allowing adequate, but not excessive, pulmonary blood flow.

Types of Surgical Shunts

Systemic to Pulmonary Artery Shunts

Systemic-to-pulmonary artery shunts are palliative procedures that increase pulmonary blood flow, thereby relieving severe cyanosis, improving functional status, and allowing for diffuse growth of small pulmonary arteries. The classic *Blalock-Taussig (B-T) shunt* redirects subclavian artery blood into the branch pulmonary artery on the side opposite the aortic arch.[295] This graft allows some growth during infancy but is unlikely to induce pulmonary vascular disease. Rather than compromise the subclavian artery and upper limb blood flow, a modified B-T shunt is now preferred using a Gortex synthetic tube graft that is interposed between the subclavian or innominate artery and the pulmonary artery. Performed either via a thoracotomy or median sternotomy, flow across the shunt is dependent upon the size of the Gortex tube (usually 3.5- or 4.0-mm diameter), the length of the tube, and site of take-off from the systemic artery. A shunt arising from the innominate artery is likely to have a higher flow because of a higher perfusion pressure than a more distally placed shunt arising from the subclavian artery. The B-T shunt is associated with low mortality and a low incidence of late postoperative complications.[296, 297] However, distortion of the pulmonary arteries may occur within a few months and seriously affect definitive repair at a later age.

The *Potts shunt* (descending aorta to left pulmonary artery) and the *Waterston shunt*[298] (ascending aorta to the right pulmonary artery) are rarely used now because the size of the shunt orifice is difficult to control precisely. These shunts may enlarge substantially with growth, become nonrestrictive, and result in excessive pulmonary flow and pulmonary vascular obstructive disease. They produce distortion and stenosis of the branch pulmonary arteries, and they also are difficult to dissect and control prior to CPB during subsequent surgery. A *central shunt* between the ascending aorta and main pulmonary artery is occasionally used when the branch pulmonary arteries are hypoplastic.

Vena Cava to Pulmonary Artery Shunt

The first cavopulmonary artery anastomosis (*Glenn shunt*) was a unidirectional shunt constructed as a palliative procedure for tricuspid atresia. A Glenn shunt provides systemic *venous* blood, instead of systemic arterial blood, to the lungs for gas exchange. The superior vena cava is disconnected from the right atrium and connected directly to the detached right pulmonary artery (i.e., superior vena cava blood perfuses the right lung and flow depends on the pressure gradient between the superior vena cava and left atrial pressure).[299] Therefore, the Glenn shunt is limited to patients with low PVR, which precludes its use in neonates. This shunt is rarely performed today because the pulmonary arteries are not in continuity and because palli-

ation is short lived due to complications such as thrombosis or occlusion of the shunt that lead to SVC syndrome, or due to progressive cyanosis that is secondary to the development of pulmonary arteriovenous collaterals.[300]

An important modification of the Glenn shunt that is now used during staged repair of single-ventricle defects involves the anastomosis of the cephalad portion of the superior vena cava to the right pulmonary artery, as in the original Glenn procedure; but pulmonary artery continuity is maintained. Therefore, blood flow is bidirectional through both right and left pulmonary arteries (hence the term *bidirectional cavopulmonary anastomosis* or *bidirectional Glenn (BDG) procedure*).[301–303] This procedure can be performed successfully in children as young as 3 to 4 months of age.[304, 305] By then, the PVR has decreased, and the effective pulmonary blood flow has increased despite reduced pulmonary artery pressures. This shunt avoids imposing the volume load on the ventricle that is associated with aortopulmonary shunts, and it minimizes the atrial distention and the high right atrial pressures inherent in a full Fontan-type operation in a high-risk patient (see below).[306]

Anesthetic Management Before and During Aortopulmonary Shunts

Complications of surgical shunts can occur immediately after surgery or years later when another surgical intervention is contemplated. Severe hypoxemia may occur in the operating room during or after creation of the shunt, implying inadequate pulmonary blood flow. Intrapulmonary shunting always must be considered in lungs that are compressed by the surgeons, but mechanical obstruction of flow into the pulmonary artery that is caused by retraction during surgery or by shunt occlusion (kinking or thrombosis) is the usual cause. An increase in PVR also may reduce flow across the shunt. Inducing an alkalosis by hyperventilation and using a high inspired oxygen concentration may minimize PVR and optimize gas exchange until shunt flow can be improved. As a note of caution, however, an increase in mean intrathoracic pressure and overinflation of the lungs during vigorous mechanical ventilation may further restrict flow across the shunt.

Systemic-to-pulmonary artery shunts are inherently inefficient because they recirculate blood to the lungs without its having reached the systemic circulation. To substantially improve arterial oxygen content, pulmonary blood flow must be several times greater than the systemic flow (Fig. 18–19). However, if the surgically created shunt is not sufficiently restrictive, pulmonary flows become excessive and cause pulmonary edema, wide pulse pressures and, occasionally, inadequate systemic perfusion. Arterial oxygen saturation is relatively high despite complete mixing of systemic and pulmonary venous blood in the left heart. Maneuvers to increase pulmonary vascular resistance (see above) can compensate to a limited degree for excessive pulmonary flow, but shunt revision may be necessary.

Anesthetic Considerations After Creation of an Aortopulmonary Shunt

In patients with systemic-to-pulmonary artery shunts, shunt flow is usually restricted by the shunt orifice and the bal-

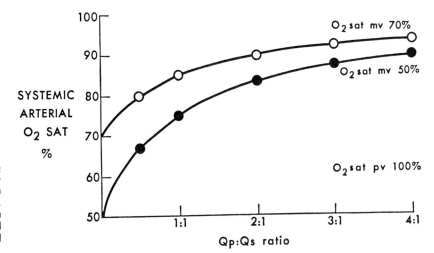

FIGURE 18-19. Changes in systemic arterial O_2 saturation with mixing lesions as the $\dot{Q}p/\dot{Q}s$ (pulmonary/systemic blood flow ratio) changes with different levels of mixed venous (mv) O_2 saturation. It presumes a pulmonary venous (pv) O_2 saturation of 100 percent. (From Rudolph AM: Congenital Diseases of the Heart. Chicago, Year Book Medical Publishers, 1974, p 79, with permission.)

ance between pulmonary and systemic vascular resistance. If the shunt is too large, excessive pulmonary blood flow will be evident by high arterial oxygen saturations, reduced systemic perfusion with increasing metabolic acidosis, low diastolic blood pressure, and pulmonary edema. The work of breathing is increased and patients may have difficulty being weaned from ventilation. If a shunt is large enough to allow excessive pressure and flow in the pulmonary vascular bed, pulmonary vascular obstructive disease may develop over time.

If the shunt is too small, arterial oxygen saturations will remain low, and pulmonary flow will be dependent on normal or increased systemic arterial pressures. Thus, hypotension seriously compromises arterial oxygenation, particularly as the shunt becomes more restrictive, and must be treated aggressively. Other causes of low oxygen saturation after shunt placement include a low mixed venous oxygen concentration that is secondary to a low cardiac output and reduced oxygen-carrying capacity from relative anemia.

An appropriately sized shunt results in a balanced circulation ($\dot{Q}p/\dot{Q}s$ approximately 1:1) with peripheral oxygen saturations between 75 to 85 percent, a normal systolic pressure, and a widened pulse pressure. Tachycardia is common immediately after the shunt is open, and blood volume replacement is usually necessary. Inotrope support with dopamine also may be necessary because the increased pulmonary blood flow imposes a volume load on the systemic ventricle. The hematocrit should be maintained between 40 and 45 percent. Afterload reduction induced with a systemic vasodilator, such as sodium nitroprusside or a phosphodiesterase inhibitor, may be indicated if the patient has poor extremity perfusion or poor systemic perfusion due to a relatively large shunt and excessive pulmonary blood flow. In general, most patients are mechanically ventilated postoperatively until blood flow is well balanced and adequate systemic perfusion is maintained.

Pulmonary Artery Banding
Pathophysiology

When pulmonary blood flow is excessive and high pressure is communicated from the ventricle to the pulmonary vasculature, surgery may be required to prevent progressive pulmonary vascular obstructive disease or to lessen symptoms of CHF. If total correction of the lesion is not possible, pulmonary blood flow can be reduced by banding the pulmonary artery.

Anesthetic Management

With induction of anesthesia for banding of the pulmonary artery, pulmonary vascular resistance occasionally decreases enough to cause massive pulmonary flow and systemic hypotension ("pulmonary steal"). If so, partial occlusion of a branch pulmonary artery with a clamp or ligature reduces pulmonary blood flow and increases peripheral perfusion until the band is applied.

Banding of the pulmonary artery is imprecise, and the hemodynamics after banding are unpredictable. Adequacy of the band is assessed in the operating room by observing a 20 to 30 percent increase in systemic blood pressure and a decrease in systemic arterial oxygen saturation. Direct measurement of the pulmonary artery pressure beyond the band may be compared with the systemic arterial pressure. It should be about 50 percent or less of the systemic pressure. Continuous monitoring of oxygen saturation is helpful for quick assessment of the adequacy of pulmonary blood flow. The oxygen saturation by pulse oximeter should be about 80 percent in common mixing lesions.[307] As hemodynamic criteria are used to assess band tightness, anesthesia is best maintained with high-dose narcotics; high concentrations of inhaled agents should be avoided. If the band is too tight, bradycardia, hypotension, and cyanosis will develop, requiring urgent band removal.

The large resistance imposed by banding the pulmonary artery stimulates hypertrophy of the ventricle supplying the banded vessel. Consequently, depression of function of that ventricle quickly reduces pulmonary blood flow, particularly if a VSD or ASD is present, allowing shunting of blood into the systemic circulation. Long-term anatomic hazards of pulmonary artery bands relate to distortion of the anatomy and hypertrophy of the ventricle.[294]

Single Ventricle and Parallel Circulation Physiology

Pathophysiology

In patients with a repaired two-ventricle heart (i.e., an "in-series" circulation whereby a separate ventricle ejects blood into the pulmonary artery and the pulmonary venous blood returns to a separate systemic ventricle), systemic oxygenation exclusively represents the efficiency of gas exchange in the lungs; lowering PVR and decreasing right ventricular afterload are important objectives when trying to increase pulmonary blood flow and correct hypoxemia in this situation. However, patients with single-ventricle anatomy represent a unique circumstance that requires physiologic interpretation of oxygenation and hemodynamics in light of the "parallel" nature of the circulation. In this circumstance, a single ventricle supplies both pulmonary and systemic blood flow, and lowering pulmonary vascular resistance in these patients may improve oxygenation but adversely affect hemodynamics in some circumstances.

There are many anatomic variations of single-ventricle or univentricular hearts. In general, both AV valves enter a single chamber. Most commonly, a small outflow chamber gives rise to one great artery, usually the aorta. Either AV valve may be atretic; subpulmonary stenosis or atresia is common. Occasionally, subaortic stenosis is present at birth or develops later.[308, 309] Therefore, in an infant with a single ventricle the anatomic variations may vary considerably, ranging from tricuspid atresia (a single left ventricle) through double-inlet left ventricle (two AV valves and one single ventricle) to mitral atresia (a single right ventricle [i.e., hypoplastic left heart]). Despite the anatomic diagnosis, virtually all patients with effective single-ventricle hearts, as shown in (Table 18–11), are amenable to a "physiologic" repair (i.e., Fontan procedure).

It is important to note, however, that an effective "parallel" circulation or physiology can exist in patients with two ventricles (Table 18–11). In these circumstances, the balance between pulmonary and systemic vascular resistance is the critical determinant of systemic perfusion and, therefore, a "balanced" circulation ($\dot{Q}p/\dot{Q}s = 1$). Much of the discussion below regarding maneuvers used to increase or decrease pulmonary blood flow apply in these patients as well prior to surgery. Examples include patients who have a large patent ductus arteriosus (left-to-right shunt across the PDA from the aorta to pulmonary artery), common ventricular outflow tract (as in truncus arteriosus), or aortic arch interruption (right-to-left flow from the pulmonary artery to the distal aorta across the PDA to maintain systemic perfusion).

For patients with single-ventricle anatomy, there is a common physiologic principle (i.e., desaturated systemic venous blood returns to the heart and mixes completely with oxygenated blood returning to the same chamber from the lungs). Common mixing of systemic and pulmonary venous blood means that the aortic O_2 saturation reflects the $\dot{Q}p/\dot{Q}s$. In the absence of lung disease (pulmonary venous desaturation), the pulmonary venous blood (oxygen saturations of 95 to 100 percent) will drain to the ventricle and mix with systemic venous blood (oxygen

TABLE 18–11
ANATOMICAL DIAGNOSES AND SURGICAL PROCEDURES THAT DEMONSTRATE PARALLEL OR BALANCED CIRCULATION PHYSIOLOGY

Defects amenable to a single ventricle repair (i.e., common mixing lesions)
  Atrioventricular valve atresia
    Tricuspid atresia
    Mitral atresia
  Ventricular hypoplasia
    Hypoplastic left heart syndrome
    Double inlet left or right ventricle
    Unbalanced atrioventricular canal
  Outflow tract obstruction
  Aortic atresia
    Shone's complex
    Pulmonary atresia and small right ventricle

Defects amenable to a two-ventricle repair
  Common ventricular outflow tract
    Truncus arteriosus
  PDA-dependent pulmonary blood flow
    Tetralogy of Fallot and pulmonary atresia
  PDA-dependent systemic blood flow
    Interrupted aortic arch

Postoperative single-ventricle palliation
  Norwood procedure for HLHS
  Modified Blalock-Taussig shunt

HLHS, hypoplastic left heart syndrome.

saturations of 55 to 60 percent or less), depending on the amount of oxygen extraction in the periphery. If pulmonary and systemic blood flows are equal (i.e., $\dot{Q}p/\dot{Q}s = 1$), the resultant "mixed" O_2 saturation measured in the systemic artery is 75 to 85 percent. As the pulmonary blood flow rises in proportion to systemic blood flow, the arterial oxygenation rises. Consequently, an arterial oxygen saturation of 90 percent is achieved at the expense of excessive pulmonary blood flow ($\dot{Q}p/\dot{Q}s > 3$) and a substantial volume load to the single ventricle, which is required to supply all systemic and pulmonary (three times systemic) blood flow. CHF ensues. If both the pulmonary artery and aorta are anatomically related to the ventricle and unobstructed, flow to the pulmonary and systemic beds will be partitioned according to the relative resistances of each circuit (i.e., parallel circulations). As the pulmonary vascular resistance decreases during the first few hours of life, pulmonary blood flow increases relative to systemic flow and systemic arterial oxygen saturation will be greater than 80 percent. Therefore, systemic oxygen saturation is a convenient marker of $\dot{Q}p/\dot{Q}s$. The effects of alterations of $\dot{Q}p/\dot{Q}s$ on systemic arterial oxygen saturation for common mixing lesions are shown in Figure 18–19.

Increased $\dot{Q}p/\dot{Q}s$

The deleterious effects of overcirculated lungs perfused at high pressure and flows, combined with the adverse effects of this volume load, will culminate in a picture of hyperdynamic CHF in which systemic perfusion is compromised and oxygen delivery is impaired despite the elevated arterial oxygen saturation (Fig. 18–20). This is especially a problem in the neonate because the neonate's heart is less capable of increasing stroke volume in re-

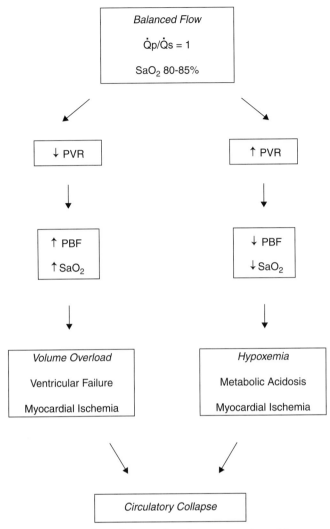

FIGURE 18–20. Effect of changes in pulmonary vascular resistance potentially contributing to circulatory collapse in patients with single ventricle physiology. $\dot{Q}p$, pulmonary blood flow; $\dot{Q}s$, systemic blood flow; SaO_2, arterial oxygen saturation; PBF, pulmonary blood flow; PVR, pulmonary vascular resistance.

sponse to increasing preload than is the mature myocardium. The myocardium of neonates who have increased $\dot{Q}p/\dot{Q}s$ ultimately cannot provide adequate systemic flow, as PVR decreases and more and more of the stroke volume is inefficiently recirculated to the lungs. Treatment is therefore directed toward raising resistance to blood flow to the lungs, balancing pulmonary and systemic blood flow ratios, and maintaining adequate systemic blood flow (Table 18–12).

PVR can be increased by producing hypoventilation and respiratory acidosis and by using a low FIO_2 to induce alveolar hypoxia. Ventilation with room air may suffice, but occasionally a hypoxic gas mixture is necessary. This is achieved by adding sufficient nitrogen to the inspired gas mixture to reduce the FIO_2 to 0.17 to 0.19. Although these maneuvers often successfully increase PVR and reduce pulmonary blood flow, it is important to remember that these patients have limited oxygen reserve, and may develop sudden and precipitous oxygen desaturation. Controlled hypoventilation in effect reduces the FRC of

the lung and the oxygen reserve, which also is compromised by the use of a hypoxic inspired gas mixture. Inotropic support often is necessary because of ventricular dysfunction secondary to the increased volume load. Systemic afterload reduction with agents such as phosphodiesterase inhibitors may improve systemic perfusion, although these drugs also may decrease PVR and thus not correct the imbalance of pulmonary and systemic flow. Patients who have continued pulmonary overcirculation with high SaO_2 and reduced systemic perfusion, despite the above maneuvers, require early surgical intervention to control pulmonary blood flow. At the time of surgery, a snare may be placed around either branch pulmonary artery to effectively limit pulmonary blood flow. Monitoring the SVC O_2 saturation as a measure of mixed venous O_2 saturation and of cardiac output, is often useful in patients with single-ventricle physiology. For instance, a patient with too much pulmonary blood flow may have an arterial O_2 saturation that is high (i.e., > 85 percent), but a low SVC O_2 saturation (i.e., < 50 percent) if systemic perfusion and cardiac output are reduced. Monitoring changes in the SVC O_2 saturation during treatment is a useful guide to the adequacy of management. In contrast, a patient who is hypoxic and has an oxygen saturation of less than 75 percent and a normal arterial–SVC O_2 saturation difference of 25 to 30 percent can be assumed to have an adequate cardiac output, and other causes for hypoxemia need to be evaluated.

Decreased $\dot{Q}p/\dot{Q}s$

Decreased pulmonary blood flow (i.e., $\dot{Q}p/\dot{Q}s$ < 1) in patients with a single ventricle and parallel circulation is reflected by hypoxemia (i.e., an SaO_2 < 80 percent). Preoperatively, this may be due to restricted flow across a small ductus arteriosus, increased PVR secondary to parenchymal lung disease, or increased pulmonary venous pressure secondary to obstructed pulmonary venous drainage or a restrictive atrial septal defect. Initial resuscitation involves maintaining patency of the ductus arteriosus with a PGE_1 infusion at a rate of 0.025 to 0.05 $\mu g/kg/min$. Most patients require tracheal intubation and mechanical ventilation, either because of apnea secondary to PGE_1 or to manipulate gas exchange to aid in balancing pulmonary and systemic flow. Systemic blood pressure, and therefore perfusion pressure across the ductus arteriosus, is maintained with volume expansion and vasopressors. Sedation, paralysis, and manipulation of mechanical ventilation to maintain an alkalosis may be effective if PVR is elevated. Nitric oxide as a specific pulmonary vasodilator also may be of use in this situation. Systemic oxygen delivery is maintained by improving cardiac output, and red blood cell transfusions are given to maintain a hematocrit greater than 40 percent. Interventional cardiac catheterization with balloon septostomy or dilation of a restrictive atrial septal defect may be necessary; however, early surgical intervention and palliation with a systemic-to-pulmonary artery shunt is usually indicated.

Anesthesia Considerations

A thorough preoperative assessment is essential to determine the balance of pulmonary and systemic flow, pres-

TABLE 18-12
PARALLEL CIRCULATION PHYSIOLOGY: MANAGEMENT CONSIDERATIONS

Clinical Circumstance	Etiology	Management
Balanced flow: $\dot{Q}p = \dot{Q}s \sim 1.0$	$\dot{Q}p = \dot{Q}s \sim 1.0$	No intervention
SaO_2 80–85% and normotensive		
Overcirculated: $SaO_2 > 90\%$ and low blood pressure	$\dot{Q}p \gg \dot{Q}s$ Low PVR Large aortopulmonary shunt size (PDA or B-T shunt)	**Raise PVR:** Controlled hypoventilation Low FIO_2 (0.17–0.19)
	Clinical signs: Wide pulse pressure Poor peripheral perfusion Congestive heart failure Oliguria	**Increase systemic perfusion:** Afterload reduction Inotrope support Treat hypertension
	Laboratory: Metabolic acidosis Low SvO_2 saturation Increased (SaO_2–SvO_2) difference	**Surgical intervention** Shunt revision
Undercirculated: $SaO_2 < 75\%$ and normal/elevated blood pressure	$\dot{Q}p < \dot{Q}s$ High PVR Small or occluded aortopulmonary shunt	**Lower PVR:** Controlled hyperventilation Alkalosis Reduce stress response Pulmonary vasodilation
	Clinical signs: Cyanosis Narrow pulse pressure Myocardial ischemia Loss of murmur (late)	**Increase cardiac output:** Raise systemic blood pressure Inotrope support
	Laboratory: Metabolic acidosis Normal (SaO_2–SvO_2) difference	**Increase mixed venous O_2:** Hematocrit > 40% Sedation/anesthesia/paralysis **Surgical intervention** Shunt revision
Low cardiac output: $SaO_2 < 75\%$ and hypotension	Ventricular failure Myocardial ischemia	**Ventricular support:** Maximize inotrope support Optimize preload Open sternum Minimize stress response
	Clinical signs: Poor peripheral perfusion Oliguria/anuria Narrow pulse pressure	**Surgical revision** Aortic arch and coronary anastomosis; transplantation
	Laboratory: Metabolic acidosis Low SvO_2 saturation Increased (SaO_2–SvO_2) difference	**Mechanical support of the circulation**

$\dot{Q}p$, pulmonary blood flow; $\dot{Q}s$, systemic blood flow; SaO_2, arterial oxygen saturation; SvO_2, SVC oxygen saturation; PVR, pulmonary vascular resistance; FIO_2, inspired oxygen concentration; PDA, patent ductus arteriosus; B-T, Blalock-Taussig; SVC, superior vena cava.

ence of cardiac failure, and possible end-organ injury from reduced systemic perfusion. A spontaneously breathing patient who has a well-balanced shunt prior to surgery, may quickly develop an unbalanced shunt after the induction of anesthesia and when the child is mechanically ventilated. The arterial oxygen saturation usually increases once the patient is anesthetized and paralyzed, due to an increase in mixed venous oxygen saturation that is caused by reduced peripheral O_2 extraction, and due to improved cardiac output that is secondary to reduced myocardial work and afterload on the ventricle. However, PVR may decrease as well, which would lead to an increase in pulmonary blood flow at the expense of systemic perfusion. Hypotension and a decreease in diastolic blood pressure may be evident. In this circumstance, it is important to maintain a low inspired O_2 concentration and ventilate the lungs with a low rate and tidal volume to maintain a mild respiratory acidosis. Close monitoring of arterial blood gases and pH is important, the ideal being a pH of

7.40, PaO_2 of 40 mm Hg, and a $PaCO_2$ of 40 mm Hg. If noninvasively monitored, an SaO_2 of 75 to 85 percent and $PETCO_2$ of 40 to 45 mm Hg is usually appropriate.

It is very important for patients to be deeply anesthetized to minimize hemodynamic changes, in particular tachycardia, in response to surgical stimulation. If the patient is over circulated (i.e., $\dot{Q}p > \dot{Q}s$) and has a low diastolic blood pressure, coronary artery perfusion may not increase sufficiently to meet the increased demand of myocardial work in response to surgical stress. Myocardial ischemia may occur and usually manifest as ST-segment changes on the ECG or the sudden onset of dysrhythmias, in particular, ventricular fibrillation.[220]

Staged Single-Ventricle Repair/Fontan Procedure

The "reparative" operation for infants with single ventricles is a modified Fontan procedure. Glenn[299] demonstrated in patients with tricuspid atresia that SVC blood could be directed into the lungs without passing through the heart, and Fontan and associates[310, 311] extended this concept to include blood returning from the inferior vena cava. Since the original description, the Fontan procedure and subsequent modifications have been successfully used to treat a wide range of simple and complex single ventricle congenital heart defects.[312, 313] The repair is "physiologic" in that the systemic and pulmonary circulations are separated, or in "series," after directing the systemic venous return directly to the pulmonary artery, and patients are no longer cyanosed. However, based on longer term outcome data, significant problems and complications may develop over time and the repair should perhaps be viewed as palliative rather than curative.[314–317]

The Fontan procedure has undergone numerous modifications since it was first described.[313] The original procedure was described by Fontan in a patient who had tricuspid atresia, and involved disconnecting the pulmonary arteries (PAs) from each other, creating a classic Glenn shunt, connecting the right atrium (RA) directly to the left pulmonary artery using a valved conduit, and placing a valve at the inferior vena cava (IVC)–RA junction.[310] It was believed the RA would function as a pumping chamber; however, following the development of echocardiography, it was apparent that the RA functioned primarily as a conduit with little pumping action contributing to pulmonary blood flow, and in the low-pressure venous system, the valves remained open. Furthermore, this procedure was complicated in the long term by a high risk of pleuropericardial effusions and atrial dysrhythmias caused by RA hypertension and distention.

An early modification involved the direct anastomosis of the RA appendage to the PA, closing the ASD and patching over the tricuspid valve.[318] This procedure, however, continued to have a high risk of complications related to RA hypertension.

Over the past 15 years, the total cavopulmonary anastomoses have become the modified Fontan procedure of preference. The SVC is anastomosed directly to the PA, and a lateral tunnel is created in the RA that baffles the IVC flow to the SVC.[319] This operation was associated with an improvement in mortality, although morbidity related to RA hypertension persisted.[313, 320, 321]

A significant advance was the creation of a fenestration or small hole in the intracardiac baffle, thereby creating an opportunity for a right-to-left atrial shunt. This fenestration can either be "fixed" in size at the time of surgery by using a small 4-mm punch or it can be made "adjustable" with a suture.[281, 322] In the event there is an increase in RA or PA pressure and reduced flow across the pulmonary vascular bed that reduces preload to the systemic ventricle, patients are able to shunt right-to-left across the fenestration. Although patients develop increased cyanosis, cardiac output is maintained. This shunt has proved very successful and enabled patients at relatively high risk to undergo a successful modified Fontan procedure.[313, 323] Although the early mortality has declined further since introduction of fenestration techniques, the most significant improvement has been in patient morbidity. The incidence of early pleuropercardial effusions, ascites, and atrial dysrhythmias has been significantly reduced (Fig.

18–21). The fenestration can be easily closed in the cardiac catheterization laboratory with a clamshell device later in the postoperative period.

More recently, the use of an external conduit baffling the IVC to the pulmonary circulation has been reported.[324] A fenestration can be created between the external conduit and RA, if necessary. The major advantage in the immediate postoperative period is that the procedure can be completed on CPB without needing to arrest the heart. In the long term, the risk for atrial dysrhythmias may be reduced because of a lower RA pressure, absence of extensive atrial suture lines, and anastomoses that are away from the sinoatrial node arterial supply.

Selection Criteria

Fontan and others originally listed a number of selection criteria considered important determinants for a successful early outcome. These included age between 4 and 15 years, low PVR (< 4 Wood units/m^2), mean pulmonary artery pressure less than 20 mm Hg, systemic ventricle ejection fraction greater than 0.6, normal sinus rhythm, normal atrioventricular valve function, and normal systemic and pulmonary venous drainage.[311] Patients with a diagnosis of tricuspid atresia who meet these criteria had a mortality rate of less than 5 percent from this procedure.[317] Modifications to these criteria have subsequently been made over the years as experience has been gained and surgical techniques have evolved.[323, 325] The modified Fontan procedure is now preferably performed in children under 2 years of age to enable earlier correction of chronic hypoxemia and to limit the potential longer term complications associated with prior palliation. The Fontan procedure also has been successfully performed in selected patients older than 15 years who have CHD and who have appropriate hemodynamics despite long-term palliation. Unobstructed flow across the pulmonary vascular bed is essential. A mean PA pressure less than 15 mm Hg and a PVR less than 2 Wood units/m^2 is preferable, as these values have been associated with a lower early mortality.[326] Diastolic dysfunction of the ventricle (i.e., an elevated end-diastolic pressure [e.g., > 12 mm Hg]) that is secondary to increased myocardial mass or outflow obstruction could increase postoperative risk. A higher SVC and PA pressure will be necessary to maintain the transpulmonary gradient and pulmonary blood flow in this situation.

Bidirectional Glenn or Cavopulmonary Connection

The benefits of a series circuit in patients with single-ventricle physiology include improved systemic oxygenation and a reduction in the obligatory diastolic load borne by the ventricle that is simultaneously asked to fill systemic and pulmonary circuits (parallel circulation). The compensatory ventricular dilation that must occur in a parallel circuit places the ventricle at an unfavorable position on the Starling curve, and this will lead to progressive ventricular dysfunction over time. As previously noted, the increase in ventricular end-diastolic volume, and eventually end-diastolic pressure, may significantly compromise the Fontan physiology and effective pulmo-

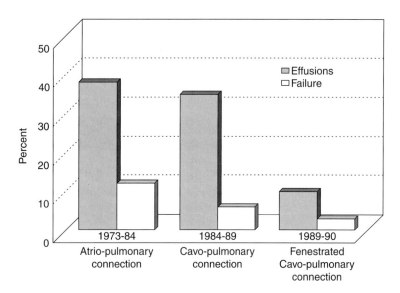

FIGURE 18–21. Incidence of pleural effusions and failure (i.e., take down or mortality) during the early surgical evolution of the modified Fontan procedure at Children's Hospital, Boston. (Modified from Castaneda AR: From Glenn to Foatan: a continuing evolution. Circulation 86:II80, 1992.)

nary blood flow.[327] Therefore, early palliation and relief of any volume load from the systemic ventricle is an important interim step in the staged management of patients with single-ventricle physiology. For most patients, this can be achieved by performing a bidirectional cavopulmonary connection or bidirectional Glenn (BDG) procedure during infancy, commonly around 6 months of age. The volume and pressure load is relieved from the systemic ventricle, but effective pulmonary blood flow is maintained, and the chance of a successful conversion to a complete cavopulmonary anastomosis or modified Fontan procedure is improved.

After a bidirectional Glenn procedure, the $\dot{Q}p/\dot{Q}s$ is reduced, as the source of pulmonary blood flow is from the superior vena cava only. At the time of surgery, the azygous vein is usually ligated to prevent decompression of venous drainage from the SVC to veins below the diaphragm and the inferior vena cava, which could contribute to a lower arterial oxygen saturation. Following the BDG, the arterial oxygen saturation should be in the 80 to 85 percent range, and preload to the systemic ventricle maintained by mixing of pulmonary venous blood with systemic venous blood returning via the inferior vena cava to the common atrium. As the volume output of the ventricle must meet only the demands of the systemic circulation, the end-diastolic volume (EDV) is substantially reduced. As the EDV decreases, an alteration in ventricular geometry takes place. In some children, the resulting small, hypertrophic ventricle exhibits diastolic dysfunction that was not present at higher EDV.[327, 328] In other children, subaortic obstruction may appear across a bulboventricular foramen that was unobstructed in the preoperative state.

The BDG is usually performed on CPB using mild hypothermia, and the heart usually is beating. The complications related to CPB and aortic cross-clamping are therefore minimal, and patients can be weaned from mechanical ventilation and have their trachea extubated in the early postoperative period.[304] Systemic hypertension is common following the BDG procedure. The etiology remains to be determined, but possible factors include improved contractility and stroke volume after the volume load on the ventricle is removed, and brain stem–

mediated mechanisms secondary to the increased systemic and cerebral venous pressure. Treatment of the hypertension with vasodilators may be necessary.

Ideal Physiology Immediately Following the Fontan Procedure

The maintenance of effective pulmonary blood flow and cardiac output following the Fontan procedure depends on the pressure gradient between the pulmonary artery and the pulmonary venous atrium. The factors contributing to a successful cavopulmonary connection are shown in Table 18–13. A systemic venous pressure of 10 to 15 mm Hg and a left atrial pressure of 5 to 10 mm Hg (i.e., a transpulmonary gradient of 5 to 10 mm Hg) are ideal.

Intravascular volume must be maintained and hypovolemia treated promptly. Venous capacitance is increased, and as patients rewarm and vasodilate following surgery, a significant amount of volume is often required. If the stated selection criteria are followed, patients undergoing a modified Fontan procedure will have a low PVR without labile pulmonary hypertension. Therefore, vigorous hyperventilation and induction of a respiratory and/or metabolic alkalosis to further reduce PVR is often of little benefit in this group of patients; conversely, the increase in mechanical ventilation requirements to induce a respiratory alkalosis may have an adverse effect on pulmonary blood flow. A normal pH and $Paco_2$ of 40 mm Hg should be the goal, and depending on the amount of right-to-left shunt across the fenestration, the arterial oxygen saturation is usually in the 80 to 90 percent range. However, PVR may increase following surgery, particularly secondary to an acidosis, hypothermia, atelectasis, hypoventilation, vasoactive drug infusions, and stress response. Any acidosis must be treated promptly. If the cause of the acidosis is respiratory, ventilation must be adjusted. A metabolic acidosis reflects poor cardiac output, and while correction with bicarbonate may be necessary in the short term to reduce the associated increase in PVR, treatment should be directed at correcting the potential causes, including reduced preload to the systemic ventricle, poor myocar-

T A B L E   1 8 – 1 3
TABLE 18–13
MANAGEMENT CONSIDERATIONS FOLLOWING A MODIFIED FONTAN PROCEDURE

	Aim	Management
Baffle pressure 10–15 mm Hg	Unobstructed venous return	→ or ↑ Preload Low intrathoracic pressure
Pulmonary circulation	PVR < 2 Wood units/m² Mean PAp < 15 mm Hg Unobstructed pulmonary vessels	Avoid increases in PVR, such as from acidosis, hypo- and hyperinflation of the lung, hypothermia, and excess sympathetic stimulation Early resumption of spontaneous respiration

Left atrium pressure 5–10 mm Hg	Sinus rhythm
	Competent AV valve
	Ventricle:
	   Normal diastolic function
	   Normal systolic function
	   No outflow obstruction
		Maintain sinus rhythm,
		→ or ↑ HR to increase CO
		→ or ↓ afterload
		→ or ↑ contractility
		
		PDE inhibitors useful because of vasodilation, inotropic and lusitropic properties

PVR, pulmonary vascular resistance; PAp, pulmonary artery pressure; AV, atrioventricular; HR, heart rate; CO, cardiac output; PDE, phosphodiesterase; →, maintain/normal; ↑, increase; ↓, decrease.

dial contractility, increased afterload, and loss of sinus rhythm.

Changes in mean intrathoracic pressure and PVR have a significant effect on pulmonary blood flow. Pulmonary blood flow is biphasic following the Fontan procedure, and earlier resumption of spontaneous ventilation is recommended to offset the detrimental effects of positive-pressure ventilation.[329] Using Doppler analysis, it has been demonstrated that pulmonary blood flow predominantly occurs during inspiration in a spontaneously breathing patient (i.e., when the mean intrathoracic pressure is subatmospheric). Therefore, the method of mechanical ventilation following a Fontan procedure requires close observation. Although it is preferable to wean the patient from positive-pressure ventilation in the early postoperative period, hemodynamic responses must be closely monitored. The use of PEEP continues to be debated. The beneficial effects of an increase in FRC, maintenance of lung volume, and redistribution of lung water need to be balanced against the possible detrimental effect of an increase in mean intrathoracic pressure. A PEEP of 3 to 5 cm H_2O, however, rarely has hemodynamic consequence, nor does it have substantial effects on effective pulmonary blood flow.

Nonspecific pulmonary vasodilators, such as sodium nitroprusside, glycerol trinitrate, PGE_1, and prostacyclin have been used to dilate the pulmonary vasculature in an effort to improve pulmonary blood flow after a Fontan procedure. The results are variable, however. Although PVR may decrease, pulmonary blood flow also could increase as a result of reduced ventricular end-diastolic pressure and improved ventricular function that occurs secondary to the reduction in systemic afterload. The response to inhaled NO also is variable, and the improvement may relate to changes in ventilation–perfusion matching rather than a direct decrease in PVR.

An elevated left atrial pressure may reflect systolic or diastolic ventricular dysfunction, atrioventricular valve regurgitation or stenosis, and loss of sinus rhythm with cannon "a" waves that raise left atrial pressure. Afterload stress is poorly tolerated after a modified Fontan procedure because of the increase in myocardial wall tension

and end-diastolic pressure. Although pulmonary blood flow is phasic to a certain extent, a substantial proportion of flow occurs during diastole as well. The diastolic or relaxation characteristics of the ventricle play a significant role in the volume of pulmonary blood flow and, hence, the preload accepted by the ventricle. Therefore, low cardiac output accompanies diastolic dysfunction. Therapeutic manipulations are not always successful in reversing this dysfunction once it is manifest. The right-sided filling pressure must be increased to maintain the transpulmonary gradient, and treatment with inotropes and vasodilators should be initiated. Despite the temptation to use them in low cardiac output states, the addition of inotropes may not improve hemodynamics and may actually worsen diastolic relaxation if large doses of drugs such as epinephrine are used. One should scrupulously maintain or augment circulating volume to avoid additional reductions in EDV. The phosphodiesterase inhibitors, milrinone and amrinone, are particularly beneficial. Besides being weak inotropes with pulmonary and systemic vasodilating properties, their lusitropic action will assist by improving diastolic relaxation and lowering ventricular end-diastolic pressure, thereby improving effective pulmonary blood flow and cardiac output. If a severe low output state with acidosis persists, takedown of the modified Fontan operation and conversion to a BDG anastomosis or other palliative procedure is lifesaving.

Early Postoperative Complications After the Fontan Procedure

Not all patients require a fenestration for a successful, uncomplicated Fontan operation. Those with ideal preoperative hemodynamics often maintain an adequate pulmonary blood flow and cardiac output without requiring a right-to-left shunt across the baffle. Similarly, not all Fontan patients who have received a fenestration will use it to shunt right-to-left in the immediate postoperative period. The hemoglobin of these patients is usually fully saturated with oxygen following surgery, and the patients may have an elevated right-sided filling pressure and an adequate cardiac output. The problem is predicting which patients are at risk for low cardiac output after a Fontan procedure, and who will benefit from placement of a fenestration; even patients with ideal preoperative hemodynamics may manifest a significant low-output state after surgery. Because of this, essentially all patients having a Fontan procedure have a fenestration created at Children's Hospital, Boston. Premature closure of the fenestration may occur in the immediate postoperative period, leading to a low cardiac output state with progressive metabolic acidosis and large chest drain losses from high right-sided venous pressures. Patients may respond to volume replacement, inotrope support, and vasodilation; however, if hypotension and acidosis persist, cardiac catheterization and removal of thrombus or dilation of the fenestration should be urgently undertaken[330] (Table 18–14).

Arterial O_2 saturation may vary substantially following a modified Fontan procedure. Common causes of persistent arterial O_2 desaturation less than 75 percent include a poor cardiac output with a low mixed venous O_2, a large right-to-left shunt across the fenestration, or additional "leak" in the baffle pathway producing more shunting. An intrapulmonary shunt and venous admixture from decompressing vessels draining either from the PA to the systemic venous circulation or from a systemic vein to the pulmonary venous system are additional causes.[331] Reevaluation with echocardiography and cardiac catheterization may be necessary.

The incidence of recurrent pleural effusions and ascites has decreased since introduction of the fenestrated baffle.[313] Nevertheless, for some patients this remains a major problem in that they develop associated respiratory compromise, hypovolemia, and possible hypoproteinemia. If there is persistent elevation of systemic venous pressure, reevaluation with cardiac catheterization may be indicated.

Atrial flutter and/or fibrillation, heart block, and less commonly ventricular dysrhythmia may have a significant impact on immediate recovery, as well as long-term outcome.[332-334] Sudden loss of sinus rhythm initially causes an increase in left atrial and ventricular end-diastolic pressure, and a decrease in cardiac output. The SVC or PA pressure must be increased, usually with volume replacement, to maintain the transpulmonary gradient. Prompt treatment with antiarrhythmic drugs, pacing, or cardioversion is necessary.

Anesthetic Considerations for Non-Cardiac Surgery Following a Fontan Procedure

There are no prospective studies that have evaluated the effects of specific anesthetic techniques and drugs in patients with Fontan physiology. Anesthetic management will vary on a case-by-case basis according to the functional and clinical status of each patient and the specific complications unique to the Fontan procedure. Intermediate to late follow-up initially demonstrated a late decline in functional status and a 15-year survival between 60 and 73 percent.[314-316, 335] However, these figures include patients operated on in the earlier surgical years; with improved surgical techniques and patient selection, subsequent survival figures have improved.

Arrhythmias, in particular atrial flutter, sick sinus syndrome, and heart block, have been reported in 20 percent or more of survivors 10 years following the Fontan procedure. The probability of freedom from atrial flutter has been reported as about 40 percent at 15 years after Fontan procedure, although these data includes patients from different surgical eras.[334] Predisposing factors to these arrhythmias include surgery involving the atrium where ex-

TABLE 18–14
CIRCUMSTANCES, ETIOLOGY AND TREATMENT STRATEGIES FOR PATIENTS WITH LOW CARDIAC OUTPUT IMMEDIATELY FOLLOWING THE FONTAN PROCEDURE

Circumstance	Etiology	Treatment
Increased TPG:		
Baffle > 20 mm Hg	Inadequate pulmonary blood flow and	Volume replacement
LAp < 10 mm Hg	preload to left atrium:	Reduce PVR
TPG increased ⩾ 10 mm Hg	Increased PVR	Correct acidosis
Clinical state:	Pulmonary artery stenosis	Inotrope support
High Sao₂/low Svo₂	Pulmonary vein stenosis	Systemic vasodilation
Hypotension/tachycardia	Premature fenestration closure	Catheter or surgical intervention
Poor peripheral perfusion		
SVC syndrome with pleural effusions and		
increased chest tube drainage		
Ascites/hepatomegaly		
Metabolic acidosis		
Normal TPG:		
Baffle > 20 mm Hg	Ventricular failure:	Maintain preload
LAp > 15 mm Hg	Systolic dysfunction	Inotrope support
TPG normal 5–10 mm Hg	Diastolic dysfunction	Systemic vasodilation
Clinical state:	AV valve regurgitation and/or stenosis	Establish sinus rhythm or AV synchrony
Low Sao₂/low Svo₂	Loss of sinus rhythm	Correct acidosis
Hypotension/tachycardia	Afterload stress	Mechanical support
Poor peripheral perfusion		Surgical intervention, including takedown to
Metabolic acidosis		BDG and transplantation

LAp, left atrial pressure; TPG, transpulmonary gradient; Sao₂, systemic arterial oxygen saturation; Svo₂, SVC oxygen saturation; SVC, superior vena cava; PVR, pulmonary vascular resistance; AV, atrioventricular; BDG, bidirectional Glenn anastomosis.

tensive suture lines are required, disrupted sinoatrial node blood supply, and chronic atrial distention. In addition, older age at Fontan operation, longer duration of follow-up, and type of surgical procedure are associated with an increased incidence of atrial flutter after the Fontan operation. Patients with recurrent arrhythmias often are treated with long-term antiarrhythmic drugs, present for repeat cardioversions, and may undergo radiofrequency ablation of reentrant flutter pathways. There are no recommendations at this time for administering prophylactic antiarrhymic drugs such as digoxin or amiodarone prior to anesthesia for noncardiac surgery. However, it is important that facilities for immediate external cardiac pacing or cardioversion are readily available in the operating room for these patients.

There is an increased incidence of thromboembolism in patients who have undergone the Fontan procedure. However, the routine use of long-term anticoagulation remains controversial. The actual incidence of thromboembolism is difficult to determine because of the heterogeneous patient population. A large retrospective review of 645 patients who underwent the Fontan procedure at Children's Hospital, Boston, between 1978 and 1993 described 17 patients (2.6 percent) who suffered a stroke following the Fontan procedure, presumably due to a thromboembolic event.[336] The nature of the Fontan circulation with its increased venous pressure and stasis of flow through the right atrial baffle, atrial dysrhythmias, alterations in pro- and anticoagulant factors, and possible increased resting venous tone in this population of patients are all contributing factors.[337] The role of prophylactic anticoagulant therapy in congenital heart disease in general, and the Fontan population in particular, is poorly defined. Antiplatelet therapy with aspirin is used commonly in the immediate and early postoperative period, although the benefit of long-term use has not been evaluated. In high-risk patients, and those who have had previous thrombus formation, Coumadin therapy for an extended period is recommended. Patients with Fontan physiology may be at increased risk for deep venous thrombosis, or thrombus formation within the Fontan baffle or atrial appendage following noncardiac surgery. Prophylactic subcutaneous heparin should be considered for older Fontan patients undergoing noncardiac procedures, and the patients should be kept well hydrated and mobilized early after surgery.

Protein-losing enteropathy (PLE) has been reported in 3 to 14 percent of Fontan patients on long-term follow-up.[335] Defined as persistent hypoalbuminemia (< 3.0 mg/dl) in the absence of liver and renal disease, associated clinical features include abdominal pain, diarrhea, edema, and ascites. Patients frequently have limited hemodynamic reserve, increased systemic venous pressure, decreased cardiac index, and increased end-diastolic ventricular pressure.

Most patients with stable single-ventricle physiology subjectively report that they are able to lead relatively normal lives with moderate exercise tolerance. Nevertheless, deterioration in function according to New York Heart Association classification has been reported over longer follow-up.[314, 315] Objective evaluation with exercise testing demonstrates the limited cardiorespiratory reserve of many Fontan patients.[338–340] The implications of these findings for subsequent anesthetics have not been studied; nevertheless, the response to exercise testing may be useful for assessing a patient's ability to tolerate the stress of anesthesia and surgery. Compared with normal control subjects, those with Fontan physiology frequently demonstrate a reduced maximal exercise work load and less endurance, take longer to recover after stopping exercise, and have a lower anaerobic threshold and maximal oxygen consumption. A decrease in arterial oxygen saturation and an increase in arteriovenous oxygen saturation difference is common because of the suboptimal increase in cardiac index.[341, 342] The inability to increase effective pulmonary blood flow and stroke volume during strenuous exercise underscores the importance of the pulmonary vascular bed in determining ventricular filling and the dependence of these patients upon heart rate to increase cardiac output.

Intraoperative monitoring during major non-cardiac surgery needs careful planning in patients with Fontan physiology. Placement of a central venous line into the SVC will enable monitoring of systemic venous return, pulmonary artery pressure, and mixed venous oxygen saturation. An important consideration, however, is the risk for thrombosis and obstruction to venous return. Cardiac catheterization may be indicated prior to surgery if there has been a change in symptoms or deterioration in function. In particular, if significant fluid shifts are anticipated during surgery, performing a hemodynamic study immediately prior to surgery is often beneficial. Besides being able to assess baseline hemodynamics, a balloon-tipped catheter can be wedged in a pulmonary artery to measure the transpulmonary gradient. Positioning the catheter using pressure waveforms alone is difficult because there is no pulsatile arterial pressure waveform and the balloon may not readily float out to a lung segment. Placement of the catheter under direct vision using fluoroscopy is preferable. Attempted measurement of cardiac output using thermodilution also will be inaccurate.

Tetralogy of Fallot

Pathophysiology

The four anatomic features of tetralogy of Fallot include a VSD, right ventricular outflow tract obstruction, over riding of the aorta, and right ventricular hypertrophy. In addition, there also may be VSDs of the muscular region of the septum and right-sided obstruction of the pulmonary valve and the main and branch pulmonary arteries.

The resistance to right ventricular outflow forces systemic venous return right-to-left across the ventricular septal defect (complex shunt) and into the aorta, producing arterial desaturation (Fig. 18–22). Pulmonary blood flow is less than systemic flow. The amount of blood that shunts right-to-left through the ventricular septal defect varies with the magnitude of the right ventricular outflow tract obstruction and with the SVR. Distal pulmonary vascular resistance is low and has minimal influence on shunting. Systemic vasodilation, in conjunction with increasing dynamic infundibular stenosis, intensifies right-to-left shunting and therefore hypoxemia, producing hypercyanotic

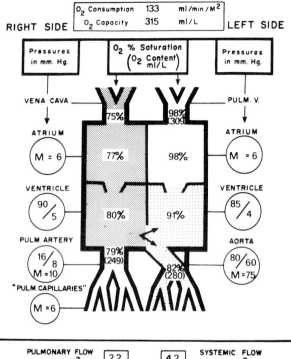

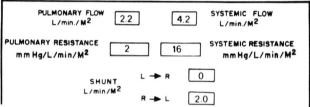

FIGURE 18–22. Catheterization findings in a patient with tetralogy of Fallot. (From Nadas AS, Fyler DC: Pediatric Cardiology. Philadelphia, WB Saunders Company, 1972, with permission.)

"spells." Such spells can occur at any time before surgical correction of the anomalies and can be life threatening. Their treatment is outlined below. Because the morbidity associated with recurrent hypercyanotic spells is significant, many physicians consider recurrent episodes of hypercyanosis an indication for corrective surgery at any age.

Anesthetic Management

TOF may be repaired either early or late. The delayed repair requires early palliation with a systemic-to-pulmonary artery shunt to prevent hypercyanotic episodes. This is followed by a transatrial and transpulmonary artery repair at 12 to 18 months of age. Excellent outcome has been achieved with this approach, and the need for a transpulmonary valve annulus outflow patch (transannular patch) at the time of surgery is reduced.[343] The risks of cyanosis and complications related to a systemic-to-pulmonary artery shunt argues for an early complete repair of TOF. This may be performed in the neonate or young infant, depending on the degree of obstruction and the arterial oxygen saturation level.[344, 345] Complete repair of this lesion in neonates and young infants more often requires a transventricular approach to close the VSD and pericardial augmentation of the RV outflow tract. A ventriculotomy is performed in the right ventricular outflow

tract and is frequently extended distally through the pulmonary valve annulus and beyond any associated pulmonary artery stenosis. The outflow tract is then enlarged with pericardium or synthetic material, and obstructing muscle bundles are resected to relieve the outflow tract obstruction.[287, 346] Being smaller and younger, these patients also may be at increased risk for complications associated with CPB and are more likely to require DHCA to facilitate surgical exposure and repair. Pulmonary regurgitation results after a transannular incision, which may compromise ventricular function in the postoperative period. In approximately 8 percent of patients, abnormalities in the origin and distribution of the coronary arteries preclude placement of the right ventricular outflow patch,[347, 348] making it necessary to bypass the stenosis by placing an external conduit from the body of the right ventricle to the pulmonary artery.[349]

Anesthetic management of these patients should maintain systemic vascular resistance, minimize pulmonary vascular resistance, and avoid myocardial depression. Hypercyanotic spells in nonanesthetized children are traditionally treated initially with 100 percent oxygen by face mask, a knee-chest position, and morphine sulfate. This regimen usually causes the dynamic infundibular stenosis to relax while maintaining systemic resistance. Deeply cyanotic and lethargic patients are given IV crystalloid infusions to augment circulating blood volume. Continued severe hypoxemia is treated with a vasopressor (e.g., phenylephrine 1 to 2 μg/kg) to increase SVR, and sometimes by judicious use of IV propranolol or esmolol to slow the heart rate; the latter allows more filling time and relaxes the infundibulum.[128] If a hypercyanotic spell persists despite treatment, immediate surgical correction of the anomaly is indicated. The child can be anesthetized with IV narcotics, and an inhalation agent such as halothane may be beneficial to reduce hyperdynamic outflow tract obstruction. Anesthetic agents that predominantly decrease SVR, such as isoflurane, should be used with caution. The pattern of mechanical ventilation is critical, as excessive inspiratory pressure or short expiratory times will increase the mean intrathoracic pressure and further reduce antegrade flow across the RV outflow.

When weaning patients from CPB following repair of a tetralogy of Fallot, the aim of therapy is to support right ventricular function and minimize afterload on the RV. This is particularly important following repair in neonates or small infants. Whereas systolic dysfunction of the RV may occur following neonatal ventriculotomy, more commonly the clinical picture is one of a "restrictive physiology" reflecting reduced RV compliance or diastolic function.[350, 351] Factors contributing to diastolic dysfunction include ventriculotomy, lung and myocardial edema following CPB, inadequate myocardial protection of the hypertrophied ventricle during aortic cross clamp, coronary artery injury, residual outflow tract obstruction, volume load on the ventricle from a residual VSD or pulmonary regurgitation, and dysrhythmias.

Patients usually separate from CPB with a satisfactory arterial blood pressure and atrial filling pressures less than 10 mm Hg on inotrope support, such as dopamine 5 to 10 μg/kg/min. However, during the first 6 to 12 hours after surgery, neonates often develop a low-cardiac-output state with increased right-sided filling pressures. This is often due to diastolic dysfunction following a right ventriculotomy. Continued sedation and paralysis usually is necessary for the first 24 to 48 hours to minimize the stress response and associated myocardial work. Preload must be maintained despite elevation of the RA pressure. In addition to high right-sided filling pressures, pleural effusions and/or ascites may develop. Significant inotrope support often is required, and a phosphodiesterase inhibitor, such as amrinone or milrinone, is beneficial because of their lusitropic properties. Because of the restrictive defect, even a relatively small volume load from a residual VSD or pulmonary regurgitation often is poorly tolerated in the early postoperative period, and it may take 2 to 3 days before RV compliance improves and cardiac output increases following surgery. Although the patent foramen ovale (PFO) or any ASD usually is closed at the time of surgery in older patients, it is beneficial to leave a small atrial communication following repair of this lesion in neonates. In the face of diastolic dysfunction and increased RV end-diastolic pressure, a right-to-left atrial shunt will maintain preload to the left ventricle, which will maintain cardiac output. Patients may be desaturated initially following surgery because of this shunting. As RV compliance and function improve, the amount of shunt decreases and both antegrade pulmonary blood flow and arterial oxygen saturation increase.

Arrhythmias following repair of a TOF include heart block, ventricular ectopy, and junctional ectopic tachycardia. It is important to maintain sinus rhythm to avoid additional diastolic dysfunction and an increase in end-diastolic pressure. Atrioventricular pacing may be necessary for heart block. Complete right bundle branch block is typical on the postoperative ECG.

Most patients recover systolic ventricular function postoperatively. However, there is a small group of patients, especially those repaired at older ages, who have persistent significant ventricular dysfunction.[352, 353] Pulmonary valve insufficiency may contribute to residual ventricular systolic dysfunction.[354] The most common cause of systolic dysfunction immediately after repair of CHD is a residual or unrecognized additional VSD,[172, 355] which causes a volume load on the left ventricle and pressure load on an already stressed right ventricle. This leads to right ventricular failure and poor cardiac output. A residual VSD, combined with a residual right ventricular outflow obstruction, is particularly deleterious.[356]

In some patients, the distal pulmonary arteries may be so hypoplastic and stenotic that they cannot be satisfactorily repaired. Suprasystemic pressure develops in the right ventricle, which in some cases can be ameliorated by partially opening the VSD to allow an intracardiac right-to-left ventricular shunt. This shunt unloads the compromised right ventricle at the expense of decreased arterial oxygen saturation.

Anesthetic Considerations After RV Outflow Reconstruction

Reconstruction of the RV outflow tract may lead to significant problems that affect RV function and risk for arrhythmias over time. Most long-term outcome data pertain to

patients following tetralogy of Fallot repair. However, similar complications and risks also are likely for those who have undergone an extensive RV outflow reconstruction. These include placement of a conduit from the right ventricle to the pulmonary artery for correction of pulmonary atresia and truncus arteriosus, and the Rastelli procedure for transposition of the great arteries with pulmonary stenosis.

Complete surgical repair of TOF has been successfully performed for over 40 years. Recent studies report a 30- to 35-year actuarial survival of about 85 percent.[357, 358] Many patients report leading relatively normal lives, but RV dysfunction may progress after repair and may only be evident on exercise stress testing or echocardiography. A spectrum of problems may develop, ranging from a dilated RV with systolic dysfunction to diastolic dysfunction from a poorly compliant RV; these problems need to be thoroughly evaluated preoperatively (Table 18–15). In addition, continued evaluation of these patients is necessary because of the increased risk for ventricular dysrhythmias and late sudden death. Factors that may adversely affect long-term survival include older age at initial repair, initial palliative procedures, and residual chronic pressure and/or volume load such as occur with pulmonary insufficiency or stenosis.

Systolic dysfunction after TOF repair that is caused by a residual volume load from pulmonary regurgitation is a predictor of late morbidity. It is reflected by cardiomegaly on chest x-ray; by increased RV end-diastolic volume by echocardiography[354]; and by exercise testing that demonstrates a reduction in anaerobic threshold, maximal exercise performance, and endurance.[359] Patients who have significant pulmonary regurgitation and reduced RV function are at potential risk for a decrease in cardiac output during anesthesia, particularly as positive-pressure ventilation may increase the amount of regurgitation. Once again, it is difficult to predict those patients who are more likely to have instability of their cardiovascular system during anesthesia for noncardiac surgery, nor is it possible to formulate a "recipe" for anesthesia that will be suited

T A B L E 1 8 – 1 5	
LONG-TERM FOLLOW-UP AFTER TETRALOGY OF FALLOT REPAIR: RIGHT VENTRICULAR FUNCTION	
Circumstance	**Clinical**
Systolic dysfunction: "nonrestrictive"	RV dilation: cardiomegaly Significant pulmonary regurgitation Volume overload: ↑ RVEDV, ↓ RV ejection fraction ↓ Maximal exercise capacity and endurance ↑ Risk for ventricular arrhythmias and possibly sudden death
Diastolic dysfunction: "restrictive"	↓ RV compliance: cardiomegaly less likely Limited pulmonary regurgitation ↑ RVEDP, contractility maintained Improved exercise capacity Lower risk for ventricular dysrhythmias

RV, right ventricle; RVEDV, right ventricle end-diastolic volume; RVEDP, right ventricle end-diastolic pressure; ↑, increased; ↓, decreased.

to all patients. Nevertheless, preoperative exercise testing may provide some insight as to hemodynamic reserve.

It is important to distinguish those patients who have restrictive physiology or diastolic dysfunction secondary to reduced ventricular compliance from those who do not. The former usually do not have cardiomegaly and demonstrate better exercise tolerance, and the risk for ventricular dysrhythmias is possibly decreased. Although the RV is hypertrophied, function is generally well preserved on echocardiography, and there is minimal pulmonary regurgitation.[350]

The incidence of significant RV outflow obstruction developing over time is low. Residual obstruction contributes to early mortality (i.e., within the first year after surgery), but the obstruction is well tolerated in the long term. A gradient more than 40 mm Hg across the RV outflow tract is uncommon, and the pressure ratio between the RV and LV is usually less than 0.5. The gradient may become more significant with time, but as the progression is usually slow. RV dysfunction occurs late.

A wide variation in the incidence of ventricular ectopy has been reported in numerous follow-up studies, including up to 15 percent of patients on routine ECG and up to 75 percent of patients on Holter monitor. Multiple risk factors, including an older age at repair, residual hemodynamic abnormalities, and duration of follow-up, have all been considered important.[360-362] In common with these factors is probable myocardial injury and fibrosis from chronic pressure and volume overload and from cyanosis. Although ventricular ectopy is common in asymptomatic patients during ambulatory ECG Holter monitoring and exercise stress testing, it is often low grade and has not identified those patients at risk for sudden death. Electrophysiologic induction of sustained ventricular tachycardia (VT), especially when monomorphic, is suggestive of the presence of a reentrant arrhythmic pathway. Although dependent on the stimulation protocol used to induce VT, the presence of monomorphic VT in a symptomatic patient with syncope and palpitations is significant and indicates treatment with radiofrequency ablation, surgical cryoablation, antiarrhythmic drugs, or placement of an implantable cardioversion-defibrillator (ICD).[363] The risk for ventricular dysrhythmias during anesthesia is unknown. Although preoperative prophylaxis with antiarrhythmic drugs is not recommended, a means for external defibrillation and pacing must be readily available during anesthesia and surgery.

Pulmonary Atresia

Pathophysiology

Atresia of the pulmonary valve or main pulmonary artery forms a spectrum of cardiac defects, the management of which depends on the extent of atresia, size of the RV and tricuspid valve (TV), presence of a VSD and collateral vessels, surface area of the pulmonary vascular bed, and coronary artery anatomy. At birth, pulmonary blood flow is derived either from a patent ductus arteriosus or from other aortopulmonary collateral blood vessels. These collaterals, which arise from the descending aorta and supply both lungs, may be extensive. The RV is usually hypertro-

phied, and a restrictive physiology is common during initial postoperative recovery.[364, 365]

At one end of the spectrum, critical pulmonary stenosis may exist with a variable degree of hypoplasia of the right ventricle, tricuspid valve, and pulmonary artery. There is no VSD. With critical pulmonic stenosis, only a pinhole orifice is present in the pulmonic valve, but the right ventricle is generally less hypoplastic than occurs with pulmonary atresia. A fixed obligatory shunt of all systemic venous return occurs from the right to the left atrium, where blood mixes completely with pulmonary venous blood. Some blood may flow into the right ventricle, but because there is no outlet, blood regurgitates back across the tricuspid valve and eventually reaches the left atrium and left ventricle. Pulmonary blood flow is derived exclusively or predominantly from a patent ductus arteriosus. These patients usually do not have extensive aortopulmonary collateral blood flow; consequently, they often become cyanotic when the patent ductus arteriosus closes after birth. Critical pulmonary valve stenosis can be effectively treated by balloon dilation in the catheterization laboratory. Antegrade flow across the RV outflow tract may not improve immediately, but gradually increases over days as RV compliance improves.

Pulmonary valve atresia or short-segment main pulmonary artery atresia, with a VSD (PA/VSD), and normal sized TV, RV, and branch pulmonary arteries, is completely repaired in the neonate. This usually requires placement of a pericardial patch to reconstruct the outflow tract. If there is long-segment pulmonary artery atresia, a homograft "conduit" is necessary to reconstruct the RV outflow. Conduits may be extrinsically compressed or kinked at the time of sternal closure, causing partial RV outflow obstruction or direct compression of a coronary artery, which leads to ischemia.

The intracardiac anatomy of tetralogy of Fallot with pulmonary atresia (TOF/PA) is similar to that of simple tetralogy of Fallot, but the right ventricular outflow tract is atretic. Because of the atretic right ventricular outflow tract, all systemic venous return courses right-to-left through the VSD. Therefore, complete mixing of pulmonary and systemic venous return occurs in the left ventricle and aorta, producing arterial hypoxemia. Infants with tetralogy of Fallot and associated pulmonary atresia regularly exhibit significant systemic-to-pulmonary collateral flow. If antegrade flow is established from the right ventricle into the main pulmonary artery by a reparative procedure, the left-to-right shunt via collateral flow will impose a diastolic load on the left ventricle. Preoperative occlusion of these collateral vessels can be accomplished by interventional techniques in the cardiac catheterization laboratory but may leave the child precariously cyanotic in the hours before operation. The most effective temporizing therapy is to reduce oxygen consumption (e.g., anesthesia, mechanical ventilation) and to increase the systemic perfusion pressure across other systemic-to-pulmonary communications.

Patients with pulmonary atresia, a ventricular septal defect, but a small RV and TV may not tolerate a complete initial repair. The RV may not be able to cope with the entire cardiac output, resulting in a low-output state and RV failure (see below). Alternative management strategies therefore include initial palliation with a shunt and/or RV outflow patch to improve pulmonary blood flow, or a repair of the outflow tract with fenestration of the VSD patch to enable a right-to-left shunt at that level. Two-ventricle repair may ultimately be limited by growth of the tricuspid valve.[364] If the right ventricle subsequently grows, the shunt and the PFO, ASD, and VSD can be closed surgically.

Patients with pulmonary atresia and an intact ventricular septum (PA/IVS) usually have a small RV and TV, which in general makes them unsuitable for a two-ventricle repair in the long term. Initial palliation with an aortopulmonary shunt is necessary; reconstruction of the RV outflow with a pericardial patch or conduit also may be considered if the RV is of sufficient size that a two-ventricle repair could be considered. Prior to surgery, the coronary anatomy should be determined, usually by cardiac catheterization. A large conal branch or aberrant left coronary artery that runs across the RV outflow tract may restrict the size of a ventriculotomy and placement of a patch or conduit. Patients with pulmonary atresia, a hypoplastic RV, and intact ventricular septum may have numerous fistulous connections between the small hypertensive RV cavity and the coronary circulation.[365, 366] A significant proportion of the myocardium may, therefore, be dependent on coronary perfusion directly from the RV. If, in addition, there are proximal coronary artery stenoses that restrict coronary perfusion from the aortic root, decompression of the RV after reconstruction of the RV outflow tract can lead to myocardial infarction.

At the worst end of the spectrum, severe pulmonary atresia may be associated with a hypoplastic RV and diminutive pulmonary arteries that are not suitable for primary repair. A palliative procedure using a B-T or central shunt is usually necessary at first to improve pulmonary blood flow. This is followed by staged single-ventricle repair (see "Managing Fontan Physiology").

Multiple aortopulmonary collateral arteries may be present and supply some or all segments of the lung. These shunts can be associated with a large left-to-right shunt, contributing to volume overload and pulmonary hypertension. Larger collateral vessels that supply significant portions of the lung can be anastomosed or "unifocalized" to the native pulmonary arteries to try and establish full antegrade pulmonary blood flow. Smaller vessels to some segments of lung can have coils injected into them in the cardiac catheterization laboratory, provided there is antegrade flow from the native pulmonary arteries to those lung segments.

When the pulmonary arteries are very diminutive, it is important to establish early antegrade flow from the right ventricle to the pulmonary artery in an effort to promote growth and establish a pathway to the pulmonary arteries for subsequent balloon dilation. A B-T shunt may be necessary to provide sufficient pulmonary blood flow if the pulmonary arteries and right ventricle are small. Initially, the VSD can be left open, and postoperative management of cyanosis or CHF will be determined by the size of and the resistance offered by the pulmonary circuit. The course in these patients can be dynamic and demanding of the most experienced practitioners. When collateral vessels are occluded in the operating room and the RV is con-

nected to diminutive pulmonary arteries, continuity is established, but cyanosis may ensue. Therapy is aimed at lowering PVR and/or (re)establishing adequate pulmonary blood flow. On the other hand, if the child is fully saturated in the aorta and has elevated pulmonary artery oxygen saturation and left atrial pressure, a left-to-right shunt through the VSD may be developing. This shunt will produce a volume load on the left ventricle and an unstable postoperative course. If this occurs, the VSD should be closed. When the hemoglobin is not fully saturated in the aorta and there is a volume-loaded left ventricle with low cardiac output and high left atrial pressure postoperatively, excessive systemic-to-pulmonary collaterals may be the culprits. Cardiac catheterization and occlusion of the vessels or immediate reoperation may be required.

Anesthetic Management

Anesthetic management of patients with pulmonary atresia is similar to that for tetralogy of Fallot, except that hypercyanotic spells do not occur in the same fashion. Maintaining patency of the ductus arteriosus is essential for the perioperative treatment of neonates who have pulmonary atresia and critical pulmonary stenosis. If the right ventricle is sufficiently well developed and the main pulmonary artery is present, it may be possible to perform a pulmonary valvotomy and provide adequate pulmonary blood flow without a supplemental systemic-to-pulmonary-artery shunt. The goal of therapy is to improve oxygenation and decrease right ventricular afterload. Because the underdeveloped noncompliant right ventricle requires high filling pressures, there may be substantial right-to-left shunting through the foramen ovale, making these infants hypoxemic during the immediate postoperative period. With growth and improved compliance of the right ventricle, the right-to-left shunting diminishes and the infant's oxygenation improves substantially. If hypoxemia persists, PGE_1 should be infused to increase pulmonary blood flow through the ductus arteriosus while arrangements are made to surgically create a pulmonary artery-to-systemic artery shunt.

In patients with long segment pulmonary atresia, the need for a conduit to bridge the gap between the right ventricle and the pulmonary artery complicates the repair. Again, right ventricular failure may occur postoperatively, especially when there is a residual VSD or a right ventricular outflow obstruction. The conduit may obstruct acutely during chest closure, further elevating pressure in the right ventricle.

After the VSD is closed and blood is flowing from the right ventricle to the pulmonary arteries, there may be excessive pulmonary blood flow ($\dot{Q}p/\dot{Q}s > 1$) as a consequence of the flow into the pulmonary arteries from the right ventricle plus the flow from the aortopulmonary collaterals described above. If this occurs, the patient develops CHF and requires intraoperative inotropic support of the heart and an extended period of postoperative mechanical ventilation. With large collateral flow, the pulse pressure is wide and diastolic pressure low. The patients may require surgery to ligate the collateral vessels, or the vessels may have to be embolized.

Anesthetic Considerations After Repair

Patients with tetralogy of Fallot and pulmonary atresia are subject to the same late problems and complications as patients with tetralogy of Fallot alone. In addition, they may develop progressive conduit obstruction after surgery; conduit obstruction is accelerated by the presence of a porcine valve in the conduit.[367, 368] Consequently, valveless conduits (unless the patient has severe pulmonary hypertension) or homografts may be preferable.[349]

Tricuspid Atresia

Pathology

In this condition, an imperforate tricuspid valve and hypoplasia of the right ventricle are present, often accompanied by a VSD of variable size and pulmonic stenosis. A fixed obligatory shunt of all systemic venous return occurs from the right atrium through the PFO or ASD into the left atrium, where complete mixing of blood takes place. The degree of hypoxemia depends on the amount of pulmonary blood flow, which is regulated by the severity of the pulmonic stenosis. The common presentation is characterized by the significant hypoxemia that is caused by the decreased pulmonary blood flow induced by either a restrictive VSD or severe pulmonic stenosis.

Anesthetic Management

The reparative operation of choice for tricuspid atresia is a modified Fontan procedure, but a palliative procedure may initially be required to improve pulmonary blood flow. A pulmonary artery band may be needed if the pulmonary blood flow is increased, or a shunt may have to be created for the severely hypoxemic child who has decreased pulmonary blood flow. The anesthetic management and complications are those discussed in the sections on shunts, banding, and modified Fontan procedures (see above). Complications of chronic hypoxemia and cyanosis are also present.

Transposition of the Great Arteries

Pathophysiology

With transposition of the great arteries (TGA), the right ventricle gives rise to the aorta (Fig. 18–23). Almost 50 percent of patients with this anomaly have a VSD; some of them have a variable degree of subpulmonic stenosis (Fig. 18–23). Oxygenated pulmonary venous blood returns to the left atrium and is recirculated to the pulmonary artery without reaching the systemic circulation. Similarly, systemic venous blood returns to the right atrium and ventricle and is ejected into the aorta again. Obviously, this arrangement is compatible with life only for a few circulation times unless there is some mixing of pulmonary and systemic venous blood via a patent ductus arteriosus or an opening in the atrial or ventricular septum at birth. The physiologic disturbance in these patients is one of inadequate mixing of pulmonary and systemic blood rather than one of inadequate pulmonary blood flow.

Mixing of blood at the atrial level can be improved by performing a balloon atrial septostomy. If dangerous levels

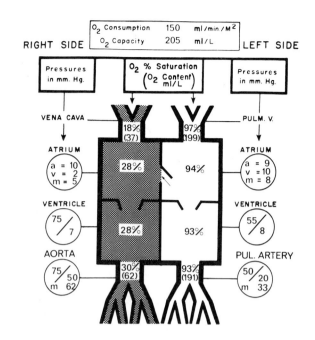

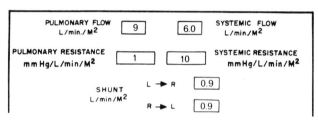

FIGURE 18–23. Catheterization findings in a patient with *d*-transposition of the great arteries and restricted pulmonary flow. (From Nadas AS, Fyler DC: Pediatric Cardiology. Philadelphia, WB Saunders Company, 1972, with permission.)

of hypoxemia persist after the septostomy and metabolic acidosis ensues, PGE_1 can be infused to maintain the patency of the ductus arteriosus, increase pulmonary blood flow (by increasing left-to-right shunting across the patent ductus arteriosus), and thereby increase the volume of oxygenated blood entering the left atrium. The volume-overloaded left atrium is likely to shunt part of its contents into the right atrium and thereby improve the oxygen saturation of aortic blood. Unlike the kinetics with other congenital heart lesions, increased shunting of blood during anesthesia improves arterial oxygen saturation before correction of the transposition.

Depending on the particular anatomy and the presence of a VSD or pulmonary stenosis, one of three corrective procedures is used. The intraoperative and postoperative problems encountered differ with each type of procedure.

Atrial Switch (Mustard and Senning Operation)

An atrial level partition of blood flow is created with a baffle. The baffle redirects pulmonary venous blood across the tricuspid valve to the right ventricle and thus to the aorta.[369–372] Systemic venous return is directed across the atrial septum to the mitral valve, into the left ventricle, and out the pulmonary artery. Although the pulmonary and systemic circuits are then connected serially instead of in parallel, this arrangement leaves the patient with a morphologic right ventricle and tricuspid valve in continuity with the aorta. This ventricle must, therefore, work against systemic arterial pressure and resistance.

One problem with atrial baffles is that they can obstruct systemic and pulmonary venous return.[373] When this occurs, the patient manifests signs and symptoms of systemic venous obstruction, as evidenced by superior vena cava syndrome or other signs of systemic venous hypertension. When the pulmonary venous pathway is obstructed, pulmonary venous hypertension may manifest themselves as respiratory failure, poor gas exchange, and pulmonary edema (seen on chest radiograph). Severe pulmonary venous obstruction is manifested in the operating room by the presence of copious amounts of bloody fluid in the endotracheal tube, low cardiac output, and frequently poor oxygenation. Residual interatrial shunts also may cause intra- or postoperative hypoxemia. Long-term rhythm disturbances, along with limitations of ventricular and atrioventricualr valve function, have made this operation nearly obsolete.

Arterial Switch Operation (ASO)

Because of the complications associated with atrial baffle procedures, Jatene and others explored whether dividing both great arteries and reattaching them to the opposite, anatomically correct ventricle, would improve survival.[374–378] This procedure requires excision and reimplantation of the coronary arteries to the neoaorta (formerly the proximal main pulmonary artery). The success of the arterial switch procedure depends on adequate preparation of the left ventricle and technical proficiency with the coronary artery transfer. Anatomic correction of transposition of the great vessels is done during the neonatal period when PVR (left ventricular afterload) and left ventricular pressure have both been high. Left ventricular pressure and mass decreases progressively after birth in infants with transposition of the great arteries and an intact ventricular septum (TGA/IVS). In such cases, the left ventricle may not tolerate the work required to perfuse the systemic vessels following the ASO. However, if the neonate has TGA and a non-restrictive VSD (TGA/VSD) the left ventricle is accustomed to high pressure and may tolerate the increase in workload at any age. In older patients who have an intact ventricular septum, banding the pulmonary artery can prepare the left ventricle to function as a systemic ventricle by increasing its afterload and muscle mass. If the left ventricle is "prepared" by banding the pulmonary artery and augmenting pulmonary blood flow with a modified Blalock-Taussig shunt, then an arterial switch procedure can usually be accomplished 1 week after hypertrophy and hyperplasia have occurred.[379] However, during this interval these patients are cyanotic and have a volume-loaded right ventricle and a pressure-loaded left ventricle. They may require considerable pharmacologic support.[5, 380]

In centers where the surgeons and anesthesiologists have considerable experience with this procedure, the incidence of mortality for neonatal repair of transposition of the great arteries is now less than 2–3 percent and may

be less than 1–2 percent for most anatomic arrangements of coronary arteries if the aortic arch is normal.[104, 381–384] Midterm follow-up of these patients shows excellent outcome. Alternative operations are reserved almost exclusively for patients with particularly difficult coronary anatomy[385, 386] or pulmonic (neoaortic) stenosis.

Myocardial ischemia or infarction may occur after mobilization and reimplantation of the coronary arteries, especially if they are stretched or kinked. Inotropic support, maintenance of coronary perfusion pressures, control of heart rate, and treatment with vasodilators may be particularly useful, as in adult patients with myocardial ischemia. Postoperative bleeding and tamponade occur more commonly with this operation because there are multiple arterial anastomoses.

Ventricular Switch (Rastelli Procedure)

The VSD of patients who have TGA, a large VSD and severe subpulmonic stenosis can be closed obliquely to direct left ventricular flow to the aorta. The pulmonary valve is oversewn and the right ventricle is connected to the pulmonary artery with a conduit.[387]

Complications of the Rastelli procedure include obstruction of left ventricular outflow due to narrowing of the subaortic region by the VSD patch. The conduit also may obstruct during or after the immediate postoperative period.[367, 368] There is a small but significant incidence of heart block in these patients, which can be a difficult postoperative problem.

Anesthetic Considerations After Repair

Patients who have a morphologic right ventricle remaining as the systemic ventricle (i.e., the atrial switch) can be regarded as having a physiologic or functional two-ventricle repair. Actuarial survival figures at 15 years have been quoted up to 85 percent; however, significant long-term functional deterioration of cardiac function is likely, and there is an increased risk for right heart failure, sudden death, and dysrhythmias.[373, 388–393] This situation is evidenced by systemic (right) ventricular dysfunction and tricuspid valve regurgitation long after the repair.[394, 395] These patients also are prone to develop significant atrial dysrhythmias, including supraventricular tachyarrhythmias and sick-sinus syndrome, later in life.[396, 397] The arrhythmias may be preceded by right ventricular dysfunction, but they also may be an isolated finding and are potentially the major cause of sudden death in these patients. A number of large follow-up series have reported the probability of a patient remaining in sinus rhythm after an atrial level repair is 50 percent 10 years and 40 percent 20 years after the repair. Function of the sinus node may be seriously impaired by atrial manipulation during surgery. Sick-sinus syndrome (requiring pacemaker insertion) may occur late in the postoperative period. The atrial baffle provides a functional repair, although many patients continue to maintain relatively active lives with few subjective symptoms despite this.[398] Objective exercise testing on intermediate and late follow-up, however, may demonstrate limited right ventricular reserve in as many as 50 percent of patients; exercise duration, peak heart rate response, and peak minute oxygen consumption all have been reported to be reduced compared with age-matched controls.[399]

One of the major advances in congenital heart surgery over the past 10 to 15 years has been the development of the arterial switch operation (ASO) to correct transposition of the great arteries. In centers with considerable experience in performing this procedure, the early hospital mortality is less than 3 percent and actuarial analyses indicate 98 percent survival rate 5 to 10 years after surgery.[384] Long-term survival data are not available because the oldest survivors are only teenagers, but based on intermediate-term follow-up data, the risk for reoperation and complications after the arterial switch operation is small.

Virtually all coronary artery patterns are amenable to the arterial switch operation. No particular pattern has been associated with late death. A recent report of coronary artery angiography in 366 patients following the ASO (median age at follow-up, 7.9 years) revealed coronary artery stenosis or occlusion in 3 percent of the patients.[400] The long-term significance of these coronary artery abnormalities is yet to be determined. Despite the angiographic findings, evaluation with serial ECG, exercise testing, and wall motion abnormalities on echocardiography rarely demonstrate evidence of ischemia.[401, 402]

After the ASO, the "native" pulmonary valve becomes the "neoaortic" valve. A 30 percent incidence of trivial to mild aortic regurgitation has been reported on intermediate-term follow-up, without significant hemodynamic changes.[403] Severe regurgitation of blood through the valve is unusual.

There appears to be a very low incidence of significant rhythm disturbances after the ASO.[404] Supravalvar pulmonary artery stenosis was an early complication, but it is now less common with the use of surgical techniques that extensively mobilize, augment, and reconstruct the pulmonary arteries. Supravalvar aortic stenosis may develop, but it is rare.

Assessment of myocardial performance using echocardiography, cardiac catheterization, and exercise testing following the ASO have demonstrated function identical to age-matched controls.[405] Based on the currently available clinical, functional, and hemodynamic data, a patient who has undergone a previous ASO with no evidence of subsequent problems should be treated as any patient with a structurally normal heart when presenting for noncardiac surgery.

Late complications of the Rastelli procedure include progressive conduit obstruction and right ventricular hypertension, residual VSDs and, occasionally, subaortic obstruction from diversion of left ventricular outflow across the VSD to the aorta.

Total Anomalous Pulmonary Venous Connection
Pathophysiology

Patients with total anomalous pulmonary venous connections are cyanotic because their pulmonary veins connect to a systemic vein and they have various degrees of pulmonary venous obstruction. The venous connection may be above the level of the heart (e.g., to the superior vena cava or the innominate or azygos vein), directly to the right atrium, or below the level of the heart and the diaphragm (e.g., to the hepatic veins). Patients with this anomaly must have a patent foramen ovale or an ASD that allows blood flow to the left side of the heart.

This anatomic arrangement provides complete mixing of all systemic and pulmonary venous blood in the right atrium. Unless there is significant stenosis of the pulmonary venous connection, most of the right atrial blood passes through the right ventricle into the pulmonary artery, which increases pulmonary blood flow. If pulmonary venous return is significantly inhibited, there is increased pulmonary venous congestion and decreased pulmonary blood flow.

Anesthetic Management

These patients may be very ill, with hypoxemia, severe pulmonary edema, and pulmonary artery hypertension. Resuscitation, including mechanical ventilation, PEEP, and inotropic support of the myocardium, is followed by early surgical intervention to relieve the pulmonary venous obstruction. Although the patients are hypoxemic, their primary pathology is caused by obstructed venous return from the lungs. Therapy that increases pulmonary blood flow (e.g., PGE_1) must be avoided. Surgical repair of total anomalous pulmonary venous connection requires attachment or redirection of the pulmonary venous confluence to the left atrium.[406]

Intraoperative and postoperative problems are often related to residual or recurrent stenosis of the pulmonary veins. In patients who had severe stenosis and pulmonary venous hypertension preoperatively, the pulmonary vascular bed is highly reactive. This reactivity may produce high pulmonary artery pressures and poor right ventricular function after bypass and during the early postoperative period. Anesthetic management of these patients following completion of the repair should emphasize inotropic support of the right ventricle, avoidance of myocardial depressant drugs, and minimizing pulmonary vascular resistance. Early extubation of the trachea usually is not feasible. Mechanical ventilation-induced hyperventilation and other postoperative therapy may be required to decrease PVR. Use of inhaled nitric oxide has been particularly useful in this population.[51]

Anesthetic Considerations After Repair

Other than the potential for late development of recurrent pulmonary venous obstruction, these patients generally do well and have good cardiovascular reserve once recovery from the surgery is complete.[407] The size of the pulmonary veins at birth may be a predictor of late recurrent pulmonary vein stenosis.[408]

Atrial Septal Defect
Pathophysiology

There are three anatomic varieties of ASD. The most common, ASD secundum, is a deficit in the septum primum, which ordinarily covers the region of the foramen ovale. ASD primum is a deficit of the inferior portion of the atrial septum (endocardial cushion) and is usually accompanied by a cleft in the anterior leaflet of the mitral valve. Sinus venous defects are located near the junction of the right atrium and the superior or inferior vena cava; they are frequently associated with a partial anomalous pulmonary venous connection.

Left-to-right shunting (simple) occurs at the atrial level, causing a low-pressure volume load to the right ventricle. Pulmonary blood flow is increased, but the increase is rarely sufficient to make these patients symptomatic during early childhood. However, later in life, as the left ventricle becomes less compliant and the left atrial pressures increase, the left-to-right shunt and volume load increase and symptoms of CHF may occur. In rare patients, the longstanding increase in pulmonary blood flows causes pulmonary vascular obstructive disease.[132]

Anesthetic Management

The defect in the atrial septum can be closed directly with sutures or, if it is sufficiently large, with a synthetic patch. Sinus venosus defects associated with partial anomalous pulmonary venous connection require a more extensive patch that also directs the partial anomalous pulmonary venous return into the left atrium.

These patients are among the healthiest encountered. Their anesthesia can be managed in many ways. Early tracheal extubation is usual. Atrial arrhythmias, including atrial flutter and atrial fibrillation, are rarely seen during the postoperative period. Mitral regurgitation may occur in patients who have undergone repair of an ASD primum. Although transient left ventricular failure has been reported, these patients rarely require inotropic support. Residual ASDs are uncommon, but occasionally failure to recognize partial anomalous pulmonary venous return results in a residual left-to-right shunt. Most patients can have their trachea extubated during the immediate postoperative period or in the operating room. With the exceptions mentioned above, these patients usually have nearly normal cardiovascular function and reserve after repair.[409]

Ventricular Septal Defect

Pathophysiology

Defects in the ventricular septum occur at several locations in the membranous and muscular partition of the septum that divides the ventricles. Simple shunting occurs across the ventricular septum. The magnitude of pulmonary blood flow is determined by the size of the VSD and the PVR (Fig. 18–24).[410] With a nonrestrictive defect, high left ventricular flows and pressures are transmitted to the pulmonary artery. Therefore, surgical repair is indicated within the first 2 years of life to prevent the progression of pulmonary vascular obstructive disease.[28, 29, 411] In patients with established pulmonary vascular disease, the pulmonary arteriolar changes may not recede when the defect is closed. In such cases, there may be progressive elevation of the PVR.[131, 412, 413] The growth and development of the pulmonary vascular bed are significant factors in the pa-

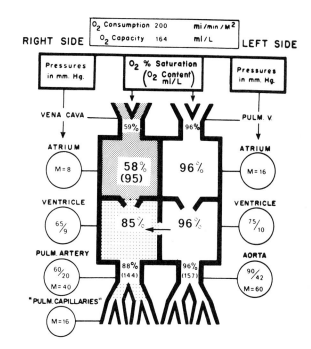

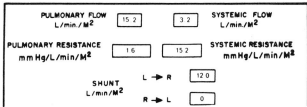

FIGURE 18–24. Catheterization findings in a patient with a VSD and pulmonary artery hypertension. (From Nadas AS, Fyler DC: Pediatric Cardiology. Philadelphia, WB Saunders Company, 1972, with permission.)

tient's ability to normalize pulmonary vascular hemodynamics after surgery.[414] When PVR approaches or exceeds systemic vascular resistance, right-to-left shunting occurs through the VSD, and the patients develop progressive hypoxemia (Eisenmenger syndrome). Closing the VSD in this circumstance adds the risk for acute right heart failure to that of progressive increases in PVR.

Anesthetic Management

Defects in the ventricular septum are closed during CPB. The most common septal defect, the membranous defect, is frequently repaired through a right atriotomy and the tricuspid valve. However, lesions in the inferior apical muscular septum or those high in the ventricular outflow tract may require a ventriculotomy. If so, postoperative ventricular function may be impaired.

Before repair, a decrease in PVR may appreciably increase left-to-right shunting in patients who have a nonrestrictive defect and may increase the degree of CHF. Postoperative ventricular failure may be a manifestation of the preoperative status of the myocardium, and also a result of surgery and CPB. Small infants who fail to thrive, who are malnourished, and who have significant CHF preoperatively may have excessive lung water and may require prolonged mechanical ventilation postoperatively.[415] Such infants may have limited intraoperative tolerance for anesthetics that depress the myocardium or for maneuvers that increase pulmonary blood flow.

Persistent CHF and an audible murmur postoperatively, evidence of low cardiac output, or the need for extensive inotropic support intraoperatively suggests that a residual or previously unrecognized additional VSD is continuing to place a volume and pressure load on the ventricles. When PVR is increased preoperatively, the increase in right ventricular afterload that is caused by closure of the VSD may be poorly tolerated, leading to the need for inotropic support of the heart and measures to decrease PVR. Occasionally, ventricular outflow tract obstruction is caused by placement of the septal patch. Aortic regurgitation that is caused by prolapse of one of the aortic valve cusps can develop in subaortic or subpulmonic VSDs. In addition, heart block may occur after closure of VSDs with a patch. A pacemaker may be needed to maintain an adequate heart rate and cardiac output.

Anesthetic Considerations After Repair

In the absence of residual VSDs, outflow obstruction, and heart block, most of these patients regain relatively normal myocardial function, especially if the VSD is repaired early.[416] However, a small percentage of patients, especially those who have had a large defect repaired late in childhood, continue to have some degree of ventricular dysfunction and pulmonary hypertension.[417-419]

Atrioventricular Canal Defects

Pathophysiology

The endocardial cushion defect or complete common AV canal, consists of defects in the atrial and ventricular septa and the AV valvular tissue. All four chambers communicate and share a single common AV valve. The atrial and ventricular shunts communicate volume and systemic pressures to the right ventricle and pulmonary artery. The ventricular shunt orifice is usually nonrestrictive (simple shunt); therefore, PVR governs the degree of excess pulmonary blood flow. Mitral regurgitation and direct LV-to-RA shunting may further contribute to atrial hypertension and total left-to-right shunting.

Anesthetic Management

Surgical repair of an atrioventricular canal consists of dividing the common AV valve and closure of the atrial and ventricular septal defect with a single patch.[420] In addition, the mitral valve (and sometimes the tricuspid valve) requires suture approximation and resuspension of the separated portions.

These patients have large left-to-right shunts. As a result of their high pulmonary blood flows, they have CHF and pulmonary hypertension. Myocardial depressants and therapy that decreases PVR while increasing shunt flow may be poorly tolerated before repair. Some patients, especially older children, may have obstructive pulmonary vascular disease. All of the potential complications of ASD and VSD closures are seen in these patients. In addition, the mitral valve may be severely regurgitant.[421] Inotropic

support for the failing heart, afterload reduction for mitral regurgitation, and measures to decrease pulmonary vascular resistance may be required intra- and postoperatively after repair.

Patients with Down syndrome frequently have an associated complete AV canal. Measures to decrease PVR and the use of prolonged ventilatory support are often necessary because the airways and pulmonary vascular beds are hyperreactive in these patients. The large tongue, upper airway obstruction, and difficult vascular access pose additional problems in these patients. The most frequent postoperative problems in Down syndrome patients are residual VSDs, mitral insufficiency,[422, 423] and pulmonary hypertension.[30]

Patent Ductus Arteriosus

Pathophysiology

The ductus arteriosus is a fetal vascular communication between the main pulmonary artery at its bifurcation and the descending aorta below the origin of the left subclavian artery. When patent, the ductus arteriosus provides a simple shunt between the systemic and pulmonary arteries. The magnitude and direction of flow between the systemic and pulmonary vessels are determined by the relative resistances to flow in the two vascular beds and the diameter (resistance) of the ductus arteriosus itself. With a large, nonrestrictive ductus and low pulmonary vascular resistance, the pulmonary blood flow is excessive and the volume load of the left heart is large. Systolic and diastolic flow away from the aorta may steal blood from vital organs (e.g., pulmonary steal) and compromise end-organ function at many sites.[424] In addition, overcirculated lungs and elevated left atrial pressure increase the work of breathing.[143, 144]

Anesthetic Management

Although the patent ductus arteriosus of premature infants often can be closed medically with indomethacin, contraindications to the use of this drug (e.g., intracranial hemorrhage, renal dysfunction, and hyperbilirubinemia) may require that the defect be closed surgically.[425] Whereas thoracotomy and surgical ligation of the ductus arteriosus are standard in older infants and children, some centers now occlude the ductus arteriosus with a percutaneously inserted vascular umbrella[426] or by using video-assisted thoracoscopic surgery (VATS).[427, 428] Advantages of VATS compared with open thoracotomy include decreased postoperative pain, shorter hospital stay, and decreased incidence of chest wall deformity.[429]

Healthy asymptomatic patients undergoing surgery can have their trachea extubated in the operating room, which allows many options for anesthetic management. However, the fragile premature infant with severe lung disease may require mechanical ventilation for protracted periods after ligation of the ductus arteriosus. Fentanyl, pancuronium, oxygen, and air constitute a common anesthetic regimen for these patients.[216] Anesthetic management of the premature infant in the operating room requires special considerations of gas exchange, hemodynamic performance, temperature regulation, metabolism, and drug and oxygen toxicity. Thoracotomy and lung retraction usually decrease lung compliance and increase oxygen and ventilatory requirements. A transient increase in systemic blood pressure with ligation of the ductus arteriosus may increase left ventricular afterload or elevate cerebral perfusion pressure to the detriment of a premature patient. Inadvertent ligation of the left pulmonary artery or descending aorta has occurred because the ductus arteriosus is often the same size or larger than the descending aorta.

The ductus arteriosus is located near the recurrent laryngeal nerve (RLN), which may be damaged during the procedure. In addition to the close relationship of the RLN to the PDA and descending aorta, the RLN has a variable course that may be difficult to identify during tissue dissection. Prior reports of PDA ligation performed by open thoracotomy indicate that the incidence of RLN injury is 1.2 to 8.8 percent.[430, 431] RLN paralysis causes hoarseness and is not detected until the endotracheal tube is removed. The incidence of RLN injury may be reduced by locating the RLN within the thorax before the DA is ligated or a clip is placed. This can be done by using direct intraoperative stimulation of the RLN and evoked electromyogram monitoring.[432] Ligation of an isolated ductus arteriosus generally results in normal cardiovascular function and reserve several months postoperatively.[433, 434]

Truncus Arteriosus

Pathophysiology

With truncus arteriosus, the embryonic truncus fails to separate normally into the two great arteries. A single great artery leaves the heart and gives rise to the coronary, pulmonary, and systemic circulations. The truncus straddles a large VSD and receives blood from both ventricles.[435]

There is complete mixing of systemic and pulmonary venous blood in the single great artery, which causes mild hypoxemia. One or two pulmonary arteries may originate from the ascending truncus; the pulmonary artery orifice is seldom restrictive. The resulting shunt (simple) produces excessive pulmonary blood flow early in life as the pulmonary vascular resistance decreases. This "pulmonary steal" may elevate the arterial oxygen saturation and decrease the systemic blood flow. In such a cases, net systemic oxygen transport decreases and lactic acidosis develops. Children with truncus arteriosus are at risk for developing early pulmonary vascular obstructive disease.[436] Regurgitation of blood through the truncal valve may place an additional volume load on the ventricles.

Anesthetic Management

Complete repair of this lesion should occur early, even in the neonatal period, before the child develops severe heart failure and irreversible pulmonary vascular changes.[13, 437] The VSD is closed with a synthetic patch and the pulmonary arteries are detached from the truncus. Vascular continuity is established between the right ventricle and the pulmonary arteries with a valved conduit.[438] The truncal valve may require valvuloplasty if a significant amount of blood regurgitates through it.

Anesthetic management centers around control of pulmonary blood flow and support of ventricular function. Pulmonary blood flow may increase further with anesthetic agents, hyperventilation, alkalosis, and oxygen administration. The increase in pulmonary blood flow results in systemic hypotension and acute ventricular failure. If measures to *increase* PVR do not decrease pulmonary flow, occlusion of one branch of the pulmonary artery with a tourniquet will limit pulmonary flow and restore the systemic perfusion pressure until CPB can be instituted. Because these patients are frequently in high-output CHF, myocardial depressants should be used with caution.

Immediately after the lesion is repaired, the combination of persistent pulmonary artery hypertension and right ventricular failure can be fatal. Hence, aggressive measures should be taken to provide normal myocardial function and to lower PVR. A residual VSD adds an additional volume and pressure load on the ventricles and may have a devastating effect on the patient's hemodynamics and oxygenation. A VSD should be suspected in patients who are not doing well postoperatively. Any residual VSD should be repaired if feasible. Truncal valve regurgitation or stenosis may induce left ventricular failure early during the postoperative period.

Anesthetic Considerations After Repair

Obstruction of the pulmonary conduit and the accompanying right ventricular hypertension may occur early or late during the postoperative course. Usually, the conduit is unable to support flow in the growing child after several postoperative years. Late development of truncal (aortic) valve regurgitation is possible. For patients who underwent repair later in childhood, residual persistent pulmonary hypertension may be a problem.

Coarctation of the Aorta

Pathophysiology

Patients with coarctation of the aorta have a narrowing of the descending aorta near the insertion of the ductus arteriosus into the aorta. Sometimes, coarctation of the aorta is associated with hypoplasia of the aortic isthmus proximal to the coarcted area. Aortic and mitral valve abnormalities, as well as VSDs, also may be present.

With severe obstruction to blood flow in the descending aorta of neonates, systemic perfusion is inadequate, causing profound metabolic acidosis. The increase in left ventricular afterload is not well tolerated, and an elevated left ventricular end-diastolic pressure (LVEDP) reflexively causes pulmonary artery hypertension. Blood flow below the coarctation then may be provided primarily by right-to-left flow from the right ventricle and pulmonary artery through the ductus arteriosus. Maintaining or reestablishing duct flow can be accomplished with a PGE$_1$ infusion, which also reduces the left ventricular afterload.

With less severe forms of aortic coarctation, the child may adapt to the obstruction by developing collateral circulation to the lower body and by increasing the left ventricular muscle mass. Upper extremity hypertension may be the only manifestation of the defect.

Anesthetic Management

Previous repairs of coarctation of the aorta in infants used the divided subclavian artery. The proximal portion of the artery was laid on the area of coarctation as a flap angioplasty. Alternative approaches recently have returned to resection of the narrowed area (including ductus arteriosus tissue) and end-to-end anastomosis of the aorta.[439] All approaches require 10 to 25 minutes of aortic cross-clamping above and below the area of coarctation. Acidosis, hypertension, or spinal cord ischemia can occur during this period.[440, 441] Paraplegia is an extremely rare but tragic complication of the procedure. Extreme upper body hypertension may compromise left ventricular function and decrease cardiac output, especially to the lower body, and must be expectantly treated. If the elevated arterial pressure in the head is transmitted to the cerebrospinal fluid (CSF), the CSF pressure may be elevated. If these elevated pressures are transmitted to the CSF below the level of the coarctation, net spinal cord perfusion pressure is decreased.[442] Alternatively, if upper body hypertension is overtreated with vasodilators during cross-clamping of the aorta, the arterial pressure may be inadequate in the vasodilated lower half of the body, which is supplied by collateral blood vessels. If this occurs, spinal cord or renal ischemia may result.[443] These complications are not so much related to changes in proximal aortic pressure or to changes in distal CSF pressure as they are to distal perfusion pressures, adequacy of arterial collaterals, and duration of cross-clamping.[444, 445] Monitoring of arterial pressures in the lower extremities may be helpful but impractical during the cross-clamp period. Hyperthermia (38° to 40°C) during cross-clamping is associated with an increased incidence of paraplegia and transient renal failure.[446] Therefore, mild hypothermia (32° to 34°C) is used in some centers during aortic cross-clamping as possible prophylaxis against these rare but tragic problems.

After the cross-clamp is removed and repair of the aorta is complete, rebound hypertension may be a problem as the patient emerges from the anesthetic. The mechanism(s) causing the hypertension have not been clearly established, but increased production of catecholamines and renin have been implicated in its pathogenesis.[447, 448] Development of abdominal pain and bowel ischemia during the postoperative period is related to insufficient blood flow in the mesenteric artery. Better control of postoperative hypertension has diminished the incidence of the severe form of this syndrome. Although propranolol, labetolol, and hydralazine may be useful for treating the moderate forms of postoperative hypertension, the more severe variety is best treated with infusions of esmolol and sodium nitroprusside during the first few hours after surgery. Captopril may be a useful oral agent for treatment of persistent hypertension. IV forms of enalapril are also available.[449]

Anesthetic Considerations After Repair

Persistent hypertension and left ventricular hypertrophy may be a problem for anesthetic management in up to 25 percent of patients after adequate repair of coarctation of the aorta.[450, 451] If the left subclavian artery was used for the repair, the left arm cannot be used for accurate blood pressure measurements. Restenosis of the coarctation is routinely balloon-dilated in the interventional catheterization laboratory. Some clinicians have advocated primary dilation of aortic coarctations in children.[452, 453]

Interrupted Aortic Arch
Pathophysiology

In some patients, the aorta is completely interrupted at one or more points along the aortic arch. A patent ductus arteriosus and a VSD are nearly always present and, in addition, left ventricular outflow obstruction may be present.[454]

Flow beyond the interrupted arch is supplied entirely by blood that is shunted right-to-left through the ductus arteriosus. Ductal closure eliminates blood flow to the lower body and leads to metabolic acidosis. Patency of the ductus arteriosus is reestablished with PGE_1.[455, 456] There is a left-to-right shunt through the VSD, which may cause excessive pulmonary blood flow and respiratory insufficiency.

Anesthetic Management

Repair of this lesion in neonates consists of a patch closure of the VSD and a direct anastomosis of the aorta (or insertion of a graft) between the ascending and descending aorta. Alternatively, the pulmonary artery is banded after the graft insertion and the VSD closure is deferred, but this palliative approach is generally discouraged.[457]

The introduction of PGE_1 has substantially improved preoperative resuscitation and perioperative morbidity of patients who have an interrupted aortic arch and has simplified anesthetic management. However, the residual effects of protracted poor perfusion may complicate the intra- and postoperative course of these patients. PGE_1 infusion should be continued until the onset of CPB. Circulatory problems after CPB that require inotropic support may be caused by a significant residual VSD, by obstruction of blood flow in the aorta, or by subaortic stenosis that is aggravated by the VSD closure and a narrow subaortic region.[458] Perioperative hypocalcemia occurs frequently in patients with interrupted aortic arch, even in infants without DiGeorge syndrome.[459]

Late problems are related to obstruction of the descending aorta with subsequent growth of the child. These problems are similar to those seen with coarctation of the aorta. Subaortic stenosis also may develop and presents considerable surgical challenges to adequate relief of obstruction.

Critical Aortic Stenosis
Pathophysiology

The aortic valves of these patients show thickening and rigidity. The valves have various degrees of fusion of the valvular commissures. In the newborn, the valve appears amorphous. There also may be evidence of endocardial fibroelastosis of the left ventricle and functional or anatomic abnormalities of the mitral valve.

Left ventricular outflow tract obstruction is poorly tolerated in the neonate because it causes left ventricular failure, poor systemic perfusion, hypotension, and pulmonary congestion. Myocardial perfusion is often borderline because the coronary perfusion pressure is relatively low and intraventricular pressure is high. Ventricular fibrillation may occur with surgical manipulation of the heart. In extreme cases, systemic blood flow may be partly supported from the right ventricle by right-to-left flow through the ductus arteriosus, provided that there is an atrial septal communication. Stabilization of the patient's condition can be aided by infusion of PGE₁ to increase systemic perfusion.

Anesthetic Management

While treatment of this anomaly includes surgical valvotomy under direction vision, in many centers, balloon angioplasty is the primary treatment. Myocardial depressants and rapid heart rates are poorly tolerated intraoperatively by these patients. A defibrillator should be available for immediate use. Preoperative resuscitation of the left ventricle is imperative, whether the aortic valve is to be traversed by surgical instruments or balloon dilation catheters. Inadequate relief of the obstruction and persistence of left ventricular failure can complicate and prolong the perioperative course.[459] Residual stenosis or other added hemodynamic burdens further reduce myocardial performance. Mitral regurgitation may continue intraoperatively, and aortic regurgitation may occur after the valvotomy is accomplished. Myocardial ischemia is not generally a problem after valvotomy. If the obstruction is adequately relieved, afterload reduction and inotropic agents may improve the poor myocardial function that is often evident postoperatively, especially when there is some degree of aortic regurgitation. In some patients, associated hypoplasia of the left ventricle or mitral valve may inhibit recovery and dictate a therapeutic approach to hypoplastic left heart.[460]

Hypoplastic Left Heart Syndrome
Pathophysiology

There has been more controversy about the treatment of hypoplastic left heart syndrome than there has been about the treatment of any other congenital heart lesion. This lesion is uniformly fatal if left untreated, but there continues to be debates over staged surgical palliation[461] versus neonatal transplantation,[462,463] versus comfort care alone.[464] The results of surgical management vary between institutions and are clearly dependent on expertise and experience, as well as the clinical condition of the neonate at presentation for surgery[465] and the degree of hypoplasia of left heart structures.[466–469]

This common example of single-ventricle physiology also represents the most severe form of an obstructive left heart lesion. An anatomic spectrum of disease is implied for the lesion, but in its most severe and common presentation there is atresia or marked hypoplasia of the aortic and mitral valves with critical underdevelopment of the left atrium, left ventricle, and ascending aorta. A 2- or

3-mm ascending aorta gives rise to the coronary circulation and the head vessels before converging with the ductus arteriosus, where the aorta becomes larger and supplies the circulation to the lower body. Pulmonary venous return arrives in the diminutive left atrium and cannot cross the atretic mitral valve; therefore, pulmonary venous flow is directed to the right atrium and right ventricle, where common mixing occurs with the systemic venous return and all blood is ejected into the pulmonary artery. Systemic blood flow is supplied from the pulmonary artery by right-to-left shunting of blood across the patent ductus arteriosus. As the PDA constricts in the neonatal period, systemic blood flow decreases and all ventricular output is directed to the lungs. The Q̇p/Q̇s ratio approaches infinity as Q̇s nears zero. Therefore, one has the paradoxical presentation of high Po₂ (70 to 150 mm Hg) despite the presence of profound metabolic acidosis. When the ductus arteriosus is reopened with PGE₁, systemic perfusion is reestablished, the acidosis resolves, and the Po₂ returns to the 40 to 60 mm Hg range, representative of a Q̇p/Q̇s ratio between 1 and 2.

Anesthetic Management

Adequate preoperative resuscitation with PGE₁ and correction of metabolic acidosis and end-organ dysfunction is crucial to the anesthetic preparation and management of patients with this lesion. Further facilitation of resuscitation can be enhanced by judicious use of inotropic agents, which can optimize cardiac output and blood flow to such organs as the kidneys. However, excessive delay in the timing of surgical intervention will result in a gradual reduction in pulmonary vascular resistance over days, with excessive pulmonary blood flow and inadequate systemic perfusion. The surgical reconstructive approach to this lesion commonly requires three operations. The ultimate aim is to provide a 2- or 3-year-old child with a reconstructed aortic arch and a Fontan type of circulation for single-ventricle physiology.[461,468,470] In the first stage of the reconstruction (Norwood operation),[161] the pulmonary artery is transected at the bifurcation and the artery is anastomosed to the ascending aorta. The ascending aorta has been surgically incised so that the aortic and pulmonary arterial confluence arises together from the single right ventricle as the neoaorta. The neoaorta is extended into the remaining native aorta using homograft material. Pulmonary blood flow is established with a modified B-T shunt that usually is 3.5 to 4 mm in diameter. The atrial septum is excised to ensure free flow of pulmonary venous return across the tricuspid valve. In addition to HLHS, the Norwood operation also is used to repair other complex single-ventricle defects with systemic outflow obstruction or hypoplasia.[471]

The anesthetic considerations are the same as those outlined in detail for patients with single-ventricle physiology (Table 18–12). The intraoperative and postoperative management require careful manipulation of PVR and SVR to provide adequate, but not excessive, pulmonary blood flow and oxygen delivery while maintaining sufficient systemic and coronary artery perfusion. The precarious nature of the coronary os, which may be extremely small and closely approximated to the suture lines, means that even small variations in hemodynamics may compromise myocardial blood flow. Myocardial depressants are poorly tolerated, and ventricular failure and tricuspid (systemic) valve regurgitation can inhibit recovery.

After CPB in the Norwood palliation procedure, the pulmonary vascular resistance may be transiently elevated and the modified B-T shunt barely adequate to sustain pulmonary blood flow and achieve adequate oxygenation. In this circumstance, hyperventilation with 100 percent oxygen and alkalosis may be required, along with inotropic support of the systemic blood pressure. However, within hours, and sometimes within minutes, pulmonary vascular resistance decreases, myocardial function is restored, and the $\dot{Q}p/\dot{Q}s$ may become excessive. Hypoventilation with room air and the use of systemic vasodilators do not always effectively reverse the pulmonary steal in this circumstance. More drastic measures, such as mechanical ventilation with hypoxic gas mixtures or with added CO_2, have been advocated by some centers and have been intermittently embraced and abandoned by others over the years.[472]

Orthotopic heart transplantation has gained acceptance as an alternative treatment for hypoplastic left heart syndrome.[473] Neonatal transplants appear to be well tolerated, and some centers have avoided maintenance steroid therapy while achieving excellent midterm results using transplantation as the sole therapeutic option for this disease.[473, 474] Others have successfully advocated a combined approach using either transplantation or staged reconstruction, depending on the pathophysiologic state of the child and the availability of a donor heart.[475] The critical shortage of donor organs markedly limits heart transplantation to correct this common congenital heart lesion. In neonates awaiting transplantation, breathing added CO_2 may help to avoid the alkalosis that is associated with the inevitable tachypnea that occurs when the PVR decreases and the pulmonary blood flow becomes excessive. Dependence on long-term mechanical ventilation, sedation, or muscle paralysis is undesirable.

It is apparent that many children have derived benefit from a completed, staged reconstruction or heart transplantation for this previously fatal illness. They are often able to lead active, productive lives and to develop normally.[476, 477] However, the long-term prognosis for this evolving therapy will not be known for several years.

REFERENCES

1. Guyer B, Hoyert DL, Martin JA, et al: Annual summary of vital statistics 1998. Pediatrics 104:1229, 1999.
2. Harmel MH, Lamont A: Anesthesia in the surgical treatment of congenital pulmonic stenosis. Anesthesiology 7:477, 1946.
3. Strong MJ, Keats AS, Cooley DA: Anesthesia for cardiovascular surgery in infancy. Anesthesiology 27:257, 1966.
4. Hickey PR, Hansen DD, Norwood WI, Castaneda AR: Anesthetic complications in surgery for congenital heart disease. Anesth Analg 63:657, 1984.
5. Wernovsky G, Giglia TM, Jonas RA, et al: Course in the intensive care unit after preparatory pulmonary artery banding and aortopulmonary shunt placement for transposition of the great arteries with low left ventricular pressure. Circulation 86(suppl II):II-133, 1992.
6. Wernovsky G, Jonas RA, Newburger JW, et al: The Boston circulatory arrest study: hemodynamics and hospital course after the arterial switch operation. Circulation 86(suppl I):I-237, 1992.
7. Wessel DL, Triedman JK, Wernovsky G, et al: Pulmonary and systemic hemodynamic effects of amrinone in neonates following cardiopulmonary bypass. Circulation 80:II-488, 1989.
8. Friedman WF, George BL: Treatment of congestive heart failure by altering loading conditions of the heart. J Pediatr 106:697, 1985.
9. Pae WE, Miller CA, Matthews Y: Ventricular assist devices for postcardiotomy cardiogenic shock. J Thorac Cardiovasc Surg 194:541, 1992.
10. Delius RE, Bove EL, Meliones JN: Use of extracorporeal life support in patients with congenital heart disease. Crit Care Med 20:1216, 1992.
11. Moler FW, Custer JR, Bartlett RH: Extracorporeal life support for pediatric respiratory failure. Crit Care Med 20:1112, 1992.
12. Duncan BW, Hraska V, Jonas RA: Mechanical circulatory support for pediatric cardiac patients. Circulation 94:173, 1996.
13. Hanley FL, Heinemann MK, Jonas RA, et al: Repair of truncus arteriosus in the neonate. J Thorac Cardiovasc Surg 105:1047, 1993.
14. Bohn DJ, Poirer CS, Demonds JF: Efficacy of dopamine, dobutamine and epinephrine during emergence from cardiopulmonary bypass in children. Crit Care Med 8:367, 1980.
15. Habib DM, Padbury JF, Anas NG: Dobutamine pharmacokinetics and pharmacodynamics in pediatric intensive care patients. Crit Care Med 20:601, 1992.
16. Berg RA, Donnerstein RL, Padbury JF: Dobutamine infusions in stable, critically ill children: pharmacokinetics and hemodynamic actions. Crit Care Med 21:678, 1993.
17. Butterworth JF: Use of amrinone in cardiac surgery patients. J Cardiothorac Vasc Anesth 7(suppl):1, 1993.
18. Rosenzweig EB, Starc TJ, Chen JM, et al: Intravenous arginine-vasopresin in children with vasodilatory shock after cardiac surgery. Circulation 100:II-182, 1999.
19. Caspi J, Coles JG, Benson LN, et al: Effects of high plasma epinephrine and Ca2+ concentrations on neonatal myocardial function after ischemia. J Thorac Cardiovasc Surg 105:59, 1993.
20. Caspi J, Coles JG, Benson LN, et al: Age-related response to epinephrine-induced myocardial stress. A functional and ulstructural study. Circulation 84(suppl III):III-394, 1991.
21. Robinson BW, Gelband H, Mas MS: Selective pulmonary and systemic vasodilator effects of amrinone in children: new therapeutic implications. J Am Coll Cardiol 21:1461, 1993.
22. Berner M, Jaccard C, Oberhänsli I: Hemodynamic effects of amrinone in children after cardiac surgery. Intensive Care Med 16:85, 1990.
23. Chang AC, Atz AM, Wernovsky G, et al: Milrinone: systemic and pulmonary hemodynamic effects in neonates after cardiac surgery. Crit Care Med 23:1907, 1995.
24. Dupuis JY, Bondy R, Cattran C, et al: Amrinone and dobutamine as primary treatment of low cardiac output syndrome following coronary artery surgery: a comparison of their effects on hemodynamics and outcome. J Cardiothorac Vasc Anesth 6:542, 1992.
25. Bailey JM, Miller BE, Lu W, et al: The pharmacokinetics of milrinone in pediatric patients after cardiac surgery. Anesthesiology 90:1012, 1999.
26. Ramamoorthy C, Anderson GD, Williams GD, Lynn AM: Pharmacokinetics and side effects of milrinone in infants and children after open heart surgery. Anesth Analg 86:283, 1998.
27. Sluysmans T, Styns-Cailteux M, Tremouroux-Wattiez M, et al: Intravenous enalaprilat and oral enalapril in congestive heart failure secondary to ventricular septal defect in infancy. Am J Cardiol 70:959, 1992.
28. Hoffman JIE, Rudolph AM, Heymann MA: Pulmonary vascular disease with congenital heart lesions: pathologic features and causes. Circulation 64:873, 1981.
29. Heath D, Edwards JE: The pathology of hypertensive pulmonary vascular disease: a description of six grades of structural changes in the pulmonary arteries with special reference to congenital cardiac septal defects. Circulation 28:533, 1958.
30. Clapp S, Perry BL, Farooki ZQ, et al: Down's syndrome, complete atrioventricular canal, and pulmonary vascular obstructive disease. J Thorac Cardiovasc Surg 100:115, 1990.
31. Del Nido PJ, Williams WG, Villamater J, et al: Changes in pericardial surface pressure during pulmonary hypertensive crises after cardiac surgery. Circulation 76(suppl III):III-93, 1987.
32. Hickey PR, Hansen DD: Pulmonary hypertension in infants: postoperative management. In Yacoub M (ed): Annual of Cardiac Surgery. London, Current Science, 1989, p 16.

33. Wheller J, George BL, Mulder DG, Jarmakani JM: Diagnosis and management of postoperative pulmonary hypertensive crisis. Circulation 70:1640, 1979.

34. Jones ODH, Shore DF, Rigby ML, et al: The use of tolazoline hydrochloride as a pulmonary vasodilator in potentially fatal episodes of pulmonary vasoconstriction after cardiac surgery in children. Circulation 64:134, 1981.

35. Drummond WH, Gregory GA, Heymann MA, Phibbs RA: The independent effects of hyperventilation, tolazoline, and dopamine on infants with persistent pulmonary hypertension. J Pediatr 98:603, 1981.

36. Bush A, Busst C, Knight WB, Shinebourne EA: Modification of pulmonary hypertension secondary to congenital heart disease by prostacyclin therapy. Am Rev Respir Dis 136:767, 1987.

37. Bush A, Busst C, Booth K, et al: Does prostacyclin enhance the selective pulmonary vasodilator effect of oxygen in children with congenital heart disease? Circulation 74:135, 1986.

38. Kirklin JW, Barratt-Boyes BG: Hypothermia, circulatory arrest, and cardiopulmonary bypass. In Cardiac Surgery. New York, Wiley Medical, 1986, p 29.

39. Meyrick B, Reid L: Ultrastructural findings in lung biopsy material from children with congenital heart defects. Am J Pathol 101:527, 1980.

40. Koul B, Willen H, Sjöberg T, et al: Pulmonary sequelae of prolonged total venoarterial bypass: evaluation with a new experimental model. Ann Thorac Surg 51:794, 1991.

41. Koul B, Wollmer P, Willen H, et al: Venoarterial extracorporeal membrane oxygenation—how safe is it? J Thorac Cardiovasc Surg 104:579, 1992.

42. Furchgott RF: The role of endothelium in the responses of vascular smooth muscle to drugs. Ann Rev Pharmacol Toxicol 24:175, 1984.

43. Furchgott RF, Zawadzki JV: The obligatory role of endothelial cells in the relaxation of arterial smooth muscle by acetylcholine. Nature 288:373, 1980.

44. Palmer RMJ, Ferrige AG, Moncada S: Nitric oxide release accounts for the biologic activity of endothelium-derived relaxing factor. Nature 327:524, 1987.

45. Ignarro LJ, Buga GM, Wood KS, et al: Endothelium-derived relaxing factor produced and released from artery and vein is nitric oxide. Proc Natl Acad Sci U S A 84:9265, 1987.

46. Ignarro LJ, Harbison RG, Wood KS, Kadowitz PJ: Activation of purified soluble guanylate cyclase by endothelium-derived relaxing factor from intrapulmonary artery and vein: stimulation by acetylcholine, bradykinin and arachidonic acid. J Pharmacol Exp Ther 237:893, 1986.

47. Wessel DL, Adatia I, Giglia TM, et al: Use of inhaled nitric oxide and acetylcholine in the evaluation of pulmonary hypertension and endothelial function after cardiopulmonary bypass. Circulation 88:2128, 1993.

48. Beghetti M, Silkoff PE, Caramori M, et al: Decreased exhaled nitric oxide may be a marker of cardiopulmonary bypass-induced injury. Ann Thorac Surg 66:532, 1998.

49. Haworth SG: Total anomalous pulmonary venous return. Prenatal damage to pulmonary vascular bed and extrapulmonary veins. Br Heart J 48:513, 1982.

50. Atz AM, Adatia I, Wessel DL: Rebound pulmonary hypertension after inhalation of nitric oxide. Ann Thorac Surg 62:1759, 1996.

51. Adatia I, Atz AM, Jonas RA, Wessel DL: Diagnostic use of inhaled nitric oxide after neonatal cardiac operations. J Thorac Cardiovasc Surg 112:1403, 1996.

52. Journois D, Pouard P, Mauriat P, et al: Inhaled nitric oxide as a therapy for pulmonary hypertension after operations for congenital heart defects. J Thorac Cardiovasc Surg 107:1129, 1994.

53. Luciani GB, Chang AC, Starnes VA: Surgical repair of transposition of the great arteries in neonates with persistent pulmonary hypertension. Ann Thorac Surg 61:800, 1996.

54. Rusell IA, Zwass MS, Fineman JR, et al: The effects of inhaled nitric oxide on postoperative pulmonary hypertension in infants and children undergoing surgical repair of congenital heart disease. Anesth Analg 87:46, 1998.

55. Roberts JD, Lang P, Bigatello LM, et al: Inhaled nitric oxide in congenital heart disease. Circulation 87:447, 1993.

56. Dukarm RC, Morin FC, Russell JA, Steinhorn RH: Pulmonary and systemic effects of the phosphodiesterase inhibitor dipyridamole in newborn lambs with persistent pulmonary hypertension. Pediatr Res 44:831, 1998.

57. Yahagi N, Kumon K, Tanigami H: Inhaled nitric oxide for the postoperative management of Fontan-type operations. Ann Thorac Surg 57:1371, 1994.

58. Miller OI, Celermajer DS, Deanfield JE, Macrae DJ: Very low dose inhaled nitric oxide: a selective pulmonary vasodilator after operations for congenital heart disease. J Thorac Cardiovasc Surg 108:487, 1994.

59. Beghetti M, Habre W, Friedli B, Berner M: Continuous low dose inhaled nitric oxide for treatment of severe pulmonary hypertension after cardiac surgery in paediatric patients. Br Heart J 73:65, 1995.

60. Leclerc F, Riou Y, Martinot A, et al: Inhaled nitric oxide for a severe respiratory syncytial virus infection in an infant with bronchopulmonary dysplasia. Intensive Care Med 20:511, 1994.

61. Thompson MW, Bates JN, Klein JM: Treatment of respiratory failure in an infant with bronchopulmonary dysplasia infected with respiratory syncytial virus using inhaled nitric oxide and high frequency ventilation. Acta Paediatr 84:100, 1995.

62. Ogura H, Cioffi WG, Offner PJ, et al: Effect of inhaled nitric oxide on pulmonary function after sepsis in a swine model. Surgery 116:313, 1994.

63. Channick RN, Newhart JW, Johnson FW, et al: Pulsed delivery of inhaled nitric oxide to patients with primary pulmonary hypertension. Chest 109:1545, 1996.

64. Ivy DD, Griebel JL, Kinsella JP, Abman SH: Acute hemodynamic effects of pulsed delivery of low flow nasal nitric oxide in children with pulmonary hypertension. J Pediatr 133:453, 1998.

65. Roberts JD, Roberts CT, Jones RC, et al: Continuous nitric oxide inhalation reduces pulmonary arterial structural changes, right ventricular hypertrophy, and growth retardation in the hypoxic newborn rat. Circ Res 76:215, 1995.

66. Atz AM, Wessel DL: Inhaled nitric oxide and heparin for infantile primary pulmonary hypertension. Lancet 351:1701, 1998.

67. Young JD, Sear JW, Valvini EM: Kinetics of methaemoglobin and serum nitrogen oxide production during inhalation of nitric oxide in volunteers. Br J Anaesth 76:652, 1996.

68. Rimar S, Gillis CN: Selective pulmonary vasodilation by inhaled nitric oxide is due to hemoglobin inactivation. Circulation 88:2884, 1993.

69. Hallman M, Bry K, Lappalainen U: A mechanism of nitric oxide-induced surfactant dysfunction. J Appl Physiol 80:2035, 1996.

70. Semigran MJ, Cockrill BA, Kacmarek R, et al: Hemodynamic effects of inhaled nitric oxide in heart failure. J Am Coll Cardiol 24:982, 1994.

71. Loh E, Stamler JS, Hare JM, et al: Cardiovascular effects of inhaled nitric oxide in patients with left ventricular dysfunction. Circulation 90:2780, 1994.

72. Bocchi EA, Bacal F, Auler JOC, et al: Inhaled nitric oxide leading to pulmonary edema in stable severe heart failure. Am J Cardiol 74:70, 1994.

73. Hare JM, Shernan SK, Body SC, et al: Influence of inhaled nitric oxide on systemic flow and ventricular filling pressure in patients receiving mechanical circulatory assistance. Circulation 95:2250, 1997.

74. Francoise M, Gouyon JB, Mercier JC: Hemodynamic and oxygenation changes induced by the discontinuation of low-dose inhalational nitric oxide in newborn infants. Intensive Care Med 22:477, 1996.

75. Lavoie A, Hall JB, Olson DM, Wylam ME: Life-threatening effects of discontinuing inhaled nitric oxide in severe respiratory failure. Am J Respir Crit Care Med 153:1985, 1996.

76. Miller OI, Tang SF, Keech A, Celermajer DS: Rebound pulmonary hypertension on withdrawal from inhaled nitric oxide. Lancet 346:51, 1995.

77. Atz AM, Wessel DL: Sildenafil ameliorates effects of inhaled nitric oxide withdrawal. Anesthesiology 91:307, 1999.

78. Brutsaert DL, Sys SU, Gillebert TC: Diastolic dysfunction in post-cardiac surgical management. J Cardiothorac Vasc Anesth 7:18, 1993.

79. Brecker SJ, Xiao HB, Mbaissouroum M, Gibson DG: Effects of intravenous milrinone on left ventricular function in ischemic and idiopathic dilated cardiomyopathy. Am J Cardiol 71:203, 1993.

80. Feneck RO: Intravenous milrinone following cardiac surgery: I. Effects of bolus infusion followed by variable dose maintenance infusion. J Cardiothorac Vasc Anesth 6:554, 1992.

81. Feneck RO: Intravenous milrinone following cardiac surgery: II. Influence of baseline hemodynamics and patient factors on therapeutic response. J Cardiothorac Vasc Anesth 6:563, 1992.

82. Remme WJ: Inodilator therapy for heart failure. early, late, or not at all? Circulation 87(suppl IV):IV-97, 1993.

83. Vincent JL, Leon M, Berre J, et al: Addition of enoximone to adrenergic agents in the management of severe heart failure. Crit Care Med 29:1102, 1992.

84. Castaneda AR, Mayer JE, Jonas RA, et al: The neonate with critical congenital heart disease: repair—a surgical challenge. J Thorac Cardiovasc Surg 98:869, 1989.

85. Anand KJS, Sippell WG, Aynsley-Green A: Randomised trial of fentanyl anaesthesia in preterm babies undergoing surgery: effects on the stress response. Lancet 1:243, 1987.

86. Reller MD, Morton MJ, Giraud GD: Severe right ventricular pressure loading in fetal sheep augments global myocardial blood flow to submaximal levels. Circulation 86:581, 1992.

87. Romero TE, Friedman WF: Limited left ventricular response to volume overload in the neonatal period: a comparative study with the adult animal. Pediatr Res 13:910, 1979.

88. Thornburg KL, Morton MJ: Filling and arterial pressure as determinants of RV stroke volume in the sheep fetus. Am J Physiol 244:H656, 1983.

89. Friedman WF: The intrinsic physiologic properties of the developing heart. Prog Cardiovasc Disease 15:87, 1972.

90. Baum VC, Palmisano BW: The immature heart and anesthesia. Anesthesiology 87:1529, 1997.

91. Mills AN, Haworth SG: Greater permeability of the neonatal lung: postnatal changes in surface charge and biochemistry of porcine pulmonary capillary endothelium. J Thorac Cardiovasc Surg 101:909, 1991.

92. Feltes TF, Hansen TN: Effects of an aorticopulmonary shunt on lung fluid balance in the young lamb. Pediatr Res 26:94, 1989.

93. Anand KJS, Phil D, Hansen DD, Hickey PR: Hormonal-metabolic stress response in neonates undergoing cardiac surgery. Anesthesiology 73:661, 1990.

94. Anand KJS, Hickey PR: Halothane-morphine compared to high-dose sufentanil for anesthesia and postoperative analgesia in neonatal cardiac surgery. N Engl J Med 326:1, 1992.

95. Fisher DJ, Heymann MA, Rudolph AM: Fetal myocardial oxygen and carbohydrate consumption during acutely induced hypoxemia. Am J Physiol 242:H657, 1982.

96. Chang AC, Hanley FL, Lock JE, Wessel DL: Management and outcome of low birth weight neonates with congenital heart disease. J Pediatr 124:461, 1994.

97. Reddy VM, McElhinney DB, Sagrado T, et al: Results of 102 cases of complete repair of congenital heart defects in patients weighing 700 to 2500 grams. J Thorac Cardiovasc Surg 117:324, 1999.

98. Anand KJS, Hickey PR: Pain and its effects in the human neonate and fetus. N Engl J Med 317:1321, 1987.

99. Shah AR, Kurth CD, Gwiazdowski SG: Fluctuations in cerebral oxygenation and blood volume during endotracheal suctioning in premature infants. J Pediatr 120:769, 1992.

100. Gruber EM, Laussen PC, Casta A, et al: Stress response in infants undergoing cardiac surgery: a randomized study of fentanyl bolus, fentanyl infusion, and fentanyl-midazolam infusion. Anesth Analg 92:882, 2001.

101. Anand K, Sippell WG, Aynsley-Green A: Randomized trial of fentanyl anesthesia in preterm neonates undergoing surgery: effects on the stress response. Lancet 1:243, 1987.

102. Hickey PR, Hansen DD, Wessel DL, et al: Blunting of stress responses in the pulmonary circulation in infants. Anesth Analg 64:1137, 1985.

103. Tabutt S, Duncan BW, McLaughlin D, et al: Delayed sternal closure after cardiac operations in the pediatric population. J Thorac Cardiovasc Surg 113:886, 1997.

104. Newburger JW, Jonas RA, Wernovsky G, et al: Perioperative neurologic effects of hypothermic arrest during infant heart surgery. The Boston Circulatory Arrest Study. N Engl J Med 329:1057, 1993.

105. Laussen PC, Reid RW, Stene RA: Tracheal extubation of children in the operating room after atrial septal defect repair as part of a clinical practice guideline. Anesth Analg 82:988, 1996.

106. Hillel Z, Thys D, Ritter S: Two-dimensional color flow Doppler echocardiography for the intraoperative monitoring of cardiac shunt flows in patients with congenital heart disease. J Cardiothorac Vasc Anesth 1:42, 1987.

107. Berman W: Cardiovascular Shunts: Phylogenetic, Ontogenetic, and Clinical Aspects. New York, Raven Press, 1985, p 399.

108. Rudolph AM: Congenital Diseases of the Heart. Chicago, Year Book Medical Publishers, 1974, p 79.

109. Peral RG, Maze M, Rosenthal MH: Pulmonary and systemic hemodynamic effects of central nervous and left atrial sympathomimetic drug administration in the dog. J Cardiothorac Vasc Anesth 1:29, 1987.

110. Abman SH, Wolfe RR, Accurso FJ: Pulmonary vascular response to oxygen in infants with severe bronchopulmonary dysplasia. Pediatrics 75:80, 1985.

111. Rudolph AM, Yuan S: Response to the pulmonary circulation to hypoxia and H+ ion changes. J Clin Invest 45:399, 1966.

112. Giglia TM, Wessel DL: Effects of oxygen on pulmonary and systemic hemodynamics in infants after cardiopulmonary bypass. Circulation 82(suppl III):III-78, 1990.

113. Morray JP, Lynn AM, Mansfield PB: Effect of pH and PCO2 on pulmonary and systemic hemodynamics after surgery in children with congenital heart disease and pulmonary hypertension. J Pediatr 113:474, 1988.

114. Chang AC, Zucker HA, Hickey PR, Wessel DL: Pulmonary vascular resistance in infants after cardiac surgery: role of carbon dioxide and hydrogen ion. Crit Care Med 23:568, 1995.

115. Peckham GJ, Fox WW: Physiologic factors affecting pulmonary artery pressure in infants with persistent pulmonary hypertension. J Pediatr 93:1005, 1978.

116. Ferrara B, Johnson DE, Chang P, Thompson TR: Efficacy and neurologic outcome of profound hypocapneic alkalosis for the treatment of persistent pulmonary hypertension in infancy. J Pediatr 105:457, 1984.

117. Bernbaum JC, Russell P, Sheridan PH, et al: Long-term follow-up of newborns with persistent pulmonary hypertension. Crit Care Med 12:579, 1984.

118. Albrecht RF, Miletich DJ, Ruttle M: The effects of prolonged hyperventilation on cerebral metabolism. Anesthesiology 61:A247, 1984.

119. West JB, Dollery NA: Distribution of blood flow in isolated lung: relation to vascular and alveolar pressures. J Appl Physiol 19:713, 1964.

120. Leffler CW, Hessler JR, Green RS: The onset of breathing at birth stimulates pulmonary vascular prostacyclin synthesis. Pediatr Res 18:938, 1984.

121. Said SI: Pulmonary metabolism of prostaglandins and vasoactive peptides. Ann Rev Physiol 44:257, 1982.

122. Hickey PR, Hansen DD, Wessel DL, et al: Pulmonary and systemic hemodynamic responses to fentanyl in infants. Anesth Analg 64:483, 1985.

123. Hickey PR, Hansen DD, Strafford MA: Pulmonary and systemic hemodynamic effects of nitrous oxide in infants with normal and elevated pulmonary vascular resistance. Anesthesiology 65:374, 1986.

124. Morray JP, Lynn AM, Stamm SJ: Hemodynamic effects of ketamine in children with congenital heart disease. Anesth Analg 63:895, 1984.

125. Berman W, Fripp RR, Rubler M, Alderete L: Hemodynamic effects of ketamine in children undergoing cardiac catheterization. Pediatr Cardiol 11:72, 1990.

126. Hickey PR, Hansen DD, Wessel DL, et al: Blunting of stress responses in the pulmonary circulation of infants by fentanyl. Anesth Analg 64:1137, 1985.

127. Vacanti JP, Crone RK, Murphy JD, et al: The pulmonary hemodynamic response to perioperative anesthesia in the treatment of high-risk infants with congenital diaphragmatic hernia. J Pediatr Surg 19:672, 1984.

128. Nudel D, Berman N, Talner N: Effects of acutely increasing systemic vascular resistance on arterial oxygen tension in tetralogy of Fallot. Pediatrics 58:248, 1976.

129. James LS, Rowe RD: The pattern of response of pulmonary and systemic arterial pressures in newborn and older infants to short periods of hypoxia. J Pediatr 51:5, 1957.

130. Haworth SG: Normal pulmonary vascular development and its disturbance in congenital heart disease. In Godman MJ (ed): Paediatric Cardiology. Vol 4. New York, Churchill Livingstone, 1981.

131. Rabinovitch MB, Haworth SG, Castaneda AR: Lung biopsy in congenital heart disease: a morphometric approach to pulmonary vascular disease. Circulation 58:1107, 1978.

132. Haworth SG: Pulmonary vascular disease in secundum atrial septal defect in childhood. Am J Cardiol 51:265, 1983.
133. Thgien G, Maxxucco A, Grisolia EF: Postoperative pathology of complete atrioventricular defects. J Thorac Cardiovasc Surg 83:891, 1982.
134. Berman W, Wood SC, Yabek SM: Systemic oxygen transport in patients with congenital heart disease. Circulation 75:360, 1987.
135. Theodore J, Robin ED, Burke CM: Impact of profound reductions of PaO2 on O2 transport and utilization in congenital heart disease. Chest 87:293, 1985.
136. Lister G, Hellenbrand WE, Kleinman CS, Talner NS: Physiologic effects of increasing hemoglobin concentration in left-to-right shunting in infants with ventricular septal defects. N Engl J Med 306:502, 1982.
137. Fouron JC, Hebert F: The circulatory effects of hematocrit variations in normovolemic newborn lambs. J Pediatr 82:995, 1973.
138. Phornphutkul C, Rosenthal A, Nadas A: Cerebrovascular accidents in infants and children with cyanotic congenital heart disease. Am J Cardiol 32:329, 1973.
139. Mauer H, McCue C, Robertson L: Correction of platelet dysfunction and bleeding in cyanotic congenital heart disease by simple red cell volume reduction. Am J Cardiol 35:831, 1975.
140. Kontras S, Sirak H, Newton W: Hematologic abnormalities in children with congenital heart disease. JAMA 195:611, 1976.
141. Ekert H, Sheers M: Preoperative and postoperative platelet function in cyanotic congenital heart disease. J Thorac Cardiovasc Surg 67:184, 1974.
142. Paul MH, Currinblay Z, Miller RA: Thrombocytopenia in cyanotic congenital heart disease. Circulation 24:1013, 1961.
143. Bancalari E, Jesse MJ, Gelband H, Garcia O: Lung mechanics in congenital heart disease with increased and decreased pulmonary blood flow. J Pediatr 90:192, 1977.
144. Gerhardt T, Bancalari E: Lung compliance in newborns with patent ductus arteriosus before and after surgical ligation. Biol Neonate 38:96, 1980.
145. Greenwood RD, Rosenthal A, Parisi L: Extracardiac abnormalities in infants with congenital heart disease. Pediatrics 55:485, 1975.
146. Greenwood RD: Cardiovascular malformations associated with extracardiac anomalies and malformation syndromes. Clin Pediatr 23:145, 1984.
147. Sanders S: Echocardiography and related techniques in the diagnosis of congenital heart defects. Echocardiography 1:185, 1984.
148. Freed MD, Miettinen OS, Nadas AS: Oximetric detection of intracardiac left to right shunts. Br Heart J 42:690, 1979.
149. Rabinovitch M: Pulmonary hypertension. In Adams FH, Emmanouilides GC (eds): Moss' Heart Diseases in Infants, Children and Adolescents. Baltimore, Williams & Wilkins, 1983, p 669.
150. Bargeron LMJR, Elliot LP, Soto B: Axial cineangiography of congenital heart disease. Radiology 56:1075, 1977.
151. Fellows KE, Keane JF, Freed MD: Angled views in cineangiography of congenital heart disease. Radiology 56:485, 1977.
152. Geva T: Introduction: magnetic resonance imaging. Pediatr Cardiol 21:3, 2000.
153. Chung T: Assessment of cardiovascular anatomy in patients with congenital heart disease by magnetic resonance imaging. Pediatr Cardiol 21:18, 2000.
154. Freed MA, Heyman MA, Lewis AB: Prostaglandin E1 in infants with ductus arteriosus-dependent congenital heart disease. Circulation 64:889, 1981.
155. Yokota M, Muraoka R, Aoshima M: Modified Blalock-Taussig shunt following long-term administration of prostaglandin E1 for ductus-dependent neonates with cyanotic congenital heart disease. J Thorac Cardiovasc Surg 90:399, 1985.
156. Lewis AB, Freed MA, Heymann MA: Side effects of therapy with prostaglandin E1 in infants with critical congenital heart disease. Circulation 64:893, 1981.
157. Donahoo JS, Roland JM, Ken J: Prostaglandin E1 as an adjunct to emergency cardiac operation in neonates. J Thorac Cardiovasc Surg 81:227, 1981.
158. Moler FW, Khan AS, Meliones JN, et al: Respiratory syncytial virus morbidity and mortality estimates in congenital heart disease patients: a recent experience. Crit Care Med 20:1406, 1992.
159. Talner NS: Heart failure. In Adams FH, Emmanouilides GC (eds): Moss' Heart Diseases in Infants, Children and Adolescents. Baltimore, Williams & Wilkins, 1983, p 708.
160. Jonas RA, Lang P, Mayer JE, Castaneda AR: The importance of prostaglandin E1 in resuscitation of the neonate with critical aortic stenosis. J Thorac Cardiovasc Surg 89:314, 1985.
161. Norwood WI, Lang P, Hansen DD: Physiologic repair of aortic atresia-hypoplastic left heart syndrome. N Engl J Med 308:23, 1983.
162. Jonas RA, Hansen DD, Cook N, Wessel D: Anatomical subtype and survival after reconstructive surgery for hypoplastic left heart syndrome. J Thorac Cardiovasc Surg 107:1121, 1994.
163. Gidding SS: Pulse oximetry in cyanotic congenital heart disease. Am J Cardiol 70:391, 1992.
164. Schmitt HJ, Schuetz WH, Proeschel PA, Jaklin C: Accuracy of pulse oximetry in children with cyanotic congenital heart disease. J Cardiothorac Vasc Anesth 7:61, 1993.
165. Haessler R, Brandl F, Zeller M, et al: Continuous intra-arterial oximetry, pulse oximetry, and co-oximetry during cardiac surgery. J Cardiothorac Vasc Anesth 6:668, 1993.
166. Tyson JE, deSa DJ, Moore S: Thromboatheromatous complications of arterial catheterization in the newborn period. Arch Dis Child 51:744, 1976.
167. Glenski JA, Beynen FM, Brady J: A prospective evaluation of femoral arterial monitoring in pediatric patients. Anesthesiology 66:227, 1987.
168. Butt WW, Gow R, Whyte H: Complications resulting from use of arterial catheters: retrograde flow and rapid elevation in blood pressure. Pediatrics 76:250, 1985.
169. Andropoulos DB, Ayres NA, Stayer SA, et al: The effect of transesophageal echocardiography on ventilation in small infants undergoing cardiac surgery. Anesth Analg 90:47, 2000.
170. DiCarlo JV, Raphaely RC, Steven JM, et al: Pulmonary mechanics in infants after cardiac surgery. Crit Care Med 20:22, 1992.
171. Gold JP, Jonas RA, Lang P, et al: Transthoracic intracardiac monitoring lines in pediatric surgical patients: a ten-year experience. Ann Thorac Surg 42:185, 1986.
172. Lang P, Chipman CW, Siden H: Early assessment of hemodynamic status after 24 hours (intensive care unit) and one year postoperative data in 98 patients. Am J Cardiol 49:1733, 1982.
173. Muhiudeen IA, Roberson DA, Silverman NH, et al: Intraoperative echocardiography for evaluation of congenital heart defects in infants and children. Anesthesiology 165:172, 1992.
174. Hsu YH, Santulli T, Wong AL, et al: Impact of intraoperative echocardiography on surgical management of congenital heart disease. Am J Cardiol 67:1279, 1991.
175. Weintraub R, Shiota T, Elkadi T, et al: Transesophageal echocardiography in infants and children with congenital heart disease. Circulation 86:711, 1992.
176. Kronik G, Mosslacher H: Positive contrast echocardiography in patients with patent foramen ovale and normal right heart hemodynamics. Am J Cardiol 49:1806, 1984.
177. Moorthy SS, Dierdorf SF, Krishna G: Transient hypoxemia from a transient right-to-left shunt in a child during emergence from anesthesia. Anesthesiology 66:234, 1987.
178. Saiman L, Prince A, Gersony WM: Pediatric infective endocarditis in the modern era. J Pediatr 122:847, 1993.
179. Levison ME, Abrutyn E: Infective endocarditis: current guidelines on prophylaxis. Curr Infect Dis Rep 1:119, 1999.
180. Dajani AS, Bisno AL, Chung KJ: Prevention of bacterial endocarditis: recommendations by the American Heart Association. JAMA 264:2919, 1990.
181. Edelman NH, Lahiri S, Braudo L: The blunted ventilatory response to hypoxia in cyanotic congenital heart disease. N Engl J Med 282:405, 1970.
182. Tanner GE, Angers DG, Barash PG: Effect of left-to-right, mixed left-to-right, and right-to-left shunts on inhalational anesthetic induction in children. Anesth Analg 64:101, 1985.
183. Anand KJS, Brown MJ, Bloom SR: Studies on the hormonal regulation of fuel metabolism in the human newborn infant undergoing anaesthesia and surgery. Horm Res 22:115, 1985.
184. Tanner G, Angers D, Barash PG: Does a left to right shunt speed the induction of inhalation anesthesia in congenital heart disease? [abstract]. Anesthesiology 57:A427, 1982.
185. Stoelting RK, Longnecker DE: The effect of right-to-left shunt on the rate of increase of arterial anesthetic concentration. Anesthesiology 36:352, 1972.
186. Hensley FA, Larach DR, Stauffer RA, Waldhausen JA: The effect of halothane/nitrous oxide/oxygen mask induction on arterial hemo-

globin saturation in cyanotic congenital heart disease. J Cardioth-orac Vasc Anesth 1:289, 1987.

187. Greeley WJ, Bushman GA, Davis DP, Reves JG: Comparative effects of halothane and ketamine on systemic arterial oxygen saturation in children with cyanotic heart disease. Anesthesiology 65:666, 1986.

188. Laishley RS, Burrows FA, Lerman J, Roy WL: Effect of anesthetic induction regimens on oxygen saturation in cyanotic congenital geart disease. Anesthesiology 65:673, 1986.

189. Friesen RH, Lichtor JL: Cardiovascular depression during halothane induction in infants: a study of three induction techniques. Anesth Analg 61:42, 1982.

190. Friesen RH, Lichtor JL: Cardiovascular effects of inhalation induction with isoflurane in infants. Anesth Analg 62:411, 1983.

191. Barash PG, Glanz S, Katz JD: Ventricular function in children during halothane anesthesia: an echocardiographic evaluation. Anesthesiology 49:79, 1978.

192. Lynch C: Differential depression of myocardial activity by halothane and isoflurane in vitro. Anesthesiology 64:620, 1986.

193. Murray PA, Stuart RS, Fraser CD Jr, et al: Acute and chronic pulmonary vasoconstriction after left lung autotransplantation in conscious dogs. J Appl Physiol 73:603, 1992.

194. Lavoie J, Walsh EP, Burrows FA, et al: The effects of propofol or isoflurane anesthesia on cardiac conduction in children undergoing radiofrequency catheter ablation for tachydysrrhythmias. Anesthesiology 82:884, 1995.

195. Zimmerman AA, Ibrahim AE, Epstein MR, et al: The effects of halothane and sevoflurane on cardiac electrophysiology in children undergoing radiofrequency catheter ablation. Anesthesiology 87:A1066, 1997.

196. Guyton RA, Andrews MJ, Hickey PR: The contribution of atrial contraction to right heart function before and after right heart ventriculotomy. J Thorac Cardiovasc Surg 71:1, 1976.

197. Moore RA, McNicholas KW, Gallagher JD: Halothane metabolism in acyanotic and cyanotic patients undergoing open heart surgery. Anesth Analg 65:1257, 1986.

198. Holzman RS, van der Velde ME, Kaus SJ, et al: Sevoflurane depresses myocardial contractility less than halothane during induction of anesthesia in children. Anesthesiology 85:1260, 1996.

199. Blayney MR, Malins AF, Cooper GM: Cardiac arrhythmias in children during outpatient general anesthesia for dentistry: a prospective randomized trial. Lancet 354:1864, 1999.

200. Sharpe MD, Cuillerier DJ, Lee JK, et al: Sevoflurane has no effect on sinoatrial node function or on normal atrioventricular and accessary pathway conduction in Wolff-Parkinson-White syndrome during alfentanil/midazolam anesthesia. Anesthesiology 90:60, 1999.

201. Ebert TJ, Muzi M: Sympathetic hyperreactivity during desflurane anesthesia in healthy volunteers. Anesthesiology 79:444, 1993.

202. Mehta M, Sokoll MD, Gergis SD: Effects of venous air embolism on the cardiovascular system and acid base balance in the presence and absence of nitrous oxide. Acta Anaesthesiol Scand 28:266, 1984.

203. Schulte-Sasse U, Hess W, Tarnow J: Pulmonary vascular responses to nitrous oxide in patients with normal and high pulmonary vascular resistance. Anesthesiology 57:9, 1982.

204. Lappas DG, Buckley MJ, Laver MB: Left ventricular performance and pulmonary circulation following addition of nitrous oxide to morphine during coronary-artery surgery. Anesthesiology 43:61, 1975.

205. Hilgenberg JC, McCammon RL, Stoelting RK: Pulmonary and systemic vascular responses to nitrous oxide in patients with mitral stenosis and pulmonary hypertension. Anesth Analg 59:323, 1980.

206. Hickey PR, Hansen DD, Strafford M, Thompson JE: Pulmonary and systemic hemodynamic effects of nitrous oxide in infants with normal and elevated pulmonary vascular resistance. Anesthesiology 65:374, 1986.

207. Lawler PGP, Nunn JF: A reassessment of the validity of the isoshunt graph. Br J Anaesth 56:1325, 1984.

208. Bokesch PM, Ziemer G, Castaneda AR, Wilson JM: The influence of right-to-left cardiac shunt on lidocaine pharmacokinetics. Anesthesiology 67:739, 1987.

209. Levin RM, Seleny FL, Streczyn MV: Ketamine-pancuronium-narcotic technique for cardiovascular surgery in infants—a comparative study. Anesth Analg 54:800, 1975.

210. Vaughan RW, Stephen MD: Ketamine for corrective cardiac surgery in children. South Med J 66:1226, 1973.

211. Gassner S, Cohen M, Aygen M: The effect of ketamine on pulmonary artery pressure: an experimental and clinical study. Anaesthesia 29:141, 1974.

212. Faithfull NS, Haider R: Ketamine for cardiac catheterization: an evaluation of its use in children. Anaesthesia 26:318, 1971.

213. Hickey PR, Hansen DD, Cramolini GM: Pulmonary and systemic hemodynamic responses to ketamine in infants with normal and elevated pulmonary vascular resistance. Anesthesiology 62:287, 1985.

214. Coppel DL, Dundee JW: Ketamine anesthesia for cardiac catheterization. Anaesthesia 27:25, 1972.

215. Lebovic S, Reich DL, Steinberg LG, et al: Comparison of propofol versus ketamine for anesthesia in pediatric patients undergoing cardiac catheterization. Anesth Analg 490:494, 1992.

216. Robinson S, Gregory GA: Fentanyl-air-oxygen anesthesia for ligation of patent ductus arteriosus in preterm infants. Anesth Analg 60:331, 1981.

217. Hickey PR, Hansen DD: Fentanyl- and sufentanil-oxygen-pancuronium anesthesia for cardiac surgery in infants. Anesth Analg 63:117, 1984.

218. Moore RA, Yang SS, McNicholas KW: Hemodynamic and anesthetic effects of sufentanil as the sole anesthetic for pediatric cardiovascular surgery. Anesthesiology 62:725, 1985.

219. Davis PJ, Cook DR, Stiller RL: Pharmacodynamics and pharmacokinetics of high-dose sufentanil in infants and children undergoing cardiac surgery. Anesth Analg 66:203, 1987.

220. Hansen DD, Hickey PR: Anesthesia for hypoplastic left heart syndrome: high dose fentanyl in 30 neonates. Anesth Analg 65:127, 1986.

221. den Hollander JD, Hennis PJ, Burm AGL, et al: Pharmacokinetics of alfentanil before and after cardiopulmonary bypass in pediatric patients undergoing cardiac surgery: part I. J Cardiothorac Vasc Anesth 6:308, 1992.

222. Yaster M: The dose response to fentanyl in neonatal anesthesia. Anesthesiology 66:433, 1987.

223. Katz R, Kelly HW: Pharmacokinetics of continuous infusions of fentanyl in critically ill children. Crit Care Med 21:995, 1993.

224. Leuschen MP, WIllett LD, Hoie EB, et al: Plasma fentanyl levels in infants undergoing extracorporeal membrane oxygenation. J Thorac Cardiovasc Surg 105:885, 1993.

225. Pokela ML, Ryhänen PT, Koivisto ME, et al: Alfentanil-induced rigidity in newborn infants. Anesth Analg 75:252, 1992.

226. Wood M, Shand DG, Wood AJ: The sympathetic response to profound hypothermia and circulatory arrest in infants. Can Anaesth Soc J 27:125, 1980.

227. Firmin RK, Bouloux P, Allen P, et al: Sympathoadrenal function during cardiac operations in infants with the technique of surface cooling, limited cardiopulmonary bypass, and circulatory arrest. J Thorac Cardiovasc Surg 90:729, 1985.

228. Koren G, Goresky G, Crean P: Pediatric fentanyl dosing based on pharmacokinetics during cardiac surgery. Anesthesiology 63:577, 1984.

229. Philips AA, McLean RF, Devitt JH, et al: Recall of intraoperative events after general anesthesia and cardiopulmonary events after general anesthesia and cardiopulmonary bypass. Can J Anaesth 40:922, 1993.

230. Dowd NP, Cheng DCH, Karski JM, et al: Intraoperative awareness in fast-track cardiac anesthesia. Anesthesiology 89:1068, 1998.

231. Lynn AM: Editorial. Remifentanil: the paediatric anaesthetist's opiate? Paediatr Anaesth 6:433, 1996.

232. Davis PJ, Wilson AS, Siewers RD, et al: The effects of cardiopulmonary bypass on remifentanil kinetics in children undergoing atrial septal defect repair. Anesth Analg 89:904, 1999.

233. Morgan P, Lynn AM, Parrot C, Morray JP: Hemodynamic and metaboic effects of two anesthetic techniques in children undergoing surgical repair of acyanotic congenital heart disease. Anesth Analg 66:1028, 1987.

234. Barankay A, Richter JA, Henze R, et al: Total intravenous anesthesia for infants and children undergoing correction of tetralogy of Fallot: sufentanil versus sufentanil-flunitrazepam technique. J Cardiothorac Vasc Anesth 6:185, 1992.

235. Ostwald P, Doenicke AW: Etomidate revisited. Anesthesiology 11:391, 1998.

236. Maunuksela EL, Gattiker RI: Use of pancuronium in children with congenital heart disease. Anesth Analg 60:798, 1981.

237. Cabal LA, Siassi B, Artal R: Cardiovascular and catecholamine changes after administration of pancuronium in distressed neonates. Pediatrics 75:284, 1985.

238. Goudsouzian NG, Liu LMP, Savarese JJ: Metocurine in infants and children. Anesthesiology 49:266, 1978.

239. Goudsouzian NG, Martyn JJA, Liu LMP, Gionfriddo M: Safety and efficacy of vecuronium in adolescents and children. Anesth Analg 62:1083, 1983.

240. Goudsouzian NG, Liu LMP, Cote CJ: Safety and efficacy of atracurium in adolescents and children anesthetized with halothane. Anesthesiology 59:459, 1983.

241. Fisher DM: Neuromuscular blocking agents in paediatric anesthesia. Br J Anaesth 83:58, 1999.

242. Lister G, Talner N: Management of respiratory failure of cardiac origin. In Gregory GA (ed): Respiratory Failure in the Child. New York, Churchill Livingstone, 1981, p 67.

243. Jenkins J, Lynn A, Edmonds J, Barker GA: Effects of mechanical ventilation on cardiopulmonary function in children after open-heart surgery. Crit Care Med 13:77, 1985.

244. Robotham JL, Lixfeld W, Holland L, et al: The effects of positive end-expiratory pressure on right and left ventricular performance. Am Rev Respir Dis 121:677, 1980.

245. Pinski MR, Summer WR, Wise RA, et al: Augmentation of cardiac function by elevation of intra-thoracic pressure. J Appl Physiol 54:950, 1983.

246. Parker JC, Hernandez LA, Peevy KJ: Mechanisms of ventilator induced lung injury. Crit Care Med 21:132, 1993.

247. Elliot MJ: Ultrafiltration and modified ultrafiltration in pediatric open heart operations. Ann Thorac Surg 56:1518, 1993.

248. Verrier EW, Boyle EM: Endothelial cell injury in cardiovascular surgery: an overview. Ann Throrac Surg 64:S2, 1997.

249. Hall RI, Smith MS, Rocker G: Systemic inflammatory response to cardiopulmonary bypass: pathophysiological, therapeutic and pharmacological considerations. Anesth Analg 85:766, 1997.

250. Wernovsky G, Wypij D, Jonas RA, et al: Postoperative course and hemodynamic profile after the arterial switch operation in neonates and infants: a comparison of low-flow cardiopulmonary bypass versus circulatory arrest. Circulation 92:2226, 1995.

251. Yndgaard S, Andersen LW, Andersen C, et al: The effect of modified ultrafiltration on the amount of circulating endotoxin in children undergoing cardiopulmonary bypass. J Cardiothorac Vasc Anesth 14:399, 2000.

252. Journois D, Israel-Biet D, Pouard P, et al: High-volume, zero-balanced hemofiltration to reduce delayed inflammatory response to cardiopulmonary bypass in children. Anesthesiology 85:965, 1996.

253. Chaturvedi RR, Shore DF, Whilte PA, et al: Modified ultrafiltration improves global left ventricular systolic function after open-heart surgery in infants and children. Eur J Cardiothorac Surg 15:742, 1999.

254. Elliot M: Modified ultrafiltration and open heart surgery in children. Paediatr Anaesth 9:1, 1999.

255. Keenan HT, Thiagarajan R, Stephens KE, et al: Pulmonary function after modified venovenous ultrafiltration in infants: a prospective, randomized trial. J Thorac Cardiovasc Surg 119:501, 2000.

256. Hickey PR, Andersen NP: Deep hypothermic circulatory arrest: a review of pathophysiology and clinical experience as a basis for anesthetic management. J Cardiothorac Anesth 1:137, 1987.

257. Fox LS, Blackstone EH, Kirklin JW, et al: Relationship of brain blood flow and oxygen consumption to perfusion flow rate during profoundly hypothermic cardiopulmonary bypass. J Thorac Cardiovasc Surg 87:658, 1984.

258. Miyamoto K, Kawashima Y, Matsuda H: Optimal perfusion flow rate for the brain during deep hypothermic cardiopulmonary bypass at 20°C. J Thorac Cardiovasc Surg 92:1065, 1986.

259. Swain JA, McDonald TJ, Griffith PK, et al: Low flow hypothermic cardiopulmonary bypass protects the brain. J Thorac Cardiovasc Surg 102:76, 1991.

260. Munoz R, Laussen PC, Palacio G, et al: Changes in whole blood lactate levels during cardiopulmonary bypass for surgery for congenital cardiac disease: an early indicator of moridity and mortality. J Thorac Cardiovasc Surg 119:155, 2000.

261. du Plessis AJ: Neurologic complications of cardiac disease in the newborn. Clin Perinat 24:807, 1997.

262. Greeley WJ, Kern FH, Ungerleider RM, et al: The effect of hypothermic cardiopulmonary bypass and total circulatory arrest on cerebral metabolism in neonates, infants and children. J Thorac Cardiovasc Surg 101:783, 1991.

263. Slogoff ST, Girgis KZ, Keats AS: Etiologic factors in neuro-psychiatric complications associated with cardiopulmonary bypass. Anesth Analg 61:903, 1982.

264. Bellinger DC, Wernovsky G, Rappaport LA, et al: Cognitive development of children following early repair of transposition of the great arteries using deep hypothermic circulation arrest. Pediatrics 87:701, 1991.

265. Kern FH, Jonas RA, Mayer JE, et al: Temperature monitoring in infants during CPB: does it predict efficient brain cooling? Ann Thorac Surg 54:749, 1992.

266. Mault JR, Ohtake S, Klingensmith ME, et al: Cerebral metabolism and circulatory arrest: effects of duration and strategies for protection. Ann Thorac Surg 103:363, 1993.

267. Rogers AT, Prough DS, Roy RC, et al: Cerebrovascular and cerebral metabolic effects of alterations in perfusion flow rate during hypothermic cardiopulmonary bypass in man. J Thorac Cardiovasc Surg 103:363, 1992.

268. du Plessis AJ, Jonas RA, Wypij D, et al: Perioperative effects of alpha-stat versus pH-stat strategies for deep hypothermic cardiopulmonary bypass in infants. J Thorac Cardiovasc Surg 114:991, 1997.

269. Jonas RA: Optimal pH strategy for cardiopulmonary bypass in neonates, infants and children. Perfusion 13:377, 1998.

270. Shin'oka T, Shum-Tim D, Laussen PC, et al: Effects of oncotic pressure and hematocrit on outcome after hypothermic circulatory arrest. Ann Thorac Surg 65:155, 1998.

271. Shin'oka T, Shum-Tim D, Jonas RA, et al: Higher hematocrit improves cerebral outcome after deep hypothermic circulatory arrest. J Thorac Cardiovas Surg 112:1610, 1996.

272. Bellinger D, Jonas RA, Rappaport L, et al: Developmental and neurologic status of children after heart surgery with hypothermic circulatory arrest or low-flow cardiopulmonary bypass. N Engl J Med 332:540, 1995.

273. Shum-Tim D, Nagashima M, Shin'oka T, et al: Post ischemic hyperthermia exacerbates neurologic injury after deep hypothermic circulatory arrest. J Thorac Cardiovasc Surg 116:780, 1998.

274. Kern FH, Morana NJ, Sears JJ: Coagulation defects in neonates during cardiopulmonary bypass. Ann Thorac Surg 54:541, 1992.

275. Manno CS, Herdberg KW, Kim HC: Comparison of the hemostatic effects of fresh whole blood, stored whole blood and components after open heart surgery in children. Blood 77:930, 1991.

276. Ruckman RN, Keane JF, Freed MD: Sedation for cardiac catheterization: a controlled study. Pediatr Cardiol 1:263, 1980.

277. Landzberg MJ, Lock JE: Transcatheter closure of cardiac defects. In Barness LA (ed): Advances in Pediatrics. St Louis, Mosby, 1993, p 247.

278. Lock JE, Keane JF, Perry SB: Diagnostic and Interventional Catheterization in Congenital Heart Disease. Norwell, MA, Kluwer Academic Publishers, 1999.

279. Rome JJ: The role of catheter directed therapies in the treatment of congenital heart disease. Annu Rev Med 46:159, 1995.

280. Wessel DL, Keane JF, Parness I, Lock JE: Outpatient closure of the patent ductus arteriosus. Circulation 77:1068, 1988.

281. Bridges ND, Lock JE, Castaneda AR: Baffle fenestration with subsequent transcatheter closure: modification of the Fontan operation for patients at increased risk. Circulation 82:1681, 1990.

282. Baker CM, McGowan FX, Keane JF, Lock JE: Pulmonary artery trauma due to balloon dilation: recognition, avoidance and management. J Am Coll Cardiol 36:1684, 2000.

283. Laussen PC, Hansen DD, Perry SB, et al: Transcatheter closure of ventricular septal defect: hemodynamic instability and anesthetic management. Anesth Analg 80:1076, 1995.

284. Tanel RE, Walsh EP, Triedman JK, et al: Five-year experience with radiofrequency catheter ablation: implications for management of arrhythmias in pediatric and young adult patients. J Pediatr 131:878, 1997.

285. Schaffer MS, Snyder AM, Morrison JE. An assessment of desflurane for use during cardiac electrophysiologic study and radiofrequency ablation of supraventricular dysrhythmias in children. Paediatr Anaesth 10:155, 2000.

286. Clarkson PM, MacArthur BA, Barratt-Boyes BG: Development progress after cardiac surgery in infancy using hypothermia and circulatory arrest. Circulation 62:855, 1980.

287. Castaneda AR, Freed MD, Williams RG: Repair of tetralogy of Fallot in infancy. J Thorac Cardiovasc Surg 74:372, 1977.

288. Parr GV, Blockstone EH, Kirklin JW: Cardiac performance and mortality early after intracardiac surgery in infants and young children. Circulation 51:867, 1975.

289. Castaneda AR, Lamberti J, Sade RM: Open-heart surgery during the first three months of life. J Thorac Cardiovasc Surg 68:719, 1974.

290. Sade RM, Williams RG, Castaneda AR: Corrective surgery for congenital cardiovascular defects in early infancy. Am Heart J 90:656, 1975.

291. Kirklin JK, Blackstone EH, Kirklin JW, et al: Intracardiac surgery in infants under age 3 months: incremental risk factors for hospital mortality. Am J Cardiol 48:500, 1981.

292. Kirklin JK, Blackstone EH, Kirklin JW, et al: Intracardiac surgery in infants under 3 months: predictors of postoperative in hospital cardiac death. Am J Cardiol 48:507, 1981.

293. Macaartney FJ, Taylor JFN, Graham GR: The fate of survivors of cardiac surgery in infancy. Circulation 62:80, 1980.

294. Malcic I, Sauer U, Stern H, et al: The influence of pulmonary artery banding on outcome after the Fontan operation. J Thorac Cardiovasc Surg 104:743, 1992.

295. Blalock A, Taussig HB: The surgical treatment of malformations of the heart in which there is pulmonary stenosis or pulmonary atresia. JAMA 128:189, 1945.

296. Edmunds LH, Stephenson LW, Gadzik JP: The Blalock-Taussig anastomosis in infants younger than 1 week of age. Circulation 62:597, 1980.

297. Arciniegas E, Farooki ZQ, Hakimi M: Classic shunting operations for cyanotic congenital heart defects. J Thorac Cardiovasc Surg 84:88, 1982.

298. Aberdeen E: The Waterston operation: ascending aorta-right pulmonary artery anastomosis. In Smith RC (ed): Operative Surgery. Vol 2: Thorax. London, Butterworth, 1968, p 234.

299. Glenn WWL: The Glenn operation: superior vena cava-pulmonary artery anastomosis. In Smith RC (ed): Operative Surgery. Vol 2: Thorax. London, Butterworth, 1968, p 240.

300. Trusler GA, Williams WG: Long-term results of the Glenn procedure for tricuspid atresia. In Kidd BSL, Rowe RD (eds): The Child with Congenital Heart Disease after Surgery. New York, Futura, 1976, p 79.

301. De Leval MR, Kilner P, Gewillig M, Bull C: Total cavopulmonary connection: a logical alternative to atriopulmonary connection for complex Fontan operations. J Thorac Cardiovasc Surg 96:682, 1988.

302. Trusler GA, Williams WG, Choen AJ, et al: The cavopulmonary shunt. Evolution of a concept. Circulation 82(suppl IV):IV-131, 1990.

303. Hopkins RA, Armstrong BE, Serwer GA, et al: Physiological rationale for a bidirectional cavopulmonary shunt. A versatile complement to the Fontan principle. J Thorac Cardiovasc Surg 90:391, 1985.

304. Chang AC, Hanley FL, Wernovsky G, et al: Early bidirectional cavopulmonary shunt in young infants: postoperative course and early results. Circulation 88:II-149, 1993.

305. Albanese SB, Carotti A, Di Donato RM, et al: Bidirectional cavopulmonary anastomosis in patients under two years of age. J Thorac Cardiovasc Surg 104:904, 1992.

306. Di Donato RM, Amodeo A, di Carlo DD, et al: Staged Fontan operation for complex cardiac anomalies with subaortic obstruction. J Thorac Cardiovasc Surg 105:398, 1993.

307. Casthely PA, Redko V, Dluzneski J, et al: Pulse oximetry during pulmonary artery banding. J Cardiothorac Vasc Anesth 1:297, 1987.

308. Gates RN, Laks H, Elami A, et al: Damus-Stansel-Kaye procedure: current indications and results. Ann Thorac Surg 56:111, 1993.

309. Freedom RM, Benson LN, Smallhorn JF, et al: Subaortic stenosis, the univentricular heart, and banding of the pulmonary artery: an analysis of the course of 43 patients with univentricular heart palliated by pulmonary artery banding. Circulation 73:757, 1986.

310. Fontan F, Baudet E: Surgical repair of tricuspid atresia. Thorax 26:240, 1971.

311. Fontan F: Repair of tricuspid atresia-surgical considerations and results. In Anderson RH, Shinebourne EA (eds): Paediatric Cardiology 1977. Edinburgh, Churchill Livingstone, 1978, p 567.

312. Gale AW, Danielson GK, McGoon DC, Mair DD: Modified Fontan operation for univentricular heart and complicated congenital lesions. J Thorac Cardiovasc Surg 78:831, 1979.

313. Castaneda AR: From Glenn to Fontan: a continuing evolution. Circulation 86:II80, 1992.

314. Fontan F, Kirklin JW, Fernandez G, et al: The outcome after a "perfect" Fontan operation. Circulation 81:1520, 1990.

315. Driscoll DJ, Offord KP, Feldt RH, et al: Five- to fifteen year follow-up after Fontan operation. Circulation 85:468, 1992.

316. Gentles TL, Mayer JE Jr, Gauvreau K, et al: Fontan operation in five hundred consecutive patients: factors influencing early and late outcome. J Thorac Cardiovasc Surg 114:376, 1997.

317. Fontan F, Deville C, Quagebeur J: Repair of tricuspid atresia in 100 patients. J Thorac Cardiovasc Surg 85:647, 1983.

318. Kreutzer GO, Florentino JV, Schlichter AJ: Atriopulmonary anastomosis. J Thorac Cardiovasc Surg 83:427, 1982.

319. Jonas RA, Castaneda AR: Atrial baffle and systemic venous to pulmonary artery anastomotic techniques. J Card Surg 3:91, 1988.

320. Nakazawa M, Nakanishi T, Okuda H: Dynamics of right heart flow in patients after Fontan procedure. Circulation 2:306, 1984.

321. Kurer CC, Tanner CS, Norwood WI, Vetter VL: Perioperative arrhythmias after Fontan repair. Circulation 82:IV-190, 1990.

322. Laks H: The partial Fontan procedure. A new concept and its clinical application. Circulation 82:1866, 1990.

323. Mayer JE, Helgason H, Jonas RA, et al: Extending the limits of modified Fontan procedures. J Thorac Cardiovasc Surg 92:1021, 1986.

324. Marcelletti CF, Hanley FL, Mavroudis C, et al: Revision of previous Fontan connections to total extracardiac cavopulmonary anastomosis: a multicenter experience. J Thorac Cardiovasc Surg 119:340, 2000.

325. Myers JL, Waldhausen JA, Weber HS, et al: A reconsideration of risk factors for the Fontan opearion. Ann Surg 211:738, 1990.

326. Mayer JE, Bridges ND, Lock JE, et al: Factors associated with marked reduction in mortality for Fontan operations in patients with single ventricle. J Thorac Cardiovasc Surg 103:444, 1992.

327. Seliem MA, Baffa JM, Vetter JM, et al: Changes in right ventricular geometry and heart rate early after hemi-Fontan procedure. Ann Thorac Surg 55:1508, 1993.

328. Penny DJ, Lincoln C, Shore DF, et al: The early response of the systemic ventricle during transition to the Fontan circulation—an acute hypertrophic cardiomyopathy? Cardiol Young 2:78, 1992.

329. Penny DJ, Redington AN: Doppler echocardiographic evaluation of pulmonary blood flow after the Fontan operation: the role of the lungs. Br Heart J 66:372, 1991.

330. Kreutzer J, Lock JE, Jonas RA, Keane JF: Transcatheter fenestration dilation and/or creation in postoperative Fontan patients. Am J Cardiol 79:228, 1997.

331. Triedman JK, Bridges ND, Mayer JE, Lock JE: Prevalence and risk factors for aortopulmonary collateral vessels after Fontan and bidirectional Glenn procedures. J Am Coll Cardiol 22:207, 1993.

332. Balaji S, Gewillig M, Bull C, et al: Arrhythmias after the Fontan procedure. Comparison of total cavopulmonary connection and atriopulmonary connection. Circulation 84(suppl III):III-162, 1991.

333. Gewillig M, Wyse RK, DeLeval MR: Early and late arrhythmias after the Fontan operation: predisposing factors and clinical consequences. Br Heart J 67:72, 1992.

334. Fishberger SB, Wernovsky G, Gentles TL, et al: Factors that influence the development of atrial flutter after the Fontan operation. J Thorac Cardiovasc Surg 113:80, 1997.

335. Cetta F, Feldt RH, O'Leary PW, et al: Improved early morbidity and mortality after Fontan operation: the Mayo Clinic experience. J Am Coll Cardiol 28:480, 1996.

336. du Plessis AJ, Chang AC, Wessel DL, et al: Cerebrovascular accidents following the Fontan procedure. Pediatr Neurol 12:230, 1995.

337. Cromme-Dijkhuis AH, Henkens CM, Bijleveld CMA, et al: Coagulation factor abnormalitites as possible thrombotic risk factors after Fontan operations. Lancet 336:1087, 1990.

338. Shachar GB, Fuhrman BP, Wang Y: Rest and exercise hemodynamics after the Fontan procedure. Circulation 65:1043, 1982.

339. Sanders SP, Wright GB, Keane JF: Clinical and hemodynamic results of the Fontan operation for tricuspid atresia. Am J Cardiol 49:1733, 1982.

340. Nir A, Driscoll DJ, Mottram CD, et al: Cardiorespiratory response to exercise after the Fontan operation: a serial study. J Am Coll Cardiol 22:216, 1993.

341. Gewillig MH, Lundstrom UR, Bull C, et al: Exercise responses in patients with congenital heart disease after Fontan repair: patterns and determinants of performance. J Am Coll Cardiol 15:1424, 1990.

342. Harrison DA, Liu P, Walters JE, et al: Cardiopulmonary function in adults late after Fontan repair. J Am Coll Cardiol 26:1016, 1995.

343. Karl TR, Sano S, Pornviliwan S, et al: Tetralogy of Fallot: favorable outcome of non-neonatal transatrial, transpulmonary repair. Ann Thorac Surg 54:903, 1992.

344. Di Donato DM, Jonas RA, Lang P, et al: Neonatal repair of tetralogy of Fallot with and without pulmonary atresia. J Thorac Cardiovasc Surg 101:126, 1991.

345. Pigula FA, Khalil PN, Mayer JE, et al: Repair of tetralogy of Fallot in neonates and young infants. Circulation 100:57, 1999.

346. Rocchini AP, Rosenthal A, Freed MD: Repair of tetralogy of Fallot. Circulation 56:305, 1977.

347. Fellows KE, Freed MD, Keane JF: Results of preoperative coronary angiography in tetralogy of Fallot. Circulation 51:561, 1975.

348. Dabizzi RP, Capriolo G, Aiazzi L: Distribution and anomalies of coronary arteries in tetralogy of Fallot. Circulation 61:95, 1980.

349. Shabbo FP, Wain WH, Ross DN: Right ventricular outflow reconstruction with aortic homograft conduit: analysis of the long-term results. Thorac Cardiovasc Surg 28:21, 1980.

350. Cullen S, Shore D, Redington AN: Characterization of right ventricular diastolic performance after complete repair of tetralogy of Fallot. Circulation 91:1782, 1995.

351. Redington AN, Penny DJ, Rigby ML: Antegrade diastolic pulmonary arterial flow as a marker of right ventricular restriction after complete repair of pulmonary atresia with intact ventricular septum and critical pulmonary valve stenosis. Cardiol Young 2:382, 1992.

352. Borrow KM, Green LH, Castenda AR: Left ventricular function after repair of tetralogy of Fallot and its relationship to age at surgery. Circulation 61:1150, 1980.

353. Reduto LA, Berger HJ, Johnstone DE: Radionuclide assessment of right and left ventricular exercise reserve after total correction of tetralogy of Fallot. J Thorac Cardiovasc Surg 85:691, 1983.

354. Bove EL, Byrum CJ, Thomas FD: The influence of pulmonary insufficiency on ventricular function following repair of tetralogy of Fallot. J Thorac Cardiovasc Surg 85:691, 1983.

355. Murphy JD, Freed MD, Keane JF: Hemodynamic results after intracardiac repair of tetralogy of Fallot by deep hypothermia and cardiopulmonary and cardiopulmonary bypass. Circulation 62:1168, 1980.

356. Guntheroth WG, Kawabori I, Baum D: Tetralogy of Fallot. In Adams FH, Emmanouilides GC (eds): Moss' Heart Disease in Infants, Children, and Adolescents. Baltimore, Williams & Wilkins, 1983, p 215.

357. Murphy JG, Gersh BJ, Mair DD, et al: Long-term outcome in patients undergoing surgical repair of tetralogy of Fallot. N Engl J Med 329:593, 1993.

358. Nollert G, Fischlein T, Bouterwek S, et al: Long term survival in patients with repair of tetralogy of Fallot: 36 year-old follow-up of the first year after surgical repair. J Am Coll Cardiol 30:1374, 1997.

359. Carvalho JS, Shineburne EA, Busst C, et al: Exercise capacity after complete repair of tetralogy of Fallot: deleterious effects of residual pulmonary regurgitation. Br Heart J 67:470, 1992.

360. Gatzoulis MA, Balaji S, Webber SA, et al: Risk factors for arrhythmia and sudden cardiac death late after repair of tetralogy of Fallot: a multicentre study. Lancet 356:975, 2000.

361. Chandar JS, Wolff GS, Garson A, et al: Ventricular arrhythmia in postoperative tetralogy of Fallot. Am J Cardiol 65:655, 1990.

362. Deanfield JE, McKenna WJ, Presbitero P, et al: Ventricular arrhythmia in unrepaired and repaired tetralogy of Fallot. Br Heart J 52:77, 1984.

363. Arie PY, Marcon F, Brunotte F, et al: Right ventricular overload and induced sustained ventricular tachycardia in operatively "unrepaired" tetralogy of Fallot. Am J Cardiol 69:785, 1992.

364. Hanley FL, Sade RM, Blackstone EH, et al: Outcomes in neonatal pulmonary atresia with intact ventricular septum. J Thorac Cardiovasc Surg 105:406, 1993.

365. Hawkins JA, Thorne JK, Boucek MM, et al: Early and late results in pulmonary atresia and intact ventricular septum. J Thorac Cardiovasc Surg 100:492, 1990.

366. Giglia TM, Mandell VS, Connor AR, et al: Diagnosis and management of right ventricle—dependent coronary circulation in pulmonary atresia with intact ventricular septum. Circulation 86:1516, 1992.

367. Silver MM, Pollock J, Silver MD: Calcification in porcine xenograft valves in children. Am J Cardiol 45:685, 1985.

368. Heck HA, Schieken RM, Lauer RM, Doty DB: Conduit repair for complex congenital heart disease. J Thorac Cardiovasc Surg 75:806, 1978.

369. Otero Coto E, Norwood WI, Lang P: Modified Senning operation for treatment of transposition of the great arteries. J Thorac Cardiovasc Surg 78:721, 1979.

370. Quaegebeur JM: Revival of the Senning operation in the treatment of transposition of the great arteries: preliminary report on recent experience. Thorax 32:517, 1977.

371. Senning A: Surgical correction of transposition of the great vessels. Surgery 45:966, 1959.

372. Senning A: Correction of the transposition of the great arteries. Ann Surg 182:287, 1975.

373. Hagler DJ, Ritter DG, Mair DD: Clinical, angiographic and hemodynamic assessment of late results after Mustard operation. Circulation 57:1214, 1978.

374. Danielson GK, Gale AW, McGraw DC: Great-vessel switch operation without coronary relocation for transposition of great arteries. Mayo Clin Proc 53:675, 1978.

375. Yacoub MH: The case for anatomic correction of transposition of the great arteries. J Thorac Cardiovasc Surg 78:3, 1979.

376. Jatene AD, Fontes VF, Souza LCB: Anatomic correction of transposition of the great arteries. J Thorac Cardiovasc Surg 83:20, 1982.

377. Castaneda AR, Norwood WI, Jonas RA: Transposition of the great arteries and intact ventricular septum: anatomical repair in the neonate. Ann Thorac Surg 38:438, 1984.

378. Pacifico AD, Stewart RW, Bargeron LM: Repair of transposition of the great arteries with ventricular septal defect by an arterial switch operation. Circulation 68:II-49, 1983.

379. Di Donato RM, Fujii AM, Jonas RA, Castaneda AR: Age-dependent ventricular response to pressure overload. Considerations for the arterial switch operation. J Thorac Cardiovasc Surg 104:713, 1992.

380. Jonas RA, Giglia TM, Sanders SP, et al: Rapid, two-stage arterial switch for transposition of the great arteries and intact ventricular septum beyond the neonatal period. Circulation 80(3 pt 1):I-203, 1989.

381. Planche C, Serraf A, Comas JV, et al: Anatomic repair of transposition of great arteries with ventricular septal defect and aortic arch obstruction. J Thorac Cardiovasc Surg 105:925, 1993.

382. Serraf A, Lacour-Gayet F, Bruniaux J, et al: Anatomic correction of transposition of the great arteries in neonates. J Am Coll Cardiol 22:193, 1993.

383. Kirklin JW, Blackstone EH, Tchervenkov CI, et al: Clinical outcomes after the arterial switch operation for transposition. Circulation 86:1501, 1992.

384. Wernovsky G, Mayer JE, Jonas RA, et al: Factors influencing early and late outcome of the arterial switch operation for transposition of the great arteries. J Thorac Cardiovasc Surg 109:289, 1995.

385. Wernovsky G, Sanders SP: Coronary artery anatomy and transposition of the great arteries. Coron Artery Dis 4:148, 1993.

386. Day RW, Laks H, Drinkwater DC: The influence of coronary anatomy on the arterial switch operation in neonates. J Thorac Cardiovasc Surg 104:706, 1992.

387. Rastelli GC, McGoon DC, Wallace RB: Anatomic correction of transposition of the great arteries with ventricular septal defect and subpulmonary stenosis. J Thorac Cardiovasc Surg 58:545, 1969.

388. Mair DD: Long-term follow-up of Mustard operation survivors. Circulation 50:II-46, 1974.

389. Williams HG, Trusler GA, Kirklin JW, et al: Early and late results of a protocol for simple transposition leading to an atrial switch Mustard repair. J Thorac Cardiovas Surg 95:717, 1988.

390. Merlo M, de Tommasi SM, Brunelli F, et al: Long term results after atrial correction of complete transposition of the great arteries. Ann Thorac Surg 51:227, 1991.

391. Graham TP, Atwood GF, Boucek RJ Jr, et al: Abnormalities of right ventricular function following Mustard's operation for transposition of the great arteries. Circulation 52:678, 1975.

392. Deanfield J, Camm J, Macartney F, et al: Arrhythmia and late mortality after Mustard and Senning operation for transposition. J Thorac Cardiovasc Surg 96:569, 1988.

393. Helbing WA, Hansen B, Ottenkamp J, et al: Long-term results of atrial correction for transposition of the great arteries. Comparison of Mustard and Senning operations. J Thorac Cardiovasc Surg 108:363, 1994.

394. Parrish MD, Graham TO, Bender HW: Radionuclide angiographic evaluation of right and left ventricular function during exercise after repair of transposition of the great arteries: comparison with normal subjects and patients with congenitally corrected transposition. Circulation 67:178, 1983.

395. Benson LN, Bonet J, McLaughlin P: Assessment of right ventricular function during supine bicycle exercise after Mustard's operation. Circulation 65:1052, 1982.

396. Gillette PC, Kugler JD, Garson A: Mechanisms of cardiac arrhythmias after Mustard operation for transposition of the great arteries. Am J Cardiol 45:1225, 1980.

397. Gelatt M, Hamilton RM, McCrindle BW, et al: Arrhythmia and mortality after the Mustard procedure: a 30 year single center experience. J Am Coll Cardiol 29:194, 1997.

398. Sagin-Saylam G, Somerville J: Palliative Mustard operation for transposition of the great arteries: late results after 15–20 years. Heart 75:72, 1996.

399. Ramsay JM, Venebales AW, Kelly MJ, et al: Right and left ventricular function at rest and with exercise after the Mustard operation for transposition of the great arteries. Br Heart J 51:364, 1984.

400. Tanel RE, Wernovsky G, Landzberg MJ, et al: Coronary artery abnormalities detected at cardiac catheterization following the arterial switch operation for transposition of the great arteries. Am J Cardiol 76:153, 1995.

401. Weindling SN, Wernovsky G, Colan SD, et al: Myocardial perfusion, function and exercise tolerance after the arterial switch operation. J Am Coll Cardiol 23:424, 1994.

402. Massin M, Hovels-Gurich H, Dabritz S, et al: Results of the Bruce Treadmill test in children after the arterial switch operation for simple transposition of the great arteries. Am J Cardiol 81:56, 1998.

403. Jenkins KJ, Hanley FL, Colan SD, et al: Function of the anatomic pulmonary valve in the systemic circulation. Circulation 84:173, 1991.

404. Rhodes LA, Wernovsky G, Keane JF, et al: Arrhythmias and intracardiac conduction after the arterial switch operation. J Thorac Cardiovasc Surg 109:303, 1995.

405. Colan SD, Boutin C, Castaneda AR, et al: Status of the left ventricle after arterial switch operation for transposition of the great arteries: hemodynamic and echocardiographic evalution. J Thorac Cardiovasc Surg 109:311, 1995.

406. Fiser B: Infradiaphragmatic total anomalous pulmonary venous drainage. J Cardiovasc Surg 20:69, 1979.

407. Raisher BD, Grant JW, Martin TC, et al: Complete repair of total anomalous pulmonary venous connection in infancy. J Thorac Cardiovasc Surg 104:443, 1992.

408. Jenkins KJ, Sanders SP, Orav EJ, et al: Individual pulmonary vein size and survival in infants with totally anomalous pulmonary venous connection. J Am Coll Cardiol 22:201, 1993.

409. Horvath KA, Burke RP, Collins JJ, Cohn LH: Surgical treatment of adult atrial septal defect: early and long term results. J Am Coll Cardiol 20:1156, 1992.

410. Collins G: Ventricular septal defect: clinical and hemodynamic changes in the first five years of life. Am Heart J 84:695, 1972.

411. Hoffman JI: Ventricular septal defect: indications for therapy in infants. Pediatr Clin North Am 18:1091, 1971.

412. DuShane JW, Kirklin JW: Late results of the repair of ventricular septal defect on pulmonary vascular disease. In Kirklin JW (ed): Advances in Cardiovascular Surgery. Orlando, FL, Grune & Stratton, 1973, p 9.

413. Friedman WF, Heiferman MF: Clinical problems of postoperative pulmonary vascular disease. Am J Cardiol 50:631, 1982.

414. Haworth SG, Sauer U, Buhlmeyer K, Reid L: Development of the pulmonary circulation in ventricular septal defect: a quantitative structural study. Am J Cardiol 40:781, 1977.

415. Vincent RN, Lang P, Elixson EM: Measurement of extravascular lung water in infants and children after cardiac surgery. Am J Cardiol 54:161, 1984.

416. Cordell D, Graham TP, Atwood GF: Left heart volume characteristics following ventricular septal closure defects in infancy. Circulation 54:417, 1976.

417. Jarmakani JM, Graham TP, Canent RV: The effect of corrective surgery on heart volume and mass in children with ventricular septal defect. Am J Cardiol 27:254, 1971.

418. Jarmakani JM, Graham TP, Canent RV: Left ventricular contractile state in children with successfully corrected ventricular septal defect. Circulation 45:I-102, 1972.

419. Jablonsky G, Hilton JD, Liu P: Rest and exercise ventricular function in adults with congenital ventricular septal defects. Am J Cardiol 51:293, 1983.

420. Mair DD, McGoon DC: Surgical correction of atrioventriular canal during the first year of life. Am J Cardiol 40:66, 1977.

421. Studer M, Blackstone EH, Kirklin JW, et al: Determinants of early and late results of repair of atrioventricular septal (canal) defects. J Thorac Cardiovasc Surg 84:523, 1982.

422. Capouya ER, Laks H, Drinkwater DC, et al: Management of the left atrioventricular valve in the repair of complete atrioventricular septal defects. J Thorac Cardiovasc Surg 104:196, 1992.

423. Rizzoli G, Mazzucco A, Maizza F, et al: Does Down syndrome affect prognosis of surgically managed atrioventricular canal defects? J Thorac Cardiovasc Surg 104:945, 1992.

424. Spach MS, Serwer GA, Anderson PAW: Pulsatile aortopulmonary pressure-flow dynamics of patent ductus arteriosus in patients with various hemodynamic states. Circulation 61:110, 1980.

425. Mahony L, Carnero V, Brett C: Prophylactic indomethacin therapy for patent ductus arteriosus in very-low-birth-weight infants. N Engl J Med 306:506, 1982.

426. Rashkind WJ, Mullins CE, Hellenbrand WE, Tait MA: Nonsurgical closure of patent ductus arteriosus: clinical application of the Rashkind PDA Occluder System. Circulation 75:583, 1987.

427. Laborde F, Noirhomme P, Karam J, et al: A new video-assisted thoracoscopic surgical technique for interruption of patent ductus arteriosus in infants and children. J Thorac Cardiovasc Surg 105:278, 1993.

428. Burke RP, Chang AC: Video-assisted throacoscopic division of a vascular ring in an infant: a new operative technique. J Card Surg 8:537, 1993.

429. Burke RP, Wernovsky G, van der Velde M, et al: Video-assisted thoracoscopic surgery for congenital heart disease. J Thorac Cardiovasc Surg 109:499, 1995.

430. Zbar RI, Chen AH, Behrendt DM: Incidence of vocal cord paralysis in infants undergoing ligation of patent ductus arteriosus. J Thorac Cardiovasc Surg 61:814, 1996.

431. Fan LL, Campbell DN, Clarke DR, et al: Paralyzed left vocal cord associated with ligation of patent ductus arteriosus. J Thorac Cardiovasc Surg 98:562, 1989.

432. Odegard KC, Kirse DJ, Del Nido PJ, et al: Intraoperative recurrent laryngeal nerve monitoring during video-assisted thorascoscopic surgery for patent ductus arteriosus. J Cardiothorac Vasc Anesth 14:562, 2000.

433. Baylen B, Meyer RA, Korfhagen J: Left ventricular performance in the critically ill premature infant with patent ductus arteriosus and pulmonary disease. Circulation 55:182, 1977.

434. Elliott LP, Anderson RH, Bargeron KM, Kirklin JK: Single or univentricular heart. In Adams FH, Emmanouilides GC (eds): Moss' Heart Disease in Infants, Children and Adolescents. Baltimore, Williams & Wilkins, 1983, p 386.

435. Mair DD, Edwards WD, Fister V: Truncus arteriosus. In Adams FH, Emmanouilides GC (eds): Moss' Heart Disease in Infants, Children, and Adolescents. Baltimore, Williams & Wilkins, 1983, p 400.

436. Marcelletti C, McGood DC, Mair DD: The natural history of truncus arteriosus. Circulation 54:108, 1976.

437. Bove EL, Lupinetti FM, Pridjian AK, et al: Results of a policy of primary repair of truncus arteriosus in the neonate. J Thorac Cardiovasc Surg 105:1057, 1993.

438. Ebert PA, Robinson SJ, Stanger P: Pulmonary artery conduits in infants younger than six months of age. J Thorac Cardiovasc Surg 72:351, 1976.

439. Gersony WM: Coarctation of the aorta. In Adams FH, Emmanouilides GC (eds): Moss' Heart Disease in Infants, Children, and Adolescents. Baltimore, Williams & Wilkins, 1983, p 188.

440. Brewer LA, Fusberg RG, Mulder GA: Spinal cord complications following surgery for coarctation of the aorta: a study of 66 cases. J Thorac Cardiovasc Surg 64:368, 1972.

441. Symbas PN, Pfaender LM, Drucker MH: Cross-clamping of the descending aorta. J Thorac Cardiovasc Surg 85:300, 1983.

442. Wadough F, Arndt CF, Metzger H: Direct measurements of oxygen tension of the spinal cord surface of pigs after occlusion of the descending aorta. J Thorac Cardiovasc Surg 89:787, 1985.

443. Gelman S, Reves JG, Fowler K: Regional blood flow during cross-clamping of the thoracic aorta and infusion of sodium nitroprusside. J Thorac Cardiovasc Surg 85:287, 1983.

444. Wadouh F, Lindemann EM, Arndt CF: The arteria radicularis magna anterior as a decisive factor influencing spinal cord damage during aortic occlusion. J Thorac Cardiovasc Surg 88:1, 1984.

445. Krieger KH, Spencer FC: Is paraplegia after repair of coarctation of the aorta due principally to distal hypotension during aortic cross clamping? Surgery 97:2, 1985.

446. Crawford FA, Sade RM: Spinal cord injury associated with hyperthermia during coarctation repair. J Thorac Cardiovasc Surg 87:616, 1984.

447. Fox S, Pierce WS, Waldhousaen JA: Pathogenesis of paradoxical hypertension after coarctation repair. Ann Thorac Surg 29:135, 1980.

448. Benedict CR, Graham-Smith PDG, Fisher A: Changes in plasma catecholamines and dopamine beta-hydroxylase after corrective surgery for coarctation of the aorta. Circulation 57:598, 1977.

449. Casta A, Conti VR, Talabi A: Effective use of captopril in postoperative paradoxical hypertension of coarctation of the aorta. Clin Cardiol 5:551, 1982.

450. Glancy DL, Morrow AG, Simon AL: Juxtaductal aortic coarctation: analysis of 84 patients studied hemodynamically, angiographically, and morphologically after age 1 year. Am J Cardiol 51:537, 1983.

451. Pollack P, Freed MD, Castaneda AR: Reoperation for isthmic coarctation of the aorta: follow up of 26 patients. Am J Cardiol 51:1690, 1983.

452. Waldman JD, Karp RB: How should we treat coarctation of the aorta? Circulation 87:1043, 1993.

453. Shaddy RE, Boucek MM, Sturtevant JE, et al: Comparison of angioplasty and surgery for unoperated coarctation of the aorta. Circulation 87:793, 1993.

454. Moulaert AJ, Bruins CC, Oppenheimer-Dekker A: Anomalies of the aortic arch and ventricular septal defects. Circulation 53:1011, 1976.

455. Elliott RB, Starling MB, Neutze JM: Medical manipulation of the ductus arteriosus. Lancet 1:140, 1975.

456. Lang P, Freed MD, Keane JF: The use of prostaglandin E1 in an infant with interruption of the aortic arch. J Pediatr 91:805, 1977.

457. Fowler BN, Lucas SK, Razook JD: Interruption of the aortic arch experience in 17 infants. Ann Thorac Surg 37:25, 1984.

458. Norwood WI, Lang P, Castaneda AR, Hougen TJ: Reparative operations for interrupted aortic arch with ventricular septal defect. J Thorac Cardiovasc Surg 86:832, 1983.

459. Jones M, Barnhart GR, Morrow AG: Late results after operations for left ventricular outflow tract obstruction. Am J Cardiol 60:569, 1982.

460. Rhodes LA, Colan SD, Perry SB, et al: Predictors of survival in neonates with critical aortic stenosis. Circulation 84:2325, 1991.

461. Jacobs ML, Norwood WI: Hypoplastic left heart syndrome. In Jacobs ML, Norwood WI (eds): Pediatric Cardiac Surgery. London, Butterworth-Heinemann, 1992, p 182.

462. Jenkins PC, Flanagan MF, Jenkins KJ, et al: Survival analysis and risk factors for mortality in transplantation and staged surgery for hypoplastic left heart syndrome. J Am Coll Cardiol 36:1178, 2000.

463. Carter C, Naftel D, Caldwell R, et al: Survival and risk factors for death after cardiac transplantation in infants. A multi-institutional study. The pediatric heart transplantation study. Circulation 96:227, 1997.

464. Oslovich H, Phillips E, Byrne P, Robertson M: Hypoplastic left heart syndrome: "to treat or not to treat." J Perinatol 20:363, 2000.

465. Kumar RK, Newburger JW, Gauvreau K, et al: Comparison of outcome when hypoplastic left heart syndrome and transposition of the great arteries are diagnosed prenatally versus when diagnosis of these two conditions is made only postnatally. Am J Cardiol 83:1649, 1999.

466. Forbess JM, Cook N, Roth SJ, et al: Ten-year institutional experience with palliative surgery for hypoplastic left heart syndrome. Risk factors related to stage I mortality. Circulation 92:II-262, 1995.

467. Donner RM: Hypoplastic left heart syndrome. Curr Treat Options Cardiovasc Med 2:469, 2000.

468. Mahle WT, Spray TL, Wernovsky G, et al: Survival after reconstructive surgery for hypoplastic left heart syndrome. Circulation 102:III-36, 2000.

469. Tchervenkov CI, Jacobs ML, Tahta SA: Congenital heart surgery nomenclature and database project: hypoplastic left heart syndrome [review]. Ann Thorac Surg 69:S170, 2000.

470. Mosca RS, Kulik TJ, Goldberg CS, et al: Early results of the Fontan procedure in one hundred consecutive patients with hypoplastic left heart syndrome. J Thorac Cardiovasc Surg 119:1110, 2000.

471. Daebritz SH, Nollert GB, Zurakowski D, et al: Results of the Norwood Stage I operation: comparisons of hypoplastic left heart syndrome with other malformations. J Thorac Cardiovasc Surg 119:358, 2000.

472. Jobes DR, Nicolson SC, Steven JM, et al: Carbon dioxide prevents pulmonary overcirculation in hypoplastic heart syndrome. Ann Thorac Surg 54:150, 1992.

473. Bailey LL, Gundry SR, Razzouk AJ, et al: Bless the babies: one hundred fifteen late survivors of heart transplantation during the first year of life. J Thorac Cardiovasc Surg 105:805, 1993.

474. Armitage JM, Fricker FJ, del Nido P, et al: A decade (1982 to 1992) of pediatric cardiac transplantation and the impact of FK 506 immunosuppression. J Thorac Cardiovasc Surg 105:464, 1993.

475. Starnes VA, Griffin ML, Pitlick PT, et al: Current approach to hypoplastic left heart syndrome. Palliation, transplantation, or both? J Thorac Cardiovasc Surg 104:189, 1992.

476. Freedom RM: Neurodevelopmental outcome after the Fontan procedure in children with hypoplastic left heart syndrome and other forms of single ventricle pathology. J Pediatr 137:602, 2000.

477. Wernovsky G, Stiles KM, Gauvreau K, et al: Cognitive development after the Fontan operation. Circulation 102:883, 2000.

19

Anesthesia for Transplantation*

GEORGE A. GREGORY
CHARLES B. CAULDWELL

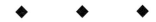

During the last decade, medical progress has made organ transplantation an accepted therapeutic modality for treating a variety of diseases affecting various organ systems in infants and children. Improvements in immunosuppressive therapy, surgical techniques, and organ preservation have permitted utilization of transplantation in a greater number of patients. Pediatric patients in particular have benefited from the growth of transplantation. In 1990, 11 percent of all solid organ transplant procedures were performed in infants, children, and adolescents; and children less than 5 years old received 12 percent of liver transplants and 6 percent of cardiac transplants.[1-4] Evolving success of solid organ transplantation has also made evident the shortage of appropriate donors for younger patients. The scope and magnitude of various transplant procedures in infants and children with underlying organ system disease will continue to challenge anesthesiologists caring for these patients.[5] In addition, as more children undergo transplantation, anesthesiologists must be prepared to care for them following transplantation, including the management of posttransplant complications and procedures.

The psychosocial adjustment following liver transplant is quite good up to the age of 8 years. For adolescent

boys, however, there may be problems of feelings of incompetence.[6]

Transplantation Technology

Recent advances in transplantation technology have facilitated increased application and survival of solid organ transplants. Most importantly, the development and refinement of immunosuppressive regimens has improved patient and graft survival in organ transplantation. Introduction of cyclosporine in 1980 produced dramatic increases in survival and decreased episodes of graft rejection for renal and liver transplant recipients. Because of side effects associated with cyclosporine (particularly nephrotoxicity, neurotoxicity, hypertension), the development of multidrug regimens was instituted and these regimens have improved the overall management of immunosuppression. Currently, combinations of cyclosporine, azathioprine, and prednisone are commonly used to maintain immunosuppression in solid organ transplantation. Compared to cyclosporine, tacrolimus has increased survival rates and reduced complication rates.[7] However, the rate of infections may be increased with the use of this drug.[8] Additional therapeutic agents are incorporated into the induction of initial immunosuppression following transplantation and the treatment of episodes of acute graft rejection. These other agents include alternative ste-

*This chapter was co-authored by Scott D. Kelley, M.D. in the previous edition. He did not participate in the revision of this chapter.

541

roid administration, antilymphocyte preparations (ATG, MALG), monoclonal antibodies (OKT3), and new experimental immunosuppressive agents (FK506, RS61443).[9] There has been a great effort to reduce or eliminate steroid administration to infants and children because administering these drugs increase the rate of infections and mortality.[10] Children on lower doses of steroids have better catch-up growth than those who require larger doses of the drug.[11]

Management of immunosuppression and episodes of rejection are critical to short- and long-term outcome for transplant recipients because episodes of rejection are extremely common in solid organ transplantation. Up to 75 percent of liver transplant recipients have evidence of rejection on weekly liver biopsies obtained in the early posttransplant period. Early diagnosis and intervention not only control most episodes of rejection, they also decrease the cost of transplantation because rejection episodes prolong hospitalization. Inadequate diagnosis or treatment of graft rejection may decrease the effectiveness of additional immunosuppression and eventually leaves retransplantation as the only therapeutic option. Because of the limited availability of organs for transplantation and decreased survival following retransplantation, efforts to manage rejection through effective immunosuppression are critical.

The introduction of Belzer's University of Wisconsin (UW) preservation solution has extended the acceptable period of cold hepatic ischemia to 24 hours and allowed most liver transplant procedures to be scheduled as urgent rather than emergent cases.[12] In many centers they are scheduled as morning procedures. In addition, longer preservation times permit the use of sophisticated "back table" surgical techniques that allow the use of reduced-size liver grafts for infants and children.[13] Renal preservation techniques, including cold storage and pulsatile perfusion methods, have extended the storage time to 36 to 72 hours in many centers. Refinements in preservation techniques for heart and lung donor organs have reduced the incidence of postpreservation organ dysfunction.[14] Organ preservation techniques are under constant evaluation and refinement. The time period from new laboratory findings to clinical application may be exceptionally short in some transplant centers. Organ procurement techniques have allowed maximal utilization of available organs from donors, thus allowing more recipients to benefit from each donor.

Hepatocellular oxidative stress is associated with a reduced survival of patients following liver transplant.[15] One-year survival is only 60 percent in patients whose serum alanine aminotransferase concentrations were 2,500 units or greater.

Another rapidly evolving area of transplantation is which criteria are to be used when selecting appropriate donors for solid organ transplantation. Early empiric limitations on donor age and coexisting disease severely restricted available donor organs. With the growing shortage of available donors compared to awaiting recipients, gradual broadening of acceptable donor criteria has occurred. Recent experience has focused on use of hepatic allografts from "marginal donors" and assessment of immediate perioperative function and long-term graft survival. Interestingly, a brief cardiac arrest has been associated with good function of the graft after transplantation.[16] Patients who undergo three or more liver transplants have approximately 71 percent of their grafts functioning well up to 23 months later.[17]

Apart from questions about donor acceptability, the distribution of available donor organs remains extremely controversial. In recent years, both the number of transplant centers and the number of waiting recipients has grown rapidly. The interactions between local organ procurement organizations and local, regional, and national transplant centers to better distribute available organs is now the focus of national attention and study. In the United States, the United Network for Organ Sharing (UNOS) is the organization responsible for matching donors and recipients for solid organ transplantation.[18]

Utilization of a stepped scale for recipient listing status has helped distribute organs on a national level to patients in greatest need. Distribution of organs to patients without critical need involve complex interactions between the various programs and organ procurement organizations, and has lead to criticism about inequalities of distribution. Because of donor shortages, the patterns of organ sharing and distribution will continue to evolve in the coming decade.

For pediatric recipients, critical donor issues remain, including defining acceptable hemodynamic support prior to donor procurement and ethical consideration of donation from anencephalic newborns.[19, 20] Neonatal donors (suffering brain death from anoxia and/or intracerebral hemorrhage) provide organs that have a degree of functional immaturity compared to older donors; despite this concern, results using these donors for liver and heart transplantation are encouraging.[21] Because of the critical donor shortage for younger patients, mortality for pediatric transplant candidates is greater than for adult candidates, and has been the impetus for expanding the donor pool by using other methods, such as reduced-size grafts in pediatric liver transplantation, and the recent introduction of live-donor techniques. In at least one center, the mortality of children awaiting liver transplant has decreased to zero due to these other methods of organ procurement.[22] Several factors affecting survival following liver transplant are retransplantation, transplantation for cancer, fewer than 20 split-liver transplants per year, and fewer than 25 liver transplants per year done in any one center; these factors significantly reduced survival.[23]

Lymphoproliferative disease occurs at a rate of approximately 1.8 per 100 patient years and is lowest in the patients primarily treated with cyclosporine and greatest in those primarily treated with tacrolimus.[24] Chemotherapy has been used successfully to treat children with lymphoproliferative disease.[25] The presence of Epstein-Barr infection increases the incidence of lymphoproliferative disease,[26, 27] as does hepatitis C.[28] One common association with lymphoproliferative disease is the occurrence of enlarged tonsils and adenoids.[29]

Anesthetic Management of Organ Transplantation: Perspective

Solid organ transplantation is most frequently utilized for management of specific organ insufficiency or failure. Pediatric transplantation also is indicated as therapy for certain metabolic disorders that cause secondary effects on other organs and tissues (e.g., α_1-antitrypsin disease, glycogen storage disease, oxalosis). In general, though, liver transplantation only occurs in patients with some degree of hepatic failure; kidney transplantation occurs in those with renal failure. Anesthetic management of these procedures requires understanding the physiologic implications of organ failure, as well as specific requirements of the transplant procedure.[30] To facilitate this discussion, issues related to the anesthetic care of children undergoing liver, renal, heart, heart–lung, lung, and multivisceral transplantation will be discussed separately. In addition, other chapters describe anesthetic care of infants and children with specific organ dysfunction who require surgery.

Perioperative anesthetic management of solid organ transplant procedures has a number of similarities. Because of the logistic constraints involving donor organ procurement and admission of patients awaiting transplantation, there is limited time available to the anesthesia team for preparation. During this time, the patient must be admitted to the hospital and an updated history and physical examination and laboratory studies must be obtained. The short period of preparation usually limits the duration of NPO status for most children, which has implications for the anesthesiologist. Anesthetic preparation and planning must incorporate the magnitude of these procedures. In most transplant procedures, the organ is transplanted in an orthotopic fashion, that is, the native organ is dissected free from surrounding structures, vessels are isolated and clamped, and the new organ is reanastomosed to the recipient vessels. Because several vascular anastomoses are required, there is significant potential for hemorrhage. Adequate vascular access, invasive monitoring, and availability of adequate quantities of blood product are required. Given the severity of underlying diseases, the physiologic alterations they cause, and the frequency of intraoperative changes in the patient's condition, arterial blood gas and pH, blood chemistry profiles, and other hematologic testing often are required during transplant procedures. When new transplantation programs are established, anesthesia departments should take an active role in defining the requirements and availability of these ancillary services to help in the care of these patients. Because of the urgent or emergent nature of most transplant cases, the resources must be available to the anesthesia team on a 24-hour, 7-days-week basis.

LIVER TRANSPLANTATION

Liver transplantation has grown rapidly in acceptance following the 1983 National Institutes of Health (NIH) Consensus Development Conference conclusion that liver transplantation offered therapeutic benefit deserving of broader application.[31] Pediatric liver transplantation has grown in parallel with transplantation in adult patients. Currently, pediatric transplants account for about 15 percent of all liver transplants in the United States, and the majority of these transplants involve children less than 5 years of age.[32] The distribution of patients for liver transplant is similar in Europe. Mortality from liver disease

decreased 58 percent in the 5 years following the NIH Consensus report and was attributed to the referral of pediatric patients for liver transplantation.[33]

Indications

A variety of hepatic diseases are amenable to liver transplantation.[34] According to this classification, indications for pediatric liver transplantation can be grouped under several categories: (1) primary liver disease expected to progress to hepatic insufficiency, (2) nonprogressive liver disease with significant morbidity, (3) liver-based metabolic disease, (4) secondary liver disease (e.g., cystic fibrosis), and (5) primary hepatic malignancy. The majority of pediatric transplants performed have attempted to correct hepatic failure or insufficiency resulting from primary liver disease, the most common cause being biliary atresia. The latter accounts for approximately 70 percent of pediatric liver transplants performed in the United States (Table 19–1).[3] Despite palliation by Kasai's procedure and other forms of biliary decompression, cirrhosis and portal hypertension usually progress and result in significant mortality in these children.[33] Liver transplantation can significantly reduce the mortality from biliary atresia.

Fulminant hepatic failure in infants and children is the result of acute viral infection and of toxic or drug-induced etiologies. Liver transplantation reduced the mortality associated with fulminant hepatic failure.[35] Treatment of acute hepatic failure in infants and children by liver transplantation has been difficult because it often is difficult to locate size-matched donors in a short period of time. This problem, together with pediatric donor shortage in general, has been the impetus for the development of reduced-size liver transplantation, including the use of "split-liver" grafts, pare-down techniques, and more recently, live-donor transplants (see below).[36]

Pathophysiology

Patients with end-stage liver disease that results from many causes manifest similar pathophysiology (Table 19–2). Although the time course of these changes and complications is variable, care of these patients requires the incorporation of the effects of this pathophysiology in the anesthetic plan.

The cardiovascular system undergoes marked changes as the child develops cirrhosis and end-stage liver disease.

T A B L E 1 9 – 1 AGE DISTRIBUTION OF PEDIATRIC LIVER TRANSPLANT RECIPIENTS		
Age Group (years)	n	%
< 1	441	29.2
1–2	419	27.8
3–4	162	10.7
5–9	255	16.9
10–15	231	15.3

Data from Belle and Detre, 1993.[32]

T A B L E   1 9 - 2
PATHOPHYSIOLOGY IN END-STAGE LIVER DISEASE

Organ System	Common Findings
Cardiovascular	Hyperdynamic circulation: increased cardiac output, decreased systemic vascular resistance, increased stroke volume and ejection fraction Expanded plasma volume Arteriovenous shunting
Pulmonary	Restrictive pulmonary function secondary to ascites Hypoxemia secondary to ventilation: perfusion mismatch, impaired hypoxic pulmonary vasoconstriction, intrapulmonary shunting Pulmonary hypertension Hepatopulmonary syndrome
Central nervous system	Encephalopathy Cerebral edema with fulminant hepatic failure
Gastrointestinal	Hepatic dysfunction: synthetic, metabolic, excretory aspects Portal hypertension (esophageal varices, portal hypertensive gastropathy) Delayed gastric emptying
Renal	Renal dysfunction from prerenal azotemia (secondary in diuretics) Hepatorenal syndrome
Hematologic	Elevated PT Thrombocytopenia Anemia Hypofibrinogenemia, dysfibrinogenemia Fibrinolysis Disseminated intravascular coagulation
Fluids, electrolytes, acid–base status	Intravascular volume depletion (secondary to diuretics) Hypokalemia, hyponatremia Metabolic alkalosis Metabolic acidosis (especially fulminant hepatic failure)

Patients with cirrhosis and portal hypertension frequently have a hyperdynamic circulation, decreased systemic vascular resistance, increased cardiac output, and a slightly decreased arterial blood pressure. The exact pathogenesis of the hyperdynamic state is controversial, but a variety of circulating vasoactive substances are thought to contribute. The hyperdynamic circulation of the patient has important implications for the anesthesiologist, including a decreased sensitivity to catecholamines and vasoconstrictors, an increased mixed venous oxygen saturation, and a decreased arteriovenous oxygen difference. Because of the vasodilated state, anesthetics may cause severe hypotension in this patient population.

Patients with end-stage liver disease also manifest significant changes in the pulmonary system and are frequently hypoxemic. A number of individual factors are likely to contribute to the hypoxemia. Intrapulmonary shunting of blood through arteriovenous fistulae causes venous admixture of oxygenated and poorly oxygenated blood in the lungs. In addition, the response of the pulmonary microvasculature to hypoxia is altered, suggesting that normal hypoxic pulmonary vasoconstriction is impaired. Impairment of hypoxic–pulmonary vasoconstric-

tion may contribute to the development of hypoxia. Many patients with chronic liver disease have abnormal pulmonary mechanics and some degree of alveolar hypoventilation. The presence of ascites and increased intra-abdominal pressure alter respiratory mechanics and often reduce functional residual capacity. In a small percentage of patients, end-stage liver disease is associated with pulmonary hypertension. Although modest elevations in pulmonary artery pressures occur due to a high cardiac output, the presence of near systemic pulmonary artery pressures usually is evidence of a specific alteration in the pulmonary vasculature. The carbon monoxide transfer coefficient was reduced frequently but the spirometric values were normal.[37] Severe pulmonary dysfunction that is associated with liver disease may be due to the hepatopulmonary syndrome, which has marked hypoxemia, clubbing, and the need for supplemental oxygen as prominent features. Several reports suggest that this syndrome improves following liver transplantation.[38] The anesthesiologist responsible must provide adequate preoxygenation and rapidly insert an endotracheal tube into the trachea following the induction of anesthesia. Positive-pressure ventilation, plus small amounts of positive end-expiratory pressure, usually produce normal oxgenation during surgery.[39] In the postoperative period, however, alveolar–arterial oxygen differences are commonly increased, particularly in children who have the hepatopulmonary syndrome.[40] Intrapulmonary shunting usually decreases after surgery, but it does so earlier the younger the patient is when he or she has a liver transplant.[41]

Central nervous system changes, especially hepatic encephalopathy, also are common in patients with end-stage liver disease. A variety of mechanisms are thought to cause the encephalopathy, and the degree of encephalopathy varies with the overall medical condition of the patient. Acute exacerbation of hepatic encephalopathy is often a sign that other complications of chronic liver disease (gastrointestinal bleeding, bacterial peritonitis, and renal dysfunction) have occurred. The anesthesiologist must be especially careful when administering preoperative sedation to patients with history of encephalopathy. Small amounts of a sedative may cause loss of consciousness and loss of protective airway reflexes. Patients with fulminant hepatic failure may develop cerebral edema and intracranial hypertension (see below). Of 10 children with an enlarged optic nerve sheath diameter (increased intracranial pressure [ICP]), 8 died.[42] Other forms of monitoring ICP have been used but are often associated with complications, such as intracranial bleeding.

The gastrointestinal system undergoes many changes when patients have end-stage liver disease, including abnormal synthetic, metabolic, and excretory functions of the liver and portal hypertension. The pathogenesis of portal hypertension is controversial but may be due to increased intrahepatic resistance or to increased blood flow to the spleen. Complications of portal hypertension include (1) altered hepatic and intestinal lymph flow and decreased plasma oncotic pressure, which facilitate the development of ascites; and (2) gastrointestinal bleeding from esophageal and gastric varices or from portal hypertensive gastropathy. Delayed gastric emptying should be suspected in patients with liver disease; a rapid sequence induction of general anesthesia and cricoid pressure should be considered.

Renal dysfunction is a common sequela of chronic liver disease and is multifactorial in origin. Alterations in the renal tubule retention and reabsorbtion of sodium appears to be a principal etiology of this dysfunction. Increased concentrations of aldosterone and decreased plasma volume are responsible for the sodium retention. Increases in circulating antidiuretic hormone (ADH) impair water diuresis. Administration of diuretics (to control ascites and edema), gastrointestinal bleeding, and mild hypotension also may contribute to relative prerenal azotemia in patients with liver disease. Severe renal dysfunction often is labeled hepatorenal syndrome. Patients with this syndrome usually have ascites, increased sodium and/or water retention, and elevated plasma renin and aldosterone activity. Treatment of the renal dysfunction with appropriate fluid administration (based on central venous pressure monitoring), renal-dose dopamine (1–3 µg/kg/min), and possibly placement of peritoneal-venous shunt may effectively reverse the renal dysfunction. Combined liver–kidney transplantation is an option for children with both liver and renal disease.[43]

Hematologic abnormalities occur with liver disease because synthesis of fibrinogen and factors II, V, VII, IX, and X decreases.[44] Because of the decreased synthesis of these factors, the prothrombin time (PT) and the partial thromboplastin time (PTT) are increased. Thrombocytopenia is common when patients develop hypersplenism in response to portal hypertension. Some patients also manifest low-grade disseminated intravascular coagulation and accelerated fibrinolysis. The altered hemostasis affects the anesthesiologist's ability to insert vascular catheters and nasogastric tubes, and increases the potential for excessive bleeding from surgical wounds. Aprotinin administration during anesthesia and surgery has significantly reduced the amount of blood loss in adults.[45, 46] Its use during surgery in infants and children is unproven, but should be just as effective.

Electrolytes and acid–base balance often are altered in chronic liver disease by renal dysfunction and/or the use of diuretics. Acid–base changes may be due to renal dysfunction or to changes in ventilation. The intravascular volume status may be difficult to assess in patients with liver disease due to the presence of ascites, peripheral edema, and anasarca. The effective plasma volume is often inadequate. Consequently, intraoperative measurement of central filling pressures is required during transplantation.

Anesthetic Management

Preoperative Evaluation

Most transplant centers utilize a multidisciplinary approach for the evaluation of patients for liver transplantation. Upon referral to the transplant center, careful assessment of the etiology and severity of the hepatic disease is initiated. Following identification of a potential candidate for liver transplantation, a stepped evaluation is initiated. In the first phase, blood typing, blood chemistries, liver and renal function tests, coagulation profiles, and viral serologies are drawn. Anatomic assessment of the native liver may include abdominal ultrasound and/or angiography. A liver biopsy may be indicated to confirm the diagnosis or severity of the liver disease. Anesthesia consultation usually includes evaluation for possible cardiopulmonary disease and instructing the family on perioperative care. Further testing, including electrocardiogram (ECG), chest x-ray, and echocardiography, is performed if indicated by the initial history and physical examinations. Care must be taken to determine if the patient has pulmonary hypertension. Careful assessment of the psychosocial and financial situation of the child's family is performed. A careful neurologic examination should be done to detect any problems present in the preoperative period. Following the initial evaluation, the patient's history and data are presented to a selection committee, which decides if the patient is a candidate for transplantation. Patients approved for transplantation are then activated on the transplant center's recipient list. In situations of acute hepatic failure or rapid decompensation of chronic liver disease, the evaluation process can be condensed to a few hours.

Referral to the transplant center and acceptance of the child as a transplant candidate allows the transplant center physicians the opportunity to optimize the patient's medical condition while the child awaits transplantation. Medical therapy to control ascites, infection, and encephalopathy is initiated. Nutritional assessment and diet modification are frequently performed. Endoscopy and sclerotherapy may be performed to treat gastrointestinal bleeding. If the patient has cardiopulmonary disease, additional studies, including arterial blood gases, response to inhaled oxygen, and cardiac catheterization may be performed to better document organ dysfunction. Vitamin K may be administered to improve hemostatic function. Prophylactic dental work or dental extraction and tonsillectomy and adenoidectomy are performed if required prior to transplantation and initiation of immunosuppression. Significant bleeding may occur following dental surgery, and blood and clotting factors may be required.

Perioperative Period

In general, patients are admitted from home when a potential donor is identified. Because of the logistic complications associated with scheduling, performing donor surgery, and transporting the donor organ to the transplant center, 8 to 12 hours' notice is often provided to the patient, family, and transplant team members. Upon admission to the hospital, interval history and physical examination are performed to seek evidence of new changes and complications since the original pretransplant evaluation. Whenever possible, the child is made NPO prior to surgery. However, because they are often frightened and may have eaten, it is best to treat each child as if he or she has a full stomach. In addition to routine blood tests, multiple additional blood samples are obtained for serologic studies, and specialized immunotesting. A peripheral intravenous (IV) line is usually started and maintenance fluids administered. If possible, the ward nurses or those in the intensive care unit arrange tours and other perioperative nursing instruction for the patient and family.

Following arrival of the donor organ at the hospital, final inspection and possible biopsy and frozen section of the liver are performed. Following notification from the transplant surgeon that the liver is appropriate for transplantation, the child is transported to a prewarmed operating room. In some children, especially those who are older, premedication may be required. If the child has an IV, sedation can be given by this route. If the child does not have an IV, nembutal 3–4 mg/kg and methadone 0.1 mg/kg can be given orally. The child will be asleep in about 20 minutes and can be transported to the operating room while breathing oxygen. Routine monitors (pulse oximetry, ECG, precordial stethoscope, arterial blood pressure) are applied prior to induction of anesthesia. One hundred percent oxygen is administered by face mask. Because of concerns that these patients have a full stomach and may aspirate gastric contents, cricoid pressure is applied and a rapid sequence induction of anesthesia performed. Since patients with significant ascites are likely to have a reduced functional residual capacity (FRC), adequate preoxygenation is required. Once the airway is secure, mechanical ventilation with an increased inspired concentration of oxygen and positive end-expiratory pressure (PEEP) is initiated.

Following tracheal intubation, vascular access is obtained and monitoring catheters are inserted. Ideally, two large-bore intravenous lines are placed in the upper extremities (18- to 20-gauge for infants, 14- to 18-gauge for a child). Adequate venous access is critical during any liver transplant procedure because the anesthesia team must be able to respond rapidly to surgical hemorrhage and prolonged periods of normal blood loss. The fluid delivery system must allow for sufficient control over the volume and rate of fluid and blood product administration in small children to prevent sudden overhydration. An arterial catheter is inserted, preferably in a radial artery, because the aorta may be clamped during reconstruction of hepatic arterial inflow. Because of the need for long-term central venous access, a 5- to 7-Fr double-lumen Broviac catheter may be inserted following the induction of anesthesia.[47] One lumen is used for central venous pressure monitoring, and the other lumen is used for infusion of medications and/or volume. In older children, a two- or three-lumen central venous catheter can be placed via the internal jugular vein. In children weighing more than 20 kg, some transplant surgeons utilize venovenous bypass; in this case, venous and arterial catheters should be placed away from the site of venous return from the bypass (axillary, subclavian vein). Perioperative management of patients with hepatopulmonary syndrome, cardiac disease, or associated pulmonary hypertension may be facilitated by measuring pulmonary artery pressures. Except for these rare cases, central venous pressure monitoring is sufficient in infants and children for liver transplant.

Anesthetic gas analysis is routine during liver transplantation. End-tidal carbon dioxide and nitrogen monitoring will aid in the detection of air embolus, a relatively common complication of liver transplant. Titration of inhalation agents may be facilitated by end-tidal gas measurements.

Particular attention is paid to maintaining normal body temperature during pediatric liver transplantation. Numerous factors facilitate development of unintentional hypothermia: exposure of the abdominal contents to air, duration of surgery, rapid administration of cool intravenous fluids and blood products, implantation of the cold liver graft and washout of the cold storage solution during reperfusion of the organ, and use of venovenous bypass. Rigorous attention is paid to warming the operating room and to the use of insulated wrapping (scalp, exposed extremities), heating blankets, heated humidifier, and warming of all intravenous fluids. In addition, forced-air warming of the lower extremities is useful in larger patients. If a cold child has a cardiac arrest, it is often necessary to open the chest and bath the heart in warm solution to resuscitate the patient. Failure to do so delays or prevents resuscitation.

No controlled studies have compared the benefits of specific types of anesthetic utilized during liver transplantation. A combination of potent inhaled anesthetic, opioid infusion, and benzodiazepine supplementation provides a relatively stable intraoperative course during liver transplantation. A technique that utilizes opioids and benzodiazepines has theoretical benefit in this patient population. Whether narcotics and benzodiazepines alter the kinetics and dynamics of inhaled agents in pediatric patients with liver disease is unknown. However, higher concentrations of inhaled anesthetics reduce splanchnic blood flow and may further decrease native liver function during the initial portion of the operation. Thus, infants with liver disease develop severe hypoglycemia if sufficient glucose is not administered during this time. A reduction in splanchnic blood flow theoretically may place the donor liver at risk for hepatotoxicity. The effect of the inhaled anesthetic on liver blood flow is both dose dependent and agent specific. Halothane, for example, causes a greater reduction in cardiac index than isoflurane and appears to inhibit hepatic arterial buffer responses to a greater degree. At one minimum alveolar concentration (MAC) of anesthesia, hepatic arterial autoregulation and hepatic oxygen delivery are better preserved by isoflurane (and enflurane) than by halothane. The impact of these changes during the early reperfusion period are unknown, but the overall goal of maximizing oxygen delivery to the native and to the donor organ appears logical. For these reasons, isoflurane usually is selected and halothane is avoided during surgery on the liver. Animal studies suggest that the newer inhalation agents, desflurane and sevoflurane, have similar effects on the splanchnic circulation to isoflurane.

Intravenous opioids have been used extensively in the anesthetic management of adult and pediatric patients undergoing liver transplant. Although end-stage liver disease is likely to affect the distribution and plasma clearance of opioids, in this particular operation, the newly transplanted liver graft may facilitate the perioperative administration of intravenous opioids. Opioid analgesics undergo hepatic biotransformation via mixed function oxidase (e.g., fentanyl) and glucuronosyltransferase (e.g., morphine). Because the hepatic extraction of morphine and fentanyl is high, plasma clearance is less affected by alterations in hepatic function than by alterations in hepatic blood flow. Morphine, fentanyl, and sufentanil appear to have unchanged plasma clearance and volumes of distribution in patients with end-stage liver disease, which may reflect the ability of the large volume of distribution to buffer any decrease in drug metabolism. In contrast, alfentanil, with its volume of distribution approximately 25 percent that of the other opioids, has a decreased plasma clearance and an increased free fraction of drug in patients with cirrhosis. The impact of large changes in and replacement of intravascular volume during the course of a lengthy liver transplant procedure is not known.

Liver disease affects the duration of action of nondepolarizing muscle relaxants. The action of pancuronium is prolonged in patients with liver disease. The duration of action of vecuronium depends on the extent of liver disease and on the dose of vecuronium. Vecuronium in a bolus of 0.1 mg/kg has the same pharmacokinetics in both patients with normal livers and those with liver disease.[48] In more advanced liver disease, a dose of 0.2 mg/kg of vecuronium may have a prolonged duration of action.[49,50] Redistribution of the drug within the body may be important for the termination of the drug's effect in patients with liver disease, but when larger doses of drug are administered, reduced hepatic clearance becomes more evident. Doxacurium, a benzisoquinolinum nondepolarizing muscle relaxant, has a long duration of action and is devoid of cardiovascular side effects at normal dosage. In one study, the pharmacokinetic values from a single dose of doxacurium administered to control patients and to those undergoing liver transplantation were similar.[51]

Because of the unique opportunity to study the effects of drug administration while the liver is out of the circulation, several studies have compared muscle relaxant requirements during different portions of the liver transplant procedure. In an early study, the duration of action of vecuronium was prolonged during the anhepatic period compared to the dissection period.[52] Infusion requirements of pancuronium and vecuronium, but not atracurium, were decreased during the anhepatic period, and returned to control values following reperfusion of the graft.[53] Atracurium infusion requirements tended to be the same or slightly decreased during the anhepatic period of clinical and experimental liver transplant procedures. However, laudanosine levels increased during the anhepatic period, suggesting that the liver does contribute to the plasma clearance of laudanosine.[54] In theory, laudanosine concentrations may increase to clinically significant levels during prolonged atracurium infusions in patients with severe liver disease or in those with a prolonged anhepatic period. No complications related to increased laudanosine concentrations in patients with liver disease have been reported.

Little information is available regarding the effect of hepatic preservation and reperfusion on the metabolism of anesthetic drugs. In one study, the appearance of morphine metabolites was documented following administration of morphine in the reperfusion period.[55] In a more detailed laboratory investigation, the hepatic extraction of morphine and fentanyl was not affected by a 24-hour period of hypothermic liver preservation; however, a transient period of decreased extraction of vecuronium was probably related to liver temperature.[56] These studies suggest that the liver graft with normal function rapidly re-

sumes its role of drug metabolism. Despite the overall uncertainty of anesthetic drug metabolism in the perioperative period following liver transplantation, delayed recovery from anesthetic drugs and neuromuscular blockade rarely poses a clinical problem. Many patients undergo a period of 8 to 16 hours of postoperative ventilatory support in the intensive care unit. During this time, termination of drug effect, either through redistribution or clearance of the drug, is observed. Because numerous factors contribute to the timing of tracheal extubation, it is rare that persistent effects of anesthesia delay the extubation of the trachea.

Surgical Procedure

Liver transplantation is usually divided into three stages: dissection, anhepatic, and reperfusion.[57] During the dissection period, the liver is mobilized via a large bilateral subcostal incision. All perihepatic adhesions are lysed, the suprahepatic vena cava, infrahepatic vena cava, and structures in the porta hepatis (portal vein, hepatic artery, and common bile duct) are identified and mobilized. Lysis of dense adhesions following a Kasai portoenterostomy or other previous surgery usually prolongs the dissection time and increases blood loss during this period. Adequate replacement of blood components during this time is essential.

Prior to implantation, the donor organ is stored in preservation solution, most commonly UW solution. Because of the high potassium content (140 mEq/L), the donor organ is perfused with a cold crystalloid or colloid solution to remove the preservation solution from the liver before the liver is implanted. In the case of reduced-size liver transplants, the partial hepatectomy of the donor liver is performed on the back table prior to implantation. The donor liver is stored in the cold preservation solution for as long as possible and usually requires additional ice applications during the dissection period. When the dissection phase is complete in the recipient, the preservation solution is flushed out of the donor liver, and it is brought onto the operative field. However, flushing the donor liver with large volumes of fluid does not always remove all of the potassium. Consequently, the serum potassium concentration of the recipient may increase significantly when the donor organ is reperfused. Occasionally, this leads to a hyperkalemic cardiac arrest at the time the donor organ is reperfused. The anhepatic stage begins with cross-clamping the suprahepatic vena cava, infrahepatic vena cava, portal vein, and hepatic artery. In some situations, the surgeons may avoid cross-clamping the vena cava by isolating the hepatic veins from the recipient vena cava and using a partial side-biting clamp on this portion of the vena cava. During the anhepatic period, the native liver is completely excised, bleeding is controlled in the retrohepatic area, and the donor liver is sutured in place. In general, vessels are anastomosed in the following order: suprahepatic vena cava, infrahepatic vena cava, and the portal vein. Following these three anastomoses, the liver is reperfused with venous inflow, which accounts for approximately 80 percent of liver blood flow. Alternatively, the hepatic artery can be anastomosed prior to restoration of blood flow. The anhepatic period ends with restoration of blood flow to the new liver.

Following restoration of blood flow into the new liver, the final stage of the operation, reperfusion, has started. Other terms for this portion of the surgery include the postanhepatic and the neohepatic period. Regardless of the term used, the surgical goals during this time include completion or revision of the hepatic artery anastomoses and establishment of biliary drainage. In infants and children, reconstruction of the hepatic arterial inflow may be more difficult and frequently includes reconstruction via a patch graft from the recipient aorta to the donor celiac trunk, hepatic artery, or aorta. Biliary drainage may occur via a direct choledochocholedochostomy, or more commonly in children, via a Roux-en-Y choledochojejunostomy. A major goal during the early reperfusion period is control of bleeding. This period requires close communication between surgeons and anesthesiologists to determine the presence of a coagulopathy (common in the early reperfusion period) as opposed to defined surgical bleeding (common following the total hepatectomy of the native liver and multiple vascular anastomoses and following previous abdominal surgery). The operating team uses a variety of clinical observations (color, texture, bile production) and laboratory measurements (prothrombin time, metabolic acidosis, ionized calcium, and glucose concentration) to document the status and quality of liver graft function. Abdominal closure may be difficult following completion of the surgical procedure. Frequently, a mild to moderate size discrepancy exists between the native, diseased liver and the donor liver. Gut distention also may compromise the available space. In addition to making the surgical closure difficult, inadequate intra-abdominal space may increase airway pressures and cause progressive difficulty with ventilation and/or oxygenation. Diuretic administration and muscle relaxation may facilitate abdominal closure; in some situations, use of a silastic silo, or Goretex patch may be required to temporarily (3 to 5 days) close the abdomen.

Occasionally, infants who have cardiac anomalies and intracardiac shunts require liver transplantation. This is especially dangerous because when the graft is reperfused there is the likelihood of air, clot, and other debris entering the systemic circulation. If this occurs, there is the danger of coronary artery or cerebral artery occlusion. It is important, therefore, to prevent this from occurring. On method that has proven effective is to leave the vena cava above the liver clamped and to open the vena cava below to allow the initial blood entering the liver from the portal vein to exit the vena cava into the abdomen. This often means that one fourth to one third of the blood volume is lost via this root. This blood must be replaced rapidly. It often is useful to have elevated the central venous pressure (CVP) to 15 to 20 cm H_2O by volume infusion just before the clamp on the portal vein is removed. Once the liver has been "flushed" with blood, the portal vein can be occluded and the vena cava can be closed. Then all clamps can be removed from the liver and the vena cava. It is helpful to have inserted an esophageal Doppler device and to record blood flow into the left atrium and ventricle at the time the clamp is removed from the vena cava superior to the liver. Our experience is that if 25 to 30 percent of the blood volume is "flushed" through the liver before the upper vena cava clamp is removed, there is no gas or debris shunted into the systemic circulation.

Intraoperative Management Issues
Hemodynamics

Periods of hemodynamic instability are common during liver transplantation.[57, 58] In the earlier portions of the anesthetic (e.g., during line placement, preparing and draping the skin), the general debilitating effects of end-stage liver disease and the reduced blood volume induced by diuresis may limit the patient's ability to compensate for the hypotensive effects of anesthetics. In response to abdominal incision and dissection around the native liver, surgical stimulation may overcome light levels of anesthesia and produce hypertension and tachycardia.

A more common scenario is development of hypotension at various points during the operation. Massive blood loss must always be entertained in the differential diagnosis for hypotension. Given the site of surgery, the presence of extensive abdominal and retroperitoneal collateral vessels, and scar tissue from previous surgeries, bleeding is frequently excessive during the dissection phase of surgery. It should always be kept in mind that splenic bleeding is a possibility. The changes in hemodynamics during the anhepatic period are frequently the most complicated to understand. With application of the venous clamps to the portal vein and to the infrahepatic and suprahepatic vena cava, there is an abrupt decrease in venous return to the right side of the heart and subsequently to the left side of the heart. Although there may be a brief period of hypotension in response to application of the clamp, infants and children appear to tolerate moderate hypovolemia and maintain normal systemic arterial pressures. Stimulation may produce hypertension and tachycardia if the anesthesia level is light. Periods of hypotension may be fewer with piggyback than with conventional techniques.[59] Reflex tachycardia, reduction in CVP, dampening of the arterial waveform during positive-pressure ventilation, and development of a metabolic acidosis are all consistent with significant hypovolemia (see Chapter 11). In adult patients, cardiac index may decrease 30 to 50 percent when the venous clamps are applied, but systemic arterial pressure is only slightly decreased because there is a compensatory increase in systemic vascular resistance. Presumably, similar physiologic changes occur in infants and children at this same time, but pulmonary artery catheters are seldom utilized in these patients because the catheters occupy a major portion of the pulmonary artery. Consequently, the exact effects of cross-clamping the inferior vena cava is poorly documented in these young patients. Volume administration during the anhepatic period is guided by central venous pressure, systemic arterial pressure, and by the arterial pressure waveform (see Chapter 11). While surgical attention is focused on the vascular anastomoses during the anhepatic period, significant bleeding may continue from areas behind the liver and at other sites of collateral flow. In rare situations, vasopressin (0.1 to 0.3 units/min IV) may be required to decrease splanchnic blood flow while the anastomoses are being completed. Fluid administration may include crystalloid, colloid, or blood products, depending upon the hemoglobin, prothrombin time, and preference of the anesthesiologist. Colloid solutions may have particular benefit during the anhepatic period and end of the dissection period. Care should be taken not to administer too much fluid during the anhepatic phase because when the blood is returned to the central circulation with unclamping the inferior vena cava, the CVP may be excessive. If the CVP is 10 to 12 cm H_2O at the time of reperfusion, there usually is little change in arterial blood pressure and the need for vasopressors is diminished. Because the portal vein is clamped during the anhepatic period, portal venous hypertension develops. In infants and small children, venovenous bypass is not used and it is used only selectively in larger children. Thus, there is no route for acute decompression of the portal venous system. Because of the increased venous pressure, there is a tendency toward fluid translocation and bowel edema during the anhepatic period. Administration of colloid solutions during the dissection and anhepatic period may reduce the amount of bowel edema that develops and facilitate closure of the abdomen at the end of the operation. In addition, the extent of bowel edema may influence the duration of impaired intestinal motility following the operation. Because large volumes of hydroxyethyl starch are associated with coagulopathy, albumin solutions are routinely utilized for colloid administration. Some clinicians prefer to use 25 percent albumin in neonates and infants up to 10 kg. If large volumes of this solution are used, serum osmolality must be determined, as the osmolality of 25 percent albumin is 305 to 315 mOsm/L.

Infants and children usually have normal urine outputs during the anhepatic period, apparently because there are other pathways by which venous blood can return to the central circulation. One possibility is that venous blood returns to the central circulation via Batson's plexus.

Completion of the anhepatic period restores venous return from the lower extremities and splanchnic bed. Despite adequate intravascular volume, hypotension is a common finding following graft reperfusion. Numerous factors are felt to contribute to the hemodynamic changes associated with reperfusion. Immediately upon reperfusion, a combination of hypotension, bradycardia, and supraventricular and ventricular dysrhythmias may develop. Prior to reperfusion, a small bolus of fluids may be administered to optimize ventricular filling. Acid–base status is checked approximately 5 to 10 minutes before reperfusion. Sodium bicarbonate is administered to achieve a pH greater than 7.25; similarly, the ionized calcium concentration is checked, and if it is decreased, additional calcium chloride is administered. Some centers have utilized prophylactic administration of atropine to prevent the bradycardia seen at reperfusion, although this may lead to ventricular arrhythmias in children. Similarly, some centers administer dopamine or phenylephrine immediately prior to reperfusion of the liver to minimize hypotension. At the moment of reperfusion, attention must be divided between the cardiac monitor and the surgical field. Evidence of life-threatening hemorrhage requires the immediate infusion of blood products while the surgeons control the bleeding. Inspection of the cardiac monitor will detect

ECG changes consistent with profound bradycardia and/or hyperkalemia. Bradycardia may result from the sudden atrial stretch occurring with restoration of normal venous return and/or influx of cold storage flush solution, with profound alterations in pH and electrolyte content. If the heart rate decreases by 30 to 40 percent, atropine should be administered, and warm solutions should be instilled into the abdominal cavity. ECG evidence of hyperkalemia includes development of peaked T waves (rare in babies), QRS widening, and sine-wave formation. Inspection of the arterial waveform trace will confirm the loss of mechanical activity. The occurrence of hyperkalemia at the time of reperfusion represents systemic toxicity of organ preservation solution that was not removed when the organ was flushed on the back table. Acute interventions for hyperkalemia include administration of calcium and bicarbonate, and circulatory support with closed chest cardiac massage and epinephrine. Because the surge in serum potassium is transient, treatment is directed towards decreasing the concentration of serum potassium and restoring the cardiac rhythm. The potassium concentration increases 0.5 to 1.5 mEq/L at the time of reperfusion in almost all patients. Because this increase in potassium is expected during reperfusion, care should be taken to prevent increases in potassium concentrations during the dissection and anhepatic periods. Forced diuresis (renal dose dopamine, diuretic administration) can help lower the potassium level. In addition, insulin and glucose administration effectively decreases the serum potassium concentration during the anhepatic period.

Other factors, including transient hypocalcemia, acidosis, and hypothermia, contribute to hypotension following graft reperfusion. There is speculation that a myocardial depressant and/or vasoactive substance accumulates during the anhepatic period in the intestinal vascular bed and exerts systemic effects at the time of reperfusion. Similarly, the ischemic hepatic graft may release metabolites or other substances into the circulation following graft reperfusion. Residual preservation solution may contribute to some changes apart from the increase in serum potassium. Studies in adult transplant patients suggest that approximately 30 to 40 percent of patients develop a "postreperfusion" syndrome consisting of decreased arterial blood pressure and profound vasodilation.[60] A study utilizing transesophageal echocardiography (TEE) suggested the possibility of right ventricular dysfunction (paradoxical motion of interventricular septum, right atrial enlargement, right-to-left interatrial deviation) following reperfusion.[61] In addition, the pulmonary circulation is known to be sensitive to acute alterations in temperature and pH, especially in infants. Perfusion of the lungs with ice-cold, hyperkalemic, acidic blood may increase pulmonary vascular resistance and cause right ventricular dysfunction. Embolization of air, clot, and cellular debris can occur at the time of graft reperfusion, as was shown by the TEE study mentioned above.[61] Despite numerous attempts, the contribution of various vasoactive substances (thromboxane, prostacyclin, prostaglandin 1-α and 2-α, kallikrein, platelet-activating factor, leukotrienes, vasoactive intestinal peptides, neurotensin) have not clearly been demonstrated to be the principal cause of the postreperfusion syndrome.

Perturbations of hemodynamics at reperfusion can affect other organs and systems. The liver graft is sensitive to increased levels of central venous and pulmonary artery pressure. Vascular engorgement of the liver is common following reperfusion of the liver, especially if the CVP was greater than about 12 cm H_2O before the liver was reperfused. Because the arterial blood supply to the liver may still be compromised (e.g., during the hepatic arterial reconstruction), excessive passive engorgement of the liver may deprive some areas of the liver of oxygen and cause poor restoration of graft function. Anesthetic management must attempt to prevent liver graft engorgement. If the systemic arterial pressure is adequate, infusion of nitroglycerin may reduce elevated central blood volumes and graft swelling or engorgement. Specific treatment for pulmonary hypertension includes increased ventilation, correction of acid–base status, and normalizing body temperature.

Hemostasis

Intraoperative hemostasis is a complex issue during orthotopic liver transplantation.[44, 57] The hemostatic system is often impaired as a result of intrinsic liver disease and as a result of the transplant procedure. Based upon preoperative diagnosis and coagulation testing, several groups have attempted to predict the risk of intraoperative bleeding during liver transplant.[62] However, a predictive score that indicates a low likelihood of bleeding is not a reason to decrease the level of preparedness. A certain amount of blood products should be immediately available to the operating room for all transplant procedures: 10 units of packed red blood cells, 10 units of fresh frozen plasma, and 6 units of platelet concentrates (i.e., six bags containing six units of platelets each) for most children. It is prudent to wash three units of packed red blood cells to remove the excess potassium present in the serum because rapid infusion of blood that has a high potassium concentration in the serum may cause a hyperkalemic cardiac arrest.[63] Other units of blood can be washed as needed during surgery. Once the initial extent of dissection and coagulopathy is determined, the need for additional crossmatching of blood and/or preparation of fresh frozen plasma, cryoprecipitate, and platelets can be determined. In the event of significant hemorrhage, the blood bank must be notified of anticipated increased requirements for blood products. The anesthesia team is responsible for maintaining adequate hemostasis during liver transplant procedures. Central to this role is the ability to rapidly monitor coagulation status intraoperatively. For the monitoring system to be effective, the anesthesiologist must have rapid access to the results of these tests so that the abnormalities can be corrected immediately. Routine coagulation testing should include measurement of prothrombin time, activated partial thromboplastin time, platelet count, hemoglobin concentration, and fibrinogen concentration. Some centers add additional tests, including clotting factor assays and measurement of euglobulin lysis times. The advent of near-patient testing has allowed certain elements of coagulation testing to be done inside the operating room. Systems are available to rapidly determine PT, PTT, fibrinogen, thrombin time, and circulating

heparin concentration at the bedside. Although it is tempting to use these systems, they require a commitment to ensure quality control and proficiency testing of their accuracy. In contrast to a 5-minute analysis time for near-patient systems, most hospital laboratories require 15 to 60 minutes to complete the standard coagulation tests. Providing rapid analysis of intraoperative coagulation tests by hospital laboratories is essential for a liver transplant program to be successful. Thromboelastography (TEG), a specific type of whole blood viscoelastic coagulation monitoring, has been used successfully by some clinicians during liver transplantation.[57] It is a test of clot strength, and requires a 30- to 60-minute recording of clot formation and lysis. The TEG gives an indication of clotting factor activity, platelet function, and fibrinolysis. Some centers have used TEG monitoring exclusively to determine the need for blood replacement and pharmacologic therapy to treat coagulopathies during liver transplantation. A particular problem with TEG is that its measurement variables do not correlate perfectly with standard hematologic test results. In favor of TEG is the fact that the test can be run in the operating room and that it attempts to measure whole blood clotting activity.

Intraoperative management of coagulopathy during liver transplantation includes the administration of blood products and of pharmacologic interventions. The principal blood product administered is fresh frozen plasma (FFP), which by virtue of the collection and storage techniques used preserves most of the clotting factors at near normal levels. When the prothrombin time is prolonged (3 to 5 seconds > control) during liver transplantation, FFP is administered to correct and maintain a PT closer to control values. Care should be taken not to overcorrect the PT (i.e., correct it to normal) in small children because this increases the likelihood of hepatic artery thrombosis. A PT of 18 is adequate at the end of surgery. Cryoprecipitate is administered when infusing FFP does not correct a low fibrinogen concentration (< 80 to 100 mg/dl). In the postreperfusion period, intravascular filling pressures may be elevated. Consequently, the decreased volume of cryoprecipitate is better tolerated.

Thrombocytopenia is a common finding during liver transplantation. Many patients have decreased platelet counts because their portal hypertension has induced hypersplenism. Intraoperative thrombocytopenia may develop or worsen due to replacement of blood loss during the dissection phase with non–platelet-containing solutions. Platelet counts decrease slightly during the anhepatic period and decrease significantly upon reperfusion of the graft. Platelet entrapment within the grafted liver has been demonstrated in a porcine model of liver transplantation; in addition, platelet activation and consumption increase following reperfusion of the graft. Platelet transfusion is indicated if thrombocytopenia is present and there is a clinical impression of abnormal hemostatic function.

Following reperfusion of the graft, multiple coagulation defects can appear due to the raw surfaces and multiple suture lines. Acute thrombocytopenia may develop as mentioned above. Circulating clotting factor concentrations may decrease abruptly secondary to hemodilution and factor consumption. A heparin effect from heparin-containing preservation and flush solution and from endogenous heparin-like activity released from the liver graft commonly is seen following reperfusion of the graft. Heparin effect can be determined by measuring the activated clotting time (ACT) in the operating room and activated partial thromboplastin time in the laboratory. Protamine administration 0.25 to 1.0 mg/kg may be used to reverse the heparin effect.

Severe postreperfusion coagulopathy occurs in some patients who undergo liver transplantation, possibly because of the reperfusion-initiated disseminated intravascular coagulation. However, normal concentrations of antithrombin III and only slight elevations in fibrin degradation products do not support this view. In contrast, several studies indicate that primary fibrinolysis may develop during liver transplantation due to changes in the circulating concentration of tissue-type plasminogen activator (t-PA). Increased hepatic secretion of t-PA and/or decreased clearance of t-PA by the allograft may increase the concentration of t-PA and cause fibrinolysis. A variety of stimuli may cause the vascular endothelium of the recipient or donor liver to secrete t-PA. Laboratory evidence of accelerated fibrinolysis is supported by abrupt changes in factor I (fibrinogen), V, and VIII following reperfusion. Additional tests that support the presence of fibrinolysis include decreased euglobulin lysis time and decreased clot lysis time, as measured by TEG or sonoclot analysis. The severity of an episode of fibrinolysis is variable. In one study of adult liver transplant patients, the use of blood products correlated with the severity of the fibrinolytic process, and patients with severe degrees of fibrinolysis had more hemodynamic instability. The relationship between accelerated fibrinolysis and overall degree of allograft dysfunction is not known. Two therapies have been utilized to pharmacologically reduce the severity of fibrinolysis during orthotopic liver transplantation. Epsilon-amino caproic acid (EACA) improves the TEG findings of fibrinolysis during liver transplantation, and administration of a test dose of the drug in the TEG has been used to determine whether the drug should be given to the patient. Prophylactic use of EACA has not been demonstrated to be of value. Administration of aprotinin, a protease-inhibitor of kallikrein, decreases the laboratory abnormalities associated with fibrinolysis and reduces transfusion requirement during liver transplantation.[64] An unblinded, uncontrolled study of t-PA administration demonstrated a significant reduction in the number of units of FFP and platelets required during surgery.[65, 45] However, a controlled trial of the use of t-PA did not show any beneficial effect of using this drug during liver transplant.[46] The difference may be that the former study did not use the piggyback technique.

The disruption of balance between coagulation and fibrinolysis continues postoperatively. In the immediate postoperative period, the balance is towards clot formation, as there is an imbalance in the synthesis of procoagulant factors and the inhibitors of coagulation. Pediatric patients may be at particular risk for thrombotic events in the immediate postoperative period due to the small size of their vessels. Hepatic artery thrombosis may cause the graft to be lost in 12 to 24 hours, and occurs with greater frequency in infants and children.[66] Hepatic artery thrombosis may result from disorders of the coagulation system and/or technical factors in hepatic arterial reconstruction.[67] Intraoperative and postoperative Doppler ultrasound examinations of the hepatic arterial and portal vein anastomoses are commonly used to assess patency of the anastomoses. Because of the potential for graft loss with vessel thrombosis, a slightly anticoagulated state is maintained in infants and small children following liver transplantation. This includes avoiding fully correcting the heparin effect in the operating room, maintaining a slightly higher prothrombin time, and early administration of aspirin.

Metabolic Control (K⁺, Ca²⁺, Acid–Base, Glucose)

Another aspect of the anesthetic management of liver transplantation is monitoring and regulation of the extracellular environment. Acute changes in acid–base status, potassium concentration, ionized calcium, and glucose are common during liver transplantation, both before and during liver transplantation. Concomitant renal dysfunction promotes acid–base changes and exacerbates electrolyte problems. Diuretic therapy can cause electrolyte imbalance (hyponatremia, hypokalemia, hypocalcemia) and prerenal azotemia. A common pattern of electrolyte changes develops in most patients. Consequently, an anticipated treatment plan can be developed. Routine intraoperative monitoring of arterial blood gases, electrolytes, and glucose concentrations will define the need for and further refine intraoperative electrolyte therapy. Because of the multiple factors contributing to hemodynamic instability in these patients, these parameters are more tightly controlled than in other operations.

Hyponatremia is common in patients presenting for liver transplantation. Consequently, there is concern that rapid increases in serum sodium associated with intraoperative administration of crystalloid and colloid solutions, blood products, and sodium bicarbonate may lead to central nervous system injury. Acute changes in serum osmolality are related to increases in serum sodium and to a tendency toward hyperglycemia. Increased administration of free water as maintenance fluids, and judicious use of bicarbonate and blood products will attenuate the increases in osmolality.

Potassium concentrations can vary greatly during the course of liver transplantation. Severe hypokalemia may be present initially because of preoperative use of diuretics, gastrointestinal fluid losses, and hyperaldosteronism. Intraoperatively, the principal concern is hyperkalemia, which may be related to blood products, especially aged red blood cells or whole blood, and influx of potassium from preservation solutions at the time of reperfusion. Washing of packed red blood cells (PRBC) prior to their administration (via the intraoperative blood salvage system, e.g., Cell Saver) will significantly reduce the amount of potassium transfused. Abrupt increases in the serum potassium concentration should be anticipated with liver reperfusion. ECG changes consistent with increasing potassium concentrations (peaked T waves, QRS changes, dysrhythmias) should be treated with calcium chloride and sodium bicarbonate. However, these T-wave changes may not be present in infants and small children. Following the abrupt increase at reperfusion, potassium concentrations tend to decrease during the remainder of the operation. Urinary losses of potassium account for some of the decrease, while potassium uptake by muscle cells and allograft liver cells also contribute to the decreases in serum potassium. Potassium administration is indicated if the serum potassium concentration decreases and the urine output is adequate in the postreperfusion period.

Patients undergoing liver transplantation are particularly susceptible to the development of ionized hypocalcemia. Although total calcium concentrations are decreased in patients with chronic liver disease, ionized calcium concentrations are normal. The latter is felt to represent the physiologically active moiety. Intraoperative administration of blood products decreases ionized calcium concentrations because citrate-based anticoagulant solutions used in collection and storage of blood products binds ionized calcium and decreases the total ionized calcium concentration. Citrate usually is metabolized rapidly by the liver. In normal patients, low ionized calcium concentrations only occur following massive and rapid administration of blood products. Patients with end-stage liver disease are particularly sensitive to the administration of citrate-containing blood products, and administration of moderate amounts of fresh frozen plasma can significantly decrease ionized calcium concentrations. Profoundly low ionized calcium concentrations, particularly during the anhepatic period, may cause myocardial depression and hypotension. Given the potential for dramatic changes in the ionized calcium concentration, direct measurement of ionized calcium is particularly useful during liver transplantation. Calcium replacement therapy during the dissection and anhepatic phases can be achieved with either bolus administration or constant infusion of calcium. Calcium chloride and calcium gluconate are equally effective in increasing the ionized calcium concentration during the anhepatic period. Calcium requirements are expected to increase (often markedly) during the anhepatic period and to quickly decrease following reperfusion of the hepatic allograft. With restoration of blood flow to the liver graft, metabolism of citrate proceeds at a much greater rate than occurred with the native liver or during the anhepatic phases. Reduction in calcium requirement following reperfusion is consistent with adequate hepatic allograft function. Consequently, development of hypercalcemia in the postreperfusion and postoperative period is common. As mentioned earlier, normal ionized calcium concentrations at the end of the anhepatic period may protect against the cardiovascular effect of abrupt increases in potassium from the reperfused liver. Measurement of ionized calcium 5 minutes before graft reperfusion and administration of calcium prior to reperfusion is suggested.

Metabolic acidosis is extremely common during orthotopic liver transplantation. Numerous factors contribute to its development, including tissue hypoperfusion; decreased or absent metabolism of lactate, citrate, and other metabolic acids by the liver; rapid administration of acidic blood products; associated renal impairment; and acidic effluent from the liver allograft. During the dissection period, development of acidosis most commonly reflects global tissue hypoperfusion. Administration of additional intravascular volume and restoration of adequate blood pressure and cardiac output often corrects the acidosis. The anhepatic period in particular is associated with rapid development of acidemia. The contribution of decreased tissue perfusion (caused by the abnormal hemodynamics associated with vena cava and portal vein occlusion) and the absence of hepatic function is unknown. Sodium bicarbonate is used to treat metabolic acidosis during the anhepatic period, and the amount of bicarbonate administered is based on the rapidity and severity of changes in acid–base balance. In general, with base deficits greater than 8–10 mEq/L, or pH less than 7.25 ($Paco_2 < 40$ mm Hg), bicarbonate should be administered to create a relatively normal pH immediately prior to reperfusion of the graft. Arterial blood gases and pH measurements obtained approximately 5 minutes prior to reperfusion will determine the amount of bicarbonate required.

Following reperfusion of the liver graft, metabolic acidosis frequently recurs. Treatment of severe metabolic acidosis at this point is indicated when there is concomitant myocardial depression and/or there are signs of persistent hyperkalemia. Normally, the exacerbation of metabolic acidosis quickly abates during the postreperfusion period; this abatement is one of the early signs that the graft is functioning. The liver allograft usually resumes metabolic function rapidly, and hepatic metabolism of lactate and citrate frequently leads to the development of a metabolic alkalosis in the later portions of the operation and in the postoperative period. Resolution of metabolic acidosis (and development of alkalosis) is indicative of adequate allograft function, although the sensitivity and specificity of these findings are not known. The extent of the metabolic alkalosis is related to the amount of intraoperative transfusion, and not to the amount of bicarbonate administered.

Glucose balance is complicated by liver transplantation. Hypoglycemia may be present in patients with fulminant liver failure or severe chronic liver disease and may necessitate preoperative administration of dextrose-containing fluids. It usually is necessary to administer glucose to these patients before the graft is reperfused. In theory, the anhepatic period should pose a greater risk of hypoglycemia because there is no liver in the circulation. Numerous factors are present that help maintain a relatively normal glucose concentration in the blood during the anhepatic period: stress response to surgery, steroid administration, dextrose-containing blood products, and reduced glucose utilization due to hypothermia. Since organ preservation solutions and flush solutions frequently contain dextrose, glucose concentrations commonly increase after reperfusion of the graft. Hyperglycemia in the reperfusion period also has been suggested as a marker for allograft function. Small infants may have markedly decreased glycogen stores when presenting for liver transplantation and are frequently at increased risk for developing hypoglycemia. Preoperative and frequent intraoperative glucose determinations are the best methods of detecting abnormal glucose levels. Dextrose should be administered if hypoglycemia is present. Hyperglycemia, glucose greater than 250 mg/dl, is treated with insulin administration. Hyperglycemia also is treated in patients who have diabetes.

Temperature Maintenance

Hypothermia is common during liver transplantation, despite utilization of multiple methods to conserve body heat. The long intra-abdominal operation, massive fluid and blood product administration, implantation of a graft that has a temperature near zero, and the use of venovenous bypass all contribute to the development of hypothermia. Infants and children have more stable temperatures during the anhepatic period when venovenous bypass is not utilized. However, there is usually a 1° to 2°C decrease in body temperature when the ice-cold donor liver is placed in the abdomen. There also may be an abrupt decreases in core temperature of 1° to 2°C with reperfusion when cold flush solution is infused into the systemic circulation. Profound hypothermia carries significant theoretic risk, including cardiac depression, arrhythmias, abnormalities in clotting function, and decreased renal function. Because of these risks, specific efforts are directed at maintaining core temperature. Heating the operating room is imperative for infants and small children. A circulating-water blanket is placed beneath the child, and the exposed extremities and scalp are wrapped with sheet-wadding or other material prior to surgical draping. Forced-air warming is useful over the legs and/or upper extremities; the position of the warming blankets will need to be adjusted if venovenous bypass is used. The forced-air warming should not include the head because if a cardiac arrest occurs, heating through the head will reduce the likelihood of successful resuscitation and, if it is successful, of having normal central nervous system (CNS) function. Intravenous fluids and blood products are warmed prior to their administration. Lowering of fresh gas flows and using a heated humidifier reduce the heat loss caused by use of cold dry inspired gases. Despite these efforts, hypothermia will develop gradually during the dissection phase. It will decrease more rapidly during the anhepatic period and immediately upon reperfusion. The above methods of heat conservation are generally effective. Core temperatures greater than 36.0°C are common at the end of the surgical procedure.

Special Techniques

Reduced-Size Grafts (Pare-Down, Split, Live-Donor Grafts)

Pediatric patients awaiting liver transplant must wait significantly longer for acceptable donors, and up to 30 percent of those patients die before an acceptable organ can be obtained. Changes in surgical management have expanded the available donor pool to provide acceptable grafts for pediatric recipients. These techniques include size reduction of an adult liver in which the donor liver is "pared-down" to provide an acceptable graft for the pediatric recipient and for an adult.[36, 68] In some situations, an adult donor graft may be split and provide two grafts for two pediatric recipients. An extension of this technique uses live donors for pediatric liver transplantation.[69] In a small number of centers, adult donors (usually a member of the patient's immediate family) undergo a partial hepatectomy (left lateral segmentectomy or left lobectomy).

Following removal of the lobe or segment from the donor, additional back table work is required to reconstruct the portal vein and hepatic arterial inflow to the liver graft. Biliary drainage is via a Roux-en-Y anastomosis. A particular anesthetic concern related to these types of transplants is the possibility of acute hemorrhage from the raw surface of the liver where the reduction technique was performed. Increased surgical blood loss should be expected at the time of graft reperfusion, and constant communication between the anesthesia and surgical teams is required during this time. Short-term outcome following reduced size liver transplants (including live donors) are similar to full size grafts in pediatric patients.[69] This technology may be particularly useful for patients with fulminant liver failure or acute decompensation of chronic liver disease when the availability of standard pediatric-size donors is limited.

Retransplantation

Hepatic retransplantation is performed to treat primary nonfunction of the allograft, allograft dysfunction resulting from thrombosis of the hepatic artery or portal vein, rejection unresponsive to aggressive medical therapy, or recurrent or primary disease in the transplanted liver. In many centers, retransplantation rates approach 15 percent of all transplants performed, and as each center matures, more and more transplant recipients are likely to require retransplantation. Because of the dense adhesions around the transplanted liver, significant hemorrhage may occur during the dissection phase. In addition, if the liver has sustained an ischemic insult, disruption of the vascular anastomoses may occur and produce catastrophic hemorrhage. There must be adequate vascular access to allow massive volume resuscitation. Sufficient blood products must be available in the operating room to rapidly instill one blood volume in the patient. Use of a rapid transfusion system (with flow rates of 1 to 2 L/min) should be considered in larger children (> 20 kg) undergoing retransplantation. An ischemic or necrotic liver may embolize necrotic cellular debris when the liver is manipulated during placement of clamps prior to the anhepatic period. Patient survival following retransplantation of the liver is worse than it is following the primary transplant.[70] Primary graft survival was 83 percent and survival following retransplant was only 66 percent in this study. This study also demonstrated that survival and complications decreased as the experience of the team increased.

Venovenous Bypass

Venovenous bypass (VVB) is an extracorporeal circuit utilized in many transplant centers to provide hemodynamic stability during the anhepatic period of liver transplantation. The bypass circuit consists of cannulae placed in the portal vein and femoral vein joined via a Y-connector. The blood is passed through a centrifugal pump and returned via a cannula in an axillary, subclavian, or internal jugular vein. During the anhepatic period, venous blood from the splanchnic bed and lower extremities is returned via the circuit to the central circulation. Compared to cases without VVB, central venous pressure and cardiac index are more stable, and there is less hypotension. Other purported benefits of VVB include a decrease in transfusion requirement, decrease in bowel edema, decrease in renal impairment, and a better environment for training transplant surgeons. Use of the VVB circuit is, however, associated with some risk. Embolic events (air, thrombus) have been reported, as have damage to brachial plexus and circuit malfunction. The duration of surgery is increased as much as 2 hours.

Size constraints have limited the application of VVB in pediatric patients. In general, VVB has not been used in infants weighing less than 10 kg. VVB has been used in selected patients weighing 10 to 20 kg. Use of VVB in larger children is dependent upon surgical preference. No outcome studies have supported the routine use of VVB in adult or pediatric patients. The use of VVB often depends on the skill and speed of the surgeon. If the surgeon can implant the new liver rapidly, there is no need for VVB. Pediatric patients in particular appear to tolerate the anhepatic period extremely well without VVB. As mentioned earlier, systemic arterial blood pressure is maintained despite a dramatic reduction in preload caused by venous clamping.

There are conflicting data regarding whether VVP is beneficial or not. Some studies suggest that the use of VVP is associated with a longer anhepatic phase of surgery and an increased need for blood. However, there was no difference in survival rates between the two groups. One study demonstrated improved oxygenation and cardiac output with a piggyback procedure (temporary portocaval shunting) versus VVP.[71] Another study demonstrated improved renal function in patients who underwent VVB.[72]

Fulminant Hepatic Failure

Fulminant hepatic failure (FHF) is present when encephalopathy develops within 8 weeks of the onset of symptoms related to liver disease in patients with previously normal hepatic function. In pediatric patients, this interval may be extremely short, often less than 2 weeks. Encephalopathy may progress in severity from grade I (mild) to moderate and severe levels (grades II and III). Development of grade IV hepatic encephalopathy with coma coincides with increasing risk for cerebral edema in patients with FHF. Because cerebral edema and intracranial hypertension are major causes for morbidity and mortality in FHF, many hepatologists aggressively monitor and treat cerebral edema during the course of FHF. Liver transplantation is one therapeutic modality in the management of FHF. Consequently, anesthesiologists must understand the pathophysiology of FHF and develop an anesthetic plan that incorporates these differences.

When a child presents with FHF, aggressive monitoring should be considered when the child passes from grade II to grade III encephalopathy. As encephalopathy progresses, protective airway reflexes may diminish, and endotracheal intubation may be required before the child becomes comatose. The use of muscle relaxants and sedatives to intubate the trachea and maintain the endotracheal tube in place will make serial neurologic examinations particularly difficult. Imaging and intracranial pressure monitoring may be the only way to evaluate neurologic status and the extent of cerebral edema. Computerized tomography scanning will detect changes in ventricular size and effacement of the sulci, which are early markers of cerebral edema. Given the logistical problems of transporting and imaging a critically ill child, scans are usually performed at 12- to 24-hour intervals. In contrast, ICP monitoring offers continuous assessment of the degree of intracranial hypertension. A variety of monitors have been utilized for this purpose in children, including subdural catheters, intraventricular catheters, and extradural fiberoptic monitors. Because of the risk for intracranial bleeding associated with placement of an ICP monitor, the prothrombin time should be aggressively corrected to near normal values with FFP, and in some situations plasmapheresis should be done before the monitor is inserted. Treatment of increased ICP from liver failure is similar to the treatment of elevated ICP in other situations: head-up positioning, head straight to facilitate venous drainage, hyperventilation, osmotic diuresis with mannitol, and the use of barbiturates. The ICP monitor reflects changes in cerebral perfusion pressure (MAP - ICP) and vasopressors may be required to support the systemic circulation. Although liver transplantation is effective in treating FHF, ICP monitoring may help select acceptable candidates for liver transplantation when a donor becomes available. When intracranial hypertension is severe and poorly controlled by maximal medical therapy, liver transplantation may be too late to prevent the adverse neurologic outcomes associated with prolonged elevated ICP.

Intraoperative ICP patterns have been described in several patients undergoing liver transplantation. Frequently, ICP changes correlate with changes in systemic hemodynamics and with manipulation of the liver. Transient increases in ICP are common at the time of liver graft reperfusion and may continue in the postreperfusion and postoperative period. Anesthetic management of FHF patients attempts to control cerebral edema and intracranial pressure. Head position, elevation of the head, and hyperventilation are continued in the operating room. To avoid the vasodilator effects of the inhaled anesthetics, anesthesia can be provided with moderate- to high-dose opioid infusion, concomitant barbiturate infusion, and low-dose (< 0.5 MAC) isoflurane. Acute increases in ICP during surgery are treated with additional barbiturate and mannitol. If the ICP is elevated at the completion of surgery, barbiturates are continued in the postoperative period and weaned as the ICP improves. Because of the combination of severe encephalopathy and prolonged administration of barbiturates, full assessment of neurologic recovery following liver transplantation for FHF may not be possible for serveral days.

Continuous Arterial Venous Hemofiltration

Renal insufficiency may develop during the course of acute or chronic liver disease. Although this frequently can be managed by trying to maintain urine output (renal dose dopamine, diuretic therapy), certain patients will develop renal insufficiency. Intervention is necessary when volume overload, hyperkalemia, metabolic acidosis, or uremic symptoms cannot be controlled with medical treatment, including hemodialysis and continuous arteriovenous hemofiltration/dialysis (CAVH/D). Conventional hemodialysis allows rapid correction of a number of metabolic abnormalities associated with renal insufficiency, but it requires specialized personnel and equipment and is associated with significant hemodynamic instability. In contrast, CAVH/D offers a more gradual correction of the metabolic abnormalities with less severe changes in hemodynamics. CAVH/D has been used in several series of patients presenting for liver transplantation. In one series, intraoperative CAVH reduced postreperfusion and postoperative cardiopulmonary dysfunction. CAVH/D has also been used to manage oliguric renal failure associated with FHF. In this setting, CAVH/D appeared to offer better control of hemodynamics and ICP than intermittent dialysis treatments. Because CAVH/D does not require dedicated personnel or specialized equipment, it can be performed at the bedside in the ICU or in the operating room. When patients with oliguric renal failure require liver transplantation, intraoperative CAVH/D can improve the ability to modulate volume status and electrolyte concentration throughout the surgery. Application of CAVH in infants and children undergoing liver transplantation is effective.

RENAL TRANSPLANTATION

Indications

Renal transplantation is the optimal therapy for children with chronic renal insufficiency (CRI) and end stage renal disease (ESRD). More specific indications for transplant include (1) uremic symptoms not responsive to dialysis, (2) failure to thrive despite aggressive nutritional therapy, (3) delayed psychomotor development, and (4) severe renal osteodystrophy.[73] Despite the availability of dialysis for children, transplantation is the preferred long-term management for children with ESRD to allow the best chance for normal growth, activity, and development. The incidence of ESRD in children 0 to 19 years of age is 15 per million.[74] The incidence increases with age and males are more likely to develop ESRD than girls secondary to the higher rate of congenital urologic anomalies. The etiologies of ESRD, and therefore the disease processes leading to transplant, differ depending on age of the patient. For children under 5 years of age, congenital lesions (renal dysplasia/aplasia, obstructive uropathy, complex urogenital malformations, and congenital nephrosis) are responsible for the majority of pediatric transplants.[75] Over 5 years of age, glomerulonephritis (e.g., focal glomerulosclerosis, membranoproliferative glomerulonephritis) and recurrent pyelonephritis are major causes of ESRD. The North America Pediatric Renal Transplant Cooperative Study (NPRTCS) registry reported that from 1987 to 1998, in over 6,500 transplants, 46 percent were over 12 years of age, 34 percent were 6 to 12 years of age, 15 percent were 2 to 5 years, and only 5 percent were under 2 years of age.[74]

Contraindications to renal transplantation are active infection and malignancy.[76, 77] Severe mental retardation, noncompliance with therapy, preexisting malignancy, and an abnormal lower urinary tract are relative contraindications and require further evaluation before placing a child on a transplant list.[78] Evaluation of retardation is complicated by encephalopathy, which is associated with uremia. Adolescents with chronic medical problems are often noncompliant with medical therapy, and failure to take immunosuppressive medications leads to graft rejection and organ failure.[78–80] Wilms' tumor is the malignancy most often associated with ESRD. Treatment of the tumor should precede the transplant by a significant period of time to ensure that the tumor has not recurred or persisted.[78] Previous bladder surgery is not a contraindication to transplant, although operations to return the bladder to an adequate size and function should occur well before the transplant itself.

Other operative procedures may be necessary prior to the transplant as well. Pretransplant nephrectomy may be needed to treat chronic infection, malignancy, uncontrolled hypertension (renovascular problems), or massive proteinuria (nephrotic syndrome).[76] Parathyroidectomy may be performed for severe renal osteodystrophy to prevent further osteomalacia.

The outcome of renal transplantation in children is encouraging. The North American Pediatric Renal Transplant Cooperative Study recently reported on 1,667 renal transplants. The overall graft survival rate for a kidney from a living related donor was 89 percent at 1 year and 80 percent at 3 years. Survival rates for cadaver kidneys were 74 percent and 62 percent.[81] Recipients less than 2 years of age and donors less than 6 years of age had increased risk of graft failure. Alexander et al. reported a graft survival of 96 percent at 1 year and 82 percent at 5 years for kidney transplant recipients less than 2 years of age and in whom cyclosporine was used for immunosuppression.[82] In that study, approximately 80 percent of the grafts came from living related donors. Others have reported similar effects of recipient and donor age.[83] Kidney transplantation is well established as an effective modality for treatment of ESRD in the pediatric population.

Pathophysiology

A patient's fluid and electrolyte balance is dramatically altered by renal failure. Hypervolemia, hypovolemia (after dialysis), hyponatremia, hyperkalemia, hypocalcemia, hyperphosphatemia, and metabolic acidosis are common. Because the failing kidney may not excrete adequate free water, hypervolemia is frequent and is a cause of hypertension. Hypovolemia can occur after aggressive dialysis. Hyponatremia occurs when water retention exceeds sodium retention, or when there is salt wasting plus an inability to concentrate urine. Hyperkalemia may be a major problem due to its effects on the cardiac conduction system, and it may require treatment before general anesthesia can be safely induced. Hypocalcemia is secondary to the hyperphosphatemia that results from the kidney's inability to excrete phosphates. Metabolic acidosis develops because the failing kidney cannot excrete the body's daily production of metabolic acids. This is due in part to inadequate synthesis of ammonia.[84]

Many organ systems are affected by ESRD. Hypertension, increased cardiac output, pericarditis, arrhythmias, and cardiomyopathy are manifestations of the altered cardiovascular system. Hypertension occurs secondary to fluid overload or to alterations in the renin-angiotensin-aldosterone system. Patients with anemia compensate for their decreased oxygen-carrying capacity by increasing their cardiac output. The use of recombinant erythropoietin has decreased the incidence of severe anemia in ESRD patients. Congestive heart failure due to hypertension and volume overload, a uremia-induced cardiomyopathy,[85] and pericardial disease[86] may complicate the management of children with ESRD. Pulmonary edema can develop as a result of fluid overload, hypoproteinemia, and altered pulmonary capillary permeability.[80]

Anemia develops due to decreased erythropoietin production and decreased erythrocyte life span, despite normal reticulocyte counts. Uremic toxins decrease RBC life span and suppress bone marrow function.[84, 87] The anemia is normocytic and normochromic, despite renal failure–induced deficiencies in folate and vitamin B_{12}. There is an increased concentration of 2,3-diphosphoglycerate (2,3-DPG), which, in conjunction with the metabolic acidosis, shifts the oxygen–hemoglobin dissociation curve to the right. This shift and an increased cardiac output partially compensate for the decreased oxygen-carrying content caused by the anemia. Administration of erythropoietin to patients with ESRD has lessened the degree of anemia.[87] However, patients on dialysis commonly receive blood transfusions, both to treat anemia and improve the outcome of transplantation.[80]

Coagulation is often altered in uremic patients by residual heparinization following dialysis and by abnormal platelet function. Platelets are usually normal in number and life span but have a reversible functional defect secondary to accumulation of guanidinosuccinic acid, which inhibits adenosine diphosphate (ADP) induced activation of platelet factor III, which is needed for normal patelet adhesion.[77] Abnormalitites in protein coagulation factors are unusual.

Renal failure induces numerous neurologic effects.[84] Uremic encephalopathy manifests as a global depression that is reversible with dialysis. Uncontrolled hypertension may lead to either focal neurologic deficits or seizures; hypertension must be controlled. Seizures may also occur with rapid electrolyte changes (e.g., hyponatremia). Peripheral neuropathies are common in patients with renal failure and usually consist of axonal degeneration with segmental demyelination. The median and common peroneal nerves are frequently involved. Autonomic dysfunction develops in children with ESRD. Baroreceptor activity may be abnormal and lead to hypotension that is unresponsive to intraoperative volume administration.

Children who have undergone hemodialysis have an increased risk of developing hepatitis due to their increased need for transfusions. This should prompt the anesthetist to take extra precautions against exposure to the patient's blood and secretions.

Nutrition is generally poor in ESRD. Uremia causes anorexia, leading to poor caloric intake and growth retardation. Despite the need for protein and calories, protein intake must be carefully controlled to prevent worsening metabolic acidosis. Renal osteodystrophy, aluminum toxicity, altered somatomedin activity, and insulin and growth hormone resistance are all associated with the growth failure.[75] Delayed gastric emptying is common in children

with renal failure. Therefore, patients undergoing a renal transplant should be considered to have a full stomach regardless of the NPO interval. It should be assumed that they are at increased risk for aspiration of gastric contents.

Preoperative Assessment and Preparation

There are two sources for kidneys for transplantation into children: cadaver and living donors. In a recent NPRTCS study of almost 2,500 pediatric transplants, 54 percent were from living donors.[88] Most of these are living-related, but there are series reporting use of living-unrelated donors in children.[89] Because living donor transplants are elective operations, there is adequate time to optimize the nutritional, hydration, and metabolic status of the patient.

Evaluation of the fluid and electrolyte status of the patient is of primary importance. If the patient has been recently dialyzed, a review of the dialysis records is often helpful. Changes in weight, blood pressure, and electrolyte concentrations before and after dialysis should be noted. The patient's dry weight is the minimum weight not associated with hypotension or cardiovascular instability; the current weight compared to the dry weight will indicate the volume status of the patient. Because there are significant changes in electrolytes (e.g., Na^+, K^+) after dialysis, serum electrolytes should be determined preoperatively. Hypertension in patients with ESRD is common and frequently indicates hypervolemia. However, many patients also require antihypertensive medications, which should be continued until the time of surgery to avoid intraoperative rebound hypertension. However, there may be a good chance that the patient is not dialyzed. In the NPRTCS study mentioned above, 25 percent of the transplants were preemptive (i.e., occurring prior to institution of dialysis).[88]

The physical examination should assess the airway and cardiopulmonary status of the patient and determine if a functioning arteriovenous shunt is present. If so, it must be protected during the operation. Patients with nephrotic syndrome or those who have been on steroids may be edematous, which could make tracheal intubation more challenging. Due to the delayed gastric emptying of patients with ESRD, the use of an antacid or anti-H_2 agent and metoclopramide may be useful before anesthesia induction.

Surgical Technique

Pediatric renal transplantation employs more than one surgical technique. In older children (weighing > 20 kg), the standard surgical approach is similar to that of adults, that is, a lower abdominal incision with extraperitoneal placement of the donor kidney in the iliac fossa. Vascular anastomoses are usually to the iliac vein (end-to-side) and iliac or hypogastric arteries (end-to-side or end-to-end). For infants and small children (weighing < 20 kg), a midline incision is made and the kidney placed intra-abdominally. The vascular connections are made to the inferior vena cava and the lower abdominal aorta. The aorta and vena cava are cross-clamped while the anastomoses are being completed. In addition, the donor organs for most small children are from adults with obvious size implications.

Anesthetic Management

Premedication is generally not necessary, but small doses of midazolam are usually safe and may allay some anxiety.[90]

Monitoring during surgery includes ECG, noninvasive blood pressure, arterial pulse oximeter, and precordial stethoscope. After induction of anesthesia, an esophageal temperature probe, peripheral nerve stimulator, and urinary catheter are placed. The urine collection device often is located where it can be seen easily by the surgeons or nurses during the operation, but the bag may not be directly visible to the anesthesiologist. CVP should be monitored by a catheter placed either percutaneously by the anesthetist or surgically (e.g., a Broviac catheter for long-term access). Because the patient's volume status is difficult to determine and may vary considerably during the operation, measurement of the CVP helps guide appropriate fluid management. The CVP catheter can also be used to obtain blood samples for laboratory tests and to administer immunosuppressants and vasoactive medications into the central circulation. An indwelling arterial catheter is not routinely used for adults or older children, but it may be quite helpful for smaller children, especially if the aorta is to be cross-clamped. One must be careful not to risk the patency of an existing arteriovenous shunt or to compromise future placement of such a shunt.

Anesthesia for renal transplantation is usually induced with intravenous drugs because the patients frequently have an IV catheter already in place. For patients without an IV catheter, inhaled induction of anesthesia is a viable alternative. The pharmacokinetics and pharmacodynamics of anesthetic drugs are altered in patients with ESRD, and this must be taken into account when administering drugs to induce anesthesia. Thiopental is a common IV induction drug used for renal transplantation. It is normally extensively plasma protein bound. Children with ESRD have decreased plasma protein concentrations. Therefore, the effects of thiopental may be greater than expected, although the greater volume of distribution found in patients with renal failure may offset some of thiopental's increased availability. Ketamine can also be used as an IV induction agent for patients with ESRD, but its sympathomimetic effects may exacerbate preexisting hypertension. Propofol is also widely used. The onset of action of propofol is only slightly slower than thiopental, but propofol does hurt when it is given into most peripheral veins. Various techniques have been tried to diminish the discomfort but generally they have mixed success. To blunt the autonomic response to laryngoscopy and tracheal intubation, opioids or lidocaine can be given intravenously. As with all sick children, careful titration of anesthetic drugs to the desired effect is always the safest approach.

The choice of muscle relaxant for tracheal intubation continues to generate discussion. Because delayed gastric emptying is common in patients with renal failure, patients undergoing renal transplantation may be at increased risk for regurgitation and possible aspiration of gastric contents. This situation makes a rapid sequence intravenous induction of anesthesia with an intravenous induction agent, cricoid pressure, and succinylcholine theoretically advantageous. However, as noted elsewhere, succinylcholine can produce several potentially serious problems, including hyperkalemia. Administration of succinylcholine may cause serum potassium concentrations to rise 0.5 to 0.75 mEq/L in normal patients.[91] A number of conditions can lead to an exaggerated rise of serum potassium and subsequent hyperkalemic arrest. Patients with ESRD are at risk for hyperkalemia if they have uremic neuropathy[92] or if they have not been dialyzed recently. An alternative to succinylcholine is to perform a modified rapid sequence intravenous induction of anesthesia using either an inhaled or intravenous agent, a nondepolarizing muscle relaxant, cricoid pressure, and controlled ventilation. The nondepolarizing muscle relaxant used should not depend on renal pathways of elimination. Two categories that fit this requirement are the atracurium/cis-atracurium family, whose elimination is by Hoffman degradation and ester hydrolysis and the steroid-based muscle relaxants that are predominantly metabolized by the liver. Atracurium has a tendency to release histamine and can lead to significant hypotension, but cis-atracurium releases considerably less histamine. Cis-atracurium's metabolism is also independent of either renal or hepatic pathways and should be an excellent choice for renal transplantation in children. The steroid-based muscle relaxants vecuronium and rocuronium have some dependence on renal excretion, perhaps 10 to 25 percent, that will lead to some prolongation of onset and duration of action of the drugs when used in patients with ESRD. Regardless of which relaxant is used for tracheal intubation and maintenance of anesthesia, a peripheral nerve stimulator should be used to assess the degree of neuromuscular blockade and the doses of muscle relaxant titrated to effect.

Maintenance of general anesthesia during renal transplantation is usually provided by a combination of potent inhaled anesthetic agents and opioids. Nitrous oxide can be used, but it may distend the intestines and make it more difficult to close the abdomen at the end of the operation. Halothane may produce an exaggerated hypotensive response in hypocalcemic patients. Sevoflurane has the theoretical problem of producing a metabolite, compound A, that has been associated with renal concentrating defects, and although useful for inhaled induction of anesthesia, should probably not be the first choice for maintenance of anesthesia, although reports of renal toxicity are rare.[93] Fentanyl is the most widely used opioid for renal transplantation. No active metabolites are excreted by the kidneys, and there is extensive experience with its use in children without significant complication. The metabolites of morphine are excreted by the kidney so probably should not be the first choice for intraoperative analgesia.

If the patient has an arteriovenous shunt, the extremity with the shunt must be positioned so that the shunt is protected and available to allow the anesthetist to periodically determine that the shunt is functional. A blood pressure cuff should not be used on that extremity. At the very least, the shunt should be checked both at the beginning and the end of the operation for a thrill or bruit and the presence of either or both documented on the anesthetic record.

Fluid management during renal transplantation is challenging owing to reduced preoperative renal function and to blood loss and third space fluid losses during the operation. Preoperative fluid status is discussed above. Interstitial fluid losses (third space) and blood losses are determined in the usual fashion (see Chapter 11). Fluid administration should be based on estimates of need and clinical criteria, including vital signs and CVP. Transplant surgeons frequently request that the CVP be maintained at levels higher than normal (e.g., 12 to 15 cm H_2O). An isotonic crystalloid solution is a suitable choice of fluid. Theoretically, lactated Ringer's solution should be avoided due to the potassium (4 mEq/L) that it contains. On the other hand, normal saline is hypernatremic (154 mEq/L) and can lead to a hypernatremic metabolic acidosis if given in large quantities. Intermittent measurements of the serum electrolyte and glucose concentrations are always suitable to follow the metabolic status of the patient. If a blood transfusion is required, washed packed red blood cells are preferred due to the small volume and the minimal amount of potassium present after washing. The blood should also be irradiated to minimize graft-versus-host reactions in an immunocompromised host.

In addition to maintaining a high CVP, the surgeons may request a higher than normal mean arterial pressure (MAP) to ensure adequate perfusion of the new kidney. Whenever a new kidney is placed into a small recipient (< 20 kg), it is possible that the aorta will be cross-clamped to perform the arterial anastomosis. When the aorta is subsequently unclamped, the blood pressure may decrease dramatically secondary to reduced afterload and the return of acidotic blood from the lower extremities. Furthermore, a large quantity of blood is diverted to the renal allograft, which will decrease the arterial blood pressure if the intravascular volume is inadequate. The anesthetist must be prepared to treat abrupt changes in arterial pressure with fluid and drugs. It must be remembered that these changes occur with patients who usually have baseline hypertension. Vascular thrombosis is a leading cause of graft failure in the smallest of recipients so the outcome may indeed depend on the reperfusion management.

The anesthetist will also be involved with the administration of immunosuppressant medications, antibiotics, diuretics, and other drugs during the operation. The surgeon or nephrologist should notify the anesthetist of the doses and timing of these medications. It is helpful to find out common side effects of these drugs that may impact anesthetic management (e.g., OKT3 can cause pulmonary edema).

At the end of the operation, a determination should be made whether the patient's trachea will be extubated. If so, residual neuromuscular blockade should be antagonized. Prolongation of the action of neuromuscular blockers is matched by prolongation of action of the reversal agents. The patient should be awake when the trachea is extubated. If there is evidence of pulmonary edema, or a relatively large kidney is placed into the abdomen of a small child or neonate, tracheal extubation can be delayed and the patient transported to a pediatric intensive care unit (ICU) and the patient's condition allowed to stabilize.

Postoperative pain control is most commonly achieved by the administration of intravenous opioids. Epidural analgesia can be used, but the association with possible hypotension has tended to limit its widespread use as well as the alterations in coagulation status of patients with ESRD.

HEART TRANSPLANTATION

Indications

Cardiac transplantation is performed in pediatric patients who have congenital or acquired heart disease. With increasing success of transplantation, indications for transplantation in neonates, infants, and children are rapidly changing. Transplantation has particular value in congenital conditions not amenable to conventional surgical correction, or in conditions where conventional methods have yielded poor results (e.g., hypoplastic left heart syndrome). Congenital or acquired heart conditions may also result in irreversible ventricular pump dysfunction in which transplantation offers the only option for long-term survival. Additional indications for transplantation include cardiomyopathies resulting from ischemia, viral infection, chemotherapy, or cryptogenic factors. Relative contraindications to cardiac transplantation include active infection, abnormal neurologic function, other end-organ dysfunction, and in particular, altered pulmonary vasculature with irreversible pulmonary hypertension. Pediatric cardiac transplant candidates must wait for availability of an appropriate donor organ: the cardiac allograft is matched to body size, blood type, and HLA antigen cross-match. Using data from the UNOS, current availability of pediatric donors is relatively well matched for patients on the waiting list. Despite this statistic, mortality of pediatric patients awaiting cardiac transplantation is significant.

Outcome

The waiting time for a heart is relatively short.[94] Ninety-three percent of patients are alive at 30 days and 81 percent are alive if the wait for an organ is 90 days. Thirty-eight percent of patients with structurally normal hearts have major complications while awaiting a heart, while only 9 percent of infants with congenital heart disease have complications.

The rate of early death following cardiac transplant is the same in adult and pediatric patients, about 8 percent.[95] The 1-year survival is about 80 percent, while the survival at 5 years has decreased to 70 percent. Risk factors adversely affecting survival include donor age and donor recipient gender mismatching. In another study, 90 percent of patients were alive at 1 year and 78 percent were alive 6 years after transplant.[96] Primary causes of death were acute rejection, lymphoproliferative disease, and infections. Preexisting elevated pulmonary vascular resistance was not predictive of early or late mortality.[97] Late complications of heart transplantation in general have been development of coronary artery disease (which is more common in patients with CMV and hepatitis C infections) cancer, and infections.[98] The risk of lymphoproliferative disease is about 10 times higher if the patient was Epstein-Barr virus (EBV) negative before and becomes positive after the transplant.[99]

Pathophysiology

Pediatric patients awaiting cardiac transplantation manifest decreased cardiac function and often have secondary impairment of other organs. Because of the variety of acquired and congenital conditions amenable to transplantation, different degrees of cardiac dysfunction may be apparent in these patients.

Neonatal orthotopic heart transplantation is indicated to treat hypoplastic left heart syndrome. After diagnosis and resuscitation, if required, prostaglandin E_1 (PGE_1) is infused to maintain the ductus arteriosus patent and to maintain systemic perfusion. Ventilatory support may be required to help maintain acid–base balance because acidosis has profound effects on pulmonary vascular resistance. The occurrence of cardiomyopathy may require ionotropic support of the failing heart, and appropriate attention must be paid to maintaining adequate intravascular volume. Young patients with congenital or acquired cardiac disease may develop adverse changes in the pulmonary vascular bed and develop pulmonary hypertension and right ventricular dysfunction (see Chapter 18).

Prior to approval for transplantation, the patient must undergo a thorough evaluation to fully assess cardiac function and reserve, other organ function, and a psychosocial assessment. Evaluation may include ECG, echocardiogram, cardiac catheterization, and trials of specific medicines and interventions. The anesthesiologist should review the data gathered during the evaluation process to gain as much knowledge about the function of the various organs of the transplant recipient. Of particular importance is the status of pulmonary circulation and the child's dependence upon a patent ductus arteriosus for pulmonary and/or systemic perfusion. Documentation of the effects of various ionotropic, chronotropic, and antiarrhythmic medications should be noted.

Anesthetic Management

Anesthetic preparation for cardiac transplantation may be hastened by the relatively short survival time of the cardiac allograft before transplant. Oftentimes, the preoperative assessment and preparation of the patients and operating room will be done in the 4 to 6 hours immediately prior to the arrival of the donor organ. Because of the time constraint, the operation on the recipient may begin before the donor organ arrives. Paramount to anesthesia preparation is ready availability of a variety of medications to support a failing heart and vascular system.[100] Prior to the induction of anesthesia, epinephrine, dopamine, dobutamine, isoproterenol, nitroprusside, and nitroglycerin should be readily available and the dosage ranges should be calculated for each child.

In coordination with the transplant surgeon, the patient is brought to the operating room near the time the donor organ is expected to arrive in the hospital. Patients dependent upon ionotropic agents and/or oxygen should be transported to the operating room with these medications being infused and the patient being adequately monitored. Monitors in the preinduction period include pulse oximetry, ECG, noninvasive blood pressure, and a precordial stethoscope. An intravenous line should be placed prior to the induction of anesthesia in order to facilitate the induction of anesthesia and provide a route for emergent administration of vasoactive medications. In children without an intravenous line, inhalation induction with halothane and nitrous oxide may reduce the stress associated with venous cannulation.[101] After the induction of anesthesia, additional monitors include direct arterial pressure, central venous pressure measurement, temperature probes (esophageal, rectal, tympanic, nasopharyngeal), capnography, and a urinary catheter. Depending on the status of the recipient's pulmonary circulation, a pulmonary artery catheter may be inserted following implantation of the cardiac allograft.

The cardiac reserve of patients requiring cardiac transplantation is marginal at best. Impaired contractile function may be particularly susceptible to the effects of anesthetic agents, alterations in acid–base status, gas exchange, arrhythmias, or electrolyte changes. Acute changes in afterload or preload may have tremendous impact on the systemic or pulmonary circulation. Premedication should be kept to a minimum, and when required, administered in a monitored setting. Because of the emergent nature of cardiac transplant procedures, a rapid sequence induction of anesthesia may be indicated. A combination of atropine 20 μg/kg, ketamine 1–2 mg/kg, and succinylcholine 1 mg/kg can be administered IV after adequate preoxygenation and application of cricoid pressure. Changes in pulmonary artery pressure seen in adult patients are not apparent in pediatric patients provided there is sufficient ventilation to maintain normal concentrations of carbon dioxide in the arteries. Another common induction technique is to administer an opioid (fentanyl 50 to 100 μg/kg; sufentanil 10 μg/kg) and pancuronium 0.1 mg/kg.[102] Potent vapors are avoided unless required briefly during inhalation induction of anesthesia; amnestic doses of a benzodiazepine can be administered. Each transplant center has a protocol used for the induction and maintenance of immunosuppression, and will usually administer one or more immunosuppressants in the operating room. The anesthesiologist should be familiar with the protocol, have the appropriate medications available, and report the time of administration in the postoperative report to the ICU.

Following induction of anesthesia and establishment of additional monitors and vascular access, the surgical procedure begins. In patients with congenital disease, a transplant may involve reopening a median sternotomy. Because of possible dense adhesions and entrapment of the cardiac structures, significant hemorrhage may occur. Therefore, adequate vascular access for rapid volume administration, blood product replacement, and emergent femoral bypass is required. In neonates and small children, cardiac transplants may be performed during circulatory arrest, whereas in larger children, hypothermic cardiopulmonary bypass may be utilized. As the final anastomoses are completed, rewarming of the patient begins and cardiopulmonary bypass is discontinued. Particular attention must be paid to strategies to reduce pulmonary vascular resistance including adequate anesthesia, slight hyperventilation, adequate oxygenation, and prevention of acidosis. Because the donor right ventricle has not been subjected to an abnormal pulmonary circulation previously, it may fail rapidly if the pulmonary artery resistance is excessively high. Additional pharmacologic interventions, such as PGE₁ or amrinone, may be required. If systemic hypotension develops, additional vasopressor(s) may be required.

Early in the postbypass period, the cardiac allograft may manifest a variety of dysrhythmias. The ECG may reveal two P waves that represent atrial activity from the donor heart and the remaining portion of recipient atria. Effective conduction occurs only from the donor sinoatrial node to the donor ventricle. Because the donor heart is denervated, the baroreceptor reflex is absent, and the donor heart rate is determined principally by concentrations of circulating catecholamines that alter the native pacemaker rate. Of therapeutic importance is the fact that the donor conduction system will respond to the direct acting chronotropic effects of the medications administered. Confirmation of the pattern of electrical activity is obtained by direct inspection of the heart. In cases of nodal rhythm, isoproterenol or temporary pacing may be required to support a heart with a fixed stroke volume. Because of the beta effects of isoproterenol, systemic arterial blood pressure may decrease, and another vasoactive medication may be required to support the circulation.

Following restitution of adequate hemodynamics and conduction activity, attention is paid to hemostasis. Protamine sulfate is required to reverse heparinization; clotting factors and platelet administration may be required as indicated by laboratory testing and clinical conditions. Closure of the chest may be difficult at the conclusion of the cardiac transplant procedure. Discrepancy in size between the donor and recipient may become apparent at the time of sternal closure. Direct compression of the heart or the pulmonary outflow tract may interfere rapidly with systemic or right ventricular function. Close inspection of the arterial blood pressure waveform and immediate notification of the surgeon that changes have occurred is required.

Following closure of the chest, the patient is transported to the ICU in a controlled and closely monitored fashion. Because of the tenuous status of the donor heart following a period of ischemic preservation and the volatility of the recipient pulmonary circulation, ready access to pharmacologic interventions is required. Normal acid–base status should be maintained in the early postoperative period, and adequate analgesia should be provided as the effects of the opioids used for anesthesia begin to wear off. Pulmonary vascular resistance must be controlled, particularly during weaning from mechanical ventilation. Despite the institution of immunosuppressent regimens, rejection of the cardiac allograft may occur in the first week following transplantation. In some centers, repeated myocardial biopsy will be required, depending upon the size of the patient.

HEART–LUNG AND LUNG TRANSPLANTATION

Indications

Combined heart–lung or isolated lung transplantation is an emerging surgical procedure in infants and children with progress reported from several centers.[103, 104] Several clinical conditions are amenable to heart–lung transplantation, including cystic fibrosis, complex congenital heart disease, Eisenmenger's syndrome, and primary pulmonary hypertension. Early results of combined heart–lung transplantation suggest survival rates similar to heart–lung transplantation in adults.[95]

Pediatric lung transplantation is also in the early phase of application for a variety of pulmonary conditions. Several centers have described single- or double-lung transplants in children with cystic fibrosis, bronchiolitis obliterans, lymphocytic interstitial pneumonitis, and diffuse pulmonary arteriovenous malformation. Neonatal lung transplantation has been considered as a potential therapy for severe pulmonary hypoplasia associated with congenital diaphragmatic hernia and cystadenomatous malformations. Whether lung transplantation can be successful in these critically ill neonates who often requiring extracorporeal membrane oxygenation remains to be seen. Reduced size lung transplantation utilizing a pulmonary lobe or segment has been proposed as a potental mechanism to address donor shortage and donor-recipient size disparity for this population of infants.

Infants listed for lung or heart–lung transplant have a high mortality before an organ can be obtained.[105] Fifty-three percent of neonates and 48 percent of older children die while awaiting an organ. Following transplant, infants had much longer hospital stays than older children. Five-year survival of patients following lung or heart–lung transplant is low. In one study it was only 33 percent.[106] One of the common causes of death is obliterative bronchiolitis and irreversible airway obstruction. Interestingly, patients who have EBV infections before transplant have better survival than those who are EBV negative and become positive after transplant.[99] The development of EBV positivity after transplant is associated with development of lymphoproliferative disease.[107]

Pediatric heart–lung and lung transplantation will be in evolution during the coming decade as the indications and contraindications are evaluated, and the success of the procedures is determined on a larger scale. It is likely, though, that these procedures will be limited by the scarcity of suitable donors, particularly for neonates. This may change as donor selection criteria undergo revision and refinement in various transplant centers, and attempts at reduced size and/or live-donor for lung transplants are undertaken.

Pathophysiology

Children requiring heart–lung or lung transplantation manifest varying degrees of cardiopulmonary dysfunction and require different procedures based upon the extent of the cardiopulmonary disease. Patients with restrictive or obstructive lung disease may benefit from single-lung transplantation, whereas many patients with primary pulmonary hypertension will benefit from combined heart–lung transplantation because of their right ventricular failure. Because of chronic infection, single-lung transplants are discouraged in patients with cystic fibrosis in favor of double-lung transplants (either sequential single-lung or en bloc double-lung transplants). Heart–lung transplants also have been utilized in patients with cystic fibrosis.

Because of the extent of their pulmonary disease, these patients are likely to manifest hypoxemia and require supplemental oxygen. They also often manifest hypercarbia at rest that is caused by their respiratory insufficiency. Right ventricular function and pulmonary artery pressures may be assessed via echocardiography and/or cardiac catheterization. Exercise studies may be performed to measure the extent of arterial desaturation as the oxygen consumption increases. Because of the complex pathophysiology involved in the underlying disease process and the additional strain of the surgical procedure, part of the evaluation process may attempt to predict the requirement for cardiopulmonary bypass during lung transplantation (see below).

Anesthetic Management

Current preservation techniques for lungs permit only 6 hours of lung ischemia time. Consequently, these cases are scheduled as semiemergent procedures and require close coordination between the organ procurement team and the transplant team. Patients are admitted from home, undergo rapid evaluation for interval changes in their condition, and are prepared for anesthesia and surgery. There is usually inadequate time to allow for a proper period of NPO. Premedication, which may be important in an anxious child or adolescent, must take into account the child's limited degree of pulmonary reserve. Most patients require supplemental oxygen at all times, including during transport to the operating room.

The recipient is brought to the operating room and routine noninvasive monitors are applied. Because of the degree of respiratory insufficiency, patients may prefer to be semirecumbent during preoxygenation and induction of anesthesia. A rapid sequence or modified rapid sequence induction of anesthesia is performed after adequate denitrogenation. Because of preexisting increased pulmonary vascular resistance, the use of ketamine should probably be avoided on the off chance that the drug will increase pulmonary vascular resistance further. The anesthetic agents and their doses should be carefully chosen to avoid excessive depressant effects on the right ventricle. Most lung transplant procedures require periods of one-lung ventilation, and particular attention is directed to providing this capability. In older adolescents, a double-lumen endotracheal tube may be utilized, whereas in smaller children, a bronchial blocker is usually used. Fiberoptic bronchoscopy will assist in the correct placement of a double-lumen endotracheal tube or endobronchial blocker for one-lung ventilation. Meticulous attention should be paid to management of ventilation. Many patients with severe emphysema and/or preexisting lung blebs are at risk for pneumothorax. Ventilation is controlled to minimize airway pressure, prevent gas trapping, and provide adequate ventilation (i.e., normal $Paco_2$ is important). In the event of sudden hemodynamic compromise, tension pneumothorax should be considered in these high-risk patients.

Routine monitoring for these procedures should include arterial and central venous pressure monitoring, and urinary catheters. Pulmonary artery catheters, considered essential in adults undergoing lung transplants, usually are used only in larger children and adolescents. Adequate vascular access for volume administration is required. End-tidal gas monitoring and arterial blood gas measurements should be available. An anesthetic regimen using moderately high doses of opioid, small amounts of benzodiazepine, and muscle relaxants usually provides stable hemodynamics. Small amounts of inhaled agents may be tolerable depending on the amount of myocardial reserve. Epidural analgesics may be provided through a lumbar or thoracic epidural catheter and may be helpful in the postoperative period. Anesthetic management for heart–lung and lung transplantation procedures is individualized to the particular recipient and the particular procedure. Initial positioning depends on the type of transplant being performed: lateral decubitus for single-lung transplant; supine for heart–lung and en bloc double-lung, and supine arms over head for sequential double-lung transplant. Placement of the endotracheal tube for one-lung ventilation should be reconfirmed following final positioning of the patient. Fluid management should be closely monitored. Blood loss is frequently minimal, and use of colloid solutions may be preferred to minimize translation of fluid into the transplanted lung. Some centers use renal-dose dopamine to facilitate urine output.

The ability of the patient to tolerate one-lung ventilation is important in the management of single-lung transplantation.[108] The ability to maintain adequate arterial oxygenation and systemic hemodynamics during one-lung ventilation and clamping of the pulmonary artery will determine the need for cardiopulmonary bypass. Strategies for improving oxygenation include increasing the inspired oxygen concentration, increasing minute ventilation, and adding positive end-expiratory pressure. Adding continuous positive airway pressure (CPAP)/PEEP to the collapsed lung is not effective because the pulmonary artery and bronchae are clamped for total pneumonectomy. Because of altered pulmonary vascular resistance, marked increases in pulmonary artery pressure may occur when the pulmonary artery clamp is applied; the rise in pressure may be sufficient to cause pulmonary hypertension and right ventricular dysfunction. Strategies to reduce pulmonary artery pressure include careful administration of vasodilators (PGE_1, nitroglycerin, nitroprusside). Inadequate oxygenation or marked pulmonary hypertension usually requires institution of partial cardiopulmonary bypass via the femoral vessels. Assessment of the patient's response to the ventilatory and hemodynamic changes associated with total pneumonectomy requires close communication between surgical and anesthesia teams, adequate availability of vasodilators and vasoactive medications, and ready availability of cardiopulmonary bypass.

Following completion of the bronchial anastomosis, ventilation of the transplanted lung is instituted before the lung is reperfused to minimize shunt through a nonventilated lung. Reperfusion of the lung may result in hemodynamic changes and sudden changes in oxygenation. Omentum may be wrapped around the bronchial anastomosis as the procedure nears completion. The double-lumen endotracheal tube is replaced with a single-lumen tube when the surgical procedure is completed. Use of an endotracheal tube changer may facilitate the tube change following a prolonged case.

INTESTINAL, MULTIVISCERAL, AND PANCREATIC TRANSPLANTATION

Indications

Successful transplantation of liver, kidneys, hearts, and lungs has led transplant surgeons to attempt to treat other illnesses affecting infants and children. In children, the short-gut syndrome, which results from necrotizing enterocolitis, intestinal malrotation and volvulus, or congenital defects (intestinal atresia, abdominal wall defects), leads to dependence on total parenteral nutrition (TPN). The long-term sequelae of TPN include steatotic liver disease and eventual hepatic failure and the complications of long-term venous access. Isolated small bowel transplants, combined small bowel–liver transplants, and extensive multivisceral transplants (liver, pancreas, gastrointestinal tract from stomach to colon) have been performed in an attempt to manage short-gut syndrome. Early attempts to perform intestinal transplants met with uniform failure due to rejection of the graft, sepsis, and the occurrence of graft-versus-host disease. With the introduction of cyclosporine, and more recently the introduction of FK506 immunosuppressive therapy, prolonged survival of the gut and return to enteral nutrition have been reported in an increasing number of patients.[109] A recent summary of worldwide experience in small bowel transplantation (in isolation or with combined liver or multivisceral transplantation) reported 23 survivors of 33 intestinal transplants.[110] Similarly, the Pittsburgh transplant center reported 10 intestinal transplants (alone or combined small bowel–liver) in children less than 5 years of age with 7 survivors.[111] The majority of these patients were discharged to home. Despite the encouraging results, intestinal and multivisceral transplantation remains experimental in children and requires prolonged hospitalization and incurs significant costs. The coming decade will further define the efficacy of this type of transplantation for treating short-gut syndrome in infants and children.

Pancreas transplantation has been utilized most commonly as combined renal and pancreas transplantation for treatment of ESRD in diabetics with other end-organ dysfunction (retinopathy, neuropathy). Because of the interval between development of insulin-dependent diabetes in children and end-organ complications, few reports of pancreas transplantation have been reported in infants and children, apart from the multivisceral procedures described above. Indications for pancreatic transplantation are changing rapidly as the success of the procedure improves. Pancreas transplantation of diabetic patients has stabilized or improved their nephropathy, retinopathy, and neuropathy. The role of early transplantation has not been proven by a large-scale study, and the utilization of this technique in pediatric diabetic patients will have to balance potential benefits of maintaining near normal control of glucose concentrations with the inherent risks of transplant surgery and lifelong immunosuppression. A potential therapy for diabetic children may be isolated pancreatic islet cell transplantation. With newer isolation techniques, relatively pure populations of islet cells can be infused into the recipient portal vein. With recent purification methods and improved immunosuppression, clinical success of the islet transplantation has yielded reduced or eliminated the need for exogenous insulin, as evidenced by C-peptide response. This form of pancreas transplant may provide the needed endocrine function to diabetic patients without the necessity for a major surgical procedure and the complications associated with exocrine function of the transplanted pancreas.

Pathophysiology

Because of the variety of disease processes necessitating intestinal or multivisceral transplantation, a spectrum of clinical presentation of patients can be expected. Despite the use of TPN, a number of the patients will be malnourished. Hepatic function may be nearly normal, display laboratory evidence of steatotic changes, or manifest frank hepatic failure and cirrhosis. Other organ systems may be involved if serious complications have resulted from the underlying disease process that produced the short-gut syndrome or from prolonged periods of TPN.

Anesthetic Management

The exact form of intestinal transplantation (i.e., isolated, combined liver–small bowel, or multivisceral transplantation) depends upon the cause of intestinal failure and associated extraintestinal organ involvement. Following identification of an appropriate donor, the recipient undergoes a regimen designed to purge and decontaminate the intestinal tract. Routine premedication is avoided, but may be required and administered under appropriate monitoring situations. Rapid sequence induction of general anesthesia and tracheal intubation is planned. Despite normal or slightly impaired hepatic function, there is a potential for extensive blood loss and hemorrhage in most of these cases. Previous abdominal surgery and extensive dissection and evisceration of the native organs prolong the dissection period and increase blood loss. Venous access sites, particularly around the central circulation, may be limited because of previous TPN catheters. Venous cutdown may be required to provided adequate access. Arterial blood pressure and central venous pressure should be monitored directly. Intraoperative management is similar to liver transplantation: hemodynamic stability may require rapid infusion of crystalloid, colloids or blood products; maintaining metabolic homeostasis requires frequent arterial blood gases and electrolyte concentration determinations. Maintenance of normothermia may be difficult despite utilization of fluid warmers, heating blankets, humidifiers, and forced-air warming.

Significant hemodynamic instability may accompany reperfusion of the transplant grafts. Because UW solution is used in the preservation process, hyperkalemia may occur following reperfusion of the organ. Hypotension is relatively common at the time of reperfusion and may reflect combined contributions of vascular filling of the grafts, release of vasoactive substances, and bleeding from the multiple anastomoses.

In multivisceral transplantation and combined pancreatic renal transplantation, particular attention is required to maintain normoglycemia. Tight intraoperative control of the glucose concentration may result in improved pancreatic allograft function. To achieve glucose concentrations of 80 to 120 mg/dl requires frequent intraoperative determinations of glucose concentration, and titration of a regular insulin infusion. A period of hyperglycemia is common following reperfusion of the pancreatic graft and requires additional insulin administration.

COMPLICATIONS FOLLOWING TRANSPLANTATION

Rejection

A common complication associated with all forms of allograft transplantation is the occurrence of rejection of the transplanted tissue by the recipient. Recent laboratory investigations and clinical correlation have provided new insight into the mechanisms of rejection. Particular cell types, frequently nonparenchymal cells within the allograft, may be the first target of acute rejection. A complex system of cell signaling and activation involving a variety of leukocytes and cytokines is responsible for initiation and propagation of organ rejection. A variety of cofactors alter the rejection process, particularly the effects of concomitant viral infection. The transition from acute to chronic rejection is often accompanied by a reduction of the lymphocytic cellular infiltrate within the allograft. Antibody-mediated rejection may result in chronic, vascular rejection and subsequent ischemic changes of the graft.

Rejection in the early posttransplant period may be a subtle process and difficult to assess by routine physical and laboratory examination. Clinical signs of rejection will vary by the transplanted organ, and are not likely to be specific. Therefore, there is need for early histologic evaluation of the organ to diagnose acute rejection. Many transplant centers routinely biopsy the organ at weekly to monthly intervals to search for evidence of acute rejection. This generally requires an invasive procedure requiring anesthesia or sedation in children. Routine immunosuppression is altered in the face of acute rejection. Steroid administration is increased first, and then the monoclonal antibody OKT3 is used. Additional options for controlling rejection include switching the primary immunosuppression to one of the newer agents, FK506, and more recently, RS61443. Progression to chronic rejection reduces the therapeutic options. As rejection progresses, function of the allograft continues to diminish, eventually producing graft failure. Other than dialysis, no organ system support can be provided for a signficant period of time, and retransplantation remains the only option.

Infection

Infections following transplantation are common because of the immunosuppression needed to prevent allograft rejection.[112, 113] A recent review of 36 pediatric liver transplant recipients revealed that 72 percent of them became infected.[114] There was an early tendency toward bacterial infections (involving the abdomen, blood stream, and surgical wound), and a later predominance of viral infection, particularly cytomegalovirus (CMV). Management of immunosuppression with prophylactic antilymphocyte antibody preparations significantly increased the risk of infection. Infectious complications caused four deaths in this small group of patients, and underscores the significance of posttransplant complications. In larger studies, CMV is the predominant pathogen causing infectious complications in transplant recipients.[115, 116] Patterns of CMV infection may include primary infection in a seronegative recipient, reactivation of the recipient's latent CMV viral infection, and superinfection of a new strain of CMV in the recipient. Although CMV disease occurs more frequently in CMV-positive recipients, the severity of CMV primary infection in seronegative recipients can be catastrophic. CMV disease presents typically in the second month following transplantation with persistent fever and a viral-like syndrome. Pneumonitis, hepatitis, and gastrointestinal manifestations may appear and herald a more serious infection. Because of the frequent occurrence of CMV disease, most transplant centers utilize antiviral prophylaxis regimens with either acyclovir or ganciclovir following solid organ transplantation.[117] For active CMV disease, ganciclovir may be a more effective treatment.

Lymphoproliferative Complications

Clinical experience has documented lymphoproliferative disorders in children following transplantation.[118] Isolated lymphomas have occurred within transplanted organs and at other sites and are associated with significant mortality. Causative factors in the development of lymphoproliferative disorders are felt to include the effects of immunosuppression and perhaps concomitant EBV and/or CMV viral infection.

Patients with Epstein-Barr viral infections can have serious complications or death. Patients with a low viral load who were treated with preemptive therapy had no evidence of lymphoproliperative disease (LD), whereas three of four who had high viral load and were not treated preemptively developed LD.[119] Two of 14 with high viral loads who were treated preemptively had LD. Therefore, it is important that early treatment be carried out. Bacteremia after intestinal transplant also is associated with an increased incidence of LD.[112]

Graft-versus-Host Disease

Graft-versus-host disease (GVHD) is a well-recognized complication of bone marrow transplantation, but recent experience is demonstrating its occurrence with solid organ transplantation. In solid organ transplantation, the amount of viable immunocompetent lymphoid tissue leads to the risk of GVHD. Small bowel transplants have been reported to have a significant incidence of GVHD, and some centers pretreat the donor with antilymphocyte preparations to reduce the occurrence of this problem. With experience, subtle manifestations of GVHD, including pancytopenia, hemolytic anemia, and cutaneous rashes, have led to an increasing awareness of this posttransplant complication. With the trend toward more extensive transplantation in younger children, recognition and control of GVHD will become more important for long-term survival.

ANESTHETIC MANAGEMENT FOLLOWING TRANSPLANTATION

Vascular Access

Following organ transplantation, pediatric patients may benefit from long-term vascular access. Frequent laboratory tests and prolonged administration of antibiotic, antiviral, antifungal, and immunosuppressive medications may be required. Indwelling catheters such as a Broviac or Hickman catheter may improve patient acceptance of the various regimens and may permit home therapy. The anesthetic care to obtain vascular access is similar to that in other children. Close attention should be directed to sterile technique in view of immunosuppression, and there should be discussion of the steroid management in the immediate perioperative period.

Diagnostic and Therapeutic Procedures (Biopsy, Interventional Radiology)

Pediatric transplant recipients also will require a number of diagnostic and therapeutic procedures. Liver, renal, or cardiac biopsy that is performed under sedation in adult recipients is likely to require general anesthesia in infants and children. A variety of posttransplant complications involving vascular structures, urinary drainage, or biliary drainage will require general anesthesia in the interventional radiology suite. Anesthetic management issues related to the care of infants and children away from the operating room are discussed in Chapter 28. It should be assumed that these sick infants and children have a full stomach and should be treated as such.

Posttransplant Surgery

Regardless of the transplant procedure, as transplant recipients age, they are likely to acquire diseases or conditions that require additional surgery. Prior to such procedures, the anesthesiologist must assess the function of the transplanted organ, review the status of the patient's immunosuppression, and perform a careful assessment of the other organ systems. Hypertension and chronic renal insufficiency are common findings in patients treated with cyclosporine. Most patients will demonstrate evidence and findings of chronic steroid administration.

Retransplantation

Retransplantation is the only effective treatment for a variety of conditions arising in solid organ transplant recipients. Technical errors and problems with preservation may result in primary nonfunction of allograft transplants. In the case of liver, heart, and lung transplantation, emergent retransplantation may offer the only chance for survival. A more common reason for retransplantation is the occurrence of chronic rejection that produces graft dysfunction or failure and is unresponsive to aggressive immunosuppression regimens. The decision to proceed with retransplantation is difficult because perioperative morbidity and mortality are greater, and the long-term results are significantly poorer than primary transplantation. With the growing discrepancy between available donor organs and waiting recipients, ethical considerations of costs and benefits to individual patients and society are often involved in the decision to retransplant.

In one study, patient survival was significantly worse following retransplantation of the liver.[120] The 1-year graft survival was only 37 percent when retransplant occurred soon after the first transplant. Graft survival was much improved when retransplant occurred later.

REFERENCES

1. Cecka JM, Terasaki PI: The UNOS Scientific Renal Transplant Registry. Clin Transpl 1, 1992.
2. The Registry of the International Society for Heart and Lung Transplantation: Ninth official report—1992. J Heart Lung Transplant 11:599, 1992.
3. Belle SH, Beringer KC, Murphy JB, Detre KM: The Pitt-UNOS Liver Transplant Registry. Clin Transpl 17, 1992.
4. Cooper JD, Patterson GA, Pohl MS: Current status of lung transplantation—report of the St. Louis International Lung Transplant Registry. Clin Transpl 77, 1992.
5. Firestone S: Special considerations for transplantation in children. Int Anesthesiol Clin 29:137, 1991.
6. Tornqvist J, Van Broeck N, Finkkenauer C, et al: Long-term psychosocial adjustment following pediatric liver transplantation. Pediatr Transplant 3:115, 1999.
7. Jain A, Mazariegos G, Kashyap R, et al: Comparative long-term evaluation of tacrolimus and cyclosporine in pediatric liver transplantation. Transplantation 70:617, 2000.
8. Reyes J, Jain A, Mazariegos G, et al: Long-term results after conversion from cyclosporine to tacrolimus pediatric liver transplantation for acute and chronic rejection. Transplantation 69:2573, 2000.
9. Tzakis AG, Reyes J, Todo S, et al: Two-year experience with FK 506 in pediatric patients. Transplant Proc 619, 1993.
10. Reding R: Steroid withdrawal in liver transplantation: benefits, risks, and unanswered questions. Transplantation 70:405, 2000.
11. Bartosh SM, Thomas SE, Sutton MM, et al: Linear growth after pediatric liver transplantation. J Pediatr 135:624, 1999.
12. Todo S, Nery J, Yanaga K, et al: Extended preservation of human liver grafts with UW solution. JAMA 261:711, 1989.
13. Stratta RJ, Wood RP, Langnas AN, et al: Effect of extended preservation and reduced-size grafting on organ availability in pediatric liver transplantation. Transplant Proc 22:482, 1990.
14. Kawauchi M, Gundry SR, de Begona JA, et al: Prolonged preservation of human pediatric hearts for transplantation: correlation of ischemic time and subsequent function. J Heart Lung Transplant 12:55, 1993.
15. Ardite E, Ramos C, Rimola A, et al: Hepatocellular oxidative stress and initial graft injury in human liver transplantation. J Hepatol 31:921, 1999.
16. Totsuka E, Fung JJ, Urakami A, et al: Influence of donor cardiopulmonary arrest in human liver transplantation: possible role of ischemic preconditioning. Hepatology 31:577, 2000.
17. Schindel DT, Dunn SP, Casa AT, et al: Pediatric recipients of three or more hepatic allografts: results and technical challenges. J Pediatr Surg 35:297, 2000.
18. Schaeffer MJ, Alexander DC: U.S. system for organ procurement and transplantation. Am J Hosp Pharm 49:1733, 1992.
19. Kawauchi M, Gundry SR, de Begona JA, et al: Utilization of pediatric donors salvaged by cardiopulmonary resuscitation. J Heart Lung Transplant 12:185, 1993.
20. Yandza T, Goulao J, Gauthier F, et al: The use in pediatric transplantation of livers from donors who died from anoxia. Transplant Proc 23:2617, 1991.

21. Yokoyama I, Tzakis AG, Imventarza O, et al: Pediatric liver transplantation from neonatal donors. Transpl Int 5:205, 1992.
22. Rogiers X, Broering DC, Mueller L, Burdelski M: Living-donor liver transplantation in children. Langenbecks Arch Surg 384:528, 1999.
23. Adam R, Cailliez V, Majno P, et al: Normalised intrinsic mortality risk in liver transplantation: European Liver Transplant Registry study. Lancet 356:621, 2000.
24. Younes BS, McDiarmid SV, Martin MG, et al: The effect of immunosuppression on posttransplant lymphoproliferative disease in pediatric liver transplant patients. Transplantation 70:94, 2000.
25. Smets F, Vajro P, Cornu G, et al: Indications and results of chemotherapy in children with posttransplant lymphoproliferative disease after liver transplantation. Transplantation 69:982, 2000.
26. Dotti G, Fiocchi R, Motta T, et al: Epstein-Barr virus-negative lymphoproliferative disorders in long-term survivors after heart, kidney, and liver transplant. Transplantation 69:827, 2000.
27. Bodeus M, Smets F, Reding R, et al: Epstein-Barr virus infection in sixty pediatric liver graft recipients: diagnosis of primary infection and virologic follow-up. Pediatr Infect Dis J 18:698, 1999.
28. Mclaughlin K, Wajstaub S, Marotta P, et al: Increased risk for post transplant lymphoproliferative disease in recipients of liver transplants with hepatitis C. Liver Transpl 6:570, 2000.
29. Huang RY, Shapiro NL: Adenotonsillar enlargement in pediatric patients following solid organ transplantation. Arch Otolaryngol Head Neck Surg 126:159, 2000.
30. Borland LM: Anesthesia for organ transplantation in children. Int Anesthesiol Clin 23:173, 1985.
31. National Institutes of Health Consensus Development Conference Statement: Liver transplantation. Hepatology 4:107S, 1984.
32. Belle SH, Detre KM: Report from the Pitt-UNOS Liver Transplant Registry. Transplant Proc 25:1137, 1993.
33. Lloyd-Still JD: Impact of orthotopic liver transplantation on mortality from pediatric liver disease. J Pediatr Gastroenterol Nutr 12:305, 1991.
34. Whitington PF, Balistreri WF: Liver transplantation in pediatrics: indications, contraindications, and pretransplant management. J Pediatrics 118:169, 1991.
35. Emond JC, Aran PP, Whitington PF, et al: Liver transplantation in the management of fulminant hepatic failure. Gastroenterology 96:1583, 1989.
36. Broelsch CE, Whitington PF, Emond JC: Evolution and future perspectives for reduced-size hepatic transplantation. Surg Gynecol Obstet 171:353, 1990.
37. Ewert R, Mutze S, Schachschal G, et al: High prevalance of pulmonary diffusion abnormalities without interstitial changes in long-term survivors of liver transplantation. Transpl Int 12:222, 1999.
38. McCloskey JJ, Schleien C, Schwarz K, et al: Severe hypoxemia and intrapulmonary shunting resulting from cirrhosis reversed by liver transplantation in a pediatric patient. J Pediatr 118:902, 1991.
39. Gunnarsson L, Eleborg L, Eriksson LS: Anesthesia for liver transplantation in patients with arterial hypoxemia. Transpl Int 3:103, 1990.
40. Itasaka H, Hershon JJ, Cox KL, et al: Transient deterioration of intrapulmonary shunting after pediatric liver transplantation. Transplantation 55:212, 1993.
41. Yonemura T, Yoshibayashi M, Uemoto S, et al: Intrapulmonary shunting in biliary atresia before and after living-related liver transplantation. Br J Surg 86:1139, 1999.
42. Helmke K, Burdelski M, Hansen HC: Detection and monitoring of intracranial pressure dysregulation in liver failure by ultrasound. Transplantation 70:392, 2000.
43. Grewal HP, Brady L, Cronin DC II, et al: Combined liver and kidney transplantation in children. Transplantation 70:100, 2000.
44. Porte RJ, Knot EAR, Bontempo FA: Hemostasis in liver transplantation. Gastroenterology 97:488, 1989.
45. Llamas P, Cabrera R, Gomez-Arnau J, Fernandez MN: Hemostasis and blood requirement in orthotopic liver transplantation with and without high-dose aprotinin. Haematologia 83:338, 1998.
46. Garcia-Huete L, Domenech P, Sabate A, et al: The prophylactic effect of aprotinin on intraoperative bleeding in liver transplantation: a randomized clinical study. Hepatology 26:1143, 1997.
47. Castaldo P, Langnas AN, Stratta RJ, et al: Long-term central venous access in pediatric liver transplantation recipients: role of percutaneous insertion of subclavian Broviac catheters. Transplant Proc 23:1991, 1991.
48. Arden JR, Lynam DP, Castagnoli KP, et al: Vecuronium in alcoholic liver disease: a pharmacokinetic and pharmacodynamic analysis. Anesthesiology 68:771, 1988.
49. Hunter JM, Parker CJ, Bell CF, et al: The use of different doses of vecuronium in patients with liver dysfunction. Br J Anaesth 57:758, 1985.
50. Lebrault C, Berger JL, D'Hollander AA, et al: Pharmacokinetics and pharmacodynamics of vecuronium (ORG NC 45) in patients with cirrhosis. Anesthesiology 62:601, 1985.
51. Cook DR, Freeman JA, Lai AA, et al: Pharmacokinetics and pharmacodynamics of doxacurium in normal patients and in those with hepatic or renal failure. Anesth Analg 72:145, 1991.
52. White JDF, Caldwell JC, Prager MC, et al: The pharmacokinetics of vecuronium during liver transplantation in humans. Anesth Analg 70:S432, 1990.
53. O'Kelly B, Jayais P, Veroli P, et al: Dose requirements of vecuronium, pancuronium, and atracurium during orthotopic liver transplantation. Anesth Analg 73:794, 1991.
54. Pittet JF, Tassonyi E, Schopfer C, et al: Plasma concentrations of laudanosine, but not of atracurium, are increased during the anhepatic phase of orthotopic liver transplantation in pigs. Anesthesiology 72:145, 1990.
55. Bodenham A, Quinn K, Park GR: Extrahepatic morphine metabolism in man during the anhepatic phase of orthotopic liver transplantation. Br J Anaesth 63:380, 1989.
56. Kelley SD, Cauldwell CB, Fisher DM, et al: Recovery of hepatic drug metabolic function following hypothermic preservation. Anesthesiology 82:251, 1995.
57. Kang Y: Liver transplantation. Int Anesthesiol Clin 29:59, 1991.
58. Carlier M, van Obbergh L, Veyckemans F, et al: Intraoperative hemodynamic modifications during pediatric orthotopic liver transplantation. Intensive Care Med 15(suppl 1):S73, 1989.
59. Nemec P, Cerny J, Hokl J, et al: Hemodynamic measurement in liver transplantation. Piggyback versus conventional techniques. Ann Transplant 5:35, 2000.
60. Aggarwal S, Kang Y, Freeman JA, et al: Postreperfusion syndrome: cardiovascular collapse following hepatic reperfusion during liver transplantation. Trans Proc 19:54, 1987.
61. Ellis JE, Lichtor JL, Feinstein SB, et al: Right heart dysfunction, pulmonary embolism, and paradoxical embolism during liver transplantation. Anesth Analg 68:777, 1989.
62. Lichtor JL, Emond J, Chung MR, et al: Pediatric orthotopic liver transplantation: multifactorial predictions of blood loss. Anesthesiology 68:607, 1988.
63. Butain SG, Pabari M: Massive transfusion and hyperkalaemic cardiac arrest in craniofacial surgery in a child. Anaesth Intensive Care 27:530, 1999.
64. Grosse H, Lobbes W, Frambach M, et al: The use of high dose aprotinin in liver transplantation: the influence on fibrinolysis and blood loss. Thromb Res 63:287, 1991.
65. Porte RJ, Molenaar IQ, Begliomini B, Groenland TH, et al: Aprotinin and transfusion requirements in orthotopic liver transplantation: a multicentre randomised double-blind study. EMSALT Study Group. Lancet 355:1303, 2000.
66. Stevens LH, Emond JC, Piper JB, et al: Hepatic artery thrombosis in infants. A comparison of whole livers, reduced-size grafts, and grafts from living-related donors. Transplantation 53:396, 1992.
67. Mazzaferro V, Esquivel CO, Makowka L, et al: Hepatic artery thrombosis after pediatric liver transplantation—a medical or surgical event? Transplantation 47:971, 1989.
68. Broelsch CE, Emond JC, Whitington PF, et al: Application of reduced-size liver transplants as split grafts, auxiliary orthotopic grafts, and living related segmental transplants. Ann Surg 212:368, 1990.
69. Emond JC, Heffron TG, Kortz EO, et al: Improved results of living-related liver transplantation with routine application in a pediatric program. Transplantation 55:835, 1993.
70. Facciuto M, Heidt D, Guarrera J, et al: Retransplantation for late liver graft failure: predictors of mortality. Liver Transpl 6:174, 2000.
71. Steib A, Saada A, Clever B, et al: Orthotopic liver transplantation with preservation of portocaval flow compared with venovenous bypass. Liver Transpl Surg 3:518, 1997.
72. Grande L, Rimola A, Cugat E, et al: Effect of venovenous bypass on perioperative renal function in liver transplantation: results of a randomized, controlled trial. Hepatology 23:1418, 1996.

73. Davis ID, Bunchman TE, Grimm PC, et al: Pediatric renal transplantation: indications and special considerations. A position paper from the Pediatric Committee of the American Society of Transplant Physicians. Pediatr Transplant 2:117, 1998.

74. Al-Akash SI, Ettenger RB: Kidney transplantation in children. *In* Danovitch GM (ed): Handbook of Kidney Transplantation. 3rd ed. Philadelphia, Lippincott Williams & Wilkins, 2001, p 332.

75. Ryckman FC, Alonso MH: Solid organ transplantation in children. *In* Ashcraft KW (ed): Pediatric Surgery. 3rd ed. Phildadelphia, WB Saunders Company, 1999, p 597.

76. Lillehei C: Renal transplantation. *In* Ashcraft K, Holder T (eds): Pediatric Surgery. 2nd ed. Philadelphia, WB Saunders Company, 1993, p 766.

77. Everts E: Anesthesia for organ transplantation. *In* Cote C, Ryan J, Todres I, Goudsouzzian N (eds): A Practice of Anesthesia for Infants and Children. 2nd ed. Philadelphia, WB Saunders Company, 1993, p 377.

78. Ettenger RB: Renal transplantation. *In* Barakat A (ed): Renal Disease in Children. New York, Springer-Verlag, 1990, p 371.

79. Arbus GS, Rochon J, Thompson D: Improved cadaveric renal transplant outcome in children. Pediatr Nephrol 5:137, 1991.

80. Grimm P, Ettenger RB: Pediatric renal transplantation. *In* Barness L (ed): Advances in Pediatrics. St Louis, CV Mosby, 1992, p 441.

81. McEnery PT, Stablein DM, Arbus G, Tejani A: Renal transplantation in children. A report of the North American Pediatric Renal Transplant Cooperative Study. N Engl J Med 326:1727, 1992.

82. Alexander SR, Arbus GS, Butt KM, et al: Renal transplantation in infants. Ann Surg 212:353, 1990.

83. Donkerwolcke RA: Survival of cadaveric renal transplant grafts from young donors and in young recipients. Pediatr Nephrol 5:152, 1991.

84. Cramolini G: Diseases of the renal system. *In* Katz J, Steward D (eds): Anesthesia and Uncommon Diseases. Philadelphia, WB Saunders Company, 1987, p 155.

85. O'Regan S, Matina D, Ducharme G, et al: Echocardiographic assessment of cardiac failure in children with chronic renal failure. Kindey Int Suppl 24:S77, 1983.

86. Bailey GL, Hampers CL, Hager EB, et al: Uremic pericarditis. Clinical features and management. Circulation 38:582, 1968.

87. Paganini EP, Miller T: Erythropoietin therapy in renal therapy. Adv Intern Med 38:223, 1993.

88. Vats AN, Donaldson L, Fine RN, et al: Pretransplant dialysis status and outcome of renal transplantation in North American children: a NAPRTCS study. Transplantation 69:1414, 2000.

89. Al-Uzri A, Sullivan EK, Fine RN, et al: Living-unrelated renal transplantation in children: a report of the North American Pediatric Renal Transplant Cooperative Study (NAPRTCS). Pediatr Transplant 2:139, 1998.

90. Vinik HR, Reves JG, Greenblatt DJ, et al: The pharmacokinetics of midazolam in chronic renal failure patients. Anesthesiology 59:390, 1983.

91. Koide M, Waud BE: Serum potassium concentrations after succinylcholine in patients with renal failure. Anesthesiology 36:142, 1972.

92. Miller RD, Way WL, Hamilton WK, et al: Succinylcholine-induced hyperkalemia in patients with renal failure? Anesthesiology 36:138, 1972.

93. Artru AA: Renal effects of sevoflurane during conditions of possible increases risk. J Clin Anesth 10:531, 1998.

94. Rosenthal DN, Dubin AM, Chin C, et al: Outcome while awaiting heart transplantation in children: a comparison of congenital heart disease and cardiomyopathy. J Heart Lung Transplant 19:751, 2000.

95. John R, Rajasinghe H, Chen JM, et al: Impact of current management practices on early and late death in more than 500 consecutive cardiac transplant recipients. Ann Surg 232:302, 2000.

96. Azeka E, Barbero-Marcial M, Jatene M, et al: Heart transplantation in neonates and children. Intermediate-term results. Arq Bras Cardiol 74:197, 2000.

97. Tenderich G, Koerner MM, Stuettgen B, et al: Pre-existing elevated pulmonary vascular resistance: long-term hemodynamic follow-up and outcome of recipients after orthotopic heart transplantation. J Cardiovasc Surg (Torino) 41:215, 2000.

98. Esposito S, Renzulli A, Agozzino L, et al: Late complications of heart transplantation: an 11-year experience. Heart Vessels 14:272, 1999.

99. Swerdlow AJ, Higgins CD, Hunt BJ, et al: Risk of lymphoid neoplasia after cardiothoracic transplantation. A cohort study of the relation to Epstein-Barr virus. Transplantation 69:897, 2000.

100. Lowe DA: Anesthetic considerations in pediatric cardiac transplantation. *In* Dunn JM, Donner RM (eds): Heart Transplantation in Children Mount Kisco, Futura Publishing, 1990, p 39.

101. Zickmann B, Boldt J, Hempelmann G: Anesthesia in pediatric heart transplantation. J Heart Lung Transplant 11:S272, 1992.

102. Hickey PR, Hansen DD: Fentanyl- and sufentanil-oxygen-pancuronium anesthesia for cardiac surgery in infants. Anesth Analg 63:117, 1984.

103. Spray TL, Mallory GB, Canter CE, et al: Pediatric lung transplantation for pulmonary hypertension and congenital heart disease. Ann Thorac Surg 54:216, 1992.

104. Spray TL: Pediatric lung transplantation. Semin Thorac Cardiovasc Surg 4:113, 1992.

105. Ro PS, Spray TL, Bridges ND: Outcome of infants listed for lung or heart/lung transplantation. J Heart Lung Transplant 18:1232, 1999.

106. Aurora P, Whitehead B, Wade A, et al: Lung transplantation and life extension in children with cystic fibrosis. Lancet 354:1591, 1999.

107. Boyle GJ, Michaels MG, Webber SA, et al: Post transplantation lymphoproliferative disorders in pediatric thoracic organ recipients. J Pediatr 131:309, 1997.

108. Conacher ID: Isolated lung transplantation: a review of problems and guide to anaesthesia. Br J Anaesth 61:468, 1988.

109. Vennarecci G, Kato T, Misiakos EP, et al: Intestinal transplantation for short gut syndrome attributable to necrotizing enterocolitis. Pediatrics 105:E25, 2000.

110. Busuttil RW, Farmer DG, Shaked A, et al: Successful combined liver and small intestine transplantation for short-gut syndrome and liver failure. West J Med 158:184, 1993.

111. Todo S, Tzakis A, Reyes J, et al: Intestinal transplantation in humans under FK 506. Transplant Proc 1198, 1993.

112. Sigurdsson L, Reyes J, Kocoshis SA, et al: Bacteremia after intestinal transplantation in children correlates temporarily with rejection or gastrointestinal lymphoproliferative disease. Transplantation 70:302, 2000.

113. Their M, Holmberg C, Lautenschlager I, et al: Infections in pediatric kidney and liver transplant patients after perioperative hospitalization. Transplantation 69:1617, 2000.

114. George DL, Arnow PM, Fox A, et al: Patterns of infection after pediatric liver transplantation. Am J Dis Child 147:924, 1992.

115. Dussaix E, Wood C: Cytomegalovirus infection in pediatric liver recipients. A virological survey and prophylaxis with CMV immune globulin and early DHPG treatment. Transplantation 48:272, 1989.

116. Fukushima N, Gundry SR, Razzouk AJ, Bailey LL: Cytomegalovirus infection in pediatric heart transplantation. Transplant Proc 25:1423, 1993.

117. Boudreaux JP, Hayes DH, Mizrahi S, et al: Decreasing incidence of serious cytomegalovirus infection using gancyclovir prophylaxis in pediatric liver transplant patients. Transplant Proc 25:1872, 1993.

118. Malatack JF, Gartner JJ, Urbach AH, Zitelli BJ: Orthotopic liver transplantation, Epstein-Barr virus, cyclosporine, and lymphoproliferative disease: a growing concern. J Pediatr 118:667, 1991.

119. Green M, Bueno J, Rowe D, et al: Predictive negative value of persistent low Epstein-Barr virus viral load after intestinal transplantation in children. Transplantation 70:593, 2000.

120. Achilleos OA, Mirza DF, Talbot D, et al: Outcome of liver retransplantation in children. Liver Transpl Surg 5:401, 1999.

20

Anesthesia for Abdominal Surgery

JOHN W. HOLL

◆   ◆   ◆

Anesthesia for surgical procedures on the gastrointestinal tract and abdominal wall of infants and children often presents formidable challenges to those who administer anesthesia to pediatric patients. Comprehensive anesthesia management begins with an understanding of the pathophysiology of the underlying disease, a thorough assessment of the patient's preoperative status, and a fundamental knowledge of the surgical goals and requirements. This information then must be integrated into a carefully formulated anesthetic plan that encompasses appropriate pharmacology, modern monitoring, technical skill, and judgment that is based on experience if the outcome is to be successful for the patient.

EMBRYOLOGY AND PATHOGENESIS

During the third week of gestation the primitive gut (archenteron) has completed separation from the notochord.[1] Incomplete separation may lead to a variety of reduplications, cysts, and nonfunctional units, and may be associated with a hemivertebra.[2] By the end of the third week of gestation, this tube, which extends from the mouth to the cloaca, is divided into the foregut, midgut, and hindgut.[3] Each division is nourished by a separate branch of the primitive aorta.[4] The paired ventral tributaries of the dorsal aortae will fuse to form the celiac artery and supply the infradiaphragmatic portion of the foregut. The ompha-

lomesenteric artery, later to be called the superior mesenteric artery, supplies the midgut, and the inferior mesenteric artery supplies the hindgut.

The foregut gives rise to the pharynx, esophagus, stomach, and the first part of the duodenum. Anomalies of the pharynx and esophagus frequently are encountered and are discussed more fully elsewhere in this volume (see Chapter 17). The stomach develops initially as a dilation of the caudal end of the foregut and then expands in size and in function. Anomalies of the body of the stomach are quite rare, but obstruction at the pyloris is common (atresia, stenosis, or a "wind sock" deformity). Although not congenital, infantile pyloric stenosis is a common surgical problem that usually manifests between the second and sixth weeks after birth. It is caused by hypertrophy of the muscularis layer of the pylorus and leads to marked swelling and obstruction.

The hepatic diverticulum arises ventrally from the foregut just distal to stomach. Three outpouchings from the diverticulum then differentiate into the liver, the gallbladder, and the ventral pancreas. Posteriorly, the dorsal pancreas arises and then rotates around the duodenum to fuse with the ventral pancreas. By the seventh gestational week all of the morphologic orientation is complete but not yet functional. Anomalous pancreatic rotation may lead to complete or partial duodenal obstruction. Hepatic caniliculi and the intrahepatic and extrahepatic bile ducts proliferate at this time and have been postulated to be very vulnerable to maternal viruses, drugs, and toxins. Intrahepatic biliary atresia may be associated with congenital heart disease.[5] Trisomy 21 (Down syndrome) is frequently associated with atresia of the first portion of the duodenum. Cystic fibrosis of the pancreas, with subsequent inspissation of meconium, may also lead to obstruction.

The midgut extends from the second portion of the duodenum to the proximal large bowel. Anomalous development of the midgut is a common cause of emergent neonatal surgery. Initially, the midgut is open ventrally to the yolk sac (Fig. 20–1). As the embryo rapidly grows, the wide-open yolk sac reduces to a relatively smaller yolk stalk (vitelline duct or omphalomesenteric duct). During the fifth to tenth weeks of fetal life the midgut grows faster than the rest of the body, so that the primitive gut is extruded into the extraembryonic coelom. The gut migrates in a counterclockwise rotation around the axis formed by the omphalomesenteric artery. Interruption of the blood supply provided by this artery may lead to bowel atresia. During the tenth week of fetal life the bowel returns to the abdomen and continues its counterclockwise rotation. When the cecum and the appendix reach the right

lower quadrant, they attach to the posterior wall of the peritoneum. Anomalous rotation and fixation may contribute to intestinal obstruction and strangulation of the gut at any time from the tenth week of gestation through adulthood. Before the bacterial colonization that occurs at birth, volvulus and strangulation of the fetal gut result in reabsorption and fibrosis of the gut.

Incomplete reabsorption of the omphalomesenteric duct results in a spectrum of anomalies that can include a patent duct, a prolapsed gastrointestinal tract, or even umbilical polyps. Meckel's diverticulum is an intraperitoneal patent tract. These diverticula contain gastric mucoa and may ulcerate. Therefore, they must be considered in the differential diagnosis of gastrointestinal bleeding and perforation at any age.

Abdominal wall defects have been classified by Moore and Stokes[6] into four categories: umbilical hernia, omphalocele, gastroschisis, and prolapse of the omphalomesenteric duct. An umbilical hernia is an outpouching of abdominal viscera through a stretched umbilical ring. Classically, it is less than 4 cm in diameter and is always covered with skin. An omphalocele represents an incomplete fetal return of the gut to the abdominal cavity be-

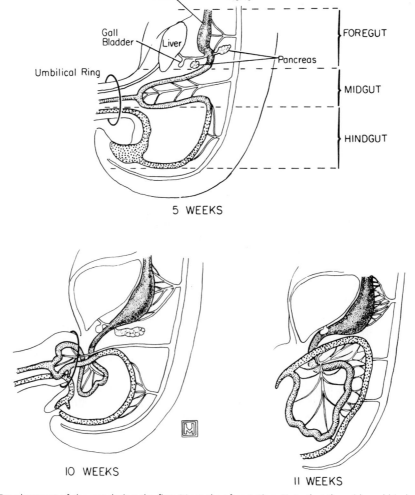

FIGURE 20–1. Development of the gut during the first 11 weeks of gestation. Note that the mid- and hindgut are present in the umbilical cord, and that these structures return to the abdominal cavity, rotate, and become fixed in position. *Finely stippled areas,* foregut; *moderately stippled,* midgut; *lightly stippled,* hindgut.

cause of a lateral fold defect of the abdominal wall.[7] The exposed viscera are covered with a thin, transparent membrane that may have perforated. The umbilical cord is inserted into the apex of the lesion. A giant omphalocele is associated with other major congenital defects and is common in patients with cranial defects. Defects of the cranial fold of the abdominal wall produce epigastric omphaloceles, which are frequently seen in combination with sternal, pericardial, diaphragmatic, and cardiac defects in the syndrome of pentalogy of Cantrell.[8] Hypogastric omphalocele is associated with extrophy of the urinary bladder and cloacal abnormalities and is thought to be caused by a faulty caudal fold of the abdominal wall.

Gastroschisis is a herniation of the bowel contents through the lateral abdominal wall, usually to the right of the umbilical cord. Because the herniated intestines are not covered by a peritoneal membrane and because the herniation may have been of long duration, considerable morphologic and functional compromise of the gut often occurs. Bowel atresia, particularly of the "apple peel" variety, is present in 10 percent of cases. Several theories have been advanced to explain the development of gastroschisis. A vascular accident to the abdominal wall, either arterial[9] or venous,[10] produces a wall defect through which intestines may freely extrude. Glick et al.[11] argue that it occurs after early fetal rupture of an omphalocele and subsequent fetal peritonitis.

Inguinal hernia and cryptorchidism, although less striking in presentation than omphalocele, gastroschisis, and extrophy, represent far more common and potentially equally dangerous pediatric surgical problems. The inguinal canal is formed by the descent of the gubernaculum through the transversalis fascia (later to become the internal inguinal ring) and the oblique aponeurosis (later to become the external inguinal ring) to the labial scrotal fold. This is followed by a fold of peritoneum known as the processus vaginalis. In the male, the testes descend through the processus vaginalis to the scrotum during the seventh to ninth months of gestation. Failure of the processus to obliterate and the inguinal ring to close provides a pathway for bowel to herniate and abdominal fluid to collect (communicating hydrocele). Incomplete closure of the ring may trap the fluid (noncommunicating hydrocele). In the female, the canal of Nuck is analogous to the processus and may also serve as a potential pathway for herniation of bowel or ovary.

From the hindgut near the allantois, the urogenital sinus, the cloaca, and the cloacal membrane arise. They are joined by the ureteric buds and unite the mesodermally derived renal system and the endodermally derived cloaca. Incomplete rupture of the cloacal membrane during the ninth week of gestation is associated with a variety of rectal and anal anomalies and with bladder exstrophy and cloacal defects.

Although isolated lesions of the lower colon (atresia, stenosis, and duplication) may occur, a more common problem is congenital aganglionic megacolon (Hirschsprung's disease), in which migration of neuroenteric ganglion cells from the neural crest is arrested before the cells reach the colonic mucosa. This arrest results in ineffective propulsion of colonic contents. Severe cases may lead to neonatal bowel obstruction, whereas others may present later as chronic constipation.

PHYSIOLOGY AND PHARMACOLOGY

The functions of the gastrointestinal tract are to ingest, digest, and selectively absorb nutrients and to excrete wastes. This process begins in a rudimentary manner shortly after the morphologic differentiation of the embryonic phase of fetal life (the first 8 weeks), becomes functional during the growth and development phase of fetal life (9 to 40 weeks), and continues maturing well into the neonatal period. Swallowing begins early in the second trimester, and coordinated intestinal motility begins in the third trimester. Enzymes that digest sucrose and maltose are present early and those that digest lactose and protein appear later. The ability of the neonatal gastrointestinal system to function solely on enteral feedings is at best marginal in the term infant and is often compromised in prematures, infants of diabetic mothers (IDM), infants with intrauterine growth retardation (IUGR), infants with respiratory distress syndrome (RDS), and asphyxiated infants. Although this fascinating area of developmental metabolism is discussed elsewhere,[12, 13] several aspects merit special emphasis for the anesthesiologist.

At birth the pH of the stomach contents is mildly acid (average pH, 6), reflecting the alkaline pH of amniotic fluid.[14] After removal or absorption of this fluid, hydrochloric acid (HCl) can be demonstrated. Although the rate of production initially is low, it rises quickly after 4 to 8 hours and reaches adult values by 24 to 48 hours.[15] There is no clear consensus, but most studies show a decrease in production of HCl between the 10th and 30th day and then a rise to adult levels by 3 months of age.[16]

Neonatal hypoglycemia is common in premature infants; in those with IDM, IUGR, RDS, and Beckwith-Wiedemann syndromes; and in stressed infants. Whole-blood glucose concentrations below 20 mg/dl in the premature, 30 mg/dl in term infants during the first 72 hours, and 40 mg/dl thereafter produce central nervous system (CNS) or systemic signs in most infants, although an occasional infant may be asymptomatic. It is better to keep the blood glucose at or above 40 mg/dl in all newborns. Overzealous dextrose replacement can be detrimental because the neonatal kidney easily spills glucose, resulting in an osmotic diuresis. All neonates and stressed infants should receive 5 percent dextrose in 0.2 percent sodium chloride (NaCl) 4 ml/kg/h or 10 percent dextrose in water ($D_{10}W$) 2 to 3 ml/kg/h, supplemented as indicated with appropriate electrolyte replacement. Infants with symptomatic hypoglycemia should have a bolus of $D_{10}W$ 2 ml/kg followed by an infusion of D_{10} 0.2 percent NaCl and frequent glucose determinations to document appropriate glucose homeostasis.

One of the most significant advances in pediatric surgery and neonatology has been the development of total parenteral nutrition (TPN). TPN makes it possible to provide adequate calories, essential proteins, lipids, vitamins, and trace elements to maintain positive nitrogen balance and to sustain normal growth and development until enteral nutrition is possible. Because of the tonicity of most intravenous (IV) alimentation fluids and the potential damage to peripheral veins, these solutions are often delivered through central venous catheters, which can be associated with a range of problems (sepsis, erosion of the vessel, extravasation of fluid, arrhythmia, and thrombosis). Metabolism of lipids provides more calories per gram at a lower respiratory quotient than metabolism of carbohydrates. This also results in lower ventilatory requirements for the infant.[17] Infants respond to the high glucose load associated with TPN by increasing insulin release. Abrupt termination of TPN may lead to sever hypoglycemia. TPN must not be used for extracellular fluid replacement during anesthesia because this leads to severe hypertonicity.

Pulmonary aspiration of gastrointestinal contents may occur as a result of vomiting or passive regurgitation.[18] Vomiting during general anesthesia most frequently occurs during the excitement phase of induction in response to hypoxia or to premature stimulation of the airway or surgical manipulation. It may also occur during emergence from anesthesia. The vomiting reflex is mediated by a vomiting center located in the chemoreceptor trigger zone on the floor of the fourth ventricle and a vomiting center in the reticular formation.[19] Stimulation, which is mediated through the autonomic nervous system, results initially in hypersalivation, reverse peristalsis, and occasionally cardiac arrhythmia. Gastric tone is decreased and duodenal tone is increased, permitting duodenal fluid to enter the stomach. Retching (glottic closure, a decrease in intrathoracic pressure, and increase in gastric and abdominal wall contractions) forces gastric contents into the lower esophagus. Vomiting then begins with an increase in intrathoracic pressure, a coordinated relaxation of pharyngoesophageal sphincter tone, an elevation of the soft palate, and the active expulsion of vomitus. In the neurologically intact person, the airway is protected during vomiting by glottic closure and forward displacement of the larynx.

Regurgitation is not a reflex act but one of passive movement of esophageal and gastric contents into the pharynx caused by a pressure gradient. In the normal, conscious patient, three areas of the esophagus impede regurgitant flow. The first, the upper esophageal (UES), is located at the junction of the pharynx and esophagus and consists of voluntary striated muscles, which are sensitive to pentothal and muscle relaxants.[20] Second, a distinct zone of high pressure in the body of the lower esophagus can be identified just cephalad to the diaphragm. Finally, the lower esophageal sphincter (LES), located caudal to the diaphragm, is the most significant of the three areas in prevention of regurgitation of stomach contents. Although the LES is not a definite anatomic structure, it functions as one because of its relation to the entrance of the esophagus into the stomach and the crura of the diaphragm. It relaxes during the terminal phase of coordinated swallowing and is affected by hormones such as gastrin, secretin, and prostaglandin, but not by muscle relaxants. Although many normal neonates exhibit discoordinated swallowing and regurgitation, persistent gastroesophageal reflux beyond 6 weeks of age is pathologic and is a well-documented cause of apneic spells, paroxysmal coughing, pneumonia, laryngospasm, and wheezing.[21] These manifestations can be improved by medical management or surgical antireflux procedures. During light inhalational anesthesia without muscle relaxants, the LES appears to be competent, as measured by esophageal pH,[22] but the resting tone decreases with deeper levels of anesthesia. Although the fasciculations caused by depolarizing muscle relaxants may[23] or may not[24] cause elevation of intragastric pressure, any positive-pressure gradient is probably counteracted by a corresponding rise in LES pressure.[25] Potentially more dangerous is the rise in abdominal pressure in response to laryngoscopy during inadequate anesthesia and incomplete diaphragmatic paralysis, but yet complete UES paralysis. This scenario is less likely to occur if adequate anesthetic and muscle relaxant are administered, cricoid pressure is skillfully applied, and sufficient time is allowed for the muscle relaxant to achieve maximal effect before laryngoscopy is attempted.

Gastric emptying time in the neonate, infant, and child is variable. Because the stomach contents are a mixture of liquid, digestible solid, and indigestible solid, it is important to consider each component separately. In the unobstructed patient, the half-life of clear isotonic fluid is between 10 and 20 minutes. Passage of digestible solids is correlated with the bulk, tonicity, pH, caloric density, and chemical composition of the gastric contents. Complex fats and fatty acids may take up to 6 to 7 hours to pass through the pylorus. Hypertonic or bulky contents must be broken down and diluted to isotonic solutions. Nondigestible solids, such as seeds or fruit pits, are cleared by "housekeeping" peristaltic waves at the end of the gastric emptying cycle. Pain, fear, anxiety, trauma, sepsis, and narcotics delay or may completely stop gastric emptying.

There has been considerable interest in the pharmacologic manipulation of gastric acid and gastric emptying time, in hopes of reducing the risk for pulmonary aspiration of gastric contents and diminishing postoperative nausea and vomiting (Table 20–1). Gastric acid secretion can be decreased by cimetidine and ranitidine, and the pH of the fluid can be raised by antacids. This may decrease the severity of aspiration pneumonia, should it occur. Metoclopramide has been advocated to speed gastric emptying, raise LES pressure, and decrease nausea, but high doses of metoclopramide may produce extrapyramidal symptoms. The clinical significance of these measures remains unclear. Because regurgitation and vomiting are uncommon in elective anesthesia of normal infants, it is difficult to justify prophylactic medication for all elective cases. However, it may be appropriate under certain circumstances, such as full stomach and known gastroesophageal reflux (GER). Pharmacologic intervention to counteract patient noncompliance with established fasting regimens is not indicated for elective cases.

Although total enteric intake and output can be easily measured, it is difficult to estimate the volume of fluid secreted by the salivary glands, stomach, liver, pancreas, and intestine that dilute and digest ingested food. For every milliliter of fluid ingested, approximately 5 ml of secretions are added by the time the food traverses the duodenum. This fluid is reabsorbed in the proximal jejunum and ileum. More water is actively absorbed in the colon, so that only 0.1 ml of the original 1 ml ingested can be recovered in the feces. After acute diarrhea or aggressive bowel preparation for surgery, this concentrat-

Anesthesia for Abdominal Surgery 571

TABLE 20-1
GASTROINTESTINAL EFFECTS OF AGENTS COMMONLY USED IN ANESTHESIA

	Lower Esophageal Pressure	Gastric Emptying Time	Gastric pH
Atropine, glycopyrrolate	↓	↑	0
Neostigmine, edrophonium	↑	↑	0
Midazolam	0	0	0
Pentothal	↓	0/↓	0
Narcotics	↓	↓ ↓	0
Succinylcholine	↑	0	0
Atracurium	0	0	0
Pancuronium	↑	0	0
Halothane, isoflurane	Dose dependent ↓	↓	0
Antacids	↑	↑	↑ ↑
Metoclopramide	↑	↑ ↑	0
Cimetidine, ranitidine	↑	0	↑

↑, increased effect; ↓, decreased effect; 0, negligible effect.
Data from Brock-Utne and Downing.[25] and Nimmo.[76]

ing mechanism is inhibited or overwhelmed so that dehydration must be suspected. IV fluids are necessary to replace intravascular volume depletion.

All of the processes that underlie the physiologic response to abdominal pathology are interrelated (Fig. 20–2). Obstruction, hemorrhage, infection, and infarction all contribute to a shock-like state in which perfusion of the bowel is compromised, further aggravating each process. Continuing evaluation and treatment of these problems form the basis of pre-, intra-, and postoperative management. Obstruction may be primary, as in congenital atresia, or secondary, as in ileus caused by peritonitis or blunt trauma. Regardless of the cause, bowel obstruction ultimately leads to vomiting, dehydration, and abdominal distention, which in turn may embarrass respiration, especially in small infants. The site of obstruction determines the nature of the fluid loss and influences the body's response to that loss.

Infection is a frequent companion to the cascade. Gram-negative organisms colonize the gastrointestinal tract within the first few days after birth. If the integrity of the bowel is compromised by ischemia or perforation, bacteria are liberated into the peritoneal cavity and ultimately into the systemic circulation. Gram-negative sepsis is complicated by the release of endotoxin, which causes vasodilation and shock. Aggressive treatment with appropriate antibiotics, fluids, and sympathomimetics must be initiated.

Bowel infarction may be caused by local compromise of blood supply or to generalized circulatory changes that result from low perfusion and redistribution of blood flow away from the gastrointestinal tract during periods of

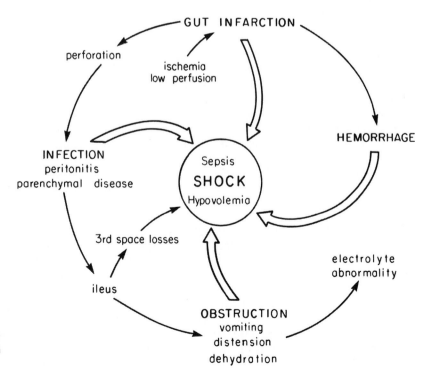

FIGURE 20–2. Physiologic cascade of a gastrointestinal insult. Note that the common factor is low perfusion of the gut.

stress. Infarction may also lead to hemorrhage and coagulopathies.

PREOPERATIVE EVALUATION AND PREPARATION

Timely, accurate diagnosis and aggressive preparation are crucial to the anesthetic management of abdominal surgery. Appropriate laboratory studies must be considered, in addition to the history and the physical examination of the patient. The anesthesiologist's role is to review these findings and to begin appropriate replacement therapy, especially in an emergency situation.

The most recent significant advances in neonatal surgery have been paralleled by advances in perinatology.[26–28] Early sonographic examination (16 to 18 weeks' gestation), indicated either because of abnormal α-fetoprotein (AFP) or by routine examination, can determine fetal age and sex, document viability, and diagnose malformations. Gastroschisis can be differentiated from omphalocele by the location of the umbilical cord and the absence of a peritoneal covering. Because of strong relationship between omphalocele and genetic abnormalities,[29,30] amniocentesis to obtain fluid to study chromosomes is indicated in patients with an omphalocele and should be offered to mothers of patients with gastroschisis. As pregnancy progresses, subsequent sonograms may be indicated to document continued growth and to explain a sudden increase in polyhydramnios. The latter may occur with fetal bowel obstruction caused by volvulus, intussusception, or bowel atresia. It is controversial whether or not early cesarean section reduces postoperative morbidity in gastroschisis.[31–34]

In the delivery room, congenital gastrointestinal obstruction should be suspected in infants with more than 20 ml gastric aspirate and those born to mothers with polyhydramnios. Intestinal obstruction must be investigated in all newborn infants who vomit after feedings and/or fail to pass meconium during the first 24 hours of life. Nonbilious vomiting is suggestive of preampullar lesions, whereas bilious vomiting suggests an intestinal site. The more distal the lesion, the later the signs of bowel obstruction become apparent and the more distended the abdomen may appear. A rectal examination should be performed to rule out anorectal malformations and to obtain a biopsy sample of mucosa ganglion cells. By far the most helpful examination is a plain radiograph of the abdomen. This may reveal air–fluid levels, failure of air to enter the colon, the "double-bubble" sign, and calcifications, which will aid in establishing the diagnosis and assessing the level of obstruction.

Estimating intravascular blood volume in the neonate is best done clinically by evaluating blood pressure, peripheral pulse quality, and urine output. Hemoglobin and hematocrit levels may reveal chronic or recent blood loss but are less useful for acute blood loss. Neonatal and early infant hemoglobin levels must be carefully interpreted with regard to the state of hydration, and the presence of cyanotic congenital heart disease. The expected decrease in hemoglobin reaches a nadir at 3 months of age in term infants.

Dehydration is best judged clinically by assessing skin turgor, capillary refill, fontanel fullness, urine output, and vital signs. Although determining serum electrolyte concentrations is useful in differentiating hypotonic from hypertonic dehydration, for documenting the results of electrolyte therapy, and for evaluating complex situations that involve renal compensation (such as the syndrome of inappropriate antidiuretic hormone [SIADH] and diabetes insipidus [DI]), values are usually normal in otherwise healthy infants and children with recent onset of gastrointestinal symptoms and are of little value in deciding what or how much solution to administer. Electrolyte concentrations should be determined in patients with protracted vomiting, such as those with congenital pyloric stenosis, bowel obstruction, and hypotonic fluid replacement, and in patients receiving diuretic therapy. Blood glucose concentrations should be determined in all neonates who require surgery.

It is very difficult to reconcile normal gastric motility studies, abnormalities caused by gastrointestinal (GI) obstruction or pathology, and medicolegal standards of anesthesia practice to arrive at appropriate NPO (nothing by mouth) orders and how they should be modified for urgent or emergent situations.[35,36] Whatever time one decides to allow the last consumption of solid food, there will be situations in which pathology or anxiety will greatly prolong gastric emptying. Therefore, all anesthetics must be managed with the contingency that the stomach will not be empty. In most cases without GI obstruction, the longer the fasting interval, the less likely the chance that significant amounts of undigested solids or liquids remain in the stomach. On the other hand, excessive deprivation of clear liquids predisposes the child to dehydration and to hypotension on induction of anesthesia. Clearly, this judgment, which is often dictated by blanket departmental rules, must be individualized to the patient and circumstance (see Chapter 5).

Preoperative preparation combines diagnosis (suspicion and confirmation) with intelligent action. Both of these actions should take place concurrently. With the exceptions of acute hemorrhage, compromised enteric circulation, or dead bowel, all of which require urgent surgery and "catch-up therapy" on the way to and during laparotomy, most obstructions and other abdominal lesions benefit from preoperative volume restoration and hydration. Volume restoration may require invasive monitoring of central venous and arterial pressure and an indwelling urinary catheter to determine urine output. Nasogastric tubes help to decrease gastric distention and respiratory embarrassment. Antibiotic administration is usually necessary. Blood products, colloid, electrolyte fluid replacement, and ionotropic agents may be required to restore blood volume and cardiac output.

ANESTHETIC MANAGEMENT

Several aspects of induction and maintenance of anesthesia for abdominal surgery deserve special emphasis. With few exceptions (e.g., the sick premature infant in whom regional anesthesia without sedation is indicated), general anesthesia is the choice for virtually all cases. This may or may not be supplemented with regional anesthesia (or vice versa). Epidural anesthesia, by the caudal or lumbar approach, is often administered shortly after induction of anesthesia to decrease anesthesia requirements, to reduce stress responses, and to provide postoperative analgesia. Alternatively, regional anesthesia can be administered at the end of the surgery solely for analgesia. Epidural anesthesia is contraindicated when hypovolemia, infection (either systemic or local), bleeding diatheses, abnormalities of the lower back, or parental request precludes it. Preservative-free morphine or fentanyl can be administered in addition to the local anesthetic (see Chapter 12). Unfortunately, large volumes of local anesthesia are necessary for upper abdominal surgery when the caudal approach is used. Some mid- and lower abdominal surgery can be accomplished with 1.25 to 1.5 ml/kg of 0.2 percent bupivacaine.[37] The lumbar approach requires less volume (0.5 to 0.75 ml/kg) and is more suited to upper abdominal procedures. A catheter can be inserted via the lumbar or caudal route for continued postoperative analgesia.

Although the choice of techniques to induce general anesthesia and produce conditions suitable for endotracheal intubation usually depends on the training, experience, and competence of the anesthesiologist, several factors related to abdominal surgery also influence this judgment. Patients presenting for abdominal surgery often have IV lines in place, which makes induction of anesthesia easy with IV pentothal 4 to 6 mg/kg, propofol 2 to 3 mg/kg, or ketamine 1 to 2 mg/kg. Hydrated patients may prefer inhalation induction of anesthesia with halothane or sevoflurane if no IV catheter is in place. Because the potential for pulmonary aspiration of gastric contents is increased, endotracheal intubation is indicated in most cases, except for some elective hernia repairs and certain diagnostic studies. Awake tracheal intubation is occasionally utilized in infants who are suspected of having anatomic abnormalities of the upper airway, extreme debilitation, or a full stomach. These patients should be preoxygenated by mask before laryngoscopy is attempted. Judicious use of nebulized topical anesthesia during a "first look," followed by a second period of mask oxygenation for 30 to 60 seconds, facilitates trachael intubation during a "second look." Concurrent oxygen administration during laryngoscopy has been described.[38] Intubation may then be facilitated by an assistant who immobilizes the head and restrains the shoulders.

Rapid-sequence induction of anesthesia, the choice of most anesthetists, includes preoxygenation by mask, administration of IV atropine (in young infants), induction doses of Pentothal, ketamine, and a short-acting muscle relaxant, such as succinylcholine 1 to 2 mg/kg, or propofol rapacuronium. Cricoid pressure is maintained during induction of anesthesia and tracheal intubation. Adequate time must be allowed for the drugs to achieve their full effect. Gastric regurgitation is stimulated in patients who are only partially anesthetized and partially paralyzed at the time of laryngoscopy. An alternative to succinylcholine is the use of nondepolarizing muscle relaxants such as mivacurium 0.2 mg/kg, rocuronium 0.1 to 0.4 mg/kg, atracurium 0.5 mg/kg, or vecuronium 0.1 to 0.2 mg/kg. Rocuronium and vecuronium in higher doses (0.4 mg/kg) lead to rapid relaxation, although not as rapid as that with

succinylcholine. The duration of action of high-dose vecuronium may be excessive (60 to 90 minutes) for brief procedures.

In some cases, anesthesiologists prefer mask induction of anesthesia with volatile anesthetics. Such cases include hydrated children in whom there is neither ileus nor gastric distention and no functional IV line. This technique requires a smooth, rapid, and closely monitored induction of anesthesia to avoid causing excessive depth of anesthesia and is aided by the presence of an experienced assistant who can start an IV line when the patient is anesthetized and apply cricoid pressure during intubation of the trachea. The rationale for this technique is that intact reflexes are present during the light levels of anesthesia when vomiting is likely to occur and that regurgitation is less likely if the stomach has been adequately decompressed via a nasogastric tube before surgery.

Patients from neonatal intensive care or trauma units often present with their trachea already intubated. In the past, some clinicians paralyzed these patients without providing anesthesia. This is not acceptable. Not only is it inhumane to perform surgery without anesthesia, it is detrimental to the patient's clinical condition. Release of increased catecholamines and other stress hormones can cause devastating changes in visceral, peripheral, and cerebral circulation. Anand et al.[39] demonstrated in preterm and term infants an association between stress-response markers and outcome. High-dose sufentanil was more effective than halothane in blunting this response during cardiac surgery,[40] although halothane was more effective than nitrous oxide plus O_2 in noncardiac neonates.[41] Fentanyl 10 to 25 μg/kg will also modify this response, and low concentrations of isoflurane (0.25 to 0.5 percent) will produce vasodilation and improve circulation.

General anesthesia can be maintained by a variety of inhalation and IV agents. Volatile general anesthics are usually well tolerated but can mask inadequate fluid replacement. Halothane is more likely to cause cardiac irritability and has been occasionally associated with hepatic dysfunction. Cardiac function is well maintained with low-dose isoflurane, and cardiac arrhythmias are uncommon. Low solubility, minimal fluoride metabolism, and potentiation of muscle relaxants make isoflurane, sevoflurane, or desflurane suitable choices for maintenance of general anesthesia. Nitrous oxide should be avoided in patients with bowel obstruction because nitrous oxide moves into a closed gas space at a rate many times faster than it moves out, owing to the greater blood solubility of nitrous oxide relative to nitrogen, hydrogen, and methane. Transfer of nitrous oxide to a gas-filled intestinal space may significantly increase the volume of the space, hamper the efforts of the surgeon, embarrass respiration by increasing intra-abdominal pressure, and decrease tissue blood flow. Narcotics such as fentanyl, sufentanil, and morphine decrease or may eliminate the need for volatile anesthetics, but may also produce hypotension and cause postoperative respiratory depression, especially in the premature or newborn infant, if fluid replacement is inadequate. Abdominal surgery is often associated with increased intra-abdominal pressure. This will decrease liver and splanchnic blood flow, thereby decreasing fentanyl biotransformation and clearance.[42]

Ventilation should be controlled during abdominal surgery for all but the most minor procedures and end-tidal carbon dioxide (P_{ETCO_2}) should be continually monitored. Inspired oxygen should be adjusted to produce a level slightly higher than necessary for full oxygen saturation, as measured by pulse oximetry. The oxygen saturation of preterm infants should be maintained between 87 and 92 percent to decrease the possibility of retinopathy of prematurity (see Chapter 14). Although operative conditions can be facilitated by judicious use of muscle relaxants, their effects should be closely monitored by electrical neurostimulation to prevent overdosing with these drugs. Concurrent administration of IV or intraperitoneal aminoglycoside antibiotics may potentiate nondepolarizing muscle relaxants. Infants, particularly neonates have low functional residual capacities during anesthesia and are prone to atelectasis. Positive end-expiratory pressure (PEEP) may prevent this.

Temperature homeostasis is especially difficult to achieve during major abdominal surgery in small infants (see Chapter 4). Exposure to a cool environment causes rapid loss of heat because of the high cardiac output and exposure of a large surface area to the cold. When the peritoneal cavity is open, a surface area equal to that of skin is exposed. The anesthetized infant is unable to compensate for the heat loss by the usual mechanisms for thermogenesis. Temperature must be maintained by warming operating rooms and prep solutions and by using warming blankets, forced air convection units, and infrared lights (but not directed to exposed bowel) particularly during induction and preparation for surgery. Intraoperatively, warm (but not hot) peritoneal irrigation and heated humidification of inspired gases are helpful.

Careful fluid balance is of utmost importance in major abdominal surgery. The rate of IV fluid administration depends on the sum of maintenance requirements, preexisting deficits, and ongoing losses (Table 20-2). In neonates, stressed infants, and patients in whom hypoglycemia is documented, or in those who have received glucose infusions of 5 to 10 percent dextrose preoperatively should receive glucose infusions until the glucose concentration is checked and found to be normal during surgery. It is convenient to run D_{5-10} 0.2 percent NaCl at maintenance rates (4 ml/kg/h) and to administer all additional fluid as balanced salt solution. However, in healthy children with adequate renal function, many anesthesiologists administer only plain lactated Ringer's (LR) solution for reasons of simplicity and expense and to avoid hyperglycemia.

In patients in whom significant blood loss is anticipated, a maximum allowable blood loss estimate (MABLE) should be calculated before surgery to produce a target hematocrit (Fig. 20-2). Actual blood loss should be carefully followed and replaced with an additional 3 ml of balanced salt solution per 1 ml of blood shed until the MABLE is reached. Once it becomes apparent that a transfusion will be required, the additional solution should be stopped and factored into the total crystalloid replacement. Packed red blood cells (RBCs) or whole blood should be filtered, warmed, and transfused in amounts sufficient to restore blood volume, maintain vital signs, and reach an acceptable hematocrit level. The quantity transfused depends on maximizing the amount of donor blood from each unit to minimize the number of donors to whom the patient is exposed. The volume replaced may exceed the measured blood loss as long as the hematocrit does not exceed 45 to 48 percent. Frequent intraoperative hematocrit determinations are helpful in this calculation. Coagulation studies are indicated when actual blood loss exceeds the estimated blood volume. Blood given to premature infants should be irradiated before it is administered; this prevents graft-versus-host reactions.

After surgery, the endotracheal tube (ETT) is left in place until the patient is awake, adequate spontaneous ventilation is demonstrated, core temperature is near normal, muscle relaxants are fully reversed, and the concentrations of narcotic and inhalational agents are sufficiently diminished so that they will not impair ventilation. Patients with large incisions, overwhelming sepsis, unstable cardiovascular systems, and CNS depression may require prolonged respiratory support. In such cases the decision not to reverse muscle relaxants and narcotics may be propitious. Such patients are best managed in a unit where intensive ventilatory and circulatory support can be provided.

SPECIAL PROBLEMS

Omphalocele and Gastroschisis

Although the embryologic origins and diagnostic ramifications of omphalocele and gastroschisis are different, the anesthetic management for the two conditions is remarkably similar. The combined incidence of these abnormalities is between 1 in 3,000 and 1 in 10,000 live births, with no predilection for race or sex. Both conditions are associated with malrotation of the gastrointestinal tract and a patent omphalomesenteric tract (Meckel's diverticulum). Gastroschisis is associated with a higher incidence of intestinal atresia, particularly of the "apple peel" variety. Omphaloceles are associated with a greater incidence of abnormalities not involving the GI tract (20 percent have congenital heart disease). In Beckwith-Wiedemann syndrome, omphalocele occurs in association with macroglossia, gigantism, organomegaly, and symptomatic hypoglycemia. Epigastric omphaloceles are associated with a high incidence of congenital heart disease and thoracic defects (pentalogy of Cantrell), whereas hypogastric omphaloceles occur more frequently with exstrophy of the bladder and genital or cloacal abnormalities. There is a greater likelihood that organs other than the intestines (e.g., liver, spleen, and urinary bladder) will be exposed in the omphalocele (Fig. 20-3). With gastroschisis, the extruded contents usually consist only of brown, leathery appearing small intestine; this is a sign of preexisting fetal peritonitis and extravasation of fluid (Fig. 20-4). During convalescence, the function of this intestine is slow to return. Outcome is more dependent on the associated pathology than on the size of the defect.

Both gastroschisis and omphalocele can be diagnosed in the first trimester of pregnancy by fetal ultrasonography and can be distinguished from each other by the presence of a peritoneal covering. Because of the high incidence of trisomies in patients with omphaloceles, early amnio-

T A B L E 2 0 – 2
INTRAVENOUS FLUID REGIMEN FOR ABDOMINAL SURGERY

Crystalloid
Maintenance (D_5/0.2–0.45% NaCl + 20 mEq KCl/L* or lactated Ringer's)

4 ml/kg/hr (<10 kg)
+ 2 ml/kg/hr (10–20 kg)
+ 1 ml/kg/hr (>20 kg)

Replacement (lactated Ringer's or 0.9% NaCl)
Dehydration[†]
Gastrointestinal drainage
Third-space loss (mild, moderate, large)
Blood loss until MABLE reached

% estimated × wt.
ml/ml
5–10–15 × EBL
3 × EBL

Blood Products
MABLE (*m*aximal *a*llowable *b*lood *l*oss *e*stimate)
EBV = Wt × %BV (0.85% newborn to 0.7% child >1 yr)

$$MABLE = EBV \times \frac{\text{(pre–blood loss Hct–target Hct)}}{\text{pre–blood loss Hct}}$$

Blood loss replacement

$$PRBC \text{ or } WB \text{ (ml)} = \frac{\text{(EBV} \times \text{target Hct)–(EBV–EBL)} \times \text{pre–blood loss Hct}}{0.7 \text{ (PRBC) or } 0.35 \text{ (WB)}}$$

Euvolemic hematocrit elevation (after equilibration or preoperatively)[‡]
PRBC or WB (ml) = Wt × (target Hct–current Hct) × 1(PRBC) or 2(WB)
(1 ml/kg [PRBC] or 2 ml/kg [WB] will raise Hct 1%)
Platelets
0.1–0.3 U/kg will raise the platelet count approximately 50,000
Note: platelets are suspended in fresh frozen plasma

BV, blood volume; EBV, estimated blood volume; EBL, estimated blood loss; D, dextrose; Hct, hematocrit (%); PRBC, packed red cells; WB, whole blood; Wt, weight (kg); U, platelets retrieved from 1 adult unit.
* Indicated in patients in whom hypoglycemia is suspect (see text).
[†] 1/2 calculated volume in first hour, 1/4 in second hour, 1/4 in third hour.
[‡] Assuming >1 year, Hct (PRBC = 0.7, WB = 0.35).
Data from Coté.[75]

centesis for chromosome evaluation should be undertaken. With gastroschisis, amniocentesis at 35 to 37 weeks' gestation can be used to establish lung maturity. If the lungs are mature, early cesarean section may diminish the changes in the extruded bowel wall, although this is challenged by some.[31–34, 43]

Immediate care at the time of birth includes wrapping the abdomen with a sterile dressing, which is then kept moist with warm saline, and placing the lower body in a plastic bag. Hypothermia must be prevented, as it leads to significant morbidity. The circumferential collar of skin and fascia surrounding the defect tends to act as a peripheral tourniquet, allowing sequestration of fluid in the exposed viscera and limiting vascular perfusion.

Corrective surgery, although urgently indicated, can be greatly aided by a few minutes of aggressive preoperative preparation. A vein and an artery should be cannulated. Often the umbilical artery can be cannulated and then translocated at the time of surgery, utilizing a technique described by Filston and Izant.[44] Initial arterial samples for

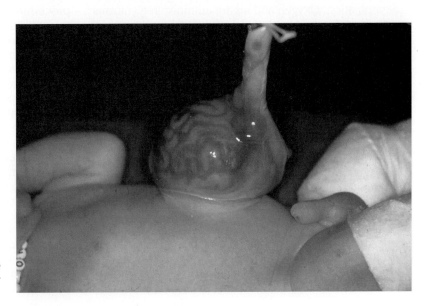

FIGURE 20–3. Moderate-sized intact omphalocele. Note the intact, glistening membrane and insertion of the umbilical cord.

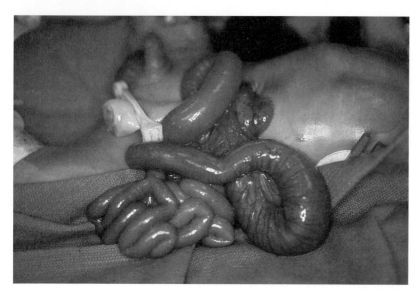

FIGURE 20–4. Ruptured gastroschisis. Note the fibrous material on the bowel.

blood gas and acid–base measurements, hematocrits, and blood glucose analyses are drawn and repeated throughout the perioperative course. It is imperative to follow blood glucose concentrations to detect and treat neonatal hypoglycemia and to avoid hyperglycemic osmotic diuresis. Because of the evaporative fluid loss from the exposed abdominal viscera and because of the vascular compromise, aggressive fluid replacement is necessary.[45] Maintenance fluid replacement is with 10 percent dextrose in 0.2 percent NaCl or Isolyte P. To this solution is added an infusion of 10 ml/kg/h warmed balanced salt solution (LR, normal saline [NS], or 5 percent albumin) and repeated boluses of 3 to 5 ml/kg of one of these solutions is added to replace third-space losses. After each bolus of fluid, arterial pressure, peripheral perfusion, and central venous pressure are reevaluated.

Anesthesia management begins in a warmed operating room with application of monitors, gastric decompression, and preoxygenation. After IV induction of anesthesia, cricoid pressure, and maximal relaxation, an ETT is inserted and secured in a manner suitable for prolonged postoperative ventilation. Oxygen and air are administered (nitrous oxide is avoided) in a suitable mixture to produce adequate oxygenation (Pa_{O_2} 50 to 70 mm Hg, Sa_{O_2} 97 to 98 percent for term infants, 87 to 92 percent for preterm infants). The oxygen requirement will vary when the surgeons attempt to replace the bowel in the abdomen. Maximal muscle relaxation is maintained throughout surgery and the initial postoperative period. Ventilation is controlled to maintain normal arterial Pa_{CO_2} or PET_{CO_2} levels. Anesthesia is provided with a low concentration of volatile anesthetic agents or fixed IV agents, such as fentanyl, morphine, or ketamine.

The surgeon can expedite reduction of the lesion by manually stretching the abdominal wall and "milking" the bowel contents proximally toward the stomach and distally through the rectum.[46] The decision then must be made as to whether the hernia can be reduced and a fascial repair accomplished or whether the bowel should be left extraperitoneally and encased in skin, synthetic mesh (silon chimney), or the Heyer-Schulte ventral wall

defect reduction silo. If either of the latter two is chosen, the hernia is reduced gradually over a period of days. Primary closure may cause ventilatory, circulatory, and renal dysfunction and bowel necrosis if the abdomen is too tense. Placing the bowel in a silon chimney is cumbersome and more likely to result in infection. However, it is also less likely to compromise other organs. After primary closure of the abdomen, increased intragastric pressure has been associated with profound decreases in cardiac index and with anuria.[47] Observing the peripheral circulation helps to determine the neonate's ability to tolerate primary closure of the abdominal wall defect. Intraoperatively, this decision is aided by draping the patient in such a way that the lower extremities can be inspected. Measuring blood pressure in the leg or following the lower extremity oxygenation with a pulse oximeter may also be helpful. If the vital signs are normal after the hernia reduction, it is usually possible to achieve adequate ventilation and oxygenation until the intra-abdominal pressure and distention diminish. If the bowel cannot be reduced or if severe lung disease is present, the more conservative procedure should be selected. During either procedure the gut must be inspected for associated atresia, malrotation, and diverticuli.

Postoperative care varies according to the magnitude of the defect, the type of repair, and the associated pathology. In healthy patients treated with a silon chimney or small primary closure, the ETT can be removed when the effects of all drugs have dissipated or have been reversed, ventilation is adequate, and body temperature is normal. In patients with large defects, particularly those with compromised circulation, muscle relaxation is continued until the abdominal pressure has decreased to the point that little respiratory or circulatory embarrassment exists.

Ventilatory care is similar to that for other neonates with respiratory distress. Fluid requirements may remain high until the abdominal venous pressure decreases, after which fluid restriction and diuresis are indicated. Inspired oxygen is adjusted to maintain a normal Sa_{O_2} (94 to 98 percent for term infants; 87 to 92 percent for preterm infants). Appropriate levels of PEEP are used to increase functional residual capacity. After decompression of the abdomen, the effects of muscle relaxants are allowed to dissipate. Patients are weaned slowly from mechanical ventilation, using intermittent mandatory ventilation. Patients with silon chimneys in place usually require no anesthesia for daily cinching of the chimney. When all the contents of the chimney have been reduced into the abdomen, the patient is returned to the operating room to repair the major fascial defect. Depending on the abdominal pressure involved, the management of anesthesia is similar to that described for total repair. Because bowel compromised by edema, manipulation, and circulatory instability is slow to resume function, TPN often is required for extended periods of time.

Bowel Surgery in the Neonate

Surgery is often required on the GI tract during the first week of life. It is essential for those who care for neonates to be vigilant to the possibility of gastrointestinal abnormalities. The diagnosis is often made by antenatal examination. Maternal serial ultrasound examinations are indicated when polyhydramnios is present, particularly when it is of sudden onset. In the delivery room one should be suspicious if a soft catheter cannot be advanced to the stomach or if more than 20 ml of gastric contents is aspirated from the stomach. The anus should be examined for patency. Meconium should be passed in the first 24 hours. Although regurgitation of gastric contents is common during the neonatal period, vomiting is not, and vomiting should be evaluated promptly to exclude surgical pathology. The presence or absence of bile should be noted.

Perhaps the most helpful diagnostic study is a plain radiograph of the abdomen to look for air–fluid levels, presence of air in the distal bowel, free peritoneal air, and calcifications.[48] A double-bubble sign is pathognomonic for duodenal atresia. Pneumotosis intestinalis and edema of the bowel wall may suggest early necrotizing enterocolitis. Free air in the abdominal cavity is associated with intestinal perforation. Calcifications are consistent with antenatal bowel perforation or meconium inspissation syndromes. Contrast studies may be necessary to define the level of obstruction. In general, the more proximal the lesion, the earlier the onset of symptoms. Bilious vomiting occurs when the obstruction is distal to the ampulla of Vater. Duodenal obstruction may be intrinsic (atresia) or extrinsic (compression). Jejunoileal obstruction may be single or multiple. Distal lesions present later and are associated with more abdominal distention. Hirschsprung's disease (congenital aganglionic megacolon) is the most common etiology of obstruction and is caused by failure of embryonic neuroganglion cells to migrate to the Meissner's and Auerbach's plexuses of the gut segment. This abnormality is usually confined to the rectosigmoid area, but in 10 percent of cases it involves the total colon. Occasionally it involves the entire large and small bowel. The diagnosis is established by rectal biopsy. If the ganglia are absent, a diverting colostomy is performed. An abdominoperineal resection is done when the infant reaches 10 kg. Meconium syndromes, including ileus, plug, and peritonitis are common presentations of cystic fibrosis.

For meconium ileus and meconium plug, an enema with hypertonic contrast material often relieves the obstruction. With early and conservative diagnosis, necrotizing enterocolitis (NEC), once considered the scourge of premature nurseries, can also be treated nonoperatively. This acquired lesion may be related to early feedings, to excessively hypertonic oral solutions, to hypoperfusion of the gut, or to infection. It is commonly associated with a patent ductus arteriosus, low systemic cardiac output, and decreased bowel perfusion. Blood in the stool, abdominal distention, low platelet count, or lower abdominal wall discoloration should be evaluated with a radiograph and treated with gastric decompression, fluids, and antibiotics. Untreated NEC progresses to bowel obstruction, perforation, and sepsis. Surgical intervention is necessary in infants who require resection of gangrenous bowel, repair of bowel perforation, and a diversionary enterostomy. These patients usually require large volumes of fluid and may develop diffuse intravascular coagulation during surgery. Intraoperative treatment of the latter may require administration of platelets, fresh frozen plasma, and cryoprecipitate. Blood transfusion is often necessary, as blood loss may be excessive.

Malrotation, hemorrhage, and perforation of the bowel are true emergencies, which deserve urgent surgical attention. Other obstructions caused by bowel atresia require surgery less urgently, and the patient may benefit from delay for diagnosis of other anomalies, preoperative preparation, availability of blood products, and a fresh, rested operating room team. Adequate venous access and gastric decompression are imperative. An arterial line is helpful for monitoring and blood sampling, and is often more helpful than a central venous line. Appropriate antibiotic therapy also is indicated.

In the operating room, monitors are applied and the stomach is decompressed in patients with bowel obstructions. The nasogastric tube is secured in a manner that allows it to be adjusted intraoperatively. After preoxygenation, anesthesia can be induced with Pentothal 4 to 6 mg/kg or propofol 2 to 3 mg/kg. Endotracheal intubation is often facilitated with muscle relaxants. The lungs are ventilated with a warmed oxygen–air mixture to which low concentrations of isoflurane or halothane are added. Intravenous fentanyl is slowly titrated to maintain normal vital signs. Nitrous oxide is avoided. Estimation and replacement of third-space extracellular fluid loss may be difficult and is aided by stable anesthesia so that changes in pulse, arterial blood pressure, and central venous pressure reflect volume and hydration status rather than light anesthesia or atropine administration. Large volumes of colloid or blood may be required. In patients with gangrenous bowel, such as those with NEC, fresh frozen plasma, cryoprecipitate, and platelets may be necessary to treat coagulation defects. Circulatory support with dopamine may augment marginal bowel perfusion.

Postoperative ventilatory management depends on the magnitude of the surgery, the type of anesthesia, the stability of the patient, the presence of other pathology, and the ability of the intensive care unit (ICU) staff to manage an intubated neonate. If endotracheal extubation is desired soon after surgery, neuromuscular blockade should be fully reversed and documented by nerve stimulation.

The patient should be awake and the stomach should be decompressed. An alternative and often safer approach in the sick neonate is to continue endotracheal intubation and ventilatory support in the neonatal ICU (NICU). If the latter course is elected, narcotics and muscle relaxants are not reversed. The patient's lungs are ventilated as long as is necessary, and then the patient is weaned from ventilation.

Biliary Tract Surgery in Infancy

Jaundice in the neonate and young infant is among the most difficult and crucial diagnoses for a pediatrician or neonatologist to make. A narrow time window exists during which correctable lesions must be differentiated from physiologic causes of hyperbilirubinemia in the neonate. Although bilirubin pigments have been demonstrated as early as 13 weeks' gestation, the major enzyme responsible for conjugation, uridine diphosphate glucuronyl transferase (UDPGT), is less than 1 percent of the adult value at term, increases dramatically in the first day, and reaches adult values at 6 weeks.[49] Prematurity, postmaturity, hemolysis, and genetics all play a role in overproduction of unconjugated bilirubin. The criteria for "physiologic" jaundice of the newborn have been well described.[50]

Extrahepatic biliary atresia and neonatal hepatitis, the two major conditions that account for conjugated (direct) hyperbilirubemia, may actually represent opposite ends of the same spectrum of the disease process.[51] Both diseases appear to be the end result of a pansclerosis during the period of ductal development rather than of ductal malformation. Sclerosis may continue to occur after birth. A variety of sophisticated tests for infection, α_1-antitrypsin deficiency, and metabolic disorders must be undertaken to differentiate hepatocellular from ductal maldevelopment. Hepatocellular maldevelopment (neonatal hepatitis) often has dismal outcome, whereas extrahepatic biliary atresia is amenable to surgical intervention (Kasai procedure) and has good outcome if the surgery is performed by an experienced pediatric surgeon before the 10th week of life.[52] Late diagnosis has led to universally bad results and frequently results in liver failure, requiring liver transplantation.

Anesthetic management of these patients is challenging. They are frequently malnourished and septic and may require anesthesia for diagnostic procedures (e.g., liver biopsy, endoscopy, placement of central venous lines or Broviac catheters) and definitive procedures (portal enterostomies, liver transplantation) (see Chapter 19). Coagulopathy and portal hypertension are often present. IV access may be extremely difficult secondary to frequent blood sampling and previous IV therapy.

Preoperatively, it is imperative that all studies and consultations be fully documented. Blood products appropriate for correction of volume loss and coagulation defects must be anticipated. A frank discussion with the parents must acquaint them with the risks and expectations associated with anesthesia and surgery. Although there have been no reports of fetal hepatic damage from maternal anesthesia with halogenated compounds or aggravation of existing neonatal hepatic dysfunction from concurrent anesthetics, it seems only prudent to avoid the highly metabolized agents, such as halothane, and to use others, such as isoflurane, only with good indication. Intramuscular ketamine or IV Pentothal or propofol are reasonable alternatives for induction of anesthesia. Anesthesia can be maintained with narcotics and nitrous oxide and supplemented with muscle relaxation. Intraoperative hemorrhage may be caused by portal hypertension, difficult surgical access to bleeding near the portal triad, proximity to the vena cava and portal vein, and coagulopathy. The anesthesiologist should be alert for hypotension secondary to vena caval compression by a surgical retractor or sponges. Arterial monitoring is helpful in identifying such changes. IV access should be located in the upper extremities. Irrigation fluids, IV solutions, and anesthetic gases should be warmed to maintain thermostasis. Because cholangitis is a frequent complication, antibiotic therapy should be coordinated with pre- and postoperative coverage and strict attention must be paid to aseptic anesthetic techniques. Postoperatively, attention is focused on whether the patient has adequate respiratory sufficiency, in light of abdominal distention and a large incision.

Inguinal Hernia

Inguinal hernia is perhaps the most common problem that confronts pediatric surgeons. Although the potential for herniation through a patent processus vaginalis (male) or canal of Nuck (female) is present in more than 90 percent of newborns, clinical herniation occurs in only 3 to 5 percent of term infants and in up to 30 percent of premature infants. Most hernias become evident during the first 6 months of life and are associated with an increased risk for bowel obstruction and gonadal injury. Surgery is indicated for the hernia, but it is not clear if and how long surgery should be delayed to optimize the patient's condition. Postponing surgery in premature infants allows them to grow and mature so that anesthesia will pose less of a risk, but this delay exposes the patient to further risk of incarceration and may make the surgical repair more difficult. This decision must be individualized to the patient and the experience of the surgeon, anesthesiologist, and the institution.

A hernia, by definition, is a protrusion of an organ or tissue through an abnormal opening. It is considered incarcerated when the hernia cannot be reduced or easily returned to its normal location. It is considered strangulated when the blood supply is compromised. Why herniation occurs in some infants with a patent processus vaginalis and not in others has not been established. The prevalence of inguinal hernias is increased in connective tissue disorders such as Ehler-Danlos syndrome, in premature infants, in patients who have ventriculoperitoneal shunts, and in those who have undergone omphalocele or bladder exstrophy repair. Males with cystic fibrosis also may have atresia of the vas deferens. Because approximately 1 percent of infant girls with bilateral inguinal or femoral hernias are diagnosed as having testicular feminization syndrome, such patients should be examined for vaginal atresia.

Inguinal hernias usually present as a lump in the groin. They should be suspected in infants with vomiting or with sudden onset of apparent abdominal pain. Unlike the adult, for whom there is concern about reducing incarcerated bowel, manual reduction of the hernia should be attempted in all cases of infant inguinal hernias. This maneuver relieves the potential bowel obstruction and enables tissue edema to subside before surgical repair of the hernia occurs. The presence or absence of testes in the scrotum should be noted. Strangulation of a testis or ovary occurs far more commonly than strangulation of bowel. After the hernia has been reduced, it is possible to rehydrate these patients orally.

There is debate about the advisability of exploring the contralateral side during repair of a unilateral hernia. Vascular compromise of the testis and damage to the vas deferens can and do occur during inguinal hernia repair. Herniagrams have been proposed to diagnose the presence of a nonclinical hernia on the contralateral side. Goldstein (R. Goldstein, personal communication) creates a pneumoperitoneum with CO_2 or air insufflation during repair of the clinically evident hernia. Appearance of creptitation on the contralateral side is an indication for surgical exploration. Excessive gas pressure may decrease lung compliance and make unsupplemented regional anesthesia difficult. CO_2 is safer if an air embolism occurs but can increase the ventilatory requirement. The volume of gas in the abdomen will expand if air is used in conjunction with inhaled nitrous oxide and may be incompletely absorbed, resulting in referred shoulder pain.

General anesthesia for elective hernia repair can be induced by inhaled anesthesia or IV injection. The decision to intubate the trachea depends on the patient's NPO status, size, the ease of airway maintenance, the expected duration of surgery, and the experience of the anesthesiologist. Because inguinal hernias are common in connective tissue disorders, muscular dystrophies, and other syndromes, the use of succinylcholine should be carefully balanced against the risk of an untoward reaction. The effects of nondepolarizing muscle relaxants and the temperature should be continuously monitored. Infiltration in the incision and around the ilioinguinal and iliohypogastric nerves with 0.25 percent bupivicaine or 0.2 percent ropivacaine may reduce the amount of anesthetic required and provide postoperative analgesia.

Spinal[53] and epidural anesthesia[54] are alternatives to general anesthesia. Spinal anesthesia with intrathecal hyperbaric tetracaine 0.4 mg/kg, 10 percent dextrose, and an epinephrine "wash" is well tolerated and provides 60 to 80 minutes of anesthesia.[55] To avoid spinal cord trauma, the needle should be inserted at the L4–L5 or L5–S1 interspace (see Chapter 12). Although epidural anesthesia is usually easy to accomplish via the caudal route, it often requires a near-maximal dose of local anesthetic and 10 to 15 minutes to be effective.

Incarcerated hernias should be treated as bowel obstructions. The patient should be rehydrated with IV balanced electrolyte solution and the stomach should be decompressed with a nasogastric tube before anesthesia is induced. Induction and management of anesthesia are accomplished in a manner similar to that described in the section on bowel obstruction. However, intra-arterial and central venous monitoring are seldom required.

Recurrent postoperative apnea has been described in neonates who present for hernia repair with a history of prematurity (born at <37 weeks' gestation), apneic episodes lasting 30 seconds or more, and chronic lung disease.[56] Liu et al.[57] recommended that if the postconceptual age is less than 46 weeks, such procedures should be done only on an inpatient basis and that the patient should be monitored postoperatively for at least 24 hours. Kurth et al.[58] recommended a cut-off date of 60 postconceptual weeks with continued monitoring for at least 12 hours after surgery. Prior hospital records should be carefully evaluated with regard to duration of tracheal intubation and ventilation, evidence of chronic lung disease, anemia, and CNS pathology. Arterial or capillary blood gas analysis and chest radiography may be indicated, in addition to routine laboratory studies. Inspired oxygen should be monitored and controlled in patients who are less than 42 weeks' postconceptual age to reduce the risk of retinopathy of prematurity. Although regional anesthesia is helpful, it may require supplemental sedation or light general anesthesia. Ketamine analgesia has been reported to depress respiratory function as much as total general anesthesia.[59] After surgery these infants must be evaluated for the "four A's": apnea, aspiration, atelectasis, and arrhythmia.

Pyloric Stenosis

Pyloric stenosis is the most frequently encountered form of infant gastrointestinal obstruction in general hospitals. Since Hirschsprung's first description in 1888 and Ramstedt's first operation in 1912, the mortality associated with this diagnosis has steadily fallen to near zero percent.

Although the usual onset of symptoms occurs between 2 and 6 weeks of age, infantile pyloric stenosis has been diagnosed as early as 36 hours after birth. Signs begin with regurgitation and progress to nonbilious projectile vomiting. The pathology involves hypertrophy of the muscular layer of the gastric outlet. Although there is no single accepted etiology, it has been suggested that milk curds move slowly through the pylorus, causing irritation, edema, and subsequent muscle hypertrophy. An olive-like mass can usually be felt in the epigastrium, slightly to the right of the midline. It is most easily palpated with the stomach emptied and the infant sucking quietly. Confirmation can be made by ultrasound examination of the abdomen. Although a barium swallow radiograph can also be done to confirm the diagnosis, this is not always necessary and adds to the morbidity by increasing the risk for aspiration of contrast material. If it is done, only water-soluble contrast should be used, and it should be removed by irrigating the stomach multiple times with saline.

Infantile pyloric stenosis has been treated medically by discontinuing feedings, administering antispasmodics, and then resuming small feedings of clear liquids. In some countries this regimen has been the sole method of treatment. Although this is only partially successful, it is the basis of prehospital treatment from the time of suspicion of diagnosis until the patient comes to the operating room. It does not provide sufficient calories but does delay and mitigate the dehydration often seen.

Surgical treatment is not an emergency, but medical resuscitation is. Because of the composition of the gastric fluid loss (hydrogen, sodium, potassium, and chloride

[Cl]), infants soon become alkalotic, hyponatremic, hypochloremic, and dehydrated.[60] The renal response is twofold. Initially, the serum pH is defended by the excretion of alkaline urine that contains sodium and potassium chloride. Later, with dehydration and depletion of sodium chloride, the kidney, in response to increased aldosterone, defends extracellular volume in preference to pH by retaining sodium chloride and secreting hydrogen ions, thus producing an acidic urine. This paradoxic aciduria worsens the already existent alkalemia. With further deterioration of the patient's condition, prerenal azotemia and shock develop. Resuscitation of these patients must include treatment of the hypovolemia and shock by rapid expansion of the intravascular volume with isotonic sodium chloride. Once urinary output is reestablished, potassium chloride should be added to the infusion. However, intracellular potassium deficits must be corrected cautiously.

Patients with pyloric stenosis present with a wide range of metabolic imbalances. Those with mild derangement (Cl more than 100 mEq/L, respiratory rate more than 20 breaths/min, current body weight more than that at the last pediatrician's visit, urine specific gravity [SG] <1.010) can be managed medically with oral glucose water, Pedialyte, or LR ad libitum until the time of surgery. Patients with moderate severity (Cl 90 to 100 mEq/L, respiratory rate 12 to 16 breaths/min, current weight equal to that at the last pediatrician's visit, urine output present with SG 1.010 to 1.020) should be given IV 5 percent dextrose in 0.45 percent sodium chloride with 20 to 40 mEq potassium chloride per liter added and administered at a rate of 10 ml/kg/h. In patients with severe derangement (Cl <90 mEq/L, sodium <120 mEq/L, respiratory rate <12 breaths/min, and no urinary output) the vascular volume should be expanded initially with balanced salt solution and/or colloid until the patient voids. Potassium should then be added to the IV fluids. Several days may be required to restore normal electrolyte values.

Intraoperative management is initiated by first aspirating the stomach with the patient in the lateral, supine, and prone positions. Monitors are applied and preoxygenation is begun. Endotracheal intubation can be achieved by rapid-sequence, awake, or inhalation techniques (see Chapter 10). Halothane and isoflurane are suitable for maintaining anesthesia. Postoperative apnea is common after pyloromyotomy, particularly in alkalotic patients. For this reason, narcotics are usually avoided. The ETT must remain in place postoperatively until the patient is awake and breathing adequately. Unless the duodenal mucosa has been violated, oral feedings of clear fluids may be resumed in 4 to 6 hours. The quantity and caloric density of these feedings are increased regularly if the feedings are well tolerated.

Gastrointestinal Examination and Endoscopic Laparoscopy

The basis for thoughtful, well-directed medical therapy and surgery is accurate diagnosis. In modern sophisticated pediatric centers, diagnosis now relies on a variety of endoscopic and radiologic procedures. In adults, most of these can be accomplished with little or no sedation. However, for infants and children it is often impossible to obtain meaningful information without deep sedation or general anesthesia.

The anesthesiologist must communicate with the radiologists, gastroenterologists, and surgeons, and must establish guidelines and appropriately equip nonoperating room locations to ensure that anesthesia can be safely provided (see Chapter 28). Anesthesiologists must be involved in hospital sedation committees and education of personnel who use these areas.

Guidelines for pediatric sedation have been well publicized by the American Academy of Pediatrics.[61] However, the need for and use of deep sedation instead of conscious sedation is often misrepresented. Amnesia with physical restraint not only may be abusive but also may be dangerous, particularly during endoscopy. Deep sedation without appropriate monitoring, airway management expertise, and understanding of the risks of sedation may be fatal.

The most common radiologic procedures requiring anesthesia or sedation are computed tomographic (CT) scanning, x-ray-guided biopsy or abscess drainage, aortography, and magnetic resonance imaging (MRI). Endotracheal anesthesia is indicated if the stomach is full, if oral radiocontrast is to be used, or if it is desired that ventilation be suspended during sequential radiographic exposures. Metoclopramide (Reglan) may advance the contrast through the bowel. Low concentrations of volatile anesthetics (halothane, isoflurane, or sevoflurane) in nitrous oxide–O_2, or low rates of propofol infusions are adequate and lead to a more prompt recovery and earlier tracheal extubation. In uncooperative patients who have been appropriately fasted and do not require oral contrast or control of breathing, sedation or brief, nonintubated general anesthesia may be employed. By use of propofol infusion or intermittent bolus Pentothal administration, sedation can be more appropriately tailored to the procedure, with prompter recovery than from traditional "lytic cocktails." Anesthesiologists are often asked to infuse IV radiocontrast agents and must monitor for allergic or hypotensive reactions.

Although most adult and many pediatric endoscopists sedate their patients for upper gastroduodenoscopy, general anesthesia offers advantages without increasing morbidity. Onset and recovery from anesthesia are much more rapid and predictable than from sedation with barbiturates and narcotics. There is less chance of traumatic injury in a nonstruggling child. Furthermore, there is another qualified individual present who can concentrate on the monitoring and safety of the patient while the gastroenterologist concentrates on the endoscopy. Preanesthetic evaluation should emphasize concurrent hepatic, hematologic, and psychological pathology. It may be prudent to avoid halothane in patients with significant hepatic dysfunction. Pentothal or propofol, in conjunction with nitrous oxide may be a wiser choice. Anemia and other bleeding disorders may coexist with GI bleeding. Major psychological disturbances are intertwined with GI complaints and require a caring approach to induction of anesthesia, with or without premedication. The anesthesiologist must be prepared to use a variety of induction techniques, including oral premedication and IV or inhalation induction of anesthesia, all with or without the parents in attendance. Endotracheal intubation, which is indicated for virtually all upper endoscopic procedures in young children, may be achieved with or without muscle relaxants. Endotracheal intubation is less often required for sigmoidoscopy and colonoscopy. Maintenance of anesthesia should be tailored to achieve easy reversibility. An area with appropriate nursing staff must be provided for postanesthetic care.

One of the most exciting areas in pediatric abdominal surgery is endoscopic laparoscopy. With technical advances in equipment, it is now possible to make diagnoses and to obtain biopsy samples of lesions through a laparoscope. In addition, one can perform a cholecystectomy, esophageal fundoplication, gastrostomy, appendectomy, closure of a bowel perforation, and sclerosing therapy for varicose veins. Many more procedures will certainly be added to this list in the future. Proponents of this technique point out that it is associated with less postoperative morbidity and lower costs.

Several anesthetic concerns are unique to laparoscopic procedures.[62] Use of an excessive gas volume to expand the abdomen elevates the diaphragm and decreases pulmonary compliance. It also may compress the vena cava, reduce blood return to the heart, and decrease cardiac output.[63] Placing the patient in the reverse Trendelenburg position to allow the bowels to fall away from the upper abdomen exaggerates the effects on venous return and cardiac output.[64] Because IV gas emboli have occurred, CO_2 is usually used as the distending gas. If nitrous oxide is used as part of the anesthetic, it will rapidly cross the peritoneum and any gas-filled bowel, enhancing abdominal distention. Nitrous oxide supports combustion that is ignited by either laser or electrocautery. Use of cool or cold gas to distend the abdomen may augment systemic hypothermia.[65] Traction on the mesentery may precipitate cardiac arrhythmias, especially when halothane is present.[66]

Although some endoscopic laparoscopic surgery is performed in adults with local anesthesia, general endotracheal anesthesia is indicated in all pediatric cases. Ventilation is controlled and may have to be increased if CO_2 is used. If a Jackson-Reese modification of the Ayres T-piece is used, it may also be necessary to increase gas flows to maintain nonrebreathing. A nasogastric tube is inserted to decompress the stomach before cannulation of the abdomen. A precordial or esophageal stethoscope and P_{ETCO_2} monitoring may aid in early detection of an embolus. Because unrecognized, hidden hemorrhage may occur, vital signs must be carefully followed intra- and postoperatively. Intraperitoneal installation of local anesthetic may help to relieve abdominal pain,[67] which is often referred to the shoulder.

Esophageal Fundoplication

Because of the increased awareness over the past two decades of GER in the pediatric patient,[68] both medical and surgical relief of this life-threatening entity has been emphasized. Although newborn infants often regurgitate during the first month of life, Carrie[69] estimated that only 1 in 500 has persistent regurgitation beyond 6 weeks of age. Ninety-eight percent of normal infants with GER will

have signs of GER by 3 months of age. The usual manifestations are repeated regurgitation and vomiting, apnea, pulmonary aspiration, reactive airway disease, hematemesis, melena, and failure to thrive. Less common presentations are stricture of the gut, Sandifer's syndrome, rumination, and a clinical picture mimicking bronchopulmonary dysplasia. GER may be present after esophageal atresia repair and gastrostomy and in developmentally delayed children who have spastic quadriplegia, hypoxic brain damage, and trisomy syndromes, in which discoordinated swallowing is present.

Although many tests have been employed to confirm GER, none is conclusive. Esophagrams are easy to perform, but there is no uniformity in the technique for doing them or in the criteria for diagnosis, and GER is not necessarily related to the presence of a hiatal hernia. Esophageal motility based on data from pressure transducers may be difficult to interpet. Esophagoscopy permits direct observation of the esophageal mucosa and allows biopsy of the esophagus to document pathology. Bronchoscopy often reveals chronic bronchial changes and allows aspiration of bronchial washings to look for lipid-laden macrophages. Monitoring the esophageal pH for 4 or more hours after an acid challenge (the Tuttle test) demonstrates episodes of acid regurgitation. More than one test may be required to make the diagnosis of GER.

Medical therapy of GER includes thickening of feedings and maintenance of the patient in an upright position. Cimetidine and ranitidine are used to decrease gastric acidity, and metoclopramide is used to increase LES pressure and to enhance gastric emptying. In 60 percent of patients, the signs of GER usually subside by the age of 18 months. In 30 percent, they persist beyond 4 years of age; 5 percent of patients experience stricture of the esophagus, and 5 percent die of complications.[57]

Patients who fail medical therapy or who have life-threatening disease are candidates for surgery. Some pediatric surgeons combine fundoplication and pyloroplasty with a permanent feeding gastrostomy, because gastrostomy alone often causes severe abnormalities of gastric motility. Preoperative anesthesia evaluation is directed toward improving the patient's pulmonary status, correcting anemia, and improving nutrition. Pneumonia should be treated and bronchospasm controlled. TPN may be indicated perioperatively. Although transfusion is often not necessary, blood should be available in case retrogastric bleeding is encountered.

Patients can be premedicated with H_2 blockers, metoclopramide, and/or antacids, but appropriate fasting is more important. Solids and formula, but not clear liquids, must be withheld for a minimum of 6 hours. After induction of anesthesia and endotracheal intubation, ventilation is controlled. The anesthesiologist must have access to the head so that the nasogastric tube and esophageal dilators can be adjusted intraoperatively without dislodging or obstructing the ETT. Central venous monitoring may be helpful, not only for monitoring but for fluid administration and parenteral nutrition after surgery. Intra-arterial pressure monitoring is used if the patient has significant pulmonary disease. Inadvertent vena caval compression by surgical retractors must be anticipated and corrected. Muscle relaxants, which improve surgical exposure, should be monitored and their effect fully reversed at the end of surgery if postoperative ventilation is not planned. Intra- or postoperative regional anesthesia may help to prevent splinting and atelectasis. Patients on high-dose steroids for severe lung disease may not tolerate aggressive fluid replacement.

After esophageal fundoplication, patients are unable to vomit. Therefore, a bowel obstruction may be a dire emergency because significant abdominal distention can compromise gut blood flow and cause bowel ischemia and death.

Appendicitis and Intussusception

Although these two disease processes are entirely distinct from each other, their anesthetic management is remarkably similar. It is instructive to compare and contrast the two entities. Although both may present over a wide age span, intussusception occurs primarily between 4 and 10 months and appendicitis most frequently between 6 and 10 years of age. Rarely does the latter occur in patients less than 1 year of age. Children with both entities present acutely in pain, often with vomiting, and they usually require urgent resolution. Both entities, if not recognized and treated promptly, may lead to serious morbidity and mortality.

Appendicitis is caused by an infectious process. During the prodromal period it is easily confused with and masked by other infections that produce fever, lethargy, and anorexia. Pain is usually localized to the right lower quadrant, but may present rectally or diffusely. The pain may resolve with perforation or antibiotic therapy, providing a false sense of security. Oral intake may have been limited for a considerable time, as reflected by a history of decreased urine output, physical signs of dry mucous membranes and poor turgor, and findings of increased urine specific gravity. Fever causes further dehydration. Anorexia and paralytic ileus are the hallmarks of appendicitis. Mechanical obstruction and distention occur late in the disease process, usually after the appendix has perforated. In many children the lesser omentum walls off the infection, creating a localized abscess; in others, generalized peritonitis rapidly develops. Diagnosis is made by history, physical exam, white blood cell count and differential examination, urinalysis (to rule out urinary infection), and rectal exam. A radiograph of the abdomen or ultrasonogram of the abdomen, which is not necessarily indicated, may reveal a fecolith. Appendicitis can be ruled out if a barium enema reveals an appendix filled with contrast solution. In patients with localized appendiceal abscess, local drainage of the abscess by the interventional radiologist or incision and drainage by the surgeon and an appendectomy at a later date are alternatives to primary appendectomy under certain circumstances. Unfortunately, both of the alternatives require general anesthesia in most children.

Intussusception is an invagination and telescoping of intestine, usually with a lead point just proximal to the ileocecal valve. With time, intussusception leads to venous obstruction and bowel edema, which obstruct and compromise vascularity. The first signs of intussusception are often pain, bloody diarrhea (often described as a currant-jelly stool) and, later, vomiting. A barium enema may be both diagnostic and therapeutic. Contrast medium under gentle hydrostatic pressure will reduce 50 to 70 percent of intussusceptions, thus obviating the need for surgery. A second attempt at hydrostatic reduction of the intussusception in the operating room after the patient is anesthetized has recently been described by Collins et al.[70] They reported an almost 90 percent success rate in reducing the intussusception.

Patients with appendicitis or intussusception may require aggressive fluid resuscitation preoperatively. The former are often more febrile and the latter more volume depleted. Both benefit from antibiotics (gentamycin 2 mg/kg, ampicillin 25 mg/kg, and metronidazole 5 mg/kg) and nasogastric decompression of the stomach if abdominal distention is significant. Although regional anesthesia is an alternative for appendectomy in adolescents, general anesthesia is routine for all appendectomies and all cases of intussusception in infants and children. Because an IV cannula is usually in place, rapid-sequence induction of anesthesia with a barbiturate is most commonly employed. In the febrile patient, the vasodilation induced by halothane or isoflurane is helpful in lowering the patient's temperature (see Chapter 4). However, these patients may be very sensitive to volatile anesthetics because of concomitant hypovolemia and hyponatremia. The latter is the result of hypotonic fluid replacement of large third-space fluid losses. Hyponatremia lowers minimum alveolar concentration (MAC).[71] Muscle relaxants should be used cautiously, particularly when intraperitoneal kanamycin or gentamycin is administered. The ETT should be left in place until the patient is fully awake and reversal of muscle relaxation has been confirmed.

Postoperative sepsis, gastrointestinal tract obstruction, and fluid replacement complicate the course of patients with generalized peritonitis. Further surgery may be required to drain subdiaphragmatic and pelvic abscesses. Prolonged ileus infrequently requires surgical reexploration of the abdomen, as the ileus usually subsides with appropriate parenteral fluid and antibiotic therapy. Monitoring of fluid replacement during and after surgery may require the use of central venous and urinary catheters as well as laboratory assessment of serum electrolytes and osmolality. In patients with ongoing sepsis, the appearance of inappropriate antidiuretic hormone (ADH) and disseminated intravascular coagulopathy may further complicate the patient's course.

LAPAROTOMY FOR MAJOR TUMOR AND BOWEL SURGERY

Anesthesia and perioperative care for elective, extensive, nontraumatic abdominal surgery share many facets in common, regardless of the etiology. These procedures include, but are not limited to, all major abdominal and retroperitoneal malignant tumors; anteroposterior colon resections for imperforate rectum and aganglionic megacolon; and organ resections such as pancreatectomy, adrenalectomy, and partial hepatectomy.

Malignant tumors are common in children. Cancer is second only to trauma as a cause of death in children.

Although advances have been made in radiotherapy and chemotherapy for cancer, surgery remains a major treatment modality for abdominal tumors. Most abdominal tumors are retroperitoneal. Wilms' tumor (nephroblastoma) and neuroblastoma are the most common solid tumors, accounting for 15 percent of all abdominal malignancies. Hodgkin's lymphoma (5 percent), non-Hodgkin's lymphoma, and teratoma are also seen in the pediatric population. Rhabdomyosarcoma often arises from the genitourinary tract. Hepatoblastoma and hepatoendotheliomas arise from the liver. All of these tumors are amenable to surgery at some time in their course, even though total excision may not be possible. The timing of surgery, chemotherapy, and radiotherapy is important and entails coordination from local multispecialty tumor boards and from national tumor registries to determine the most up-to-date treatment protocol for that specific tumor. Pheochromocytoma usually arises from the adrenal gland but may be found elsewhere in the abdomen. This tumor causes increased catecholamine production and increased vanillylmandelic acid (VMA) excretion. Erratic changes in blood pressure should be treated with α-adrenergic blockers, such as phentolamine, and β-adrenergic blockers, such as propanolol or esmolol. Neuroblastomas, which may arise at any place along the neural crest and occasionally regress spontaneously, may also produce elevated VMA and catecholamines, although less so than pheochromocytoma.

Anteroposterior (AP) colon resections are the definitive surgery for both high imperforate anus and aganglionic megacolon (Hirschsprung's disease). A diverting and staging colostomy is performed in the neonatal period, and an AP resection is usually performed when the patient reaches 10 kg. In the latter case, multiple biopsies are required to establish the level of bowel at which normal myenteric plexi are present.

The specific anesthetic concerns for surgical resection of various organs depend on the organ to be removed. Patients scheduled for splenectomy for congenital spherocytosis are usually anemic and unresponsive to transfusion before resection. Resection of the tail of the pancreas in a nondiabetic patient is well tolerated, but resection of the head of the pancreas or total pancreatic resection induces diabetes mellitus and requires diabetic management. Total hepatectomy and transplantation are discussed elsewhere (see Chapter 19).

All of the above procedures require a disciplined approach and demand the utmost attention of the anesthesiologist. Many of these children have had multiple hospitalizations and encounters with health care personnel on all levels. A thorough chart review of all previous anesthetics, as well as communication with relevant consultants, will familiarize the anesthesiologist with the treatment plan and the information previously conveyed to the patient and family. The anesthesiologist must be sensitive to the emotional and psychological needs of both parents and patient, from the preoperative interview through the postoperative visit.

Patients who present for major abdominal surgery must be evaluated for anemia and hypovolemia. The latter is of special concern when a surgical bowel preparation has been performed. Concurrent IV fluid administration may

be advisable. Transfusion therapy must be anticipated. Discussion of and consent for alternative methods, such as directed donor acquisition of blood, preoperative autologous blood donation, blood scavenging, and deliberate hypotension-hypothermia-hemodilution (see Chapter 13) must be completed before appropriate blood and blood products are ordered. The coagulation system should be assessed because hemorrhage is a potential problem, particularly when liver function is compromised or if massive transfusions are administered.

The anesthesiologist should be prepared to replace large fluid losses with warmed balanced salt solution, colloid, and blood products. Access to central venous and arterial vessels is necessary. Broviac catheter insertion should be considered if chemotherapy and/or TPN will be necessary postoperatively. Compression or interruption of the inferior vena cava or abdominal aorta often occurs as a result of the pathology or the surgery. The surgeon must be prepared to halt active dissection temporarily and to tamponade bleeding while the blood volume is restored. Urinary catheterization is required to assess urine output. Muscle relaxants and controlled ventilation help to provide a quiet, relaxed surgical field. All anesthetic gases, peritoneal irrigation, and transfusions should be warmed to prevent intraoperative hypothermia. Continuous epidural anesthesia, usually instituted after induction of anesthesia, will provide good muscle relaxation, reduce requirements for general anesthetics, possibly reduce the stress response to major surgery, and allow better postoperative pain control. Blood loss may be difficult to accurately measure because of diffuse "ooze," irrigation, and concealed blood loss. Much reliance must be placed on the observation of moment-to-moment changes in parameters such as direct arterial pressure, pulse, and central venous pressure. Innovative techniques may be necessary, such as resection of infant liver tumors utilizing hypothermic circulatory arrest.[72]

ABDOMINAL TRAUMA

Management of abdominal trauma must be understood by all who undertake anesthesia in children. Ideally, all cases of acute pediatric trauma should be referred to a pediatric trauma center or, if this is not possible, to a center with the facility and experience to deal systematically with trauma in children. Airway management and vascular access, two areas in which the anesthesiologist is ideally suited, remain the first priority. Ninety percent of abdominal trauma in children under 14 years of age is blunt rather than penetrating.[73] Abdominal trauma must be suspected and investigated when a child sustains a major deceleration injury, when a conscious child complains of abdominal pain, when there are visible marks (e.g., tire tracks, abrasions) on the overlying skin of the abdomen, and when the unconscious child has an expanding abdomen and/or failing vital signs. Baseline chemistry determinations for serum enzymes and amylase should be obtained. Visualization of free air on an AP radiographic examination of the abdomen suggests perforated bowel or pneumothorax/pneumomediastinum. CT scanning is the sine qua non of head injury. It is relatively simple to extend the CT examination to the chest, abdomen, and pelvis, and to look for ruptured organs such as liver, spleen, and kidney.

The two major indications for exploratory laparotomy are perforated viscus (free air) or hemorrhage that cannot be stabilized with reasonable fluid volume replacement. With rare exceptions, most relatively major injuries in children can be watched expectantly and aggressively monitored in an ICU. This is particularly important in spleen trauma,[74] where preservation of the spleen can avoid a lifetime of prophylactic antibiotics for postsplenectomy sepsis.

Anesthesiologists who deal with pediatric abdominal trauma are involved in four typical scenarios: (1) a diagnostic CT scan; (2) nonabdominal surgery such as orthopedic, neuro-, or ophthalmologic surgery in a patient with a concomitant nonoperative abdominal lesion; (3) failed conservative management; and (4) operating room (OR) resuscitation. The latter is more fully addressed elsewhere[75] (see Chapter 7).

Trauma patients who undergo CT scanning range from moderately unstable with multiple-system injury to cooperative, alert patients with an injury to a single organ system. In the latter, reassurance and no medication or minimal sedation (midazolam 0.05 mg/kg or Pentothal 3 to 5 mg/kg) may be all that is required. Patients with abdominal distention, vomiting, or those who require oral contrast material should undergo tracheal intubation after a rapid-sequence induction of anesthesia. Patients who undergo tracheal intubation in the field or on arrival at the hospital can be lightly anesthetized with Pentothal, fentanyl, and/or minimal concentrations of inhaled anesthetics, and should be paralyzed until their condition is stabilized in the ICU.

Patients with multisystem injuries who are to undergo nonabdominal procedures should be draped so that the abdomen can be examined and the abdominal girth measured during surgery. The general surgeon should be available to reevaluate the patient if changes occur in the abdominal examination, vital signs, or hematocrit. The anesthesiologist must be suspicious that significant head injury may coexist with abdominal and peripheral pathology. Based on postinjury history and physical examination, cerebral CT scanning may be indicated before surgery. If any of these tests indicate intracranial hypertension and decreased cerebral perfusion, an intracranial pressure monitor should be inserted and continuously monitored during anesthesia. Postoperatively, these patients should be returned directly to the ICU, where they can be observed and monitored closely. Patients with continuing abdominal hemorrhage who fail conservative management usually do so with enough forewarning that the operating room can be prepared in an orderly manner. The department of anesthesiology, the department of surgery, and the OR staff must rehearse these emergency preparations in anticipation of emergent laparotomy rather than improvising them on the spot. Adequate blood products and equipment such as blood pumps, warmers, and blood retrieval systems must be available in the operating theater. The entire surgical team and extra anesthesia staff should be present before the skin incision. Once the peritoneum is entered and the effective tamponade is released, major hemorrhage may occur. The surgeon must quickly expose and control the source of the hemorrhage. Radical procedures, such as a temporary shunt for major vena caval lacerations, aortic cross-clamping for severe arterial hemorrhage, and cardiopulmonary bypass for concomitant thoracic and cardiac injury, may be life saving. Once bleeding is controlled, blood volume must be restored and evaluated by assessment of arterial and central venous pressures and urinary output. Catecholamines may be required to treat cardiac failure. As tolerated, the concentration of anesthesia agents is increased and maintained. Postoperatively, continued controlled ventilation in an ICU is indicated.

REFERENCES

1. Arey LB: Developmental Anatomy. A Textbook and Laboratory Manual of Embryology. 7th ed. Philadelphia, WB Saunders Company, 1965.
2. Milla PJ: Development of intestinal structure and function. In Tanner MS, Stockes RJ (eds): Neonatal Gastroenterology Contemporary Issues. Newcastle on Tyne, Intercept, 1984, p 2.
3. Gray SW, Skandalakis JE: Embryology for the Surgeons. Philadelphia, WB Saunders Company, 1972.
4. Hamlon WJ, Boyd JD, Mossman HW: Human Embryology. 3rd ed. Baltimore, Williams & Wilkins, 1962.
5. Alagille D, Odievrer M, Gautier EJ: Hepatic ductular hypoplasia associated with characteristic facies, vertebral malformations, retarded physical, mental, and sexual development, and cardiac murmur. J Pediatr 86:63, 1975.
6. Moore TC, Stokes GE: Gastroschisis report of two cases treated by modification of Gross operation for omphalocoel. Surgery 33:112, 1953.
7. Duhamel B: Embryology of exomphalos and allied malformations. Arch Dis Child 38:142, 1963.
8. Cantrell JR, Haller JA, Ravitch MM: A syndrome of congenital defects involving the abdominal wall, sternum, diaphragm, pericadium, and heart. Surg Gynecol Obstet 107:602, 1958.
9. Hoyme HE, Higginbotton MC, Jones KL: The vascular pathogenesis of gastroschisis: intrautcrine interruption of the omphalomesenteric artery. J Pediatr 98:228, 1981.
10. deVries PA: The pathogenesis of gastroschisis and omphalocele. J Pediatr Surg 15:245, 1980.
11. Glick PL, Harrison MR, Adzick NS, et al: The missing link in the pathogenesis of gastroschisis. J Pediatr Surg 20:406, 1985.
12. Kleigman RM, Fanaroff AA: Developmental metabolism and nutrition. In Gregory GA (ed): Pediatric Anesthesia. 2nd ed. New York, Churchill Livingstone, 1989, p 201.
13. Grand RJ, Watkins JB, Torti FM: Development of the human gastrointestinal tract: a review. Gastroenterology 70:790, 1976.
14. Avery GB, Randolph JG, Weaver T: Gastric acidity in the first day of life. Pediatrics 37:1005, 1966.
15. Wershil BK: Gastric function. In Walker WA, Durie PR, Hamilton JR, et al (eds): Pediatric Gastrointestinal Disease, Pathophysiology, Diagnosis, Management. Philadelphia, BC Decker, 1991, p 258.
16. Grand RJ, Watkins JB, Torti FM: Development of the human gastrointestinal tract. Gastroenterology 70:790, 1976.
17. Askanazi J, Nordenstrom J, Rosenbaum S, et al: Nutrition for the patient with respiratory failure: glucose vs fat. Anesthesiology 54:373, 1981.
18. Salem MR, Wong AY, Collins VJ: The pediatric patient with a full stomach. Anesthesiology 39:435, 1973.
19. Davenport HW: Physiology of the Digestive Tract. 4th ed. Chicago, Year Book Medical Publishers, 1977.
20. Vanner RG, Pryle BJ, O'Dwyer JP, et al: Upper oesophageal sphincter pressure and the intravenous induction of anaesthesia. Anaesthesia 47:371, 1992.
21. Berquist WE, Rachelefsky GS, Kadden M, et al: Gastroesophageal reflux-associated recurrent pneumonia and chronic asthma in children. Pediatrics 68:29, 1981.

22. Fasano M, Kofke WA, Keamy MF: Continuous hypopharyngeal pH during mask anesthesia [abstract]. Anesthesiology 65:A172, 1986.

23. Muravchuck S, Burkett L, Gold M: Succinylcholine-induced fasciculations and intragastric pressure during induction of anesthesia. Anesthesiology 55:180, 1981.

24. Salem MR, Wong AY, Eln YH: The effect of suxamethonium on the intragastric pressure in infants and children. Br J Anaesth 44:166, 1972.

25. Brock-Utne JG, Downing J: The lower oesophageal sphincter and the anesthetist. S Afr Med J 70:170, 1986.

26. van de Geijn, Van Vugt JM, Sollie JE, et al: Ultrasonographic diagnosis and perinatal management of fetal abdominal wall defects. Fetal Diagn Ther 6:2, 1991.

27. Calisti A, Manzoni C, Perrelli L: The fetus with an abdominal wall defect: management and outcome. J Perinat Med 15:105, 1987.

28. Kurjak A, Gogolja D, Kogler A, et al: Ultrasound diagnosis and perinatal management of surgically correctable fetal malformations. J Ultrasound Med Biol 10:4343, 1984.

29. Mann L, Ferguson-Smith M, Desai M, et al: Prenatal assessment of anterior abdominal wall defects and their prognosis. Prenat Diagn 4:427, 1984.

30. Nyberg DA, Fitzsimmons J, Mack L, et al: Chromosome abnormalities in fetuses with omphalocele, Significance of omphalocele contents. J Ultrasound Med 8:299, 1989.

31. Moretti M, Khoury A, Rodriguez J, et al: The effect of mode of delivery on the perinatal outcome in fetuses with abdominal wall defects. Am J Obstet Gynecol 163:833, 1990.

32. Lewis DF, Towers CV, Garite TJ, et al: Fetal gastroschisis and omphalocele: is cesarean section the best mode of delivery? Am J Obstet Gynecol 163:770, 1990.

33. Sipes SL, Weiner CP, Sipes II, et al: Gastroschisis and omphalocele: does either antenatal diagnosis or route of delivery make a difference in perinatal outcome? Obstet Gynecol 76:195, 1990.

34. Hagberg S, Hokegard KH, Rubenson A, et al: Prenatally diagnosed gastroschisis—a preliminary report advocating the use of elective caesarean section. Z Kinderchir 43:419, 1988.

35. Coté C: Aspiration: an overrated risk in elective patients. Adv Anesth 9:1, 1992.

36. Morrison JE, Lockhart CH: Preoperative fasting and medication in children. Anesthesiol Clin North Am 9:731, 1991.

37. Spear RM: Dose-response in infants receiving caudal anaesthesia with bupivacaine. Paediatr Anaesth 1:47, 1991.

38. Todres ID, Crone RK: Experience with a modified laryngoscope in sick infants. Crit Care Med 9:544, 1981.

39. Anand KJ, Hansen DD, Hickey PR: Hormonal-metabolic stress responses in neonates undergoing cardiac surgery. Anesthesiology 73:670, 1990.

40. Anand KJ, Hickey PR: Halothane-morphine compared with high-dose sufentanil for anesthesia and postoperative analgesia in neonatal cardiac surgery. N Engl J Med 326:1, 1992.

41. Anand KJ, Sippel WG, Schofield NM, et al: Does halothane anaesthesia decrease the metabolic and endocrine stress responses of newborn infants undergoing operation? BMJ 296:668, 1988.

42. Yaster M, Nicholar E, Maxwell LG: Opioids in pediatric anesthesia and in the management of childhood pain. Anesthesiol Clin North Am 9:750, 1991.

43. Moretti M, Khoury A, Rodriguez J, et al: The effect of mode of delivery on the perinatal outcome in fetuses with abdominal wall defects. Am J Obstet Gynecol 160:833, 1990.

44. Filston HC, Izant RJ: Translocation of umbilical artery to the lower abdomen: an adjunct to the postoperative monitoring of arterial blood gases in major abdominal wall surgery. J Pediatr Surg 10:225, 1975.

45. Philippart AL, Canty TG, Filler RM: Acute fluid volume requirements in infants with anterior abdominal wall defects. J Pediatr Surg 7:553, 1972.

46. Canty TG, Collins DL: Primary fascial closure in infants with gastroschisis or omphalocele. J Pediatr Surg 18:707, 1983.

47. Yaster M, Scherer TL, Stone MM, et al: Prediction of successful primary closure of congenital abdominal wall defects using intraoperative measurements. J Pediatr Surg 24:1217, 1989.

48. Flake AW, Ryckman FC: Selected anomalies and intestinal obstruction. In Fanaroff AA, Martin RJ (eds): Neonatal-Perinatal Medicine. St. Louis, CV Mosby, 1992, p 1038.

49. Kawade N, Onishi S: The prenatal and postnatal development of UDP-glucuronyl transferase activity toward bilirubin and the effect of premature birth on this activity in human liver. Biochem J 196:257, 1981.

50. Maisels MJ: Neonatal jaundice. In Avery GB (ed): Neonatology Pathophysiology and Management of the Newborn. 3rd ed. Philadelphia, JB Lippincott, 1987, p 554.

51. Oski FA: Obstructive jaundice due to biliary atresia and neonatal hepatitis. In Taeush HW, Ballard RA, Avery MA (eds): Schaffer and Avery Disease of Newborns. 6th ed. Philadelphia, WB Saunders Company, 1992, p 772.

52. Kasai M, Suzuki H, Ohashi E, et al: Technique and results of operative management of biliary atresia. World J Surg 2:571, 1978.

53. Abajian JC, Mellis PW, Browne AE, et al: Spinal anesthesia for surgery in the high risk infant. Anesth Analg 63:359, 1984.

54. Spear RM, Deshpande JK, Maxwell LG: Caudal anesthesia in the awake, high-risk infant. Anesthesiology 69:407, 1988.

55. Blaise G, Roy L: Spinal anesthesia in pediatric surgery. Anesth Analg 64:196, 1985.

56. Gregory GA, Steward DJ: Life-threatening perioperative apnea in the ex-"premie." Anesthesiology 59:495, 1983.

57. Liu LM, Coté CJ, Ryan J, et al: Life-threatening apnea in infants. Anesthesiology 59:506, 1983.

58. Kurth CD, Spitzer AR, Broennle AM, et al: Postoperative apnea in former preterm infants [abstract]. Anesthesiology 63:A475, 1985.

59. Welborn LG, Rice LJ, Broadman LM, et al: Postoperative apnea in former preterm infants: prospective comparison of spinal and general anesthesia. Anesthesiology 71:347, 1989.

60. Winters RW: The Body Fluid in Pediatrics. Boston, Little, Brown, 1973.

61. American Academy of Pediatrics, Committee on Drugs: Guidelines for monitoring and management of pediatric patients during and after sedation for diagnostic and therapeutic procedures. Pediatrics 89:1110, 1992.

62. Marco AP, Yeo CJ, Rock P: Anesthesia for a patient undergoing laparoscopic cholecystectomy. Anesthesiology 3:1268, 1990.

63. Kelman GR, Swapp GH, Smith I, et al: Cardiac output and arterial blood gas during laparoscopy. Br J Anaesth 44:1155, 1972.

64. Johannsen G, Andersen M, Juhl B: The effect of general anesthesia on the haemodynamic events during laparoscopy with CO_2 insufflation. Acta Anaesthesiol Scand 33:132, 1989.

65. Ott DE: Correction of laparoscopic insufflation hypothermia. J Laparoendosc Surg 1:183, 1991.

66. Myles PS: Bradyarrhythmias and laparoscopy: a prospective study of heart rate changes with laparoscopy. Aust N Z J Obstet Gynecol 31:171, 1991.

67. Helvacioglu A, Weis R: Operative laparoscopy and postoperative pain relief. Fertil Steril 57:548, 1992.

68. Herbst JJ: Gastroesophageal reflux. J Pediatr 98:859, 1981.

69. Carrie IJ: The natural history of the partial thoracic stomach ("hiatal hernia") in children. Arch Dis Child 34:344, 1959.

70. Collins DL, Pinckney LE, Miller KE, et al: Hydrostatic reduction of ileocolic intussusception: a second attempt in the operating room with general anesthesia. J Pediatr 115:204, 1989.

71. Tanifuji Y, Eger El II: Brain sodium, potassium and osmolality: effects on anesthetic requirement. Anesth Analg 57:404, 1978.

72. Ward CF, Arkin DB, Benumof JL: The use of profound hypothermia and circulatory arrest for hepatic lobectomy in infancy. Anesthesiology 47:473, 1977.

73. Pokorny WJ: Abdominal Trauma. In Raffensperger JG (ed): Swenson's Pediatric Surgery. 8th ed. Norwalk, CT, Appleton, 1990, p 274.

74. Touloukian RJ: Splenic injury. In Touloukian RJ (ed): Pediatric Trauma. 2nd ed. St. Louis, Mosby Year Book, 1990, p 332.

75. Coté C: Blood, colloid, and crystalloid therapy. Anesthesiol Clin North Am 9:869, 1991.

76. Nimmo WS: Pharmacology of agents that affect gastric secretion, emptying and vomiting. Can J Anaesth 37:899, 1990.

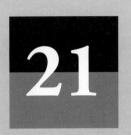

Anesthesia for Genitourinary Surgery

FREDERIC A. BERRY
BARBARA A. CASTRO

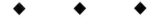

The kidney is a resilient organ capable of maintaining normal function from moderate challenges of trauma, disease, or surgery. It usually takes a series of superimposed iatrogenic misfortunes for the otherwise normal renal system to decompensate. However, when there is a severe fluid challenge or when a mild to moderate fluid challenge is superimposed on a background of varying degrees of renal disease, the renal system needs fine tuning, otherwise it will decompensate. In this situation, the renal system needs the same degree of supportive care that is usually provided for the cardiovascular and pulmonary systems. Anticipatory and supportive care can be provided more effectively when the anesthesiologist understands renal function. Consequently, the first half of this chapter provides a working knowledge of the physiology of the renal system.

EMBRYOLOGY

The field of embryology is concerned with prenatal life.[1, 2] It encompasses two main time periods. The first, the *embryonic period,* lasts from conception through the eighth week of gestation, by which time the main organ systems have developed. At this point, the developing embryo enters the *fetal period,* and the major changes that occur from the 9th to the 40th week are growth and further tissue differentiation. These changes are not abrupt but occur as a gradual transition, with overlapping of the embryonic and fetal periods.

The embryology of the renal system is described here, with some mention of the genital system because of the intimate and sometimes inseparable origin and development of the two systems. Both arise from a common mesodermal ridge called the urogenital ridge. Early in development, the excretory ducts of both systems empty into the cloaca. As the two systems continue to develop and differentiate, separate anatomic pathways develop. However, particularly in the male, some overlapping of the two systems remains despite entirely different functions.

Development of the Renal System

The renal system consists of an interface between the vascular system and a selective excretory organ, which results in a continuous process of renal activity (i.e., a selective processing system to conserve essential material and a conduit to discharge the waste materials into a holding area from which they can leave the body). At the vascular end there is contact with a vascular tuft called a glomerulus, which filters part of the renal blood flow. This structure is connected to a reabsorptive and secretory tubule capable of clearing metabolites and other material from the circulation. The tubule is, in turn, connected to

587

an excretory duct for discharging wastes. The basic renal unit therefore consists of three parts: a vascular system to supply blood flow, a conservation and excretory system for processing the blood, and a collecting system for collecting and discharging waste.

During fetal life there are three overlapping renal systems. The first to develop is the pronephros, or head kidney; the second is the mesonephros, or middle kidney; and the third is the metanephros, or permanent kidney. The names of the various renal systems describe not only their anatomic locations but also their order of cephalocaudal development.

Development of the Permanent Kidney

The metanephros, or permanent kidney, begins to develop during the fifth gestational week. The collecting system is derived from the ureteric bud, which is an outgrowth of the mesonephric duct just before the duct enters the cloaca. Differentiation of the ureteric bud results in formation of the collecting system, which is composed of the collecting tubules, papillary ducts, minor calyces, major calyces, renal pelvis, and ureter. This differentiation occurs by repeated divisions and branchings of the ureteric bud.

Differentiation of the metanephric tissue, or excretory system, is induced by the collecting tubules, which penetrate the metanephric blastema. These newly formed tubules induce division of the metanephrogenic tissue so that a small mass of tissue covers each tubule. The tissue

formed becomes a renal vesicle, which gives rise to a small tubule that forms the nephron, the metanephric excretory unit (Fig. 21–1). One end of the excretory unit, or tubule, joins a vascular tuft to form the glomerulus, and the other end of the excretory tubule joins the collecting system. The vascular end becomes Bowman's capsule. The continued lengthening and differentiation of the tubule lead to the development of the proximal convoluted tubule, the loop of Henle, and the distal convoluted tubule. This process of differentiation continues through the 34th gestational week. The most recently formed nephrons are in the outer cortex of the kidney and are referred to as cortical nephrons. The oldest nephrons are nearest the medulla and are referred to as juxtamedullary nephrons. In the mature neonate the cortical nephrons predominate at a ratio of 8:1; however, in the more immature newborns (i.e., those under 34 weeks' gestational age) there is a greater proportion of juxtamedullary nephrons. There are anatomic and functional differences between these two types of nephrons (see below). The birth of an infant at 28 weeks' gestation does not accelerate new nephron formation. It takes approximately 34 weeks' gestation for nephrons to develop, regardless of whether the infant is inside or outside the uterus. Each kidney produces 1 million nephrons. After the 34th week, all increases in renal size result from the continued enlargement and growth of the nephrons rather than from the formation of new nephrons.

Development of the renal system occurs in both a cephalocaudad and a caudocephalad direction. Interestingly,

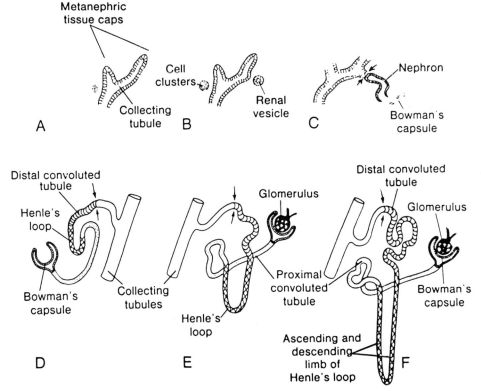

FIGURE 21–1. Development of a metanephric excretory unit. *Arrows* indicate the place where the excretory unit established an open communication with the collecting system, thus allowing for the flow of urine from the glomerulus into the collecting ducts. (From Langman J: Medical Embryology. Baltimore, Williams & Wilkins, 1981, with permission.)

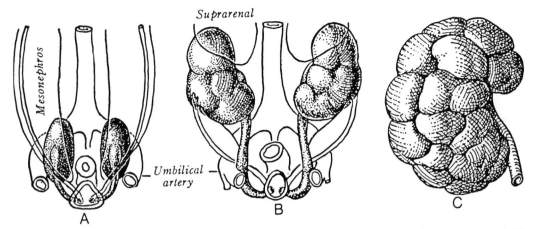

FIGURE 21–2. Ascent and lobation of the human kidney. *A* and *B,* Shift in position between 6 and 9 weeks, and early lobation (× 25). *C,* External lobation at birth. (From Arey LB: Developmental Anatomy. 3rd ed. Philadelphia, WB Saunders Company, 1934, with permission.)

however, migration of the permanent kidney occurs in a cephalad direction (Fig. 21–2), as a result of several interrelated factors. First is the marked growth and development of the lumbar and sacral regions. Second, the degree of the body curvature of the fetus is reduced; as the fetus grows, it tends to straighten. However, there is actual migration of the kidneys, so that at 8 weeks their position is at the level of the future second lumbar vertebra. In addition, the kidney rotates 90 degrees. Initially its hilum faces in a ventral direction, but at the end of rotation it assumes a medial position. Certain congenital anomalies of the kidney occur because of this migration.

Development of the Lower Urinary Tract

The embryologic development of the kidney and genital system is closely interwoven, particularly regarding development of the cloaca. From the fourth to seventh weeks, a wedge of mesenchyme migrates caudally as the urorectal septum, to fuse with the cloacal membrane and divide the cloaca into a ventral bladder and a dorsal anorectal canal. The perineal body is formed where this fusion occurs. The superior aspect of the bladder, the urachus, is continuous at the umbilicus with the remnant of the allantois (Fig. 21–3).

Formation of Fetal Urine and Amniotic Fluid

The metanephric, or permanent, kidney begins to develop at 5 weeks' gestation and produces urine by the ninth week. During the ninth week the ureter also opens into the bladder as the membrane that separates them regresses. If this membrane partially or completely fails to regress, partial or complete ureterovesticular obstruction occurs. The renal tubules develop steadily, so that by the 14th week the loop of Henle is functioning and tubular reabsorption is taking place.

Urine formation is important in the hydrodynamics of amniotic fluid, but it does not play an important role in removing waste material from the fetus; the placenta performs this function adequately. Fetal urine is a hypotonic ultrafiltrate of fetal plasma. It is both sugar- and protein-free. Part of the amniotic fluid comes from fetal lung, but most is produced by the amnion.

The amniotic fluid acts as a protective cushion—a shock absorber to equalize pressure, to prevent adherence of the amnion, and to allow changes in fetal position. In addition, amniotic fluid is necessary for normal growth and maturation of the lung.[3] By the 20th week the fetus is swallowing amniotic fluid, which is absorbed from the gastrointestinal tract into the vascular system. It is filtered

FIGURE 21–3. *A,* Development of the urogenital sinus into the urinary bladder, the pelvic part of the urogenital sinus, and the definitive urogenital sinus. *B,* In the male the definitive urogenital sinus develops into the penile urethra. The prostate gland is formed by outbudding of the urethra, whereas the seminal vesicles are formed by an outbudding of the ductus deferens. (From Langman J: Medical Embryology. Baltimore, Williams & Wilkins, 1981, with permission.)

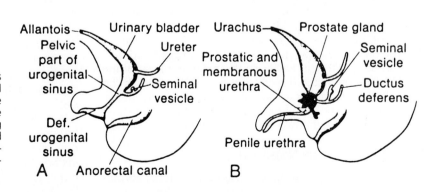

through the kidney and contributes to the formation of urine. As urine empties from the bladder into the amniotic cavity, it contributes to the amniotic fluid. The turnover of amniotic fluid at term is approximately 500 ml/day (150 ml/kg/day).[4]

BASIC ANATOMY OF THE RENAL SYSTEM

At birth, embryologic movement of the kidney (upward migration of the kidneys out of the pelvis into the retroperitoneal space) is complete. In the mature state, the right kidney is located at a somewhat lower level than the left, and the superior pole of the right kidney lies opposite the L12 vertebra and is protected posteriorly by the 12th rib. The right kidney extends down to the level of the L3 vertebra. The superior pole of the left kidney, which is approximately 1.5 cm higher than the right, lies a little above the T12 vertebra and extends down to the L2 vertebra. With changes in position and on deep inspiration, the kidneys may move as much as 2 cm in position, extending down to the iliac crest on deep inspiration. The kidney bed is formed posteriorly by the quadratus lumborum muscle. The lateral border of the bed is formed by the aponeurosis of the transversus abdominis muscle, and the medial border by the psoas muscle. The abdominal component of the diaphragm covers the upper third of the kidney.

The position of the great vessels and their relation to the kidney is of interest. The left kidney is located approximately 2.5 cm from the aorta, which is just anterior to the vertebral column. The right kidney almost touches the vena cava, as it is located to the right of the aorta and slightly to the right of the midline. The celiac plexus and the ganglia of the autonomic nervous system lie in close apposition to the aorta and approximately between the kidneys. The duodenum and the hepatic flexure of the colon are immediately adjacent to the right kidney. The tail of the pancreas and the splenic flexure of the colon are adjacent to the left kidney. Even though the adrenal glands are immediately adjacent anatomically (i.e., superiorly and medially), the supporting fascial structures are entirely separate, so that the adrenal glands do not participate in the full movement experienced by the kidney during respiration and changes in position.

The ureters originate from the more interior aspects of the renal pelvis and travel retroperitoneally. They cross the pelvic rim anterior to the iliac artery and veins and enter the bladder wall posteriorly. The ureter is lined with a mucous membrane that is continuous with the mucous membrane of the bladder. The ureter enters the bladder in an oblique direction, which creates a valve-like effect.

The bladder is a pelvic organ located anterior and inferior to the peritoneal cavity. In the male, the base of the bladder is connected directly to the prostate gland; in the female the bladder rests directly on the muscular pelvic floor. The trigone of the bladder is formed by three structures, or orifices: the two ureters and the urethral orifice.

Anatomy of the Nephron

The renal unit, or nephron, is composed of a renal corpuscle, the distal and proximal convoluted tubules, the loop

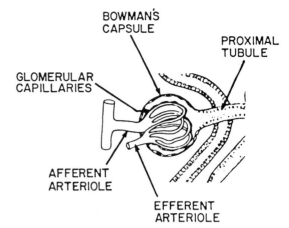

FIGURE 21–4. Anatomy of the glomerulus, illustrating the arrangement of capillary lobules, derived from the expanded chamber of the afferent arteriole. The lower section illustrates the foldings of the glomerular basement membrane. (From Smith HW: The Kidney. New York, Oxford University Press, 1951, with permission.)

of Henle, and the collecting duct. The renal corpuscle consists of the glomerulus and Bowman's capsule. Bowman's capsule is invaginated on one side by the capillary tufts of the glomerulus, with its afferent and efferent arterioles. Because of this invagination, the capillaries of the glomerulus are covered by one layer of Bowman's capsule; the other layer is continuous with the basement membrane of the tubule. This continuity results in the familiar structure of the renal corpuscle, with the blood supply entering one side of Bowman's capsule and the proximal tubule extending from the other side (Fig. 21–4).

The classic concept of the anatomy of the nephron is that the proximal convoluted tubule descends toward the medulla of the kidney, where it becomes the thin loop of Henle, which makes a hairpin turn. The ascending loop of Henle becomes the distal convoluted tubule, which ascends adjacent to the proximal convoluted tubule. The distal convoluted tubule passes by the glomerulus at the hilum of the entrance of the afferent arteriole and the exit of the efferent arteriole. This area is called the juxtaglomerular apparatus (see below). The distal tubule joins a collecting duct. The collecting ducts then merge and form straight collecting ducts, which descend into the renal medulla. The ducts unite to form larger ducts that continue to unite with each other and finally form the papillary ducts of Bellini, which empty into the renal pelvis. The lengths of the tubules and of the loop of Henle vary with the location of the nephron. The cortical nephrons have short tubules and loops of Henle, and the juxtamedullary nephrons have long tubules and loops of Henle. The classic diagram has been greatly simplified to facilitate understanding. The proximal convoluted tubule may extend a relatively large distance toward the capsule of the kidney before making its sojourn toward the medulla of the kidney, particularly nephrons of the subcortical zone and the juxtamedullary nephrons. The loops of Henle of the latter group of nephrons are long compared with the relative length pictured in Figure 21–5.

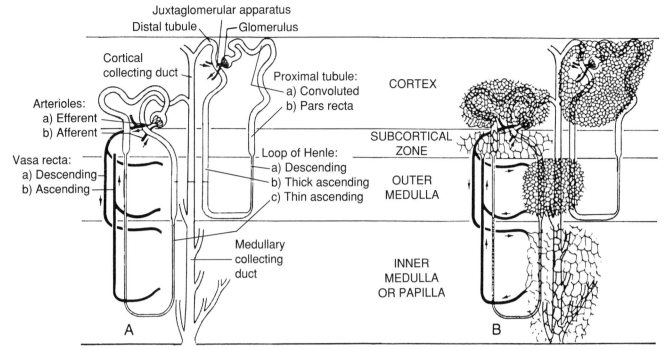

FIGURE 21–5. *A,* Superficial cortical and juxtamedullary nephrons and their vasculature. The glomerulus and the surrounding Bowman's capsule are known as the renal corpuscle. The beginning of the proximal tubule (the urinary pole) lies opposite the vascular pole, where the afferent and efferent arterioles enter and leave the glomerulus. The early distal tubule is always closely associated with the vascular pole belonging to the same nephron; the juxtaglomerular apparatus is located at the point of contact. *B,* Capillary networks have been superimposed on the nephrons illustrated in *A.* Note that the capillary network, which is interposed between the descending and ascending vasa recta, primarily surrounds the collecting duct and the ascending limb of Henle. In the outer and inner medulla the vasae rectae run in bundles, closely associated with the descending limb of Henle. (From Valtin H: Renal Function: Mechanisms Preserving Fluid and Solute Balance in Health. Boston, Little, Brown, 1973, with permission.)

RENAL PHYSIOLOGY

Although the kidney is an amazing organ, it is hardly noticeable under normal conditions. It is only at times of stress and challenge that the physician takes note of its function and its limitations. The section below deals with the normal physiology of the mature kidney and discusses the physiology of the immature kidney and the process of maturation.

Renal Blood Flow and Its Distribution

The kidneys in the lean adult are about 0.5 percent of body weight but receive 20 to 25 percent of the cardiac output. This enormous blood flow is necessary because of the function and resulting high oxygen requirement of the kidney. In the fetal state the renal blood flow is quite low, because it only needs to deliver nutrition to the kidney for the purposes of growth and development. However, within the first several days after birth there is a tremendous increase in renal blood flow and glomerular filtration and an improvement in renal function. This increase is thought to result from both a decrease in renal vascular resistance and an increase in systemic blood pressure.

One of the most significant aspects of renal flow is the mechanism for its redistribution that occurs with anesthesia, heart failure, drugs, shock, and various other pathophysiologic states and their treatment. Redistribution is part of the "stress response." When a decrease in blood pressure results in the release of endogenous vasopressors, not only may there be a reduction in total renal blood flow, but blood flow within the kidney may be redistributed, thereby greatly altering renal function.

During normal circulation, approximately 80 to 90 percent of renal blood flow goes to the cortical nephrons, approximately 10 percent perfuses the medulla, and 1 to 2 percent perfuses the papilla. During periods of hypotension and hypoxia, intrarenal redistribution of blood flow occurs; the outer cortex becomes relatively ischemic, and more of the renal blood flow is shunted to the medullary areas. The renin–angiotensin system is thought to play a major role in this redistribution, as the outer cortex has a high content of renin, whereas the renin content of the juxtamedullary area is low.

Autoregulation of Renal Blood Flow

Most anesthesiologists are well versed in the concepts of autoregulation of blood flow because of the interest that has developed in the area of cerebral autoregulation. Autoregulation refers to a control system that ensures that blood flow is relatively independent of systemic pressure. The concept is that the control of the blood flow resides wholly within the organ described. It must be independent of both extrinsic neurologic control and blood-borne hormones. The kidney has a well-developed system of autoregulation that results in little change in blood flow and glomerular filtration rate as the systemic pressure is varied over a range of 70 to 180 mm Hg. Figure 21–6 depicts the concept of autoregulation. As can be seen, there are parallel changes in glomerular filtration rate and renal plasma flow, suggesting that the afferent arteriole is the most likely effector site for renal autoregulation.

FUNCTIONAL ASPECTS OF THE RENAL SYSTEM

The kidney can be thought of as a physiologic regulator with two main functions: (1) excretion of body and drug metabolites; and (2) maintenance of the volume and composition of the fluid compartments of the body. Excretion of endogenous and exogenous metabolites is one of the main functions of the kidney. During anesthesia and surgery the kidney is challenged with a vast array of exogenous pharmaceutical agents. The endogenous metabolites are primarily urea, creatinine, sulfate, and phosphate, which help to compose what is often referred to as the solute load.

The fluid compartments of the body are intracellular, extracellular, and transcellular. Transcellular fluid refers to a specialized type of extracellular fluid that includes cerebrospinal, pleural, peritoneal, intraocular, and synovial fluids, as well as digestive secretions. Transcellular fluid is similar to extracellular fluid in terms of its electrolyte content. Digestive fluid accounts for approximately 1 to 3 percent of body weight. In the normal state it is a rather insignificant amount of fluid, although in the context of a volume challenge it may become considerable. Vomiting and diarrhea may cause large losses of transcellular fluid with high electrolyte content. In intestinal obstruction, the transcellular fluid space may easily double or triple to 4 to 8 percent of body weight.

Intracellular fluid is found within a rather diverse group of cells (e.g., muscle and red blood cells [RBCs]). It represents approximately 40 percent of the total body weight. This percentage is stable from birth through maturation. Extracellular fluid consists of interstitial fluid and plasma. The electrolyte contents of intracellular and extracellular fluids are compared in Table 21–1. The major difference between plasma and interstitial fluid is the relative lack of plasma proteins within the interstitial space. However, the plasma proteins do leak into the interstitial fluid through the capillary walls; they are returned to the plasma by lymphatic vessels. At birth the extracellular fluid volume of term infants is 40 percent of body weight. In immature premature neonates, the extracellular fluid volume may be as much as 52 percent of body weight, whereas it approximates 20 percent in infants at 18 months of age. The change in extracellular fluid volume from birth to 18 months represents one of the major physiologic changes in body composition (Fig. 21–7). The other changes are those of muscle mass and fat. The newborn infant has relatively little fat and muscle mass, but the amount of both changes rather rapidly. The mechanisms for maintaining normal body composition are discussed below.

Conservation and Excretion

Approximately 25 percent of the cardiac output goes through the kidneys. In a 70-kg person this represents a blood flow of approximately 1,300 ml/min entering the two kidneys through the renal arteries. The normal urine flow is approximately 1 ml/min so that 1,299 ml of blood per minute leaves through the renal veins. The daily renal turnover of water, sodium, bicarbonate, and chloride is given in Table 21–2. It can be seen that more than 99 percent of the filtered load is reabsorbed. Therefore, small changes in the reabsorption of any of these substances can bring about enormous changes in the composition of the body compartments. It is obvious that an enormous amount of conservation must occur within the renal system to maintain homeostasis. Therefore, the physiology of the kidney is presented in the context of conservation of essential material and excretion of metabolites. The basic renal mechanisms are glomerular filtration and vary-

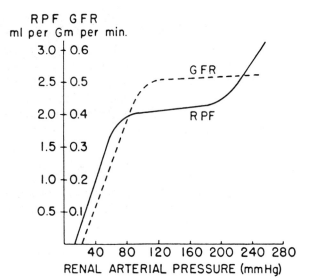

FIGURE 21–6. Autoregulation of glomerular filtration rate and renal plasma flow in the dog.

Ion Species	Plasma (mEq/L)	Interstitial Fluid (mEq/L)	Intracellular Fluid (mEq/L H₂O)
Na	142	144.0	±10
K	4	4.0	160
Ca	5	2.5	
Mg	3	1.5	35
Total cations	154	152.0	
Cl	103	114.0	±2
HCO₃	27	30.0	±8
PO₄	2	2.0	140
Protein	16	0.0	55
Total anions	148	146.0	

T A B L E   2 1 – 1
ELECTROLYTE CONTENT OF INTRACELLULAR AND EXTRACELLULAR FLUID

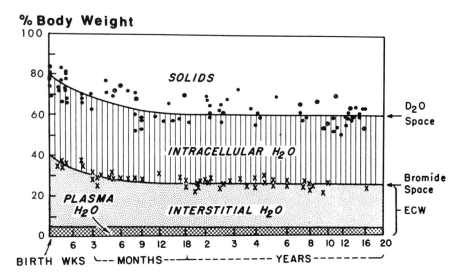

FIGURE 21–7. Percent body weight of the various body compartments with age. (From Talbot NB, Richie RH, Crawford JD: Metabolic Homeostasis. Cambridge, MA, Harford University Press, 1959. Copyright 1959 by The Commonwealth Fund, with permission.)

ing degrees of reabsorption and secretion in the proximal tubule, loop of Henle, distal tubule, and collecting duct.

Glomerular Filtration

Glomerular filtration allows separation of the plasma water and its constituents from blood cells and plasma proteins with molecular weights less than 70,000. Molecules of 15,000 to 70,000 molecular weight are filtered to varying degrees. The capillary membrane is permeable to small proteins with molecular weights of 15,000 or less.

The product of glomerular filtration is an ultrafiltrate of plasma that is relatively protein-free except for small amounts of albumin. Albumin is reabsorbed in the proximal convoluted tubules. The amount of filtration is referred to as the glomerular filtration rate (GFR) of plasma. Approximately 1,300 ml of whole blood per minute perfuses the kidneys of a normal 70-kg man (i.e., approximately 700 ml of plasma perfuses the kidneys per minute). Inulin clearance is the classic method for measuring GFR. This compound fulfills all the criteria for an ideal clearance substance: it is freely filtered by the glomerular capillaries, is biologically inert, is neither reabsorbed nor secreted by tubules, and can be accurately measured in plasma and urine.

Filtration Fraction

The filtration fraction is the ratio of the ultrafiltrate to total plasma flow. The normal value is 0.20, which means that 20 percent of the plasma flowing through the kidneys is

filtered by the glomerular capillaries. Even though the physical forces governing capillary flow are the same in the kidney as in other capillary beds, the volume of glomerular ultrafiltrate is greater than the volume of filtrate in the other beds. Several factors are responsible.

1. The pores of the glomerular capillaries are 25 to 60 percent larger than those of muscle capillaries.
2. The glomerular capillary pressures are considerably higher than those in the muscle capillaries.
3. The capillary area per gram of tissue is greater. The capillary area of skeletal muscle has been estimated at 7,000 cm^2/100 g of muscle, whereas glomerular capillary area has been estimated to range from 10,000 to 15,000 cm^2/100 g of renal tissue.
4. Glomerular capillaries may be up to 100 times more permeable than muscle capillaries to water and crystalloid.[1, 3]

Tubular Reabsorption

The tubules are the primary organs of conservation. Approximately 70 percent of the glomerular ultrafiltrate is absorbed in the proximal tubule, and reabsorption is isosmotic. The 70-kg man (surface area 1.73 m^2) is usually given as the index for the normal processes of the body. The GFR figures for the 70-kg woman are somewhat smaller: 125 ml/min/1.73 m^2 in men versus 100 ml/min/1.73 m^2 in women. The difference is thought to be because of the higher percentage of strategically located fat in women.

TABLE 21 – 2
DAILY RENAL TURNOVER OF H_2O, Na^+, HCO_3^-, AND Cl^- IN ADULTS

Measurement	Filtered	Excreted	Reabsorbed	Filtered Load Reabsorbed (%)
H_2O (L/day)	180	1.5	178.5	99.2
Na^+ (mEq/day)	25,000	150	24,850	99.4
HCO_3^- (mEq/day)	4,500	2	4,498	99.9
Cl^- (mEq/day)	18,000	150	17,850	99.2

Limited Tubular Reabsorptive Mechanisms

All of the constituents of extracellular fluid, with the exception of high-molecular-weight proteins, are freely filtered by the glomerular capillaries. The conservation process requires selective reabsorption to restore the essential constituents to the circulation. The tubules have a limited ability to actively reabsorb many substances; this limit is called the tubular maximal reabsorption capacity (Tm). Reabsorption of glucose, which is electrically neutral and unbound to protein, best exemplifies the concept of Tm. Under normal conditions glucose is readily filtered by the glomerular capillaries and is completely reabsorbed by the proximal tubular cells. However, if the amount of glucose in the plasma is increased above the Tm, glucose appears in the urine. The maximal rate of glucose reabsorption (TmG) has a remarkably constant value in a given individual. The average value in men is 375 mg/min/1.73 m² surface area; in women it is slightly less, 303 mg/min/1.73 m². In the full-term infant these values are approximately 180 to 200 mg/dl. Premature infants spill sugar at levels considerably below this figure, 125 mg/dl. The concepts of Tm are schematized in Figure 21–8. There are several other substances for which a Tm exists, including phosphate, sulfate, uric acid, amino acids, and probably albumin. In the case of inorganic phosphate, the Tm is normally exceeded, and the presence of small amounts of phosphate in the urine is therefore normal.

Passive Reabsorption Mechanisms

Two substances in the glomerular filtrate, water and urea, are passively reabsorbed. Passive reabsorption in itself does not require direct work or energy, but creation of the gradient does. Indirect energy is provided by the energy required to reabsorb sodium. It creates osmotic, electrical, and concentration gradients that encourage passive reabsorption of these substances. Water and urea are thought to be passively reabsorbed along the length of the nephron.

Tubular Secretion

Substances are removed from the bloodstream by glomerular filtration, tubular secretion, or a combination thereof.

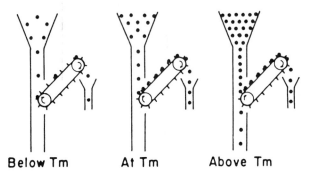

FIGURE 21–8. Mechanical model of a reabsorptive mechanism that exhibits limitation of transport capacity. (From Pitts RF: Physiology of the Kidney and Body Fluids. 3rd ed. Chicago, Year Book Medical Publishers, 1974, with permission.)

Tubular secretion refers to the process whereby substances are transported from the peritubular blood, interstitium, or tubular cell into the tubular lumen. Substances that are secreted include organic acids (such as penicillin, Diodrast, and para-aminohippuric acid [PAH]), strong organic bases (such as histamine), and other substances (such as urea).

Conservation of Sodium, Chloride, and Water

The most important element of conservation by the kidney consists of reabsorption of salt and water. Approximately 60 to 70 percent of the filtered sodium load is reabsorbed in the proximal tubule. The reabsorption of sodium is isosmotic. Water is reabsorbed along with the sodium. The active reabsorption of sodium ions and the passive diffusion of chloride ions develop an osmotic force so that water is reabsorbed passively. Because water can diffuse readily in both directions across the proximal tubular epithelium, there is effectively no osmotic pressure gradient. This reabsorption of sodium is because of the presence of a sodium pump. The energy for the pump is thought to be provided by enzymatic hydrolysis of adenosine triphosphate (ATP). The enzyme is called sodium-dependent, potassium-dependent adenosine triphosphatase (Na^+, K^+-ATPase). It acts as a carrier molecule at the cytoplasmic border of the peritubular membrane to combine with a sodium ion and release it at the extracellular or peritubular fluid border. Figure 21–9 outlines ion transport in a proximal tubular cell.

When the GFR is reduced and the filtered load in the proximal tubule is reduced, a higher percentage of the filtered sodium is reabsorbed in the proximal tubule. As the tubular fluid approaches the loop of Henle, approximately 35 percent of the filtered sodium remains in the tubular fluid in an isosmotic fluid concentration. Chloride is also reabsorbed in the proximal tubule.

Loop of Henle

Henle's loop plays an important role in the concentrating and diluting mechanisms of the urine. Sodium reabsorption does not take place in the thin loop of Henle, but in the ascending limb of Henle's loop the active transport of sodium results in secondary reabsorption of chloride. A sodium "pump" is thought to be the mechanism for sodium reabsorption. This segment of the loop of Henle also has low permeability to water. The reabsorption of sodium, chloride, and urea and the low permeability to water account for the dilution of urine that occurs in the ascending loop of Henle. Approximately 25 to 40 percent of the filtered load is reabsorbed in Henle's loop.

Distal Convoluted Tubule

The distal convoluted tubule is presented with approximately 10 percent of the filtered load. Because of the impermeability to water of the ascending loop of Henle, the fluid entering the distal convoluted tubule is hypoosmotic. Sodium transport in this region occurs in the presence of a high electrochemical gradient and requires

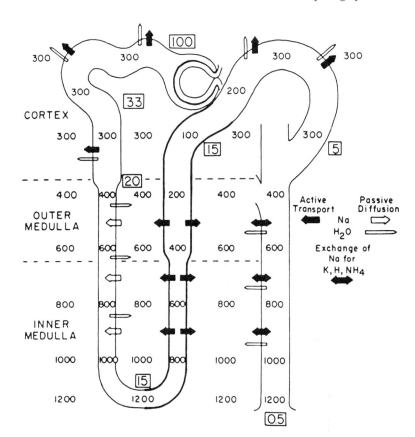

FIGURE 21–9. Summary of passive and active exchanges of water and ions in the nephron in the course of elaboration of hypertonic urine. Concentrations of tubular urine and peritubular fluid are given in milliosmoles per liter; the large, boxed numerals are estimated percentages of glomerular filtrate remaining within the tubule at each level. Evidence indicates that chloride is actively transported by the ascending limbs of Henle's loop. (From Pitts RF: Physiology of the Kidney and Body Fluids. 3rd ed. Chicago, Year Book Medical Publishers, 1974, with permission.)

a great deal of energy. The hormone aldosterone, which is part of the renin–angiotensin system, acts in the terminal part of the distal tubule to enhance the rate of sodium reabsorption. In addition to aldosterone, angiotensin II may also enhance sodium reabsorption. Chloride reabsorption is thought to be passive in the distal tubule.

Collecting Duct

Less than 5 percent of the filtered load of sodium is still present by the time the tubular fluid arrives at the collecting duct. However, this area plays an important role in regulating urinary excretion of salt. Up to this point, 95 to 97 percent of the filtered sodium has been reabsorbed. In this area the concentration gradients are high. Aldosterone enhances reabsorption of sodium in this area. Antidiuretic hormone (ADH) also acts in this area to enhance water reabsorption (see below).

Potassium Reabsorption and Secretion

Potassium is filtered in the glomerulus and is largely reabsorbed in the proximal tubule. Some absorption of potassium also occurs in the loop of Henle. The major area of potassium flux, however, is in the distal tubular epithelium, where secretion into the distal tubule and collecting duct may occur. Diets high in potassium lead to increased distal tubular potassium secretion, and those low in potassium to reduced secretion. The acid–base status can affect potassium secretion. Alkalosis stimulates potassium secretion through changes in the cellular pH, whereas acidosis depresses potassium secretion.

In summary, the proximal tubule and the loop of Henle are responsible for most of the routine reabsorption of the various constituents of the filtrate, such as sodium, water, and chloride. The distal nephron, consisting of the distal convoluted tubule and collecting duct, is responsible for the "fine tuning" of the conservation and excretion of the various elements (e.g., sodium, water, urea, potassium, and ammonia).

Urea Clearance

Urea is the major end-product of protein metabolism. In addition to its role as a metabolite, it is important in the countercurrent system that provides a method of conserving water by concentrating the urine. The rate of urea formation depends directly on the diet and on normal liver function. Urea is filtered in the glomerulus and is then reabsorbed along the renal tubule. Normally, passive reabsorption of urea leads to its accumulation in the medullary interstitial fluid. This accumulation increases the total solute content of the renal medulla, thereby increasing the osmotic forces that promote water reabsorption in the distal tubule and collecting duct. Urea clearance varies with urine flow. A reduction in fluid intake results in fluid conservation and reduced urine output. The urea clearance decreases sharply when urine flow falls below 1 to 2 ml/min in a 70-kg man. This decrease may lead to an increase in blood urea nitrogen (BUN) if the urine output remains low. Such an increase is referred to as *prerenal azotemia* and is the result of inadequate fluid volume rather than renal damage.

Renal Control of the Fluid Volumes of the Body

The control of extracellular fluid (ECF) volume and content is one of the main responsibilities of the renal system. The renin–angiotensin–aldosterone (RAA) system responds to fluctuations in dietary salt intake to maintain normal concentrations of sodium, potassium, and water, as well as normal blood pressure.

There are many devices within the body for sensing changes in ECF volume and content, including the baroreceptors in the right atrium, carotid sinus, and aortic arch, the hypothalamic osmoreceptors, and those intrinsic to the kidney (e.g., the macula densa). The ECF volume is determined mainly by the sodium content of the body. A decrease in total body sodium results in a decrease in ECF. These decreases may occur as a result of dietary restriction, humoral changes such as those in Addison's disease, or ECF losses. Such losses occur mainly through bleeding, tissue trauma from injury or surgery, and gastrointestinal pathology. Two factors determine the response of the compensatory mechanisms of the body: the speed with which fluid is lost and the amount and type of fluid lost. The severity of the losses evokes graded responses from the compensatory mechanisms. Table 21–3 lists the electrolyte concentrations of various body fluids. All the fluids listed are part of what is referred to as transcellular fluid, which can be thought of as a specialized type of extracellular fluid. Transcellular fluid is separated from the blood plasma, not only by the capillary endothelium but also by a layer of epithelial cells that modify the composition of the fluid. The important point, however, is that loss of these fluids is comparable to loss of ECF.

Compensatory Mechanisms for Fluid Conservation

For the sake of discussion, the compensatory mechanisms for the restoration of fluid loss are divided into definitive and temporary mechanisms (Table 21–4). The definitive mechanism restores the actual fluid lost, in terms of electrolyte content and volume, and is controlled by the RAA system. The main effector organs for the definitive compensatory mechanisms of the body are the kidney and the gastrointestinal (GI) tract. The GI tract plays an important role early in the course of fluid loss when there is no

TABLE 21 – 4
COMPENSATORY MECHANISMS

Definitive compensatory mechanisms
   Renal
   Gastrointestinal

Temporary compensatory mechanisms
   Renal
   Transcapillary refill
   Endogenous vasopressors
      Angiotensin II
      Vasopressin (ADH)
      Sympathetic amines

interference with the oral intake. The anesthesiologist is usually involved with surgical situations in which the GI mechanism for compensation is not operative, either because oral intake is stopped or because a GI tract disorder is the primary cause of the surgical problem. Therefore, emphasis is placed on the kidney.

For the kidney to function properly, perfusion volumes must be normal and pressure must be within the range of autoregulation. The function of the temporary compensatory mechanisms is to maintain the circulatory status of the body, first, for survival and second, to maintain threshold circulation in the kidney until the definitive mechanisms can compensate for the volume challenge.

The Renin–Angiotensin–Aldosterone System

The RAA system enhances the reabsorption of chloride, sodium, and water. Renin is secreted by the juxtaglomerular cells of the afferent arteriole. The stimulus for renin release is decreased renal perfusion or a reduced sodium concentration in the distal tubule. The sensing device for these changes is the macula densa. Renin is released into the afferent arteriole.[5] Renin substrate is converted to angiotensin I, which has no significant renal activity; angiotensin I is converted to angiotensin II by the converting enzyme. The effects of angiotensin II are four-fold: (1) release of aldosterone from the adrenal cortex; (2) systemic vasoconstriction; (3) stimulation of the release of ADH from the pituitary; and (4) compensatory responses from the GI system.

The last mechanism is discussed first, and only briefly, as it usually either is inoperative during surgery or is the primary cause of the problem. The absorptive and secretory processes of the intestine occur simultaneously; absorption is quantitatively greater than secretion. Angiotensin II has several effects on the GI tract, including induction of thirst and an appetite for salt, and it affects the transport of sodium and water. Low doses of angiotensin II interact with sympathetic nerve endings that are in close proximity to the transport epithelial cells. The release of norepinephrine leads to an α-adrenergic response that facilitates transport of sodium and water into the serosal cells of the GI system. High doses of angiotensin II interact with receptors of the transport epithelial cells to stimulate production of prostaglandins. Prostaglandins decrease absorption, increase secretion of sodium and water, or both.[6, 7] The

TABLE 21 – 3
ELECTROLYTE CONCENTRATIONS IN VARIOUS BODY FLUIDS

Source	Na (mEq/L)	K (mEq/L)
Saliva	60	20
Gastric	60 ± 30	9.1 ± 4
Bile	145 ± 15	5.1 ± 1.2
Ileum	125 ± 20	5.0 ± 2.1
Diarrhea	60 ± 30	30 ± 15
CSF	140 ± 5	4.5 ± 1
Sweat	30 ± 10	

overall effect of a moderate sympathetic response is to inhibit secretion and increase absorption. At a very high-level sympathetic response, absorption is inhibited and secretion is increased. High-level sympathetic activity may occur with any form of stress.

Aldosterone released from the adrenal cortex circulates to the kidney, specifically to the distal tubule and collecting duct, where it stimulates sodium transport. The systemic vasoconstrictive effects of angiotensin II help to maintain systemic pressure and tissue perfusion while specific replacement therapy is given, and the definitive mechanisms for sodium reabsorption restore the ECF volume to normal. It is obvious that angiotensin II is both a temporary and definitive compensatory mechanism. Clinical evaluation of a patient with a fluid volume deficit who is being supported by these compensatory mechanisms reveals (1) a reduction in urine sodium and urine output and (2) systemic vasoconstriction. Angiotensin II is a potent vasoconstrictor used to support the circulation at times of volume reduction. If adequate sodium and fluid are intravenously administered to the patient so that the definitive mechanisms can restore the ECF volume and sodium content to normal, the compensatory mechanisms are turned off. If adequate sodium and volume levels are not maintained, additional compensatory mechanisms are activated, including transcapillary refill, the secretion of ADH, and activation of the sympathetic nervous system.

Sometimes the system overresponds. The homeostatic systems of the body are extremely sensitive to changes in dietary salt. Severe salt restriction for a period of days may cause the RAA system to "overshoot" when salt is again added to the diet. In one study, 9 days of severe salt restriction followed by excessive dietary sodium resulted in a net gain of 270 mEq of sodium, which resulted in a 2-kg gain in body weight.[8] An analogous situation may occur in the surgical patient who has been on diuretics or several days of bowel preparation, or who, alternatively, may have been losing ECF through bleeding or trauma. In an attempt to protect the blood pressure and ECF volume, the RAA system may "overshoot" and temporarily increase body weight during the postoperative period.

Temporary Compensatory Mechanisms

Transcapillary Refill

When the fluid deficit exceeds the definitive replacement capability, the temporary compensatory mechanism of transcapillary refill is activated and interstitial fluid is translocated to the plasma volume to maintain a normal circulating blood volume. The loss of interstitial fluid results in loss of skin turgor and, in the infant, sinking of the eyeballs and the fontanelles. Clinically, these findings indicate a severe deficit of sodium and water.

Appropriate Secretion of ADH

Normally, ADH maintains plasma osmolality within a narrow range (280 to 290 mOsm/L). In the face of a fluid deficit, ADH (vasopressin) is released. When a fluid deficit is replaced with a balanced salt solution, there is appropriate restoration of fluid volume to normal. There is little

free water with balanced salt solutions to be reabsorbed and there is little effect of ADH. However, if hypotonic fluid is administered (0.25 percent normal saline), free water will be reabsorbed and hypotonic expansion of the extracellular fluid volume will occur. A volume deficit is a stronger stimulus than changes in osmolality, so that ADH decreases the permeability of the distal tubule and collecting duct to increase free water absorption. This leads to dilutional hyponatremia.

In addition, the stress of anesthesia and surgery releases ADH. When ADH release is combined with hypotonic fluid administration, dilutional hyponatremia may occur. When hyponatremia develops rapidly (i.e., over 12 to 24 hours) the patient may develop cerebral edema as water moves from the hypotonic ECF into normotonic brain cells. The degree and rapidity of this fluid shift lead to various symptoms, ranging from confusion, disorientation, lethargy, nausea, and vomiting to seizures.[9] The latter is a medical emergency and requires immediate treatment with hypertonic saline (i.e., 2 ml/kg of $NaHCO_3$ [equivalent to a 6 percent sodium solution]). When hyponatremia develops over days to weeks, the body has time to compensate for these changes. The treatment is fluid restriction and slow restoration of electrolyte balance to minimize the dangers of developing the osmotic demyelination syndrome.[10]

Appropriate ADH release should not be confused with the syndrome of inappropriate ADH release (SIADH). SIADH is associated with central nervous system (CNS) disorders such as infection, intracranial tumors, head trauma, with tumors of the lung and duodenum, and with pulmonary disorders, such as tuberculosis and pneumonia and other forms of chronic infection.[11] All too often, hyponatremia is diagnosed as SIADH when the problem is appropriate ADH release. Clinical history and laboratory findings differentiate the two. With appropriate ADH the hyponatremia is associated with a marked reduction in urine sodium. With SIADH the urine contains normal or increased amounts of sodium. Urine output is not particularly helpful in the differential diagnosis because administration of a very hypotonic solution in the face of a sodium deficit stimulates urine output, as does dilution of serum sodium by reabsorption of extra free water.

Activation of the Sympathetic Nervous System

The final compensatory mechanism for maintaining circulation in the face of severe volume loss is activation of the sympathetic nervous system, which occurs when ECF losses compromise the normal circulating blood volume. Activation of the sympathetic nervous system results in release of epinephrine and norepinephrine.

Atrial Natriuretic Peptide

The RAA system tightly maintains and defends normal sodium and potassium balance and arterial blood pressure. It also defends against excessive losses of ECF volume and hypotension. The atrial natriuretic factor is activated after excess sodium ingestion or administration and when the blood pressure is elevated. The response time of the atrial natriuretic peptide (ANP) system is slower than that of RAA system.

The body responds to excessive sodium administration or to a hypertensive state by releasing a peptide(s) from the atria in response to increasing atrial pressure and atrial stretch.[12, 13] ANP has several actions. It increases the GFR and the filtration fraction without increasing renal blood flow, thereby markedly increasing sodium excretion. It may also decrease tubular reabsorption of sodium without increasing GFR. The reduction in arterial blood pressure is because of the vasodilating properties of ANP, a reduction in ECF volume, and effects on the RAA system. There are four antirenin system actions of ANP: (1) reduction of renin excretion; (2) blocking of aldosterone secretion; (3) blocking of sodium-retaining actions of aldosterone; and (4) blocking of the vasoconstrictive effects of angiotensin II.

ANP is present in both premature and full-term infants, but its concentration increases during the first 2 days of life in response to the relatively large ECF volume of the newborn (which decreases significantly during the first year or so of life). Premature infants have a larger ECF volume than full-term infants.[14] Mechanically ventilated infants with respiratory distress syndrome (RDS) also have high levels of ANP,[15] perhaps in part because positive-pressure ventilation increases pressure in the atria and stimulates the release of ANP. The role of ANP in sodium and water excretion in the infant has not as yet been fully studied. ANP is increased in children with chronic renal failure and volume expansion.[16]

Mechanism for Concentrating and Diluting Urine

One of the major functions of the kidney is to maintain the osmolality of the extracellular fluid within a narrow range (280 to 290 mOsm/L) to optimize cellular function. As the ultrafiltrate passes down the proximal tubule, approximately 60 to 70 percent is absorbed isosmotically. The loop of Henle has been pinpointed as one of the two areas at which a major alteration in the osmolality of the urine occurs. The other structures concerned with concentrating and diluting urine are the collecting ducts. The concept of the countercurrent mechanism greatly enhanced the explanation of how the kidney is able to eliminate the normal osmotic load generated by the body.[17, 18] Two basic processes are responsible for the countercurrent mechanism. Countercurrent multiplication occurs in the loop of Henle and a countercurrent exchange occurs in the medullary blood vessels. The major difference between the two systems is that the countercurrent multiplication system in the loop of Henle requires energy and is an active process, whereas the countercurrent exchange system in the medulla is a passive system.

The final step in the ability to either concentrate or dilute urine occurs in the collecting duct under the influence of ADH. ADH works through two interrelated mechanisms: It diminishes the flow of blood through the vasa recta, and it alters the permeability of the collecting ducts to water. An elevation in plasma osmolality indicates a relative lack of water. This change in osmolality is sensed by the hypothalamic osmoreceptor, leading to release of

ADH. The supraoptic nuclei of the hypothalamus produce ADH, which descends along the nerve fibers to the neurohypophysis for storage and then release. The stimulus for release is either osmotic, as described above, or the presence of low blood volume, which stimulates thoracic and carotid volume receptors. The volume receptors for ADH release require a greater stimulus than the osmotic change, and such stimulation occurs only at times of moderately severe volume challenge. ADH acts in the collecting duct to alter the duct's permeability to water and urea. As permeability increases, water freely diffuses into the interstitium along osmotic pressure gradients. ADH is inhibited in the presence of low plasma osmolality and a high blood volume, thereby reducing the permeability of the collecting duct to water. Water in the collecting duct remains in the collecting system and is excreted through the ureter. This enhanced excretion of water increases plasma osmolality and decreases blood volume.

Acid–Base Balance

Normal daily activities include oxidative metabolism, which produces 13,000 mEq of carbonic acid per day. The lungs remove this "volatile" acid by excreting CO_2. Other acids derived from the catabolism of proteins and phospholipids are called "fixed" acids because they have no volatile component. To minimize body pH changes from the constant endogenous infusion of these fixed acids, the body has developed three lines of defense: (1) the buffer system, which is immediately activated when fixed acids come in contact with the buffers; (2) alterations in alveolar ventilation in response to alterations in pH (this mechanism is activated within minutes); and (3) renal mechanisms that alter the excretion of H^+ and the absorption of bicarbonate. These mechanisms are rapidly activated but take hours to become significant.

The buffer systems of the body include not only the buffers present in the blood, such as hemoglobin and bicarbonate, but those of the intracellular and extracellular volumes as well. The phosphate buffer system is an example.

Renal Mechanisms that Compensate for Alterations in Acid-Base Balance

The kidney is responsible for eliminating fixed (nonvolatile) acids and bases and for maintaining the extracellular concentration of bicarbonate ions. The renal tubules play the primary role in acid–base regulation through the mechanisms of bicarbonate reabsorption, titratable acid excretion, and ammonia secretion.

Bicarbonate Reabsorption

The daily filtered load of bicarbonate in a 70-kg man amounts to approximately 4,500 mEq. One of the basic responsibilities of the kidney is to conserve essential material. Figure 21–10 outlines the reabsorption of sodium bicarbonate. In the normal situation, 99.9 percent of the filtered bicarbonate is reabsorbed, approximately 90 percent of which is reabsorbed in the proximal tubule. Four factors can modify the rate of reabsorption of bicar-

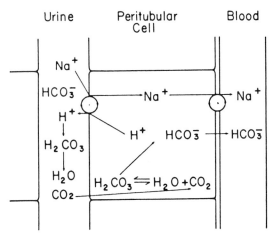

Urine   Peritubular   Blood
             Cell

FIGURE 21–10. Proximal tubular bicarbonate reabsorption. (From Bevan DB: Renal Function in Anesthesia and Surgery. Orlando, FL, Grune & Stratton, 1979, with permission.)

bonate: (1) the $Paco_2$; (2) the concentration of potassium; (3) the concentration of chloride; and (4) the presence of steroids. An increase in $Paco_2$ decreases pH and reduces the reabsorption of bicarbonate. Elevated body stores of potassium increase the excretion and thus reduce the plasma concentration of bicarbonate. Conversely, when potassium levels decrease, bicarbonate reabsorption is increased. There is a reciprocal relation between the plasma concentration of chloride and bicarbonate. The mechanism is thought to be related to the ECF volume. When ECF volume is low, reabsorption of bicarbonate is increased and chloride concentration is decreased. Likewise, when the ECF volume is excessive, reabsorption of bicarbonate is depressed and chloride concentration is elevated. Increased plasma corticosteroid concentrations are associated with increased reabsorption of bicarbonate. There are two possible mechanisms: a direct effect of the corticosteroids and an indirect response that is a consequence of alterations in sodium and potassium balance.

Titratable Acid and Ammonium Excretion

Dietary acids (e.g., sulfuric and phosphoric acids) are neutralized by sodium bicarbonate. Conservation of sodium bicarbonate conserves sodium and conserves bicarbonate for the buffering systems. This is accomplished by the tubular secretion of hydrogen ions in exchange for sodium.

The body excretes hydrogen ions by excretion of titratable acid and ammonium. Phosphate is the main urinary buffer. In chronic renal disease and in neonates, both forms of fixed acid excretion (i.e., acidification of urine and NH_4^+ secretion) are reduced. With renal disease, the reduction in the NH_4^+ pathway is much greater than it is for titratable acid. Normally, approximately 75 percent of the daily load of fixed acid is excreted as NH_4^+ and the remainder as titratable acid. The NH_3 that produces NH_4^+ is generated by renal cells. This adaptive mechanism is greatly reduced when the quantity of renal tissue is reduced.

Renal Maturation

Older infants, children, and adults with renal problems usually have acquired or congenital renal disease. Neonates have the additional problem of renal immaturity. Very-low-birth-weight (VLBW) infants (defined as infants weighing <1 kg and having a gestational age of <30 weeks) have two problems with renal function. First, the number of glomeruli are not yet maximal, which occurs at about 34 weeks of gestational age. Second, the renal blood flow is low and the renal vascular resistance is high. Consequently, VLBW infants may have very limited renal function for weeks. It is important to use the correct physiologic basis to compare the renal function of the neonate with that of the older infant and child. The usual basis is 1.73 m^2 of surface area. On this basis, "adult" renal maturation is not achieved until 12 to 18 months. The ability of the infant's kidney to increase performance under stress suggests that this criterion does not provide an accurate picture of the maturation of the infant's kidney. McCance and Widdowson[19] suggested that comparison of renal function should be based on total body water, since the infant has relatively more body water than the adult. The total body water of infants under 6 months of age is 69 to 77 percent of body weight, whereas that of an older infant or adult is 60 percent. This water is primarily interstitial fluid. When values for renal function are calculated per unit of total body water, rather than per 1.73 m^2 of body surface, the values for renal function mature much more rapidly and approach mature values at an earlier age (Table 21–5).

Glomerular Filtration Rate

The GFR remains constant until approximately 34 weeks' gestational age, after which it increases rapidly.[20] It has been suggested that this sudden increase occurs because glomerulogenesis is completed. (In terms of body size, a gestational age of 34 weeks means that the normal fetus or premature infant weighs at least 2,000 g.)

Major circulatory changes occur at the time of birth. Renal and pulmonary vascular resistance decrease and systemic blood pressure increases. This results in a remarkable increase in renal blood flow (RBF). Regardless of gestational age, the first 2 to 3 days of extrauterine life are

T A B L E 2 1 – 5				
COMPARISON OF RENAL FUNCTION IN INFANTS				
		Urea Clearance		GFR	
Age (days)	No. of Infants	Per 1.73 m^2	Per Unit Body Water	Per 1.73 m^2	Per Unit Body Water
2–8	4	17	42	34	82
3–13	7	34	78	48	109
2–22	11	29	71	49	122
8–28	4	34	77	51	116
38–356	12	55	104	100	

Modified from Roy RN, Chance GW, Raddle IC, et al: Late hyponatremia in very low birth weight infants. Pediatr Res 10:526, 1976, with permission.

characterized by an increase in arterial blood pressure, a decrease in renal vascular resistance, and an increase in RBF, which results in a dramatic increase in GFR.

Certain medical maneuvers or conditions at birth may alter the RBF. Studies of early versus late clamping of the umbilical cord have demonstrated significant differences in urine flow, inulin clearance, PAH clearance, and high sodium excretion.[21] Infants whose cords were clamped early had lower blood volumes and systolic pressures than those whose cords were clamped later; late clamping of the umbilical cords led to a higher blood volume and systolic blood pressure and to increased RBF and GFR. RBF and GFR are reduced with asphyxia and hypoxia, because of a decreased arterial pressure plus cardiac and renal ischemia.

Tubular Function

Glucosuria and proteinuria and low tubular capacities for phosphate and bicarbonate are evidence of tubular immaturity at birth.[22] In premature infants, glucosuria was present in 13 percent of infants who were less than 34 weeks' gestational age, when the blood glucose level was less than 100 mg/dl. This suggests that immature infants have a decreased tubular reabsorptive capacity for glucose. After 34 weeks' gestational age, glucosuria usually occurs only with hyperglycemia. Glucosuria may act as an osmotic diuretic and cause sodium and water loss. In the mature kidney, albumin is filtered by the glomerulus and completely reabsorbed from the tubules. With tubular immaturity, some degree of proteinuria may be present, particularly in premature infants. Proteinuria occurs in 16 to 21 percent of premature infants.[20]

Maturation of the Concentrating and Diluting Mechanisms

The more immature the kidney, the less it is able to concentrate or dilute urine. Full-term newborn infants also have limited ability to perform these functions, but to a lesser degree than premature neonates. During the transition period, the diuretic response to a water load is sluggish

in all infants. However, by 5 days of age the kidney responses of term neonates are similar to those of the mature kidney. However, the rate of free water excretion in these infants is still reduced, which increases the risk of overzealous administration of water. Neonates can usually concentrate their urine to a level approximately half that of the adult because the medullary concentration of urea in the immature kidney is low, resulting in a reduced osmotic gradient and the concentrating ability of the collecting duct.

Acid–Base Balance

The neonate has a lower bicarbonate level than the older infant (21 to 23 mEq/L vs. 25 to 27 mEq/L).[22] The explanation for the lower plasma bicarbonate concentration is that the kidneys have a lower threshold for excretion of bicarbonate. The result is that during the early postnatal period there is a limited ability to acidify urine. Within the first several months this level increases to the normal values. The limitation in the infant's ability to excrete a hydrogen ion load is the low concentration of buffers, such as ammonia and phosphate, in the urine. It takes approximately 1 year for the production of ammonia to reach mature levels.

Reabsorption of Sodium in Infants

As infants begin to grow, their sodium requirement remains high owing to sodium losses in the urine and to the need for sodium for bone. In one study, 30 percent of healthy premature infants became hyponatremic by 2 to 6 weeks of age when an adequate amount of sodium was not provided.[23] After the initial transition period, neonates have increased sodium retention, and the proximal tubule responds appropriately to the normal sodium load. It has been postulated that the positive sodium balance after the transition period is stimulated by growth. Sodium is deposited in various growing tissues, particularly bone, which results in a continuous stimulus for renin-release activation of the RAA system.

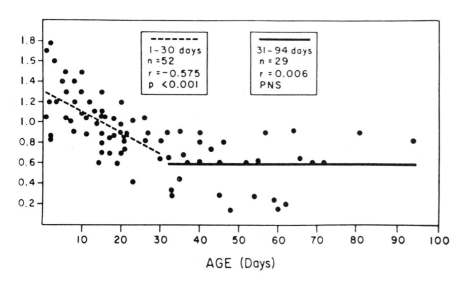

FIGURE 21–11. Plasma creatinine values (mg/dl) during the first 3 months in low-birth-weight infants. (From Stonestreet BS, Oh W: Plasma creatinine in low birth weight infants during the first three months of life. Pediatrics 61:789, 1978, with permission.)

Maturational Changes in Specific Renal Function Tests and Creatinine

At birth, the creatinine concentrations of term infants are the same as those of the mother and are 0.6 to 1.2 mg/dl. Within a month they decrease to 0.1 to 0.2 mg/dl. Low-birth-weight infants have relatively high serum creatinine concentrations compared with term infants (Fig. 21–11). This decrease is believed to be because of an increase in GFR and a decrease in tissue catabolism during the first 10 postnatal days. Normal creatinine values for the pediatric patient population are listed in Table 21–6.

Evaluation of Renal Function in Children

Evaluation of the child with renal disease includes the triad of history, physical examination, and laboratory determinations. The three clinical situations in which evaluation of renal function is a priority are the child with a stable history of renal disease for elective surgery; the child with acute alterations in renal function that are caused by cardiovascular disease, renal disease, and/or hypovolemia; and the child with a history of renal disease who has a superimposed acute problem. A 50 to 60 percent reduction in functional nephrons is required for clinical renal disease to be evident. For that reason, history and physical examination are usually unremarkable early in the disease. An elevated arterial blood pressure may be the only finding. Younger infants may present with a history of poor feeding, lethargy, and pallor. Older children, because of hypertension, may complain of headache and malaise. The hemolytic-uremic syndrome may present after an episode of diarrhea. Children with nephrosis may present with periorbital or generalized edema. A careful history of the volume of urine output is very useful when evaluating hydration. The remarkable thing is that urine output is very similar at all ages. The first voiding occurs during the first 24 hours of postnatal life, regardless of gestational age. Thereafter, the normal urine output is 1 to 2 ml/kg/h. Dehydration and renal disease are often followed by decreased urine output. Oliguria is a sign of renal impairment, caused by either dehydration or renal disease, and is defined as a urine output of less than 1 ml/kg/h. Anuria is defined as a urine output of less than 1.5 ml/kg/day.

Urinalysis

Urine specific gravity is quite useful in evaluating renal function, since the ability to concentrate urine depends on tubular function. After an overnight fast, a specific gravity of 1.018 or greater, in the absence of sugar or protein, indicates normal tubular function. A persistent urine specific gravity of 1.010, which is the specific gravity of plasma, indicates isosthenuria and severe renal damage. Patients with isosthenuria are unable to dilute or concentrate their urine.

Blood Chemistries

Blood chemistry values are found in the various tables in this chapter. As a rough guideline, a 50 percent decrease

TABLE 21 – 6
CREATININE AND BUN CONCENTRATIONS FOR MALE AND FEMALE SUBJECTS

Age (Years)	Female Subjects: Creatinine		Male Subjects: Creatinine		Female Subjects: BUN		Male Subjects: BUN	
	$\overline{X}$	SD	$\overline{X}$	SD	$\overline{X}$	SD	$\overline{X}$	SD
1	0.35	0.05	0.41	0.10	11.04	2.72	10.8	3.8
2	0.45	0.07	0.43	0.12	13.9	5.5	11.0	4.7
3	0.42	0.08	0.46	0.11	11.4	2.9	11.4	3.5
4	0.47	0.12	0.45	0.11	10.2	4.6	10.7	3.1
5	0.46	0.11	0.50	0.11	10.5	3.0	12.4	3.9
6	0.48	0.11	0.52	0.12	10.8	3.7	11.8	3.5
7	0.53	0.12	0.54	0.14	10.5	3.1	12.2	3.9
8	0.53	0.11	0.57	0.16	11.3	3.6	10.9	3.8
9	0.55	0.11	0.59	0.16	11.6	4.1	12.6	6.0
10	0.55	0.13	0.61	0.22	10.5	4.1	12.4	6.7
11	0.60	0.13	0.62	0.14	10.1	3.6	11.3	3.8
12	0.59	0.13	0.65	0.16	9.4	2.6	11.6	3.3
13	0.62	0.14	0.68	0.21	10.8	3.8	11.8	3.7
14	0.65	0.13	0.72	0.24	12.1	4.9	11.4	4.2
15	0.67	0.22	0.76	0.22	10.9	4.7	12.0	3.6
16	0.65	0.15	0.74	0.23	11.0	3.6	11.6	3.3
17	0.70	0.20	0.80	0.18	10.2	3.7	12.7	3.7
18–20	0.72	0.19	0.91	0.17	12.2	3.3	12.2	2.8

Modified from Schwartz GJ, Haycock GB, Edelmann CM, et al: A simple estimate of glomerular filtration rate in children derived from body length and plasma creatinine. Pediatrics 58:259, 1976, with permission.

in renal function results in a doubling of the creatinine concentration. The blood urea concentration is more variable than the creatinine concentration, since the urea concentration may be caused by renal or other problems (e.g., GI bleeding). Because the amount of creatinine produced by the muscle every day is relatively constant, the serum creatinine concentration is an excellent reflection of the state of renal function.

Diuretics

Diuretics are classified according to their site of action in the nephron (Fig. 21–12). This classification is somewhat oversimplified, because diuretics usually have several pharmacologic effects involving more than one specific enzyme system or anatomic location. Our knowledge of the pharmacologic effects of these drugs is far from complete. All diuretics have desirable and undesirable effects.

The carbonic anhydrase inhibitor acetazolamide (Diamox) is the most frequently used diuretic that affects proximal sodium excretion. Acetazolamide is used primarily to reduce intraocular tension, decrease cerebrospinal fluid production, and alkalinize the urine. Carbonic anhydrase inhibition blocks reabsorption of sodium bicarbonate and water in the proximal tubule, resulting in an alkaline urine. The effects of this diuretic are relatively short-lived and are offset by the compensatory mechanisms of the kidney to retain sodium.

Theophylline also works on the proximal tubule to decrease sodium reabsorption. In addition, it increases cardiac output, which increases renal blood flow, GFR, and the rate of sodium excretion.

The most commonly used diuretics (furosemide [Lasix] and ethacrynic acid [Edecrin]) are loop diuretics, so called because they inhibit the transport of sodium and chloride in the ascending limb of Henle's loop. These drugs usually have no effect on renal blood flow, but in certain situations they produce renal vasodilation and increase blood flow to the superficial renal cortex. They may have a slight, nonpharmacologically significant effect in the proximal tubule. Their major action is thought to be depression of the sodium pump in the ascending limb of Henle's loop. Because chloride is passively reabsorbed with sodium, these drugs inhibit chloride reabsorption as well. During diuresis, sodium-potassium and sodium-hydrogen ion exchange are accelerated, and the loss of potassium and hydrogen ion is increased. This loss leads to hypokalemia and metabolic alkalosis. In patients also being treated with digitalis, the resulting hypokalemia may lead to digitalis toxicity.

The thiazide diuretics are thought to inhibit reabsorption of sodium and chloride in the distal tubule. Potassium secretion is also increased, and hypokalemia may occur in patients given these drugs. In humans and dogs, thiazides reduce GFR and renal plasma flow by 20 percent.

Other diuretics (spironolactone [Aldactone] and triamterene [Dyrenium]) work in the distal nephron to cause potassium retention and enhanced sodium excretion. Spironolactone competitively inhibits aldosterone in the distal nephron. Aldosterone increases reabsorption of small amounts of sodium in the distal nephron and accelerates sodium exchange with potassium and hydrogen ions in the distal tubules and collecting ducts, which is the primary site for aldosterone's modulating effect. Although the acute effect of blocking aldosterone may be modest, the cumulative effects of chronic administration may be substantial. Triamterene (Dyrenium) antagonizes the renal effects of aldosterone and inhibits distal tubular sodium reabsorption. The side effects of these drugs include occasional hyperkalemia. These drugs are often used in conjunction with the other diuretics to diminish the excretion of hydrogen ion and potassium by the other agents.

Osmotic Diuretics

Osmotic diuretics are used for two general purposes: to decrease the ECF volume in head trauma and to attempt to increase urine output after a renal insult. Mannitol is a low-molecular-weight sugar that increases the osmolality of the ECF. Water moves passively from the intracellular space into the interstitial and intravascular spaces to reduce the increased osmolality. This movement temporarily increases blood volume and renal blood flow. Because of its low molecular weight, mannitol is freely filtered in the kidney by the glomerulus, but it is not absorbed. Therefore, mannitol and water are eliminated in the urine. The transient increase in blood volume may increase arterial blood pressure and cerebral blood flow, and in patients with a cerebral insult the intracranial pressure (ICP) may be temporarily increased. The increase in blood volume might also result in congestive heart failure.

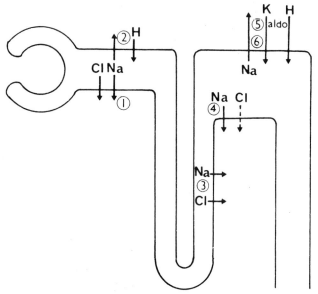

FIGURE 21–12. Sites of action of diuretic agents on the kidney. *1,* Inhibition of proximal sodium reabsorption (furosemide, ethacrynic acid). *2,* Carbonic anhydrase inhibitors (acetazolamine). *3,* Inhibition of salt reabsorption from loop of Henle (furosemide, ethacrynic acid, mannitol, mercurials). *4,* Inhibition of sodium reabsorption from cortical diluting site (thiazides). *5,* Aldosterone antagonists (spironolactone). *6,* Nonaldosterone sodium-potassium exchange (triamterene, amiloride). (From Bevan DB: Renal Function in Anesthesia and Surgery. Orlando, FL, Grune & Stratton, 1979, with permission.)

RENAL FAILURE

Renal failure is a frequent cause of hospitalization among pediatric patients. The causes of renal failure may be either relatively transient, with no residual effects, or may be fulminant, resulting in death or in a prolonged period of combined medical and surgical management that may ultimately lead to renal transplantation. An understanding of the causes and management of acute and chronic renal failure in the pediatric patient is essential to establishing an appropriate anesthetic course for such patients.

Definition of Terms

Acute renal failure (ARF) is defined as an acute decline in normal renal function that results in the accumulation of nitrogenous waste. Anuria is arbitrarily defined as urine excretion of less than 1.5 ml/kg/day. The prognosis for patients with anuria is ominous. Oliguria is defined as urine excretion of less than 1 ml/kg/h, which is the minimal amount of urine required to excrete the normal daily solute load. The diagnosis of ARF is usually not made until urine output falls below 0.5 to 1.0 ml/kg/h.

Acute renal failure can be divided into four stages:

Stage 1. Oliguric or nonoliguric renal failure lasting 7 to 12 days. Progressive azotemia is present.

Stage 2. Early diuresis in cases of oliguric renal failure. It lasts 4 to 7 days. BUN concentration continues to rise.

Stage 3. Late diuretic period. BUN and creatinine concentration begin to decrease.

Stage 4. Recovery. BUN and creatinine concentration continue to decrease and usually stabilize. This stage may last for many months.

ARF may be reversible to some degree and in some cases complete recovery is possible.

Acute Renal Failure

Acute renal failure is traditionally divided into three classifications depending on whether the etiology of the ARF is prerenal, postrenal, or the result of intrinsic renal disease (Table 21–7). Intrinsic renal disease can be further subdivided according to renal structure(s) primarily affected (i.e., glomeruli, tubules, interstitium, and the vascular supply). It is also important to consider the age of the patient, neonate versus child or adolescent, when discerning the etiology of ARF in the pediatric patient.

Prerenal ARF

Prerenal ARF is usually caused by mild to moderate hypoperfusion of the kidney. The most common cause of hypoperfusion in the pediatric patient is a reduction in extracellular fluid volume. Hypoperfusion reduces GFR which, along with increased reabsorption of the glomerular filtrate, leads to increased absorption of urea and water. This, in turn, leads to an increased plasma urea content and a decreased urine volume. The fractional reabsorption of sodium is also increased and the urine sodium content is reduced. Creatinine, which is not reabsorbed, continues to be filtered and excreted normally. Thus, the increase in the plasma BUN/creatinine ratio is important in the diagnosis of prerenal azotemia.

TABLE 21–7
CAUSES OF ACUTE RENAL FAILURE

Prerenal (hypovolemia/hypotension/hypoperfusion)
 Dehydration or hemorrhage
 Burns
 Septic shock
 Pancreatitis, peritonitis, ascites
 Cardiac surgery
 Major trauma
 Osmotic diuresis associated with diabetes mellitus
 Respiratory distress syndrome
 Diabetes insipidus
 Hepatorenal syndrome
Renal (intrinsic)
 Prolongation of prerenal factors
 Primary glomerular diseases
  Acute poststreptococcal nephritis
  Membranoproliferative glomerulonephritis
  Rapidly progressive glomerulonephritis of unknown cause
 Systemic disease with renal involvement
  Systemic lupus erythematosus
  Hemolytic–uremic syndrome
  Bacterial endocarditis
  Vasculitides
  Henoch-Schönlein purpura
 Metabolic/drugs/toxins
  Hypersensitivity reactions
  Antibiotics (aminoglycosides, methicillin, amphotericin)
  Metals or chelating agents (lead, gold, platinum, ethylenediamine tetraacetic acid)
  Organic solvents (carbon tetrachloride, ethylene glycol, methanol, toluene)
  Oxalic acid, uric acid
  Massive hemolysis (hemoglobinuria)
  Rhabdomyolysis (myoglobinuria)
  Radiocontrast dyes
  Antihypertensive medications (captopril)
 Infiltrating diseases
  Tumor
  Pyelonephritis
 Vascular
  Renal artery thrombosis or embolus
  Renal vein thrombosis
Postrenal (either bilateral ureteral or bladder outlet obstruction)
 Obstruction from stone, blood clots, tumor
 Congenital obstructive uropathy

From Feld LG, Springate JE, Fildes RD: Acute renal failure. I. Pathophysiology and diagnosis. Pediatrics 109:401, 1986, with permission.

The incidence of ARF in the neonate population may be as high as 3 to 10 percent. This highlights the fact that the maturing kidney is highly susceptible to injury. The majority of cases of prerenal ARF in neonates can be attributed to perinatal asphyxia. However there are a number of clinical situations in the neonatal intensive care unit that may contribute to development of prerenal ARF including respiratory distress syndrome requiring mechanical ventilation or extracorporeal membrane oxygenation (ECMO), neonatal sepsis, and volume depletion following surgery to repair major cardiac or congenital defects.[24, 25]

In older children the etiology of prerenal ARF is extracellular volume depletion secondary to trauma, burn management, sepsis, and gastrointestinal losses. With appropriate fluid and electrolyte management, the prognosis in these children is very good.[25]

Postrenal ARF

Postrenal ARF is the result of incomplete or complete urinary tract obstruction. Early in acute obstruction, GFR is reduced. Flow of glomerular filtrate is slowed and salt and water reabsorption is enhanced, leading to excretion of small volumes of highly concentrated urine that contain little sodium, similar to prerenal azotemia. The urinary tract obstruction must be bilateral for this picture to develop. If partial obstruction is sustained, intrinsic renal damage and altered renal function occur. Renal damage decreases the amount of glomerular filtrate reabsorbed; a decreasing volume of sodium-rich, relatively isotonic (or mildly hypotonic) urine is excreted. The GFR is often decreased, and the plasma BUN and serum creatinine levels increase. When the urinary tract obstruction is complete, no urine is formed.

Congenital malformations of the urinary tract and kidney are often diagnosed on prenatal ultrasonic examinations. However, congenital obstructive uropathy, such as posterior urethral valves, may present in the neonate as oliguric renal failure with an abdominal mass. The relief of the obstruction in the neonate may result in the appearance of normal renal function initially; however, it is not unusual for some degree of chronic renal insufficiency to persist in the long term.[25]

In older children and adolescents the cause of urinary tract obstruction is similar to adults (i.e., nephrolithiasis, tumor, and blood clots). The timely relief of such obstruction usually results in the complete recovery of renal function.

Intrinsic Renal Failure

The pathogenesis of intrinsic renal failure may be a progression of prerenal or postrenal ARF, a systemic disease with renal involvement, or a process that directly involves the kidney (e.g., glomerulonephritis) or renal toxins (e.g., aminoglycosides). The primary renal injury may be glomerular or tubular. Intrinsic renal disease interferes with normal renal function and the kidneys cannot conserve salt and water. It may be associated with oliguria caused by a reduced amount of functional tissue. This results in a relatively low volume of urine, a relatively high concentration of urine electrolytes, and a urine osmolality that approaches or exceeds that of plasma (260 to 350 mOsm/L). The urine specific gravity is that of serum, between 1.010 and 1.012. Tubular injuries occur with ischemia or nephrotoxins. The tubular walls may become damaged and obstructed, leading to reduced renal blood flow, tubular back-leak, tubular damage, and a reduced glomerular capillary ultrafiltrate.

A neonate who presents with acute renal failure may have a genetic renal disease such as autosomal recessive polycystic kidney disease or an inborn error of metabolism leading to Fanconi's syndrome (panproximal tubular dysfunction). More common causes of intrinsic ARF in the neonate are the toxic nephropathies. Many commonly used drugs in the neonatal intensive care unit (NICU) are nephrotoxic, including indomethacin for closing of a patent ductus arteriosus (PDA) and aminoglycoside antibiotics for treatment of life-threatening infections. Even medications used during pregnancy, such as angiotensin-converting enzyme (ACE) inhibitors, can lead to renal disease in the neonate. An uncommon complication of umbilical artery catheterization is renal artery thrombosis, which may lead to ARF in the neonate.[25]

Two of the more common causes of intrinsic ARF in children are glomerulonephritis and hemolytic-uremic syndrome (HUS). In the already hospitalized child, ARF may develop in the setting of sepsis, subsequent to bone marrow or liver transplantation, or as a result of tumor lysis syndrome following treatment of childhood leukemia or lymphoma.[25] A number of therapeutic agents used in the hospitalized child may be nephrotoxic; including intravenous immunoglobulin (IVIG), nonsteroidal anti-inflammatory agents (ibuprofen and ketorolac), chemo-therapeutic agents, immunosuppressive agents (cyclosporine and tacrolimus), antihypertensive drugs (ACE inhibitors), and antiviral agents (acyclovir).[24]

Management of ARF

Treatment of prerenal and postrenal ARF is aimed at reversing the inciting event in an attempt to prevent progression to intrinsic ARF. The extracellular volume depletion leading to hypoperfusion of the kidney in prerenal ARF is treated with vigorous fluid resuscitation using isotonic crystalloid or colloid based on body mass or surface area. Once circulating volume is established, careful attention to replacement of ongoing losses (gastrointestinal, insensible, and urinary) is mandatory. When gastrointestinal losses are high it may be necessary to replace potassium and bicarbonate despite abnormal renal function.[25] The relief of obstruction in postrenal ARF is essential to preventing irreversible renal damage. In the setting of prolonged partial obstruction, some degree of chronic renal insufficiency is likely despite complete resolution of the obstruction.

Once the ARF is established to be intrinsic in nature, conservative therapy is initiated. The major goal of conservative therapy is avoidance of the life-threatening complications of fluid overload, hyperkalemia, or intractable metabolic acidosis. Careful monitoring of body weight, serum electrolytes, and intake and output of fluid is crucial to determining appropriate fluid management. Hyperkalemia may need to be treated acutely using calcium gluconate or continuous albuterol inhalation or less urgently using insulin/glucose infusion or sodium polystyrene resin. Alkali supplementation, oral or intravenous, may be necessary to correct metabolic acidosis.[24]

Conservative management does not always obviate the need for renal replacement therapy. Once it is determined that renal replacement therapy should be initiated, the modality chosen depends on age and size of the patient, the cause of ARF, cardiovascular status, and institutional resources. The modalities available to the pediatric population include peritoneal dialysis, intermittent hemodialysis, continuous arteriovenous hemofiltration, and continuous venovenous hemofiltration with or without dialysis.[24]

Mention should be made of some of the adjunctive therapies of ARF. The use of low-dose dopamine to preserve renal perfusion and induce a modest natriuresis and diuresis remains controversial. It may have a role in certain circumstances; however, routine use is discouraged.[24] Children with ARF have increased metabolic needs and are usually catabolic. Aggressive nutritional support, enteral or parenteral, is recommended, although complications such as electrolyte disturbances and fluid overload can develop. Hypertension may develop in the setting of ARF. If the patient is symptomatic, an infusion of an easily titratable antihypertensive such as nitroprusside should be instituted. The asymptomatic patient can be treated with any number of antihypertensive agents.

Outcome of ARF

Morbidity and mortality from ARF in the pediatric population remains high despite numerous advances in renal replacement therapy. Mortality rates of 35 to 73 percent are reported. Factors that tended to increase mortality include the presence of anuria, the need for dialysis, history of cardiac surgery, multiple organ failure, associated respiratory and neurological complications, and delayed referral. Of note, children with primary renal disease as opposed to extrarenal disturbances leading to ARF have better outcomes.[26]

Chronic Renal Failure

End-stage renal disease (ESRD) in children is reported to occur in 11 cases per million each year. The overall mortality rate is 4.8 percent, with younger children having a poorer prognosis than older children.[27] The primary cause of ESRD in the pediatric population is glomerulonephritis followed by the congenital obstructive uropathies and the congenital hypoplasia/dysplasia syndromes.[27, 29, 32]

Progressive renal disease can be viewed as a developing process with five stages: loss of renal reserve, chronic renal insufficiency (CRI), chronic renal failure (CRF), uremia, and finally ESRD. Patients progress through these phases at variable rates. The "gold standard" for estimating renal failure is measurement of GFR. However, since the techniques used to measure GFR are too cumbersome to perform on a routine basis, in clinical practice determinations of serum creatinine, creatinine clearance, and the reciprocal serum creatinine are used for monitoring the progression of renal disease.[28] Creatinine is a product of muscle metabolism, and its concentration in plasma is usually stable from day to day. It is filtered by the kidney and it is not reabsorbed. The serum creatinine level reflects creatinine production and GFR. At birth, the neonate's creatinine concentration is the same as the mother's (0.8 to 0.9 mg/dl). The normal serum creatinine concentration ranges from 0.2 mg/dl after several weeks of life to 0.9 mg/dl in teenagers. The serum creatinine concentration varies with the GFR and remains normal if the GFR is 40 to 50 percent of normal or higher. For every subsequent 50 percent reduction in GFR, the serum creatinine concentration doubles. A complete cessation of glomerular flow increases serum creatinine by approximately 0.5 mg/dl/day. An elevated but stable serum creatinine concentration indicates a stable state of chronic renal insufficiency.

Renal Replacement Therapy

Renal replacement therapy refers to the supportive care of patients with renal failure. The goal of renal replacement therapy is maintenance of fluid, electrolyte, and acid–base homeostasis until the underlying problem is resolved, kidney function recovers, or renal transplantation is performed.

Indications for dialysis in acute renal failure are fluid overload, symptomatic electrolyte/acid–base disturbances (hyperkalemia, metabolic acidosis, hyperphosphatemia, hypocalcemia, hyperuricemia, hyperammonemia), and removal of exogenous toxins.[30] In children with chronic renal failure and ESRD the ultimate goal for the best quality of life is a well-functioning renal transplant. However, dialysis is frequently required as a bridge to transplantation. There are no set levels of serum creatinine or BUN to justify initiation of dialysis. In practice, dialysis is usually initiated at a creatinine clearance of 5 to 10 ml/min/1.73 m^2 or 10 percent of normal renal function for age. Nonspecific symptoms such as decreased appetite, nausea, fatigue, poor growth, and declining renal function may signal the need for dialysis. Early initiation of dialysis may help avoid some of the complications of chronic renal failure.[27, 30]

The choice of dialysis modality must be individualized and depends on a variety of factors including age and size of patient, etiology of renal failure, cardiovascular stability of patient, and institutional resources and experience. Following is a brief description of the modalities available and their advantages and disadvantages. Peritoneal dialysis remains the most commonly used modality in pediatric patients, with approximately 65 percent of all dialysis patients using some form of peritoneal dialysis compared with 35 percent who undergo hemodialysis.[27]

Peritoneal Dialysis

Peritoneal dialysis refers to the instillation of an aqueous solution (dialysate) into the peritoneal space and subsequent diffusion of solutes along an electrochemical gradient across the serous membrane of the peritoneum. Thus, toxic molecules can be removed from the blood stream and electrolytes that are deficient can be replenished. In addition, by adding an osmotic agent such as glucose, ultrafiltration can be achieved.

The technique requires the insertion of a catheter into the peritoneal space. When dialysis is needed acutely and is anticipated to be required for only 3 to 5 days, a rigid catheter without a cuff can be placed percutaneously at the bedside. However, for chronic peritoneal dialysis a Tenckhoff catheter with one or two cuffs is inserted surgically. The cuffs help prevent bacterial migration.

Most families are taught to provide peritoneal dialysis at home with ease. Continuous ambulatory peritoneal dialysis (CAPD) uses gravity to instill individualized bags of dialysate into the peritoneal cavity 4 to 5 times per day with dwell times of 4 to 8 hours. The advantages of this mode are excellent extracellular fluid control and great mobility for patients. The major disadvantages are the risk of infection with multiple exchanges and the time requirement for each exchange. Continuous cycler-assisted peritoneal dialysis (CCPD) uses an automated cycler to instill and drain individualized dialysate overnight. This reduces both the risk of infection and the time commitment.

The advantages of peritoneal dialysis are stable metabolic control, fewer fluid and dietary restrictions, more stable blood pressure control, less anemia, and technical ease. The most common complication of peritoneal dialysis is infection. It is estimated that patients experience one episode of peritonitis per year. If treated early, antibiotics can be given intraperitoneally at home and hospitalization can be avoided. Other complications of peritoneal dialysis include development of abdominal hernias, leakage of peritoneal fluid through the diaphragm into the pleural space, and decreased appetite.[25, 27, 30]

Hemodialysis

Hemodialysis refers to the use of extracorporeal perfusion to transfer fluids and solutes by diffusion and ultrafiltration between the blood and dialysate. Continual countercurrent flow of blood and dialysate separated by a semipermeable membrane creates a concentration gradient. Solutes are removed from the blood by diffusion along the concentration gradient, and fluid is removed by ultrafiltration. In pediatric patients, the dialysate and blood lines are chosen to maintain the total dialysis circuit volume at less than 10 percent of the child's estimated blood volume. Available equipment now allows for infants as small as 4 kg to be hemodialyzed. The typical patient undergoes hemodialysis three times per week with each session lasting 3 to 4 hours.

Vascular access is essential to provide extracorporeal blood flow. In the acute setting, uncuffed double-lumen catheters can be placed percutaneously into the subclavian, internal jugular, or femoral vein. In young children, adequate blood flow is possible only when the catheter tip is in the right atrium. For chronic hemodialysis, a surgically placed tunneled catheter is placed into the subclavian or internal jugular vein. The most commonly used vascular access in adults, the arteriovenous fistula, can be created in pediatric patients weighing more than 20 kg. Complications of arteriovenous (AV) fistulas include thrombosis, stenosis, and infection.

The complications of hemodialysis include hypotension, muscle cramps, seizures, and disequilibrium syndrome. Hypotension is the most common complication, occurring in up to 30 percent of patients. It usually presents as the sudden onset of nausea, vomiting, abdominal cramping, and tachycardia. It is treated with bolus infusion volume expanders. The pathogenesis of muscle cramping is unclear. However predisposing factors include dialysis-induced hypotension, ultrafiltration below the patient's dry weight, and the use of sodium-poor dialysate. Treatment includes increasing dialysate sodium concentration or hypertonic saline or glucose infusion. Disequilibrium syndrome may occur during or shortly after dialysis. Early symptoms are nausea, vomiting, irritability, headache, blurred vision, and lethargy. Severe cases may progress to tremors, seizures, coma, and death. It is believed to be related to the rapid correction of uremia leading to acute cerebral edema. It is best prevented by decreasing the rate of solute removal and shortening dialysis times. Prophylactic mannitol has been used prior to dialysis in some patients. Seizures occur in 8 to 50 percent of dialyzed children. Predisposing factors are young age, prior seizure history, cardiopathy, CNS lesions, and uremic encephalopathy. Treatment is aimed at correcting underlying electrolyte abnormalities.[25, 27, 30, 31]

Continuous Renal Replacement Modalities

Critically ill children may benefit from the use of continuous hemofiltration/hemodiafiltration. These techniques allow for greater hemodynamic stability and can be performed in both the neonatal and pediatric intensive care units. The four basic modalities available are continuous arteriovenous hemofiltration (CAVH), continuous arteriovenous hemodiafiltration (CAVHD), continuous venous hemofiltration (CVVH), and continuous venous hemodiafiltration (CVVHD). A detailed description of each modality is beyond the scope of this chapter.[25, 30]

COMPLICATIONS OF ESRD

Anemia

Children with chronic renal failure develop a normocytic, normochromic, hypoproliferative anemia. The major cause of the anemia is inadequate secretion of erythropoietin by the kidney. Therapy with recombinant human erythropoietin has been successful in correcting the anemia as well as reducing the need for transfusion and improving overall quality of life. Current recommendations are to raise the hematocrit to 31 to 36 percent. Subcutaneous administration is preferred because it most closely mimics the endogenous erythropoietin concentrations and is effective at lower doses. The initial dose is usually 50 to 100 U/kg three times per week until target hematocrit is achieved then maintenance dose of 50 to 75 U/kg once a week is sufficient. EMLA cream is often used to decrease the pain at the injection site. The stimulation of erythropoiesis increases iron requirements, and it is recommended that supplemental iron be given to maintain serum ferritin concentrations greater than 100 mg/ml and transferrin saturation greater than 20 percent. The most significant adverse reaction to erythropoietin therapy is hypertension. Patients should be monitored closely and antihypertensive therapy should be initiated or increased if necessary.[27–29, 31]

Growth Retardation

Growth retardation is common in children with CRF. Contributing factors include age at onset of disease, cause of primary renal disease, malnutrition, metabolic acidosis, renal osteodystrophy, and infection. Growth hormone concentrations are elevated in children with CRF; however, patients demonstrate end-organ hyporesponsiveness. Growth hormone (GH) therapy has been shown to increase height velocity in children with CRF. The goal of such therapy is to have the child attain their genetic potential for height. Early concerns about GH therapy causing a state of glomerular hyperfiltration and leading to further deterioration of renal failure have been disproven. The potential adverse effects include hyperglycemia, hypothyroidism, glucosuria, hyperkaluria, headache, and mild transient edema.[28, 29]

Renal Osteodystrophy

The kidney plays a major role in bone and mineral homeostasis; calcium, phosphorous, and magnesium levels are balanced; parathyroid hormone (PTH) and aluminum are cleared via the kidney; and calcitriol (1,25-dihydroxyvitamin D_3) and 24,25-dihydroxyvitamin D_3 are synthesized in the kidney. Deterioration of renal function leads to hyperphosphatemia, hypocalcemia, and hyperparathyroidism. The symptoms of renal osteodystrophy include bone pain, muscle weakness, skeletal deformities, extraskeletal calcification, and growth retardation. The goals of therapy are to maintain calcium and phosphorous levels within normal limits and parathyroid hormone level two to three times the upper limit to allow for normal bone development. Treatment includes the use of phosphate binders (usually calcium acetate or carbonate) and vitamin D sterol supplementation (oral calcitriol). Aluminum-containing phosphate binders should be avoided because of the impaired elimination of aluminum in renal failure and the potential for neurotoxicity. Maintenance of normal plasma bicarbonate concentrations is also associated with better control of secondary hyperparathyroidism and stimulation of bone turnover. The patient with chronic acidosis may require bicarbonate supplementation with citrate solutions or sodium bicarbonate tablets.[28, 29]

Hypertension

Blood pressure initially rises in patients with CRF because of intravascular volume expansion and then is sustained by elevated vascular resistance. Hypertension has been shown to accelerate the rate of decline in renal function in children. The goal of antihypertensive therapy is to decrease blood pressure slowly to below the 95th percentile for age and gender, to treat with as few drugs as possible, and to use drugs that work on different systems when monotherapy fails.

The first line of therapy involves lifestyle modification including dietary sodium restriction (except children with salt-losing nephropathy), weight loss, and exercise. Diuretics are the next step in patients whose GFR is greater than 10 to 15 ml/min/1.73 m^2. Thiazide diuretics are less effective when GFR falls below 30 to 40 ml/min/1.73 m^2. Potassium-sparing diuretics should be avoided. Subsequent antihypertensive therapy is aimed at lowering peripheral vascular resistance. ACE inhibitors have become the preferred agents because of their ability to reduce proteinuria and preserve renal function. Adverse reactions are rare in children and include rash, neutropenia, taste disturbances, angioedema, and hyperkalemia. Caution must be exercised when initiating therapy with ACE inhibitors, since they have been shown to worsen renal insufficiency. Calcium channel blockers have been shown to exert renal protective effects similar to that of ACE inhibitors. Their mechanism of action is through vasodilation. They do not require dosage adjustment in ESRD and are

not significantly removed with dialysis. Other available antihypertensive agents include β-blockers, α-adrenergic blocking agents, centrally acting agents, and vasodilators.[27-29]

ANESTHESIA FOR GENITOURINARY SURGERY

Specific Genitourinary Abnormalities

Genitourinary problems are of three main types: congenital, hereditary, and acquired. A congenital anomaly is present at birth and may be hereditary or acquired. Hereditary anomalies are genetically transmitted and are important for future genetic counseling of the parents.

In Utero Diagnosis of Urinary Tract Abnormalities: Diagnostic and Treatment Possibilities

Ultrasonography of the pregnant patient has opened up many areas of potential diagnosis and treatment of fetal and early postnatal disease. Fetal urinary tract abnormalities are detected by ultrasonography in approximately 1 in 2,000 live births. Even though the kidney and bladder can be identified by 22 weeks of age, some urinary tract abnormalities are not evident until after 28 weeks of gestational age. One hope of ultrasonography is to identify bilateral ureteral obstructive disease and to decompress the urinary tract in utero to prevent further progression of renal disease and perhaps to allow recovery of renal function before birth. Initially, creation of bilateral cutaneous ureterostomies in the fetus offered some hope that the relief of the obstruction would accomplish the hoped-for goals. However, it soon became clear that this was not the case. A report from the International Fetal Surgery Registry in 1986 revealed that a total of 73 replacements of such shunts had occurred in patients with fetal obstructive uropathy. Fourteen of the pregnancies were terminated by elective abortion. Of the 59 live births, 30 survived. Of the 29 neonatal deaths, 27 were because of pulmonary hypoplasia. Therefore, it is evident that the issue is not merely the relief of urinary tract obstruction but also the need for amniotic fluid, which is required for development of the normal pulmonary system. Of the survivors, many later had severe renal disease. In the future it will be important to have a means for determining the degree of impairment of the fetal renal tissue as well as the type of urinary tract anomaly. If the kidneys are already severely damaged at the time of fetal surgery, the hysterotomy and the very expensive and difficult surgery for the mother will be of no avail. Attempts to assess fetal renal function have been difficult, but include an evaluation of fetal urine. Normal fetal urine is hypotonic. Discovery of an isotonic fetal urine would suggest considerable damage, very poorly functioning fetal kidneys, and a very poor prognosis.

Postnatal Renal Evaluation

The other advantage of ultrasonography is to evaluate renal function of neonates with suspected renal disease.

Furthermore, does early diagnosis of renal disease make any difference in outcome? At the present time, no studies prove this hypothesis one way or the other. One potential benefit, however, of knowing that renal disease is present would be the ability to initiate antibiotic prophylaxis to prevent infection and septicemia from occurring. It is evident that fetal surgery and the use of ultrasonography to diagnose and treat fetal and neonatal renal disease is in its early stages. Both techniques may have great potential for the treatment of fetal and neonatal anomalies and for counseling of parents in the future.

CONGENITAL ANOMALIES

Congenital anomalies are those that are usually recognized at birth or shortly thereafter. They may or may not be inherited. For discussion purposes, the prenatal period of growth and development is divided into two time periods. The embryonic period, from conception to approximately 8 to 9 weeks' gestation, is the time of organ formation. The fetal period, from the end of the embryonic period to birth, is the time of organ differentiation. This division is obviously simplistic, as the two periods overlap considerably.

Anomalies Occurring During the Embryonic Period

In general, the earlier and the more severe the interruption of normal growth and development, the greater the problem. An early and serious embryologic defect may cause a problem that affects not only the renal system but several others as well. Potter's syndrome, for example, is characterized by bilateral absent kidneys, hypoplastic lungs, characteristic facies, skeletal anomalies, and GI anomalies.[33-35] Interruption of normal development later in the embryologic period may result in various anomalies of the genitourinary system.[36]

Renal Dysplasia

One of the renal anomalies associated with this time period is caused primarily by abnormal metanephric and ureteric bud differentiation, resulting in various degrees of renal dysplasia.[37] Specifically, renal dysplasia refers to maldevelopment of the renal parenchyma and is evidenced by abnormal secretory and collecting ducts. Some authors report that 50 to 60 percent of patients with renal dysplasia have other urinary tract anomalies. The anomalies consist of various degrees of obstruction of the ureters and lower urinary tract. These lesions run the gamut from a small segmental area of dysplasia in one kidney, with few clinical implications, to total bilateral disruption of renal structure and function, resulting in fetal death. Early in embryologic development, when the ureter joins the bladder, the ureter is not patent. Partial or complete failure of a lumen to develop results in obstruction of the upper system and various degrees of dysplasia. Bilateral vesicoureteral obstruction leads to bilateral renal dysplasia.

Urethral Obstruction– Malformation Complex

Another area of potential obstruction is the proximal or distal urethra, particularly in male infants. Such congenital obstruction may lead to the "urethral obstruction–malformation complex."[35] When the proximal urethra is involved, the problem is caused by posterior urethral valves. When the distal, or penile, urethra is involved, it usually is obstructed by diverticuli or strictures. This anomaly results in decreased production of amniotic fluid, leading to the potential development of the oligohydramnios–deformation complex and obstruction of urine flow leading to bladder distention.

The oligohydramnios–deformation complex consists of several problems. The first is decreased production of amniotic fluid, in this case caused by obstruction of urine flow into the amniotic cavity. This occurs when urinary obstruction is severe enough to cause renal dysplasia, renal insufficiency, and decreased urine production. The implications and results of oligohydramnios are far-reaching. Amniotic fluid is produced by the amnion, lung, and kidney. Normal growth and development of the lung depend on a critical volume of amniotic fluid from these sources. Both polyhydramnios and oligohydramnios have been associated with pulmonary hypoplasia.[38] In addition, the decreased amniotic fluid may result in fetal compression, which has been associated with pulmonary hypoplasia, limb positioning defects, and Potter's facies.

The second problem of the urethral obstruction–malformation complex stems from the hydrostatic effect of the obstructed urethra. The hydrostatic pressure distends the bladder. As seen in Figure 21–13, there is a potential cascade of developmental pathology. The entire urinary tract is eventually subjected to hydrostatic backpressure that results in renal dysplasia. It may lead to abnormal differentiation, arrested development, or regressive changes in previously normal nephrons. Survival of the neonate usually depends on the degree of pulmonary and renal involvement. The bladder distention can cause other local pressure problems. For example, distention of the abdomen caused by the enlarged bladder and kidneys can lead to dystrophic abdominal muscles. The triad of renal anomalies, deficiency of abdominal muscles, and undescended testes is known as the "prune belly" syndrome. At times, the hydrostatic pressure in the bladder results in a patent urachus and urine empties through the umbilicus. The urachus develops from the vertex of the bladder and is usually a rudimentary structure, except when the lower urinary tract is involved. However, even as a rudimentary structure, the urachus persists in 25 percent of adults as a muscular tube with a minute opening.

Other potential sequelae of the bladder distention are (1) cryptorchidism secondary to the presence of the distended bladder, which obstructs the usual descent of the testes; (2) malrotation of the gut, which occurs because the large bladder prevents normal gut rotation and fixation of the mesentery; and (3) lower limb deficiencies. There are also various degrees of pulmonary and renal dysfunction, as well as minimal abdominal muscle tone. Infants with these abnormalities require intensive postoperative

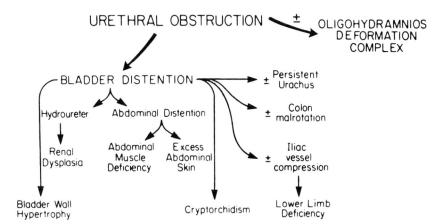

FIGURE 21-13. Development of pathology of the more severe degree of the urethral obstruction malformation complex is interpreted as the secondary effects of bladder distention on the surrounding tissues. (From Pagon RA, Smith DW, Shepard TH: Urethral obstruction malformation complex: a cause of abdominal muscle deficiency and the "prune belly." J Pediatr 94:900, 1979, with permission.)

airway management because of the involvement of their respiratory and abdominal muscles.

Vesicoureteral Reflux

Urinary tract infections are a frequent and, at times, a surgical problem in the pediatric patient.[39] Various studies have revealed that approximately 50 percent of children presenting with a urinary tract infection (UTI) will have some type of abnormality of the genitourinary tract. Abnormalities are often congenital and are often associated with vesicoureteral reflux (VUR). The types of reflux are usually divided into primary reflux where the problem is caused by an incompetent ureterovesicular valve. The normal valve mechanism is created by an oblique entry of the ureter into the bladder where the ureter goes through a normal tunneling mechanism within the bladder. The main factor determining the effectiveness of the valve mechanism is the ratio of the ureteral diameter to the length of the ureter in the submucosal tunnel within the bladder. Secondary reflux occurs because of urethral obstruction, which means that it is virtually limited to males with posterior urethral valves or in children with a neurogenic bladder.

In the presence of urinary tract infections, renal parenchymal damage is likely to occur when the reflux extends into the renal pelvis, causes renal parenchymal infection, and leads to scarring and parenchymal fibrosis. Poor renal growth is another sequela. With adequate medical or surgical treatment, renal growth may be normal. It is unclear whether renal growth rate differs if the treatment is medical or surgical. The major sequelae of VUR is that in a small number of patients the VUR may lead to scarring of the kidney. VUR associated with scarring may result in hypertension. Early studies of VUR and renal scarring reveal an incidence of hypertension in 10 to 20 percent of the patients. At times, the hypertension developed even after surgical correction of the VUR but in some patients did not appear for many years following surgery. There have been concerted efforts to evaluate these patients with long-term studies.[39]

Medical management of VUR consists of continuous low-dose chemoprophylaxis. Surgical management consists of reimplantation of the ureter or ureters. The anesthesiologist may deal with these patients for diagnostic studies or for surgical treatment of VUR. Children with recurrent urinary tract infections used to undergo various diagnostic procedures that required anesthesia. These procedures included cystoscopy, and the like. However, current diagnostic techniques are much more accurate and do not require the use of anesthesia. These include renal ultrasound, radiologic cystograms, and other relatively noninvasive renal diagnostic tests.

Exstrophy (Epispadias Complex)

Some bladder anomalies are not associated with obstruction. Exstrophy of the bladder is a major, but fortunately rare, congenital anomaly that arises during the fifth and sixth weeks of embryonic life. An abnormally large cloacal membrane hinders normal mesodermal movement in the infraumbilical area and prevents midline fusion of the musculoskeletal elements of the infraumbilical anterior abdominal wall. Because fusion fails to occur, the rectus abdominus muscles and the pubic arch are separated. The cloacal membrane dehisces normally, but the dehiscence results in an absence of the anterior wall of the bladder. The remaining posterior bladder wall everts, and the urinary tract is open and everted from the urinary meatus to the umbilicus, hence the name *exstrophy–epispadias complex*. If the dehiscence occurs before the urorectal septum has fused with the cloacal membrane, exstrophy of the lower gastrointestinal tract may be present. This anomaly is referred to as cloacal exstrophy. The defect may also involve the spinal canal and result in meningomyelocele. Other anomalies may also be present.

The surgical repair of this defect, particularly if the bony pelvis is involved, is traumatic, and the anesthesiologist will require large-caliber intravenous (IV) lines for administration of blood and fluids.

Hypospadias

Hypospadias is a common genitourinary anomaly. Although it is associated with hernias and hydroceles, it does not appear to be associated with an increased risk of upper urinary tract anomalies. An enormous number of potential psychological problems are associated with the surgical repair of this condition. This potential problem, along with the concerns of toilet training, favors surgical repair by about 1 year of age. The recently increased interest in combined general and regional anesthesia for children, both for the surgical procedure and for postoperative pain relief, is especially applicable for children with hypospadias.

Circumcision

The controversy regarding whether routine circumcision should be done in the neonatal period continues to smolder, and it is obvious that it will be decades, if ever, for there to be a consensus on the issue.[40, 41] There is evidence that uncircumcised male children do have a higher incidence of urinary tract infections and there is evidence that children who have urinary tract infections on a recurrent basis may develop renal parenchymal damage. The anesthesiologist may well be consulted at two time periods about the types of anesthesia for circumcision. The first of these is in the neonatal period where circumcision is often done within a day or two after delivery. The simplest technique for anesthesia for circumcision is the use of a subcutaneous ring of anesthetic placed at the base of the penis using a very small needle (#27) and small quantities of 0.2% ropivacaine or 0.25% bupivacaine. This nerve block is far superior to the more invasive penile block, which has the potential danger of a hematoma and ischemia of the penis. Circumcisions that are done later in life in children require a general anesthetic and, for the initial postoperative analgesia, the ring block is an excellent choice.

Anomalies in Rotation and Position of the Kidney

During the embryonic period the normal kidney rotates and ascends from the pelvis to become an abdominal organ. The hilum, which initially faces ventrally, eventually rotates to a medial position in the fetus. Several potential rotational anomalies may occur. First, the kidney may fail to rotate or may rotate in the wrong direction; second, it may rotate excessively. With anomalies of rotation, the kidney fails to ascend to its normal position. Compression of the ureter is the main consequence of this failure, but only rarely is the obstruction complete.

Even with normal rotation, anomalies of kidney position, referred to as ectopia, may occur. The kidney may fail to ascend (pelvic kidney), may ascend into the thorax (thoracic kidney), or may cross to the other side (crossed ectopia). Ectopia of the kidney is often associated with other anomalies, such as meningomyelocele and imperforate anus. Ectopic kidneys are also subject to ureteral obstruction and may be associated with continuing problems.

Anomalies of Renal Fusion

A horseshoe kidney results when an isthmus of kidney crosses the midline, fusing the two kidneys in a horseshoe shape. The position of the kidney is often lower than normal, with an arterial blood supply that originates farther down the aorta. There is potential for obstruction of the ureters because of the malrotation of the kidneys and the altered anatomy. Occasionally, the two kidneys fuse completely into a single kidney, which ascends into the normal position within the abdomen. One ureter crosses the midline. This is referred to as crossed ectopia with fusion. As with all of the other anomalies of renal fusion, this anomaly is associated with malrotation, anomalous vasculature, and the potential for obstruction of the ureters.

Associated Congenital Defects

In any neonate with a documented congenital anomaly there is a high risk for other such anomalies. Therefore, any neonate with an anomaly of the genitourinary system must be carefully evaluated for anomalies of the cardiovascular and pulmonary systems.

INHERITED DISORDERS

The list of inherited disorders is long. It includes some rather common disorders, such as the nephropathy of the sickle cell disorders and the rare familial nephrotic syndrome. This section discusses several of the more common disorders.

Sickle Cell Disease and the Kidney

Sickle cell disease, in patients homozygous for sickle cell hemoglobin, was first described in 1910.[42] Abnormalities of the urine, slightly increased urine volume, and low specific gravity were mentioned in the first clinical description. Sickle cell anemia is caused by an alteration in the molecular structure of the hemoglobin molecule.[43] Sickle cell patients are susceptible to hypoxia, acidosis, and hyperosmolality. There is a morphologic change in the hemoglobin, which undergoes tactoid formation and gelling. These changes in the hemoglobin molecule alter the shape of the erythrocyte into an elongated sickle form. The structural changes increase blood viscosity and interfere with microcirculation, causing intravascular aggregation of RBCs, ischemia, and infarction. In addition, the altered shape of the RBC membrane increases permeability of the membrane and hemolysis. Any form of sickle cell hemoglobin can be associated with renal abnormalities, even sickle cell trait (hemoglobin AS). Although sickle cell trait, in which patients have only a single copy of the abnormal gene (heterozygosity), is usually a benign condition, it may be associated with renal problems, including decreased concentrating capacity (isosthenuria) and episodic hematuria.

All patients with sickle cell hemoglobin have a diminished ability to concentrate urine. In patients with sickle cell hemoglobin, the normally low medullary blood flow and altered viscosity cause structural alterations of the RBCs, which further reduce blood flow and produce local hypoxia and small areas of infarction in the renal papillae. The most conspicuous signs of established sickle cell nephropathy are focal scarring and patchy interstitial fibrosis in the inner medulla and papillae. This necrosis reduces the number of functional juxtamedullary nephrons that concentrate the urine. Therefore, the concentrating defect in sickle cell anemia is a result of the sickling process itself. The inability to achieve maximally concentrated urine is the most consistent feature of sickle cell nephropathy and occurs in both the homozygous (SS) and the heterozygous state (AS). Sickle cell patients who are more than 10 years old have reduced their urinary concentrating ability to approximately 400 mOsm/L, where it remains. In patients with hemoglobin SC disease, the ability to concentrate urine decreases more slowly. By the age of 15 the defect is irreversible. The practical aspects of this inability to concentrate the urine are seen in patients subject to dehydration because of inadequately replaced excessive fluid losses. The kidney's ability to dilute urine is not affected. The other major clinical manifestation of sickle cell nephropathy is hematuria, which occurs in both homozygous and heterozygous patients. In approximately 90 percent of cases, the hematuria is unilateral, and the left kidney is involved four times more often than the right. As patients with sickle cell disease age, they are more susceptible to pyelonephritis, papillary necrosis, and proteinuria, and they occasionally develop the nephrotic syndrome. The progression of renal disease is slow and does not usually occur in pediatric patients. The need for dialysis and transplantation usually occurs in older patients with sickle cell disease.

Polycystic Renal Disease

There are two basic forms of polycystic renal disease: a hereditary and a nonhereditary form. The hereditary form is divided into infantile and adult forms. Polycystic disease is diffuse and bilateral and is associated with various degrees of renal damage. The most common form does not become manifest until the third or fourth decade. Infantile polycystic disease may become evident shortly after birth and may be associated with liver abnormalities. The infantile form of the disease may not become manifest until adolescence or late teens. The degree of involvement of the kidneys and the liver determines the rate of survival. The basic pathology consists of multiple renal cysts and interference with normal renal function. The disease may present in many ways, including abdominal pain, hypertension, and urinary abnormalities (hematuria and proteinuria). The major considerations for anesthesia are the degree of renal and liver damage. A recent study of a large group of children with multicystic dysplastic kidney disease revealed that 39 percent of the patients had contralateral disease.[44] The most common abnormality identified was VUR, which occurred in approximately half of the patients with bilateral disease. Ureteral pelvic junction obstruction was present in about a third of the patients with bilateral disease. Associated urologic abnormalities occurred in 51 percent.

Acquired Cystic Kidney Disease

Acquired cystic kidney disease (ACKD) is a frequent complication of renal insufficiency. It occurs in approximately 50 percent of adult patients undergoing hemodialysis. In addition, there is an association between ACKD and renal cancer in adult patients. One study evaluated the kidneys of children with end-stage renal disease by high-resolution ultrasonography.[45] Eighty-three percent of the children had a functioning renal transplant with a 3-year survival time. ACKD was found in 29 percent of the patients and a solitary cyst in 33 percent. One child, who had received hemodialysis for 12 years, had renal cell carcinoma diagnosed after bilateral nephrectomy. This study strongly suggests that all patients with end-stage renal disease who are on dialysis should be regularly monitored by ultrasonography or other techniques for the presence of ACKD.

Congenital Adrenal Hyperplasia

Congenital adrenal hyperplasia is an inherited disease of the adrenal cortex that leads to medical and genital problems at birth or in later life.[46] It is the most frequent adrenal disorder of childhood. Sixty percent of infants have a severe salt-losing crisis, which may be life threatening. The normal synthesis for cortisol occurs in the adrenal cortex, and deficiency of the five enzymes required for cortisol biosynthesis lead to subsequent underproduction of cortisol and aldosterone. In 90 to 95 percent of the cases, 21-hydroxylase is involved and in approximately 5 percent 11β-hydroxylase is deficient. The result of insufficient cortisol production is increased production of adrenocorticotropic hormone (ACTH). Increased amounts of ACTH lead to increased levels of hormones that do not require the deficient enzymes for their production. There is overproduction of testosterone. If this inherited defect is present before the eighth week of fetal life, it will cause major problems in development of the genitalia. In the male fetus, testosterone causes the urogenital groove to fuse and form the penis and scrotum. Excessive testosterone in the male leads to early virilization. Excessive testosterone in the female causes various degrees of fusion of the vaginal introitus and enlargement of the clitoris. At birth, gender assignment may be difficult. Surgery may be required to correct the enlarged clitoris and the fused vaginal outlet.

The deficiency of aldosterone causes a salt-losing state in approximately 60 percent of patients. Because aldosterone is responsible for tubular reabsorption of sodium and excretion of potassium, aldosterone deficiency results in hyponatremia and hyperkalemia. If a salt-losing crisis occurs, it usually does so between 10 and 20 days after birth. Symptoms of hyponatremia include vomiting, lethargy, and poor feeding.

No other congenital anomalies are associated with congenital adrenal hyperplasia. Most of these infants are receiving oral steroid replacement. Administration of excessive steroids may cause sodium retention and hypertension. Intramuscular administration of steroids during anesthesia results in slower release and a stable blood level of cortisol; IV administration of steroids results in high blood levels of cortisol, but its half-life is relatively short.

Wilms' Tumor

Wilms' tumor, also known as nephroblastoma, is the most common abdominal malignancy of childhood, with neuroblastoma a close second. Nephroblastoma is usually recognized between 6 months and 5 years of age. It usually presents as a large abdominal mass, which can extend into the inferior vena cava or renal vein. The lung is the most common site of metastasis. Wilms' tumor is congenital. It is thought to be caused by anomalous metanephric differentiation of the renal blastema. The renal blastema may develop into either a benign metanephric hamartoma or a Wilms' tumor.

Wilms' tumor has been associated with other genitourinary anomalies, such as horseshoe kidneys, duplication of the urinary tract, aplastic or hypoplastic kidneys, urethral anomalies, and hypospadias. It has been reported to occur in successive generations and in siblings. It has also been associated with hemihypertrophy and congenital aniridia.

The current treatment for Wilms' tumor consists of surgery, radiation therapy, and chemotherapy. If the tumor has metastasized to the lungs, Adriamycin and cyclophosphamide may be added. Adriamycin is associated with cardiac toxicity when the total dose exceeds 300 mg/m^2. Prognosis is favorable if the tumor is encapsulated, the infant is under 2 years of age, and there is no evidence of tumor extension.

The major problems that face the anesthesiologist during resection of a Wilms' tumor are intravascular volume loss and maintenance of normal renal function and thermoregulation. These tumors may be relatively large and may be associated with preoperative anemia and extension of the tumor into the vena cava and renal vein. These factors increase the likelihood that large blood transfusions will be needed. The potential for relatively uncontrolled severe hemorrhage is very high. Therefore, two large-bore IV catheters should be placed, along with an arterial and a central line. If both kidneys are involved, as happens in approximately 3 percent of cases, renal function may be adversely affected, especially if the tumors involve most of the kidney.

Neuroblastomas

Neuroblastomas are the most common retroperitoneal tumors and may alter renal function because of their location and size. They arise from the postganglionic adrenergic cells of the sympathetic nervous system, most frequently from the adrenal glands and the sympathetic ganglia (abdominal, thoracic, and cervical). Seventy-five percent of these tumors secrete catecholamines, which may result in hypertension.[47] Von Recklinghausen's disease (neurofibromatosis) is associated with both neuroblastomas and pheochromocytomas. All of these conditions may cause hypertension, either by compression of renal circulation and renal hypertension or by the release of catecholamines. The preoperative history may not reveal the potential for catecholamine release in hypertension, however. In a recent review of 20 years' experience with neuroblastomas, only 8 percent of the children had signs or symptoms that would have suggested increased catecholamine secretion.[48] These included flushing, diaphoresis, diarrhea, and hypertension. Eighty to 90 percent of patients with one of these tumors had elevated catecholamine levels. Many of these patients have hypertension on routine blood pressure monitoring. The authors reported a very small incidence of intraoperative hypertension (<3 percent). A major problem in patients with increased concentrations of catecholamines is the occurrence of hypo-

tension after tumor resection. The hypotension can be treated with volume replacement and, at times, vasopressor support.

ACQUIRED RENAL DISEASE

This section discusses some of the major causes of acquired renal disease. For example, the perinatal asphyxia syndrome occurs in newborns who have undergone severe intrapartum asphyxia and at birth have severe metabolic acidosis and hypoxia.[49] This leads to myocardial depression and often to congestive heart failure, which may present as RDS. The result is a decrease in cardiac output and renal ischemia. In its broadest sense, this is a congenital disease because the infant is born with it. At the same time, it can be considered acquired disease because it is caused by circulatory insufficiency of the fetal–placental unit.

Glomerulonephritis and some other intrinsic renal diseases fall into the category of acquired renal disease. (Acute or chronic renal failure are discussed under that heading.) The same is true for renal failure associated with trauma and surgery. Acquired renal disease also includes the various immunologic disorders, such as the nephrotic syndrome.

The Hemolytic-Uremic Syndrome

The HUS caused by *Escherichia coli* 0157:H7 is now recognized as one of the most common causes of acute renal failure in childhood. The disease process consists of gastroenteritis with severe diarrhea and a hemorrhagic colitis in 95 to 100 percent of the patients.[50–52] The period of illness is followed several days later by the triad of HUS, consisting of microangiopathic hemolytic anemia, thrombocytopenia, and acute nephropathy. The age group most frequently affected is that between 6 months and 5 years, but HUS can occur in older children and adults. Multiple systems are affected in 50 to 60 percent of patients. The CNS is frequently involved, characterized by seizures, coma, and occasionally cerebral infarction. Pancreatitis occurs in 20 percent and acute respiratory distress syndrome (ARDS) in 3 percent. The mortality rate of HUS is approximately 3 percent and occurs as a result of pulmonary hemorrhage, respiratory insufficiency, cardiac arrest, and cerebral edema associated with increased intracranial pressure. Approximately 50 to 60 percent of children with HUS will need dialysis. One epidemic in the United States was caused by eating rare or undercooked beef.

Anesthesiologists become involved with patients with HUS during the acute presentation of the syndrome to obtain access for peritoneal or vascular dialysis, or later when the child has chronic renal disease. The long-term sequelae of HUS include residual hypertension and chronic renal disease. The residual pathophysiology of the kidney appears to be glomerulosclerosis and progressive loss of nephrons. Some of these children have end-stage renal disease and require dialysis and/or transplantation.

Miscellaneous Diseases: Renal Vascular Disease in Children

Renal vascular disease (RVD) is more commonly a cause of hypertension in children than in adults,[53] and the pathophysiology of the process differs between the two age groups. In adolescence, the primary pathology is fibromuscular dysplasia, whereas in adults it is most often caused by atherosclerosis. Children more often have generalized vascular disease than adults, as well as bilateral disease, intrarenal disease, and disease of the aorta and cerebral vessels. For that reason, angioplasty has not been as successful in hypertensive children with renal disease as in adults. In carefully selected cases, such as that reported by Chevalier,[54] 19 of 32 cases were successfully treated by angioplasty. Only 4 of the 19 had bilateral disease. In one report of a group of untreated children with significant and sustained hypertension, renal artery stenosis was the third most common diagnosis after renal scarring and glomerular disease.[53] It is evident from these studies that children with undiagnosed hypertension should be evaluated for renovascular disease, because there is a potential for cure or amelioration of the problem by surgery, angioplasty, and antihypertensive medication.

Renal Transplantation in Small Children

Please see Chapter 19.

RENAL AND URETERAL CALCULI

Renal and ureteral calculi are relatively rare in infants and children. When they occur they are usually caused by immobilization, hypercalcemia, or urinary tract infection. The ability to break up these calculi noninvasively by lithotripsy has been a giant boon to these patients. The resulting "sand" is washed out of the urinary tract by the normal urine flow. However, a very small number of patients require cystoscopy to remove the debris. In some instances bacteria are liberated from the disintegrated stones, and the patient develops septicemia.

Even though lithotripsy is noninvasive, it causes tissue trauma. Considerable trauma may be sustained by the kidney when multiple shocks are required to disrupt a large stone. There may be posttreatment hematuria and discomfort.

Regional anesthesia is often used for lithotripsy in adults because the patients may require cystoscopy and placement of ureteral stents to identify the stone and this may necessitate moving the patient from one location to another. General anesthesia is the preferred technique in children. A plan for rapidly removing the patient from the water bath is needed because these patients occasionally require resuscitation.

ANESTHETIC IMPLICATION IN DIFFERENT AGE GROUPS

Small infants present special problems, including management of their postoperative pain. Even the smallest infant perceives pain. The mainstay of postoperative pain management is regional anesthesia. Regional anesthesia is useful intraoperatively to reduce and eliminate the need for narcotics and muscle relaxants as well as reduce the concentrations of volatile anesthetics required. This allows a lighter level of anesthesia to be used for maintenance, so that the infant and/or child can be more rapidly extubated at the end of surgery. Postoperatively, caudal or lumbar epidural techniques are very appropriate for the management of postoperative discomfort. This is covered in more detail in other chapters. Infants under 2 months of age have an increased sensitivity to the hydrophilic narcotics such as morphine, and for this reason the clinician needs to be very aware of the prolonged half-life and decreased clearance of narcotics such as morphine.[55] In addition, the small infant has a great variability in the response to narcotics, along with the increased sensitivity. There is a potential for renal failure to magnify this problem, since active metabolites of narcotics may accumulate during renal failure.

Toddlers

Toddlers and preschool children present a particular challenge. Separation from their parents is a major problem. The needs for various lab tests as well as being NPO (nothing by mouth) for surgery are difficult to explain to children between 3 and 6 years of age. At this age, children are trying to develop and maintain some degree of self-control and courage. They are developing concepts of time and space and, because of their newly acquired ability for imagination, tend to exaggerate the impact of their illnesses. Korsch described it beautifully: "These young children have no assurance that painful experiences will ever stop, that assaults by caretakers have any reliable limit, or that the dreary lonely nights in the hospital will definitely come to an end."[56] A major change has occurred since the publication of this article. That change has been a revolution in visiting hours for parents and family members both on the routine ward as well as on intensive care units.

At approximately 6 years of age, children usually have the ability to communicate. Many can understand and participate in the decisions about their anesthetic care. The anesthesiologist can allow them to decide if they want premedication and also, as far as the induction of anesthesia, whether or not they want to hold the mask, or when allowed, if the parent can hold the mask, and so forth. The introduction of parents into the induction process has become a much more humane way of inducing anesthesia both for the child and for the parents. Modern medicine requires outcomes research, which is very important for the progress and development of anesthetic and various other therapeutic techniques. As far as allowing parents to be present for the induction of anesthesia, attempts are being made to decide whether or not it is of value to allow parents to be there, either for the benefit of the child or for the benefit of the parents. Various parameters are being examined, such as stress levels and immediate postoperative behavioral problems. It is these authors' opinion that we are not really looking at the correct issues as far as allowing parents to be present for the induction of anesthesia. The issues are not short term but long term. The parent–child relationship is one that develops over the lifetime of the child and is very difficult to define in any 2-week period. After having allowed parents to be present for induction for over two decades, even though they may have had stress, and often cry during or immediately after the induction, when questioned if they would like to be there the next time their child has anesthesia, the overwhelming response is "yes, I wouldn't do it otherwise."

Adolescents

Adolescence creates a different set of problems. On the one hand, adolescents are extremely sensitive and conscious of their growing bodies. On the other, they feel indestructible. Many also need to tell adults that they do not really understand anything about this growing up process in modern times. The additive effects of the problems of normal adolescence and those of chronic disease sometimes makes it difficult for parents and health care workers to provide these particular patients with what they need. Giving them choices, such as regional or general anesthesia or IV induction versus inhalation induction, can greatly enhance communication and cooperation.

CHRONIC RENAL DISEASE AND THE FAMILY UNIT

Sometimes the technical aspects of a disease process and medical science compete, making it difficult for the physician, the child, and the family to cope with the psychological problems of chronic disease. In this age of medical "miracles," more and more children and their families must contend with chronic illness.[57] The superb review by Korsch,[56] on the psychological complications of renal disease during childhood, is timeless and highlights many of the acute and chronic problems of the child and family. Because the child returns for multiple hospitalizations and anesthetic experiences, it is comforting for the child and the family to be able to identify with a small group of anesthesiologists.

The greatest single stress for children and parents with chronic disease is the many separations from parents that may be necessitated by medical and surgical treatments. Enormous strides have been made in liberalizing visiting hours, so that the parents may be there to support their child. However, many parents, either because of the distances that need to be traveled or because of job obligations or of the single-parent family, are not able to be there at all times for their child. These times of isolation and/or separation are very difficult for the child as well as the parent and often leave the parent with a guilt feeling because they cannot be there. There are no easy answers to this problem, but the opportunity for the anesthesiologist to show concern, empathy, and understanding should not be missed.

Genitourinary disease has special problems not typical of other chronic illnesses. A major problem is the anatomic location. Diseases of the genitourinary tract carry with them enormous amounts of emotional overlay and embarrassment, which are difficult for even the most intelligent adult or child to deal with. Loss of bladder and bowel control and fear of sexual impotence are often present. Other problems include those of special diets, dialysis, and medication. The normal parent–child conflicts can be severely magnified by the parent or child who uses control of diet, medication, and dialysis as a weapon.

As the patient with chronic renal failure approaches transplantation, new problems arise. The first is finding a donor. The use of living related donors has brought about many ethical decisions that add additional stress to the family unit. New opportunities for guilt feelings arise. After surgery, multiple anxieties concerning rejection of the kidney and the enormous expense of the whole procedure can be a burden for the family. On the other hand, renal transplantation provides a new degree of independence for the child and the family and an opportunity to develop more normally.

Acknowledgment

The authors again gratefully acknowledge the assistance of Mr. Robert Bland in preparing this chapter for publication.

REFERENCES

1. Langman J: Medical Embryology. Baltimore, Williams & Wilkins, 1981.
2. Patten BM: Human Embryology. 3rd ed. New York, McGraw-Hill, 1968.
3. Arey LB: Developmental Anatomy. 3rd ed. Philadelphia, WB Saunders Company, 1934.
4. Inselman LS, Mellins RB: Growth and development of the lung. J Pediatr 98:1, 1981.
5. Cook WF: Cellular localization of renin. In Fischer JW (ed): Kidney Hormones. New York, Academic Press, 1971, p 117.
6. Levens NR, Peach MJ, Carey RM, et al: Response of rat jejunum to angiotensin II: role of norepinephrine and prostaglandins. Am J Physiol 240:G17, 1981.
7. Levens NR, Peach MJ, Carey RM: Interactions between angiotensin peptides and the sympathetic nervous system mediating intestinal sodium and water reabsorption in the rat. J Clin Invest 67:1197, 1981.
8. Sealey JE, Båhler FR, Laragh JH, et al: Aldosterone excretion: physiological variations in man measured by radioimmunoassay or double-isotope dilution. Circ Res 31:367, 1972.
9. Arieff AI: Hyponatremia, convulsions, respiratory arrest, and permanent brain damage after elective surgery in healthy women. N Engl J Med 314:1529, 1986.
10. Sterns RH, Riggs JE, Schochet SS: Osmotic demyelination syndrome following correction of hyponatremia. N Engl J Med 314:1535, 1986.
11. Decaux G, Waterlot Y, Genette F, et al: Treatment of the syndrome of inappropriate secretion of antidiuretic hormone with furosemide. Med Intell 304:329, 1981.
12. Laragh JH: Atrial natriuretic hormone, the renin-aldosterone axis, and blood pressure-electrolyte homeostasis. N Engl J Med 313:1330, 1985.
13. Schwab TR, Edwards BS, DeVries WC, et al: Atrial endocrine function in humans with artificial hearts. N Engl J Med 315:1398, 1986.
14. Tulassay T, Rascher W, Seyberth HW, et al: Role of atrial natriuretic peptide in sodium homeostasis in premature infants. J Pediatr 109:1023, 1986.
15. Schaffer SG, Geer PG, Goetz KL: Elevated atrial natriuretic factor in neonates with respiratory distress syndrome. J Pediatr 109:1028, 1986.
16. Rascher W, Tulassay T, Lang RE: Atrial natriuretic peptide in plasma of volume-overloaded children with chronic renal failure. Lancet 2:303, 1985.
17. Gottschalk CW, Mylle M: Micropuncture study of the mammalian urinary concentrating mechanism: evidence for the countercurrent hypothesis. Am J Physiol 196:927, 1959.

18. Gottschalk CW: Micropuncture studies of tubular function in the mammalian kidney. Physiologist 4:35, 1961.

19. McCance RA, Widdowson EM: The correct physiological basis on which to compare infant and adult renal function. Lancet 2:860, 1952.

20. Arant BS Jr: Developmental patterns of renal functional maturation compared in the human neonate. J Pediatr 92:705, 1978.

21. Oh W, Oh MA, Lind J: Renal function and blood volume in newborn infants related to placental transfusion. Acta Paediatr Scand 56:197, 1966.

22. Edelmann CM Jr, Soriano JR, Boichis II, et al: Renal bicarbonate reabsorption and hydrogen ion excretion in normal infants. J Clin Invest 46:1309, 1967.

23. Roy RN, Chance GW, Raddle IC, et al: Late hyponatremia in very low birth weight infants. Pediatr Res 10:526, 1976.

24. Flynn JT: Causes, management approaches, and outcome of acute renal failure in children. Curr Opin Pediatr 10:184, 1998.

25. Mendley SR, Langman CB: Acute renal failure in the pediatric patient. Adv Ren Replace Ther 4(Suppl 1):93, 1997.

26. Arora P, Kher V, Rai PK, et al: Prognosis of acute renal failure in children: a multivariate analysis. Pediatr Nephrol 11:153, 1997.

27. Smith PS: Management of end-stage renal disease in children. Ann Pharmacother 32:929, 1998.

28. Rahman M, Smith MC: Chronic renal insufficiency: a diagnostic and therapeutic approach. Arch Intern Med 158:1743, 1998.

29. Saborio P, Hahn S, Hisano S, et al: Chronic renal failure: an overview from a pediatric perspective. Nephron 80:134, 1998.

30. Evans ED, Greenbaum LA, Ettenger RB: Principles of renal replacement therapy in children. Pediatr Clin North Am 42:1579, 1995.

31. Uribarri J: Past, present and future of end-stage renal disease therapy in the United States. Mt Sinai J Med 66:14, 1999.

32. ERSD in children. Am J Kidney Dis 18(5 suppl 2):79, 1991.

33. Thomas IT, Smith DW: Oligohydramnios, cause of the nonrenal features of Potter's syndrome, including pulmonary hypoplasia. J Pediatr 84:811, 1974.

34. Pramanik AK, Altshuler G, Light IJ, Sutherland JM: Prune-belly syndrome associated with Potter syndrome. Am J Dis Child 131:672, 1977.

35. Pagon RA, Smith DW, Shepard TH: Urethral obstruction malformation complex: a cause of abdominal muscle deficiency and the "prune belly." J Pediatr 94:900, 1979.

36. Bernstein J: The morphogenesis of renal parenchymal maldevelopment (renal dysplasia). Pediatr Clin North Am 18:395, 1971.

37. Atiyeh B, Husmann D, Baum M: Contralateral renal abnormalities in multicystic-dysplastic kidney disease. J Pediatr 121:65, 1992.

38. Inselman LS, Mellins RB: Growth and development of the lung. J Pediatr 98:1, 1981.

39. Levitt SB, Duckett J, Spitzer A, et al: Report of the International Reflux Study Committee: medical versus surgical treatment of primary vesicoureteral reflux. Pediatrics 67:392, 1981.

40. Setzer N: Circumcision questions [letter to the editor]. Pediatrics 93:1021, 1994.

41. Wiswell TE, Tencer HL, Welch CA, Chamberlain JL: Circumcision in children beyond the neonatal period. Pediatrics 92:791, 1993.

42. Herrick JB: Peculiar elongated and sickle shaped red blood corpuscles in a case of severe anemia. Arch Intern Med 6:517, 1910.

43. Murayama M: Molecular mechanism of red cell "sickling." Science 153:145, 1966.

44. Atiyeh B, Husmann D, Baum M: Contralateral renal abnormalities in multicystic-dysplastic kidney disease. J Pediatr 121:65, 1992.

45. Querfeld U, Schneble F, Wradzidlo W, et al: Acquired cystic kidney disease before and after renal transplantation. J Pediatr 121:61, 1992.

46. Swerdlow AJ, Higgins CD, Brook CGD, et al: Mortality in patients with congenital adrenal hyperplasia: a cohort study. J Pediatr 133:516, 1998.

47. Cramolini GM: Diseases of the renal system. In Katz J, Steward DJ (eds): Anesthesia and Uncommon Pediatric Diseases. Philadelphia, WB Saunders Company, 1987, p 155.

48. Haberkern CM, Coles PG, Morray JP, et al: Intraoperative hypertension during surgical excision of neuroblastoma: case report and review of 20 years' experience. Anesth Analg 75:854, 1992.

49. Cabal LA, Devaskar U, Siassi B, et al: Cardiogenic shock associated with perinatal asphyxia in preterm infants. J Pediatr 96:705, 1980.

50. Siegler RL: Spectrum of extrarenal involvement in postdiarrheal hemolyticuremic syndrome. J Pediatr 125:511, 1994.

51. Brandt JR, Fouser LS, Watkins SL, et al: Escherichia coli O157:H7-associated hemolytic-uremic syndrome after ingestion of contaminated hamburgers. J Pediatr 125:519, 1994.

52. Boyce TG, Swerdlow DL, Griffin PM: Escherichia coli O157:H7 and the hemolytic-uremic syndrome. N Engl J Med 333:364, 1995.

53. Deal JE, Snell MF, Barratt TM, Dillon MJ: Renovascular disease in childhood. J Pediatr 121:378, 1992.

54. Chevalier RL, Tegtmeyer CJ, Gomez RA: Percutaneous transmural angioplasty for renovascular hypertension in children. Pediatr Nephrol 1:89, 1987.

55. Kart T, Christrup LL, Rasmussen M: Recommended use of morphine in neonates, infants and children based on a literature review: part 1—pharmacokinetics. Paediatr Anaesth 7:5, 1997.

56. Korsch BM: Psychological complications of renal disease in childhood. In Edelmann CA (ed): Pediatric Kidney Disease. Boston, Little, Brown, 1978, p 342.

57. Shidler NR, Peterson RA, Kimmel PL: Quality of life and psychosocial relationships in patients with chronic renal insufficiency. Am J Kidney Dis 32:557, 1998.

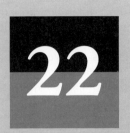

22

Anesthesia for Orthopedic Surgery

M. RAMEZ SALEM

ARTHUR J. KLOWDEN

Infants and children of all ages and stages of development require anesthesia for orthopedic procedures. Pathology includes congenital anomalies, deformities, infection, and trauma. At one end of the spectrum is the otherwise healthy child who, with proper treatment, soon returns to totally normal function. Many of these surgical procedures are now being performed on an outpatient basis. At the other end is the child with multiple congenital anomalies, with impairment of the cardiovascular or other systems. In many instances, anesthetic management varies little from those applicable to other children. However, certain disease states may present challenges with airway management, positioning, hemodynamic control, blood loss, and maintenance of body temperature.

Some children undergo repeated hospitalizations and anesthetics. Some undergo prolonged immobilization. Absence from school, separation from parents, and physical handicaps can lead to deeply rooted psychiatric problems, including overwhelming fear and apprehension, and even hostility to medical personnel. Disorders of the cardiovascular, respiratory, hematopoietic, endocrine, or neuromuscular systems may be present. Body casts may limit postoperative movements. Mentally retarded patients may become difficult to handle; efforts should be made to render their hospital stay as tolerable as possible. These patients benefit from psychological as well as pharmacologic preparation. The requirements for each child should be decided on an individual basis.

These children may present special problems to the anesthesiologist, who should be familiar not only with the issues pertaining to pediatric anesthesia but also with the pathophysiology of the lesions present. The management of critically ill children allows no margin for error. Cooperation among the anesthesiologist, orthopedic surgeon, and other personnel involved in their care is essential for a successful outcome.

SCOLIOSIS

The term *scoliosis* is derived from a Greek word meaning crooked or curvature. Deformities of the spine have been recognized since the stone age.[1] Cave drawings provide evidence that scoliosis afflicted early humans. Hippocrates, in about 400 B.C., was the first to note that patients with spinal deformities have concomitant respiratory pathology and often die young. He also developed methods of bracing to treat patients afflicted with the disease, but with poor results.[2] In 1914, Russell Hibbs performed the first spinal fusion for scoliosis, and in 1946 the Milwaukee brace was designed by Blout and Schmidt.[1,2] With these developments, great progress was made in the management of scoliosis.

Since the introduction of poliomyelitis vaccine, surveys largely reflect the incidence of idiopathic scoliosis. In one

617

survey of school children in the United Kingdom, the overall incidence was 1.8 per 1,000.[3] The incidence was much higher in girls (3.9 per 1,000) than in boys (0.3 per 1,000). In a radiographic survey in the United States, a higher incidence was found (4 per 1,000) because of the inclusion of more mild degrees of scoliosis.[4] Approximately 80 percent of all patients requiring surgery are females.

The cause of scoliosis remains obscure in most cases, hence the term *idiopathic scoliosis*.[1, 5] Idiopathic forms are by far the most common; approximately 90 percent of all cases of idiopathic scoliosis are probably genetic, and thus the two terms sometimes are used synonymously. It is not unusual to see families in which four or five children have some form of scoliosis.[1, 5] In such cases, genes carrying scoliosis are present on both sides of the family. It can be predicted that if a person with scoliosis has children, approximately one third of all offspring will have scoliosis.[1] Most children who develop idiopathic scoliosis are genetically programmed much as a computer might be, with a message to be printed out years later. The scoliotic genetic message manifests itself during the juvenile or early adolescent years and progresses to a predetermined severity unless the course is interrupted by proper treatment.[1]

Structural scoliosis is a complicated deformity with both lateral curvature and vertebral rotation, as well as variable deformity of the rib cage.[1, 6] The pathologic anatomy of scoliosis is shown in Figure 22–1. As the disease progresses, the vertebrae and spinous processes in the area of the major curve rotate toward the concavity of the curve. The vertebral body becomes distorted toward the convex side. The rotating vertebrae push the ribs on the convex side of the curve posteriorly, forming a characteristic posterior angle (rib hump) and a narrower thoracic cage. On the concave side, the posterior angles of the ribs are flattened, and these ribs become prominent anteriorly. The ribs are close together on the concave side of the curve but widely separated on the convex side. The disks and vertebral bodies become wedge-shaped and are narrower in the concavity. In addition, the pedicles and laminae are shorter and thicker on the convex side of the curve and the vertebral canal is narrower on the concave side. Scoliosis is sometimes associated with kyphosis (hunchback) and lordosis (swayback). The pathology may vary somewhat between paralytic and congenital forms. Generally, in the paralytic curve that is caused by severe muscle imbalance (as in poliomyelitis), the ribs assume an almost vertical position on the convex side.

The thoracic and lumbar regions are the most frequent sites of the primary curve.[7] The most popular method to measure the curve is that described by Cobb (Fig. 22–2).[7] This method relies on accurate determination of the upper and lower end-vertebrae of the curve. The end-vertebrae are those that tilt most severely toward the concavity of the curve. A horizontal line is drawn at the superior border of the highest vertebral body, and another is drawn at the inferior border of the lowest vertebral body. Perpendiculars to these lines are drawn, and the intersecting angles are measured. The more severe the scoliosis, the larger the angles. The Cobb method tends to yield consistent measurements even when the angles are measured by different examiners.[7]

A simplified classification of scoliosis is shown in Table 22–1.[5] Idiopathic scoliosis has three well-marked periods of onset corresponding to periods of rapid growth, and therefore is classified into three age groups: infantile (up to 4 years), juvenile (4 to 9 years), and adolescent (10 years to the age of skeletal maturity). Infantile idiopathic scoliosis is commonly noticed during the first year of life. It usually occurs in boys and generally results in a left thoracic curve. Most of these curves resolve spontaneously, but some progress to severely rigid curves. Juvenile idiopathic scoliosis is evenly distributed between the sexes, and most patients have right thoracic curves. Adolescent scoliosis exists predominantly in girls, and most curves are to the right. Idiopathic scoliosis may or may not progress during growth. Usually, the younger the child when the structural curves develop, the less favorable the prognosis.[1, 4]

Congenital scoliosis is probably the result of some form of trauma to the zygote or embryo during the early formative period.[3, 8] Because many organ systems develop simultaneously, children with congenital scoliosis almost always have a concomitant cardiac or urinary tract defect and should be examined for these anomalies. The vertebral type of scoliosis can be either open or closed.[1, 5] The open type caused by myelomeningocele can be severe and is usually associated with partial or complete neurologic deficit.[1, 5] Congenital scoliosis is often severe, rigid, and difficult to treat. In the worst forms the spine deteriorates rapidly, and patients may come to surgery at 3 years of age.

A wide variety of neuromuscular diseases is associated with scoliosis (Table 22–1).[1, 5, 9] Scoliosis that is a sequela of poliomyelitis is usually seen within 2 years after the onset of the disease. Factors that determine the prognosis include muscle function, severity of imbalance, site of the curve, and the age of the child.[1, 5, 9] Because the curvature increases more after cessation of growth than it does with idiopathic scoliosis, the prognosis of paralytic scoliosis is worse than that of a comparable idiopathic curve.[1, 5, 9]

The diagnosis of syringomyelia is based on dissociated sensory loss (loss of pain and temperature sensations with preservation of sense of touch), amyotrophy, and thoracic scoliosis. The disease is caused by a cavity that occupies the central part of the spinal cord in the cervical region but may extend cephalad or caudad. The cavity progressively replaces the gray matter of the posterior and anterior horns of the spinal cord. Symptoms may begin during late childhood or adolescence. Scoliosis may appear after other evidence of the disease is established.

Friedreich's ataxia is the classic form of hereditary ataxia. The clinical features result from involvement of the spinocerebellar pathways (ataxia, intention tremor, and scanning speech), pyramidal tract degeneration (extensor plantar reflexes), peripheral neuropathy (absent tendon reflexes), impairment of the senses of position and vibration and, in some patients, other sensory loss and optic atrophy. The progressive muscle weakness involves the respiratory muscles.

Neurofibromatosis (von Recklinghausen's disease), a genetic disorder affecting the nervous system, has both cutaneous and subcutaneous manifestations. Peculiar cafe au lait skin pigmentations with smooth borders, which

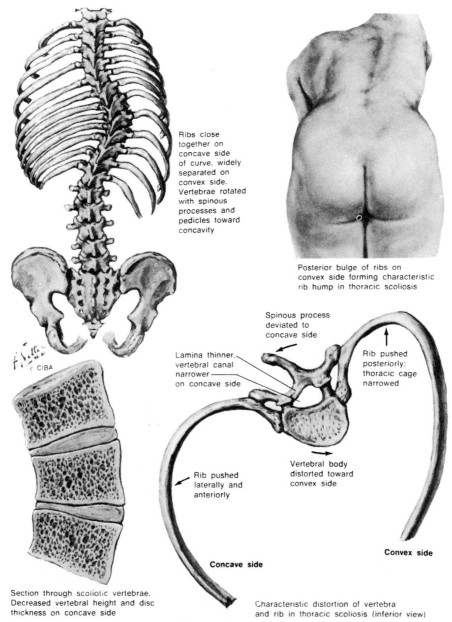

Ribs close together on concave side of curve, widely separated on convex side. Vertebrae rotated with spinous processes and pedicles toward concavity

Posterior bulge of ribs on convex side forming characteristic rib hump in thoracic scoliosis

Spinous process deviated to concave side

Lamina thinner, vertebral canal narrower on concave side

Rib pushed posteriorly; thoracic cage narrowed

Rib pushed laterally and anteriorly

Vertebral body distorted toward convex side

Convex side

Concave side

Section through scoliotic vertebrae. Decreased vertebral height and disc thickness on concave side

Characteristic distortion of vertebra and rib in thoracic scoliosis (inferior view)

FIGURE 22–1. Deformity and characteristic distortion of vertebra and rib in thoracic scoliosis. (From Keim HA: Scoliosis. Ciba Foundation Symposium. Vol 1. Summit, NJ, Ciba, 1978, with permission.)

are most prominent over the trunk, are characteristic of the disease. The incidence of severe kyphosis associated with scoliosis is about 10 percent. The spinal deformity is not anatomically related to the neurofibromas but is usually a thoracic kyphoscoliotic curve with a sharp angle. Neurofibromas tend to enlarge the foramina between the vertebral bodies and to cause dumbbell-shaped tumors. Most of the neurofibromas are asymptomatic, but in certain locations they create abnormalities by compressing adjacent structures, including spinal roots, the cerebellopontine angle, and the medulla oblongata. The deformities progress during growth and, when severe, often lead to neurologic symptoms. The progression of curves is insidious, and the curves must be treated aggressively. The incidence of pheochromocytoma in these patients is higher than in the general population.[10] An abnormal re-

sponse to muscle relaxants has also been reported, with resistance to succinylcholine and sensitivity to nondepolarizing muscle relaxants, similar to the response in patients with myasthenia gravis.[11]

The myopathic forms are caused by either a progressive or a static disorder. The progressive disorders are best typified by the muscular dystrophies.[1, 5] The severe X-linked recessive form is usually manifested during the second or third year of life.[1, 5, 8] The pelvic-femoral muscles are involved early, causing muscle imbalance. Later the shoulder and trunk muscles become involved. Scoliosis curves are long and C-shaped.[1, 5] The spines of some of these children seem almost to collapse when they assume the erect posture.[1, 5, 9] Cardiac involvement is usually observed late in the disease and may be manifested by tachycardia, arrhythmias, conduction block, S-T segment changes, and

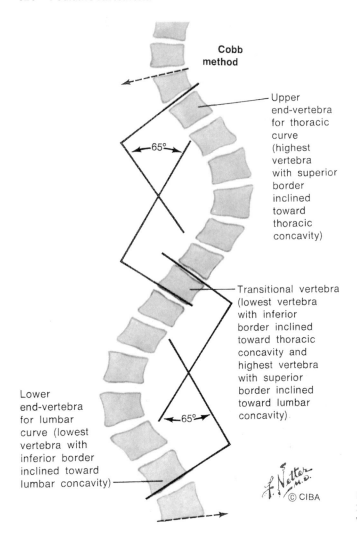

Cobb method

Upper end-vertebra for thoracic curve (highest vertebra with superior border inclined toward thoracic concavity)

Transitional vertebra (lowest vertebra with inferior border inclined toward thoracic concavity and highest vertebra with superior border inclined toward lumbar concavity)

Lower end-vertebra for lumbar curve (lowest vertebra with inferior border inclined toward lumbar concavity)

65°

65°

FIGURE 22–2. Measurement of the curve in scoliosis. (From Keim HA: Scoliosis. Ciba Foundation Symposium. Vol 1. Summit, NJ, Ciba, 1978, with permission.)

mitral valve prolapse.[9, 12] Respiratory or cardiac failure may occur during the second decade of life. Pulmonary function studies in these patients facilitate the early detection of impending respiratory failure. The prognosis in these children is always guarded, although some can be helped by judicious bracing and surgery. Hypercapnia in the absence of infection is indicative of a poor prognosis. A large series of patients with Duchenne muscular dystrophy have had spinal fusion for scoliosis with safety, including no instance of malignant hyperthermia.[12] One patient died intraoperatively of a dystrophic cardiomyopathy. Although there may be no lasting improvement in pulmonary function postoperatively, wheelchair seating and comfort are improved.[12]

Respiratory Function

Two main factors significantly affect respiratory function in scoliosis patients: the degree of the curve and the association of a neuromuscular disease.[9] Marked changes in respiratory function are seldom a feature in cases of idiopathic scoliosis in which the curve is less than 65 degrees. As curvature increases, rotation progresses, causing the chest cavity to narrow (Fig. 22–1).[1, 9, 13] The most common pulmonary function abnormality is restriction of the lung volume parameters (vital capacity, functional residual capacity, and total lung volume).[9] The greatest reduction is in the vital capacity.[9, 13] Pulmonary function values in patients with scoliosis computed on the basis of the patient's height may underestimate the magnitude of lung restriction, because the deformity makes measured height less than the true height.[9] A formula using arm span has been proposed,[14] although for all practical purposes vertical height is as useful as any index for prediction of lung volumes. The lung volumes and the compliance of the total respiratory system and of the chest wall are inversely related to the degree of the curve.[9]

The primary abnormality in pulmonary gas exchange is ventilation–perfusion maldistribution.[9, 15] Both the alveolar–arterial oxygen tension difference ($P[A–a]O_2$) and the dead space/tidal volume ratio (V_D/V_T) are increased.[15] Both ventilation and pulmonary blood flow, as measured by ^{133}Xe, lack the gravity-dependent gradients seen in normal healthy subjects. The most common blood gas abnormality is a slight decrease in arterial oxygen tension (PaO_2) with a normal arterial carbon dioxide tension ($PaCO_2$).[13, 16] The increased maldistribution increases the ventilatory requirements, and hypercapnia is a manifestation of the failure to meet these requirements.[9] The reduced ventilatory response to CO_2 associated with severe scoliosis im-

T A B L E   2 2 – 1
CLASSIFICATION OF STRUCTURAL SCOLIOSIS

Idiopathic (genetic) scoliosis (approximately 70% of all cases of
  scoliosis; classified by age of onset)
Congenital scoliosis (probably not genetic)
  Vertebral
    Open—with posterior spinal defect
      With neurologic deficit (e.g., myelomeningocele)
      Without neurologic deficit (e.g., spina bifida occulta)
    Closed—no posterior element defect
      With neurologic deficit (e.g., diastematomyelia with spina
        bifida)
      Without neurologic deficit (e.g., hemivertebra, unilateral
        unsegmented bar)
  Extravertebral (e.g., congenital rib fusions)
Neuromuscular scoliosis
  Neuropathic forms
    Lower motor neuron disease (e.g., poliomyelitis)
    Upper motor neuron disease (e.g., cerebral palsy)
    Others (e.g., syringomyelia)
  Myopathic forms
    Progressive (e.g., muscular dystrophy)
    Static (e.g., amyotonia congenita)
    Others (e.g., Friedreich's ataxia, unilateral amalia)
Neurofibromatosis (von Recklinghausen's disease)
Mesenchymal disorders
  Congenital (e.g., Marfan's syndrome, Morquio's disease, amyoplasia
    congenita, various types of dwarfism)
  Acquired (e.g., rheumatoid arthritis, Still's disease)
  Others (e.g., Scheuermann's disease, osteogenesis imperfecta)
Trauma
  Vertebral (e.g., fracture, irradiation, surgery)
  Extravertebral (e.g., burn, thoracic surgery)

pairs the ventilatory compensation for ventilation–perfusion maldistribution and contributes to hypoxemia and hypercapnia. These functional abnormalities and the interaction of other associated impairments of respiratory function may culminate in respiratory failure (Fig. 22–3). In longstanding cases, pulmonary hypertension may be present. Several mechanisms contribute to the increase in pulmonary vascular resistance. First, the number of

vascular units per unit volume of lung is less than that of normal lungs.[17] Second, in the regions compressed by the rib cage deformity, blood flows in extra-alveolar vessels, which have increased resistance. The third is the presence of hypoxemia and hypercapnia,[18] and the fourth is the uncommon presence of congenital heart disease.[19]

The majority of patients with idiopathic scoliosis who present for surgery do not have marked impairment of pulmonary function. Changes in pulmonary function occur when the curve progresses beyond 65 degrees in idiopathic scoliosis, but may be seen in congenital scoliosis with curves of less than 65 degrees.[9, 15] In patients with vital capacities above 35 percent of predicted values, surgery is usually well tolerated and the trachea is often extubated the same day.[20] If the vital capacity is below 30 percent of normal, particularly in the presence of neuromuscular disease, the patient usually needs overnight mechanical ventilation postoperatively.[20]

A number of mechanical factors contribute to the respiratory function abnormalities present in scoliosis associated with neuromuscular disease.[9] These include deformity, abnormalities in central respiratory control and innervation of the motor neurons of the respiratory muscles, and loss of motor function. Impairment of the defense mechanism (e.g., coughing) and respiratory infections are additional factors. The inspiratory and vital capacities are reduced as a result of the loss of inspiratory muscle force. When associated with impaired control of ventilation or marked inspiratory weakness, hypoventilation, hypercapnia, and hypoxemia become major contributory factors to respiratory failure. When respiratory control is impaired, there is extreme sensitivity to central nervous system (CNS) depressants such as general anesthetics, sedatives, and opioids.[9]

Surgical Treatment

Scoliosis surgery may be performed via a posterior approach, an anterior approach or in a combined antero-

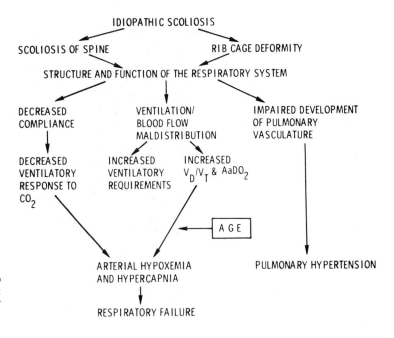

FIGURE 22–3. Factors in idiopathic scoliosis that contribute to respiratory function abnormalities and failure. (From Kafer ER: Respiratory and cardiovascular functions in scoliosis. Bull Eur Physiopathol Respir 13:299, 1977, with permission.)

posterior procedure. The posterior approach is far more common and has undergone evolution since the first spinal fusion was performed.[1, 21, 22] The technique used since 1962 was spinal fusion with implantation of a Harrington rod (Fig. 22–4).[1, 21, 22] With this technique, incisions are made through the skin, fascia, and supraspinal ligament. Spinal musculature is then reflected subperiosteally. A Harrington hook is notched into a facet joint of an upper vertebra. Spinous processes and intraspinal ligaments are removed. The soft tissues can be stretched and the curve corrected by installing an outrigger. The vertebrae are decorticated and all facet joints are destroyed. The Harrington rod, a distraction rod that jacks the spine into a

straight line, is inserted on the concave side of the curve and maximally extended. A bone graft is obtained from the iliac crest, cut into matchstick-sized strips, and placed along the entire fusion area, mainly on the concave side of the curve.

Among the important modifications of the Harrington rod technique is the Luque procedure.[23, 24] This is a system of segmental spinal instrumentation with multiple levels of interlocking vertebral component fixation. First used with a Harrington rod, Luque later developed his own more flexible L-rods to be attached with sublaminar wiring at each spinal level. However, the same sublaminar wires that create stability when passed through the epidural

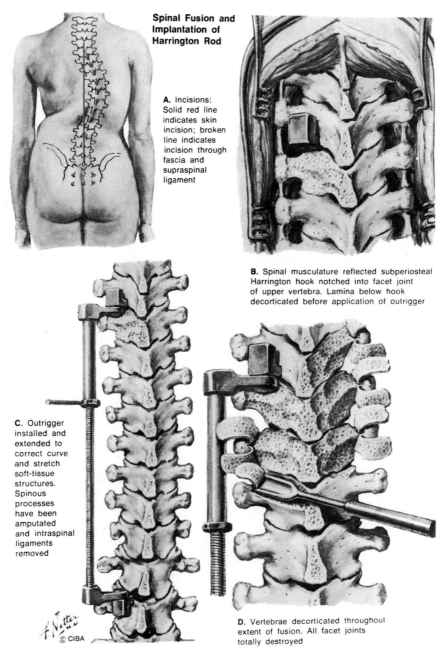

Spinal Fusion and Implantation of Harrington Rod

A. Incisions: Solid red line indicates skin incision; broken line indicates incision through fascia and supraspinal ligament

B. Spinal musculature reflected subperiosteal Harrington hook notched into facet joint of upper vertebra. Lamina below hook decorticated before application of outrigger

C. Outrigger installed and extended to correct curve and stretch soft-tissue structures. Spinous processes have been amputated and intraspinal ligaments removed

D. Vertebrae decorticated throughout extent of fusion. All facet joints totally destroyed

FIGURE 22–4. *A–H,* Steps of spinal fusion and implantation of the Harrington rod. (From Keim HA: Scoliosis. Ciba Foundation Symposium. Vol 1. Summit, NJ, Ciba, 1978, with permission.)

Illustration continued on opposite page

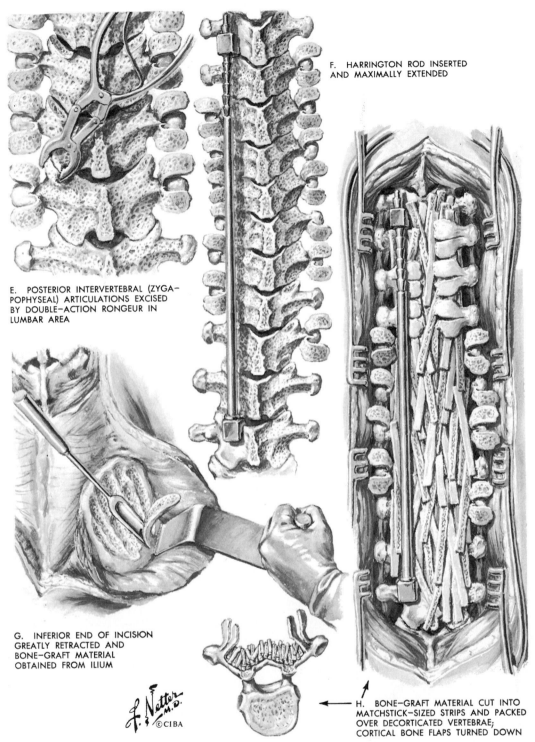

E. POSTERIOR INTERVERTEBRAL (ZYGA-POPHYSEAL) ARTICULATIONS EXCISED BY DOUBLE-ACTION RONGEUR IN LUMBAR AREA

F. HARRINGTON ROD INSERTED AND MAXIMALLY EXTENDED

G. INFERIOR END OF INCISION GREATLY RETRACTED AND BONE-GRAFT MATERIAL OBTAINED FROM ILIUM

H. BONE-GRAFT MATERIAL CUT INTO MATCHSTICK-SIZED STRIPS AND PACKED OVER DECORTICATED VERTEBRAE; CORTICAL BONE FLAPS TURNED DOWN

FIGURE 22–4. (*Continued*).

space anterior to each lamina also increase the risk of neurologic complications by virtue of their approximation to the spinal cord and nerves.[25] The advantages significantly outweigh the risks in children with preexisting neurologic disorders, such as myelomeningocele, or those with neuromuscular- or osteogenesis imperfecta–associated scoliosis.[26] The main advantage of the Luque technique is increased stability. The rod–wire–bone inter-

face is not stable in all cases, however, and the rods sometimes migrate, leading to the loss of correction. Attempts to correct this problem with a rigid plate implant for cross-bracing were recently introduced as the Texas Scottish Rite Hospital Crosslink System.[27]

A combination of the Luque contoured rod and a Harrington rod has been used in an attempt to minimize the disadvantages and maximize the advantages of both systems.[26] This Wisconsin system adds segmental wiring through each spinous process. Although the neurologic risk is less than with the Luque system, the clinical results are similar to that of the Harrington rod, with increased stability but no correction of a sagittal curve.[26]

Another important form of instrumentation was devised by Cotrel and Dubousset.[28, 29] The rods used can be formed to produce a more natural spine curvature. The fusion does not have to extend as far above and below the curvature as previously, thus leading to a less painful and faster recovery. The Cotrel-Dubousset design[30] involves screws and hooks that can be fixed at any level or position to apply either compression or distraction forces. The rods can be bent at any part of their length, and can restore the sagittal curve of the spine and correct three-dimensional deformities. Transverse traction devices are used to firmly lock the two separated rods together as a stable framework (Fig. 22–5). Although the correction achieved is in three planes, it is technically more difficult and neurologically more compromising; a threefold increase in the risk of

neurologic complications has been reported compared with a Harrington rod insertion.[25] The actual bulk of the system negates its use in small, malnourished patients, and it is not appropriate for very large curves. It rapidly became the predominant technique preferred for most patients with idiopathic scoliosis.

Recent additions to the hardware armamentarium include the Isola, Horizon, and Moss-Miami techniques. The Moss-Miami instrumentation system[31–33] (Fig. 22–6) is a current favorite. Developed as an extension of the system created by Cotrel and Dubousset, it advocates a segmental approach to the three dimensions of spinal instrumentation. This necessitates an analysis of each motion segment and the placement of implants at virtually all spinal levels. Since clinical trials began in 1993, alterations and additions have been made to correct some of the early problems of hardware breakage, loss of correction, and pseudoarthrosis. The system can be used for all conditions requiring instrumentation.

The anterior approach, popularized by Dwyer in 1969, is usually reserved for cases in which posterior fusion is not possible (e.g., myelomeningocele).[34] The vertebral column is approached laterally on the convex side of the curve. A thoracotomy is performed with the patient in the lateral or semilateral position. The diaphragm is divided near its peripheral attachments to gain access to the retroperitoneal and retropleural vertebrae. Bolts are inserted transversely through each vertebral body. The bolts are then crimped onto a titanium cable, which is applied to the convex side of the curve. By removing the intervertebral disks between adjacent vertebrae in the curve and pulling the vertebrae together, a dramatic correction can be obtained. The pleural flap is reattached to cover the bolts and cable. The chest is closed in a routine fashion and the pleural cavity is drained by a chest tube connected to underwater drainage.

Unfortunately, the Dwyer implant has certain disadvantages,[35] including difficulty in producing proper spinal derotation, postinstrumentation kyphosis, and the inability to vary segmental correction. Instrumentation devised by Zielke and Pellin[36] has replaced the Dwyer implant in many institutions. They used a flexible rod system, threaded nuts at all screw sites, and a derotating bar. Although the anterior approaches can achieve some axial and frontal correction, they are biomechanically weak and should be followed by a body cast. Currently, an anterior approach is most often used to improve the flexibility of the spine before the more corrective and definitive posterior spine instrumentation, which is performed 1 to 2 weeks later.

Recently, some surgeons have undertaken a combined anterior and posterior approach in the same operation. The anterior approach is done in the lateral thoracotomy position and the patient is then turned prone for the posterior approach. This two-in-one procedure is quite lengthy and may be associated with significant blood loss and increased postoperative pain. Nonetheless, some surgeons feel that it is the preferred technique for specific patients, reducing the psychological aspects and nutritional problems encountered with two separate surgical procedures requiring two anesthetics 1 or 2 weeks apart.

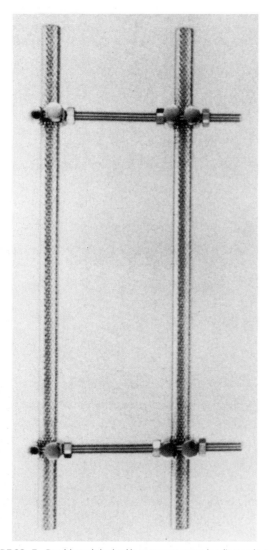

FIGURE 22–5. Double rods locked by two transverse loading rods, resulting in strong framelike setup. (From Cotrel Y, Dubousset J: New segmental posterior instrumentation of the spine. Orthop Trans 9:118, 1985, with permission.)

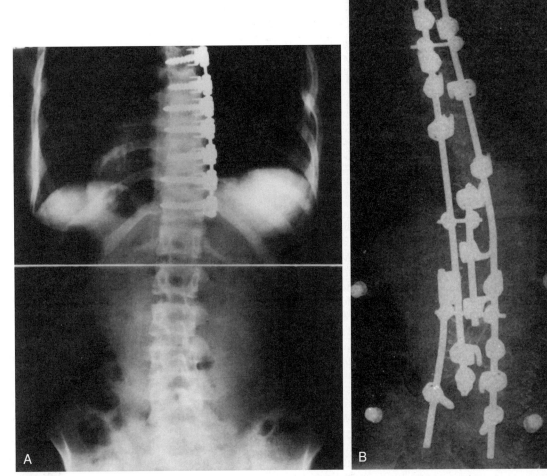

FIGURE 22–6. *A,* Posterior AP radiograph of a girl with a 48-degree thoracic curve instrumented with anterior instrumentation from T5 to T11. The rod is a 3.2-mm threaded rod with a 6-mm vertebral body screw through a four-prong staple (Harms-Moss) anterior instrmentation. (From Betz RB, Harms J, Clements DH, et al: Anterior instrumentation for thoracic idiopathic scoliosis. Semin Spine Surg 9:141, 1997, with permission.) *B,* Miami-Moss instrumentation in a patient with paralytic scoliosis after anterior fusion without structural grafts and posterior sacral fixation using an intrasacral rod technique. (From Shufflebarger HL: Moss-Miami spinal instrumentation system: methods of fixation of the spondylopelvic junction. *In* Margulies JY, et al [eds]: Lumbosacral and Spinopelvic Fixation. Philadelphia, Lippincott-Raven, 1996, with permission.)

Blood Loss

Scoliosis surgery is an extensive operative procedure that is often accompanied by substantial blood loss (Table 22–2).[37, 38] Profuse bleeding may occur when the erector spinae muscles are stripped from the spinous processes, laminae, and transverse processes. Severe oozing may occur from the large area of exposed cancellous bone. The amount of blood loss is related to the length of time required for instrumentation.[37, 38]

The vertebral venous system provides channels into which blood may be diverted from the lower parts of the body if the inferior vena cava (IVC) becomes obstructed.[37, 38] In the prone position, any rise in intra-abdominal pressure is transmitted to the IVC. Consequently, blood is diverted into the vertebral venous plexuses, causing excessive blood loss.[39] A rise in intra-abdominal pressure may be caused by increased muscle tone of the abdominal muscles, external pressure by sandbags or operating table

mattresses, gastric inflation, coughing and bucking, and increased airway pressure.

Various methods have been suggested to reduce blood loss (Table 22–3). The surgical technique is of utmost importance in decreasing bleeding. Subperiosteal dissection, pressing the wound edge firmly with approximated fingertips, the use of packs when feasible, and the use of retractors provide a certain degree of hemostasis.[37–40] Meticulous attention should be given to positioning the patient correctly so that the adverse effects of the prone position are minimized. Probably no modification has had a greater impact on minimizing blood loss than the use of special support frames. The Relton-Hall operation frame consists of four sturdy, well-padded supports arranged in two V-shaped pairs.[37, 39] The superior pair supports the anterolateral aspects of the upper thoracic cage and the inferior pair supports the anterolateral aspects of the pelvic girdle. The patient's abdomen is truly free of any pressure, and pressure on the IVC is thus minimized. The anterolat-

T A B L E　2 2 - 2
FACTORS AFFECTING BLOOD LOSS DURING SCOLIOSIS SURGERY

Surgical factors
　Extent of dissection and number of vertebrae to be fused
　Length of operation
　Site and size of bone graft and phase of operation in which it is
　　obtained
　Previous spinal fusion
　Surgical technique
Anesthetic factors
　Increased arterial pressure
　Increased venous pressure
Postural factors
　Increased abdominal wall tension
　Increased intra-abdominal pressure　　} Intermittent positive-
　Extrinsic pressure　　　　　　　　　　pressure ventilation
Respiratory factors　　　　　　　　　　Increased pressure
　　　　　　　　　　　　　　　　　　　in inferior vena cava
　　　　　　　　　　　　　　　　　　　and diversion of
　　　　　　　　　　　　　　　　　　　blood into vertebral
　　　　　　　　　　　　　　　　　　　venous plexus

eral supports tend to facilitate stability of the patient during the procedure. Furthermore, avoidance of abdominal pressure helps in maintaining functional residual capacity (FRC) at a near-normal level, which tends to prevent atelectasis and hypoxemia during anesthesia and surgery (Fig. 22–7). Other frames are also available. The CHOP frame allows individual adjustments of each post's height and position.

Several factors combine to make intermittent positive-pressure ventilation (IPPV) necessary during scoliosis surgery. These include the prone position, the effects of anesthetic drugs and techniques, and the presence of respiratory disability. IPPV causes a rise in the mean intrathoracic pressure, impeding the venous return to the right side of the heart and increasing the peripheral venous pressure. The increase in IVC pressure causes diversion of blood into the vertebral venous plexuses, as well as increased bleeding. In theory, this effect could be minimized by applying a negative phase between inflations (no more than –5 cm H_2O).[37] However, the use of a negative expiratory phase may increase the incidence of air embolism

T A B L E　2 2 - 3
SUGGESTED METHODS OF BLOOD CONSERVATION FOR SCOLIOSIS SURGERY

Reduction of blood loss
　Proper anesthetic and surgical techniques
　Proper positioning—use of frame
　Complete muscle relaxation
　Infiltration with epinephrine
　Hypotensive anesthesia
　Early management of DIC
　Desmopressin?
Autologous blood transfusion
　Preoperative blood donation
　Acute normovolemic hemodilution
　Blood salvage procedures
Combination of techniques
Oxygen-carrying blood substitutes

and airway closure and is therefore contraindicated. Controlled hyperventilation ($Paco_2$ 25 to 30 mm Hg) has been advocated to contribute to a reduction in blood loss by producing peripheral vasoconstriction.[37] However, hypocapnia is undesirable during scoliosis surgery, especially during induced hypotension,[41, 42] as low $Paco_2$ causes a marked decrease in spinal cord blood flow (SCBF).[41]

Complete relaxation of the diaphragm and the abdominal musculature decreases the intra-abdominal pressure and the pressure on the IVC.[37] Straining, coughing, bucking, and airway obstruction increase bleeding and should be avoided. Gastric inflation as a result of bag-and-mask ventilation before intubation, especially when excessive airway pressures are used, may cause a significant rise in intra-abdominal pressure. This can be prevented by applying gentle cricoid pressure during bag-and-mask ventilation and by using appropriate airway pressures.[43] If gastric inflation is suspected, decompression may be done by inserting a gastric tube or a suction catheter before the patient is turned to the prone position.

Bleeding from the skin edges, subcutaneous tissues, and muscles is significantly reduced by infiltrating the operative site with a large volume of 1:500,000 epinephrine solution (up to 500 ml).[44] Probably both the local vasoconstrictive effect of the drug and the hydrostatic pressure exerted by the fluid bulk contribute to the effectiveness of this method.[37] It is well known that certain anesthetics (e.g., halothane) sensitize the myocardium to exogenous catecholamines.[45] The dosage of epinephrine needed to produce arrhythmias is therefore lower in halothane-anesthetized patients than in those who are awake. It has been suggested[45] that a 1:100,000 epinephrine solution in a dosage of 0.15 ml/kg per 10-minute period, not to exceed 0.45 ml/kg of the same solution per hour, is safe. Although this claim has not been challenged, a larger dose may be permitted if one of the newer inhalation drugs is used instead of halothane, as they are less sensitizing to the myocardium.[46] The maximal dosages of epinephrine for subcutaneous infiltration for adult patients that are recommended as unlikely to produce arrhythmias with halothane, isoflurane, and enflurane are 1.0, 3.5, and 5.5 μg/kg, respectively. During desflurane or sevoflurane anesthesia, the maximal recommended dosages of epinephrine are similar to that of isoflurane.[47, 48]

Children appear to have a much lower incidence of arrhythmias after epinephrine infiltration. No arrhythmias occurred during a variety of pediatric operations utilizing cutaneous infiltration of 1:100,000 epinephrine (2 to 15 μg/kg), with a wide range of end-tidal halothane concentrations and a normal or lowered $Paco_2$. Epinephrine, at a dose of at least 10 μg/kg, could safely be used in the presence of a normal or lower than normal $Paco_2$.[49] Furthermore, the addition of lidocaine to the epinephrine solution increases the margin of safety. If a larger dose of epinephrine is used (rarely justified), a β-adrenergic blocking drug such as propranolol (up to 0.06 mg/kg) or esmolol (0.5 mg/kg/min for 2 to 4 minutes) can be given as a prophylactic measure.

Goldstein[50] suggested in 1966 that the use of hypotensive anesthesia might reduce the continuing problem of blood loss during scoliosis surgery. In 1974, McNeil et al.[38] and Bennett et al.[40] found that the use of hypotensive anesthe-

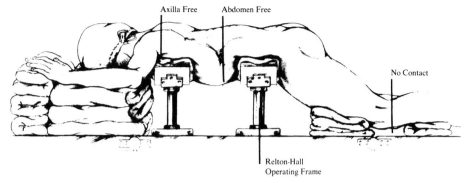

FIGURE 22–7. Position of patient on Relton-Hall frame. (From Schwentker EG: Posterior fusion of the spine for scoliosis. Surg Rounds October, 1978, p. 12, with permission.)

sia decreased blood loss by an average of 40 percent. The mean amount of blood transfused in patients with normal blood pressure was 2.27 L, whereas in the hypotensive group the mean amount was 1.38 L. No complications directly related to the hypotensive technique were noted. The average operating time was reduced by more than 30 minutes.[38, 40] These findings led to the widespread use of induced hypotension for scoliosis surgery. Other studies have reconfirmed these findings.[51-53] In addition, the use of hypotensive anesthesia has allowed scoliosis correction to be performed in Jehovah's Witnesses without blood transfusion.[54]

Induced Hypotension in Scoliosis Surgery

Important factors govern the success and safety of induced hypotension during scoliosis surgery. The benefits gained from the use of induced hypotension depend on the skill of the surgeon. In this regard, hypotensive anesthesia is not the answer to poor surgical technique; as Enderby put it, "Good surgical technique skillful enough to match the high standards of hypotensive anesthesia is essential if any real advantages are to accrue to the patient."[55]

Dry Operative Field

Some controversy surrounds the relative importance of arterial pressure and blood flow in producing a "drier" operative field.[56] Although some investigators believe that the dry field often correlates with the reduction in blood pressure,[57] evidence indicates that the improved operating conditions accompanying hypotension in scoliosis surgery are related to a reduction in cardiac output. It has been reported[58] that the onset of a dry operative field during deliberate hypotension in children in the supine position was accompanied by a significant reduction in cardiac output. Other investigators[44, 59] have also found a positive correlation between blood loss and left ventricular stroke work index during hypotensive anesthesia for surgical correction of scoliosis. These findings may explain the variations in reported data regarding blood loss during scoliosis surgery. Greater reduction in blood loss with pentolinium than with sodium nitroprusside was also reported.[40] The latter drug tends to increase cardiac output. In operations in which most bleeding is of venous origin (e.g., orthope-

dic operations), blood loss was less with nitroglycerin than with sodium nitroprusside at comparable levels of hypotension.[60] It is possible that the lower venous pressure associated with the use of nitroglycerin was partly responsible for the decreased blood loss. These findings, however, could not be confirmed in children[61] or adults[53] undergoing posterior spinal fusion.

A relatively dry operative field and improved operative conditions may not be achieved at a predetermined hypotensive level. The skillful anesthesiologist should ascertain that hypotensive anesthesia has achieved its objectives. A lower level of blood pressure or other hemodynamic adjustments (decreased heart rate) may be needed to improve the operative field.

Techniques for Inducing Hypotension

Hypotension is initiated only after tracheal intubation is performed, a steady anesthetic state is achieved, and the patient is placed in the prone position.[56] Light anesthesia can be maintained either with opioid/nitrous oxide/oxygen supplemented by a muscle relaxant or with a low concentration of a volatile anesthetic. The hypotensive drug is administered at least 10 minutes before the incision is made. Further decreases in arterial pressure can be obtained by a gradual increase in the anesthetic concentration. Drugs with vagolytic or sympathomimetic actions, such as atropine and pancuronium, are better avoided.

Some anesthesiologists prefer to use the inhalational anesthetics as the sole means of inducing and maintaining hypotension.[62] Such a practice should be discouraged during scoliosis correction for the following reasons: (1) impairment of the contractile function of the myocardium occurs with increasing concentrations of the anesthetic, (2) blood pressure control may be unsatisfactory with deep anesthesia alone, (3) sluggish return of blood pressure to normal level may be encountered when the anesthetic is discontinued, (4) longer time may be needed to perform the wake-up test, and (5) high anesthetic concentrations may interfere with sensory evoked potentials.

Hypotension induced by a ganglion-blocking or direct-acting drug is frequently accompanied by reflex tachycardia mediated through the baroreceptors,[56] which tends to increase the cardiac output and counteract the fall in pressure. Tachyphylaxis or failure to maintain the required hypotensive state with repeated administration of a hypotensive drug is more often seen in children than adults.[42, 58] Resistant hypotension is not a unique feature of one particular drug and has been reported with most hypotensive drugs.[61]

Resistance to hypotensive drugs has been attributed to several mechanisms, including stimulation of both the sympathetic and the renin–angiotensin system. The relative importance of these mechanisms may differ with the various hypotensive drugs. Sodium nitroprusside-induced hypotension is associated with increases in heart rate, cardiac output, activation of the renin–angiotensin system, and release of catecholamines.[63-67] Conversely, ganglion blockade results in a lesser increase in catecholamines and no activation of the renin–angiotensin axis.[59, 66] The increase in heart rate with the use of ganglion-blocking drugs is probably the result of parasympathetic blockade. It may be more prominent in children because of their increased vagal tone.[58, 66]

Stimulation of the sympathetic and renin-angiotensin systems may adversely affect the operative course of patients undergoing induced hypotension.[59] First, there may be difficulty controlling the blood pressure. Second, even when blood pressure is controlled the cardiac output may remain elevated, making it difficult to decrease bleeding. Finally, rebound hypertension[68] and its possible sequelae of bleeding, cerebral edema, and cerebral vascular accidents are undesirable complications.

Nicardipine is a dihydropyridine calcium channel blocking drug with potent systemic and coronary artery vasodilatory effects, without negative chronotropic, inotropic, or dromotropic effects. Although its half-life is approximately 1 hour, accumulation during an infusion slows its elimination and increases the half-life to 1 to 8 hours. A study comparing it to sodium nitroprusside in 20 pediatric patients for scoliosis correction demonstrated significantly less blood loss with nicardipine (761 ml vs. 1,297 ml), but a much longer time to return to baseline pressures (26.8 minutes vs. 7.3 minutes).[69] Nicardipine may not be the ideal hypotensive drug because of its inability to promptly restore blood pressure toward normal when its infusion rate is reduced or stopped.

Prevention of tachycardia can be simply achieved by administering a β-adrenergic blocking drug. It is preferable to give the β-adrenergic blocking drug before, rather than after administering the hypotensive drug, when a much larger dose may be required. Treatment with a β-adrenergic blocking drug prevents increases in heart rate, cardiac output, plasma renin activity, and catecholamines, and facilitates the control of blood pressure without the need for a high inhalational anesthetic concentration. In addition, it obtunds rebound hypertension after cessation of a sodium nitroprusside infusion,[65, 67, 68] and decreases the dose requirements of sodium nitroprusside by approximately 40 percent.

Propranolol can be given slowly in small increments up to a total dosage of 0.06 mg/kg before or after administration of the hypotensive drug. The advantages of esmolol are rapid onset, short and titratable action, and cardioselectivity. It can be given in a loading dose of 500 μg/kg/min for 2 to 4 minutes and continued by constant infusion at a rate of 300 μg/min. Failure to maintain the hypotensive

state has also been attributed to excessive fluid therapy.[56] Labetalol, has both α_1- and β-adrenoceptor antagonist properties.[70] In anesthetized patients, labetalol reduces blood pressure by decreasing systemic vascular resistance (SVR) without an increase in heart rate or cardiac output.[70, 71] Its action is characterized by gradual onset, prolonged duration (2 to 3 hours), and slow return of blood pressure to normal. The recommended dosage for induced hypotension is 0.3 mg/kg followed by 0.15-mg/kg increments. A background inhalational anesthetic should be used with labetalol. Labetalol is proving to be a useful hypotensive drug during the surgical correction of scoliosis, when prolonged hypotension is required.

It may be reasonable to withhold intraoperative fluids until hypotension is achieved, after which fluids can be given as required. Intravenous (IV) fluids can be administered to correct profound hypotension and to reverse the hypotensive state when it is no longer needed.

Onset and Degree of Hypotension

Hypotension should be induced slowly over a period of 10 to 15 minutes.[72] Time is needed for the cerebral, coronary, and renal vasculature to dilate maximally so as to maintain adequate perfusion in the face of a lowered head of pressure. The desired level of hypotension depends on the age and condition of the patient and the requirements of surgery. In general, a systolic pressure of approximately 75 mm Hg may be sufficient to yield good operative conditions for scoliosis surgery. In young children, a lower systolic pressure may be necessary in some patients to achieve a relatively bloodless field.[58] An excessively dry operative field, dark venous blood, and deterioration of sensory evoked potentials are important warning signs and should be considered an indication to raise the blood pressure. If the blood pressure drifts too low, attempts should be made to raise it by lightening the level of anesthesia and speeding up the IV infusion. Vasoactive substances are better avoided unless the fall in pressure is uncontrollable.

Frequent and accurate recording of the arterial pressure is essential during induced hypotension (see Chapter 11). Arterial cannulation can be used for continuous monitoring and for analysis of arterial blood pH and gases. Because cardiac arrest is often fatal if it occurs when the patient is in the prone position (e.g., time is wasted in turning the patient), profound hypotension should be avoided and continuous monitoring of arterial pressure is required. Noninvasive devices such as ultrasonic Doppler, oscillotonometers, and other automated devices can be used as backup systems and for comparison of measurements.

Acid–Base Balance and Oxygenation

Maintaining a near-normal Pa_{CO_2} is recommended during deliberate hypotension for scoliosis in order to maintain a near-normal acid–base balance and SCBF. Earlier studies[73] suggested that the alveolar dead space may increase to as much as 80 percent of the tidal volume in the hypotensive adult patient in the head-up position and with increased airway pressure. Further investigations demonstrated that the increase in alveolar dead space is less than was previously thought,[74] and that in contrast to adults, the alveolar dead space does not increase during induced hypotension in chidren.[42, 75] If vigorous ventilation is applied to compensate for the theoretically increased dead space, hypocapnia with its possible sequelae may result. Measurement of end-tidal carbon dioxide ($PETCO_2$) provides a reliable estimate of $PaCO_2$ during hypotensive anesthesia in normal children.[42, 75] The only exception is in infants weighing less than 8 kg when a Mapelson D system is used or when positive end-expiratory pressure (PEEP) is added.[76]

An increase in $P(A-a)O_2$ may result during induced hypotension.[77, 78] Two possible mechanisms have been proposed to explain this phenomenon.

1. Increased intrapulmonary shunt ($\dot{Q}_{sp}/\dot{Q}_t$): changes in FRC and closing volume during anesthesia and surgery contribute to airway closure, trapping of gas distal to the closure and alveolar collapse. This local alveolar hypoxia is normally offset (to a degree) by reflex pulmonary vasoconstriction (HPV), which directs blood from hypoxic areas of the lung to adequately ventilated alveoli. Blunting or inhibition of this reflex has been noted with hypocapnia, inhalational anesthetics, and vasodilators.[79] Although inhibition of HPV occurs with all vasodilators, it is greater with sodium nitroprusside than with nitroglycerin, causing an increase in $\dot{Q}_{sp}/\dot{Q}_t$ from 5 percent to 9 percent.[78]

2. Contribution of cardiac output: a decrease in cardiac output is accompanied by increased extraction of oxygen by the tissues, resulting in a decrease in mixed venous oxygen tension (PvO_2) and mixed venous oxygen content (CvO_2). Any portion of this decreased CO that passes through nonventilated areas ($\dot{Q}_{sp}/\dot{Q}_t$) causes a greater decrease in PaO_2 than when the cardiac output is normal.[80] Therefore, a reduction in cardiac output during deliberate hypotension results in a decrease in PaO_2. However, these changes are significant only in the presence of regional atelectasis.[80] Because of the great oxygen demand in children and the possible increase in $P(A-a)O_2$, a high inspired oxygen fraction (FIO_2) is recommended during hypotension.[42] Although the oxygen delivery is only slightly increased with the use of an $FIO_2 > 0.5$, the increase may be critical during profound hypotension.[81]

Provided that adequate oxygenation and a near-normal $PaCO_2$ are maintained, metabolic acidemia is not a feature of induced hypotension. The acidemia seen with sodium nitroprusside overdose results from depressed oxygen uptake caused by cyanide formation.[82]

Anesthetic Requirements and Deliberate Hypotension

It has been observed that the anesthetic requirement is decreased during induced hypotension. In a study on dogs, the minimal alveolar concentration (MAC) of halothane decreased by approximately 30 percent during in-

duced hypotension, irrespective of the drug used.[83] On return to normotension, MAC returned to control values in dogs given pentolinium or trimethaphan but remained at the hypotensive level in dogs given nitroprusside.[83] These findings have implications in scoliosis surgery. Concentrations of inhalational anesthetics should be reduced during hypotension, or delayed awakening may occur. Similarly, inhaled anesthetics should be turned off sooner if an intraoperative awakening is planned.

Autologous Blood Transfusion in Scoliosis Surgery

Three categories of autologous transfusion can be utilized for scoliosis correction: (1) preoperative blood donation, (2) acute normovolemic hemodilution, and (3) intraoperative or postoperative blood salvage procedures.

Preoperative Autologous Blood Donation

The ideal patient for preoperative autologous blood donation (PABD) is one who is healthy enough to undergo elective surgery, is likely to need a transfusion during or after surgery, has 2 or more weeks before surgery, and has a hemoglobin level greater than 11 g/dl.[84] Some medical centers now accept slightly lower hemoglobin values, especially when there is a strong need for PABD.

PABD is ideally suited for use in adolescents, since isoimmunization during youth can complicate future transfusion needs. Successful PABD programs for orthopedic surgery have been extended to adolescents and to children. However, technical problems and lack of cooperation often make young children unlikely candidates for donation. Withdrawal of amounts equal to 10 to 12 percent of their estimated blood volumes is usually well tolerated.[85] American Association of Blood Bank standards recommend a minimal 4-day interval between phlebotomies, and the last donation should be completed at least 3 days before surgery.[84] The commonly used schedule is one donation per week. The shelf-life of red blood cells with conventional storage can be prolonged to 42 days when additive solutions (Adsol, AS-1) are used; with this extended shelf-life, one donation per week will result in the collection of sufficient amounts of blood before surgery in most patients.

Despite its obvious advantages, PABD also has some disadvantages and limitations. Transient vasovagal reactions occur in 2.5 percent of patients, but a higher incidence is found among first-time donors (13 percent) and female donors.[86] These reactions consist of lightheadedness caused by transient hypotension and bradycardia; in 10 percent of these reactions, patients lose consciousness. It is possible that IV replacement with crystalloids and monitoring of cardiovascular function during preoperative donation may decrease the incidence of reactions. Other disadvantages include delay of the surgical procedure, inconvenience to the patient, and cost. Furthermore, PABD does not completely eliminate the possibility that allogeneic transfusion will be needed, and it is not applicable to patients of the Jehovah's Witnesses faith. Certain controversial issues, such as testing of blood intended for autologous use, release of infectious units, and crossover into the allogeneic blood supply, are still being debated.[87] Contraindications to PABD include bacteremia, decreased oxygen delivery (low fixed cardiac output, anemia, and hypoxemia), and young age because of technical difficulties.

Although PABD provides an inherent and powerful endogenous erythropoietic stimulus to counteract the decrease in hemoglobin levels, the response may not be sufficient to cause maximal marrow erythropoiesis. The ability of recombinant human erythropoietin combined with iron therapy to enhance the procurement of autologous blood is now unquestioned.[88] Studies have shown that red blood cell (RBC) volume donated by patients who received erythropoietin and iron therapy was 40 percent greater than the volume donated by patients who did not receive the therapy.[88] One would expect that procuring more autologous blood before surgery would greatly reduce or even eliminate the need for allogeneic blood transfusion. Erythropoietin is most useful when relatively large donations are needed and when maximal collection of blood is needed in a short period (2 to 3 weeks).

Various regimens for the administration of recombinant erythropoietin have been recommended. Initially, 600 U/kg IV was recommended at each visit for blood collection (twice weekly). This required repeated visits to the hospital. Kulier et al.[89] advocated a single weekly dose of erythropoietin (400 U/kg) given subcutaneously once a week starting 4 weeks before surgery. They found that this simple protocol provided a constant and efficient stimulus for erythropoiesis and adequately compensated for the hemoglobin decrease after the weekly donation.

Acute Normovolemic Hemodilution

Acute normovolemic hemodilution (ANH) refers to the intentional decrease of hemoglobin concentration by withdrawal of a calculated volume of the patient's blood, after anesthetic induction and before critical phases of surgery are started, accompanied by simultaneous replacement with a cell-free substitute to maintain near-normal blood volume. The patient's own fresh blood is reinfused near the end of the surgical procedure after major blood loss has ceased. This technique has been extended to children undergoing spinal fusion and instrumentation.[90, 91] Although moderate ANH to a hematocrit level of 20 percent has been recommended as the lowest acceptable hematocrit, profound hemodilution has been used, especially when avoiding allogeneic blood transfusion is vital. Fontana et al.[92] showed that healthy children undergoing scoliosis surgery can be safely hemodiluted to an average hemoglobin of 3 g/dl without signs of global hypoxia or impairment of global cardiac performance. However, that study was limited to children with normal cardiac function and performed under very controlled conditions. The use of extreme ANH for scoliosis surgery should be limited to specialized centers. The physiologic effects of ANH and techniques are described in Chapter 13.

Combined Deliberate Hypotension and Hemodilution

Because deliberate hypotension can decrease blood loss and ANH minimizes the need for allogeneic blood transfu-
sion, the combination of the two techniques has been advocated.[93] Such combined use requires experience and vigilance and should never be taken lightly.

In adult patients, it was found that when ANH and hypotension were combined, intraoperative allogeneic blood replacement was decreased twofold compared with blood replacement when hypotensive anesthesia was used. Observations with the combined use of the two techniques indicate that cardiac output tends to decrease significantly after ANH when the blood pressure falls below 60 mm Hg. Therefore, it is advisable to limit hypotension and to monitor blood pressure accurately. Short-acting hypotensive drugs are preferable to long-acting drugs so that blood pressure can be easily restored in case of hemodynamic instability. Because decreases in blood pressure can be achieved easily in hemodiluted patients, the dose of hypotensive drug should be decreased to avoid precipitous hypotension.

Animal studies of the hemodynamic responses to the combination of ANH and hypotension have shown that maintenance of oxygen delivery to critical tissue beds may be at risk.[94-96] However, these findings should not detract from the value of the technique. The combination of ANH and controlled hypotension is designed to aid in minimizing blood loss when severe hemorrhage is likely and to avoid massive blood transfusion; both are known to cause a substantial reduction in oxygen delivery. It is probable that decreases in oxygen delivery to critical tissue beds when the combined technique is used are far less than those associated with massive blood loss. These animal studies should lead us to emphasize the importance of preoperative evaluation of these patients, vigilance and experience, use of high FIO_2, and continuous monitoring of arterial pressure, electrocardiogram (ECG), arterial blood gases, blood loss, body temperature, and urine output when hypotension and ANH are combined.[93]

Blood Salvage Procedures

Salvage and reinfusion of blood shed during surgery is the commonest form of autologous blood transfusion.[97-101] Hematologically and biochemically superior to stored blood, salvaged RBCs are immediately available, type-specific, compatible, and normothermic, without the risks associated with allogeneic blood transfusion.[102, 103] The indications for blood salvage in children (weighing >10 kg) include an anticipated blood loss of 20 percent or more of the estimated blood volume, and procedures in which more than 10 percent of patients are transfused with more than one unit.[103, 104] Blood salvage in infants and in small children (<10 kg) is rarely indicated, since an anticipated blood loss of 1 to 1.5 times their estimated blood volume is required before currently available blood salvage procedures are practicable.[104] Recent experience with intraoperative blood salvage for spinal fusion in both adults and children has demonstrated that intraoperative blood salvage alone (or used in conjunction with PABD blood) can significantly reduce perioperative allogeneic blood requirements by about 50 percent.[97-101] Therefore, although blood salvage can sometimes provide all the necessary replacement RBCs during a surgical procedure, it should be considered an adjunct to, rather than a substitute for, allogeneic blood transfusion.

Intraoperatively, blood salvaging is commonly accomplished by cell processing. Shed blood is aspirated from the surgical field, mixed with anticoagulant, and stored in a cardiotomy reservoir. When a sufficient amount of blood has collected, it is pumped into a spinning (approximately 5,000 rpm) centrifuge bowl, which separates blood components on the basis of density. As the bowl fills with higher density RBCs, other constituents of blood are continually displaced and spilled over into the waste container. A wash cycle rinses away all residual contaminants and anticoagulants and suspends the RBCs to any desired hematocrit (usually 50 to 70 percent).[104] The trauma imposed by suction, centrifugation, washing, and reinfusion appears to have negligible effects on RBC survival.[102] For optimal results and safety, a trained operator whose only responsibility is to recycle shed blood should operate these systems.[103–106] Since only 50 to 70 percent of shed RBCs are salvageable and a minimum 250- to 350-ml volume of captured shed blood is necessary to fill a pediatric-sized (125 to 175 ml) centrifuge bowl, blood salvaging is usually practical only in children weighing over 10 kg. Therefore, adequate stores of allogeneic blood should be available for use when RBC harvest through blood salvaging is inadequate.

The volume of blood lost postoperatively can be significant[106] and is salvageable, usually by filtration apparatus. Situated between a vacuum source and the wound drains, a reservoir with an internal 150- to 170-μm filter collects sanguinous wound drainage. This blood is either continuously reinfused or is allowed to collect for a period of time (<6 hours) before reinfusion through a fine filter (10- to 50-μm). Anticoagulation is usually not required, as this blood has been totally defibrinogenated through extensive contact with wound surfaces. Reinfusion of 15 percent of the blood volume of this filtered blood has been shown to be safe.

Since processing removes virtually all blood components except RBCs, colloid or fresh frozen plasma administration may be indicated, particularly during replacement of massive blood loss with salvaged RBCs. Although coagulopathy, characterized by thrombocytopenia, hypofibrinogenemia, and platelet dysfunction, has occurred during autotransfusion of salvaged blood, this is usually associated with massive autotransfusion (>3,000 ml) and is probably the result of dilution of platelets and coagulation factors rather than a consumptive process (i.e., disseminated intravascular coagulation [DIC]).[103–105]

Various contraindications to the use of blood salvage have been suggested. Extravasated blood older than 6 hours and excessively hemolyzed blood should not be reinfused. Shed blood contaminated with bowel contents, malignant cells, microfibrillar collagen hemostat, and wound sterilizing or antibiotic wash solutions should not be salvaged. Many Jehovah's Witnesses patients will not permit the use of blood salvage techniques during orthopedic procedures. Not enough is known about sickle cell disease to suggest these patients as candidates for blood salvage.

Disseminated Intravascular Coagulation

DIC has been reported in a few patients undergoing scoliosis surgery who had normal preoperative coagulation profiles.[107–109] Generalized oozing and sudden massive bleeding occurred soon after decortication of spinous processes and facet joints and obtaining bone grafts. It has been suggested that the massive raw surface secondary to decortication or chipping at the bone, primarily spine or iliac crest, may provide the surface contact needed to stimulate the intrinsic system of the coagulation cascade, thus triggering defibrination. The coagulation profile reveals decreased platelets, plasma coagulation factors, and fibrinogen, in association with elevated fibrin split products. Although washout of coagulation factors by massive replacement may contribute to the abnormal coagulation profile, the sudden onset of bleeding, hypofibrinogenemia, and high fibrin split products all point to defibrination as the cause for the bleeding episode. This type of DIC is self-limited and usually ends with the completion of the operation. Whereas mortality from DIC (due to all causes) in most series is greater than 50 percent, there were no deaths in the orthopedic procedures reported.

The main therapy is adequate replacement to control the hemorrhagic diathesis by using fresh frozen plasma, cryoprecipitate, and platelets, as well as blood.[109] Although heparin has been suggested as a therapeutic modality, it is not recommended in DIC occurring during scoliosis surgery because (1) this type of defibrination is self-limited and is adequately controlled by replacement therapy, (2) the use of heparin carries a significant risk of increased bleeding, and (3) heparin therapy in DIC remains controversial, since there have been no controlled trials supporting its efficacy.

Pharmacologic Enhancement of Hemostatic Activity

In the last decade, drugs that can modulate the coagulation cascade have been introduced to decrease blood loss during major operations. These drugs include desmopressin (DDAVP), aprotinin, tranexamic acid, and ε-aminocaproic acid. In contrast to the plethora of studies demonstrating the transfusion-sparing efficacy of these drugs in cardiac, aortic, knee, and hip operations and orthotopic liver transplantation, only a few studies have focused on the use of DDAVP in scoliosis correction.

Desmopressin is an analogue of the natural hormone vasopressin. Deamination of cysteine in position 1 allows for an increase in the antidiuretic, or V_2 effect. Desmopressin, through its V_2 effects, causes endothelial cells to release von Willebrand's factor, tissue-type plasminogen activator, and certain prostaglandins. An increase in the release of von Willebrand's factor accounts for the hemostatic activity of DDAVP in certain diseases by promoting platelet adhesion to the vascular endothelium. Although it has been reported that a single dose of 10 μg/m^2 of DDAVP after induction of anesthesia could reduce intraoperative bleeding by 30 percent in patients undergoing spinal fusion with normotensive anesthesia,[110] others have found that it does not reduce surgical bleeding in patients without a known bleeding diathesis.[111] In a randomized double-blinded study on 21 pediatric patients who were treated for neuromuscular scoliosis with spinal infusion and instrumentation, there was no difference in blood loss between the group that received DDAVP and the group that did not.[112] Certain side effects of DDAVP, including its vasodilator property and the release of tissue-type plasminogen activator, producing fibrinolysis, may have offset the otherwise beneficial rise in the release of von Willebrand's factor.[111] It is also possible that bleeding from bone is particularly difficult to control and may not be readily influenced by substances that modify hemostasis, since blood vessels in bone are noncollapsible structures and consequently remain open when the bone is cut. Until further studies document the beneficial effects of DDAVP, its routine use during scoliosis surgery should be guarded. Its use can be hazardous because its V_2 effects may worsen the syndrome of inappropriate antidiuretic hormone secretion (SIADH), which may already be present.

Spinal Cord Function and Operative Correction of Scoliosis

A 1975 survey conducted by the Scoliosis Research Society[113] determined that the incidence of acute neurologic complications resulting from the treatment of scoliosis was 0.72 percent in a series of 7,885 cases. However, the report stated that the true incidence is probably higher. A total of 74 major complications involving the spinal cord were reported, one half of them complete paraplegia and one half partial paraplegia.[113] One third recovered completely, one third had partial recovery, and one third had no return of function. In addition, 13 minor complications involving cranial and peripheral nerves were reported. The report also indicated that certain conditions are associated with an increased risk of neurologic injury: kyphosis, severe congenital scoliosis, and preexisting neurologic deficit.[113] Certain procedures also increase the risk of neurologic injury: skeletal traction, spinal osteotomy, and the use of Harrington instrumentation. The prognosis for recovery from spinal cord complications is better for incomplete than for complete lesions, and can be further improved by removing the rod within 3 hours. A survey of spine surgeons in 1987 indicated that 1.84 percent of cases had some form of neurologic injury postoperatively.[25] Injury to the spinal cord was noted in 0.23 percent of cases after Harrington instrumentation; this percentage increased to 0.6 percent for Cotrel-Dubousset instrumentation and to 0.86 percent when sublaminar (Luque) wiring was used. Complete recovery was seen in only 52 percent of the cases, even when cord decompression and/or removal of instrumentation took place; an additional 41 percent had partial improvement.

Blood Supply of the Spinal Cord

The arterial blood supply of the spinal cord in humans is segmental in nature.[114] Three main arteries traverse the length of the cord: a single anterior artery and two posterior arteries. The anterior spinal artery originates from the confluence of two small branches that arise from the vertebral arteries just before the latter join to form the basilar artery. The vessel descends along the anterior surface of the spinal cord and in most patients contains markedly narrowed segments along its course.[114] Occasionally, the anterior spinal artery is completely interrupted at one or more places as it descends on the surface of the cord. The two posterior spinal arteries, which also arise from

the vertebral arteries, descend on the posterior surface of the cord. These vessels are much smaller and play a much less important role as a source of blood supply than the anterior spinal artery. The anterior and posterior spinal arteries intercommunicate through a series of minute circumflex arteries that encircle the cord.

The spinal arteries receive most of the blood in a segmental manner from the radicular arteries, which are the main sources of blood supply to the spinal cord.[114] These arteries arise from the vertebral, ascending cervical, intercostal, lumbar, and iliolumbar arteries. Radicular branches to the anterior spinal artery are the main feeding branches. Usually, there are 4 to 10 large radicular arteries, with at least 1 arising in the cervical, 2 in the thoracic, and 1 in the lumbar region. The largest, located in the lower part of the thoracic and upper part of the lumbar regions, is known as the arteria radicularis magna or artery of Adamkiewicz.[114] This artery originates as a branch of one of the lower intercostal or lumbar arteries, between the levels of T8 and L4 (Fig. 22–8).

The three functional zones of the spinal cord are the cervical enlargement, which is essentially ganglionic; the thoracic zone, in which the longitudinal tracts (white matter) predominate; and the region of the lumbar enlargement, essentially ganglionic.[125] The ganglionic areas of the cord are metabolically more active than the white matter

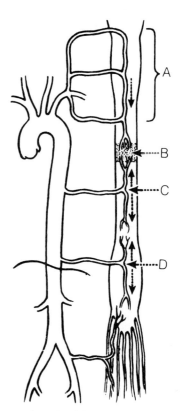

FIGURE 22–8. Arterial supply of the spinal cord. *A,* Cervical and upper thoracic cord supplied by radicular branches of vertebral, ascending cervical, and superior intercostal arteries. *B,* Watershed. *C,* Midthoracic cord supplied from a single intercostal artery. *D,* Thoracolumbar region supplied by a large vessel near the diaphragm (arteria magna) and cauda equina supplied from lower lumbar, iliolumbar, and lateral sacral arteries, which occasionally also supply the distal part of the cord. (From Pasternak BM, Boyd DP, Ellis FH: Spinal cord injury after procedures on the aorta. Surg Gynecol Obstet 135:29, 1972, with permission.)

area and are more richly supplied with blood vessels.[115] The number and size of the cervical and lumbar feeders are greater than those in the thoracic cord, which depends largely on proximal and distal sources for its blood supply. For this reason the thoracic cord circulation has been described as a "watershed," and it is in this region that the vascular supply is least generous.[115] This critical zone extends from T4 to T9, and it is at these levels that special care should be taken during surgery. Narrow segments or even complete interruption of the artery can be found in the areas between the major radicular arteries in these watershed zones. The anastomoses across the watershed zones are poor whenever the arteria radicularis magna has an infrarenal origin; blood flow to the cord depends, in these situations, on the many well-distributed radicular vessels (Fig. 22–8).[114, 115]

There is a misconception that preserving the artery of Adamkiewicz ensures the integrity of the blood supply of the spinal cord.[115] There are several other medullary feeder arteries at various levels, and these may be equally important in maintaining the circulation of the cord. Dwyer and Schafer[34] have reported anterior spinal fusion procedures in which 4 to 16 segmental arteries (thoracic and lumbar) were ligated without ill effects. It is to the preservation of the three longitudinal arterial trunks that the efforts of the spinal surgeon should be directed, in order to prevent neurologic deficit, as total ischemia results in irreversible damage accompanied by central necrosis.[34, 115]

The canine SCBF exhibits well-functioning autoregulation between mean pressures of 50 and 150 mm Hg (Fig. 22–9).[41, 116] This allows normal function of spinal cord energy metabolism in the face of decreased arterial pressure. Above and below the autoregulation range, SCBF becomes directly dependent on the perfusion pressure. Spinal cord injury may lead to impairment or loss of this autoregulation. In this situation, hypotension may further compromise SCBF. Similar to cerebral blood flow, SCBF is highly sensitive to changes in Pa_{CO_2}.[41]

Monitoring Spinal Cord Function During Spinal Fusion and Instrumentation

Early warning of potential damage to the spinal cord is highly desirable. Three methods are currently available. In 1973, Vauzelle et al.[117] described waking the patient during the operation to test motor function. That same year, Hardy et al.[118] described monitoring somatosensory cortical evoked potentials. Recently, the monitoring of motor evoked potentials has been introduced.

Intraoperative Awakening

The method commonly used is a modification of that of Vauzelle and associates, in which an opioid and/or an inhalational agent/nitrous oxide/relaxant anesthetic technique is used and the patient is awakened after the rod (or rods) are placed, and asked to move the feet on command.[119] Patients should be informed about the procedure during the preanesthetic visit. They are told that when the rod is in place they will be awakened momentarily and asked to move their hands and then their feet, and that as soon as they do so they will be reanesthetized. They are also informed that they probably will not remember the event and that, even if they do, they will not feel pain.[119]

The start of the awakening process depends on good communication between the surgeon and the anesthesiologist. At least 20 minutes of advance warning before the wake-up test is desirable so that no additional opioids or relaxants are given in the interim. If an inhalational anesthetic is being used, it is discontinued at least 10 minutes before the desired time of awakening, while nitrous oxide is continued. In this regard, sevoflurane and desflurane may result in faster awakening than halothane or isoflurane, by virtue of their lower blood-gas partition coefficients. If deliberate hypotension is used, it may be necessary to turn off the inhaled anesthetic even sooner. When it is time to perform the test, nitrous oxide is turned off and the patient ventilated with 100 percent oxygen.

We do not routinely give reversal drugs. If the muscle relaxant has been given appropriately, and particularly after the introduction of short- and intermediate-acting muscle relaxants given by either IV infusion techniques or intermittent injection, the patient should have sufficient muscle strength to perform the test. If needed, small increments of atropine and edrophonium can be given. We do not wait for or require the resumption of spontaneous respiration, although in most patients spontaneous respiration returns within 5 minutes. Similarly, the use of opioids in appropriate amounts and timing usually negates the need for their reversal. If it becomes necessary to reverse the respiratory depressant effect of the opioids, naloxone in increments of 0.02 to 0.04 mg can be given. The dose of naloxone is kept small so that it does not completely reverse the analgesic and sedative effects of the opioid. Another approach is to use small doses of doxapram 0.25 to 0.5 mg/kg, up to 1 to 1.5 mg/kg for its analeptic effects.[120]

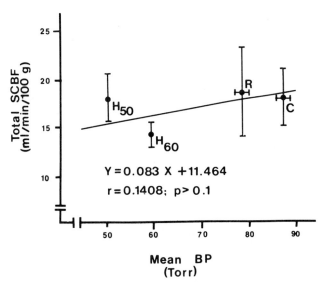

$$Y = 0.083 \, X + 11.464$$
$$r = 0.1408; \; p > 0.1$$

FIGURE 22–9. Linear regression analysis indicating independence of total spinal cord blood flow (SCBF) against mean arterial blood pressure (BP) for 44 data pairs. Regression equation, correlation coefficient, and p value are shown. H_{50}, MAP 50 mm Hg; H_{60}, MAP 60 mm Hg; R, reestablishment of normotension; C, control blood pressure. (From Jacobs HK, Lieponis JV, Bunch WH, et al: The influence of halothane and nitroprusside on canine spinal cord hemodynamics. Spine 7:35, 1982, with permission.)

This is almost always effective and tends to provide a less abrupt and stormy wake-up. It is important that the patient should not be too awake and that the anesthesiologist, with the help of an assistant, hold the head and arms in place. Excessive struggling may result in tracheal extubation and may jeopardize the fixation of the rods.

The intraoperative awakening test is a gross test of spinal motor function.[117, 119] It is unreliable in patients with paresis of the lower limbs, uncooperative patients, the mentally retarded, and the very young. However, this simple test makes it possible to identify patients at risk at the earliest possible moment and to ensure that the opportunity for recovery of neural function is optimal. In a study of 166 consecutive patients, three were discovered to have a neural deficiency when they were awakened intraoperatively.[119] These deficits disappeared immediately on release of the distracting force. In one series of 150 patients who were questioned retrospectively about their anesthetic experience, only 12 remembered awakening and none had any pain during the test period.[119]

The actual wake-up process must be rehearsed sequentially at least the day before surgery and again on the morning of surgery. It is preferable to have the same person rehearse and perform the wake-up test with the patient, using the same vocal inflection and word sequence. The sequence usually followed states, "[Name]—it's time for the wake-up test. Squeeze my hand. Harder. Now let go. Now move your feet [or toes] up and down. Now move your feet in and out like windshield wipers. Very good. Now don't move, and go back to sleep." It is important that the surgeons stop all painful manipulations when the test is being attempted, since pain may contribute to possible recall. Just as significantly, moreover, it can disrupt the wake-up test by causing the patient to react with confusing, random, nonpurposeful movements. An observer must be stationed under the drapes at the patient's feet to observe and report movements. The room should be comparatively quiet (e.g., radio off) so that communication between the anesthesiologist and patient, as well as between the anesthesiologist and surgeons and the anesthesiologist and observer ("he's moving his feet up and down now") is enhanced. Good hand control should be established before the patient is asked to move the feet. If there is a definite absence or weakness of movement of one or both feet, but the patient can move both hands on command, an attempt can still be made to improve both motor power and wakefulness over the next few minutes. If there is failure to improve, the distraction of the rod is decreased and the test is repeated. On completion of the test, the patient is quickly reanesthetized with thiopental (1 to 1.5 mg/kg) or propofol (0.5 to 0.75 mg/kg) and nitrous oxide is restarted. Midazolam can be given for amnesia. Additional opioids can be given and the inhalational anesthetic is resumed.

When a non–English-speaking patient requires a wake-up test, one of three methods can be employed: (1) an appropriate translator is brought into the operating room, (2) the words for the wake-up test are written out in transliteration (e.g., by an English-speaking friend or relative of the patient), and (3) a tape recording can be used. We have used a familiar voice (e.g., mother, father) speaking in their native tongue directly to the patient in a personal manner with good results.

Ankle Clonus Test

In addition to the wake-up test and monitoring of somatosensory evoked potentials, a third test to evaluate the integrity of the spinal cord during scoliosis surgery has been proposed. Although not yet in widespread use, the ankle clonus test has been recommended as a test with both high sensitivity and high specificity.[121] The ankle clonus test is performed bilaterally by applying rapid dorsiflexion to the feet, followed by an eased dorsiflexion that is sustained for a period of time. Rhythmic gastrocnemius contractions and the resultant plantar flexion are a normal response for a brief time, early in the recovery phase from general anesthesia. However, they are not found in the normal awake patient, except possibly in some patients with neuromuscular scolioisis.

Following curve correction, at the same time that a wake-up test might be performed, the clonus test is initiated. It must be done continuously as anesthesia is lightened, to ensure that this transient occurrence is not overlooked. Any clonus, even a few beats, are considered a normal response indicating spinal cord integrity. The complete absence of transient ankle clonus, called a positive result, represents a possible neurologic deficit, and should be followed by a wake-up test. Continuous monitoring of somatosensory evoked potentials is also recommended for maximum safety.

Sensory Evoked Potentials

Compared to the electroencephalogram (EEG), which is a collection of spontaneous electrical potentials generated by the cerebral cortex, sensory evoked potentials (SEPs) are specific electrical potentials generated by the CNS in response to brief discrete sensory stimuli. These potentials reflect the functional integrity of the afferent sensory pathways from the stimulation site to the sensory cortex.[122, 123] SEPs are obtained by stimulating a peripheral sensory nerve and recording the resultant electrical potentials at various sites along the sensory pathways. Because of the very low amplitude of SEPs (0.1 to 20 μV), it is not usually possible to distinguish them from the background EEG activity. To extract SEPs from the EEG, computer signal averaging or summation is used. SEPs have been defined as near-field and far-field potentials, cortical and subcortical (arising from the spinal cord and brain stem) potentials, short and long latency potentials, primary cortical and secondary cortical potentials, and initial and delayed waves.

From 100 to more than 1,000 successive responses can be averaged to produce a tracing that represents time (in milliseconds) versus voltage (in microvolts). SEPs are quantitated by measuring the poststimulus latency and interpeak amplitude in the waveform. Deflections below the baseline are labeled positive (P) and those above the baseline are labeled negative (N). Standard identification of waveforms is by a letter designating the direction of deflection (P or N), followed by a number representing the poststimulus latency of the waveform. Normal values should be established for each laboratory and may differ slightly from those of other laboratories. SEPs used for diagnostic procedures and perioperative monitoring include somatosensory evoked potentials (SSEPs), brain stem auditory evoked potentials (BAEPs), and visual evoked potentials (VEPs). For monitoring spinal cord function during scoliosis correction, SSEPs are used. The pathways involved in the generation of SSEPs include sensory nerves with their cell bodies in the dorsal root ganglia and central processes traveling rostrally in the ipsilateral dorsal column of the spinal cord, synapsing in the dorsal column nuclei at the cervicomedullary region; second-order fibers crossing to the contralateral thalamus via the medial lemniscus; and third-order fibers to the frontoparietal sensory cortex.

The commonest peripheral sensory nerves stimulated are the median and posterior tibial nerves. The nerves are stimulated with a surface electrode using monopolar, constant current, square-wave pulses of 0.2 to 2 msec duration at a rate between 1 and 2 Hz. The stimuli are set to produce visible but painless stimulation at 20 mA. For recording SSEPs after median nerve stimulation, recording electrodes are placed at Erb's point (just above the clavicle overlying the brachial plexus), at the posterior midline of the neck at C2, and on the scalp overlying the contralateral sensory cortex. With posterior tibial nerve stimulation, electrodes are placed over the lower lumbar spine and the contralateral cortex. Subcortical SSEPs are recorded by electrodes placed into bone ligaments or in the epidural space during surgery.

Normally, after median nerve stimulation, certain peaks representing specific neural generators are observed: N9 (brachial plexus at Erb's point); N11 (posterior columns or spinal roots); N13/P13 (dorsal column nuclei); N14, 15 (brain stem or thalamus); and N19/P22 (parietal sensory cortex). With posterior tibial nerve stimulation, absolute latencies are increased because of the longer distance the stimuli must traverse. The initial cortical wave after posterior tibial nerve stimulation usually occurs at 30 to 40 msec. Interpeak latencies can be used to assess central conduction times.

Various pharmacologic, physiologic, and pathologic factors, as well as instrumentation, influence SSEPs.

Pharmacologic Factors

Inhalational anesthetics have similar effects on cortical SSEPs.[123, 124] A dose-dependent increase in latency (reflecting an increase in conduction time) and a decrease in amplitude have been observed with all inhalational anesthetics. However, up to 0.5 to 1 MAC of an inhalation anesthetic in the presence of nitrous oxide is compatible with adequate monitoring of cortical SSEPs (Fig. 22–10). Since subcortical potentials are less affected by anesthetics compared with cortical potentials, there has been an increasing tendency to monitor subcortical rather than cortical SSEPs intraoperatively. Nitrous oxide 50 percent, alone or in combination with an opioid or inhalational anesthetic, causes decreases in amplitude without changes in latency. The following points need to be emphasized if inhalational anesthetics are used during SSEP monitoring[123]: (1) Higher concentrations cause disappear-

ance of the waveform and, therefore, should be avoided; (2) individual variations exist, and it is possible to observe elimination of the waveform at low concentrations in some patients and preservation of the waveform at higher concentrations in others; and (3) anesthetic concentrations should not be altered during critical periods if SSEPs are to reflect changes resulting from operative manipulations.

Thiopental causes a dose-dependent increase in latency and a decrease in amplitude of waveforms during SSEP monitoring.[123, 125, 126] Changes in cortical or "later" potentials are more pronounced than changes in subcortical or "earlier" potentials. This may be related to the preferential effect of barbiturates on synaptic transmission rather than axonal conduction. Adequate SSEP monitoring, however, can be achieved with doses of thiopental far in excess of those that produce an isoelectric EEG. Propofol increases latency similar to the barbiturates, but has minimal effects on amplitude. Both etomidate and ketamine produce an increase in amplitude of SSEPs (Fig. 22–11).[127, 128] This effect has been exploited to enhance cortical SSEP monitoring and detection of intraoperative events that affect spinal cord function. Whereas etomidate causes an increase in latency, ketamine has no effect. However, when nitrous oxide is added, the ketamine-enhanced cortical amplitude is reduced by approximately 50 percent.[128] Midazolam results in a decrease in amplitude without a change in latency.

Although the effect of opioid drugs on SSEPs may be similar to that of inhalational anesthetics and barbiturates, the magnitude of change is minimal. Higher doses of opioids are compatible with reproducible SSEPs.[123, 129] Therefore, it is possible to monitor cortical SSEPs with the use of up to 60 μg/kg of fentanyl. Meperidine results in an increase in latency but, unlike other opioids, may cause an increase in amplitude.[130] Droperidol tends to cause an increase in latency and a decrease in amplitude.[131] Despite the ability to monitor SSEP accurately while a relatively high dose of opioids is used, bolus doses of opioids and other sedatives should be avoided during critical stages of surgery to exclude the effects of these drugs on SSEPs and thus ascertain the influence of surgical intervention on spinal cord function.[123] Table 22–4 summarizes the effect of anesthetic drugs on SSEPs.

Physiologic Factors

Various physiologic factors, including blood pressure, Pao$_2$, pH, hematocrit, and temperature, can influence SSEPs.[123, 132, 133] These changes are brought about by decreases in cerebral or SCBF, decreases in oxygen delivery, or increases in oxygen consumption by the neural structures. The changes seem to be more pronounced in cortical than in subcortical SSEPs. A decrease in mean arterial pressure below the autoregulation level, caused by blood loss or hypotensive drugs, results in a progressive decrease in amplitude until the waveform disappears without a change in latency. Similarly, hypoxemia adversely affects SSEPs.[133] At hematocrits below 15 percent, isovolemic hemodilution causes progressive increases in latency and variable changes in amplitude.[123, 134] Hypothermia leads to increases in latency and decreases in amplitude. Loss of waveforms occurs at 25 degrees to 27 degrees C.[123, 135]

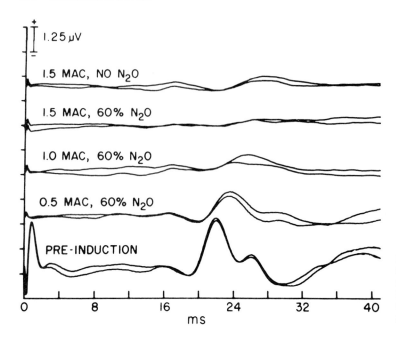

1.25 μV

1.5 MAC, NO N₂O

1.5 MAC, 60% N₂O

1.0 MAC, 60% N₂O

0.5 MAC, 60% N₂O

PRE-INDUCTION

ms

FIGURE 22–10. Representative SSEP cortical responses (C-3′ or C-4″ - FPz) at various MAC levels of isoflurane with 60 percent nitrous oxide, and at 1.5 MAC without nitrous oxide. (From Peterson DO, Drummond JC, Todd MM: Effects of halothane, enflurane, isoflurane, and nitrous oxide on somatosensory evoked potentials in humans. Anesthesiology 65:35, 1986.)

Hyperthermia is also accompanied by decreases in amplitude and loss of waveforms at 42 degrees C.[123] Cold or warm fluids used to irrigate the brain or spinal cord can cause changes in SSEPs in the presence of normal core temperature; therefore, irrigating fluids should be warmed to body temperature before use.[136]

Pathologic Factors/Instrumentation

Injury along pathways involved in the generation of evoked potentials or impairment of their blood supply will result in abnormal SSEPs. In normotensive cats, spinal distraction to the point of marked alterations in evoked

response caused a 50 percent decrease in SCBF at and caudal to the distraction site.[137] Additional distraction produced total abolition of SCBF at the distraction site and for a considerable distance rostral and caudal to it.[137]

With the popularity of induced hypotension for the correction of scoliosis, there has been concern that hypotension may decrease SCBF and predispose the spinal cord to injury, particularly when it is distracted during instrumentation.[41, 138] What may be an insignificant decrease in perfusion pressure to most of the spinal cord could represent a marked reduction in the perfusion pressure in the watershed zones. It has been suggested that the effects of hypotension and direct pressure on the spinal cord are

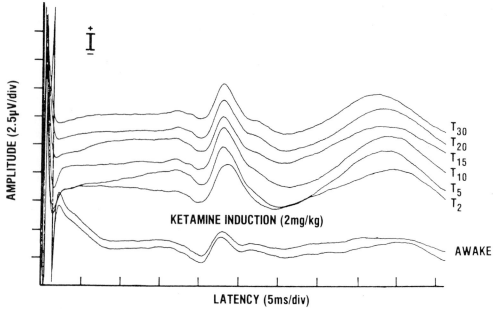

FIGURE 22–11. Example of SSEP wave forms before and after induction with ketamine. (From Schubert A, Licina MG, Lineberry PJ: The effect of ketamine on human somatosensory evoked potentials and its modification by nitrous oxide. Anesthesiology 72:33, 1990.)

TABLE 22–4
ANESTHETIC DRUG EFFECTS ON SOMATOSENSORY EVOKED POTENTIALS

Drug	Latency	Amplitude
Sevoflurane, desflurane, isoflurane, enflurane, halothane	↑	↓
Barbiturates, droperidol, diazepam	↑	↓
Propofol	↑	0
Fentanyl, morphine	↑	↓
Sufentanil, alfentanil	0	↓
Meperidine	↑	↑ ↓
Nitrous oxide, midazolam	0	↓
Etomidate	↑	↑
Ketamine	0	↑

↑, increased; ↓, decreased; 0, no change. See text for details.

additive in producing impairment of spinal cord function. In anesthetized cats, neither spinal cord compression nor reduction of the aortic pressure (by clamping the thoracic aorta) altered spinal cord function when these were applied individually.[138] However, when both procedures were applied simultaneously, spinal cord function, as evidenced by changes in SSEPs, was reversibly altered.[138] Hypotension worsened the effects of compression, and intentional hypertension reversed SSEP changes caused by compression. In a feline distraction model, SSEP changes occurred at less distraction during deliberate hypotension than during normotension, suggesting ischemia as the main mechanism of injury.[139]

In a canine model, sodium nitroprusside-induced hypotension initially decreased SCBF, but the flow returned to normal by 30 minutes.[140] Spinal distraction applied during sodium nitroprusside- or nitroglycerin-induced hypotension did not reduce SCBF. In contrast, trimethaphan decreased SCBF throughout the entire hypotensive period.[141] Although the superimposed distraction did not lead to further reduction in SCBF, that study suggested that trimethaphan may not be the drug of choice for deliberate hypotension during scoliosis surgery, despite its apparently favorable hemodynamic and hormonal responses.[141] Cautious extrapolation of these findings to the clinical setting is advisable, as the effects of trimethaphan may be different in humans.

Changes in SSEPs at systemic pressures within the normal range have been observed in patients undergoing spinal distraction.[123] These changes resolved with slight increases of blood pressure. Ponte[142] reported that, in two patients who developed paraplegia after hypercorrection of scoliosis, partial recovery of neurologic function occurred when blood was infused to correct hypovolemic hypotension in preparation for removal of Harrington rods. These reports do not document any deleterious effects of well-conducted induced normovolemic hypotension on spinal cord function during scoliosis correction. However, they emphasize that hemorrhagic hypotension could result in a severe reduction in SCBF and alteration of spinal cord function; spinal distraction (even without hypotension) may result in alteration of spinal cord function; changes in SSEPs noted during hypotension may return to normal after increases in blood pressure; and monitoring spinal cord function is essential whenever the spinal cord

is potentially at risk for injury or interruption of its blood supply.[121]

SSEP Monitoring During Scoliosis Surgery

Equipment for recording SSEPs provides a display of data on an oscilloscope and also storage and printing of such data. However, inadequate intraoperative SSEPs have been reported to occur in 0 to 41 percent of patients.[122, 123] These problems are related to artifacts and electrical interference, abnormal preoperative SSEPs, inaccessible sites for stimulation and recordings, and sensitivity of cortical SSEPs to various physiologic and pharmacologic factors.

A common system of SSEP monitoring during scoliosis surgery involves stimulation of at least two sensory nerves, one above and one below the area of potential spinal cord injury. The posterior tibial nerve at the ankle and the median nerve at the wrist are often utilized.[122, 123, 143] SSEP changes related to depth of anesthesia should be seen in both posterior tibial and median nerve stimulation. However, injury to the spinal cord during posterior fusion and instrumentation alters SSEPs evoked by stimulating the posterior tibial nerve, whereas those induced by stimulating the median nerve remain unchanged. Impulses along the dorsal column are sensitive to anterior spinal artery ischemia even though their blood supply arises from the posterior spinal arteries.[144] Traumatic myelopathy usually affects multiple tracts, and therefore SSEPs often reflect the degree of injury. Because the blood supply to the dorsal column is primarily from the posterior spinal arteries and that of the anterior motor tracts is predominantly from the anterior spinal artery, concerns have been raised about the validity of using SSEP monitoring to assess the viability of the motor tracts.

The reliance on SSEPs is based on the assumption that impairment of motor function is unlikely to occur in the absence of changes in SSEPs.[120] However, there are reports documenting cases in which SSEPs were judged to be normal or insignificantly altered, and yet the patients awakened with motor deficits.[123, 145–147] Since the potential exists for failure to identify isolated motor damage during spinal surgery, SSEPs may never replace the wake-up test as an index of motor viability. In fact, the combined use of the wake-up test and SSEP monitoring has been advocated in some centers, as neither test alone is totally reliable.

SSEP monitoring has the following advantages over intraoperative awakening: it can be performed continually; the risks introduced by awakening the patient, such as dislodgment of the tracheal tube, dislocation of orthopedic instrumentation, and air embolism with deep inspiration, are avoided; and it can be performed in uncooperative, mentally retarded children, those with muscle paresis of the lower limbs, and those with a language barrier. Furthermore, recordings can be made repeatedly, both intraoperatively and postoperatively, and can be compared with preanesthetic recordings.

Intraoperative changes in SSEPs (decreased amplitude, increased latency, and loss of waveform) indicate surgical trespass or spinal cord ischemia (Fig. 22–12).[123, 146, 148] These changes should warn the surgeon and anesthesiologist either to lessen the degree of spinal distraction or to improve the SCBF. SSEP changes have been noted in 2.5 to 65 percent of patients undergoing surgical procedures on the spine or spinal cord.[123] When these changes were reversed by surgical or anesthetic interventions, the patients had preserved neurologic function postoperatively. Both false-negative and false-positive results have been reported with SSEP monitoring; patients with intact SSEPs intraoperatively had new postoperative neurologic deficits, and patients with substantial intraoperative SSEP changes had normal postoperative neurologic function.[149] Nevertheless, the reliability of SSEP monitoring for prediction of postoperative neurologic outcome has been regarded as excellent.[122, 123]

The reliability of SSEPs for detection of intraoperative neurologic dysfunction during scoliosis surgery has been widely accepted.[144, 149] One study examined 395 patients in whom SSEP monitoring was attempted during surgery on the spinal cord or spinal column.[150] Of these patients, 105 underwent spinal instrumentation for scoliosis. One third of the patients showed SSEP changes intraoperatively, although some of these changes were technical in nature. The highest percentage of SSEP changes occurred

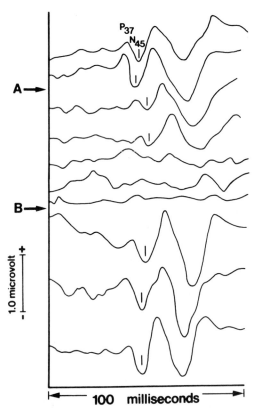

FIGURE 22–12. Serial SSEP tracings illustrating altered spinal cord function during anterior cervical spinal fusion. The tracings were taken during posterior tibial nerve stimulation from beginning of surgery (*top*) through surgical closure (*bottom*). *A,* Complete loss of recognizable cortical evoked responses is seen after placement of anterior neck retractor. *B,* These responses return after replacement of the retractor. The monitoring peaks of interest are marked by P_{37} and N_{45}. (From Sloan TB, Ronai AK, Kohte A: Reversible loss of somatosensory evoked potentials during anterior certical spinal fusion. Anesth Analg 65:96, 1986, with permission.)

in scoliosis patients. In 14 cases, surgically induced SSEP changes were reversed without neurologic sequelae, but eight other cases had irreversible SSEP changes and suffered neurologic deficits. Of the eight, three were patients undergoing scoliosis surgery.

Motor Evoked Potentials

The limitations of the intraoperative wake-up test have led investigators to explore the possibilities of monitoring motor evoked potentials (MEPs).[155] This would be highly desirable in surgery close to the spinal cord, in conjunction with SSEPs. Compared to SSEPs, which monitor primarily the ascending sensory tracts, MEPs assess the functional integrity of the descending motor tracts and pathways. MEPs can be produced by direct (epidural) or indirect (transosseous) stimulation of the motor neurons in the spinal cord and brain, respectively. Transosseous stimulation can be accomplished by electrical or magnetic means. Transcranial magnetic stimulation (TMS) is performed by placing a magnetic coil over the motor cortex. Impulses descend through the ventral motor tracts, producing contralateral peripheral nerve potentials, electromyographic action potentials, or visible limb movements. TMS is noninvasive, painless, does not require direct contact with the scalp, and is probably without hazards. Current guidelines for TMS recommend intermittent rather than continuous stimulation, and cautious use in patients with a history of seizures, skull lesions or fractures, patients with implantable devices (pacemakers), and patients with central venous catheters.[152]

Various studies have demonstrated that, compared with SSEPs, MEPs are markedly depressed by inhalational anesthetics.[153–155] Even 70 percent nitrous oxide produces significant alterations in MEPs, including threshold elevation, amplitude depression, and delay in latency.[154] However, in concentrations of less than 50 percent, nitrous oxide is compatible with MEP monitoring. Findings similar to those of the effect of inhalational anesthetics have been noted in the presence of nonpharmacologic factors, including spinal cord compression, distraction, or ischemic injury. MEP changes also occur with hypoxemia, hypotension, and hypothermia. This may be related to the unique sensitivity of motor neurons or motor-dependent facilitatory circuits to structural or metabolic insults.

Anesthetic and other adjuvant drugs with central inhibitory action (thiopental, propofol, and midazolam) tend to cause marked changes in MEPs and therefore should be carefully titrated. Although the combination of droperidol and low-dose fentanyl (or other opioids) produces noticeable changes in MEP threshold, amplitude, and latency, MEP monitoring is feasible.[156] Careful titration of a continuous infusion tends to alleviate the magnitude of MEP alterations commonly seen with bolus injections of opioids.

Anesthetic drugs with a central excitatory effect, such as ketamine and etomidate, exert a less adverse effect on MEPs compared with those that have a central depressant action.[157, 158] In primates receiving ketamine 15 and 35 mg/kg, amplitude depression and latency prolongation were noted but without any changes in brain stimulation threshold. However, measurable MEPs can be recorded with high doses of ketamine (up to 50 mg/kg) and etomidate.

The use of these drugs has proved advantageous for intraoperative MEP monitoring.

In addition to ketamine and etomidate, all other intravenous anesthetic drugs have been utilized for anesthesia, while allowing the successful monitoring of MEPs. Some drugs, however, seem to preserve MEPs more effectively than others. A continuous infusion of either methohexital or etomidate preserved MEPs better than propofol or thiopental.[159] However, in another study, even propofol allowed successful monitoring of MEPs in 86 percent of cases.[160] A combination of intravenous anesthetics was noted to improve the elicitation of distinct MEPs from 8 percent (1 of 13 patients) obtained with nitrous oxide and isoflurane to 88 percent (15 of 17 patients) with propofol and alfentanil.[161]

Neuromuscular blocking drugs obviously affect electromyographic responses. However, by continuous infusion techniques using short-acting muscle relaxants such as atracurium or mivacurium and preservation of one to two twitches in a train-of-four, reliable MEPs can be monitored.

Anesthetic Regimen for Intraoperative MEP Recording

The marked influence of anesthetic drugs on MEPs demands the use of a rather rigid protocol.[162] The regimen described below has been used with success in some centers for simultaneous monitoring of MEPs and SSEPs. Such a protocol has helped to expand the use of MEP monitoring during scoliosis surgery.

Premedication should be light or avoided. For induction of anesthesia, short-acting drugs and short- or intermediate-acting muscle relaxants are used. As supplemental drugs, alfentanil 0.005 to 0.02 mg/kg or equivalent doses of other short-acting opioids can be added. Maintenance of anesthesia is performed with less than 50 percent nitrous oxide and/or inhalational anesthetic of less than 0.25 MAC. Continuous infusion of etomidate 0.01 to 0.02 mg/kg/min, ketamine 0.03 to 0.09 mg/kg/min, or propofol 0.1 to 0.2 mg/kg/min can be used. Alfentanil 0.02 to 0.1 mg/kg/h or equivalent doses of other short-acting opioids are used. Muscle relaxant infusion (atracurium or mivacurium) can be used to maintain at least one twitch in the train-of-four.

Anesthetics should be discontinued 30 to 45 minutes before monitoring and anesthesia maintained with etomidate and/or ketamine infusion using a minimum dose. Two to three twitches in the train-of-four can be maintained by titrating the infusion. A titratable infusion of droperidol–fentanyl is another alternative; fentanyl dose is limited to a minimum. Hypertension and tachycardia can be avoided or treated by nitroglycerin and esmolol infusions.

Preanesthetic Assessment

Accurate preoperative assessment of the cardiovascular, respiratory, neuromuscular, and renal systems is important. An increased association of scoliosis in children with congenital heart disease is well documented.[26] In children with congenital cardiac disease, there is a 12 percent incidence of scoliosis with deformities; this is three times more common in patients with cyanotic heart disease. The incidence of mitral valve prolapse in patients with scoliosis is about 25 to 28 percent, compared with 0.3 to 10 percent in the overall childhood population.[163, 164] Antibiotic prophylaxis may be indicated in some of these patients. Certain other congenital deformities, particularly those of the upper limbs and genitourinary systems, seem to have a specific association with scoliosis.[19]

A careful history of birth, growth, and development often gives an indication of the presence of congenital anomalies and other conditions from which the patient is suffering, such as neurofibromatosis and neuromuscular disease. A history of drug therapy is important. Steps should be taken to correct coagulation defects before surgery. Unless otherwise indicated, acetylsalicylic acid should be discontinued 1 week before surgery. A history of previous spinal fusion should alert the anesthesiologist to the possibility of profuse bleeding during a second operation. A history suggestive of respiratory failure and cardiac disease should be sought. Findings such as pigeon chest, elongated fingers, and ocular changes are suggestive of Marfan syndrome. In patients with cardiac disease, the cardiovascular system may be evaluated by a cardiologist and echocardiography may be indicated. A neurologic examination should be performed and any deficits recorded. Technical problems that might influence the management of anesthesia (e.g., use of a body cast or traction) should be noted, and a plan should be formulated that takes these problems into consideration. Anatomic problems that might interfere with tracheal intubation should be sought. Special techniques that have been described for patients with a difficult airway may be required.[165]

A quantitative estimate of the severity of scoliosis is necessary. Laboratory investigations are dependent on the severity of the associated medical conditions, as well as the severity of the scoliosis. Healthy children with idiopathic scoliosis might only require a complete blood count (CBC). However, laboratory workup for children with medical disorders should be more extensive. In addition to a CBC, their clinical conditions may warrant a urinalysis, electrocardiogram (ECG), chest radiograph, coagulation profile, creatine phosphokinase (CPK), serum glutamic pyruvate transaminase (SGPT) and serum glutamic-oxaloacetic transaminase (SGOT) liver enzyme studies, blood urea nitrogen (BUN), and creatinine for renal evaluation, as well as pulmonary functions tests. Pulmonary function tests should include vital capacity, forced expiratory volume and its derivatives, response to aerosol bronchodilators, and resting arterial blood gases. Pulmonary physiotherapy can be started several days before surgery when the need for postoperative respiratory support is anticipated. In very young or retarded children, pulmonary function tests may be impossible to obtain.[166] In such cases, a careful history eliciting information about exercise tolerance is mandated. Additional tests can be performed, as necessary. Allen's test is performed to assess the adequacy of circulation to the hand before arterial cannulation.

Psychological preparation is of the utmost importance. If intraoperative awakening is planned, it should be fully explained to the patient. The exact sequence of commands and movements of the hands and feet should be rehearsed during the preanesthetic visit. If postoperative ventilatory support is a possibility, the patient is told what to expect. The patient is informed about the oral or nasal endotracheal tube, inability to talk, and mechanical ventilation. The plans for reduction of blood loss and blood replacement are responsibilities shared by the anesthesia and orthopedic teams. Although a combination of blood-saving methods has an augmentative effect in decreasing the use of allogeneic blood, the anesthesia and surgical teams should use those techniques with which they are most experienced.[97] An adequate amount of compatible blood should be available before surgery. The choice of premedicant drugs depends on the anesthesiologist's preference, the condition of the patient, and the anesthetic technique. Anticholinergic drugs can be omitted or reduced if deliberate hypotension is planned, to avoid tachycardia. Relative contraindications to deliberate hypotension include a marked reduction in the delivery of oxygen to the tissues (anemia, low fixed cardiac output, low oxygen saturation); sickle cell disease or uncorrected polycythemia; and cerebral, renal, or cardiac disease (right-to-left intracardiac shunt). The patient may be admitted to the hospital before surgery or may arrive to the hospital on the day of surgery.

Anesthetic Management and Postoperative Care

Anesthesia for posterior spinal fusion is preferably induced with the patient on the transport stretcher rather than on the operating table. Most older children prefer IV induction of anesthesia. Drugs that tend to raise the arterial pressure (e.g., ketamine) should be avoided. Even in the absence of specific contraindications to succinylcholine (e.g., patients who are paralyzed, those with neurologic or neuromuscular disease, and those known or suspected to have malignant hyperthermia), most anesthesiologists prefer to use a nondepolarizing drug for both tracheal intubation and the maintenance of muscle paralysis. Atracurium in a dose of 0.5 mg/kg IV or vecuronium in a dose of 0.1 to 0.15 mg/kg IV allows tracheal intubation in less than 3 minutes, whereas rocuronium (0.6 to 0.9 mg/kg IV) results in good intubating conditions in less than 90 seconds. Continuous infusion or repeated intermittent boluses of these drugs can be used for maintenance of muscle relaxation. It is important to maintain adequate muscle relaxation during the operation because increases in muscle tone can raise venous pressure and increase bleeding. As some of these patients are children who prefer or require a mask induction of anesthesia, the dose of relaxant can be reduced when moderately deep levels of inhalational agent have been achieved. A tracheal tube of an appropriate size is placed, its position confirmed, and then taped securely. Suctioning of salivary secretions from the mouth and pharynx, and the application of tincture of benzoin or other adhesive, help to prevent loosening of the tape around the tube when the patient is turned to the prone position.

Two anesthetic techniques have been popularized for scoliosis surgery: an opioid/nitrous oxide/oxygen/relaxant technique or an inhalational anesthetic in oxygen, with or without nitrous oxide, opioid, and relaxants. Continuous infusion of an opioid (fentanyl, alfentanil, or sufentanil)

has been used to provide optimal conditions for SSEP monitoring. Alternatively, intermittent injections of opioid can be given. Doses of morphine can be given at the start of the case (to a total dose of 0.1 to 0.25 mg/kg) and additional doses of fentanyl used (to a total dose of 7 to 15 μg/kg), or a fentanyl infusion can be given (e.g., 2 to 4 μg/kg/h). A low dose of an inhalational anesthetic (e.g., isoflurane 0.5 percent) can be used with the opioid even when SSEPs are to be monitored. Intermittent positive-pressure ventilation (IPPV) with zero end-expiratory pressure is routinely used. The stomach can be decompressed after tracheal intubation. It is preferable to insert two large IV cannulas. An arterial line can be started before or after anesthetic induction. The ETT should be temporarily disconnected to avoid dislodgment when the patient is turned to the prone position. The ECG cables, blood pressure cuff tubing, and arterial line may be "prepositioned" for the prone position or temporarily disconnected to avoid tangling. Continuity of monitoring can be maintained via an esophageal stethoscope. Turning of the patient to the prone position may require several individuals at the start and the conclusion of surgery. The patient should be properly positioned on the frame used and the head, arms, and legs supported (Fig. 22–7). Vital signs and the position of the tracheal tube should be rechecked after the patient is turned to the prone position. Care should be taken to avoid pressure areas around the elbows and knees to prevent ulnar and peroneal nerve injury. Hyperextension of the arms and pressure on the eyeballs should be avoided. The application of an ophthalmic ointment (e.g., Lacri-Lube) and taping of the eyes are important protective measures. Oval eye pads and/or the newer foam-and-plastic eye cups are also suggested. Parameters to be monitored include ECG, breath sounds, heart sounds (esophageal stethoscope), temperature, blood pressure, PETCO$_2$ monitoring, SpO$_2$, arterial pH and blood gases, and urine output. In some patients, the central venous pressure (CVP) may be monitored. Transesophageal echocardiography or measurement of pulmonary capillary wedge pressure may provide useful information in some patients with cardiac disease or pulmonary hypertension. In patients with myelomeningocele, the dural veins may proliferate over the defect, which may result in excessive blood loss and risk of venous air embolism. In these cases, venous air embolism precautions, including CVP, precordial Doppler, and PETCO$_2$ monitoring, are helpful.

A β-adrenergic blocking drug may be given slowly if deliberate hypotension is contemplated. If epinephrine is used for infiltration, the maximum calculated dose should not be exceeded; otherwise, propranolol or esmolol may be given to guard against dysrhythmias. Blood loss should be quantified and should be replaced with warm blood and fluids. The anesthesiologist should be alert for possible early evidence of malignant hyperthermia.[167, 168] This includes inadequate relaxation, hypertonicity, a rise in temperature, tachycardia, ventricular arrhythmias, and hypercapnia. The key to successful management is early cessation of inhalation anesthetics; cooling; administration of dantrolene; and supportive respiratory and cardiovascular procedures (see Chapter 4). In one review of malignant hyperthermia, 6 of the 89 patients who experienced an episode of malignant hyperthermia with rigidity had idiopathic scoliosis.[167] By contrast, body temperature may fall 2 degrees to 3 degrees C during correction of scoliosis. Factors that contribute to heat loss include a cold operating room, transfusion of cold blood and fluids, a large open wound, and suspension of the body by the frame. A forced-air patient warming system is helpful to maintain normal body temperature. Blood and fluids should also be warmed. Other potential intraoperative problems during scoliosis surgery include potassium release,[169] and myoglobinuria after succinylcholine administration[170] and cardiac arrhythmias (myocardial involvement in muscular dystrophy).[171]

Assessing and adequately replacing blood loss are major problems during scoliosis surgery. Sponges should be weighed as soon as they are removed from the field to avoid errors caused by evaporation. Volumes of irrigating fluid should be measured accurately. Blood on gowns, drapes, and the floor should be taken into consideration. In addition, third-space losses may require the infusion of crystalloid up to 10 ml/kg/h. Urine output should be closely monitored via a urinary catheter, but the reduction in glomerular filtration rate and renal blood flow during deliberate hypotension may reduce this output dramatically. Although 0.5 ml/kg/h or higher is desirable, urine output may fall to minimal levels and may not reliably reflect hydration. If deliberate hypotension is induced, the blood pressure should be allowed to return to a near-normal level before closure of the wound is begun. Fresh frozen plasma (FFP) may be added if a massive blood transfusion is given. A coagulation profile may be necessary to determine whether FFP, cryoprecipitate, or platelets are required. At the end of surgery, the patient is turned to the supine position with extreme care. Residual neuromuscular blockade should be reversed unless postoperative mechanical ventilation is planned. Respiratory depression due to opioids can be reversed with naloxone. Adequacy of ventilation is carefully assessed. Patients with a preoperative vital capacity of less than 30 to 40 percent of the predicted value usually require ventilatory assistance during the early postoperative period. Serial measurements of arterial pH, blood gases, hemoglobin, glucose, and electrolyte concentrations are continued. Pneumothorax is a recognized complication of spinal fusion that is caused by nicking of the pleura; a chest radiograph after surgery may confirm its presence. It is important not to extubate the trachea of these patients prematurely.

Once awake, many of these patients complain of severe pain. Analgesics are tailored to the individual needs of each patient. The commonest measure used is patient-controlled analgesia (PCA), which may be needed for several days. Additionally, caudal or epidural opioids and/or bupivacaine have been used with success in patients after scoliosis correction (see Chapter 25). Because of their effect on platelet function, nonsteroidal anti-inflammatory drugs (NSAIDs), such as ketorolac, are better avoided for the first postoperative day, until bleeding has ceased. Oxygen by mask is given during the first few hours after extubation and may be required for longer periods in patients with impaired pulmonary function.

Cycloplegia that results in pupillary dilation and lack of accommodation after ganglion blockade (trimethaphan) may be noted during the early postoperative period. Pa-tients should be assured that "they will be able to see better." Hemoglobin concentrations should be determined after surgery and serially thereafter. The amount of blood loss from the drain should be repeatedly assessed. A fall of 3 g/dl hemoglobin may occur during the first postoperative week because of oozing into the tissue spaces, destruction of transfused cells, and fluid shifts. Blood transfusion should be given as needed. After scoliosis correction, all children should be cared for in an intensive care environment.

For corrective surgery by the anterior (Dwyer) approach, the anesthetic methods described for the posterior approach are modified by the requirement for an open chest. Bleeding is usually not as excessive as that seen with the posterior approach. However, wedge excision of abnormal vertebrae with a spinal osteotomy can lead to significant blood loss because of the nearby epidural and vertebral plexuses. Full muscle relaxation and use of a high FIO_2 are important considerations. Selective one-lung ventilation of the dependent lung can be performed in older children and is advantageous in providing improved access to the vertebral column, particularly for correction of high curvatures. Serial blood gas determinations are recommended during one-lung ventilation. It may be advisable to interrupt surgery at regular intervals to allow full expansion of the lung. Postoperative care is similar to that for a thoracotomy (see Chapter 17). Postoperative hypoventilation, secretion retention, atelectasis, and pain are more severe after anterior fusion via a thoracotomy than after procedures involving a posterior approach.

Respiratory Function After Correction of Scoliosis

Lung volumes are decreased during the first 10 postoperative days after major surgery, and scoliosis correction is no exception.[166] The magnitude of these changes is related not only to the site and type of surgery but also to the preoperative respiratory function. In a study of five adolescents[182] who underwent scoliosis correction, there was a slight decrease in PaO_2 in the first 2 days without changes in pH and $PaCO_2$. Total lung volume, vital capacity, and FRC were 61 percent, 44 percent, and 81 percent of preoperative values, respectively, and residual volume increased by 124 percent. After the fifth postoperative day, FRC returned to preoperative values. Although total lung capacity and vital capacity increased slightly, they remained below the preoperative values for some time after surgery. These changes are brought about by the immediate effects of surgery on the configuration of the rib cage and the mechanical properties of the chest wall (pain, increased rib cage elastic forces due to altered configuration, chest wall edema, and impaired respiratory muscle performance), by alteration of the mechanical properties of the lungs (increased lung water, increased surface tension, and atelectasis), and by dynamic factors that alter neuromotor control of the diaphragm and intercostal muscles. In patients with abnormal preoperative pulmonary function, further reduction in vital capacity may be associated with hypoxemia, lessened ability to cough, and inhibited periodic large breaths. Additional pulmonary complications and infections can lead to further impairment of the pulmonary defense mechanisms and may culminate in respiratory failure. This reaffirms the importance of thorough preoperative evaluation and preparation of these patients.[166]

Long-term changes in respiratory function have been studied after correction of spinal deformity.[15] Although lung volume was unaltered after correction, gas exchange improved. Physiologic dead space (mainly the alveolar component) was reduced by 40 percent, hypoxemia was relieved, and the ventilatory equivalent (the minute ventilation required to achieve the resting oxygen consumption) was reduced by 20 percent, primarily because wasted ventilation (physiologic dead space) was decreased. This implies that the relation between ventilation and blood flow improved after correction, an assumption confirmed by a rise in Pao_2 and a fall in $P(A-a)O_2$.

Regional distribution of ventilation and blood flow, as studied by the ^{133}Xe technique,[15] remained normal after correction of scoliosis in patients with normal lung volumes (curves less than 65 degrees) and failed to improve in any particular lung zone in those with greater curves. In fact, the gradient of blood flow was even less after correction, especially in the right lung. Alteration in extraalveolar pulmonary blood vessels, particularly toward the bottom of the lung, might account for these changes. The initial alteration may reflect the decreased retractile effect of elastic tissue on extra-alveolar vessels that results from the deformity, as well as a reduction in thoracic size. This effect appears to be greater in the right lower lung zone, where crowding of the lung is more significant. The ribs are elevated to the extent that they can no longer create a negative transpulmonary pressure during inspiration, and therefore the tethering effect on vessels is less. A persistently abnormal distribution of blood flow in the lungs of those with greater curves suggests that permanent pulmonary vascular changes occurred before correction. This finding may indicate that correction should be done early, before the curve exceeds 65 degrees.[15]

SPECIAL PEDIATRIC ORTHOPEDIC PROBLEMS

There are many orthopedic problems that are associated with significant problems during anesthesia (Table 22–5). These are discussed below.

Use of Pneumatic Tourniquets

Pneumatic tourniquets are used in about 40 percent of pediatric orthopedic procedures.[172] The use of tourniquets provides a bloodless operative field and decreases blood loss. The tourniquet is placed over the arm, thigh, or leg (depending on the site of surgery) over cotton padding. After raising the limb, an Esmarch bandage is applied tightly to exsanguinate that portion of the limb distal to the tourniquet. The tourniquet is then inflated to a pressure 100 mm Hg above systolic pressure for a lower extremity and 50 mm Hg above systolic pressure for an upper extremity. The size of the cuff is important; the width should be greater than half the limb's diameter. The main concerns associated with the use of tourniquets include hemodynamic, metabolic, and respiratory changes as a result of

inflation and deflation; tourniquet pain; and potential injury to nerves and muscles if inflation is prolonged.

After tourniquet inflation, progressive decreases in venous pH and Po_2 and increases in Pco_2, lactate, intracellular enzymes, and potassium occur. Creatine phosphate and nicotinamide adenine dinucleotide stores decrease in muscles within 30 to 60 minutes. When the tourniquet is deflated, products of anaerobic metabolism enter the circulation, causing a transient state of reactive hyperemia and a mixed respiratory and metabolic acidosis. Mixed venous oxygen saturation may fall 20 percent in 1 minute. The accumulated acid metabolites are buffered by plasma bicarbonate, resulting in the release of CO_2 and an increase in $Paco_2$ (and $Petco_2$). After tourniquet deflation, the time for clearance of the increased metabolites depends on the duration of inflation, the levels of metabolites before deflation, the extremity exsanguinated (upper vs. lower and one vs. both), the efficacy of the buffering capacity, the patient's circulatory status, ventilation (spontaneous or controlled), and the patient's response to the extra load of metabolites. The maximum increase in $Petco_2$ is about 3 mm Hg after release of an upper extremity tourniquet and about 9 mm Hg after release of a lower extremity tourniquet.[173] The time to maximal increase in $Petco_2$ is 1.5 to 2.5 minutes.

Tourniquet inflation times of 2 to 3 hours have been reported as free of hemodynamic and metabolic consequences in adult patients. Because of the greater oxygen consumption and higher metabolic rate in infants and children, it was thought that tourniquet hemostasis might result in greater accumulation of ischemic metabolites and that physiologic compensation might not be sufficient. Lynn et al.[172] found that children tolerated tourniquet release with fewer hemodynamic changes than have been reported in adults. A slight decrease in systolic blood pressure (8 to 10 mm Hg), lasting less than 10 minutes with no change in heart rate, was noted. The potassium levels increased slightly with tourniquet deflation but remained within the normal range. The respiratory acidosis was quickly compensated, but the metabolic acidosis persisted for more than 10 minutes after tourniquet release. Large increases in lactate were seen with longer tourniquet inflation times (>75 minutes) and with bilateral tourniquets. The greatest decrease in pH was seen when bilateral tourniquets were deflated simultaneously.

Healthy patients who have adequate spontaneous ventilation usually respond to the extra CO_2 load upon tourniquet deflation by increasing their minute ventilation, regardless of the anesthetic given. To minimize the systemic and metabolic effects after tourniquet deflation, the following recommendations are suggested for pediatric patients[172, 174]: (1) when possible, inflation times should be limited to less than 75 minutes; (2) $Petco_2$ should be closely monitored before and after release of the tourniquet; and (3) if controlled ventilation is used, minute ventilation should be increased by about 50 percent just before and 5 minutes after tourniquet deflation. If a Mapleson D circuit is being used, an increase in fresh gas flow may also be necessary to maintain $Petco_2$ at a near-normal level after tourniquet deflation. These measures are of importance with long tourniquet inflation times (>75 minutes), and when bilateral tourniquets are deflated simultaneously or within 30 minutes of each other.

T A B L E   2 2 - 5
ORTHOPEDIC SYNDROMES WITH POTENTIAL ANESTHETIC IMPLICATIONS

Syndrome	Potential Anesthetic Implications	Syndrome	Potential Anesthetic Implications
Achondroplasia	Chronic respiratory infection, hydrocephalus, long narrow mouth w/high arched palate, limited head extension, prominent mandible and forehead, constrictive thoracic cage, cyanotic and apneic episodes, dwarfism	Lesch-Nyhan	Self-mutilation, airway distortion 2 degrees to scarification, mental retardation, spasticity, choreoathetosis, seizures, contractures, hypertension, aspiration pneumonia
Apert's	Facial, limb and cardiac anomalies, hydrocephalus, choanal atresia, craniosynostosis	Marfan's	Joint laxity, vertebral and ocular anomalies, mitral valve prolapse, dilatation or dissection of ascending aorta with aortic valve insufficiency
Arnold-Chiari	Vocal cord paralysis, stridor, respiratory distress, apnea, abnormal swallowing, recurrent aspiration pneumonia, possible ↑ intracranial pressure, unstable blood pressure, weakness → paralysis	Möbius'	Microstomia, micrognathia, limb and brain anomalies, cranial nerve palsies
		Morquio's	Odontoid hypoplasia, vertebral anomalies, growth deficiency, aortic valve insufficiency, joint contractures
Cri du chat	Microcephaly, micrognathia, facial asymmetry, high vaulted palate, cleft lip/palate, feeding and swallowing difficulties w/chronic aspiration, congenital heart defects, seizures, severe retardation	Neurofibromatosis	Brain, vertebral, dermal and cardiac anomalies, subcutaneous tumor w/tendency to malignancy, mental deficiency, kyphoscoliosis
Crouzon's	Facial and ocular anomalies, upper airway obstruction, choanal atresia, seizures, craniosynostosis, mental retardation	Noonan's	Facial, vertebral and cardiac anomalies, micrognathia, mental deficiency, pectus evacatium
Cornelia de Lange	Facial and cardiac anomalies, micrognathia, seizures, choanal atresia, contractures, hypertonia	Radial aplasia-thromocytopenia (Tar)	Facial, vertebral, cardiac and renal anomalies, micrognathia, severe thrombocytopenia, anemia, intracranial hemorrhage
Ehlers-Danlos	Joint laxity, fragile blood vessels, cardiac valvular prolapse, glaucoma	Robin's (Pierre-Robin)	Severe micrognathia, cleft palate, laryngeal anomalies, mandibular growth improves w/age during infancy
Ellis-van Creveld	Facial and cardiac anomalies, small thorax		
Freeman-Sheldon	"Whistling facies" w/microstomia, ↑ muscle tone, vertebral anomalies, myotonia	Treacher Collins	Severe micrognathia (not improving during infancy), facial, auricular and cardiac anomalies, choanal atresia, microstomia, airway hypoplasia
Goldenhar's	Laryngeal, ocular, cardiac and renal anomalies, cervical spine fusion, hemifacial micrognathia, glaucoma, encephalocele	Trisomy 21 (Down's)	Odontoid hypoplasia, macroglossia, cardiac defects, joint laxity, mild mental deficiency
Holt-Oram	Cardiac, vertebral and upper limb and shoulder girdle anomalies, hypoplasia of distal blood vessels	Turner (XO)	Micrognathia, short neck, growth retardation, cardiac anomalies
		VATER Association	Vertebral, cardia, renal and limb anomalies, TE fistula, esophageal atresia, congenital scoliosis, imperforate anus
Hurler's	Facial anomalies, macroglossia, chronic respiratory infections, growth and mental deficiencies, joint stiffness, cardiac failure, hydrocephalus		

Modified from Benumof JL: Anesthesia and Uncommon Diseases. 4th ed. Philadelphia, WB Saunders Company; and Katz J, Stewart DJ: Anesthesia and Uncommon Pediatric Disease. 2nd ed. Philadelphia, WB Saunders Company, 1993, with permission.

A dull aching pain may occur 45 minutes after tourniquet inflation in awake children undergoing limb surgery, despite a successful regional anesthetic. The pain becomes unbearable with time, but subsides immediately after tourniquet deflation. Attempts to relieve upper extremity tourniquet pain by stellate ganglion block, intercostobrachial nerve block, or IV opioids are usually ineffective. Although the etiology is unclear, tourniquet pain has been related to the sensory level, type of regional anesthetic technique, the local anesthetic, and the dose given. It has been proposed that small unmyelinated C fibers are more resistant to neural blockade than the larger myelinated A-delta fibers. With the decrease of local anesthetic concentration with time, the C fibers recover before the A fibers, thus transmitting the sensation of tourniquet pain. Another explanation is based on the finding that local anesthetic activity is enhanced by increasing the frequency of nerve stimulation. However, this effect of local anesthetics varies with regard to frequency-dependant nerve blockade, bupivacaine being the most potent. This may explain why the incidence of tourniquet pain (as a result of increased rate of firing of nociceptive fibers) is less when bupivacaine is used for neural blockade, compared with other anesthetics. Regardless of the etiology, prophylaxis includes a high level of spinal or epidural anesthesia (for the lower extremity) and the addition of an opioid to the local anesthetic used for neural blockade. Therapy includes general anesthesia or tourniquet deflation.

A progressive increase in the temperature of pediatric patients (0.4° to 1.6°C) can occur during prolonged leg tourniquet inflation (90 minutes), and a greater increase (1.1° to 2.3°C) occurs with bilateral leg tourniquets.[175, 176] This slight hyperthermia may be related to a reduction in the effective heat loss from the skin and an altered distribution of heat within the body. Therefore, during prolonged leg tourniquet inflation, attention should be given to the patient's temperature and routine warming may be avoided.[176]

Prolonged ischemia results in mitochondrial swelling, myelin degeneration, depletion of glycogen storage, Z-line lysis, and tissue edema. Thromboxane is released with disruption of endothelial integrity. Within 30 minutes of inflation, nerve conduction ceases, reflecting ischemia or direct extrinsic pressure on the nerves by the tourniquet. If prolonged inflation (>90 minutes) is required, the tourniquet should be deflated periodically every 75 to 90 minutes to minimize the risk of postoperative neurapraxis.

On theoretical grounds, the use of tourniquets in patients with sickle cell disease has been discouraged for fear that it may lead to circulatory stasis, acidosis, and hypoxemia, the triad known to induce sickling. Clinical experience and recent studies suggest that the use of tourniquets in these patients is not associated with harmful effects provided that oxygenation and mild hyperventilation are maintained.[177] Therefore, patients with sickle cell disease should not be denied the benefits of tourniquets when indicated. The usual precautions for tourniquet use should be adopted.

Congenital Hip Dislocation

Congenital dislocation of the hip[178] is a displacement of the femoral head out of the acetabular socket. It can be present at birth or may occur shortly afterward. Two main classifications are recognized. Teratogenic hip dislocation can represent either an independent abnormality or one that is associated with other congenital deformities, such as arthrogryposis. Laxity of the ligaments and the capsule and malposition in utero (breech presentation) may be predisposing factors. Typical hip dislocation is characterized by its postnatal appearance.

The incidence has been reported as 1 to 15 per 1,000 live births, with girls affected six to eight times more often than boys. Dislocation of the left hip occurs three times more frequently than the right, but in 25 percent of cases the dislocation is bilateral. Treatment in the newborn consists of manipulative reduction and splinting. The major complications are avascular necrosis of the ossification center of the femoral head and cessation of growth of the proximal femoral epiphysis. Skeletal traction or open reduction and osteotomy may be required to obtain a normal hip.

An inhalational anesthetic is usually given for closed manipulation of the hip. This can be done with face mask, laryngeal mask airway (LMA), or endotracheal anesthesia. Open reduction may require blood replacement. To prepare for this possibility, a reliable IV line should be in place. The application of hip spica casts at repeated intervals after surgery may impose anesthetic problems. The infant is suspended by one support under the coccyx and another under the shoulders. The patient's perineum is held against the vertical strut between the legs. Because infants are diaphragmatic breathers, an adequate space is provided within the spica for the infant to breathe. A "belly pad" of stockinette or a small towel is placed over the abdomen and kept there until the cast is completed. Its removal at the end of the procedure should allow adequate diaphragmatic movement. Anesthesia for the change of a cast should never be taken lightly. Airway patency should be maintained by an LMA or tracheal intubation. Routine monitoring, with particular attention to temperature and breath sounds, should be performed. The need for fluoroscopy and placement on a spica cast-

ing table involves patient repositioning and can lead to accidental extubation or misplacement of the LMA. It may be necessary to temporarily disconnect the anesthesia circuit when the position is changed.

The Ilizarov Procedure

Professor G.A. Ilizarov popularized a revolutionary new technique for bone lengthening by combining a cortical bone osteotomy with slow external distraction, usually without bone grafting. This corticotomy preserves the medullary and periosteal blood supply and allows for new osseous tissue formation. This long, technically demanding procedure has numerous potential problems and complications, but has permitted many patients with congenital and/or acquired limb disorders to lead more normal lives. There are no specific anesthetic variances for this procedure.[179]

Arthrogryposis (Amyoplasia Congenita)

Arthrogryposis multiplex congenita is a clinical syndrome rather than a pathologic entity. It is characterized by multiple symmetric contractures that develop in utero. These contractures often interfere with parturition. Although the joint tissues may be thickened and fibrotic, the contractures in most cases are caused by shortening of the flexor muscles. Congenital ankylosis has been reported in rare instances.

Signs of the disease are manifest either at birth or during the first few months of life. The postpartum cases have usually been associated with a myopathy that simulates progressive muscular dystrophy and is characterized by unusual muscle shortening and contracture. The infant lies supine with the head turned to one side, the shoulders rotated internally, the hips rotated externally, and the arms and legs in partial flexion. The decreased muscle mass causes the limbs to appear spindly with large, fusiform joints, and the skin looks wrinkled. In advanced cases, muscle fibers are almost lacking and are replaced by collagenous scar tissue. The patients have been described as looking like thin wooden dolls.[180]

This complex of symptoms has been divided into two groups: those that are neuropathic in origin and those that are myopathic. The former is the result of intrauterine neuromyopathy. The articular contractures may be due to lack of movement during early development in utero, instituted by neuronal lesions and leading to muscle changes. Conceivably, other developmental defects in the motor nervous system might be at fault. The spinal cord is narrow and the neural canal deficient in approximately one half of patients with arthrogryposis. There is degeneration and a reduction in the size and number of anterior horn cells in the CNS. Pyramidal tracts and motor roots are demyelinated, and axons in the peripheral nerves are decreased. Elevated levels of creatine phosphokinase and 1,6-diphosphofructoaldolase have been reported. The myopathic type is proposed to represent the result of intrauterine progressive muscular dystrophy. In these cases, no CNS lesions can be demonstrated and the only attribution is to a primary muscle disease. Lack of embryonic movement may lead to joint deformities.

Other anomalies are present in more than two thirds of children. Rigidity of the temporomandibular joints and mandibular hypoplasia may make mask ventilation, visualization of the larynx, and endotracheal intubation difficult. Airway assessment is important. If a difficult intubation is anticipated, a technique for intubating the difficult airway may be required. Scoliosis, rib-cage deformities with altered pulmonary mechanics, and hip dislocation are common. Ten to 26 percent of affected patients have associated congenital heart disease, including patent ductus arteriosus, aortic stenosis, coarctation of the aorta, and cyanotic congenital heart disease.[181] Malformations of the genitourinary tract are frequently seen. If closed reduction and casting fail to improve the deformity, surgery is indicated. Multiple operations are usually necessary in the severe quadrimelic type of arthrogryposis.

These patients may be prone to respiratory depression, hypotension, and "sensitivity" to anesthetics. IV access may be very difficult because veins are both sparse and tiny. An association with malignant hyperthermia has been suggested but not confirmed.[182] Hyperpyrexia in a child with "a tentative diagnosis of arthrogryposis" had been reported[168] and malignant hyperthermia was reported in one child "confirmed" by muscle biopsy.[183] However, a 1986 review of 32 years' experience on 67 patients undergoing 398 anesthetics[184] revealed no episodes of malignant hyperthermia, despite many varied exposures to known triggering agents. Patients with arthrogryposis seem to be susceptible to a nonmalignant hyperthermia related to hypermetabolic responses to anesthesia and surgery.[185] This hyperthermia responds readily to active cooling and occurs even in the presence of nontriggering agents, similar to osteogenesis imperfecta.

Camptomelic Dysplasia Syndrome

Although reports of camptomelic dysplasia syndrome first appeared during the 1950s, it was not until the 1970s that it became more widely recognized. Maroteaux utilized the term *campomelique*, from the Greek for "bent limb," to characterize the syndrome.[186] The subtitle "short life span dwarfism with respiratory distress, hypotonia, peculiar facies, and multiple skeletal and cartilaginous deformities" managed to succinctly characterize the syndrome. The mode of inheritance is autosomal recessive.

The patients are of low-normal weight and are usually full-term newborns with disproportionately large heads, often containing a large brain with gross cellular disorganization in the cerebral cortex, thalamus, and caudate nucleus, which leads to severe mental retardation. The child's face is clearly abnormal, with cleft palate, small mouth, micrognathia, flat nasal bridge, narrow palpebral fissures, and abnormal ears. There is often incomplete cartilaginous development of the airway with tracheobronchomalacia. The chest is small and bell-shaped and the abdomen is relatively large and protuberant. There is disproportionate shortness, particularly of the lower extremities, with pretibial dimpling, vertically narrow ileal bones, and talipes equinovarus. There may also be hypoplastic cervical vertebrae, nonmineralized thoracic pedicles, absent or hypoplastic scapulas, kyphoscoliosis, hip dislocations, XY gonadal dysgenesis, short proximal phalanges, hypoplastic olfactory bulbs, hydronephrosis (38 percent), and congenital cardiac defects (21 percent).

Most patients die during the first month of life from respiratory insufficiency. Those who survive into early infancy have feeding difficulties, failure to thrive, hypotonia, apneic episodes, cyanosis, and other evidence of serious CNS deficiency. A few have now survived longer but have been severely mentally retarded. Some patients have radiographic evidence of a trachea with several abnormal bends and small-appearing lungs. A large head, which the patient cannot support, frequent upper respiratory infections, severe tracheomalacia, and no attempts at vocalization may be seen. Fluoroscopy has revealed significant narrowing of the subglottic trachea to about 1 mm in diameter on maximal inspiration. There is a question as to the appropriateness of medical intervention in these cases; anesthetic and postanesthetic management may be very difficult.

Congenital Constriction Bands (Streeter's Dysplasia)

Streeter's dysplasia is a rare abnormality that manifests as ring-like concentric bands in the upper or lower limbs and occasionally in the trunk. The exact cause is unknown.[178] These bands are probably the result of germ plasm defects. They are not due to "amniotic bands," as was formerly believed.

The constrictions may be shallow, including only the skin and the subcutaneous tissue, or deep, extending to the fascia and as far as the bone. Deep bands may interfere with the venous and lymphatic return, causing peripheral edema. If local circulation is markedly disrupted, the part of the limb distal to the constriction may undergo autoamputation in utero. Distal parts of the limbs (e.g., the fingers, toes, forearms, and legs) are affected more often than the thigh or upper arm. Bands that interfere with circulation or lymphatic drainage require surgical division, ordinarily in two or three successive stages to minimize circulatory embarrassment. IV lines may be difficult to secure if the disease is extensive, and one may have to resort to the head or neck for intravenous access.

Limb Dysplasias

Syndactyly is the most common anomaly of the hand. The simplest form is an incomplete web between the fingers, without bone or joint deformity. Severe webbing of all fingers may be accompanied by incomplete segmentation of bony parts and multiple joint deformities. The incidence is approximately 1:2,000 and is higher in male infants. Syndactyly occurs as an isolated anomaly or is associated with other anomalies of the extremities or with craniofacial dysostosis (Apert syndrome).

Absence of the radius may be complete or partial. In approximately one half of cases the radius is totally absent. The deformity is bilateral in one half of these cases. With partial absence of the radius, it is frequently the distal portion that has failed to develop; the proximal radius may be hypoplastic and fused to the ulna. In severe cases the hand may form an angle of 90 degrees with the forearm. In the affected limb, diffuse muscle involvement is usually present. The neurovascular structures may also be involved. The radial nerve usually terminates at the elbow, and sensory innervation to the radial aspect may be provided by the median nerve. The radial artery may be displaced or not palpable, and radial artery cannulation may be impossible. A number of congenital deformities are associated with congenital absence of the radius (i.e., cleft lip, cleft palate, clubfoot, hydrocephalus, absence of fusion of ribs, aplasia or collapse of the lung, and hemivertebrae).

Three specific entities are worthy of mention. The Holt-Oram syndrome (cardiac-limb syndrome) consists of atrial or ventricular septal defects, arrhythmias, and malformations of the upper extremities. Patients with this syndrome are usually acyanotic. Various conduction blocks may be present. Radial aplasia-thrombocytopenia syndrome is usually recognized during infancy when the child presents with petechiae, purpura, melena, hematuria, and signs of easy bruising. Bone marrow examination reveals absent, diminished, or inactive megakaryocytes. A congenital cardiac defect is present in approximately 25 percent of these patients. Fanconi syndrome consists of pancytopenia and abnormalities of the thumb or radius. The reasons for the association are not understood, but the systems involved undergo embryonic differentiation during the same period, between 25 and 34 days of fetal life. Most babies are premature, and postnatal growth retardation is the rule. Renal anomalies are present in one third of the patients. Bleeding, pallor, and recurrent infections begin between 5 and 10 years of age.

Anesthetic problems in these children include difficulty in maintaining airway patency, difficulty in introducing a nasal airway (choanal atresia), and the necessity for using a smaller endotracheal tube because of glottic narrowing (Apert syndrome). Anemia, pancytopenia, and coagulation defects may be present. The use of LMA may be helpful. Preoperative assessment of cardiac function and care in the use of muscle relaxants are important considerations.[204]

The Amelic Child

Congenital absence of all extremities is rare. Complete amelia may be present in 1 of 3.5 million births.[188, 189] Idiopathic scoliosis was noted in 48 percent of a series of patients with upper extremity anomalies.[188] Amelic patients present an obvious challenge to the anesthesiologist in terms of both monitoring and fluid infusion. The additional challenge presented by the desire to perform induced hypotension for a spinal fusion has been documented.[189]

Because of an absence of superficial veins, venous cannulation may be performed via a subclavian or jugular approach. If a percutaneous approach fails, a venous cutdown is mandated. Obtaining blood for laboratory tests, as well as for typing and crossmatching, may have to be done in the operating room after venous cannulation has been accomplished. Intramuscular ketamine may be used for sedation when needed.

Monitoring of blood pressure can be attempted using a superficial temporal artery[207] with a Doppler probe and a long tourniquet cuff, at least 1.5 times the circumference of the head and fixed firmly in the fronto-occipital plane; the values obtained are within ±15 mm Hg of values in the arm using the conventional Riva-Rocci method. For continuous blood pressure readings or blood gas determinations, an arterial line is desirable. A method of cannulation via cutdown of a superficial temporal artery has been described.[191] An excellent correlation between the values obtained from the left superficial temporal artery and those from the right radial artery was reported.[191] IV ketamine may prove useful for the uncomfortable and time-consuming arterial cutdown.

Talipes Equinovarus (Clubfoot)

Talipes equinovarus is one of the more common congenital deformities of the foot and has been recognized since ancient times. It occurs in approximately 1 per 1,000 live births and is twice as common in boys as in girls. Approximately 12 percent of the children have other congenital anomalies as well. The exact cause has not been determined, but it is thought to be an arrest in the development of the foot during embryonic life.

Soft tissue procedures, such as Achilles tendon lengthening and capsulotomy, can be undertaken in cases resistant to conservative measures. Surgery is now being performed on infants as young as 3 to 4 months of age in the prone position. Routine anesthetic measures are needed, with careful attention to temperature monitoring and control.[187] An association with malignant hyperthermia has been suggested but not documented.[192] In a recent study,[193] 17 infants having clubfoot correction also had muscle biopsies done, 12 of which were abnormal. One showed mild congenital muscular dystrophy; two, congenital myotonic dystrophy; one, mild spinal muscular atrophy; and four, nonspecific congenital myopathy. In addition, another four showed a congenital type I fiber predominance. The authors warn of the need to take precautions to prevent malignant hyperthermia–related problems.

Septic Arthritis

The onset of septic arthritis may be preceded by a variety of infections, such as otitis media, pharyngitis, infected skin lesions, or upper respiratory infection. The highest incidence occurs between 1 and 2 years of age. The hip is the most commonly affected joint. The usual causative organism is *Staphylococcus aureus*, although the incidence of infection due to *Haemophilus influenzae* is increasing. Irritability, poor feeding, and pseudoparalysis of the affected limb are early manifestations. Although satisfactory drainage can often be accomplished with arthrocentesis, severe cases may require arthrotomy. It is often necessary to anesthetize a toxic, febrile child in a hypermetabolic state. Anticholinergic drugs should not be administered IV to such patients. In addition to the institution of measures to control temperature after anesthesia is induced, fluids must be given to combat dehydration, and ventilation is increased by 10 percent for every 1°C rise in temperature.[187] Careful PET_{CO_2} monitoring is important because of the increase in metabolic activity. If a Mapleson D circuit is used, an increase in fresh gas flow may be required to compensate for the excessive CO_2 production.

Fractures

Greenstick fractures and epiphyseal injuries are confined to the pediatric age group because their bone growth is incomplete. Growing bone responds to open surgical intervention by overgrowth, absorption, nonunion, and excessive formation of callus. Children sustain fractures of long bones from inconsequential trauma. The possibility of deliberately inflicted trauma must be borne in mind. Radiographic evidence of fractures in various stages of healing, and multiple soft tissue injuries, particularly cigarette burns, are pathognomonic of the battered child syndrome. Affected children are usually under 2 years of age.[178]

Fractures of the distal forearm are common, usually the result of a fall on the outstretched hand. When closed reduction is required, it need not be performed as an emergency procedure. The arm should be splinted and elevated and ice should be applied; analgesics help to lessen the pain. Fractures around the elbow require immediate treatment, and all but minimally displaced fractures require reduction under anesthesia.[178]

Multiple trauma is common in children, often resulting from automobile accidents. Management is directed toward establishing and maintaining the airway, preventing aspiration of gastric contents, replacing lost blood and fluids, and immobilizing fractures to prevent further injury (see Chapter 27). Careful examination may reveal evidence of head, neck, and thoracic or abdominal injuries. The incidence of fat embolism in pediatric orthopedic patients is unknown. Its occurrence in healthy children, who have a relatively less fatty bone marrow than adults, seems to be rare.[194] In addition, marrow fat in children contains palmitin and stearin.[194] These triglycerides are less fluid than is olein, which is found in large amounts in adult marrow.

THE EMERGENCY PATIENT

Delayed gastric emptying may follow a recent injury or trauma; therefore, the emergency pediatric orthopedic patient should be considered at risk of aspiration of gastric contents.[195-197] Brachial plexus or regional IV anesthesia can be used in the older, cooperative child for upper extremity surgery (see Chapter 12). There are three convenient levels at which the brachial plexus can be blocked by a single injection technique.[198] The extent of anesthesia after a block depends primarily on the level at which the anesthetic was injected and the volume of anesthetic injected at that level. Height rather than age seems to be the most important single factor in determining the correct volume (in milliliters)[198]; this is approximately related to one half the height (in inches). In general, the total mepivacaine or lidocaine dose should not exceed 5 to 6 mg/kg. IV regional anesthesia can be accomplished with 0.5 percent lidocaine. A dosage of approximately 2 to 2.5 mg/

kg is effective when preceded by a 20-minute period of preinjection ischemia, and a maximal dosage of 3 to 4 mg/kg should not be exceeded.

Delaying the operative procedure, if feasible, helps to reduce the intragastric pressure before anesthesia is induced.[197] Cimetidine 6 to 7 mg/kg or ranitidine 2.5 mg/kg[199] or metoclopramide 0.1 to 0.2 mg/kg can be given in pediatric patients to reduce gastric acidity and enhance gastric emptying.

Awake tracheal intubation after IV sedation (with midazolam and/or opioid) and topical anesthesia may be the method of choice in near-moribund children and in children with anatomic problems that may render intubation difficult. If topical anesthesia is used, the larynx is continuously visualized until intubation is accomplished to avoid silent regurgitation.

Rapid sequence induction and intubation is the commonest technique used for children who are at risk of aspiration of gastric contents. In this technique, anesthesia is induced with either intravenous thiopental 3 to 6 mg/kg, propofol 1.5 to 3 mg/kg or other induction drugs, and is immediately followed by a full paralyzing dose of a muscle relaxant. Tracheal intubation is performed once paralysis is complete. The essential components of this technique are preoxygenation, the proper use of a muscle relaxant, and cricoid pressure. Preoxygenation for approximately 2 minutes in children has become an integral component of this technique, and is particularly important if (1) manual ventilation is not desirable prior to intubation, (2) difficulty with ventilation or intubation is suspected, and (3) when the patient's FRC is decreased or oxygen requirements are increased. Fall in Sa_{O_2} during induction should alert the clinician to the need to establish airway patency and lung ventilation.

For years succinylcholine has been the most popular muscle relaxant used to facilitate rapid tracheal intubation. Its rapid onset and short duration remain unsurpassed. Satisfactory conditions occur in less than 60 seconds. Various treatment regimens have been suggested to attenuate succinylcholine fasciculations; the most effective has been the use of a subparalyzing dose of a nondepolarizing muscle relaxant. Pretreatment (at least 2 minutes before succinylcholine) with d-tubocurarine 0.05 to 0.07 mg/kg or pancuronium 0.01 to 0.015 mg/kg attenuates muscle fasciculations, prevents the increase in intragastric pressure, and decreases postoperative muscle pain. However, this pretreatment also antagonizes the paralyzing effect of succinylcholine, delays the onset of paralysis and may result in coughing, bucking, and even vomiting due to inadequate relaxation. Therefore, it is important that whenever pretreatment is given, the dose of succinylcholine be increased to 2 mg/kg. Because the intragastric pressure does not increase after the administration of succinylcholine to infants and children, pretreatment with a nondepolarizing relaxant may not be advisable. Even if there is a rise in intragastric pressure with succinylcholine, there is a corresponding increase in lower esophageal sphincter tone, so that the net effect on the barrier pressure is a small increase. Therefore, succinylcholine does not increase the tendency to regurgitation in patients with normal gastroesophageal function.

Because of the other side effects of succinylcholine (even with pretreatment) including increased intraocular and intracranial pressure, postoperative myalgia, hyperkalemia, cardiac arrhythmias, hemodynamic effects, masseter muscle rigidity, myoglobinuria, and the potential for triggering malignant hyperthermic and myotonic responses in susceptible patients, substitution with a nondepolarizing relaxant has been advocated. A plethora of studies attempted to shorten the time of onset of paralysis and enhance intubating conditions using nondepolarizing muscle relaxants. These include megadosing, the priming and timing principle, and the use of newer nondepolarizing relaxants (see Chapter 3). Considerable evidence has accumulated in recent years showing excellent intubating conditions in less than 60 seconds in children when rocuronium 0.9 to 1.2 mg/kg is used. In some institutions, rocuronium has replaced succinylcholine for rapid-sequence induction and intubation. The nondepolarizing muscle relaxant, rapacuronium, has been suggested as the best replacement for succinylcholine. Given in a dose of 2.0 mg/kg, intubation is usually possible in 50 seconds.[200]

Before induction of anesthesia, the cricoid cartilage is palpated and lightly held between the second finger and the thumb, and the index finger is placed on its anterior surface. As consciousness is lost after anesthetic induction, pressure is increased by the index finger maintaining the cricoid in its central position, while the head is kept extended. Cricoid pressure can also be correctly accomplished in the sniffing position, which also facilitates visualization and intubation. The pressure is maintained until intubation and cuff inflation are done. This simple maneuver results in occlusion of the upper esophagus by backward pressure of the cricoid ring against the bodies of the cervical vertebrae to prevent gastric contents from reaching the pharynx should regurgitation occur. Traditionally, manual ventilation of the lungs is avoided before intubation during rapid sequence induction. The rationale being that inflation of the lungs can lead to gastric distention, a potential cause for regurgitation. With the use of adequate preoxygenation and a rapidly acting muscle relaxant, manual ventilation before intubation is not usually required. However, when the oxygen reserves may be insufficient (delayed or failed intubation, decreased FRC), when oxygen consumption is increased, or when the onset of paralysis is slow, manual ventilation may become necessary. Studies confirmed that cricoid pressure actually prevents gastric inflation even when higher inflation pressures are used, provided the airway is patent. Thus, manual inflation of the lungs need not be withheld before intubation as long as cricoid pressure is performed. However, improper application of cricoid pressure may occlude the airway and may interfere with visualization of the larynx. Cricoid pressure is also effective in sealing the esophagus around the nasogastric tube.[195] Therefore, a nasogastric tube already in place should not be withdrawn before rapid sequence induction. If a rise in intragastric pressure occurs during anesthetic induction, an unoccluded nasogastric tube will act as a "blow-off" valve, while cricoid pressure will prevent gastric contents from reaching the pharynx. Contraindications to cricoid pressure include suspected airway injury especially at the cricotracheal junction, unstable cervical spine, and foreign body in either the esophagus or the airway.

Extubation should be carried out after infants and children are fully awake and have regained adequate reflexes. Airway obstruction may result if these patients are extubated prematurely. It is preferable to remove the tube while maintaining 20 to 30 cm H_2O positive airway pressure. This "pseudocough" maneuver helps to prevent inhalation of material present in the pharynx during extubation[197] (see Chapter 10).

Fat Embolism

Fat embolism probably occurs to a minor degree in almost all patients with long bone fractures. Ten to 15 percent of these patients seem to develop a fat embolism syndrome, particularly after fractures of the tibia and femur, especially when fixation of the bones is delayed and extensive medullary canal reaming occurs.[201] Patients become symptomatic within 72 hours and may present with hypoxemia (including adult respiratory distress syndrome), tachypnea, diffuse patchy pulmonary infiltrates, tachycardia, hypotension, confusion, and agitation, which may progress into stupor and coma, cerebral edema, and petechiae on the axilla, upper thorax, and conjunctiva. The pathogenesis includes the aggregation of circulating free fatty acids and the direct release of fat globules from the fractured bone into the circulation; some fat globules may be found in the urine. Breakdown of capillary endothelium leads to brain and lung hemorrhagic exudates. Treatment is primarily supportive with early recognition being vital. Oxygen supplementation, careful fluid management, continuous positive airway pressure, and vasopressors are recommended when indicated. The use of high-dose corticosteroids is controversial.

Volkmann's Ischemia

Since Volkmann's description of the injury in 1881, numerous investigators have attempted to elucidate the pathophysiology of Volkmann's ischemia.[178, 202] Warning signs are pain, pallor (or cyanosis), absent pulse, paresthesia, and paralysis. A characteristic finding is exaggeration of pain on passive extension of the fingers. Within 6 to 12 hours, progressive swelling and firmness develop in the volar compartment of the forearm. The radial pulse may be present or absent. Various degrees of sensory loss are always present, the median nerve is almost always involved, and the ulnar nerve is paralyzed in most cases. The destructive process develops fully within 12 to 24 hours. Within 5 to 10 days, the swelling and sensitivity gradually subside, and the muscles of the flexor compartment become hard. Gradual fibrosis of the muscles produces a fixed contracture deformity.

Although Volkmann's ischemia can occur after fractures of both bones of the forearm or injuries of the soft tissue around the elbow, it is most often associated with supracondylar fractures of the humerus. Brachial artery entrapment at the fracture site, contusion and spasm of the artery, or compression due to rapidly progressive swelling in a taut fascial compartment may cause arterial occlusion. Ischemia produces anoxia in the muscles, which, in turn, increases capillary permeability, and intramuscular edema develops, causing an increase in intrinsic tissue pressure. Circular unyielding dressings on the limb and limited expansion in a taut fascial envelope increase the venous compression, which further increases tissue pressure. Reflex generalized vasospasm occurs and a destructive ischemia–edema cycle develops. Necrosis of the muscle with secondary fibrosis and calcification is the terminal phase of the pathologic process.

The acute ischemic stage should be terminated immediately by removal of tight bandages, reduction of the fracture, and extension of the elbow. If ischemia cannot be relieved within 6 to 12 hours, arteriography is performed. If the brachial artery is in spasm, a stellate ganglion block is performed. If circulation is not improved within 30 minutes, fasciotomy, epimysiotomy of the forearm, and exploration of the brachial artery are required.

Osteogenesis Imperfecta

Osteogenesis imperfecta (OI) is a connective tissue disorder that primarily affects bone (Fig. 22–13).[203,204] The inner ear, sclerae, tendons, fascia, ligaments, and skin are often involved. It is usually inherited as an autosomal dominant trait, although on occasion the congenital type may be manifested as the result of an autosomal recessive trait. The primary problems are easily fractured osteoporotic bones and spine deformities.

The first description of patients with abnormal bone brittleness and multiple fractures was in 1678, the first description of a family with inherited softness or fragility of bones was in 1788, and the term *osteogenesis imperfecta* was coined in 1849. An Egyptian mummy was discovered, dating from about 1000 B.C., which had findings of OI and

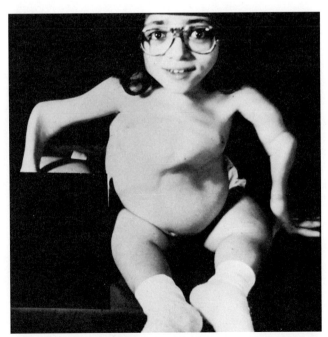

FIGURE 22–13. Multiple fractures eventually produce severe deformities in osteogenesis imperfecta. This patient also shows significant evidence of kyphoscoliosis with rib cage deformities. (Photograph courtesy of Shriner's Hospital for Children, Chicago Unit.)

thus appears to represent the earliest known existence of the disease. The incidence is reported as from 1 in 20,000 to 1 in 60,000 live births. The basic defect appears to be in the maturation of collagen that has an abnormally high proline content. The osteoblasts either lack the normal enzymes or are refractory to the normal stimuli of stress. The severe form, osteogenesis imperfecta congenita, is evidenced at birth by the occurrence of multiple fractures during delivery, deformity of the limbs, and a soft skull. Intracranial hemorrhage is the most common cause of death during the neonatal period. If the neonate survives, severe thoracic deformity often leads to early respiratory failure and death. Osteogenesis imperfecta tarda is much less severe, with delayed walking often the main presenting sign. The forehead is broad, with prominent parietal and temporal bones and a hanging occiput. Faciocranial disproportion may also exist. Blue sclerae are a distinctive manifestation of the disease, but fragility of the bones is the most outstanding feature. Fractures occur during infancy and childhood, but improvement may occur after puberty, presumably because of the influence of sex hormones on bone matrix formation. Fractures have been reported from minimal manipulation, including application of a blood pressure cuff or changing a diaper.

Many congenital and acquired anomalies have been reported to be associated with OI. Among these anomalies are dentinogenesis imperfecta with brittle, discolored (often slightly gray-blue), and sometimes opalescent teeth; cleft palate; hydrocephalus; umbilical and inguinal hernias; hyperhidrosis; spina bifida; kyphoscoliosis; premature arteriosclerosis; emphysema; otosclerosis with deafness; and lax ligaments with recurrent joint dislocation. Ventilation–perfusion abnormalities are documented when severe scoliosis is present, and hypoxemia may ensue. The classic triad of multiple fractures in a patient with deafness and blue sclerae does not occur frequently, as deafness is present only in about 10 percent of patients.[205] Congenital cardiac defects have been documented, including abnormalities of the chordae tendineae, cystic medial necrosis of the aorta, and dilation of the valvular annulus leading to both mitral and aortic regurgitation.[206] Antibiotic prophylaxis should be considered in patients with heart disease. A recognized but ill-defined platelet dysfunction may occur, sometimes leading to a bleeding diathesis; platelet counts are usually within normal limits, but platelet aggregation may be abnormal[207] and easy bruising has been noted.

Although the basic defect is in the connective tissue, some investigators have found enough evidence to convince them that OI is a generalized metabolic disease.[208] The platelet disturbance would then represent one component of a high-energy phosphate metabolism disturbance. Other abnormalities include increased oxygen consumption, elevated serum thyroxine levels, increased heart and respiratory rates, and a significant elevation of body temperature, particularly in prepubertal children. Most OI patients dress more lightly and sleep in cooler surroundings then non-OI patients; they are frequently diaphoretic and mildly hyperthermic. Although originally reported during anesthesia, we have seen increased temperatures on many occasions before anesthesia, often with but also without atropine. These children are intelligent, verbal, and often aware of their possible demise. Some are easily stressed. It is postulated that excess thyroid hormone leads to the uncoupling of oxidative phosphorylation; part of the energy usually trapped during adenosine triphosphate synthesis may be lost as heat, leading to the temperature elevation.[209] It is, however, a nonmalignant hyperthermia that is readily controlled with surface cooling, cold IV solutions, and a decrease in ambient temperature.[204, 209]

Although medical management has been attempted with anabolic steroids, sodium fluoride, and calcitonin, it has been virtually useless. Surgical management consists of fragmentation, realignment, and fixation of the long bones by the use of rods.[210, 211] The technique involves subperiosteal exposure of the entire shaft of a long bone, osteotomy through the proximal and distal metaphyses, and removal of the shaft. The shaft is cut into several pieces, which are then threaded onto a steel rod. The realigned shaft (similar to a shish kebab) is replaced between the metaphyses. The operation is usually done in children between 2 and 8 years of age but can also be performed during infancy and in older patients. The exact order of bone fragments is not critical, as they serve only as a framework, or scaffolding, holding the periosteum in the shape of what is hoped will be the newly generated bone. Sofield and Millar[210, 211] performed more than 1,000 of these procedures, helping to prevent recurrent fractures and allowing significant mobilization of patients.

Because of the frequent fractures and gross deformities, anesthetic management may be complicated. Careful preoperative documentation is vital, as well as questioning or reexamining the child in the operating room before induction of anesthesia, seeking new fractures. All movements, positioning, monitoring applications, IV line placement, and steps in airway control must be done judiciously. Endotracheal intubation has been reported to be complicated by the fragile, brittle teeth and in an occasional patient with a short neck. Odontoid hypoplasia and cervicomedullary compression are rarely seen, even in severe cases, but must be kept in mind. In theory, excessive traction and hyperextension during intubation could result in fracture of the cervical spine. These children are usually small for their age, and all equipment, tubes, and drugs must be appropriately adjusted. Although often playful and even euphoric, it is not uncommon for them to come to surgery asking, "Is today the day I'm going to die?" They require careful, supportive emotional handling as well as careful, supportive physical handling.

Succinylcholine has been described as relatively contraindicated because of the danger of fasciculation-induced fractures. Intermediate-duration nondepolarizing muscle relaxants, atracurium, vecuronium and rocuronium have proven useful for intubation in these children. In our experience at the Shriner's Hospital in Chicago, neither intubation nor case management has proven unusually difficult. Nonetheless, fiberoptic bronchoscopy should be available if needed and may be helpful in difficult cases.

Klippel-Feil Syndrome

Fusion of cervical vertebrae has been found in an Egyptian mummy dating from about 500 B.C. The association of massive fusion of cervical vertebrae, severe shortness of the neck with painless limitation of head movement, and a low posterior hairline was described as early as the sixteenth century. However, the first complete clinical and pathologic description was published in 1912 by Klippel and Feil,[212] who discovered a complete fusion of the cervical vertebrae at postmortem examination of one of their patients. Additional cases, including some with only partial fusions, were reported.

The complete classic triad is present only in about 50 percent of patients with Klippel-Feil syndrome (Fig. 22–14).[213] The syndrome refers to all individuals with congenital fusion of the cervical vertebrae. The frequency is about 1 per 42,000 births, and 65 percent of patients are females. Usually a sporadic occurrence of unknown etiology, autosomal dominant and autosomal recessive[214] inheritance with variable expression have been noted in rare cases. The syndrome results from a failure of normal segmentation of the cervical somites during weeks 3 to 8 of gestation. The entire fetus can be influenced, resulting in widespread symptomatology because of the close fetal spatial relationship and growth disturbances in the embryologic precursors of the heart, genitourinary system, cervical spine, and CNS. Many "hidden" abnormalities are more detrimental to the patient than the obvious neck deformity.

Among the reported clinical findings are congenital high scapula (Sprengel's deformity) in 25 to 35 percent of cases,[213] severe webbing of the neck (pterygium colli),

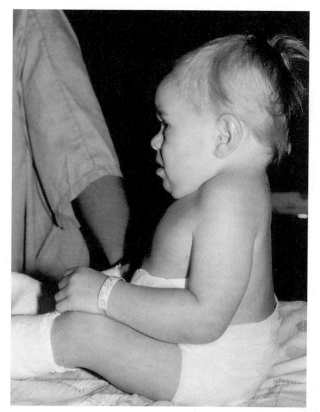

FIGURE 22–14. A classic profile of a boy with Klippel-Feil syndrome, whose "head rests on his shoulders." The rigid spine and probable difficult intubation are evident. (Photograph courtesy of Shriner's Hospital for Children, Chicago Unit.)

and facial asymmetry and mild torticollis (20 percent); there is a 60 percent incidence of significant scoliosis, and 45 percent have posterior spina bifida. About 35 percent have renal anomalies, most commonly the absence of one kidney.[215] Congenital heart disease is noted in 4.2 to 14 percent, most commonly a ventricular septal defect.[216] Hearing impairment, deafness, and speech retardation are reportedly associated in 30 percent.[217] Synkinesia consists of involuntary paired movements of the hands (mirror motions) in 20 percent of Klippel-Feil patients. Other less common abnormalities include rib anomalies, pectus excavatum, syndactyly, facial nerve palsy, lateral rectus palsy, ptosis, hypoplastic thumbs or upper extremities, cleft or high arched palate, congenital absence of the uterus and upper vagina, skull asymmetry, and micrognathia.[218]

Neural deficits have been noted in Klippel-Feil patients, including paresthesias and episodic weakness. These are usually a direct result of cervical nerve root entrapment or irritation.[219] Trauma or progressive instability may lead to spinal cord compression; quadriplegia has been reported after minor trauma.[220] Syncopal attacks may be initiated by sudden rotary neck movements.[221] Because potentially unstable cervical spines do occur, many patients are advised to avoid contact sports and other stressful physical activity. Some patients may require traction and even spinal fusion. Congenital spinal stenosis has been reported in conjunction with Klippel-Feil syndrome.[222]

Pulmonary disability is uncommon but has been reported.[223] The restricted ventilation occasionally seen in the syndrome seems to be due to deformed costovertebral joints inhibiting chest motion, the degree of kyphoscoliosis present with absent vertebrae and lessened thoracic space, and abnormal spacing of ribs with rib fusion, decreasing rib cage expansion and elevation.[223] Scoliosis in the thoracic area should not be allowed to progress beyond 55 degrees if seriously compromised pulmonary function is to be avoided. The spondylothoracic dwarf represents a severe form of this disease that leads to respiratory failure and early death. A relation between craniovertebral anomalies and occult respiratory dysfunction has also been noted,[224] with apparent cerebrospinal fluid disturbances, intrinsic CNS malformations, and traction or bony impingement on the brain stem.

Although some of these patients have been anesthetized with little difficulty, many patients should have a consultation with the anesthesiologist preoperatively because of anticipated problems during intubation.[225] Cleft palate, mandibular malformations, micrognathia, and limited neck extension have been described,[226] and sleep-induced ventilatory disturbances can occur in patients with intrinsic CNS dysfunction.[227] A subgroup of patients have no detectable motion and fixed hyperextension of their neck, usually associated with absence of the posterior cervical laminae; if associated with an enlarged foramen magnum, this condition is termed *iniencephaly*.[228] Manipulation of the neck during intubation or positioning should be minimized and done cautiously to avoid possible neurologic injury. The problems encountered with airway management obviously depend on the degree of neck fixation and "bull neck" status, and on the extent of micrognathia

or jaw protrusion. Fiberoptic-aided intubation (in the awake or anesthetized state) may be safer in these patients. The laryngeal mask airway may be useful for management of the difficult airway. Extubation should be performed when the patient is fully awake and adequate laryngeal reflexes have returned. These patients should be watched carefully postoperatively.

Rheumatoid Arthritis in Children (Still's Disease)

Juvenile rheumatoid arthritis (RA) is a generalized systemic disease in which arthritis is but one manifestation. It is an autoimmune disease in which a macroglobulin (an antibody-like factor) is produced and a rheumatoid factor is deposited within the joint, causing release of lysosomal enzymes; accelerated release of this factor initiates damage to the joint. It has been suggested that approximately 3 new cases occur per year per 100,000 children under 15 years of age; 70 percent of the children are female. The onset is most commonly between 2 and 4 years of age, but it may be earlier. Multiple joint involvement similar to that in the adult is most common. Fever, rash, joint redness, leukocytosis, and an increased erythrocyte sedimentation rate are prominent features. The extreme form of the disease is characterized by polyarthritis, lymphadenitis, and splenomegaly.[178, 229, 230]

Rheumatoid arthritis is a systemic disease of mesenchymal tissues and may affect collagen and connective tissue of any organ. The possible involvement of the heart should be kept in mind. Echocardiographic evidence of pericarditis has been found in 36 percent of children with RA. Abnormalities predisposing to difficult airway management include temporomandibular ankylosis, mandibular hypoplasia, and cricoarytenoid arthritis. Atlantoaxial or low cervical subluxation may occur. A microcytic hypochromic anemia is often present and is refractory to hematinics. The vertebrae may fail to grow, and ankylosis of the apophyseal joints may result.

The anesthesiologist is confronted with a chronically ill, anemic child with possible cardiac involvement. Difficulty in maintaining airway patency and inability to intubate the trachea are the most serious anesthetic problems in these children.[165, 229–232] The availability of small fiberoptic bronchoscopes has revolutionized the airway management of these children. Fiberoptic-aided intubation can safely be performed in the awake or anesthetized state (see Chapter 23).

The Myotonias

Increased muscle tension transiently outlasting voluntary muscle contraction is the characteristic symptom of a group of diseases called myotonias.[233] Myotonia may also appear as part of other syndromes, including polymyositis, periodic paralysis, and hypothyroidism.[233] The myotonias include recessive generalized myotonia (Becker's), chondrodystrophic myotonia (Schwartz-Jampel syndrome), and the three described below. Myotonia is intensified by all drugs that can directly or indirectly (via the end-plate) depolarize the muscle fiber or membrane. The relationship to malignant hyperthermia has been studied with somewhat inconclusive results. Although the myotonias are probably not associated with an increased susceptibility to malignant hyperthermia, it has been suggested that nontriggering agents be used and that the anesthesiologist be prepared for an "anesthetic-induced reaction" in these cases.[233]

Myotonia Dystrophica (Steinert's Disease)

Myotonia dystrophica is an autosomal dominant inherited disease with an incidence of 5 per 100,000 births. The patients may show one or more of the following symptoms: weakness and wasting of the facial, cervical, and proximal limb muscles; frontal baldness; cataracts; gonadal atrophy; thyroid nodules; endocrine failure; mental retardation; and voluntary and percussion myotonia.[234, 235] The endocrine failure appears to be a failure of the end-organ, as the pituitary is intact. The clinical feature common to all myotonic disorders is myotonia, a state of sustained contraction or delayed relaxation of the skeletal muscles. Studies suggest that the fundamental problems may be a reduction in the chloride conductance of the muscle membrane and a reduced ability of the sodium channels to inactivate[233]; these result in repetitive firing of action potentials in response to mechanical, chemical, or electrical stimulation. The electromyogram (EMG) shows continuous low-voltage activity, with higher voltage, fibrillation-like potential bursts. A mechanical stimulus evokes a burst of rhythmic activity of 90 to 100 per second, which eventually slows to low-voltage activity. An acoustic amplification of the EMG gives a characteristic sound likened to a dive-bomber or a motorcyclist taking off at a high speed.

Cardiac involvement is characterized by defects in the conduction system and abnormalities of the contractile mechanism. Conduction defects are present in approximately 50 percent of these patients. The incidence of demonstrable conduction defects is increased to 90 percent with recordings made of the bundle of His. Respiratory involvement appears to result from both skeletal muscular weakness and oropharyngeal involvement, which leads to frequent aspiration and pneumonia.

The disease usually begins during the second to fourth decades as myotonia, which progresses to atrophy in later years. The histologic manifestations are combined nerve terminal and muscle degeneration. The disease usually progresses to death during the sixth decade from bulbar involvement or cardiorespiratory failure.

The overall mortality under anesthesia of patients with myotonia dystrophica is higher than the normal rate. These patients exhibit a marked sensitivity to barbiturates, which is manifested as respiratory depression. Preoperative medication should be minimal and the use of opioids is best avoided. In addition to the apnea reported after thiopental and opioids, these patients are also sensitive to diazepam and inhalational anesthetics.[236] Attempts to maintain the airway or intubate the patient can mechanically trigger a myotonic response, which may further prevent adequate airway maintenance and ventilation. Because of muscle weakness, the jaw may easily be dislocated during attempts to maintain the airway. The prevalence of cardiac

irregularities requires close monitoring of cardiac function.

Generalized myotonia has been reported after administration of succinylcholine.[237] After succinylcholine, there is a decrease in evoked twitch height, and a contracture proportional to the dose administered develops (Fig. 22–15). When myotonia is present, contractures can be elicited repeatedly by chemical, electrical, or mechanical stimulation. Therefore, if general anesthesia is accompanied by endotracheal intubation, intubation is best accomplished without the use of succinylcholine. When applicable, regional or local anesthetic techniques are preferred. If localized myotonia develops in the abdominal muscle wall during abdominal surgery, it is best controlled by injecting a local anesthetic into the affected muscle. Administering muscle relaxants systemically will probably not relieve this localized myotonia. The development of contracture is not usually prevented by spinal or regional block. Similarly, the use of a nondepolarizing relaxant does not totally prevent mechanically stimulated contractures.

Patients with myotonia appear to react normally to nondepolarizing muscle relaxants in many cases, but advanced cases with muscle wasting may be sensitive. The dose of relaxant may need to be reduced, and careful monitoring must be done. Reversal of a nondepolarizing block by anticholinesterases may be hazardous because of cholinergic overactivity. However, Mitchell and associates[236] did give neostigmine to two of their patients without triggering a contracture. The newer nondepolarizing relaxants, atracurium, vecuronium, rocuronium, and mivacurium, can be utilized. With appropriate dosage and monitoring, reversal may not be necessary. The relaxant of choice for many patients with muscle disease is now atracurium. Its brief duration, its ability to "self-destruct" by an alternative pathway, and its safety in the presence of either hepatic or renal disease make it efficacious. Mivacurium may also prove to be a relaxant to consider in these patients.[238] A single dose of 0.08 mg/kg of mivacurium was reported to be effective for a 90-minute surgery. Mechani-

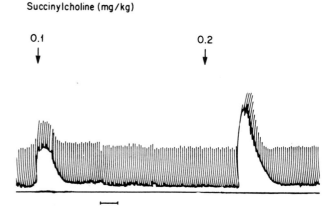

Succinylcholine (mg/kg)

0.1   0.2

FIGURE 22–15. The myotonic response to succinylcholine. Evoked thumb adduction in response to stimulation of the ulnar nerve at 0.15 Hz. Note the upward baseline shift (contracture) and the decrease in the amplitude of the twitch height. Time scale 1 minute. (From Koht A, Schütz W, Schmidt G, et al: Effects of etomidate, midazolam, and thiopental on median nerve somatosensory evoked potentials and the additive effects of fentanyl and nitrous oxide. Anesth Analg 67:435, 1988, with permission.)

cal ventilation until adequate postoperative recovery is demonstrated is another option.

Myotonia Congenita (Thomsen's Disease)

Myotonia congenita is an inherited autosomal dominant disease characterized by the early onset of muscle hypertrophy. The patient appears "muscle bound."[239] Mechanical and electrical myotonia may be elicited, and the electromyogram demonstrates the "dive-bomber" effect. The myotonia is most severe after rest and tends to decrease with exercise.[239, 240] There is no dystrophic change and no involvement of heart muscle. The disease runs a benign course, with no systemic involvement. Generalized rigidity after administration of succinylcholine has been reported.[239] Anticholinesterases have been reported to enhance myotonia. Rather than attempting reversal with neostigmine, it is preferable to ventilate these patients mechanically until spontaneous respiration is adequate. Shivering should be avoided, as it may increase myotonia.

Paramyotonia Congenita (Eulenburg's Disease)

Paramyotonia congenita is another rare inherited disease in which myotonia is usually followed by paresis. It is commonly induced by exposure to cold. No other systems appear to be involved.[234] Generalized severe increases in muscle tone lasting for 30 minutes and interfering with ventilation have been noted after administration of succinylcholine.[234] The use of succinylcholine should be avoided in these patients.

Muscular Dystrophies

Myopathies are primary diseases involving striated muscle, with combinations of neurophysiologic, biochemical, and morphologic changes. Dystrophies are hereditary myopathies with weakness and muscle degeneration, usually progressive.[241] Included in this group of primary muscle diseases are a number of hereditary syndromes characterized by microscopic degeneration of muscle fibers with abundance of fatty and fibrous tissue. There is no evidence of denervation in these diseases.[241]

Progressive muscular dystrophy affects not only skeletal muscle but also cardiac muscle and smooth muscle of the alimentary tract. Because these patients have a tendency to tachycardia, administration of atropine may not be advisable. For anesthesia, thiopental should be used with caution, if at all. Because of the generalized muscle weakness, muscle relaxant dosage must be carefully monitored. These patients may be sensitive to nondepolarizing relaxants.[242] Succinylcholine may cause hyperkalemia, arrhythmias, rhabdomyolysis, myoglobinuria, malignant hyperthermia,[243] and cardiac arrest.[244, 245] It should probably never be administered to these patients.[246] Gastric dilation frequently develops in these patients postoperatively because of the effects of the disease on smooth muscle.[234, 243] Aspiration pneumonia is a common complication, in part because of the patients' poor esophageal motility. A rapid-sequence induction has been advocated, treating these children as if they had a full stomach.[247]

The *Duchenne type* of muscular dystrophy (DMD) is the most common and most severe. It is an inherited, X-linked, recessive disease that predominantly affects male infants. The incidence is reported as 3 per 10,000 births. The gene for DMD has been isolated, with its locus at position 21 on the short arm of the X chromosome. It is a huge gene, prone to a high rate of mutation. The DMD gene product, dystrophin, is absent or nonfunctional in these patients.[248] The onset is early (2 to 6 years), with weakness of the pelvic girdle followed by atrophy of the proximal muscles. The atrophy is preceded by pseudohypertrophy, usually in the calf muscles. In the early stages of the disease plasma levels of CPK, SGOT, LDH, SGPT, and aldolase are elevated; these elevations are believed to result from permeability of the cell membrane to sarcoplasmic constituents. The levels drop with the development of atrophy. Patients are usually in a wheelchair by their early teens. Cardiac abnormalities, in the form of tachyarrhythmias or heart block, are observed in almost all patients. The ECG is abnormal in up to 90 percent of patients.[249] Cardiac conduction defects occurred in 50 percent of one series.[250] Although most cardiac arrests have been attributed to hyperkalemia and rhabdomyolysis,[251] a recent report noted bradydysrhythmia possibly due to an electrical conduction problem, or primary myocardial muscle failure.[252] Progressive myocardial necrosis may occur,[253] and in late stages degeneration of cardiac muscle may be manifest as papillary muscle dysfunction with mitral regurgitation and decreased myocardial contractility.[254] Respiratory muscle weakness causes these patients to be prone to respiratory infection. Death occurs late in the second decade, usually (90 percent) from respiratory complications.

Except for acute cardiac problems that occur during anesthesia, the main problems with these patients are related to postoperative pulmonary complications. The recommended regimen calls for light premedication and light levels of general anesthesia. Preoperative instruction in the pulmonary physiotherapy that will be conducted during the postoperative period may be worthwhile. Opioids, both intra- and postoperatively, must be used cautiously because of the susceptibility to respiratory depression. Hypotensive anesthesia has been successfully performed for scoliosis correction.[255]

The *fascioscapulohumeral*, or *Landouzy-Dejerine type*, is another syndrome of muscular dystrophy. It is an autosomal dominant trait, affecting male and female infants equally. It tends to appear later than the Duchenne type, usually occurring in adolescents. In addition, it is characterized by less cardiovascular and respiratory involvement. Respiratory difficulty, when it occurs, is caused by weakness of the accessory muscles of respiration. When general anesthesia is required, special efforts should be made to avoid respiratory complications.

In the *limb girdle type* of muscular dystrophy, whether shoulder (*ERB's*) or pelvic (*Leyden Möbius*), onset occurs between the first and third decades. Cardiac involvement in the form of sinus tachycardia and bundle-branch block is common. The respiratory difficulty is similar to that of Landouzy-Dejerine muscular dystrophy.

The *distal type* of dystrophy is an inherited autosomal dominant disease with an onset around the third decade. It has been described only in Swedes.

Familial Periodic Paralysis

Familial periodic paralysis (FPP) is an inherited autosomal dominant disorder with a high degree of penetrance in male infants. Three types of the disease, characterized by the serum potassium level, have been described. In the most common type, the onset of paralysis is associated with a low serum potassium level, whereas in the other two types the serum potassium levels may be either normal or elevated during the attacks.[234, 241, 246, 256]

In the *hypokalemic type* of FPP, the first manifestation is usually in the second decade; attacks can be precipitated by high carbohydrate or salt intake, cold, a period of rest after very strenuous exercise, mental stress, trauma, surgical stress, or menstruation. The paralysis is variable and is commonly asymmetric, affecting primarily the upper and lower limbs, neck, and trunk. The flaccid paralysis can be severe and can persist for up to 36 hours. It rarely affects the diaphragm or cranial muscles. The blood pressure usually rises, and arrhythmias are common during the attack. The ECG shows evidence of hypokalemic changes. Although serum potassium levels may fall to 2 to 3 mEq/L, the levels do not correlate well with the severity of the weakness. The electromyogram shows abnormal lengthening of the action potential until paralysis ensues, at which time the action potentials are replaced by electrical silence. Diaphoresis and diuresis terminate the attack, with the serum potassium level returning to normal before the electromyogram. There are nonspecific changes in the microscopic appearance of the muscle, consisting of vacuoles in the sarcoplasmic reticulum that increase in number during the attack. A thyrotoxic variety of paralysis resembles the hypokalemic type, except that in the former a much greater decrease in the serum potassium concentration occurs, the incidence is higher in male infants, and the paralytic episodes end when the patient becomes euthyroid.[241, 256]

Preanesthetic evaluation should include advising the patient to avoid a high carbohydrate intake the night before surgery. Because mental stress can precipitate attacks, alleviating anxiety during the preoperative period may be important. The serum electrolytes should be carefully evaluated. Glucose administration should be limited, and potassium should be supplemented to avoid hypokalemia. Because changes in pH can have a profound effect on serum potassium levels, alkalosis should be avoided. Cold can precipitate an attack and special efforts should therefore be made to keep the patient in a comfortable environment, including a warm operating room. Monitoring during surgery should include an ECG for evaluation of changes suggestive of hypokalemia. Monitoring of cardiac function is essential, as cardiac failure is known to occur during episodes of paralysis. Muscle relaxants, unless absolutely necessary, should be avoided, as the effects of the drugs are not certain. If muscle relaxants have been used and the patient appears paralyzed at the end of surgery, a differential test of extremity versus facial muscle activity can be tried. The test depends on the observation that facial muscles are much less affected by the disease than are those of the extremities, and both are similarly blocked by relaxant drugs. Postoperative respiratory support may be necessary in patients with this condition.

In the *hyperkalemic* form of FPP, onset is usually before the age of 10 years; the attacks occur spontaneously after muscular exercise and are not related to carbohydrate intake. The paralytic attacks are of shorter duration than in the hypokalemic variety (a matter of hours rather than days). Paralysis starts in the lower extremities and gradually involves the remainder of the body, including the facial muscles but, like that in the hypokalemic variety, usually spares the respiratory muscles. The serum potassium level may increase in the range of 20 percent, yet may still be within the normal range. During the attack, some patients exhibit mechanical myotonia of the tongue and hypothenar muscles, similar to that in paramyotonia congenita. In this variety, the preparations for anesthesia are the reverse of those followed for the hypokalemic variety (i.e., avoidance of carbohydrate depletion, use of a potassium-free diet, and administration of glucose during the operation). An ECG should be used to monitor cardiac performance and detect signs of hyperkalemia. Muscle relaxants should be avoided because of their uncertain effect.

The *normokalemic* form occurs mostly in children, with severe and prolonged attacks precipitated by the same predisposing factors as in the hypokalemic variety. In this type, multifocal ventricular ectopic foci are usually seen on the ECG. General endotracheal anesthesia is usually preferred, with ECG monitoring for arrhythmias.

Cerebral Palsy

Cerebral palsy can be defined as a nonprogressive central motor deficit caused by events during the perinatal period. Many children with cerebral palsy require corrective orthopedic procedures. The incidence of cerebral palsy is approximately 7 per 100,000 births. Of these seven, one child dies before the age of 6, two require custodial care, one is severely handicapped, two are moderately handicapped and capable of improvement, and one is mildly handicapped. The underlying pathology appears to be damage to the upper motor neurons in the spinal cord or brain. Symptoms include incoordination, lack of balance, mental retardation, convulsions, and speech defects. Surgical procedures are designed to release contractures, to facilitate bracing, to increase range of motion, to improve gait, and to minimize deformity. The most common procedures performed include heel-cord lengthening, adductor myotomy, and hamstring lengthening. Tendon transfers are also performed to improve hand function. Because of the various degrees of involvement in patients with cerebral palsy, the choice of anesthetic drugs should be tailored to the individual need and surgical requirement. Severely affected children may have gastroesophageal reflux and problems with pharyngeal coordination. This may make them vulnerable to aspiration during induction and extubation, and should mandate a cautious approach to these potentially anemic, malnourished children.[26] Although denervated muscles exhibit an exaggerated potassium efflux after succinylcholine, cerebral palsy patients have successfully received succinylcholine without development of hyperkalemia.[257] The response to nondepolarizing muscle relaxants appears to be normal.

Epidermolysis Bullosa

Epidermolysis bullosa is a rare genetic disorder of the skin characterized by formation of blisters; the blisters usually occur at the sites of pressure or friction but may also occur spontaneously in the more severe forms of the disease (Fig. 22–16). There are four main varieties: simplex, hyperplastic (dystrophic), polydysplastic (dystrophic), and lethalis.[258–260]

In the *simplex* variety, which is autosomal dominant, bullae are noted early in life and are subepidermal. They appear at sites of friction, especially in warm weather, usually on the hands and feet. Blisters develop as a result of liquefaction degeneration of the basal and suprabasal layers of the epidermis.

In the *hyperplastic, dystrophic* variety (also autosomal dominant), bullae usually follow trauma but may arise spontaneously. Recurrent episodes lead to mutilating deformities, particularly of the hands and feet. The mucous membranes are involved in approximately one fifth of the cases, and leukoplakia may follow.

The *polydysplastic* form is inherited as a recessive trait and is far more severe than the others. Large, spontaneous bullae appear at birth or during early infancy. The digits may stick together, forming glove-like hands and feet. The mucosal surfaces are usually involved, and the mouth, pharynx, esophagus, and larynx are therefore affected.[261] Esophageal stricture may occur. With this variety the teeth, hair, and nails show dystrophic changes. Affected children are usually underdeveloped, and survival beyond the second decade is unlikely.

The *lethalis* variant, inherited as a recessive trait, is the most severe form. The digestive and respiratory systems are markedly involved. Survival beyond a few months is rare. There has been a report describing anesthesia for two patients with what is now termed the *JEB variety* (junctional epidermolysis bullosa) (formerly called lethalis).[262] Some of these patients are now surviving into childhood and may require anesthesia in the future.

In addition to these four main varieties, three rarer forms are also classified: a nonhereditary acquired form, first seen in adolescence or adulthood; an autosomal dominant variation involving only the hands and feet (Weber-Cockayne disease); and a rare form with localized absence of the skin, nail dystrophy, and mouth erosions (Bart syndrome).[263] All are characterized by skin that is particularly susceptible to shearing forces. Even minimal shearing or friction can rapidly produce bullae in the stratified squamous epithelium that have some of the characteristics of burns.[263]

Cutaneous infection occurs, especially with the severe forms. In some forms, malignant changes are also present. Prevention of trauma, pressure, and friction is essential. Administration of systemic steroids to suppress formation of bullae may be lifesaving in early infancy. With the dystrophic forms, various plastic and orthopedic procedures may be indicated to correct deformities.

Patients with the severe forms may show all the sequalae of a generalized, debilitating disease. Ulcers in the mouth and nasopharynx may lead to malnutrition, anemia, and electrolyte imbalance. Secondary infections and fever are always a possibility. The high incidence of associated porphyria has been stressed, and urine should therefore be tested to rule out the presence of porphyrins.

A careful preoperative evaluation should be done, and a consultation with the dermatologist may be helpful. Touching the skin may be painful to the patient. Application of devices such as the blood pressure cuff; adhesive tape; monitoring electrodes; airways; oropharyngeal; esophageal; or rectal probes; and urinary catheters carries the risk of contaminating and severely traumatizing the skin and the mucosa and should be used only when they are absolutely essential. If so, they are applied gently, and when possible the skin is well protected with cotton (cuffs and tourniquets). Pressure is a lesser hazard than friction. For example, a spring-loaded pulse oximeter probe is used rather than one requiring an adhesive. Premedication and induction with barbiturates should probably be avoided because of the potential that porphyria is present. Airway manipulation should be avoided whenever possible. Application of the face mask and artificial airways may excoriate, blister, or cross-contaminate the skin and the mucosa, leading to facial injuries, supraglottic airway obstruction, and pulmonary infections. When airways are necessary, gentle introduction and close observation for bulla formation and airway obstruction is mandatory. The eyes should not be taped but should be protected with an ophthalmic ointment. When tracheal intubation is per-

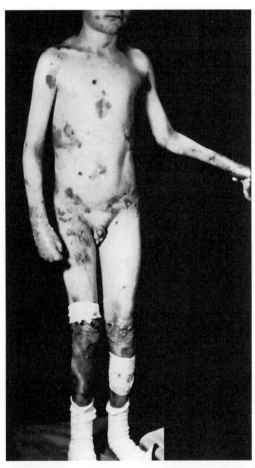

FIGURE 22–16. This teenage boy shows a rather severe form of epidermolysis, including advanced changes in the hands. Intravenous sites may be sparse, and all skin contacts are painful. (Photograph courtesy of Shriner's Hospital for Children, Chicago Unit.)

formed, it must be atraumatic; an undersized, well-lubricated endotracheal tube should be used. If a tight mask fit becomes essential, the face must be protected with cotton or foam padding.

Nondepolarizing relaxants have been considered relatively contraindicated because disused and dystrophic muscles may exhibit unpredictable sensitivity. A short-acting drug such as rapacuronium may prove useful, as may low-dose atracurium with its unique metabolism. Extensive tissue injury could conceivably produce hyperkalemia after administration of succinylcholine. Adhesions that involve the tongue could result in airway problems. Esophageal strictures increase the incidence of regurgitation and aspiration.

Regional anesthesia was not considered suitable in the past because of the likelihood of infection, contractures, and trauma to the skin. In recent years, however, spinal, epidural, and regional anesthesia have all been successfully performed in these patients.[263–266]

Anesthesia can be provided with a potent inhalational drug delivered by mask. In some cases the mask is held close to, but not touching, the face. The laryngeal mask airway may prove useful for some of these patients. Despite its potential disadvantages, ketamine appears to be a viable alternative, as it usually requires no airway manipulation; it has been used, without intubation, with good results. A retrospective report[260] reviewed the experience with endotracheal intubation on 131 occasions in patients with epidermolysis bullosa dystrophica. The authors found no laryngeal or tracheal complications. They indicated that the hazards of intubation in these patients have been overemphasized and advocated its more routine use.[260] It should be noted, however, that in several patients in this series tracheal intubation was difficult and, in fact, 17 of 33 (51 percent) of the patients had gross dental problems and/or restriction of mouth opening sufficient to make intubation a challenge; two of these patients could not be intubated. The study also found new oral lesions in some patients, even in those without tracheal lesions. Laryngeal stenosis has also been reported in a few patients who were never intubated.[261] Because many of these patients are receiving steroids before surgery, routine preparation and postoperative therapy with such drugs are indicated. Transfer of these patients from the gurney to the operating table, and vice versa, must be done with meticulous care. Monitoring in the recovery room should be limited to the essential monitors. General anesthesia has been used for up to 12 hours in a patient with dystrophic epidermolysis bullosa, while still avoiding either airway trauma or disruption of skin integrity.[276] An association with neuromuscular diseases (muscular dystrophy[268] and myasthenia gravis[269]) has been reported.

Sotos Syndrome

Sotos syndrome is cerebral gigantism associated with dilated ventricles, macrocephaly, acromegalic features, and mental retardation; this prenatal onset of accelerated growth appears to be transmitted as an autosomal dominant trait,[270] although a recessive inheritance has also been suggested.[271] Hypotonia, high-arched palate, cardiac abnormalities, lipid storage myopathy, increased secretion of growth hormone, hydrocephalus with increased intracranial pressure, emotional disorders, and aggressive behavior have been reported. Scoliosis is reported to occur in 4 percent of these patients, and successful posterior spinal fusion has been performed with continuous SSEP monitoring and induced hypotension.[272]

Rett Syndrome

Rett syndrome is a recently described[273] syndrome of progressive higher brain-function deterioration, seen only in females. After an initial normal period of development lasting 4 to 18 months, rapid regression begins, characterized by severe autism; dementia; axial hypotonia; limb spasticity; movement disorders including dystonia; myoclonic jerking, and choreoathetosis; stereotyped hand movements; progressive diffuse muscle wasting; microcephaly; growth retardation; and thoracic deformity. Abnormal patterns of respiration occur, including periods of disorganized ineffective respiratory efforts mixed with periods of apnea while awake, hypoxemia, loss of consciousness, and upper airway obstruction.[274, 275] These patients may be at risk for recurrent aspiration pneumonia and impaired respiratory function. Frequent desaturation may cause permanent hypoxic damage and may contribute to cerebral deterioration. Other findings include vasomotor disturbances with cool limbs, tropic changes, and profuse sweating. Elevated ammonia levels were reported by Rett but are not found consistently; increased lactic acid levels have been noted. A reduction in dopamine and norepinephrine metabolites has been discovered.[276] It is estimated that Rett syndrome, although still not widely known, may account for 25 percent of all severely retarded females.[277] Most are wheelchair-bound by their teens, and few survive past 30 years. Scoliosis occurs in approximately 50 percent of patients. Harrington rod spinal fusion for scoliosis has been reported in these patients.[278] Anesthetic management may be complicated by their inability to cooperate preoperatively (for pulmonary function testing) and postoperatively (e.g., for coughing, deep breathing, incentive spirometry). Their irregular respiratory pattern, excessive secretions, weak cough, and aspiration history suggest the need for careful extubation and postoperative ventilation in an intensive care environment. The anesthetic management of three patients for scoliosis correction was reported in 1996.[279] One 11-year-old died suddenly 1 month after discharge with acute heart and lung failure. Sudden death is noted in 22 percent of Rett syndrome patients. Although a lengthened QT interval had been noted,[280] it was not seen in another report.[278]

REFERENCES

1. Keim HA: Scoliosis. Ciba Foundation Symposium. Vol 1. Summit, NJ, Ciba, 1978.
2. Moe JH: Historical aspects of scoliosis. In Bradford DS, Lonstein JE, Moe JH, et al (eds): Moe's Textbook of Scoliosis and Other Spinal Deformities. 2nd ed. Philadelphia, WB Saunders Company, 1987, p 1.
3. Wynne-Davies R: Familial (idiopathic) scoliosis: a family survey. J Bone Joint Surg Br 50:24, 1968.
4. Shands AR, Esiberg HB: The incidence of scoliosis in the state of Delaware. J Bone Joint Surg Am 37:1243, 1955.

5. Goldstein LA, Waugh TR: Classification and terminology of scoliosis. Clin Orthop 93:10, 1973.
6. Roaf R: Rotation movements of the spine with special reference to scoliosis. J Bone Joint Surg Br 40:312, 1958.
7. Cobb JR: Outline for the study of scoliosis. AAOS Instruct Course Lect 5:261, 1948.
8. Wynne-Davies R: Heritable Disorders in Orthopedic Practice. Oxford, Blackwell Scientific Publications, 1973.
9. Kafer ER: Respiratory and cardiovascular functions in scoliosis and the principles of anesthetic management. Anesthesiology 52:339, 1980.
10. Layzer RB: Degenerative diseases of the nervous system. In Wyngaarden J, Smith LH Jr, McDermott W (eds): Textbook of Medicine. 18th ed. Philadelphia, WB Saunders Company, 1988.
11. Baraka A: Myasthenic response to muscle relaxants in von Recklinghausen's disease. Br J Anaesth 46:701, 1974.
12. Shapiro F, Sethna N, Colan S, et al: Spinal fusion in Duchenne muscular dystrophy: a multidisciplinary approach. Muscle Nerve 15:604, 1992.
13. Kafer ER: Respiratory and cardiovascular functions in scoliosis. Bull Eur Physiopathol Respir 13:299, 1977.
14. Hepper NAG, Black LF, Fowler WS: Relationships of lung volume and height and arm span in normal subjects and in patients with spinal deformity. Am Rev Respir Dis 91:356, 1965.
15. Shannon DC, Riseborough EJ, Valenca LM, et al: The distribution of abnormal lung function in kyphoscoliosis. J Bone Joint Surg Am 52:131, 1970.
16. Bergofsky EH, Turino GM, Fishman AP: Cardiorespiratory failure in kyphoscoliosis. Medicine 38:263, 1959.
17. Davies G, Reid I: Effect of scoliosis on growth of alveoli and pulmonary arteries and on the right ventricle. Arch Dis Child 46:623, 1971.
18. Rudolph AM, Yuan S: Response of the pulmonary vasculature to hypoxia and hydrogen ion concentration changes. J Clin Invest 45:399, 1966.
19. Roth A, Hall JE, Mizel M, et al: Scoliosis and congenital heart disease. Clin Orthop 93:95, 1973.
20. Jenkins JG, Bohn DJ, Edmonds JF, et al: Evaluation of pulmonary function in muscular dystrophy patients requiring spinal surgery. Crit Care Med 10:645, 1982.
21. Harrington PR: Treatment of scoliosis correction and internal fixation by spinal instrumentation. J Bone Joint Surg Am 44:591, 1962.
22. Harrington PR, Dickson JH: An eleven year clinical investigation of Harrington instrumentation—a preliminary report on 578 cases. Clin Orthop 93:113, 1973.
23. Luque ER, Cardoso A: Segmental correction of scoliosis with rigid internal fixation. Orthop Trans 1:136, 1977.
24. Luque ER: Segmental spinal instrumentation for correction of scoliosis. Clin Orthop 163:192, 1982.
25. Lowe T: Morbidity and mortality committee report, Scoliosis Research Society. Read at 22nd Annual Meeting, Vancouver, BC, Canada, 1987.
26. Cohen DE, Steven JM: Anesthesia for orthopedic surgery. In Motoyama EK, Davis PJ (eds): Smith's Anesthesia for Infants and Children. 5th ed. St Louis, CV Mosby, 1990, p 611.
27. Ashman RB, Herring JA, Johnston CE II: Texas Scottish Rite hospital instrumentation system. In Bridwell KH, DeWald RL (eds): The Textbook of Spinal Surgery. Philadelphia, JB Lippincott, 1991, p 219.
28. Cotrel Y, Dubousset J: New segmental posterior instrumentation of the spine. Orthop Trans 9:118, 1985.
29. Cotrel Y, Dubousset J, Guillaumat M: New universal instrumentation in spinal surgery. Clin Orthop 227:10, 1988.
30. Chopin D, Morin C: Cotrel-Dubousset instrumentation for adolescent and pediatric scoliosis. In Bridwell KH, DeWald RL (eds): The Textbook of Spinal Surgery. Philadelphia, JB Lippincott, 1991, p 183.
31. Shufflebarger HL: Moss-Miami spinal instrumentation system: methods of fixation of the spondylopelvic junction. In Margulies JY, et al (eds): Lumbosacral and Spinopelvic Fixation. Philadelphia, Lippincott-Raven, 1996.
32. Betz RB, Harms J, Clements DH, et al: Anterior instrumentation for thoracic idiopathic scoliosis. Semin Spine Surg 9:141, 1997.
33. Shufflebarger HL: Moss-Miami spinal instrumentation. In Bridwell K (ed): The Textbook of Spinal Surgery. Vol 2. Philadelphia, JB Lippincott, 1996.
34. Dwyer AF, Schafer MF: Anterior approach to scoliosis: results of treatment in fifty-one cases. J Bone Joint Surg Am 56:218, 1974.
35. Dwyer AF, O'Brien JP, Seal PP, et al: The late complications after the Dwyer anterior spinal instrumentation for scoliosis. J Bone Joint Surg Br 59:117, 1977.
36. Zielke K, Pellin B: Neue instrumente und implantate zur erganzung des Harrington systems. Z Orthop Chir 114:534, 1976.
37. Relton JES: Anesthesia in the surgical correction of scoliosis. In Risenborough EJ, Herndon JH (eds): Scoliosis and Other Deformities of the Axial Skeleton. Boston, Little, Brown, 1975, p 309.
38. McNeil TW, DeWald RL, Kuo KN, et al: Controlled hypotensive anesthesia in scoliosis surgery. J Bone Joint Surg Am 56:1167, 1974.
39. Relton JES, Hall JE: An operation frame for spinal fusion: a new apparatus designed to reduce haemorrhage during operation. J Bone Joint Surg Br 49:327, 1967.
40. Bennett EJ, Salem MR, Sakul P, et al: Induced hypotension for spinal corrective procedures. Mid East J Anesth 4:177, 1974.
41. Jacobs HK, Lieponis JV, Bunch WH, et al: The influence of halothane and nitroprusside on canine spinal cord hemodynamics. Spine 7:35, 1982.
42. Salem MR, Wong AY, Bennett EJ, et al: Deliberate hypotension in infants and children. Anesth Analg 53:975, 1974.
43. Salem MR, Wong AY, Mani M, et al: Efficacy of cricoid pressure in preventing gastric inflation during bag-mask ventilation in pediatric patients. Anesthesiology 40:96, 1974.
44. Phillips WA, Hensinger RN: Control of blood loss during scoliosis surgery. Clin Orthop 229:88, 1988.
45. Katz RL, Bigger JT: Cardiac arrhythmias during anesthesia and operation. Anesthesiology 33:193, 1970.
46. Johnston RR, Eger EI II, Wilson C: A comparative interaction of epinephrine with enflurane, isoflurane, and halothane in man. Anesth Analg 55:709, 1976.
47. Hayashi Y, Sumikawa K, Tashiro C, et al: Arrhythmogenic threshold of epinephrine during sevoflurane, enflurane, and isoflurane anesthesia in dogs. Anesthesiology 69:145, 1990.
48. Weiskopf RB, Eger EI II, Holmes MA, et al: Epinephrine-induced premature ventricular contractions and changes in arterial blood pressure and heart rate during I-653, isoflurane, and halothane anesthesia in swine. Anesthesiology 70:293, 1989.
49. Karl HW, Swedlow DB, Lee KW, et al: Epinephrine-halothane interactions in children. Anesthesiology 58:142, 1983.
50. Goldstein LA: Surgical management of scoliosis. J Bone Joint Surg Am 48:167, 1966.
51. Patel N, Patel B, Paskin S, et al: Induced moderate hypotensive anesthesia for spinal fusion and Harrington rod instrumentation. J Bone Joint Surg Am 67:1384, 1985.
52. Lawhon SM, Kahn A III, Crawford AH, et al: Controlled hypotensive anesthesia during spinal surgery: a retrospective study. Spine 9:450, 1984.
53. Porter SS, Asher M, Fox DK: Comparison of intravenous nitroprusside, nitroprusside-captopril, and nitroglycerin for deliberate hypotension during posterior spine fusion in adults. J Clin Anesth 1:87, 1988.
54. Brodsky JW, Dickson JH, Erwin WD, et al: Hypotensive anesthesia for scoliosis surgery in Jehovah's Witnesses. Spine 16:304, 1991.
55. Enderby GEH: Postural ischaemia and blood pressure. Lancet 2:1097, 1954.
56. Salem MR: Therapeutic uses of ganglionic blocking drugs. Int Anesthiol Clin 16:171, 1978.
57. Sivarajan M, Amory DW, Everett GB, et al: Blood pressure, not cardiac output, determines blood loss during induced hypotension. Anesth Analg 59:203, 1980.
58. Salem MR, Toyama T, Wong AY, et al: Haemodynamic responses to induced arterial hypotension in children. Br J Anaesth 50:489, 1978.
59. Knight PR, Lane GA, Nicholls MG, et al: Hormonal and hemodynamic changes induced by pentolinium and propranolol during surgical correction of scoliosis. Anesthesiology 53:127, 1980.
60. Fahmy NR: Nitroglycerin as a hypotensive during general anesthesia. Anesthesiology 49:17, 1978.
61. Yaster M, Simmons RS, Tolo VT, et al: A comparison of nitroglycerin and nitroprusside for inducing hypotension in children: a double-blind study. Anesthesiology 65:175, 1986.
62. Prys-Roberts C, Lloyd JW, Fisher A, et al: Deliberate profound hypotension induced with halothane: studies of haemodynamics and pulmonary gas exchange. Br J Anaesth 46:105, 1974.
63. Miller ED, Ackerly JA, Vaughan ED, et al: The renin-angiotensin system during controlled hypotension with sodium nitroprusside. Anesthesiology 47:257, 1977.

64. Rawlinson WAL, Loach AB, Benedict CR: Changes in plasma concentration of adrenaline and noradrenaline in anaesthetized patients during sodium nitroprusside-induced hypotension. Br J Anaesth 50:937, 1978.

65. Khambatta HJ, Stone JG, Kahn E: Propranolol alters renin release during nitroprusside induced hypotension and prevents hypertension on discontinuation of nitroprusside. Anesth Analg 60:569, 1981.

66. Knight PR, Lane GA, Hensinger RN, et al: Catecholamine and renin-angiotensin response during hypotensive anesthesia induced by sodium nitroprusside or trimethaphan camsylate. Anesthesiology 59:248, 1983.

67. Fahmy NR, Mihelakos PT, Battit GE, et al: Propranolol prevents hemodynamic and humoral events after abrupt withdrawal of nitroprusside. Clin Pharmacol Ther 36:470, 1984.

68. Khambatta HJ, Stone JG, Khan E: Hypertension during anesthesia on discontinuation of sodium nitroprusside-induced hypotension. Anesthesiology 51:127, 1979.

69. Hersey SL, O'Dell NE, Lowe S, et al: Nicardipine versus nitroprusside for controlled hypotension during spinal surgery in adolescents. Anesth Analg 84:1239, 1997.

70. Fahmy NR, Bottros MR, Charehaflieh J, et al: A randomized comparison of labetalol and nitroprusside for induced hypotension. J Clin Anesth 1:409, 1989.

71. Green DW: Techniques for deliberate hypotension: pharmacological blockade. In Enderby GEH (ed): Hypotensive Anaesthesia. London, Churchill Livingstone, 1985, p 109.

72. Salem MR: Deliberate hypotension is a safe and accepted anesthetic technique. In Eckenhoff JE (ed): Controversy in Anesthesiology. Philadelphia, WB Saunders, 1979, p 95.

73. Eckenhoff JE, Enderby GEH, Larson A, et al: Pulmonary gas exchange during deliberate hypotension. Br J Anaesth 35:750, 1963.

74. Askrog VF, Pender JW, Eckenhoff JE: Changes in physiological deadspace during deliberate hypotension. Anesthesiology 25:744, 1964.

75. Salem MR, Paulissian R, Joseph NJ, et al: Effect of deliberate hypotension on arterial to peak expired carbon dioxide tension difference. Anesth Anagl 67:S194, 1988.

76. Badgwell JM, Heavner JE, May WS, et al: End-tidal PCO_2 monitoring in infants and children ventilated with either a partial rebreathing or a non-rebreathing circuit. Anesthesiology 66:405, 1987.

77. Stone JG, Khambatta HJ, Matteo RS: Pulmonary shunting during anesthesia with deliberate hypotension. Anesthesiology 45:508, 1976.

78. Casthely PA, Lear S, Cottrell JE, et al: Intrapulmonary shunting during induced hypotension. Anesth Analg 61:231, 1982.

79. Benumof JL, Wahrenbrock EA: Blunted hypoxic pulmonary constriction by increased lung vascular pressure. J Appl Physiol 38:846, 1975.

80. Cheney FW, Colley PS, Peter PS: The effect of cardiac output on arterial blood oxygenation. Anesthesiology 52:496, 1980.

81. Salem MR, Kim Y, Shaker MH: Effect of alteration of inspired oxygen concentration on jugular bulb oxygen tension during deliberate hypotension. Anesthesiology 33:358, 1970.

82. Tinker JH, Michenfelder JD: Sodium nitroprusside: pharmacology, toxicology and therapeutics. Anesthesiology 45:340, 1976.

83. Rao TLK, Jacobs K, Salem MR, et al: Deliberate hypotension and anesthetic requirements of halothane. Anesth Analg 60:513, 1981.

84. Widman FK: Standards for Blood Banks and Transfusion Services. 14th ed. Arlington, VA, American Association of Blood Banks, 1991.

85. Cowell HR, Swickard JW: Autotransfusion in children's orthopaedics. J Bone Joint Surg Br 56:908, 1974.

86. Stehling LC: Predeposited autologous blood donation. Acta Anaesthesiol Scand Suppl 32:58, 1988.

87. Silvergleid AJ: Preoperative autologous donation: what have we learned? Transfusion 31:99, 1991.

88. Goodnough LT, Wasman J, Corlucci K, et al: Limitation to donating adequate autologous blood prior to elective orthopedic surgery. Arch Surg 124:494, 1989.

89. Kulier AH, Gombotz H, Fuchs G, et al: Subcutaneous recombinant human erythropoietin and autologous blood donation before coronary artery bypass surgery. Anesth Analg 76:102, 1993.

90. Kafer ER, Collins ML: Acute intraoperative hemodilution and perioperative blood salvage. Anesth Clin North Am 8:543, 1990.

91. Wong KC, Webster LR, Coleman SS, et al: Hemodilution and induced hypotension for insertion of a Harrington rod in a Jehovah's Witness patient. Clin Orthop 152:237, 1980.

92. Fontana JL, Welborn L, Mongan PD, et al: Oxygen consumption and cardiovascular function in children during profound intraoperative normovolemic hemodilution. Anesth Analg 80:1000, 1995.

93. Fahmy NR: Techniques for deliberate hypotension: haemodilution and hypotension. In Enderby GEH (ed): Hypotensive Anaesthesia. London, Churchill Livingstone, 1985, p 164.

94. Plewes JL, Farhi LE: Cardiovascular responses to hemodilution and controlled hypotension in the dog. Anesthesiology 62:149, 1985.

95. Crystal GJ, Rooney MW, Salem MR: Myocardial blood flow and oxygen consumption during isovolemic hemodilution alone and in combination with adenosine-induced hypotension. Anesth Analg 67:538, 1988.

96. Crystal GJ, Salem MR: Myocardial and systemic hemodynamics during isovolemic hemodilution alone and combined with nitroprusside-induced controlled hypotension. Anesth Analg 72:227, 1991.

97. Lisander B, Jonsson R, Nordwall A: Combination of blood-saving methods decreases homologous blood requirements in scoliosis surgery. Anaesth Intensive Care 24:555, 1996.

98. Lehner JT, Van Peteghem PK, Leatherman KD, et al: Experience with an intraoperative autogenous blood recovery system in scoliosis and spinal surgery. Spine 6:131, 1981.

99. Flynn JC, Metzger CR, Csencsitz TA: Intraoperative autotransfusion (IAT) in spinal surgery. Spine 7:432, 1982.

100. Kruger LM, Colbert JM: Intraoperative autologous transfusion in children undergoing spinal surgery. J Pediatr Orthop 5:330, 1985.

101. Lennon RL, Hosking MP, Gray JR, et al: The effects of intraoperative blood salvage and induced hypotension on transfusion requirements during spinal surgical procedures. Mayo Clin Proc 62:1090, 1987.

102. Ray JM, Flynn JC, Bierman AH: Erythrocyte survival following intraoperative autotransfusion in spinal surgery. An in vivo comparative study and 5 year update. Spine 11:879, 1986.

103. Williamson KR, Taswell HF: Intraoperative blood salvage. In Taswell HF, Pineda AA (eds): Autologous Transfusion and Hemotherapy. Boston, Blackwell Scientific, 1991, p 122.

104. Zauder HL: Intraoperative and postoperative blood salvage devices. In Stehling LC (ed): Perioperative Autologous Transfusion. Arlington, VA, American Association of Blood Banks, 1991, p 25.

105. American Association of Blood Banks: Guidelines for Blood Salvage and Reinfusion in Surgery and Trauma. Arlington, VA, American Association of Blood Banks, 1990.

106. Blevins FT, Shaw B, Valeri CR, et al: Reinfusion of shed blood after orthopaedic procedures in children and adolescents, J Bone Joint Surg Am 75:363, 1993.

107. Demirjian Z, Sara M, Steinberg D, et al: Disseminated intravascular coagulation in patients undergoing orthopedic surgery. Clin Orthop 102:174, 1974.

108. Hassman GC, Keim HA: Disseminated intravascular coagulation in orthopedic surgery. Clin Orthop 103:118, 1974.

109. Raphael BG, Lackner H, Engler GL: Disseminated intravascular coagulation during surgery for scoliosis. Clin Orthop 162:41, 1982.

110. Kobrinsky NL, Letts RM, Patel LR, et al: 1-desamino-8-D-arginine vasopressin (desmopressin) decreases operative blood loss in patients having Harrington rod spinal fusion surgery. Ann Intern Med 107:446, 1987.

111. Guay J, Reinberg C, Poitras B, et al: A trial of desmopressin to reduce blood loss in patients undergoing spinal fusion for idiopathic scoliosis. Anesth Analg 75:405, 1992.

112. Theroux MC, Corddry DH, Tietz AE, et al: A study of desmopressin and blood loss during spinal fusion for neuromuscular scoliosis: a randomized, controlled, double-blinded study. Anesthesiology 87:260, 1997.

113. MacEwen GD, Bunnell WP, Sriram K: Acute neurological complications in the treatment of scoliosis: a report of the Scoliosis Research Society. J Bone Joint Surg Am 57:404, 1975.

114. Pasternak BM, Boyd DP, Ellis FH: Spinal cord injury after procedures on the aorta. Surg Gynecol Obstet 135:29, 1972.

115. Dommissee GF: The blood supply of the human spinal cord: a critical vascular factor in spinal surgery. J Bone Joint Surg Br 56:225, 1974.

116. Hickey R, Albin MS, Bunegin B, et al: Autoregulation of spinal cord blood flow: is the cord a microcosm of the brain? Stroke 17:1183, 1986.

117. Vauzelle C, Stagnara P, Jouvinroux P: Functional monitoring of spinal cord activity during spinal surgery. Clin Orthop 93:173, 1973.
118. Hardy RW, Nash CL, Brodkey JS: Experimental and clinical studies in spinal cord monitoring: the effects of pressure, anoxia, and ischemia on spinal cord function. J Bone Joint Surg Am 55:435, 1973.
119. Hall JE, Levine CR, Sudhir KG: Intraoperative awakening to monitor spinal cord function during Harrington instrumentation and spine fusion. J Bone Joint Surg Am 60:533, 1978.
120. Ben-David B, Haller GS, Taylor PD: Anesthesia for surgery of the spine. In Bradford DS, Lonstein JE, Moe JH, et al (eds): Moe's Textbook of Scoliosis and Other Spinal Deformities. 2nd ed. Philadelphia, WB Saunders Company, 1987, p 607.
121. Hoppenfeld S, Gross A, Andrews C, Lonner B: The ankle clonus test for assessment of the integrity of the spinal cord during operations for scoliosis. J Bone Joint Surg Am 79:208, 1997.
122. Grundy BL: Intraoperative monitoring of sensory-evoked potentials. Anesthesiology 58:72, 1983.
123. Black S, Cucchiara RF: Neruologic monitoring. In Miller RD (ed): Anesthesia. 3rd ed. New York, Churchill Livingstone, 1990, p 1185.
124. Peterson DO, Drummond JC, Todd MM: Effects of halothane, enflurane, isoflurane, and nitrous oxide on somatosensory evoked potentials in humans. Anesthesiology 65:35, 1986.
125. Drummond JC, Todd MM, Sang H: The effect of high dose sodium thiopental on brain stem auditory and median nerve somatosensory evoked responses in humans. Anesthesiology 63:249, 1982.
126. Koht A, Schütz W, Schmidt G, et al: Effects of etomidate, midazolam, and thiopental on median nerve somatosensory evoked potentials and the additive effects of fentanyl and nitrous oxide. Anesth Analg 67:435, 1988.
127. Sloan TB, Ronai AK, Toleikis JR, et al: Improvement of intraoperative somatosensory evoked potentials by etomidate. Anesth Analg 67:582, 1988.
128. Schubert A, Licina MG, Lineberry PJ: The effect of ketamine on human somatosensory evoked potentials and its modification by nitrous oxide. Anesthesiology 72:33, 1990.
129. Pathak KS, Brown RH, Cacorbi HF, et al: Effects of fentanyl and morphine on intraoperative SCEP. Anesth Analg 63:833, 1984.
130. Grundy BL, Brown RH: Meperidine enhances SCEP's. Electroencephalogr Clin Neurophysiol 50:177, 1980.
131. Grundy BL, Brown RH, Clifton PC: Effect of droperidol on SCEP. Electroencephalogr Clin Neurophysiol 50:1581, 1980.
132. Eng DY, Dong WK, Bledsoe SW, et al: Electrical and pathological correlates of brain hypoxia during hypotension. Anesthesiology 53:592, 1980.
133. Grundy BL, Heros RC, Tung AS, et al: Intraoperative hypoxia detected by evoked potential monitoring. Anesth Analg 60:437, 1981.
134. Nagao S, Roccaforte P, Moody RA: The effects of isovolemic hemodilution and reinfusion of packed erythrocytes on SEP and visual evoked potentials. J Surg Res 25:530, 1978.
135. Stockard JJ, Sharbrough FW, Tinker JA: Effects of hypothermia on the human brainstem auditory response. Ann Neurol 3:368, 1978.
136. Bendo AA: Monitoring the nervous system. Prob Anesth 7:115, 1993.
137. Dolan EJ, Transfeldt EE, Tator CH, et al: The effect of spinal distraction on regional spinal cord blood flow in cats. J Neurosurg 53:756, 1980.
138. Brodkey JS, Richards DE, Blasingame JP, et al: Reversible spinal cord trauma in cats: additive effects of direct pressure and ischemia. J Neurosurg 37:591, 1972.
139. Yeoman PM, Gibson MJ, Hutchinson A, et al: Influence of induced hypotension and spinal distraction on feline somatosensory evoked potentials. Br J Anaesth 63:315, 1989.
140. Kling TF, Fergusson NV, Leach AB, et al: The influence of induced hypotension and spine distraction on canine spinal cord blood flow. Spine 10:878, 1985.
141. Kling TF, Wilton N, Hensinger RN, et al: The influence of trimethaphan (Arfonad)-induced hypotension with and without spine distraction on canine spinal cord blood flow. Spine 11:219, 1986.
142. Ponte A: Postoperative paraplegia due to hypercorrection of scoliosis and drop of blood pressure. J Bone Joint Surg Am 56:444, 1974.
143. Engler GL, Spielholtz NI, Bernhard WN, et al: Somatosensory evoked potentials during Harrington instrumentation for scoliosis. J Bone Joint Surg Am 60:528, 1978.
144. Rowed DW, McLean JAG, Tator CH: Somatosensory evoked potentials in acute spinal cord injury: prognostic value. Surg Neurol 9:203, 1978.
145. Ginsberg H, Shetter A, Raudzens P: Postoperative paraplegia with preserved intraoperative SEP's. Orthop Trans 8:161, 1984.
146. Koht A, Sloan TB, Ronai AK, et al: Intraoperative deterioration of evoked potentials during spinal surgery. In Schramm J, Jones SJ (eds): Spinal Cord Monitoring. Berlin, Springer-Verlag, 1985.
147. Diaz JH, Lockhart CH: Postoperative quadriplegia after spinal fusion for scoliosis with intraoperative awakening. Anesth Analg 66:1039, 1987.
148. Sloan TB, Ronai AK, Koht A: Reversible loss of somatosensory evoked potentials during anterior cervical spinal fusion. Anesth Analg 65:96, 1986.
149. McCallum JE, Bennett MH: Electrophysiologic monitoring of spinal cord function during intraspinal surgery. Surg Forum 26:469, 1975.
150. Schmitt EW: Neurological complications in the treatment of scoliosis, a sequential report of the Scoliosis Research Society 1971 through 1979. Reported at the 17th Annual Meeting of the Scoliosis Research Society, Denver, 1981.
151. Maccabee PJ, Amassian VE, Cracco RQ, et al: Stimulation of the human nervous system using the magnetic coil. J Clin Neurophysiol 8:38, 1991.
152. Agnew WF, McCreery DB: Considerations for safety in the use of extracranial stimulation of motor evoked potentials. Neurosurgery 20:143, 1987.
153. Drummond JC, Tung HC, Bickford RG: The effects of sedative agents on magnetic motor evoked potentials. J Clin Neurophysiol 4:366 1988.
154. Zentner J, Ebner A: Nitrous oxide suppresses the electromyographic response evoked by electrical stimulation of the motor cortex. Neurosurgery 25:60, 1989.
155. Ghaly RF, Stone JL, Levy WJ, et al: The effect of an anesthetic induction dose of midazolam on motor potentials evoked by transcranial magnetic stimulation in the monkey. J Neurosurg Anesthesiol 3:20, 1991.
156. Ghaly RF, Stone JL, Levy WJ, et al: The effect of neuroleptanalgesia (droperidol-fentanyl) on motor potentials evoked by transcranial magnetic stimulation in the monkey. J Neurosurg Anesthesiol 3:117, 1991.
157. Ghaly RF, Stone JL, Aldrete JA, et al: Effects of incremental ketamine hydrochloride doses on motor evoked potentials (MEPs) following transcranial magnetic stimulation: a primate study. J Neurosurg Anesthesiol 2:79, 1990.
158. Ghaly RF, Stone JL, Levy WJ, et al: The effect of etomidate on motor evoked potentials induced by transcranial magnetic stimulation in the monkey. Neurosurgery 27:936, 1990.
159. Taniguchi M, Nadstawek J, Langenbach U, et al: Effects of four intravenous anesthetic agents on motor evoked potentials elicited by magnetic transcranial stimulation. Neurosurgery 33:407, 1993.
160. Jelline K, Platt M, Jewkes D, et al: Effects of nitrous oxide on motor evoked potentials recorded from skeletal muscle in patients under total anesthesia with intravenously administered propofol. Neurosurgery 29:558, 1991.
161. Pechstein U, Nadstawek J, Zentner J, Schramm J: Isoflurane plus nitrous oxide versus propofol for recording of motor evoked potentials after high frequency repetititve electrical stimulation. Electroencephalogr Clin Neurophysiol 108:175, 1998.
162. Ghaly RF, Stone JL, Levy WJ: A protocol for intraoperative somatosensory (SEP) and motor evoked potentials (MEP) recordings. J Neurosurg Anesthesiol 4:68, 1992.
163. Hirschfeld SS, Rudner C, Nash CL, et al: The incidence of mitral valve prolapse in adolescent scoliosis and thoracic hypokyphosis. Pediatrics 40:451, 1982.
164. Priamiano FP, Nussbaum E, Hirschfeld SS, et al: Early echocardiographic and pulmonary function findings in idiopathic scoliosis. J Pediatr Orthop 3:475, 1983.
165. Benumof JL: Management of the difficult adult airway: with special emphasis on awake tracheal intubation. Anesthesiology 75:1087, 1990.
166. Schur MS, Brown JT, Kafer ER, et al: Postoperative pulmonary function in children: comparison of scoliosis with peripheral surgery. Am Rev Respir Dis 130:46, 1984.
167. Britt BA, Kalow W: Malignant hyperthermia: a statistical review. Can Anaesth Soc J 17:293, 1970.
168. Relton JES, Creighton RE, Johnston AE, et al: Hyperpyrexia in association with general anaesthesia in children. Can Anaesth Soc J 13:419, 1966.

169. Gronert GA, Theye RA: Pathophysiology of hyperkalemia induced by succinylcholine. Anesthesiology 43:89, 1975.

170. Moore WE, Watson RL, Summary JJ: Massive myoglobinuria precipitated by halothane and succinylcholine in a member of a family with elevation of serum creatinine phosphokinase. Anesth Analg 55:680, 1976.

171. Miller ED Jr, Saunders DB, Rowlingson JC, et al: Anesthesia-induced rhabdomyolysis in a patient with Duchenne's muscular dystrophy. Anesthesiology 48:146, 1978.

172. Lynn AM, Fischer T, Brandford HG, et al: Systemic responses to tourniquet release in children. Anesth Analg 65:865, 1986.

173. Dickson M, White M, Kinney W, et al: Extremity tourniquet deflation increases end-tidal PCO_2. Anesth Analg 70:457, 1990.

174. Lee T-L, Tweed WA, Singh B: Oxygen consumption and carbon dioxide elimination after release of unilateral lower limb pneumatic tourniquets. Anesth Analg 75:113, 1992.

175. Mostello LA, Casey WF, McGill WA: Does the use of a surgical tourniquet induce fever in infants? Anesth Analg 72:S191, 1991.

176. Bloch EC, Ginsberg B, Binner RA Jr, et al: Limb tourniquets and central temperature in anesthetized children. Anesth Analg 74:486, 1992.

177. Adu-Gyamfi Y, Sankarankutty M, Marwa S: Use of a tourniquet in patients with sickle-cell disease. Can J Anaesth 40:24, 1993.

178. Tachidijian MO: Pediatric Orthopedics. 2nd ed. Philadelphia, WB Saunders Company, 1990.

179. Paley D: The correction of complex foot deformities using Ilizarov's distraction osteotomies. Clin Orthop 293:97, 1993.

180. Friedlander HL, Westin GW, Wood WL Jr: Arthrogryposis multiplex congenita. J Bone Joint Surg Am 50:89, 1968.

181. Oberoi GS, Kaul HL, Gill IS, et al: Anaesthesia in arthrogryposis multiplex congenita: case report. Can J Anaesth 34:288, 1987.

182. Honda N, Konno K, Itohda Y, et al: Malignant hyperthermia and althesin. Can Anaesth Soc J 24:514, 1977.

183. Baudendistel L, Goudsouzian N, Coté CJ, et al: End-tidal CO_2 monitoring. Its use in the diagnosis and management of malignant hyperthermia. Anaesthesia 39:1000, 1984.

184. Baines DB, Douglas IO, Overton JH: Anaesthesia for patients with arthrogryposis multiplex congenita: what is the risk of malignant hyperthermia? Anaesth Intensive Care 14:370, 1986.

185. Hopkins PM, Ellis FR, Halsall PJ: Hypermetabolism in arthrogryposis multiplex congenita. Anaesthesia 46:374, 1991.

186. Maroteaux P, Spranger J, Opitz JM, et al: Le syndrom campomélique. Presse Med 79:1157, 1971.

187. Stehling L: Anesthesia for children requiring orthopedic surgery. Anesthesiol Rev 5:19, 1978.

188. Makey JT, Heiple KG: Scoliosis associated with congenital deficiencies of the upper extremity. J Bone Surg 52:279, 1970.

189. Heyman HJ, Ivankovich AD, Shulman M, et al: Intraoperative monitoring and anesthetic management for spinal fusion in an amelic patient. J Pediatr Orthop 2:299, 1982.

190. Thiagarajah S, Girnar DS, Park K, et al: Blood pressure monitoring using the superficial temporal artery and a Doppler ultrasonic flow detector. Anesth Analg 58:526, 1979.

191. Davis NL, Williams W, Tamer DF, et al: Intraoperative monitoring of left temporal and right radial arterial pressures during aortic arch surgery. Anesthesiology 44:62, 1976.

192. Smith RJ: Preoperative assessment of risk factors. Br J Anaesth 60:317, 1988.

193. Zanette G, Manani G, Pittoni G, et al: Prevalence of unsuspected myopathy in infants presenting for clubfoot surgery. Paediatr Anaesth 5:165, 1995.

194. Wilkins KE: Fat embolism in anesthesia for orthopedic surgery. In Zauder HL (ed): Anesthesia for Orthopedic Surgery. Philadelphia, FA Davis, 1980, p 147.

195. Salem MR, Wong AY, Lin YH: The effect of suxamethonium on the intragastric pressure in infants and children. Br J Anaesth 44:166, 1972.

196. Salem MR, Wong AY, Fizzotti GF: Efficacy of cricoid pressure in preventing aspiration of gastric contents in pediatric patients. Br J Anaesth 44:401, 1972.

197. Salem MR, Wong AY, Collins VJ: The pediatric patient with a "full" stomach. Anesthesiology 39:435, 1973.

198. Salem MR, Wong AY, Mani M, et al: Premedicant drugs and gastric juice pH and volume in pediatric patients. Anesthesiology 44:216, 1976.

199. Goudsouzian N, Coté CJ, Liu MP, et al: The dose-response effects of oral cimetidine on gastric pH and volume in children. Anesthesiology 55:533, 1981.

200. Fisher DM: Neuromuscular blocking agents in paediatric anaesthesia. Br J Anaesth 83:58, 1999.

201. Zuckerman JD, Skovron ML, Koval KJ, et al: Postoperative complications and mortality associated with operative delay in older patients who have a fracture of the hip. J Bone Joint Surg Am 77:1551, 1995.

202. Eaton RG, Green WT, Stark HA: Volkmann's ischemic contracture. J Bone Joint Surg Am 47:1289, 1965.

203. Shoenfeld Y: Osteogenesis imperfecta: review of the literature with presentation of 29 cases. Am J Dis Child 129:679, 1975.

204. Solomons CC, Myers DN: Hyperthermia of osteogenesis imperfecta and its relationship to malignant hyperthermia. In Gordon RA, Britt BA, Kalow W (eds): International Symposium on Malignant Hyperthermia. Springfield, IL, Charles C Thomas, 1973, p 319.

205. King JD, Bobechko WP: Osteogenesis imperfecta: an orthopedic description and surgical review. J Bone Joint Surg Br 53:72, 1971.

206. Heppner RL, Babitt HI, Bianchine JW, et al: Aortic regurgitation and aneurysm of the sinus of Valsalva associated with osteogenesis imperfecta. Am J Cardiol 31:654, 1973.

207. Hathaway WE, Solomons CC, Ott J: Abnormalities of platelet function in osteogenesis imperfecta. Clin Res 18:209, 1970.

208. Cropp GV, Myers DN: Physiological evidence of hypermetabolism in osteogenesis imperfecta. Pediatrics 49:375, 1972.

209. Stehling LC: Anesthesia for congenital anomalies of the skeletal system. In Stehling LC, Zauder HL (eds): Anesthetic Implications of Congenital Anomalies in Children. East Norwalk, CT, Appleton-Century-Crofts, 1980.

210. Sofield HA, Millar EA: Fragmentation, realignment, and intramedullary rod fixation of deformities of the long bones in children (a 10 year appraisal). J Bone Joint Surg Am 41:1371, 1959.

211. Millar EA: Observation on the surgical management of osteogenesis imperfecta. Clin Orthop 159:154, 1981.

212. Klippel M, Feil A: Un cas d'absence des vertebres cervicales. Nouv Iconog Salpetriere 25:223, 1912.

213. Hensinger RN, Lang JR, MacEwen GD: Klippel-Feil syndrome: a constellation of associated anomalies. J Bone Joint Surg Am 56:1246, 1974.

214. da Silva EO: Autosomal recessive Klippel-Feil syndrome. J Med Genet 19:130, 1982.

215. Moore WB, Matthews TJ, Rabinowitz R, et al: Genitourinary anomalies associated with Klippel-Feil syndrome. J Bone Joint Surg Am 57:355, 1975.

216. Morrison SG, Perry LW, Scott LP III: Congenital brevicollis and cardiovascular anomalies. Am J Dis Child 115:614, 1968.

217. Stark EW, Bartan TE: Hearing loss and the Klippel-Feil syndrome. Am J Dis Child 123:233, 1972.

218. Nagib MG, Maxwell RE, Chou SN: Identification and management of high-risk patients with Klippel-Feil syndrome. J Neurosurg 61:523, 1984.

219. Van Kerckhoven MF, Fabry G: The Klippel-Feil syndrome: a constellation of deformities. Acta Orthop Belg 55:2:107, 1989.

220. Elster AD: Quadriplegia after minor trauma in the Klippel-Feil syndrome. J Bone Joint Surg Am 66:1473, 1984.

221. Naguib M, Farag H, Ibrahim AEL: Anaesthetic consideration in Klippel-Feil syndrome. Can Anaesth Soc J 33:66, 1986.

222. Prusick UR, Samberg LC, Wesolowski OP: Klippel-Feil syndrome associated with spinal stenosis. J Bone Joint Surg Am 67:161, 1985.

223. Baga N, Chusid EL, Miller A: Pulmonary disability in the Klippel-Feil syndrome. Clin Orthop 67:105, 1969.

224. Kreiger AJ, Rosomopp HL, Kuperman AS, et al: Occult respiratory dysfunction in a craniovertebral anomaly. J Neurosurg 31:15, 1969.

225. Holinger LD, Weiss KS: Diagnosis and management of airway obstruction in craniofacial anomalies. Otolaryngol Clin North Am 14:1005, 1981.

226. Hemi C, Pruzansky S: Craniofacial and extracranial malformations in the Klippel-Feil syndrome. Cleft Palate J 17:65, 1980.

227. Chung F, Crago RR: Sleep apnea syndrome and anaesthesia. Can Anaesth Soc J 29:439, 1982.

228. Sherk HH, Shut L, Chung S: Iniencephalic deformity of the cervical spine with Klippel-Feil anomalies and congenital elevation of the scapula. J Bone Joint Surg Am 56:1254, 1974.

229. Eisele JH: Connective tissue diseases. In Katz J, Benumof JL, Kadis LB (eds): Anesthesia and Uncommon Diseases: Pathophysiologic

and Clinical Correlations. 3rd ed. Philadelphia, WB Saunders Company, 1990, p 645.

230. Jenkins LC, McGraw RW: Anaesthetic management of patients with rheumatoid arthritis. Can Anaesth Soc J 16:407, 1969.

231. Davies JAH: Blind nasal intubation using doxapram hydrochloride. Br J Anaesth 40:361, 1968.

232. Salem MR, Mathrubhutham M, Bennett EJ: Difficult intubation: current concepts. N Engl J Med 295:879, 1976.

233. Lehmann-Horn F, Knorr-Held S: Muscle diseases relevant to the anaesthetist. Acta Anaesth Belg 41:113, 1990.

234. Sokoll MD, Gergis SD: Anesthesia and neuromuscular disease. Anesthesiol Rev 2:20, 1975.

235. Dalal FY, Bennett EJ, Prithul RP, et al: Dystrophica—a multisystem disease. Can Anaesth Soc J 19:436, 1972.

236. Aldridge LM: Anesthetic problems in myotonic dystrophy. Br J Anaesth 57:1119, 1985.

237. Mitchell MM, Ali HH, Savarese JJ: Myotonia and neuromuscular blocking agents. Anesthesiology 49:44, 1978.

238. Watt NA, Scott RPF: Mivacurium chloride and myotonic dystrophy. Br J Anaesth 75:498, 1995.

239. Patterson IS: Generalized myotonia following suxamethonium. Br J Anaesth 34:340, 1962.

240. Kaufman L: Anesthesia in dystophica myotonia. Proc R Soc Med 53:183, 1960.

241. Duncan PG: Neuromuscular diseases. In Katz J, Steward DJ (eds): Anesthesia and Uncommon Pediatric Diseases. 2nd ed. Philadelphia, WB Saunders Company, 1987, p 509.

242. Ririe DG, Shapiro F, Sethna NF: The response of patients with Duchenne's muscular dystrophy to neuromuscular blockade with vecuronium. Anesthesiology 88:351, 1998.

243. Kelfer HM, Singer WD, Reynolds RN: Malignant hyperthermia in a child with Duchenne muscular dystrophy. Pediatrics 71:118, 1983.

244. Smith RB, Grenvik A: Cardiac arrest following succinylcholine in patients with central nervous system injuries. Anesthesiology 33:558, 1970.

245. Rosenberg H, Gronert GA: Intractable cardiac arrest in children given succinylcholine. Anesthesiology 77:1054, 1992.

246. Azar I: The response of patients with neuromuscular disorders to muscle relaxants. Anesthesiology 61:173, 1984.

247. Hall S: Anesthetic considerations. In Tachdijian MO (ed): Pediatric Orthopedics. 2nd ed. Philadelphia, WB Saunders Company, 1990, p 67.

248. Morris P: Duchenne muscular dystrophy: a challenge for the anaesthetist [editorial]. Paediatr Anaesth 7:1, 1997.

249. Slucka C: The electrocardiogram in Duchenne progressive muscular dystrophy. Circulation 38:933, 1968.

250. Sanyal SK, Johnson WW: Cardiac conduction abnormalities in children with Duchenne progressive muscular dystrophy. Circulation 66:853, 1982.

251. Sethna NF, Rockoff MA, Worthen HM, et al: Anesthetic-related complications in children with Duchenne muscular dystrophy. Anesthesiology 68:462, 1988.

252. Irwin MG, Henderson M: Cardiac arrest during major spinal scoliosis surgery in a patient with Duchenne's muscular dystrophy undergoing intravenous anaesthesia. Anaesth Intensive Care 23:626, 1995.

253. Perloff JK, deLeon AC, Doherty D: The cardiomyopathy of progressive muscular dystrophy. Circulation 33:625, 1966.

254. Sanyal SK, Johnston WW, Dische MR, et al: Dystrophic degeneration of papillary muscle and ventricular myocardium. Circulation 62:430, 1980.

255. Fox HJ, Thomas CH, Thompson AG: Spinal instrumentation for Duchenne's muscular dystrophy. Experience of hypotensive anesthesia to minimize blood loss. J Pediatr Orthop 17:750, 1997.

256. Levitt LP, Rose L, Dawson D: Hypokalemic periodic paralysis with arrhythmia. N Engl J Med 286:253, 1972.

257. Dierdorf SF, McNiece WL, Rao CC: Effect of succinylcholine on plasma potassium in children with cerebral palsy. Anesthesiology 62:88, 1985.

258. Rook A: Epidermolysis bullosa. In Rook A, Wilkinson DS, Ebling FJG (eds): Textbook of Dermatology. 3rd ed. Oxford, Blackwell Scientific Publications, 1972, p 1444.

259. Lee C, Nagel EL: Anesthetic management of a patient with recessive epidermolysis bullosa dystrophica. Anesthesiology 43:122, 1975.

260. James I, Wark H: Airway management during anesthesia in patients with epidermolysis bullosa dystrophica. Anesthesiology 56:323, 1982.

261. Thompson JW: Epidermolysis bullosa dystrophica of the larynx and trachea—acute airway obstruction. Ann Otol Laryngol Rhinol 69:428, 1980.

262. Holzman RS, Worthen HM, Johnson KL, et al: Anesthesia for children with functional epidermolysis bullosa (lethalis). Can J Anaesth 34:395, 1987.

263. Hurwitz S: Clinical Pediatric Dermatology. Philadelphia, WB Saunders Company, 1981.

264. Spielman FJ, Mann ES: Subarachnoid and epidural anesthesia for patients with epidermolysis bullosa. Can Anaesth Soc J 31:549, 1984.

265. Kelly RE, Koff HD, Rothaus KO, et al: Brachial plexus anesthesia in eight patients with recessive dystrophic epidermolysis bullosa. Anesth Analg 66:1318, 1987.

266. Sopchak AM, Thomas PS, Clark WR: Regional anesthesia in a patient with epidermolysis bullosa. Reg Anaesth 18:132, 1993.

267. Yonker-Sell AE, Connolly LA: Clinical reports: twelve hour anaesthesia in a patient with epidermolysis bullosa. Can J Anaesth 42:735, 1995.

268. Niemi K-M, Sommer H, Kero M, et al: Epidermolysis bullosa simplex associated with muscular dystrophy with recessive inheritance. Arch Dermatol 124:551, 1988.

269. Fine J-D, Stenn J, Johnson L, et al: Autosomal recessive epidermolysis bullosa simplex. Arch Dermatol 125:931, 1989.

270. Winship IM: Sotos' syndrome. Clin Genet 28:243, 1985.

271. Boman H, Nilsson D: Sotos' syndrome in two brothers. Clin Genet 18:421, 1980.

272. Suresh D: Posterior spinal fusion in Sotos' syndrome. Br J Anaesth 66:728, 1991.

273. Rett A: Ueber ein eigenartiges hirnatropisches Syndrome. Wien Med Wochenschr 116:723, 1966.

274. Glaze DG, Frost JD Jr, Zoghbi HY, et al: Rett syndrome: characterization of respiratory patterns and sleep. Ann Neurol 21:377, 1987.

275. Cirignotta F, Lugaresi E, Montagna P: Breathing impairment in Rett syndrome. Am J Med Genet 24(Suppl 1):167, 1986.

276. Zoghbi HY, Percy AK, Glaze DG, et al: Reduction of biogenic amine levels in the Rett syndrome. N Engl J Med 313:921, 1985.

277. Hagberg B: Rett's syndrome: prevalence and impact on progressive severe mental retardation in girls. Acta Paediatr Scand 74:405, 1985.

278. Maguire D, Bachman C: Anaesthesia and Rett syndrome: a case report. Can J Anaesth 36:478, 1989.

279. Dearlove DR, Walker RWM: Case Report: anaesthesia for Rett syndrome. Paediatr Anaesth 6:155, 1996.

280. Sekwl EA, Moak JP, Schultz RJ, et al: Electrocardiographic findings in Rett syndrome. An explanation for sudden death? J Pediatr 125:80, 1994.

23

Eyes, Ears, Nose, Throat, and Dental Surgery

CLAIRE M. BRETT
MAURICE S. ZWASS

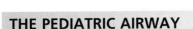

THE PEDIATRIC AIRWAY

The Normal Airway

Assessing pediatric patients for ears, nose, and throat (ENT) surgery is particularly challenging because the site of surgery often involves the upper airway and directly affects the anesthetic plan and its risks. Preoperatively, the anesthesiologist must meticulously assess all aspects of the airway and the cardiorespiratory systems; he or she must also develop plans for intubating the trachea, for intraoperative airway management, and for postoperative recovery. Flexibility and back-up plans are essential.

A clear understanding of the anatomy and physiology of the upper airway must precede any discussion of anesthesia and surgery to treat upper airway pathology. Maintaining upper airway patency is an "active" and complicated process.[1] The upper airway is almost always open, but it is potentially collapsible, especially during airway surgery. The fact that there are anatomic differences in the airway of infants, older children, and adults must be understood and taken into account.

The upper airway is exposed to potentially collapsing negative pressure during inspiration, but the pharynx is kept open by the upper airway muscles, in particular the genioglossus. The pharynx is particularly prone to collapse because negative pressure pulls the tongue against the

pharynx. The genioglossus is the principal muscle that dilates the pharynx. This muscle receives feedback from the central nervous system (CNS) via the hypoglossal nerve and from the lower airway via the vagus nerve.[1] Hypoxia and hypercarbia increase the dilating activity of the genioglossus.[2, 3] General anesthesia depresses activity of the upper airway muscles (probably through effects on the CNS). This commonly results in oropharyngeal obstruction. The contribution of the tongue to airway obstruction is exaggerated in infants because they have large tongues relative to the total size of their mouths. Infants or children with small upper airway secondary to craniofacial anomalies, neuromuscular or CNS disorders, tumors or hemangiomas, or an upper respiratory infection are especially prone to pharyngeal obstruction by the tongue.

The importance of head position in maintaining upper airway patency during anesthesia is well recognized. Postmortem studies show that flexing the head of the human infant causes the upper airway to collapse more readily.[4] This fact is particularly important during the induction of anesthesia in children with abnormal upper airways. Also, neonates (especially the premature neonate) have small, soft, and easily collapsible airways, particularly if the neck is flexed. Extending or keeping the neck in a neutral position while applying positive pressure during bag-and-mask ventilation, especially during induction of general anesthesia, is vital.

Other unique anatomic features of the upper airway of infants are important. The larynx of the infant is higher in the neck (C3–4) than in the adult (C4–5).[5] The infant's epiglottis is large, but it is narrow and short. Because of these anatomic features, the straight laryngoscope blade generally allows better visualization of the larynx of the normal infant. When laryngeal anatomy is complicated further by craniofacial anomalies (e.g., micrognathia or midface hypoplasia), direct visualization of the larynx may be impossible, and alternative methods of securing the airway should be available (see section "The Difficult Airway," below).

The vocal cords of infants are slanted so that the posterior commissure is more cephalad than the anterior commissure. Consequently, the anterior sublaryngeal airway is more susceptible to trauma from an endotracheal tube. The subglottic area also is prone to traumatic injury from an endotracheal tube because the narrowest portion of the infant's larynx is at the cricoid cartilage. In adults, the narrowest portion is the glottic rim. Thus, an endotracheal tube that easily passes through the vocal cords of an infant or child may fit snugly in the subglottis and cause subglottic edema and symptoms of increased airway resistance after tracheal extubation. This increased resistance is usually reversible, but subglottic stenosis may occur following prolonged tracheal intubation with an oversized endotracheal tube.

Before inducing anesthesia for surgery involving the upper airway, the anesthesiologist must understand the effects of the surgery on the physiology of the airway. The airway of each patient should be carefully examined. Indirect examinations, including scans and radiographs, should be reviewed with the appropriate consultants. Finally, a bed should be reserved in the pediatric intensive care unit (PICU) for patients who are likely to require monitoring or postoperative ventilatory support.

The Difficult Airway

When a patient has a difficult airway, the anesthesiologist must formulate a carefully constructed, flexible plan to maximize success and minimize risk to the patient. A thorough history and physical examination must be part of the evaluation. The goals are to avoid surprises, identify airway difficulties, and be prepared for their management. Difficult tracheal intubations generally occur when the larynx is easily visualized by direct laryngoscopy but a lesion in the supraglottic, glottic, or subglottic region prevents insertion of the usual-sized tracheal tube, or when facial or oral pathology prevents visualization of the larynx. Circumstances that may result in a difficult tracheal intubation may be organized by anatomic location and include congenital, inflammatory, traumatic, metabolic, and neoplastic disorders.

When a difficult tracheal intubation is anticipated, it is important to have available an individual experienced in performing pediatric bronchoscopy, and, in some cirumstances, a practitioner skilled in cricothyrotomy and/or tracheostomy. Preoperatively, the patient's parents should be informed of the risks and the potential need for a tracheostomy. In some situations it may be less traumatic to proceed with a tracheostomy to ensure an airway rather than persist with multiple unsuccessful attempts to intubate the trachea.[6]

The American Society of Anesthesiologists has published *Practice Guidelines for Management of the Difficult Airway*.[7] These guidelines, although not directed towards pediatric patients, offer a general approach to the difficult airway. The guidelines were produced to "facilitate management of the difficult airway and to reduce the likelihood of adverse outcomes." The guidelines also provide an algorithm for the management of the difficult airway (Fig. 23–1).

Intubation of the Nonvisualized Larynx

Inability to visualize the larynx presents an enormous challenge to the anesthesiologist and requires patience and a "bag of tricks" to accomplish an essentially blind intubation. Lesions commonly associated with difficult visualization of the larynx include the craniofacial dysmorphologies (e.g., Pierre Robin sequence, Treacher-Collins [mandibulofacial dysostosis], Goldenhar's [oculoauriculovertebral dysplasia], Hallermann-Streiff [oculomandibulodyscephaly], Möbius', and Cornelia de Lange's syndromes.[6, 8–22] All are characterized by mandibular hypoplasia, micrognathia, and glossoptosis. Mechanical obstruction is caused by the posteriorly displaced tongue and relative macroglossia.[8] The macroglossia associated with glycogen storage diseases[23] or a cystic hygroma of the tongue often prevents direct visualization of the larynx. There are case reports of nonvisualization of the trachea and difficult tracheal intubation in children with fetal alcohol syndrome and familial osseous dysplasia (cherubism).[12, 24, 25] Children with hemifacial syndromes often have their glottis pulled to one side, and this may make tracheal intubation diffcult.[26] Congenital craniofacial syndromes are frequently accompanied by developmental delay or severe mental retardation, which complicates anesthesia and airway management.[27, 28]

A patient with a cystic hygroma of the tongue is of special concern.[29] This fluid-containing multilocular lesion may involve the tongue sufficiently to fill the oral cavity. The tongue often protrudes outside the mouth and prevents its closure, making the maintenance of an airway during anesthesia difficult or impossible (Fig. 23–2).[30] Respiration in children with this lesion often becomes completely obstructed during induction of anesthesia, and ventilation is nearly impossible, as is direct laryngoscopy. A nasopharyngeal airway may provide some airway patency. Children with a huge tongue and an unstable natural airway should not undergo induction of anesthesia until a patent airway is ensured, by awake blind nasotracheal intubation, an elective tracheostomy under local anesthesia, awake nasotracheal fiberoptic intubation over a fiberoptic bronchoscope[10] (see below), or by the use of a laryngeal mask airway if one can be inserted. Following partial resection of a cystic hygroma of the tongue, a tracheostomy may be necessary until the child grows and further resection of the tumor results in a patent oral airway. These tumors often recur.

Micrognathia, glossoptosis, or macroglossia are frequently associated with inability to visualize the glottis by direct laryngoscopy and inability to insert an oral endotra-

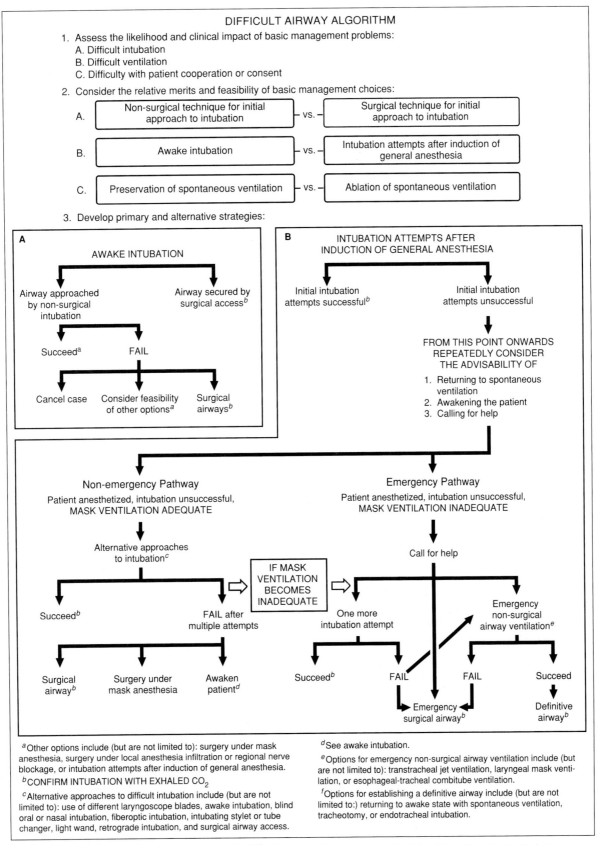

DIFFICULT AIRWAY ALGORITHM

1. Assess the likelihood and clinical impact of basic management problems:
   A. Difficult intubation
   B. Difficult ventilation
   C. Difficulty with patient cooperation or consent

2. Consider the relative merits and feasibility of basic management choices:

   A. Non-surgical technique for initial approach to intubation — vs. — Surgical technique for initial approach to intubation

   B. Awake intubation — vs. — Intubation attempts after induction of general anesthesia

   C. Preservation of spontaneous ventilation — vs. — Ablation of spontaneous ventilation

3. Develop primary and alternative strategies:

A AWAKE INTUBATION

Airway approached by non-surgical intubation / Airway secured by surgical access[b]

Succeed[a]   FAIL

Cancel case   Consider feasibility of other options[a]   Surgical airways[b]

B INTUBATION ATTEMPTS AFTER INDUCTION OF GENERAL ANESTHESIA

Initial intubation attempts successful[b] / Initial intubation attempts unsuccessful

FROM THIS POINT ONWARDS REPEATEDLY CONSIDER THE ADVISABILITY OF
1. Returning to spontaneous ventilation
2. Awakening the patient
3. Calling for help

Non-emergency Pathway
Patient anesthetized, intubation unsuccessful, MASK VENTILATION ADEQUATE

Alternative approaches to intubation[c]

IF MASK VENTILATION BECOMES INADEQUATE

Succeed[b]   FAIL after multiple attempts

Surgical airway[b]   Surgery under mask anesthesia   Awaken patient[d]

Emergency Pathway
Patient anesthetized, intubation unsuccessful, MASK VENTILATION INADEQUATE

Call for help

One more intubation attempt   Emergency non-surgical airway ventilation[e]

Succeed[b]   FAIL   FAIL   Succeed

Emergency surgical airway[b]   Definitive airway[b]

---

[a]Other options include (but are not limited to): surgery under mask anesthesia, surgery under local anesthesia infiltration or regional nerve blockage, or intubation attempts after induction of general anesthesia.

[b]CONFIRM INTUBATION WITH EXHALED CO_2

[c]Alternative approaches to difficult intubation include (but are not limited to): use of different laryngoscope blades, awake intubation, blind oral or nasal intubation, fiberoptic intubation, intubating stylet or tube changer, light wand, retrograde intubation, and surgical airway access.

[d]See awake intubation.

[e]Options for emergency non-surgical airway ventilation include (but are not limited to): transtracheal jet ventilation, laryngeal mask ventilation, or esophageal-tracheal combitube ventilation.

[f]Options for establishing a definitive airway include (but are not limited to:) returning to awake state with spontaneous ventilation, tracheotomy, or endotracheal intubation.

FIGURE 23–1. Algorithm for use in patients with difficult airways. (From American Society of Anesthesiologists Task Force on Guidelines for Management of the Difficult Airway: Caplan RA [Chairman]: Practice guidelines for management of the difficulty airway. Anesthesiology 78:597, 1993, with permission.)

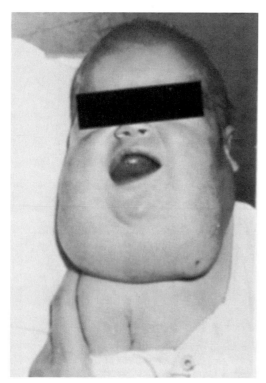

FIGURE 23–2. Massive bilateral cervical submandibular cystic hygroma in a newborn that involves the tongue and the retromandibular, pharyngeal, and retropharyngeal areas. Awake intubation was followed by N₂O/O₂/halothane anesthesia for tracheostomy, feeding gastrostomy, and partial resection of the tumor.

cheal tube. Therefore, alternate means of tracheal intubation should be planned so that excessive attempts to intubate the trachea with conventional techniques are avoided. Intubation over a fiberoptic bronchoscope is ideal,[31] and is commonly planned to provide an airway for an infant or child with an abnormal upper airway. This skill should be acquired in structured courses under the supervision of experienced practitioners.

The literature has advocated a number of alternate techniques or "tricks" for accomplishing tracheal intubation, and although the success with them frequently is low, they are worthy of mention.

Awake Nasotracheal Intubation

Awake nasotracheal intubation requires adequate preoxygenation by mask and cautions use of sedation or analgesia, such as intravenous fentanyl 1 to 2 μg/kg, or midazolam 0.1 to 0.2 mg/kg, and topical anesthesia of the nasal mucosa and larynx.[32] A painless nasotracheal intubation is essential to ensure the patient's cooperation and to prevent gagging, coughing, and swallowing. Cotton swabs (Q-tips) moistened with 1 to 4 percent cocaine or a fine mist spray of the drug from a nebulizer provides excellent topical anesthesia and vasoconstriction of the nasal mucosa. Alternatively, Grose et al.[33] advocated the use of topically applied 3:1 mixture of 4 percent lidocaine and 1 percent phenylephrine. They found this combination to be as effective and potentially less toxic than 4 percent cocaine for nasotracheal intubation.

Topical laryngeal block requires knowledge of the sensory nerve supply to the larynx.[34] Sensation to the pharynx, tonsil, and posterior tongue is supplied by the glossopharyngeal nerve; the vagus nerve innervates the supraglottic structures to the level of the false cords through the internal laryngeal branch of the superior laryngeal nerve. The vagus nerve also innervates the remainder of the larynx and upper trachea through the inferior laryngeal nerve (called "recurrent" on the left).[32, 34]

A lidocaine spray, when directed to the posterior tongue and deep posterior pharynx, anesthetizes these areas. A gauze pad moistened with lidocaine, blocks the internal laryngeal branch of the superior laryngeal nerve, which runs just underneath the mucosa.[32, 35] Puncturing the cricothyroid membrane with a 25-gauge needle and injecting 1 ml of lidocaine directly into the trachea anesthetizes the mucous membranes that are supplied by the inferior laryngeal nerve.[27, 30]

Topical anesthesia to the upper airway of most older children is an effective technique if combined with intravenous sedation, but success is less predictable in the young child. An alternate means of applying topical anesthesia to the upper airway is by nebulizing lidocaine and oxygen and inhaling the drugs through a clear plastic face mask.[36] This technique is simple, noninvasive, and painless and can be used in the young child.

Lidocaine is rapidly absorbed from the mucous membranes. Consequently, no more than 4 to 5 mg/kg should be used.[35] Pelton et al.[37] found lidocaine concentrations of approximately 3.0 μg/ml in the plasma of children following aerosol application of 3 mg/kg lidocaine. This concentration is below the toxic plasma level of lidocaine, 6 to 10 μg/ml, at which signs of CNS excitability are occasionally seen.[38] (Likewise, the total calculated dose of cocaine should not exceed 3.0 mg/kg and that of tetracaine, 1 mg/kg.[35]) Patients weighing between 10 and 15 kg may be given 1.0 to 1.5 ml of 4 percent lidocaine diluted in 2 ml of normal saline; infants weighing 15 to 20 kg can be given 1.5 to 2.0 ml of 4 percent lidocaine diluted in 2 ml of normal saline. The volume of solution (4 percent lidocaine in 2 ml of saline) may be increased to 3 to 4 ml for children 20 to 30 kg. Diluting the 4 percent lidocaine is unnecessary for larger children (>35 kg), who can receive 3 to 4 ml of 4 percent lidocaine.

Following application of the topical anesthetic, the patient's head should be placed in an optimal position for tracheal intubation. The axes of the mouth, pharynx, and larynx are aligned when the head is extended at the atlanto-occipital joint and the neck is flexed at the cervical spine; it is commonly called the "sniffing position" and is ideal for tracheal intubation.[39] The relatively large occiput of the infant and young child provides for this ideal position; older children should be positioned with a small pillow under the head. Blind nasotracheal intubation is performed by manipulating the endotracheal tube and the patient's head while listening for maximal breath sounds. When the breath sounds are loudest, the tip of the endotracheal tube is advanced into the glottis.[40] Occasionally, it is necessary to move the larynx so that it is positioned in front of the endotracheal tube. To do this, gentle pressure is applied over the hyoid bone. Moving the thyroid cartilage does little to move the glottis. A curved endotracheal tube can be ensured if it is packed for a few minutes in a round basin of ice; the tube returns to the original shape as the plastic warms. Several tubes may be necessary if several attempts at tracheal intubation are required. Use of the laryngoscope may help in maneuvering the tube into the midline, even though the laryngeal structures are not visualized; the pediatric Magill forceps may be used to advance the tip of the endotracheal tube into the glottic opening.[40]

On occasion, all maneuvers to manipulate the nasotracheal tube into the larynx fail, and the tube continues to enter the esophagus. Berry[41] advocates use of a stylet for nasotracheal intubation. He first places the nasotracheal tube into position and then introduces the stylet. By bending the lubricated stylet with a short 30-degree angle on the distal end, the stylet may be gently introduced down the tube after it is in the nasopharynx. The proximal portion of the tube and stylet are gently maneuvered posteriorly, resulting in an anterior movement of the distal stylet and tube into the trachea.[41]

Tactile Intraoral Endotracheal Tube Placement

A variant of blind nasotracheal intubation has been described for use in a child with Treacher-Collins syndrome.[15] A nasotracheal tube is placed into the pharynx, and inhalation anesthesia is induced during spontaneous respiration. The anesthesiologist's second and third fingers are inserted into the mouth and over the anesthetized child's tongue; the epiglottis is palpated, and the tube is directed between the two fingers into the glottis.[15]

This same technique has also been successful to direct a nasotracheal tube into the larynx of patients with severe flexion contracture of the neck from burn scarring and in partial traumatic loss of the mandible.

Nasopharyngeal Airway for Induction of Anesthesia

The following improvisation was prompted by an inability to place a face mask on a child who had a 27 × 8-cm tumor in the midline of the face. The child had frontonasal dysplasia, a meningoencephalocele, and only one nostril; awake tracheal intubation was also impossible.[42]

An endotracheal tube was inserted nasally as far as the posterior pharynx. The tube was utilized for an inhalational induction of anesthesia. With the child's mouth closed, positive pressure was easily achieved. Succinylcholine allowed uncomplicated oral-tracheal intubation.

Laryngeal Trachea Anesthesia Introducer Used as a Stylet

A laryngeal tracheal anesthesia (LTA) kit has facilitated the insertion of an orotracheal tube under general anesthesia.[33, 43, 44] The stylet of the LTA kit is inserted through the eye of an endotracheal tube, directing it midline (under partial direct vision) underneath the epiglottis toward the glottis. Using the LTA stylet as a guide, the tube is advanced into the trachea.[43, 44]

Retrograde Translaryngeal Catheter

Occasionally, tracheal intubation can be accomplished over a catheter that is placed retrograde through the cricothyroid membrane. This may be a useful technique for older children who are awake and cooperative. After placing a subcutaneous wheal, a transtracheal spray of local anesthetic (see section "Awake Nasotracheal Intubation," above) can be given. Supplemental sedation should be titrated, depending on the overall status of the patient. A small pillow placed under the shoulders is essential to extend the head on the neck.

An epidural catheter is passed through an appropriately sized needle or vascular catheter that has been placed into the trachea through the cricothyroid membrane. The epidural catheter is advanced between the vocal cords to the pharynx.[46] A tracheal tube changer or stiff ureteral stent is threaded over the catheter, which has been advanced out the mouth or nose (for nasotracheal intubations) to be used as a stent for the tracheal tube. The endotracheal tube can be passed over this catheter or stent and advanced into the trachea.[32, 46]

After the endotracheal tube has entered the proximal trachea, the catheter is cut near the skin and pulled out through the connector end of the endotracheal tube while holding caudad pressure on the endotracheal tube.[46]

This technique is generally contraindicated if the airway is so narrowed that it may become more obstructed by traumatic edema, there is infection in the pretracheal area, or if a significant coagulopathy has been identified. Some authors have recommended that this technique not be used in infants,[18] but data to support this recommendation in any age group are absent. Although pediatric patients, especially infants, have smaller airways, congenital anomalies that may make it difficult to identify airway anatomy, and associated medical problems that need to be carefully evaluated (e.g., asthma), this technique has been successfully used in infants as young as 1 day old. In infants and children, the retrograde technique is often combined with fiberoptic guidance.[47] That is, a needle cricothyrotomy was performed with a 22-gauge polytetrafluoroethylene (Teflon) catheter over a needle. When gas was freely aspirated, the needle was removed, and the catheter was advanced towards the larynx. A 100-cm-long, 0.018-inch-diameter Teflon-coated guidewire was passed through the catheter and advanced cephalad until it exited a nostril. The catheter was passed into the suction port of a 2.8-mm outer diameter intubating bronchoscope. An endotracheal tube had been loaded onto the bronchoscope. The bronchoscope was advanced over the wire until the vocal cords were identified. The endotracheal tube was then placed into the trachea and advanced to the appropriate depth. Twenty patients were reported in this series, eight of which were 24 months of age or younger. Oxygen was insufflated throughout the procedure.

Borland et al.[47] described puncturing the cricothyroid membrane with a 20-gauge needle attached to a saline-filled syringe. Confirmation of intratracheal placement of the needle was made when air was aspirated into the saline-filled syringe. A 0.021-inch, extra-long, flexible-tipped guidewire was then threaded through the needle superiorly into the trachea, larynx, and posterior pharynx and retrieved from the mouth. A 16-gauge red-rubber catheter was inserted nasally and retrieved from the mouth. The wire and catheter were tied together with a suture and the wire was withdrawn through the naris. The wire was threaded through the sidehole of a well-lubricated small endotracheal tube, and while maintaining tension on both ends of the wire, the nasal endotracheal tube was advanced until it was within the trachea at the site of the cricothyroid membrane puncture. At that point, the guidewire was withdrawn (not cut, because it will unravel) and the nasotracheal tube was advanced farther into the trachea.[47]

Bullard Laryngoscope

The Bullard laryngoscope (Fig. 23–3A) allows direct visualization of the laryngeal inlet, via a fiberoptic sidearm. The fiberoptic sidearm courses around a blade that has a 90-degree bend that functions like a laryngoscope blade. This instrument allows visualization of structures that are around a corner, such as occurs in patients whose glottic opening is at an exaggerated angle with respect to the tongue (Pierre Robin, Treacher-Collins, etc.). To intubate the trachea, the blade is inserted into the mouth with the handle parallel to the patient's body and then rotated through 90 degrees (Fig. 23–3B). It allows the curved blade to be positioned so the larynx can be visualized through the fiberoptic sidearm. Then the trachea can be intubated directly with a styleted tracheal tube or with the grasping forceps supplied with the instrument. The grasping forceps are inserted into the appropriate channel and emerge from the distal end of the scope where they can be used to grasp the Murphy eye of the tube. The endotracheal tube is advanced into the larynx under direct vision.[48] As with other methods, facility with this technique requires practice in patients with normal airway anatomy.

Light Wand

The *light wand* is a malleable lighted stylet that is a useful adjunct in managing difficult pediatric airways.[49–51] Hemodynamic responses to the light wand are similar to those occurring with standard laryngoscopy.[52] To use the wand, its malleable portion is bent into a curve that would be expected to successfully pass into the laryngeal inlet. An endotracheal tube, without its 15-mm connector, is passed over a lubricated light wand. The light wand is introduced into the patient's mouth along the curvature of the tongue. As the device passes downward, a diffuse light may be appreciated in the neck. Proper positioning of the light wand produces a sharp, well-defined, bright circle of light directly in the midline on the skin of the neck at the level of the cricothyroid membrane. The endotracheal tube is gently advanced off the stylet once proper positioning of the stylet is ensured.[50] This technique is particularly useful in patients with normal anatomy but with limited mobility in their neck and jaw. For example, in patients with cervical spine fractures, tracheal intubation can be accomplished without moving the neck.[51] Disposable and nondisposable tracheal light wands (Rush, Inc.) now are made in infant (ETT, 2.5 to 4.0) and child (ETT, 4.0 to 6.0) sizes. The infant version is less stiff, and, therefore, may be more difficult to manipulate into position.[53] Since this technique is "blind," several attempts may be required to intubate the trachea; with experience, the success rate increases.[50] Consequently, clinicians should initially use this device in children with normal anatomy to become proficient

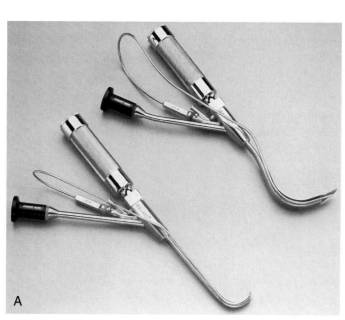
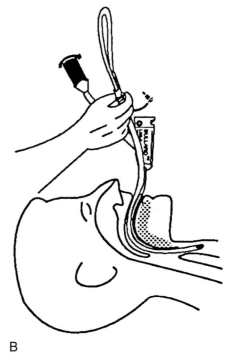

FIGURE 23–3. *A,* The adult (*above*) and pediatric (*lower*) Bullard laryngoscopes. *B,* Using the Bullard laryngoscope. (Courtesy of Circon Corporation.)

in its use before attempting to use it for a child with a difficult airway.

Fiberoptic Bronchoscope

Fiberoptic bronchoscopy is no longer an "exotic" technique. It has become integral to the practice of anesthesia, often the first-line approach to facilitating a difficult oral or nasal intubation in adults, children, and infants.[39, 40, 54, 55] Congenital anomalies of the face and mandible, of the temporomandibular joints, and of the tongue should alert the clinician to the possibility that intubation of the trachea may be difficult. Masses, tumors, trauma, cervical instability, and infectious processes may distort airway anatomy. In general, a fiberoptic intubation of the trachea should be considered for any infant or child who has craniofacial anomalies that may be associated with difficulty managing the airway (e.g., Goldenhar's, Smith-Lemli-Optiz, Treacher-Collins, Carpenter's, Apert's, Crouzon's, Pfeiffer's, and orofaciodigital syndromes), either because of poor mask fit or difficult visualization of the larynx. Syndromes that result in macroglossia (e.g., Beckwith-Wiedemann, trisomy 21) or deposition of accumulated by-products (e.g., Hurler's, Pompe's, Morquio's) may make airway management difficult. In addition, patients with cervical instability (e.g., Klippel-Feil, post-trauma) should be considered for fiberoptic airway management when intubation of the trachea is indicated.

When using a fiberoptic bronchoscope, the anesthesiologist must be familiar with the bronchoscope used, the handling of the scope and its shortcomings. Guidelines for flexible fiberoptic bronchoscopy have been developed by the American Thoracic Society and the American Lung Association.[56] A variety of "workshops" and "courses" introduce the novice to the technique in a controlled environment, but clinical experience in the presence of experts is an essential part of achieving competence in this technique.

Current available fiberoptic scopes range in size from 1.8 mm to 5.5 mm, but the devices most commonly used by anesthesiologists to intubate the trachea of pediatric patients are 2.1 to 4.0 mm. The smallest fiberoptic scope with a directable tip is 2.1 mm in diameter (LF-P), which accommodates a 3.0-mm endotracheal tube. The larger scopes (2.8, 3.5, 4.0 mm) offer more directional control, have a suction channel to facilitate removal of secretions that can obscure one's view, provide a route for administration of local anesthetics or insufflation of oxygen, or for placement of a flexible guidewire (see above). However, the smaller ultrathin scopes have revolutionized securing an airway in small infants with abnormal upper airway anatomy.[55, 57] The larger endotracheal tubes may be stiff relative to smaller fiberoptic scopes and may increase the difficulty of using the fiberoptic scope.[58] For example, the maximum size endotracheal tube that should be used with the 2.7 mm scope is 4.5 mm.

The specific technique of fiberoptic bronchoscopy varies with the patient, the size of the bronchoscope available, and the specific needs of the case. The usual technique for fiberoptic bronchoscopy involves placing a lubricated, appropriate-sized, endotracheal tube through the nose into the posterior pharynx. A lubricated bronchoscope is

passed through the nose and beyond the distal tip of the tube. Under direct vision, the bronchoscope is advanced through the vocal cords and into the midtrachea. The endotracheal tube is then slid off the fiberscope and the position of the tube is confirmed by direct visualization through the scope, auscultation of the chest, observation of chest rise and fall, and end-tidal carbon dioxide. In small patients, even the smaller fiberoptic bronchoscopes can significantly obstruct the upper trachea and endotracheal tube. Therefore, the scope must be removed as soon as possible.[59]

Fiberoptic bronchoscopy and intubation can be performed on awake patients whose airway is anesthetized with topical or nebulized local anesthetics (see section "Awake Nasotracheal Intubation," above), or who are anesthetized with inhaled anesthetics, or intravenous agents such as ketamine or propofol. Providing supplemental oxygen and monitoring oxygen saturation during these procedures is essential, because the airways are often compromised for brief periods during the endoscopy. Supplemental oxygen can be delivered by cannula, face mask, or insufflation into the opposite naris and, with some broncoscopes, via the channel provided for this purpose. Some practitioners administer atropine or glycopyrolate before the bronchoscopy to dry secretions that may coat the lens of the scope and interfere with visualization of the airway.

Intubation of the trachea and examination of the airway by fiberoptic bronchoscopy can be performed via face mask when a patient is anesthetized and breathing spontaneously. The endotracheal tube (without the 15-mm adapter) and fiberscope are placed through an adapter or diaphragm on the mask adaptor or through a small hole in the mask that allows passage of the scope and endotracheal tube. The scope is inserted into the naris or mouth and directed into the pharynx and airway. The nasal route may be preferable, because the bronchoscope may be more stable and provide a better angle of approach to the larynx versus the acute angle provided with an oral approach.[58] A special oral airway may ensure that the scope remains in the midline when the oral approach is used.

Many modifications of the standard technique of fiberoptic bronchoscopy have been used for pediatric patients. Some clinicians visualize the larynx through a bronchoscope that is placed into one naris. The endotracheal tube is then inserted through the other naris and a low, constant flow of oxygen is delivered through the endotracheal tube. The larynx is visualized through the fiberscope, and an assistant extends, flexes, or elevates the patient's head, and the tube is advanced into the trachea.[60] Stiles[61] described using an adult fiberoptic bronchoscope to intubate the trachea of infants and small children. The fiberoptic bronchoscope is inserted orally in an anesthetized, spontaneously breathing patient and the vocal cords are visualized. A flexible guidewire is passed through the suction port of the scope and threaded into the lower airway. The bronchoscope is then removed and a cardiac catheter or tube exchanger is passed over the wire. The endotracheal tube is then advanced over the catheter into the airway, and the catheter and wire are removed while leaving the endotracheal tube in the trachea. Care must be taken to avoid applying excessive downward pressure on the wire or catheter to prevent injury to the airway or lung.

A laryngeal mask airway (LMA) also can be used to facilitate fiberoptic airway endoscopy in children.[56, 62–74] With this technique, a larger fiberscope can be used. The larynx and trachea are not obscured by an endotracheal tube.[65, 66] A variation of this technique uses an endotracheal tube that easily passes through the LMA. The LMA can be used to anesthetize the patient; then the LMA can be used as a conduit for directing the bronchoscope.[59–62] The LMA also has been used to facilitate placement of a stylet into the airway over which an endotracheal tube can be passed.[63, 64] LMAs have also been used for blind tracheal intubations.[73, 74]

The fiberoptic bronchoscope is an essential tool for the evaluation and control of potentially difficult pediatric airways. An individual proficient in the use of this instrument often can complete the procedure in approximately 60 seconds, which is comparable to the time required for a laryngoscopic intubation.[59]

Upper Respiratory Infection

Frequently, anesthesiologists are asked to evaluate children with signs and/or symptoms of an upper respiratory infection (URI). Children with URIs are more likely to be scheduled to undergo procedures of the head and neck than children without a URI.[75] Several studies have defined the risks of anesthesia in children who present for surgery with a URI or a history of a recent URI. Anesthesiologists generally agree that elective surgery should be postponed if the infant or child has a fever and purulent secretions, which implies a medical problem beyond an "uncomplicated URI." Tait and Knight[76, 77] have pointed out, however, that children with uncomplicated URIs who undergo myringotomy and placement of tubes, which usually takes less than 10 minutes and is done without placement of an endotracheal tube, are at no increased risk from general anesthesia. Aside from these two situations, there is still significant controversy concerning the risks of elective surgery and anesthesia for children with a current or recent URI.

For elective surgery, the nature of the procedure may affect the anesthesiologist's decision to proceed or not proceed with surgery if the child has a URI. For example, a twofold increase in laryngospasm was reported in patients with a URI who were undergoing "airway surgery."[78] Similarly, data from the Children's Hospital of Winnipeg suggest that children with URIs are more likely to have a "respiratory-related adverse event" in the perioperative period than children who do not have a URI.[75] Rolf and Cote[79] reported a higher frequency of minor desaturation episodes and an increased risk of bronchospasm following tracheal intubation in children with URIs. The risk of postoperative oxygen desaturation associated with a URI has also been described, suggesting that children with an acute URI or a recent history of a URI should receive supplemental oxygen and be carefully monitored by pulse oximetry in the immediate postoperative period.[80]

Understanding the pathophysiology of viral infection on the airway may provide a framework for making rational decisions about when to cancel surgery for patients with a URI. Although the specific mechanism for the perioperative respiratory complications associated with a URI is not entirely defined, it is clear that there are two main pathophysiologic effects on the respiratory system: peripheral airway abnormalities and airway hyperreactivity.

Although the term "URI" implies that the infection is limited to the upper airway, the lower airway also can be markedly affected. The effects on the lower airways are likely to be the main source of hypoxemia and compromised pulmonary function. In patients with a URI, it should be anticipated that pulmonary complications may be more significant during or after a long procedure, a procedure that requires intra- and postoperative mechanical ventilation, a procedure associated with extensive surgical trauma to the lung parenchyma, or when the patient has underlying pulmonary abnormalities (e.g., cystic fibrosis, steroid-dependent asthma).

Peripheral Airway Abnormalities

Studies describing diminished diffusion capacity,[81] abnormal frequency dependence of compliance[82, 84] and resistance,[83] and increased closing volumes[84] have been reported in adults, but equivalent data are not available for infants and young children. However, qualitative similarities seem probable. That is, decreased diffusion capacity, increased closing volume, and airway dysfunction are likely to occur in children and predispose them to intrapulmonary shunting and hypoxia.

Parainfluenza infection (PI-3) had a dramatic effect on intrapulmonary shunt and Po_2 in both awake and anesthetized (halothane/nitrous oxide) adult sheep.[85] This virus causes bronchiolitis of the terminal airways, sloughing of epithelial cells, and subsequent hyperplasia. An interstitial injury of the alveolar septa is also present.

Apneic, anesthetized children with a URI demonstrated a more rapid decrease in their oxygen saturation to 95 percent than similar children without a URI, suggesting that a URI has effects on the functional residual capacity (FRC) and/or closing volume of children during anesthesia.[86] This would be consistent with studies that document the effects of a URI on the spirometry of awake children.[87]

Clinical reports of "pulmonary collapse" (i.e., atelectasis) associated with general anesthesia and surgery are not difficult to find in the literature.[88, 89] One report describes the recognition of pneumonia (later identified as *Haemophilus influenzae*) by detecting asymmetric chest movement and hypoxemia during surgery to repair a laceration of an upper lip.[90] A viral infection may affect mucociliary function and contribute significantly to the occurrence of hypoxemia in the perioperative period.

Thus, the concept that an *upper respiratory* infection has diffuse effects on the *lower respiratory* epithelial function is clinically relevant. The effects of viral inoculation on airway function of rats and other experimental animals could explain the atelectasis and hypoxemia seen in surgical patients with URIs.

Airway Hyperactivity

Bronchospasm can be a significant complication during anesthesia and surgery. The role of intubation of the trachea in causing "respiratory events" in anesthetized children with a URI is not clear. Several studies have demonstrated that the incidence of respiratory complications in children with a URI is not altered when the inhaled anesthetic is delivered via a mask. However, it is higher in tracheally intubated children.[75] Data from the Children's Hospital of Winnipeg suggests children with a URI who required tracheal intubation had an 11-fold increase in risk for a respiratory complication.[75] No age group was at higher risk than another age group, except that children less than 1 year old with a URI had very high relative risk for postoperative croup. Similarly, Rolf and Cote[91] reported a higher frequency of minor desaturation episodes in children with URIs. Tracheal intubation of patients with URIs was associated with a higher incidence of bronchospasm.[91] Tracheal intubation was also shown to elicit a potent airway reflex that enhances the decrease in FRC induced by anesthesia[92] (see section "Peripheral Airway Abnormalities," above).

Patients with bronchospastic disease can manifest significant airway hyperreactivity during anesthesia, which is caused by the intense physical and pharmacologic stimulation of the airway during surgery. Even patients without underlying bronchospastic disease may develop a temporary increase in airway reactivity during viral infections. Although the precise mechanism of this phenomenon has not been totally defined, there is evidence that the immunologic and inflammatory consequences of viral infection release a variety of mediators that cause bronchospasm. Abnormal neural responses to tachykinins (i.e., sensitization of airway receptors secondary to epithelial damage), other mediators, and increased vagal reactivity may increase airway reactivity and can be inhibited by atropine.[93] However, a more selective anticoholinergic agent would have advantages. Atropine blocks the effect of acetylcholine on the smooth muscle but also increases the release of acetylcholine from the vagus nerve endings.[94] A better strategy with a more selective agent would be to block the M_3 receptor (stimulation of which causes bronchoconstriction) but not the M_2 receptor (which inhibits acetylcholine release at nerve terminals).

The role of noncholinergic bronchoconstriction in causing airway reactivity associated with viral infections may be important. For example, substance P (a tachykinin) is present in the neurons of the lung and causes the airways to contract. Capsaicin releases substance P from the lung and mimics the effects of substance P. The contractile effects of both substance P and capsaicin were enhanced in bronchial ring segments taken from guinea pigs infected with parainfluenza 3. Pretreatment with H_1, H_2, muscarinic, serotonergic, and α-adrenergic blockers did not obliterate the effect of substance P.[95]

Studies of the effects of various substances produced by viruses also have contributed to our understanding of the mechanisms of hyperreactivity of the airway during a URI. Parainfluenza and influenza viruses contain an enzyme, neuraminidase, which cleaves sialic acid residues present on the M_2 muscarinic receptor agonist binding site. Inhibition of the M_2 inhibitory site increases acetylcholine release. Studies in guinea pigs have demonstrated alteration of high-affinity agonist binding (carbachol) in lung membrane preparations in response to either neuraminidase or parainfluenza virus. In addition, a neuraminidase-blocking agent inhibited viral-induced changes.[96]

Thus, the effect of a URI can be quite profound. That bronchospasm can be exacerbated during airway manipulation during anesthesia and surgery is not surprising. The precise role of viral infection in the responses of the airway during anesthesia and surgery may vary considerably from one patient to another and with different viruses. Consequently, anticipating intraoperative "adverse respiratory events," planning for vigorous therapy of bronchospasm, and meticulous monitoring of oxygenation both intra- and postoperatively is mandatory in patients with a URI who must undergo surgery and anesthesia.

Whether having a URI at the time of surgery contributes to overall morbidity of anesthesia remains controversial. However, it seems reasonable that a recent or current URI increases the risk for pulmonary complications in the perioperative period, especially if the trachea must be intubated. Available data do not specifically define the risks when major surgical procedures last more than 1 to 2 hours. However, it is reasonable to believe that prolonged and complicated procedures might increase the risk for airway obstruction or bronchospasm (especially if suctioning the trachea is impossible during surgery). Although emergent procedures are performed in the presence of significant medical problems, elective procedures should be undertaken cautiously.

Some experts propose that the increase in airway reactivity associated with a URI lasts 4 to 6 weeks. Empey demonstrated a 200 percent increase in airway resistance after inhaled histamine in adults who had a URI, compared with a 30 percent increase in controls.[97] The increased airway reactivity persisted as long as 6 weeks after the URI ended. Nandwani studied the upper airway reflex sensitivity of nonsmoking, healthy adult patients who inhaled ammonia vapor.[98] Airway reactivity was 2 to 2.5 times normal, but had returned to baseline 2 weeks after the URI ended. There are many children who have 6 to 10 URIs per year. If the symptoms persist for 5 to 7 days, some young children may have as little as 2 to 4 weeks between infections. This does not leave much time to schedule surgery if the surgeon and anesthesiologist insist on a child being completely free of URI symptoms for 4 to 6 weeks before elective surgery is undertaken.

Avoiding unnecessary risk during elective anesthesia and surgery in an otherwise healthy child must be balanced against the frustration of scheduling and rescheduling surgery, which has serious consequences for working families with complicated schedules, busy operating rooms, and physicians with limited "open" time. Thus, it may not be possible to have an asymptomatic period of 4 to 6 weeks after an acute URI. In such cases, surgery may have to be done, and the anesthesiologist must have heightened awareness of possible intra- and perioperative respiratory complications. The anesthesiologist should be prepared to treat bronchospasm aggressively, deliver supplemental oxygen to patients during transport from the operating room to the recovery room, and carefully monitor oxygen saturation in the recovery room to ensure adequate oxygenation before discharge home or to the ward. In other words, treat the child with a URI as if he has "reactive airways disease," because he probably does.

Although "URI" is considered a single disease process, often with a common set of presenting symptoms, there may be enormous variability in the pathophysiologic effects of a particular virus, and these effects may vary depending on the stage of the illness (e.g., initial symptoms, height of symptoms, recovery phase). Therefore, there will always be a need for subjective interpretation of a particular patient's clinical signs, symptoms, and past history when surgery is proposed.

Other aspects of preoperative assessment will be discussed with each specific surgical procedure.

ANESTHESIA FOR SPECIFIC SURGICAL PROCEDURES

Myringotomy and Tympanostomy Tubes

Abnormal eustachian tube function is probably the mechanism for otitis media, a common ailment of infancy and childhood. Hypertrophied tonsils or adenoids may obstruct eustachian tubes. More commonly, abnormal opening and closing of the eustachian tube in response to increased compliance or congenital malformation results in edema, inflammation, and an effusion.[99] Chronic serous otitis media is manifested by decreased mobility of the tympanic membrane. Chronic serous otitis media may be followed or preceded by an episode of acute suppurative otitis media. Acute suppurative otitis is frequently accompanied by fever, irritability, and feeding intolerance. The tympanic membrane is red and has decreased mobility. Antimicrobial agents are used to treat acute suppurative otitis media when a bacterial infection is suspected. Placement of tympanostomy tubes is usually reserved for treatment of recurrent and chronic otitis media. Antibiotic therapy effectively treats an episode of acute otitis media, but the underlying eustachian tube dysfunction causes the problem to recur. When it does, establishing sustained ventilation of the middle ear via tympanostomy tubes is the only adequate treatment.

Infants who have their first episode of otitis media before the age of 3 months are prone to recurrent infection and frequently present for myringotomy and placement of tympanostomy tubes. Often, these patients are 15 to 36 months of age when surgery is performed. Since these patients may also have adenotonsillar hypertrophy, careful perioperative evaluation of their upper airway is important. A history of snoring or sleep apnea should prompt reevaluation of whether to delay the surgery, since 10 to 15 percent of these children have upper airway obstruction during a general anesthetic.[100] Delaying surgery may be important to establish whether a tonsillectomy and/or adenoidectomy should be performed at the same time as placement of tympanostomy tubes. For example, a formal sleep study to quantitate the degree and frequency of obtructive sleep apnea may be indicated. Consideration for hospitalization, rather than "come-and-go" surgery, may be necessary (see section "Tonsillectomy/Adenoidectomy," below) in the setting of airway obstruction. Some patients, such as children with craniofacial anomalies (e.g., trisomy 21 or Apert's syndrome) or those with an acute upper respiratory infection (see sections "Upper Respiratory Infection," above and "Tonsillectomy/Adenoidectomy," below), may be predisposed to airway obstruction or other airway complications.

An operating microscope is frequently used to perform a myringotomy and to place bilateral tympanostomy tubes. The procedure is usually completed within 10 to 20 minutes. Consequently, most children undergoing myringotomy and tube placement are not premedicated and are anesthetized with an inhalation anesthetic. They seldom require tracheal intubation, and usually do not have an intravenous catheter placed. Before deciding to proceed without intubating the trachea, it is important to determine that the airway is adequate when the head is turned to the side so the surgeons can perform the surgery. Frequently, the surgeon will manually examine the adenoids after the tympanostomy tubes are placed. Consequently, the level of anesthesia must be sufficiently deep to permit the surgeon to do this without inducing laryngospasm.

Usually, there are few postoperative complications, and the child is discharged home within 15 to 30 minutes of being admitted to the recovery room. If the patient has a complicated medical history (e.g., cyanotic heart disease, a chromosomal abnormality) or he or she has associated upper airway anomalies, the anesthetic technique might require modification, and a longer postoperative course (or hospitalization) should be anticipated.

Nitrous oxide is not contraindicated during simple myringotomy and tube placement. However, if extensive reconstruction of the tympanic membrane is planned, nitrous oxide should be avoided, because the high blood gas partition coefficient (34 times that of air) increases the gas pressure of the inner ear. If that space is compliant, the volume of the area increases. If it is noncompliant, the pressure of the area increases. The middle ear is relatively noncompliant. Pressure in the middle ear increases during nitrous oxide anesthesia, and pressure peaks after nitrous oxide has been administered for 30 minutes.[101] The pressure returns to preanesthetic values 45 minutes after the nitrous oxide is discontinued. If eustachian tube function is normal, the middle ear periodically decompresses. With chronic otitis media, this does not reliably occur, and the increased pressure may cause temporary or permanent hearing loss.[101] Although nitrous oxide may be used during the induction of anesthesia, it should be discontinued at least 30 to 45 minutes before a graft is placed onto the tympanic membrane because increased inner ear pressure will displace the graft. If a myringotomy is not planned and a patient is known to have eustachian tube dysfunction, nitrous oxide should be avoided, because increased pressure in the middle ear space may rupture the tympanic membrane.

Tonsillectomy/Adenoidectomy
Preoperative Assessment

Tonsillectomy, with or without adenoidectomy, accounts for at least 340,000 operations per year in the United States. Greater than 95 percent of patients have no postoperative problems. However, some children have serious coexisting medical problems. Therefore, careful evaluation of the child's underlying medical problems is essential. In particular, hematologic abnormalities, immunosuppression, and obstructive sleep apnea are indications of possible intra- and postoperative complications.

Children less than 3 years of age require special consideration because the primary indication for adenotonsillectomy is airway obstruction induced by adenotonsillar hypertrophy. As a consequence, these children often have obstructive sleep apnea syndrome. That hypertrophied tonsils and adenoids cause intermittent airway obstruction, obstructive sleep apnea, chronic alveolar hypoventilation, and cor pulmonale was first reported more than 20 years ago. This pathophysiology may be reversible if the problem is diagnosed and treated early.

Although the cardiopulmonary sequelae of pulmonary hypertension only develop in a few children, many children have upper airway obstruction. Severely affected children have at least 30 apneic episodes per night that last 10 seconds or more. They commonly snore, have sleep disturbances, daytime hypersomnolence, decreased school performance, personality changes, recurrent enuresis, hyponasal speech, growth disturbances, and short stature.

Special Problems

Patients with craniofacial disorders may have other medical problems that have implications for anesthetic management for tonsillectomy and/or adenoidectomy. For example, patients with mucopolysaccharidosis I (Hurler's syndrome) and II (Hunter's syndrome) have diffuse infiltration of their upper airway and larynx with abnormal mucopolysaccharides. This predisposes them to upper airway obstruction and difficult tracheal intubation, even without tonsillar hypertrophy. Cardiac valvar and myocardial involvement may be present, especially with Hurler's syndrome; coronary artery disease can be present at an early age. Kyphoscoliosis develops, especially in Hunter's syndrome, and can result in pulmonary abnormalities.

Trisomy 21 is another common and important syndrome in which craniofacial problems are prominent. These children are predisposed to significant upper airway obstruction when adenotonsillar hypertrophy is added to their midfacial hypoplasia (i.e., narrow oral and nasal passages). In addition, they have a high incidence of congenital heart lesions and excessive pulmonary blood flow, which predispose them to pulmonary hypertension. Thus, patients with mucopolysaccharidosis or trisomy 21 may have underlying pathophysiology that may exaggerate the effects of adenotonsillar hypertrophy.

Patients with sickle cell disease who have recurrent tonsillitis have an increased risk for sepsis. Sleep apnea-induced hypoxia may increase the incidence of sickle cell crises. Thus, frequent tonsillitis (more than six episodes per year) or adenotonsillar hypertrophy resulting in upper airway obstruction should be treated aggressively in these patients.

Although the risk of acquiring human immunodeficiency virus (HIV) infection or hepatitis from a blood transfusion is of concern, the risk of increased postoperative morbidity from a sickle cell crisis (e.g., acute chest crisis) in nontransfused patients must be weighed against the infectious risk of giving heterologous blood products preoperatively. Before major surgery, the hematocrit is sometimes raised above 35 percent by a simple transfusion in patients with sickle cell disease. More commonly, a partial exchange transfusion is performed to increase the hematocrit and to decrease the percentage of hemoglobin S (HbS) to less than 30 percent. If the surgery is elective and simple, patients frequently will receive a packed red blood cell transfusion once a week for 3 to 4 weeks. This depresses sickle cell hemoglobin production. During both surgery and recovery, adequate hydration, oxygenation, and a normal body temperature must be maintained to minimize inducing a sickle cell crisis.

Coagulation Status

Coagulation status must be carefully evaluated before a tonsillectomy or adenoidectomy. Routine laboratory work is not necessary unless the medical or family history is suspicious for easy bruising, excessive menstruation, gingival bleeding, or excessive bleeding during prior surgery or extraction of teeth. A careful history for drug ingestion (e.g., acetylsalicylic acid [ASA], or aspirin) is important. If there is a history of recent ASA ingestion, surgery should be postponed until platelet function is normal.[102] Parents should be told to avoid ASA and ASA-containing products for at least a week before surgery. If the ASA is administered for a particular medical problem (e.g., to maintain patency of a Blalock-Taussig shunt), the doctor who recommended administering the ASA should be consulted, and a plan should be made with the ENT surgeon.

If there is a suspicious history of bleeding, a bleeding time and platelet function should be evaluated. A platelet count plus a prothombin time (PT) and a partial thomboplastin time (PTT) test constitute an appropriate initial evaluation. If von Willebrand's disease is suspected, a specific evaluation should be initiated.

Von Willebrand's disease is a hereditary disorder characterized by a prolonged bleeding time. Patients frequently give a history of skin and mucous membrane bleeding (e.g., nosebleeds). Although there are variant forms of von Willebrand's disease, all have a common pattern: (1) decreased von Willebrand factor concentration, (2) decreased ristocetin cofactor activity, and (3) decreased factor VIII activity. Von Willebrand factor is a plasma glycoprotein which facilitates platelet adhesion and is the plasma carrier for factor VIII. Perioperative treatment may include factor VIII concentrate or cryoprecipitate or, in some cases, the use of 1-desamino-8-D-arginine vasopressin (DDAVP) (usually type I von Willebrand's disease). The diagnosis of a mild disorder can be difficult. If this diagnosis is suspected, consultation with a pediatric hematologist is indicated.

Intraoperative Management

Anesthesia for tonsillectomy/adenoidectomy can be accomplished with a combination of inhaled and intravenous agents. Special care must be taken with patients who have a history of upper airway obstruction. Atropine is not routinely used at our institution.

An oral RAE (named for Ring, Adair, and Elwyn who originally described these ETT), a molded preformed endotracheal tube has the advantages of being easily stabilized in the self-retaining mouth gag, and the preformed bend in the tube allows the connector to be positioned away from the site of surgery (Fig. 23–4). The disadvantage of RAE tubes is that the length of the endotracheal tube beyond the bend of the tube is fixed. If a patient requires an endotracheal tube that is smaller than normal for age, the length of the RAE tube may be too short to place the tip of the tube in the midtrachea, increasing the chance of accidental tracheal extubation. In such cases, the trachea should be intubated with a straight endotracheal tube. A reinforced endotracheal tube is a good alternative to an oral RAE tube. Reinforced tubes limit the possibility of compression and obstruction of the tube by the mouth gag. In all cases, meticulous attention should be paid to preventing movement and pinching of the endotracheal tube by the mouth gag (Fig. 23–5). Breath sounds, chest excursion, peak airway pressure, end-tidal carbon dioxide, and oxygen saturation should be monitored at all times.

There can be significant postoperative pain following adenotonsillectomy. Therefore, administration of a narcotic intraoperatively should be considered (e.g., 0.1 mg/kg of morphine intravenously). Infiltrating the tonsillar beds with a local anesthetic may effectively provide short-term pain control if an adenoidectomy is not performed. Treatment of pain with depressant drugs must take into account preoperative assessment of the airway and the intraoperative course.

Before extubating the trachea, the surgeon and anesthesiologist should examine the posterior pharynx for evidence of ongoing bleeding or the presence of lymphoid tissue, blood clots, or other foreign material that can be aspirated into the lungs. The endotracheal tube is commonly removed after the patient is awake, preferably with the patient in the lateral and head-down position.

Fluid management may be challenging during a tonsillectomy/adenoidectomy. Commonly, 5 to 10 percent (or more) of the blood volume is lost. Allowable blood loss should be calculated preoperatively (see Chapter 6). The "minimum allowable hematocrit" depends on many factors, but it is certainly lower than the often-stated 30 percent in most patients. In the absence of significant cardiopulmonary disease, children tolerate a hematocrit as low as 20 percent. Following tonsillectomy and/or adenoidectomy, some blood loss may not be apparent because the blood is swallowed. Placement of a throat pack during surgery may reduce hidden blood loss. When the throat pack is removed, it should be examined to assess blood loss. Postoperative losses are also frequently difficult to assess secondary to swallowed blood.

Since fluid and blood may have to be administered rapidly, an appropriate size IV catheter should be placed and secured well to prevent intra- or postoperative loss of the catheter. Patients may awaken thrashing about and restless. If the IV catheter is not secure, it can be dislodged. Placing an IV catheter into a hypovolemic, "excited" postoperative patient is a difficult and usually avoidable emergency. A well-functioning IV catheter is necessary in the postoperative period to facilitate pain control, to deliver fluid/blood as needed, and to induce general anesthesia if reoperation is required for postoperative hemorrhage.

Postoperative Management

Much attention has been directed to the occurrence of early and late postoperative hemorrhage following adenotonsillectomy. The bleeding often occurs over several hours. Pallor and tachycardia develop gradually. Continued blood loss results in restlessness and hypotension.

Postoperative hemorrhage often requires surgical reexploration. Such children require prompt volume resuscitation and are at risk for aspiration of swallowed blood. In older children, a thorough examination of the posterior pharynx and placement of a nasal pack may be possible. However, in most cases, a general anesthetic is required.

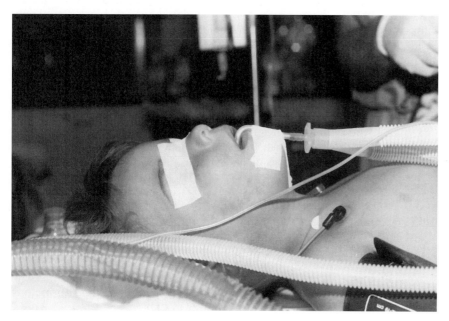

FIGURE 23–4. Patient is positioned for tonsillectomy and/or adenoidectomy. The oral RAE tube is stabilized to the lower lip and thereby positioned away from the site of surgery.

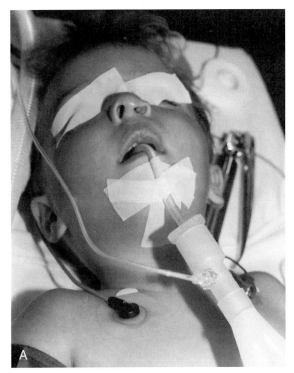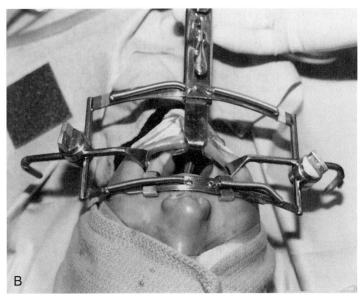

FIGURE 23–5. Patient is positioned for tonsillectomy and/or adenoidectomy (*A*). Note the position of the endotracheal tube in the mouth retractor used to hold the mouth open (*B*). The retractor must be carefully placed to avoid kinking or dislodging the endotracheal tube.

To replace blood volume, the child should be given a combination of crystalloid and colloid (e.g., fresh frozen plasma, packed red blood cells [PRBCs]) depending on the hematocrit, the clotting status, and the medical history. In most cases, bleeding following tonsillectomy is not brisk or massive. Consequently, surgery can be delayed for a short time until volume resuscitation is adequate. When the patient's condition is stabilized, general anesthesia can be induced. Ideally, the stomach should be aspirated before the induction of anesthesia. However, this is almost always met with resistance and can increase blood pressure and bleeding. If the stomach contents cannot be aspirated preoperatively, a large tube can be inserted into the stomach intraoperatively to remove as much of the gastric contents as possible. *This does not guarantee that the stomach is empty.*

Multiple laryngoscopes and suctioning devices should be immediately available, and all patients should be preoxygenated with 100 percent oxygen before inducing anesthesia. Some experts advocate a rapid sequence induction of anesthesia when patients have a full stomach and airway compromise, whereas others advocate an inhalation induction while holding cricoid pressure. Either technique can be appropriate. The key issues are assessing the airway and ensuring that intravascular volume is adequate. If a patient has respiratory distress before the induction of anesthesia, using inhalation anesthesia and an F_{IO_2} of 1.0 will allow the anesthesiologist to determine if positive-pressure ventilation can be administered before delivering a muscle relaxant. In the absence of respiratory distress and the absence of distorted airway anatomy (e.g., tracheal deviation), a rapid sequence induction of anesthesia also may be safe. In the end, the technique chosen

to secure the airway will depend on the experience of the anesthesiologist and the physiologic and airway status of the patient. The trachea should be extubated only when the child is awake.

The anesthesiologist may choose to use a cuffed endotracheal tube in patients undergoing an adenotonsillectomy or reexploration for posttonsillectomy hemorrhage. If so, a cuffed tube should be chosen that is 0.5 to 1.0 mm smaller in diameter than the appropriate-sized uncuffed tube. The cuff allows the gas leak around the endotracheal tube to be adjusted to avoid trauma to the trachea and to decrease the leak if vomiting occurs. Using a cuffed endotracheal tube may decrease the risk of pulmonary aspiration in such high-risk patients.[103]

Twelve to 27 percent of patients less than 3 years old have upper airway obstruction following adenoidectomy or tonsillectomy.[104] Removing hypertrophied tonsils/adenoids often has dramatic effects on the anatomy of the upper airway, resulting in a "floppy" collapsible upper airway and airway obstruction Although adjustment to this "new space" usually occurs over several days, the immediate postoperative period can be characterized by continued upper airway obstruction and hypoxemia, especially in patients less than 3 years old.[105] Postoperative edema and the effect of this surgery on the support system of the airway combine to make airway obstruction more common in this age group. Patients with any evidence of airway obstruction should receive supplemental oxygen in a monitored setting in the immediate postoperative period. An "overnight" (23-hour) admission is frequently recommended, since upper airway problems may lead to reintubation of the trachea and admission to the PICU. In one study, respiratory compromise occurred as late as 14 hours after surgery.[105] If an outpatient procedure is planned, at least 6 hours of monitoring in a recovery room is recommended.

Although uncommon, some patients with upper airway obstruction have cor pulmonale preoperatively.[106] This diagnosis should be considered and cardiac evaluation sought in patients with a history of severe airway obstruction and sleep apnea. Some experts recommend postoperative ventilatory support for 1 to 3 days for patients with a preoperative diagnosis of cor pulmonale. Patients with cor pulmonale may be particularly prone to postobstructive pulmonary edema, especially if laryngospasm or upper airway obstruction occurs after tracheal extubation.

Peritonsillar Abscess

The presence of pus between the capsule of the tonsil and the fascia of the superior constrictor muscle can cause upper airway obstruction. Patients frequently present with fever, severe sore throat, dysphagia, and trismus. Although it would be ideal to drain such an abscess while preserving the cough reflex to prevent pulmonary aspiration of pus, a local anesthetic is not likely to be successful in young children.

Similar to the considerations for induction of anesthesia for surgical treatment of posttonsillectomy hemorrhage, the choice of an inhalational agent versus a rapid sequence induction in patients with peritonsillar abscess depends on the severity of upper airway obstruction and the expertise of the anesthesiologist. Inducing anesthesia in the head-down tilt position with the head turned toward the side of the abscess is ideal if ventilation is adequate. If there is significant airway compromise, the ability to deliver adequate positive-pressure ventilation must be ensured before a muscle relaxant is administered. If mechanical ventilation is easy via a mask, administering a muscle relaxant may facilitate atraumatic intubation of the trachea. Avoiding rupturing the abscess during the induction of anesthesia is essential and requires gentle use of suction devices and meticulous placement of the laryngoscope. An FiO2 of 1.0 should be administered until the trachea is intubated. The patient should be fully awake before the trachea is extubated.

The anesthesiologist may choose to use a cuffed endotracheal tube in patients with a peritonsillar abscess. Although not proven, doing so may decrease the risk of pulmonary aspiration in these patients.[103]

Tracheostomy

Placement of a tracheostomy in young infants is associated with more complications than in adults. Infants with congenital anomalies of the airway and exnpremature infants require a tracheostomy with some frequency to alleviate upper airway obstruction and to facilitate long-term mechanical ventilation for the treatment of respiratory insufficiency. Chronic lung disease is a common residual problem in very-low-birth-weight premature infants that may require ventilatory support for several months or more. Long-term ventilatory support is easier via a tracheostomy, especially if the child is to be ventilated at home or in a chronic care facility. The specific timing of and the indications for tracheostomy in infants with chronic lung disease vary among medical centers. Expremature infants who develop glottic or subglottic stenosis following prolonged mechanical ventilation are sometimes not candidates for definitive surgical treatment. Therefore, a tracheostomy may be required to bypass an area of tracheal obstruction. In some cases, laryngeal reconstruction is possible at a later time.

Tracheobronchomalacia is another cause of upper airway obstruction that may be effectively and more efficiently treated by a tracheostomy in infants. Infants with this problem often require continuous positive pressure for months to years, and home therapy is possible with a tracheostomy. Although parenchymal lung disease is the most common etiology for prolonged mechanical ventilation in the expremature infant, intrinsic tracheobronchial abnormalities, such as tracheobronchomalacia, should always be considered when a baby cannot be weaned from the ventilator.[107]

Severe upper airway obstruction accompanies a variety of congenital anomalies, including subglottic hemangiomas, congenital subglottic stenosis, and congenital laryngeal paralysis.[108] Upper airway obstruction also may occur with micrognathia, which characterizes many complex syndromes (including Pierre Robin anomalad, Crouzon's disease, Goldenhar's syndrome, Meckel's syndrome, Silver's syndrome, Smith-Lemli-Opitz syndrome, and Treacher-Collins syndrome). Some of these infants require a tracheostomy until adequate mandibular growth occurs.

Children with severe neurologic compromise or neuromuscular degenerative problems may require a tracheostomy to allow suctioning of secretions and to protect the airway. After facial or airway burns, or after traumatic injuries to the larynx, a tracheostomy may provide the safest and most secure route for airway support.

Anesthetic Considerations

When an endotracheal tube is in place in a well-oxygenated patient, placement of a tracheostomy is relatively safe. Ideally, tracheostomy should be done only when an endotracheal tube or a bronchoscope is in place, particularly in young infants. In an emergency, it may be necessary to intubate the trachea while the patient is awake. Inhalation of halothane or sevoflurane (FiO2 of 1.0) during spontaneous ventilation provides a safe means inducing anesthesia in most patients. If the airway is clear and unobstructed, a muscle relaxant may be used to facilitate tracheal intubation.

Once the trachea is incised, the anesthesiologist must pull the endotracheal tube back to the upper end of the tracheal incision. However, the endotracheal tube should not be removed from the trachea until it is certain that the tracheostomy tube is in place and functioning and that the lungs can be ventilated via the tracheostomy tube. The tracheostomy tube often must be larger than the endotracheal tube that was in place, because the trachea is larger than the subglottic area (Table 23–1 compares inside and outside diameters of endotracheal and tracheostomy tubes).

The surgeon should leave "stay sutures", on each side of the trachea, to allow the tracheal stoma to be pulled

T A B L E   2 3 – 1
ENDOTRACHEAL TUBES COMPARED TO TRACHEOSTOMY TUBES*

	Endotracheal Tubes		Shiley[†]		Holinger[†]	
	ID	OD	ID	OD	ID	OD
Premature	2.5	3.5			2.5	4.0
Newborn–3 mo	3.0	4.2	3.1	4.5	3.5	5.0
3–10 mo	3.5	4.9	3.4	5.0	3.5	5.5
10–24 mo	4.0	5.5	3.7	5.5	4.0	6.0
2–4 yr	4.5	6.1	4.1	6.0	4.5	7.0
4–5 yr	5.0	6.8	4.8	7.0	5.0	8.0
5–6 yr	5.5	7.4	5.0	8.5	5.5	9.0
6–7 yr	6.0	8.0			6.0	10.0
8–9 yr	6.5	8.7				
10–12 yr	7.0	9.5	7.0	10.5		

* The internal diameter (ID) is the number which, by convention, is used to describe the size of the endotracheal or tracheostomy tube. The tube size recommended is an approximation, and the appropriate size for a given age varies by at least 0.5 to 1.0 mm.
[†] Tracheostomy tube.

up to the skin surface if the trachea is accidentally decannulated in the early postoperative period. The tracheostomy tube must be secured in place before leaving the operating room.

Complications

Tracheostomy in infants and children has been more hazardous than in adults in the immediate postoperative period and afterwards. However, over the last 10 to 20 years, improved surgical and anesthetic techniques, improved monitoring, and training of hospital personnel and families has reduced the danger dramatically. A recent report from England reviewed the outcome of 57 tracheostomies in 56 children less than 12 years old (40 children were <1 year of age).[109] Only 11 complications were identified in the 91 years accumulated experience. These authors attributed this success to postoperative intensive care, careful education of parents, and home visits by nurses specially trained in the care of tracheostomies.

Young infants (e.g., expremature infants) who require a tracheostomy are at particular risk.[110] However, a recent review of tracheostomy in the first year of life[111] reported a mortality rate of 1.6 percent, suggesting that the procedure can be accomplished safely when performed in a controlled environment by an experienced surgeon. In general, complications can be divided into those that occur intraoperatively, those that occur in first 7 postoperative days, and those that occur after the first postoperative week. Early postoperative complications (tube obstruction, pulmonary edema, sepsis, atelectasis, air leak) occurred almost twice as often in preterm infants than in full-term infants, reflecting the overall seriously ill state of the preterm infants. All children, but especially the infants less than 1 year of age, should be monitored in an intensive care unit (PICU or neonatal ICU [NICU]) for at least 24

hours postoperatively. Since the earliest postoperative complications include pneumomediastinum, pneumothorax, and subcutaneous air, it is important to obtain a chest radiograph shortly after the patient arrives in the intensive care unit.

Late complications (granulation tissue, obstructed tracheostomy tube, tracheitis, skin breakdown, tracheal stenosis, tracheomalacia, aspiration) were more common in patients in whom the tracheostomy was placed to treat upper airway obstruction than in patients who required long-term mechanical ventilation for respiratory insufficiency. This is probably related to the fact that patients with upper airway obstruction are healthier and live longer. That is, the late complications were related to the longer duration of tracheostomy. It is noteworthy that, although the mortality rate secondary to the tracheostomy placement itself is low, the overall mortality rate of infants who undergo tracheostomy placement in the first year of life is between 25 and 75 percent,[110–112] reflecting the serious nature of their illnesses. The more severely ill infants die of their underlying illnesses.

Although the complications following tracheostomy can be life threatening, they are preventable or treatable if recognized promptly. Therefore, monitoring in a PICU or step-down unit is indicated until a stable tract forms after 7 to 10 days. The essential need is for careful monitoring of ventilation and oxygenation and the ability to provide ready translaryngeal intubation if the tracheostomy is accidentally dislodged and cannot be replaced quickly. Meticulous attention to humidification of inspired gases, careful suctioning of the airway, and prompt treatment of a tension pneumothorax and tube obstruction improve outcome.

Supraglottitis

Supraglottitis is a life-threatening infection that produces such severe edema of the supraglottic structures that there is a significant risk for complete airway obstruction. Supraglottitis is a more appropriate term for this infection than epiglottitis, because the process is not limited to the epiglottis. The differential diagnosis for this disease includes laryngotracheobronchitis (croup) and tracheitis (Table 23–2). Tracheitis can present with symptoms similar to those of supraglottitis. Because supraglottitis is frequently caused by *Haemophilus influenzae*, there should be a strong suspicion that tracheitis is the cause of respiratory distress in children who present with upper airway distress and a history of receiving the anti–*Haemophilis influenzae* type B (HIB) polysaccharide vaccine.

Before the routine immunization of children with HIB, supraglottitis was most commonly caused by *Haemophilus influenzae* type B and occurred in children between the ages of 2 and 6 years. However, a changing pattern of disease has occurred.[113, 114] Conjugate vaccines were licensed for use in children 15 months of age or older in 1989 and for use in children 2 months of age or older in 1990. During 1987 through 1995, the incidence of invasive *Haemophilus influenzae* disease among children less than 5 years of age decreased 96 percent in the United States[115–117] and Europe.[118] Although fulminant infectious supraglottitis still does occur, *Neisseria meningitidis*,[119]

T A B L E   2 3 — 2
SUPRAGLOTTITIS, LARYNGO-
TRACHEOBRONCHITIS, TRACHEITIS

	Supraglottitis	Laryngotracheobronchitis	Tracheitis
Age	2–6 yr	2 mo–3 yr	2–6 yr
Onset	Fulminant	Gradual	Gradual
Etiology	Bacterial	Viral	Bacterial
Presentation			
Voice	Muffled	Bark	Bark
Secretions	Drooling	Drooling	None
Fever	>38.5°C	37°–38°C	>38.5°C
Distress	Anxious, sitting	Normal	Toxic, sitting

group A *Streptococcus*,[120] and *Candida albicans*[121] are now the primary cause of meningitis and epiglottitis in the postimmunization years.

The incidence of disease has remained constant in older children and has increased in adults, whereas the incidence has decreased in children less than 5 years of age.[122] Immunization with the current polysaccharide vaccine does not protect against the "nontypable" *Haemophilus influenzae*. Nonetheless, to date, neither the incidence of nontypable *Haemophilus influenzae* invasive disease nor the carriage rate of this organism among children less than 5 years old has increased.[123]

Because a patient with supraglottitis is at risk for sudden and complete airway obstruction, a multidisciplinary team is generally involved in managing these patients from the time of their initial presentation to an emergency room or clinic. It is essential to have this coordinated approach established and all services available immediately. Most centers do not rely on medically managing these young patients, because of the risk of sudden airway obstruction. Thus, when the diagnosis of supraglottitis is made or strongly suspected, the goal is to secure the airway in a controlled, prompt manner. Because endotracheal intubation is a safe and efficacious alternative to tracheostomy, endotracheal intubation is the preferred method of supportive airway care. The following approach is consistent with that reported in other centers.[124]

A pediatrician, an anesthesiologist skilled in pediatric airway problems, and a surgeon skilled in placing a tracheostomy in an infant or child should be notified and and should be present when, or shortly after, the child arrives in the emergency room. A thorough, rapid cardiopulmonary history and assessment are made. Examination of the airway is limited to noting respiratory rate, observing the pattern of breathing, and assessing the work of breathing and level of respiratory distress. At most, the heart and lungs should be examined. No manipulation or examination of the mouth or oropharynx should be performed, because this may precipitate acute airway obstruction, especially if the child becomes agitated. No arterial blood gas sampling or venipuncture are done and an intravenous catheter is not inserted. Instead, the child remains sitting up on a parent's (or other familiar caretaker's) lap and receives supplemental oxygen. Oxygen saturation is monitored with a pulse oximeter, while the child is observed closely by the medical personnel.

If the child is not in marked respiratory distress, obtaining a single lateral radiograph of the neck to confirm the diagnosis may be considered. In this case, the child must receive supplemental oxygen while being transported sitting up to the radiography machine. He or she must be accompanied by someone who can emergently intubate the trachea. If the child is in significant respiratory distress or the diagnosis is made clinically, the child should be promptly transported, sitting up, to the operating room while receiving oxygen and being monitored (i.e., no radiography). He must be accompanied by personnel skilled in pediatric airway management and cardiopulmonary resuscitation (CPR).

The tracheostomy tray is open and the surgeon is present when the patient arrives in the operating room. In the past, anesthesia was induced with halothane and 100 percent oxygen while the child sat on the lap of a parent or other familiar caretaker. Sevoflurane can also be used because it allows a smooth induction of anesthesia with minimal airway irritation.[125] The appropriateness of parental or other caregiver presence during induction of anesthesia needs to be assessed for each patient.

With the onset of anesthesia, the patient is placed in the supine or semisitting position, often while continuous positive pressure is applied via the mask to overcome upper airway obstruction. When the depth of anesthesia is adequate, an IV infusion is started. Carefully evaluating the depth of anesthesia is vital to avoid precipitating laryngospasm during laryngoscopy and insertion of an endotracheal tube. The endotracheal tube should be approximately 0.5 to 1.0 mm smaller in diameter than is appropriate for the age and size of the patient. The orotracheal tube is changed to a nasotracheal tube by some anesthesiologists because they believe that the tube is more secure and the patient is more comfortable.

Blood and laryngeal cultures should be obtained during anesthesia, and appropriate antibiotics should be administered intravenously. The selection and dose of antibiotics will vary depending on the organisms seen in a specific geographic area and in a specific patient (e.g., immunocompromised, HIV infection). If the diagnosis of supraglottitis is ruled out when the upper airway is examined, and if the diagnosis is thought to be bacterial tracheitis, the antibiotic chosen may differ from that chosen to treat supraglottitis. Consulting with the pediatric infectious disease service in each medical center is appropriate.

Medically managing young patients who have supraglottitis is not recommended, because it is difficult to clinically assess the degree of upper airway obstruction present. The morbidity from 24 to 48 hours of tracheal intubation is minimal with excellent nursing care. Most centers prefer the use of an endotracheal tube over performing a tracheostomy to treat airway obstruction. The pediatricians, surgeons, and anesthesiologists must have previously agreed on the treatment so that treatment is not delayed because of controversy about the best way to secure the airway.

OTHER TRACHEAL SURGERY

Anterior Cricoid Split Procedure

Long-term endotracheal intubation allowed prolonged respiratory support of infants during the early 1970s.[126] Improved ventilatory support salvaged low-birth-weight infants, and the periods of tracheal intubation were extended with excellent results. Preterm infants tolerated intubation better than full-term neonates or older infants. However, retrospective studies have documented laryngotracheal injury as a complication of endotracheal intubation in as many as 2.5 percent of patients.[127] In many of these patients, the underlying disease may improve, but the endotracheal tube cannot be removed because of glottic or subglottic airway compromise. A careful endoscopic evaluation of the airway must be performed to differentiate upper from lower respiratory compromise.[127] Subglottic lesions are more frequent and more serious than glottic lesions.[126]

Treatment options include tracheostomy or tracheal reconstruction. The cricoid split procedure described by Cotton and Seid in 1980 is one alternative to prolonged tracheostomy for those infants who meet the following stringent criteria.[128-130]

1. Failed tracheal extubation two or more times
2. Weight more than 1,500 g
3. Failed extubation secondary to endoscopically proven laryngeal stenosis
4. No assisted ventilation for 10 days or more
5. Supplemental oxygen requirement less than an $F_{IO_2} = 0.35$
6. No congestive heart failure for the previous month
7. No acute respiratory infection
8. Hypertension under medical control (R. T. Cotton and C. Myer, personal communication)

The procedure is performed over an endotracheal tube. A midline vertical cartilaginous incision is made 2 mm from the thyroid notch inferiorly through the second tracheal ring. Stay sutures are placed through the cricoid ring as in a tracheostomy, and the skin incision is closed. The endotracheal tube often is left in place for approximately 2 weeks before tracheal extubation is attempted.

The goal is to decompress the area of the subglottic space enclosed by the cricoid ring, the only complete cartilaginous ring of the airway. The endotracheal tube temporarily stents the incision open, which allows fibrous ingrowth and prevents airway obliteration with granulation tissue. The 2-week period allows time for mucosal healing.

Laryngeal Reconstruction

The care of congenital and acquired subglottic stenosis in infants and children has been particularly perplexing for pediatric and ENT surgeons. A tracheostomy is required for about 50 percent of patients with congenital subglottic stenosis and for an even higher percentage of patients with severe acquired subglottic stenoses.[131] The advent of procedures such as an anterior cricoid split may prevent some infants from developing severe subglottic stenosis or may reduce the number of patients requiring tracheostomy.[132]

Tracheostomy significantly changes the quality of life, and although a tracheostomy is often life-saving, it can be associated with a significant risk of morbidity and mortality. This morbidity and mortality have led to development of reconstructive therapy that allows early decannulation of the trachea.[133] Surgical therapies include dilation of the lesion, with or without endoscopic excision of tissue, laser excision of tissue with or without stenting of the airway, and interposition grafts of auricular cartilage, hyoid bone, costal cartilage, or composite nasal septum. The sporadic and unique characteristics of each lesion have made studies difficult to do. A proposal was made to standardize reporting.[134-136] Laryngotracheoplasty with costal cartilage grafting is often the surgical technique used in children. Two major advantages of the costal cartilage graft laryngotracheoplasty are minimal alteration in donor and recipient site growth and the excellent survival of this autologous tissue in the contaminated airway. A tracheostomy often is required during the postoperative period.

Laryngotracheoplasty is performed through a horizontal skin incision with midline dissection from the cartilage of the thyroid notch superiorly to the third or fourth tracheal rings inferiorly (Fig. 23–6). A vertical median anterior incision is made into the stenotic lumen. Posterior subglottic or posterior commissure stenoses may require a midline posterior cartilaginous incision to increase the posterior lumen. Sculpted segments of costal cartilage are sutured into the midline incisions, thereby increasing the airway lumen. A solid stent may be necessary to provide support during the postoperative period. This stent may be wired to the tracheostomy tube. Either inhalation or IV anesthesia is used. Ventilation with humidified inspiratory gases is accomplished through the tracheostomy. Patients with a tracheostomy are particularly dependent on meticulous postoperative airway care.

After allowing an appropriate period for stable healing of the grafts, the stents may be removed and the intraluminal granulation tissue excised. Further operative procedures may be required to remove granulation tissue to allow the epithelium to cover the grafts and operative sites. Decannulation occurs when an adequate airway lumen has been obtained.

Although surgical thyrotracheal anastomosis has been performed in adults with few complications, surgeons have been hesitant to adapt this technique to patients who require laryngeal growth after the operation. Recently, several reports have documented a high success rate in

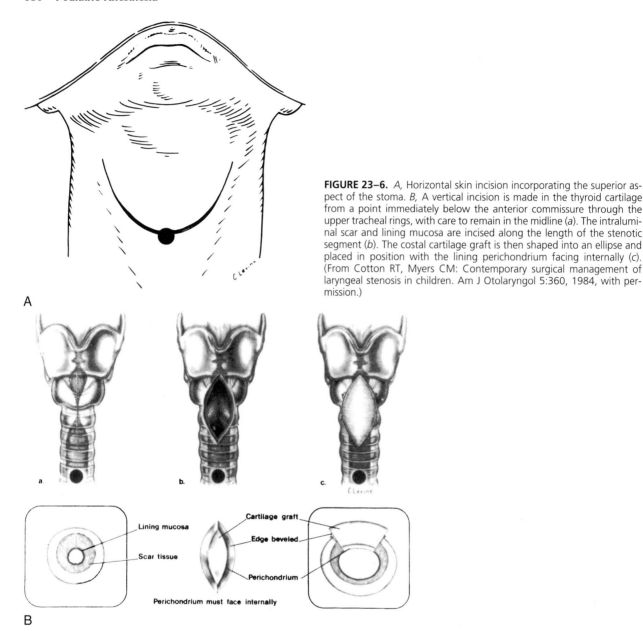

FIGURE 23–6. *A,* Horizontal skin incision incorporating the superior aspect of the stoma. *B,* A vertical incision is made in the thyroid cartilage from a point immediately below the anterior commissure through the upper tracheal rings, with care to remain in the midline (*a*). The intraluminal scar and lining mucosa are incised along the length of the stenotic segment (*b*). The costal cartilage graft is then shaped into an ellipse and placed in position with the lining perichondrium facing internally (*c*). (From Cotton RT, Myers CM: Contemporary surgical management of laryngeal stenosis in children. Am J Otolaryngol 5:360, 1984, with permission.)

children, and normal laryngotracheal growth after this procedure. Overall, a success rate in relieving the subglottic stenosis has been approximately 97 percent following this single open procedure.[137–140] Since this surgery seems to have no significant affect on the laryngeal growth of young children, this surgical treatment of subglottic stenosis may provide earlier and less traumatic decannulation from tracheotomy.

ENDOSCOPY

A common feature of both diagnostic and therapeutic endoscopic procedures is that the anesthesiologist must share the airway with the endoscopist and must provide adequate alveolar ventilation while maintaining a clear view and appropriate access for the surgeon. Regardless of whether the indication for endoscopy is diagnostic or therapeutic, most patients have some degree of compromise of either the upper or lower airway.

Some of the lesions commonly diagnosed endoscopically include laryngomalacia or tracheomalacia, vascular anomalies causing tracheobronchial compression, congenital or acquired subglottic stenosis, vocal cord palsies, papillomas, hemangiomas, cysts, granulomas, and foreign bodies.[141–143] Therapeutic bronchoscopy is used either to extract foreign bodies or to selectively aspirate thick, tenacious plugs from bronchi to resolve atelectasis, as in cystic fibrosis.[143]

Preoperative evaluation of the airway requires a careful history of the degree of airway obstruction that occurs during sleeping, crying, or feeding. Information is also required about the amount of respiratory distress (use of accessory muscles of respiration, tachypnea, and improvement following position changes or airway manipulations). Further definition of the airway problem can be obtained from chest radiographs, head and neck computed tomographic scans, magnetic resonance imaging scans, pulmonary function tests, or arterial blood gas determinations.[144, 145]

Direct Laryngoscopy

On rare occasions, mild sedation and topical anesthesia are sufficient to allow laryngoscopy in infants or older children. Most commonly, pediatric patients require general anesthesia for either laryngoscopy or any endoscopic examination of the tracheobronchial tree.

Preoperative sedatives and opiates should be given gingerly to any child with airway compromise, and then only with appropriate monitoring and by a person who is skilled in advanced airway management. Some experts recommend an antisialogue to minimize secretions.[146–148]

Sedation/anesthesia can be induced with midazolam, thiopental, propofol, or with inhaled anesthetics, usually halothane or sevoflurane, in an F_{IO_2} of 1.0. The larynx and trachea may also be anesthetized with local anesthetics (2 to 4 percent lidocaine, 3 to 5 mg/kg [total dose]). This will usually allow observation of vocal cord movement and provide adequate jaw relaxation, and satisfactory anesthesia for initial airway endoscopy.[8, 43, 146] Propofol (150 to 200 μg/kg/min) is an alternative technique that produces adequate conditions for laryngoscopy. Inhalation agents are often needed in addition. After the status of the airway is known, intermittent doses of rocuronium, rapacuronium, or vecuronium may be introduced to facilitate bronchoscopy. Because of the availability of multiple effective, safe, short-acting nondepolarizing muscle relaxants, few pediatric anesthesiologists still use succinylcholine in this setting.

Jet Ventilation: Without an Endotracheal Tube

Since the late 1960s, jet ventilation through the sidearm of a bronchoscope or directly into the trachea via a specially adapted laryngoscope has been used to ventilate the lungs of patients during endoscopy when the surgeon requires a totally unobstructed view of the upper airway. The Sanders device delivers oxygen through a 14- to 16-gauge cannula at 50 psi down an open bronchoscope. The Venturi effect created entrains sufficient gas during delivery of the jet of oxygen at high pressure to provide ventilation. The system also depends on gas escaping through an open glottis during an unobstructed expiratory phase of respiration. If expiration is obstructed, gas trapping and barotrauma can occur. Dangerously high inflation pressures may be present when the 3- and 4-mm bronchoscopes are used. Pediatric patients are less likely to have a significant gas leak around the bronchoscope, particularly very small patients, and higher inflation pressures may develop.[146] A variety of modifications of the Sanders device have been introduced, which attempt to reduce the incidence of barotrauma during endoscopy procedures while maintaining adequate ventilation.

Jet ventilation is associated with a number of complications besides barotrauma. Tumor (e.g., papilloma), blood, or tissue may be forced into the airway. To be effective, the jet ventilation laryngoscope must be aligned carefully with the glottic opening. If this does not occur, poor ventilation, inadequate oxygenation, and/or gastric dilatation may result. The system also does not allow precise control of F_{IO_2} nor does it allow measurement of end-tidal carbon dioxide, or peak or end-expiratory airway pressure. An F_{IO_2} of 1.0 is usually administered, since entrainment of air by the Venturi jet dilutes the oxygen. The volume of air entrained may be 10 to 20 times that delivered by the jet itself. Even in the era of pulse oximetry, the use of jet ventilation requires that the anesthesiologist have a clear view of the patient's chest at all times to ensure that appropriate chest wall movement occurs with each breath.

Miyasaka et al.[147] reported that in 6-month- to 3-year-old children, maximal inflation pressures and the volume of ventilation are vulnerable to small alterations in such variables as the size of the jet and the bronchoscope, the length and angle of the jet, the shape of the bronchoscope (tapered or straight), and the introduction of a suction cannula. Tidal volumes in excess of 10 ml/kg were achieved with driving pressures of 24 to 45 psi. However, the results of this study are applicable only when the Sanders No. 19 adapter is used. Any modifications should be carefully assessed.[147]

Patients with underlying pulmonary disease and poor lung or chest wall compliance are not ideal candidates for jet ventilation. Patients with abnormal airways may be particularly susceptible to barotrauma.

Total intravenous anesthesia is the usual anesthetic delivered for jet ventilation via a laryngoscope or bronchoscope. Fentanyl or alfentanil, or remifentanil in combination with propofol or thiopental, are commonly used to blunt airway reflexes. Since movement, especially, coughing, can cause severe complications, muscle relaxation is frequently employed during the procedure.

Rigid Bronchoscope

The rigid pediatric ventilating bronchoscope is equipped with an optical telescope and a fiberoptic light source (Fig. 23–7). The Hopkins rod lens optical telescope, when used with the Storz pediatric bronchoscope, gives superior resolution, magnification, and a wide-angle view.[143] Miniaturized grasping or biopsy forceps can be manipulated through the instrument channel. A closed system is maintained, which permits ventilation while the viewing telescope is in place.[143, 148] A larger foreign body forceps may be placed through the main channel of the scope if the telescope magnification is removed. A sidearm makes it possible to attach the ventilating bronchoscope to any anesthetic system to maintain anesthesia, oxygenation, and assisted or controlled manual ventilation.

The optical telescope used with these systems occupies nearly the entire internal lumen of the smaller bronchoscopes. This reduces the area for gas flow, markedly increases airflow resistance, and retards passive expiration. If passive expiration is impeded, hyperinflation and/or hypoventilation may occur.[149, 150] If intrathoracic pressure is sufficiently increased, cardiac output can be impaired, and the risk of barotrauma increases.[150] Maintaining adequate expiratory time is essential to allow complete expiration. A 2.8-mm telescope in a 3.5-mm bronchoscope allows

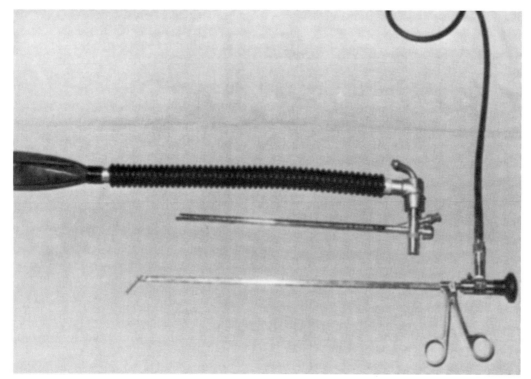

FIGURE 23–7. The 4.0 (ID) Storz ventilating bronchoscope and optical telescope with foreign body grasper. Note 1-inch nail removed from the left main-stem bronchus (nailhead peripheral) of a 3-year-old child.

adequate exhalation and prevents hyperinflation of the lungs, even during positive-pressure ventilation.[148] When using smaller scopes intermittently, the endoscopist can remove the telescope, occlude the orifice of the scope, and allow the anesthesiologist to deliver a brief period of unobstructed manual hyperventilation.[149, 150] For long bronchoscopic examinations, intermittent determinations of $Paco_2$ will confirm the adequacy of ventilation. When a 2.5-mm bronchoscope is required to evaluate the airway of small infants, the surgeons must remove the telescope more frequently to permit adequate ventilation and complete passive exhalation.

Any rapid deterioration of cardiac function during bronchoscopy should make one highly suspicious that a tension pneumothorax has developed.[151] Clinical findings of a pneumothorax alone justify thoracostomy before obtaining a chest radiograph. Vocal cord movement may be evaluated by laryngoscopy as the patient awakens from anesthesia. Care must be taken to avoid inducing laryngospasm during this time.

AIRWAY FOREIGN BODIES

Foreign Body Aspiration

In the absence of a history of trauma or infection, the onset of respiratory distress in a toddler who has no underlying airway abnormalities should raise suspicion of an acute aspiration of a foreign body. In addition, a chronic abnormality on physical examination and/or persistent abnormality on chest radiography should raise suspicion of pneumonia caused by airway obstruction induced by a foreign body. Aspiration of foreign bodies continues to be a major source of morbidity and mortality in children less than 5 years old.[156] Anesthesia and bronchoscopy to remove a foreign body from the airway of a young child also can be life threatening. Avoiding mishaps demands skill, communication, and teamwork between the endoscopist and anesthesiologist. Most reports of foreign body removal from pediatric patients include at least one death.[152–154, 157]

Nature of Aspirated Objects

Most patients who have aspirated objects have a positive history of aspiration.[154, 157] Foreign body aspiration occurs most commonly in 1- to 3-year-old toddlers, who often place small objects in their mouths and who lack molars for grinding hard food.[153, 154] Commonly inhaled objects are organic foods such as seeds, popcorn kernels, chunks of carrots, bones, and especially nuts and peanuts. Coins, toy parts, jewels, batteries, or sharp objects such as needles and pins[153, 154, 157–160] are less commoly aspirated. Aspirated partially chewed nuts often are distributed widely in the lung.[153] Peanuts, if retained for any period of time, cause mucosal irritation, edema, and a greater incidence of pneumonia distal to the bronchial obstruction than most other foreign bodies.[161] An aspirated peanut or bean softens and swells and can be easily fragmented when grasped by a forceps in the airway.[152, 161] This fragmentation may cause a child's death, if during the course of removal, the pieces occlude both main-stem bronchi and prevent ventilation.[152] A report from the Office of the Medical Examiner of Cook County, Chicago, reviewed deaths over a

10-year period from foreign body aspiration in children younger than 14 years of age. The most common cause of fatal aspiration was a toy balloon.[162] Other studies have found similar high risk of death from aspirating balloons in children older than 3 years of age.[163] As a result of their increasing prevalence in the household, aspiration of plastic objects is increasing. The American Academy of Pediatrics and a leading toy manufacturer, Mattel, have developed a radiopaque marker to place in plastic toys, which is available to all toy manufacturers.[164] Use of this marker could prevent more than 10 percent of deaths from aspiration of foreign bodies in this age group.[163]

Clinical Findings

The degree of respiratory distress following foreign body aspiration is related to the size, location, and nature of the object. Objects lodged in the larynx or trachea are associated with high mortality rates. When an object is lodged in one main bronchus or in a more distal airway, typical signs and symptoms of aspiration include choking or gagging followed by a cough, stridor, dyspnea, occasionally cyanosis, and unilateral decreased air entry or wheezing on chest auscultation.[153, 154, 157, 165–167] Signs and symptoms that eventually lead to investigation of the cause of these symptoms also include hoarseness, recurrent croup, cyanotic attacks, tachypnea, persistent cough, and hemoptysis. Laryngeal obstruction may cause aphonia.[166] In one study, 51 percent of the patients had transient symptoms at the moment of ingestion, such as retrosternal pain, cyanosis, and dysphasia.[159] The predictive value of various signs and symptoms, the clinical history, and radiographs to demonstrate the presence of a foreign body have been investigated. Only the "choking crisis" had significant sensitivity and specificity, emphasizing the critical need for obtaining a thorough history.[168]

Children usually are brought to the hospital soon after aspiration has occurred, but occasionally symptoms become worrisome to the parents days, weeks, or months after the event. In one review, 12 to 26 percent of patients had an asymptomatic period that delayed diagnosis longer than 1 week.[169] A long history of recurrent or intractable pneumonia (despite therapy) or unexplained atelectasis or emphysema should alert physicians to the possible presence of an aspirated foreign body.[152, 154, 157] Possible sequelae of this condition include massive hemoptysis, lung abscess, and bronchiectasis.[161] Other serious complications from chronically retained foreign bodies include bronchoesophageal fistula, mediastinitis, esophageal diverticulum, and lobar atelectasis. One patient died from an aortoesophageal fistula. Some chronically retained foreign bodies may require a thoracotomy for their removal.[170] In one series, six patients required lung resection to treat bronchiectasis caused by foreign bodies that had been in the bronchial tree for years.[171]

Chest Radiographs

Because many inhaled objects are radiolucent, signs of complete or partial airway obstruction are the only radiographic clues to the location of the aspirated object. When bronchial obstruction is complete, air is absorbed beyond the obstruction and atelectasis is observed on the chest radiograph.[154] Most commonly, the bronchial obstruction is partial, air can enter around the foreign body on inspiration when the bronchus dilates, but bronchial constriction occurs during expiration, and the airway is completely obstructed. The foreign body behaves as a unidirectional value.[153, 154] The radiograph demonstrates obstructive emphysema with unilateral hyperaeration, a depressed and flattened diaphragm, and shift of the mediastinum away from the affected side (Fig. 23–8).[153] Chest radiographs should be obtained during both inspiration and expiration, as the latter is more likely to demonstrate obstructive emphysema (overinflation).[155] Fluoroscopy has also been advocated to demonstrate mediastinal movement during rapid (crying) respiration[154, 157, 158], this technique is rarely utilized currently.

Commonly, chest radiographs taken following foreign body aspiration are normal, especially when they are obtained within the first 24 hours after the aspiration occurs.[153, 154, 172] For example, in one study of 293 bronchoscopies, 265 revealed foreign bodies. Of these 265 patients, 225 had a history of choking. The radiograph was normal in 110 of these patients; nine had atypical findings on chest radiography.[173] Consequently, the sensitivity and specificity of the imaging studies in identifying the presence of a foreign body in the airway were 73 percent and 45 percent, respectively.[174] Thus, a positive history plus clinical symptoms of aspiration are sufficient to justify endoscopy for diagnosis and retrieval of the foreign body. Conventional radiographic imaging should not alter the decision for surgical intervention, provided there is a well-equipped endoscopic team familiar with the care of children with airway foreign bodies.

Laryngotracheal foreign bodies (in contrast to bronchial foreign bodies) can best be diagnosed with posteroanterior and lateral neck radiographs, which reveal a subglottic density or swelling in more than 90 percent of cases. Therefore, radiographic examination of both the chest and lateral aspects of the neck should occur when a laryngeal foreign body is suspected and the patient's condition is stable.[166, 175]

Emergency or Elective Removal

The urgency to proceed with anesthesia and bronchoscopic removal of a foreign body is dictated by the severity of respiratory distress, and the location and nature of the aspirated material. Typically, objects retained in the larynx or trachea cause considerably more distress and are associated with higher mortality than objects lodged peripherally.[166, 175–177] Foreign bodies can move from one part of the airway to another and cause sudden complete airway occlusion. According to one study, the diagnosis of laryngotracheal foreign body was made within the first 24 hours of aspiration in only slightly more than one half the patients. The remaining patients were diagnosed following failure of medical management for croup or reactive airway disease, usually within 1 week of aspiration. Children diagnosed late either did not respond to therapy or their condition deteriorated despite appropriate medical therapy, which led to endoscopy for a possible laryngotracheal foreign body.[166, 175] Even in the absence of marked respira-

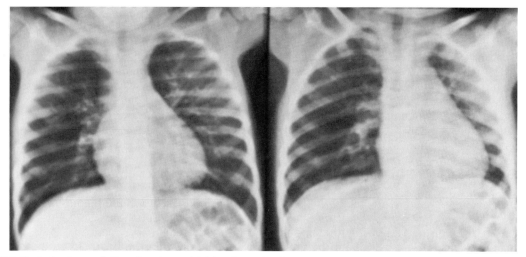

FIGURE 23–8. Inspiratory (*left*) and expiratory (*right*) radiographs of a 3-year-old child who aspirated a peanut. The expiratory film demonstrates air trapping in the right lung because the peanut acts as a check valve in the right main-stem bronchus. There is a leftward shift of the mediastinum.

tory distress, objects such as peanuts, which can fragment, or sharp objects should be aggressively removed. Similarly, objects located at precarious sites, such as the carina, demand prompt attention, even if the patient is minimally symptomatic.

Fortunately, objects retained in the upper airway that require urgent removal are relatively uncommon. However, foreign bodies located within a main-stem bronchus or more distally often require urgent removal. Ideally, the foreign body is removed very shortly after aspiration to minimize the occurrence of pneumonia or other complications. When possible, removal of the object should be done as an urgent, not emergent, procedure in a well-prepared patient.[157, 158, 161] An initial trial of bronchodilators, postural drainage, and chest physiotherapy to dislodge and expel the foreign body before attempting bronchoscopy is no longer recommended.[172]

Bronchoscopic removal of a foreign object is successful 95 to 98 percent of the time, but a small number of patients may need repeated bronchoscopies because the foreign body either was not found or it was removed incompletely.[157, 161] Rarely, thoracotomy and bronchotomy are necessary.[161, 178]

Foreign Body Removal: Anesthetic Management

The general principles of anesthetic management of pediatric patients for bronchoscopy/laryngoscopy are applicable for bronchoscopic removal of a foreign body. The anesthesiologist must be prepared to promptly treat total airway obstruction. Ventilation and oxygenation must be ensured and a depth of anesthesia must be maintained that allows bronchoscopy without coughing, laryngospasm, or uncontrolled dislodging of the foreign body. Sedation/premedication may be indicated to treat or to prevent agitation, but only after oxygenation is normal. Even when the oxygenation is adequate, treating agitation with sedation should be done cautiously and only when oxygenation is monitored with pulse oximetry. There must be

a clear plan of action for treatment of airway obstruction (i.e., equipment, drugs, and personnel immediately available). The anesthesiologist must determine if parental presence during the induction of anesthesia will be beneficial. In some cases, the presence of parents is an excellent alternative to sedation.

Virtually every aspect of anesthetizing children for removal of an airway foreign body is controversial. Arguments for and against inhalation induction, intravenous induction, spontaneous ventilation, controlled ventilation, and the use and avoidance of muscle relaxation have been made repeatedly. After careful assessment of the patient, an anesthetic plan can be developed with backup plans if a "surprise" occurs. An inhalation induction allows the anesthesiologist to avoid positive-pressure ventilation and the possibility of moving the foreign body. However, if the child has a "full stomach," spontaneous ventilation offers little protection from aspiration of gastric contents. Few anesthesiologists would advocate a rapid sequence induction of anesthesia in an infant if there is respiratory distress and no absolute delineation of the current location of a foreign body. Most would follow a "middle course," allowing a child to breathe oxygen and a potent inhaled anesthetic until it can be established that gentle positive-pressure ventilation adequately expands the chest. At that point, the decision about muscle relaxation can be made. If the decision is made to avoid muscle relaxants, a deep level of anesthesia is required to permit bronchoscopy without coughing. The addition of topical anesthesia is advantageous.

Ideally, spontaneous ventilation should be preserved, at least until the nature and location of the foreign body have been identified by bronchoscopy,[152, 154] particularly if the object could not be localized radiographically. Even if the position of the foreign body was determined radiographically, the anesthesiologist must always be aware that the position of the foreign body may change.

A child admitted with a history of aspirating a foreign body and signs of severe inspiratory and expiratory obstruction should continuously breathe 100 percent oxygen. A person skilled in advanced airway management should be with the child at all times and the child should be taken directly to the operating room for removal of the foreign body.[154, 161] The use of nitrous oxide in such patients is contraindicated in most cases because it reduces the F_{IO_2}. Also, if significant air trapping is present, nitrous oxide could increase the gas volume and pressure in the affected lung. Rapid bronchoscopy usually allows rapid removal of the foreign body. On occasion, the bronchoscope may dislodge a tracheal foreign body and push it peripherally into a main-stem bronchus with improvement in ventilation and relief of the immediate crisis.[143, 176]

If the child has aspirated vegetable matter, it may be fragmented during removal. Therefore, the endoscopist should consider working with the patient in the lateral position, affected side down. If this is not possible, thoracotomy instruments and a surgeon skilled in pediatric thoracic surgery should be immediately available, because a fragmented object may acutely occlude both main-stem bronchi.[152] A Fogarty No. 3 embolectomy balloon catheter may help dislodge impacted foreign bodies.[143, 158]

Occasionally, the size of the foreign body exceeds the internal diameter (ID) of the bronchoscope. When this occurs, the foreign body, the forceps, and bronchoscope must be removed together through immobile vocal cords.[158] Administering a small dose of a short-acting nondepolarizing muscle relaxant allows adequate, brief relaxation to permit removal of the bronchoscope and foreign body. If the foreign body is lost during its attempted removal, the pharynx should be immediately inspected. If the object is not found, the bronchoscope should be reintroduced, and the larynx or trachea reexamined. If tracheal obstruction occurs and the object cannot be immediately removed, it may be necessary to push the object back to its original location to allow ventilation of the lungs. If possible, the foreign body should be returned to the affected lung and not to the unaffected lung because placing it in the unaffected lung could result in unreliable ventilation of either lung.[152] Following removal of the foreign body, the endoscopist must reexamine the airway to look for additional multiple or fragmented foreign bodies and to remove secretions that are distal to the obstruction.

The bronchoscope often must be reinserted several times before the foreign body and secretions are successfully removed. This may produce mucosal edema and respiratory distress after bronchoscopy. Administration of steroids, humidified oxygen, nebulized racemic epinephrine and, rarely, tracheal reintubation for 1 or 2 days may be required until the edema subsides.[179–181] Initial doses of 0.5 to 1.5 mg/kg of dexamethasone (and smaller doses for 2 to 3 days) may minimize the subglottic swelling caused by repeated insertion of the bronchoscope.[179] Racemic epinephrine (2.25 percent) may be given in a 1:6 to 1:10 dilution through a nebulizer and clear plastic face mask for 10-minute periods while monitoring the electrocardiogram (ECG). Treatment is repeated as necessary every 2 hours.[180] Some patients treated with recemic epinephrine develop "rebound" edema. Patients who respond to recemic epinephrine should be monitored carefully for at least 3 to 4 hours after each dose of the drug to determine if "rebound" edema occurs.

Although prompt removal of a foreign body through an open rigid bronchoscope is the mainstay of treatment for removal of a tracheal foreign body, diagnostic flexible bronchoscopy also may have a role.[182–184] Flexible bronchoscopy is not recommended when respiratory distress is present. If a foreign body aspiration is clearly evident by history, physical examinations, and radiography, most physicians would proceed to a rigid bronchoscopic examination of the airway. If the patient's condition is stable and the evidence of a foreign body aspiration less clear, some people suggest that diagnostic flexible bronchoscopy under local anesthesia and sedation is less traumatic to the patient and his or her airway.[183] If a foreign body is identified, the patient then must undergo a rigid bronchoscopy. The decision to utilize fiberoptic bronchoscopy for diagnostic evaluation for foreign body aspiration depends on the skills and services available at each medical center. The risks of possibly having to undergo two procedures should be carefully considered.

Endotracheal intubation and airway protection should precede foreign body extraction from the esophagus. Accidentally dropping an esophageal foreign body into an unprotected larynx can cause a disaster.[175] Endoscopic removal of foreign bodies from the upper gastrointestinal inlet is successful in greater than 98 percent of cases.[184] Frequently, foreign bodies in the small and large intestine pass through the gastrointestinal tract spontaneously. Surgical intervention is rarely needed.[185] As with chronic airway foreign bodies, retained esophageal foreign bodies can be treacherous. Complications include bronchoesophageal fistula, aortoesophageal fistula, mediastinitis, esophageal diverticulum, and lobar atelectasis. These retained foreign bodies may require a thoracotomy to remove them.[170]

LASER MICROLARYNGEAL SURGERY

Lasers

Development of fiberoptic instrumentation, the operating microscope, and the carbon dioxide laser has provided a precise method for surgical excision and ablation of tissue.[186] Laser light energy can be aimed, calibrated, and used as a surgical tool.[187] The CO_2 laser's light waves are absorbed by all biologic tissues and rapidly vaporize intracellular water.[188] The energy is rapidly dissipated in tissues with a high water content. The surrounding tissue is unaffected. Because the radiation is absorbed, injury to the eyes is limited to the cornea. The CO_2 laser has been used with excellent results for treating such lesions as papillomas of the nose, oral cavity, or larynx; subglottic stenosis; subglottic hemangioma; glottic webs; choanal atresia; postintubation granuloma; vocal cord nodules; and lymphangiomas.[186, 189] Advantages of the CO_2 laser for surgery of the small pediatric airway include excellent hemostasis, minimal postoperative edema and scarring (tracheostomy is rarely needed), and rapid healing and preservation of voice quality.[186, 190] This form of therapy is applicable to patients of all ages, including neonates, as long as the patient can tolerate a general anesthetic.[190] The precision of this instrument is such that lesions as small as 2 mm can be accurately treated through a binocular microscope.

The argon and the ruby laser are primarily used in ophthalmologic surgery. The argon laser also has applications in plastic and dermatologic surgery. The neodymium:yttrium-aluminum-garnet (Nd:YAG) laser is used to treat gastrointestinal bleeding and to excise endobronchial lesions. The disadvantage of this instrument, compared to the CO_2 laser, is that tissue penetration is less controllable.

Safety Precautions

To prevent thermal injury to the cornea or retina from the laser beam, the operating room personnel must wear glasses and the patient's eyes must be protected with moist gauze pads or protective goggles.[186, 190] Although the CO_2 laser does not penetrate the cornea, emissions from the Nd:YAG and argon lasers can do so. In fact, the argon beam can penetrate the cornea and lens, and cause severe retinal injury. Since the Nd:YAG and the argon lasers penetrate glass, operating rooms with windows should cover glass surfaces with an appropriate material.

Areas of healthy tissue that might come in contact with the laser beam should be covered with wet sponges to effectively absorb the laser energy. Vital structures some distance from the operative site can be injured by overshoot of the laser beam or by reflection of the beam off of a polished instrument. This caused tracheal laceration in a child undergoing resection of recurrent laryngeal papillomas. The tracheal tear became evident in the recovery room as bilateral pneumothoraces and subcutaneous emphysema. Constant vigilance by recovery room nurses is important to observe and detect laser-induced pneumothoraces.[191]

Both paper and cloth drapes are combustible. Therefore, minimal draping is important when lasers are used. Severe burns to patients have occurred and, because the burning of disposable drapes produce profuse smoke, inhalation injury can also occur to the patient and to operating room staff.[192] People operating the laser should be constantly aware that the laser beam can reflect off polished, shiny surfaces. Any instrument off which the beam is reflected can become hot and burn tissue that comes in contact with the hot instrument. The laser should be maintained in the "pulse" mode to minimize the energy emitted.

Unfortunately, latex, rubber, silicone, and plastic endotracheal tubes also can absorb CO_2 laser energy and ignite.[190, 192–194] Wrapping the endotracheal tube in aluminum foil tape causes the laser beam to be deflected off the metal. This protects the endotracheal tube from thermal damage. Various metallic tapes have been evaluated. Venture copper foil tape and 3M No. 425 aluminum tape are both protective, whereas the Radio Shack tape No. 44-1155 and 3M tape No. 1430 and 433 do not protect the endotracheal tube.[195] Similar results were obtained when the Nd:YAG laser was tested using the same brands of tape. Other protective devices have been introduced to reduce the risk of combustion in the airway during laser surgery. Laser-Guard (Merocel, Mystic, CT) is a protective coating that provides an effective barrier to laser energy.[196]

The foil is covered with a moist sponge layer that absorbs any heat generated. This outside sponge layer also provides a smooth surface that minimizes trauma to the airway. Although the shafts of the endotracheal tube can be covered with protective material, the endotracheal tube cuff is vulnerable to the effects of laser radiation. Filling the cuff with saline rather than air is recommended. Deflation of a saline-filled cuff took longer after perforation and the incidence of combustion was less, when subjected to 40 w from a carbon dioxide laser.[197] These same investigators recommend positioning saline-soaked pledgets above the endotracheal tube cuff during laser surgery.

In addition to the risk for combustion, foil-wrapped tubes may kink, irritate the tracheal mucosa, obstruct the airway if the foil separates from the tube and, on occasion, permit the laser beam to penetrate and ignite unprotected portions of the tube.[189, 190, 195, 198]

The mixture of gases delivered into the endotracheal tube may affect the risk for combustion during general anesthesia and laser surgery of the airway. For example, halothane (2 percent) plus 40 percent oxygen and 60 percent helium decreased the time to ignition of polyvinyl chloride endotracheal tubes by carbon dioxide laser radiation from 43 ± 5.4 seconds to 25.3 ± 1.9 seconds.[199] When compared with red rubber, silicone, and Xomed Laser-Shield I (Xomed, Jacksonville, FL) endotracheal tubes, polyvinyl chloride tubes had a higher index of flammability. Although helium impedes combustion during carbon dioxide laser surgery, the differences between nitrogen and helium on combustibility are not clinically, significant.[200] In a previous study, nitrous oxide and oxygen were shown to be additive in their ability to sustain combustion.[201]

The Xomed Laser-Shield I endotracheal tube (Xomed-Treace, Jacksonville, FL) is a silicone rubber tube that was designed for use with a carbon dioxide laser in the pulse-only mode. However, laboratory studies demonstrated that this endotracheal tube is combustible and provides no advantages over appropriately wrapped polyvinyl endotracheal tubes when a high-energy carbon dioxide laser energy was used. Sosis noted that when carbon dioxide laser radiation was directed perpendicularly to the shaft of the tube, a fire started immediately, and the tube disintegrated within 3 seconds. The fire was difficult to extinguish.[202] Similarly, the Bivona (Gary, IN) laser endotracheal tube is significantly combustible and has a blowtorch response to the high-energy output of a CO_2 laser. In contrast, the Mallinckrodt Laser-Flex (Glens Falls, NY) endotracheal tube, with a stainless steel shaft, offered considerable protection from combustion when direct laser energy was applied. During prolonged exposure to high-energy output from a CO_2 laser (35 w, beam diameter of 0.6 mm), continuous mode, one of five of these tubes demonstrated blowtorch combustion. In the presence of human blood, Mallinckrodt Laser-Flex tubes ignited. The manufacturer recommends inflating the cuff with saline. In adolescents, a foil-wrapped long 4-mm ID endotracheal tube that has been fitted with a standard size cuff can be used.[203]

Venturi ventilation can be used during laryngoscopic procedures by securing an injection needle to a straight blade laryngoscope.[9, 204] While observing chest expansion, oxygen or an oxygen/air mixture is intermittently forced through a needle by high pressure (50 psi). This entrains room air. Intravenous anesthetics and muscle relaxants are used to provide anesthesia. The Venturi ventilation technique allows adequate ventilation and oxygenation while providing an unobstructed view for the endoscopist by eliminating the endotracheal tube.[9, 204] There is a potential for barotrauma if exhalation becomes obstructed (see sections "Laryngeal Papillomas," below and "Jet Ventilation," above).[190]

In an effort to improve existing Venturi jet techniques, Brooker et al. developed a subglotic ventilation anesthesia system.[205] The Hunsaker Mon-Jet tube is a laser-safe subglottic jet tube that allows monitoring of tracheal pressure and end-tidal CO_2. The device aligns the jet away from the tracheal mucosa to prevent injecting gas into the submucosa. The device also uses an automatic jet ventilator with an adjustable rate, inspiratory to expiratory (I:E) ratio, and flow rate. Peak inspiratory and peak end-expiratory airway pressure are monitored. If the limits are exceeded, the device shuts off.

All the above methods—wrapped tubes, metal tubes, insufflation without a tube, or jet ventilation—are intended to decrease the hazard of fire, but each method has its own set of problems. If, despite all precautions, ignition of the endotracheal tube should occur, immediately discontinue the flow of oxygen and disconnect the endotracheal tube from the gas source. Most materials do not readily burn in air.[190] The endotracheal tube must be removed immediately. Therefore, the anesthesiologist must have direct access to the tube at all times. Ensure that the entire tube has been removed from the airway. A chest radiograph should be obtained and bronchoscopy should be performed to reveal the extent of the injury to the lung and trachea caused by direct burn, smoke inhalation, or retention of a foreign body. Complications are treated according to the severity of the injury and may include steroids, humidification of inspired gases, tracheostomy, and assisted ventilation. Tracheal stenosis can be a late complication.[190]

Surgical Requirements

Surgical requirements for suspension laryngoscopy include hyperextension of the neck and a motionless surgical field (i.e., relaxed vocal cords) so that the lesion may be ablated without injury to the surrounding healthy tissue.[188] There must be rapid recovery of consciousness and protective airway reflexes at the conclusion of surgery.

Laryngeal Papillomas

The CO_2 laser is most frequently used to ablate laryngeal papillomas, the most common benign tumor of the pediatric larynx. Treatment of this disease, and its distal extension, also have been treated with argon plasma coagulation technique (APC).[206] With APC, carbonization and vaporization are minimal. Laser resection is not a cure; the virus-induced warty lesions reappear at the glottis or any portion of the airway. Consequently, many operative resections are often necessary to maintain a patent airway. Children with laryngeal papillomas present initially with a history of hoarseness, which may progress to aphonia and respiratory distress. Severe obstruction by vocal cord and supraglottic growths may cause chronic airway obstruction. However, the clinical course of children with recurrent respiratory papillomatosis varies.

Most children are infected with human papilloma virus type 6 or 11. In some series, herpes simplex virus type II (HSV-II) infection is associated with aggressive disease that requires tracheostomy.[207] In this series, tracheostomy was not associated with poor prognosis; the tracheas of eight of the nine children were eventually decannulated.

In the past, tracheostomy was viewed as a treacherous undertaking because it was thought to cause seeding of the papillomas or to predispose the tracheobronchial tree to spread of the lesions.[32] However, experience at Children's Hospital of Pittsburgh differs with this philosophy. Thirteen of 35 patients with more widespread disease treated between 1984 and 1994 underwent tracheostomy placement. Although spread of the disease did occur, it was limited to the tracheostomy site. Complications from the tracheostomy were rare. It was concluded that tracheostomy is life-saving for these patients and is not associated with increased morbidity from spread of the disease into the distal airway.[208]

Early anecdotal studies indicated that interferon therapy might be beneficial for treatment of laryngeal papillomas, but long-term follow-up is required.[204] The only effective way to keep the airway free of papillomas is by repeated endoscopic and laser excision of the papillomas until puberty, when they tend to regress.[209] Laser microsurgery is associated with increased risk for anesthesia complications (15 percent) in pediatric patients. This is especially true when the laryngotracheal disease is extensive, the children are less than 3 years of age, and they have laryngeal papillomatosis and do not have a tracheostomy.[210]

Children who have undergone multiple surgeries for laryngeal papillomas may be very apprehensive and anxious.[187] Judicious use of sedatives and, most importantly, a reassuring preoperative visit by the anesthesiologist helps to allay fears. A child with significant airway obstruction should only receive preoperative sedation while being monitored and when oxygen, positive-pressure ventilation, and suction are available. An anesthesiologist or other person skilled in advanced airway intervention must be present at all times.

Anesthesia may be induced either by inhalation or by small IV doses of thiopental or propofol. Spontaneous ventilation should be maintained until the extent of airway obstruction is known.[32, 187] A partially obstructed airway may become completely obstructed with the onset of anesthesia, and positive-pressure ventilation may be impossible, even when spontaneous ventilation was adequate before anesthesia began.[211] It is often helpful to maintain 5 to 10 cm of positive end-expiratory pressure in the anesthetic system to distend the hypopharynx and to facilitate mask ventilation. Muscle relaxants should be used only after positive-pressure ventilation by mask is possible. When there is significant obstruction, it may be preferable to intubate the trachea after inducing anesthesia with halothane or sevoflurane in oxygen. Difficulty ventilating the lungs after intubating the trachea may occur if a papilloma is released into the trachea or obstructs the endotracheal tube.

After the airway has been secured with a small endotracheal tube, immobility of the airway and vocal cords for

TABLE 23 – 3
COMMONLY USED OPHTHALMOLOGIC DRUGS AND THE ANESTHETIC EFFECT

Drug	mg/drop	Ophthalmologic Effect	Anesthetic Implication
Atropine (1%)	0.5	Mydriasis Cycloplegia	Tachycardia, flushing
Cocaine (1%)	0.5	Vasoconstriction	Hypertension, dysrhythmia, hyperthermia
Cyclopentolate (1%)	0.5	Mydriasis Cycloplegia	Not common Convulsions
Echothiophate (0.25%)	0.1	Antiglaucoma	Anticholinesterase, long acting
Epinephrine (0.25%)	0.1	Antiglaucoma	Hypertension, dysrhythmias
Phenylephrine (2.5%)	1.2	Mydriasis Vasoconstriction Decongestion	Hypertension
Scopolamine (0.5%)	0.25	Mydriasis Cycloplegia	CNS excitement
Timolol (0.25%)	0.1	Antiglaucoma	β-Blockade, nonselective

the laser surgery can be ensured with deep inhalation anesthesia, intravenous narcotics, or an intravenous infusion of propofol, with or without nondepolarizing muscle relaxants.

EYE SURGERY

Providing appropriate anesthesia care for pediatric patients during eye surgery requires a basic understanding of intraocular pressure and its control, pharmacology of drugs used by the ophthalmologist, and the potential for drug interactions with anesthetics (Table 23–3). Also, the anesthesiologist must be aware that several medical problems are associated with congenital and acquired eye anomalies and pathology and that many anesthetic drugs and procedures have profound effects on ocular physiology.

Intraocular Pressure and its Control

Both the anterior and the posterior chambers of the eye are filled with aqueous humor. Two thirds of the aqueous humor is produced in the posterior chamber by active secretion, filtration, and diffusion from the blood supply to ciliary body (Fig. 23–9). The aqueous humor passes from the ciliary body behind the iris to the front of the lens, then through the pupil into the anterior chamber (Fig. 23–10). The most lateral portion of the anterior chamber, called the angle, contains a meshwork of tissue that filters the aqueous humor before it reaches the canal of Schlemm and eventually drains into the episcleral veins (Fig. 23–10). Aqueous humor is considered to be the "blood supply" for the lens and cornea, which are avascular. This fluid contains no blood cells and only 1 percent of the concentration of protein found in plasma. Thus, the aqueous humor is clear and allows transmission of light to the retina.[212]

Normal intraocular pressure (IOP) is maintained between 10 and 21 mm Hg by a balance between the production and drainage of aqueous humor. Interestingly, IOP is higher than intracranial and mean venous pressure and is necessary to maintain normal refractive function of the cornea and its stroma.[213] A sudden increase in intraocular pressure can precipitate acute glaucoma and damage vision. If the globe is open, an increase in intraocular pressure can cause the vitreous to be extruded, the lens to prolapse, and/or hemorrhage from blood vessels. Thus,

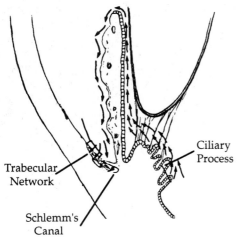

FIGURE 23–9. Magnified view of the ciliary body showing aqueous humor production and flow pattern.

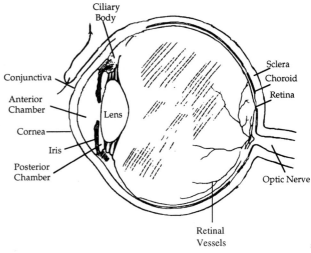

FIGURE 23–10. Anatomy of the anterior chamber of the eye.

the anesthesiologist must attempt to prevent changes in IOP during surgery.

Intraocular pressure increases dramatically during coughing, vomiting, and straining. During these events, the pressure may rise as high as 40 mm Hg. Laryngoscopy and intubation of the trachea also can increase intraocular pressure.[214] Although this effect of laryngoscopy is transient and of no serious consequence in the patient with normal intraocular physiology, these increases in pressure may be very significant for patients with glaucoma or other eye pathology. Extraocular events (e.g., extraocular muscle contracture after succinylcholine administration or orbicularis muscle contraction) also may increase intraocular pressure. Nondepolarizing muscle relaxants, on the other hand, decrease pressure on the globe and may decrease intraocular pressure.

Several metabolic or acid–base derangements may occur during general anesthesia and can affect intraocular pressure. Hypoxia and hypercarbia cause retinal venodilatation and can increase intraocular pressure.[215] Mild hypo- or hypercarbia produce clinically insignificant effects.[216] Hypothermia decreases intraocular pressure by decreasing the rate of aqueous humor production. Arterial pressure changes have little effect on intraocular pressure.[217] Venous hypertension (e.g., during coughing), however, can have dramatic effects on the intraocular pressure because venous hypertension increases the intraocular blood volume.

Intraocular Pressure and Anesthetics

Most CNS depressants, such as barbiturates, narcotics, sedatives, and inhalation and neuroleptic anesthetics decrease intraocular pressure. All these agents are appropriate for pre- and intraoperative use. Providing a deep plane of anesthesia before intubating the trachea is essential in patients with high intraocular pressure and in patients with an "open eye" (see below). Retrobulbar block also effectively decreases intraocular pressure. The head-up position (even slight), osmotic diuretics, and carbonic anhydrase inhibitors, such as acetazolamide (Diamox), can also decrease intraocular pressure.

Ketamine's effects on intraocular pressure are controversial. Corssen and Hoy[218] reported that ketamine increased intraocular pressure, even when the depth of anesthesia was adequate. In unpremedicated children the increase in pressure may last 30 minutes following a 5-mg/kg dose of ketamine intramuscularly.[219] Intraocular pressure was determined by Schiotz tonometry, which measures corneal compressibility. Subsequent studies in both adults[220] and children[221] reported that ketamine does not increase intraocular pressure. In these studies, intraocular pressure was measured by "applantation tonometry," a method that is believed to more accurately measure intraocular pressure. Because of its possible detrimental effects on intraocular pressure and because it causes nystagmus and blepharospasm, ketamine probably has little place in the current practice of pediatric anesthesia for eye surgery.

Intraocular Pressure and Neuromuscular Blockers

Nondepolarizing muscle relaxants do not increase and may decrease intraocular pressure.[222] Succinylcholine, a depolarizing muscle relaxant, raises intraocular pressure about 7 mm Hg in normal eyes.[223] This modest increase is transient and of little consequence to normal eyes. However, if a patient has high intraocular pressure, the increase in intraocular pressure following succinylcholine may be greater. Any rise may be significant. In the case of an open globe, an increase in pressure could result in loss of vitreous humor. No technique has been identified that prevents ocular hypertension after the administration of succinylcholine. Some investigators have reported that small doses of nondepolarizing agents given before a paralyzing dose of succinylcholine prevent the rise in intraocular pressure.[224] Other investigators have claimed that pretreatment is not effective.[225] The method of measuring pressure may partly explain these differences (i.e., indentation[224] vs. applantation[225]). Until the controversy is settled, succinylcholine probably should not be used during intraocular surgery. Currently, the large number of nondepolarizing agents available allow other options for paralyzing patients with a penetrating eye injury (i.e., "open eye") and a "full stomach."

Anesthesia: "Full Stomach" and "Open Eye"

Traumatic eye injury occurs commonly in children. The best chance to salvage the eye requires that the wound be surgically explored to remove foreign material and the laceration closed within several hours of the injury. After penetrating trauma, the pressure inside the eye is atmospheric. External pressure on the eye or an increase in internal pressure can prolapse the lens, iris, or vitreous and markedly reduce the chance of recovery of vision. The goal preoperatively and during the induction of anesthesia is to prevent coughing, crying, and vomiting because these activities increase intraocular venous blood volume. Increasing intraocular venous blood volume and intraocular pressure may cause the ocular contents to extrude.

Preventing an increase in intraocular pressure is important, but difficult to accomplish. Preoperatively, the child should remain flat and quiet, and the eyes should be patched to minimize eye movements (which can be scary and confusing to young children). Sedating the child before patching the eyes is essential if the child is too young to cooperate and cannot understand a careful, gentle explanation of the procedure. Giving a young child pentobarbital (4 to 5 mg/kg, maximum 120 mg), diazepam (0.2 mg/kg), or midazolam (0.5 to 0.75 mg/kg) orally may provide sufficient sedation to allow insertion of an IV catheter. After the sedative has been given, EMLA (eutectic mixture of local anesthetics) cream should be applied to several sites where veins are visible (or likely to be present); the EMLA is covered with an occlusive dressing, such as Tegaderm. Forty-five to 60 minutes later, the skin should be numb enough to allow painless insertion of an IV catheter. Once an IV catheter is in place, titrating subsequent doses of sedatives is simplified.

After the IV catheter is in place, a rapid sequence induction of anesthesia can be easily accomplished. The anesthesiologist should assume that all children who present with a penetrating eye injury have a full stomach. After trauma, stomach emptying is so erratic and unpredictable that delaying surgery for 6 to 8 hours does not decrease reliably the risk of aspirating gastric contents. Tracheal intubation should not be attempted until paralysis is complete. This prevents coughing and its potentially catastrophic effect on intraocular pressure.

In the presence of an open eye, the anesthesiologist must carefully preoxygenate the patient while being meticulous not to allow the mask to press on the injured eye. Preoxygenation is followed by injection of an anesthetic and a nondepolarizing muscle relaxant into a rapidly flowing IV catheter, preferably directly into an injection port at the site of the catheter. Some anesthesiologists give a dose of lidocaine (2 mg/kg),[256] fentanyl (2 to 3 μg/kg), or morphine sulfate (0.05 to 0.1 mg/kg) before administering thiopental (4 to 6 mg/kg) or propofol (2 mg/kg), to minimize the effects of laryngoscopy and intubation on intraocular pressure. Administration of the anesthetic is immediately followed by a dose of a nondepolarizing muscle relaxant (pancuronium [0.1 mg/kg], vecuronium [0.15 to 0.2 mg/kg], rocuronium [0.8 to 1.5 mg/kg], or rapacuronium [1.2 to 2.0 mg/kg]). These doses of muscle relaxants allow tracheal intubation to be accomplished within 45 to 60 seconds. The newer, nondepolarizing agents may cause a slightly quicker onset of paralysis, compared with pancuronium and vecuronium.[227] Rocuronium (0.8 to 1.5 mg/kg) offers advantages over atracurium and succinylcholine because rocuronium provides rapid onset of neuromuscular blockade and a decrease in intraocular pressure without side effects. Rapacuronium also is an excellent choice to provide complete neuromuscular blockade rapidly.

Neuromuscular blockade should be monitored during the induction of anesthesia to ensure that paralysis is complete before laryngoscopy is attempted. Sufficient cricoid pressures should be applied to occlude the esophagus and prevent passive regurgitation of stomach contents into the lungs. Cricoid pressure should be maintained until the airway is secured. The application of cricoid pressure also may decrease the likelihood of stomach dilation if gentle positive-pressure ventilation is required before the trachea is intubated.

If a child has an open eye and a full stomach, inserting an IV catheter after administration of oral sedation and numbing the skin with local anesthesia allows rapid sequence induction of anesthesia. However, for the normal, chubby toddler who has no visible veins, the risk of crying, struggling, and raising intraocular pressure while an IV catheter is being inserted may be a greater risk than the risk of aspiration during induction of anesthesia with inhaled anesthetics and cricoid pressure. Such a toddler could benefit from oral premedication or from a rectally administered barbiturate. Intranasal midazolam may cause crying and agitation and, therefore, should be avoided in this setting.

Anesthesia for Specific Ophthalmologic Procedures

Strabismus

Malalignment of the visual axes, *strabismus,* can be congenital or acquired. The congenital or infantile type is probably caused by an abnormality of innervation. The incidence of strabismus in patients with meningomyeloceles, traumatic cranial nerve palsies, and congenital myopathy is high. Infantile strabismus virtually always requires surgery. The outcome of this surgery is excellent when the surgery occurs early in life.

The primary considerations for anesthesiologists caring for children having strabismus surgery are cardiovascular effects of medications placed in the eye, the oculocardiac reflex, malignant hyperthermia, and postoperative nausea.

Phenylephrine is placed in the eye(s) to produce mydriasis and hemostasis. However, absorption of the phenylephrine can cause profound systemic vasoconstriction and hypertension. To prevent systemic hypertension, only 1.0 to 2.5 percent (not 10 percent) phenylephrine should be used and only one drop should be put into each eye.[228, 229] Other agents (0.5 percent cyclopentolate, 0.5 percent tropicamide) can be used to induce mydriasis without causing hypertension.

Surgery for strabismus often requires traction on the extraocular muscles, which produces vagal stimulation via the trigeminal-vagal reflex. The most common effect of vagal stimulation is sinus bradycardia. Junctional rhythm, ectopic atrial rhythm, bigeminy, multifocal premature ventricular contractions, and ventricular tachycardia have been reported.[230] Stimulation of the oculocardiac reflex seems to be related to the degree of tension applied to the muscle[230] and can usually be prevented by a delicate surgical technique. The heart rate increases rapidly when tension on the muscle decreases. Treatment of the bradycardia depends on the severity and the underlying condition of the patient. If the cardiovascular effect is minimal and transient, observation alone is sufficient. The changes in rhythm may decrease during the surgery, since the reflex may fatigue or diminish with continued intermittent traction. If the patient has underlying cyanotic congenital heart disease, a rhythm disturbance such as bradycardia may cause severe hemodynamic effects that require treatment. In the absence of significant cardiovascular compromise, atropine is an appropriate therapy. Epinephrine is the appropriate treatment for cardiovascular collapse. Lidocaine may be indicated for the treatment of ventricular dysrhythmias. A retrobulbar block may prevent the oculocardiac reflex by blocking the afferent limb of the trigeminal-vagal reflex.

The LMA provides an alternative to endotracheal intubation in normal children scheduled for elective strabismus surgery.[231] In the absence of gastroesophageal reflux, an LMA provides an excellent airway for patients who can sustain spontaneous ventilation for the duration of eye muscle surgery.

Strabismus and Malignant Hyperthermia

Malignant hyperthermia is a genetic disease[232–238] of muscle that is often triggered by surgery and anesthesia. The molecular biology of this disease is complicated and much remains to be clearly defined, especially in the context of the characteristics of the disease among various populations. Often the result is a fulminant and life-threatening hypermetabolic state[239] (see Chapter 4). Patients who are susceptible to malignant hyperthermia have a generalized muscle disorder. Consequently, it is not surprising that patients undergoing ptosis or strabismus surgery have a higher incidence of malignant hyperthermia.[239] Other generalized muscle diseases with a strong association with malignant hyperthermia include myotonia congenita, Duchenne's muscular dystrophy, central core disease, and arthrogryposis. Some investigators claim that patients who have osteogenesis imperfecta also have a higher than usual incidence of malignant hyperthermia.

Occult myopathies have been linked to episodes of cardiac arrest. In one report, 25 apparently healthy children (age <18) had a cardiac arrest within 24 hours of surgery.[240] Of these 25, 92 percent were scheduled for minor surgery and had been anesthetized with an inhalation anesthetic. Seventy-two percent of these children received succinylcholine. Hyperkalemia was detected in 72 percent of patients in whom it was measured (13 of 18) at the time of the cardiac arrest. Previously unrecognized Duchenne's or other muscular dystrophy was diagnosed in 48 percent of these patients. Similarly, another report describes two apparently healthy boys who developed rhabdomyolysis after a general anesthetic that included succinylcholine.[241] One child was subsequently diagnosed with Becker's dystrophy. The authors noted that 74 percent of 66 other cases of anesthesia-induced rhabdomyolysis were related to unrecognized congenital muscle disorders, and 21 percent occurred in children susceptible to malignant hyperthermia. Succinylcholine had been used in 43 of these 66 patients.[240, 241] The molecular and cellular link between myopathy and malignant hyperthermia has not been clearly defined, but the significance of occult myopathy, particularly in male children, and the increased risk for malignant hyperthermia should be considered in patients undergoing strabismus surgery.[239]

Approximately 30 percent of malignant hyperthermia cases occur during a second or third general anesthetic. Therefore, a negative history of prior problems does not negate a patient's susceptibility for developing malignant hyperthermia. In the Danish Malignant Hyperthermia Register, of 127 patients with clinical evidence of malignant hyperthermia, 37 percent had received a prior anesthetic that included trigger agents (inhaled agents and/or succinylcholine) without developing malignant hyperthermia.[242] A positive family history for malignant hyperthermia should be specifically sought, when evaluating all patients preoperatively.

Clinically, malignant hyperthermia can present in several forms.[243] The classic disease occurs intraoperatively and results in a rapid rise in temperature, muscle rigidity, dysrhythmias, rhabdomyolysis, acidosis, and hyperkalemia. However, some patients develop an unexplained tachycardia; temperature elevation is a late sign of malignant hyperthermia in these patients. Approximately one half of patients who develop masseter muscle rigidity following succinylcholine are susceptible to malignant hyperthermia by the muscle biopsy contracture test. If masseter muscle spasm occurs after succinylcholine, it is important to obtain a creatine phosphokinase (CPK) level. If the concentration of CPK exceeds 20,000 IU, malignant hyperthermia susceptibility is strongly suggested.[244] If masseter spasm occurs, a muscle biopsy and contracture test is indicated.

Agents that can trigger malignant hyperthermia include depolarizing muscle relaxants and all potent inhaled anesthetics, including desflurane.[245] Both amide and ester local anesthetics are nontriggering. General anesthesia can be safely provided for malignant hyperthermia–susceptible patients with barbiturates, narcotics, nitrous oxide, and nondepolarizing muscle relaxants. However, there are a few reports of jaw rigidity after use of a nondepolarizing muscle relaxant.[246] Two of the three patients reported were nonsusceptible and the third was susceptible to malignant hyperthermia when tested by standard methods.

Although there is less experience with propofol, this agent appears to be a nontriggering anesthetic.[247] Propofol does not activate calcium efflux via channels of the ryandidine receptor,[248] a well-described effect of inhalation agents in malignant hyperthermia–susceptible swine.[249] Propofol has not triggered malignant hyperthermia in patients who were potentially susceptible, and is considered to be a nontriggering agent.[250, 251]

Treatment of malignant hyperthermia is discussed in Chapter 4.

Strabismus and Postoperative Nausea and Vomiting

Nausea and vomiting after strabismus surgery occurs in 50 to 80 percent of patients[252–254] and may delay the patient's discharge from the hospital or ambulatory surgical center. The mechanism for this high incidence of vomiting is not known. However, it may be secondary to altered visual perception and a different afferent input postoperatively or may be secondary to an oculoemetic reflex, which is analogous to the oculocardiac reflex. Prevention of the oculocardiac reflex during strabismus surgery by prophylactic treatment with anticholinergic agents (atropine or glycopyrrolate) did not reduce the incidence of nausea and/or vomiting.[255]

Various prophylactic therapies have been recommended to decrease the incidence of postoperative nausea and vomiting, but none have been a cure. The topic continues to attract attention, in that the list of papers addressing postoperative nausea and vomiting after eye surgery never seems to dissipate. In spite of a plethora of studies, no totally effective method of eliminating postoperative nausea and vomiting has been found. The results from one study sometimes contradict the results from another. A variety of agents are partially effective, but no single agent, combination of agents, or anesthetic technique has eliminated postoperative vomiting following strabismus surgery.

To decrease postoperative vomiting, it is commonly recommended that administration of narcotics be avoided. Acetaminophen (10 to 40 mg/kg, per rectum) or ketorolac frequently provide adequate pain control. Recently, propofol plus nitrous oxide was reported to lessen postoperative vomiting in pediatric outpatients following strabismus surgery, compared with patients who received halothane, nitrous oxide, and droperidol.[256] Similarly, propofol caused less nausea and a more normal level of consciousness and activity postoperatively than halothane/thiopental anesthesia.[257] Another study reported that propofol/sufentanil anesthesia caused less nausea and vomiting than isoflurane/nitrous oxide.[258] Postoperative nausea and vomiting were absent after thiopental/isoflurane or propofol anesthesia in 5- to 14-year-old children who underwent strabismus surgery. All children received glycopyrrolate, vecuronium, fentanyl, and nitrous oxide/oxygen.[259]

Both droperidol and metoclopramide are thought to antagonize dopaminergic sites and thereby reduce nausea and vomiting.[260, 261] Droperidol often is used to treat perioperative nausea and vomiting, since currently this drug is much less expensive than the serotonin antagonists. Droperidol 15 to 75 μg/kg, when given before or during surgery, has been shown to be an effective antiemetic.[262, 263] However, droperidol produces sedation that may be very protracted.

For years, metoclopramide has been recommended to treat perioperative nausea and vomiting. Broadman et al. reported an incidence of vomiting after metoclopramide of 37 percent compared with 59 percent when no antiemetic was given.[264] Another study documented that metoclopramide 0.25 mg/kg was as effective as droperidol 0.75 mg/kg in decreasing postoperative vomiting. Both study groups had shorter but equal recovery and discharge times than the control group.[265] When compared with ondansetron, metoclopramide (0.15 mg/kg) had no effect on the incidence of nausea and vomiting in pediatric patients undergoing either tonsillectomy and adenoidectomy or strabismus surgery.[266]

Over the last few years, serotonin antagonists such as ondansetron and granisetron have been used to treat and prevent perioperative nausea and vomiting. Many studies have addressed the effectiveness of these drugs, either alone or in combination with other agents in preventing nausea and vomiting. For example, children given granisetron (20 μg/kg) orally before the induction of anesthesia with halothane (isoflurane for maintenance of anesthesia; ketorolac or acetaminophen for analgesia) reduced the incidence of nausea and vomiting compared with placebo.[267] Another study reported that prophylactic ondansetron given to children before strabismus surgery effectively decreased the frequency and severity of postoperative vomiting.[268] Others found that a combination of droperidol and granisetron for children undergoing strabismus surgery was more effective than either droperidol (50 μg/kg) alone, or granisetron (40 μg/kg) alone.[269]

As the expense of the serotonin antagonists decreases, these agents are likely to become the mainstay of treatment for perioperative nausea and vomiting, especially in high-risk patients (e.g., strabismus surgery, tonsillectomy/adenoidectomy, laparoscopic surgery).

Strabismus and Succinylcholine

Some authorities suggest that succinylcholine should be avoided during surgery on the eye because this drug causes sustained contracture of the extraocular muscles rather than paralysis. Contracture of these muscles may affect the forced duction test performed by the ophthalmologist during surgery to estimate the amount of restriction in movement of the extraocular muscles. France et al.[270] quantitated the magnitude and duration of this effect of succinylcholine on the forced duction test and com-

pared the results with those induced by pancuronium. The force required to rotate the globe increased after succinylcholine and remained elevated for 15 minutes. In contrast, pancuronium decreased the rotational forces needed to perform the forced duction test. From a practical standpoint, there seems to be variability from ophthalmologist to ophthalmologist in the importance of performing this intraoperative test on the outcome of strabismus surgery. Therefore, communication with the surgeon is essential. The other reason to avoid using succinylcholine during strabismus surgery is the increased incidence of malignant hyperthermia; currently, many nondepolarizing, short-acting muscle relaxants are available.

Cataracts

Surgery for congenital cataracts is generally performed within the first few weeks of life to provide the optimal chance for a good visual outcome. Congenital cataracts are of two main types: idiopathic and those associated with syndromes. Various in utero infections (rubella, toxoplasmosis, cytomegalovirus, herpes simplex) frequently are associated with cataract formation. Metabolic diseases, such as galactosemia, and chromosomal abnormalities, such as trisomy 21, are also associated with the presence of cataracts. Several syndromes (e.g., Stickler's, Hallermann-Steiff, Laurence-Moon-Biedl, Lowe, Conradi's, cerebrotendinous xanthomatosis) are associated with a high incidence of cataracts.

A maximally dilated pupil is essential for successful cataract surgery. Although several mydriatics are available and are applied preoperatively (1 percent cyclopentolate, 2.5 percent phenylephrine), epinephrine (1 : 200,000) is usually infused continuously through a needle placed in the anterior chamber. Although epinephrine is aspirated from the anterior chamber during surgery, when the lens and anterior and posterior capsules are removed, there is the potential for systemic absorption of the drug. Some epinephrine may drain through Schlemm's canal and be absorbed into veins, or the epinephrine may spill onto the conjunctiva and be absorbed. The risk of hemodynamically significant effects is small, especially since children have a much higher threshold from dysrhythmias following epinephrine absorption for surgical sites. For example, 2 to 15 μg/kg of epinephrine (injection into mucosa or skin) did not cause premature ventricular contractions during halothane anesthesia in young patients.[271, 272]

As in all surgical cases, anesthesia for cataract surgery must take into account the individual patient's coexisting medical problems. If congenital cataracts are part of a syndrome, a complete knowledge of cardiorespiratory, hematologic, and neurologic status of the patient should be available and understood, so an appropriate intra- and postoperative anesthetic plan can be developed. For example, if cataracts are associated with retinitis of prematurity, the anesthesiologist must be familiar and facile with the care of premature and expremature infants. If the patient has Marfan's syndrome, associated cardiovascular anomalies must be evaluated. If a patient has homocystinuria, care must be taken to prevent thromboembolic lesions of the pulmonary, cerebral, coronary, and renal vessels. Patients with homocystinuria are frequently maintained on aspirin and are, therefore, susceptible to prolonged bleeding. Because hypoglycemia is common in these patients, serum glucose concentration should be monitored intraoperatively.

A deep plane of anesthesia is required for all patients to minimize the chance of coughing or straining to prevent losing vitreous or other intraocular contents after the globe is incised. If a patient's cardiovascular system cannot tolerate a deep plane of anesthesia, neuromuscular blockade should be established. Complete paralysis is necessary because a patient will be able to cough if he or she has recovered partial diaphragmatic function. Since the diaphragm generally recovers before the peripheral muscles, it is essential that complete paralysis of the peripheral muscles be maintained so that diaphragmatic function will be inadequate to allow coughing. After the globe is incised, succinylcholine should not be administered, because contraction of the extraocular muscles for 15 to 20 minutes can potentially increase intraocular pressure sufficiently to extrude the ocular contents through the surgical incision.

Ideally, the patient who has had cataract surgery should not cry excessively or struggle postoperatively. Sedation is usually used to achieve this goal during the recovery period. Droperidol may be useful because it has antiemetic and sedative effects. Diazepam or midazolam may also be effective. Often, acetaminophen or a nonsteroidal agent can provide adequate pain control and may eliminate the need for narcotics, which can cause nausea. Some children, other than young expremature infants, may undergo cataract extraction on a come-and-go basis. The analgesia/sedation regimen should reflect this possibility.

Glaucoma

If outflow of aqueous humor is obstructed for any reason, intraocular pressure increases and causes glaucoma. As with cataracts, glaucoma can be an isolated primary congenital disorder or it can be part of a syndrome (e.g., Sturge-Weber syndrome, rubella, mesodermal dysgenesis). A late or juvenile form of congenital glaucoma presents after 6 years of age, often in families with a strong history of open-angle glaucoma.

Successful surgical treatment of infantile glaucoma requires early recognition of the problem. Confirming the diagnosis in infants who present with a history of excessive tearing, photophobia, irritability, and buphthalmos usually requires measuring the intraocular pressure during a general anesthetic. The eye examination and pressure measurement can be followed by surgery if the diagnosis is confirmed. The initial surgery usually consists of goniotomy or trabeculotomy to create a route for the exit of aqueous humor via Schlemm's canal. If unsuccessful, cryotherapy is sometimes used to destroy the ciliary body and decrease aqueous humor production.

Anesthetic considerations for patients during glaucoma surgery include awareness of associated medical problems, especially if a syndrome has been diagnosed, and a knowledge of how to manage intraocular pressure (see section "Intraocular Pressure and its Control," above).

Retinoblastoma

Radiation therapy is a primary treatment for retinoblastoma, a congenital malignancy that usually is diagnosed and treated during the first 3 years of life. Radiation therapy is administered over a 4- to 6-week period, often four to five times per week. During each session, the head must remain absolutely motionless for 45 to 90 seconds. Patients are unattended during the treatment to avoid exposing medical personnel to excessive radiation. Postanesthesia sedation should be minimal to avoid disrupting the infant's feeding and sleeping schedules, so that he or she continues to grow and develop normally during these 4 to 6 weeks.

A wide range of techniques have been described to permit repeated radiation treatment of retinoblastoma. Brett et al.[273] described an insufflation technique. After an inhalation induction of anesthesia via a mask, a soft 8- to 10-Fr catheter (or an endotracheal tube) is inserted into a naris and attached to a source of halothane or sevoflurane and nitrous oxide in oxygen. The catheter is advanced into the posterior pharynx a distance equal to that measured from the patient's nose to the tragus of the ear. The catheter must be carefully positioned to avoid entering the esophagus and causing gastric distention. At least 5 to 10 cm H_2O of positive pressure should be maintained in the anesthetic circuit to prevent the patient from breathing room air rather than the anesthetic mixture of gases and awakening prematurely. During delivery of the radiation, the patient and the pulse oximeter attached to the patient are observed via a closed-circuit television camera, which transmits data to a monitor outside the treatment room. This method of administering anesthesia provides immobility for a predictable, short period of time, avoids maintaining a heparin lock or central line, and avoids repeated needle sticks and tracheal intubation. It also allows the patient to awaken quickly after the procedure and to go home without the expense of a stay in the postanesthesia recovery room.

If the infant has an indwelling central line to facilitate delivery of chemotherapy, propofol can provide an adequate depth of anesthesia that quickly and predictably abates, which allows prompt recovery and discharge home. Often, a single bolus of 2 mg/kg of propofol is sufficient to allow a single 1 to 2 minutes of radiation treatment. Although intramuscular ketamine was recommended to anesthetize infants for radiation therapy in the 1970s and 1980s, this drug is seldom used now. The nystagmus that accompanies ketamine anesthesia is less than ideal for radiation treatment of a retinoblastoma.

DENTAL PROCEDURES

The majority of pediatric dental procedures are performed on an outpatient basis. In normal children, local anesthesia, with or without sedation, is sufficient to accomplish most procedures. However, when extensive dental restoration is required and/or a child is severely retarded or has serious behavior problems, significant coexisting disease (e.g., congenital heart disease), a family or a personal history of malignant hyperthermia, or a history of severe reaction to medications that may be administered during the procedure, special monitoring and deep sedation/general anesthesia may be required.[274, 275]

Considerations for Dental Surgery

The dentist or oral surgeon should determine the young patient's physical and emotional status as part of the preoperative preparation. Then a decision can be made whether he or she requires conscious sedation, deep sedation, or general anesthesia. Most pediatric dental procedures are performed in the office using behavior-modification techniques, parental support, and local anesthesia. However, life-threatening situations can occur when local anesthetics are combined with premedication and other drugs.[276–278] Adverse events usually occur when combinations of drugs and relatively higher than usual doses of local anesthetics, sedatives, or analgesics are administered with inadequate monitoring or insufficiently skilled personnel available. Consequently, the physiologic status of the patient, the consequences of the medication administered, and the appropriate location for the procedure and/or sedation must be considered carefully.

Severely Retarded Children and Children with Serious Behavior Disturbances

Patients with mental retardation or serious behavioral disturbances can pose difficulties because of poor motor control and involuntary movements, spasticity, and aggressive behavior (screaming, biting, kicking), particularly when they are frightened by a strange environment.[279] This behavior may result in difficulty placing and securing an intravenous catheter or in performing an inhalational induction of anesthesia. Ketamine, 3 to 5 mg/kg intramuscularly mixed with atropine (10 to 20 μg/kg), has been useful for the induction of anesthesia in some of these patients.[280, 281] After the injection of this mixture of drugs, sedation or a "catatonic state" will develop, and the patient can be moved, intravenous access obtained, general anesthesia induced, the patient's trachea intubated, and anesthesia maintained with a technique of choice. Many patients in this category have seizure disorders and should receive their anticonvulsant medications on the day of the procedure. Ketamine can be employed in patients with seizure disorders.[281] Doing so neither precipitates nor aggravates seizures.

Children with Congenital Heart Disease

Many children with congenital heart disease require dental care under general anesthesia. These children may be uncooperative because of past hospital experiences. The anesthesiologist must understand the patient's cardiovascular anatomy and prior surgical intervention and the hemodynamic and physiologic implications to provide optimal care for these patients (see Chapter 18). For example, direction and magnitude of intracardiac shunts,

whether pulmonary blood flow is increased or decreased, the current general status (patient's height and weight compared with normal children), level of and tolerance for feeding and activity, previous surgical procedures (related to cardiac condition and otherwise), medications, baseline hemoglobin and oxygen saturation, and electrolytes all should be considered. Reports of recent chest radiographs, ECGs, and/or echocardiograms should be obtained. Reviewing these findings with the patient's cardiologist to determine if the patient is presently in optimal condition for the procedure and if the patient needs prophylaxis for bacterial endocarditis (see Appendix A) may be appropriate. Ensuring that a pediatric cardiologist is available for intra- and/or postoperative consultation may be critical. Some cyanotic patients with hematocrits greater than 65 percent may benefit from red cell phoresis or partial reverse exchange transfusion. In general, most medications administered for hemodynamic stability should be continued pre- and postoperatively.

Patients with cyanotic congenital heart disease may have a hyperviscosity syndrome with an associated coagulation disorder caused by an acquired defect in platelet aggregation.[282, 283] Decreasing the patient's hematocrit to the high 50 to low 60 percent range with an isovolemic exchange transfusion corrects the bleeding tendency associated with the hyperviscosity syndrome.[282, 284] If present, consideration should be given to elective preoperative hematocrit reduction to avoid problems associated with hyperviscosity.[284]

Monitoring patients with congenital heart disease during general anesthesia must be tailored to the diagnosis and the general status of the patient. The standard monitors (ECG, arterial blood pressure, temperature, pulse oximetry, and end-tidal CO_2) may need to be supplemented with intra-arterial or central venous monitoring. Every precaution must be taken to prevent gas bubbles from entering intravascular lines if patients have intracardiac communications, especially if the shunt is right to left (i.e., from the pulmonary to the systemic side of the circulation).

No single anesthetic regimen is necessarily better than any other. However, the anesthesiologist should attempt to maintain preload, pulmonary and systemic vascular resistances, heart rate, and contractility within the patient's normal range. Knowledge of the anatomy of a patient's lesion allows one to provide an anesthetic that achieves this goal.[284] For example, a 4-year-old who has a small ventricular septal defect that appears to be closing, is hemodynamically stable, and requires no medication needs no monitoring other than that used for a normal patient. Prophylaxis for subacute bacterial endocarditis (SBE) and careful attention to avoiding air bubbles in the intravenous infusion are necessary.

SBE Prophylaxis

Bacteremia occurs after 65 percent of dental extractions, after 16 percent of dental restorations,[285] and after 16 percent of nasotracheal intubations,[286] presumably through traumatized mucosa. The bacteremia is generally transient and rarely persists for more than 15 minutes.[285] However, 14 percent of patients[287] with "transient bactermia" had positive blood cultures in the recovery room. Patients with poor dental hygiene or periodontal infections may experience bacteremia even in the absence of dental procedures. Individuals at risk for developing bacterial endocarditis should establish and maintain the best possible oral health to reduce the potential for bacterial seeding. Hemolytic streptococci (*Streptococcus viridans*) and *Staphylococcus aureus* are the most common organisms causing subacute bacterial endocarditis in pediatric patients who have heart disease.[286, 288, 289] The American Heart Association (Table 23–4) suggests that patients at risk for developing infective endocarditis should receive antibiotic prophylaxis for dental procedures that cause gingival bleeding, including professional cleaning.[290] An exception is shedding of primary teeth, for which there are no data supporting an increased risk for bacteremia. Similarly, oral endotracheal intubation is not an indication for antibiotic prophylaxis unless it is associated with another procedure for which prophylaxis is recommended.

Children with cyanotic congenital heart disease are at risk for infective endocarditis following most reparative and all palliative surgical procedures; this includes patients with palliative systemic artery–to–pulmonary artery shunts.[288, 290] These patients should receive antibiotic prophylaxis throughout their lifetime for all procedures that place them at risk for sepsis. Patients with an isolated

secundum atrial septal defect; patients who have surgical repair without residua of an atrial septal defect, a ventricular septal defect, or a patent ductus arteriosus; or patients with physiologic, functional, or innocent heart murmurs do not require prophylaxis with antibiotics. Previous Kawasaki disease or rheumatic fever without valvar dysfunction, cardiac pacemakers, and implanted defibrillators; mitral valve prolapse without valvar regurgitation; or previous coronary artery bypass surgery also do not require prophylaxis.[290] Since antibiotic prophylaxis failure is possible, any unexplained fever following dental surgery in a child at risk for infective endocarditis warrants thorough evaluation, and antibiotics should be administered as needed.

Issues for Dental Anesthesia

Opinions vary whether tracheal intubation is necessary to protect the airway of patients receiving general anesthesia for dental procedures.[274] Most believe that the decision to insert an endotracheal tube should depend on the type and duration of the procedure planned. For brief procedures (usually extractions lasting less than 3 minutes), a nasal mask (Goldman nosepiece), nasopharyngeal airway,[291–293] or a laryngeal mask airway are sufficient. Longer dental rehabilitative procedures are best managed with tracheal intubation. Most anesthesiologists and dental surgeons prefer nasotracheal rather than orotracheal intubation for dental procedures, but in some patients this is not practical. Securing and maintaining an orotracheal tube during dental anesthesia requires uncompromising vigilance. Oral tubes are usually secured to one side of the mouth and then carefully resecured on the other side when necessary.

Patients with epidermolysis bullosa can form blisters in response to pressure, friction, or minor trauma. When these patients require tracheal intubation, placement of an oral tracheal tube is preferred. The tube can be sutured to the mouth, teeth, or tongue, or the tube can be secured around the patient's head with a fabric tube holder. It should not be taped to the skin. The stability of an oral tube is potentially a problem and requires constant attention to prevent the tube from being accidentally removed.

Nasotracheal Intubation and Dental Surgery

Most dental surgeons working in the mouth prefer naso- rather than orotracheal intubation; this allows the surgeon to use a rubber dam.[274] Nasotracheal intubation can be achieved using several techniques. In most children, the endotracheal tube can be inserted under direct vision without difficulty. The vocal cords usually can be visualized easily. Then the endotracheal tube can be directed through the vocal cords, usually without the use of Magill forceps.

Many anesthesiologists use nasal RAE endotracheal tubes for dental surgery. The fixed bend helps stabilize the endotracheal tube, decreases the likelihood of kinking the tube, and allows a low profile for maximum surgical convenience when the bend is situated at the opening of the naris. There are two disadvantages of these tubes that

---

TABLE 23–4
RECOMMENDED PROPHYLACTIC ANTIBIOTIC REGIMEN FOR DENTAL, ORAL, OR UPPER RESPIRATORY TRACT PROCEDURES

Drug	Dosing Regimen* Standard Regimen
Amoxicillin	50 mg/kg orally 1 h before procedure, then 25 mg/kg 6 h after initial dose. For IM or IV dosing: 50 mg/kg 30 min before procedure, then 25 mg/kg IM or IV 6 h after initial dose.
Amoxicillin/Penicillin-Allergic Patients	
Erythromycin or clindamycin	Erythromycin ethylsuccinate 20 mg/kg or erythromycin stearate 20 mg/kg orally 2 h before procedure; then half initial dose 6 h after initial dose. Clindamycin 10 mg/kg orally 1 h before procedure or IV clindamycin 10 mg/kg 30 min before and 5 mg/kg (orally or IV) 6 h after initial dose.
High-Risk Patients	
Ampicillin, gentamicin, and amoxicillin	IV or IM administration of ampicillin 50 mg/kg plus gentamicin 2.0 mg/kg (not greater than 80 mg) 30 min before procedure; followed by amoxicillin 25 mg/kg orally 6 h after initial dose; or IV regimen can be repeated 8 h after initial dose.
High-Risk Patients Allergic to Ampicillin Amoxicillin, or Penicillin	
Vancomycin	IV vancomycin 20 mg/kg over 1 h, starting 1 h before procedure; no repeated dose necessary.

* Total pediatric dose should not exceed total adult dose.
Modified from Dajani AS, Bisno AL, Chung KJ, et al: Prevention of bacterial endocarditis. Recommendations by the American Heart Association. JAMA 264:2919, 1990. Copyright 1990 American Medical Association, with permission.

are related to this bend. If the tube is positioned correctly, the distance from the bend to the distal end of the tube is fixed. This allows endobronchial intubation to occur in some patients. In others, the tip of the endotracheal tube barely extends beyond the vocal cords. The bend also makes suctioning difficult.

Selection of the correct tube size is achieved using routine methods. A slight leak of gas from around the tube is desired during positive-pressure ventilation. By initially inserting the tube orally, the correct tube size can be determined without repeated reintubation via the nasopharynx. Limiting the number of nasotracheal intubations may decrease the incidence of epistaxis. Epistaxis can make nasotracheal intubation more difficult because it severely limits visualization of the larynx. In older children, a cuffed nasal RAE tube eliminates the need to first intubate the trachea orally. An undersized endotracheal tube can be inserted, decreasing trauma to the nasal mucosa. Then sufficient air can be inserted into the endotracheal tube cuff to permit a leak to occur at approximately 20 cm H_2O peak airway pressure. An air leak at 20 cm H_2O confirms that the endotracheal tube is appropriately sized, reducing the incidence and severity of postintubation stridor or croup.[154] Despite careful tube selection, children undergoing long dental procedures still can experience postintubation croup, possibly secondary to surgical manipulation of the jaw against the endotracheal tube during the surgery. When croup occurs, treatment is supportive with humidified oxygen. Nebulized racemic epinephrine also can be used to treat severe croup. A child who has been treated with racemic epinephrine must be monitored for at least several hours after the treatment to ensure that airway obstruction does not recur when the effects of the drug dissipate. Occasionally, steroids may be indicated to treat croup. In some cases, hospital admission and overnight observation are required. Despite thorough topicalization of the nose and pharynx, an occasional patient will have severe bleeding from a partial adenoidectomy that occurs when a nasotracheal tube is inserted into the pharynx. Care must be taken to vasoconstrict the naris and pharynx thoroughly and to adequately lubricate the endotracheal tube to minimize the incidence of this serious complication.

Sedation Versus Anesthesia

When the decision is made to use general anesthesia for a child's dental procedure, much of the care is simplified. His or her airway and level of consciousness will be monitored and managed by an individual skilled in advanced airway support. When sedation rather than general anesthesia is used, the dentist is responsible for ensuring that the standards for monitoring the child are appropriate for the level of sedation provided.

Published guidelines for monitoring and caring for pediatric patients during and after sedation stress that monitoring during "deep sedation and general anesthesia are virtually inseparable."[294, 295] Specifically,

the state of deep sedation, regardless of how it is achieved, requires that there must be one person available whose *only responsibility* is to constantly observe the patient's vital signs,

airway patency, and adequacy of ventilation, and to either administer drugs or direct their administration. At least one individual must be present who is trained in and capable of providing pediatric basic life support and who is *skilled in airway management* and cardiopulmonary resuscitation; training in pediatric advanced life support is strongly encouraged.

Of particular note are the statements concerning monitoring. For example: "Vital signs, including oxygen saturation and heart rate, must be documented at least every 5 minutes in a time-based record."

Conscious sedation is a medically controlled state of depressed consciousness that allows protective reflexes to be maintained, retains the patient's ability to maintain a patent airway independently and continuously, and permits *appropriate* response by the patient to physical stimulation or verbal command (e.g., "open your eyes," "what is your name").[296] Some pediatric anesthesiologists state that the term "conscious sedation" is an oxymoron when applied to children, because a child must be in a state of "pharmacologic coma" to tolerate a painful procedure.[297] This state is equivalent to general anesthesia and requires meticulous monitoring of respiratory status, especially during the setting of dental surgery, where the surgery may interfere with the airway.

These guidelines should be carefully reviewed before recommending "sedation" for children for dental procedures. The same dose of medication given to two different children may result in different levels of sedation. Depth of consciousness can rapidly move into the realm of deep sedation/general anesthesia when additional sedation is administered. Monitoring requirements for sedated children apply to every practitioner in every setting in both inpatient and outpatient facilities.

Complications Associated with Dental Procedures

The major complications associated with dental surgery and anesthesia are problems with airway maintenance (both with and without an endotracheal tube), dysrhythmias, and subcutaneous emphysema.

Extraction-Associated Dysrhythmias

Unpremedicated children undergoing dental extractions during halothane/nitrous oxide/oxygen anesthesia occasionally had cardiac dysrhythmias.[298-301] They have been attributed to light anesthesia, elevated endogenous catecholamines, and trigeminal nerve stimulation.[275, 287, 300, 302] Both the incidence and the severity of ventricular dysrhythmias can be reduced by deepening the anesthetic level or by blocking afferent surgical stimulation from the fifth nerve with a local anesthetic.[299, 300]

Subcutaneous Emphysema

Although rare, air-driven (20 to 30 psi) ultrahigh-speed dental instruments can cause subcutaneous emphysema of the face and cervical areas that may extend into the mediastinum and cause a pneumothorax, a pneumomediastinum, a pneumopericardium, or an intravascular air embolism.[303-306] Air also may cause the patient's tongue or oral tissues to swell and obstruct the airway. The air probably enters along the mandibular periosteum at the operative site.

The use of clear drapes allows the patient's face to be observed intraoperatively and to detect gas-induced swelling early. Discontinuing the use of nitrous oxide as soon as subcutaneous emphysema is noted decreases expansion of the gas volume. A chest radiograph should be obtained to detect and follow intrathoracic extension of the gas; the trachea should be intubated when necessary.[306] Prophylactic antibiotic administration may be justified because of the possibility of cellulitis occurring if organisms from the mouth are carried interstitially with the air.

COMMON PROBLEMS: PEDIATRIC ANESTHESIA

Laryngospasm

Laryngospasm is usually a transient, life-threatening event in which either the true vocal cords or the true and false vocal cords oppose in the midline and close the glottis. This closure of the glottis by the intrinsic laryngeal muscles is involuntary.[307] The lateral cricoarytenoid and the thyroarytenoid muscles (adductors of the glottis) and the cricothyroid muscles (a tensor of the vocal cords) are the primary muscles involved in laryngospasm.

The exact incidence of laryngospasm is difficult to determine. Olsson and Hallen[308] reported the incidence of laryngospasm during 156,064 anesthetics delivered to 136,929 patients. The overall incidence was 1,232 episodes of laryngospasm in 1,197 patients (overall incidence = 0.8 percent or 7.9 events per 1,000 anesthetics or 8.7 events per 1,000 patients). The overall incidence of laryngospasm in children 0 to 9 years of age was 17.4 per 1,000 patients; for patients between 0 and 3 months of age, the incidence was 28.2 per 1,000 patients. In this study, asthma and respiratory infections were associated with an increase in the incidence of laryngospasm in children. The increased incidence of laryngospasm in patients who have a URI has been described recently.[78]

The LMA provides an alternative to endotracheal intubation for a variety of procedures. Some people have proposed that this device may reduce airway complications in patients who have a URI. However, LMAs were associated with a similar incidence of cough, breath-holding, excessive secretions, and laryngospasm, as occurred with endotracheal tubes.[309] Patients whose airways were managed with an LMA had a lower incidence of mild bronchospasm and a lower incidence of oxygen desaturation during placement of the airway than those treated with an endotracheal tube. Treatment of bronchospasm and laryngospasm that developed during use of an LMA was not addressed in this study. Both may be more difficult to treat because high peak airway pressure cannot be delivered through an LMA.

The rapid wash-in and wash-out of desflurane and sevoflurane may be associated with a lower incidence of laryngospasm, since reliable swift wake-up is possible. Similarly, if deep tracheal extubation is indicated, rapid deepening of anesthesia is possible with these agents. Both desflurane[310] and sevoflurane[311] permitted tracheal extubation without an increased incidence of laryngospasm or other airway complications. Because the incidence of laryngospasm is related to the depth of anesthesia (not a particular anesthetic), the trachea should be extubated when the patient is fully awake or fully anesthetized.

Airway obstruction associated with laryngospasm may be partial or total. Gas exchange via a partially obstructed airway causes noisy airway sounds that vary in intensity and tone but usually resemble a high-pitched squeak. During anesthesia and surgery, laryngospasm is most commonly associated with airway manipulation (e.g., intubation or extubation of the trachea), with foreign material in the larynx (e.g., secretions), or with light anesthesia in a nonintubated patient. In general, laryngospasm is unlikely if the anesthetic depth is sufficiently deep during extubation and intubation of the trachea or if the patient is fully awake before the endotracheal tube is removed. There is seldom a need to perform laryngoscopy to make the diagnosis. Laryngoscopy wastes time and further stimulates the airway.

Intravenous lidocaine (2 mg/kg) prevents or controls laryngospasm in both children[312] and adults[313] undergoing tonsillectomy. Topical lidocaine also is thought to effectively decrease the incidence of laryngospasm by suppressing laryngeal mucosal neuroreceptors without affecting central neural reflex. In piglets, topical lidocaine decreased both the laryngeal chemoreflex and mechanoreflex without decreasing the superior laryngeal nerve adductor reflex.[314] Intravenous lidocaine had no effect on laryngeal mucosal reflexes.[312] Lidocaine probably provides a sufficient increase in the depth of anesthesia to decrease the occurrence of laryngospasm.

Specific treatment of laryngospasm depends on the severity of the episode and on the initial response of the patient to treatment. The first step in its treatment is to deliver steady positive pressure to the airway plus an F_{IO_2} of 1.0. The laryngospasm often breaks after 30 to 45 seconds and the patient can resume spontaneous ventilatory efforts or the anesthesiologist can resume positive-pressure ventilation. If the laryngospasm continues despite positive pressure and if the oxygen saturation begins to decrease, the anesthesiologist may need to administer a muscle relaxant to break laryngospasm and allow immediate ventilation with oxygen. A small dose of succinylcholine 0.5 to 1.0 mg/kg is effective. However, if the child is hypoxemic, administering succinylcholine may precipitate profound bradycardia and further worsen oxygen delivery. If succinylcholine is to be given to a hypoxemic child, approximately 20 μg/kg of atropine should also be given. Short-acting nondepolarizing muscle relaxants may provide an alternative to succinylcholine.[315] For instance, rapacuronium given intravenously (1.2 mg/kg in children[316] and 1.5 mg/kg in adults)[316] or intramuscularly (2.8 mg/kg to infants and 4.8 mg/kg to children)[317] provided good to excellent intubating conditions approximately 3 minutes after the drug was administered. However, succinylcholine does so in 1.1 to 1.3 minutes.[317] Of note, a shorter period of time is needed to provide adequate conditions for ventilation by mask than is needed to provide adequate conditions for tracheal intubation.

Acute pulmonary edema is often associated with acute upper airway obstruction caused by trauma,[318] masses,[318] croup, epiglottitis,[319] and laryngospasm.[320–322] It is believed that attempted ventilation against a closed glottis, which generates 30 to 60 cm H_2O intrapleural pressure, plus the immediate decrease in airway pressure that occurs with relief of laryngospasm induces pulmonary edema.[319] The increased negative intrapleural pressure and increased venous return (i.e., increased preload) may injure the microvasculature (i.e., increased permeability). The combination of the preload and the increased vascular permeability allows fluid movement out of the vasculature and produces interstitial edema and pulmonary edema. In addition, negative intrathoracic pressure increases left ventricular transmural pressure (i.e., afterload)[323] and affects cardiac performance.

Laryngospasm-induced pulmonary edema is most effectively managed by prompt tracheal intubation and application of continuous positive airway pressure or positive end-expiratory pressure with positive-pressure ventilation. Diuretics, morphine, and sedatives are also effective adjuncts. If the patient has no underlying cardiorespiratory problems, the pulmonary edema resolves quickly, allowing the trachea to be extubated within several hours.

Stridor

Stridor is noisy breathing caused by turbulent flow through the narrowed lumen of an airway. It is a symptom of many different problems that produce a narrowed, partially obstructed airway. Inspiratory stridor generally is caused by anomalies that narrow the airway above the thoracic inlet (e.g., cysts or masses, laryngomalacia, vocal cord paralysis, hemangiomas, laryngoceles, papillomas), adenotonsillar hypertrophy, midfacial hypoplasia, and croup. Expiratory stridor is most commonly associated with airway obstruction below the thoracic inlet (e.g., cysts, hemangiomas, vascular rings, foreign bodies).[323, 324] Biphasic stridor is common and is characteristic of midtracheal abnormalities secondary to tracheomalacia and tracheal stenosis. Laryngoscopy and fiberoptic and/or rigid bronchoscopy and a variety of imaging procedures are often required to determine the etiology of stridor. To accomplish these procedures, deep sedation or general anesthesia usually is required. Therefore, the anesthesiologist should understand the physiology and clinical implications of stridor.

Inspiration through a partially obstructed extrathoracic airway reduces the intraluminal pressure of the extrathoracic airway below atmospheric pressure. The transluminal pressure gradient narrows the lumen further, increasing the stridor. During expiration, the extrathoracic intraluminal pressure is positive and greater than atmospheric, dilating the lumen and decreasing stridor. In contrast, inspiration through a partially obstructed intrathoracic airway reduces extraluminal pressure below intraluminal pressure and dilates the airway. During expiration, the reverse occurs, and the expiratory noise (wheezing) worsens.[323, 324]

A careful medical history of the degree and duration of symptoms, age and acuteness of onset, and a history of previous tracheal intubation is important. For example, the newborn with severe stridor is likely to have a congenital anomaly of the airway as the etiology for stridor. A 3-year-old with sudden onset of severe stridor is more likely to have a foreign body or an infectious etiology as the cause of stridor. The child in the recovery room or intensive care unit who develops stridor following tracheal extubation is likely to have airway edema as the cause of stridor. The severity and rapidity of progression of the symptoms defines the diagnostic and treatment plan.

Approximately 45 to 60 percent of stridor (except postextubation stridor) in the young infant is because of laryngomalacia[324, 325] Symptoms of laryngomalacia generally are present from birth and must be differentiated from other congenital anomalies that cause stridor. Babies with laryngomalacia usually do not have feeding difficulties, but children with glottic or oropharyngeal lesions or a tracheoesophageal fistula commonly do have these symptoms. The noise is usually worse in babies when they are agitated, and they sometimes improve when placed in the prone position. They worsen in the supine position. Although many of these infants do well and improve as they grow, their stridor often persists for 4 to 5 years.[325]

Although infants and children with laryngomalacia do not have a higher incidence of upper or lower respiratory infections, their upper airway obstruction often worsens when an upper respiratory infection occurs.[325] A child with laryngomalacia and an upper respiratory tract infection who presents for anything but emergency surgery should prompt careful evaluation and thought before proceeding with a general anesthetic, especially one that requires endotracheal intubation. If the surgery is emergent, care should be taken to use an endotracheal tube that allows an audible air leak when a positive pressure of 20 to 25 cm H_2O is generated. In addition, the patient should be monitored postoperatively in a PICU, where prompt ventilatory support can be provided.

Although uncommon, an infant with neurologic abnormalities may present with stridor. Laryngeal nerve paralysis may be caused by birth trauma or cardiac malformations that affect the left recurrent laryngeal nerve. Frequently, the etiology of the injury is unclear. Unilateral vocal cord paralysis commonly is the result of a peripheral nerve lesion and often improves with growth. Infants with unilateral cord paralysis commonly have stridor or hoarseness and feeding difficulties. Infants with bilateral vocal cord paralysis often have central nervous system disease (e.g., hydrocephalus, an Arnold-Chiari malformation, a Dandy-Walker cyst, an encephalocele, posterior fossa hematomas, child abuse).[326–330] Some people relate the stridor to vocal cord paralysis that is caused by stretching the vagus nerve over the jugular foramen. However, it is often unclear why stridor occurs and why it persists after the increased intracranial pressure is normalized. Children who have bilateral vocal cord paralysis and serious respiratory obstruction or recurrent aspiration pneumonia often require a tracheostomy.

Anesthetic considerations for children who are stridorous are similar, regardless of the etiology of the obstruction. Maintaining continuous positive airway pressure during spontaneous ventilation via a face mask can reverse the upper airway pressure gradient and decrease or eliminate the obstruction. It is vital to have a wide range of endotracheal tubes available, since lesions such as cricoid ring stenosis, webs, cysts, hemangiomas, epiglottitis, and croup usually necessitate the use of a smaller than normal endotracheal tube. Other lesions, such as vocal cord paralysis, usually do not narrow the airway. Meticulous care should be taken to ensure that the endotracheal tube chosen does not cause further injury to the trachea (i.e., ensure a leak at 20 to 25 cm H_2O airway pressure).

Postextubation stridor is a significant problem because children who have undergone a surgical or diagnostic procedure involving the upper airway or who have had mechanical ventilatory support are at high risk for laryngeal/tracheal edema, narrowing of the airway, and stridor. The mucosa of the subglottic area of children is vascular and consists of loose areolar tissue. The cricoid cartilage is the narrowest area in the airway of children less than 5 years old. Swelling caused by a tight endotracheal tube, burns, or other trauma causes inflammation and narrowing of the internal diameter of the airway, because the cartilage prevents edema from being displaced outward. Consequently, this area is particularly prone to edema.[331]

Inhaled racemic epinephrine (0.5 ml of 2.25 percent solution nebulized in 2.5 ml of normal saline) may reduce the edema. The drug can be administered repeatedly if heart rate is less than 200 beats/min. Oxygen saturation should be monitored during treatment. If the patient requires multiple racemic epinephrine treatments, an arterial blood gas should be obtained to ensure that ventilation is adequate, especially if the patient has increased work of breathing.

Some clinicians have used heliox (70 percent helium and 30 percent oxygen) to facilitate ventilation in patients with stridor. However, the patient must have a low oxygen requirement if hypoxia is to be avoided.[332] The low density of helium decreases work of breathing. If reintubation of the trachea is required, the endotracheal tube should be at least 0.5 mm smaller than the tube used intraoperatively (or previously in the PICU).

In the setting of a postoperative patient, the possible negative effect of steroids (e.g., on wound healing) needs to be balanced against the possible benefit of steroids on the airway. If tracheal extubation is not possible after several attempts, and there is no other clear etiology for the failure to permanently extubate the trachea, a 48-hour course of steroid therapy may lessen airway edema and allow successful tracheal extubation.

REFERENCES

1. Mathew OP: Maintenance of upper airway patency. J Pediatr 106:863, 1985.
2. Onal E, Lapota M, O'Connor TD: Diaphragmatic and genioglossal electromyogram responses to isocoapnic hypoxia in humans. Am Rev Respir Dis 124:215, 1981.
3. Onal E, Lapota M, O'Connor TD: Diaphragmatic and genioglossal responses to CO_2 rebreathing in humans. J Appl Physiol 50:1052, 1981.
4. Wilson SL, Thach BT, Brouillette RT, Abu-Osba YK: Upper airway patency in the human infant: influence of airway pressure and posture. J Appl Physiol 48:500, 1980.
5. Eckenhoff JE: Some anatomic considerations of the infant larynx influencing endotracheal anesthesia. Anesthesiology 12:401, 1951.
6. Stehling L: Goldenhar syndrome and airway management. Am J Dis Child 132:818, 1978.
7. American Society of Anesthesiologists Task Force on Guidelines for Management of the Difficult Airway: Caplan RA (Chairman): Practice guidelines for management of the difficulty airway. Anesthesiology 78:597, 1993.
8. Maze A, Bloch E: Stridor in pediatric patients. Anesthesiology 50:132, 1979.
9. Crockett DM, McCabe BF, Scamman FL, et al: Venturi jet ventilation for microlaryngoscopy: technique, complications, pitfalls. Laryngoscope 97:1326, 1987.
10. Wilson RS, Putman L, Phillips MT, et al: Anesthetic problems in surgery for varying levels of respiratory obstruction in infants and children. Anesth Analg 53:878, 1974.
11. Berry FA, Tompkins MJ: Anesthesia for congenital anomalies of the head and neck. In Stehling LC, Zauder HL (eds): Anesthetic Implications of Congenital Anomalies in Children. Norwalk, CT, Appleton-Century-Crofts, 1980.
12. McIntyre JWR: Continuing medical education article: the difficult tracheal intubation. Can J Anesthesiol 34:204, 1987.
13. Ravindran R, Stoops CM: Anesthetic management of a patient with Hallermann-Streiff syndrome. Anesth Analg 58:254, 1979.
14. Ross EDT: Treacher Collins syndrome. Anaesthesia 18:350, 1963.
15. Sklar GS, King BD: Endotracheal intubation and Treacher-Collins syndrome. Anesthesiology 44:247, 1976.
16. Divekar VM, Sircar BN: Anesthetic management in Treacher-Collins syndrome. Anesthesiology 26:692, 1965.
17. Feingold M, Baum J: Goldenhar's syndrome. Am J Dis Child 132:136, 1978.
18. Levin RM: Anesthesia for cleft lip and cleft palate. Anesth Rev 6:25, 1979.
19. Rasch DK, Browder F, Barr M, Greer D: Anaesthesia for Treacher Collins and Pierre Robin syndromes: a report of three cases. Can Anesth Soc J 33:364, 1986.
20. Miyabe M, Dohi S, Homma E: Tracheal intubation in an infant with Treacher-Collins syndrome—pulling out the tongue by a forceps. Anesthesiology 62:213, 1985.
21. Populaire C, Lundi JN, Pinaud M, Souron R: Elective tracheal intubation in the prone position for a neonate with Pierre Robin syndrome. Anesthesiology 62:214, 1985.
22. Ferguson S: Moebius syndrome: a review of the anaesthetic implications. Paediatr Anaesth 6:51, 1996.
23. Tobias JD: Anesthetic care for the child with Morquio syndrome: general versus regional anesthesia. J Clin Anesth 11:242, 1999.
24. Finucane BT: Difficult intubation associated with the foetal alcohol syndrome. Can Anaesth Soc J 27:574, 1980.
25. Maydew RP, Berry FA: Cherubism with difficult laryngoscopy and tracheal intubation. Anesthesiology 52:810, 1985.
26. Nargozian C, Ririe DG, Bennun RD, Mulliken JB: Hemifacial microsomia: anatomical prediction of difficult intubation. Paediatr Anaesth 9:393, 1999.
27. Dernedde G, Pendeville P, Veyckemans F, et al: Anaesthetic management of a child with Marshall-Smith syndrome. Can J Anaesth 45:660, 1998.
28. Antila H, Laitio T, Aantaa R, et al: Difficult airway in a patient with Marshall-Smith syndrome. Paediatr Anaesth 8:429, 1998.
29. Weller RM: Anaesthesia for cystic hygroma in a neonate. Anaesthesia 29:588, 1974.
30. MacDonald DJF: Cystic hygroma. Anaesthesia 21:66, 1966.
31. Ovassapian A, Dykes MHM: Difficult pediatric intubation—an indication for the fiberoptic bronchoscope. Anesthesiology 56:412, 1982.
32. Donlon JV: Anesthetic management of patients with compromised airways. Anesth Rev 7:22, 1980.
33. Gross JB, Hartigan ML, Schaffer DW: Suitable substitute for 4% cocaine before blind nasotracheal intubation. Anesth Analg 63:915, 1984.
34. Vandam LD: Functional anatomy of the larynx. Weekly Anesthesiology Update, Lesson 5, 1:1, Princeton, NJ, 1977.
35. Webster AC: Anesthesia for operations on the upper airway. Int Anesthesiol Clin 10:61, 1972.
36. Vuckovic DD, Rooney SM, Goldiner PL, et al: Aerosol anesthesia of the airway using a small disposable nebulizer. Anesth Analg 59:803, 1980.

37. Pelton DA, Daly M, Cooper PD, et al: Plasma lidocaine concentrations following topical aerosol application to the trachea and bronchi. Can Anaesth Soc J 17:250, 1970.

38. Appendix II. *In* Gilman AG, Goodman LS, Gilman A (eds): The Pharmacological Basis of Therapeutics. New York, Macmillan, 1985.

39. Salem MR, Mathrubhuthan M, Bennett EJ: Difficult intubation. N Engl J Med 295:879, 1976.

40. Ament R: A systemic approach to the difficult intubation. Anesthesiol Rev 7:12, 1978.

41. Berry FA: Use of a stylet in blind nasotracheal intubation. Anesthesiology 61:469, 1984.

42. Marquex X, Roxas RS: Induction of anesthesia in an infant with frontonasal dysplasia and meningoencephalocele: a case report. Anesth Analg 56:736, 1977.

43. Rita L, Seleny FL: A new pediatric laryngotracheal spray. Anesth Rev 5:37, 1978.

44. Rosenberg MB, Levesque PR, Bourke DL: Use of the LTA kit as a guide for endotracheal intubation. Anesth Analg 56:287, 1977.

45. Lopez NR: Mechanical problems with the airway. Clin Anesth 3:8, 1968.

46. Audenaert SM, Montgomery CL, Stone B: Retrograde-assisted fiberoptic tracheal intubation in children with difficult airways. Anesth Analg 73:660, 1991.

47. Borland LM, Swan DM, Leff S: Difficult pediatric endobronchial intubation: a new approach to the retrograde technique. Anesthesiology 55:577, 1981.

48. Borland LM, Casselbrant M: The Bullard laryngoscope: a new indirect oral laryngoscope (pediatric version). Anesth Analg 70:105, 1990.

49. Ellis DG, Jakymec A, Kaplan RM, et al: Guided orotracheal intubation in the operating room using a lighted stylet: a comparison with direct laryngoscopic technique. Anesthesiology 64:823, 1986.

50. Holzman RS, Nargosian CD, Florence B: Lightwand intubation in children with abnormal upper airways. Anesthesiology 69:784, 1988.

51. Fox DJ, Matson MD: Management of the difficult pediatric airway in an austere environment using the lightwand. J Clin Anesth 2:123, 1990.

52. Knight RG, Castro T, Rastrelli AJ: Arterial blood pressure and heart rate response to lighted stylet or direct laryngoscopy for endotracheal intubation. Anesthesiology 69:269, 1988.

53. Krucylak CP, Schreiner MS: Orotracheal intubation of an infant with hemifacial microsomia using a modified lighted stylet. Anesthesiology 77:826, 1992.

54. Tahir AH: Use of fiberoptic endoscope in difficult orotracheal intubation. Anesthesiol Rev 3:16, 1976.

55. Finer NN, Muzyka D: Flexible endoscopic intubation of the neonate. Pediatr Pulm 12:48, 1992.

56. Medical Section of the American Lung Association, American Thoracic Society: Flexible endoscopy in the pediatric airway. Am Rev Respir Dis 145:233, 1992.

57. Roth AG, Wheeler M, Stevenson GW: Comparison of the use of a rigid laryngoscope with the ultrathin fiberoptic laryngoscope for intubation of infants. Can J Anaesth 41:1068, 1994.

58. Wood RE, Course Director: Pediatric Flexible Bronchoscopy—A Postgraduate Course. The University of California at Davis and the University of North Carolina at Chapel Hill, September 1986.

59. Rucker RW, Silva WJ, Worcester CC: Fiberoptic bronchoscopic nasotracheal intubation in children. Chest 76:56, 1979.

60. Alfery DD, Ward CF, Harwood IR, Mannino FL: Airway management for a neonate with congenital fusion of the jaws. Anesthesiology 51:340, 1979.

61. Stiles CM: A flexible fiberoptic bronchoscope for endotracheal intubation of infants. Anesth Analg 53:1017, 1974.

62. Selim M, Mowafi H, Alp-Ghamdi A, Adu-Gyamfi Y: Intubation via IMA in pediatric patients with difficult airways. Can J Anesth 46:891, 1999.

63. Hasan MA, Black AE: A new technique for fibreoptic intubation in children. Anaesthesia 49:1031, 1994.

64. Asai T, Fujise K, Uchida M: Use of the laryngeal mask in a child with tracheal stenosis. Anesthesiology 75:903, 1991.

65. Maekawa H, Mikawa K, Tanaka O, et al: The laryngeal mask may be a useful device for fiberoptic airway endoscopy in pediatric anesthesia [letter]. Anesthesiology 75:169, 1991.

66. Walker RW, Murrell D: Yet another use for the laryngeal mask airway [letter]. Anesth Analg 46:591, 1991.

67. Benumof JL: Use of the laryngeal mask airway to facilitate fiberoptic-aided tracheal intubation [letter]. Anesth Analg 74:313, 1992.

68. Silk JM, Hill HM, Calder I: Difficult intubation and the laryngeal mask. Eur J Anaesthesiol 4:47, 1991.

69. Kadota Y, Oda T, Yoshimura N: Application of a laryngeal mask to fiberoptic bronchoscope-aided tracheal intubation [letter]. J Clin Anesth 4:503, 1992.

70. Hasham F, Kumar CM, Lawler PG: The use of the laryngeal mask airway to assist fiberoptic orotracheal intubation [letter]. Anaesthesia 46:891, 1991.

71. McCrirrick A, Pracilio JA: Awake intubation, a new technique. Anaesthesia 46:661, 1991.

72. Smith JE, Sherwood NA: Combined use of the laryngeal mask airway and fiberoptic laryngoscope in difficult intubation [letter]. Anaesth Intensive Care 19:471, 1991.

73. Heath ML: Endotracheal intubation through the laryngeal mask—helpful when laryngoscopy is difficult or dangerous. Eur J Anaesthesiol 4:41, 1991.

74. Heath ML, Allagian J: Intubation through the laryngeal mask. A technique for unexpected difficult intubation. Anaesthesia 46:545 1991.

75. Cohen MM, Cameron CB: Should you cancel the operation when a child has an upper respiratory tract infection? Anesth Analg 72:282, 1991.

76. Tait AR, Knight PR: The effect of general anesthesia on upper respiratory infections in children. Anesthesiology 67:930, 1987.

77. Tait AR, Knight PR: Intraoperative complications in patients with upper respiratory tract infections. Can J Anaesth 34:300, 1987.

78. Schreiner MS, O'Hara I, Markakis DA, Politis GD: Do children who experience laryngospasm have an increased risk of upper respiratory tract infection? Anesthesiology 85:475, 1996.

79. Rolf N, Cote CJ: Frequency and severity of desaturation events during general anesthesia in children with and without upper respiratory infections. J Clin Anesth 4:200, 1992.

80. DeSoto H, Patel RI, Soliman IE, Hannallah RS: Changes in oxygen saturation following general anesthesia in children with upper respiratory infection signs and symptoms undergoing otolaryngological procedures. Anesthesiology 68:276, 1988.

81. Horner GJ, Gray FD: Effect of uncomplicated presumptive influenza on the diffusing capacity of the lung. Am Rev Respir Dis 108:866, 1973.

82. Picken JJ, Niewohner DE, Chester EH: Prolonged effects of viral infections of the upper respiratory tract upon small airways. Am J Med 52:738, 1972.

83. Hall WJ, Douglas RG Jr, Hyde RW, et al: Pulmonary mechanics after uncomplicated influenza A infection. Am Rev Respir Dis 113:141, 1976.

84. Fridy WW, Ingram RH, Hierholzer JC, Coleman MT: Airways function during mild viral respiratory illnesses. Ann Intern Med 80:150, 1974.

85. Dueck R, Prutow R, Richman D: Effect of parainfluenza infection on gas exchange and FRC response to anesthesia in sheep. Anesthesiology 74:1044, 1991.

86. Kinouchi K, Tanigami H, Tashiro C, et al: Duration of apnea in anesthetized infants and children required for desaturation of hemoglobin to 95%. Anesthesiology 77:1105, 1992.

87. Collier AM, Pimmel PL, Hasselblad V: Spirometric changes in normal children with upper respiratory infections. Am Rev Respir Dis 117:47, 1978.

88. McGill WA, Coveler LA, Epstein BS: Subacute upper respiratory infection in small children. Anesth Analg 58:331, 1979.

89. Williams OA, Hills R, Goddard JM: Pulmonary collapse during anaesthesia in children with respiratory tract symptoms. Anaesthesia 47:411, 1992.

90. Campbell NN: Respiratory tract infection and anaesthesia. Anaesthesia 45:561, 1990.

91. Rolf N, Cote CJ: Frequency and severity of desaturation events during general anesthesia in children with and without upper respiratory infections. J Clin Anesth 4:200, 1992.

92. Bickler PE, Dueck R, Prutdow RJ: Effects of barbiturate anesthesia on functional residual capacity and ribcage/diaphragm contributions to ventilation. Anesthesiology 66:147, 1987.

93. Aquilina AT, Hall WJ, Douglas RG, Utell MJ: Airway reactivity in subjects with viral upper respiratory infections: the effects of exercise and cold. Am Rev Respir Dis 122:3, 1980.

94. Fryer AD, Maclagan J: Muscarinic inhibitory receptors in parasympathetic nerves in the guinea pig. Br J Pharmacol 83:973, 1984.

95. Saban R, Dick EC, Fishleder RI, Buckner CK: Enhancement by parainfluenza 3 infection of contractile responses to substances P and capsaicin in airway smooth muscle from the guinea pig. Am Rev Respir Dis 136:586, 1987.

96. Fryer AD, El-Fakahany EE, Jacoby DB: Parainfluenza virus type 1 reduces the affinity of agonists for muscarinic receptors in guinea-pig lung and heart. Eur J Pharmacol 181:51, 1990.

97. Empey DW, Laitinen LA, Jacobs L, et al: Mechanisms of bronchial hyperreactivity in normal subjects after upper respiratory tract infections. Am Rev Respir Dis 113:131, 1976.

98. Nandwani N, Raphael JH, Langton JA: Effect of an upper respiratory tract infection on upper airway reactivity. Br J Anaesth 78:352, 1997.

99. Paradise JL: Otitis media in infants and children. Pediatrics 65:917, 1980.

100. Markowitz-Spence L, Brodsky L, Syed N, et al: Anesthetic complications of tympanostomy tube placement in children. Arch Otolaryngol Head Neck Surg 116:809, 1990.

101. Patterson ME, Bartlett PC: Hearing impairment caused by intratympanic pressure changes during general anesthesia. Laryngoscope 86:399, 1976.

102. Davies DW, Steward DJ: Unexpected excessive bleeding during operation: role of acetylsalicylic acid. Can Anaesth Soc J 24:452, 1977.

103. Berry FA: Post-tonsillectomy bleeding. In Stehling LC (ed): Common Problems in Pediatric Anesthesia. Chicago, Year Book Medical Publishers, 1982, p 246.

104. Tom LWC, DeDio RM, Cohen DE, et al: Is outpatient tonsillectomy appropriate for young children? Laryngoscope 102:277, 1992.

105. McColley SA, April MM, Carroll JL, et al: Respiratory compromise after adenotonsillectomy in children with obstructive sleep apnea. Arch Otolaryngol Head Neck Surg 118:940, 1992.

106. Brown OE, Manning SC, Ridenour B: Cor pulmonale secondary to tonsillar and adenoidal hypertrophy: management considerations. Int J Pediatr Otorhinolaryngol 16:131, 1988.

107. Doull IJ, Mok Q, Tasker RC: Tracheobronchomalacia in preterm infants with chronic lung disease. Arch Dis Child Fetal Neonatal Ed 76:F203, 1997.

108. Narcy P, Contencin P, Viala P: Surgical treatment for laryngeal paralysis in infants and children. Ann Otol Rhinol Laryngol 99:124, 1990.

109. Shinkwin CA, Gibbin KP: Tracheostomy in children. J R Soc Med 89:4:188, 1996.

110. Kenna MA, Reilly JS, Stool SE: Tracheotomy in the preterm infant. Ann Otol Rhinol Laryngol 98:68, 1987.

111. Markus NJ, Schild JA, Holinger PH: Tracheostomy in the first year of life. Trans Am Acad Ophthalmol Otol 82:466, 1976.

112. Gibson R, Byrne JET: Tracheotomy in neonates. Laryngoscope 82:643, 1972.

113. Ryan M, Hunt M, Snowberger T: A changing pattern of epiglottitis. Clin Pediatr 21:532, 1992.

114. Phillips-Emmerson SG, Richman B, Spahn T: Changing patterns of epiglottitis in children. Otolaryngol Head Neck Surg 104:287, 1991.

115. Lee AK, Crutcher JM: Oklahoma notes decline in Haemophilus influenzae: invasive Haemophilus influenzae disease among children aged <5 years—Oklahoma, 1990–1997. J Okla State Med Assoc 92:276, 1999.

116. Centers for Disease Control and Prevention: Haemophilus influenzae invasive disease among children aged <5 years—California, 1990–1996. MMWR Morb Mortal Wkly Rep 47:737, 1998.

117. Hickerson SL, Kirby RS, Wheeler JG, Schutze GE: Epiglottitis: a 9-year case review. South Med J 89:487, 1996.

118. Peltola H: Haemophilus influenzae type b disease and vaccination in Europe: lessons learned. Pediatr Infect Dis J 17(Suppl):S126, 1998.

119. Schwam E, Cox J: Fulminant meningococcal supraglottitis: an emerging infectious syndrome? Emerg Infect Dis 5:464, 1999.

120. Wenger JK: Supraglottitis and group A Streptococcus. Pediatr Infect Dis J 16:1005, 1997.

121. Gonzalez Valdepena H, Wald ER, Rose E, et al: Epiglottitis and Haemophilus influenzae immunization: the Pittsburgh experience—a five-year review. Pediatrics 96:424, 1995.

122. Madore DV: Impact of immunization on Haemophilus influenzae type b disease. Infect Agents Dis 5:8, 1996.

123. Centers for Disease Control and Prevention: Haemophilus influenzae invasive disease among children aged <5 years—California, 1990–1996. MMWR Morb Mortal Wkly Rep 47:737, 1998.

124. Crockett DM, McGill TJ, Healy GB, Friedman EM: Airway management of acute supraglottitis at the Children's Hospital, Boston, 1980–1985. Ann Otol Rhinol Laryngol 97:114, 1988.

125. Spalding MB, Ala-Kokko TI: The use of inhaled sevoflurane for endotracheal intubation in epiglottitis. Anesthesiology 89:1025, 1998.

126. Hawkins DB: Hyaline membrane disease of the neonate, prolonged intubation in the management and effects on the larynx. Laryngoscope 88:201, 1978.

127. Pransky SM, Grundfast KM: Differentiating upper from lower airway components in neonates. Ann Otol Rhinol Laryngol 94:509, 1985.

128. Cotton RT, Seid AB: Management of the extubation problem in the premature child. Ann Otol Rhinol Laryngol 89:508, 1980.

129. Grundfast KM, Coffman AC, Milmoe G: Anterior cricoid split: a "simple" surgical procedure and a potentially complicated care problem. Ann Otol Rhinol Laryngol 94:445, 1985.

130. Cotton RT: Prevention and management of laryngeal stenosis in infants and children. J Pediatr Surg 20:845, 1985.

131. Cotton RT, Myers CM: Contemporary surgical management of laryngeal stenosis in children. Am J Otolaryngol 5:360, 1984.

132. Cotton RT: Management of subglottic stenosis in infancy and childhood: review of a consecutive series of cases managed by surgical reconstruction. Ann Otol 87:649, 1978.

133. Healy GB: An experimental model for the endoscopic correction of subglottic stenosis with clinical applications. Laryngoscope 92:1103, 1982.

134. Morgenstein KM: Composite auricular graft in laryngeal reconstruction. Laryngoscope 82:844, 1972.

135. Toohil RJ: Composite nasal septal graft in the management of advanced laryngotracheal stenosis. Laryngoscope 91:233, 1981.

136. Grundfast KM, Morris MS, Bernsley C: Subglottic stenosis: retrospective analysis and proposal for standard reporting system. Ann Otol Rhinol Laryngol 96:101, 1987.

137. Kanchanarak C, Waisayanand C: Thyrotracheal anastomosis in children: 1989–1996. J Otolaryngol 27:132, 1998.

138. Monnier P, Lang F, Savary M: Partial cricotracheal resection for severe pediatric subglottic stenosis: update of the Lausanne experience. Ann Otol Rhinol Laryngol 107(11 pt 1):961, 1998.

139. Thome R, Thome DC: Posterior cricoidotomy lumen augmentation for treatment of subglottic stenosis in children. Arch Otolaryngol Head Neck Surg 124:660, 1998.

140. Stern Y, Gerber ME, Walner DL, Cotton RT: Partial cricotracheal resection with primary anastomosis in the pediatric age group. Ann Otol Rhinol Laryngol 106:891, 1997.

141. Lines V: Anaesthesia for laryngoscopy and microlaryngeal surgery in children. Anaesth Intensive Care 1:507, 1973.

142. Holinger LD: Etiology of stridor in the neonate, infant and child. Ann Otol 89:397, 1980.

143. Johnson DG: Bronchoscopy. In Welch KJ, Randolph JG, Ravitch MM, et al (eds): Pediatric Surgery. 4th ed. Chicago, Year Book Medical Publishers, 1986, p 619.

144. Rosenfield NS, Peck DR, Lowman RM: Xeroradiography in the evaluation of acquired airway abnormalities in children. Am J Dis Child 132:1177, 1978.

145. Joseph PM, Berdon WE, Baker DH, et al: Upper airway obstruction in infants and small children. Pediatr Radiol 121:143, 1976.

146. Sloan IAJ, McLeod ME: Evaluation of the jet injector in paediatric fiberoptic bronchoscopes. Can Anesth Soc J 32:79, 1985.

147. Miyasaka K, Sloan IA, Foroese AB: An evaluation of the jet injector (Sanders) technique for bronchoscopy in paediatric patients. Can Anaesth Soc J 27:117, 1980.

148. Woods AM: Pediatric endoscopy. In Berry FA (ed): Anesthetic Management of Difficult and Routine Pediatric Patients. 2nd ed. New York, Churchill Livingstone, 1990.

149. Widlund B, Walczak S, Motoyama E: Flow-pressure characteristics of pediatric Storz-Hopkins bronchoscopes. Anesthesiology 57: A417, 1982.

150. Woods AM, Gal TJ: Decreasing airflow resistance during infant and pediatric bronchoscopy. Anaesth Analg 66:457, 1987.

151. Gallagher MJ, Muller BJ: Tension pneumothorax during pediatric bronchoscopy. Anesthesiology 55:685, 1981.

152. Ward CF, Benumof JL: Anesthesia for airway foreign body extraction in children. Anesth Rev 4:13, 1977.
153. Baraka A: Bronchoscopic removal of inhaled foreign bodies in children. Br J Anaesth 46:124, 1974.
154. Kim IG, Brummitt WM, Humphry A, et al: Foreign body in the airway: a review of 202 cases. Laryngoscope 83:347, 1973.
155. Hawkins DB, Kahlstrom EJ, MacLaughlin EF, et al: Foreign bodies of the right nostril and left bronchus. Pediatrics 59:303, 1977.
156. Tariq M, Beg MH: A foreign body in the bronchus still presents problems. Int J Clin Pract 53:81, 1999.
157. Blazer S, Naveh Y, Fredman A: Foreign body in the airway. Am J Dis Child 134:68, 1980.
158. Pyman C: Inhaled foreign bodies in children: a review of 230 cases. Med J Aust 1:62, 1971.
159. Hachimi-Idrissi S, Corne L, Vandenplas Y: Management of ingested foreign bodies in childhood: our experience and review of the literature. Eur J Emerg Med 5:319, 1998.
160. Cataneo AJ, Reibscheid SM, Ruiz Junior RL, Ferrari GF: Foreign body in the tracheobronchial tree. Clin Pediatr 36:701, 1997.
161. Law D, Kosloske AM: Management of tracheobronchial foreign bodies in children: a reevaluation of postural drainage and bronchoscopy. Pediatrics 58:362, 1976.
162. Lifschultz BD, Donoghue ER: Deaths due to foreign body aspiration in children: the continuing hazard of toy balloons. J Forensic Sci 41:247, 1996.
163. Rimell FL, Thome A Jr, Stool S, et al: Characteristics of objects that cause choking in children. JAMA 274:1763, 1995.
164. Greensheer J, Holroyd JH: Aspiration of newer radiopaque plastic parts. Am Acad Pediatr News 4:3, 1984.
165. Bodart E, de Bilderling G, Tuerlinckx D, Gillet JB: Foreign body aspiration in childhood: management algorithm. Eur J Emerg Med 6:21, 1999.
166. Esclamado RM, Richardson MA: Laryngotracheal foreign bodies in children. Am J Dis Child 141:259, 1987.
167. Burton EM, Brick WG, Hall JD, et al: Tracheobronchial foreign body aspiration in children. South Med J 89:195, 1996.
168. Metrangelo S, Monetti C, Meneghini L, et al: Eight years' experience with foreign-body aspiration in children: what is really important for a timely diagnosis? J Pediatr Surg 34:1229, 1999.
169. Fitzpatrick PC, Guarisco JL: Pediatric airway foreign bodies. J La State Med Soc 150:138, 1998.
170. Gilchrist BF, Valerie EP, Nguyen M, et al: Pearls and perils in the management of prolonged, peculiar, penetrating esophageal foreign bodies in children. Pediatr Surg 32:1429, 1997.
171. Cataneo AJ, Reibscheid SM, Ruiz Junior RL, Ferrari GF: Foreign body in the tracheobronchial tree. Clin Pediatr 36:701, 1997.
172. Daniilidis J, Symeonidis B, Triandis K, Kouloulas A: Foreign body in the airways. Arch Otolaryngol 103:570, 1977.
173. Zarella JT, Dimler M, McGill LC, Pippus KJ: Foreign body aspiration in children: value of radiography and complications of bronchoscopy. J Pediatr Surg 33:1651, 1998.
174. Silva AB, Muntz HR, Clary R: Utility of conventional radiography in the diagnosis and management of pediatric airway foreign bodies. Ann Otol Rhinol Laryngol 107:834, 1998.
175. Healy GB: Foreign bodies of the air and food passages in children. Am J Dis Child 141:249, 1987.
176. Young LW, Seibert RW, Seibert JJ: Radiological case of the month. Am J Dis Child 133:749, 1979.
177. Esclamado RM, Ricardson MA: Laryngotracheal foreign bodies in children. J Dis Child 141:259, 1989.
178. Causey AL, Talton DS, Miller RC, Warren ET: Aspirated safety pin requiring thoracotomy: report of a case and review. Pediatr Emerg Care 13:397, 1997.
179. Hawkind DB: Corticosteroids in the management of laryngotracheobronchitis. Otolaryngol Head Neck Surg 88:207, 1980.
180. Koka BV, Jeon IS, Andre JM, et al: Postintubation croup in children. Anesth Analg 56:501, 1977.
181. Downes JJ, Godinez RI: Acute upper-airway obstruction in children. In Hershey SG (ed): ASA Refresher Courses in Anesthesiology. No. 8. Philadelphia, JB Lippincott, 1980, p 29.
182. Prakash UB, Midthun DE, Edell ES: Indications for flexible versus rigid bronchoscopy in children with suspected foreign-body aspiration. Am J Respir Crit Care Med 156 (3 pt 1):1017, 1997.
183. Godfrey S, Avital A, Maayan C, et al: Yield from flexible bronchoscopy in children. Pediatr Pulmonol 23:261, 1997.
184. Martinot A, Closset M, Marquette CH, et al: Indications for flexible versus rigid bronchoscopy in children with suspected foreign-body aspiration. Am J Respir Crit Care Med 155:1676, 1997.
185. Kim JK, Kim SS, Kim JI, et al: Management of foreign bodies in the gastrointestinal tract: an analysis of 104 cases in children. Endoscopy 31:302, 1999.
186. Healy GB, McGill T, Simpson GT, et al: The use of carbon dioxide laser in the pediatric airway. J Pediatr Surg 14:735, 1979.
187. Snow JC, Kripke BJ, Strong MS, et al: Anesthesia for carbon dioxide laser microsurgery on the larynx and trachea. Anesth Analg 53:507, 1974.
188. Kalhan SB, Cascorbi HF: Anesthetic management of laser microlaryngeal surgery. Anesth Rev 8:23, 1981.
189. Healy GB, McGill T, Strong S: Surgical advances in the treatment of lesions of the pediatric airway: the role of carbon dioxide laser. Pediatrics 61:380, 1978.
190. Hermans JM, Bennett MJ, Hirshman CA: Anesthesia for laser surgery. Anesth Analg 62:218, 1983.
191. Ganfield RA, Chapin JW: Pneumothorax with upper airway laser surgery. Anesthesiology 56:398, 1982.
192. Sliney DH: Laser safety. Lasers Surg Med 16:215, 1995.
193. Hirshman CA, Leon D, Porch D, et al: Improved metal endotracheal tube for laser surgery of the airway. Anesth Analg 59:789, 1980.
194. Cozine K, Stone JG, Shulman S: Ventilatory complications of carbon dioxide laryngeal surgery. J Clin Anesth 3:20, 1991.
195. Kaeder CS, Hirshman CA: Acute airway obstruction: a complication of aluminum tape wrapping of tracheal tubes in laser surgery. Can Anaesth Soc J 26:138, 1979.
196. Sosis MB: Evaluation of five metallic tapes for protection of endotracheal tubes during carbon dioxide laser surgery. Anesth Analg 68:392, 1989.
197. Sosis MB, Braverman B: Evaluation of foil coverings for protecting plastic endotracheal tubes from the potassium-titanyl-phosphate laser. Anesth Analg 77:589, 1993.
198. Snow JC, Norton ML, Saluga TS, et al: Fire hazard during CO_2 laser microsurgery on the larynx and trachea. Anesth Analg 55:146, 1976.
199. Pashayan AG, Gravenstein JS: Helium retards endotracheal tube fires from carbon dioxide lasers. Anesthesiology 62:274, 1985.
200. Simpson JI, Schiff GA, Wolf GL: The effect of helium on endotracheal tube flammability. Anesthesiology 73:538, 1990.
201. Wolf GL, Simpson JI: Flammability of endotracheal tubes in oxygen and nitrous oxide enriched atmospheres. Anesthesiology 67:236, 1987.
202. Sosis MB: Which is the safest endotracheal tube use with the CO_2 laser? A comparative study. J Clin Anesth 4:217, 1992.
203. Torres LE, Reynolds RC: Experiences with a new endotracheal tube for microlaryngeal surgery. Anesthesiology 52:357, 1980.
204. Gross G: Therapy of human papilloma virus infection and associated epithelial tumors. Intervirology 40:368, 1997.
205. Brooker CR, Hunsaker DH, Zimmerman AA: A new anesthetic system for microlaryngeal surgery. Otolaryngol Head Neck Surg 118:55, 1998.
206. Bergler W, Honig M, Gotte K, et al: Treatment of recurrent respiratory papillomatosis with argon plasma coagulation. J Laryngol Otol 111:381, 1997.
207. Rimell FL, Shoemaker DL, Pou AM, et al: Pediatric respiratory papillomatosis: prognosis of viral typing and cofactors. Laryngoscope 107:915, 1997.
208. Shapiro AM, Mimmell FL, Shoemaker D, et al: Tracheotomy in children with juvenile-onset recurrent respiratory papillomatosis: the Children's Hospital of Pittsburgh experience. Ann Otol Rhinol Laryngol 105:1, 1996.
209. Hawkins DB, Udall JN: Juvenile laryngeal papillomas with cardiomegaly and polycythemia. Pediatrics 63:156, 1979.
210. Leon DA, Hirshman CA: Pediatric laser microsurgery: some problems and solutions. Anesthesiology S53:344, 1980.
211. Theroux MC, Grodecki V, Reilly JS, Kettreick RG: Juvenile laryngeal papillomatosis: scary anaesthetic! Paediatr Anaesth 8:357, 1998.
212. Weinstein GW, Raju VK, Schwab L, et al: Normal growth and development. In Key Facts in Ophthalmology. New York, Churchill Livingstone, 1984, p 16.
213. Aboul-Eish E: Physiology of the eye pertinent to anesthesia. In Smith RB (ed): Anesthesia in Ophthalmology. Vol 13. Ophthalmology Clinics. Boston, Little, Brown, 1973, p 1.

214. Joshi C, Bruce DL: Thiopental and succinylcholine: action on intraocular pressure. Anesth Analg 54:471, 1975.

215. Duncalf D, Weitzner SW: Ventilation and hypercapnia on intraocular pressure during anesthesia. Anesth Analg 42:232, 1963.

216. Ausinsch B, Graves SA, Munson ES, Levy NS: Intraocular pressure in children during isoflurane and halothane anesthesia. Anesthesiology 42:167, 1975.

217. Cunningham AJ, Barry P: Intraocular pressure—physiology and implications for anaesthetic management. Can Anaesth Soc J 33:195, 1986.

218. Corssen G, Hoy JE: A new parenteral anesthetic—CI-581: its effect on intraocular pressure. J Pediatr Ophthalmol 4:20, 1967.

219. Yoshikawa K, Murai Y: The effect of ketamine on intraocular pressure in children. Anesth Analg 50:199, 1971.

220. Peuler M, Glass DD, Arens JF: Ketamine and intraocular pressure. Anesthesiology 43:575, 1975.

221. Ausinsch B, Rayburn RL, Munson ES, Levy NS: Ketamine and intraocular pressure in children. Anesth Analg 55:773, 1976.

222. Litwiller RW, Difazio CA, Rushia EL: Pancuronium and intraocular pressure. Anesthesiology 42:750, 1975.

223. Donlon JV: Anesthesia factors affecting intraocular pressure. Anesthesiol Rev 8:13, 1981.

224. Miller RD, Way WL, Hickey RF: Inhibition of succinylcholine-induced increased intraocular pressure by nondepolarizing muscle relaxants. Anesthesiology 29:123, 1968.

225. Meyers EF, Krupin T, Johnson M, Zink H: Failure of non-depolarizing neuromuscular blockers to inhibit succinylcholine-induced increased intraocular pressure, a controlled study. Anesthesiology 48:149, 1978.

226. Warner LO, Balch DR, Davidson PJ: Is intravenous lidocaine an effective adjuvant for endotracheal intubation in children undergoing induction of anesthesia with halothane-nitrous oxide? J Clin Anesth 9:270, 1997.

227. Vinik HR: Intraocular pressure changes during rapid sequence induction and intubation: a comparison of rocuronium, atracurium, and succinylcholine. J Clin Anesth 11:95, 1999.

228. Borromeo-McGrail V, Bordiuik JM, Keitel H: Systemic hypertension following ocular administration of 10% phenylephrine in the neonate. Pediatrics 51:1032, 1973.

229. Solosko D, Smith RB: Hypertension following 10 percent phenylephrine ophthalmic. Anesthesiology 36:187, 1972.

230. Blanc VF, Hardy JF, Milot J, Jacob JL: The oculocardiac reflex: a graphic and statistical analysis in infants and children. Can Anaesth Soc J 30:36, 1983.

231. Ates Y, Alanoglu Z, Uysalel A: Use of the laryngeal mask airway during ophthalmic surgery results in stable circulation and few complications: a prospective audit. Acta Anaesthesiol Scand 42:1180, 1998.

232. McCarthy TV, Healy JMS, Heffron JJA, et al: Localization of the malignant hyperthermia susceptibility locus to human chromosome 19q12-13.2. Nature 343:562, 1990.

233. Gillard E, Otsu K, Lfujii J, et al: A substitution in the human skeletal muscle calcium release channel cosegregates with malignant hyperthermia. Anesth Analg 75:441, 1992.

234. Fujii J, Otsu K, Zorzato F, et al: Identification of a mutation in porcine ryanodine receptor associated with malignant hyperthermia. Science 253:448, 1991.

235. Deufel T, Golla A, Iles D, et al: Evidence for genetic heterogeneity of malignant hyperthermia susceptibility. Am J Hum Genet 50:1151, 1992.

236. Stewart SL, Rosenberg H, Fletcher JE: Failure to identify the ryanodine receptor G1021A mutation in a large North American population with malignant hyperthermia. Clin Genet 54:358, 1998.

237. Serfas KD, Bose D, Patel L, et al: Comparison of the segregation of the RYR1 C1840T mutation with the segregation of the caffeine/halothane contracture test results for malignant hyperthermia susceptibility in a large Manitoba Mennonite family. Anesthesiology 84:322, 1996.

238. Vita GM, Olckers A, Jedlicka AE, et al: Masseter muscle rigidity associated with glycine 1306-to-alanine mutation in the adult muscle sodium channel alpha-subunit gene. Anesthesiology 82:1097, 1995.

239. Britt BA: Malignant hyperthermia: a pharmacogenetic disease of skeletal and cardiac muscle. N Engl J Med 290:1140, 1974.

240. Larach MG, Rosenberg H, Gronert GA, Allen GC: Hyperkalemic cardiac arrest during anesthesia in infants and children with occult myopathies. Clin Pediatr 36:9, 1997.

241. Pedrozzi NE, Ramelli GP, Tomasetti R, et al: Rhabdomyolysis and anesthesia: a report of two cases and review of the literature. Pediatr Neurol 15:254, 1996.

242. Bendixen D, Skovgaard LT, Ording H: Analysis of anaesthesia in patients suspected to be susceptible to malignant hyperthermia before diagnostic in vitro contracture test. Acta Anaesthesiol Scand 41:480, 1997.

243. MacLennan DH, Phillips MS: Malignant hyperthermia. Science 256:789, 1992.

244. Rosenberg H, Gletcher JE: Masseter muscle rigidity and malignant hyperthermia susceptibility. Anesth Analg 65:161, 1986.

245. Allen GC, Brubaker CL: Human malignant hyperthermia associated with desflurane anesthesia. Anesth Analg 86:1328, 1998.

246. Albrecht A, Wedel DJ, Gronert GA: Masseter muscle rigidity and nondepolarizing neuromuscular blocking agents. Mayo Clin Proc 72:329, 1997.

247. McKenzie AJ, Couchman KG, Pollock N: Propofol is a safe anesthetic agent in malignant hyperthermia susceptible patients. Anaesth Intensive Care 20:165, 1992.

248. Fruen BR, Mickelson JR, Roghair TJ, et al: Effects of propofol on Ca2+ regulation by malignant hyperthermia-susceptible muscle membranes. Anesthesiology 82:1274, 1995.

249. Louis CF, Zualkernan K, Roghair T, Mickelson JR: The effects of volatile anesthetics on calcium regulation by malignant hyperthermia-susceptible sarcoplasmic reticulum. Anesthesiology 77:114, 1992.

250. Price SR, Currie J: Anesthesia for a child with centronuclear myopathy. Pediatr Anaesth 5:1155, 1995.

251. Cheam EW, Critchley LA: Anesthesia for a child with complex I respiratory chain enzyme deficiency. J Clin Anesth 10:524, 1998.

252. Hardy JF, Charest J, Girouard G, Lepage Y: Nausea and vomiting after strabismus surgery in preschool children. Can Anaesth Soc J 33:57, 1986.

253. Cohen MM, Cameron CB, Duncan PG: Pediatric anesthesia morbidity and mortality in the perioperative period. Anesth Analg 70:160, 1990.

254. Karlsson E, Larsson LE, Nilsson K: Postanaesthetic nausea in children. Acta Anaesthesiol Scand 34:515, 1990.

255. Chisakuta AM, Mirakhur RK: Anticholinergic prophylaxis does not prevent emesis following strabismus surgery in children. Paediatr Anaesth 5:97, 1995.

256. Watca MF, Simeon RM, White PF, Stevens JL: Effect of propofol on the incidence of postoperative vomiting after strabismus surgery in pediatric outpatients. Anesthesiology 75:204, 1991.

257. Serin S, Elibol O, Sungurtekin H, Gonullu M: Comparison of halothane/thiopental and propofol anesthesia for strabismus surgery. Ophthalmologica 213:224, 1999.

258. Standl T, Wilhelm S, von Knobelsdorff G, Schulte am Esch J: Propofol reduces emesis after sufentanil supplemented anaesthesia in paediatric squint surgery. Acta Anaesthesiol Scand 40:729, 1996.

259. Humunen K, Vaalamo MO, Maunuksela EL: Does propofol reduce vomiting after strabismus surgery in children? Acta Anaesthesiol Scand 41:973, 1990.

260. Stewart DJ: Cancer therapy, vomiting, and antiemetics. Can J Physiol Pharmacol 68:304, 1990.

261. Sanger GJ: New antiemetic drugs. Can J Physiol Pharmacol 68:314, 1990.

262. Abramowitz MD, Oh TH, Epstein BS, et al: The antiemetic effect of droperidol following outpatient strabismus surgery in children. Anesthesiology 59:579, 1983.

263. Lerman J, Eustis S, Smith DR: Effect of droperidol pretreatment on postanesthetic vomiting in children undergoing strabismus surgery. Anesthesiology 65:322, 1986.

264. Broadman LM, Ceruzzi W, Patane PS, et al: Metoclopramide reduces the incidence of vomiting following strabismus surgery in children. Anesthesiology 72:245, 1990.

265. Lin DM, Furst SR, Rodarte A: A double-blinded comparison of metoclopramide and droperidol for prevention of emesis following strabismus surgery. Anesthesiology 76:357, 1992.

266. Munro HM, D'Errico CC, Lauder GR, et al: Oral granisetron for strabismus surgery in children. Can J Anaesth 46:45, 1999.

267. Shende D, Mandal NG: Efficacy of ondansetron and metoclopramide for preventing postoperative emesis following strabismus surgery in children. Anaesthesia 52:496, 1997.

268. Lawhorn CD, Kymer PJ, Stewart FC, et al: Ondansetron dose response curve in high-risk pediatric patients. J Clin Anesth 9:637, 1997.
269. Fujii Y, Saitoh Y, Tanaka H, Toyooka H: Combination of granisetron and droperidol for the prevention of vomiting after paediatric strabismus surgery. Paediatr Anaesth 9:329, 1999.
270. France NK, France TD, Woodburg JD: Succinylcholine alteration of the forced duction test. Ophthalmology 87:1282, 1980.
271. Smith RB, Douglas H, Petruscak J: Safety of intraocular adrenaline with halothane anaesthesia. Br J Anaesth 44:1314, 1972.
272. Karl HW, Swedlow DB, Lee KW: Epinephrine-halothane interactions in children. Anesthesiology 58:142, 1983.
273. Brett CM, Wara WWM, Hamilton WK: Anesthesia for infants during radiotherapy: an insufflation technique. Anesthesiology 64:402, 1986.
274. Scott JG, Allan D: Anaesthesia for dentistry in children; a review of 101 surgical procedures. Can Anaesth Soc J 17:391, 1970.
275. Vermeulen M, Vinckier F, Vandenbroucke J: Dental general anesthesia: clinical characteristics of 933 patients. J Dent Child 58:27, 1991.
276. Granoff DM, McDaniel DB, Borkowf SP: Cardiorespiratory arrest following aspiration of chloral hydrate. Am J Dis Child 122:170, 1971.
277. Aubuchon RW: Sedation liabilities in pedidontics. Pediatr Dent 4:171, 1982.
278. Goodson JM, Moore PA: Life threatening reactions after pediatric sedation: an assessment of narcotic, local anesthetic, and antiemetic drug interaction. J Am Dent Assoc 107:329, 1983.
279. Weis FR, Cho CH: Ketamine for induction of anesthesia in the severely retarded. Anesthesiol Rev 4:35, 1977.
280. Sobczak OM: Use of ketamine in pediatric dentistry. Anesth Analg 54:248, 1975.
281. Celesia GG, Chen R, Bamforth BJ: Effects of ketamine in epilepsy. Neurology 25:169, 1975.
282. Maurer HM, McCue CM, Robertson LW, et al: Correction of platelet dysfunction and bleeding in cyanotic congenital heart disease by simple red cell volume reduction. Am J Cardiol 35:831, 1975.
283. Ekert H, Sheers M: Preoperative and postoperative platelet function in cyanotic congenital heart disease. J Thorac Cardiovasc Surg 67:184, 1974.
284. Moore RA: Anesthesia for the pediatric congenital heart patient for noncardiac surgery. Anesthesiol Rev 8:23, 1981.
285. Berry FA, Yarbrough S, Yarbrough N, et al: Transient bacteremia during dental manipulation in children. Pediatrics 51:476, 1973.
286. Berry FA, Blankenbaker WL, Ball CG: A comparison of bacteremia occurring with nasotracheal or orotracheal intubation. Anesth Analg 52:873, 1973.
287. Shulman ST, Amren DP, Bisno AL: Prevention of bacterial endocarditis. Am J Dis Child 139:232, 1985.
288. Kaplan EL, Rich H, Gersony W, et al: A collaborative study of infective endocarditis in the 1970's. Circulation 59:327, 1979.
289. Johnson CM, Rhodes KH: Pediatric endocarditis. Mayo Clin Proc 57:85, 1982.
290. Dajani AS, Bisno AL, Chung KJ, et al: Prevention of bacterial endocarditis. Recommendations by the American Heart Association. JAMA 264:2919, 1990.
291. Bell JM: Dental anesthesia in children. Anaesth Intensive Care 1:540, 1973.
292. Boralessa H, Holdcroft A: Methohexitone or etomidate for induction of dental anaesthesia. Can Anaesth Soc J 27:578, 1980.
293. Berkowitz RJ, Smith RM: Anesthesia for dentistry in children. In Smith RB (ed): Anesthesia for Infants and Children. St Louis, CV Mosby, 1980.
294. American Academy of Pediatrics, Committee on Drugs: Guidelines for monitoring and management of pediatric patients during and after sedation for diagnostic and therapeutic procedures. Pediatrics 89:1110, 1992.
295. Committee on Drugs, Section on Anesthesiology, American Academy of Pediatrics: Guidelines for the elective use of conscious sedation, deep sedation, and general anesthesia in pediatric patients. Pediatrics 76:317, 1985.
296. Cote CJ: Sedation for the pediatric patient. A review. Pediatr Clin North Am 41:31, 1994.
297. Coté CJ: Monitoring guidelines: Do they make a difference? AJR Am J Roentgenol 165:910, 1995.
298. Thurlow AC: Cardiac dysrhythmias in outpatient dental anaesthesia in children. Anaesthesia 27:429, 1972.
299. Thurlow AC: Cardiac dysrhythmias during minor oral surgery in children. In Abstracts of Scientific Papers, ASA Annual Meeting, 1976.
300. Plowman PE, Thomas WJW, Thurlow AC: Cardiac dysrhythmias during anesthesia for oral surgery. Anaesthesia 29:571, 1974.
301. Rollason WN, Hall DJ: Dysrhythmias during inhalational anesthesia for oral surgery. Anaesthesia 28:139, 1973.
302. Miller JR, Redish CH, Fisch C, et al: Factors in arrhythmias during dental outpatient general anesthesia. Anesth Analg 49:701, 1970.
303. Rosenberg MB, Wunderlich BK, Reynolds RN: Iatrogenic subcutaneous emphysema during dental anesthesia. Anesthesiology 51:80, 1979.
304. Milne B, Katz H, Rosales J, et al: Subcutaneous facial emphysema complicating dental anesthesia. Can Anaesth Soc J 29:71, 1982.
305. Trummer MJ, Fosburg RG: Mediastinal emphysema following use of high-speed air-turbine dental drill. Ann Thorac Surg 9:378, 1970.
306. Hunt RB, Sahler OD: Mediastinal emphysema produced by air turbine-dental drills. JAMA 205:101, 1968.
307. Rex M: A review of the structural and functional basis of laryngospasm and discussion of the nerve pathways involved in the reflex and its clinical significance in man and animals. Br J Anaesth 42:891, 1970.
308. Olsson GL, Hallen B: Laryngospasm during anaesthesia. A computer-aided incidence study in 136,929 patients. Acta Anaesthesiol Scand 28:567, 1984.
309. Tait AR, Pandit UA, Voepel-Lewis T, et al: Use of the laryngeal mask airway in children with upper respiratory tract infections: a comparison with endotracheal intubation. Anesth Analg 86:706, 1998.
310. Wilhelm W, Berner K, Grundmann U, et al: Desflurane or isoflurane for paediatric ENT anaesthesia. A comparison of intubating conditions and recovery profile. Anaesthetist 47:975, 1998.
311. Inomata S, Suwa T, Toyooka H, Suto Y: End-tidal sevoflurane concentration for tracheal extubation and skin incision in children. Anesth Analg 87:1263, 1998.
312. Baraka A: Intravenous lidocaine controls extubation laryngospasm in children. Anesth Analg 57:506, 1978.
313. Gefke K, Anderson LW, Friesel E: Lidocaine given intravenously as a suppressant of cough and laryngospasm in connection with extubation after tonsillectomy. Acta Anaesthesiol Scand 27:111, 1983.
314. McCulloch TM, Flint PW, Richardson MA, Bishop MJ: Lidocaine effects on the laryngeal chemoreflex, mechanoreflex, and afferent electrical stimulation reflex. Ann Otol Rhinol Laryngol 10:1583, 1992.
315. Mazurek AJ, Rae B, Hann S, et al: Rocuronium versus succinlycholine: are they equally effective during rapid-sequence induction of anesthesia? Anesth Analg 87:1259, 1998.
316. Fleming NW, Chung F, Glass PSA, et al: Comparison of the intubation conditions provided by rapacuronium (ORG 9487) or succinylcholine in humans during anesthesia with fentanyl and propofol. Anesthesiology 91:1311, 1999.
317. Reynolds LM, Infosino A, Brown R, et al: Intramuscular rapacuronium in infants and children. Anesthesiology 91:1285, 1999.
318. Oswalt CE, Gates GA, Holmstrom FMG: Pulmonary edema as a complication of acute airway obstruction. JAMA 238:1833, 1977.
319. Travis KW, Todres DI, Shannon DC: Pulmonary edema associated with croup and epiglottitis. Pediatrics 59:695, 1977.
320. McGonagle M, Kennedy TL: Laryngospasm induced pulmonary edema. Laryngoscope 94:1583, 1984.
321. Jenkins JG: Pulmonary edema following laryngospasm. Anesthesiology 60:611, 1984.
322. Lee KWT, Downes JJ: Pulmonary edema secondary to laryngospasm in children. Anesthesiology 59:347, 1983.
323. Buda AJ, Pinsky MR, Ingels NB, et al: Effect of intrathoracic pressure on left ventricular performance. N Engl J Med 301:453, 1979.
324. Holinger LD: Etiology of stridor in the neonate, infant, and child. Ann Otol Rhinol Laryngol 89:397, 1980.
325. Friedman EM, Vastola AP, McGill TJI, Healy GB: Chronic pediatric stridor: etiology and outcome. Laryngoscope 100:277, 1990.
326. Vandertop WP, Asai A, Hoffman HJ, et al: Surgical decompression for symptomatic Chiari II malformation in neonates with myelomeningocele. J Neurosurg 77:541, 1992.

327. Grundfast KM, Harley E: Vocal cord paralysis. Otolaryngol Clin North Am 22:569, 1989.
328. Hesz N, Wolraich M: Vocal cord paralysis and brainstem dysfunction in children with spina bifida. Dev Med Child Neurol 27:522, 1985.
329. Myer CM III, Fitton CM: Vocal cord paralysis following child abuse. Int J Pediatr Otorhinolaryngol 15:217, 1988.
330. Chaten FC, Lucking SE, Young ES, Mickell JJ: Stridor: intracranial pathology causing postextubation vocal cord paralysis. Pediatrics 87:39, 1991.
331. Quartararo C, Bishop MJ: Complications of tracheal intubation: prevention and treatment. Semin Anesth 11:119, 1990.
332. Kemper KJ, Izenberg S, Marvin JA, Heimbach DM: Treatment of postextubation stridor in a pediatric patient with burns: the role of heliox. J Burn Care Rehabil 11:337, 1990.

24

Anesthesia for Plastic Surgery

BARBARA W. PALMISANO

LYNN M. RUSY

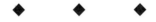

General anesthesia has been administered for surgical procedures that correct disfiguring lesions in infants and children since anesthesia was first introduced in the middle of the nineteenth century. Cleft lip and palate reconstruction was among the earliest surgical procedures for which general anesthesia was used for pediatric patients.[1] John Snow published the first report of giving ether to a 7-year-old boy for cleft lip reconstruction in *Lancet* in 1847. He gave chloroform for lip reconstruction 147 times between 1847 and 1858, mostly to infants between 3 and 6 weeks of age. Cleft lip and palate procedures have also been an impetus for innovations in anesthesia care for infants. This includes Ivan Magill's first use of endotracheal anesthesia for an infant in 1924 and Philip Ayre's introduction of the T-piece circuit in 1937.[2] Modern developments in anesthesia and plastic surgery are permitting increasingly complex attempts at reconstruction of the disfigured infant and child. The past decade has seen major advances in the understanding of anomalous development as well as evolution of diagnostic and therapeutic technology. This chapter focuses on the anesthetic challenges of two areas of pediatric plastic surgery: major craniofacial reconstruction (including cleft lip and palate repair) and burn reconstruction.

MAJOR CRANIOFACIAL RECONSTRUCTION

Craniofacial Embryology: Normal Development[3, 4]

The basic structures of the fetus are formed during the embryonic period of gestation (postconceptual weeks 2 to 8). The skeleton of the head is composed of the neurocranium (calvaria or cranial vault), the viscerocranium (facial skeleton), and the cranial base. These structures are highly integrated, and their formation and development are closely interwoven. The cranial base is the foundation of the skull, and its formation and development greatly influence the morphology of the other components. Embryologically, the cranial base and facial complex are derived from neural crest tissues, whereas the neurocranium is from mesoderm.

The neural tube closes by the third week of gestation (see Chapter 14). Its dorsal crests are composed of multipotent tissue that migrates widely into adjacent mesenchyme between the diencephalon and the cardiac swelling. Translocated neural crest cells undergo differentiation into a wide variety of cell types and form cartilage, bone,

707

ligaments, muscles, and arteries of the cranial base and facial regions.

Cranial Base

The cranial base extends from the foramen magnum to the frontonasal junction and consists of the sphenoid, petrous portion of the temporal bone, and cranial surfaces of the ethmoid bones. Phylogenetically, it is the oldest portion of the skull, and its development appears to be strongly genetically determined. The bony structure is preceded by a cartilaginous structure, the chondrocranium, which first appears in the sixth week of gestation. Before chondrification, there is establishment of blood vessels, cranial nerves, and the spinal cord between the brain and extracranial sites. Centers of ossification appear during the eighth week of gestation. In contrast to the largely intramembranous bone of the cranial vault (laid down by direct ossification of mesenchyme—the osteogenic membrane), the cranial base is endochondral bone (formed from cartilaginous prototype) and its sutures are cartilaginous joints, synchondroses, which grow by chondrocyte mitosis. The spheno-occipital synchondrosis is the principal site of growth in the cranial base during childhood.

The cranial base is an important shared junction between the cranial vault and face. Its inner surface relates to the brain and its outer surface relates to the nasopharynx and facial complex. Its shape and size strongly influence the final calvarial morphology. The primary stimulus to growth of the cranial base is growth of the brain. The size and alignment of the floor of the cranial base (anterior and middle cranial fossae) are determined by the ventral parts of the frontal and temporal lobes.[5] The cranial base is, in turn, the template on which the upper face develops. Various junctures between the cranial base and facial bones, especially in the nasomaxillary complex, determine the influence of the cranial base on facial growth. The anterior cranial fossa is spatially related to the nasomaxillary complex. The middle cranial fossa is similarly related to the pharyngeal space and airway. The interposition of three sets of space-occupying sense organs complicates the attachment of these two skull components to each other and influences the growth of the facial skeleton in particular.

Cranial Vault

The mesenchyme that precedes the cranial vault or neurocranium is derived from paraxial mesoderm and is at first arranged as a capsular membrane around the developing brain. Ossification of intramembranous calvarial bones depends on the presence of the brain. According to the *functional matrix* concept, bone growth is in response to functional demands. The sutures of the calvaria can be considered an interosseous ligament connecting opposing surfaces of bone. The bones of the calvaria are displaced outward by the expanding brain and respond by depositing new bone at the contact edges of the sutures.[5] The ultimate size and shape of the cranial vault are therefore determined by internal hydrostatic pressures exerted by the expanding brain on the cranial sutures, which stimulate compensatory sutural bone growth. The cranial vault

consists of the frontal, parietal, temporal, and occipital bones.

Face

The face is formed between the fourth and tenth weeks of gestation by the fusion of five facial swellings: the single frontal prominence and paired maxillary and mandibular prominences (Fig. 24–1). They surround a central depression, which is the stomodeum or future mouth.

The frontal prominence encloses the forebrain from which pairs of thickened ectodermal surface placodes (nasal and optic) are derived. The nasal placodes invaginate to form the nasal passages. The surface ridges (nasomedial and nasolateral processes) give rise to the nose, the philtrum of the upper lip, and the primary palate. The nasal complex is formed from merging of the frontal prominence with the nasal capsule, which is part of the cranial base. The nasal capsule surrounds the olfactory organs and forms the cartilages of the nostrils and the nasal septum. Septal cartilage intervenes between the cranial base above and the palate below and plays a major role in subsequent growth of the midface. The optic placodes, which ultimately develop into eyes, are induced by lateral optic diverticula from the forebrain. Expansion of the cerebral hemispheres produces medial migration to a frontal position.

The maxillary and mandibular prominences are derived from the first branchial arch. The branchial arches are five segmented bilateral swellings of the pharyngeal foregut, consisting of a mesodermal core surrounded by neural crest tissue. The arches are separated by branchial grooves externally and pharyngeal pouches internally. The cartilaginous skeleton of the first arch, Meckel's cartilage, provides a template for development of the mandible. The ear and auditory apparatus are derived from the first and second arches and from the first groove and pouch. The external ear components migrate from an initial cervical location. The internal ear components arise from the otic placode, which is induced by the vestibulocochlear nerve. The rest of the branchial arches, grooves, and pouches form various parts of the pharynx and laryngeal apparatus.

The facial prominences and their contents of skeletal cartilage, mesenchyme, and neurovascular bundles undergo cell proliferation, swelling, migration, and fusion in a critically timed series of events. Fusion of the paired mandibular prominences in the midline provides continuity of the lower jaw and lip. Fusion of the maxillary and mandibular prominences laterally creates the commissures of the mouth. Fusion of the nasomedial processes and maxillary prominences provides continuity of the upper jaw and lip and separation of the stomodeal chamber into separate oral and nasal cavities. Fusion of the nasomedial processes in the midline forms the central upper lip, the tip of the nose, and the primary palate (Figs. 24–1 and 24–2).

The secondary palate is formed from palatine shelves that initially grow inferiorly from the maxillary prominences downward into the stomodeum and lateral to the tongue. Initially, these palatal shelves are widely separated from the primary palate owing to their vertical orientation on either side of the tongue (Fig. 24–2). During the eighth

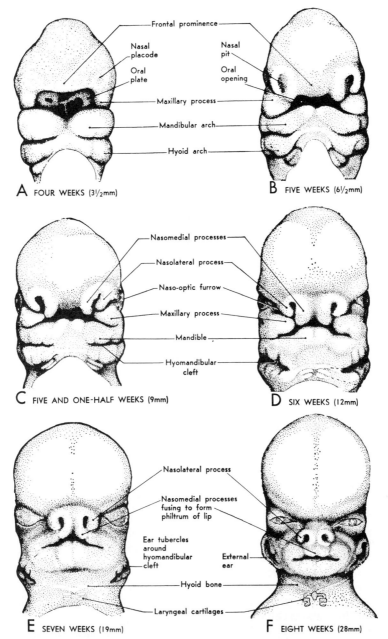

FIGURE 24–1. Stages in the embryologic development of the face. The median and paramedian structures from upper lip to forehead derive from the frontal prominence. The maxillary, and mandibular regions, the ear, and the pharyngeal, and laryngeal structures derive from the branchial arches. (From Patten BM: Human Embryology, 3rd ed. New York, McGraw-Hill, 1968, p 346. The McGraw-Hill Companies, with permission.)

week of gestation, coincident with withdrawal of the tongue from between the shelves, the lateral palatal shelves rotate to a horizontal position and fuse with each other. The nature of the "intrinsic shelf force" responsible for this reorientation is unknown, although mouth-opening reflexes, which involve withdrawal of the face from against the heart prominence, have been implicated in the withdrawal of the tongue from between the vertical palatal shelves. Forward growth of the mandible relocates the tongue more anteriorly. Successful fusion of the components of the palate by the 12th week requires a complicated synchronization of shelf movements with with-

drawal of the tongue and growth of the mandible. By this time the face takes on a human appearance.

Anomalous Development

Various genetic and environmental factors cause anomalous craniofacial development.[6] Genetically based malformations may be caused by single-gene deficiencies or by chromosomal aberrations. Genes for several autosomal dominant craniofacial malformations have recently been defined.[7] Environmental factors include congenital infections, irradiation, and exposure to chemical teratogens,

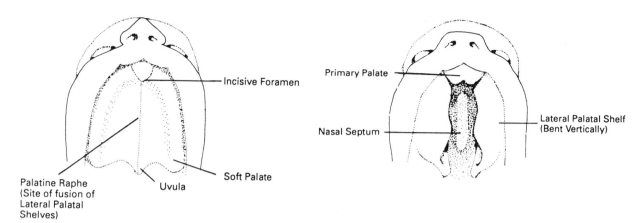

FIGURE 24–2. Lines of fusion of the embryological primordia of the palate (*left*). Schematic view of the three primordia of the palate in a 7.5-week-old embryo (*right*). (From Sperber GH: Craniofacial Embryology, 4th ed. London, Butterworth Scientific, 1989, p 134, with permission.)

such as phenytoin, vitamin A analogs, and alcohol. For many malformations, the etiology is unknown.

Maldevelopment can occur through several mechanisms. Malformations that develop during the embryonic period are distinct from deformations that occur later in the fetal period and may be self-correcting with postnatal catch-up growth.[6] Malformations can originate in anomalies of neural crest cells that may be deficient in number, may not complete migration, or may fail in cytodifferentiation. Neural crest tissues also form much of the cardiac conotruncal septum, and there is an association between craniofacial and cardiovascular malformations in syndromes in which neural crest defects play a role.[8, 9] Examples are retinoic acid syndrome, DiGeorge syndrome, the CHARGE association, and some variants of hemifacial microsomia. Malformations can also be caused by intrauterine compression of the embryo early in gestation. For example, in the amnion rupture sequence, early rupture of the amnion leads to defective morphogenesis secondary to compression of the embryo. In addition, adherence of amniotic bands to developing embryonic structures may interfere with normal development and result in simple to bizarre malformations that are not associated with embryologic lines of fusion. Malformations can be a result of intrauterine vascular accidents. For example, a shift in the blood supply of the face from the internal to the external carotid artery occurs during the seventh week of gestation as a result of normal atrophy of the stapedial artery. This shift occurs at a critical time of midface and palate development and provides the potential for deficient blood supply and consequent defects of the midface, upper lip, and palate. Malformations can also be secondary to defects in brain development because all components of the skull depend on the brain development. Comprehensive references are available that describe craniofacial malformations.[6, 10, 11] Several syndromes are described below.

Craniosynostosis and Craniosynostosis Syndromes

The precocious development of the brain is reflected by rapid enlargement of the head, beginning in early gesta-

tion and continuing through the first postnatal year. *Craniosynostosis*, or premature closure of the cranial sutures, results in arrested growth of the skull. Isolated synostosis produces characteristic skull distortions as a result of redirection of growth toward patent sutures (Table 24–1). The degree of skull deformity depends on the number of sutures involved and the time of onset of premature fusion. The earlier the synostosis, the greater the deformity.

Several different mechanisms are responsible for craniosynostosis.[6] Intrauterine fetal head constraint is a cause for isolated nonfamilial craniosynostosis. A genetic defect is responsible for familial simple craniosynostosis and for most craniosynostosis syndromes with known genesis. Several specific genetic defects have recently been identified (Table 24–2). Crouzon's, Apert's, Pfeiffer's, and Jackson-Weiss syndromes, once thought to be separate but overlapping entities, have been found to result from different mutations of the same gene.[12] Craniosynostosis can also be secondary to metabolic and hematologic disorders and to microcephaly due to defective brain growth. Known teratogens that cause craniosynostosis are diphenylhydan-

T A B L E 2 4 – 1 NOMENCLATURE OF CRANIOSYNOSTOSIS		
Affected Suture	**Traditional Name**	**Literal Translation**
Sagittal	Scaphocephaly	Boat skull
Metopic	Trigonocephaly	Triangle skull
Unilateral coronal	Plagiocephaly*	Oblique skull
Bicoronal	Brachycephaly	Short skull
Multiple sutures	Acrocephaly[†]	Topmost skull
	Turricephaly[†]	Tower skull
	Oxycephaly	Sharp skull
	Kleeblattschädel	Cloverleaf skull

* Plagiocephaly is not necessarily synonymous with unilateral coronal synostosis.
[†] Some authors use acrocephaly and/or turricephaly synonymously with brachycephaly to indicate bicoronal synostosis.
Adapted from Marsh JL: Comprehensive Care for Craniofacial Deformities. St. Louis, CV Mosby, 1985, p 123, with permission.

T A B L E 2 4 – 2		
CRANIOSYNOSTOSIS SYNDROMES		
Syndrome	Chromosome Localization	Gene
Apert's Syndrome	10q25.3-q26	*FGFR2*
Crouzon's Syndrome	10q25.3-q26	*FGFR2*
Jackson-Weiss syndrome	10q25.3-q26	*FGFR2*
Beare-Stevenson cutis gravata syndrome	10q25.3-q26	*FGFR2*
Pfeiffer's syndrome	10q25.3-q26	*FGFR2*
	8p11.2-p12	*FGFR1*
Thanatophoric dysplasia	4p16	*FGFR3*
Crouzonodermoskeletal syndrome	4p16	*FGFR3*
Muenke's craniosynostosis	4p16	*FGFR3*
Craniosynostosis, Boston type	5qter	*MSX2*
Saethre-Chotzen syndrome	7p21-p22	*TWIST*

Courtesy of M.M. Cohen, Jr.

toin, aminopterin and methotrexate, retinoic acid, oxymetazoline, and valproic acid.

Craniosynostosis may be an isolated deformation or part of a malformation syndrome. Isolated nonsyndromic craniosynostosis occurs in 6 in every 10,000 births.[6] Sagittal synostosis is most common (57 percent), coronal synostosis occurs less frequently (18 to 29 percent), and metopic and lambdoidal synostoses occur least frequently. Calvar-ial synostosis may also be part of a widespread craniofacial malformation that involves the cranial base and face.

Apert's Syndrome (Acrocephalosyndactyly)

Apert's syndrome is the most severe of several craniosynostosis syndromes in which the malformation involves all the craniofacial structures: calvaria, cranial base, and face. Apert's syndrome occurs in approximately 16 per 1 million births as a result of mutations in the FGFR2 gene on chromosome 10.[12] Although there is an autosomal dominant mode of transmission, most cases are sporadic. Apert's syndrome is characterized by craniosynostosis, midface hypoplasia/retrusion, and symmetric syndactyly of the hands and feet (Fig. 24–3). The dysmorphic features are listed in Table 24–3.

Craniosynostosis in Apert's syndrome involves multiple cranial sutures but most commonly the coronal sutures, resulting in brachycephaly, usually with a flattened occiput. The cranial base is malformed, having a broad, flat, and short contour with premature synostosis. The anterior cranial fossa is markedly shortened, which constrains the area within which the nasomaxillary complex can develop. The nasal cavity, palate, and maxilla are shortened, narrowed, and retropositioned. Midface hypoplasia and brachycephaly lead to proptosis because the orbits are too shallow to house the globe. The middle cranial fossa is rotated to a more vertical position than normal, which secondarily diminishes the dimensions of the pharynx. The interorbital space is always large and the orbits may be malaligned. The shortened cranial base results in a vaulted cranium with deep forehead. A significant number

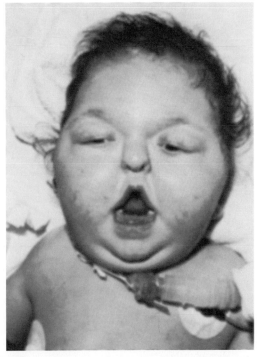
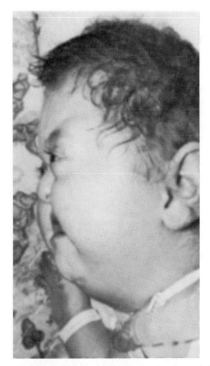

FIGURE 24–3. Young child with Apert's syndrome demonstrating craniosynostosis, exorbitism, midface retrusion, hypertelorism, cupid's lips, and syndactyly. She has a tracheostomy because of airway obstruction and chronic lung disease. She also has congenital heart disease.

TABLE 24-3
FEATURES OF APERT'S SYNDROME

Craniofacial dysmorphology
  Craniosynostosis
    Coronal synostosis most common
    Steep full forehead (frontal bossing)
    Flat occiput
    ± Hydrocephalus
  Maxillary retrusion (midface hypoplasia)
    Flat facies
  Shallow orbits
    Exorbitism or proptosis
  Relative mandibular prognathism
  Variable facial asymmetry
  Supraorbital horizontal groove
  Hypertelorism
  Down-slanting palpebral fissures
  Strabismus
  Parrot-beaked nose
  Depressed nasal bridge
  Cleft palate or bifid uvula
  Trapeziodal-shaped (cupid's) lips
  High arched palate
  V-shaped maxillary dental arch
  Severe tooth crowding
  Dental malocclusion
  Reduced nasopharyneal dimensions

Limb dysmorphology
  Syndactyly
    Osseous and/or cutaneous
    Fingers and toes
    Digits 2, 3, 4 always
    Symmetric
  Thumb and great toe malformations

Occasional abnormalities
  Cardiovascular
    Atrial septal defect
    Overriding aorta
    Ventricular septal defect
    Pulmonic stenosis
    Coarctation of aorta
    Endocardial fibroelastosis
    Pulmonary artery atrophy
  Skeletal
    Aplasia or ankylosis of joints
    Synostosis of radius and humerus
    Short humerus
    Cervical spine fusion
  Pulmonary
    Pulmonary aplasia
    Cartilaginous anomalies
    Tracheoesophageal fistula
  Gastrointestinal
    Pyloric stenosis
    Ectopic anus
  Renal
    Polycystic kidney
    Hydronephrosis
  CNS
    Mental retardation
    Hearing deficit

Facial Anomalies: Branchial Arch Malformations

Branchial arch anomalies are symptom complexes caused by deficient development of the branchial arches. They are etiologically and pathogenetically heterogeneous.[6] Wide variability in expression is characteristic. External ear deficiencies, auricular tags, and persistent branchial clefts or cysts are common branchial arch anomalies. Micro- or macrostomia results from abnormal merging of the maxillary and mandibular prominences, and are examples of severe first-arch anomalies. Micrognathia, also a first-arch anomaly, is the result of retarded mandibular development by any mechanism. It may be an intrinsic malformation or a deformation secondary to late gestational constraint, as may occur with the chin being compressed against the chest.

Treacher-Collins Syndrome (Mandibulofacial Dysostosis)

Treacher-Collins syndrome involves structures derived from the first and second branchial arch region.[6] The facial bones are absent or hypoplastic due to deficiencies of maxillary and branchial arch mesenchyme. The syndrome is an autosomal dominant disorder with variable expressivity, but over 50 percent of cases are new mutations. The responsible gene has been mapped to chromosome 5q31-34. The mutation leads to aberrant expression of a nucleolar protein named treacle. The abnormalities are bilateral,

TABLE 24-4
FEATURES OF TREACHER-COLLINS SYNDROME

Facial dysmorphia
  Skeletal hypoplasia/aplasia
    Malar and zygomatic bones
    Supraorbital ridges
    Mandible
  Facial muscle hypoplasia/hypoplasia
  Eye
    Lower lid coloboma or notching
    Partial absence of lower eyelashes
    Antimongoloid slant to palpebral fissures
  Ears
    Auricle malformation, misplacement
    Ear canal defects, conductive deafness
    Inner ear malformations
    Nonpneumatized mastoid
  Pharyngeal hypoplasia
  Dental malocclusion
  High arched palate
  Projection of scalp hair onto lateral cheek
  Blind fistulas, dimples, or tags between the ears and angle of the
    mouth

Occasional abnormalities
  Macrostomia
  Microstomia
  Cleft palate
  Velopharyngeal incompetence
  Upper eyelid coloboma
  Choanal atresia
  Microphthalmia
  Absence of parotid gland
  Congenital heart disease
  Mental deficiency not common

of patients are mentally retarded, which may be secondary to malformations of the central nervous system.

Other craniosynostosis syndromes include Crouzon's, Pfeiffer's, Saethre-Chotzen, Jackson-Weiss, and Carpenter's syndromes.

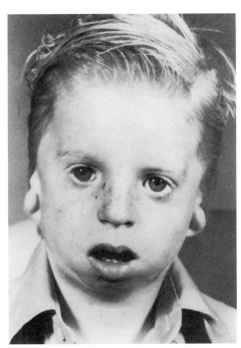

FIGURE 24–4. Five-year-old boy with Treacher-Collins syndrome. He has malar deficiencies, microtia, lower lid colobomas, and a retrognathic mandible. (From Jackson IT, Munro IR, Salyer KE, Whitaker LA [eds]: Atlas of Craniomaxillofacial Surgery. St. Louis, CV Mosby, 1982, p 582, with permission.)

usually symmetric, and confined to the craniofacial complex (Table 24–4 and Figs. 24–4 and 24–5). The characteristic facial appearance is the product of the relationship between an abnormal cranial base with a dysmorphic mandible and maxillary-malar complex.[13] The face is narrow, with down-sloping palpebral fissures, depressed cheekbones, and large down-turned mouth. There is a reduced cranial base angle (nasion-sella-basion angle), which positions the posterior pharynx forward. The dimensions of the pharynx are reduced in all dimensions by the combination of hypoplastic skeletal elements.[13-15] Some patients also exhibit a discrete area of constriction near the base of the tongue, such as one 11-year-old patient who had a pharyngeal lumen width of 5 mm.[14] There is little correlation between the degree of pharyngeal hypoplasia and the severity of the facial deformity. The malar (cheek) bone is hypoplastic and the orbital wall is deficient. The mandible is disfigured in all dimensions.

Nager's and Miller's syndromes are characterized by a facial features similar to those of Treacher-Collins with additional limb deformities.

Robin Sequence

The Robin sequence (retrognathia combined with cleft palate and glossoptosis) is a branchial arch anomaly in which early mandibular retrognathia is the primary defect. The sequence may be isolated or part of a syndrome (e.g., Stickler's, velocardiofacial, Treacher-Collins, and fetal alcohol syndromes).[16] In a "sequence," some anomalies are caused secondarily by a primary anomaly, whereas in a syndrome multiple anomalies have a single pathogenesis. The etiology and pathogenesis of the Robin sequence are diverse, but the common feature is failure of mandibular development with secondary failure of the tongue to descend from between the palatal shelves. In cases in which this is an isolated finding, intrauterine mandibular constraint may be responsible for the deformity. The mandible is intrinsically normal and will undergo catch-up growth postnatally.[6] If the Robin sequence is associated with a syndrome that includes intrinsic mandibular hypoplasia, the mandible will remain small.

Oculo-auriculo-vertebral Spectrum: Goldenhar's Syndrome and Hemifacial Microsomia

The oculoauriculovertebral spectrum is also known as the first and second branchial arch syndrome, hemifacial

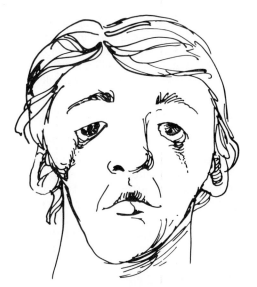
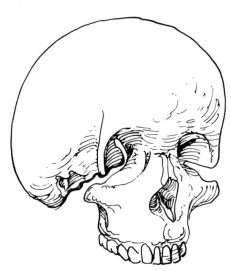

FIGURE 24–5. Treacher-Collins syndrome: facial clefts 6, 7, and 8. (From Jackson IT, Munro IR, Salyer KE, Whitaker LA [eds]: Atlas of Craniomaxillofacial Surgery. St. Louis, CV Mosby, 1982, p 225, with permission.)

microsomia, Goldenhar's syndrome, or facioauriculover-
tebral syndrome. This condition, which represents maldevelopment of the first and second branchial arches, is
complex and heterogeneous (Table 24–5 and Figs. 24–6
and 24–7). There is defective facial development involving
the ear, eye, zygomatic bone, mandible, parotid gland,
tongue, and facial muscles. Maldevelopment is not limited
to facial structures: cardiac, renal, skeletal, and other
anomalies also occur. The abnormalities present in various combinations, tend to be asymmetric, and 70 percent
are unilateral.[10] The constellation of anomalies suggests
that they originate at approximately 30 to 45 days of gestation. It has been suggested that disturbances in the
branchial arches or in neural crest cells impede development of adjacent tissues. A vascular pathogenesis secondary to hematoma formation at the time of development
of the stapedial artery system has been demonstrated in
animals.[17] In this model, focal hemorrhage with expanding
hematoma formation results in destruction of tissues in
the ear and jaw area. Three unrelated children have been

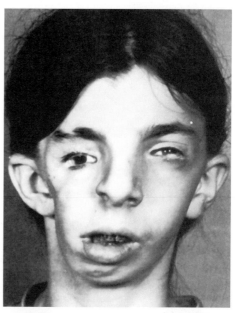

FIGURE 24–6. Severe craniofacial microsomia with epibulbar dermoids, colobomas, preauricular pits, low-set ears, short mandibular rami, and anterior open bite. The deficiencies are more severe on the right. (From Converse JM [ed]: Reconstructive Plastic Surgery. Philadelphia, WB Saunders Company, 1977, p 2361, with permission.)

TABLE 24–5
FEATURES OF THE OCULOAURICULOVERTEBRAL SPECTRUM OF ANOMALIES (GOLDENHAR'S SYNDROME AND HEMIFACIAL MICROSOMIA)

Features are highly variable, asymmetric, and commonly unilateral

Facial dysmorphia
  Skeletal hypoplasia
    Malar
    Maxillary
    Temporal
    Mandibular
  Facial musculature hypoplasia
    Muscles of mastication
    Muscles of facial expression
  Macrostomia
    Lateral cleft-like extension of mouth
  Salivary gland hypoplasia
  Ear anomalies
    Malformed and misplaced ears
    Accessory ear tags
    Middle ear anomalies
    Variable deafness
  Tongue and soft-palate anomalies

Goldenhar's syndrome
  Epibulbar dermoid
  Vertebral anomalies, commonly cervical
  Occasional abnormalities
    Eye anomalies
    Micro- or anophthalmos
    Colobomas
    Epibulbar dermoid
  Cleft lip
  Cleft palate
  High arched palate
  Mental deficiency
  Hypoplasia or aplasia of lung
  Laryngeal anomalies
  Renal anomalies
  Limb and rib anomalies
  Cerebral anomalies
  Cranial nerve anomalies
  Skull defects
  Congenital heart disease
    Tetralogy of Fallot
    Ventricular septal defect
  Other malformations

reported with similar unilateral craniofacial defects and
other structural abnormalities with known disruptive vascular pathogenesis.[18] The frequency of occurrence is estimated to be 1 in every 3,000 to 5,000 births. The condition
is usually sporadic, although familial instances have been
reported. Several chromosomal anomalies have been associated with this condition, and it has been reported
in infants born to mothers who had taken thalidomide,
primidone, or retinoic acid. It is usually discordant in
monozygotic twins.

Maxillary, mandibular, and auricular hypoplasia are the
primary features. Macrostomia is the result of a lateral
facial cleft from the commissure of the mouth. Mandibular
condyle deformities, present in all patients, range from
slight hypoplasia of the condyle to its complete absence
with agenesis of the ascending ramus. When accompanied
by epibulbar dermoid and vertebral anomalies, it is called
the Goldenhar syndrome, and when it occurs predominantly unilaterally it is called hemifacial microsomia. Most
of these patients have normal intelligence.

Facial Anomalies

Hypertelorism and Orbital Malposition

Orbital malposition may occur in any direction and may
be in different directions in each orbit. The bones and
sutures composing the walls of the orbits may be primarily
involved, or malposition may be secondary to craniosynostosis or craniofacial clefting. It may be associated with
encephalocele, tumor, or other cranio-orbital malformation. Isolated orbital hypertelorism is a skeletal deformity
that consists of lateralization of the bony orbit with enlargement of the ethmoid sinuses. The nose may be slightly
involved or severely distorted, and the nasal deformity
may be the most difficult to correct. Dysfunction of the

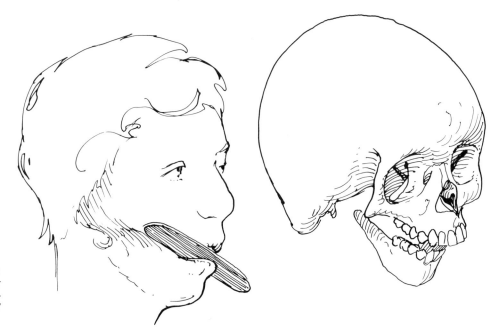

FIGURE 24–7. Craniofacial microsomia: cleft 7. (From Jackson IT, Munro IR, Salyer KE, Whitaker LA [eds]: Atlas of Cranio-maxillofacial Surgery. St. Louis, CV Mosby, 1982, p 226, with permission.)

upper eyelid, extraocular muscles, and lacrimal system frequently occur. Orbital hypotelorism is uncommon and does not occur as an isolated anomaly.

Facial Clefts

Clefting occurs when there is any interruption of skeleton or soft tissue. Failure of facial prominences to merge results in developmental clefts. Clefts that cannot be explained embryologically may be the result of disruptive factors.[6] The causes of most clefts are unknown, and the majority occur sporadically. Skeletal and soft tissue hypoplasia or aplasia are the anatomic defects of craniofacial clefts. Any part of the cranium or face may be involved. Various combinations of eye, ear, and central nervous system (CNS) deformities are associated.

Tessier devised an anatomic and descriptive classification that correlates clinical appearance with surgical anatomic findings.[19] This system designates 15 locations (numbered 0 through 14) for clefts and describes their respective courses through bone and soft tissue (Fig. 24–8). Many syndromes that include hypoplastic facial dysmorphology are categorized as clefts. Treacher-Collins syndrome includes clefts 6, 7, and 8 in its complete form (Fig. 24–5) and cleft 6 in its incomplete form. Cleft 6 accounts for the eyelid coloboma; cleft 7 explains the absence of the zygomatic arch, anterior displacement of the scalp hair, and mandibular deformities; and cleft 8 is represented by defects in the lateral orbital rim. The oculoauriculovertebral spectrum (hemifacial microsomia, Goldenhar's) is cleft 7 (Fig. 24–7).

Facial Anomalies: Cleft Lip and Cleft Palate

Cleft lip and/or palate are the most frequent of the congenital craniofacial malformations. It occurs in 1 in 700 births in the United States, and there is a marked racial predilection. The highest rates are in Native Americans and Asians, and the lowest rate is in African-Americans.[6] Clefts may be isolated, familial, or part of a syndrome. More than 300 syndromes involve cleft lip, cleft palate, or both, but more syndromes are associated with cleft palate than with cleft lip. They constitute a heterogeneous group of malformations with great variability in degree of cleft formation (Fig. 24–9). The etiology of clefting is multifactorial, with both genetic and environmental influences.

Clefting of the upper lip and nostril results from failure of the nasomedial process to merge with the maxillary prominences (lateral cleft lip, either uni- or bilateral) or from failure of the two nasomedial processes to merge (rare median cleft lip or bifid nose). Hypoplasia of the palatal shelves or mistiming of palatal shelf elevation results in cleft palate. Problems with tongue removal from between the shelves and problems with shelf elevation and contact probably account for most cases of human cleft palate.[9] There may be a critical time beyond which the palatal shelves cannot meet and fuse. If there is delay in elevation of the palatal shelves from the vertical to horizontal while the head is continuously growing, a widening gap is produced between the shelves so that they cannot meet. Clefting of the palate may or may not be associated with cleft upper lip, as the two conditions are separate developmental entities. However, failure of lip fusion may impair subsequent closure of the palatal shelves.

Physiologic Sequelae of Craniofacial Malformations

Hydrocephalus and Intracranial Pressure

In a retrospective review of 1,727 patients treated over 20 years, the occurrence of hydrocephalus in patients with nonsyndromic craniosynostosis (1,447 patients) was similar to that observed in the normal population (0.3 percent).[20] In patients with syndromic craniosynsotosis (280

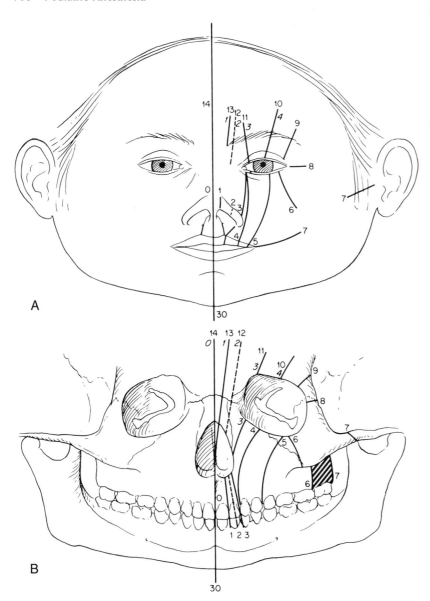

FIGURE 24–8. Tessier classification of facial clefts. *A,* Location of clefts on the face. *B,* Skeletal pathways. (From Converse JM [ed]: Reconstructive Plastic Surgery. Philadelphia, WB Saunders Company, 1977, p 2129, with permission.)

patients), the frequency was 12 percent and patients with kleeblattschädel deformity and Crouzon's syndrome were more likely to have hydrocephalus than those with other syndromes. Jugular foramen stenosis and crowding of the posterior fossa are two primary factors responsible for hydrocephalus in syndromic craniosynostosis.[20] Fusion of cranial base synchondroses produces alterations in the skull base and stenosis of the jugular foramen. The resulting venous hypertension leads to increased cerebrospinal fluid (CSF) hydrostatic pressure. If calvarial sutures (coronal and sagittal) are open, there will be progressive head enlargement with dilation of ventricles and subarachnoid spaces. If calvarial sutures are fused, intracranial pressure will increase but ventriculomegaly may not occur until after surgery to release the synostosis. When the posterior fossa is small and crowded, especially if the lambdoidal suture is fused, cerebellar tonsillar herniation or compression of the basal cistern can occur and produce obstructive hydrocephalus.

Intracranial pressure may be elevated without hydrocephalus in patients with craniosysostosis. Presumably, a restrictive cranium is a factor. Renier[21] monitored intracranial pressure during sleep in 350 patients with unoperated craniosynostosis and without hydrocephalus (Table 24–6). The patients ranged in age from 6 weeks to 15 years, and 44 percent were less than 1 year. The overall rate of intracranial hypertension was 23 percent, but the proportion varied by type of craniosynostosis and age. For single sagittal synostoses (trigono- and scaphocephaly), the rates of intracranial hypertension were 6 and 8 percent, respectively. The rate was higher, 12 percent, for single synostoses of a coronal suture (plagiocephaly). Other authors have also reported elevated intracranial pressure with single-suture synostosis, which provides a rationale, in addition to cosmetics, for surgical correction.[22, 23] In Renier's study, 26 percent of patients with synostoses of both coronal sutures (brachycephaly excluding Apert's and Crouzon's syndromes) had intracranial hypertension.

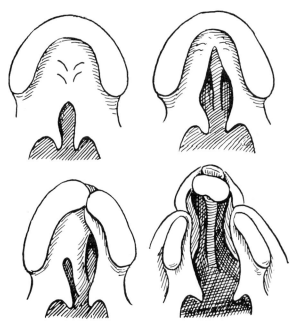

FIGURE 24–9. Various degrees of cleft palate and lip. *A,* Cleft of the soft palate only. *B,* Cleft of the soft and hard palate as far forward as the incisive foramen. *C,* Complete unilateral alveolar cleft, usually involving the lip. *D,* Complete bilateral alveolar cleft, usually associated with bilateral clefts of the lip. (From McCarthy JG, Cutting CB, Hogan VM: Introduction to facial clefts. *In* McCarthy JG [ed]: Plastic Surgery, Vol 4, Cleft Lip & Palate and Craniofacial Anomalies. Philadelphia, WB Saunders Company, 1990, p 2443, with permission.)

In extensive synostoses, usually involving both coronal and sagittal sutures (oxycephaly), the rate of intracranial hypertension was highest, at 54 percent.

In Renier's study, the incidence of intracranial hypertension also increased with age. After 1 year of age, the incidence of intracranial hypertension was four times greater for scaphocephaly and doubled for plagiocephaly. With brachycephaly, intracranial hypertension was more precocious: 22 percent of children under 1 year of age had intracranial hypertension compared with 31 percent over 1 year. Oxycephaly is usually not seen before 3 years of age, and 85 percent of children had intracranial hypertension at that age.

Clinical signs and symptoms of elevated intracranial pressure were uncommon. Intracranial volume measurements calculated from computed tomography (CT) scans did not give a reliable indication of intracranial pressure (ICP), although markedly reduced intracranial volume did increase the likelihood of intracranial hypertension.[22]

In nonsyndromic forms of craniosynostosis where the abnormality is confined to the calvarium, the effects of cranial vault expansion are predictable. In complex craniosynostosis, however, the effects are less certain. In Renier's series, 54 patients had postoperative ICP measurements. Whereas before surgery 74 percent had elevated and 11 percent had borderline ICP, after surgery 7 percent had elevated and 20 percent still had borderline ICP. In another series in which 22 patients had ICP monitored postoperatively, 45 percent had elevated ICP and 32 percent were borderline.[24] In this series, magnetic resonance imaging (MRI) was also used to evaluate 34 patients with complex craniosynostosis up to 8 years following surgery. Cerebellar tonsillar herniation was found in 52 percent and hydrocephalus was found in 41 percent, over half of whom developed the hydrocephalus after surgery. Another report covering a 20-year period noted the incidence of postoperative hydrocephalus to be 45 percent for patients with syndromes versus 4 percent for patients with isolated craniosynostosis, and the incidence of shunt placement to be 22 percent versus 1 percent.[25, 26]

Upper Airway Obstruction

Malformations involving the face and cranial base often reduce upper airway dimensions, resulting in various degrees of airway obstruction. A reduced cranial base angle produces anteroposterior shortening of the nasal and oral airway by positioning the pharyngeal wall forward.[15] In addition, it may draw the temporomandibular joint posteriorly so that the mandible is positioned retrusively.[16] When the mandible is small and retrognathic, the tongue is placed posteriorly and impinges in the oro- and hypopharynx.[13] Midface hypoplasia and retroposition also diminish the dimensions of the nasal airway. Neurologic dysfunction, such as pharyngeal hypotonia or incoordination, compounds airway obstruction in children with abnormal anatomy.[27] Other skeletal abnormalities, such as turbinate hypertrophy, septal deviation, and choanal narrowing or atresia, contribute to upper airway obstruction.

Upper airway obstruction, especially obstructive sleep apnea, is common in craniofacial syndromes.[14, 15, 28–31] Sher and colleagues[28] used flexible fiberoptic nasopharyngoscopy in patients with obstructive sleep apnea to identify the mechanisms of pharyngeal obstruction. Four mechanisms were identified:

1. Posterior movement of the tongue to the posterior pharyngeal wall (Fig. 24–10).
2. Tongue movement posteriorly compressing the soft palate or cleft palatal tags posteriorly against the posterior pharyngeal wall so that there is a meeting of tongue, velum, and posterior pharyngeal wall in the upper oropharynx.

TABLE 24–6
INTRACRANIAL PRESSURE BEFORE SURGERY

	Total No. of Patients	Baseline ICP (mm Hg)		
		≤10	11–15	>15
Trigonocephaly	31	21	8	2
Scaphocephaly	118	76	33	9
Plagiocephaly	65	40	17	8
Brachycephaly	34	17	8	9
Oxycephaly	66	23	7	36
Crouzon's syndrome	9	3	0	6
Apert's syndrome	16	3	6	7

Modified from Renier D: Intracranial pressure in craniosynostosis: pre- and postoperative recordings-correlation with functional results. *In* Persing JA, Edgerton MT, Jane JA (eds): Scientific Foundations and Surgical Treatment of Craniosynostosis. Baltimore, Williams & Wilkins, 1989, p 264, with permission.

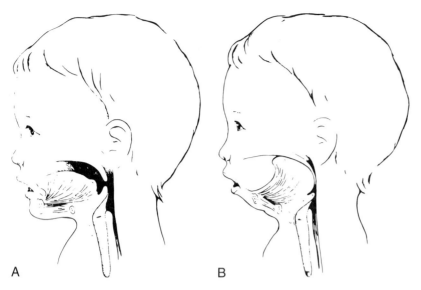

FIGURE 24-10. Anatomic features of the larynx. *A,* Normal child. *B,* Child with mandibular hypoplasia. Posterior placement of tongue makes the larynx appear to be more anteriorly situated than normal. (From Handler SD, Keon TP: Difficult laryngoscopy/intubation: the child with mandibular hypoplasia. Ann Otol Rhinol Laryngol 92:401, 1983, with permission.)

3. Movement of the lateral pharyngeal walls medially apposing each other.
4. Pharyngeal constriction in a circular or sphincteric manner.

Some patients can be successfully managed with nasal continuous positive airway pressure (CPAP) during sleep.[30] For others, airway obstruction may be severe enough to require tracheostomy. In a retrospective review of 251 patients with craniofacial anomalies who had surgery over a 5-year period, 20 percent required tracheostomy either to relieve chronic airway obstruction or to manage the airway in the perioperative period.[32] Patients with craniofacial synostosis (Crouzon's, Pfeiffer's, or Apert's syndromes) had the highest rate of tracheostomy (48 percent). Those with mandibular facial dysostosis (Treacher-Collins or Nager's syndromes) had the next highest rate (41 percent). Twenty-two percent of patients with oculoauriculovertebral sequence (Goldenhar's and hemifacial microsomia) required tracheostomy. The mean duration of cannulation for patients who had tracheostomy in infancy or early childhood was 4 years, whereas for patients who had tracheostomy after 4 years of age, the mean duration of cannulation was less than 6 months, with 60 percent having decannulation after 1 week.

With the Robin sequence, especially nonsyndromic, placement of a nasopharyngeal airway or glossopexy (suturing the tongue to the mandible and lower lip) may relieve significant airway obstruction during the first months of life while the mandible grows and the airway expands.[27, 33] In some syndromes (e.g., Treacher-Collins and Apert's), because the anatomic interrelationships become progressively distorted, the obstruction may not improve with age or may actually worsen.[13, 29, 34]

Associated Anomalies

With syndromic craniofacial anomalies, many systems may be malformed, particularly the CNS, and the cardiac and pulmonary systems. Cranial sensory and speech organs may also be malformed, so that hearing, vision, or speech may be impaired. Cervical spine anomalies, including intervertebral fusion, are well known in Goldenhar's syndrome but are also common with craniosynostosis syndromes such as Crouzon's, Apert's, and Pfeiffer's.[35-37]

Craniofacial Reconstruction: Surgical Procedures

Major craniofacial surgery was introduced in 1967 by Dr. Paul Tessier in Paris, when he presented the first craniofacial dysjunction procedures in which the face was cleaved away from the base of the cranium with techniques that employed both an intracranial and an extracranial approach.[38, 39] Over the past 30 years, these techniques have been expanded to cover a variety of complex congenital and acquired (traumatic and neoplastic) deformities of the face and cranium.[40] A coordinated interdisciplinary approach is essential. The reasons for operating are to improve physical function (neurologic, ocular, nasal, dental, and phonetic) and to improve appearance and psychologic function ("obviating the stigmata of a monster").[41] The basic objective of craniofacial surgery is to correct skeletal deformity, with soft tissue correction following. The deformed skeleton is cut, disjoined, mobilized, repositioned, augmented, and fixed. Wide exposure of the skeleton is required. Therefore, the soft tissues, including the orbital contents, are extensively dissected and mobilized away from their bony attachments. Intracranial and extracranial approaches are utilized and scalp, preauricular, and intraoral incisions are made to avoid scars on the face. For intracranial and upper and midface procedures, the surgical approach is through a bicoronal scalp incision that extends from ear to ear and from which the soft tissues of the scalp and face are reflected forward over the facial mass (Figs. 24-11 and 24-12). This gives wide exposure of the facial skeleton down to the maxillary alveolus. The anterior cranial base or fossa is exposed through a frontal craniotomy, with retraction of the frontal lobes of the brain (Figs. 24-13 and 24-14). A prerequisite to providing anesthesia for major craniofacial surgery is a clear under-

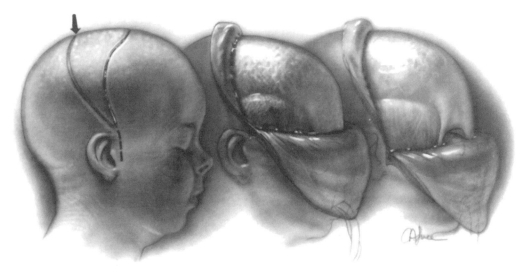

FIGURE 24–11. Bicoronal incision for intracranial and upper and midface procedures extends from ear to ear. Peeling back the face provides wide exposure to the facial skeleton. (From Persing JA, Jane JA, Edgerton MT: Surgical treatment of craniosynostosis. *In* Persing JA, Jane JA [eds]: Scientific Foundations and Surgical Treatment of Craniosynostosis. Baltimore, Williams & Wilkins, 1989, p 136, with permission.)

standing of the lesion and the proposed surgical procedure.

Cranial and Facial Remodeling

Strip craniectomy improves craniofacial contour only in isolated sagittal synostosis. For other synostoses, cranial remodeling follows basic principles of removing, reshaping, and repositioning bone. Cranial remodeling may involve any part of the cranium, or the entire cranial vault (Fig. 24–15). For complex craniosynostoses in which the cranial base and face are also involved, the sutures involved are commonly those of the anterior cranial vault (coronal, sagittal, or metopic sutures) as well as the ante-

rior cranial base (frontosphenoidal, frontoethmoidal, and sphenozygomatic sutures). The surgical approach aims to release sutures and to advance the face forward away from the cranial base. The principal functional objectives are to open the cranium to allow normal brain expansion, to open the nasopharyngeal airway, to provide greater support and protection for the eyes, and to achieve proper alignment of the upper and lower dental arches. This is usually undertaken in at least two steps: (1) frontocranial remodeling, with release of the synostosis and advancement of the frontal-supraorbital area, and (2) midface advancement. Additional procedures are required for correction of orbital malposition and reconstruction of facial clefts. Some patients with craniofacial syndromes will re-

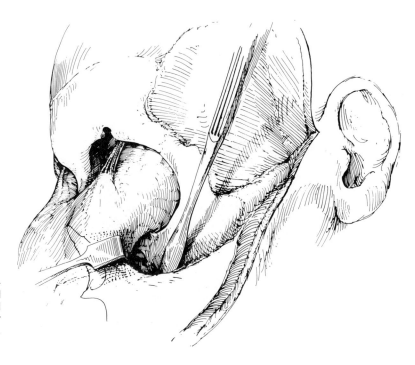

FIGURE 24–12. Soft tissues of the scalp and face, including the orbital contents when necessary, are peeled forward to expose the skeleton. Here a periosteal elevator is used to separate tissue layers. (From Jackson IT, Munro IR, Salyer KE, Whitaker LA [eds]: Atlas of Craniomaxillofacial Surgery. St. Louis, CV Mosby, 1982, p 44, with permission.)

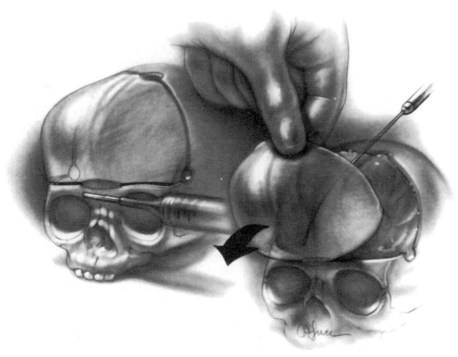

FIGURE 24–13. Many craniofacial procedures that employ an intracranial approach begin with a frontal craniotomy. (From Persing JA, Jane JA, Edgerton MT: Surgical treatment of craniosynostosis. *In* Persing JA, Jane JA [eds]: Scientific Foundations and Surgical Treatment of Craniosynostosis. Baltimore, Williams & Wilkins, 1989, p 140, with permission.)

lapse and undergo multiple procedures due to syndrome-related limited growth potential in the anterior cranial base and midface.[42]

Frontocranial Remodeling

Release of craniosynostosis and frontal-supraorbital advancement is generally undertaken during the first 3 to 6 months of life to accommodate rapid growth of the brain during the first year. The entire frontal aspect of the cra-

nium is detached to allow the forces of the growing brain to remodel the cranium into a more normal configuration (Fig. 24–16). A frontal craniotomy, with removal of a frontal bone flap, is performed first. A separate supraorbital skeletal segment may be mobilized by extending the osteotomy through the lateral orbital walls, across the orbital roofs, and across the nasal bridge. This segment is contoured and then advanced. The frontal bone flap is returned, either as a solid piece or cut into multiple fragments that are rearranged into a more normally shaped

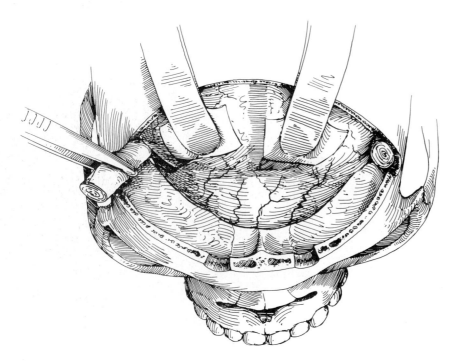

FIGURE 24–14. With the dura and frontal lobes retracted posteriorly, the floor of the anterior fossa is widely visible. (From Jackson IT, Munro IR, Salyer KE, Whitaker LA [eds]: Atlas of Craniomaxillofacial Surgery. St. Louis, CV Mosby, 1982, p 69, with permission.)

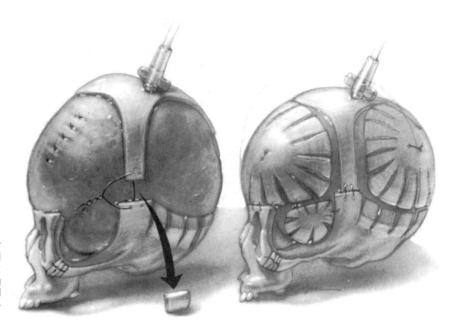

FIGURE 24–15. Total cranial vault remodeling for turribrachycephaly secondary to bilateral coronal synostosis. (From Persing JA, Jane JA, Edgerton MT: Surgical treatment of craniosynostosis. *In* Persing JA, Jane JA [eds]: Scientific Foundations and Surgical Treatment of Craniosynostosis. Baltimore, Williams & Wilkins, 1989, p 183, with permission.)

forehead. The segments are fixed in place with wires or miniplates and bone grafts are used to fill gaps, or the forehead may be left "floating" with a wide osseous defect.

Midface Advancement

Craniofacial dysjunction and midface advancement are delayed until the patient is at least 4 or 5 years old. Certain indications or personal preferences will lead the surgeon to select a specific operative procedure, which usually includes a Le Fort osteotomy (Fig. 24–17). At the beginning of the twentieth century a French surgeon, Reń Le Fort, found that the maxilla, naso-orbital complex, and zygomas fracture in predictable ways at weak points or *linea minoris resentiae*.[43] These fracture lines have been

modified into controlled osteotomies for the correction of skeletal anomalies.

The Le Fort I osteotomy corrects malocclusion due to underdevelopment of the maxilla (Fig. 24–18). This procedure is performed through an intraoral incision. A horizontal cut is made across the nasal floor, the anterior maxilla, and through the pterygomaxillary junction. The maxilla is mobilized downward, advanced, and fixed. Bone grafts are used to fill the spaces.

The Le Fort II osteotomy is used to advance the lower maxilla and entire nose forward (Fig. 24–19). A bicoronal scalp incision, with soft tissue reflection to expose the midface, is combined with an intraoral incision. The osteotomy passes across the nasal bridge, then bilaterally down the lateral nasal bones, through the inferior orbital

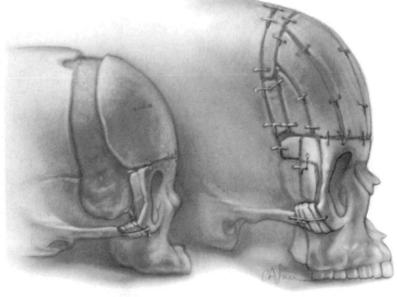
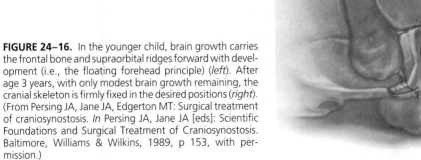

FIGURE 24–16. In the younger child, brain growth carries the frontal bone and supraorbital ridges forward with development (i.e., the floating forehead principle) (*left*). After age 3 years, with only modest brain growth remaining, the cranial skeleton is firmly fixed in the desired positions (*right*). (From Persing JA, Jane JA, Edgerton MT: Surgical treatment of craniosynostosis. *In* Persing JA, Jane JA [eds]: Scientific Foundations and Surgical Treatment of Craniosynostosis. Baltimore, Williams & Wilkins, 1989, p 153, with permission.)

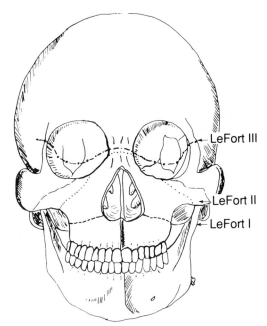

FIGURE 24–17. Le Fort I, II, and III osteotomies.

rim, and across the maxilla to the pterygomaxillary junction. The segment is mobilized and advanced, the defects are filled with bone grafts, and the entire segment is fixed with rigid miniplates or wire. Intermaxillary fixation is not needed when rigid internal fixation plates are used.

The Le Fort III osteotomy (Fig. 24–20) is used for complete underdevelopment of the midface, typical of Apert's, Crouzon's, and similar syndromes. It permits advancement of the nose, maxilla, and orbits after dysjunction of the entire midface. A bicoronal scalp incision is made, the soft tissues are reflected forward over the midface, and the orbital contents are dissected free. The basic osteotomy starts at the frontozygomatic suture, then passes through the orbits below the supraorbital rim and across the nasal bridge. The pterygomaxillary junctions are separated with an osteotome passed behind the maxilla from above (Fig. 24–21). Likewise, an osteotome is passed downward through the nasal bridge to separate the nasal

septum from the skull base. The facial block is advanced after forceful mobilization with disimpaction forceps, which involves a down-fracture and side-to-side and rotary manipulations (Fig. 24–20). The spaces are filled with bone grafts and the bones are fixed. The use of rigid internal fixation plates precludes the need for intermaxillary fixation.

Monoblock frontofacial advancement, in which frontal and orbitofacial blocks are advanced simultaneously, is performed by some surgeons. The supraorbital area is included en bloc with the facial mass for mobilization and advancement, and the frontal bone flap is remodeled when necessary.

Various combinations and modifications of these osteotomies are performed either simultaneously or in stages. The transverse maxillary osteotomies (Le Fort I and II) are usually delayed until adolescence to avoid disruption of the unerupted permanent dentition.

Surgical Correction of Hypertelorism and Orbital Malposition

Surgical correction of orbital malposition is performed to facilitate correction of strabismus, to normalize facial appearance, and to possibly achieve binocular vision. Surgery is usually performed at about 5 years of age unless there are mitigating factors. The orbit can be thought of as a box housing the eye. To correct hypertelorism or other orbital malposition, the box is freed from contiguous bone and repositioned (Fig. 24–22). In moderate and severe degrees of hypertelorism, an intracranial approach is employed: a bicoronal scalp incision is made; soft tissues, including orbital contents and nasal mucosa, are reflected down to midface; a frontal craniotomy is performed; and the frontal lobes of the brain are retracted to expose the anterior cranial fossa. Intra- and extraorbital osteotomies convert the anterior orbit into a mobile box (Fig. 24–22). A central block of bone (frontal, nasal, ethmoidal) is removed from between the orbits. The orbits, with the globe and other soft tissues, are then moved medially and fixed in place (Fig. 24–23). Bone grafts are inserted into the gaps created at the lateral orbital walls. The nose is rebuilt with bone grafts if necessary. For minor degrees of hyper-

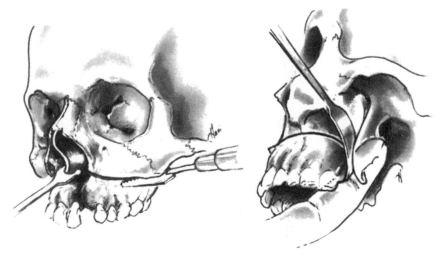

FIGURE 24–18. Le Fort I osteotomies. (From Bardach J, Salyer KE: Surgical Techniques in Cleft Lip and Palate, 2nd ed. St. Louis, Mosby Year Book, 1991, p 251, with permission.)

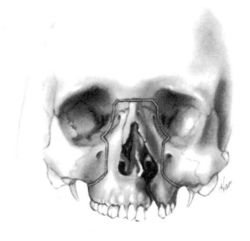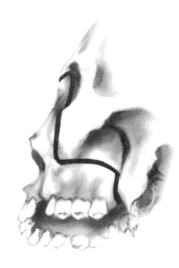

FIGURE 24–19. Le Fort II osteotomies. (From Bardach J, Salyer KE: Surgical Techniques in Cleft Lip and Palate, 2nd ed. St. Louis, Mosby Year Book, 1991, p 255, with permission.)

telorism, an extracranial approach is possible, which eliminates the frontal craniotomy and brain retraction. There is still extensive soft tissue dissection, but the osteotomies are less extensive. There is also danger of piercing the cribriform plate with resulting CSF leakage.

Reconstruction of Facial Clefts: Major Facial and Mandibular Malformations

Skeletal and soft tissue hypoplasia are the anatomic defects of the major facial and mandibular malformation syndromes. Hypoplasia may involve any part of the face and cranium. Multiple staged surgical procedures are often required for craniofacial reconstruction. The skeleton must be normalized, the soft tissues augmented, ears and nose reconstructed, and sometimes the face must be reanimated. For the hypoplastic skeleton, displacement osteotomies reposition the bones into more normal positions, and calvarial bone grafts are used to augment surfaces and fill spaces.

Soft tissue hypoplasia can involve skin, subcutaneous tissue, cartilage, and the muscles of mastication and facial

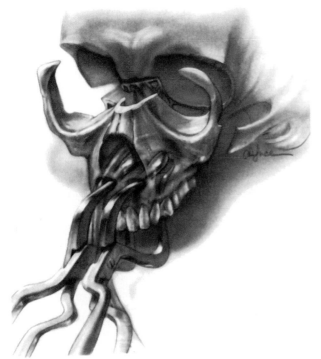

FIGURE 24–20. Le Fort III osteotomy. Rowe disimpaction forceps are used to "down-fracture" the posterior maxillary wall and allow advancement of the midface. (From Persing JA, Jane JA, Edgerton MT: Surgical treatment of craniosynostosis. *In* Persing JA, Jane JA [eds]: Scientific Foundations and Surgical Treatment of Craniosynostosis. Baltimore, Williams & Wilkins, 1989, p 229, with permission.)

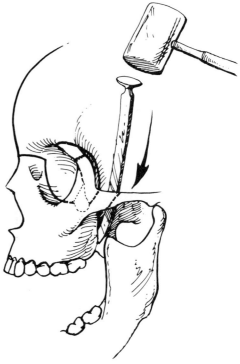

FIGURE 24–21. Osteotome is placed in the pterygomaxillary fissure. Gentle taps with a hammer separate the maxillary tuberosity from the pterygoid plates. (From Jackson IT, Munro IR, Salyer KE, Whitaker LA [eds]: Atlas of Craniomaxillofacial Surgery. St. Louis, CV Mosby, 1982, p 203, with permission.)

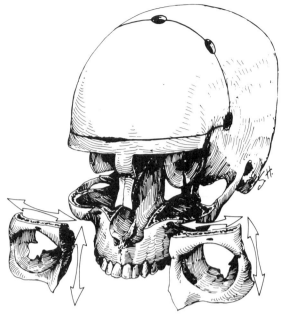

FIGURE 24–22. Orbits can be considered as boxes containing the eye. Each orbit can be moved in any plane. (From Jackson IT, Munro IR, Salyer KE, Whitaker LA [eds]: Atlas of Craniomaxillofacial Surgery. St. Louis, CV Mosby, 1982, p 329, with permission.)

expression. Various approaches can be taken to augment and restructure soft tissues. Skin and mucosal flaps from local or distant sites may be used. To add bulk and appropriate contours, dermis-fat grafts from the groin can be introduced subcutaneously. Additional contour can be gained with inlay bone grafts. Temporal muscle transfers to the face also add bulk. These procedures may require extensive dissection of soft tissue. Facial nerve palsy can be compensated for with nerve transfer from the motor branch of cranial nerve V or, if the malformation is unilateral, cross-face nerve grafts and microneuromuscle transfers can be attempted.

Traditionally, mandibular reconstruction has followed the same principles as other craniofacial procedures: cut, mobilize, reposition, augment, and fix. The mandible was mobilized through the intraoral route with bilateral sagittal osteotomies and rotated and advanced into a normalized position. Distraction osteogenesis is now replacing the traditional method (see below) in many cases. New mandibular parts are constructed from costochondral rib grafts or split cranial grafts. This is usually done before eruption of the permanent teeth.

Distraction Osteogenesis

Distraction osteogenesis is a process of inducing a bone callus (by osteotomy) and then distracting the proximal and distal ends. It has been used for many years by orthopedic surgeons to lengthen limbs but did not gain widespread clinical acceptance because of associated morbidity. In 1988, Illizarov, a Russian orthopedic surgeon, described a technique for distraction osteogenesis involving only corticotomy with minimal disruption of the periosteum and endosteum, which reduced the incidence of complications and allowed wider application of the technique.[44]

The principal application in craniofacial surgery has been in mandibular lengthening. The first use of distraction osteogenesis to lengthen the mandible was reported in four children in 1992.[45] The technique consisted of percutaneous insertion of pins into the mandible proximal and distal to a corticotomy (Figs. 24–24 and 24–25). The pins were attached to an external fixator lengthening device and the mandible was lengthened 1 mm/day by turning a bolt. The authors reported mandibular lengthening of 18 to 24 mm.

The procedure is minimally invasive compared with traditional methods of mandibular reconstruction. It is associated with less blood loss, less surgical time, and less tissue exposure, and the requirement for bone grafting is reduced. It may produce greater bone lengthening and allow procedures to be performed on younger children. Several authors believe that facial soft tissue growth is observed after mandibular distraction.[45-47] The major complication is the production of hypertrophic scars as the pins migrate through the skin.

Since the original description, mandibular distraction has become increasingly popular for treatment of mandibular hypoplasia and asymmetry.[46-48] Endoral (internal) devices have been developed that eliminate scars on the face and are at less risk for loosening or dislodgement. Mandibular distraction has been used successfully to alleviate symptoms of respiratory distress and obstructive sleep apnea, and allow tracheostomy decannulation. It has been applied to infants as young as 14 weeks.[48]

The technique is being applied experimentally to other facial bones with both internal and external lengthening devices.

Cleft Lip and Cleft Palate Reconstruction

Surgical reconstruction of the lip, palate, and nose is undertaken for cosmetic, psychological, and functional pur-

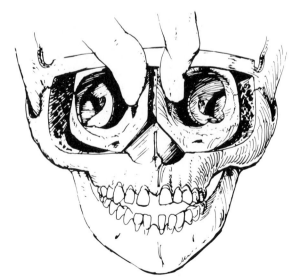

FIGURE 24–23. After osteotomies and removal of a central block of bone, the orbits are shifted medially. (From Jackson IT, Munro IR, Salyer KE, Whitaker LA [eds]: Atlas of Craniomaxillofacial Surgery. St. Louis, CV Mosby, 1982, p 357, with permission.)

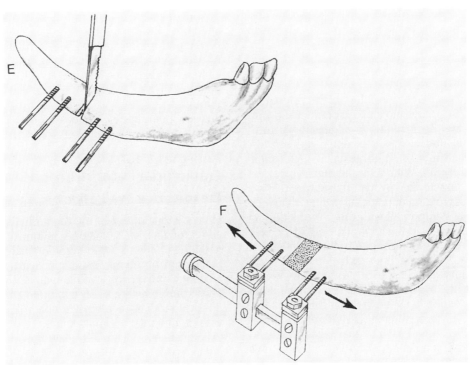

FIGURE 24–24. The technique of mandibular distraction. *E,* The pins have been inserted and the osteotomy is completed with a mechanical saw. *F,* Commencement of distraction with the appliance in position. The *arrows* designate the movement of the mandibular segments with formation of bony regenerate in the resulting gap. (From McCarthy JG: Craniofacial microsomia. A primary or secondary surgical treatment program. Clin Plast Surg 24:459, 1997, with permission.)

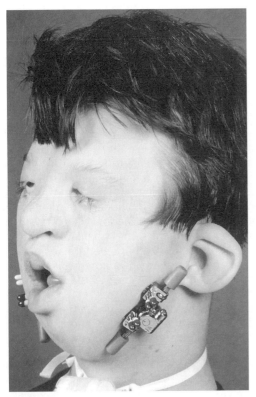

FIGURE 24–25. Nine-year-old boy with Treacher-Collins syndrome and bilateral mandibular distraction devices in place. A partial turn of the screw will advance the mandible 1 mm each day.

poses. Functional aims are to separate the nasal and oral cavities, to improve speech and swallowing mechanisms, to prevent middle ear disease, to improve hearing, and to provide normal dental occlusion. Primary procedures for cleft lip reconstruction are usually performed at 3 months of age and for cleft palate reconstruction at 12 to 18 months before the normal development of speech. Tissue deficiency and displacement contribute to anatomic defects. Surgical reconstruction of soft tissues involves dissecting, undermining, and creating flaps for rotation and advancement. Reconstruction of the bony palate involves bone or mucoperiosteal flaps and bone grafting. For example, bone flaps can be made from the palatal shelves and positioned medially to fill the cleft. Mucoperiosteal flaps can also be turned off the vomer and joined to the edge of the bony cleft to close it. If the cleft is sufficiently narrow, paring of the medial palatal edges with elevation of nasal and palatal mucosa may accomplish closure. Free bone grafting is required for some deficiencies, especially of the alveolar ridge. Bone is taken from ribs, iliac crest, or skull.

Secondary procedures are performed to revise residual defects, such as velopharyngeal incompetence (see below), oronasal fistulae, dental malocclusion, and residual cosmetic deformities. When dental malocclusion is severe, osteotomy and repositioning of the maxilla or mandible is performed in much the same manner as for craniofacial surgery. Bone grafts are used to fill deficiencies in the alveolar ridge and improve the contour of hypoplastic maxillae. Secondary procedures for cosmetic improvement and fistulae repair involve scar excision, soft tissue rearrangement, and occasionally skin grafting. The nose is often the most difficult area to reconstruct to normal appearance.

Pharyngeal Flap

Velopharyngeal incompetence is failure of the velum (soft palate) and posterior pharynx to close or contact appropriately for speech and swallowing. It occurs in 25 to 30 percent of patients after cleft palate repair and can also occur with any anatomic or neuromuscular abnormality of the palate or pharynx. With velopharyngeal incompetence, speech is characterized by hypernasality and misarticulation, and nasal regurgitation occurs with swallowing. Diagnosis has greatly improved with the use of video nasoendoscopy, which provides a dynamic view of the velopharynx. Surgical correction is commonly attempted with a pharyngeal flap procedure, in which flaps of mucosa and muscle are raised from the posterior pharynx and attached to the velum (Fig. 24–26). This results in a permanent midline connection between the palate and posterior pharynx. Alternatively, a sphincter pharyngoplasty can be performed, in which small lateral pharyngeal flaps are tucked under a wide medial flap to create a bulky transverse roll in the posterior pharynx, thus narrowing the pharynx and allowing contact with the velum.

The result of these procedures is a narrowed nasopharyngeal vault with potential for obstructed nasal airflow. Obstructive sleep apnea is not uncommon after a pharyngeal flap procedure, especially with the Robin sequence.[49–52] Velocardiofacial syndrome, the most common syndrome causing palatal clefting and velopharyngeal insufficiency, is associated with medially displaced carotid arteries that may render pharyngoplasty unsafe.[53] This condition can be identified with nasoendoscopy but not with endoral examination. Obviously, blind nasal tracheal intubation or passage of a nasogastric tube should not be attempted in a patient with a pharyngeal flap. Kopp reported performing nasotracheal intubation in the presence of a pharyngeal flap by first passing a flexible suction catheter to explore the patency of each nares and the pharyngeal flap passages.[54] When the catheter emerges through the ostium, it is grasped with a clamp and the endotracheal tube gently passed over it.

Anesthesia for Craniofacial Reconstruction

Preoperative Evaluation

Many factors influence the emotional state of the patient and family who face major craniofacial surgery.[55–58] Many pediatric patients with craniofacial anomalies have behavorial problems associated with poor self-concept, anxiety, introversion, and negative social experiences. These problems are rarely profound and represent limitations rather than severe psychopathology.[55] Most children with craniofacial anomalies make social and psychological adjustments to their appearance and are not functioning in a psychosocially deviant range. The time of surgery is stressful for the patient and parents.[59] There is fear of pain and physical jeopardy because the surgery is extensive and potentially life-threatening. Older children may also fear loss of identity because of the impending alteration in their appearance. Parents may be particularly protective. Many patients undergo multiple surgical procedures over the course of many years, and the child and family have great emotional investment in the process.

It is important to establish rapport and to gain the confidence and acceptance of the patient and parents. One can be sensitive yet open and candid in discussing the anomalies. It helps to encourage the child and parents to express their concerns and expectations. The child may have communicative disorders involving sight, hearing, or speech, and these must be accommodated during the preoperative preparation. Various hospital activities may help to prepare the child, such as puppet plays, movies, storybooks, and other play therapy designed to introduce the child to the coming events.

It is appropriate to be reassuring, because the procedure offers hope and there is a high degree of satisfaction with the surgical results. Eighty-seven percent of patients report subjective improvement in appearance after surgery.[60] In addition to increased satisfaction with body image and emotional improvement, some patients also have improvement in behavior and school performance. Ninety-one percent of parents of small children and 77 percent of adolescents would repeat the decision to undergo surgery.[56, 61]

A complete preoperative medical evaluation is required. Patients with craniofacial anomalies often have anomalies of other systems, and many can be classified into recognized syndromes. Comprehensive references to syndromes are available.[6, 10] Associated CNS, pulmonary, and cardiac anomalies are especially noteworthy. Because of the nature of the surgery, a careful history of bleeding tendencies should be taken and special attention must be paid to evaluation of the airway.

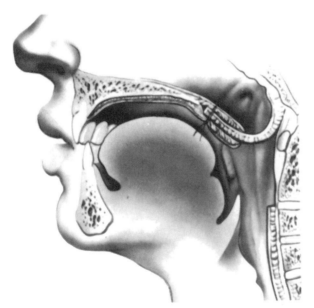

FIGURE 24–26. Pharyngeal flap. A flap of mucosa and muscle is raised from the posterior pharyngeal wall and attached to the soft palate. (From Shprintzen RJ, Lewin ML, Croft CB, et al: A comprehensive study of pharyngeal flap surgery: tailor made flaps. Cleft Palate J 16:50, 1979. From the American Cleft-Craniofacial Association, with permission.)

Airway Anomalies

Twenty to 37 percent of patients undergoing major craniofacial surgery have airway problems.[62, 63] Sixty-five percent of patients with mandibular dysostosis (Treacher-Collins, Goldenhar's, or hemifacial microsomia syndrome) and 53 percent of patients with craniofacial synostosis have problems with airway management. It is extremely important to make a thorough and comprehensive evaluation of the airway because, although many anomalies are grossly evident, not all are readily apparent. Patients often undergo multiple procedures, so a history of airway problems and how they were previously managed can be reviewed. If airway management is expected to be difficult and the possibility of performing a tracheostomy exists, this should be discussed with the patient and parents before surgery.

Certain facial, upper airway, and neck anomalies make airway management (both mask and tracheal intubation) difficult. Facial asymmetry, malar hypoplasia, and nasal deformities may make it difficult to fit a mask to the face with a good seal. Anatomic anomalies such as choanal atresia or stenosis, macroglossia, micrognathia, and diminished nasopharyngeal spaces may produce airway obstruction. Small air passages can be further obliterated by secretions or adenoidal hypertrophy. Signs of airway obstruction, such as mouth breathing, may be present when the patient is awake. Other signs, such as snoring, noisy breathing, and apnea may be present only during sleep. Obstructive sleep apnea is evidenced by snoring with frequent sleep arousals, abnormal movements during sleep, daytime somnolence, nocturnal enuresis, and morning headaches. A history of sleep apnea can be elicited by asking whether the child snores and holds the breath between snores. Poor attention span and school performance, as well as personality and behavioral changes, are also symptoms of obstructive sleep apnea. In severe cases, the child may be underweight and have pulmonary artery hypertension or cor pulmonale. Patients with upper airway obstruction during sleep may have airway obstruction in several perioperative circumstances: with somnolence from premedication, during mask induction of anesthesia, and during the postoperative period after extubation.

Airway anomalies may render direct visualization of the larynx difficult or impossible. Mandibular hypoplasia or micrognathia is a well-known cause of this problem, but microstomia, macroglossia, trismus, and restriction of temporomandibular joint movement may also cause difficulty with laryngoscopy. Certain anatomic features should be carefully examined, such as shape, size, and symmetry of the mandible, anteroposterior distance from the chin to the hyoid bone, size of the tongue, shape of the palate, movement of temporomandibular joints both to open the mouth and to be displaced anteriorly, and size of the mouth (interincisor distance) when open. Range of motion of the neck, especially extension, should be examined. Vertebral anomalies, such as cervical vertebral fusion that is seen with Goldenhar's, Apert's, Crouzon's, and other craniosynostosis syndromes, may limit neck motion.[35–37, 64]

Laboratory Evaluation

When large blood loss is expected, minimal laboratory testing in an otherwise healthy child usually consists of hemoglobin or hematocrit and crossmatching blood. Tests of coagulation (e.g., prothrombin and partial thromboplastin times, platelet count, and bleeding time) should be considered especially in young infants. Other laboratory evaluations, such as, chest x-ray, electrocardiography (ECG), pulmonary function tests, arterial blood gases, and serum electrolytes, are based on the patient's coexisting conditions.

Preoperative Medication

Preoperative medication can be used to augment but should not substitute for psychological preparation. The decision to use preoperative medication is balanced between the need for sedation and the presence of coexisting conditions and airway anomalies. For example, patients with increased intracranial pressure or potential airway obstruction may not safely tolerate respiratory depressants. Optimal sedation should smooth the induction process. Oral benzodiazepines are generally well tolerated. Benzodiazepines, pentobarbital, and chloral hydrate can be given orally and rectally. Fentanyl can be administered in a transmucosal form. Painful intramuscular injections should be avoided when possible. Antisialagogues can be included in the oral premedication if desired.

Intraoperative Anesthetic Management

Successful anesthetic management requires close communication between surgeon and anesthesiologist, especially when the surgeon is working near the airway and when blood loss is rapid. Management of anesthesia is influenced by the patient's coexisting conditions and airway anomalies and by particular features of the craniofacial procedure.

Associated Conditions

Associated respiratory, cardiac, and neurologic anomalies or disorders will influence anesthetic management. The presence of cervical vertebral anomalies may influence head positioning for the procedure. If the patient has complex craniosynostosis, consideration must be given to the potential for raised ICP as previously discussed. Signs and symptoms of elevated ICP are uncommon, and even when ICP is normal, intracranial compliance may be reduced if the cranial vault is not accommodative in all dimensions. Anesthetic induction and maintenance with techniques and agents that decrease ICP are appropriate for these patients.

Airway Anomalies

In considering airway management during the induction of anesthesia, be forewarned that difficulties may be encountered unexpectedly, that physical appearance is not always a reliable guide, and that past uneventful anesthetic courses do not preclude current problems, especially when a cleft palate or pharyngeal flap procedure has been performed in the interim. When difficulty with the airway is anticipated, a general plan should be formulated ahead of time with the understanding that no single technique is foolproof. The plan should include provisions for several alternative techniques, and a variety of equipment should be available, especially laryngeal mask airways and small endotracheal tubes. It is advisable to proceed cautiously with induction of anesthesia, remembering that spontaneous ventilation offers a margin of safety. Airway catastrophes can be avoided by permitting the patient to maintain spontaneous breathing until it is verified that controlled ventilation is possible and easy to reestablish after laryngoscopy or other manipulations.

Difficulty with fitting the mask to the patient's face can be overcome by building up the face with gauze, applying a large mask to the entire face, and using high gas flow. Clear masks with moldable air cushions may fit best. Some patients develop upper airway obstruction at light levels of anesthesia. This can be prevented or attenuated by clearing the nasal passages of secretions before induction and by applying the usual physical maneuvers: maintaining the "sniffing" position, opening the mouth, applying gentle positive airway pressure (5 to 10 cm H_2O), and employing the "jaw thrust" when the patient is sufficiently anesthetized to tolerate it. Nasopharyngeal and oral airways may also be useful.

With mandibular hypoplasia and other oral and cervical malformations, direct laryngoscopy may be impossible or possible only with unconventional maneuvers. In patients with mandibular hypoplasia, the larynx is often described as "anteriorly placed." The larynx is actually in normal position with respect to other cervical structures, but the tongue, which is attached to the hypoplastic mandible, is more posterior than normal and overhangs the larynx, giving the impression that the larynx is anteriorly placed.[65] It is often impossible to open the mouth wide enough to displace the tongue sufficiently to allow visualization of the larynx.

Laryngeal mask airway (LMA) and fiberoptic bronchoscopy have become important tools in airway management for infants and children with craniofacial malformations. The LMA can be inserted in awake infants (with topical anesthesia), or after induction of anesthesia in infants and children to direct blind or fiberoptic-guided tracheal intubation.[66–68]

There are many reports of difficulty with airway management in patients with craniofacial malformations, such as with Treacher-Collins syndrome, hemifacial microsomia, the Robin sequence, and others.[62, 65–79] Prior to use of LMA and fiberoptic bronchoscopy, some unconventional maneuvers were described, such as pulling the tongue out forcefully with a suture, forceps, or custom-made retractors, and use of a Jackson anterior commissure laryngoscope with an "optical stylet." Blind or tactile tracheal intubation, with and without lighted guides, has also been described.

For some patients, a tracheostomy may be required for airway management. Some centers perform elective tracheostomy when extensive facial osteotomies are planned in small children or when the airway would be difficult to manage if intraoperative reintubation were necessary.[63, 80] With the use of rigid internal fixation with plates rather than intermaxillary fixation, tracheostomy can sometimes be avoided. Some patients may have a tracheostomy tube already in place because of severe respiratory obstruction. The anesthesiologist must be aware of the complications and hazards of tracheostomy in pediatric patients: accidental decannulation, obstruction, hemorrhage, and air leaks (the most dangerous of which include pneumothorax and pneumomediastinum, but also subcutaneous emphysema).

Features of the Craniofacial Procedure

Several features of craniofacial surgical procedures will influence anesthetic management: (1) the procedure may be long with extensive tissue exposure; (2) massive blood loss may occur; (3) the procedure may be intracranial; and (4) the airway may be part of the surgical field.

Long Procedure with Wide Tissue Exposure. Major craniofacial procedures average 4 to 5 hours but can last for over 12 hours. Operating time is reduced with an experienced surgical team.[80, 81] Meticulous attention must be paid to protecting the anesthetized patient during prolonged operating time. This includes proper positioning with the joints comfortably flexed, peripheral nerves protected, and pressure points, including the head, adequately padded. The patient may be in a supine, prone, or modified prone position (Fig. 24–27).

During a long period of wide tissue exposure, the patient loses a great amount of body heat. Careful attention must be paid to maintaining temperature homeostasis by employing measures to conserve and provide heat (see Chapter 4). Such measures include minimizing the time of whole-body exposure to cold air before draping, warming the room to 23° to 24°C, and using a heat lamp during exposure. A warming blanket or forced-air warmer should be used, along with passive insulation (plastic or cloth covers) around the body. Irrigation and intravenous fluids and blood should be warmed, and airway gases should be heated and humidified. When large portions of the cranium are exposed, the skull should be repeatedly bathed in warm irrigation fluid.

Excessive Blood Loss. The magnitude of blood loss is related to the extent and duration of the surgical procedure and may equal multiples of the patient's blood volume for major craniofacial surgery. Blood loss reportedly decreases with greater experience of the team.[81–83] In one study of 115 patients undergoing repair of craniosynostosis, mean estimated red cell volume loss was 91 percent of total (range, 5 to 400 percent).[84] Percentage red cell volume loss was greater for infants less than 6 months of age, for complex versus simple synostosis, and for complex vault remodeling versus forehead reconstruction versus strip craniectomy. Infants undergoing strip craniectomy lose an average of 60 percent of their blood volume.[84, 85]

For intracranial procedures, blood loss starts with the initial scalp incision. Infiltration with a dilute vasoconstrictor solution (epinephrine 1:200,000 to 1:400,000 up to 10 $\mu g/kg$ mixed with 0.25 to 1 percent lidocaine)[86] may decrease blood loss from skin and mucosal incisions. Bleeding from the osseous venous plexus is generally continuous throughout osteotomy and bone mobilization, and may be quite brisk. Rapid loss of large volumes of blood

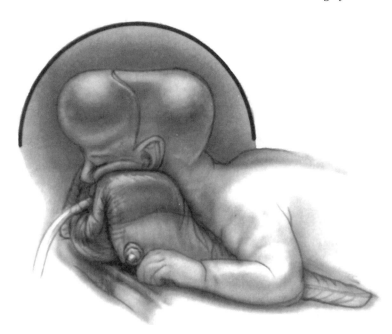

FIGURE 24–27. Modified prone position, with chin support in a padded "bean bag" to allow simultaneous access to the anterior and posterior skull. (From Persing JA, Jane JA, Edgerton MT: Surgical treatment of craniosynostosis. *In* Persing JA, Jane JA [eds]: Scientific Foundations and Surgical Treatment of Craniosynostosis. Baltimore, Williams & Wilkins, 1989, p 134, with permission.)

can occur from uncontrolled arterial bleeding or inadvertent entrance into a dural sinus. For example, the internal maxillary artery may be divided during mandibular osteotomy, and likewise the palatine artery may be cut during a Le Fort I procedure.[80] The severed artery may be difficult to identify and clamp if it retracts to an inaccessible location. Irregularities in the internal surface of the cranium (e.g., bone spurs invaginating the dural sinuses) promote dural sinus tears and hemorrhage that cannot be rapidly controlled. Other sources of major bleeding are the major extradural veins and pharyngeal veins. The presence of scarring and adhesions makes persistent bleeding greater and major arterial, sinus, and venous bleeding more likely in repeat operations.

For infants, blood loss should be aggressively replaced milliliter for milliliter. It is unwise to fall behind in its replacement, as sudden, rapid loss may occur. For larger children and adolescents, initial blood loss can be replaced with appropriate volumes of crystalloid or colloid solutions until a reasonable level of hemodilution is achieved. Much of the blood loss is unmeasurable because it is obscured in the surgical field and drapes. Close communication with the surgeon about the pace of bleeding and close monitoring of the patient's intravascular volume are necessary. Normovolemia should be maintained, and fresh whole blood is the ideal replacement. At least two relatively large-bore intravenous (IV) catheters should be in place for swift delivery of blood. Blood transfusion may be rapid and massive, with all the attendant problems (e.g., hypocalcemia, hyperkalemia, and coagulopathy).[87, 88] When blood replacement exceeds one blood volume, coagulation factors, especially platelets, may need replenishment.[89] Osteotomies, especially of the maxilla, may continue to ooze during the postoperative period, so the child should leave the operating room with an adequate hematocrit.

Induced hypotension can be used to limit blood loss and create a drier surgical field (see Chapter 13). There is no consensus on the utility of this technique and no objective data to support its use in cranial surgery.[90–93] Cerebral hypoxia is a hazard with induced hypotension and also with hyperventilation.[94] Therefore, it is probably unwise to combine the two. Regional brain ischemia can occur even when global perfusion is normal (e.g., when the frontal lobes are retracted). For these reasons, deliberate hypotension may be better suited to extracranial rather than intracranial procedures, although it has been used for both.[80] Several studies have reported decreased blood loss and improved operating conditions with hypotensive anesthesia in young adults undergoing orthognathic surgery.[95–97] One also demonstrated a reduction in the number of patients who required transfusion.[96]

Other techniques that have been used in craniofacial surgery to reduce or eliminate homologous blood transfusion include preoperative use of erythropoietin and intraoperative autologous blood salvage.[98–100] The cost of erythropoietin treatment makes it prohibitive for routine use. The usefulness of intraoperative autologous blood salvage in small children is limited because transfusion is usually started before a full reservoir of autologous blood can be collected.

Intracranial Procedures. For intracranial procedures, anesthetic techniques that decrease intracranial volume should be employed (see Chapter 16). In fronto-orbital procedures, the brain is manipulated and retracted to provide adequate exposure of the anterior cranial fossa and facial bones. Reduction of brain bulk decreases the amount of retraction necessary. Therefore, anesthetic agents such as halothane, enflurane, and ketamine, which increase intracranial volume, should be avoided. Narcotics, benzodiazepines, thiopental, propofol, isoflurane, sevoflurane, and desflurane in combination with mild hyperventilation are preferred. Brain retraction should be released for a few minutes every 30 to 60 minutes to minimize the incidence of brain ischemia.[101] Other measures to decrease intracranial volume include positioning with the head up 20 to 30 degrees and use of diuretics (mannitol and furosemide). The respiratory pattern should not inhibit intracranial cerebrospinal and venous drainage. Therefore, positive end-expiratory pressure (PEEP) should be avoided and mean airway pressure should be kept low by using a long expiratory time, if possible.

Potential hazards during intracranial procedures include dural sinus tears, cerebral edema, and venous air embolism. Dural sinus tears may produce rapid, massive blood loss. There is the risk of cerebral injury and edema when the brain is manipulated and retracted. Air embolism through open venous channels is possible because the open cranium is usually positioned higher than the central circulation.[102, 103] Meticulous surgical technique may prevent this complication.

Intraoperative Airway Management. During Le Fort midface advancement procedures, the surgeon must work intimately around the airway. With maxillary osteotomy and down-fracturing maneuvers, the nasotracheal tube may be lacerated, transected, or dislodged from the trachea. Pilot tubes for endotracheal tube cuffs are easily cut. A plan should be formulated ahead of time between the surgeon and anesthesiologist for endotracheal tube replacement should this be necessary. Usually, the surgical field is quickly covered with sterile drapes to allow the anesthesiologist access to the airway for reintubation. Replacement tubes, catheter guides, and other appropriate equipment for reintubation must be readily available.

When the airway is in the surgical field, an adequate airway must be maintained despite lack of access to the face. The circuit should be lightweight, with all connectors well secured. The head of the operating table may be turned 180 degrees from the anesthesia machine, and the airway circuit must have adequate length to allow this. If the surgeon will move the head during the procedure, the endotracheal tube and circuit must be unencumbered. Care must be taken in initially positioning the endotracheal tube to avoid either extubation when the neck is extended or the maxilla advanced, or endobronchial intubation when the neck is flexed. The maxilla or mandible can be advanced by as much as 3 cm. The tube should be secured by wiring or suturing to facial structures such as teeth, nasal septum, mandible, or alveolar ridge. A nasal tube is required when the procedure is intraoral or when intermaxillary fixation will be done. Armor tubes are useful to prevent compression of the airway by surgical manipulation. The hypopharynx should be packed to prevent intraoperative aspiration of blood, bone chips, and tissue fragments. At the end of the procedure, the nose, mouth, and pharynx should be cleared and the stomach aspirated.

Postoperative swelling of the face and scalp may be severe. After bilateral midface and mandibular osteotomies, postoperative swelling of structures surrounding the upper airway may dictate that the endotracheal tube remain in place for 12 to 48 hours. This is especially true when intermaxillary fixation and occlusive intraoral prostheses limit access to the airway. Persistent oropharyngeal bleeding, cerebral edema, or pulmonary disease may also delay extubation. Extubation should be done when the patient is fully awake and able to follow commands with intact airway reflexes and the stomach empty. Immediate provisions for reestablishing an artificial airway (including

wire cutters to release intermaxillary fixation wires) should be readily available.

Other Anesthetic Considerations

Specific anesthetic drugs should be chosen on the basis of the preceding considerations. Depth of anesthesia can be balanced with muscle relaxation to prevent coughing, bucking, or patient movement with erratic surgical stimuli. Preferably, the patient should be awake and comfortable at the end of the procedure so that neurologic assessment can be made. This can be accomplished by using a potent narcotic or "balanced" technique or by titrating narcotic when the patient is emerging from anesthesia. Extracranial bone graft sites (rib or iliac crest) may contribute more to postoperative pain than cranial sites.

Fluids should be administered to provide maintenance requirements, replace interstitial and evaporative losses, and maintain urine output at approximately 0.5 ml/kg/h. The exact amount of fluid required will depend on the extent of tissue dissection and exposure. For small infants, maintenance fluids should contain an amount of glucose based on intraoperative monitoring of blood glucose levels. A urinary bladder catheter should be placed to prevent bladder distention and as an adjunct to intravascular volume monitoring. Serial blood analyses must be made of arterial pH and blood gases, hemoglobin, electrolytes, ionized calcium, glucose, and coagulation parameters.

A high level of physiologic monitoring is required. Routine anesthesia monitors, such as ECG leads, precordial or esophageal stethoscope, pulse oximeter, central thermometer, and airway gas and pressure monitors, are used. An intra-arterial catheter allows direct blood pressure monitoring and blood sampling. The arterial blood pressure and waveform are good indicators of intravascular volume. A broad-based wave with dicrotic notch and little or no variation with respiration is a good indicator of normovolemia. A central venous catheter is a useful adjunct for monitoring intravascular volume. During intracranial procedures, it is necessary to monitor for venous air embolism because the open cranium is generally elevated above the central circulation. This can be accomplished with a capnograph or precordial Doppler. A central venous catheter may be useful for aspiration of entrained air, although early detection and prevention of further entrainment may be more important than aspiration.

Perioperative Hazards and Complications

Although reports of 20-year series of major craniofacial surgery attest to its relative safety, significant morbidity and mortality can result.[25, 26] Intraoperative death has been reported from massive blood loss and air embolism.[84, 103–106] Postoperative death has resulted from cerebral, respiratory, and circulatory causes (e.g., cerebral edema, massive extradural hemorrhage, respiratory arrest, respiratory obstruction at extubation, tracheostomy blockage, and hemorrhage).[80, 91, 107]

Major intraoperative complications not resulting in death have also been reported. Cardiac arrest has occurred from severe blood loss, air embolism, and pneumoperitoneum (a complication of tracheostomy).[102, 105, 108]

Other reported complications are pneumothorax during rib graft procurement, subdural hematoma, and bradycardia from the oculocardiac reflex.[83, 91, 103, 109] Fifteen cases (including adults) of sudden bradycardia or asystole during craniomaxillofacial surgery were reported in a 13-year period.[110] Stimulation of any sensory branch of the fifth cranial nerve (maxillary and mandibular as well as ophthalmic) is believed to elicit reflex bradycardia and asystole. This reflex has also been noted during maxillofacial and temporomandibular surgery.[110, 111]

Several complications related to the endotracheal tube have been reported, such as intraoperative extubation (usually during midface advancement), endotracheal tube blockage from kinking (also during midface advancement), and endotracheal tube laceration.[63, 82, 83, 109] Pilot tubes for cuffed endotracheal tubes have also been lacerated. There are several reports of emergent endotracheal tube replacement intraoperatively. Complications of tracheostomy have also been reported, including tube kinking, laceration of the posterior tracheal wall, esophageal perforation, and cardiac arrest from pneumoperitoneum.[63, 80, 108, 112]

Postoperative complications not resulting in death have included respiratory obstruction at extubation, pulmonary edema, cerebral edema, extradural hematoma, subgaleal hemorrhage, and seizures.[25, 63, 82, 83, 105, 106] Infection, blindness, CSF leak, facial nerve damage, bone resorption, and hydrocephalus are other major surgical complications.

Anesthesia for Cleft Lip and Cleft Palate Reconstruction

Preoperative Evaluation

The anesthesiologist's approach to the patient with cleft lip and palate is similar to that described in the preceding section for patients with other craniofacial deformities. In this case, however, the surgical procedure is not as extensive. By the time the infant with cleft lip comes for the first operation at 3 months of age, the parents have usually overcome their initial reactions of shock to their malformed infant and are hopeful that surgery will help to restore normal appearance and function.[58] Preoperative preparation must accommodate the older child with cleft palate who may have communication problems because of poor speech and hearing. Many children require multiple procedures, and great effort should be expended to ensure that the anesthetic experience is not unpleasant for parent or child.

A complete medical evaluation should be made, with special attention to the presence of other anomalies. All patients with cleft palate have eustachian tube dysfunction and usually have chronic serous otitis with clear rhinorrhea. Acute infections should be resolved before surgery. Preoperative sedation is appropriate for the child who does not have airway compromise.

Intraoperative Management of Anesthesia

Induction

Most patients with isolated cleft lip or palate present no difficulty with airway management. The reported inci-

dence of difficult laryngoscopy was 3 percent in 800 patients anesthetized over a 10-year period for repair of cleft lip and palate.[113] Extensive clefts, retrognathia, and age less than 6 months were associated with difficult laryngoscopy. With extensive bilateral clefts of lip and alveolus, the laryngeal view was sometimes obstructed by a protruding premaxilla. The incidence of failed intubation was only 1 percent. However, since a problem occasionally arises, it is wise to induce anesthesia with the patient spontaneously breathing. The ease of airway management can then be assessed before the patient is rendered apneic. Airway obstruction may occur if the tongue is impacted against a palatal cleft. This is easily remedied if recognized. If the premaxilla is protruding, care must be taken to avoid injuring it with the laryngoscope. Antisialagogue medication is useful for oral procedures. Oral intubation with a preformed curved tube that lies flat against the face minimizes the potential for tube kinking and dislodgment. The RAE tube[114] is commercially available (Fig. 24–28), and a stylet can be used to facilitate insertion if necessary. The tube should be placed in the midline, with the lip immobile and not distorted.

Maintenance

There are several special anesthetic considerations for cleft lip and palate reconstruction procedures. The first is that the airway is shared with the surgeon. The endotracheal tube must be well secured to prevent inadvertent dislodgment. Adequacy of the airway should be assessed continuously, especially after patient positioning and placement of a mouth gag or pharyngeal packs. For palate

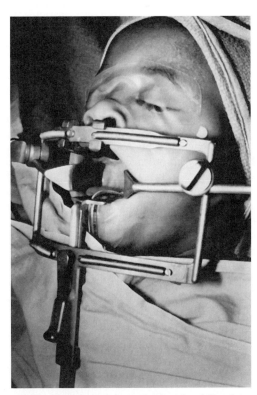

FIGURE 24–28. Dingman mouth gag in place for cleft palate repair. A preformed RAE endotracheal tube is also in place.

and pharyngeal procedures, correct positioning may require exaggerated extension of the neck, which may bring the endotracheal tube up and out of the trachea. A mouth gag is placed to provide surgical exposure and stabilize the tube (Fig. 24–28). Pharyngeal packs are placed to prevent aspiration of blood. Compression or kinking of the tube is a potential hazard with these maneuvers.

For hemostasis, epinephrine-containing local anesthetic solutions (0.25 to 1 percent lidocaine with 1:200,000 to 1:400,000 epinephrine) are injected before incision. Cardiac arrhythmias may result, especially with halothane anesthesia.[115] In normocarbic children, epinephrine with lidocaine can be safely infiltrated to doses of 10 μg/kg during halothane anesthesia.[86] The use of local vasoconstrictors are reported to significantly reduce blood loss in palatoplasty.[116]

Other anesthesia considerations are routine. Fluid and temperature homeostasis must be maintained. Blood loss is rarely enough to require transfusion, although occasionally this becomes necessary in palate and pharyngeal procedures. Inhalation anesthesia is commonly used, but the choice of anesthetic agent is not crucial as long as the considerations outlined here are accommodated.

Postoperative Management

The most common acute postoperative problems are bleeding and airway obstruction.[116, 117] At the conclusion of palate and pharyngeal surgery, the pharynx should be inspected for bleeding and the presence of pharyngeal packs. Placing the infant or child in the lateral position permits drainage of blood and secretions from the pharynx. Extubation should be delayed until the patient is fully awake and has regained normal neuromuscular function to minimize the potential for airway obstruction from either anatomic causes or bleeding. Airway manipulation with mask or artificial airways may damage a lip or nose repair, so it is advisable to delay extubation until the patient is able to maintain a patent airway without assistance. After lip procedures, infants are restrained with straight sleeves to prevent them from disrupting the repair.

After palatoplasty or pharyngoplasty, the infant or child will awaken from anesthesia with a totally altered upper airway. The presence of constricting flaps and nasopharyngeal edema will compromise the nasal airway and the child will be abruptly converted to a mouth-breather. After pharyngoplasty, 10 percent or more of patients experience temporary obstructive sleep apnea.[51, 52] This was completely eliminated in a series of 200 patients by modifying the surgical technique and keeping a nasopharyngeal airway in place for 48 hours postoperatively.[118] Years after surgery, 57 percent of patients who have undergone palatoplasty or pharyngoplasty are predominately or exclusively mouth-breathers.[119] The rate is as high as 72 percent for those who have undergone pharyngoplasty.

Pharyngeal anomalies, which are common with craniofacial syndromes, place the patient at high risk for airway obstruction, especially after pharyngoplasty.[118] The anomalies may be structural, such as pharyngeal narrowing related to malformation of the basicranium (as seen with Treacher-Collins syndrome) or mandible (as with the Robin sequence).[118, 120, 121] Or, they may be functional, such

as pharyngeal hypotonia as seen with the velocardiofacial syndrome.[118] Death occurred in one such patient 4 weeks after surgery.[122]

Acute postoperative airway obstruction after palatoplasty has also been reported secondary to massive lingual swelling.[123–125] The mouth and tongue should be carefully inspected before extubation, particularly if the mouth gag has been in place for more than 2 to 3 hours.

Local anesthesia infiltration will decrease postoperative analgesia requirements. Nonnarcotic analgesics are preferred, but when narcotic supplementation is required it should be titrated in small doses with close supervision. Infraorbital nerve block performed while the patient is asleep has been used to provide postoperative analgesia after cleft lip surgery.[126, 127]

BURNS

Burns are the leading cause of fatal injury for children in the home and are a frequent cause of nonfatal injury.[128] Over 1,000 children in the United States die each year from fire/burns.* Eighty percent of fatalities result from house fires, with most occurring at the scene due to smoke inhalation.[129, 130] Between 1968 and 1985, an average of 1,800 children per year were admitted to specialized burn units in the United States.[128] Over 50 percent of these children were under 5 years old, and the majority of their injuries were the result of hot liquid scalds. Between 5 and 18 years, flame burns were the most common form of thermal injury. Burns are also caused by electricity, chemicals, and radiation.

Burns are classified by the percent of total body surface area (BSA) affected and by depth. An estimate of the percent BSA burned is made from charts based on the work of Lund and Browder,[131] which adjust surface-area proportions for age (Fig. 24–29). The head is relatively larger and the limbs are relatively smaller in children compared with adults. Burn depth is classified as superficial (first degree), partial-thickness (second degree), or full-thickness (third degree). Superficial burns involve only the outer epidermal layer. Although the area is erythematous, there is minimal tissue damage and the protective functions of the skin remain intact. Partial-thickness burns involve the entire epidermis and variable portions of the dermis. There is blistering, weeping transudates, and excruciating pain. A superficial partial-thickness burn involves only the upper part of the dermis. It heals quickly, with minimal scarring, from repopulation by the epithelial cells that lie in hair follicles, sweat glands, and other skin appendages anchored deep in the dermis. A deep partial-thickness burn extends farther into the dermal layer, with few viable epidermal cells remaining. Reepithelialization is very slow, and scarring occurs if the wound is not grafted. The local response to burn injury involves not only direct coagulation of burned tissue but also microvascular reactions in the surrounding dermis, with progressive vasoconstriction and thrombosis. Survival of the surrounding dermis and epidermal appendages is dependent on opti-

---

* Statistics for 1993–1996, from National Center for Injury Prevention and Control.

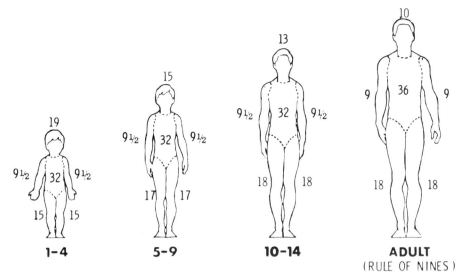

FIGURE 24–29. Burn assessment chart with body proportions. Numbers under figures indicate age; other numbers indicate percent body surface. (Modified from Carvajal HF: Burn injuries. *In* Behrman RE, Kliegman RM, Nelson WE, Vaughan VC III [eds]: Nelson Textbook of Pediatrics, 14th ed. Philadelphia, WB Saunders Company, 1992, p 235, with permission.)

mal conditions. Factors that may lead to progressive dermal ischemia are residual heat, mechanical trauma, vasoactive mediators, and dehydration.[132] Fluid losses and the metabolic effects of deep dermal burns are similar to those of full-thickness burns. A full-thickness burn involves destruction of the entire epidermis and dermis, leaving no residual epidermal cells to repopulate. The skin takes on a dry, leathery, firm consistency with charring or pearly white discoloration.[132] The tissue is avascular and a zone of ischemia exists between the dead tissue above and deeper living tissue below. Survival of this marginally viable tissue is also dependent on optimal conditions. Prevention of conversion of viable tissue to eschar is a major goal during the resuscitation period.

Major burns in children warrant referral to specialized burn care centers with expertise in pediatrics. Major burns are defined as second- and third-degree burns greater than 10 percent total BSA (20 percent for children over 10 years); third-degree burns greater than 5 percent total BSA; second- and third-degree burns involving the face, hands, feet, perineum, and major joints; electrical and chemical burns; burns with inhalation injury; and burns in anyone with preexisting medical disorders.[133] Morbidity and mortality increase with increasing size and depth of the burn. Older children, ages 13 to 18 years, have the best survival rates (50 percent survival with 70 percent BSA burns), and survival is progressively worse the younger the child (only 20 percent survival for infants under 3 years with 70 percent BSA burns).[128] A more recent report notes survival with more than 85 percent BSA burns to be 43 percent for children under 2 years, 72 percent for those 3 to 10 years, and 84 percent for those 11 to 18 years.[134] Advances in the care of thermally injured patients have markedly improved survival in children. These advances include an understanding of resuscitation, hypermetabolic support, wound coverage, infection control, and support of inhalation injury.[135–141]

Acute Resuscitation

Priorities in management of major thermal burns are similar to those for any major trauma: *a*irway, *b*reathing, and *c*irculation (ABC). Establishment of an adequate airway and assessment of inhalation injury are first priority. Fluid resuscitation is instituted and examination is made for associated injuries. The burn wound is assessed and escharotomy performed if necessary. The wound is not locally managed until these more urgent concerns have been addressed.

Airway and Respiratory Management

There are several sources of airway and respiratory compromise in patients with major burns: edema and obstruction of the upper airway, chemical injury to the lung from inhalation of smoke, asphyxia from oxygen deprivation and inhalation of toxic gases, and restriction of respiratory movements by constricting eschar.

Direct thermal injury to the hypopharynx or glottis produces swelling and inflammation, which can rapidly cause life-threatening airway obstruction. Cutaneous burns of the head and neck may also produce progressive swelling that compromises the upper airway. Any burn on the head or neck, singeing of the eyebrows and nasal hair, or soot in the oral pharynx should prompt inspection of the upper airway. If there is stridor or any evidence of upper airway burns, it is best to secure the airway very early before progressive edema obscures normal anatomy.

House fires are responsible for 80 percent of burn-related deaths in children, and most of these deaths are caused by smoke inhalation.[129, 130] Thermal injury below the vocal cords is uncommon unless caused by steam. Inhalation of toxic chemical and particulate constituents of smoke directly injures the tracheobronchial mucosa and pulmonary parenchyma, resulting acutely in bronchospasm and pulmonary edema. Signs that should make one suspicious of inhalation injury include burns of the face or inside the mouth, singeing of the eyebrows and nasal hair, soot in the oral pharynx, and carbonaceous sputum. A history of confinement in a burning environment ("closed space injury") also increases the risk of inhalation injury. Hypoxia, hypercapnia, wheezing, dyspnea, cough, tachypnea, rales, and rhonchi may be present. Changes in ventilation-perfusion matching and intrapulmonary shunt result in an early decrease in arterial oxygenation. Because patients with inhalation injury can decompensate rapidly, endotracheal intubation and supportive ventilation with PEEP should be initiated early. Fiberoptic bronchoscopy can be useful in the evaluation of inhalation injury. Erythema, edema, ulceration, or hemorrhagic necrosis may be seen in the tracheobronchial tree. Carbonaceous secretions and debris may also be present, and bronchoscopy is useful in removing debris and inspissated secretions.

Asphyxia is the most acute serious consequence of fires. The fire consumes oxygen and produces asphyxiating and toxic gases (e.g., CO_2, carbon monoxide, and hydrogen cyanide). Carbon monoxide (CO) is a major cause of death in fires. CO, which has over 200 times greater affinity for hemoglobin than oxygen, displaces oxygen from hemoglobin-binding sites and diminishes oxygen delivery to tissues. Arterial Po_2 and oxygen saturation measured by pulse oximetry (Spo_2) may be normal, although oxygen content of blood is severely depressed. Carboxyhemoglobin (COHb) level in blood is elevated and is useful in evaluating the extent of CO intoxication. With mild CO intoxication there is irritability, headache, weakness, nausea, and dyspnea. More severe intoxication is associated with confusion, seizures, cardiac dysrythmias, coma, and death. The half-time of CO elimination is 4 hours, but this can be shortened to 40 to 80 minutes by hyperventilation in 100 percent oxygen, and to 20 to 25 minutes by use of hyperbaric oxygen. Use of hyperbaric oxygen has been advocated for patients with cardiovascular or neurologic symptoms or COHb level greater than 40 percent.[142] However, the availability of this therapy is limited and the logistics of delivering acute burn care to patients within the confines of a hyberbaric oxygen chamber are formidable.

Cyanide poisoning also causes asphyxiation in fires and should be suspected whenever there is smoke inhalation.[143] An elevated plasma lactate level is a useful indicator of cyanide toxicity when there are no other factors (e.g., hypotension or circulatory shock) to explain it. A carboxyhemoglobin level greater than 15 percent measured within 3 hours of fire exposure identifies patients most likely to have high cyanide levels.[144] Blood cyanide levels are not helpful in making the diagnosis, as the half-life of cyanide in blood is short (approximately 1 hour) and measurements are not readily available. A dose of sodium thiosulfate, which enhances hepatic metabolism of cyanide, can safely be given immediately to all patients with smoke inhalation injury. If the patient is critically ill, with findings suggestive of cyanide intoxication (e.g., coma, seizures, cardiac dysrhythmias, acidemia, or hypotension), sodium nitrite can be administered with careful monitoring of blood pressure. Sodium nitrite converts hemoglobin to methemoglobin, which binds cyanide avidly, but hypotension may occur secondary to vasodilation and

there is also risk of diminished oxygen delivery from an increase in non–oxygen-carrying hemoglobin.[145] Hydroxocobalamin, which is considerably less toxic than sodium nitrite, is also used as a cyanide antidote.[146]

Circumferential burns of the thorax or abdomen can produce constricting eschar that restricts respiratory movement and may precipitate respiratory failure. Full-thickness escharotomy extending the length of the eschar will release the restriction. This is performed at the bedside and does not require anesthesia.

Fluid Resuscitation

Major advances in resuscitation of burn victims have been made since the need to infuse large quantities of salt-containing fluids has been recognized.[147] After a major burn, there is rapid reduction of plasma volume owing to the loss of barrier functions of the skin and development of edema. Within burned tissues there is increased microvascular permeability, impaired cell membrane function and cell swelling, and increase in tissue osmotic pressure leading to interstitial fluid accumulation.[148, 149] Edema of nonburned tissues is initially due to transient endothelial injury from systemic inflammatory mediators and later secondary to hypoproteinemia. Loss of plasma volume is greatest during the first 4 to 6 hours after injury and decreases substantially by 18 to 24 hours if adequate perfusion has been maintained. Protein loss is greatest during the first 8 hours but continues until the wounds are completely grafted. Adequate initial volume resuscitation is critical to survival of the patient and also to prevent conversion of viable but ischemic deep thermal burns to nonviable eschar.[148]

Some controversy exists as to quantity and composition of fluids required and appropriate guidelines for monitoring hydration. Overzealous attempts at restoring blood volume may result in excessive burn edema which, although less lethal than shock, can result in serious morbidity. Massive burn wound edema may impair the availability of cellular oxygen and increase the ischemic insult. The goal of fluid resuscitation is to restore and maintain both perfusion and tissue oxygen delivery at optimal levels to protect the zone of ischemia in burned tissue.[150] Restoration of plasma volume should be accomplished without overloading the circulation, preferably over a 24-hour period. Formulas for fluid replacement such as the Parkland formula or the modified Brooke formula, which use single calculations based on burn size (e.g., 4 ml/kg/percent body burn), tend to underhydrate pediatric patients. Better estimates of fluid requirements for children are made by calculating burn-related requirements and maintenance requirements separately. To do this using the Parkland formula for the first 24 hours, lactated Ringer's solution is administered in an amount equal to maintenance requirements plus burn requirements of 4 ml/kg/percent body burn.[151] A recommendation with the modified Brooke formula is for children less than 20 kg to administer maintenance fluids plus an additional 2 to 3 ml/kg/percent body burn.[136] The only formula developed specifically for children is the Galveston formula, which uses body surface area for all calculations.[152] The rationale for this approach is that burn-related fluid losses are proportional to burn edema and evaporative fluid losses, which are both proportional to surface area burned. This avoids underhydration of small children and overhydration of larger children and children with large burns that occurs with formulas based on weight.[153] BSA burned is calculated by multiplying percent burn times total BSA. Total fluid requirements for the first day are estimated as 5,000 ml/m^2 BSA burned (burn-related losses) plus 2,000 ml/m^2 total BSA (maintenance fluids). Half of the 24-hour fluid allowance is administered during the first 8 hours and the other half during the subsequent 16 hours. In this program, an isotonic glucose-containing solution with added albumin is used for the first 24 hours. The solution consists of 50 ml of 25 percent human serum albumin (12.5 g) mixed with 950 ml of 5 percent dextrose in lactated Ringer's solution. For infants less than 1 year of age, the concentration of sodium is lowered to prevent hypernatremia. No potassium is added during the first 12 to 24 hours after the burn or before normal kidney function has been demonstrated. Hypertonic salt solutions have been used in adults to limit the total amount of fluid administered and minimize edema. The risks of hypernatremia and hyperosmolality with intracellular dehydration make this alternative less attractive for children.

The addition of colloid to initial hydrating solutions is controversial. The concern is that protein administration during the first 24 hours may increase protein accumulation in the interstitium and may thereby accentuate and prolong edema. There is transient systemic endothelial injury and capillary leakage after major burns mediated by proinflammatory cytokines, complement, arachidonic acid metabolites, and oxygen free radicals.[154] Thereafter, the edema that occurs in nonburned tissues does not appear to be due to altered protein permeability but rather to the severe hypoproteinemic state of the burned patient.[155] Early colloid infusion has been shown to minimize edema in nonburned tissues and to increase blood volume better than crystalloid.[147] In children, it has been reported that when albumin is added to fluids from the onset of resuscitation, serum albumin levels can be maintained within the normal range.[156]

Formulas for fluid requirements provide only estimates of the quantity of fluid needed. Monitoring the results of fluid therapy and making appropriate adjustments represent a significant challenge. Many authors recommend adjusting fluids to a rate that will maintain a urine output of 0.5 to 1 ml/kg/h. Carvajal[152] cautions that no single criterion predicts the state of hydration consistently or accurately and that as many predictors as possible should be correlated before making decisions to adjust fluid administration. The hourly urine volume alone is not a good monitor because the kidneys are under the influence of exaggerated hormonal responses (i.e., antidiuretic hormone) which, for the most part, correlate poorly with the state of hydration. Urine output and the ability to concentrate the urine should be demonstrated.[153] Urine output should be evaluated over 4-hour periods, with 120 ml/m^2 considered an adequate amount. Other signs of adequate hydration are a progressive decline in the high hematocrit seen in the immediate postburn period and a normal or improving blood pH. Rate of fluid administration should be adjusted up or down as needed, but

fluid pushes should be avoided because rapid expansion of the intravascular compartment and increased venous pressure may increase fluid losses into the interstitium. Because vital signs and urine output do not reliably predict adequacy of resuscitation, in high-risk patients invasive monitoring with a pulmonary artery catheter may be necessary.[157] Serial determinations of cardiac index and oxygen delivery are the most sensitive indices of adequate volume status and perfusion.

After the first day, fluid losses occur primarily through burn exudate and evaporation from denuded areas. Maximal weight gain and edema occur at 2 to 3 days afterburn. Thereafter, a diuresis ensues and the patient returns to preburn weight at approximately 14 days.[156] Fluid requirements decrease after the first day afterburn, and the Galveston program advocates that requirements be estimated as 3,750 ml/m^2 BSA burned/day plus 1,500 ml/m^2 total BSA/day. The albumin-containing solution described previously is used. However, the sodium content is reduced to 50 mEq/L for children and 35 to 40 mEq/L for infants.[152] With the Parkland formula, colloid is also administered after the first day (0.5 ml/kg of 5 percent albumin over 6 to 8 hours) plus D_5 0.25 percent saline at a rate sufficient to maintain urine output at 1 ml/kg/h.[151] Protein loss in burn exudate remains significant until all burn wounds are grafted and healing.

Acute Burn Wound Management

The burn wound can be adversely affected by desiccation and infection. It is cleaned and debrided and soluble antibiotics (e.g., 1 percent silver sulfadiazine) are applied to the surface of deep burns. The wound is covered with moist and then with dry gauze. Edema and inelastic eschar that form with circumferential burns may compromise the vascular supply of the extremities or restrict respiratory motions of the chest wall or abdomen. Escharotomy is performed as a bedside procedure by incising the insensitive eschar to release the restriction. Rarely, fasciotomy is required to prevent a compartment syndrome.

Acute Resuscitation: Physiology

Hypovolemia and the acute neurohormonal stress response account for most of the acute physiologic changes that occur with major burn injury. Fluid losses occur from direct transudation of fluid from the wound and from both local and systemic capillary leakage. Cardiac output is significantly reduced within minutes of injury.[158] Systemic vascular resistance increases two- to threefold. Pulmonary vascular resistance increases even more. The mediators of this intense vasoconstriction appear to be catecholamines, vasopressin, and thromboxane A_2. Depressed cardiac contractility, derangements of ventricular contractility, and pathologic increases in afterload contribute to depression of cardiac output. A myocardial depressant factor has been identified in animals, and high levels of the same inflammatory mediators implicated in myocardial depression in septic shock have been found in burned patients.[158] These include tumor necrosis factor, the interleukins, vasopressin, and oxygen free radicals. Myocardial depression is generally rapid in onset and short in duration, resolving in a period of hours to days. Responses to endogenous and exogenous catecholamines are attenuated and suggest that the adrenergic receptors are either maximally stimulated or desensitized. Experimentally, after burn injury myocardial β-adrenergic receptors have decreased affinity for ligands, impaired receptor-mediated signal transduction, and decreased adenylate cyclase activity resulting in decreased cyclic adenosine monophosphate (cAMP) production.[159, 160]

Initially the hematocrit is typically elevated, owing to hemoconcentration from loss of plasma. With extensive deep burns there may be hemolysis, free plasma hemoglobin, and hemoglobinuria. Activation of clotting and consumption of clotting factors within the wound may occur. Spontaneous bleeding is uncommon, even though clotting factors are depleted in patients with massive burns.

Renal function depends on the state of the circulation and on the hormonal and toxic influences on the kidneys. Glomerular filtration rate is initially depressed because of hypovolemia. Vasopressin and aldosterone promote retention of water and sodium, although tubular function may be impaired by circulatory or toxic (hemoglobinuria or myoglobinuria with electrical burns) insults. An osmotic diuresis and tubular dysfunction may be seen, similar to that seen with nonoliguric renal failure. Increased nonreabsorbable colloid from destroyed tissues may also promote an osmotic diuresis.[161] Measurement of plasma osmolality is helpful in determining if plasma water content is normal. Careful control of electrolyte and fluid balance and administration of adequate water to excrete the osmolar load from injured tissue are required.

The goal of resuscitation is to restore circulating blood volume and minimize the early stress response. This is accomplished with adequate fluid resuscitation, correction of hypoxia and ventilatory disturbances, prevention of hypothermia, and adequate control of pain and anxiety.[148]

Special Circumstance: Electrical Burns

High-voltage (greater than 1,000 V) electrical burns are associated with deep and extensive tissue destruction, especially of muscle.[162] The body surface area involved is usually relatively limited, but the injury on the surface may be only the "tip of the iceberg." Electrical burns are caused by conversion of electrical energy into heat, which is the principal mediator of tissue injury.[163] The amount of heat generated is a function of voltage drop and current flow per unit cross-sectional area. This dependence on cross-sectional area accounts for the high frequency of severe injury to the extremities. The skin is burned or charred at points of current entry and exit where current density is greatest. Electrical paths between entrance and exit points place any structure in the body at risk for injury.

Electrical burns produce extensive deep muscle injury, and injury to remote parts of the CNS and the thoracic and abdominal cavities.[163] Instant death probably results from cardiac arrest, fibrillation, or massive CNS injury. Cardiac arrhythmias or electrocardiographic changes occur in 10 to 30 percent of patients, but myocardial infarction or direct myocardial injury is not common. Acute renal failure may occur secondary to serum free hemoglobin, myoglobin, and denatured proteins from the exten-

sively injured muscle. Major amputations comprise the most common complication. Spinal cord damage may be acute or delayed. Associated injuries (e.g., fractures, head injury, and other traumatic injuries) occur in a substantial number of patients who are thrown or fall.

Electrical burns cause considerably more tissue damage than is apparent on the body surface and require more fluids for resuscitation than is calculated by formulas based on burned body surface area. Fluids should be calculated by overestimating the burn area by 25 to 50 percent.[152] Prevention of renal insufficiency also takes precedence over minimizing tissue edema. A forced diuresis, aimed at flushing the renal tubules of myoglobin and hemoglobin by-products, can be induced with mannitol 0.5 g/kg or furosemide 1 mg/kg. Because acidosis promotes tubular precipitation of hemochromogens, alkalization of the urine by sodium bicarbonate administration may protect the kidneys.[163] The patient may require acute surgical intervention in the operating room for debridement of dead and devitalized tissues, fasciotomies of deep muscle compartments, or management of associated injuries.

Hypermetabolic Phase: Physiology

After the acute phase of injury and initial resuscitation, a hypermetabolic state ensues, which lasts until the wounds are closed and healing. The metabolic response to burns is similar to that of sepsis and trauma and is characterized by protein and lipid catabolism, total body protein loss, peripheral insulin resistance, increased energy expenditure and stimulated synthesis of acute phase proteins.[164] Mediators of the neuroendocrine response, such as catecholamines, glucagon, and glucocorticoids, and agents released by the immune system including pro- and antiinflammatory cytokines, interact in the regulation of the metabolic response. The magnitude of the response is proportional to the size and depth of the burn.[165, 166] Body temperature and the zone of thermal neutrality rise. Five to 8 hours after burn injury there is inhibition of heat-losing mechanisms and a rapid increase in heat storage in children.[167] The hypothalamic thermoregulatory "set-point" is reset to a higher-than-normal body temperature (approximately 38.5°C).[168] In the milieu of these anti-insulin hormones, serum glucose and insulin are also elevated.[169] Endogenous processes are geared to production of energy substrates by catabolism of fat and protein stores. High caloric and nitrogen intake to support a high metabolic state, prevent protein breakdown, and promote wound healing is essential for survival.[170, 171] There is also evidence that good nutrition attenuates the inflammatory and metabolic responses.[164] Several pharmacologic means to alter the hypermetabolic, catabolic response to burn injury are under investigation: β-blockers (propranolol), cyclooxygenase inhibitors (ibuprofen), and anabolic agents (growth hormone and submaximal insulin dose).[172-174] The response can be minimized by providing a warm environment (28° to 32°C), and by use of occlusive dressings to minimize evaporative heat loss.[165] Adequate treatment of pain and anxiety are also important in minimizing the stress response.

In the hypermetabolic state, heart rate is elevated and cardiac output is increased in direct relation to oxygen consumption. Hypertension is common and must be effectively treated to prevent hypertensive encephalopathy.[175-177] Ventilatory requirements are greater than normal because metabolic rate, and therefore oxygen consumption and CO_2 production, are high. Patients with 50 percent body surface burns consume oxygen at twice the normal rate by the end of the first week.

Respiratory function may be impaired due to injury to the respiratory tract. Chemical tracheobronchitis is manifest by edema, disturbed ciliary function, retained secretions, sloughing of airway mucosa, atelectasis, and bronchospasm. Lung parenchymal injury is manifest as pulmonary edema and surfactant deficiency. The clinical picture can vary from one of mild pulmonary edema to one of severe respiratory distress syndrome. The injury may appear immediately after the burn or have a subtle onset 3 or 4 days later. This delayed pattern of pulmonary injury may occur with or without direct smoke inhalation injury. Scald burns involving 25 to 30 percent BSA can produce respiratory distress syndrome, even in the absence of smoke inhalation.[178, 179] This suggests that inflammatory mediators and perhaps perfusion shock play a role in its genesis. Pulmonary complications may also be due to infection. Respiratory failure is the most frequent form of organ failure found in burned patients, and patients with respiratory failure have a high incidence of multiorgan failure and mortality.[179, 180] Patients with inhalation injury have a much higher incidence (73 percent) of respiratory failure than those without inhalation injury (5 percent).[179] The management of inhalation injury consists of supportive care: humidified oxygen, bronchodilator drugs, good pulmonary toilet (chest physiotherapy, bronchoscopic suctioning), and mechanical ventilation with PEEP, pressure support, or high-frequency modalities.

During the acute phase of injury the patient is at risk for acute renal failure secondary to circulatory insufficiency or toxins. The occurrence of acute renal failure shows a binomial distribution, with one peak occurring during the first week after burn and another approximately 3 weeks after the burn.[181] Renal failure that occus immediately after burns is generally due to hypovolemia and delay in fluid resuscitation. Elevated levels of stress hormones also produce renal ischemia, which results in tubular necrosis. The later appearance of renal failure is mainly associated with systemic sepsis.[181] The mortality rate in burned children with acute renal failure has decreased from 100 percent prior to 1983 to 56 percent after 1984.[181] Even without frank renal failure, renal tubular dysfunction may persist into the postresuscitative hypermetabolic stage, with impairment of both concentrating and diluting mechanisms. When this occurs, urine osmolality approaches that of plasma.[182] The glomerular filtration rate is increased in the hypermetabolic stage, and drugs that are cleared by glomerular filtration are rapidly eliminated.

The CNS can be injured by anoxia, with resulting cerebral edema and increased ICP. CNS dysfunction may also manifest as burn encephalopathy, which consists of altered sensorium and seizures.[183] Neurologic dysfunction, especially seizures, occur secondary to other complications of burn injury (e.g., electrolyte imbalances, fever, and hypertension).[184]

Many hematologic alterations occur after burn injury. The red blood cell (RBC) half-life is decreased from 22 days to 6 days and there is an ongoing nonautoimmune hemolytic anemia.[182] Ongoing blood loss also contributes to anemia. The platelet count may decrease to thrombocytopenic levels during the first week after the burn and return to supranormal levels thereafter. Subsequent thrombocytopenia may be an early indicator of sepsis.[185] Prothrombin and partial thromboplastin times may be elevated during the first week after injury, and then slowly return to normal. Fibrin-split products are elevated for the first few days. Fibrinogen concentrations increase two- to threefold after the second day, which increases plasma viscosity. Factors V and VIII also are markedly elevated. White blood cell (WBC) counts are typically elevated, although transient leukopenia may be caused by silver sulfadiazine.

Gastrointestinal function is initially diminished, and ileus and acute gastric distention are common. During the hypermetabolic phase, stress ulcers are common in children unless specific measures are taken to prevent them, such as antiulcer medications and frequent feedings when tolerated. The gastrointestinal (GI) tract is viewed as a reservoir of microorganisms which, under the conditions of transient ischemia, can translocate across the intestinal wall and produce sepsis.[186] Enteral nutrition, use of limited-spectrum antibiotics, and judicious use of medications that limit motility promote favorable regulation of GI microflora and maintain the integrity of the mucosal barrier.

The skin normally acts to conserve heat and fluids and to protect against infection. The loss of skin in burn injury means the loss of these vital functions. Fluid and electrolyte intake must balance usual losses plus additional losses of exudate and evaporation from the wound. Patients are prone to electrolyte imbalances; in particular, hypocalcemia can persist for weeks. Magnesium depletion may exist even with normal serum levels and may be a contributing factor to the pathogenesis of postburn hypocalcemic hypoparathyroidism and parathyroid hormone resistance.[187] Infection is a major cause of death in severely burned patients. Burned patients are at high risk for local wound infection and for systemic sepsis. Dysfunction of various components of the immune system occurs after major burn injury. Chronically elevated temperature and WBC counts make these parameters less reliable indicators of infection.[188, 189] A falling platelet count and feeding intolerance may be the earliest indicators of systemic infection. Leukopenia (not associated with silver sulfadiazine) is an ominous sign. Aggressive nutritional support and early excision and grafting of burned tissue are important in reducing the risk of infection in burned patients.

Surgical Reconstruction of Burns: Early Excision and Grafting

Surgical reconstruction of major burns is performed in both the acute and chronic stages of injury. Primary excision of eschar and grafting of the wound are started when the patient's condition has stabilized, usually within 2 to

4 days after injury. Secondary reconstruction of scars and contractures may be necessary later.

Early excision of eschar and skin grafting are generally believed to improve survival of children with major burns.[190, 191] Two types of excisions are done, tangential and fascial. With tangential excision, the eschar is shaved in sequential thin slices until a bleeding viable matrix is reached on which to lay a graft. This procedure is very bloody and is generally limited to 15 percent total body surface area (or less in very young children). Excision to the muscle fascial plane is faster and associated with much less blood loss. However, because fat and lymphatics are removed the cosmetic results are less favorable. Fascial excision is therefore reserved for burn wound sepsis and when it is desirable to limit operating time and blood loss (e.g., when the area to be excised is very large or the patient is unstable or otherwise at risk for operative complications).[192, 193] For large burns, total fascial excision can be done early or serial tangential excision can be performed every 3 to 7 days. The wound is closed with autogenous skin grafts. In large burns, the amount of unburned skin available for grafting may be inadequate. Temporary cadaver allografts, porcine xenografts, synthetic membranes, or semibiologic skin substitutes are applied until autografting is possible.[132] The use of cultured autologous epidermal cells has been disappointing because of exorbitant cost and low engraftment rate.

Anesthesia for Excision and Grafting of the Burn Wound

Altered Pharmacology

Major burn injury causes profound alterations in the clinical pharmacokinetics of many drugs,[194, 195] secondary to the many physiologic changes.[196] In the acute phase, cardiac output and blood flow to tissues are diminished. Later, in the postresuscitative or hypermetabolic phase, these parameters are increased. Glomerular filtration rate and creatinine clearance are increased in the hypermetabolic phase, but hepatic phase I drug metabolism (oxidation, reduction, and hydroxylation) is decreased. Albumin (which binds acidic and neutral drugs, e.g., diazepam) is decreased, whereas α_1-acid glycoprotein (which binds basic drugs, e.g., lidocaine, propranolol, bupivacaine, fentanyl, and alfentanil) is increased. In addition, neural and hormonal mechanisms, as well as other circulating mediators, also affect drug disposition and action.

Perhaps the most profound pharmacologic changes involve muscle relaxants. Burned patients are supersensitive to succinylcholine and hyposensitive to nondepolarizing muscle relaxants.[197] The use of succinylcholine is contraindicated because it can cause lethal hyperkalemia. This response is related to dose and time elapsed after burn injury, although the exact time of onset is unknown. The response may last as long as 2 years, and it has been recommended that succinylcholine be avoided until at least several months after complete healing of wounds.[197] Resistance to nondepolarizing muscle relaxants develops 1 week after injury and is related to the magnitude of the burn.[198] The dosage of nondepolarizing muscle relaxants must be increased by two- to fivefold the normal dose in patients with greater than 20 percent BSA burns. Several

studies have demonstrated resistance to nondepolarizing muscle relaxants in children.[198–201] Although the exact duration of this effect is unknown, resistance to d-tubocurarine has been documented in a child more than 1 year after complete healing of burn wounds.[202] Antagonist drugs should be used in normal doses. The mechanism for these alterations in response to neuromuscular blocking drugs is believed to be a denervation-like phenomenon in which acetylcholine receptors are increased (up-regulation) in number and are located in extrajunctional locations in the muscle membrane.[197] Other factors, such as changes in acetylcholinesterase activity and receptor affinity, may also alter responses to neuromuscular blocking drugs.

Changes in the pharmacokinetics of benzodiazepines have been documented in burned patients.[195] Hepatic clearance of diazepam and chlordiazepoxide is reduced and the elimination half-life of diazepam is doubled (from 36 hours to 72 hours). Although the duration of action of a single dose is short owing to rapid uptake by tissues, repeated administration of diazepam saturates the tissues and termination of its effect then depends on biotransformation, which is prolonged in burned patients. Impaired clearance may be due to impaired hepatic oxidative metabolism or to concomitant administration of other medications such as cimetidine, which reduces hepatic blood flow and inhibits diazepam clearance. Lorazepam metabolism is unimpaired in burned patients and is not affected by concomitant cimetidine administration.

Cimetidine elimination is increased, and higher than usual plasma concentrations are required to control gastric pH in burned children.[195] Ranitidine is the preferred H_2-blocker because of its lack of side effects and interference with metabolism of other drugs. The dosage should be guided by serial measurements of gastric fluid pH.

Cardiovascular responses to adrenergic agents are greatly diminished in the hypermetabolic stage of burn injury. Topical application of epinephrine at the time of wound excision is well tolerated and produces minimal cardiovascular changes.[195] It infrequently causes arrhythmias, even with halothane anesthesia. As noted above, after burn injury myocardial β-adrenergic receptors have been shown to have decreased affinity for ligands, impaired receptor-mediated signal transduction, and decreased adenylate cyclase activity resulting in decreased cAMP production.[159, 160]

Ketamine and halothane have been extensively used in burned patients, and repeated administration of halothane has been shown to be safe. Total IV anesthesia with propofol and alfentanil has also been reported.[203] Oxygen consumption and hyperdynamic cardiovascular variables (cardiac output, heart rate, and blood pressure) decrease during anesthesia with enflurane and isoflurane but return to preanesthetic values when anesthesia is discontinued.[204] Dosage requirements for thiopental are elevated in burned children for at least 1 year after injury. The induction dose for a normovolemic child is 7 to 8 mg/kg.[205]

Narcotics are the most common form of analgesic therapy, and requirements are high in burned patients.[206] In acutely burned children, volume of distribution and elimination half-life of morphine are markedly shortened and the rate of clearance is increased.[206] In contrast, in adults elimination of morphine, meperidine, and alfentanil is diminished.[195, 207, 208] High-dose morphine has been shown to reduce the hypermetabolic response.[209] Long-term infusion of morphine, ketamine, and midazolam has been reported for a single pediatric patient.[210]

Preoperative Evaluation

Preoperative evaluation of patients with major burns focuses on assessment of the extent and location of the burn, physiologic derangements, and current drug therapy. If the patient has burns of the head or neck, management of the airway may be difficult. The airway must be thoroughly assessed, including inspection for edematous structures and demonstration of ability to open the mouth, displace the temporomandibular joint forward, and extend the neck. If difficulty with conventional airway maneuvers is anticipated, alternative plans must be made. Tracheostomy should be avoided because of the high mortality from sepsis when a tracheostomy is placed in burned tissue.[211] Burns on the face may make fitting a mask uncomfortable and securing the endotracheal tube difficult. Clear, air-cushioned masks may be most acceptable. Tape should not be applied to burned or grafted areas. The endotracheal tube can be secured with umbilical ties secured around the head or, if this interferes with the surgical field, the tube can be sutured or wired to facial structures.[212, 213] Alternatively, a nasotracheal tube can be split to near the point of entrance to the nose and the split ends can act as flanges to which the ties can be attached.[214]

When the surgical procedure involves the face, it may be a challenge to avoid the surgical field with airway equipment. Preformed, curved tubes (oral and nasal RAE tubes) that angle the circuit cephalad or caudad may be useful. If there are extensive burns on the back, positioning and airway management may be difficult, and suitable plans and alternatives should be formulated with the surgeon preoperatively.

In the preoperative assessment, past medical history and the presence of other injuries must not be overlooked. Physiologic derangements should be corrected before anesthesia and surgery. Intravascular volume, acid–base status, oxygenation, electrolytes, glucose, and coagulation parameters should all be normalized.

Patients with extensive burns undergo multiple surgical procedures at frequent intervals. Special care must be taken so that the operative experience is neither psychologically nor physiologically disruptive. Adequate analgesia and sedation should be provided preoperatively (for transport) and postoperatively. Care must be taken to minimize heat loss during transport by covering the patient with warm blankets. If the patient is taking enteral feedings, the perioperative fasting period should be minimized to maintain vital caloric intake. To prevent infection, antiseptic technique should be used at all times by all personnel in contact with the burned patient. Personnel should wear gloves, caps, masks, and gowns. All equipment should be clean and anything that contacts the wound should be sterile. Invasive procedures must be performed with sterile technique.

Intraoperative Management

The greatest challenges during excision and grafting procedures are heat conservation and blood loss. Ongoing communication between surgeon and anesthesiologist about blood loss and temperature maintenance is essential.

When surfaces of denuded tissue are exposed, the patient rapidly becomes hypothermic if measures to prevent this are not taken. General anesthetics block thermoregulation, and although heat production increases during the operative period it is not sufficient to counterbalance heat loss.[215] Burned patients have a higher-than-normal core temperature (38° to 39°C) and are most comfortable in a higher-than-normal ambient temperature (30° to 31°C).[166] The operating room should be as warm as can be tolerated by personnel and should be draft-free. Radiant warmers can be placed above the patient. A warming blanket or forced-air warmer, along with passive insulation (plastic or cloth covers), should be placed around nonoperative sites. All fluids that come in contact with the patient, including IV and irrigation fluids and blood products, should be warmed. Inspired gases should be warmed and humidified. Operative time is minimized by a well-coordinated team effort. For example, one team can excise eschar while another harvests grafts. This allows wounds to be covered as expeditiously as possible. Most procedures should be limited to approximately 1.5 hours.

Blood loss is rapid and massive in all but the most limited excisions. It is commonly estimated that 3.5 to 5 percent of blood volume is lost for every 1 percent of the body surface excised.[135] Scalp is a particularly bloody donor site. Administration of desmopressin (dDAVP) does not reduce the blood loss.[216] For small children, blood replacement with whole blood that is as fresh as possible should start when blood loss begins. Because blood loss is difficult to estimate, accurate measurements of the patient's intravascular volume must be available. This can be provided by direct arterial blood pressure and perhaps by central venous pressure monitoring. Several measures can be taken to limit blood loss with tangential excision: tourniquets can be applied to the extremities; epinephrine (1:10,000)-soaked sponges can be applied to the bleeding surface with minimal systemic side effects; thrombin and collagen pads can be applied topically; and excision can be limited to 10 to 15 percent of total body surface area.

The complications of massive transfusion must be anticipated, especially acute citrate intoxication. Burned patients are chronically hypocalcemic, and hypotension commonly occurs with rapid infusion of blood products containing citrate. Simultaneous administration of $CaCl_2$ 5 mg/kg blunts this hypotensive response.[88] Halothane accentuates myocardial depression and hypocalcemia during infusion of citrated blood products.[217] Coagulation parameters, especially platelet count, should be monitored, and clotting factors and platelets should be administered as needed. Prophylactic administration of fresh frozen plasma or platelets is not indicated because of the higher-than-normal preoperative levels of platelets, fibrinogen, and factor VIII and the slower-than-normal washout of platelets and factor IX.[218] As stated above, ongoing communication between surgeon and anesthesiologist about blood loss and temperature maintenance is essential.

Because of the hypermetabolic state, requirements for alveolar ventilation are higher than normal. Usually the patient's trachea is intubated and ventilation controlled for all but very short, limited procedures. If the patient has pulmonary injury and respiratory distress syndrome, the anesthesia ventilator may not be adequate to deliver appropriate tidal volume, inspiratory pressure, and PEEP. An intensive care unit ventilator or manual ventilation may be required. Patients with pulmonary injuries who require PEEP should be transported with ventilatory systems that can provide it (such as a Mapleson system with valve).

Maintenance fluid requirements are higher than normal and should be continued through the operative period. The surgeon may infiltrate normal saline subcutaneously to facilitate harvesting of donor skin. This usually constitutes a significant amount of fluid and must be compensated for by decreasing IV fluids. If the patient is receiving parenteral alimentation with a high concentration of glucose, a similar amount of glucose should be delivered during the operative period to prevent hypoglycemia. Serum glucose concentrations should be monitored to avoid hyperglycemia and hyperosmolar dehydration.

Monitoring and vascular access may be difficult if the area of burned tissue is extensive. ECG leads can be placed on any intact skin, a "back pad" can be placed under dependent parts, or an esophageal lead can be used. If these are not possible, alligator clips or needle electrodes can be applied or pads can be stapled on after anesthesia is induced. Intra-arterial access for monitoring and blood sampling is necessary for all but very limited procedures. Continuous display of arterial blood pressure and wave form is necessary for continuous assessment of intravascular volume. Central venous pressure monitoring is also helpful for tracking intravascular volume. Pulse oximeter probes can be placed on the tongue, as an adjunct to peripheral oximetry, in children with extensive thermal injury.[219] Blood sampling should be done as necessary to monitor arterial pH and blood gases, glucose, electrolytes, and coagulation parameters. A urinary catheter should be placed to monitor urine output. At least two relatively large-bore IV lines are required for rapid infusion of blood products. Femoral vessels are frequently used because this area is commonly spared from injury. In some cases, temporary lines must be placed through burned tissue for the duration of the surgical procedure, but these lines should be promptly removed postoperatively because of the risk of infection. Cut-downs should be avoided because they increase the risk of infection. Pressure bags or other devices for rapid infusion of blood should be available.

Hypermetabolic burned patients who have normal intravascular volumes require higher doses of anesthetic, narcotic, and sedative drugs. The inclusion of narcotics and sedatives in the anesthetic plan provides some degree of postoperative analgesia and smoothes emergence from anesthesia. A smooth emergence from anesthesia without shivering is important to avoid dislodgment of grafts and the tremendous increase in oxygen consumption that occurs with shivering. Shivering can also be prevented by administration of meperidine, 0.3 mg/kg, and warming the patient before emergence.

Anesthesia for Secondary Burn Reconstruction

The principal late complications of burn injuries are hypertrophic scars and contractures. Hypertrophic scars are treated surgically by excision or shaving, followed by primary closure or skin grafting. Contractures may involve any joint. Release of contractures commonly involves skin grafting and local flaps. Airway management may be particularly hazardous when neck contractures are present (Fig. 24–30). Fiberoptic intubation of the trachea of the awake or sedated patient may be required, or the contractures can be released with local anesthesia before induction of general anesthesia. Alternatively, if the airway can be managed with a mask the contractures can be released under IV or inhalational anesthesia delivered by mask or by a laryngeal mask airway.

Burn Pain

Pain associated with burns is severe and persists until the wounds are well healed. In children, pain increases with size and depth of the burn.[220] Experimentally, cutaneous burn injury results in local inflammatory changes manifest as redness, lowered pain thresholds (allodynia), and enhanced pain response to noxious stimuli (hyperalgesia).[221, 222] Hyperalgesia may be due to changes in C-polymodal nociceptors that develop a decreased threshold and increased rate of firing.[223] Intense C-fiber stimulation also induces a state of central hypersensitivity in dorsal horn neurons of the spinal cord.[224]

Pain associated with burns can be clinically differentiated into background (constant) pain and procedural pain related to dressing changes and wound debridement. Success in managing background pain has been reported

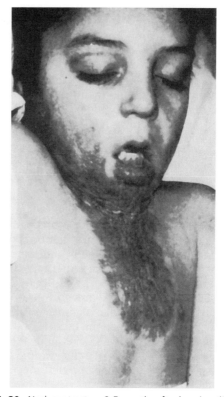

FIGURE 24–30. Neck contracture 2.5 months after burning. (From Evans AJ: The treatment of burn in infants and children. *In* Mustardé JC [ed]: Plastic Surgery in Infancy and Childhood. Edinburgh, Churchill Livingstone, 1979, p 599, with permission.)

with scheduled acetaminophen (10 to 15 mg/kg every 4 hours) and oral or intravenous morphine (every 4 hours).[220] Administration of morphine via patient-controlled analgesia regimen is ideal for patients able to participate. Requirements for escalating doses of narcotics, perhaps related to tolerance, and difficulty in maintaining pain control are common problems with large burns that require prolonged care. Successful use of methadone in two morphine-tolerant burned children has been reported.[225] The use of topical and intravenous lidocaine for management of burn pain has been reported in adults.[226,227] A neuropathic-like pain may be due to abnormalities in newly regenerated nerve endings or to central mechanisms. Low dosages of tricyclic antidepressants can significantly improve this type of burn pain. Other related problems may require attention, such as, anxiety, puritis, and acute and posttraumatic stress symptoms.[220] Medications such as lorazepam, diphenhydramine and antidepressants are useful in alleviating these symptoms and improving pain control. Other forms of pain management such as transcutaneous nerve stimulation and psychological interventions can be useful. Distractive strategies and cognitive interventions such as mental imagery, relaxation training, and even hypnotherapy can be used as supplemental pain therapy in patients able to use such interventions.[228]

Wound debridement and frequent dressing changes are required for proper wound healing. Procedural pain associated with these activities can be excruciating. Ketamine, opioids and benzodiazepines are commonly used for sedation/analgesia, which can range from conscious sedation to general anesthesia. In the burn injury model the analgesic effects of ketamine, an NMDA receptor antagonist that reduces spinal hypersensitivity, can be distinguished from that of opioids and local anesthetics, which act peripherally.[224] Ketamine is commonly used because it provides intense analgesia with minimal respiratory depression. It can be administered intravenously, rectally, or orally. A long-acting opioid, such as morphine, that provides adequate analgesia during a dressing change may be overly sedative when the painful stimulus is over and the patient returns to the hospital ward. A combination of ketamine and opioid provides intense analgesia while reducing untoward effects. Fentanyl is useful due to its potency and short half-life. Oral transmucosal fentanyl (10 μg/kg, Oralet, Abbott Laboratories, North Chicago, IL) has been used successfully to manage procedural pain for burn wound care in children in the convalescent phase of injury when burn size was less than 15 percent BSA.[220] It is currently under investigation for use in other phases of burn wound care. Benzodiazepines are an important adjunct to management of procedural pain. Oral lorazepam in low dose has been shown to improve pain scores of patients with high baseline pain treated with opioids during burn wound care.[229] Benzodiazepines are also useful to control the dysphoric effects of ketamine. Oral or IV midazolam is commonly used.

REFERENCES

1. Jones RG: A short history of anesthesia for hare-lip and cleft palate repair. Br J Anaesth 43:796, 1971.
2. Ayre P: Endotracheal anesthesia for babies: with special reference to hare-lip and cleft lip operations. Anesth Analg 16:330, 1937.
3. Sperber GH: Craniofacial Embryology. 4th ed. London, Butterworth Scientific, 1989.
4. Larsen WJ: Human Embryology. 2nd ed. New York, Churchill Livingstone, 1997.
5. McCarthy JG, Epstein FJ, Wood-Smith D: Craniosynostosis. In McCarthy JG (ed): Plastic Surgery, Cleft Lip & Palate and Craniofacial Anomalies, Vol 4. Philadelphia, WB Saunders Company, 1990, p 3013.
6. Gorlin RJ, Cohen MMJ, Levin LS: Syndromes of the Head and Neck. 3rd ed. New York, Oxford University Press, 1990.
7. Scheuerle AE: Recent advances in craniofacial genetics. J Craniofac Surg 6:440, 1995.
8. Morriss-Kay G, Tucket F: Early events in mammalian craniofacial morphogenesis. J Craniofac Genet Dev Biol 11:181, 1991.
9. Johnston MC, Bronsky PT: Animal models for human craniofacial malformations. J Craniofac Genet Dev Biol 11:227, 1991.
10. Jones KL: Smith's Recognizable Patterns of Human Malformation. 4th ed. Philadelphia, WB Saunders Company, 1988.
11. Cohen MM: The Child with Multiple Birth Defects. 2nd ed. Oxford Monographs on Medical Genetics No. 31. New York, Oxford University Press, 1997.
12. Gorlin RJ: Fibroblast growth factors, their receptors and receptor disorders. J Craniomaxillofac Surg 25:69, 1997.
13. Arvystas M, Shprintzen RJ: Craniofacial morphology in Treacher Collins syndrome. Cleft Palate Craniofac J 28:226, 1991.
14. Shprintzen RJ, Croft C, Berkman MD, et al: Pharyngeal hypoplasia in Treacher-Collins syndrome. Arch Otolaryngol 105:127, 1979.
15. Shprintzen RJ: Palatal and pharyngeal anomalies in craniofacial syndromes. Birth Defects 18:53, 1982.
16. Shprintzen RJ: The implications of the diagnosis of Robin sequence. Cleft Palate Craniofac J 29:205, 1992.
17. Poswillo D: Hemorrhage in development of the face. Birth Defects 11:61, 1975.
18. Robinson LK, Hoyme HE, Edwards DK, et al: Vascular pathogenesis of unilateral craniofacial defects. J Pediatr 111:236, 1987.
19. Tessier P: Anatomical classification of facial, cranio-facial and latero-facial clefts. J Maxillofac Surg 4:69, 1976.
20. Cinalli G, Sainte-Rose C, Kollar EM, et al: Hydrocephalus and craniosynostosis. J Neurosurg 88:209, 1998.
21. Renier D: Intracranial pressure in craniosynostosis: pre- and postoperative recordings-correlation with functional results. In Persing JA, Edgerton MT, Jane JA (eds): Scientific Foundations and Surgical Treatment of Craniosynostosis. Baltimore, Williams & Wilkins, 1989, p 263.
22. Gault DT, Renier D, Marchac D, et al: Intracranial pressure and intracranial volume in children with craniosynostosis. Plast Reconstr Surg 90:377, 1992.
23. Thompson DN, Malcom GP, Jones BM, et al: Intracranial pressure in single-suture craniosynostosis. Pediatr Neurosurg 22:235, 1995.
24. Thompson DN, Jones BM, Harkness W, et al: Consequences of cranial vault expansion surgery for craniosynostosis. Pediatr Neurosurg 26:296, 1997.
25. McCarthy JG, Glasburg SB, Cutting CB, et al: Twenty-year experience with early surgery for craniosynostosis: I. Isolated craniofacial synostosis—results and unsolved problems. Plast Reconstr Surg 96:272, 1995.
26. McCarthy JG, Glasber SB, Cutting CB, et al: Twenty-year experience with early surgery for craniosynostosis: II. The craniofacial synostosis syndromes and pansynostosis—results and unsolved problems. Plast Reconstr Surg 96:284, 1995.
27. Sher AE: Mechanisms of airway obstruction in Robin sequence: implications for treatment. Cleft Palate Craniofac J 29:224, 1992.
28. Sher AE, Shprintzen RJ, Thorpy MJ: Endoscopic observations of obstructive sleep apnea in children with anomalous upper airways: predictive and therapeutic value. Int J Pediatr Otorhinolaryngol 11:135, 1986.
29. Mixter RC, David DJ, Perloff WH, et al: Obstructive sleep apnea in Apert's and Pfeiffer's syndromes: more than a craniofacial abnormality. Plast Reconstr Surg 86:457, 1990.
30. Jarund M, Lauritzen C: Craniofacial dysotosis: airway obstruction and craniofacial surgery. Scand J Plast Reconstr Surg Hand Surg 30:275, 1996.

31. Perkins JA, Sie KC, Milczuk H, et al: Airway management in children with craniofacial anomalies. Cleft Palate Craniofac J 34:135, 1997.

32. Sculerati N, Gottlieb MD, Zimbler MS, et al: Airway management in children with major craniofacial anomalies. Laryngoscope 108:1806, 1998.

33. Argamaso RV: Glossopexy for upper airway obstruction in Robin sequence. Cleft Palate Craniofac J 29:232, 1992.

34. McGill T: Otolaryngologic aspects of Apert Syndrome. Clin Plast Surg 18:309, 1991.

35. Anderson PJ, Hall C, Evans RD, et al: The cervical spine in Crouzon syndrome. Spine 22:402, 1997.

36. Kreiborg S, Barr JM, Cohen JMM: Cervical spine in the Apert syndrome. Am J Med Genet 43:704, 1992.

37. Hemmer KM, McAllister WH, Marsh JL: Cervical spine anomalies in the craniosynostosis syndromes. Cleft Palate J 24:328, 1987.

38. Tessier P, Guiot G, Rougerie J: Osteotomies cranio-naso-orbito-faciales. Ann Chir Plast 12:103, 1967.

39. Tessier P: Ostostomies totales de la face: syndrome de Crouzon, syndrome d'Apert, oxycéphalies, scaphophalies, turricéphalies. Ann Chir Plast 12:273, 1967.

40. Posnick JC: Paediatric craniofacial surgery: historical perspectives, recent advancements and refinements. Br J Oral Maxillofac Surg 33:343, 1995.

41. Tessier P: Cranio-facial dysostosis. In Mustardé JC (ed): Plastic Surgery in Infancy and Childhood. 2nd ed. Edinburgh, Churchill Livingstone, 1979, p 277.

42. Reinhart E, Mühling J, Michel C, et al: Craniofacial growth characteristics after bilateral fronto-orbital advancement in children with premature craniosynostosis. Childs Nerv Syst 12:690, 1996.

43. Tessier P: The classic reprint: experimental study of fractures of the upper jaw. 3. Rene Le Fort, M.D., Lille, France. Plast Reconstr Surg 50:600, 1972.

44. Davies J, Turner S, Sandy JR: Distraction osteogensis—a review. Br Dent J 185:462, 1998.

45. McCarthy JG, Schreiber J, Karp N, et al: Lengthening the human mandible by gradual distraction. Plast Reconstr Surg 89:1, 1992.

46. Molina F, Monasterio FO: Mandibular elongation and remodeling by distraction: a farewell to major osteotomies. Plast Reconstr Surg 96:825, 1995.

47. Carls FR, Sailer HF: Seven years clinical experience with mandibular distraction in children. J Craniomaxillofac Surg 26:197, 1998.

48. Cohen SR, Simms C, Burstein FD: Mandibular distraction osteogenesis in the treatment of upper airway obstruction in children with craniofacial deformities. Plast Reconstr Surg 101:312, 1998.

49. Witt PD, Marsh JL, Muntz HR, et al: Acute obstructive sleep apnea as a complication of sphincter pharyngoplasty. Cleft Palate Craniofac J 33:183, 1996.

50. Abramson DL, Marrinan EM, Mulliken JB: Robin sequence: obstructive sleep apnea following pharyngeal flap. Cleft Palate Craniofac J 34:256, 1997.

51. Orr WC, Levine NS, Buchanan RT: Effect of cleft palate repair and pharyngeal flap surgery on upper airway obstruction during sleep. Plast Reconstr Surg 80:226, 1987.

52. Shprintzen RJ: Pharyngeal flap surgery and the pediatric upper airway. Int Anesthesiol Clin 26:79, 1988.

53. Ross DA, Witzel MA, Armstrong DC, et al: Is pharyngoplasty a risk in velocardiofacial syndrome? An assessment of medially displaced carotid arteries. Plast Reconstr Surg 98:1182, 1996.

54. Kopp VJ, Rosenfeld MJ, Turvey TA: Nasotracheal intubation in the presence of a pharyngeal flap in children and adults. Anesthesiology 82:1063, 1995.

55. Pertschuk MJ, Whitaker LA: Psychosocial adjustment and craniofacial malformations in childhood. Plast Reconstr Surg 75:177, 1985.

56. Phillips J, Whitaker LA: The social effects of craniofacial deformity and its correction. Cleft Palate J 16:7, 1979.

57. Padwa BL, Evans CA, Pillemer FC: Psychosocial adjustment in children with hemifacial microsomia and other craniofacial deformities. Cleft Palate Craniofac J 28:354, 1991.

58. Clifford E: Psychologic considerations: patients with clefts and craniofacial malformations. In Serafin D, Georgiade NG (eds): Pediatric Plastic Surgery. St. Louis, CV Mosby, 1984, p 259.

59. Marsh JL: Comprehensive Care for Craniofacial Deformities. St. Louis, CV Mosby, 1985.

60. Lefebvre A, Barclay S: Psychosocial impact of craniofacial deformities before and after reconstructive surgery. Can J Psychiatry 27:579, 1982.

61. Pertschuk MJ, Whitaker LA: Psychosocial outcome of craniofacial surgery in children. Plast Reconstr Surg 82:741, 1988.

62. Delégue L, Guilbert M: Management of airway problems during the repair of craniofacial anomalies in children. In Caronni EP (ed): Craniofacial Surgery. Boston, Little, Brown, 1985, p 141.

63. Handler SD, Beaugard ME, Whitaker LA, et al: Airway management in the repair of craniofacial defects. Cleft Palate J 16:16, 1979.

64. Sherk HH: Facial malformations and spinal anomalies. Spine 7:526, 1982.

65. Handler SD, Keon TP: Difficult laryngoscopy/intubation: the child with mandibular hypoplasia. Ann Otol Rhinol Laryngol 92:401, 1983.

66. Markakis DA, Sayson SC, Schreiner MS: Insertion of the laryngeal mask airway in awake infants with the Robin sequence. Anesth Analg 75:822, 1992.

67. Rabb MF, Minkowitz HS, Hagberg CA: Blind intubation through the laryngeal mask airway for management of the difficult airway in infants. Anesthesiology 84:1510, 1996.

68. Inada T, Fujise K, Tachibana K, et al: Orotracheal intubation through the laryngeal mask ariway in paediatric patients with Treacher-Collins syndrome. Paediatr Anaesth 5:129, 1995.

69. Ross EDT: Treacher Collins syndrome—an anesthetic hazard. Anaesthesia 18:350, 1963.

70. Maclennan FM, Robertson GS: Ketamine for induction and intubation in Treacher-Collins syndrome. Anaesthesia 36:196, 1981.

71. Rasch DK, Browder F, Barr M, et al: Anaesthesia for Treacher Collins and Pierre Robin syndromes: a report of three cases. Can Anaesth Soc J 33:364, 1986.

72. Divekar VM, Sircar BN: Anesthetic management in Treacher-Collins syndrome. Anesthesiology 26:292, 1965.

73. Sklar GS, King BD: Endotracheal intubation and Treacher-Collins syndrome. Anesthesiology 44:247, 1976.

74. Miyabe, M, Dohi S, Homma E: Tracheal intubation in an infant with Treacher-Collins syndrome—pulling out the tongue by a forceps. Anesthesiology 62:213, 1985.

75. Dinner M, Goldin EZ, Ward R, et al: Russell-Silver syndrome: anesthestic implications. Anesth Analg 78:1197, 1994.

76. Gallagher DM, Hyler RL, Epker BN: Hemifacial microsomia: an anesthetic airway problem. Oral Surg Oral Med Oral Pathol 49:2, 1980.

77. Sutera PT, Gordon GJ: Digitally assisted tracheal intubation in a neonate with Pierre Robin syndrome. Anesthesiology 78:983, 1993.

78. Krucylak CP, Schreiner MS: Orotracheal intubation of an infant with hemifacial microsomia using a modified lighted stylet. Anesthesiology 77:826, 1992.

79. Przybylo HJ, Stevenson GW, Vicari FA, et al: Retrograde fibreoptic intubation in a child with Nager's syndrome. Can J Anaesth 43:697, 1996.

80. Munro IR, Sabatier RE: An analysis of 12 years of craniomaxillofacial surgery in Toronto. Plast Reconstr Surg 76:29, 1985.

81. Whitaker LA, Broennle AM, Kerr LP, et al: Improvements in craniofacial reconstruction: methods evolved in 235 consecutive patients. Plast Reconstr Surg 65:561, 1980.

82. Scholtes JL, Thauvoy C, Moulin D, et al: Craniofaciosynostosis: anesthetic and perioperative management. Report of 71 operations. Acta Anaesthesiol Belg 36:176, 1985.

83. Murray JE, Swanson LT, Strand RD, et al: Evaluation of craniofacial surgery in the treatment of facial deformities. Ann Surg 182:240, 1975.

84. Meyer P, Renier D, Arnaud E, et al: Blood loss during repair of craniosynostosis. Br J Anaesth 71:854, 1993.

85. Kearney RA, Rosales JK, Howes WJ: Craniosynostosis: an assessment of blood loss and transfusion practices. Can J Anaesth 36:4, 1989.

86. Karl HW, Swedlow DB, Lee KW, et al: Epinephrine-halothane interactions in children. Anesthesiology 58:142, 1983.

87. Brown KA, Bissonette B, MacDonald M, et al: Hyperkalaemia during massive blood transfusion in paediatric craniofacial surgery. Can J Anaesth 37:401, 1990.

88. Coté CJ, Drop LJ, Hoaglin DC, et al: Ionized hypocalcemia after fresh frozen plasma administration to thermally injured children: effects of infusion rate, duration, and treatment with calcium chloride. Anesth Analg 67:152, 1988.

89. Coté CJ, Liu LMP, Szyfelbein SK, et al: Changes in serial platelet counts following massive blood transfusion in pediatric patients. Anesthesiology 62:197, 1985.

90. Ousterhout DK: Craniofacial surgery: recent advances. *In* Habal M (ed): Advances in Plastic and Reconstructive Surgery. Chicago, Year Book Medical Publishers, 1984, p 21.

91. Whitaker LA, Munro IR, Salyer KE, et al: Combined report of problems and complications in 793 craniofacial operations. Plast Reconstr Surg 64:198, 1979.

92. Jackson IT: Craniofacial dysostosis. *In* Serafin D, Georgiade NG (eds): Pediatric Plastic Surgery. St. Louis, CV Mosby, 1984, p 440.

93. Christianson L: Anesthesia for major craniofacial operations. Int Anesthesiol Clin 23:117, 1985.

94. Harp JR, Wollman H: Cerebral metabolic effects of hyperventilation and deliberate hypotension. Br J Anaesth 45:256, 1973.

95. Chan W, Smith DE, Ware WH: Effects of hypotensive anesthesia in anterior maxillary osteotomy. J Oral Surg 38:504, 1980.

96. Lessard MR, Trepanier CA, Baribault JP, et al: Isoflurane-induced hypotension in orthognathic surgery. Anesth Analg 69:379, 1989.

97. Schaberg SJ, Kelly JF, Terry BC, et al: Blood loss and hypotensive anesthesia in oral-facial corrective surgery. J Oral Surg 34:147, 1976.

98. Helfaer MA, Carson BS, James CS, et al: Increased hematocrit and decreased transfusion requirements in children given erythropoietin before undergoing craniofacial surgery. J Neurosurg 88:704, 1998.

99. Velardi F, Di Chirico A, Di Rocco C, et al: "No allogeneic blood transfusion" protocol for the surgical correction of craniosynostoses. II. Clinical application. Childs Nerv Syst 14:732, 1998.

100. Jimenez DF, Barone CM: Intraoperative autologous blood transfusion in the surgical corection of craniosynostosis. Neurosurgery 37:1075, 1995.

101. Bruce DA, Sutton LN, Schut L: Neurosurgical considerations in cranio-orbital surgery. Clin Plast Surg 14:187, 1987.

102. Harris MM, Strafford MA, Rowe RW, et al: Venous air embolism and cardiac arrest during craniectomy in a supine infant. Anesthesiology 65:547, 1986.

103. Vercauteren M, van Vyve M, Janssen L, et al: Craniostenosis: the importance of the anesthesiologist. Acta Anaesthesiol Belg 36:168, 1985.

104. Shillito J, Matson DD: Craniosynostosis: a review of 519 surgical patients. Pediatrics 41:829, 1968.

105. Converse JM, Wood-Smith D, McCarthy JG: Report on a series of 50 craniofacial operations. Plast Reconstr Surg 55:283, 1975.

106. Edgerton MT, Jane JA, Berry FA: Craniofacial osteotomies and reconstructions in infants and young children. Plast Reconstr Surg 54:13, 1974.

107. Marchac D, Renier D: Craniofacial surgery for craniosynostosis improves facial growth: a personal case review. Ann Plast Surg 14:43, 1985.

108. Diaz JH, Henling CE: Pneumoperitoneum and cardiac arrest during craniofacial reconstruction. Anesth Analg 61:146, 1982.

109. Davies DW, Munro IR: The anesthetic management and intraoperative care of patients undergoing major facial osteotomies. Plast Reconstr Surg 55:50, 1975.

110. Blanc VF: Trigeminocardiac reflexes. Can J Anaesth 38:696, 1991.

111. Lang S, Lanigan DT, van der Wal M: Trigeminocardiac reflexes: maxillary and mandibular variants of the oculocardiac reflex. Can J Anaesth 38:757, 1991.

112. Whitaker LA, Munro IR, Jackson IT, et al: Problems in cranio-facial surgery. J Maxillofac Surg 4:131, 1976.

113. Gunawardana RH: Difficult laryngoscopy in cleft lip and palate surgery. Br J Anaesth 76:757, 1996.

114. Ring WH, Adair JC, Elwyn RA: A new pediatric endotracheal tube. Anesth Analg 54:273, 1975.

115. Johnston RR, Eger EI II, Wilson C: A comparative interaction of epinephrine with enflurane, isoflurane, and halothane in man. Anesth Analg 55:709, 1976.

116. Doyle E, Hudson I: Anaesthesia for primary repair of cleft lip and cleft palate: a review of 244 procedures. Paediatric Anaesth 2:139, 1992.

117. Lees VC, Pigott RW: Early postoperative complications in primary cleft lip and palate surgery—how soon may we discharge patients from hospital? Br J Plast Surg 45:232, 1992.

118. Shprinten RJ, Singer L, Sidoti EJ, et al: Pharyngeal flap surgery: postoperative complications. Int Anesthesiol Clin 30:115, 1992.

119. Hairfield WM, Warren DW, Seaton DL: Prevalence of mouth-breathing in cleft lip and palate. Cleft Palate J 25:135, 1988.

120. Lynch M, Underwood S: Pulmonary oedema following relief of upper airway obstruction in the Pierre-Robin syndrome: a consequence of early palatal repair? Br J Anaesth 66:391, 1991.

121. Roa NL, Moss KS: Treacher-Collins syndrome with sleep apnea: anesthetic considerations. Anesthesiology 60:71, 1984.

122. Kravath RE, Pollak CP, Borowiecki B, et al: Obstructive sleep apnea and death associated with surgical correction of velopharyngeal incompetence. J Pediatr 96:645, 1980.

123. Bell C, Oh TH, Loeffler JR: Massive macroglossia and airway obstruction after cleft palate repair. Anesth Analg 67:71, 1988.

124. Lee JT, Kingston HG: Airway obstruction due to massive lingual oedema following cleft palate surgery. Can Anaesth Soc J 32:265, 1985.

125. Patane PS, White SE: Macroglossia causing airway obstruction following cleft palate repair. Anesthesiology 71:995, 1989.

126. Ahuja S, Datta A, Krishna A, et al: Infra-orbital nerve block for relief of postoperative pain following cleft lip surgery in infants. Anaesthesia 49:441, 1994.

127. Bösenberg AT, Kimble FW: Infraorbital nerve block in neonates for cleft lip repair: anatomical study and clinical application. Br J Anesth 74:506, 1995.

128. East MK, Jones CA, Feller I, et al: Epidemiology of burns in children. *In* Carvajal HF, Parks DH (eds): Burns in Children: Pediatric Burn Management. Chicago, Year Book Medical Publishers, 1988, p 3.

129. Anonymous: Fatal injuries to children—Unites States, 1986. MMWR Morb Mortal Wkly Rep 39:442, 1990.

130. Rivara FP, Grossman DC, Cummings P: Injury prevention. Second of two parts. N Engl J Med 337:613, 1997.

131. Lund CC, Browder NC: The estimation of areas of burns. Surg Gynecol Obstet 79:352, 1944.

132. Barone CM, Yule GJ: Pediatric Thermal Injuries. *In* Bentz ML (ed): Pediatric Plastic Surgery. Stamford, CT, Appleton & Lange, 1998, p 595.

133. Anonymous: Hospital and prehospital resources for optimal care of patients with burn injury: guidelines for development and operation of burn centers. American Burn Association. J Burn Care Rehabil 11:98, 1990.

134. Wolf SE, Rose JK, Desai MH, et al: Mortality determinants in massive pediatric burns. An analysis of 103 children with ≥ 80% TBSA burns (≥ 70% full-thickness). Ann Surg 225:554, 1997.

135. Sheridan RL: The seriously burned child: resuscitation through reintegration—1. Curr Probl Pediatr 28:105, 1998.

136. Sheridan RL: The seriously burned child: resuscitation through reintegration—2. Curr Probl Pediatr 28:139, 1998.

137. Wolf SE, Debroy M, Herndon DN: The cornerstones and directions of pediatric burn care. Pediatr Surg Int 12:312, 1997.

138. Rose JK, Barrow RE, Desai MH, et al: Advances in burn care. Adv Surg 30:71, 1996.

139. Nguyen TT, Gilpin DA, Meyer NA, et al: Current treatment of severely burned patients. Ann Surg 223:14, 1996.

140. Rose JK, Herndon DN: Advances in the treatment of burn patients. Burns 23(Suppl 1):S19, 1997.

141. Muller MJ, Herndon DN: The challenge of burns. Lancet 343:216, 1994.

142. Ilano AL, Raffin TA: Management of carbon monoxide poisoning. Chest 97:165, 1990.

143. Baud FJ, Barriot P, Toffis V, et al: Elevated blood cyanide concentrations in victims of smoke inhalation. N Engl J Med 325:1761, 1991.

144. Clark CJ, Campbell D, Reid WH: Blood carboxyhaemoglobin and cyanide levels in fire survivors. Lancet 1:1332, 1981.

145. Kulig K: Cyanide antidotes and fire toxicology. N Engl J Med 325:1801, 1991.

146. Beasley DM, Glass WI: Cyanide poisoning: pathophysiology and treatment recommendations. Occup Med 48:427, 1998.

147. Demling RH: Burns. N Engl J Med 313:1389, 1985.

148. Demling RH: Pathophysiological changes after cutaneous burns and approach to initial resuscitation. *In* Martyn JAJ (ed): Acute Management of the Burned Patient. Philadelphia, WB Saunders Company, 1990, p 12.

149. Lund T, Wiig H, Reed RK: Acute postburn edema: role of strongly negative interstitial fluid pressure. Am J Physiol 255:H1069, 1988.

150. Carvajal HF: Controversies in fluid resuscitation and their impact on pediatric populations. *In* Carvajal HF, Parks DH (eds): Burns in Children: Pediatric Burn Management. Chicago, Year Book Medical Publishers, 1988, p 51.

151. Finkelstein JL, Schwartz SB, Madden MR, et al: Pediatric burns. An overview. Pediatr Clin North Am 39:1145, 1992.

152. Carvajal HF: Resuscitation of the burned child. *In* Carvajal HF, Parks DH (eds): Burns in Children: Pediatric Burn Management. Chicago, Year Book Medical Publishers, 1988, p 78.

153. Carvajal HF: Fluid resuscitation of pediatric burn victims: a critical appraisal. Pediatr Nephrol 8:357, 1994.

154. Crum RL, Dominic W, Hansbrough JF, et al: Cardiovascular and neurohumoral responses following burn injury. Arch Surg 125:1065, 1990.

155. Demling RH, Kramer G, Harms B: Role of thermal injury-induced hypoproteinemia on fluid flux and protein permeability in burned and nonburned tissue. Surgery 95:136, 1984.

156. Carvajal HF: A physiologic approach to fluid therapy in severely burned children. Surg Gynecol Obstet 150:379, 1980.

157. Dries DJ, Waxman K: Adequate resuscitation of burn patients may not be measured by urine output and vital signs. Crit Care Med 19:327, 1991.

158. Carleton SC: Cardiac problems associated with burns. Cardiol Clin 13:257, 1995.

159. Kaufman TM, Horton JW: Burn-induced alterations in cardiac β-adrenergic receptors. Am J Physiol 31:H1585, 1992.

160. Wang C, Jeevendra Martyn JA: Burn injury alters b-adrenergic receptor and second messenger function in rat ventricular muscle. Crit Care Med 24:118, 1996.

161. Herrin JT: Renal function in burns. *In* Martyn JAJ (ed): Acute Management of the Burned Patient. Philadelphia, WB Saunders Company, 1990, p 239.

162. Burke JF, Quinby WC Jr, Bondoc C, et al: Patterns of high tension electrical injury in children and adolescents and their management. Am J Surg 133:492, 1977.

163. Remensnyder JP: Acute electrical injuries. *In* Martyn JAJ (ed): Acute Management of the Burned Patient. Philadelphia, WB Saunders Company, 1990, p 66.

164. Hasselgren PO: Burns and metabolism. J Am Coll Surg 188:98, 1999.

165. Caldwell FT: Etiology and control of postburn hypermetabolism: the 1991 Presidential Address to the American Burn Association. J Burn Care Rehabil 12:385, 1991.

166. Wilmore DW, Mason AD Jr, Johnson DW, et al: Effect of ambient temperature on heat production and heat loss in burn patients. J Appl Physiol 38:593, 1975.

167. Childs C, Stoner HB, Little RA: Cutaneous heat loss shortly after burn injury in children. Clin Sci 83:117, 1992.

168. Wilmore DW, Orcutt TW, Mason AD Jr, et al: Alterations in hypothalmic function following thermal injury. J Trauma 15:697, 1975.

169. Wolfe RR, Herndon DN, Jahoor F, et al: Effect of severe burn injury on substrate cycling by glucose and fatty acids. N Engl J Med 317:403, 1987.

170. Hildreth MA, Herndon DN, Desai MH, et al: Current treatment reduces calories required to maintain weight in pediatric patients with burns. J Burn Care Rehabil 11:405, 1990.

171. Henley M: Feed that burn. James Ellsworth Laing prize-winning essay for 1989. Burns 15:351, 1989.

172. Ferrando AA, Chinkes DL, Wolf SE, et al: A submaximal dose of insulin promotes net skeletal muscle protein synthesis in patients with severe burns. Ann Surg 229:11, 1999.

173. Ramirez RJ, Wolf SE, Barrow RE, et al: Growth hormone treatment in pediatric burns: a safe therapeutic approach. Ann Surg 228:439, 1998.

174. Baron PW, Barrow RE, Pierre EJ, et al: Prolonged use of propranolol safely decreases cardiac work in burned children. J Burn Care Rehabil 18:223, 1997.

175. Popp MB, Friedberg DL, MacMillen BG: Clinical characteristics of hypertension in burned children. Ann Surg 191:473, 1980.

176. Popp MB, Silberstein EB, Srivastava LS, et al: A pathophysiologic study of the hypertension associated with burn injury in children. Ann Surg 193:473, 1981.

177. Falkner B, Roven S, DeClement FA, et al: Hypertension in children with burns. J Trauma 18:213, 1978.

178. Strongin J, Hales CA: Pulmonary disorders in the burn patient. *In* Martyn JAJ (ed): Acute Management of the Burned Patient. Philadelphia, WB Saunders Company, 1990, p 25.

179. Hollingsed TC, Saffle JR, Barton RG, et al: Etiology and consequences of respiratory failure in thermally injured patients. Am J Surg 166:592, 1993.

180. Saffle JR, Sullivan JJ, Tuohig GM, et al: Multiple organ failure in patients with thermal injury. Crit Care Med 21:1673, 1993.

181. Jeschke MG, Barrow RE, Wolf SE, et al: Mortality in burned children with acute renal failure. Arch Surg 133:752, 1998.

182. Davies JWL: Physiological Responses to Burning Injury. Orlando, FL, Academic Press, 1982.

183. Mohnot D, Snead OC, Benton JW Jr: Burn encephalopathy in children. Ann Neurol 12:42, 1982.

184. Mukhdomi GJ, Desai MH, Herndon DN: Seizure disorders in burned children: a retrospective review. Burns 22:316, 1996.

185. Housinger TA, Brinkeroff C, Warden GD: The relationship between platelet count, sepsis, and survival in pediatric burn patients. Arch Surg 128:65, 1993.

186. Epstein MD, Banducci DR, Manders EK: The role of the gastrointestinal tract in the development of burn sepsis. Plast Reconstr Surg 90:524, 1992.

187. Klein GL, Nicolai M, Langman CB, et al: Dysregulation of calcium homeostasis after severe burn injury in children: possible role of magnesium depletion. J Pediatr 131:246, 1997.

188. Parish RA, Novack AH, Heimbach DM, et al: Fever as a predictor of infection in burned children. J Trauma 27:69, 1987.

189. Childs C: Fever in burned children. Burns 14:1, 1988.

190. Herndon DN, Barrow RE, Rutan RL, et al: A comparison of conservative versus early excision. Therapies in severely burned patients. Ann Surg 209:547, 1989.

191. Tompkins RG, Remensnyder JP, Burke JF, et al: Significant reductions in mortality for children with burn injuries through the use of prompt eschar excision. Ann Surg 208:577, 1988.

192. Parks DH, Wainwright DJ: The surgical management of burns. *In* Carvajal HF, Parks DH (eds): Burns in Children: Pediatric Burn Management. Chicago, Year Book Medical Publishers, 1988, p 156.

193. Briggs SE: Rationale for acute surgical approach. *In* Martyn JAJ (ed): Acute Management of the Burned Patient. Philadelphia, WB Saunders Company, 1990, p 118.

194. Martyn J: Clinical pharmacology and drug therapy in the burned patient. Anesthesiology 65:67, 1986.

195. Martyn J: Clinical pharmacology and therapeutics in burns. *In* Martyn JAJ (ed): Acute Management of the Burned Patient. Philadelphia, WB Saunders Company, 1990, p 180.

196. Bonate PL: Pathophysiology and pharmacokinetics following burn injury. Clin Pharmacokinet 18:118, 1990.

197. Martyn JA, White DA, Gronert GA, et al: Up-and-down regulation of skeletal muscle acetylcholine receptors. Anesthesiology 76:822, 1992.

198. Mills AK, Martyn JAJ: Neuromuscular blockade with vecuronium in pediatric patients with burn injury. Br J Clin Pharmacol 28:155, 1989.

199. Martyn JA, Liu LMP, Szyfelbein SK, et al: The neuromuscular effects of pancuronium in burned children. Anesthesiology 59:561, 1983.

200. Martyn JA, Goudsouzian NG, Matteo RS, et al: Metocurine requirements and plasma concentrations in burned paediatric patients. Br J Anaesth 55:263, 1983.

201. Hagen J, Martyn JA, Szyfelbein SK, et al: Cardiovascular and neuromuscular responses to high-dose pancuronium-metocurine in pediatric burned and reconstructive patients. Anesth Analg 65:1340, 1986.

202. Martyn JA, Matteo RS, Szyfelbein SK, et al: Unprecedented resistance to neuromuscular blocking effects of metocurine with persistence after complete recovery in a burned patient. Anesth Analg 61:614, 1982.

203. Reyneke CJ, James MFM, Johnson R: Alfentanil and propofol infusions for surgery in the burned patient. Br J Anaesth 63:418, 1989.

204. Gregoretti S, Gelman S, Dimick A, et al: Hemodynamic changes and oxygen consumption in burned patients during enflurane or isoflurane anesthesia. Anesth Analg 69:431, 1989.

205. Coté CJ, Petkau AJ: Thiopental requirements may be increased in children reanesthetized at least one year after recovery from extensive thermal injury. Anesth Analg 64:1156, 1985.

206. Osgood PF, Szyfelbein SK: Management of burn pain in children. Pediatr Clin North Am 36:1001, 1989.

207. Furman WR, Munster AM, Cone EJ: Morphine pharmacokinetics during anesthesia and surgery in patients with burns. J Burn Care Rehabil 11:391, 1990.

208. Macfie AG, Magides AD, Reilly CS: Disposition of alfentanil in burns patients. Br J Anaesth 69:482, 1992.

209. Taylor JW, Hander EW, Skreen R, et al: The effect of central nervous system narcosis on the sympathetic response to stress. J Surg Res 20:313, 1976.

210. Cederholm I, Bengstsson M, Bjorkman S, et al: Long term high dose morphine, ketamine and midazolam infusion in a child with burns. Br J Clin Pharmacol 30:901, 1990.

211. Eckhauser FE, Billote J, Burke JF, et al: Tracheostomy complicating massive burn injury. A plea for conservatism. Am J Surg 127:418, 1974.

212. Wade EJ, Purdue GF, Hunt JL: A modified technique for securing oro-nasal tubes. J Burn Care Rehabil 11:244, 1990.

213. Goudsouzian N, Szyfelbein SK: Management of upper airway following burns. In Martyn JAJ (ed): Acute Management of the Burned Patient. Philadelphia, WB Saunders Company, 1990, p 46.

214. Galvis AG, Mestad PH: Modified endotracheal tube for airway management of children with facial burns. Anesth Analg 60:116, 1981.

215. Crabtree JH, Bowser BH, Campbell JW, et al: Energy metabolism in anesthetized children with burns. Am J Surg 140:832, 1980.

216. Haith LR, Patton ML, Goldman WT, et al: Diminishing blood loss during operation for burns. Surg Gynecol Obstet 176:119, 1993.

217. Coté CJ: Depth of halothane anesthesia potentiates citrate-induced ionized hypocalcemia and adverse cardiovascular events in dogs. Anesthesiology 67:676, 1987.

218. Cullen JJ, Murray DJ, Kealey GP: Changes in coagulation factors in patients with burns during acute blood loss. J Burn Care Rehabil 10:517, 1989.

219. Coté CJ, Daniels AL, Connolly M, et al: Tongue oximetry in children with extensive thermal injury: comparison with peripheral oximetry. Can J Anaesth 39:454, 1992.

220. Atchison NE, Osgood PF, Carr DB, et al: Pain during burn dressing change in children: relationship to burn area, depth and analgesic regiments. Pain 47:41, 1991.

221. Petersen KL, Brennum J, Dahl JB: Experimental evaluation of the analgesic effect of ibuprofen on primary and secondary hyperalgesia. Pain 70:167, 1997.

222. Moiniche S, Dahl JB, Kehlet H: Time course of primary and secondary hyperalgesia after heat injury to the skin. Br J Anaesth 71:201, 1993.

223. Lundell JC, Silverman DG, Brull SJ, et al: Reduction of postburn hyperalgesia after local injection of ketorolac in healthy volunteers. Anesthesiology 84:502, 1996.

224. Ilkjaer S, Petersen KL, Brennum J, et al: Effect of systemic N-methyl-D-aspartate receptor antagonist (ketamine) on primary and secondary hyperalgesia in humans. Br J Anaesth 76:829, 1996.

225. Williams PI, Sarginson RE, Ratcliffe JM: Use of methadone in the morphine-tolerant burned paediatric patient. Br J Anaesth 80:92, 1998.

226. Jönsson A, Cassuto J, Hanson B: Inhibition of burn pain by intravenous lignocaine infusion. Lancet 338:151, 1991.

227. Brofeldt BT, Cornwell P, Doherty D, et al: Topical lidocaine in the treatment of partial-thickness burns. J Burn Care Rehabil 10:63, 1989.

228. Pal SK, Cortiella J, Herndon D: Adjunctive methods of pain control in burns. Burns 23:404, 1997.

229. Patterson DR, Ptacek JT, Carrougher GJ, et al: Lorazepam as an adjunct to opioid analgesics in the treatment of burn pain. Pain 72:367, 1997.

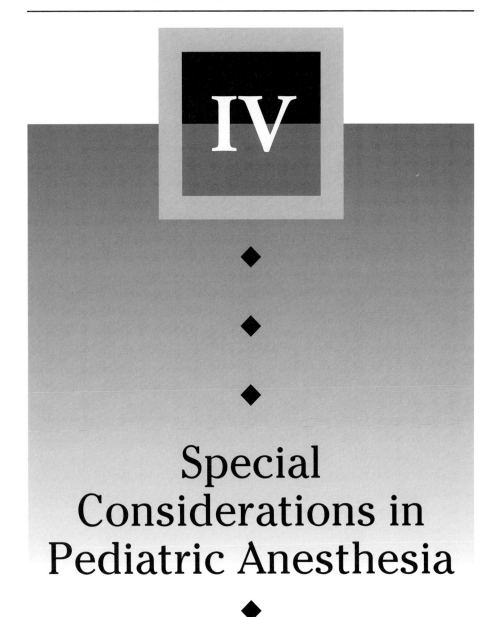

SECTION

IV

Special
Considerations in
Pediatric Anesthesia

Pediatric Pain Management

CHRISTINE D. GRECO
CONSTANCE S. HOUCK
CHARLES B. BERDE

◆　　◆　　◆

All anesthesiologists caring for infants and children should regard pain management as a central aspect of their mission as physicians. In this chapter, we will review: (1) the developmental neurobiology of pain, (2) challenges associated with pain assessment, (3) analgesic pharmacology in infants and children, (4) approaches to pediatric acute pain management, and (5) common chronic and recurrent pain syndromes in children.

Through the second trimester of human gestation, there is progressive maturation of peripheral, spinal, and supraspinal pathways that convey sensation of tissue damage or inflammation. The term *nociception* refers to this process of encoding and sensing tissue injury and inflammation. The term *pain* refers to both the sensory and emotional experience of noxious events, which may be caused by tissue injury or inflammation, or by abnormal nerve excitability. *Neuropathic pain* refers to forms of pain that persist due to abnormal nerve excitability as inflammation subsides or injured tissues heal. The term *suffering* refers to experience of pain and other forms of distress in the context of perceived harm to the person's integrity.[1]

Preterm and term neonates respond to tissue injury or inflammation with withdrawal reflexes, distress behaviors, autonomic arousal, and hormonal-metabolic stress responses.[2] The general architecture of the sensory nervous system is established by midgestation, but there are some differences in that patterns of connections and functions mature over the first months of life.[3] Among premature infants compared with term neonates and older infants, withdrawal reflexes are evoked by stimuli of lower intensity, and the withdrawal occurs more rapidly. In neonatal animals, myelinated A fibers (that carry nonnoxious input in the mature nervous system) synapse in both deep and superficial laminae in the spinal cord; these connections to superficial lamina second-order cells are "pruned" during development.[4, 5] In very young premature infants, both noxious and nonnoxious stimuli evoke limb flexion. Sensory innervation in premature infants also involves greater overlapping of cutaneous receptive fields.[4, 5] Spinal dorsal horn neurons involved in nociception receive inputs from a comparatively greater portion of the body surface in neonatal animals, compared with older animals.[6]

Studies in infant rats suggest that, whereas afferent transmission of nociceptive information occurs comparatively early, descending pathways in the spinal cord involved in modulation or inhibition of pain sensation develop comparatively later. For example, the dorsolateral funiculus is a descending spinal tract whose function appears to develop later.[7]

Despite these delays in development of spinal descending pathways and neurotransmitters, α_2-adrenergic agonists and opioids administered into the cerebrospinal fluid

(CSF) exert analgesic effects in newborn animals[8] and humans.

In a previous era in which analgesics and anesthetics were commonly withheld from neonates, one of the rationalizations given was that, even if newborns experienced pain, painful experiences would not be remembered and therefore they would produce no lasting harm. (Even if this were true, many would still regard it as ethically unacceptable to permit preventable experiences of pain regardless of whether or not they can be recalled or produce lasting effects.) Recent studies have examined in both animals and humans whether untreated pain in neonates has persistent consequences. Taddio and co-workers examined behavioral and physiologic indices of distress following injections for immunizations in male infants performed at 4 to 6 months of age.[9] These infants were chosen from a cohort who had received circumcision with or without a topical local anesthetic, EMLA, and from a comparison group who had not undergone circumcision. Group differences in several distress measures were reported. Ruda and co-workers recently demonstrated that adult rats who had received persistent inflammatory stimuli as neonates showed long-term changes in dorsal horn synaptic organization and nociceptive functioning.[10]

Pain assessment is an essential part of pain treatment. Pain should be assessed in terms of its mechanisms, causes, and exacerbating or alleviating factors. Pain assessment is not limited to numerical measures of intensity alone, but rather should be broad-based and take into account the social and emotional factors that modify suffering. Pain measurement should employ self-report scales, whenever possible, for children ages 4 and older, using either visual analog scales, or scales that involve drawings of faces or color analog scales. Behavioral measures have been developed for neonates, young children, and children with motor or cognitive impairments. For a detailed discussion of pain assessment and measurement issues, see Finley and McGrath, 1998.[11] Recently in the United States, the Joint Commission on Accreditation of Health Care Organizations has taken a role in mandating universal pain assessment in hospitals and outpatient centers.

PREVENTION AND TREATMENT OF ACUTE PAIN IN CHILDREN

Developmental Issues in Analgesic Pharmacology

Although most of the major organ systems are anatomically well developed at birth, their functional maturity is often delayed. In the first months of life in both preterm and full-term newborns, these systems rapidly mature, most approaching a functional level similar to adults before 3 months of age. General principles of newborn physiology and its effects on the pharmacology of opioids and local anesthetics are summarized below:

1. Most analgesics (including opioids and local anesthetics) are conjugated in the liver. Newborns, and especially premature infants, have delayed maturation of the enzyme systems involved in drug conjugation, including sulfation, glucuronidation, and oxidation. Several of these hepatic enzyme systems, including cytochrome P-450 subtypes, and the mixed-function oxidases, mature at varying rates over the first 1 to 6 months of life.[12]
2. Glomerular filtration rates are diminished in the first week of life, especially in premature infants,[13] but generally are sufficiently mature to remove medications and metabolites by 2 weeks of age.
3. Newborns have a higher percentage of body weight as water and less as fat than older patients. Water-soluble drugs, therefore, often have larger volumes of distribution.
4. Newborns have reduced plasma concentrations of both albumin and α_1-acid glycoprotein than older children and adults. For some drugs, this may lead to greater unbound drug concentrations and greater drug effect or drug toxicity.
5. There may be increased passage of some drugs across the blood–brain barrier in newborns, which previously has been cited as a reason for the increased relative potency and respiratory depressant effects of morphine in the neonate. This hypothesis has been supported by some animal studies, but other studies imply alternative explanations.[14, 15] Recent research has indicated that passage of drugs into the central nervous system (CNS) is not solely a passive process involving degrees of "leakiness" of intercellular junctions. In addition, there are several membrane proteins that actively either extrude drugs or facilitate their uptake into the CNS.[16] One particular example is P-glycoprotein, which actively extrudes most opioids from the CNS.[17]
6. Newborns, and especially premature infants,[18] have diminished ventilatory responses to hypoxemia[19] and hypercarbia. These ventilatory responses are further impaired in newborns and infants with a range of conditions, including chronic lung disease and myelomeningocele.[20]

Nonopioid Analgesics

Acetaminophen

Acetaminophen is the most commonly used analgesic agent in pediatric practice. It is an effective analgesic for mild to moderate pain, and it is rational to combine acetaminophen with opioids for patients with moderate to severe pain. It has very good safety in neonates, provided clinicians adhere to dosing guidelines, as summarized below. Infants preferentially conjugate acetaminophen to the sulfate metabolite rather than the glucuronide metabolite.[21] Over early childhood, the sulfation accounts for a greater fraction of acetaminophen's metabolism, reaching mature glucuronide/sulfate ratios by around age 12.

Acetaminophen is available by the oral route in several tablet and liquid formulations. Clinicians should be cautioned that commonly used liquid and "dropper" formulations use different concentrations. Oral dosing of 10 to 15 mg/kg is commonly recommended, though single oral doses of 20 mg/kg appear quite safe in children. Plasma concentrations for analgesia in a dose–response study appeared similar to those reported previously for fever control. Daily maximum oral dosing is recommended not to exceed 100 mg/kg for children, 75 mg/kg for term neonates, and 40 mg/kg for premature infants less than 32 weeks gestation.

Rectal dosing of acetaminophen may be the preferred route for a subset of patients perioperatively, especially among selected infants and toddlers who do not cooperate with oral dosing. A series of studies has confirmed that rectal absorption is slow, somewhat variable, and comparatively inefficient. Single rectal doses of 30 to 45 mg/kg produced plasma concentrations that were generally in the effective range, and never in a range associated with hepatotoxicity.[22,23] Following these large rectal doses, there is a comparatively slow decline in plasma concentrations of the drug. Based on a 24-hour kinetic study, it was recommended that initial doses of 35 to 40 mg/kg be followed by subsequent doses of 20 mg/kg, with the dosing interval extended to at least 6 hours.[23] If a large rectal dose is to be followed by oral dosing, it is also recommended that a first oral dose be given no sooner than 6 hours after the initial dose. Dosage guidelines for acetaminophen and the most commonly used nonsteroidal anti-inflammatory drugs (NSAIDs) in children can be found in Table 25–1.

Nonsteroidal Anti-Inflammatory Drugs

NSAIDs provide excellent analgesia with a good safety margin in many contexts. NSAIDs act by reversible inhibition of cyclooxygenases, enzymes that convert arachidonic acid to prostanoids. Except in the newborn period, when the half-life after administration is significantly longer, the pharmacodynamics and pharmacokinetics of the NSAIDs in children are not much different than in adults. Children appear to have a lower incidence of renal and gastrointestinal side effects[24,25] than adults, even with chronic administration of the drug.[26]

NSAIDs are more similar than they are different. Adult clinical trials, outcome studies, and systematic reviews indicate that there is no unique effectiveness of the parenteral route; oral and rectal NSAIDs are equally effective.[27] There are no NSAIDs that possess uniquely greater analgesic effect than others, particularly when comparisons are made with equitoxic doses. Choice among these drugs may be governed by cost, general availability, desired route of administration, and duration of action.

Ibuprofen is frequently chosen to treat mild to moderate pain in the United States because the drug is available in a liquid form, allowing for easy administration to younger children. Since it has recently become available as an over-the-counter medication for fever reduction as well as pain relief, there is a large amount of clinical experience in infants and children with this drug. A review of short-term ibuprofen use in a large cohort of children revealed no increase in clinically significant renal or gastrointestinal side effects compared with acetaminophen.[24] Since it is available as a rectal preparation in Canada, it has also been used as a "prophylactic" analgesic for postoperative pain, reducing the need for additional opioid analgesics by approximately 30 percent.[28]

Several NSAIDs, such as etodolac, and modified salicylates have been used in recent years with a moderately reduced risk of gastric upset or, in the case of choline magnesium trisalicylate (Trilisate), a decreased risk of platelet dysfunction. With the advent of more selective cyclooxygenase isoenzyme-2 (COX-2) inhibitors (see below), utilization of these drugs is likely to diminish.

Ketorolac is an NSAID available for parenteral use in the United States; in other countries there is extensive experience with other parenteral NSAIDs, especially diclofenac.[29] Ketorolac has been used both as an adjuvant to opioid analgesia and as a single agent for the treatment of postoperative pain in children and adolescents.[30,31] Vetter and Heiner demonstrated that the administration of a single dose of 0.8 mg/kg of ketorolac reduced the need for self-administered opioid analgesia by approximately 30 percent in the first 12 hours after surgery.[32] This led to a significant reduction in urinary retention compared with opioid analgesia alone. A preliminary study at our institution suggested that ketorolac significantly reduced the incidence and severity of postoperative bladder spasms.[33] Dosage recommendations have been reduced in the last few years to 0.25 to 0.5 mg/kg every 6 hours with no requirement for a loading dose.

NSAIDs do not produce tolerance or physical or psychological dependence, and are not associated with sedation or respiratory depression. They are, therefore, particularly

TABLE 25–1
ORAL DOSING GUIDELINES FOR COMMONLY USED NONOPIOID ANALGESICS

Drug	Dose (mg/kg) (<60 kg)	Dose (mg) (>60 kg)	Interval (hours)	Daily Maximum Dose (mg/kg) (<60 kg)	Daily Maximum Dose (mg) (>60 kg)
Acetaminophen	10–15	650–1000	4	100*	4,000
Ibuprofen	6–10	400–600[†]	6	40[†‡]	2,400[†]
Naproxen	5–6[†]	250–375[†]	12	24[†‡]	1,000[†]
Aspirin[§]	10–15[†§]	650–1000[†]	4	80[†‡§]	3,600[†]

* Maximum daily doses for acetaminophen in term neonates and infants, should be reduced to 75 mg/kg, and to 40 mg/kg in preterm neonates.
[†] Dosing guidelines for neonates and infants have not been established.
[‡] Higher doses may be used in selected cases for treatment of rheumatologic conditions in children.
[§] Aspirin carries a risk of provoking Reye's syndrome in infants and children. If other analgesics are available, aspirin use should be restricted to indications where antiplatelet or anti-inflammatory effect is required, rather than as a routine analgesic or antipyretic in neonates, infants, or children. Dosing guidelines for aspirin in neonates have not been established.
Adapted from Berde CB, Sethna NF: Analgesics in the treatment of pain in children. N Engl J Med (in press) 2001; and World Health Organization: Cancer Pain and Palliative Care in Children. Geneva, WHO Publications, 1998.

useful for patients whose opioid use is limited by respiratory depressant effects. NSAIDs may cause nausea, gastrointestinal bleeding, platelet dysfunction, and nephropathy, though the incidence of renal impairment when used on a short-term basis appears to be very low. NSAIDs cause greater renal impairment during conditions of reduced renal blood flow; adequate fluid replacement and maintenance of cardiac output and intravascular volume can reduce the risk of renal injury. A review of the short-term use (48 hours) of intravenous ketorolac in over 1,700 children at this institution demonstrated a low rate of complications. Four children (0.2 percent) demonstrated hypersensitivity reactions (urticaria and/or bronchospasm), two children (0.1 percent) had evidence of renal impairment (though both had other underlying problems that could account for the renal insufficiency), and one child (0.05 percent) had melena at the completion of a 48-hour course of the drug.[34]

Two major cyclooxygenase isoenzymes, COX-1 and COX-2, have been identified and shown to mediate a different spectrum of biologic effects.[35] COX-1 is expressed constitutively and contributes to maintenance of gastric mucosal integrity and barrier function, platelet aggregation, and some aspects of distribution of renal blood flow. COX-2 expression is induced by inflammation or tissue injury, with levels of expression in peripheral and central neurons and in leukocytes. Several selective COX-2 inhibitors have been introduced into clinical practice in the past several years. Studies in adults have found that, in comparison with traditional NSAIDs, several COX-2 inhibitors produced a significantly lower incidence of gastritis or ulcers,[36] and excellent preservation of platelet function. The risk of nephrotoxicity from currently available COX-2 inhibitors appears similar to that of conventional NSAIDs.[37] Available pediatric data on COX-2 specific inhibitors at the time of this writing are largely limited to the drug nimesulide,[38] which is not available in the United States. COX-2 inhibitors may be particularly attractive as analgesics for types of surgery for which bleeding risks of NSAIDs are a particular concern, including tonsillectomy and neurosurgical procedures.

Recent retrospective case series and some preliminary animal studies have raised a concern that NSAIDs may impair bone healing or bone graft formation.[39] There has been some dispute regarding whether the dosing regimens or duration of application in some animal studies are relevant to predicting the effects of short-term (e.g., 2- to 3-day) postoperative use with recommended doses. This area is controversial at present, and there is a great need for proper animal studies and large-scale controlled, prospective human studies to address these issues.

Opioid Analgesics

Opioids are the most commonly used analgesic agents for moderate to severe acute pain. For the vast majority of children, opioids produce excellent analgesia with a wide margin of safety. There is, however, marked individual variation in opioid dose requirements and doses must be adjusted to effect. For the treatment of acute pain, the correct dose of opioid is that which treats the pain, yet does not result in excessive somnolence or respiratory depression.

Several physiologic and pharmacokinetic factors influence opioid action in neonates. In the first week of life, the elimination half-life of morphine is more than twice as long in newborns than in older children or adults, and even longer in premature infants. This appears to be due to several factors, most important of which is the immaturity of the newborn infant's hepatic enzyme systems. Clearance of morphine is dependent on conjugation of the drug to the metabolites morphine-3-glucuronide and the morphine-6-glucuronide; the latter contributes a substantial fraction of morphine's analgesic effects. This reaction is catalyzed by mixed function oxidases and the cytochrome P-450 system which, though present, have attained only a portion of their full function. Fentanyl and sufentanil also have diminished hepatic metabolism in premature and term neonates. Glomerular filtration is reduced in the first week of life, leading to slower elimination of morphine's active metabolites.

Infant animals have not yet given a consistent picture of the age dependence of opioid-induced analgesia and respiratory depression. Some of these discrepancies may be due to species differences or differences in study design, including the choice of a tonic or phasic pain stimulus.[40] For example, whereas one study found similar analgesic weight-scaled dose–response of several opioids in newborn rats compared with older rats,[40] another reported that newborn rats were less sensitive to the analgesic effects of morphine but more sensitive to its respiratory depressant effects than older rats.[41] These age-related effects were ascribed to developmental changes in the number and subtypes of μ receptors.[41] A prevalent view has been that the increased respiratory sensitivity of the newborn to opioids was due to increased blood–brain barrier permeability, leading to increased brain entry. Two studies in neonatal dogs disputed this view,[14, 15] using pharmacokinetic-pharmacodynamic modeling to argue that morphine has greater intrinsic respiratory depressant actions in the newborn, not more rapid brain entry. Studies in monkeys found no evidence for greater respiratory depression from morphine in newborns compared with older animals, even at morphine plasma concentrations that would produce respiratory depression in adult humans.[42]

Ventilatory responses to hypoxia and hypercarbia develop over the first 3 to 6 months of life. Premature and former premature infants with chronic lung disease continue to show depressed hypoxic drive for several months. This has led to the recommendation for cardiorespiratory monitoring and careful observation whenever opioids are administered to infants less than 2 to 3 months of age. In our practice, inpatients receiving parenteral opioids receive continuous apnea monitoring and hourly respiratory observations.

Opioids can be administered by a number of routes, including orally, intravenously, intramuscularly, subcutaneously, rectally, transdermally, or transmucosally. Oral administration is generally the easiest and can lead to relatively constant drug levels with regular administration. After minor and less painful surgery, oral opioids are usually well tolerated and provide excellent postoperative pain relief. If immediate onset of pain relief is required for severe pain, or if a patient is not yet tolerating oral intake, then parenteral administration of the drugs is recommended.

Codeine is available in an elixir form and is, therefore, the most commonly administered oral opioid in young children. It is often given in combination with acetaminophen. In fact, this combined form is not only more effective than the single drug alone, but also may, unlike most opioids in the United States, be prescribed over the phone. The commercially available acetaminophen/codeine elixir contains the two drugs in a 10 : 1 ratio (acetaminophen 120 mg with codeine 12 mg/5 ml). Since the currently recommended doses are in a 20 : 1 to 30 : 1 ratio (10 to 15 mg/kg acetaminophen and 0.5 mg/kg codeine), we recommend basing the elixir dosage on the codeine dose and administering additional acetaminophen. Dosage guidelines for this and other opioid analgesics can be found in Table 25–2. Although codeine is convenient and readily available, its analgesic effects when given in the recommended doses are comparatively weak. Clinicians should not hesitate to prescribe "strong" opioids if combinations of codeine, acetaminophen, and NSAIDs do not provide adequate pain relief. In pooled analyses of studies in adults, 45 to 60 mg of codeine with acetaminophen is no more effective than 600 to 800 mg of ibuprofen.[43]

The analgesic effects of codeine derive from its metabolic conversion to morphine. A significant fraction of the general population (ranging from 3 to 14 percent in different ethnic groups) lacks the enzyme that o-demethylates codeine to generate morphine.[44] Thus, if a patient fails to show an analgesic effect from standard dosing of codeine, consideration should be given to substituting a second opioid, in order to circumvent this pharmacogenetic barrier.

Oxycodone is frequently combined with acetaminophen or aspirin, though it is now more commonly available as a single drug, either by tablet, elixir, or sustained-release tablet.

Methadone is an opioid that is useful in several contexts, though it requires individualized dose titration and frequent assessment of its effects. Oral absorption is efficient, with bioavailability generally ranging from 60 to 90 percent. Methadone's clearance is slow, but highly variable. In chronic dosing, it is frequently feasible to use dosing intervals ranging from 6 to 12 hours. Oral elixir formulations are available, which permit methadone, unlike sustained-release morphine, to be a long-acting medication among patients unable to swallow pills whole.

Methadone is also unique in that it is supplied as a racemic mixture, and the two enantiomers have distinct and complementary actions: the l-isomer is a μ-opioid agonist, whereas the d-isomer is an antagonist at the N-methyl-D-aspartate (NMDA) subgroup of glutamate receptors.[45] In both animals and humans, NMDA receptor antagonists have been shown to prevent or antagonize tolerance to opioids. The consequence of this is that methadone's relative potency compared with morphine and other μ-agonists appears much greater in opioid-tolerant subjects compared with opioid-naive subjects. Thus, although the commonly cited intravenous (IV) single-dose potency ratio for methadone and morphine is roughly 1 : 1, in morphine-tolerant oncology patients, methadone may pro-

vide equal analgesia with daily milligram dosing ranging from one third to less than one tenth of the daily morphine milligram dose.[46] Methadone's slow but variable clearance, and the aforementioned incomplete cross-tolerance, both can make its dose response unpredictable. Methadone should be prescribed with caution and with frequent assessment to detect early signs of sedation or hypoventilation.

A technologically simple regimen involving loading doses (usually 0.1 to 0.2 mg/kg)[47] and small bolus doses of methadone was shown to be very effective for postoperative analgesia. As noted earlier, intravenous bolus dosing of other opioids, such as morphine, fentanyl, or hydromorphone, on a 4-hourly schedule produces excessive fluctuations in plasma concentrations of the drug. In contrast, methadone's long duration of action permits fairly constant effect with a 4-hourly dosing schedule. A practical and simple method of administration of methadone is sometimes referred to as a "reverse prn" method. Patients are assessed by the nursing staff at intervals not exceeding 4 hours. A "sliding scale" adjusts the intravenous methadone dose according to the nurse's assessment of the child's pain as either severe (0.07 mg/kg), moderate (0.05 mg/kg), or mild (0.03 mg/kg). This method is convenient and inexpensive, and permits easy adjustment of dosing to patients' variable requirements.

Opioids are generally administered to children postoperatively via the intravenous route. Because of the multiple injections that children receive in the first year of life, many children have a tremendous fear of "shots." If offered an injection for pain relief, most children will deny that they are in pain to avoid receiving a shot and many are willing to endure a great deal of pain if intramuscular injections are all that are offered for postoperative pain relief.

Though intermittent boluses of morphine, meperidine, hydromorphone, or fentanyl can provide rapid pain relief, their duration of action is short, resulting in marked fluctuations in serum opioid concentrations during the dosage period. When bolus injections are chosen, it is recommended that the dosing interval should not be greater than every 2 hours. Continuous opioid infusions and patient-controlled anesthesia (PCA) are commonly used to circumvent these fluctuations in plasma concentrations and thereby provide a more steady analgesic effect.

Continuous Opioid Infusions

Continuous intravenous infusions of opioids (most commonly morphine, hydromorphone, or fentanyl) can provide effective analgesia for infants and children following surgery[48, 49]; as with all methods of opioid administration, peripheral opioid side effects are common.[50] Since effective plasma opioid concentrations vary widely among individuals, provisions should be available to permit supplemental bolus dosing and increases or decreases in infusion rate as indicated by clinical signs. Initial loading doses to achieve analgesic concentrations are administered either intraoperatively or in the postanesthesia care unit (PACU).

For toddlers and children, commonly recommended initial morphine infusion rates are roughly 0.025 mg/kg/h. Due to the pharmacokinetic and pharmacodynamic factors described above, initial infusion rates in newborns

T A B L E   2 5 – 2

OPIOID ANALGESIC INITIAL DOSAGE GUIDELINES*

Drug	Equianalgesic Doses		Usual Starting IV or SC Doses and Intervals		Parenteral/ Oral Dose Ratio	Usual Starting Oral Doses and Intervals	
	Parenteral	Oral	Child <50 kg	Child >50 kg		Child <50 kg	Child >50 kg
Codeine	120 mg	200 mg	N/R	N/R	1:2	0.5–1 mg/kg every 3–4 hours	30–60 mg every 3–4 hours
Morphine	10 mg	30 mg (chronic) 60 mg (single dose)	Bolus: 0.1 mg/kg every 2–4 hours Infusion 0.03 mg/kg/h	Bolus 5–8 mg every 2–4 hours Infusion 1.5 mg/h	1:3 (chronic) 1:6 (single dose)	Immediate Release: 0.3 mg/ kg every 3–4 hours Sustained Release: 20–35 kg: 10–15 mg every 8–12 hours 35–50 kg: 15–30 mg every 8–12 hours	Immediate Release: 15–20 mg every 3–4 hours Sustained Release: 30–45 mg every 8–12 hours
Oxycodone	N/A	15–20 mg	N/A	N/A	N/A	0.1–0.2 mg/kg every 3–4 hours	5–10 mg every 3–4 hours
Methadone†	10 mg	10–20 mg	Bolus: 0.1 mg/kg every 4–8 hours	1:2	1:2	0.2 mg/kg every 4–8 hours	10 mg every 4–8 hours
Fentanyl	100 μg (0.1 mg)	N/A	Bolus: 0.5–1 μg/kg every 1–2 hours Infusion: 0.5–2 μg/kg/h	Bolus: 25–50 μg every 1–2 hours Infusion: 25–100 μg/h	N/A	N/A	N/A
Hydromorphone	1.5–2 mg	6–8 mg	Bolus: 0.02 mg every 2–4 hours Infusion: 0.006 mg/ kg/h	Bolus: 1 mg Every 2–4 hours Infusion: 0.3 mg/h	1:4	0.04–0.08 mg/kg every 3–4 hours	2–4 mg every 3–4 hours
Meperidine‡ (pethidine)	75–100 mg	300 mg	Bolus: 0.8–1 mg/kg every 2–3 hours	Bolus: 50–75 mg every 2–3 hours	1:4	2–3 mg/kg every 3–4 hours	100–150 mg every 3–4 hours

* Doses refer to patients >6 months of age. In infants <6 months of age, initial doses/kg should begin at roughly 25 percent of the doses/kg recommended here. All doses are approximate and should be adjusted according to clinical circumstances.

† Methadone requires additional vigilance, because it can accumulate and produce delayed sedation. If sedation occurs, doses should be withheld until sedation resolves. Thereafter, doses should be substantially reduced and/or the dosing interval should be extended to 8–12 hours.

‡ Meperidine should generally be avoided if other opioids are available, especially with chronic use, because its metabolite can cause seizures.

Adapted from Berde CB, Sethna NF: Analgesics in the treatment of pain in children. N Engl J Med (in press) 2001; and World Health Organization: Cancer Pain and Palliative Care in Children. Geneva, WHO Publications, 1998.

and infants are recommended as 0.01 mg/kg/h and 0.015 mg/kg/h, respectively.[49] Prematures and infants with respiratory or cardiac diseases may in some cases require even lower initial infusion rates (e.g., 0.005 mg/kg/h). Adjustment of these rates is then based on clinical signs of either inadequate pain relief or increased somnolence.

Patient-Controlled Analgesia

PCA is widely used for postoperative pain relief in both children and adults. With appropriate preoperative teaching and encouragement, children as young as 6 to 7 years of age can independently use the PCA pump to provide good postoperative pain relief.[51] Children between the ages of 4 and 6, however, generally require encouragement from their parents and nursing staff to push the button before anticipated painful movements or procedures. Even with encouragement, the failure rate among 4- and 5-year-olds with PCA appears quite high.

The traditional notion for adults is that the inherent safety in PCA is that the patient will stop pushing the button when they become sleepy, and thereby the plasma concentration will always remain in a safe range. Nurse-controlled analgesia (NCA)[52] is widely used to permit small titrated dosing of opioids for infants and children who are unable to use the PCA button; this technique appears to have very good safety. Although some have advocated use of parent-controlled analgesia,[52] we believe that it may pose some risk in the setting of opioid-naive postoperative patients. If hospitals make a choice to use parent-controlled analgesia postoperatively, we would advocate a formal program for parent teaching and standards for frequent nursing observation. Conversely, we believe that parent-controlled analgesia has a very useful role in the management of ongoing pain or palliative care due to cancer, acquired immunodeficiency syndrome (AIDS), and other life-threatening diseases.

PCA may be administered either alone or in conjunction with a low-dose continuous infusion. Initial parameters for the most commonly used agents can be found in Table 25–3. Morphine, hydromorphone, and fentanyl have all been used; there are insufficient data to recommend one of these agents as uniquely preferable to the others. Meperidine is generally not recommended where other opioids are available because of the potential for seizures due to its metabolite, normeperidine.

The issue of whether to use a background infusion of opioids, along with PCA, to allow for longer periods of uninterrupted sleep has been a controversial one especially in opioid-naive postoperative patients. Basal infu-

TABLE 25–3
TYPICAL STARTING PARAMETERS FOR PCA

Drug	Bolus Dose (μg/kg)	Continuous Rate (μg/kg/h)	4-Hour Limit (μg/kg)
Morphine	20	4–15	300
Hydromorphone	5	1–3	60
Fentanyl	0.25	0.15	4

Lockout interval = 7 minutes.

sions may improve sleep quality, though brief self-limited episodes of hypoxemia can be more frequent.[53-55] Alternatively, PCA may be used in bolus-only mode together with round-the-clock administration of NSAIDs and acetaminophen.

For children with acute pain associated with chronic illness, such as cancer or vaso-occlusive crisis in sickle cell disease, a larger basal infusion is preferred to adequately control disease-related pain. For tumor-related pain or palliative care, we commonly aim to provide roughly two thirds of the overall opioid requirement from the basal infusion.

Opioids by Other Routes

For patients with cancer or AIDS who are unable to take oral opioids and have no intravenous access, the subcutaneous administration of opioids has proven to be very effective.[56] Morphine and hydromorphone are well suited to this method of administration and are available in more concentrated solutions. This route can be used for continuous infusion, intermittent boluses, or PCA. Though usually well tolerated, itching and redness often occur at the insertion site and may be bothersome to some children. Needle insertion sites usually need to be changed as needed (usually every 3 to 5 days).

Transdermal fentanyl has been used effectively for treatment of cancer pain in children.[57] Since there is considerable lag before therapeutic blood concentrations are reached and elimination is slow, transdermal fentanyl is more useful for persistent pain than for pain with marked fluctuations in intensity. Supplemental opioids are often needed for acute exacerbations of pain in these patients. Transdermal fentanyl is not recommended for routine postoperative pain management in opioid-naive children.

Transmucosal fentanyl, the "fentanyl lollipop," has been investigated as an analgesic and sedative agent prior to painful procedures in children.[58] The onset of effect is usually noted in 10 to 30 minutes, so "titration" of this agent is possible. Though readily accepted by children, nausea and vomiting and facial pruritus are common.

LOCAL ANESTHETICS AND REGIONAL ANESTHESIA

Local Anesthetics in Infants and Children

Local anesthesia has some unique risks and concerns in infants and children. Test-dosing is recommended, though its reliability is reduced during general anesthesia.[59] All dosing for major regional blockade should be fractionated, and administered with continuous monitoring of electrocardiogram (ECG) and frequent blood pressure measurements. The dose to block a nerve varies more weakly with body size than the dose that produces systemic toxicity, so that smaller subjects have a narrower therapeutic index.[60,61] Infants clear amide local anesthetics more slowly than children and adults,[62] so that lower infusion rates are permitted, and repeated dosing is more likely to produce systemic accumulation of the drug and toxicity. Chloroprocaine can be administered at high infusion rates even in neonates.[63] We also use fractionated dosing of chloroprocaine to reconfirm the position of an epidural catheter in the PACU or on the postoperative wards.

Topical Anesthesia for Cut Skin

The stratum corneum of the epidermis presents a permeability barrier to local anesthetics. A variety of strategies have been used to circumvent this barrier. Formulations combining tetracaine, epinephrine, and cocaine (TAC) were shown to provide analgesia when applied to cut skin, in order to facilitate laceration repair.[64] Subsequent studies showed that cocaine was not essential for these mixtures; combinations of tetracaine and phenylephrine were equally effective.[65] TAC and its variants should be avoided in the vicinity of end-arteries, since ischemic complications can result. Application near mucosal surfaces should be avoided, since efficient systemic absorption can produce seizures or death. New topical anesthetics along with modalities of transdermal drug delivery such as iontophoresis have proven to be both safe and effective for a number of painful procedures routinely performed in children.

Topical Anesthesia for Intact Skin

EMLA

EMLA (a eutectic mixture of the local anesthetics lidocaine and prilocaine) was one of the first topical anesthetics commercially available for use on intact skin and has been the most extensively used and studied.[66, 67] The physicochemical feature of this type of mixture is that it permits higher aqueous solubility of the uncharged (base) forms. This physical feature permits a higher effective concentration at the stratum corneum and increases the rate of uptake.

The effectiveness of EMLA can be increased by applying a thicker layer and increasing the duration of application to 90 to 120 minutes. Application times of less than 45 minutes result in a high failure rate. A new patch delivery system may simplify the application process and make it easier for parents to apply the cream at home prior to outpatient procedures.

Clinical trials have shown effectiveness of EMLA in reducing the pain or distress of a number of common pediatric procedures including venous cannulation, venipuncture, lumbar puncture, circumcision, urethral meatotomy and adhesion release, immunizations, arterial cannulation, dermatologic procedures, allergy testing, accessing implanted central venous access catheters, and laceration repair.

Iontophoresis

Iontophoresis employs an electrical field to drive local anesthetics in their charged ionic form across the stratum corneum. Iontophoresis has a much shorter onset time in providing cutaneous anesthesia (10 to 25 minutes); it has

become popular for analgesia prior to painful procedures in children.

The most common anesthetic used by this route is 2 percent lidocaine with 1:100,000 epinephrine. Though there is a mild tingling sensation during drug delivery, this is generally well tolerated.[57, 58] Iontophoresis appears to result in deeper levels of dermal anesthesia and may penetrate deeply enough to numb both skin and veins, allowing for less painful venous cannulation compared with EMLA. The duration of application of iontophoresis to achieve sufficient analgesia is dependent on the amount of current used. With higher currents (i.e., 4 mA), there is more tingling of the skin, but analgesia can be achieved in approximately 10 minutes. Longer application times (approximately 25 to 30 minutes) are needed when lower currents are used, but the tingling sensation can be made almost undetectable. Many centers have allowed older children to adjust the current themselves based on their tolerance of the electrical current.

Amethocaine

Amethocaine (Ametop) is a topical preparation of tetracaine, formulated as either a gel[68] or a patch.[69] It is widely available in Europe and Canada, but not available in the United States at present. It has three distinct advantages over EMLA cream: (1) cutaneous analgesia can be achieved in only 30 minutes, (2) duration of analgesia after removal of the drug is significantly longer, and (3) it vasodilates (whereas EMLA constricts), facilitating venous cannulation.

Liposomal Lidocaine

Lidocaine can be dispersed in liposomes to facilitate transcutaneous delivery. This formulation appears to provide skin anesthesia within 30 minutes in recent studies.[70]

Vapocoolant Spray

Vapocoolant sprays (primarily ethyl chloride) have been used for the treatment of myalgic pain since the 1950s. Recent studies have suggested that these sprays also can provide inexpensive, rapid, and effective analgesia for short-duration procedures such as venipuncture and immunization.[71] Due to the concern regarding inhalation of these agents, especially in small children, the vapocoolant may also be placed on a cotton ball and directly applied to the injection site for 15 seconds. The vapocoolant is allowed to dry for 1 to 2 seconds and then the procedure is performed as quickly as possible.

The advantages of this technique are the rapid onset time and the low cost (approximately $0.50 per application). Skin reactions have been noted with agents containing ethyl chloride but, because of the rapid evaporation of these agents, appear to be quite rare.

Infiltration of Local Anesthetics

When topical local anesthesia is not feasible because of time constraints in urgent or emergent situations, infiltration of 1 percent lidocaine to an intended puncture site can significantly reduce the pain associated with venous or arterial cannulation. Intradermal injection pain can be significantly lessened by the use of a smaller needle and buffering of the local anesthetic with the addition of sodium bicarbonate (9 ml lidocaine mixed with 1 ml sodium bicarbonate).

Regional Anesthesia and Analgesia

Recently there has been increased interest in the use of regional anesthetic techniques to decrease general anesthetic requirements and aid in postoperative pain management in children and adolescents. These techniques range from local infiltration of the wound edges, blockade of peripheral nerves, plexus blocks, and epidural and subarachnoid blocks or infusions. Single-shot caudal injections of local anesthetics and peripheral nerve blocks have proven to be easy to perform and can provide significant pain relief after many common outpatient pediatric operations. Details regarding the indications and performance of these blocks are described in Chapter 12. We present here only a few selected opinions about techniques and drug selection.

Epidural Analgesia

Epidural analgesia can provide excellent postoperative analgesia in infants and children undergoing thoracic, abdominal, perineal, and lower extremity surgery. We recommend use of loss-of-resistance to saline, rather than air; for lumbar placement; we favor continuous advancement using Bromage's grip. Our preference is for 18-gauge short needles and 20-gauge catheters even in infants. Several thinner needles and catheters are available; some are difficult to thread or generate excessive resistance during infusions.

The epidural space may be approached at any level, but is most frequently approached via the lumbar or caudal route in children. For upper abdominal or thoracic procedures, a direct thoracic epidural approach may be used in selected circumstances, but performance of thoracic puncture under general anesthesia should be performed only by very experienced personnel and with careful consideration of potential benefits and risks. In older children, sedated awake thoracic epidural placement is quite feasible. Catheters can be advanced via the caudal route to thoracic levels in neonates and younger infants; success rates vary among published series[72] and failure rates are greater for infants larger than 5 kg. Blind lumbar-to-thoracic placement has a higher failure rate. In selected cases, catheters can be advanced from lumbar or caudal routes under fluoroscopic guidance, and catheter tip positions can be confirmed by a contrast epidurogram. We prefer this technique whenever epidurals are placed for management of chronic pain or pain due to advanced cancer.[73] In our experience, lumbar-to-thoracic placement of catheters is more successful if placement occurs at L1-L2 rather than lower levels, and with the epidural needle angled in a cephalad direction, rather than directly perpendicular to the axis of the spine. Recently, Tsui and coworkers have described a high success rate for cephalad advancement of wire-wrapped epidural catheters to tho-

racic levels by use of electrical stimulation.[74] This method appears quite promising, and awaits replication by other groups. For extensive thoracic and abdominal procedures, especially among high-risk patients, our belief is that thoracic catheter placement can provide optimal analgesia[75] both at rest and with movement.

Epidural drug selection should be individualized and varies with site of surgery, site of epidural catheter tip, and patient-specific risk factors. In general, we recommend infusion of local anesthetics in combination with either opioids or clonidine or both,[76] rather than alone. Clonidine appears to be an attractive adjunct in epidural infusions and in single-shot caudal blocks,[77] because it intensifies the analgesia from local anesthetics, but it does not generate a number of the side effects of opioids, including itching, nausea, ileus, or urinary retention. Even at doses that produce sedation, it appears to have much less risk of respiratory depression than opioids.[77, 78]

When the surgery is very extensive or when the catheter is placed at lumbar levels for upper abdominal or thoracic surgery, our preference is to use hydromorphone, which spreads rostrally in the neuraxis, but produces less pruritus than morphine.[79] We require continuous electronic monitoring for patients receiving hydrophilic opioids, and generally avoid their use in neonates. Further studies are needed to determine the optimal dosing for continuous infusions of hydromorphone in children. (See Table 25–4 for representative guidelines for epidural infusions.)

Continuous epidural anesthesia/analgesia can be safely administered on the surgical and medical wards if there

| TABLE 25–4 |
| REPRESENTATIVE PEDIATRIC EPIDURAL INFUSIONS |

Solution	Suggested Rates in ml/kg/h	Comments
Children and infants > 2–3 months		
Bupivacaine 0.1% with fentanyl 2 µg/ml	0.2–0.4	
Bupivacaine 0.1% with fentanyl 2 µg/ml and/or clonidine 0.8 µg/ml	0.2–0.3	
Bupivacaine 0.1% with hydromorphone 5-10 µg/ml	0.1–0.2	Electronic monitoring is strongly recommended. Especially useful for thoracic or upper abdominal surgery. See text for precautions.
*Neonates and infants < 2–3 months		
1.5% 2-chloroprocaine with clonidine 0.1 µg/ml	0.5–0.7	See text for precautions.
Bupivacaine 0.1% with fentanyl 0.5 µg/ml and/or clonidine 0.1 µg/ml	0.1–0.2	See text for precautions.

* Recommendations for neonates and young infants are provisional and not based on extensive safety studies.

is proper observation and a management protocol. The nursing staff must be educated about the potential complications that may arise with these infusions and the appropriate measures to take if such complications arise. Choice among methods of electronic monitoring and frequencies of clinical assessment vary among centers. Our practice is to require frequent clinical assessment of level of consciousness and respiratory rate and depth by the nursing staff for all patients receiving parenteral opioids, PCA, or epidural infusions. We require electronic monitoring for subgroups of patients including, but not limited to, all infants less than 6 months receiving either parenteral opioids or any epidural infusion (i.e., any combination of local anesthetics, opioids, or clonidine), all patients receiving hydrophilic epidural opioids, and patients with medical conditions that produce an increased risk of apnea or hypoventilation. Electronic monitors with audio alarms that are heard in a patient's room, but not in the hallways and nurses' station, may generate a false sense of security, and may fail to alert staff to critical incidents.

PAINFUL PROCEDURES

In the last 10 years, as the number of nonoperative diagnostic and therapeutic procedures for children has grown, pediatric caregivers have been searching for ways to make these procedures more acceptable to children and their parents. The increasing use of sedative and analgesics for children grew out of the popularity of the use of "conscious sedation" in adults to make invasive procedures more comfortable and less stressful. There has been increasing availability of sedation services staffed by pediatric anesthesiologists and others, using either locations near the operating room or remote sites.

There is considerable controversy regarding which forms of sedation should be administered under which circumstances to which child. Our view is that most hospitals caring for children will adopt a two-tiered approach. A subgroup of procedures can be performed by pediatric subspecialists, especially pediatric radiologists, gastroenterologists, and emergency room physicians, using a set of guidelines that restrict drug selection, maximum dosing, and criteria for assessment. Included are procedures that are comparatively brief, do not require absolute immobility, and involve only moderately painful interventions, which can be facilitated by local anesthesia. It is improbable that most institutions can provide anesthesiologists for all circumstances for which children require sedation. The safety track record of sedation protocols done by some pediatric subspecialists according to American Academy of Pediatrics (AAP) guidelines appears quite good. Examples of these include sedation for radiologic procedures[80] and for pediatric oncology procedures. Adverse events continue to occur at a significant incidence, and are often associated with failure to follow AAP guidelines, including use of oximetry and continuous observation, as well as inadequate patient assessment.[81] For younger infants; for children with airway, respiratory, neurologic, or cardiac conditions that increase risk; and for more extensive procedures or procedures that require complete immobiliza-

tion (e.g., radiation therapy for orbital tumors), sedation or anesthesia by anesthesiologists appears preferable.[82]

CHRONIC PAIN IN CHILDREN

The majority of anesthesiologists caring for children will not necessarily be involved in chronic pain management on a regular basis. Nevertheless, a number of patients coming to the operating room will have chronic conditions that produce persistent or recurrent pain, and these conditions may have impact on perioperative management. In addition, because of their expertise in analgesic pharmacology, conscious sedation, and regional anesthesia, pediatric anesthesiologists may be called on for consultation regarding application of these approaches to treatment of children with chronic pain or cancer pain, and an appreciation of the relevant issues will help to ensure optimal involvement.

Pain can become recurrent or persistent for a number of reasons. With some conditions, tissue injury or inflammation persists for long periods of time, generating ongoing nociceptive signaling. Pain due to joint inflammation in rheumatoid arthritis or due to vaso-occlusion and distal ischemia in sickle cell disease are examples of persistent or recurrent *nociceptive* pain.

Some forms of pain persist even as tissues heal and inflammation subsides. Injury to the central or peripheral nervous system can result in abnormal patterns of spontaneous or evoked impulse generation, leading to *neuropathic* pain. Examples of this include posttraumatic neuralgias, phantom pain following amputation, diabetic neuropathy, and so forth.

For both acute and chronic pain, the experience of pain and suffering as well as the consequences of pain on behavior and functioning depend on a complex interplay of tissue injury, disease-related factors, inherent biologic/psychological factors, and social factors. Pain experience, behavioral manifestations of pain, and impact of pain on daily activities can be influenced by social reinforcers.[83] This statement should not be interpreted to suggest that pain is largely "psychogenic" or "not real." True malingering, faking, or psychogenic pain are comparatively uncommon, and should not be invoked lightly or as an excuse for clinicians' failure to find a straightforward mechanism for the patient's pain.

The Common "Benign Recurrent Pains" of Childhood

Chronic persistent pains are relatively common among adults, but comparatively uncommon in children. Several common types of pain in childhood involve episodic painful episodes interspersed with pain-free periods in a child who appears otherwise generally well, and who is growing and reaching normal developmental milestones. These conditions are exceedingly common in general pediatric practice.

Chronic Headaches

Recurrent headaches are a common problem in school-age children; depending on the inclusion criteria and population studied, the prevalence may range from 5 to 15 percent of school children. Although the vast majority of headaches are not associated with serious structural and organic diseases, a chronic progressive headache can be a worrisome sign of a pathologic process and neuroimaging is indicated in these cases. On initial evaluation, all children with headaches should have a thorough general physical exam, a complete neurologic exam, and careful funduscopic examination. A small subgroup of children with recurrent headaches will have a range of specific and treatable diagnoses for which clues may be offered on the history and physical exam, including dental conditions, impaired visual acuity, acute or chronic sinusitis, endocrine or metabolic disorders, and systemic or intracranial hypertension or hypotension.

The most common types of headaches that occur in children are tension headaches, migraine, and mixed tension-migraine headaches. Migraine headaches are slightly more common in boys before the age of puberty but become more common in girls after menarche. There is often a strong family history of migraines, and almost 60 percent of adults with vascular headaches report onset of symptoms during childhood.[84] Many children with migraines may not describe the classic visual or auditory auras, but may instead report fatigue, irritability, dizziness, or nausea prior to development of the headache. Typically, children describe throbbing unilateral or frontal headaches that are frequently associated with photophobia, nausea, and vomiting. Over 90 percent of children obtain relief of the migraine from sleep.[84] Tension headaches are frequently described as a squeezing pain that occurs bilaterally, circumferentially, or in the occipital region. Tension headaches show no sex predominance and are rarely associated with nausea, vomiting, photophobia, or auras. Children with combined headaches experience chronic tension-like headaches often related to stress and anxiety, and acute recurrent migraine headaches. The majority of children with pain in the temporomandibular region do not have structural pathology of the temporomandibular joint; many have pain associated with sensitization of the muscles of mastication, including the masseters and pterygoids.

Treatment for headaches in children without underlying pathology involves a combination of pharmacologic agents, biobehavioral techniques, and lifestyle changes that promote functional and adaptive behavior. Reassurance should be provided to patients and parents that a more serious etiology is not the underlying cause. A diary that records frequency and intensity of headaches; associated symptoms; pain medications; and precipitating factors such as certain foods, stress, and menstruation can help recognize causative factors as well as help guide therapy.

If a child has chronic daily headache, one should carefully evaluate psychosocial stressors or factors that may reinforce or amplify the symptoms, and one should consider whether medication-induced rebound headaches are involved. Medication-induced "rebound" headache is common among adults with chronic daily headache, either from excessive use of NSAIDs or from combination medications such as Fioricet. Intermittent opioid use should be avoided in most cases.

In drug therapy of migraine, a distinction is made between drugs given to interrupt an ongoing episode (abortive therapy) and drugs given to prevent or reduce the frequency of headaches (preventive or prophylactic therapy). NSAIDs are often the first-line abortive drug therapy for migraine, tension, and combined headaches[85]; there are probably few important differences among the NSAIDs in effectiveness for headache treatment. Ibuprofen is widely used and can be administered in tablet form or suspension in doses of 6 to 10 mg/kg orally. Injectable NSAIDs such as ketorolac or diclofenac can be used if there is persistent vomiting and inability to take oral opioids, though, as noted above, injectable NSAIDs are no more effective than oral NSAIDs. Sumatriptan is a 5-HT serotonin antagonist that is used as abortive migraine therapy and for treatment of acute migraines in adult patients. Although additional safety and efficacy studies are needed in children, some studies have shown headache reduction with sumatriptan in children with severe migraines[86, 87]; others have given equivocal results.[88] Sumatriptan can be administered orally, nasally, or intramuscularly, which may be convenient for patients who experience significant vomiting with migraines.

β-Blockers, anticonvulsants, and antidepressants are the most frequently used drugs for prophylactic migraine therapy. Propranolol doses of 1 to 2 mg/kg daily are typically used; however, controlled trials of propranolol in pediatric headache management show equivocal results.[89] Several placebo-controlled studies have shown benefit with calcium channel blockers.[90, 91] Low-dose tricyclic antidepressants such as nortriptyline may also provide effective migraine prophylaxis. Initial starting doses of 0.2 mg/kg orally are used at bedtime and are slowly titrated based on therapeutic response and side effects, often to around 1 mg/kg/day. Trazodone has been shown to be more effective than placebo in a crossover trial.[92] Pediatric neurologists commonly prescribe the antihistaminic cyproheptadine for migraine prophylaxis. Cyproheptadine is generally safe; weight gain is a common side effect. Despite its widespread use, no controlled trials of its efficacy in pediatric migraine have been reported.

Evidence supports the effectiveness of cognitive-behavioral methods in the treatment of certain types of chronic headaches in children. Outcome studies of management of chronic headaches in children provide stronger evidence of effectiveness for biobehavioral treatments than for any specific pharmacologic treatment.[89, 93] These methods are also useful because children can generalize them to new situations. Relaxation training, alone or assisted by biofeedback, is commonly used for headache therapy. In learning these skills, patients can use progressive muscle relaxation, imagery, and biofeedback to reduce stress and anxiety and to help modulate pain. Structured counseling is provided regarding development of coping skills and avoidance of triggers of maladaptive responses. Through behavioral modification and cognitive behavioral therapy, children and their parents can learn a more proactive approach that emphasizes wellness, and avoidance of catastrophizing or assumption of a sick role.

Abdominal Pain

Recurrent abdominal pain is a common problem among school-age children. Studies have shown that as many as 10 to 25 percent of school-age children experience recurrent abdominal pain.[94] In the majority of these cases, no clear-cut etiology can be found. Apley and others have found that only 10 percent of all cases of recurrent abdominal pain in children have an organic cause.[94] Common features of nonorganic recurrent abdominal pain include pain that is episodic that rarely awakens the child at night, and is often periumbilical without signs suggestive of systemic disease. A thorough history, physical examination, and review of systems is crucial in determining organic causes of abdominal pain. A psychosocial history is also mandatory, particularly to understand how the child and family cope with pain, as well as to explore any behavior suggesting school avoidance and social isolation. Children who have a history of recurrent fevers, weight loss, bloody stools, or other signs of possible systemic illness require additional laboratory and radiologic studies. An initial complete blood count, urinalysis, and stool guaiac test are reasonable initial screening studies. However, without clinical findings on history and physical exam, extensive diagnostic tests in children with recurrent abdominal pain are generally of low yield. For example, there is little benefit from screening gastrointestinal barium studies or ultrasound studies in children with recurrent abdominal pains that appear benign from history and physical exam. Other studies examining the use of abdominal ultrasound as a screening tool in the evaluation of abdominal pain has also shown little or no benefit.

Recent studies have sought to identify subgroups of children with recurrent abdominal pain who might have more specific etiologies not disclosed by a standard history and examination. Some children without a clear history of constipation improve with introduction of dietary fiber.[95] Another subgroup of children with no clinical history of lactose intolerance show positive lactose breath hydrogen tests, and improvement with either elimination of dietary lactose or lactose enzyme supplementation.[96] A cohort of children with recurrent abdominal pain associated with bloating, cramps, or dyspepsia were compared with normal control children using a noninvasive ultrasonographic method of examining gastric motility following a test meal.[97] The children with recurrent abdominal pain had impaired gastric relaxation after a meal, suggesting that altered motility may contribute to the condition in some cases. Longitudinal studies suggest that a subset of children with recurrent abdominal pain will have persistent symptoms in adulthood, in some cases evolving into irritable bowel syndrome. Recurrent episodic abdominal pain should be distinguished from recurrent persistent (i.e., daily) abdominal pain. In two selected series of children with chronic persistent pain, laparoscopy disclosed treatable diagnosis in a high percentage of cases.[98, 99]

Reassurance should be given to parents and children that although no organic etiology appears likely based on the initial evaluation, clinical reassessment will be ongoing, especially if symptoms change. Treatment strategies should emphasize improved pain coping skills through biobehavioral approaches with a goal of maintaining school attendance and other normal activities. The routine use of pain medications should be avoided.

Local anesthetic blockade may be useful in a small percentage of cases. Infiltration of local anesthetic may help diagnose pain as a result of nerve entrapment or neuromas involving abdominal surgical scars. Celiac plexus blockade using local anesthetic may help to differentiate visceral from somatic sources of abdominal pain, though all anesthesiologists should be aware of the fact that all forms of diagnostic nerve blockade are prone to false-positive and false-negative results.[100]

Chest Pain

Chest pain is a frequent complaint among children and adolescents, accounting for at least 650,000 physician visits annually.[101] Although a symptom of chest pain is often quite worrisome for patients and families, especially in cases where an adult family member has had chest pain and serious cardiac disease, the incidence of cardiac etiologies for chest pain in this age group is extremely low. The most common etiologies of chest pain include musculoskeletal conditions (particularly costochondritis and muscle pain from coughing) and conditions that receive no final diagnosis. Selbst et al. studied over 400 children presenting to emergency rooms with a complaint of chest pain. Initially, 13 percent of these patients were thought to have idiopathic chest pain, 16 percent had musculoskeletal causes, 9 percent had psychogenic pain, and 9 percent had costochondritis as a cause of chest pain.[102] At 2-year follow-up, the diagnosis of idiopathic chest pain increased to 34 percent, and in 54 percent of patients the chest pain had resolved at the time of follow-up.[102] Fyfe and Moodie studied 67 patients who were referred to a pediatric cardiology clinic for the evaluation of chest pain. Six percent of these patients were found to have underlying cardiac disease.[103]

A broad-based history and physical examination is the first step in evaluating a child with chest pain. Based on results of several studies, Selbst suggests that organic causes of chest pain is more likely in younger children or if there are any abnormal findings on physical exam.[104] In general, cardiac causes are usually suggested by history, physical exam, and family history. Abdominal and gastroesophageal disease such as reflux esophagitis, esophageal spasm, or gastritis may present as referred chest pain. Costochondritis, coughing, slipped rib syndrome, and muscle spasm and other musculoskeletal conditions are also causes of chest pain in children and adolescents.[105, 106]

Reassurance that cardiac disease is extremely unlikely has been shown to be of benefit in ultimate improvement in symptoms.[103, 107] Many children and adolescents with chest pain experience relief with such nonpharmacologic treatments as TENS unit, heat therapy, exercise, and stress relaxation techniques. Nonsteriodal anti-inflammatory drugs may be helpful for a musculoskeletal pain such as costochrondritis.

Neuropathic Pain

Over 35 percent of referrals to our pain clinic at Children's Hospital in Boston are due to neuropathic pain, primarily as a result of extremity trauma, postsurgical nerve injury, nerve involvement of tumor, metabolic neuropathy, and congenital and traumatic paraplegia. Children and adolescents often describe neuropathic pain as "strange," "burning," or "pins and needles." A history, physical examination, and a careful and systematic neurologic exam is important, even in cases where the cause seems apparent. The term *allodynia* refers to pain evoked by light touch of the skin. Without obvious skin pathology, allodynia implies an alteration in normal sensory processing and excessive excitability of nerves, and should point clinicians to consider neuropathic pain disorders. Nerve conduction studies need not be abnormal among patients with neuropathic pain. Nerve conduction velocities detect compound action potentials in A alpha-beta fibers, and are insensitive to abnormalities in C-fiber and A-delta fiber functioning. A noninvasive method of assessment of thermal and vibratory thresholds called quantitative sensory testing is under investigation as a means of quantifying sensory abnormalities in patients with neuropathic pain.[108]

Pharmacotherapy of Neuropathic Pain

The use of medications for the treatment of neuropathic pain in children has been extrapolated from adult studies. Randomized, controlled studies in adult patients show the usefulness of tricyclic antidepressants in diabetic neuropathy and postherpetic neuralgia as well as a spectrum of other neuropathic pain conditions.[109, 110]

Tricyclics are commonly used in the treatment of neuropathic pain in children, although there are no prospective pediatric clinical trials available. Nortriptyline and amitriptyline are the most commonly used in children and they can also be useful in improving sleep disturbances common to these patients. Our general preference is to begin with nortriptyline, because of a somewhat better side-effect profile.[111] Because children metabolize tricyclics more efficiently than adults, twice-daily dosing is often needed, though even in these patients, we still prescribe at least two thirds of the daily dose in the evening. There have been very rare case reports of sudden death in patients on tricyclic antidepressants, presumably due to cardiac arrhythmias. In addition to a thorough cardiac history and physical exam, we obtain a baseline screening ECG. Patients who have abnormalities on the initial evaluation are referred to a pediatric cardiologist prior to starting tricyclics.

Like tricyclic antidepressants, there are no prospective clinical trials of anticonvulsants in the treatment of neuropathic pain in children. Studies have shown the beneficial use of anticonvulsants such as carbamezepine, phenytoin, and gabapentin[112, 113] in adults with neuropathic pain. Gabapentin is an anticonvulsant that has been increasingly used for children with neuropathic pain. Unlike phenytoin, gabapentin is not associated with hypersensitivity reactions or hepatic and hematologic toxicities, and monitoring of serum levels is not needed. Limiting side effects of gabapentin are usually somnolence and dizziness. Although gabapentin has been increasingly used for neuropathic pain in children and adults,[114] there are no controlled trials showing its effectiveness for the treatment of reflex sympathetic dystrophy (RSD) in adults or children.

There is no evidence that anticonvulsants in general and gabapentin in particular are better than tricyclics in the treatment of neuropathic pain.[115]

There is a longstanding controversy regarding the effectiveness of opioids in the treatment of certain types of neuropathic pain. There are many patients with neuropathic pain who either fail to achieve analgesia with standard dosing, or who find analgesia only at doses that produce intolerable sedation. Conversely, other patients find useful analgesic effects at nonsedating doses.[116] For patients with neuropathic pain due to cancer, it is worthwhile trying opioids with generous dosing and aggressive treatment of opioid side effects.[117]

Chronic use of opioids for patients with pain not due to cancer or other life-threatening illnesses is also a subject of controversy.[118] We prescribe opioids on a long-term basis for a small subgroup of children with chronic pain as part of a multidisciplinary approach that combines psychological interventions, physical rehabilitation, and maintenance of normal activities, including school or work.

Reflex Sympathetic Dystrophy

RSD (also known as complex regional pain syndrome type 1 [CRPS1]) is characterized by persistent limb pain and allodynia, with cyanosis, mottling, coldness, increasing sweating, atrophy, or other signs of autonomic dysfunction. Radiographs often show osteopenia in the affected limb. The term *causalgia* (CRPS2) is used for a similar syndrome associated with definable injury to a major nerve trunk.

The clinical presentation of RSD/CRPS in children differs from that in adults. Wilder et al.[119] reported findings in 70 pediatric patients with RSD. The majority of patients were female, and their RSD involved a lower extremity. All patients were able to identify a specific injury; however, some patients developed RSD in a second extremity without additional injury. Some patients also experienced eating disorders and family dysfunction. A significant percentage of patients were involved in highly competitive and stressful sports, ballet, or gymnastics.

Anesthesiologists who treat chronic pain in adults often emphasize early and aggressive use of sympathetic blockade as a primary treatment for adults with RSD, in order to improve limb perfusion, relieve pain, "break a cycle," and facilitate mobilization. In contrast, results of several pediatric case series suggest that a majority of children with RSD/CRPS can have resolution or marked improvement in their signs and symptoms by a noninvasive regimen that emphasizes active physical therapy and cognitive-behavioral interventions.[120–122] Others have emphasized that transcutaneous electrical nerve stimulation (TENS) and sympathetic blockade are beneficial.[123] In the Wilder study, a conservative approach with physical therapy, biobehavioral treatment, and TENS was effective in reducing overall pain scores and improving function in over 50 percent of patients.[119] In those patients who did not respond to a conservative approach, sympathetic blocks were beneficial in many, but not all, cases. There was no association between the onset of symptoms and the therapeutic benefit of sympathetic blockade.

Based on this experience and literature review, our approach has evolved over the years as a "hybrid" of the treatment models common among pediatric rheumatologists and adult anesthesiologists. After an initial assessment, we have an extended patient and family education session, or "day-1 talk" regarding the nonprotective character of neuropathic pain, and the need to mobilize the affected extremity. Regular school attendance is strongly encouraged. Many patients or parents have read about the condition prior to coming to the clinic, and based on materials derived from adult series, they may come with an overly pessimistic view of the condition and its prognosis. We strongly emphasize that the overwhelming majority of children and adolescents who take a positive and active role in their treatment will return to normal functioning and to partial or complete resolution of pain.

Patients then receive an initial trial of outpatient physical therapy and cognitive-behavioral treatment. The approach to physical therapy is very active, and emphasizes return to weight-bearing, desensitization, and a trial of TENS. Cognitive-behavioral treatment is individualized, and may include relaxation training and biofeedback training, teaching adaptive patterns of coping, and individual or family counselling. If there is improvement in weight-bearing, circulation, and involvement in daily activities, then this program is continued.

Medications commonly tried for RSD/CRPS include tricyclics, anticonvulsants, and oral vasodilators; results are quite variable and difficult to predict. Our impression is that for the majority of patients with RSD, opioids do not provide clinically important analgesic benefit at doses that permit alertness and daily functioning. Patients and parents should be clear that medication trials are best done in a methodical, systematic fashion. Evaluation of results can be facilitated by a home diary that tracks pain reports, side effects, and functional status.

Sympathetic blockade is used for the subset of patients who do not progress with a very good trial of physical therapy, or those with severe circulatory impairment and ischemic complications. In order to minimize the number of needle procedures and to facilitate an intensive inpatient rehabilitative program, we commonly perform sympathetic blockade in children using continuous catheter infusion techniques during a 5- to 10-day inpatient admission. Prospective clinical trials of both physical therapy and sympathetic blockade are in progress.

Over the past 15 years, over 500 children and adolescents have been treated in our clinic for RSD. Over 85 percent have had a reduction in pain intensity and good recovery of limb function. Less than 5 percent of patients have received trials of spinal cord stimulation or implanted spinal infusion pumps; results of these trials are too limited to draw conclusions regarding indications and outcomes among children. Several patients had received neurodestructive sympathectomy prior to treatment at our center. In the past 15 years, only five patients in our center (<1 percent overall) have received operative or chemical sympathectomy. In all cases, the indication was for preservation of limb perfusion rather than for pain relief, and in no case did neurodestructive sympathectomy per se produce dramatic long-lasting relief of pain.

Pain after Amputation

Children undergo limb amputations for reasons such as cancer, infection, trauma, and congenital deformities. Worldwide, injuries due to land mines are the most common indication for amputations in children. Two case series found that most pediatric amputees experienced phantom limb sensations, and a majority of patients experienced phantom limb pain, which was often described as severe.[124, 125] It has been a common belief that children who have limb amputations at an early age or who have congenital absence of a limb experience little or no phantom sensations. However, one report found that 20 percent of a cohort of patients with congenital limb absence and 50 percent with amputations at an early age experienced phantom limb sensations.[126] In general, phantom limb sensations are described as a variety of sensory qualities, such as itching, tingling, and pain referred to the absent limb. There is some evidence to suggest an association between the perioperative use of chemotherapeutic agents and the development of phantom limb pain.[127]

There are few data on best treatments for phantom pain in children or adults. TENS, tricyclic antidepressants, anticonvulsants, cognitive-behavioral therapy, and physical rehabilitation, including early use of a prosthesis,[128] have been beneficial for some patients. Some studies suggest that the use of preoperative neural blockade may help to prevent the development of phantom limb pain[129]; others have reported no benefit.[130]

Cancer

Children and adolescents with cancer frequently experience acute or persistent pain.[131] Fortunately, pediatric malignancies are often responsive to initial aggressive induction chemotherapy, and tumor therapy is a major pain-relieving modality in many cases. Pain experienced by children with malignancies can be a result of the tumor itself or of the treatment.

Treatment-Related Pain

In contrast to adults, treatment-related pain is more prevalent in children than tumor-related pain. Procedures such as bone marrow biopsies and aspirates and lumbar punctures are common sources of distress and pain. Treatment of brief needle procedures should involve individualized use of cognitive-behavioral interventions, conscious sedation, local and topical anesthesia, and brief general anesthesia.

Mucositis due to high-dose chemotherapy or radiation is a common and troublesome problem. Parenteral opioids are commonly used. PCA and NCA are useful to permit dose-titration and treatment of episodic pain exacerbations,[132, 133] though all parenteral opioid regimens, including PCA, fail to achieve good analgesia in some patients.[134] Topical therapies are widely used, but evidence for their effectiveness is weak.[135] Biologic therapies,[136] including colony-stimulating factors,[135] may reduce the incidence and severity of this problem in the future. Neuropathic pain can be caused by surgical resection of limb sarcomas or chest wall tumors. Neuropathies induced by chemotherapy and irradiation can be troublesome.

Tumor-Related Pain

Tumors may produce pain by pressure or stretch of bone, viscera, soft tissues, and major nerves. Bone pain is a common tumor-related pain, which can occur from bone marrow involvement such as in leukemia or from metastasis of solid tumors to localized areas. A burning or shock-like quality to pain may indicate tumor involvement of peripheral nerves, plexuses, or the epidural space. Capsular stretch of the solid viscera can produce severe pain.

A focused and thorough but sensitive evaluation will help define the location, quality, and etiology of pain and may help guide treatment strategies.

Pain in children with cancer should be viewed not as an isolated concern, but rather must be seen in the context of a condition that produces fear, anxiety, grief, loss, isolation, and suffering.[1, 137] Pharmacologic treatment of pain and other symptoms should be accompanied by psychosocial support.

The World Health Organization (WHO) has proposed an ''analgesic ladder'' to help guide pharmacologic treatment of cancer pain that has been successfully used in several series in adults. A monograph[138] adapting this program for children is available through the WHO or by contacting the authors. Nonopioid analgesics such as acetaminophen and NSAIDs are recommended as the initial treatment of mild pain. If platelet dysfunction is of concern, choline magnesium trisalicylate or a COX-2 inhibitor may be considered instead of NSAIDs. If this is ineffective, the ''second step'' is commonly to use codeine or lower-dose oxycodone, though there are some who regard the ''weak'' and ''strong'' opioid distinction as artificial, and who would recommend instead progressing directly to the ''third step'' with stronger opioids such as morphine in graded doses. Mixed μ-agonist/antagonists and/or κ-agonists such as butorphanol, nalbuphine, pentazocine, or buprenorphine are generally not recommended. These agents may produce dysphoria, they may precipitate withdrawal in opioid-tolerant subjects, they may have flatter dose–response curves with escalation to high doses, and there is little evidence for any unique benefit relative to μ-agonists. Their use may be recommended only as a best available alternative in parts of the world where government restrictions currently make other opioids unavailable.

Opioid use for cancer pain requires proactive treatment of side effects. Constipation is nearly universal, but readily prevented by the use of stimulant laxatives; stool softeners and bulk forming agents are inadequate. The use of dextroamphetamine or methylphenidate in morning and midday doses can be very effective in antagonizing sedation from opioids, allowing patients to be more alert and interactive during the day, as well as providing some additional analgesia. Nausea also occurs commonly and can be treated with ondansetron, metoclopramide, or phenothiazines. Pruritus is sometimes responsive to antihistamines such as diphenhydramine or hydroxyzine. Switching to a different opioid may also be helpful, since in some cases, patients experience fewer side effects with one opioid versus another. For example, some patients experience less pruritus with fentanyl compared with morphine.

Oral dosing of opioids for cancer pain is recommended where possible. Short-acting oral morphine tablets or elixir dosed every 4 hours provides effective pain relief in many cases. Unlike acute postoperative pain, chronic cancer pain medications should generally be given on a round-the-clock basis to avoid repeated periods of breakthrough pain. Sustained-release morphine,[139] hydromorphone, or oxycodone preparations can be convenient for providing prolonged effect. For children who will benefit from a longer acting opioid but who are unwilling or unable to swallow tablets, methadone elixir can be used. The problem of incomplete cross-tolerance was discussed in an earlier section.

There are a significant number of children who are unable to tolerate oral opioids due to a variety of issues such as refractory vomiting, painful swallowing from severe mucositis, or delirium associated with terminal disease. In these cases, either IV or subcutaneous routes are appropriate. Many patients with cancer have indwelling, tunneled venous catheters for long-term use, making IV opioid administration convenient and for the most part, painless. PCA is commonly used to treat cancer pain in children, for both inpatient and outpatient therapy. Portable PCA devices are convenient for outpatients. PCA is especially useful for patients who have wide fluctuations in pain intensity and can also be useful during brief painful procedures. Nurse-controlled and parent-controlled anesthesia have been used successfully in infants, toddlers, and older patients who are unable to use PCA. The addition of a basal infusion appears to provide more consistent overall pain relief for disease-related pain and, when used at night, may help to promote more restful sleep. For patients without intravenous access, subcutaneous opioid infusions with and without a bolus capability can provide effective pain relief.[56, 140, 141] Typically, a 22-gauge catheter is placed in the subcutaneous tissue of the thigh, abdomen, or chest and secured. Concentrated morphine or hydromorphone solutions allow small infusion volumes and are well tolerated by most patients. Although redness and itching can occur around the insertion site, subcutaneous needles only need to be changed every 3 to 5 days or as needed. Transdermal fentanyl patches[57] are available that provide doses as low as 25 μg/h and may obviate the need for venous access in some patients, though they do not permit dose titration with fluctuating pain intensity. Steady state is typically reached at 12 to 24 hours.

A study of the terminal course of 199 children and adolescents managed according to the WHO guidelines showed good analgesic effect of standard-opioid dose escalation in most cases.[142] Five percent of these patients required more than 100-fold dose escalation beyond standard initial dose recommendations (i.e., escalation to the equivalent of intravenous morphine at 3 mg/kg/h). Most of these patients had solid tumors metastatic to spine, central nervous system, and peripheral nerves, and many had symptoms of neuropathic pain. Myoclonus can occur when enormous opioid infusion rates are used, which may be responsive to clonazepam or other benzodiazepines. For selected patients with intractable pain or intolerable side effects despite aggressive opioid dose escalation, epidural or subarachnoid infusions of local anesthetics and opioids may provide excellent analgesia.[73] Our preference is to use the subarachnoid route for patients whose pain is largely below the umbilicus, and to use thoracic epidural placement for patients with pain in thoracic and upper abdominal dermatomes. Catheters are tunneled at initial placement to facilitate skin care and fixation. Invariably, neuraxial opioids alone are not sufficient, and dermatomally applied local anesthetics are required to produce an adequate therapeutic index. The subarachnoid route is therefore useful, because one can escalate local anesthetic dosing to much greater effect without producing toxic plasma concentrations. Neurolytic blockade is infrequently performed in children, although it may have a limited role for treatment of pain due to upper abdominal visceral malignancies.

Optimal pain management for children with cancer involves an individualized approach for each patient with consideration of complex issues such as patient and family wishes with respect to degree of sedation, nature and origin of the pain, and other forms of discomfort such as air hunger, relentless vomiting, and pruritus.[143] These issues must be considered in the context of patient and family grief, anxiety, fear of dying, and isolation. Efforts to facilitate palliative care in the home environment should be encouraged.[137] Anticipatory management can help prevent many home care pain emergencies by providing adequate availability of opioids to anticipate rapid escalation in dose requirements. Whereas much of the writing on pediatric palliative care has focused on children with malignancy, more attention needs to be directed to children with a range of other life-shortening illnesses, especially neurodegenerative disorders.

Cystic Fibrosis

Patients with cystic fibrosis may experience recurrent or persistent pain, especially headache and chest pain.[144] Other causes of chronic pain in patients with cystic fibrosis include back pain due to musculoskeletal causes and compression fractures, arthritis pain,[145] and abdominal pain.[146]

The incidence of chronic pain increases as these patients age and develop more severe lung disease. Chest pain appears commonly due to chest wall muscle fatigue or muscle strain. Severe coughing may produce overt rib fractures or areas of point tenderness over a rib that may represent periosteal tears. COX-2 inhibitors may have a useful role in providing analgesia without respiratory depression, sedation, or constipation, with less risk of exacerbating hemoptysis than conventional NSAIDs.

In severe or persistent cases, thoracic epidural anesthesia can be helpful to facilitate coughing. Thoracic epidural analgesia is preferred over intercostal blockade, because the duration of effect of intercostal blocks is too short to be clinically useful, and because the risk of pneumothorax is considerable. Headaches may be due to a range of causes. Muscle contraction headaches are common, and may be exacerbated by intense contraction of accessory muscles of respiration with coughing. Sinus disease is ubiquitous in patients with cystic fibrosis, and may contribute to headache in many cases. Hypoxia and hypercarbia contribute to headaches in patients with advanced disease. In selected patients, systemic opioids may provide

analgesia with a reasonable risk–benefit ratio.[144] Patients with cystic fibrosis have a very high incidence of constipation due to opioids, especially with perioperative use. Aggressive use of laxatives should be used before ileus ensues.

Sickle Cell Pain

Sickle cell disease is characterized by both acute, recurrent pain and chronic pain. Vaso-occlusive episodes produce severe ischemia pain, particularly in the extremities, chest, and abdomen. These painful episodes account for the majority of emergency room visits and hospital admissions. Most vaso-occlusive episodes are effectively managed at home through the use of NSAIDs and opioids; day-treatment programs offer a useful alternative to emergency room visits and hospital admissions in many cases.[147] However, because of the wide range of severity and frequency of painful episodes,[148] some patients require more frequent hospitalization. Oral therapy with NSAIDs and opioids should be used when possible; there should be little hesitation regarding titrating opioids as needed for analgesia; parenteral opioids are indicated when rapid titration is needed for severe pain, or when the oral route is not feasible. Excessive concerns regarding addiction have often led to inadequate pain treatment for these patients. PCA offers the advantage of control and self-titration, since pain episodes are often unpredictable and fluctuate in intensity. Continuous epidural infusions have been used for higher risk patients with acute chest syndrome, with good analgesia and maintenance of ventilatory drive.[149] The unresolved question is how often to choose this route of analgesia for patients with a recurrent and long-term illness.

A comprehensive approach to patients with pain from sickle cell disease has been suggested by several centers.[147] This model emphasizes education and communication for patients and families regarding coping mechanisms,[150] effective pain assessment measures, and maintenance of normal activities before maladaptive behaviors are learned. A clear and consistent plan for medication use is helpful, particularly for the management of painful episodes at home. Biobehavioral techniques such as stress relaxation, hypnosis, and family therapy have also been successful, particularly when introduced during pain-free periods.

Poorly Understood Conditions: Fibromyalgia, Diffuse Musculoskeletal Pains, Chronic Fatigue, Chronic Orthostatic Hypotension

Children frequently present to pediatric pain clinics with a spectrum of complaints related to myalgia, fatigue, dizziness, impaired mental concentration, or related complaints.[151] In some patients, the signs and symptoms are consistent with a discrete diagnosis; in others, there is overlap with several diagnostic entities, or there are coexisting diagnoses, including headache, abdominal pain, or depression. Approaches to treatment should emphasize maintenance of normal activities, moderate exercise, return to regular school attendance, improved sleep hygeine, and use of cognitive-behavioral interventions. Selected patients may improve with antidepressants or, in the case of chronic hypotension, with agents that affect blood pressure, intravascular volume, or baroreceptor responses. However, in general, medication trials should not be the central aspect of treatment.

TENS

TENS is a device that emits a small electrical impulse across the skin to peripheral sensory nerves. Electrodes are placed as close as possible to the peripheral nerve distribution in the affected site or electrodes may be placed at acupuncture sites. The pain-relieving effect of TENS unit has been rationalized by the gate-control theory of Melzack and Wall.[152] According to this theory, stimulation of large myelinated A fibers by TENS inhibits the transmission of pain and other noxious stimuli through smaller unmyelinated C fibers to the dorsal horn.

Although some children experience a slight tingling sensation, TENS is well tolerated by most children. Side effects are relatively few; the most common side effect is local skin irritation and hypersensitivity. Contraindications are very few: placement over the anterior neck has rarely caused hypotension and bradycardia, and there is a theoretical concern for interference with pacemakers and other implanted devices. TENS is widely used as an adjuvant to chronic pain treatment programs in children. Controlled trials have given mixed results, and suggest a considerable aspect of placebo effect in some settings. Additional randomized, clinical trials are needed to better define the efficacy of TENS in chronic pain conditions.[153]

Cognitive-Behavioral Treatment

Psychological techniques such as biofeedback, guided imagery, and others are an integral part of most chronic pain treatment plans. Cognitive-behavioral interventions have been shown to be effective in the treatment of chronic headaches[154] and are widely used in other chronic pain conditions such as neuropathic pain and recurrent abdominal pain.[155] Through *progressive muscle relaxation training*, patients are taught progressive relaxation of certain muscle groups. Often, relaxation training is taught in combination with diaphragmatic breathing exercises and guided imagery to enhance a state of relaxation. *Biofeedback* is a technique where patients are taught to control a physiologic response such as peripheral blood flow or muscle tension; this is a useful adjunct to relaxation training in the management of headaches and neuropathic pain. *Hypnosis* is a condition characterized by focused attention and physical relaxation in which patients can be treated by positive suggestion. Cognitive oriented interventions such as thought-stopping and cognitive restructuring have been used for such chronic pain conditions as headache and recurrent abdominal pain where patients are taught more effective ways to deal with negative thoughts and life stressors that may alter their perception of pain. In general, children are especially eager and enthusiastic subjects for biobehavioral approaches to pain. Children under the age of 7 typically require coaching and assistance from adults to implement biobehavioral strategies due to cognitive and developmental function.

Psychiatric and Psychological Treatment of Pain and Pain-Associated Disability[83]

Children with chronic pain can experience associated depression, anxiety, and fear that may perpetuate and intensify their overall pain experience. In some cases, a child's emotional distress or preexisting psychological condition may interfere with biobehavioral treatment, physical therapy, and other pain management strategies. Through individual and/or family therapy, psychiatric or psychological consultation can help to identify and treat psychological issues and maladaptive coping skills in order to promote improved functioning with respect to chronic illness and pain. Patients and families are at times reluctant to consider psychological or psychiatric treatment for fear of attributing symptoms to a psychological origin. Education may be necessary to highlight and normalize the relationship between cognitive and emotional factors and physiologic functioning, and to clarify that the effectiveness of psychological therapy does not imply a psychological origin to pain.

In caring for children with chronic pain, it is crucial to examine the impact on family functioning and school attendance and performance. School absenteeism has several analogies to work absenteeism as a pattern of disability in adults with chronic pain. Return to regular school attendance is a central aspect of pain treatment for children. Home tutoring is not an adequate substitute for the regular school environment.

Complementary and Alternative Medicine (CAM)

The use of acupuncture, herbs, and other forms of alternative medicine has been increasing among pediatric patients and providers. In a recent survey, over 70 percent of pediatric pain clinics in the United States offer patients at least one form of alternative medicine. Acupuncture is a method of treatment from traditional Chinese medicine that involves placement of tiny sterile needles in points on skin denoted as acupuncture points. Acupuncture is now practiced widely in the United States for a range of medical conditions including gynecologic pain, nausea, and headaches, and appears to have a very good safety record.[156] A number of proposed mechanisms for the therapeutic effect of acupuncture have received preliminary study.[157]

Herbal remedies are increasingly used among pediatric patients, particularly adolescent girls.[158] Over 40 percent of patients with chronic medical illnesses such as cancer or cystic fibrosis report using CAM. Common conditions for which patients use CAM (in particular, herbs) include gynecologic disorders, urinary tract infections, and fatigue. Because many herbal remedies can be bought over the counter and are naturally occurring products, many patients do not feel the need to list these supplements as a medication. Many of the herbal preparations, however, do have pharmacologic properties that could potentially interact with other medications.

Our view is that physicians should become knowledgeable about complementary and alternative practice, both to advise their patients regarding safety and also to make informed judgments about integration of aspects into their own practice. Clinical trials in this area are difficult to perform and easily confounded by placebo effects, but it is crucial that these practices be evaluated critically. Open-mindedness should not lead to uncritical acceptance of these approaches.

CONCLUSION

Children of all ages should receive compassionate and effective pain treatment. Anesthesiologists caring for children should continue to take a role of advocacy and leadership in this area. Analgesics should be used in effective doses, but pain and symptom management and supportive care should not be limited to medical therapies alone.

REFERENCES

1. Cassell EJ: The nature of suffering and the goals of medicine. N Engl J Med 306:639, 1994.
2. Anand KJS, Hickey PR: Pain and its effects in the human neonate and fetus. N Engl J Med 317:1321, 1987.
3. Andrews K, Fitzgerald M: Cutaneous flexion reflex in human neonates: a quantitative study of threshold and stimulus-response characteristics after single and repeated stimuli. Dev Med Child Neurol 41:696, 1999.
4. Fitzgerald M: The development of activity evoked by fine diameter cutaneous fibres in the spinal cord of the newborn rat. Neurosci Lett 86:161, 1988.
5. Fitzgerald M, Butcher T, Shortland P: Developmental changes in the laminar termination of A fibre cutaneous sensory afferents in the rat spinal cord dorsal horn. J Comp Neurol 348:225, 1994.
6. Fitzgerald M, Jennings E: The postnatal development of spinal sensory processing. Proc Natl Acad Sci U S A 96:7719, 1999.
7. Fitzgerald M, Koltzenburg M: The functional development of descending inhibitory pathways in the dorsolateral funiculus of the newborn rat spinal cord. Dev Brain Res 24:261, 1986.
8. Marsh D, Dickenson A, Hatch D, Fitzgerald M: Epidural opioid analgesia in infant rats II: responses to carrageenan and capsaicin. Pain 82:33, 1999.
9. Taddio A, Katz J, Ilersich A, Koren G: Effect of neonatal circumcision on pain response during subsequent routine vaccination. Lancet 349:599, 1997.
10. Ruda MA, Ling QD, Hohmann AG, et al: Altered nociceptive neuronal circuits after neonatal peripheral inflammation. Science 289:628, 2000.
11. Finley GA, McGrath PJ (eds): Measurement of Pain in Infants and Children. Seattle, IASP Press, 1998.
12. Tateishi T, Nakura H, Asoh M, et al: A comparison of hepatic cytochrome P450 protein expression between infancy and postinfancy. Life Sci 61:2567, 1997.
13. van den Anker J: Pharmacokinetics and renal function in preterm infants. Acta Paediatr 85:1393, 1996.
14. Luks AM, Zwass MS, Brown RC, et al: Opioid-induced analgesia in neonatal dogs: pharmacodynamic differences between morphine and fentanyl. J Pharmacol Exp Ther 284:136, 1998.
15. Bragg P, Zwass MS, Lau M, Fisher DM: Opioid pharmacodynamics in neonatal dogs: differences between morphine and fentanyl. J Appl Physiol 79:1519, 1995.
16. Henthorn TK, Liu Y, Mahapatro M, Ng KY: Active transport of fentanyl by the blood-brain barrier. J Pharmacol Exp Ther 289:1084, 1999.
17. Thompson SJ, Koszdin K, Bernards CM: Opiate-induced analgesia is increased and prolonged in mice lacking P-glycoprotein. Anesthesiology 92:1392, 2000.
18. Martin RJ, DiFiore JM, Jana L, et al: Persistence of the biphasic ventilatory response to hypoxia in preterm infants. J Pediatr 132:960, 1998.
19. Cohen G, Malcolm G, Henderson-Smart D: Ventilatory response of the newborn infant to mild hypoxia. Pediat Pulmonol 24:163, 1997.
20. Petersen MC, Wolraich M, Sherbondy A, Wagener J: Abnormalities in control of ventilation in newborn infants with myelomeningocele. J Pediatr 126:1011, 1995.
21. Miller RP, Roberts RJ, Fischer LJ: Acetaminophen elimination kinetics in neonates, children, and adults. Clin Pharmacol Ther 19:284, 1976.
22. Montgomery CJ, McCormack JP, Reichert CC, Marsland CP: Plasma concentrations after high-dose (45 mg · kg^{-1}) rectal acetaminophen in children. Can J Anaesthesia 42:982, 1995.
23. Birmingham PK, Tobin MJ, Henthorn TK, et al: Twenty-four-hour pharmacokinetics of rectal acetaminophen in children: an old drug with new recommendations. Anesthesiology 87:244, 1997.
24. Lesko S, Mitchell A: An assessment of the safety of pediatric ibuprofen. A practitioner-based randomized clinical trial. JAMA 273:929, 1995.
25. Lesko SM, Mitchell AA: Renal function after short-term ibuprofen use in infants and children. Pediatrics 100:954, 1997.
26. Szer IS, Goldenstein-Schainberg C, Kurtin PS: Paucity of renal complications associated with nonsteroidal antiinflammatory drugs in children with chronic arthritis. J Pediatr 119:815, 1991.
27. Tramer MR, Williams JE, Carroll D, et al: Comparing analgesic efficacy of non-steroidal anti-inflammatory drugs given by different routes in acute and chronic pain: a qualitative systematic review. Acta Anaesthesiol Scand 42:71, 1998.
28. Maunuksela EL, Ryhanen P, Janhunen L: Efficacy of rectal ibuprofen in controlling postoperative pain in children. Can J Anaesth 39:226, 1992.
29. Romsing J, Ostergaard D, Drozdziewicz D, et al: Diclofenac or acetaminophen for analgesia in paediatric tonsillectomy outpatients. Acta Anaesthesiol Scand 44:291, 2000.
30. Rusy LM, Houck CS, Sullivan LJ, et al: A double-blind evaluation of ketorolac tromethamine versus acetaminophen in pediatric tonsillectomy: analgesia and bleeding. Anesth Analg 80:226, 1995.
31. Bean-Lijewski JD, Hunt RD: Effect of ketorolac on bleeding time and postoperative pain in children: a double-blind, placebo-controlled comparison with meperidine. J Clin Anesth 8:25, 1996.
32. Vetter T, Heiner E: Intravenous ketorolac as an adjuvant to pediatric patient-controlled analgesia with morphine. J Clin Anesth 6:110, 1994.
33. Park JM, Houck CS, Sethna NF, et al: Ketorolac suppresses postoperative bladder spasms after ureteral reimplantation. Anesth Analg 91:11, 2000.
34. Houck CS, Wilder RT, McDermott JS, et al: Safety of intravenous ketorolac therapy in children and cost savings with a unit dosing system. J Pediatr 129:292, 1996.
35. Needleman P, Isakson PC: The discovery and function of COX-2. J Rheumatol 24:6, 1997.
36. Simon LS, Weaver AL, Graham DY, et al: Anti-inflammatory and upper gastrointestinal effects of celecoxib in rheumatoid arthritis: a randomized controlled trial. JAMA 282:1921, 1999.
37. Swan SK, Rudy DW, Lasseter KC, et al: Effect of cyclooxygenase-2 inhibition on renal function in elderly persons receiving a low-salt diet. A randomized, controlled trial. Ann Intern Med 133:1, 2000.
38. Pasquale G, Scaricabarozzi I, D'Agostino R, et al: An assessment of the efficacy and tolerability of nimesulide vs paracetamol in children after adenotonsillectomy. Drugs 46:234, 1993.
39. Reikeraas O, Engebretsen L: Effects of ketoralac tromethamine and indomethacin on primary and secondary bone healing. An experimental study in rats. Arch Orthop Trauma Surg 118:50, 1998.
40. McLaughlin CR, Dewey WL: A comparison of the antinociceptive effects of opioid agonists in neonatal and adult rats in phasic and tonic nociceptive tests. Pharmacol Biochem Behav 49:1017, 1994.
41. Pasternak GW, Zhang A, Tecott L: Developmental differences between high and low affinity opiate binding sites: their relationship to analgesia and respiratory depression. Life Sci 27:1185, 1980.
42. Lynn AM, McRorie TI, Slattery JT, et al: Pharmacokinetics and pharmacodynamics of morphine in infant monkeys. Dev Pharmacol Ther 16:41, 1996.

43. McQuay H, Moore A: Comparing analgesic efficacy of non-steroidal anti-inflammatory drugs given by different routes in acute and chronic pain. *In* McQuay H, Moore A (eds): An Evidence-Based Resource for Pain Relief. Oxford, Oxford Medical Publications, 1998, p 94.

44. Caraco Y, Sheller J, Wood AJ: Impact of ethnic origin and quinidine coadministration on codeine's disposition and pharmacodynamic effects. J Pharmacol Exp Ther 290:413, 1999.

45. Davis AM, Inturrisi CE: d-Methadone blocks morphine tolerance and N-methyl-D-aspartate-induced hyperalgesia. J Pharmacol Exp Ther 289:1048, 1999.

46. Ripamonti C, Groff L, Brunelli C, et al: Switching from morphine to oral methadone in treating cancer pain: what is the equianalgesic dose ratio? J Clin Oncol 16:3216, 1998.

47. Berde CB, Beyer JE, Bournaki MC, et al: Comparison of morphine and methadone for prevention of postoperative pain in 3- to 7-year-old children. J Pediatr 119:136, 1991.

48. Lynn A, Opheim KE: Morphine intravenous infusions and effects of PaCO2 in infants and toddlers following cardiac surgery. J Pain Symptom Manage 6:207, 1996.

49. Lynn A, Nespeca MK, Bratton SL, et al: Clearance of morphine in postoperative infants during intravenous infusion: the influence of age and surgery. Anesth Analg 86:958, 1998.

50. Esmail Z, Montgomery C, Courtm C, et al: Efficacy and complications of morphine infusions in postoperative paediatric patients. Paediatr Anaesth 9:321, 1999.

51. Berde CB, Lehn BM, Yee JD, et al: Patient-controlled analgesia in children and adolescents: a randomized, prospective comparison with intramuscular administration of morphine for postoperative analgesia. J Pediatr 118:460, 1991.

52. Monitto CL, Greenberg RS, Kost-Byerly S, et al: The safety and efficacy of parent-/nurse-controlled analgesia in patients less than six years of age. Anesth Analg 91:573, 2000.

53. McNeely JK, Trentadue NC: Comparison of patient-controlled analgesia with and without nighttime morphine infusion following lower extremity surgery in children. J Pain Symptom Manag 13:268, 1997.

54. Doyle E, Harper I, Morton NS: Patient-controlled analgesia with low dose background infusions after lower abdominal surgery in children. Br J Anaesth 71:818, 1993.

55. Doyle E, Mottart KJ, Marshall C, Morton NS: Comparison of different bolus doses of morphine for patient-controlled analgesia in children. Br J Anaesth 72:160, 1994.

56. Miser AW, Davis DM, Hughes CS, et al: Continuous subcutaneous infusion of morphine in children with cancer. Am J Dis Child 137:383, 1983.

57. Collins JJ, Dunkel IJ, Gupta SK, et al: Transdermal fentanyl in children with cancer pain: feasibility, tolerability, and pharmacokinetic correlates. J Pediatr 134:319, 1999.

58. Schechter NL, Weisman SJ, Rosenblum M, et al: The use of oral transmucosal fentanyl citrate for painful procedures in children. Pediatrics 95:335, 1995.

59. Desparmet J, Mateo J, Ecoffey C, Mazoit X: Efficacy of an epidural test dose in children anesthetized with halothane. Anesthesiology 72:249, 1990.

60. Hu D, Hu R, Berde CB: Neurologic evaluation of infant and adult rats before and after sciatic nerve blockade. Anesthesiology 86:957, 1997.

61. Kohane DS, Sankar WN, Shubina M, et al: Sciatic nerve blockade in infant, adolescent, and adult rats: a comparison of ropivacaine with bupivacaine. Anesthesiology 89:1199, 1998.

62. Larsson BA, Lonnqvist PA, Olsson GL: Plasma concentrations of bupivacaine in neonates after continuous epidural infusion. Anesth Analg 84:501, 1997.

63. Henderson K, Sethna NF, Berde CB: Continuous caudal anesthesia for inguinal hernia repair in former preterm infants. J Clin Anesth 5:129, 1993.

64. Bonadio WA, Wagner V: Efficacy of tetracaine-adrenaline-cocaine topical anesthetic without tetracaine for facial laceration repair in children. Pediatrics 86:856, 1990.

65. Smith G, Strausbaugh S, Harbeck-Weber C, et al: New non-cocaine-containing topical anesthetics compared with tetracaine-adrenaline-cocaine during repair of lacerations. Pediatrics 100:825, 1997.

66. Maunuksela E, Korpela R: Double-blind evaluation of a lignocaine-prilocaine cream (EMLA) in children. Effect on the pain associated with venous cannulation. Br J Anaesth 58:1242, 1986.

67. Benini F, Johnston CC, Faucher D, Aranda JV: Topical anesthesia during circumcision in newborn infants. JAMA 270:850, 1993.

68. Lawson R, Smart N, Gudgeon A, Morton N: Evaluation of an amethocaine gel preparation for percutaneous analgesia before venous cannulation in children. Br J Anaesth 75:282, 1995.

69. Doyle E, Freeman J, Im NT, Morton NS: An evaluation of a new self-adhesive patch preparation of amethocaine for topical anaesthesia prior to venous cannulation in children. Anaesthesia 48:1050, 1993.

70. Bucalo BD, Mirikitani EJ, Moy RL: Comparison of skin anesthetic effect of liposomal lidocaine, nonliposomal lidocaine, and EMLA using 30-minute application time. Dermatol Surg 24:537, 1998.

71. Zappa SC, Nabors SB: Use of ethyl chloride topical anesthetic to reduce procedural pain in pediatric oncology patients. Cancer Nur 15:130, 1992.

72. Bosenberg A, Bland B, Schulte-Steinberg O, et al: Thoracic epidural anesthesia via the caudal route in infants. Anesthesiology 69:265, 1988.

73. Collins JJ, Grier HE, Sethna NF, et al: Regional anesthesia for pain associated with terminal pediatric malignancy. Pain 65:63, 1996.

74. Tsui BC, Tarkkila P, Gupta S, Kearney R: Confirmation of caudal needle placement using nerve stimulation. Anesthesiology 91:374, 1999.

75. Meignier M, Souron R, Leneel J: Postoperative dorsal epidural analgesia in the child with respiratory disabilities. Anesthesiology 59:473, 1983.

76. Curatolo M, Petersen-Felix S, Scaramozzino P, Zbinden AM: Epidural fentanyl, adrenaline and clonidine as adjuvants to local anaesthetics for surgical analgesia: meta-analyses of analgesia and side-effects. Acta Anaesthesiol Scand 42:910, 1998.

77. Constant I, Gall O, Gouyet L, et al: Addition of clonidine or fentanyl to local anaesthetics prolongs the duration of surgical analgesia after single shot caudal block in children. Br J Anaesth 80:294, 1998.

78. Dupeyrat A, Goujard E, Muret J, Ecoffey C: Transcutaneous CO2 tension effects of clonidine in paediatric caudal analgesia. Paediatr Anaesth 8:145, 1998.

79. Chaplan SR, Duncan SR, Brodsky JB, Brose WG: Morphine and hydromorphone epidural analgesia. A prospective, randomized comparison. Anesthesiology 77:1090, 1992.

80. Egelhoff JC, Ball WS Jr, Koch BL, Parks TD: Safety and efficacy of sedation in children using a structured sedation program. AJR Am J Roentgenol 168:1259, 1997.

81. Cote CJ, Notterman DA, Karl HW, et al: Adverse sedation events in pediatrics: a critical incident analysis of contributing factors. Pediatrics 105:805, 2000.

82. Means LJ, Ferrari L, Mancuso TJ, et al: The pediatric sedation unit: a mechanism for safe pediatric sedation. Pediatrics 103:199, 1999.

83. Bursch B, Walco GA, Zeltzer L: Clinical assessment and management of chronic pain and pain-associated disability syndrome. J Dev Behav Pediatr 19:45, 1998.

84. Rothner AD: Headaches in children and adolescents. Child Adolesc Psychiatr Clin N Am 8:727, 1999.

85. Hamalainen M, Hoppu K, Valkeila E, Santavuori P: Ibuprofen or acetaminophen for the acute treatment of migraine in children: a double-blind, randomized, placebo-controlled, crossover study. Neurology 48:103, 1997.

86. Linder S: Subcutaneous sumatriptan in the clinical setting: the first 50 consecutive patients with acute migraine in a pediatric neurology office practice. Headache 36:419, 1996.

87. Ueberall MA, Wenzel D: Intranasal sumatriptan for the acute treatment of migraine in children. Neurology 52:1507, 1999.

88. Hamalainen M, Hoppu K, Santavuori P: Sumatriptan for migraine attacks in children: a randomized placebo-controlled study. Do children with migraine respond to oral sumatriptan differently from adults? Neurology 48:1100, 1997.

89. Olness K, MacDonald J, Uden D: Comparison of self-hypnosis and propranolol in the treatment of juvenile classic migraine. Pediatrics 79:593, 1987.

90. Lutschg J, Vassella F: The treatment of juvenile migraine using flunarizine or propranolol. Schweiz Med Wochenschr 120:1731, 1990.

91. Sorge F, Marano E: Flunarizine v. placebo in childhood migraine. A double-blind study. Cephalalgia 5(Suppl 2):145, 1985.

92. Battistella P, Ruffilli R, Cernetti R, et al: A placebo-controlled crossover trial using trazodone in pediatric migraine. Headache 33:36, 1993.

93. Sartory G, Muller B, Metsch J, Pothmann R: A comparison of psychological and pharmacological treatment of pediatric migraine. Behav Res Ther 36:1155, 1998.

94. Apley J, Naish N: Recurrent abdominal pains: a field survey of 1,000 school children. Arch Dis Child 33:165, 1958.

95. Feldman W, McGrath P, Hodgson C, et al: The use of dietary fiber in the management of simple, childhood, idiopathic, recurrent, abdominal pain. Results in a prospective, double-blind, randomized, controlled trial. Am J Dis Child 139:1216, 1985.

96. Webster RB, DiPalma JA, Gremse DA: Lactose maldigestion and recurrent abdominal pain in children. Dig Dis Sci 40:1506, 1995.

97. Olafsdottir E, Gilja OH, Aslaksen A, et al: Impaired accommodation of the proximal stomach in children with recurrent abdominal pain. J Pediat Gastroenterol Nutr 30:157, 2000.

98. Stylianos S, Stein JE, Flanigan LM, Hechtman DH: Laparoscopy for diagnosis and treatment of recurrent abdominal pain in children. J Pediat Surg 31:1158, 1996.

99. Stringel G, Berezin SH, Bostwick HE, Halata MS: Laparoscopy in the management of children with chronic recurrent abdominal pain. J Soc Laparoendosc Surg 3:215, 1999.

100. Hogan Q, Abram S: Neural blockade for diagnosis and prognosis. A review. Anesthesiology 86:216, 1997.

101. Ezzati T: Ambulatory care utilization patterns of children and young adults: National Ambulatory Medical Care Survey United States, January–December 1975. Vital & Health Statistics—Series 13: Data from the National Health Survey 1978, p 1.

102. Selbst SM, Ruddy R, Clark BJ: Chest pain in children. Follow-up of patients previously reported. Clin Pediatr 29:374, 1990.

103. Fyfe DA, Moodie DS: Chest pain in pediatric patients presenting to a cardiac clinic. Clin Pediatr 23:321, 1984.

104. Selbst SM: Consultation with the specialist. Chest pain in children. Pediatr Rev 18:169, 1997.

105. Mooney DP, Shorter NA: Slipping rib syndrome in childhood. J Pediatr Surg 32:1081, 1997.

106. Taubman B, Vetter VL: Slipping rib syndrome as a cause of chest pain in children. Clin Pediatr 35:403, 1996.

107. Lababidi Z, Wankum J: Pediatric idiopathic chest pain. Mo Med 80:306, 1982.

108. Zaslansky R, Yarnitsky D: Clinical applications of quantitative sensory testing (QST). J Neurol Sc 153:215, 1998.

109. McQuay H, Tramer M, Nye B, et al: A systematic review of antidepressants in neuropathic pain. Pain 68:217, 1996.

110. Sindrup SH, Jensen TS: Efficacy of pharmacological treatments of neuropathic pain: an update and effect related to mechanism of drug action. [review]. Pain 83:389, 1999.

111. Watson CP, Vernich L, Chipman M, Reed K: Nortriptyline versus amitriptyline in postherpetic neuralgia: a randomized trial. Neurology 51:1166, 1998.

112. Backonja MM: Gabapentin monotherapy for the symptomatic treatment of painful neuropathy: a multicenter, double-blind, placebo-controlled trial in patients with diabetes mellitus. Epilepsia 40:S57, 1999.

113. Rowbotham M, Harden N, Stacey B, et al: Gabapentin for the treatment of postherpetic neuralgia: a randomized controlled trial. JAMA 280:1837, 1998.

114. Mellick GA, Mellick LB: Reflex sympathetic dystrophy treated with gabapentin. Arch Phys Med Rehabil 78:98, 1997.

115. Morello CM, Leckband SG, Stoner CP, et al: Randomized double-blind study comparing the efficacy of gabapentin with amitriptyline on diabetic peripheral neuropathy pain. Arch Intern Med 159:1931, 1999.

116. Dellemijn PL, van Duijn H, Vanneste JA: Prolonged treatment with transdermal fentanyl in neuropathic pain. J Pain Symptom Manag 16:220, 1998.

117. Mercadante S, Fulfaro F, Casuccio A, Barresi L: Investigation of an opioid response categorization in advanced cancer patients. J Pain Symptom Manage 18:347, 1999.

118. Portenoy RK: Current pharmacotherapy of chronic pain. J Pain Symptom Manage 19:S16, 2000.

119. Wilder RT, Berde CB, Wolohan M, et al: Reflex sympathetic dystrophy in children. Clinical characteristics and follow-up of seventy patients. J Bone Joint Surg Am 74:910, 1992.

120. Bernstein BH, Singsen BH, Kent JT, et al: Reflex neurovascular dystrophy in childhood. J Pediatr 93:211, 1978.

121. Sherry DD, Wallace CA, Kelley C, et al: Short- and long-term outcomes of children with complex regional pain syndrome type I treated with exercise therapy. Clin J Pain 15:218, 1999.

122. Stanton RP, Malcolm JR, Wesdock KA, Singsen BH: Reflex sympathetic dystrophy in children: an orthopedic perspective. Orthopedics 16:773, 1993.

123. Kesler RW, Saulsbury FT, Miller LT, Rowlingson JC: Reflex sympathetic dystrophy in children: treatment with transcutaneous electric nerve stimulation. Pediatrics 82:728, 1988.

124. Krane E, Heller EB: The prevalence of phantom sensation and pain in pediatric amputees. J Pain Symptom Manag 10:21, 1995.

125. Wilkins KL, McGrath PJ, Finley GA, Katz J: Phantom limb sensations and phantom limb pain in child and adolescent amputees. Pain 78:7, 1998.

126. Melzack R, Israel R, Lacroix R, Schultz G: Phantom limbs in people with congenital limb deficiency or amputation in early childhood. Brain 120:1603, 1997.

127. Smith J, Thompson JM: Phantom limb pain and chemotherapy in pediatric amputees. Mayo Clin Proc 70:357, 1995.

128. Weiss T, Miltner WH, Adler T, et al: Decrease in phantom limb pain associated with prosthesis-induced increased use of an amputation stump in humans. Neurosci Lett 272:131, 1999.

129. Elizaga AM, Smith DG, Sharar SR, et al: Continuous regional analgesia by intraneural block: effect on postoperative opioid requirements and phantom limb pain following amputation. J Rehabil Res Dev 31:179, 1994.

130. Nikolajsen L, Ilkjaer S, Christensen JH, et al: Randomised trial of epidural bupivacaine and morphine in prevention of stump and phantom pain in lower-limb amputation. Lancet 350:1353, 1997.

131. Miser AW, Dothage JA, Wesley M, Miser JS: The prevalence of pain in a pediatric and young adult cancer population. Pain 29:73, 1987.

132. Collins JJ, Geake J, Grier HE, et al: Patient-controlled analgesia for mucositis pain in children: a three-period crossover study comparing morphine and hydromorphone. J Pediatr 129:722, 1996.

133. Zucker TP, Flesche CW, Germing U, et al: Patient-controlled versus staff-controlled analgesia with pethidine after allogeneic bone marrow transplantation. Pain 75:305, 1998.

134. Chapman CR, Donaldson GW, Jacobson RC, Hautman B: Differences among patients in opioid self-administration during bone marrow transplantation. Pain 71:213, 1997.

135. Symonds RP: Treatment-induced mucositis: an old problem with new remedies. Br J Cancer 77:1689, 1998.

136. Anderson PM, Ramsay NK, Shu XO, et al: Effect of low-dose oral glutamine on painful stomatitis during bone marrow transplantation. Bone Marrow Transplant 22:339, 1998.

137. Goldman A: Home care of the dying child. J Palliative Care 12:16, 1996.

138. World Health Organization: Cancer Pain and Palliative Care in Children. Geneva: World Health Organization, 1998.

139. Hunt A, Joel S, Dick G, Goldman A: Population pharmacokinetics of oral morphine and its glucuronides in children receiving morphine as immediate-release liquid or sustained-release tablets for cancer pain. J Pediatr 135:47, 1999.

140. Bruera E, Brenneis C, Michaud M, et al: Continuous sc infusion of narcotics using a portable disposable device in patients with advanced cancer. Cancer Treat Rep 71:635, 1987.

141. Bruera E, Brenneis C, Michaud M, et al: Patient-controlled subcutaneous hydromorphone versus continuous subcutaneous infusion for the treatment of cancer pain. J Natl Cancer Inst 80:1152, 1988.

142. Collins JJ, Grier HE, Kinney HC, Berde CB: Control of severe pain in children with terminal malignancy. J Pediatr 126:653, 1995.

143. Wolfe J, Grier HE, Klar N, et al: Symptoms and suffering at the end of life in children with cancer. N Engl J Med 342:326, 2000.

144. Ravilly S, Robinson W, Suresh S, et al: Chronic pain in cystic fibrosis. Pediatrics 98:741, 1996.

145. Schidlow DV, Goldsmith DP, Palmer J, Huang NN: Arthritis in cystic fibrosis. Arch Dis Child 59:377, 1984.

146. Littlewood JM: Abdominal pain in cystic fibrosis [review]. J R Soc Med 88:9, 1995.

147. Benjamin LJ, Swinson GI, Nagel RL: Sickle cell anemia day hospital: an approach for the management of uncomplicated painful crises. Blood 95:1130, 2000.

148. Platt OS, Thorington BD, Brambilla DJ, et al: Pain in sickle cell disease. Rates and risk factors. N Engl J Med 325:11, 1991.

149. Yaster M, Tobin JR, Billett C, et al: Epidural analgesia in the management of severe vaso-occlusive sickle cell crisis. Pediatrics 93:310, 1994.
150. Gil KM, Carson JW, Sedway JA, et al: Follow-up of coping skills training in adults with sickle cell disease: analysis of daily pain and coping practice diaries. Health Psychol 19:85, 2000.
151. Breau LM, McGrath PJ, Ju LH: Review of juvenile primary fibromyalgia and chronic fatigue syndrome. J Dev Behav Pediatr 20:278, 1999.
152. Melzack R, Wall PD: Pain mechanisms: a new theory. Science 150:971, 1965.
153. McQuay HJ, Moore RA, Eccleston C, et al: Systematic review of outpatient services for chronic pain control. Health Technol Assess 1:1, 1997.
154. McGrath PJ, Humphreys P, Goodman JT, et al: Relaxation prophylaxis for childhood migraine: a randomized placebo-controlled trial. Dev Med Child Neurol 30:626, 1988.
155. Scharff L: Recurrent abdominal pain in children: a review of psychological factors and treatment. Clin Psychol Rev 17:145, 1997.
156. Ulett GA, Han J, Han S: Traditional and evidence-based acupuncture: history, mechanisms, and present status. South Med J 91:1115, 1998.
157. Hui KK, Liu J, Makris N, et al: Acupuncture modulates the limbic system and subcortical gray structures of the human brain: evidence from fMRI studies in normal subjects. Hum Brain Map 9:13, 2000.
158. Eisenberg DM, Davis RB, Ettner SL, et al: Trends in alternative medicine use in the United States, 1990–1997: results of a follow-up national survey. JAMA 280:1569, 1998.

26

Outpatient Anesthesia

RAAFAT S. HANNALLAH

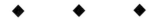

Children are excellent candidates for outpatient (ambulatory, short-stay or same-day) surgery. They rarely have severe systemic diseases and are good anesthesia risks. In addition, many common surgical procedures, such as herniotomy and myringotomy, are simpler to perform in children than in adults and are associated with a shorter, less complicated convalescence period.

It is therefore not surprising that up to 60 percent of pediatric surgical procedures in the United States today are performed safely on an outpatient basis.[1] The popularity of outpatient surgery has created new challenges and rewarding opportunities for the pediatric anesthesiologist. This chapter reviews fundamental concepts concerning the safe practice of pediatric outpatient anesthesia. It is based on a review of the literature, and on the author's personal and institutional experience.

ADVANTAGES

Some of the reasons for performing surgery on an outpatient basis are identical in children and adults. These include reducing the cost of medical care, increasing the availability of hospital beds for those who need more complex surgical procedures, and offering a level of care comparable to that received by the inpatient, without the inconveniences and potential hazards of hospitalization.

Outpatient surgery has several distinct advantages that are unique to the pediatric patient. Most beneficial is the fact that separation from the parent is minimized. This is particularly beneficial for the preschooler, who still depends on his or her mother as the ultimate security object

during times of stress. The child's feeding schedule is less disrupted, and hospital-acquired infections are reduced.

LIMITATIONS

Although the advantages are striking, pediatric outpatient surgery presents potential problems. Unfortunately, there is a tendency to associate outpatient surgery with "minor procedures" and "healthy patients," and to treat all children about to undergo minor operations as though they are medically fit and psychologically well adjusted. This attitude does a disservice to those who require special consideration.

Assuming that all outpatients are a medically uniform group is a common practice that may lead to problems. These problems occur when patients have undiagnosed acute diseases, such as upper respiratory tract infections or diarrhea, or when asymptomatic patients arrive with a previously diagnosed or even undiagnosed chronic condition, such as heart disease. Unfortunately, even when a prior consultation has been sought, the report containing the diagnosis and recommendations for therapy may not always be available. This can lead to delays and hard feelings between physicians and parents.

Another potential problem results from the stipulation that one or both parents remain with the child throughout their stay in the facility. This may require that the parent(s) take leave from work and that siblings who are at home must be cared for by others. In some cases this inconvenience and out-of-pocket expense to the parents may be greater than the cost of hospitalization. In addition, some parents are apprehensive about caring for their child who has undergone surgery at home after discharge, particularly when the child is very young or when any problems have arisen during recovery. The lack of privacy of outpatient accommodations and the potential necessity for extra visits to the hospital for preoperative screening and consultations pose other problems for pediatric surgical outpatients. A long distance between the home and the surgical facility causes many inconveniences, especially when the procedure is scheduled early in the morning and the family is required to leave several hours earlier.

The question of reducing the cost of medical care to a given patient versus the overall increased cost to an institution or community whose inpatient census declines because of the advent of outpatient surgery is yet another complex issue that has generated great debate.

ORGANIZATION OF PEDIATRIC OUTPATIENT FACILITIES

Outpatient surgery can be performed in different types of facilities: (1) hospital-sponsored ambulatory care facilities, which include hospital satellites, short-stay units within the hospital, and the general surgical suite of a hospital; (2) freestanding facilities that are not affiliated with a hospital; or (3) in a physician's office. In combined adult/pediatric facilities, separate secretarial services, a waiting room, operating rooms, and a recovery area for children are desirable, regardless of whether or not the outpatient surgical facility is affiliated with a hospital. The operating and recovery rooms and the anesthetic and monitoring equipment should not differ from those required for hospitalized patients. To make the entire process function smoothly, personnel and facilities should be dedicated solely for outpatient surgery. Secretaries, clerks, nurses, and physicians who have an understanding of the special needs of patients who are undergoing outpatient surgery tend to provide unique care that is frequently not possible when outpatients are mixed with inpatients. In addition, some studies suggest a higher incidence of cross-infection when outpatients are not separated from inpatients.

However, space may not always be available for a separate unit. In addition, local, regional, state, and governmental regulatory agencies may not approve construction of a new facility or even the modification of an existing one. Under such circumstances, it is perfectly reasonable for outpatients, and inpatients to share the same operating room suite. This may even be beneficial if it allows more efficient use of existing equipment and personnel. At a minimum, a waiting area for patients, as well as dressing rooms, bathrooms, and a separate recovery area for outpatients are essential for proper care and comfort.

Playrooms for both preoperative pediatric patients and those recovering after surgery make the environment more comfortable. Facilities for progressive care and feeding should also be available.

In a self-sufficient unit that is not affiliated with a hospital or one that functions independently, other facilities must be available. These include a laboratory; areas for sterilizing, packaging, and maintaining equipment; and a place to file and retrieve records. In a free-standing unit, arrange-

ments for potential admission of patients who develop complications that need overnight hospitalization are made by prior agreement between the institutions involved or by requiring that each physician with privileges at the outpatient facility also have admitting privileges at a nearby hospital. A protocol for transferring a patient to the hospital and the capacity for performing cardiopulmonary resuscitation within the facility are also required.

The hours during which a facility is staffed by nurses and other support personnel determines how patients are scheduled for surgery. For example, a unit that closes at 6:00 P.M. and has an expected recovery time from a given procedure of 3 hours might require that such operations be completed by 3:00 P.M. Many free-standing units schedule procedures requiring longer recovery early in the day, and those usually associated with prompt recovery (e.g., myringotomies and examinations under anesthesia) towards the end of the day. Special arrangements are made more easily in hospital-based units, which may handle late patients in the main recovery area or may temporarily transfer nurses to the short-stay unit. Requirements for the presence of medical personnel in the short-stay unit are discussed below.

Office-Based Anesthesia

A recent trend in outpatient surgery is to perform many surgical procedures in the physician's office. It is expected that office anesthesia may account for up to 10 percent of all anesthetics in the near future. Since office-based anesthesia is an extension of free-standing outpatient practice, all applicable management guidelines should apply equally to both practice locations. One of the major requirements for safe management of children in the office setting is the anesthesiologist's high level of comfort, which is based on both training and experience, with the child's age, medical condition, and proposed surgical procedure. The other is the availability of an environment that is designed and equipped to cater to the special needs of children.[2]

Since most children undergoing surgery require general anesthesia or a deep level of sedation, and since most children prefer not to be stuck with needles while they are awake, the availability of an anesthesia machine is an important factor in determining the type of pediatric procedures that can be readily performed in the office (e.g., bone marrow transplantation).

The child should be in good health; if not, any systemic disease must be under good control. An understanding of the underlying pathophysiology and thorough preoperative evaluation will help guide the anesthesiologists as to the appropriateness of choosing the office setting in each individual patient.

Although an absolute minimal age for otherwise healthy infants undergoing outpatient surgery cannot be rigidly suggested, it is probably prudent to limit the selection of office procedures to mature infants who have successfully transitioned from the neonatal period (i.e., age 3 to 6 months).

The planned surgical procedure should be associated with only minimal bleeding and minor physiologic derangements. Brief and superficial procedures such as herniorrhaphy, myringotomy, and circumcision are selected most often. When scheduling children for surgery in an office-based setting, the need to send the children home quickly must be balanced with the desire to have the anesthesiologist leave soon after the last patient recovers from anesthesia. This may mandate that the patients who have longer procedures or who may need longer observation be scheduled earlier in the day so that their recovery coincides with the recovery of the last quick cases on the schedule.

Preoperative screening and preparation are usually done in association with the surgeon and his or her office staff. It is very desirable to have the anesthesiologist contact the parents by phone or any other convenient way before the day of surgery to introduce him/herself, obtain a good history, explain the need for preoperative fasting, and discuss the anesthetic and recovery plans.

Pediatric Perioperative Environment

A recent publication by the Section on Anesthesiology of the American Academy of Pediatrics introduced specific guidelines for patient care facilities and their medical staff who wish to provide pediatric anesthesia care.[3] The document emphasized important facility-based issues such as the experience and training of the health care team and the resources committed to the care of infants and children throughout the perioperative period. The ability of the staff in addressing such issues as airway management, fluid administration, temperature regulation, monitoring, vascular catheter insertion, and postoperative pain are as important as the skill and experience of the individual anesthesiologist in determining the type of patient and/or procedure to be performed in any specific outpatient facility.

FACTORS IN SELECTION OF PATIENTS

The criteria for selecting patients and procedures for outpatient surgery vary greatly among institutions. These criteria are usually influenced by the condition of the patient, the attitude of the parents, the type of surgical procedure, and any special considerations for anesthetic management and recovery. Because the surgeon initiates the entire process, he or she must cooperate with and completely understand the overall process.

The Patient

The child should be in good health; if a systemic disease is present, it should be well evaluated and controlled. Some anesthesiologists still restrict outpatient surgery to patients classified as American Society of Anesthesiologists (ASA) Physical Status (PS) I and II (which is appropriate for the office setting). Others accept ASA class III or even IV patients under special circumstances.[4] The latter usually require prior consultation with a member of the anesthesia staff and a current written statement from the attending physician regarding the nature of illness and recommended therapy. Patients with a controlled convulsive disorder or well-regulated diabetes, for example,

might be acceptable, whereas those with a bleeding tendency, liver insufficiency, incipient heart failure, uncontrolled diabetes, or infectious diseases are not. Many children with chronic disease benefit substantially from outpatient treatment.[4] Hospital-acquired infections are a special risk to these children, as is the emotional trauma of repeated hospitalization. A child with leukemia or one who is receiving immunosuppressant medication is a particularly suitable candidate for outpatient care. Physically handicapped, psychologically disturbed, or mentally retarded children benefit tremendously from the physical presence and continued support of a parent or guardian, possibilities that are usually fostered in outpatient facilities.

The age of the child is usually not a limiting factor when surgery is scheduled on an outpatient basis at our institution and at most others.[4] Most anesthesiologists prefer not to perform outpatient anesthesia during the neonate's first week of life because the transition from fetal to neonatal physiology is still incomplete. Moreover, some recent reports have described postoperative apneic episodes after anesthesia and surgery in otherwise healthy full-term young infants.[5, 6] Because of these and similar anecdotal reports, many anesthesiologists are reluctant to schedule even a previously healthy full-term infant of less 2 to 4 weeks of age on an outpatient basis. Neonates considered for surgery should ideally be scheduled early in the day so that the period of postoperative observation can be extended for as long as clinically indicated.[5]

Prematurely born infants (gestational age at birth <37 weeks) who undergo general anesthesia during the first months of life are at increased risk for respiratory and/or cardiovascular complications during the perioperative period.[7] Among the most common and most serious of these complications are apnea, periodic breathing, and/or bradycardia.[8-12]

The age at which the premature infant attains physiologic maturity and no longer presents an increased risk for postoperative apnea must be considered individually, with attention given to such factors as growth, persistent problems during feeding, and time needed to recover from upper respiratory infections. It is generally considered that infants younger than 46 weeks' postconceptual age (PCA) with a preoperative history of apnea are at greatest risk,[10-12] although some investigators have reported apnea in infants as old as 60 weeks PCA.[11]

As the child matures, the tendency toward apnea greatly diminishes; however, the age at which all prematurely born infants can be safely anesthestized on an outpatient basis is unknown. Many of the current recommendations are based on data derived from retrospective review of complications, prospective evaluation of a small number of patients, or from studies in which infants with preexisting disease who underwent complex surgical procedures are included.

Until more extensive, prospective studies are performed, it seems prudent to admit to a hospital or to a 23-hour recovery unit, all expremature infants less than 46 weeks' PCA so that they can be monitored for apnea, bradycardia, and oxygen desaturation. The choice of this (or any other) particular age is rather arbitrary and is not universally accepted.[13, 14] It is best to individualize this decision and, when in doubt, to err on the conservative side. If the infant is anemic,[14, 15] has bronchopulmonary dysplasia (BPD), or has other neonatal problems, this period may need to be extended. Should any question arise, inpatient care and postoperative monitoring are recommended.

The Child with a Runny Nose

A child who presents with a runny nose may have a completely benign, noninfectious condition (e.g., seasonal or vasomotor rhinitis), in which case elective surgery may be performed. On the other hand, the runny nose may be a symptom of an upper respiratory tract infection (URI), in which case elective surgery may need to be postponed. Since an estimated 20 to 30 percent of all children have a runny nose a significant part of the year, every child with a runny nose must be evaluated on an individual basis.[1]

Although the definitive preanesthetic assessment of these patients requires a complete history, a physical examination, and occasionally the interpretation of certain laboratory data, the history is the most important element in the differential diagnosis. Specifically, allergic problems should be actively sought. The general assessment of the child (e.g., fever, fatigue, lack of sleep, loss of appetite) can help differentiate an acute illness from a chronic condition. Parents can usually tell whether their child's runny nose is "the usual runny nose" or something different that may require cancellation of elective surgery. Parents of outpatients can be instructed to call-in on the morning of surgery if the child develops URI symptoms so the findings can be reviewed, and, if a decision to cancel surgery is made, they are spared a wasted trip to the hospital.

If surgery is postponed because of simple nasopharyngitis, it can usually be rescheduled in 1 to 2 weeks. If the child has a flu-like syndrome that involves both the upper and lower respiratory tracts, surgery should be postponed for at least a month after the child has recovered.

Asthma

Asthma is the most common chronic disease of childhood, affecting 5 to 10 percent of children in the United States, and the incidence of this diseasse is on the rise. It is not, therefore, unusual for patients with asthma to present for what is usually a minor surgical procedure in an outpatient setting.[1] The decision to accept and proceed with surgery in such patients depends on the severity and frequency of symptoms and the adequacy of pharmacologic control. A good history, which is an important part of a well-organized screening process, can help establish the severity of asthma. Children with mild asthma who have infrequent symptoms and do not require continuous medications are excellent candidates for outpatient surgery. When children with moderate asthma (those who require daily medications to control their symptoms) are scheduled for outpatient surgery, they should be instructed to continue their medications through the morning of surgery.[16] A β-agonist should be administered in the holding area via nebulizer to young children or via inhaler to older patients. If the patient is wheezing, has a coexisting URI, persistent cough or tachypnea on the day of surgery, it is best to delay the procedure and reschedule it. Children

with severe asthma (i.e., those who always wheeze) usually require aggressive perioperative medical management, and are not good candidates for outpatient surgery.

The choice of a specific anesthetic technique in an asthmatic child is usually dictated by the nature of the surgical procedure. Most anesthetics available today have been used successfully in asthmatics. If an endotracheal tube must be inserted, sufficient depth of anesthesia must be established first. Intravenous lidocaine and/or a β-agonist inhalant may be administered just before extubation of the trachea. Deep extubation of the trachea should be considered when possible.

Patients with asthma may leave the facility when the usual discharge criteria are met. Children should not have any signs of wheezing when discharged. Adequate hydration should be ensured.

Malignant Hyperpyrexia

Although the question is still controversial, children with known or suspected susceptibility to malignant hyperpyrexia (MH) can be scheduled for outpatient surgery.[17] Use of nontriggering agents is mandatory, and a somewhat longer period of observation may be required after surgery. It is important, however, to emphasize that this practice is contingent on the assumption that any outpatient unit that provides general anesthesia has the ability to monitor end-tidal carbon dioxide (P_{ETCO_2}), arterial blood gases, and electrolytes, and should be able to treat the rare but unexpected case of MH. Dantrolene must be immediately available to treat suspected MH, if it occurs.

The Parents

In the past, the choice of outpatient care has been largely influenced by the parents' wishes and the experience of friends and family. Third-party payers, however, are now unlikely to comply with parents' demands for hospitalization of a healthy child who is having a relatively minor, superficial operation. Parents of pediatric outpatients; however, should be capable of understanding and willing to follow specific instructions related to ambulatory surgery. In most cases it is up to the physicians and nurses to educate the parents and make them feel secure and comfortable caring for their child following surgery.

The Procedure

The planned surgical procedure should be of short duration and should be associated with minimal bleeding and minor physiologic derangements. Reed and Ford stated that almost any operation that does not require a major intervention into the cranial vault, abdomen, or thorax can be considered.[18] Superficial procedures are selected most often. Septic patients are rarely considered because of the need for separate recovery areas.

Insurance guidelines in many states require that certain surgical procedures (e.g., myringotomy, hernia repair) be performed on an outpatient basis unless there are factors that prohibit this form of care. If these procedures are performed as inpatient surgery, the hospital is not reimbursed for room and board charges. Special, individual consideration may be given, however, under certain conditions. These may include patients with medical conditions (e.g., severe diabetes or heart disease) that require hospitalization for postoperative observation and care, patients who will simultaneously undergo an unrelated procedure that requires hospitalization, patients for whom there is a possibility that another surgical procedure could follow the initial procedure, or documentation of complications requiring hospital services and care for events occurring during surgery or the recovery period.

Representative procedures that are commonly performed on an outpatient basis at Children's National Medical Center (CNMC) are shown in Table 26–1. Of these, the five most commonly performed operations are herniorrhaphy, myringotomy, adenoidectomy with or without myringotomy, circumcision, and eye muscle surgery.

TABLE 26–1
EXAMPLES OF PROCEDURES SUITABLE FOR OUTPATIENT SURGERY

General surgery
  Hernia repair
  Excision of cyst, ganglion, skin lesion, breast mass
  Suture of lacerations, removal of sutures
  Dressing change
  Muscle biopsy
  Sigmoidoscopy, bronchoscopy, esophagoscopy, dilation
  Incision and drainage of abscess
  Proctologic and vaginal procedures

Otolaryngology
  Adenoidectomy
  Myringotomy and insertion of tubes
  T&A unless contraindicated
  Removal of foreign body from ear
  Frenulectomy
  Laryngoscopy
  Closed reduction of nasal fracture

Ophthalmology
  Examination under anesthesia
  Eye muscle surgery
  Lacrimal duct probing
  Excision of chalazion
  Insertion of lens or prosthesis

Dentistry
  Extraction
  Restoration

Orthopedics
  Cast change
  Arthroscopy
  Closed reduction of fracture
  Manipulation

Urology
  Cystoscopy
  Meatotomy
  Orchiopexy
  Circumcision
  Hydrocelectomy
  Testicular biopsy
  Hypospadias repair

Plastic surgery
  Otoplasty
  Scar revision

Because of the increased risk of hemorrhage, a debate continues regarding the advisability of performing tonsillectomy, with or without adenoidectomy, in an outpatient setting. However, recent experience indicates that outpatient tonsillectomy and adenoidectomy (T&A) is safe and cost-effective and that there is little benefit in keeping these patients in the hospital more than a few hours after surgery. They only need to remain in hospital long enough to ensure adequate hydration and absence of bleeding.[19] Children who bleed while in the recovery room, however, are a high-risk subgroup for recurrent bleeding, and may need to be admitted to hospital.[19] Chiang and associates reported 40,000 outpatient T&A procedures without a single death.[20] These authors emphasized careful selection of patients and careful preoperative evaluation of the patients to eliminate patients with bleeding tendencies and cardiopulmonary disease. To decrease the risk of hemorrhage, no patients with allergies underwent surgery during the pollen season, and no operation was performed until 4 to 5 weeks after an acute attack of tonsillitis.

Recently there have been reports of postoperative apnea and/or airway obstruction in children after tonsillectomy.[21] Most of those patients were young (<3 years old) and had a documented history of preoperative obstructive sleep apnea syndrome (OSAS) or other obstructive phenomena during sleep. These patients have a diminished ventilatory response to CO_2 rebreathing and are at increased risk of postoperative respiratory compromise.[22] In extreme cases the airway obstruction can result in pulmonary hypertension and cor pulmonale. Most of these children continue to suffer from the same symptoms in the immediate postoperative period. Therefore, it is very important that the indication for tonsillectomy (repeated infections vs. obstructive symptoms) be carefully reviewed, especially in young patients. Postoperative observation in a 23-hour recovery facility is appropriate for patients with mild obstructive symptoms. Inpatient care, or even intensive care unit (ICU) admission for airway support may be indicated in those with documented OSAS.[23] Management of posttonsillectomy pain and vomiting continues to be a clinical challenge, and will be discussed later in this chapter.

PREOPERATIVE REQUIREMENTS AND SCREENING

One of the rewards of outpatient anesthesia and surgery is the increased involvement of the anesthesiologist in the planning and management of the preoperative period. In fact, many day-surgery units are successfully managed by anesthesiologists. Regardless of who bears administrative responsibility for the unit, full cooperation among surgeons, hospital staff, and parents is an essential requirement for the successful outcome of such endeavors.

From the anesthesiologist's point of view, the essential preoperative requirements for safe conduct of anesthesia in outpatients are the same as those for inpatients. The standard requirements are a complete history and physical examination (H&P), appropriate laboratory tests and consultations when indicated, an appropriate fasting period, and a chance to personally evaluate the child so that rapport can be established with both child and his or her parents. The special challenge in outpatient anesthesia, however, is to accomplish as many of these steps as possible before the patient arrives in the hospital for surgery and therefore to minimize delays and last-minute cancellations. Meeting that challenge requires proper planning and organization.

Because the surgeon is the first member of the team the parents meet when outpatient surgery is scheduled, the smoothness and success of the entire experience depend on the conduct of that first encounter. The procedure must be explained and as many of the parent's questions as possible answered in the surgeon's office. Assured, relaxed parents are more supportive and reassuring of the child. Detailed written instructions must be given with regard to fasting; where and when to report the day of surgery; and who should be called for further instructions if the child develops a cold, fever, or any unexpected illness before surgery. Arrangements for any indicated preoperative laboratory testing can be made at this time. Many surgeons find it useful to even review some of the postoperative instructions, and prescribe some routine postoperative medications (e.g., analgesics, antiemetics, and antibiotics) at this time.

The laboratory data required and the duration of time for which the results remain acceptable before surgery vary among facilities.[24] In the past, the traditional standing orders included a complete blood count and urinalysis. Hospital or state rules may govern whether or not this is still a requirement. The analysis of specimens may be performed at the outpatient facility, or a written report of results from an accredited outside laboratory also may be acceptable. Some institutions allow these tests to be completed as early as 30 days before surgery, provided there is no change in the child's physical condition, whereas others require that tests be done within a more limited time frame, such as 48 hours before surgery.

A recent trend in outpatient anesthesia, however, has been to question whether any routine preoperative testing really adds to the safety of anesthesia and whether these tests influence outcome or whether they are performed simply as a ritual.[25] For example, studies have shown that the incidence of anemia in healthy children is extremely low[25, 26] and does not usually require modification of the anesthetic management.[26] Accordingly, most pediatric anesthesiologists now believe that healthy pediatric patients, especially those over 1 year of age, do not require routine hemoglobin determinations before elective surgery.[26] Moreover, most pediatric institutions either do not require urinalysis or request it only when there is a specific indication, such as a history of genitourinary disease. It is unfortunate, however, that many of us still practice under jurisdictions in which legislation requires such routine preoperative testing.[24]

Busy outpatient units cannot rely on the surgeon alone to present the units consistently with a fully evaluated and prepared child. This is especially true when a large number of surgeons with varying interests and attitudes have privileges to practice in the unit. To expedite the evaluation process and ensure some degree of uniformity in the pre-

operative preparation of the children, personnel in some of the units have found it useful to participate in the preoperative screening process. The degree of involvement varies from a simple phone call to the parents by the unit clerk a day or two before surgery, to the establishment of a formal screening clinic to evaluate all patients before their admission to the operating suite.

At CNMC, surgeons select and schedule patients for outpatient surgery in accordance with set guidelines under which ASA PS I or II patients are considered routine candidates for outpatient surgery. A consultation is requested before an ASA PS III patient is scheduled. A list of suggested ambulatory surgical procedures is provided to the surgeons and is updated periodically.[27]

Once the child's surgery is scheduled, preoperative screening is accomplished by obtaining a detailed medical history by a telephone call made through the AM Surgical Admission Center (AMSAC) 3 to 7 days before surgery (Appendix 26–1). A printed questionnaire designed to elicit information about anesthesia-related risk factors is used. Parents are asked specific questions about history of prematurity and about cardiac, pulmonary, renal, endocrine, and other anesthesia-related risks.[27] The AMSAC is under the medical direction of the department of anesthesiology, and is staffed by registered nurses (RNs), a licensed practical nurse (LPN), and admission clerks. The telephone calls are made by the RN during the day or by the LPN during the evening. The RN reviews all calls made by the LPN. If preexisting medical problems, such as history of prematurity or asthma, are discovered in the course of the telephone call, the case is reviewed by a staff anesthesiologist. When warranted by the medical history, an appointment is made for the child to have an examination by an anesthesiologist a few days before surgery. Further consultations and tests are arranged according to the anesthesiologist's recommendations. The appropriateness of ambulatory surgery for these patients is reviewed, and surgeons are contacted if a change in admission status is contemplated.

A second telephone call to detect acute illnesses is made to the parents on the evening before surgery by the evening-shift nurses of a short-stay recovery unit. Such calls are made after 5 P.M., when the time required for direct patient care has decreased. During this call, the nurse inquires about acute illnesses, such as upper respiratory infection or diarrhea. Instructions about arrival time, fasting, and practical matters related to parking, what to bring to the hospital, and expected duration of stay are reinforced.

Our experience with this telephone screening process has been extremely favorable. By using this system, the number of children whose surgery had to be canceled or rescheduled has significantly decreased.[27] Although all screening techniques should achieve similar results, telephone screening has the distinct advantage that it does not require a separate preoperative visit to the hospital by children if their history does not suggest the presence of a coexisting medical condition.

On the day of surgery all patients are evaluated for acute illness and NPO status. Vital signs are recorded. Any consultation reports are evaluated, and the need for special preoperative psychological or pharmacologic treatment is considered before the child arrives in the operating room area.

PREPARING THE CHILD FOR OUTPATIENT SURGERY

Psychological Preparation

From a psychological point of view, anesthesia and surgery on an outpatient basis can be a mixed blessing. The short stay in the hospital or surgical facility has the definite advantage of minimizing or even eliminating the trauma of separating child and parent; however, other emotional problems may occur. Many of these problems stem from the child's lack of familiarity with the hospital environment and the brief exposure to this environment before the induction of anesthesia. In many centers, the child may be taken to the operating room within 30 or 45 minutes of admission to the outpatient facility—hardly enough time for the child to become familiar with the new surroundings or to establish rapport with the staff. For this reason, many institutions offer preparation programs that begin a few days before surgery with a visit to the hospital, a tour of the facility, and a movie or a puppet show that illustrates the entire procedure in a language the child understands.

At CNMC, the children and parents are invited for a preoperative visit to the hospital. A puppet show or video is followed by a short tour of the hospital. The tour is conducted by a staff member who is trained to answer all questions honestly and who can familiarize the child and parents with what will happen on the day of surgery. The tour is oriented to the child and is conducted in a friendly, playful fashion with special attention paid to the areas where children will be staying before and after surgery.

The tour guide must carefully ascertain that the child knows he or she will be coming to the hospital for surgery. The admission procedure is explained and the need for laboratory tests, identification bands, and the use of hospital gowns is stressed. Finally, the waiting area or playroom where child (and parents if appropriate) will go on the day of surgery is visited. The children are encouraged to bring along a favorite toy or comforter. Some children want to try on a hospital gown at this time. (For many young children, having to undress and wear that strange gown is one of the worst memories about the day of surgery.)

The children are shown either a special operating or induction room or a set-aside anesthesia machine. They are allowed to handle the machine, breathing circuits, masks, syringes, and other equipment. Although it is often difficult to spot an unusually fearful child at this time, any such patient should be brought to the attention of the department of anesthesiology for "extra-special handling."

Both the recovery room and the location where the child will stay until fit for discharge are then visited. The fact that the child may have pain following surgery is mentioned, with the reassurance that measures will be taken to minimize the discomfort. Special equipment (e.g.,

intravenous [IV] lines, oxygen tubing, and thermometer) is shown and explained. The child is told where and at what time he or she will meet his or her parents, and the fact that a return home will take place on the same day is always emphasized. Videotape viewing is used to reinforce the ideas presented in person. This has been shown to facilitate preoperative preparation and reduces anxiety.[28]

Although there is general agreement that this kind of preparation program is useful, few studies document its value. Rosen et al.[29] studied anesthesia induction in 500 unpremedicated children between the ages of 2 and 12 years. They found that children who attended a preadmission orientation program (including a puppet show) did significantly better during induction of anesthesia than those who did not attend. Care is needed, however, when these results are interpreted. Parental motivation, traveling distance, socioeconomic conditions, and the child's age are some of the factors that motivate the parents to bring their children to the program. These factors may in themselves lead to better cooperation. In addition, children who have undergone previous anesthesia rarely returned to attend the program, and these children were shown to have a poorer cooperation rating. It would be desirable to have different preoperative programs for adolescents who may be insulted by terms such as "magic gas" that are often used to explain anesthesia induction to preschool children.

Pharmacologic Premedication

The use of premedication in pediatric outpatients has come full circle from the early years when it was routine to administer heavy sedation, and the 1970s and 1980s when patients were usually not premedicated. At the present time, the use of selective preinduction sedation is the norm.[30] Historically, premedication of children was thought to be a necessity for safe administration of general anesthesia. With modern anesthetic agents and techniques, it is possible to safely anesthetize an unpremedicated struggling, screaming child within a few minutes. As a result, premedication has now assumed more value for the emotional protection of the child than as an adjunct to anesthesia. Although most authors state that if the child has been properly prepared premedication is not necessary or is even undesirable if it prolongs recovery and delays discharge home, others believe that some form of sedation is advantageous[31] to facilitate the induction of anesthesia.

One major problem of applying the results of premedication studies to clinical practice is that most authors merely compare the effects of different premedication regimens or a placebo on a mixed population of children. Although it is usually possible to demonstrate that a particular regimen is superior to another, almost all regimens have a 10 to 20 percent failure rate. The results cannot be used to predict that a desired effect will occur in the individual child who would benefit the most (e.g., one who is unusually apprehensive or disturbed).

Our own belief is that when children are properly prepared psychologically, rapport with the anesthesiologist is established and separation from parents is minimized up to and even during the induction of anesthesia, so that most children do not require preoperative sedation. However, some (up to 20 percent of all children) do require it, often because their parents are anxious and transmit their anxiety to their child.

If a patient is to undergo repeated painful procedures, is known to be apprehensive, or is too young to benefit from verbal reassurances, premedication should be administered before the induction of anesthesia begins. Intramuscular (IM) injections, as a route for routine premedication, should be avoided whenever possible in children. Although many combinations of drugs and routes of drug administration have been used to administer preanesthetic sedation, the oral route is the least threatening method of doing so.[32] Oral midazolam 0.5 mg/kg is a safe and effective route for administering preanesthetic medication in pediatric outpatients if the drug is administered 30 to 45 minutes before anesthesia is induced. The use of oral midazolam in this dose did not alter the recovery times from anesthesia, even after surgical procedures lasting less than 30 minutes.[32] If premedication is not used routinely, the anesthesiologist should be prepared to handle the occasional difficult or extremely frightened child by using a combination premedicant-induction agent such as rectal methohexital (Brevital) or occasionally IM ketamine.[33] This is especially important when a mask induction is planned. The possibility of a slightly prolonged recovery from anesthesia is a small price to pay for avoiding the potential psychological trauma of a stormy induction of anesthesia.

Preinduction Techniques

Low-dose (2 mg/kg) IM ketamine can be used to sedate young children who do not cooperate with other methods of anesthetic induction. The onset time is short (2 to 3 minutes), and recovery is not prolonged. When ketamine is followed by an inhaled anesthetic, there is minimal likelihood of delirium or bad dreams during recovery from anesthesia.[33]

Rectal administration of methohexital is sometimes used in preschool children. A dose of 25 mg/kg (10 percent solution) has an onset time of 6 to 10 minutes and produces enough sedation to peacefully separate an upset child from his or her parents.[34] Rectal midazolam 1 mg/kg has the same onset time as oral administration of the drug, improves separation from parents, and does not delay discharge home.[35] Intranasal administration of midazolam 0.2 mg/kg also has been reported to produce anxiolysis and sedation in preschool children. The onset of sedation is rapid (5 to 10 minutes), and there is no evidence of delayed recovery.[36]

Parental Presence During Induction of Anesthesia

Since one of the main reasons for administering routine premedication, or for having to administer premedication to patients, is to facilitate separation of the child from the parents, some anesthesiologists find that they can reduce or even eliminate the need for such agents by allowing the parents to stay with the child during the induction of anesthesia.[37] Although still controversial,[38] this approach

is gaining a lot of supporters, and is being requested by many parents. Some institutions have specially built induction rooms where the parents can be present when anesthesia is induced without the parents having to wear special operating room attire. Others allow selected parents to wear a coverall gown or scrubs and walk with the child into the actual operating room. Studies have shown that children are less upset when the parents are present.[37] Parent selection and education are essential for parental presence during the induction of anesthesia to be successful, since anxious parents can make their children even more upset.[39]

ANESTHETIC AGENTS AND TECHNIQUES

Despite the current popularity of outpatient surgery, there is still no agreement among anesthesiologists as to what constitutes the best way to ensure a smooth induction of and a rapid and comfortable recovery from anesthesia without compromising safety. Since no single approach will be effective for all children in all situations, the anesthesiologist must be familiar with and have confidence in many methods of anesthetic induction. A particular agent or technique should be chosen and tailored to fit the needs of the individual child, not used merely because it is the routine in a particular institution or is the only method with which the anesthesiologist is comfortable. The choice of an anesthetic technique for the pediatric outpatient should ensure a smooth induction of anesthesia, and quick emergence from anesthesia at the end of surgery. It also should ensure prompt recovery in the postanesthesia care unit (PACU) and rapid discharge home with no or minimal pain and/or postoperative nausea or vomiting (PONV). Although many of the newer anesthetic agents and techniques that were developed to meet these goals in outpatients are now the standard in most patients, and are familiar to all anesthesiologists, it is important to review the rationale for the selection of these agents and techniques.[1]

Inhalational Induction of Anesthesia

Inhalation induction of anesthesia has long been favored by children and pediatric anesthesiologists. Successful inhalational induction of anesthesia, however, requires the child's cooperation and acceptance of the face mask, especially in unpremedicated outpatients. Such cooperation can be encouraged in a variety of ways. For example, a transparent mask can be used, or the inside of the mask can be painted with a flavor or a smell of the child's choice. The child can be allowed to sit up during the induction of anesthesia, and he or she can be allowed to hold his or her mask during the induction of anesthesia. At times it is useful for the parents to hold the mask during the induction of anesthesia, especially if the patient is a "frequent flyer." Placing a mask directly on the face of a child is often frightening to the child. Holding the mask slightly off of the face is less frightening. If the flow-rate of the inspired gas is 10 L, this rate exceeds that of the child. Therefore, the child will quickly go to sleep without the sensation of being smothered. When the child loses consciousness, the mask can be applied tightly to his or her face.

For over three decades, halothane was the standard inhalational induction agent in pediatrics. It offered reasonably fast loss of consciousness with minimal airway irritation. Despite some concerns over its tendency to slow the heart rate and, in the presence of hypercarbia, to predispose the child to arrhythmias, it was and is the "gold standard" against which other inhalational agents are compared.

The rate of early postoperative recovery following short outpatient procedures compares favorably with that of *isoflurane*. With the recent introduction of sevoflurane in the United States, after years of experience in Japan, sevoflurane has replaced halothane as the induction agent of choice.

Sevoflurane has solubility characteristics closer to those of desflurane and nitrous oxide than to halothane or isoflurane. The drug has a very pleasant smell and is the least irritating inhalational induction agent available.[40] Sevoflurane can be used for both induction and for maintenance of anesthesia in children. Clinical experience with sevoflurane in Japan, the United States, and Europe has shown that the drug causes a smooth induction of anesthesia with no airway irritation. Emergence and recovery from anesthesia also are faster when compared with halothane.[41] Sevoflurane undergoes metabolic breakdown in the body, and this breakdown results in release of free fluoride ions. The clinical significance of this breakdown appears to be negligible, especially in children undergoing short outpatient surgical procedures. Sevoflurane considerably improves the ease of inhalation induction in pediatric outpatients. However, there are conflicting data whether sevoflurane speeds the induction of anesthesia, especially if the concentration of drug is increased gradually.[42] In a recent multicenter comparative study, the time to loss of eyelash reflex with sevoflurane was only 0.3 minute faster than with halothane.[43] In practice, however, patients readily accept 8 percent sevoflurane in the inspired gas, once they are comfortable with face mask application. The anesthetic uptake and the loss of consciousness are extremely rapid (15 to 20 seconds) with no or minimal resistance or irritation and less bradycardia or arrhythmias than with halothane. The availability of sevoflurane has reduced the need for preoperative sedation and the use of alternate induction techniques in pediatric outpatients. However, the cost of sevoflurane far exceeds that of halothane or isoflurane. Consequently, many clinicians induce anesthesia with sevoflurane and switch to one of the other agents as soon as the patient is anesthetized.

In recent studies, early recovery following sevoflurane anesthesia was reported to be 33 percent more rapid than halothane.[43] The time to discharge from hospital, however, was similar for both anesthetics. This may be due to the fact that the incidence of agitation attributable to sevoflurane was almost threefold greater than that attributable to halothane necessitating more frequent use of sedation during recovery. These recovery advantages of sevoflurane over halothane, however, were not shown in a different study that compared it with both halothane and desflurane.[44] Patients who received desflurane anesthesia following induction of anesthesia with halothane had faster emergence and recovery from desflurane anesthesia than did those who received halothane or sevoflurane. Emergence and recovery from anesthesia following halothane and sevoflurane were not significantly different. Again, the times to discharge from the hospital were essentially similar for the three agents. It is the author's conclusion that sevoflurane is the clear choice for inhalational induction of anesthesia in the typically unpremedicated pediatric outpatient. If predictably rapid emergence is desired (e.g., ear, nose, and throat [ENT] surgery), then maintenance of anesthesia with desflurane (in a low-flow gas mixture to reduce cost) may be preferable.

Desflurane has chemical and physical characteristics that are potentially attractive for outpatient surgical patients. Desflurane's low blood–gas partition coefficient (0.42) should theoretically result in rapid alveolar uptake of the gas. However, early experience with desflurane in pediatric patients demonstrated that desflurane resulted in an unacceptably high incidence of airway irritation and moderate to severe coughing and laryngospasm that resulted in arterial oxygen desaturation. Desflurane is not, therefore, indicated for induction of anesthesia in children.[45] Desflurane, however, can be easily introduced following other induction agents, typically sevoflurane or halothane. Welborn et al. reported that a brief period of halothane inhalation for the induction of anesthesia, followed by desflurane for maintenance of anesthesia, resulted in the same rapid emergence and recovery from anesthesia seen when desflurane was used for both induction and maintenance of anesthesia.[46] Maintenance of anesthesia with desflurane also resulted in significantly faster emergence and recovery from anesthesia than occurred when halothane alone was used. This approach is particularly useful in patients undergoing ENT procedures, such as tonsillectomy and/or adenoidectomy, when the timing of the end of surgery cannot be accurately predicted, and when rapid emergence from anesthesia and return of airway reflexes is desirable. Recovery following unsupplemented desflurane (and to a slightly lesser degree, sevoflurane) anesthesia has been associated with a higher incidence of excitement than occurred when halothane was used.[47] Attempts to modify the emergence agitation that is frequently seen with these agents have not been completely successful. Attention must be given to ensure adequate analgesia in these patients. Even when there is complete absence of pain, as usually occurs in children who have a functional regional block, agitation still occurs. Recent experience indicates that administering 2 to 3 μg/kg of fentanyl effectively reduces this emergence phenomenon without delaying emergence from anesthesia or discharge from the hospital when desflurane is used in pediatric ENT patients.[48]

Intravenous Techniques

Intravenous induction of anesthesia is the method of choice in many older children, especially when EMLA is used to prevent the pain of venipuncture. The use of EMLA in outpatients requires careful planning, since the drug must be applied to the skin for at least 1 hour for the drug to exert its full effect. The parents should be encouraged to apply EMLA at home before they go to the hospital, especially since EMLA is now available as a prepackaged "EMLA patch." In most cases, EMLA should be applied to two potential IV sites so a back-up site is available in case the first venipuncture is unsuccessful.

When *thiopental sodium* is used in healthy unpremedicated children, a relatively large dose (5 to 6 mg/kg) may be required to ensure smooth and rapid transition to general inhalational anesthesia. Children who receive barbiturate for the induction of anesthesia tend to be sleepier and require more airway support for the first 15 minutes of recovery from anesthesia than those who received halothane. This difference disappears by 30 minutes of recovery.[49]

Studies of the use of propofol in children indicate that it results in smooth induction of anesthesia with a smaller incidence of side effects and faster recovery from anesthesia than thiopental does. Propofol 2.5 to 3.5 mg/kg is sufficient for induction of anesthesia in children who accept venipuncture. Pain on injection of propofol can be minimized or prevented by using the large antecubital veins for the drug administration. If the hand veins must be used, lidocaine (1 to 2 mg lidocaine/1 ml of propofol) can be mixed with propofol immediately prior to its injection, with excellent results. Alternatively, propofol infusion can be started following a brief period of inhaled anesthesia and establishing IV access. Because of the higher volume of distribution and increased clearance of propofol (see Chapter 3), children require a higher infusion rate (125 to 250 μg/kg/min) of propofol than adults. This is especially true for younger children and during the early part of the maintenance phase of anesthesia.

Propofol anesthesia consistently has been shown to be associated with an extremely low incidence of postoperative vomiting, even after surgical procedures that normally result in vomiting (e.g., strabismus surgery[50]), or when administered with ondansetron during tonsillectomy.[51] The absence of vomiting results in faster discharge home compared with halothane.[49]

Methohexital

Methohexital 1.5 to 2 mg/kg offers the distinct advantage of a significantly shorter recovery time for outpatients than does an equivalent single dose of thiopental.[52] However, induction of anesthesia with methohexital is followed by an appreciable incidence of involuntary muscle movements, hiccough, and coughing episodes that can sometimes be troublesome. A severe burning sensation often develops along the course of the vein into which the drug is administered, which is particularly undesirable in children because it promotes hand movement. This movement can dislodge the needle from the vein. Pain can be avoided by mixing a small amount of lidocaine (1 mg/ml) with the methohexital. Methohexital also has been reported to induce epileptiform convulsions in susceptible patients.

Etomidate

Etomidate, a nonbarbiturate hypnotic agent, has been used extensively for IV induction of anesthesia in Europe.

When used in a dose of 0.2 mg/kg in children, etomidate produces sleep rapidly and safely, with negligible cardiovascular system side effects and little respiratory depression.

Pain is common after injection of etomidate and, unlike methohexital, the pain is not prevented by adding lidocaine to the solution. Myoclonia also is seen after injection of this drug. Using an analgesic (e.g., fentanyl) for premedication or with the induction of anesthesia can reduce these problems. Some authors, however, find that the combination of etomidate and fentanyl frequently is associated with nausea and vomiting, which may delay discharge of the patient from the hospital.[53]

Intraoperative Use of Narcotics

Narcotics can be used in outpatients as a part of a balanced anesthesia technique with nitrous oxide/oxygen/muscle relaxants to maintain anesthesia or to supplement a "light" inhalational anesthetic technique. By reducing the amount of potent inhalational or IV agents needed (and absorbed in fat for later release), narcotics may actually contribute to more rapid awakening from anesthesia.[54] The residual analgesia may eliminate or reduce the need for further potent pain medication during the recovery period. If ultra-short-acting agents are used (e.g., remifentanil), provision must be made for ensuring adequate postoperative analgesia by administering a small dose of a longer acting opioid or by administering a regional block before the child is allowed to recover from anesthesia.[55]

AIRWAY MANAGEMENT

Mask Anesthesia

Many outpatient procedures are of short duration and do not invade a body cavity. For these procedures, anesthesia can usually be administered via a mask. Intubation of the trachea for convenience may unnecessarily complicate the anesthetic. In seeking to achieve good intubating conditions in these patients, one may come dangerously close to administering an overdose of drug if a volatile agent is used, or prolonged muscle paralysis may occur if a muscle relaxant is administered that would otherwise not be indicated.

LMA

As with adult patients, the use of laryngeal mask airways (LMAs) is gaining popularity in pediatric outpatient practice. This has been a little slower, however, mainly because of the delay in introduction of a full spectrum of mask sizes. In many European countries today, flexible LMAs are routinely used for T&A surgery.

Endotracheal Intubation

Outpatient anesthesia per se is not a contraindication for using an endotracheal tube. At many centers, a large number of pediatric ambulatory surgery patients have had their tracheas intubated without serious complications. The indications and techniques of endotracheal intubation are the same as for inpatients.

Traditionally, the endotracheal tube size selected should enable full expansion of both lungs and normal lung inflation while allowing a leak of gas with airway pressure of 20 to 25 cm H_2O. More recently, however, some authors have advocated the use of cuffed endotracheal tubes in smaller and smaller children to allow the use of lower fresh gas flows and save on the cost of newer expensive volatile agents.[56] It is thought that the seal produced by these cuffed tubes occurs in the trachea where the cartilaginous rings are not complete, and distention can occur without compromising the vascularity of the mucosa. This is a more physiologic state when compared with the seal that can result from using a large uncuffed tube that compresses the mucosa in the cricoid area.

The most significant risk associated with the use of an endotracheal tube in outpatient surgery is the possibility that a child may develop postintubation croup during recovery from anesthesia, especially after discharge from the hospital.[57] However, with careful technique during intubation of the trachea and the use of proper sized, implant tested tubes, the incidence should be very small (<1 percent). Of special importance is the time at which "significant" croup develops. Most patients who develop postintubation croup will have symptoms of the problem within 1 hour of tracheal extubation; thus, many centers allow pediatric patients whose tracheas have been intubated to be discharged after 1 hour has passed. Parents must be advised to observe and report to a previously designated physician or service any respiratory difficulties that develop after discharge. If the child develops croup and requires treatment with racemic epinephrine, he or she must be observed for a longer period (2 to 3 hours) to ensure that rebound edema does not develop.

PERIOPERATIVE FLUID MANAGEMENT

The need for routine of intravenous fluid administration during pediatric outpatient anesthesia is controversial. Children undergoing very brief surgical procedures (e.g., myringotomies) may not need any parenteral fluid administration, provided they are not excessively starved preoperatively, and if it is expected that they will be able to ingest and retain oral fluids soon after they are awake from anesthesia. For most other children, intraoperative maintenance fluid administration can be calculated based on the child's body weight according to standard formulae.

Administering intravenous fluid therapy during and after surgery is specifically indicated in longer operations (over 30 to 60 minutes), in procedures known to be associated with a high incidence of postoperative nausea and vomiting (e.g., strabismus surgery), and in young children who have been fasting for a prolonged period of time. If continuing postoperative fluid loss is anticipated (vomiting or inability to tolerate oral intake), it is advisable to correct the anticipated deficit early on so that the child is well hydrated when ready to go home. This avoids delaying discharge of the child home while "catch-up" fluid administration is instituted. Adequate parenteral hydration also obviates the need for forcing children to ingest oral fluids before the children are allowed to go home. Recent studies confirm that children who are forced to drink before leaving the facility have a higher incidence of vomiting, and are discharged home later than children who are allowed to drink only when they are thirsty enough to request a drink.[58]

Many anesthesiologists prefer to have an IV infusion of fluid started in every child undergoing surgery to guarantee a ready route for emergency administration of drugs. Apart from the extra expense and time involved and the occasional need for an extra pair of hands, there is no real objection to this practice unless it requires repeated attempts at venipuncture in a healthy, well-hydrated chubby child who has a patent airway and will have a brief, painless procedure. It is reassuring to remember that the only two emergency drugs that are likely to be needed in the healthy day-surgery child are succinylcholine and atropine. In the absence of an infusion or visible veins, both drugs are rapidly effective when given IM in a dose twice that used for IV administration. However, when these drugs are given IM to a child whose cardiac output is reduced, absorption of the drug from the injection site may be markedly delayed.

POSTOPERATIVE ANALGESIA

Successful management of outpatient anesthesia requires that the anesthesiologist carefully evaluate and provide for the child's need for postoperative pain. The need for analgesics following surgery depends on the nature of the procedure and the pain threshold of the patient. *It does not depend on whether the child is an outpatient or an inpatient.* Many young children do very well postoperatively with small amounts of oral analgesics or no analgesic whatsoever. However, many others ambulate better when they are given appropriate doses of a more potent analgesic.[59] Certainly every child deserves individual consideration of whether he or she requires analgesics. It is unfortunate that many anesthesiologists and surgeons deny an appropriate dose of a narcotic to a child who is in pain because "in their own experience" the procedure "usually" does not warrant it or the surgeon or anesthesiologist fears that giving narcotics will delay discharge from the hospital.

Regional blocks or local infiltration of local anesthetics should be used whenever possible to supplement general anesthesia and to limit the need for narcotic administration during recovery from anesthesia. Postoperative pain or discomfort can be managed by one or more of the following methods.

Nonnarcotic Analgesics

Acetaminophen 10 to 15 mg/kg orally (PO) is the most commonly used mild analgesic for pediatric outpatient patients. For young children, the initial dose of actaminophen often is administered rectally (up to 45 mg/kg) prior to awakening from anesthesia.[60] Supplemental doses are given orally every 4 to 6 hours (not PRN) to maintain adequate blood levels and effective analgesia.[61] The maximum daily dose of this drug in children should not exceed 100 mg/kg/day. Acetaminophen can be combined with codeine for more effective control of moderately severe pain and/or discomfort. Acetaminophen with codeine elixir contains 120 mg acetaminophen and 12 mg codeine per 5 ml. The usual dose is 5 ml for children 3 to 6 years, and 10 ml for those who are 7 to 12 years old.

Tramadaol is a centrally acting synthetic analgesic. It is believed to have two mechanisms of action; binding to μ-opioid receptors and weak inhibition of the reuptake of norepinephrine and serotonin. Its role in pediatric outpatient pain management is currently under investigation.

Nonsteroidal Anti-inflammatory Drugs

Conventional nonsteroidal anti-inflammatory drugs (NSAIDs) (e.g., ketorolac) are effective in relieving postoperative pain following minor operations in children. Early administration of ketorolac immediately following induction of anesthesia seems to provide optimal postoperative analgesia. Several studies have demonstrated the analgesic and opioid-sparing effects of ketorolac, which may reduce the incidence of opioid-related adverse effects such as respiratory depression, nausea, and vomiting. Ketorolac, however, like many other NSAIDs, has some troubling side effects. There are reported instances of decreased bone repair after osteotomy, bronchospasm, acute renal failure, and possibly increased surgical bleeding secondary to altered platelet function.[62] Several recent articles reported an increased incidence of postoperative hemorrhage in patients who received ketorolac. Some, however, did not find increased bleeding when ketorolac was given at the end of the procedure. More studies are required to determine the optimal dose and route of administration of ketorolac, as well as its efficacy as an analgesic following more painful outpatient surgical procedures in children. It is expected that newer NSAIDs that target cyclooxygenase isoenzyme 2 (COX-2) without inhibiting COX-1, when given in therapeutic doses, will soon be available for intravenous as well as oral administration and that these drugs will selectively block pain receptors and have minimal side effects. These should be extremely valuable in pediatric outpatients.

Potent Narcotic Analgesics

When narcotics are indicated during recovery from anesthesia, a short-acting drug should be chosen. Intravenous use allows more accurate titration of the dose and avoids the use of "standard" dosages based on weight, which may lead to a relative overdose of narcotic in some patients. If remifentanil is used intraoperatively, planning for postoperative analgesia must be started before the patient awakens for anesthesia. Fentanyl, up to a dose of 2.0 μg/kg, is our drug of choice for intravenous use. Meperidine (0.5 mg/kg) and codeine (1.0 to 1.5 mg/kg) can be used intramuscularly if no intravenous route is available. IM codeine tends to result in less vomiting than other opioids, especially morphine.[63] Nasal administration of fentanyl results in an analgesic blood level of drug comparable to that following IV administration of the drug,[64] which makes it useful when the child does not have, or has lost IV access.[65]

Regional Analgesia

Although regional anesthesia alone is usually not used in pediatric outpatients, many simple nerve blocks can be combined with light general anesthesia to provide excellent postoperative pain relief and early ambulation, with minimal or no need for narcotics (see Chapter 12). However, plans should be made before discharging the patient home for providing analgesia when the block is no longer effective and the patient is at home.

Regional blocks or infiltration of the surgical site with a local anesthetic can be combined with light general anesthesia to provide excellent intraoperative and postoperative pain relief and early ambulation, with minimal or no need for narcotics.[66] If the block is performed before surgery starts, but after the child is asleep, one can reduce the requirement for general anesthesia during surgery, which in turn may result in a more rapid recovery from anesthesia, earlier discharge home, more rapid return of normal appetite, and less nausea and vomiting.[1]

The types of nerve blocks that can be used safely in pediatric outpatients are limited only by the skill and interest of the anesthesiologist. Generally, the block chosen should be simple to perform, have minimal or no side effects, and should not interfere with motor function and early ambulation.

Ilioinguinal and iliohypogastric nerve block can be performed by infiltration of 0.25 percent bupivacaine solution (in doses up to 2 mg/kg) in the region medial to the anterior superior iliac spine. This block has been used successfully to provide excellent postoperative analgesia for pediatric outpatients following elective inguinal herniorrhaphy or orchiopexy.

The *dorsal nerve of the penis* can blocked by simple injection of 1 to 4 ml of 0.25 percent bupivacaine without epinephrine deep to Buck's fascia 1 cm from the midline. This provides over 6 hours of analgesia following circumcision. Alternate approaches to penile block are a midline injection or subcutaneous infiltration (ring block), which presumably blocks the nerve after it has ramified into the subcutaneous tissue. Topical application of lidocaine on the incision site at the conclusion of surgery also has been shown to be effective.

Caudal block provides excellent postoperative analgesia following a wide variety of surgical procedures such as circumcision, hypospadias repair, orchiopexy, and herniorrhaphy. By using a 0.25 percent bupivacaine solution in a dose of 0.5 to 0.7 ml/kg, no motor paralysis is produced. If a larger volume (1 to 1.5 ml/kg) is indicated, the use of a 0.125 percent bupivacaine or 0.2 percent ropovacaine is recommended to avoid motor weakness.[67] Caudal block has been used extensively in our outpatient surgical unit, with most children discharged home free of pain between 1 and 2 hours postoperatively. Analgesia (as measured by subsequent need of a mild oral analgesic) lasts 4 to 6 hours with this technique. Although voiding may be slightly delayed in children who receive a caudal block, catheterization of the bladder is never needed, and children can be allowed to go home before voiding.

Multimodal Analgesia

A multimodal analgesic approach involves the use of combined analgesic regimens to achieve sufficient analgesia through the additive or synergistic effects of different analgesics. There is a reduction in the number of side effects that occur because of the use of lower doses of analgesics and because of the differences in side-effect profiles. A possible model of a multimodal strategy for postoperative pain relief in pediatric outpatients is the combination of a regional block with acetaminophen. Another is the possible opioid-sparing effect of combining a peripheral acting analgesic such as a COX-2–inhibiting NSAID with a smaller dose of opioids when regional analgesia is not possible (e.g., following tonsillectomy).

POSTOPERATIVE NAUSEA AND VOMITING

PONV can be a significant problem in pediatric outpatients. Contributing factors include the type of surgical procedure, the presence of pain, the use of opioid analgesics, a history of motion sickness, and sudden movement. Certain surgeries are particularly prone to induce emesis: tonsillectomy, strabismus repair, orchiopexy, hernia repair, ear surgery, and laparoscopy. Tramer et al. reviewed 27 randomized clinical trials involving a total of 2,033 children and found an average incidence of 54 percent of early (<6 hours) and a 59 percent incidence of late (up to 24 hours) emesis when prophylaxis was not used.[68]

A recent multicenter trial of 429 children concluded that intravenous ondansetron prophylaxis (0.1 mg/kg; maximum 4 mg) was more effective than placebo in preventing postoperative vomiting in children during both the 0- to 2-hour and 0- to 24-hour study periods (89 vs. 70 percent and 68 vs. 39 percent, respectively).[69] Intravenous ondansetron (0.1 mg/kg) also was found to be effective in treating established postoperative emesis in yet another multicenter trial of 2,720 pediatric outpatients.[70]

Although intravenous ondansetron is an effective prophylactic antiemetic, many authors continue to compare it with other less expensive alternatives.[1] Davis et al. compared the effects of ondansetron (0.1 mg/kg), droperidol (75 μg/kg), and placebo on the incidence of emesis in children undergoing dental surgery where anesthesia was maintained with N_2O/O_2 and alfentanil.[71] The 24-hour incidence of emesis was significantly less with ondansetron (9 percent) than with placebo (35 percent) or droperidol (32 percent). Ondansetron-treated patients had significantly shorter hospital stays than the droperidol-treated patients.

As previously stated, the combination of propofol and ondansetron is extremely effective in providing pain relief and in reducing the incidence of vomiting in children following tonsillectomy.[51] It is interesting to note that a recent meta-analysis of published randomized clinical trials concluded that ondansetron and droperidol were more effective than metoclopramide in preventing postoperative vomiting.[72] However, although ondansetron and droperidol were equally effective in adults, ondansetron was more effective than droperidol in preventing vomiting in children.

Granisetron is a selective 5-hydroxytryptamine$_3$ receptor antagonist, which has a more potent and longer activity against vomiting associated with chemotherapy than ondansetron. In a randomized, double-blind study of 97 pediatric outpatients, Cieslak et al. found that 40 μg/kg of granisetron given as prophylaxis for vomiting decreased postoperative vomiting from 42 percent to 9 percent when compared with a group of patients who were given a placebo.[73] Although this dose of drug is much higher than the dose recommended for chemotherapy-induced emesis, a lower dose (10 μg/kg) was not effective.

The fact that there are many approaches to the management of PONV indicates that there is no one answer to the problem.[74] It appears, however, that a combination antiemetic regimen, possibly combined with the intraoperative use of dexamethasone, is the most effective treatment of this problem yet. It is probably fair to say, however, that even now, many anesthesiologists continue to base their choice of antiemetics on personal experience and anecdotal evidence. Even when scientific data strongly suggest that one drug, or a combination of drugs, is (are) superior to all others, the cost factor must be taken into consideration.[1] The price tag one puts on the comfort and satisfaction of patients, however, is beyond the scope of this discussion. Nevertheless, it is expected that any new treatment modality of PONV in the future will have to prove pharmacoeconomic as well as pharmacodynamic superiority to existing protocols.

For patients with persistent postoperative vomiting, our current approach is to stop offering oral fluids and ensure adequate intravenous hydration. Intravenous ondansetron 0.1 mg/kg is administered. In the absence of an IV line, or if vomiting occurs after the IV line is removed, ondansetron can be placed over the tongue for quick absorption without the need for swallowing. Occasionally, rectal promethazine 0.5 mg/kg (Phenergan 12.5 to 25 mg) or prochlorperazine 0.1 mg/kg (Compazine 2.5 to 5 mg) is administered in the hospital and/or given to the parents to administer at home.[1]

RECOVERY AND DISCHARGE CRITERIA

The key to understanding why certain anesthetic agents and techniques are selected, modified, or avoided in outpatient surgery is related to recovery. Rapid recovery and early ambulation after surgery are major objectives in pediatric outpatient surgery. However, the anesthesiologist must not rely solely on early return of consciousness or stabilization of vital signs as indices of full recovery. The return of consciousness does not ensure full recovery of the nervous system any more than the return of blood pressure to normal implies complete recovery of the circulatory system. In addition, individual variation exists among patients, even after identical procedures. When caring for outpatients, we must guarantee both safe discharge from the recovery room and from the hospital. There is no second opportunity to transfer care of the outpatient to other medical or paramedical personnel, and there is no further period of observation, monitoring, and treatment.[75]

Facilities for postoperative care vary among institutions. Patients in some centers go to the main recovery room and then to a short-stay (phase 2 recovery) area from which they are discharged home. Others are discharged home directly from the recovery room. In a free-standing unit, the patient goes directly to the short-stay recovery area until discharge home. The following discussion compares the criteria for discharge home from the recovery room with those of the short-stay recovery unit.

Recovery Room

In general, criteria for discharge from the recovery room are the same as those for inpatients and depend on achieving stability of vital signs. Absence of bleeding, presence of sufficient reflexes to prevent aspiration of vomitus, orientation by the patient to time and place, and ability of the patient to maintain a safe position in bed also are criteria for discharge from the hospital.

Efforts have been made to standardize the evaluation of recovery with use of a scoring system. The first quantitative scoring system to evaluate patient recovery was developed by Aldrete and Kroulik.[76] Using the Apgar scoring system as a model, they assigned a score of 0, 1, or 2 to each of five signs: activity, respiration, circulation, consciousness, and color (Table 26-2). According to this system, which is used by many centers today, when the patient achieves a total score of 8 or more, he or she is ready for discharge from the recovery room.

In 1975, Steward[77] suggested that patient color is difficult to interpret consistently and that blood pressure has little constant relation to recovery from general anesthesia in children. The simplified Postanesthesia Recovery Score was suggested as a more sensitive and reliable measure of recovery (Table 26-3).

Some anesthesiologists have used data obtained from pulse oximetry instead of "color" in recovery scores.[78]

TABLE 26 – 2
ALDRETE POSTANESTHETIC RECOVERY SCORE

Patient Sign	Criterion	Score
Activity	Able to move 4 extremities	2
	Able to move 2 extremities	1
	Able to move 0 extremities	0
Respiration	Able to deep-breathe and cough	2
	Limited breathing, good airway	1
	Apneic, obstructed	0
Circulation	SBP ± 20% preop	2
	SBP ± 20–50% preop	1
	SBP ± 50% preop	0
Consciousness	Awake (answers questions)	2
	Arousable (by name)	1
	Nonresponsive	0
Color	Pink	2
	Pale, dusky, blotchy, jaundiced	1
	Cyanotic	0

From Aldrete JA, Kroulik D: A post anesthetic recovery score. Anesth Analg 49:924, 1970, with permission.

TABLE 26 – 3
STEWARD POSTANESTHETIC RECOVERY SCORE

Patient Sign	Criterion	Score
Consciousness	Awake	2
	Responding to stimuli	1
	Not responding	0
Airway	Coughing on command or crying	2
	Maintaining good airway	1
	Airway requiring maintenance	0
Movement	Moving limbs purposefully	2
	Moving limbs nonpurposefully	1
	Not moving	0

From Steward DJ: A simplified scoring system for the postoperative recovery room. Can J Anaesth 22:111, 1975, with permission.

Initial observations, however, suggest that recovery scores do not correlate with postoperative hypoxemia in children.[79] Still, pulse oximetry is the only quantitative method of assessing oxygenation during recovery from general anesthesia. The ASA's standards for postanesthesia care include the use of pulse oximetry during the initial phase of recovery.[80] Most anesthesiologists would ordinarily expect a reasonably normal oxygen saturation to be present before the patient is released into the second phase of recovery.

We believe that more uniformity is provided on discharge when all personnel within a facility use the same criteria. In addition, when scoring is done on the written recovery record, it provides the basis for observing trends and is useful for medicolegal purposes. We use a modified Aldrete system; however, a patient is not usually discharged before a score of 10 is achieved. If the patient is released before this time, the physician must state the reason in writing on the recovery record.

Short-Stay (Phase 2) Recovery Unit

Discharge of the child from the hospital cannot be based on criteria used for adults (e.g., ability to make decisions). However, the patient must at least have reached a maximum on the recovery room scoring system, appear to be fully awake, have no or readily controllable pain and vomiting, and have no evidence of surgical or anesthetic complications.

In an effort to provide uniform care, to make it possible to compare data within and between institutions, and to ensure a complete legal record, some institutions have developed discharge criteria. Unlike a scoring system, *all* criteria must be met. At the CNMC, discharge from the short-stay unit is guided by, but not necessarily limited to, the following:

1. Appropriateness and stability of vital signs.
2. Ability to swallow oral fluids and cough or demonstrate a gag reflex.
3. Ability to ambulate consistent with the developmental age of the child.
4. Absence of nausea, vomiting, and dizziness, preferably including the ability to retain oral fluids.
5. Absence of respiratory distress.

6. Attainment of a state of consciousness appropriate to the developmental level (for a complete description and guidelines for use of discharge criteria, see Appendix 26–2).

In our institution, the attending physician may write a discharge order in advance so that, provided specific discharge criteria are met, the patient is authorized to be released without further evaluation by a physician at the time of discharge. A registered nurse documents the status of the patient, acts only as an observer to document that *all* criteria are met, and makes no decisions independently. Two exceptions to this policy are patients who have had endotracheal intubation and whose recovery time is less than 3 hours, and patients who have received depressant medication for relief of pain, vomiting, or dizziness within the previous 90 minutes. In these two situations, and when a patient is discharged before all six formal criteria are met, the physician must personally evaluate and authorize discharge of the patient and must write a note on the permanent record to that effect.

We have been satisfied with the ability of our physicians and nursing staff to use this system successfully. One of the questions that remain, however, is that of adherence to the criterion that the patient be able to tolerate oral fluids. Some patients may vomit repeatedly when fluids are offered to them. If they are otherwise well hydrated, we may be creating a problem that otherwise would not exist.[58]

Role of Parents During the Recovery Period

Postanesthesia Recovery Room

Many parents want to be with their children as soon as the operation is terminated. In addition to confirming that the child has indeed survived the procedure, parents correctly believe that their child relates to them better than to other, unfamiliar faces at a time when anxiety could result from separation. Unfortunately, most recovery rooms are not large enough or properly designed to enable parents to participate in this aspect of care. In addition, many recovery room nurses fear that participation of the parents at this level may be detrimental to the care of their child and perhaps to that of other children as well. Parent participation in recovery of handicapped children has proven useful in our institution in selected cases, especially for deaf, blind, and retarded children whose ability to communicate with anyone other than the parent or guardian is compromised. Parents should not have access to the recovery room until the child's vital signs have stabilized, airway obstruction is no longer a threat, and awakening has begun. The parents must understand that should the child's condition deteriorate or for any reason it seems prudent for them to leave the unit at any time, they must do so promptly and without arguing.

Short-Stay Unit

Parents are encouraged (or may even be required) to participate in the child's care in the short-stay (i.e., postre-covery) unit. Parents can care for and hold, cuddle, and feed the child, and their involvement may reduce the need for a high nurse/patient ratio.

Fast Tracking

With the availability of newer anesthetic agents and techniques that allow more rapid emergence from anesthesia, it is possible to have patients completely awake in the operating room, and to transfer them directly to a phase 2 recovery area, thus completely bypassing the PACU. The number of adult patients who received general anesthesia and went directly to phase 2 recovery varied from 14 to 42 percent in one recent study.[81] Experience with fast tracking in children is still limited. Patel reported success in bypassing the PACU in children undergoing a limited variety of procedures including myringotomies and hernia repairs.[78] Parents were extremely satisfied with the earlier union with their children. The children were discharged home faster, had less need for analgesics, and experienced less PONV than those who had the traditional stay in PACU.

DISCHARGE HOME

Every child, regardless of age, must have an escort home, preferably by private car or taxicab. The escort should be provided with written instructions regarding the home care of the child and should be provided with a telephone number to call for further advice or to report complications. Such service is essential in the outpatient unit. In addition to counseling the parent of each child about postoperative care, most units have designed handouts that specify the care to be provided and the signs that might herald a complication. For convenience, the handout is usually limited to postoperative instructions for a specific operative procedure. An example of such a pamphlet for patients who undergo circumcision is shown in Appendix 26–3.

Role of the Physician in the Discharge Process

The role of the physician in the discharge of short-stay patients has been described in documents that address guidelines for care.[82, 83] These guidelines have been formulated to provide uniform care and to detect and treat complications appropriately.

In all of the guidelines, the discharge of the patient from an ambulatory surgical facility is the responsibility of a licensed independent practitioner (LIP),* usually a physician. Ideally, the physician (or LIP) should evaluate the patient at the time of discharge from the facility. One accrediting organization, the Accreditation Association for Ambulatory Health Care, Inc. (AAAHC), requires that patients who have received anesthesia are evaluated by the

---

* A licensed independent practitioner (LIP) is defined as any individual who is permitted by law and by the organization to provide patient care services without direction or supervision within the scope of the individual's license and in accordance with individually granted privileges.

operating surgeon, anesthesiologist, or dentist after recovery from anesthesia and before discharge home. The Joint Commission on the Accreditation of Healthcare Organization guidelines allow the use of "discharge criteria" to determine the readiness of the patient for discharge (Table 26–4).[83]

Regardless of whether the ambulatory surgical facility is hospital affiliated or free-standing, an LIP, preferably an anesthesiologist, must be in attendance in the facility at all times during patient treatment and recovery, and until medical discharge.[83]

COMPLICATIONS AND ADMISSIONS

Complications

Although life-threatening complications after outpatient anesthesia are rare, discomfort that prolongs or complicates recovery is common.[84] The most commonly reported complications before discharge home are sore throat, headache, muscle pains, nausea and vomiting, and postoperative pain. Methods of reducing postoperative pain of patients who have undergone herniorrhaphy and circumcision are outlined in Chapter 25. Sore throat has been related to endotracheal intubation, and its incidence has been reported to be as high as 59 percent. Sore throat also was observed in 24 percent of patients in whom an oropharyngeal airway was used, compared with 6 percent in whom it was not. Headache has been reported in 12 percent of children after surgery. Both sore throat and headache are usually treated easily and successfully with nonnarcotic analgesics.

Aside from pain, the most difficult common complication to prevent or treat is protracted vomiting, which is most commonly associated with tonsillectomy and adenoidectomy and with strabismus surgery. Vomiting is twice as common after operations that last more than 20 minutes than with those that last less than 20 minutes. The frequency of vomiting in intubated, unmedicated children who receive nitrous oxide/halothane anesthesia for strabismus surgery has been reported to be as high as 80 percent.[85]

Admissions

Complications that result in admission of the patient to a hospital following outpatient surgery are usually the same types of problems discussed previously, but they occur with either greater frequency or greater severity. In a well-formulated program, the admission rate is usually less than 2 percent in a modern institution. At our institution, the admission rate for surgical outpatients is 0.9 percent.[84]

The most common reasons for admission of patients operated on in our unit are shown in Table 26–5. These can be subgrouped into anesthetic (e.g., protracted vomiting or severe croup), surgical, and social/administrative reasons.

Severe postoperative vomiting is the most common anesthesia-related reason for unanticipated overnight admission after outpatient surgery in our hospital and most other hospitals. Contributing factors include the type of surgical procedure, the presence of pain, the use of opioid analgesics, history of motion sickness, and sudden movement. As mentioned previously, forcing children to drink after surgery may induce vomiting, which may even result in an overnight admission to the hospital. We currently admit patients who continue to vomit spontaneously in spite of withholding oral fluids and administering antiemetic therapy. Patients who vomit only when challenged to drink are allowed to go home while still NPO as long as they received adequate IV hydration during surgery and recovery in the PACU.

Although croup is uncommon after endotracheal intubation of pediatric patients, it does occur. Fortunately, croup that is severe enough to cause respiratory distress almost always occurs during the recovery phase from anesthesia rather than after discharge home. At CNMC, patients are not discharged home within 1 hour of tracheal extubation unless they have been examined by the anesthesiologist. Treatment of croup with racemic epinephrine is highly effective. Nevertheless, we do not recommend discharging the patient home unless the physician believes that the croup is mild, the parents have observed this problem in their child previously and are not alarmed, the parents live close to the hospital, and the child no longer requires epinephrine to alleviate symptoms. In general, the smaller

---

TABLE 26–4
DISCHARGE REQUIREMENTS

SA.1.17 A licensed independent practitioner who has appropriate clinical privileges and who is familiar with the patient is responsible for the decision to discharge a patient.

SA.1.17.1 When the responsible licensed independent practitioner is not personally present to make the decision to discharge or does not sign the discharge order,

SA.1.17.1.1 The name of the licensed independent practitioner responsible for the discharge is recorded in the patient's medical record; and

SA.1.17.1.2 Relevant discharge criteria that are approved by the medical staff are rigorously applied to determine the readiness of the patient for discharge.

SA.1.17.2.1 The discharge criteria are approved by the licensed independent practitioner staff.

From Joint Commission on Accreditation of Healthcare Organizations: Surgical and Anesthesia Services, Accreditation Manual for Ambulatory Health Care. Oak Brook Terrace, IL, JCAHO, 1992, with permission.

TABLE 26–5
REASONS FOR ADMISSION TO THE HOSPITAL FROM THE SHORT-STAY RECOVERY UNIT AT CNMC

Reason	Number	Percent
Protracted vomiting	30	33
Croup	8	9
Family request	6	7
Fever	6	7
Bleeding	3	3
Complicated surgery	15	17
Sleepiness	2	2
Others	20	22
Total	90	100

From Patel RL, Hannallah RS: Anesthetic complications following pediatric ambulatory surgery: a 3-yr Study. Anesthesiology 69:1009, 1988.

the child with croup, the more likely the possibility of admission. Croup can be a life-threatening complication. If any doubt exists concerning its severity and course, admission to the hospital is indicated.

Surgery-related reasons for admission can be the result either of an unexpected complication (e.g., postoperative bleeding after tonsillectomy) or of more extensive surgery than originally scheduled.

Unplanned overnight admission also may be necessary if it becomes apparent that the parents are unable to or cannot be relied on to take care of the child at home.

FOLLOW-UP

Telephone calls or mailed questionnaires are necessary to determine the frequency of posthospitalization problems. A large percentage of parents have reported that their child continued to have an upset stomach, sleepiness, and so on after the return home (Table 26–6). Fortunately, most of the complications reported are mild and require no treatment. A questionnaire should be designed that detects problems of the child and the satisfaction of the parents with the care their child received. There also should be a section that requests suggestions for improvement of the care.

Any short-stay unit should collect and analyze data for trends that might indicate ways to correct deficiencies and eventually to improve patient care. Design and modification of policy are better done by prospective review rather than by reacting to mishaps. The former method leads to more uniform, safer care and minimizes the potential for medicolegal actions.

ACKNOWLEDGMENT

The author acknowledges Burton S. Epstein, MD, Seymour Albert Professor Emeritus of Anesthesiology, George Washington University Medical Center, Washington, DC, a teacher, mentor and friend. Dr. Epstein authored, then coauthored this chapter in the first three editions of this volume. His criticism and advice continue to influence its current format.

REFERENCES

1. Hannallah RS: Outpatient anesthesia. In Coté C, Todres D (eds): A Practice of Anesthesia in Infants and Children. 3rd ed. Philadelphia, WB Saunders Company, 2001, pp 55–67.
2. American Society of Anesthesiologists: Office-based anesthesia: considerations for anesthesiologists in setting up and maintaining a safe office anesthesia environment. 2000.
3. American Academy of Pediatrics, Section on Anesthesiology: Guidelines for the pediatric perioperative anesthesia environment. Pediatrics 103:512, 1999.
4. Steward DJ: Anaesthesia for day-care surgery; a symposium (IV): anaesthesia for paediatric outpatients. Can J Anaesth 27:412, 1980.
5. Coté CJ, Kelly DH: Postoperative apnea in a full-term infant with a demonstrable respiratory pattern abnormality. Anesthesiology 72:559, 1990.
6. Tetzlaff JE, Annand DW, Pudimat MA, Nicodemus HF: Postoperative apnea in a full-term infant. Anesthesiology 69:426, 1988.
7. Welborn LG: Postoperative apnea in the former preterm infant—a review. Paediatr Anaesth 2:37, 1992.
8. Steward DJ: Preterm infants are more prone to complications following minor surgery than are term infants. Anesthesiology 56:304, 1982.
9. Gregory GA, Steward DJ: Life-threatening perioperative apnea in the ex-"premie." Anesthesiology 59:495, 1983.
10. Liu LMP, Cote CJ, Goudsouzian NG, et al: Life-threatening apnea in infants recovery from anesthesia. Anesthesiology 59:506, 1983.
11. Kurth CD, Spitzer AR, Broennle AM, Downes JJ: Postoperative apnea in preterm infants. Anesthesiology 66:483, 1987.
12. Welborn LG, Ramirez N, Oh TH, et al: Postanesthesia apnea and periodic breathing in infants. Anesthesiology 65:658, 1986.
13. Melone JH, Schwartz MZ, Tyson KRT, et al: Outpatient inguinal herniorrhaphy in premature infants: is it safe? J Pediatr Surg 27:203, 1992.
14. Coté CJ, Zaslavsky A, Downes JJ, et al: Postoperative apnea in former preterm infants after inguinal herniorrhaphy. Anesthesiology 82:809, 1995.
15. Welborn LG, Hannallah RS, Luban NL, et al: Anemia and postoperative apnea in former preterm infants. Anesthesiology 74:1003, 1991.
16. Lindeman KS: Anesthesia, airways, and asthma. Semin Anesth 14:221, 1995.
17. Yentis SM, Levine MF, Hartley EJ: Should all children with suspected or confirmed malignant hyperthermia susceptibility be admitted after surgery? A 10-year review. Anesth Analg 75:345, 1992.
18. Surgicenter—a new idea for one day surgery. Resident Staff Physician 15:65, 1973.
19. Rakover Y, Almog A, Rosen G: The risk of postoperative haemorrhage in tonsillectomy as an outpatient procedure in children. Int J Pediatr Otorhinolaryngol 41:29, 1997.
20. Chiang TM, Sukis AE, Ross DE: Tonsillectomy performed on an outpatient basis: report of a series of 40,000 cases performed without a death. Arch Otolaryngol 88:307, 1968.
21. Tom LWC, DeDio RM, Cohen DE, et al: Is outpatient tonsillectomy appropriate for young children? Laryngoscope 102:277, 1992.
22. Strauss SG, Lynn AM, Bratton SL, Nespeca MK: Ventilatory response to CO2 in children with obstructive sleep apnea and adenotonsillar hypertrophy. Anesth Analg 89:328, 1999.
23. Patel R, Hannallah R: Ambulatory tonsillectomy. Ambul Surg 1:89, 1993.
24. Patel RI, Hannallah RS: Laboratory tests in children undergoing ambulatory surgery: a review of clinical practice and scientific studies. Ambul Surg 8:165, 2000.
25. Steward DJ: Screening tests before surgery in children [editorial]. Can J Anaesth 38:693, 1991.
26. Roy WL, Lerman J, McIntyre BG: Is preoperative haemoglobin testing justified in children undergoing minor elective surgery? Can J Anaesth 38:700, 1991.

T A B L E   2 6 – 6
POSTHOSPITALIZATION COMPLICATIONS REPORTED BY PARENTS AFTER OUTPATIENT SURGERY ($n = 4,998$)

Complications	No. of Patients	Percent
Vomiting (frequency)		
1–2	359	7.2
3–4	64	1.2
>4	24	0.5
Vomiting (total)	447	8.9
Cough	324	6.5
Sleepiness	297	5.9
Sore throat	257	5.1
Fever	235	4.7
Hoarseness/mild croup	168	3.4
Total	1,728	34.5

From Patel RL, Hannallah RS: Anesthetic complications following pediatric ambulatory surgery: a 3-yr study. Anesthesiology 69:1009, 1988.

27. Patel RI, Hannallah RS: Preoperative screening for pediatric ambulatory surgery: evaluation of a telephone questionnaire method. Anesth Analg 75:258, 1992.
28. Cassady JF, Wysocki TT, Miller KM, et al: Use of a preanesthetic video for facilitation of parental education and anxiolysis before pediatric ambulatory surgery. Anesth Analg 88:246, 1999.
29. Rosen DA, Rosen KR, Hannallah RS: Preoperative characteristics which influence the child's response to induction of anesthesia [abstract]. Anesthesiology 63:A462, 1985.
30. Ullyott SC: Paediatric premedication. Can J Anaesth 39:533, 1992.
31. Kain ZN, Mayes LC, Wang SM, Hofstadter MB: Postoperative behavioral outcomes in children: effects of sedative premedication. Anesthesiology 90:758, 1999.
32. Weldon BC, Watcha MF, White PF: Oral midazolam in children: effect of time and adjunct therapy. Anesth Analg 75:51, 1992.
33. Hannallah RS, Patel RI: Low dose intramuscular ketamine for anesthesia pre-induction in young children undergoing brief outpatient procedures. Anesthesiology 70:598, 1989.
34. Goresky GV, Steward DJ: Rectal methohexitone for induction of anaesthesia in children. Can Anaesth Soc J 26:213, 1979.
35. Spear RM, Yaster M, Berkowitz ID, et al: Preinduction of anesthesia in children with rectally administered midazolam. Anesthesiology 74:670, 1991.
36. Karl HW, Keifer AT, Rosenberg JL, et al: Comparison of safety and efficacy of intra-nasal midazolam or sufentanil for preinduction of anesthesia in pediatric patients. Anesthesiology 76:209, 1992.
37. Hannallah RS: Who benefits when parents are present during anesthesia induction in their children. Can J Anaesth 71:271, 1994.
38. Kain ZN, Mayes LC, Wang SM, et al: Parental presence during induction of anesthesia versus sedative premedication: which intervention is more effective? Anesthesiology 89:1147, 1998.
39. Bevan JC, Johnston C, Haig MJ, et al: Preoperative parental anxiety predicts behavioural and emotional responses to induction of anaesthesia in children. Can J Anaesth 37:177, 1990.
40. Doi M, Ikeda K: Airway irritation produced by volatile anaesthetics during brief inhalation: comparison of halothane, enflurane, isoflurane and sevoflurane. Can J Anaesth 40:122, 1993.
41. Greenspun J, Hannallah R, Welborn L, Norden J: Comparison of sevoflurane and halothane in children undergoing outpatient ear, nose, and throat surgery. J Clin Anesth 7:398, 1995.
42. Goresky GV, Muir J: Inhalation induction of anaesthesia [editorial]. Can J Anaesth 43:1085, 1996.
43. Lerman J, Davis PJ, Welborn LG, et al: Induction, recovery, and safety characteristics of sevoflurane in children undergoing ambulatory surgery. Anesthesiology 84:1332, 1996.
44. Welborn LG, Hannallah RS, Norden JM, et al: Comparison of emergence and recovery characteristics of sevoflurane, desflurane, and halothane in pediatric ambulatory patients. Anesth Analg 83:917, 1996.
45. Zwass MS, Fisher DM, Welborn LG, et al: Induction and maintenance characteristics of anesthesia with desflurane and nitrous oxide in infants and children. Anesthesiology 76:373, 1992.
46. Welborn LG, Hannallah RS, McGill WA, et al: Induction and recovery characteristics of desflurane and halothane anaesthesia in paediatric outpatients. Paediatr Anaesth 4:359, 1994.
47. Davis PJ, Cohen IT, McGowan FX, Latta K: Recovery characteristics of desflurane versus halothane for maintenance of anesthesia in pediatric ambulatory patients. Anesthesiology 80:298, 1994.
48. Cohen I, Hannallah R, Hummer K: The minimal effective dose of fentanyl to prevent emergence agitation following desflurane anesthesia in children. Anesth Analg 88:S292, 1999.
49. Hannallah RS, Britton JT, Schafer PG, et al: Propofol anaesthesia in paediatric ambulatory patients: a comparison with thiopentone and halothane. Can J Anaesth 41:12, 1994.
50. Martin TM, Nicolson SC, Bargas MS: Propofol anesthesia reduces emesis and airway obstruction in pediatric outpatients. Anesth Analg 76:144, 1993.
51. Barst SM, Leiderman JU, Markowitz A, et al: Ondansetron with propofol reduces the incidence of emesis in children following tonsillectomy. Can J Anesth 46:359, 1999.
52. Kortilla K, Linnoila M, Ertama P, et al: Recovery and simulated driving after intravenous anesthesia with thiopental, methohexital, propanidid, or alphadione. Anesthesiology 43:291, 1975.
53. Craig J, Cooper GM, Sear JW: Recovery from day-case anesthesia: comparison between methohexitone, Althesin and etomidate. Br J Anaesth 54:447, 1982.
54. Epstein BS, Levy ML, Thein MH, et al: Evaluation of fentanyl as an adjunct to thiopental-nitrous oxide-oxygen anesthesia for short surgical procedures. Anesthesiol Rev 2:24, 1975.
55. Davis PJ, Finkel JC, Orr RJ, et al: A randomized, double-blind study of remifentanil versus fentanyl for tonsillectomy and adenoidectomy surgery in pediatric ambulatory surgical patients. Anesth Analg 90:863, 2000.
56. Khine H, Corddry D, Kettrick R, et al: Comparison of cuffed and uncuffed endotracheal tubes in young children during general anesthesia. Anesthesiology 86:627, 1977.
57. Koka BV, Jeon IS, Andre JM, et al: Post intubation croup in children. Anesth Analg 56:501, 1977.
58. Schreiner MS, Nicolson SC, Martin T, Whitney L: Should children drink before discharge from day surgery? Anesthesiology 76:528, 1992.
59. Hannallah RS: Postoperative analgesia in the pediatric patient. Can J Anaesth 29:641, 1992.
60. Montgomery CJ, McCormack JP, Reichert CC, Marsland CP: Plasma concentrations after high-dose (45 mg · kg-1) rectal acetaminophen in children. Can J Anaesth 42:982, 1995.
61. Anderson BJ, Holford NH, Woollard GA, et al: Perioperative pharmacodynamics of acetaminophen analgesia in children. Anesthesiology 90:411, 1999.
62. Hall SC: Tonsillectomies, ketorolac, and the march of progress. Can J Anaesth 43:544, 1996.
63. Semple D, Russell S, Doyle E, Aldridge LM: Comparison of morphine sulphate and codeine phosphate in children undergoing adenotonsillectomy. Paediatr Anaesth 9:135, 1999.
64. Galinkin JI, Fazi LM, Cuy RM, et al: Use of intranasal fentanyl in children undergoing myringotomy and tube placement during halothane and sevoflurane anesthesia. Anesthesiology 93:1378, 2000.
65. Finkel JC, Cohen IT, Hannallah RS, et al: The effects of intranasal fentanyl on the emergence characteristics following sevoflurane anesthesia in children undergoing surgery for bilateral myringotomy tube (BMT) placement. Anesth Analg 92:1164, 2001.
66. Wong AK, Bissonnette B, Braude BM, et al: Posttonsillectomy infiltration with bupivacaine reduces immediate postoperative pain in children. Can J Anaesth 42:770, 1995.
67. Da Conceicao MJ, Coelho L, Khalil M: Ropivacaine 0.25 % compared with bupivacaine 0.25 percent by the caudal route. Paediatr Anaesth 9:229, 1999.
68. Tramer M, Moore A, McQuay H: Prevention of vomiting after paediatric strabismus surgery: a systematic review using the numbers-needed-to-treat method. Br J Anaesth 75:556, 1995.
69. Patel RI, Davis PJ, Orr RJ, et al: Single-dose ondansetron prevents postoperative vomiting in pediatric outpatients. Anesth Analg 85:538, 1997.
70. Khalil S, Rodarte A, Weldon BC, et al: Intravenous ondansetron in established postoperative emesis in children. Anesthesiology 85:270, 1996.
71. Davis PJ, McGowan FX Jr, Landsman I, et al: Effect of antiemetic therapy on recovery and hospital discharge time—a double-blind assessment of ondansetron, droperidol and placebo in pediatric patients undergoing ambulatory surgery. Anesthesiology 83:956, 1995.
72. Domino KB, Anderson EA, Polissar NL, Posner KL: Comparative efficacy and safety of odansetron, droperidol, and metoclopramide for preventing postoperative nausea and vomiting: a meta-analysis. Anesth Analg 88:1370, 1999.
73. Cieslak GD, Watcha MF, Phillip MB, Pennant JH: The dose-response relation and cost-effectiveness of granisetron for prophylaxix of pediatric postoperative emesis. Anesthesiology 85:1076, 1996.
74. Baines D: Postoperative nausea and vomiting in children. Paediatr Anaesth 6:7, 1996.
75. Epstein BS: Recovery from anesthesia. Anesthesiology 43:285, 1975.
76. Aldrete JA, Kroulik D: A post anesthetic recovery score. Anesth Analg 49:924, 1970.
77. Steward DJ: A simplified scoring system for the postoperative recovery room. Can J Anaesth 22:111, 1975.
78. Patel RI, Verghese ST, Hannallah RS, et al: Fast-tracking children following ambulatory surgery. Anesth Analg 92:918, 2001.
79. Soliman IE, Patel RI, Ehrenpreis MB, Hannallah RS: Recovery scores

do not correlate with postoperative hypoxemia in children. Anesth Analg 67:53, 1988.

80. American Society of Anesthesiologists' Standards for Postanesthesia Care (approved by the House of Delegates on October 12, 1988 and last amended on October 21, 1992).

81. Apfelbaum JL, Grasela TH, Walawander CA, Baresh P, SAFE Study Team: Bypassing the PACU: a new paradigm in ambulatory surgery [abstract]. Anesthesiology 87:A32, 1997.

82. American Society of Anesthesiologists' Guidelines for Ambulatory Anesthesia and Surgery (Approved by the House of Delegates on October 11, 1973 and last amended on October 21, 1998), Park Ridge, IL.

83. Joint Commission on Accreditation of Healthcare Organizations: Surgical and Anesthesia Services, Accreditation Manual for Ambulatory Health Care. Oak Brook Terrace, IL, JCAHO, 1992.

84. Patel RL, Hannallah RS: Anesthetic complications following pediatric ambulatory surgery: a 3-yr study. Anesthesiology 69:1009, 1988.

85. Abramowitz MD, Oh TH, Epstein BS, et al: The antiemetic effect of droperidol following outpatient strabismus surgery in children. Anesthesiology 59:579, 1983.

Appendix 26 – 1

Preoperative Telephone Screening at CNMC

Children's
National Medical Center

AMSAC
PRE-OPERATIVE TELEPHONE SCREENING   Patient's Name: _____

DATE SCHEDULED FOR SURGERY:	HOME PHONE:	WORK PHONE:
SURGEON/DENTIST:	DATE AND TIME OF CALL:	DISPOSITION:
CHIEF COMPLAINT: *(TYPE OF SURGERY):*		AGE:
RESPONDANT:	RELATIONSHIP	

SUBJECTIVE FINDINGS:

	CHECK (✓) BOX		
	YES	NO	COMMENTS

Does your child have or ever had:

Asthma _____ ☐ ☐ _____

Breath-holding spells *(apnea)* _____ ☐ ☐ _____

Croup/Bronchitis/Pneumonia _____ ☐ ☐ _____

Heart problems, heart murmurs *(Rheumatic)* ____ ☐ ☐ _____

Hepatitis *(Hepatitis B Carrier/liver disease)* ____ ☐ ☐ _____

Kidney Disease _____ ☐ ☐ _____

Bleeding disorders *(bruises easily)* ____ ☐ ☐ _____

Diabetes _____ ☐ ☐ _____

Sickle Cell Disease or Trait _____ ☐ ☐ _____

Seizures or convulsions _____ ☐ ☐ _____

Allergies to medicines, food, environmental factors ____ ☐ ☐ _____

Prematurity _____ ☐ ☐ _____

Was O₂ or ventilator required ☐ ☐ _____

History of Apnea/Bradycardia _____ ☐ ☐ _____

Is your child currently on any medications _____ ☐ ☐ _____

Has your child ever had:

Previous hospitalization/surgery _____ ☐ ☐ _____

If the child had previous surgery:

Problems with anesthesia _____ ☐ ☐ _____

(delayed awakening, unexplained fever, MH, jaundice/vomiting/difficult intubation) ____ ☐ ☐ _____

Does anyone in your family have a history of

Bleeding disorders _____ ☐ ☐ _____

Muscle disease _____ ☐ ☐ _____

Trouble with anesthesia/M.H. _____ ☐ ☐ _____

Does your child wear any prosthesis _____ ☐ ☐ _____

Glasses/Braces/Bridges/Hearing aid/Trach/Wheelchair/Crutches _____ ☐ ☐ _____

Does your child have:

Any developmental delays/learning disabilities ____ ☐ ☐ _____

Is your child prepared for surgery _____ ☐ ☐ _____

Will you bring your child in on the day of surgery?
If NO, who will? _____ ☐ ☐ _____

Does your child have any problems I have not mentioned? ____ ☐ ☐ _____

Adolescents:

History of smoking _____ ☐ ☐ _____

Drug/alcohol use _____ ☐ ☐ _____

Chance of being pregnant _____ ☐ ☐ _____

PLANS: (1) Counsel:

	CHECK (✔) BOX YES	NO	COMMENTS
Phone call from Admissions Counselor, RN will call day before with food instructions, time of surgery, time to arrive _____	☐	☐	_____
Puppet show and why prepare _____	☐	☐	_____
Explain NPO and why _____	☐	☐	_____
Any questions parent has _____	☐	☐	_____
Rules of SSRU/Surgical Unit _____	☐	☐	_____

_____
_____
_____

AMSAC/SSRU
DAY BEFORE SURGERY TELEPHONE CALL

Signature: _____

DATE AND TIME OF CALL:	DISPOSITION:	RESPONDANT:	RELATIONSHIP:
DATE OF SURGERY:		ARRIVAL TIME TO AMSAC:	
TIME OF SURGERY:	NPO TIME:FULL		CLEAR:

SUBJECTIVE FINDINGS:

	CHECK (✔) BOX YES	NO	COMMENTS
Does your child now have:			
Cold symptoms/sore throat/cough _____	☐	☐	_____
GI symptoms (diarrhea) _____	☐	☐	_____
Fever _____	☐	☐	_____
Rashes/cold sores _____	☐	☐	_____
Loose teeth, tooth aches, dental problems _____	☐	☐	_____
Has your child been exposed to: Chicken pox, German measles, measles, mumps in the past 3 weeks _____	☐	☐	_____
Is your child now taking any medications? _____	☐	☐	_____
Did you and your child attend the Puppet Show or Is your child prepared for surgery? _____	☐	☐	_____
Are there any other medical problems not discussed? _____	☐	☐	_____
Does your child have any nicknames _____	☐	☐	_____

ASSESSMENT: _____
_____
_____

PLANS: (1) Counsel:

	CHECK (✔) BOX YES	NO	COMMENTS
Times as above _____	☐	☐	_____
Reinforce What and Why NPO (No tooth-brushing, gum) _____	☐	☐	_____
Review rules of SSRU/Surgical Unit _____	☐	☐	_____
Other (Trach protocol, crutches, etc.) _____	☐	☐	_____
Any questions parents have? _____	☐	☐	_____

Signature: _____

ASSESSMENT: _____
_____
_____

CHNMC 144.1/144.2

(From Children's National Medical Center, Washington, D.C., with permission.)

Appendix 26-2

◆ ◆ ◆

Guidelines for Use of Discharge Criteria
(Children's National Medical Center)

Ideally, a physician is available personally to discharge all surgical patients. However, short-stay surgical patients may be released by a nurse when the patient meets discharge criteria established by hospital policy. (Physicians may discharge patients who do not meet criteria only after a personal evaluation of the patient and by a discharge order.) The physician indicates those patients who may be discharged, utilizing the discharge criteria stamp by writing the following provisional discharge order at the time of the surgical procedure: "[Patient's name] may be discharged when discharge criteria are met." However, the following two circumstances require special consideration:

1. Patients whose anesthesia management has included endotracheal intubation must remain in the hospital a minimum of 1 hour (time in recovery room plus time in short-stay recovery unit) even in the absence of respiratory distress. A patient who meets the discharge criteria but has had less than 1 hour of combined recovery time may be discharged by the anesthesiologist after the anesthesiologist has personally evaluated the patient.
2. Patients who receive depressant medication for relief of pain, vomiting, or dizziness must be observed in the hospital at least 30 minutes after the depressant medication was administered.

When patients meet each of the discharge criteria, it is noted in the nurse's notes. When all the criteria are met, the discharge stamp is entered on the progress note, along with the current time. The nurse then signs the discharge stamp and the patient may be discharged home at that time. To avoid confusion over the interpretation of some portions of the discharge criteria, the following guidelines have been proposed.

Criterion 1: vital signs. These include temperature, pulse, respirations, and arterial blood pressure. Postoperative vital signs are taken every 15 minutes in the recovery room, twice at 30-minute intervals and once at 60 minutes until the vital signs are stable, and then at 4-hour intervals on the unit. Vital signs are stable if over the period of 1 hour after transfer from the recovery room they are appropriate for age and are consistent with the patient's preanesthesia vital signs and those in the recovery room.

Criterion 2: ability to swallow, cough, and gag. The patient must demonstrate the ability to swallow oral fluids and to cough or to demonstrate a gag reflex.

Criterion 3: ability to ambulate. The patient must demonstrate the ability to perform movement consistent with the developmental age level and usual movement patterns (as determined during the nursing admission history).

Criterion 4: minimal nausea, vomiting, dizziness. The patient must demonstrate the ability to swallow and maintain sips of fluids for 1 hour. (Because maintenance fluids are provided intravenously during the surgical procedure, the patient need not retain more than sips of fluid.) If vomiting is persistent (more than three times in 1 hour), notify the anesthesia department or the resident in the appropriate department. If dizziness is present, the patient must still be able to perform movements consistent with age. Parents should be taught to manage their child's fluid intake the remainder of the day after discharge. Initial fluids offered should be water, cola, or ginger ale at room temperature. Small amounts of fluids should be offered in an amount the child accepts.

Criterion 5: absence of respiratory distress. The patient may not present any of the signs of respiratory distress: snoring, cyanosis, or dyspnea. If these signs are present, call the anesthesia department as soon as possible so that the patient can be evaluated and, if necessary, treated.

Criterion 6: state of consciousness. The patient must be alert and oriented to person, place, and time as appropriate for the developmental level. Consult parents when evaluating state of consciousness.

The discharge criterion policy does not require that a patient void before discharge from the PACU unless specifically noted in the physician's orders. If voiding is required, but has not occurred, the attending physician or resident should be consulted by phone before the patient is discharged home.

Appendix 26–3

Home Care Instructions Following Circumcision at CNMC

► *Circumcision: Home Care Instructions*

Note

For _____

If you have printed instructions from your private doctor, please follow those and use this as a supplement.

Activity

• May begin quiet activities.

No strenuous activity such as running, skating, jumping, or using straddle toys (walker, tricycle, bicycle) or playground equipment for 1 week.
• May return to school in 2-4 days when child is comfortable.
• May sleep on stomach.

Diet

Progress slowly to a regular diet.
• Give clear liquids (apple juice, carbonated drinks, water, popsicles, Jello).
 * Breastmilk is considered a clear liquid.

• Then give full liquids and soft foods (soups, pudding, apple sauce, soft cereal, milk and milk products).
• Then give solid foods (regular diet).

Babies:
• Give 1/2 strength formula (mix 4 ounces of water with 4 ounces of formula) for the first feeding.
• Then give full strength formula as tolerated.

Vomiting

If vomiting occurs:
• Stop feeding for 1 hour.
• Then give ice chips or sips of clear liquids.
• Then progress slowly to a regular diet.

Medications

Give your child Acetaminophen (ie., Tylenol, Tempra or Panadol) ____mg. every ____hours for discomfort. Don't give aspirin or products containing aspirin since they may cause bleeding. Acetaminophen was last given at _____.

Important Things You Should Know & Do

- Give plenty of clear liquids which will increase urine production. Urine may be blood tinged the first time your child urinates.
- If there is a gauze dressing on the penis, take it off as instructed by your doctor.
- Stitches will fall out (dissolve) on their own; they don't need to be removed.
- Some redness and swelling is normal.
- Don't put any medicines, ointments, vaseline or powder on the penis unless told to do so by your doctor.
- If the skin slips over the head of the penis during the first week after surgery, gently pull the skin back down with your fingers. If you can't pull the skin back, call your doctor.
- Use loose diapers and clothes for several days for greater comfort.

Bathing

Your child may have a sponge bath.
No tub bath or shower for _____days.

Call the Doctor

If your child has:
- any bright red bleeding which doesn't stop after applying continuous pressure for 5 minutes (Take your child to the nearest Emergency Room)
- fever over 102° F when taken by mouth that doesn't go down with Acetaminophen
- swelling that doesn't lessen (the swelling should be gone in 1 week)
- drainage (pus) from the incision
- pain not relieved by Acetaminophen

Special Instructions for Post-Op Anesthesia

If your child has any trouble breathing (ie., shortness of breath, wheezing, nasal flaring) or can't hold down any clear liquids (vomited more than 4 times at home), call the Short Stay Recovery Unit at (202) 745-5122 or the Anesthesiologist- on-call. An anesthesiologist can be reached 24 - hours - a - day through the hospital operator at (202) 745-5000.

If Questions, Call

Short Stay Recovery Unit (202) 745-5122 (8:00 am to 11:00 pm Monday - Friday)
In an emergency, call:
—— Doctor _____Phone _____
—— Private Doctor _____ (all other times)
—— _____on-call (202) 745-5000 (all other times)
Make a follow-up appointment with _____in _____days/weeks.

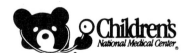

111 Michigan Avenue, N.W., Washington, D.C. 20010-2970   (202) 745-5000

18930

(From Children's National Medical Center, Washington, D.C., with permission.)

27

Anesthesia for Trauma in the Pediatric Patient

THEODORE W. STRIKER

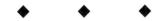

Pediatric patients who sustain major trauma present a challenge to the anesthesiologist, who must cope with possibly life-threatening physiologic disturbances. Such patients often require all available resources for their treatment. The techniques for diagnosis, monitoring, and treatment are variations of those used for adults, but these techniques have unique associated problems that are peculiar to infants or children. The treatment selected may ultimately determine if the child returns to normal health and life. Despite all efforts, the toll exacted by accidental trauma is high.

A leading cause of morbidity and mortality among infants and children is trauma. Despite the best efforts of a wide range of interested parties, the incidence of trauma continues to escalate. Accidents continue to be the major cause of death in infants, children, and young adults from birth to 24 years of age.[1] Motor vehicle deaths account for most fatal accidents during childhood, particularly for children less than 6 months of age.[2]

Accidents involving serious head injury were associated with the most morbidity and mortality.[3] Patients who sustained head injury had a 16 percent mortality rate compared with a 6 percent mortality rate among patients without head injury. Furthermore, the combination of head injury and multiple trauma was associated with death or a vegetative state 2.5 times more often than either head injury or multiple trauma alone. The mortality rate (6.7 percent) was not affected by the number of organ systems involved but was directly related to the presence or absence of head injury. "Fourteen of seventeen deaths resulted from head injury."[3]

It is incumbent on the anesthesiologist who cares for patients with either isolated or multiple trauma to initiate decisive action that will minimize the chances for acute and long-term morbidity or mortality. The anesthesiologist must ensure that the airway and ventilation are adequate, hemorrhage is detected and treated, perfusion is adequate, and the patient's physiologic status is stable. In addition, special care must be taken to prevent further damage to patients with obvious or potential cervical spine trauma.

The use of premedication for trauma patients is a subject that is seldom addressed dispassionately. Data on this subject are nonexistent. The best method of reducing anxiety in trauma patients is to reduce the time taken to perform definitive procedures, but the liberal use of analgesics can be both safe and beneficial. After adequate general and neurologic evaluation and determination that the patient's condition allows it, intravenous (IV) narcotics can be used to effectively provide needed analgesia. Assuming that blood volume is adequate, morphine 0.05 to 0.1 mg/kg or fentanyl 2 to 4 μg/kg provides significant and immediate relief of pain. Both drugs should be given slowly to achieve the desired effect (pain relief) without causing obtundation. The fact that narcotics are respiratory depressants should not preclude their use. Atropine

0.01 to 0.02 mg/kg can be given as a premedicant or when anesthesia is induced.

ASSESSING TRAUMA IN PEDIATRIC PATIENTS

The preoperative state of patients who require surgical intervention for trauma must be assessed. Ruddy and Fleisher[4] described a series of indices based on type of trauma and body region or organ system involved to facilitate initial work-up of the injured child.

Assessment of the traumatized patient includes an organized approach to the various systems that may be injured and that may play a significant role during the intra- and postoperative periods. Patients with head injuries constitute a significant proportion of pediatric trauma patients. Teasdale and Jennett[5] designed the Glasgow Coma Scale to provide uniformity for evaluating levels of consciousness in injured patients (Table 27-1).

The initial assessment and score obtained with the Glasgow Coma Scale provide a baseline against which subsequent changes can be evaluated. Bruce and coworkers[6] determined the prognostic significance of the Glasgow Coma Scale and showed it to be helpful in predicting ultimate outcome. The main benefit of using this scale is that it provides a means to evaluate the progression of neurologic damage. Allowance must be made for the effects of drugs given previously.

A patent airway must be ensured early in the care of traumatized patients. All appropriate measures should be taken to clear the airway of foreign material and to eliminate soft tissue, pharyngeal, and supraglottic obstruction. Measures should be taken to facilitate effective alveolar ventilation, with or without assistance. Mandibular fractures and other intraoral trauma are common in pediatric patients. An effort must be made to prevent aspiration of blood, dental fragments, and other tissue whenever possible. Immediate tracheal intubation is recommended

as the most reliable means of maintaining a patent airway. It must be recognized that the larynx and trachea of small children and infants are vulnerable to injury and that postanesthetic sequelae resulting from iatrogenic tracheal trauma may be significant.

Injuries to the neck necessitate a thorough evaluation of the airway to determine the presence or absence of tracheal or laryngeal injury and the extent of the injury. In recent years, the use of fiberoptic endoscopic techniques for intubation of the trachea has increased. Such techniques facilitate the placement of an endotracheal tube, either by the nasal or oral route, with minimal manipulation of the head and neck. Facility with this technique allows the anesthetist to secure the airway with minimum change of patient position, and minimum hazard of progression of cervical spinal injury, should one be present.[7] In addition, the use of radiographic assistance to insert an airway has been advocated, but has not been widely accepted.[8] Endoscopic manipulation of the airway, whether for tracheal intubation or for diagnosis of tracheal trauma, must be done judiciously, especially if injury to the cervical spine is suspected. Although awake nasotracheal intubation is routine in the adult, such maneuvers are both physically and psychologically traumatic to small children and infants and should be employed only as a last resort. Furthermore, nasotracheal intubation causes significant bleeding if a portion of the adenoid is dislodged during the procedure. Placement of an orotracheal tube is recommended to avoid complication of basal skull fracture.

Assessment of the patient's neurologic status and determination of whether intracranial hypertension is present provides important information that aids in the choice of anesthetic technique and the decision of which drugs to include and which to exclude. The use of computed tomographic (CT) scans to determine the extent of head injury is standard. It is important to take steps early to reduce or minimize elevation of intracranial pressure (ICP). Such steps include the use of hyperventilation ($Paco_2$ 25 to 30 mm Hg) and the administration of osmotic or loop-active diuretic agents such as mannitol and furosemide.

The best assessment of functional blood volume may be assessment of right heart function. In contrast to adults with arteriosclerotic heart disease, healthy pediatric patients show little if any biventricular disparity in cardiac function. Therefore, tests of right heart function give a much better indication of cardiac output in infants or children than in adults. The use of central venous pressure as an indicator of circulating blood volume and preload is helpful in patients with large blood volume shifts or significant hemorrhage. Percutaneous cannulation of major veins is feasible by many routes. Subclavian vein cannulation is frequently used in children over 10 kg, but in smaller infants it should be undertaken cautiously because there is an increased risk for pneumothorax. In infants and children, internal jugular vein cannulation has achieved wide use; femoral vein cannulation has likewise seen a resurgence in popularity. The availability of disposable prepackaged cannulas and Seldinger wires makes the technique an attractive one. There has also been a resurgence in the use of intraosseous infusion of drugs and fluids in patients with difficult venous access.[9, 10]

| T A B L E   2 7 - 1 |
| GLASGOW COMA SCALE* |

Criteria	Points
Motor response (eye movement)	
Spontaneously	4
Speech	3
Pain	2
None	1
Best verbal response	
Oriented	5
Confused	4
Inappropriate	3
Incomprehensible	2
None	1
Best motor response	
Obeys commands	5
Localized pain	4
Flexion to pain	3
Extension to pain	2
None	1

* The lower the score, the more serious the injury.
From Teasdale G, Jennett B: Assessment of coma and impaired consciousness: a practical scale. Lancet 2:81, 1974 Copyright 1974 The Lancet Ltd., with permission.

Although arterial blood pressure measurements were rarely made in infants and children until recently, they are now routine. Blood pressure is an indicator of adequacy of cardiac output, as it is in adults. The standard methods for measuring arterial pressure (Riva-Rocci and oscillometry) have been refined by the addition of Doppler and subsonic devices. However, it is still necessary to employ invasive techniques for pressure measurement if tissue perfusion is poor enough to preclude measurement of blood pressure by indirect methods. The development of small, reliable percutaneous catheters has facilitated the use of radial artery cannulation in almost all infants. Todres and co-workers[11] have successfully used percutaneous arterial catheterization in newborn and premature infants.

Pulse oximetry and infrared CO_2 analysis make possible breath-by-breath determination of oxygen saturation and end-tidal CO_2 ($PETCO_2$) tension. These excellent indicators of perfusion and pulmonary function may be particularly useful for the adjustment of cerebral blood flow.

As in adults, gastric contents pose a hazard to obtunded infants and children with decreased reflexes and to the safe induction of anesthesia. The problem is compounded by gastric distention caused by aerophagia or ingested food. Decompression of the distended stomach is not always feasible, nor does it guarantee that the stomach is empty. Occasionally, attempts at gastric decompression are frustrating and traumatic. If so, they should be discontinued.

Induction of anesthesia in patients with suspected full stomachs can be accomplished by a variety of techniques. Rapid intubation of the trachea while the Sellick maneuver is performed has been advocated by many authors and is a standard technique in adults. Head-up position, application of cricoid pressure, head-down, and head-down-lateral position have all been advocated as appropriate positions for induction of anesthesia in patients with a full stomach. Most authors recommend rapid intubation of the trachea and inflation of the endotracheal tube cuff in patients in whom cuffed endotracheal tubes are appropriate.[12-14]

Is there an alternative to using a rapid-sequence ("crash") induction to induce anesthesia? A commonly used alternative is an inhalation induction of anesthesia with spontaneous ventilation after the stomach is decompressed. Cricoid pressure is often applied. An adequate depth of anesthesia allows the trachea to be intubated smoothly, even by trainees and anesthesiologists who do not routinely anesthetize children. There are few reports of aspiration of gastric contents in this age group, which may be attributable to the decreased gastric motility associated with the relatively large doses of atropine (0.01 to 0.02 mg/kg) employed in infants and children. The use of inhalational anesthetics for induction of anesthesia should not supplant rapid IV induction but, rather, provides a safe alternative to it.

PHYSIOLOGIC RESPONSE TO STRESS OF TRAUMA

Patients who sustain major trauma are almost always in an altered metabolic state when they are seen in the emergency or operating room, owing to the accelerated catabolic state induced by trauma. Nitrogen metabolism is markedly deranged, and nitrogen-sparing is decreased.[15]

Administration of glucose is of little if any benefit in reversing trauma-induced catabolism. In addition to its lack of effect on nitrogen metabolism, exogenous glucose exaggerates the hyperglycemia often present in traumatized individuals. Hyperglycemia, although tolerated in adults, may cause a hyperosmolar state in small children and infants that is poorly tolerated, particularly when there are other metabolic derangements. It can cause hyperosmolar diuresis and hypovolemia. Glucose intolerance is probably caused by extensive liberation of catecholamines, which have an inhibitory effect on pancreatic function and on insulin receptors. In the traumatized infant or child, it is tempting to administer glucose-containing solutions to preserve glycogen stores, but this temptation should be resisted in view of the deleterious effects of an exogenous glucose load.

In light of the known alterations in nitrogen, amino acid, and glucose metabolism associated with trauma, blood glucose concentrations should be monitored throughout the intraoperative and immediate postoperative period. It is advisable to administer a balanced electrolyte solution and to give potassium after urine output is ensured. This should sustain patients until the postoperative period, when appropriate parenteral alimentation can be initiated with essential amino acids, fats, and electrolytes. Glucose can be added if hypoglycemia is present.

The blood volume of healthy infants is well described (Table 27–2). Pediatric patients respond adversely to small blood losses that are not detrimental to adults. Therefore, it is common for patients, particularly infants sustaining severe trauma, to require transfusion with two or three times their normal blood volume. Steward[16] reported that patients with thoracoabdominal trauma often require transfusion of 300 percent of their estimated blood volume (Table 27–3). Significant hypovolemia may occur before hypotension and tachycardia appear. Sudden changes in perfusion may occur without advance warning.

TABLE 27–2
BLOOD VOLUME RELATED TO AGE

Age (y)	Blood Volume (ml/kg)
0–2	80
2–16	70
>16	55–60

TABLE 27–3
BLOOD REPLACEMENT AFTER ABDOMINAL TRAUMA IN CHILDREN

Injury	Volume Transfused (% of EV)		
	n	Average	Range
Ruptured spleen	9	52	20–100
Lacerated liver	5	119	14–285

From Steward DJ: Manual of Pediatric Anesthesia. New York, Churchill Livingstone, 1979, with permission.

Small changes in blood volume are usually well tolerated in otherwise healthy children, but a hemorrhage of more than 20 percent of the predicted blood volume is frequently associated with poor peripheral perfusion. During the initial assessment, if it is found that significant hemorrhage has occurred and blood is not available for the patient, an initial bolus colloid solution 5 to 10 ml/kg (e.g., 5 percent plasma) should be administered initially and repeated as needed until the heart rate decreases or the arterial pressure rises. At the same time, a balanced electrolyte solution should be administered as a maintenance solution. Attention should be paid to the osmotic activity of the IV solution to prevent hyper- or hypo-osmotic states (Table 27–4).

Transfusion of more than one blood volume is accompanied by problems inherent to transfusion per se. If it is anticipated that large volumes of blood and fluid will be necessary, all fluids and blood products should be warmed to reduce the incidence of hypothermia. Infusion of large volumes of blood or fluid, particularly through a central line, may cause severe, catastrophic arrhythmias. Alterations in clotting can arise from a number of sources. Transfusion of old blood that is deficient in clotting factors can reduce the patient's clotting factor levels. Changes in the overall clotting function are determined by measuring the prothrombin time and partial thromboplastin time. Fresh frozen plasma or whole, freshly donated blood can be used to improve the clotting status. Platelet function may be qualitatively or quantitatively disturbed. If platelet dysfunction is detected, replacement of platelets may be needed. Transfusion of large amounts of blood often alters the cation concentrations of blood, especially calcium and potassium. The concentration of both ions may be seriously reduced, although rapid infusion of large volumes of blood may raise the potassium concentration of the patient's blood to dangerous levels. If needed, both calcium and potassium should be given in sufficient amounts to return their serum concentrations to normal. Whether to use calcium chloride or calcium gluconate to replace calcium losses is irrelevant. Ionized calcium is the important product needed. Calcium chloride yields twice the amount of elemental calcium per aliquot administered as calcium gluconate. Both are effective when given in the correct dosage.

When large volumes of fluid are administered, the function of the right side of the heart should be evaluated. Although volume overload is difficult to achieve in healthy patients when only crystalloid solution is used, it is a constant hazard in patients who have reduced perfusion, uncertain blood volume, or altered renal function, and in those who are receiving colloid infusion. The volume of fluid required can best be determined by observing the patient's vital signs, particularly the central venous pressure and urine volume. A urine output of 0.5 to 2 ml/kg/h usually indicates adequate renal perfusion unless the patient is having an osmotic diuresis.

TECHNIQUES OF GENERAL ANESTHESIA FOR TREATMENT OF PATIENTS WITH TRAUMA

Anesthesia for Treatment of Head Injury

After adequate resuscitation in the emergency room, patients brought to the operating room for treatment of severe head injury require the most complete monitoring available (see Chapter 16). The anesthesiologist should search for physiologic changes that can alter or be altered by the central nervous system (CNS) injury.

Provision of a patent airway is of paramount importance. Although the airway may not be compromised by the injury, it is important that the trachea be intubated before operation to control airway secretions and ventilation during the intra- and postoperative periods. When CNS trauma is present, tracheal intubation must be accomplished with minimal manipulation of the head and cervi-

T A B L E   2 7 – 4
CONTENTS OF COMMONLY USED INTRAVENOUS SOLUTIONS

Contents	Solution						
	Ringer's lactate	Normosol-R, pH 7.4	0.9% Saline	5% Dextrose in Water	10% Dextrose in Water	5% Dextrose in Half-Strength Saline	5% Dextrose in Quarter-Strength Saline
Dextrose (g/L)	—	—	—	50	100	50	50
Na (mEq/L)	130	140	154	—	—	77	38.5
Cl (mEq/L)	109	98	154	—	—	77	38.5
K (mEq/L)	4	5	—	—	—	—	—
Ca (mEq/L)	3	—	—	—	—	—	—
Mg (mEq/L)	—	3	—	—	—	—	—
Lactate (mEq/L)	28	—	—	—	—	—	—
Cal/L	9	18	—	170	340	170	170
pH	6.7	7.4	5.7	5.0	4.9	4.9	4.7
Tonicity	Iso	Iso	Iso	Hypo	Hyper	Hyper	Hyper
mOsm/L	273	295	308	253	505	407	330

cal spine to avoid further trauma. Stabilization of the head by an assistant or by sand bags is helpful in all cases, but particularly when cervical and spinal cord trauma are suspected. Stabilization of the head should be augmented by applying traction. Although muscle relaxants facilitate tracheal intubation, they also reduce resistance to head movement. Therefore, care should be taken to prevent excessive head movement.

The use of a depolarizing muscle relaxant (succinylcholine 1 to 2 mg/kg) should be preceded by a nondepolarizing muscle relaxant to minimize fasciculation and increase in ICP.[17] Atropine 0.01 to 0.02 mg/kg should precede the use of succinylcholine to reduce the likelihood of dysrhythmias. If nondepolarizing muscle relaxants are used exclusively, pancuronium 0.1 to 0.2 mg/kg can be employed to achieve rapid muscle relaxation without fasciculation. After securing the airway, modest hyperventilation ($Paco_2$ 25 to 30 mm Hg) should be instituted.

Coincident with the induction of anesthesia or securing of the airway, monitoring is initiated. Radial artery cannulation should be instituted for continuous monitoring of blood pressure and frequent blood gas determinations. Alternate sites for arterial cannulation include the dorsalis pedis and posterior tibial arteries. If possible, a central venous catheter is inserted to facilitate assessment of right heart filling pressures and to permit rapid infusion of fluids or transfusion of blood.

The bladder should be catheterized in head-injured patients (1) to facilitate assessment of renal perfusion, (2) to permit continuous monitoring of urine output after administration of diuretics and estimation of the adequacy of fluid administration, and (3) to allow frequent determination of urine specific gravity.

Temperature should be monitored carefully to detect changes that may indicate hypothalamic dysfunction. This determination is particularly important in smaller children and infants because their immature thermoregulatory mechanisms may be further impaired by brain injury.

Many authors believe that balanced "anesthesia" with oxygen and muscle relaxants is the technique of choice for children who require general anesthesia to permit surgical treatment of head injury. If the patient does not have an elevated ICP, the addition of nitrous oxide is desirable. In the presence of moderate to severe intracranial hypertension, nitrous oxide may further elevate the patient's ICP.

For immobilization during surgery, a nondepolarizing muscle relaxant is usually employed. Each of the three most commonly used nondepolarizing relaxants—atracurium, vecuronium, and pancuronium—has its adherents and detractors. Michenfelder[18] considered that pancuronium is the relaxant of choice and should be used with nitrous oxide, thiopental, and narcotics. The use of intermediate-duration, nondepolarizing drugs such as atracurium and vecuronium has been advocated by some authors because these drugs lack cardiovascular effects, but there is no evidence that either drug is superior to any of the other nondepolarizing agents.

During surgery, light anesthesia can be deepened with narcotics. Fentanyl 1 to 4 μg/kg is a potent narcotic that induces few changes in the cardiovascular system of patients with normal blood volumes. It should be recalled, however, that the respiratory depression induced by fen-

tanyl is dose related and may last for 3 to 4 hours after the drug is given intravenously, despite the brevity of its analgesic and sedative effects.[19]

Although halothane and enflurane are commonly used inhaled anesthetics for routine general anesthesia, their use in patients with head injuries is of questionable value. Stullken and co-workers[20] showed that cerebral metabolism was equally affected by halothane, enflurane, isoflurane, and thiopental. Isoflurane increased cerebral blood flow at all concentrations tested. Halothane and enflurane caused maximal cerebral blood flow during the induction of anesthesia; thiopental decreased the cerebral blood flow during induction of anesthesia (Table 27–5). Jennett and co-workers[21] showed that halothane increased ICP even when the patient was hypocapnic. This finding was later challenged by Adams and coworkers,[22] who demonstrated that the rise of ICP associated with halothane administration could be blocked by hypocapnia if the hypocapnia was induced before halothane was administered.

It is believed that all inhaled anesthetic agents increase ICP in a nonlinear fashion and that anesthetizing patients with these agents should be avoided when possible in patients whose neurologic status is unstable.

During anesthesia for patients with head injury, it may be necessary to actively lower ICP. Currently, four modalities are utilized for this purpose: hyperventilation, dexamethasone, diuretics, and barbiturates. Hyperventilation ($Paco_2$ 25 mm Hg) can reduce ICP because lowering the $Paco_2$ reduces the cerebral blood flow and cerebral blood volume. Administration of dexamethasone 1 mg/kg minimizes edema and helps to "stabilize membranes." Dexamethasone also decreases the volume of cerebrospinal fluid, which may be beneficial postoperatively. Diuretics are employed acutely to reduce brain water content. Mannitol 0.5 to 1 g/kg, an osmotic diuretic, is most frequently used. One author[16] recommended mannitol at a dose of 2 g/kg. Furosemide 1 mg/kg is also recommended, and the combination of mannitol and furosemide may minimize the rebound intracerebral hypertension sometimes seen after administration of mannitol alone. The use of barbiturates to minimize increases in ICP has been advo-

TABLE 27–5
EFFECTS OF ANESTHETIC DRUGS ON CEREBRAL BLOOD FLOW

Drugs	CBF
Barbiturates	↓ ↓
Narcotics	↓ or →
Ketamine	↑ ↑ ↑
Athesin	↓ ↓
Nitrous oxide	→
Halothane	↑ ↑
Methoxyflurane	↑
Enflurane	↑ or →
Isoflurane	↑

From Michenfelder JD: Anesthesia for intracranial surgery: physiologic considerations. ASA Refresher Course Lectures. Chicago, American Society of Anesthesiologists, 1975, with permission.

cated by many authors, but this point is controversial. There is no question that thiopental can reduce ICP. Therefore, it is recommended for the induction of anesthesia. A more extensive discussion of barbiturate use can be found in Chapter 16.

Anesthesia for Trauma to the Thorax and Abdomen

Patients who sustain trauma to the trunk have problems pertaining to the thoracic wall and to organs of the thoracic and abdominal cavities. The most frequent problem seen with thoracoabdominal injuries is serious hemorrhage caused by disruption of major vessels or by laceration or avulsion of organs or viscera. In this situation, it is important to insert at least one (and preferably two) large-bore venous catheters into vessels located proximal to the site of hemorrhage. If the infant or child is large enough, access can be secured via the subclavian, internal jugular, or cephalic vein.

Initial therapy for these patients is directed toward early restoration of intravascular volume, usually with a balanced electrolyte solution (e.g., lactated Ringer's solution). It also can be accomplished with isotonic saline and supplemental potassium. Replacement with whole blood or blood products is initiated as soon as cross-matched blood is available. In cases of severe hemorrhage, immediate securing of the airway and operative control of blood loss are paramount.

In patients with isolated or suspected serious thoracic trauma, the presence of pneumothorax or hemopneumothorax must always be suspected. In addition, disruption of the trachea or esophagus must be considered. Tension pneumothorax constitutes the greatest immediate risk to the patient. The airway must be secured immediately and 100 percent oxygen administered. Appropriate steps to evacuate the pleural cavity must take precedence over all other therapeutic maneuvers and should proceed once the airway is secured. Simultaneous with the institution of electrocardiographic and arterial monitoring, appropriate venous access (percutaneous or venesection) should be obtained. In patients with a lacerated lung or bronchus, anesthesia should be induced and maintained with 100 percent oxygen, ketamine, and pancuronium to provide minimal obtundation and immobilization. In the absence of a pneumothorax, anesthesia is maintained with nitrous oxide, oxygen, and a nondepolarizing muscle relaxant such as pancuronium 0.1 to 0.2 mg/kg.

Anesthesia for Early Treatment of Burns

Infants and children who sustain major burns (more than 15 percent of body surface area or involving the airway) require immediate surgery and almost always require general anesthesia. If there is evidence of airway involvement or severe smoke inhalation, it is mandatory that an endotracheal tube be inserted to secure the airway. Singed hair in the nares and eyebrows, erythema or blistering of the face and lips, ashes or burned particles around the face, and coughing indicate airway and possible pulmonary involvement regardless of whether frank airway obstruc-

tion is present. Nasotracheal intubation is desirable if the nares and nasal passages are not involved in the burn. It should be anticipated that edema and distortion of the tongue and the parapharyngeal and supraglottic tissues and the airway may be present and hinder tracheal intubation. When the airway is compromised, early tracheostomy may be necessary.

An additional hazard in seriously burned patients is gastric dilation and paralytic ileus. Attempts should be made to decompress the stomach before induction of anesthesia.

Sites for IV catheters are scarce in badly burned patients. Occasionally, it is necessary to utilize venesection under local anesthesia to establish appropriate infusion routes before anesthesia is induced.

Burn patients are subject to multiple problems related to the extensive destruction of skin. Of immediate concern are large fluid losses, protein extravasation, and loss of thermoregulation. Blood volume must be restored before induction of anesthesia. This is best accomplished by infusing crystalloid or colloid 5 to 15 mg/kg to maintain normal venous pressures. Continuous monitoring of temperature is necessary to detect the rapid heat loss associated with large burned areas. Adjustment of environmental temperature is the most effective method of maintaining normal core temperature.

After the blood volume has been restored, induction of anesthesia with nitrous oxide, oxygen, and halothane and maintenance of spontaneous ventilation allows intubation of the trachea without undue risk to the patient. The use of muscle relaxants in patients with extensive airway involvement and potential airway obstruction is hazardous. Humidification of gases in these patients is helpful during and after anesthesia.

With respect to the burned patient, the use of narcotics, particularly fentanyl, has been advocated as a program of initial treatment and as other procedures are required, the type of narcotic can be supplemented with such drugs as ketamine and methadone and has been reviewed by Beushausen and Mucke.[23]

Anesthesia for Management of Musculoskeletal Injuries

Most injuries to the musculoskeletal system of infants and children are readily apparent to the examiner. Early in the evaluation of patients with trauma, such injuries should be detected and immobilized until definitive therapy can be initiated. Although the injury itself is usually evident, the magnitude of the associated hemorrhage may not be obvious. It is difficult to gauge the volume of hematoma around a fracture site until the fracture is directly exposed. Long-bone fractures are notorious for the large, concealed hemorrhages associated with them. Liberal use of replacement fluid, either crystalloid or whole blood, is in order. In the patient with multiple trauma sites, it is easy to underestimate the contribution of a fracture to overall blood loss. Attention should be paid to this aspect of volume loss in patients who do not respond appropriately to therapy.

Patients with extensive muscle and musculoskeletal trauma are subject to other, less frequent, but no less threatening problems. Myoglobinuria and altered renal function are occasionally seen. Although fat embolism is usually a late event after trauma, it may occur early. Disruption of major blood vessels may also enhance thrombus formation. The presence of a pulmonary embolus should be suspected in any patient in whom catastrophic cardiovascular collapse occurs without explanation.[24]

Patients with musculoskeletal injuries that can be treated in the emergency room or in other treatment locations can be greatly comforted by the increasing injection of local anesthetics into the hematoma at the site of a fracture. This has been advocated by several authors who have found adequate pain relief and were able to make patients comfortable for bony manipulations.[25, 26]

The use of nitrous oxide in fixed quantities in the emergency room situation is a widely discussed technique that seems not to be frought with the complications initially anticipated by anesthetists. It is not the position of this author to advocate or disparage the technique.[27, 28]

ANESTHESIA FOR MINOR TRAUMA

Anesthesia for most patients who experience trauma is simple and straightforward. Most injuries are not life threatening and bodily function is seldom seriously deranged. In addition, most traumatized children were healthy before the trauma occurred. Other systems are not compromised by preexisting chronic disease. The major difference in treating minor and treating life-threatening trauma is one of approach rather than of specific techniques. The usual vigilance of the anesthesiologist is required in both cases, but the intensity and extent of monitoring may differ. Although the techniques of general anesthesia described above are applicable for all types of trauma, there is more latitude in the management of patients with less severe trauma than there is in critically injured children. Regional anesthesia is appropriate for patients whose specific injury warrants it, particularly when general anesthesia might be less desirable or deferred because of a full stomach. IV administration of fentanyl 2 to 4 μg/kg effectively provides analgesia and sedation. With reassurance, the anesthesiologist can usually persuade even a young child to cooperate and participate during regional anesthesia.

Infants and children who sustain major or minor trauma require integrated, rational therapy. The following is one approach to these patients. It is not exhaustive, but should serve as a guide for establishment of appropriate therapy.

I. Evaluation
   A. First priority
      1. Airway integrity
      2. Ventilatory adequacy
      3. Perfusion
   B. Secondary priority
      1. Neurologic status
         a. Intracranial function
         b. Spinal cord function
      2. Blood volume
II. Initial treatment
   A. Establishment of airway

1. Position of head and jaw
2. Insertion of naso-oropharyngeal airway
3. Intubation of trachea
4. Tracheotomy
   B. Ventilation
      1. Elevated F_{IO_2}
      2. Assisted or controlled ventilation
   C. Blood volume
      1. Infusion sites
         a. Central
         b. Peripheral (optimally it is proximal to the trauma site)
   D. Fluid
      1. Crystalloid
      2. Lactated Ringer's solution; glucose only when indicated
III. Initial monitoring and laboratory studies
   A. Monitoring
      1. Electrocardiography (ECG)
      2. Blood pressure
         a. Indirect
         b. Arterial cannulation
            1) Blood pressure
            2) Blood sampling
      3. Oxygen saturation
      4. P_{ETCO_2}
   B. Laboratory studies
      1. Hemoglobin, hematocrit
      2. Blood gases
      3. Blood type and crossmatch
      4. Electrolytes
IV. Definitive treatment
   A. Anesthetic
      1. Technique
         a. Barbiturate with normal blood volume
         b. Narcotic
            1) Fentanyl 1 to 4 μg/kg
            2) Morphine 0.1 mg/kg
         c. Relaxant
            1) Pancuronium 0.1 to 0.2 mg/kg
            2) d-Tubocurarine 0.6 to 0.8 mg/kg
      2. Induction
         a. Suspect all patients of having a full stomach
         b. Rapid induction; cricoid pressure following barbiturate and relaxant
         c. Gas induction; initial decompression of stomach (stomach may *not* be empty)
         d. Awake intubation; mask oxygenation with spontaneous ventilation, smooth intubation
      3. Monitoring
         a. Precordial stethoscope
         b. ECG
         c. Blood pressure cuff or arterial cannulation, depending on severity
         d. O_2 saturation
         e. P_{ETCO_2}
         f. Temperature
         g. Urine 0.5 to 2 mg/kg/h
      4. Laboratory studies
         a. Frequent arterial blood gases
         b. Frequent hemoglobin and hematocrit
         c. Electrolytes, particularly Na^+ and K^+

d. Osmolarity (serum and urine)
e. Platelet and clotting studies with large-volume transfusions

The anesthesiologist's participation in postoperative care varies with the institution. Problems encountered before and during anesthesia are seldom static. All physiologic variations can occur during the postoperative period and should be anticipated. Patients with major trauma require intensive care after surgical intervention. The primary site of trauma may be responsible for postoperative problems (e.g., recurrent hemorrhage or disturbed organ function). Secondary problems of major proportion may also arise de novo. Thus, a patient with hemorrhage from a fracture site or organ laceration may develop postoperative pulmonary insufficiency or renal failure. Most problems associated with trauma are largely reversible. The lack of degenerative disease greatly enhances the patient's potential for recovery. Therefore, the stakes are high. The effort expanded on behalf of infants or children who have suffered trauma of any kind provides great reward, and maximal participation is warranted.

REFERENCES

1. Accident Facts. Chicago, National Safety Council, 1986
2. Baker SP: Motor vehicle occupant deaths in young children. Pediatrics 64:860, 1979.
3. Colombiani PM, Buck JR, Dudgeon DL, et al: One-year experience in a regional pediatric trauma center. J Pediatr Surg 20:8, 1985.
4. Ruddy RM, Fleisher GR: Pediatric trauma: an approach to the injured child. Pediatr Emerg Care 1:151, 1985.
5. Teasdale G, Jennett B: Assessment of coma and impaired consciousness: a practical scale. Lancet 2:81, 1974.
6. Bruce DA, Schut L, Bruno LA, et al: Outcome following severe head injuries in children. J Neurol 48:679, 1978.
7. Wheeler M, Ovassapian A: Pediatric fiberoptic intubation. In Ovassapian A (ed): Fiberoptic Endoscopy and the Difficult Airway. 2nd ed. Philadelphia, Lippincott-Raven Publishers, 1996, p 105.
8. Morell RC, Colonna DM, Mathes DD, et al: Fluoroscopy-assisted intubation of a child with an unstable subluxation of C1/C2. J Neurosurg Anesthesiol 9:25, 1997.
9. Hodge D: Intraosseous infusions: a review. Pediatr Emerg Care 1:215, 1985.
10. Fiser DH: Intraosseous infusion. N Engl J Med 322:1579, 1990.
11. Todres ID, Rodgers MC, Shannon DC, et al: Percutaneous catheterization of the radial artery in the critically ill neonate. J Pediatr 387:273, 1975.
12. Salem MR, Wong AY, Lin YH: The effect of suxamethonium on the intragastric pressure in infants and children. Br J Anaesth 44:166, 1972.
13. Sellick BA: Cricoid pressure to control regurgitation of stomach contents during induction of anaesthesia. Lancet 2:404, 1961.
14. Salem MR, Wong AY, Fizzotti GF: Efficacy of cricoid pressure in preventing aspiration of gastric contents in pediatric patients. Br J Anaesth 44:401, 1972.
15. Shaw JH, Wolf RR: An integrated analysis of glucose, fat and protein metabolism in severely traumatized patients. Studies in the basal state and the response to total parenteral nutrition. Ann Surg 209:63, 1989.
16. Steward DJ: Manual of Pediatric Anesthesia. New York, Churchill Livingstone, 1979.
17. Minton MD, Grosslight K, Stirt JA, Bedford RF: Increases in intracranial pressure from succinylcholine: prevention by prior non-depolarizing blockage. Anesthesiology 65:165, 1986.
18. Michenfelder JD: Anesthesia for intracranial surgery: physiologic considerations. ASA Refresher Course Lectures. Chicago, American Society of Anesthesiologists, 1975.
19. Harper MH, Hickey RF, Cromwell TH, et al: The magnitude and duration of respiratory depression produced by fentanyl and fentanyl plus droperidol in man. J Pharmacol Exp Ther 199:466, 1976.
20. Stullken EH Jr, Milde JH, Michenfelder JD: The non-linear responses of cerebral metabolism to low concentrations of halothane, enflurane, isoflurane and thiopental. Anesthesiology 46:28, 1977.
21. Jennett WB, Baker J, Fitch W, et al: Effect of anaesthesia on intracranial pressure in patients with space-occupying lesions. Lancet 1:61, 1969.
22. Adams RW, Gronert GA, Sundt TM, et al: Halothane, hypocapnia, and cerebrospinal fluid in neurosurgery. Anesthesiology 37:510, 1972.
23. Beushausen T, Mucke K: Anesthesia and pain management in pediatric burn patients. Pediatr Surg Int 12:327, 1997.
24. Limbird TJ, Ruderman RJ: Fat embolism in children. Clin Orthop 136:267, 1978.
25. Alioto RJ, Furia JP, Marquardt JD: Hematoma block for ankle fractures: a safe and efficacious technique for manipulations. J Orthop Trauma 9:113, 1995.
26. Furia JP, Alioto RF, Marquardt JD: The efficacy and safety of the hematoma block for fracture reduction in closed, isolated fractures. Orthopedics 20:423, 1997.
27. Hennrikus WL, Shin AY, Klingelberger CE: Self-administered nitrous oxide and a hematoma block for analgesia in the outpatient reduction of fractures in children. J Bone Joint Surg Am 77:335, 1995.
28. Gregory PR, Sullivan JA: Nitrous oxide compared with intravenous regional anesthesia in pediatric forearm fracture manipulation. J Pediatr Orthop 169:187, 1996.

28

Anesthesia Outside the Operating Room

STEVEN C. HALL

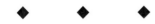

Providing anesthetic services outside the traditional operating room environment is not a new concept. The first known pediatric anesthetic administered in the United States was administered by Crawford Long of Athens, Georgia. He anesthetized an 8-year-old boy with sulfuric ether on July 3, 1842, to amputate the boy's toe.[1] This was done in Dr. Long's private office, by a physician (Dr. Long) who did not have extensive training in administering anesthesia. It was the beginning of a long tradition of providing anesthetic services in nontraditional settings. Currently, the majority of pediatric general anesthetics are delivered in well-equipped and well-staffed operating rooms in hospitals that ensure uniform and strictly controlled conditions.[2] However, anesthesiologists are increasingly asked to provide sedation or general anesthesia outside the traditional operating room environment.

Anesthesiologists are requested to provide services for three basic circumstances. First, the procedure must be performed in a special setting because of equipment restrictions (e.g., balloon dilatation of an aortic valve performed in the catheterization suite). Second, sedation or general anesthesia is requested to control patient behavior in a nonsurgical setting (e.g., the uncooperative child who needs a magnetic resonance imaging [MRI] study). And third, because of an emergency (e.g., emergency opening of the chest of patient in the intensive care unit [ICU] who previously has undergone a thoracotomy). Recently, however, anesthesiologists have been requested to pro-

vide services or advice in a fourth circumstance. It has been recognized that sedation and pain relief have been underutilized in pediatric patients. This has led parents, pediatricians, emergency room physicians, radiologists, surgeons, intensivests, and a wide variety of others to demand that the benefits of sedating children and relieving their pain for procedures be readily available to children. Consequently, anesthesiologists are asked to assist in either providing the service themselves or in making recommendations about institutional use of sedative and analgesic drugs.[3, 4]

Anesthesiologists are uniquely trained to provide sedative and anesthetic services outside the operating room based on our focused evaluation of patients, appropriate monitoring, understanding of the proper choice and administration of drugs, and continued care of the patient until the drug effects are gone. Because of this systematic and complete approach, anesthesiologists are able to provide safe and superior conditions for a variety of painful or uncomfortable procedures. By providing these services efficiently, an anesthesiologist can actually decrease the total time needed to perform some procedures by rendering the child cooperative or immobile. Physicians responsible for procedures such as cardiac catheterization, MRI examinations, invasive radiography, trauma, emergency room care, and other procedures are asking anesthesiologists to help provide humane service and advice about reasonable alternatives to sedation and general anesthesia. For an anesthesia department to respond to these requests in a timely and appropriate fashion, the department must have a clear plan about providing services in nontraditional environments.

A RATIONAL APPROACH TO CARE

Anesthesiologists have developed methods of care for patients in the operating room and ICU that are easily transferable to other settings. By using the same principles used in the operating room and ICU, it is possible to practice high-quality medicine in new locations. Our focus on preanesthetic evaluation and preparation, fasting requirements, medication selection, monitoring, postanesthetic care, and continuous quality management can be directly applied to care in non–operating room settings. These fundamental aspects of care cannot be compromised when care is provided in distant locations.

Our first challenge in providing care outside the operating room is to understand the needs and baseline practice of the physicians and other health professionals who have asked us to help them. Our comprehensive approach to a patient needing sedation or anesthesia may be foreign to these physicians, especially if they have had little interaction with anesthesiologists. Our insistence on proper evaluation of the patient before proceeding with the anesthetic, for instance, may not be duplicated in a busy radiologic practice where the radiologist may never see the child who has received sedation for a procedure. The anesthesia service must clearly introduce our principles and methods to these physicians when we become involved in new ventures. By establishing protocols and including lines of communication before actively providing anesthesia or sedation in a new location, we can define the care and coverage we can provide, as well as what is required to provide that care safely. There is a potentially significant secondary benefit to this process. As other physicians witness how anesthesiologists systemically provide safe and efficient service, they may incorporate some of these practices into their own care of children.

Establishing Protocols

Experience has demonstrated the need to establish protocols related to several aspects of providing anesthetic care outside the operating room. The first step is to survey the needs of the new service or procedure and the setting in which it will occur. After reviewing the proposed procedure and the facilities, several protocols should be developed in conjunction with the physician, nursing, and technical staffs involved. The benefits of careful evaluation, preparation, and development of consensus between all those involved in delivering care is that this preparation will decrease the number of errors, conflicts, and the amount of patient/family and physician dissatisfaction with the service.[5] In addition, it will increase reorganization of efforts of everyone involved.

Site Survey

Although each new procedure and each institution is different, there are specific issues that almost always must

be addressed whenever anesthetic care is to be delivered to children.[6, 7] The first issue usually is the site of the proposed procedure. Each site has its own unique challenges. It is important to view the site to understand how much room is available for equipment, what equipment can be moved, and how easy it will be to access equipment and patients. It is important to know if the door is of adequate size to allow equipment to be moved in and out of the room. It also is important to know where patient preparation and recovery will occur. If there is little room to maneuver or gain access to the patient, consideration should be given to removing extraneous equipment from the area. No matter how spacious an area initially appears, it will seem confined once all of the equipment and personnel are present for the procedure.

Although it is possible to provide sedation and general anesthesia with completely portable equipment, it is much more convenient and safer if piped oxygen, nitrous oxide, suction, and anesthetic gas scavenging are available. There must be adequate electrical outlets and circuits to power ventilators, monitors, pumps and, if necessary, suction devices. If the equipment used for the procedure requires multiple electrical outlets, the institution's biomedical department should be consulted to determine whether the remaining outlets are adequate for the anesthesia equipment. Electrical outlets should be located so that the use of long extension cords is avoided. This minimizes the potential for unsuspecting personnel tripping over the cords. Lighting is often a problem and must be addressed early during the survey of an area. Anesthesiologists require sufficient lighting to adequately observe, evaluate, and treat patients; additional lighting may have to be provided.

The table on which the patient will lie should be examined. Ability to have adequate access to the patient should be determined, as well as the ability to move the table and to place it in the Trendelenburg position. The anesthesiologist must not only be able to gain physical access to the patient, he or she also must be able to observe the patient easily. The physician performing the procedure usually will see nothing of the patient except the area under study and treatment. Under deep sedation or general anesthesia, patients cannot protect their airways to the same degree as when they are awake. The anesthesiologist must be able to position the patient comfortably and to prevent injury caused by pressure. The patient's arms should not be overflexed or extended, to reduce the risk of developing nerve palsies. Adequate padding must be provided, especially for long procedures. Lastly, if the table is not the same as the one used for induction and emergence from anesthesia, a roller or similar device should be available for moving the occasional obese or heavy patient.

One requirement often overlooked is the need to provide temperature regulation for younger patients undergoing long procedures. Most areas outside the operating room do not permit the room temperature to be increased or decreased. Constant air conditioning may be necessary to prevent overheating of equipment, such as radiology machines. Patient protective coverings, heating blankets and lights, or heated humidifiers or fluid warmers may be needed to prevent hypothermia. The use of portable forced air warming blankets is particularly useful for maintaining a stable temperature.[8, 9]

A means of communicating with the outside (telephone or intercom) should be readily available in the area in case help or additional equipment or supplies are required. Those responsible for providing equipment and supplies should be familiar with the area in which the procedure is being performed so that additional supplies can be brought to the area without disrupting the procedure.

Equipment needs should be established and provided before the anesthesiologist agrees to work in a new setting. If anesthesia services will be required frequently in a given location, it is preferable to have anesthesia equipment permanently based there. Disposable equipment and drugs can either be brought to the area for each case or routinely stocked on site. Since the cost of providing permanent equipment for the site may be significant, discussions with those buying the equipment—usually the institution—must demonstrate that the equipment will be used frequently enough to make the expenditure cost-effective. Equipment and supplies left on-site must be kept in secure and locked facilities when not in use to prevent theft or abuse and to guarantee availability of the equipment during emergency use of the area. Although it is reasonable to keep some drugs in a locked cabinet, it is prudent to store controlled substances and those that require refrigeration in the main anesthesia supply area and to take them to the area when needed.

If an anesthesia machine is brought to the site, there is a potential hazard for top-heavy machines to either tip over or to collide with personnel, walls, and other equipment. Wheels on the machines can easily get caught in gaps between elevators and the floor and can jump when they run over expansion joints in the floor. A machine going up or down an incline can gain momentum and move in unexpected directions at unexpected speeds. In our institution, we modified the anesthesia machines used outside the operating room by widening the wheel base and installing larger wheels to increase stability and control. However, we found that it is better to purchase additional machines and dedicate them to a site where anesthesia services are required and avoid moving anesthesia machines whenever possible.

Adequate facilities should be provided for patients and their families to sit and relax while waiting for their child who is undergoing a procedure. Operating rooms provide adequate facilities for privacy for changing clothes and waiting with family members, which decreases the psychological trauma of being in the hospital. The same consideration should be provided outside the operating room. Private changing and waiting areas, as well as a conference or examination area where matters can be discussed with the family, are important. During the procedure, the child should not be exposed to other procedures or to traffic. Lastly, parents or others who are waiting during the procedure should be informed about where nearby telephones and restrooms are located and where to purchase food and obtain water.

Patient Selection

After the site survey has been completed, the anesthesia service should establish protocols with the requesting service that clearly define patient selection and preparation. Patients having anesthesia outside the operating room must receive the same evaluation and preparation as those going to the operating room. Is the patient going to have the procedure and anesthetic as an outpatient? Will this procedure only be performed on healthy patients or will it be performed for patients who have significant underlying medical problems that necessitate the procedure? If the patient has significant medical problems, who will be responsible for ensuring that the child is in the best possible condition before admission to the hospital? Does the anesthesia department have special requirements that the managing service should know about, such as mandatory overnight admission and monitoring of some former preterm infants?

These are complex questions that should be fully explored. The considerations for anesthetizing these patients are the same as those for patients undergoing the same operation in the operating room. In some instances, the managing service will be aware of the usual requirements of the anesthesia department. However, many physicians, such as radiologists, usually are not involved in determining the overall medical status of patients. Preanesthetic evaluation by the child's pediatrician or other physician may be an appropriate routine to guarantee that the child is in the best possible general medical condition before the procedure is accomplished. In many institutions, a preprocedure history and physical examination is required before general anesthesia is administered, and there must be a separate evaluation by an anesthesiologist. The anesthesia and managing services must decide who is qualified and responsible for performing this evaluation. In our own institution, medical staff bylaws were changed to allow a single history and physical examination to be used for noninvasive diagnostic radiologic procedures under general anesthesia, and the physician (nonradiologist) requesting the procedure provides a brief, appropriate note about the patient's medical condition. If the patient's condition is clear, based on this note, the anesthesia service provides the only history and physical examination, since it is the anesthesiologist who will use this information for patient management. Complicating this process is the increased demand by insurance carriers that patients have procedures on an outpatient basis when possible. There must be a concerted effort by the anesthesia service to educate the managing service about the need for proper preprocedure preparation.

A simple solution to many of these challenges has been used in several institutions. Patients having general anesthesia for procedures outside the operating room are admitted through the operating room's ambulatory care area. The nursing staff includes these patients in their normal routine for surgical candidates. This can include instructions to the family before the day of the procedure, a call the night before to check on the child's condition, reinforcement of fasting instructions, and confirming the time of arrival for the day of the procedure. The advantage of this approach is that this nursing staff is usually very adept at detecting problems and communicating with the appropriate service before the day of the procedure. If further testing or consultation is needed, this is done before the patient arrives at the institution. These functions also can be performed by staff at each individual area outside the operating room if these individuals understand the need to communicate with both the managing and the anesthesia services.

Scheduling

The issue of providing care outside the operating room is complicated by having the appropriate personnel available to provide the services required at the time they are required. As the amount of time committed and number of sites covered outside the operating room increases, there is increased stress placed on the anesthesia service. If only a few areas are covered, arrangements made with these services can be straightforward, especially if those services schedule cases far enough in advance so that adjustments can be made in the anesthesia coverage in other areas. If coverage is requested on short notice, this is much more difficult to arrange. In our institution, services that desire coverage on a regular basis are incorporated into our weekly schedule. These services are offered a day or two of coverage each week or every other week. This coverage is monitored and altered as usage increases or decreases. It is expected that if a day of coverage is offered, enough cases will be scheduled to fill the allotted time. It is then the responsibility of the anesthesia service to do those cases as expeditiously as possible in the time available. Experience has demonstrated that some services increase their use of anesthesia services after they determine that "throughput" is increased by our presence. Other services do not provide the volume they anticipated. The governing principle is that routine coverage is provided only if there is a continuing volume of patients that is sufficient to justify continuing the coverage. For coverage on nonscheduled days, the requesting services understand that the department will provide personnel, but it may be at the end of the workday. Scheduled commitments have first priority for elective work. Emergency cases are covered the same as other emergencies in the institution.

What about the request to "run up to the clinic and give just a little anesthesia or light anesthesia for a short procedure?" One of the important educational aspects of providing care outside the operating room is to communicate to our colleagues the nature, risks, and benefits of providing sedative and anesthesia services. Although it is good medicine and good politics to be available to help provide humane services throughout the institution, those requesting the service must understand the requirements of the anesthesia service. We should keep in mind, however, that the child may receive either inadequate sedation or analgesia if we are not available or that the requesting service may provide sedation or analgesia on their own without providing the same safeguards that the anesthesia service feel are in the child's best interest.

Fasting

When anesthesia is administered in a nontraditional setting, the same rules regarding preanesthetic fasting apply.[10, 11] The criteria for adequate preanesthetic fasting have changed dramatically for pediatric patients in the last few years.[12–14] Fasting policies are designed to balance the need for adequate hydration and provision of glucose against the danger of a full stomach and aspiration of gastric contents during the anesthetic or sedation. Recent studies have demonstrated that in healthy children, gastric emptying of clear liquids occurs at a relatively rapid rate.[15, 16] This has led to most pediatric institutions allowing the child to drink clear liquids on the day of anesthesia up until 2 to 3 hours before induction of anesthesia or administration of sedative drugs.[17] There is no restriction on the volume of clear liquids the child can drink. However, even with this liberal policy, some radiologic procedures can pose problems for the anesthesiologist. To obtain satisfactory abdominal computed tomographic (CT) scan examinations, as many as half the patients must be sedated and must drink significant quantities of oral contrast agents.[18] If the sedated patient has lost all or part of their ability to protect their airway, the patient is at risk for aspirating gastric contents. Obviously, the more profound the sedation, the greater the risk that the child will lose these reflexes. Should these patients all have their airway secured before they receive oral contrast materials? There is no evidence in the literature that aspiration has been a problem in this setting. However, the physician in charge of the sedation must closely monitor the patient's condition and be aware of the risks of sedation in patients who have a full stomach.

Postanesthetic Discharge

The anesthesiologist must be aware that physicians from the managing service may have little experience with the normal course of a child's recovery from anesthesia. If there is no residual problem related to the procedure, the determining factor for discharging a patient from a recovery area or from the institution is often best made by the anesthesiologist. If the anesthesiologist is not the one who will discharge the patient after anesthesia/ sedation, there should be a clear mechanism for both determining discharge suitability and responding to problems. The standard for discharge should be the same as that for discharging patients following administration of an anesthetic in the operating room. Protocols should be established to guarantee that the family is given instructions about postprocedure and postanesthetic care. The family also should be given a telephone number that they can call at any time if they have questions. The family must be clearly instructed under which conditions they should immediately bring the child back to the institution for evaluation. If the normal procedure for surgical patients is that the family be contacted by telephone the following day, the same should be done for these patients. Also, anesthetics given outside the operating room should be part of the same continuing quality assurance program that is used for surgical procedures.

SPECIFIC CHALLENGES OUTSIDE THE OPERATING ROOM

Anesthetic care outside the operating room presents multiple challenges to the anesthesiologist. These challenges fall into four generic classes of problems, although additional site-specific problems may be encountered at any location. The anesthesiologist should develop experience and strategies for dealing with these problems.

Equipment and Procedure-Related Challenges

Many procedures require a unique equipment that alters the environment in which the anesthesiologist works (e.g., MRI scanning). Because of the intense magnetic field and the need to eliminate extraneous radiofrequency interference, the anesthesiologist often must use modified equipment and techniques. One mistake often made by institutions is to put old, outdated equipment in remote locations where anesthesia is required. This is not acceptable. The equipment used in these areas should be as good or better than that used in the operating room because there is less help available in remote locations if the equipment fails.

Patient-Related Medical Challenges

Patients may require a specific procedure because they have significant physiologic impairment that is undiagnosed (e.g., cardiac catheterization for congenital heart disease). Patients requiring cardiac catheterization, for instance, may have poor cardiac reserve that will make the administration of anesthesia especially challenging.

Anesthetic/Sedative Technique Challenges

Not all patients having procedures need general anesthesia for the procedure to be successfully and humanely performed. For many procedures, judicious sedation may be an effective alternative to anesthesia. One example is the uncooperative child who must remain still for a relatively short CT scan.[19, 20] The increased use of sedation by nonanesthesiologists makes it important to ensure that all patients have adequate preanesthetic evaluation and intraoperative monitoring and treatment. It also is important to ensure that there is a complete record kept of drug doses, vital signs, and complications each time a child is sedated.

Administrative and Political Challenges

To be successful, an ongoing program that provides care outside the operating room must have established policies and procedures that guarantee efficient care and meet the needs of both the managing service and the anesthesia department. This requires not only the participation of physicians, nurses, and technicians but also the participation and cooperation of the institution's administration. In addition, there are regulatory considerations that define the requirements for providing anesthesia and sedation services in accredited institutions. Both physicians providing care to the patients and the institution's administration must ensure that the systems of care they have established comply with relevant regulations.

Various elements of these different challenges will be part of the discussions of specific procedures.

SPECIFIC PROCEDURES

The Radiology Suite

Anesthesiologists spend more time in the various radiology suites providing off-site anesthesia than in any other part of the hospital. Therefore, it is especially important for anesthesiologists to be aware of the challenges associated with providing care in these locations. There are problems related to specific equipment, space, and anesthetic technique that are unique to each area. There also are challenges common to all off-site locations.

Computed Tomographic Scanning

Use of CT scanning in children is common and provides important information for both elective and emergency cases. Elective CT scanning is used for evaluations of a wide variety of conditions, including the brain and spinal cord, facial bone structure, thoracic masses, abdominal masses, and potential knee injuries. Emergency scans are especially useful in identifying problems in the central nervous system (CNS) and in the abdomen.[21] CT evaluation of the CNS is used to identify increased intracranial pressure (e.g., ventriculoperitoneal shunt malfunction), or the presence of space-occupying lesions, such as a subdural hematoma or intracranial tumor. Abdominal CT examinations, along with abdominal ultrasound, have revolutionized the treatment of blunt abdominal trauma. When a liver, spleen, or kidney injury has been identified by one of these techniques, surgeons now observe the patient instead of immediately operating on the injured organ.[22]

Sedation Versus General Anesthesia

CT scanning is used in pediatric patients of all ages. In many children, no sedation is needed to accomplish the scans.[23] With modern scanners and software, the time of each scan has decreased dramatically. It is possible to complete many examinations in less than 15 minutes, with each set of data taking only 2 to 3 minutes to collect. Most newborns and small infants can be coaxed into remaining still if they are given a sugar water–covered pacifier or even a bottle to suck on. Older infants and children may require no sedation, and patients who are unconscious or critically ill often do not require sedation. A skilled technologist can often time the scan to those times an otherwise fussy child is quiet. If the child is immobilized, the patient must be monitored to ensure that ventilation is not impeded and that the airway is unobstructed.

However, CT scanning does require a still patient in a confined area. Because of this, some children require sedation to remain quiet during scanning.[24] Also, some studies take a considerable amount of time (e.g., three-dimensional reconstruction of facial bones), or require an uncomfortable position (e.g., coronal sections). Sedation may be useful in these situations.

Monitoring. If the patient requires sedation, he or she must be closely monitored. Fortunately, the commonly available monitors used for this purpose are accurate and work well in the CT scanner without modification. Pulse oximeters, invasive blood pressure cuffs, capnographs, and electrocardiograms (ECGs) can all be used without difficulty. Although supplemental oxygen can easily be administered to sedated patients through nasal prongs, there has been some hesitancy on the part of radiologists to use supplemental oxygen.[25] As long as the patient's oxygen saturation is monitored closely by pulse oximetry, it is probably safe to use oxygen only when the patient's oxygen saturation decreases below an acceptable level. Pulse oximetry, however, does not detect hypoventilation and subsequent hypercarbia. Although supplemental oxygen does not prevent this, it does moderate the danger of the hypoxemia and hypercarbia associated with hypoventilation.

Although monitoring is relatively straightforward for sedated patients in the CT scanner, it is not always used. In 1990, a large-scale survey was made of U.S. hospitals and their sedation practices for CT scanning. Of the hospitals surveyed, 450 reported using sedation for some of their pediatric patients undergoing CT scanning.[18] The radiologist was responsible for ordering the sedation in 47 percent of the cases, with the primary care physician responsible for 37 percent of the cases. (Anesthesiologists were responsible in 3 percent of the cases.) The significance of this is that the radiologist, someone with little personal knowledge of the patient, routinely took responsibility for the sedation in this setting. The hospitals varied somewhat in their prescribing patterns, but reported that the use of "deep" sedation or general anesthesia was relatively rare, from a low of 7 percent in young infants (as a group) to 23 percent in older infants (in pediatric hospitals). One of the most disturbing aspects of this survey was the monitoring reported. With both light and deep sedation, the person in attendance was most likely to be the CT technician performing the study. The radiologist was present in a little over half of the institutions where sedation was used. The most common monitoring technique employed was visual inspection of the patient from the control room of the scanner. With light sedation, intermittent blood pressure measurement was used in 25 percent of the hospitals and an electrocardiogram, respiratory monitor, pulse oximeter, or automated blood pressure machine was used in 5 percent or less of the reporting institutions. With deep sedation, electrocardiography was used in 45 percent of the hospitals, respiratory monitoring in 25 percent, pulse oximetry in 20 percent, and automated blood pressure in 15 percent. In recent years, there has developed increased sophistication in the understanding of sedation and the need for monitoring among radiologists,[26] but the need to emphasize basic principles of evaluation, monitoring, and drug administration continues.

Sedation Regimens. There is extensive experience with several different sedative regimens for pediatric patients. Sedative drugs are normally administered to patients in the CT scanning area by radiology personnel. Chloral hydrate and the barbiturates have been especially popular,[23, 27–33] though other regimens have depended on various combinations of opioids, benzodiazepines and, more recently, propofol.[30, 34]

For children under 1 year of age, chloral hydrate alone appears to be the most commonly used agent,[18, 27, 28, 31, 35, 36] though children under 1 month of age usually are not sedated.[23, 27, 28] A standard first dose of oral chloral hydrate of 50 to 75 mg/kg usually is given, with an upper limit of 100 mg/kg or 2 g. With higher doses of the drug, there are occasional complications. For example, Greenberg et al. reported vomiting in 4 percent of patients, hyperactivity in 1 percent, and respiratory complications in 1 percent.[27] This study is typical of others in the radiology literature "demonstrating" the safety of sedation. Chloral hydrate is repeatedly praised as being relatively free from ventilatory depression and other respiratory complications. Although it is true that there is less ventilatory depression with chloral hydrate than with barbiturates or opioids, respiratory complications do occur. In the Greenberg et al. series, there were four episodes labeled as respiratory complications: one patient developed wheezing, one patient had copious secretions, and two patients developed upper airway obstruction that required tracheal intubation! Even with the chloral hydrate, significant airway obstruction can occur.

There has been concern expressed about chloral hydrate and a risk of cancer. The basis of the recent interest is a letter to the editor in the journal *Science* in 1990. This letter was written by a lay person and expressed concern that "chloral hydrate is a toxic metabolite of the rodent carcinogen trichloroethylene and is a mutagen and chromosome damaging agent."[37] Large quantities of chloral hydrate have been used for many years by pediatricians, radiologists, dentists, and others without any evidence of carcinogenicity. Also, the U.S. Food and Drug Administration (FDA) has not issued a recommendation against its use. The carcinogenic potential of chloral hydrate continues to be evaluated without evidence of significance mutagenic risk.[38, 39] Some practitioners have decreased their use of the drug because of uncertainty about this issue, but many others have continued to use the drug.[23]

Beyond 1 year of age, various combinations of chloral hydrate,[40] midazolam,[41, 42] opioids,[36, 43] and barbiturates[29, 31, 32, 44, 45] are used for sedation in both the CT and MRI scanners. These medications are given either intramuscularly or intravenously, though rectal administration is occasionally used.[42, 45–48] There is greater risk of complications when these more potent drugs are used.[23, 36, 49] The most common problems are ventilatory depression and upper airway obstruction. Patient monitoring must be directed to these potential problems. Both physician and technical personnel in the radiologic suites should be well educated about the signs of airway obstruction and hypoventilation and about proper treatment of these problems if they occur. A variety of factors, including temperament, previous sleep, and prior experiences in the hospital can affect the amount of sedation induced by a given regimen.[50]

General Anesthesia. The anesthesiologist providing sedation or general anesthesia uses a variety of techniques that generally are used by the radiologist. Rectal barbiturates, ketamine, or combinations of midazolam and fentanyl, and intravenous barbiturates, benzodiazepines, or propofol are commonly used techniques. Because the anesthesiologist is well trained and experienced in the use of these drugs and has responsibility only for sedation or anesthesia during the procedure, it is possible for him or her to provide exceptional conditions for the radiologist to perform needed studies. Because of the anesthesiologist's skill in the use of these agents, techniques such as intravenous thiopental can be used to provide deep sedation or anesthesia, often without intubating the patient's trachea.[24]

However, there has been a significant change in recent years. Radiologists have become much more aggressive in administering intravenous medications in relatively high doses to obtain suitable conditions.[49, 51] A good example is propofol, whose characteristics of quick onset of action and emergence, good upper airway maintenance, and minimal coughing and minimal nausea make it tempting for them and others to use.[52–54] Propofol infusions have been used to provide deep sedation or general anesthesia in children.[55–58] For nonpainful procedures, the infusion of propofol provides adequate conditions without the need for adjuncts; for painful procedures, such as invasive radiology, supplemental analgesia is needed. Anesthesiologists have found propofol especially useful for cases outside the operating room because of its controllability and rapid emergence characteristics. Radiologists and others have recognized the potential for this drug in their areas.[58–60]

In a controversial article, Bloomfield et al. published experience using either intravenous pentobarbital or intravenous propofol for sedation during radiologic imaging.[60] The propofol was given by bolus (2 mg/kg), followed by an infusion (6 mg/kg/h). Although recovery in the propofol group was faster, the decreases in heart rate and oxygenation were also greater. Of particular interest in this report are the personnel administering the drug. When the study was initiated, anesthesiologists were jointly involved with drug administration, though their role with subsequent patients was minimized. The authors noted that this regimen is only suitable for selected patients and requires constant physician supervision. However, an accompanying editorial by Cauldwell and Fisher questioned the safety of administration of anesthetic agents by nonanesthesiologists.[61] They point out not only the safety issues but also the potential liability of using drugs when the manufacturer's package insert states the drug is to be used only by personnel trained in administration of general anesthesia. A follow-up letter by Bloomfield stressed the involvement of anesthesiologists in all uses of propofol in their institution.[62] However, administration of propofol and other potent, short-acting drugs by nonanesthesiologists has become increasingly common in the radiologic suite and elsewhere.

Should radiologists or other nonanesthesiologists use propofol or ketamine or some of the other potent drugs that anesthesiologists use in these situations? This is a complex and controversial medical and legal issue that must be addressed by each institution. Each institution must establish general sedation policies and guidelines. This will be addressed more specifically later in the chapter.

As a practical matter, much of the sedation given children can be ordered, administered, and monitored by nonanesthesiologists. Personnel who take this responsibility should be working under reasonable and comprehensive guidelines to ensure the safety of the pediatric patient. If the radiology department cannot provide adequate, safe conditions, the anesthesia department must make efforts to assist in providing care for these patients.

Magnetic Resonance Imaging

MRI is unique among radiologic procedures because it does not use ionizing radiation.[63] The patient is placed in the middle of a strong electromagnetic coil that produces a field of fixed strength, usually 1.5 T (tesla). (The strength of a magnetic field is reported in tesla units. One T is 10,000 to 20,000 times stronger than the earth's magnetic field at the surface.[64]) This field induces a net orientation of protons, specifically hydrogen ions, along the long axis of the patient.[65] Oscillating magnetic pulses are then induced, which change the orientation of the protons. When the pulse ends, the protons return to their original orientation, releasing an electrical signal. This signal is detected by a receiver coil.[21] The MRI picture is based on averaging data from multiple signals. Any movement of the patient during the scanning process can produce an artifact because the emitted signal comes from a different point in space for that short period of time. Also, external radiofrequency signals, such as those from electronic equipment, also will distort the weak signal.

MRI has the unique advantage, compared with CT scanning, of being able to differentiate white and gray matter in the central nervous system. Because the intensity of the signal depends on the changes in the hydrogen ions in tissue water, small differences in tissue structure are detected.[65] This allows acute ischemia of the brain to be identified by MRI, as well as the ability to distinguish between acute and resolving phases of intracerebral hemorrhage. There is an absence of artifact secondary to bone, as occurs with CT scanning. This is especially important in detecting subdural and subarachnoid hemorrhages, as well as delineating posterior fossa abnormalities. Images of the thoracic and abdominal regions, as well as joints, are demonstrated with high fidelity. Current research is focused on using MRI not only to obtain static images but also to spectroscopically analyze tumors and to detect metabolic defects.

MRI also is increasingly used to evaluate the cardiovascular system.[67, 68] Blood flowing through the heart and the rest of the cardiovascular system generates very little MRI signal. Because of this, there is a large contrast between the blood filling the chambers of the heart and blood vessels and the tissue surrounding the blood. The ability of MRI to differentiate tissues without the use of contrast makes it useful for investigating cardiac anatomy. However, motion of the heart or blood vessels decreases the effective signal. To compensate for movement of the heart or other blood vessels, the R wave of the ECG is used to synchronize the cardiac cycle, allowing beat-to-beat evaluation of signals. With this gating of the signals, it is possible to detect thrombi, aneurysms, valve abnormalities, and thinning of the ventricular wall, as occurs after a myocardial infarction.[66–68] With rapid imaging and processing, it is also possible to use repetitive images to develop a cine evaluation not only of static anatomy but also of wall motion.

The presence of a powerful magnetic field is an important consideration when treating patients in the MRI scanning room.[63] The patient scanning area is a cylindrical space, a little over 6 feet long, in the center of the electromagnet. Ferromagnetic objects can be drawn into the center of this core, injuring the patient or anyone else in the path of the object.[65, 69] One manufacturer of these machines shows a training film where a wall of bricks is placed in front of the magnet. A hammer is then released. It crashes through the wall and is held motionless in the middle of the magnet's core. The attractive power for ferromagnetic objects falls off dramatically as distance increases from the magnet. Ferromagnetic objects should be kept at least 5 m away from the magnet, if at all possible, though the absolute safe distance depends both on the strength of the magnet and on its shielding.[70, 71] The magnetic field can interfere with the function of some equipment, such as monitors, infusion pumps, and personal objects like pens or keys, which can be drawn into the magnet. The magnetic field can demagnetize analog watches (digital watches function normally) and destroy the magnetic information included on credit cards and magnetic tapes.[72]

Any object that can induce a radiofrequency signal can disrupt the patient's signal and produce an inadequate image. Because of the multiple challenges in providing anesthesia and monitoring in the MRI scanning room, the anesthesiologist must be familiar with the various considerations related to the equipment and monitors. If there is question about the ferromagnetic content of an object, a magnet, such as a pacemaker magnet, should be placed next to be object to determine if there is noticeable attractive force. When this object is brought into the scanning room for the first time, the anesthesiologist should carefully observe the object to ensure that it is not attracted to the magnet. On the other hand, any device (e.g., electronic monitor) that can induce a radiofrequency signal into the system can disrupt the signal from the patient (because the detected signals from the patient are of very low power) and produce an inadequate image.

The magnetic field can displace or alter ferromagnetic devices located inside a patient. Patients with cardiac pacemakers are usually prohibited from undergoing MRI because the magnetic field can either convert the pacemaker to the asynchronous mode or inactive the pacemaker.[69, 73–76] Deaths related to pacemaker malfunction have been reported.[76] Ferromagnetic cerebral vessel clips can be detached from vessels by the magnetid field, causing intracranial hemorrhage.[69, 76, 77] This is less likely to occur with hemostatic clips in other parts of the body because a fibrotic scar is more likely to develop around these clips.[78] Although there was concern about prosthetic heart valves that contain metal, modern valves are not at risk for damage by the magnet.[79, 80] In addition, nonferromagnetic hemostatic clips are increasingly used and are safe during MRI.[81]

Patients should be queried about implants of all types, including pacemakers, neurostimulators, cochlear implants,[82] and infusion pumps, as part of preprocedure evaluation.[76] If there is any doubt about the ferromagnetic content of an implanted object, it is possible to place a magnet next to an example of the object to see if the magnet attracts the object. If it does, it may be appropriate not to proceed with the MRI. Aluminum, nickel, high-grade stainless steel, tantalum, and most other alloys are not attracted by magnets.[83]

The radiofrequency energy used to induce a signal can produce core body heating, but this is not a problem with currently used machines.[69] There is concern when field strengths above 2.0 T were used. Although there is a theoretical danger of heating implanted metallic prostheses, current evidence does not indicate that it is a problem.[84]

Planning of a New Unit

An anesthesiologist should be involved when a new MRI unit is being planned and built.[63, 71, 85] This will enable anesthesia requirements to be addressed so they can be provided for before the structure is built. When many of the first MRI units were built, there was little concern about whether anesthesia services would be required in the scanning room. Although there might not be a perceived need for general anesthesia at the time of planning, experience at most centers has shown that sedation and anesthesia are needed for some patients. This has led to the inclusion of the anesthesia department in the planning of newer units.

Discussions with the manufacturers of the MRI scanners have provided important information for anesthesiologists. The manufacturers' engineers and sales representatives are important sources of information about the requirements and limitations of the installation. They also are often a valuable source of advice about providing monitoring and anesthesia services, based on their experiences at other institutions.

The scanning suite should have piped medical gases installed in both the scanning room itself and in the anteroom if the anteroom will be used for clinical care. This enables the administration of oxygen without the danger of ferromagnetic cylinders in the room. Piped-in nitrous oxide also is useful. If medical-grade air is routinely used for the patients scheduled for MRI (i.e., preterm newborns), it should be provided as a piped source. If an anesthesia machine is used in the scanning room, backup supplies of oxygen and nitrous oxide in aluminum cylinders are needed. Lastly, piped high-pressure suction also should be provided. This suction can be used for both patient suctioning and anesthetic gas scavenging.

There should be a designated area outside the scanning room for patient preparation and for recovery from anesthesia/sedation. Even if the anesthesia machine is used inside the scanning room, an area outside the scanning room is useful for preinduction preparation and postprocedure recovery. When recovery from anesthesia/sedation is planned for another area, such as the operating rooms' postanesthesia care unit (PACU), the patient may require stabilization of his or her condition before transport to the PACU. In many institutions, it is safer for patients to recover in the MRI area than to transport a semiconscious patient long distances without the availability of suction and adequate help. This designated area should have monitors, piped medical gases and suction, as well as adequate electrical outlets and lighting. A resuscitation cart and defibrillator should be provided. A frequently overlooked need in the MRI suite is adequate lighting. A portable high-intensity light source is useful for small procedures, such as inserting intravenous catheters when patients have difficult venous access.

The MRI scanner is often a long distance from the areas normally frequented by the anesthesiologist. For this reason, it is useful to maintain a store of items commonly used by the anesthesia service in the area instead of transporting all needed equipment to the scanner area each time an anesthetic is to be administered. A locked cabinet can be used to store extra intravenous fluids and tubing, cannulae, suction catheters, endotracheal tubes, laryngoscopes, and batteries. If drugs and other dated products are kept in the area, there should be someone assigned who regularly checks the stock and replaces outdated drugs and equipment. An inventory list that is checked periodically will preserve the usefulness of the storage by ensuring that the stock is maintained.

Location of the Anesthesia Equipment

There are, in general, three choices about where the anesthesia machine can be placed relative to the MRI scanner.[86] The first choice is to use an anesthesia machine and, if needed, a ventilator that is safe for use in the scanner. The second choice is to use a standard anesthesia machine outside the scanning room and lead the tubing into the scanner room through a shielded conduit. The third choice is to not use an anesthesia machine and to depend on other drugs to produce anesthesia that can be administered by nonferromagnetic equipment, such as infusion pumps.

Machine in the Scanning Room. If an anesthesia machine is to be used inside the scanning room, the two most important considerations are the nature of the machine and the distance from the magnet. The farther the machine is from the magnetic field, the less attraction the magnet has on ferromagnetic components of the machine. A machine with ferromagnetic components can be pulled toward the magnet, potentially striking and injuring either the patient or other people. Also, ferromagnetic material or unshielded electronic equipment can potentially distort the image. The magnet also may cause equipment with ferromagnetic components to malfunction because valves may fail to open or close.

By keeping the machine 8 to 9 m away from the magnet, machines that contain some ferromagnetic parts have been used safely.[83] It should be remembered when evaluating reports of successful use of equipment near an MRI magnet, the distance of the equipment from the scanner and the strength of the magnetic field must be known. Studies on earlier MRI machines with low-tesla fields may not be applicable to the current MRI machines. Most machines currently being installed are 1.5 T. Manufacturers have developed MRI-compatible anesthesia machines, such as the Ohmeda Excel 210.87. This machine has less than 1 percent ferromagnetic material by weight. Ferromagnetic materials have been replaced with either stainless steel or aluminum. Either piped medical gases or aluminum cylinders can be used as a gas source with this machine. The usual safety features of modern anesthesia machines have been maintained, including an oxygen supply pressure alarm, recessed oxygen flush, and hypoxic mixture guard. The machine also is equipped with manufacturer-supplied vaporizers that are accurate, even when placed close to the magnet.

There has been great interest in developing mechanical ventilators that function normally inside the scanner. As with anesthesia machines, the two concerns are adequate functioning of the ventilator and lack of degradation of the scanning image.[88] Some ventilators, such as the Monaghan 225 (Monaghan Medical Corporation, Plattsburgh, NY), are promoted as MRI compatible, based on elimination of internal electronic components and replacing them with fluidic controls.[89] It also has been proposed that many ventilators function well if ferromagnetic parts are replaced with nonferromagnetic parts.[90] Many models of standard ventilators also can be used in proximity to 1.5-T scanners, including Air-Shield (Hill Rom Air-Shield, Hatboro, PA), Siemens (Siemens, Solna, Sweden), and Ohmeda (Datex-Ohmeda, Madison, WI) models, without modification.[87, 90-93]

Machine Outside the Scanning Room. When the scanning room is built, the inside wall is sheathed with copper sheeting to provide a "Faraday cage" that drains off external electromagnetic radiation, such as radio and television signals. This material is then covered with drywall. When the wall is being built, a copper tube can be placed through the wall into the console room. When this conduit is covered with a copper cap, the Faraday cage is intact, and there is no leakage of external signals that affect the MRI. It also is possible to place anesthesia machine and monitoring tubing through this conduit to the patient and to keep the Faraday cage intact by covering the tubing opening with copper foil. With this arrangement, a standard anesthesia machine and ventilator with ferromagnetic elements can be positioned outside the scanner and used to provide gases, vapors, and mechanical ventilation. The function of the machine and mechanical ventilator can be monitored and changed by an anesthesiologist who is located outside the scanning room. The additional ventilator tubing required for this arrangement does not cause a significant decrement in the anesthesiologist's ability to deliver anesthetic gases and oxygen.[94] A scanning room can easily be retrofitted to allow use of a standard anesthesia machine and mechanical ventilator by inserting a conduit in the door to the control room.

Anesthesia Without an Anesthesia Machine. Although we commonly use anesthesia machines when providing anesthesia, it is not absolutely necessary to do so. One alternative to using an anesthesia machine is to mount a compatible vaporizer on the wall of the scanner; gas is delivered to the scanner from an oxygen flowmeter to administer inhaled anesthetics to patients.[95] The other alternative is not to use inhaled anesthetics. Either intermittent boluses or continuous infusion of other anesthetic agents can be used. Total intravenous anesthesia is increasingly popular with anesthesiologists for a wide variety of situations and can be used in the scanning room as well. Anesthesia can be provide with an unprotected airway during spontaneous ventilation.[73] If the trachea is intubated, plastic and nonferrous circuits, such as the Mapleson D, can be used to provide oxygen, and ventilation can be assisted or manually controlled. When total intravenous anesthesia is used in the scanning room, the drugs are usually delivered by an infusion pump(s). However, not all pumps presently available work accurately in this setting. Because of potential inaccuracy in the amount of drug delivered by some pumps, only pumps that are known to be accurate and to not interfere with the MRI signal should be used.[96]

Location of Anesthesia Personnel

The role and need for an observer inside the scanning room is controversial. There is an absence of data that suggest that having an observer in the room adds information not available from the other monitors, especially when a small child is barely visible in the bore of the magnet.[97] The scanning room is usually dimly lit with incandescent lights to avoid radiofrequency interference from fluorescent lighting. Although solid-state television cameras have been focused on the patient, the image does not provide the close observation anesthesiologists are used to providing in the operating room environment.

Is it dangerous for anesthesia personnel to remain in the scanning room to observe the patient? Although there is no ionizing radiation, some people have expressed concern about exposure to a strong electromagnetic field.[98] For instance, Gangarosa et al. advised caution in exposing pregnant women during the first trimester of pregnancy to the magnet for extended periods, but these authors gave no specific guidelines for safe or unsafe exposure.[69] Outside of the medical environment, similar concerns have been expressed about living close to high-tension electrical wires. The current evidence does not support any adverse effect from exposure to MRI fields.[99, 100] In vitro and in vivo studies of the carcinogenic and teratogenic potential of MRI did not show any relationship between exposure to MRI and any of the above abnormalities.[101, 102] Epidemiologic evidence has not shown evidence of increased disease in human workers.[103] The FDA has not considered this a serious enough problem to issue safety recommendations for total MRI exposure. Despite extensive investigation, there is no reproducible scientific study that shows a health hazard associated with exposure to magnetic fields, nor is there evidence of problems associated with prolonged exposure to these fields.[100] It has been suggested that the lack of adverse outcomes following exposure to strong magnetic fields is because of the small value of the magnetic susceptibility of human tissues and to the lack of ferromagnetic components in these tissues.[100]

It is a tradition in anesthesiology that the patient is closely observed by the anesthesiologist. However, when the patient is in the scanning cylinder, direct visualization of the patient is not possible. The patient should be observed periodically between scanning runs and any time the patient's position is changed, whether the anesthesiologist stays in the scanning room at all times or not.

Monitoring Equipment

There are unique problems with monitoring the condition of patients who are in the MRI scanning room. Cathode ray displays are often ineffective because the electron beam that produces the image is distorted by the magnetic field. Electrical activity and connections within the monitors can be distorted by the magnetic field, making the monitor unusable. Wires and leads from the monitor can, by forming a loop, act as an antenna. This antenna not only can absorb signal intended for the MRI receiver, but current induced in the loop can heat and burn the patient's skin.[104] Leakage of radiofrequency energy from a monitor can degrade the scanner's signal and distort the accumulated image.

Several general measures can be taken to minimize interference caused by the monitor. The monitor should be placed as far from the center of the magnetic field as possible.[105] Monitors containing a low amount of ferromagnetic material are preferable. Several manufacturers now use nonferromagnetic components, filters, and shielding to produce a variety of monitors suitable for use in the MRI scanning room. Some manufacturers offer single monitors, whereas others offer entire systems that include noninvasive blood pressure, electrocardiogram, pulse oximetry, capnography, and respiratory plethysmography. Several manufacturers work with the MRI scanner manufacturers to ensure compatibility of their monitors.

Electrocardiography has been a difficult monitoring modality to use during MRI. The electrocardiograph can be a source of patient injury (burn) and signal degradation. The electrocardiograph also may not function accurately if not properly shielded. Concern has been expressed about using conventional ECG monitoring during MRI.[106] The concern is related to the wires used to attach the electrodes to the cable.[107] Because the wires are ferromagnetic, they can cause significant distortion of the ECG signal by the strong magnetic field. It is possible to improve the ECG by using telemetric leads and a base station.[73] This is not widely used. Another concern is the risk of burns. If the wires form a loop, a current can be induced in this loop, the wire can overheat, and thermal injury can occur.

Several suggestions have been made that can minimize both patient injury and signal degradation.[108, 109] Based on advice from the engineers who installed the MRI machine in our own institution, several changes in the orientation of the ECG leads were made. Using these recommendations, none of our patients have had visible burns. The suggestions are:

1. Use a four-lead system instead of a three-lead system. The fourth lead is used as a second ground. All leads are kept close to the center of the patient's trunk. The incidence of ECG artifacts has been significantly lower than with a three-lead system. The wires are checked before each use to ensure that no fraying of the insulation has occurred.

2. Place a cloth beneath the four wires. A folded sheet is placed on the patient's skin and the lead wires so that the wires attached to the electrodes do not come in contact with the patient's skin. Even if the lead wires become hot, there is a buffer between them and the patient's skin.

3. Braid the wires together as soon as possible. The reason for this is to prevent a loop, with subsequent induction of current, from forming.

4. When the patient is moved, the position of the wires is rechecked. Moving the patient into or out of the scanner may cause the wires to coil and form a loop. The only way to ensure that the arrangement of wire has not changed is to visibly check all wires each time the patient is moved. If the patient is sedated, but not anesthetized, there is the constant risk that the patient will move and cause the wires to form a loop. The patient must be observed closely for signs of movement and a change in the configuration of the wires. This is more easily done if the anesthesiologist remains in the scanner with the patient during the scan.

An alternative to the ECG is pulse monitoring. For instance, there is a fiberoptic-based system that detects capillary blood flow. A laser Doppler probe can be placed on either an earlobe or lip to measure capillary blood flow and, by measuring fluctuations in the capillary blood volume, detect changes in the cardiac cycle. Because the signal is transmitted from the probe by a fiberoptic cable, the strong magnetic field has no effect on the cable or the signal.[66]

Pulse oximetry is a valuable and crucial monitor for both sedated and anesthetized patients. Early models were susceptible to interference from the magnetic field and were a source of interference for the MRI signal. Currently available models provide accurate, continuous determinations of SaO_2 in the scanning room. Models are available from many manufacturers that are reliable, including Invivo Research (Orlando, FL), Nonin Medical (Plymouth, MN),[106] Datex-Ohmeda (Madison, WI),[92] and Criticare (Pewaukee, WI). These monitors rely on a low ferromagnetic content, heavy insulation, and periodic filters to produce an accurate signal. The oximeter probe is placed as far from the center of the magnet as possible to minimize interference. As with ECG wires, a loop in the cable can act as an antenna that can cause heat buildup and a burn.[110] A loop in the cable also can cause the monitor to act as a source of radiofrequency signals that can interfere with the MRI signal and degrade the image.[111] Because of the importance of pulse oximetry, anesthesiologists anesthetizing patients for MRIs should only use oximeters that work well in this environment.

Arterial blood pressure can be measured by standard cuffs and manometers.[64] Some manometers contain sufficient ferromagnetic material that the manometer must be placed 7 to 10 m from the bore of the magnet. Extra-long tubing must be used so this can be accomplished. Automated cuffs from several manufacturers, such as Critikon (Tampa, FL),[92] Invivo Research (Orlando, FL),[112] and Datascope (Paramus, NJ),[113] can be used in the scanning room without artifact or inaccurate results. These cuffs are used with extra-long tubing to allow the unit to be observed through the console window and to keep the base unit as far from the magnet as possible. Alternatively, the data can be transmitted to a monitor outside the scanning room in some integrated systems. Intra-arterial pressure can be measured, if necessary. Long, low-compliance arterial line tubing allows transducers to be placed as far as possible from the magnet, decreasing the chance of causing artifacts in the measurements.[114]

Capnography can be used in the MRI scanning room. Commercially available units use a long plastic sampling catheter so the base of the unit can be placed several meters from the magnet.[92, 115] Capnography is used to "fine tune" ventilation in the anesthetized patient, as well as to detect apnea or circuit disconnects. The long tubing delays the gas sample from reaching the base unit, though this delay can be minimized by using low-compliance tubing with a small diameter. The tracing also may be damped, giving more of a mean value instead of the clear expiratory pattern usually seen in the operating room. Capnography also can be used in nonintubated sedated or anesthetized patients. A nasal cannula connected to the monitor will give reliable readings, even if the other channel of the nasal cannula is used to deliver oxygen.

Precordial and esophageal stethoscopes can be used in the scanning room if they are made of plastic.[83] However, these devices are of limited use during scanning because of the noise the scanner makes when active. For this reason, stethoscopes are most useful for intermittent evaluation of breath and heart sounds, especially if there is a question about endotracheal tube placement or if there is difficulty with the other monitoring equipment. It is possible to use an amplified microphone to increase the usefulness of this monitor.[116]

Advances in electronics and engineering have produced a variety of improvements in monitoring devices that improve our ability to monitor the condition of infants and children in the difficult environment of the MRI scanning room. We now have available the capability to monitor the same parameters that we do in the operating room. Working closely with the radiologists during the planning phase when new scanners are being installed will ensure that proper monitors are available when needed for patients in the MRI scanner. When deciding which monitors to use in the MRI scanner, one factor to consider is whether it is better to purchase individual monitors (automated blood pressure, pulse oximeter, capnograph) or to purchase an integrated system. Individual monitors have the advantage of portability and low individual purchase price, whereas an integrated system has the advantage of displaying all covered functions in a single display, usually in the control room. An integrated system also can be networked into the hospital's information system for access in other locations or permanent record keeping. The needs of both the radiologist and anesthesiologist should be considered when making this decision.

Anesthetic Technique

As with CT scanning, there are a variety of ways to provide adequate scanning conditions, including nonpharmacologic methods that provide immobility,[117, 118] though most young children require some sedation to accomplish the procedure. In many institutions, sedation is administered by the radiologists.[51, 119–121] The rates for successful sedation of patients who require MRI scanning vary. Some radiologists find that they are able to provide adequate sedation in the vast majority of procedures without the need for excessive sedation.[28, 49, 51, 122, 123] If the radiology service is unable to provide adequate conditions using regimens they are comfortable with, the anesthesia department may be asked to anesthetize the patient.

There has been a recent trend for radiologists to develop sedation services for their patients that are heavily dependent on nurses.[124, 125] These services are based on protocol-driven approaches to sedation, with the nursing service having varying degrees of autonomy.[126] Radiologists who have published their experiences with a nurse-based service often are very enthusiastic about the level of sedation and throughput of patients. However, because the radiologists are ultimately responsible for all activities of the supervised nurses, a nurse-based service must be constantly evaluated by the responsible physicians and not be used as a means to avoid involvement with sedated patients.

In other institutions, the anesthesia department provides deep sedation or general anesthesia for most or all children having an MRI scan. Because the incidence of anesthesia department involvement in the MRI suite varies dramatically by institution, it is difficult to give guidelines about how often the anesthesia department should be participating in the MRI suite. This must be worked out between each radiology and anesthesia department.[127]

The primary goal of the anesthesiologist providing care in the MRI scanning room is to ensure that good imaging conditions are provided in a safe, humane, and expeditious fashion.[127] Because the MRI scan is composed of summated data, the patient must be immobile for relatively long periods (up to 20 minutes per scan). Patients, especially children, are not comfortable lying still for such long periods. Also, the child is placed in a confined space, with no contact with parents or others, for this time. Lastly, MRI is very noisy (up to 95 dB).[69] To put this in perspective, the Occupational Safety and Health Administration guidelines for maximal noise exposure limit daily exposure at this level to 2 hours a day.[128] The use of ear plugs or headphones minimizes the exposure of awake or sedated patients and of anesthesiologists to the noise.

For short scans, a single dose of ketamine, rectal methohexital, or other similar regimen has been used by some practitioners. However, most examinations last longer than the effects of a single dose of these drugs. Intravenous anesthesia has been accomplished with a variety of agents[129, 130] and inhalation techniques.[131] A wide variety of sedative and anesthetic techniques have been used for patients undergoing MRI. However, there is no evidence that one technique is superior to others. Despite this, individual anesthesiologists have developed regimens for the procedure that they feel work well in their circumstance.

"Open" MRI scanners are now available that make it unnecessary to place the child in a closed cylinder. It is possible that these scanners and those with faster imaging times will reduce the need for sedation and/or anesthesia.[132] Because it is possible to have a parent present when using "open" scanners, the question of parental presence

during sedation may become an issue. Although there is little information about parental presence during sedation for MRI scanning, our experience with parental presence for induction of anesthesia may provide a guide for deciding about the appropriateness of parental presence in this setting.[133, 134]

When anesthetizing children outside the operating room, special attention should be paid to ensuring an expeditious awakening of the patient at the end of the procedure. For this reason, propofol infusion has been used frequently to provide an adequate level of anesthesia and quick awakening and recovery from anesthesia.[129, 135] As mentioned earlier, there are infusion pumps available that can be used effectively and safely in the scanning room, making the continuous infusion of propofol a viable anesthetic technique for this purpose. It has been suggested that children who do not have increased intracranial pressure or a full stomach do not always require tracheal intubation when propofol is infused continuously.[136]

When deep sedation or general anesthesia is administered without a protected airway in the MRI scanner, the anesthesiologist must ensure patency of the airway. Once the desired depth of sedation or anesthesia is achieved, the child is positioned to minimize upper airway obstruction. The head is supported by rolls and a foam "donut" is placed under the occiput to prevent lateral movement of the head. Some patients may benefit from inserting a roll under the patient's shoulders. Flexion of the neck or extension of the head may be required to provide a clear airway. There is evidence that a chin lift is the best maneuver to open the airway of sedated or anesthetized patients.[137] If there is doubt about stability of the cervical spine, these maneuvers must be done in consultation with the child's neurosurgeon or neurologist. Occasionally, it will be necessary to secure the head in the desired position with a strip of adhesive tape. In the sedated patient, administration of supplemental oxygen can be accomplished using nasal prongs or taping a gas hose near the patient's mouth.

Although an unprotected airway can be used for many patients who are sedated or anesthetized, this may not be wise when sedating/anesthetizing several types of patient. Because the patient is hard to see in the scanner, the practitioner must be confident that the patient's upper airway is unobstructed or hypoventilation will develop during the scan. Patients that have a history of airway obstruction, obesity, or gastroesophageal reflux may benefit from securing the airway. Critically ill patients (increased intracranial pressure, cardiopulmonary instability, or altered level of consciousness) are at risk for hypoventilation and hypoxemia in this setting and would benefit from having a secured airway.[138] Patients in whom it is necessary to induce short periods of apnea (e.g., those undergoing MRI scans of the lung) will benefit from tracheal intubation because they will require hyperventilation to induce apnea.

In our institution, most infants who receive general anesthesia have their tracheas intubated and their lungs ventilated. This enables us to establish a level of ventilation that is relatively constant throughout the scan. If tracheal intubation is accomplished outside the scanning room, a standard laryngoscope can be used. If trachel intubation is performed in the scanning room, a standard metal laryngoscope is not used because it can be drawn into the magnet. In the magnet room, plastic laryngoscopes with the ferromagnetic batteries replaced with lithium batteries are used to prevent the scope from being drawn into the magnet.[71, 139] Capnography is used to monitor both the adequacy of ventilation and the possibility of airway obstruction or other changes in the pattern of ventilation. When the patient is in the scanner, he or she is effectively removed from observers. Intermittent movement of the patient during scanning poses a significant risk for disconnection of the breathing circuit from the endotracheal tube. The use of both a ventilator disconnect alarm and a capnograph allows early detection of airway disconnections. Because the trachea is intubated and the lungs are ventilated, any anesthetic agent can be used. The specific regimen depends on the status of the patient[113, 114]; critically ill children who have the potential for increased intracranial pressure, for instance, receive the same anesthetic they would receive in the operating room. If support measures such as inotropic infusions, elevated positive end-expiratory pressure (PEEP), or high inspired oxygen levels were required before arriving in the MRI suite, these measures must be continued during the scan.

The laryngeal mask airway (LMA) has proven to be very useful in the management of the airway in this setting.[140, 141] The mask is easy to insert and, in most patients, provides a good airway for both spontaneous and controlled ventilation.[142–144] Relatively "light" levels of anesthesia can be used without the patient coughing or breath-holding. However, because experience is required to properly insert and evaluate the mask airway, practitioners should gain experience with it in the operating room, before using it in a situation where the patient is physically removed from observation.

Cardiopulmonary Resuscitation

There should be a policy that is clearly understood by both the radiology and anesthesia staffs about where cardiopulmonary resuscitation will take place. Should resuscitation be attempted in the scanning room or should the patient be moved to the waiting area outside? The advantage of initial resuscitation inside the scanning room is that full efforts are initiated as soon as the child is removed from the magnet tunnel. The advantage of moving the child outside the room is the ability to use standard resuscitation equipment in an area that has more capacity than the scanning room. There is at least one report of a defibrillator with ferromagnetic batteries failing in the presence of the strong magnetic field.[145] Also, personnel responding to the arrest do not have to be concerned about removing all ferromagnetic materials from their persons before entering the area for resuscitation. In the rush to resuscitate the patient, someone may enter the magnet room with metal in their pocket, which may injure the patient or others if the metal object is drawn into the magnet. If resuscitation is carried out outside the scanning room, basic life support measures should be started as soon as the patient is removed from the magnet tunnel. Because of the special nature of the scanning area, mock

resuscitations should be practiced so that the personnel assigned to the area are familiar with their expected roles.

Surgery in the MRI Suite

One recent advance is the use of MRI to guide the surgeon and to help him or her evaluate the effectiveness of surgical procedures.[85, 146–150] Percutaneous needle biopsies of the brain or other parts of the body, tumor resections, evacuation of cyst, and laminectomies are among the procedures performed in MRI scanners. Two different approaches have been used for these procedures. The first involves performing the surgical procedure adjacent to the scanner where the field strength is low and then inserting the patient into the scanner when imaging is required.[149] The second approach requires construction of a unit that specifically enables surgery to be accomplished while the patient is in the scanner on a movable bed or when the scanner moves.[146–148] The MRI scanners used for this work are of lower strength (0.5 T) than conventional scanners. Thus, there are fewer problems related to the attractive potential of the magnet.

Because of the close proximity between the anesthesiologist, the anesthesia equipment, and the scanner, all anesthesia equipment must be MRI-compatible. Because of the potential for problems occurring during anesthesia and surgery when the patient is in the scanner, it is especially important that the anesthesia service be involved in the design of the operating suite to ensure that the anesthesiologists understand the limitations of the suite and that the requirements for safe patient management are met.[85] Since many of the procedures that will be performed in this setting will require general anesthesia, it is reasonable that any new anesthesia equipment required to safely accomplish anesthesia for these cases should be part of the budget of the new unit.

Recovery

For at least two reasons, postanesthetic recovery is more of a problem with MRI than with other sites outside the operating room. First, patients that require MRI often have significant CNS disease or other problems. Therefore, knowledge and expertise in caring for these particular patients is required. Second, the MRI suite is often a long distance from the PACU, where most other patients recover from anesthesia. Transfer to a recovery area without supplemental oxygen can result in hypoxemia.[151] Transfer of patients over long distances without adequate monitoring or supplemental oxygen may increase this risk. For these reasons, many institutions provide postanesthetic care on-site. If the latter is the choice, the same facilities and nursing that are provided in the PACU (and demanded by local and state statute) should be provided in the MRI area.[152] This requires that the nurses be trained in proper monitoring and recovery procedures. Because of the relatively long scan times required for an MRI scan compared with a CT scan, more sedation is required and recovery takes longer.[163]

Several issues complicate recovery from general anesthesia of patients who have undergone MRI. Not all MRI units have full-time nursing staff assigned to the area. If recovery from anesthesia/sedation is to be accomplished locally, the nursing staff must be available and must not have responsibilities that take them away from the recovering patient. Unless there is a significant volume of patients who require sedation/anesthesia, hiring additional nurses to provide coverage of these areas during recovery from anesthesia/sedation may not be considered cost-effective. Because these areas usually are isolated, there is less support from other nurses and physicians if an emergency arises. Lastly, physician responsibilities for supervision of recovery from anesthesia/sedation and discharge from the MRI suite must be clearly delineated. This is especially important if the patient is leaving the institution instead of returning to a bed in the hospital. Is the anesthesiologist responsible for discharge of the patient or is it the responsibility of the radiologist? More importantly, does a physician have to see the patient before discharge? In some institutions, if the child meets specific criteria for alertness and recovery, such as a recovery score, the nurse can discharge the patient from the unit. In other institutions, a physician must see the patient before discharge. There are few good data in the literature to support either approach. The anesthesia and radiology departments must decide what they will do and involve the institution's legal department if necessary. The guiding principle must be that patients only can be discharged when the nurses and physicians are sure that it is safe for the patient to leave the institution.

Angiography and Embolization

Angiography is performed for a variety of reasons, but diagnosis of cerebral tumors or vascular malformations is the most common reason an anesthesiologist is required during angiography. Patients undergoing angiography have pain when percutaneous catheters are inserted and when dye is injected. If the patient moves during the injection of dye, subsequent images may be inadequate.

Before providing sedation or anesthesia for cerebral angiography, the anesthesiologist must assess the patient's medical condition. If there is evidence that the patient has increased intracranial pressure, the monitoring and the anesthetic techniques must be equivalent to those used were the patient having a surgical procedure. Hypertension induced by laryngoscopy or other maneuvers must be avoided to minimize the danger of causing intracranial hemorrhage, especially if the patient has an aneurysm or a vascular malformation.[106, 154] Ventilation should be controlled.[70, 115] Mild hyperventilation will prevent further increases in intracranial pressure and slow the passage of dye through the brain. This improves the quality of the study. Spontaneous ventilation plus anesthesia using a volatile anesthetic may increase cerebral blood flow and volume, which is undesirable if the intracranial pressure is already increased.

The most common problems the anesthesiologist encounters during cerebral angiography occur when the contrast media is injected. Contrast agents are divided into two types, the older high-osmolality agents (1,400 to 1,500 mOsm/L) and the newer low-osmolality agents (600 to 700 mOsm/L).[156] The older (and less costly) agents have a higher incidence of adverse reactions.[157] Contrast agents

have direct myocardial depressant, arrhythmogenic, and vasodilating properties. They often cause transient hypertension followed by hypotension when these drugs are injected. These changes may be significant in patients who have the potential for bleeding or ischemia. The dye also can induce seizures and cerebral edema. Because of its osmolality, the dye induces a diuresis. For long procedures, a urinary catheter should be inserted to both empty the bladder and to guide volume administration. Unfortunately, these dyes are nephrotoxic in large doses.[158] For these reasons, a running total of the amount of dye injected should be kept. The volume of dye administered is usually limited to 4 ml/kg in a healthy child under 1 year of age and 6 ml/kg in older children.[159]

Some patients develop significant systemic reactions following injection of the dye. These reactions are related to chemotoxic responses, such as histamine release and complement activation.[21, 160] Reactions as mild as nausea, vomiting, and flushing may occur, but bronchospasm, angioneurotic edema, and anaphylaxis also occur and can be immediately life threatening. Treatment of these reactions is the same as that with other allergic reactions. Useful agents include diphenhydramine, steroids, oxygen, fluids and, if necessary, epinephrine.[161] Patients with a history of previous allergic reactions to contrast media may benefit from prophylactic steroids and antihistamines.[162, 163]

The total dose of radiation a patient receives during a long angiographic procedure can be significant.[164] The anesthesiologist is often situated near the patient. Consequently, he or she must be very careful to stay behind protective shielding as much as possible and to inform the angiographer whenever he or she (the anesthesiologist) is not protected with lead. If the anesthesiologist frequently provides care for patients in a setting where he or she is repeatedly exposed to ionizing radiation, he or she should wear a radiation monitoring badge so the total exposure to ionizing radiation can be kept within a safe level.[165]

Angiography of renal, adrenal, hepatic, or peripheral vessels is occasionally performed in children. There is usually no specific indication or contraindication to the type of anesthetic used. However, the anesthesiologist must be familiar with the intended procedure and its possible complications. For instance, if the study is being performed to detect a pheochromocytoma, the anesthesiologist must evaluate the child before proceeding to determine if aggressive medical pretreatment of hypertension and volume depletion is required before angiography is performed. When the child is properly prepared, the anesthesiologist must be prepared to quickly treat sudden hypertension, which often occurs when the dye is injected into the circulation of the suspected tumor. In addition, the patient may have significant physiologic abnormalities that are related to the underlying problem (e.g., liver failure) for which the angiogram is being obtained. These problems can influence the anesthetic management. The anesthesiologist must clearly understand the patient's current medical status before proceeding.

Angiography may be combined with embolization to treat arteriovenous malformations. These malformations may occur in the periphery or in internal organs (e.g., liver).[166] The patient must be evaluated before anesthesia is induced to ensure that the patient's cardiovascular system is stable. Persistent bleeding from the malformation may have left the patient hypovolemic. Newborns and infants who have large arteriovenous malformations may be in high-output cardiac failure at the time they present for angiography.[167] The patient's condition should be stabilized as much as possible before proceeding with anesthesia.[168] Embolization is usually accomplished with materials such as Gelfoam pledgets, wire coils, or cyanoacrylates. Occasionally, toxic chemicals, such as alcohol, are used. Complications such as bleeding or migration of the embolic material to a distal site may require surgical intervention. This usually entails taking the anesthetized patient to the operating room as an emergency so the surgeons can widely expose the area at risk. These complications occur rarely, but the ability to aggressively treat them must be available.

Radiation Oncology Therapy

Patients with radiosensitive tumors require multiple, short radiation therapy treatments.[169] Treatment of these children present two challenges to the anesthesiologist. First, the child must remain very still for the short duration of the treatment. It is crucial that the child not move during the treatment. Because the ambient radiation in the room is high, the anesthesiologist cannot remain in the room with the patient during treatment. The second challenge is that the treatments occur every day or every few days for several weeks.[170, 171]

Because the anesthesiologist cannot remain in the room during the treatment, an adequate level of anesthesia is induced by one of several means, and the anesthesiologist then must leave the room. The child's condition is monitored by using cameras to observe the patient and the monitor displays.[172] The quality of image is not always high grade, but it is usually adequate to clearly see the pulse oximeter readings.

The anesthetic technique used should ensure a few minutes of safe sleep. Because of the shortness of the procedure, it is rare that tracheal intubation or LMA insertion is required.[173] Rectal barbiturates are useful for short procedures like this if the patient is amenable.[171, 174] Rectal methohexital 25 to 35 mg/kg has been used for radiotherapy; awakening following the procedure has been rapid,[171] though tachyphylaxis may develop after repeated administrations of the drug to some patients.[170] Induction of anesthesia with a volatile agent administered through a face mask, followed by a short period during which inhaled anesthetic is insufflated, also has been used.[175, 176] Emergence from anesthesia is usually very rapid after short exposures to inhaled anesthetics. Many oncology patients will have an indwelling central venous catheter. Intravenous injection of ketamine[177] or a propofol infusion[178, 179] is a reasonable alternative in these patients. Because of the short nature of the anesthetic exposures, the technique should be tailored to ensure rapid emergence from anesthesia. These children are usually outpatients and benefit from quick emergence from anesthesia and discharge to home.

Gamma Knife

Gamma knife stereotactic radiotherapy is increasingly used for a wide variety of conditions, including intra-cranial tumors, vascular malformations, and epileptic foci.[180–184] This form of therapy has some of the same features as radiation oncology treatments. An accurate and powerful radiation beam from ^{60}Co sources is delivered[185] for a short period of time. The patient must be in a room without an observer. A television camera is used to view the monitors and the patient during the procedure. The difference between gamma knife therapy and radiation therapy is the amount of time required to complete each treatment.

A stereotactic head frame is applied to the patient's cranium and a CT scan is obtained. Local anesthesia and sedation or general anesthesia is used while the frame is secured to the head. After the CT scan is completed, computations are made to ensure that the beam will be directed to the appropriate part of the brain. These calculations take several hours. The patient also may have an angiogram obtained at this time. Older children can be sent to a bed on a ward to wait, and usually do not require sedation. However, younger or more anxious children require sedation while the calculations are being done. Most of our patients wait in the recovery room while the calculations are done. These children usually receive a continuous infusion of midazolam and fentanyl to maintain a sedative state.[186] Although it may be necessary to secure the airway with an endotracheal tube or LMA for these procedures, it often is not necessary to do so.

The time required to complete gamma knife radiotherapy is on average just over 7 hours in our medical center. The child must be transported from the CT scanner to angiography, to a waiting area (such as the recovery room), and then to the treatment area. The majority of this time is spent in the recovery room. Each institution must decide if an anesthesiologist must remain with each sedated patient throughout the wait in the PACU or if it is adequate for the recovery room staff to do so.

The most common complications related to gamma knife therapy are vomiting and seizures. Seizures occur in less than 5 percent of the cases; prophylactic seizure medication and steroids can be used to reduce the risk.[185] Nausea and vomiting occurs in less than 10 percent of patients and are usually self-limited.

Myelography

Most myelograms are obtained without general anesthesia unless the patient is uncooperative. Because the patient is initially prone, the anesthesiologist must ensure that nerves and bony prominances are adequately padded and that the endotracheal tube is taped securely. After the spinal tap is completed and the dye is injected, the patient usually is moved into various positions to move the dye to different areas of the neuraxis. During these maneuvers, there is a risk of dislodging the endotracheal tube or of stretching nerves and causing nerve palsies. If the dye ascends above the tentorium, seizures may occur. Although pneumoencephalography is now rarely performed, it can be associated with significant postprocedure headache, nausea, and vomiting.[159]

After the myelogram, it is common for a CT scan to be obtained. This may entail transporting the patient and moving an anesthesia machine to another site. Instead of transporting the anesthesia machine with the patient to the CT scanner (possibly in another building), we find it more useful to maintain anesthesia with intravenous agents while the patient is being moved and to have a second anesthesia machine waiting for us at the CT scanner.

THE CARDIOLOGY LABORATORY

Diagnostic Catheterization

Anesthesiologists are now spending a lot of time in the cardiac catheterization laboratory. As the cardiologists perform more complex procedures on patients with significant physiologic impairments, there is need for greater control of the child's physiologic parameters. Although cardiologists traditionally have sedated children for cardiac catheterization, there is an increasing need to ensure quiet conditions during these new procedures. Therefore, anesthesiologists are being asked to anesthetize and to monitor the sickest of these patients.

Children undergoing cardiac catheterization are a good example of the challenges that face anesthesiologists when children must be anesthetized outside the operating room. Children presenting for cardiac catheterization present us with the same challenges of uncorrected congenital heart disease we face when these children go to the operating room for operative repair of their heart disease. However, the anesthesiologist in the cardiac catheterization laboratory must face these challenges without the benefits of the well-lighted and well-equipped operating room. The catheterization laboratory is not designed with anesthesia or with anesthesiologists in mind. There often is a paucity of room, lights, electrical outlets, or personnel available to assist in the administration of anesthesia. Before anesthesia is provided in the cardiac catheterization laboratory, it is important to ensure that adequate facilities are available to safely provide anesthesia for these sick patients and that we will have adequate access to the patient. Close communication between the cardiologist and anesthesiologist is essential to ensure successful and expeditious patient care. As a practical matter, the technical staff of the catheterization laboratory are the people most likely to provide help to the anesthesiologist during the anesthetic. Before the procedure begins, they should understand what is expected of them in terms of assisting the anesthesiologist, running blood gases and other laboratory tests, and helping with transport of the patient to and from the catheterization laboratory.

Unlike cardiac surgery, cardiac catheterization is often performed for diagnostic purposes; there usually is no improvement in the patient's condition at the end of the procedure.[187] Because anesthetic management can significantly alter the patient's hemodynamics, it is crucial to understand the patient's current clinical status and probable anatomic lesion. Children with congenital heart disease will present with one of three conditions: uncorrected, palliated or partially repaired, or repaired cardiac lesions. These three conditions represent a wide variety of functional states. The cardiac lesion may have been anatomically repaired, but the child still may have severe functional limitations, as well as a circulatory pattern that is anatomically abnormal and confusing to the anesthesiologist.

A precatheterization diagnosis usually is based on the clinical examination and the echocardiogram. Important aspects of the preanesthetic evaluation of the patient parallel the evaluation performed before anesthesia is administered for an operative procedure.[188] Evaluation of the patient must determine several aspects of the patient's current condition. A simple checklist to help the anesthesiologist determine the significance of the child's heart disease includes the following:

I. Anatomy
   A. The probable cardiac lesion
   B. The presence of intracardiac shunts
      1. Magnitude and direction of flow
      2. Causes of variations in shunting
   C. The presence of obstructive lesions
      1. Magnitude of obstruction
      2. Dynamic versus fixed obstruction
   D. The presence of valvar lesions
   E. Previous palliative or corrective surgery
      1. Response to anesthetics
      2. Success of repair
      3. Course in intensive care unit and hospital

II. Physiology
   A. Heart failure, now or in the past
   B. Adequacy of current cardiac output
      1. Adequacy of right and left ventricles in size and function
      2. Evidence of inadequate function, such as tachycardia, dyspnea, sweating, loss of weight or appetite
   C. Known cardiac rhythm disturbances
   D. Recent changes in exercise tolerance

III. Pharmacology
   A. Current medications
      1. Electrolyte, digoxin levels
   B. Medications required in the past
   C. Allergies
   D. Known useful or ineffective medications, especially antidysrhythmics

Based on this evaluation, the anesthesiologist can make an assessment of the patient's current status and functional reserve. Clarifying these findings with the cardiologist allows the anesthesiologist to prepare for potential difficulties.

Current experience with anesthesia for children who have congenital heart disease has demonstrated that it is possible to anesthetize virtually all patients safely.[187, 189] A wide variety of anesthetic agents can be used, including ketamine, volatile anesthetics, propofol, and opioids.[190–196] Extensive experience has demonstrated that the method of monitoring and administration of medications is what is important in children with congenital heart disease, not the particular agent used. However, some agents may be better suited to an individual patient, depending on the patient's anatomic lesion, degree of shunting, and reserve.[187, 189, 197, 198]

Who should administer anesthesia to these patients? For the anesthesiologist to be effective and safe when caring for these patients outside the operating room, he or she should have the same knowledge, skills, and experience expected of the anesthesiologist who will care for the patient when he or she undergoes cardiac surgery. The anesthesiologist must be familiar with the physiologic alterations caused by each anesthetic agent and titrate these drugs against changes in the patient's condition[199, 200] (see Chapter 18). Two important caveats must be remembered. First, anesthesia should not be induced in children with congenital heart disease unless rapid access to resuscitative drugs, such as inotropes, is available. This is especially true in the catheterization laboratory, where less help is available than in the operating room; the anesthesiologist should prepare inotrope and vasopressor infusions before the induction of anesthesia if it is likely that they will be needed. Second, sudden deterioration in the patient's condition can occur if the patient has uncorrected airway obstruction, hypoventilation, hypovolemia, hypervolemia, or hypothermia. Meticulous attention to anesthetic management and to monitoring will make the course of the patient smoother.

The most common complications of cardiac catheterization that directly affect the anesthesiologist are blood loss and dysrhythmias. The cardiologist uses the femoral vessels for vascular access. Although efforts are made to prevent excessive blood loss, infants and small children can lose enough blood from vessel bleeding and blood gas samples to require blood transfusion. They also can lose significant amounts of blood into the retroperitoneal space if there is a tear or multiple holes in the femoral vessels. The anesthesiologist must aggressively monitor and replace these losses. Dysrhythmias occur commonly during manipulation of intracardiac catheters. The anesthesiologist must closely monitor the physiologic significance of dysrhythmias and keep the cardiologist informed of significant changes. Less commonly, blood vessel or heart rupture, anaphylactic reactions to contrast media, seizures, and embolic/thrombotic events can occur.

Balloon Dilatation

Cardiologists are increasingly treating lesions in the cardiac catheterization laboratory that once were treated in the operating room. To do so, they insert catheters to treat stenotic lesions and they place devices that occlude septal defects. Balloon dilatation has been used successfully to nonsurgically treat pulmonic stenosis,[201] aortic stenosis,[202] and coarctation of the aorta.[203, 204] These procedures cause sudden cessation of blood flow during the short time the balloon is inflated and may disrupt forward flow of blood sufficiently to cause hypotension. This period of absent cardiac output usually is well tolerated. However, it may cause significant cardiac decompensation in some patients, such as in infants with critical aortic stenosis and a small left ventricle. Rupture of the vessel is a rare but real concern. After dilation of a native coarctation of the aorta, there is a significant rate of recurrence of the stenosis and of aneurysm formation. Because of the potential risks of these procedures, different centers view the advisability of balloon dilatation of coarctation of the aorta with varying degrees of enthusiasm. Because there is the potential for hypotension, malignant dysrhythmias, or cardiac arrest during manipulation of the catheter, anesthesiologists are increasingly asked to provide deep sedation or general anesthesia for these infants. The cardiologist must tell the anesthesiologist when he or she is about to dilate the stenosis. It is prudent to decrease any myocardial depressant medication and to be prepared to treat sudden hypotension or dysrhythmias if they occur.

Umbrella Insertion

Another exciting advance in cardiac catheterization is transcatheter closure of an atrial septal defect,[205, 206] ventricular septal defect,[207] patent ductus arteriosus,[208] and a fenestrated Fontan using a clamshell-like device. The device is introduced through the femoral vein and positioned across the septal defect. After ensuring proper placement by transesophageal echocardiography or fluoroscopy,[205] the device is secured, obliterating the defect. Complications seen with this procedure have included dysrhythmias, significant cardiac decompensation, and embolism. These devices occasionally have become dislodged and embolized to the right ventricle and aorta or to distal vessels. Rarely, it is necessary to rapidly proceed to an operating room to extract the device under direct vision. As with balloon dilatation of stenotic vessels, the anesthesiologist must plan the anesthetic based on both the underlying cardiac anomaly and the intended procedure.[199]

A relatively new procedure in the catheterization laboratory is the transcatheter radiofrequency ablation of aberrant conduction pathways. This technique consists of mapping the conduction system within the heart, stimulating dysrhythmias by pacing or isoproterenol infusion, and then destroying the pathways with radiofrequency energy. This procedure presents several unique challenges to the anesthesiologist, including maintaining adequate blood pressure and cardiac output despite prolonged periods of tachycardia and using an anesthetic technique that does not prevent initiation of the aberrant dysrhythmia. Multiple anesthetic techniques have been described as providing the best conditions,[209–211] but considerable modification of any technique may be needed for an individual patient to provide adequate anesthetic depth and the ability to induce the dysrhythmia.

The Neonatal Intensive Care Unit: Patent Ductus Closure, Laparotomy, and Repair of Diaphragmatic Hernia

In many pediatric and tertiary hospitals, the number of surgical procedures performed in the neonatal ICU (NICU) has increased dramatically because relatively straightforward procedures can be performed there without having to transport the infant to the operating room. There has been concern that transporting critically ill children, especially the small-for-gestational age and preterm neonates, puts the child at risk for accidental tracheal extubation, inadequate ventilation or PEEP, accidental removal of vascular lines, inadequate monitoring, or the development of hypothermia.[212]

When transport of critically ill children is possible, the anesthesia department should have a clear policy about the minimum number of people required for the transport. The number and expertise of these people should be adequate to deal with emergencies like tracheal extubation or depression of the cardiopulmonary systems if they occur during the transport. This usually involves having an experienced physician in attendance throughout the transport. It is necessary to monitor vital functions and to ventilate the lungs with both air and oxygen. In our institution, we have three lightweight carts that we use during transport of patients to other facilities. These carts have a blender to mix air and oxygen from tanks containing medical grade gases, a flowmeter, extra airway equipment (self-inflating resuscitation bags, different size bags, masks, airways), and a portable monitor that displays pulse oximetry, ECG, capnography, and one intravascular pressure channel. This cart is attached to the front of the bed so that the person guiding the bed and cart has a clear view of the monitors. Appropriate drugs required for resuscitation and for muscle relaxation, laryngoscope handles and blades, and endotracheal tubes are added to the cart at the time of transport.

A wide variety of surgical procedures can be performed in the ICU, including several that traditionally have been performed in the operating room. Initial successes with closure of a patent ductus arteriosus in the neonatal ICU led to an appreciation that other surgery could be performed in the ICU.[213, 214] Procedures performed in our own institution have included patent ductus arteriosus ligation, repair of congenital diaphragmatic hernia, closure of gastroschisis, and exploratory laparotomy for necrotizing enterocolitis. These procedures share the common features that all are relatively simple to perform, but they have the potential for sudden blood loss, hypotension, and cardiac arrest. These procedures also can be completed in a relatively short period of time, with most of them taking much less than an hour to complete. The anesthetic preparation and management of these patients are not different from those required when the surgery is performed in the operating room. Blood must be available in the ICU and must be checked before the surgery begins; resuscitative drugs should be immediately available; all of the instruments used in the operating room must be available; all personnel must understand their responsibilities for both routine and emergency conditions.

Performing surgery and providing anesthesia in the ICU involves several logistic challenges. Space for equipment and patient access are limited. Most neonatal units have several patients and their related personnel sharing the room in which the surgery will be done. A few units have a "mini-operating room" in the area, but this is rare. The room temperature cannot be manipulated as easily as in the operating room. Infection control is a concern because of the nature of the room, including the exposure from more than one patient area. Lastly, the unit's nursing staff is not trained and does not practice in the same manner as operating room nurses.

Dealing with personnel outside the traditional operating room environment can involve political and interpersonnel difficulties. ICU nursing staff may not be particularly enthusiastic about having surgical procedures performed in what is viewed as "their area." If both the ICU nursing and physician staff are not positive about the arrangement, the process will not go smoothly. Consequently, the willingness of the ICU staff to participate in these procedures should be clearly understood before implementing new procedures. Conversely, if the nursing staff is enthusiastic, as they are in my institution, they provide a tremendous amount of help during these procedures. Questions about space, staffing, infection control, and responsibility for ordering of blood and drugs should be resolved before agreeing to anesthetize patients in this setting. If the ICU staff is not agreeable and committed to having procedures performed in their area, it may be wise to reevaluate the advisability of performing surgery there.

Anesthetic management in the neonatal ICU is similar to that in the operating room. Because an anesthesia machine is not usually present, volatile agent–based anesthesia is seldom used. Most anesthetics given in the ICU consist of high-dose fentanyl. High-dose fentanyl is associated with cardiovascular stability and with diminution or elimination of the stress response in most patients.[215–219] In modern ICUs, it is now standard practice for many mechanically ventilated patients to receive infusions of muscle relaxants, usually pancuronium or vecuronium, and an opioid, usually fentanyl. Although these infusions can be used as a base for an anesthetic, they will not provide adequate anesthesia for surgery. These drugs, and any additional drugs administered by nonanesthesia personnel, should be discussed with the ICU staff and understood by the anesthesiologist. There may be a temptation on the part of the neonatal staff, once they are comfortable with having surgical procedures performed in their unit, to just "turn up the drips" so that a procedure can be performed without an anesthesiologist being present. However, the risks of inadequate stress relief and lack of experience in responding to sudden blood loss, surgical compression of the lungs or great vessels, accidental tracheal extubation, and all of the other complications anesthesiologists are used to handling should be discussed to dissuade these activities. As in the operating room, attention must be paid not only to cardiopulmonary stability, but also to temperature maintenance, prevention of hyperoxia, adequate padding of nerves and pressure points, positioning of the patient, and maintenance of adequate glucose and fluid administration.[219, 220]

Emergency Department and Patient Floors: Fracture Reduction, Suturing, Bone Marrow Aspiration, and Spinal Tap

It is increasingly recognized that sedation and pain relief have been underutilized in pediatric patients. Pediatricians, emergency room physicians, radiologists, surgeons, intensivists, and a wide variety of others have come to understand the benefits of sedating children. The need to provide both adequate pain relief and humane conditions to perform procedures distressful to children has become a priority for many clinicians. The child in the emergency room with a fracture or laceration, the child needing routine bone marrow aspirations, and children needing extensive dental care are some of the candidates for more aggressive sedation. Anesthesiologists are asked to assist in either providing the service or making recommendations about institutional use of sedative and analgesic drugs. There are several aspects of doing so that must be understood.

Sedation and analgesia are not necessarily the same process. They often require different drugs, goals, and methods of evaluating their effects. It is important that practitioners who undertake these activities understand the differences between sedation and anesthesia and apply this understanding to their practice. Sedation is the process of decreasing the level of consciousness to the degree that a patient is cooperative for a procedure. Drugs used for sedation have different actions and side effects. Barbiturates and chloral hydrate are commonly used to provide sedation. The benzodiazepines are properly classed as anxiolytics, and the phenothiazines are antipsychotics. Most of these drugs can induce general anesthesia if given in large enough doses. Monitoring of patients given these drugs should be consistent with their expected actions. There will be increasing loss of control and consciousness with administering increased doses of the drugs. The increased loss of consciousness may be associated with loss of airway patency and a decreased pulmonary ventilation.[23, 137, 221-224]

Opioids, especially fentanyl, are used frequently in pediatric patients. They often are combined with sedative drugs to enhance the overall effect of these drugs.[225-229] Monitoring children given opioids should take into consideration the unique effects of these drugs. Opioids produce dose-dependent depression of ventilation, but the sedative properties of the opioids are less well defined. Opioids can also produce sudden onset of chest wall rigidity and hypoventilation.[222, 224] The dose-dependent depression of ventilation caused by opioid administration is diminished by anything that increases central nervous system (CNS) stimulation, such as pain, agitation, or excitement. Therefore, a patient who is undergoing a painful procedure or is being actively stimulated is less likely to hypoventilate than the patient who is pain-free and undisturbed. A patient may have adequate ventilation during the painful part of a procedure, but may hypoventilate and become hypoxemic when the stimulation ceases. Two other aspects of fentanyl respiratory depression must be understood by those who prescribe it: (1) ventilatory depression is enhanced in patients who are sedated by other drugs, and (2) the hypoxic ventilatory response, an important safety measure, is decreased by both opioids and sedatives.[221, 222, 224]

The side effects of different drugs are important components of their safety profile. A popular regimen used to produce profound sedation in children is widely known as "DPT." This consists of meperidine (Demerol, Winthrop, New York), promethazine (Phenergan, Wyeth-Ayerst, Philadelphia), and chlorpromazine (Thorazine, Smith Kline and French, Philadelphia). Both promethazine and chlorpromazine are very-long-acting drugs. Because of this, there can be profound sedation and analgesia at the time the procedure is performed, and the sedation and respiratory depression may persist for several hours afterwards.[225, 228-231] Also, chlorpromazine can induce seizures in those patients who are prone to seizures. This combination, as well as some of the older "cocktails" used to heavily sedate children, has been associated with multiple adverse reactions, leading many institutions to either restrict the use of combinations of potent sedative drugs or to require physicians to take an active role in monitoring these patients.

SEDATION: WHO, HOW, AND UNDER WHAT RESTRICTIONS?

The rational and safe use of sedation for children is a complex problem. We now have drugs that allow an unprecedented improvement in the care delivered to children. Sedation and analgesia can be provided in circumstances where both were ignored or inadequately delivered before. Our pediatric, dental, and surgical colleagues have witnessed the advances we have made with a wide variety of drugs and approaches for both pain relief and preanesthetic sedation.[232-235] These drugs and techniques have been adopted in a variety of settings, such as children undergoing dental restorations,[236-242] painful procedures,[243-247] and nonpainful examinations.[248-256] Conversely, there continues to be evidence that sedation can cause significant mortality and morbidity if these drugs are not used judiciously.[257-259]

Multiple articles from nonanesthesiologists have proposed giving significant doses of sedative and analgesic medications for sedation.[260-263] These articles recommend the use such diverse drugs as midazolam, fentanyl, and ketamine in oncology patients.[243, 248, 250, 264] Propofol has been recommended for dental procedures,[265, 266] and emergency departments have recommended the use of propofol, fentanyl, and ketamine in a "safe" manner for a wide variety of sedation and analgesic needs.[228, 267-275] The levels of potent medications proposed in some of these studies approach those used for general anesthesia,[276] especially when combinations of drugs are used.[277] What is the role of the anesthesia department in an institution in guaranteeing safe and effective use of these potent drugs for the care of children needing analgesia and sedation?

It may be possible for the anesthesia departments of some institutions to provide analgesia and sedation for all pediatric patients who require these services. This can be expedited by having readily available and scheduled procedure rooms, as well as a designated group of anesthesiologists who have responsibility for this area and are easily identifiable and available. For instance, an active acute pain service can make valuable contributions to the management of children who have both acute and chronic pain.[278] The availability of trained anesthesia personnel may be especially valuable in institutions where those desiring the service have little experience with sedation of pediatric patients.

The potential demands on an anesthesia department can be staggering. Although the anesthesia service will not provide all of the pediatric analgesia and sedation provided in the institution, requests for assistance increase as other departments understand how an anesthesia-based service can make them more efficient. Two recent national manpower studies[279, 280] have recognized this potential demand and the lack of current personnel to meet it. As anesthesia departments strive to serve all those who request their service, the departments must balance the need to provide care themselves with the need to help other departments develop their own capabilities to provide safe sedation.

Anesthesia departments can contribute to the safety of pediatric sedation by participating in the development of institutional guidelines that can be followed by different departments. The Joint Commission on the Accreditation of Healthcare Organizations (JCAHO) has published rules for the development of guidelines within institutions they accredit. The JCAHO has stated that when medications are given that can result in loss of consciousness, there should be mechanisms or processes specified for evaluating and monitoring these activities, as well as establishing guidelines for safe administration of these drugs.[281] The director of the organized anesthesia services in that institution has a responsibility to participate with services that administer these drugs in developing the process of establishing guidelines. A clarification from the JCAHO emphasized the role of the director of anesthesia services; the director has a responsibility to participate in development of guidelines, but it is the responsibility of the department or service providing the sedation that has ultimate responsibility for both the guidelines and the care delivered.[282] In recent comments, the JCAHO noted that although no JCAHO standard directly addresses "conscious" sedation, standards that apply when sedation is used include those about informed consent, staff competence, data collection for processes that involve risk, and procedures that place patients at risk, among others.[283] JCAHO clearly states that each institution should develop criteria for competence of practitioners who desire to administer sedation in their institution.

What criteria should be used to identify competence and proper practice of sedation? Different organizations[284-288] have developed standards and guidelines to encourage safe care of sedated patients. In addition, many departments have developed their own structured programs.[289, 290] These standards and guidelines are usually concerned with evaluation, monitoring, and general care instead of "cook book" formulas for specific agents. The American Society of Anesthesiologists (ASA) has published standards for basic intraoperative care,[291] as well as for sedation and analgesia by nonanesthesiologists.[288] Other groups also have published guidelines oriented to the sedated, not anesthetized, patient.[285, 292, 293] The American Academy of Pediatrics (AAP) guidelines for sedation of children,[286] revised in 1992, have been particularly popular and have become the basis for institutional guidelines in several instances. Why so many different guidelines instead of just one set that everyone can agree to?[294] There are substantive differences between the guidelines regarding the degree of monitoring required for specific types and levels of sedation. The AAP and ASA guidelines closely mirror the general approach to sedation that anesthesiologists traditionally take.

The AAP and ASA guidelines[286, 288] discuss the distinction between conscious sedation and deep sedation. Conscious sedation is a state of depressed consciousness in which the child retains a patent airway and protective reflexes and is arousable by verbal command or physical stimulation. Deep sedation is any state from which the child is not easily aroused or does not maintain an adequate airway. This distinction is a difficult one for anesthesiologists to make because the sedative state is often fluid, moving from one level of depression to another. In addition, there is now a distinction being made between sedation and sedation/analgesia, a state induced by using more than one class of drug.

The general guidelines for both conscious and deep sedation have several points in common.[286, 288] First, equipment requirements include (onsite and available) a positive-pressure oxygen delivery system that can administer at least 90 percent oxygen for at least 60 minutes. An emergency kit containing drugs, laryngoscopes, and endotrcheal tubes must be available, as well as monitors and a suction device. Second, documentation for the sedation should include a presedation health evaluation, informed consent, records of medication given, vital signs, recovery parameters, and instructions at discharge to the responsible person. Third, for conscious sedation, there must be a person in addition to the practitioner performing the procedure to monitor the child's condition. Monitoring should include continuous measurement of oxygen saturation and heart rate and intermittent respiratory rate and blood pressure. For deep sedation, the person monitoring the patient should have that monitoring as their only responsibility. The capability for ECG monitoring and insertion of vascular catheters must be available. ECG monitoring is exempted from monitoring requirements in MRI because of potential thermal injury. Also, with deeper levels of sedation, capnography can be very useful in detecting hypoventilation and airway obstruction.[295-297] Lastly, the discharge criteria used to ensure that the patient is fit for discharge should be documented before the child leaves the treatment area or facility.

The ASA and AAP guidelines are provided as suggestions for care, not absolute standards. On the other hand, they are an attempt to provide a framework to guide sedation by nonanesthesiologists. As each anesthesia department participates in developing their own institution's parameters, these guidelines may be of help. The additional support that each anesthesia department provides in terms of coverage of procedures requiring sedation, though not necessarily anesthesia, should be clarified. This will enable other services to determine their needs for development of sedation mechanisms.

SUMMARY

Providing anesthesia outside the operating room is an exciting and challenging aspect of the care anesthesiologists deliver. Equipment, space, transport, and personnel needs are the major focus of anesthesiologists when leaving our traditional environment. These areas of focus are important when attempting to provide safe care in what may be relatively hostile environments. However, several other aspects of these endeavors also are important. By providing service outside the operating room, anesthesiologists can bring a quality of humane care not previously available. By efficiently providing adequate conditions for diagnostic or therapeutic procedures, anesthesiologists can make other practitioners more efficient. By providing quality patient evaluation, monitoring, and care, anesthesiologists can decrease the risk of children being exposed to poorly monitored sedation. By providing education, anesthesiologists can increase the level of expertise of others within the institution. Lastly, by being available, anesthesiologists are "good citizens" of their institution, enhancing the level of service and care to its patients.

REFERENCES

1. Faulconer A, Keys TE: Foundations of Anesthesiology. Springfield, IL, Charles C Thomas, 1965, p 310.
2. Rae BR, Hall SC: The pediatric patient. In Morell RC, Eichhorn JH (eds): Patient Safety in Anesthetic Practice. New York, Churchill Livingstone, 1997, p 129.
3. Hall SC: Ambulatory anesthesia outside the operating room. In Twersky RS (ed): The Ambulatory Anesthesia Handbook. St. Louis, CV Mosby, 1994, p 361.
4. Hall SC: Sedation techniques. In White PF (ed): Ambulatory Anesthesia and Surgery. London, WB Saunders Company, 1997, p 595.
5. Hall SC: Pediatric anesthesia outside the operating room: the anesthesiologist as pioneer. Int Anesthesiol Clin 14:385, 1996.
6. American Academy of Pediatrics, Section on Anesthesiology: Guidelines for the pediatric perioperative anesthesia environment. Pediatrics 103:512, 1999.
7. Gilbertson LI: Hospital standards and requirements. Int Anesthesiol Clin 37:1, 1999.
8. Kurz A, Kurz M, Poeschl G, et al: Forced-air warming maintains intraoperative normothermia better than circulating-water mattresses. Anesth Analg 77:89, 1993.
9. Murat I, Berniere J, Constant I: Evaluation of the efficacy of a forced-air warmer (Bair Hugger) during spinal surgery in children. J Clin Anesth 6:425, 1994.
10. Litman RS: Sedation and anesthesia outside the operating room: answers to common questions. Semin Pediatr Surg 8:34, 1999.
11. Morton NS, Oomen GJ: Development of a selection and monitoring protocol for safe sedation of children. Paediatr Anaesth 8:65, 1998.
12. Splinter WM, Schaffer JD, Zunder IH: Clear fluids three hours before surgery do not affect the gastric fluid contents of children. Can J Anaesth 37:498, 1990.
13. Schreiner MS, Triebwasser A, Keon TP: Ingestion of liquids compared with preoperative fasting in pediatric outpatients. Anesthesiology 72:593, 1990.
14. Kallar SK, Everett LL: Potential risks and preventive measures for pulmonary aspiration: new concepts in preoperative fasting guidelines. Anesth Analg 77:171 1993.
15. Splinter WM, Schreiner MS: Preoperative fasting in children. Anesth Analg 89:80, 1999.
16. Ferrari LR, Rooney FM, Rockoff MA: Preoperative fasting practices in pediatrics. Anesthesiology 90:978, 1999.
17. Warner MA, Caplan RA, Epstein BS, et al: Practice Guidelines for preoperative fasting and the use of pharmacologic agents to reduce the risk of pulmonary aspiration: Application to healthy patients undergoing elective procedures. Anesthesiology 90:896, 1999.
18. Keeter S, Benator RM, Weinberg SM, Hartenberg MA: Sedation in pediatric CT: national survey of current practice. Radiology 175:745, 1990.
19. Pappas JN, Donnelly LF, Frush DP: Reduced frequency of sedation of young children with multisection helical CT. Radiology 215:897, 2000.
20. Kaste SC, Young CW, Holmes TP, Baker DK: Effect of helical CT on the frequency of sedation in pediatric patients. AJR Am J Roentgenol 168:1001, 1997.
21. Gordon I: Diagnostic Imaging in Paediatrics. London, Chapman & Hall, 1987, p 11.
22. Cosentino CM, Luck SR, Barthel MJ, et al: Transfusion requirements in conservative nonoperative management of blunt splenic and hepatic injuries during childhood. J Pediatr Surg 25:950, 1990.
23. Boyer RS: Sedation in pediatric neuroimaging: the science and the art. AJNR Am J Neuroradiol 13:777, 1992.
24. Spear RM, Waldman JY, Canada ED, et al: Intravenous thiopentone for CT and MRI in children. Paediatr Anaesth 3:29, 1993.
25. Fisher DM: Sedation of pediatric patients: an anesthesiologist's perspective. Radiology 175:613, 1990.
26. Frush DP, Bisset GS, Hall SC: Pediatric sedation in radiology: the practice of safe sleep. Am J Radiol 167:1381, 1996.
27. Greenberg SB, Faerber EN, Aspinall CL: High dose chloral hydrate sedation for children undergoing CT. Comput Assist Tomogr 15:467, 1991.
28. Temme JB, Anderson JC, Matecko S: Sedation of children for CT and MRI scanning. Radiol Technol 61:283, 1990.
29. Merrick PA, Case BJ, Jagjivan B, Stackman TJ: Care of pediatric patients sedated with pentobarbital sodium in MRI. Pediatr Nurs 17:34, 1991.
30. Malviya S, Voepel-Lewis T, Eldevik OP, et al: Sedation and general anaesthesia in children undergoing MRI and CT: adverse events and outcomes. Br J Anaesth 84:743, 2000.
31. Kao SC, Adamson SD, Tatman LH, Berbaum KS: A survey of post-discharge side effects of conscious sedation using chloral hydrate in pediatric CT and MR imaging. Pediatr Radiol 29:287, 1999.
32. Sanderson PM: A survey of pentobarbital sedation for children undergoing abdominal CT scans after oral contrast medium. Paediatr Anaesth 7:309, 1997.
33. Alp H, Guler I, Orbak Z, et al: Efficacy and safety of rectal thiopental: sedation for children undergoing computed tomography and magnetic resonance imaging. Pediatr Int 41:538, 1999.
34. Conners GP, Sacks WK, Leahey NF: Variations in sedating uncooperative, stable children for post-traumatic head CT. Pediatr Emerg Care 15:241, 1999.
35. Thompson JR, Schneider S, Ashwal S, et al: The choice of sedation for computed tomography in children: a prospective evaluation. Radiology 143:475, 1982.
36. Cook BA, Bass JW, Nomizu S, Alexander ME: Sedation of children for technical procedures: current standard of practice. Clin Pediatr 31:137, 1992.
37. Smith MT: Chloral hydrate warning [letter]. Science 19:359, 1990.
38. Harrington-Brock K, Doerr CL, Moore MM: Mutagenicity of three disinfection by-products: di- and trichloroacetic acid and chloral hydrate in L5178Y/TK +/− (−)3.7.2C mouse lymphoma cells. Mutat Res 413:265, 1998.
39. Steinberg AD, DeSesso JM: Have animal data been used inappropriately to estimate risks to humans from environmental trichloroethylene? Regul Toxicol Pharmacol 18:137, 1993.
40. Greenberg SB, Faerber EN, Radke JL, et al: Sedation of difficult-to-sedate children undergoing MR imaging: value of thioridazine as an adjunct to chloral hydrate. AJR Am J Roentgenol 163:165, 1994.
41. Diament MJ, Stanley P: The use of midazolam for sedation of infants and children. AJR Am J Roentgenol 150:377, 1988.
42. Coventry DM, Martin CS, Burke AM: Sedation for paediatric computerized tomography—a double-blind assessment of rectal midazolam. Eur J Anaesthesiol 8:29, 1991.
43. Glanville JN: Nalbuphine hydrochloride (Nubain, DuPont) as premedication for radiologic procedures. Clin Radiol 42:212, 1990.
44. Strain JD, Campbell JB, Harvey LA, Campbell JB: IV Nembutal: safe sedation for children undergoing CT. AJR Am J Roentgenol 151:975, 1988.
45. Burckart GJ, White TJ, Seigle RL, et al: Rectal thiopental versus an intramuscular cocktail for sedating children before computerized tomography. Am J Hosp Pharm 37:222, 1980.
46. Audenaert SM, Montgomery CL, Thompson DE, Sutherland J: A prospective study of rectal methohexital: efficacy and side effects in 648 cases. Anesth Analg 81:957, 1995.
47. Manuli MA, Davies L: Rectal methohexital for sedation of children during imaging procedures. AJR Am J Roentgenol 160:577, 1993.
48. Glasier CM, Stark JE, Brown R, et al: Rectal thiopental sodium for sedation of pediatric patients undergoing MR and other imaging studies. Am J Neuroradiol 16:111, 1995.
49. Allan MW, Laurence AS, Gunawardena WJ: A comparison of two sedation techniques for neuroradiology. Eur J Anaesthesio 6:379, 1989.
50. Voepel-Lewis T, Malviya S, Prochaska G, Tait AR: Sedation failures in children undergoing MRI and CT: is temperament a factor? Paediatr Anaesth 10:319, 2000.

51. Shepherd JK, Hall-Craggs MA, Finn JP, Bingham RM: Sedation in children scanned with high-field magnetic resonance; the experience at The Hospital for Sick Children, Great Ormond Street. Br J Radiol 63:794, 1990.
52. Martin TM, Nicolson SC, Bargas MS: Propofol anesthesia reduces emesis and airway obstruction in pediatric outpatients. Anesth Analg 76:144, 1993.
53. Runcie CJ, MacKenzie SJ, Arthur DS, Morton NS: Comparison of recovery from anaesthesia induced in children with either propofol or thiopentone. Br J Anaesth 70:192, 1993.
54. Kain ZN, Gaal DJ, Kain TS, et al: A first-pass cost analysis of propofol versus barbiturates for children undergoing magnetic resonance imaging. Anesth Analg 79:1102, 1994.
55. Marsh B, White M, Morton N, Kenny GNC: Pharmacokinetic model driven infusion of propofol in children. Br J Anaesth 67:41, 1991.
56. Hannallah RS, Baker SB, Casey W, et al: Propofol: effective dose and induction characteristics in unpremedicated children. Anesthesiology 74:217, 1991.
57. Levati A, Colombo N, Arosio EM, et al: Propofol anaesthesia in spontaneously breathing paediatric patients during magnetic resonance imaging. Acta Anaesthesiol Scand 40:561, 1996.
58. Merola C, Albarracin C, Lebowitz P, et al: An audit of adverse events in children sedated with chloral hydrate or propofol during imaging studies. Paediatr Anaesth 5:375, 1995.
59. Valtonen M: Anaesthesia for computerized tomography of the brain in children: a comparison of propofol and thiopentone. Acta Anaesthesiol Scand 33:170, 1989.
60. Bloomfield EL, Masaryk TJ, Caplin A, et al: Intravenous sedation for MR imaging of the brain and spine in children: pentobarbital versus propofol. Pediatr Radiol 186:93, 1993.
61. Cauldwell CB, Fisher DM: Sedating patients: is propofol a panacea? Radiology 186:9, 1993.
62. Bloomfield EL: Propofol for sedation of pediatric patients. Radiology 186:580, 1993.
63. Hall SC: Monitoring in radiology. In Lake CL (ed): Clinical Monitoring for Anesthesia and Critical Care. 2nd ed. Philadelphia, WB Saunders Company, 1994, p 395.
64. Nixon C, Hirsch NP, Ormerod IEC, Johnson G: Nuclear magnetic resonance imaging. Anesthesiology 62:80, 1985.
65. Menon DK, Peden CJ, Hall AS, et al: Magnetic resonance for the anaesthetist. Part 1: physical principles, application, safety aspects. Anaesthesia 47:240, 1992.
66. Higgins CB, Lanzer P, Stark D, et al: Imaging by nuclear magnetic resonance in patients with chronic ischemic heart disease. Circulation 69:523, 1984.
67. Neubauer S, Horn M, Hahn D, Kochsiek K: Clinical cardiac magnetic resonance spectroscopy—present state and future directions. Mol Cell Biochem 184:439, 1998.
68. Bottomley PA: MR spectroscopy of the human heart: the status and the challenges. Radiology 191:593, 1994.
69. Gangarosa RE, Minnis JE, Nobbe J, et al: Operational safety issues in MRI. Magn Reson Imaging 5:287, 1987.
70. Brown TCK, Fisk GC: Anaesthesia for Children. 2nd ed. London, Blackwell Scientific Publication, 1992, p 291.
71. Peden CJ, Menon DK, Hall AS, et al: Magnetic resonance for the anaesthetist. Part II: anaesthesia and monitoring in MR units. Anaesthesia 47:508, 1992.
72. Fowler JR, TerPenning B, Syverud SA, et al: Magnetic field hazards. N Engl J Med 314:1517, 1986.
73. Roth JL, Nugent M, Gray JE, et al: Patient monitoring during magnetic resonance imaging. Anesthesiology 62:80, 1985.
74. Pavlicek W, Geisinger M, Castle L, et al: The effects of nuclear magnetic resonance on patients with cardiac pacemakers. Radiology 147:149, 1983.
75. Erlebacher JA, Cahill PT, Pannizzo F, et al: Effect of magnetic resonance imaging on DDD pacemakers. Am J Cardiol 57:437, 1986.
76. CDRH Magnetic Resonance Working Group: A Primer on Medical Device Interactions with Magnetic Resonance Imaging Systems. Rockville, MD, U.S. Department of Health and Human Services, 1997.
77. Dujovny M, Kossovsky N, Kossowsky R, et al: Aneurysm clip motion during magnetic resonance imaging: in vivo experimental study with metallurgical factor analysis. Neurosurgery 17:543, 1985.
78. Gold JP, Pulsinelli W, Winchester P, et al: Safety of metallic surgical clips in patients undergoing high-field-strength magnetic resonance imaging. Ann Thorac Surg 48:643, 1989.

79. Soulen RL, Budinger TF, Higgins CB: Magnetic resonance imaging of prosthetic heart valves. Radiology 154:705, 1985.
80. Shellock FG, Curtis JS: MR imaging and biomedical implants, materials, and devices: an updated review. Radiology 180:541, 1991.
81. Pride GL Jr, Kowal J, Mendelsohn DB, et al: Safety of MR scanning in patients with nonferromagnetic aneurysm clips. J Magn Reson Imaging 12:198, 2000.
82. Teissl C, Kremser C, Hochmair ES, Hochmair-Desoyer IJ: Magnetic resonance imaging and cochlear implants: compatibility and safety aspects. J Magn Reson Imaging 9:26, 1999.
83. Patteson SK, Chesney JT: Anesthetic management for magnetic resonance imaging: problems and solutions. Anesth Analg 74:121, 1992.
84. Davis PL, Crooks L, Arakawa M, et al: Potential hazards in NMR imaging: heating effects, of changing magnetic fields and RF fields on small implants. AJR Am J Roentgenol 137:857, 1981.
85. Manninen PH, Kucharczyk W: A new frontier: magnetic resonance imaging-operating room. J Neurosurg Anesthesiol 12:141, 2000.
86. Manninen PH: Anaesthesia outside the operating room. Can J Anaesth 38:R126, 1991.
87. Rao CC, Krishna G, Emhardt J: Anesthesia machine for use during magnetic resonance imaging. Anesthesiology 73:1054, 1990.
88. Dunn V, Coffman CE, McGowan JE, et al: Mechanical ventilation during magnetic resonance imaging. Magn Reson Imaging 3:169, 1985.
89. Ramsay JG, Gale L, Sykes MK: A ventilator for use in nuclear magnetic resonance studies. Br J Anaesth 58:1181, 1986.
90. Williams EJ, Jones NS, Carpenter TA, et al: Testing of adult and paediatric ventilators for use in a magnetic resonance imaging unit. Anaesthesia 54:969, 1999.
91. Klein AS, Blanch PB: Evaluation of six ventilators within the MRI environment. Anesthesiology 75:A403, 1991.
92. Karlik SJ, Heatherley T, Pavan F, et al: Patient anesthesia and monitoring at a 1.5-T MRI installation. Magn Reson Med 7:210, 1988.
93. Mirvis SE, Borg U, Belzberg H: MR imaging of ventilator-dependent patients: preliminary experience. AJR Am J Roentgenol 149:845, 1987.
94. Rotello LC, Radin EJ, Jastremski MS, et al: MRI protocol for critically ill patients. Am J Crit Care 3:187, 1994.
95. Kross J, Drummond JC: Successful use of a Fortec II vaporizer in the MRI suite: a case report with observations regarding magnetic field-induced vaporizer aberrancy. Can J Anaesth 38:1065, 1991.
96. Williams EJ, Tam YC, Kendall IV, et al: Infusion pump performance in an MR environment. Eur J Anaesthesiol 16:468, 1999.
97. Shellock FG, Crues JV: MRI: safety consideration in magnetic resonance imaging. Magn Reson Imaging Decis 2:25030, 1988.
98. McBrien ME, Winder J, Smyth L: Anaesthesia for magnetic resonance imaging: a survey of current practice in the UK and Ireland. Anaesthesia 55:737, 2000.
99. Shellock FG: Biological effects of MRI: a clean safety record so far. Diagn Imaging 9:96, 1987.
100. Schenck JF: Safety of strong, static magnetic fields. J Magn Reson Imaging 12:2, 2000.
101. Geard CR, Osmak RS, Hall EJ, et al: Magnetic resonance and ionizing radiation: a comparative evaluation in vitro of oncogenic and genotoxic potential. Radiology 152:199, 1984.
102. Osbakken M, Griffith J, Taczanowsky P: A gross, morphologic, hematologic, and blood chemistry study of adult and neonatal mice chronically exposed to high magnetic fields. Magn Res Med 3:502, 1986.
103. Budinger TF, Bristol KS, Yen CK: Biologic effects of static magnetic fields [abstract]. New York, Society of Magnetic Resonance in Medicine, 1984, p 118.
104. Hall SC, Stevenson GW, Suresh S: Burn associated with temperature monitoring during magnetic resonance imaging [letter]. Anesthesiology 76:152, 1992.
105. McArdle CB, Nicholas DA, Richardson CJ, Amparo EG: Monitoring of the neonate undergoing MR imaging: technical considerations. Radiology 159:223, 1986.
106. Cote CJ: Anesthesia outside the operating room. In Cote CJ, Ryan JF, Todres ID, Goudsouzian NG (eds): A Practice of Anesthesia for Infants and Children. 2nd ed. Philadelphia, WB Saunders Company, 1993.
107. Kanal E, Shellock FG, Talagala L: Safety considerations in MR imaging. Radiology 176:593, 1990.

108. Wendt RE, Rokey R, Vick GW, et al: Electrocardiographic gating and monitoring in NMR imaging. Magn Reson Imaging 6:89, 1988.
109. Dimick RN, Hedlund LW, Herfkens RJ, et al: Optimizing electrocardiographic electrode placement for cardiac-gated magnetic resonance imaging. Invest Radiol 22:17, 1987.
110. Shellock FG, Slimp GL: Severe burn of the finger caused by using a pulse oximeter during MR imaging. AJR Am J Roentgenol 153:1105, 1989.
111. Sellden H, De Chateau P, Ekman G, et al: Circulatory monitoring of children during anaesthesia in low-field magnetic resonance imaging. Acta Anaesthesiol Scand 34:41, 1990.
112. Shellock FG: Monitoring during MRI. An evaluation of the effect of high-field MRI on various patient monitors. Med Electronics 17:93, 1986.
113. Smith DS, Askey P, Young ML, et al: Anesthetic management of acutely ill patients during magnetic resonance imaging. Anesthesiology 65:710, 1986.
114. Tobin JR, Spurrier EA, Wetzel RC: Anaesthesia for critically ill children during magnetic resonance imaging. Br J Anaesth 69:482, 1992.
115. Shellock FG: Monitoring sedated pediatric patients during MR imaging. Radiology 177:586, 1990.
116. Henneberg S, Hok B, Wiklund L, Sjodin G: Remote auscultatory patient monitoring during magnetic resonance imaging. J Clin Monit 8:37, 1992.
117. Lawson GR: Controversy: sedation of children for magnetic resonance imaging. Arch Dis Child 82:150, 2000.
118. Rosenberg DR, Sweeney JA, Gillen JS, et al: Magnetic resonance imaging of children without sedation: preparation with simulation. J Am Acad Child Adolesc Psychiatry 36:853, 1997.
119. Cohen MD, Weetman RW, Provisor AJ, et al: Efficacy of magnetic resonance imaging in 139 children with tumors. Arch Surg 121:522, 1986.
120. Ringertz HG, Brasch RC, Gooding CA: Artifacts, variants, and factors degrading image quality in pediatric magnetic resonance imaging. Pediatr Radiol 15:173, 1985.
121. Hollman GA, Elderbrook MK, VanDenLangenberg B: Results of a pediatric sedation program on head MRI scan success rates and procedure duration times. Clin Pediatr 34:300, 1995.
122. Marti-Bonmati L, Ronchera-Oms CL, Casillas C, et al: Randomised double-blind clinical trial of intermediate- versus high-dose chloral-hydrate for neuroimaging of children. Neuroradiology 37:687, 1995.
123. Ronchera-Oms CL, Casillas C, Marti-Bonmati L, et al: Oral chloral hydrate provides effective and safe sedation in paediatric magnetic resonance imaging. J Clin Pharm Ther 19:239, 1994.
124. Sury MR, Hatch DJ, Deeley T, et al: Development of a nurse-led sedation service for paediatric magnetic resonance imaging. Lancet 353:1667, 1999.
125. Beebe DS, Tran P, Bragg M, et al: Trained nurses can provide safe and effective sedation for MRI in pediatric patients. Can J Anaesth 47:205, 2000.
126. Keengwe IN, Hegde S, Dearlove O, et al: Structured sedation programme for magnetic resonance imaging examination in children. Anaesthesia 54:1069, 1999.
127. Porche VH: Anesthetic considerations in radiologic procedures performed outside the operating room. Int Anesthesiol Clin 36:9, 1998.
128. Braver R: Noise: thresholds of danger. Safety Standards, July–August:2, 1972.
129. Martin LD, Pasternak LR, Pudimat MA: Total intravenous anesthesia with propofol in pediatric patients outside the operating room. Anesth Analg 74:609, 1992.
130. Browne BL, Prys-Roberts C, Wolf AR: Propofol and alfentanil in children: infusion technique and dose requirement for total i.v. anaesthesia. Br J Anaesth 69:570, 1992.
131. Rejger VS, Cohn BF, Vielvoye GJ, De Raadt FB: A simple anaesthetic and monitoring system for magnetic resonance imaging. Eur J Anaesthesiol 6:373, 1989.
132. Ba-Ssalamaha A, Schick S, Heimberger K, et al: Ultrafast magnetic resonance imaging of the brain. Magn Reson Imaging 18:237, 2000.
133. Kain ZN, Mayes LC, Wang SM, et al: Parental presence during induction of anesthesia versus sedative premedication: which intervention is more effective? Anesthesiology 89:1147, 1998.
134. Kain ZN, Mayes LC, Wang SM, et al: Parental presence and a sedative premedicant for children undergoing surgery: a hierarchical study. Anesthesiology 92:939, 2000.
135. Manninen PH, Chan AS, Papworth D: Conscious sedation for interventional neuroradiology: a comparison of midazolam and propofol infusion. Can J Anaesth 44:26, 1997.
136. Frankville D, Spear R, Fisher B, Sheehan P: Is routine endotracheal intubation necessary when using intravenous anesthesia for MRI? Anesthesiology 77:A1165, 1992.
137. Reber A, Wetzel SG, Schnabel K, et al: Effect of combined mouth closure and chin lift on upper airway dimensions during routine magnetic resonance imaging in pediatric patients sedated with propofol. Anesthesiology 90:1617, 1999.
138. Barnett GH, Ropper AH, Johnson KA: Physiological support and monitoring of critically ill patients during magnetic resonance imaging. J Neurosurg 68:246, 1988.
139. Geiger RS, Cascorbi HF: Anesthesia in an NMR scanner. Anesth Analg 63:622, 1984.
140. Goudsouzian NG, Denman W, Cleveland R, Shorten G: Radiologic localization of the laryngeal mask airway in children. Anesthesiology 77:1085, 1992.
141. Brimacombe J: Does the laryngeal mask have a role outside the operating theatre? Can J Anaesth 42:258, 1995.
142. Benumof JL: Laryngeal mask airway. Indications and contraindications. Anesthesiology 77:843, 1992.
143. Haynes SR, Morton NS: The laryngeal mask airway: a review of its use in paediatric anaesthesia. Paediatr Anaesth 3:65, 1993.
144. Grebenik CR, Ferguson C, White A: The laryngeal mask airway in pediatric radiotherapy. Anesthesiology 72:474, 1990.
145. Snowdon SL: Defibrillator failure in a magnetic resonance unit. Anaesthesia 44:359, 1989.
146. Kaibara T, Saunders JK, Sutherland GR: Advances in mobile intraoperative magnetic resonance imaging. Neurosurgery 47:131, 2000.
147. Alexander E, Moriarty TM, Kikinis R, et al: The present and future role of intraoperative MRI in neurosurgical procedures. Stereotact Funct Neurosurg 68:10, 1997.
148. Merkle EM, Lewin JS, Aschoff AJ, et al: Percutaneous magnetic resonance image-guided biopsy and aspiration in the head and neck. Laryngoscope 110:382, 2000.
149. Rubino GJ, Farahani K, McGill D, et al: Magnetic resonance imaging-guided neurosurgery in the magnetic fringe fields: the next step in neuronavigation. Neurosurgery 46:643, 2000.
150. Hall WA, Liu H, Martin AJ, et al: Safety, efficacy, and functionality of high-field strength interventional magnetic resonance imaging for neurosurgery. Neurosurgery 46:632, 2000.
151. Chripko D, Bevan JC, Archer DP, Bherer N: Decreases, in arterial oxygen saturation in paediatric outpatients during transfer to the postanaesthetic recovery room. Can J Anaesth 36:128, 1989.
152. Hall SC: Special considerations for the pediatric patient. In Brown M, Brown E (eds): Comprehensive Postanesthesia Care. Baltimore, Williams & Wilkins, 1997, p 437.
153. Malviya S, Voepel-Lewis T, Prochaska G, Tait AR: Prolonged recovery and delayed side effects of sedation for diagnostic imaging studies in children. Pediatrics 105:E42, 2000.
154. Hood JB, Wallace CT, Mahaffey JE: Anesthetic management of an intracranial arteriovenous malformation in infancy. Anesth Analg 56:236, 1977.
155. Dallas SH, Moxon CP: Controlled ventilation for cerebral angiography, Br J Anaesth 41:597, 1969.
156. King BF, Harmtan GW, Williamson B, et al: Low-osmolality contrast media. A current perspective. Mayo Clin Proc 64:976, 1989.
157. Cohan RH, Dunnick NR: Intravenous contrast media: adverse reactions. AJR Am J Roentgenol 149:665, 1987.
158. Brezis M, Epstein FH: A closer look at radiocontrast-induced nephropathy. N Engl J Med 320:179, 1989.
159. Kassner EG: Iatrogenic Disorders of the Fetus, Infant, and Child. Volume 1. New York, Springer-Verlag, 1985.
160. Goldberg M: Systemic reactions to intravascular contrast media. Anesthesiology 60:46, 1984.
161. Cohan RH, Dunnick NR, Bashore TM: Treatment of reactions to radiographic contrast material. AJR Am J Roentgenol, 1988.
162. Lasser EC: Pretreatment with corticosteroids to prevent reactions to IV contrast material: overview and implications. AJR Am J Roentgenol 150:257, 1988.
163. Greenberger PA, Patterson R, Tapio CM: Prophylaxis against repeated radiocontrast media reactions in 857 cases. Arch Intern Med 145:2197, 1985.

164. Aldridge HE, Chisholm RJ, Dragatakis L, Roy L: Radiation safety in the cardiac catheterization laboratory. Can J Cardiol 13:459, 1997.

165. Henderson KH, Lu JK, Strauss KJ, et al: Radiation exposure of anesthesiologists. J Clin Anesth 6:37, 1994.

166. Allison DJ, Hordan H, Hennessy O: Therapeutic embolization of the hepatic artery: a review of 75 procedures. Lancet 1:595, 1985.

167. Holden AM, Fyler DC, Shillito J, et al: Congestive heart failure from intracranial arteriovenous fistula in infancy: clinical and physiologic considerations in eight patients. Pediatrics 49:30, 1972.

168. Ishak B, Gutierrez F, Seleny F: Anesthetic management of arteriovenous malformations of the brain in infants and children. Anesthesiol Rev 5:23, 1978.

169. Lo JN, Buckley JJ, Kim TH, et al: Anesthesia for high-dose total body irradiation in children. Anesthesiology 61:101, 1984.

170. Griswold JD, Vacanti FX, Goudsouzian NG: Twenty-three sequential out-of-hospital halothane anesthetics in an infant. Anesth Analg 67:779, 1988.

171. Foesel TEH, Schrimer U, Wick C: Repeated rectal methohexitone as the sole anaesthetic agent for radiotherapy. Paediatric Anaesth 2:329, 1992.

172. Bashein G, Russell AH, Momii ST: Anesthesia and remote monitoring for intraoperative radiation therapy. Anesthesiology 64:804, 1986.

173. Glauber DT, Audenaert SM: Anesthesia for children undergoing craniospinal radiotherapy. Anesthesiology 67:801, 1987.

174. Goresky GV, Steward DJ: Rectal methohexitone for induction of anaesthesia in children. Can Anaesth Soc J 26:213, 1979.

175. Fisher DM, Robinson S, Brett GM, et al: Comparison of enflurane, halothane, and isoflurane for diagnostic and therapeutic procedures in children with malignancies. Anesthesiology 63:647, 1985.

176. Brett CM, Wara WM, Hamilton WK: Anesthesia for infants during radiotherapy: an insufflation technique. Anesthesiology 64:402, 1986.

177. Bennett JA, Bullimore JA: The use of ketamine hydrochloride anaesthesia for radiotherapy in young children. Br J Anaesth 45:197, 1973.

178. Aldridge LM, Gordon NH: Propofol infusions for radiotherapy. Paediatr Anaesth 2:133, 1992.

179. Martin LD, Pasternak LR, Pudimat MA: Total intravenous anesthesia with propofol in pediatric patients outside the operating room. Anesth Analg 74:609, 1992.

180. Boyd TS, Mehta MP: Stereotactic radiosurgery for brain metastases. Oncology 13:1397, 1999.

181. Regis J, Bartolomei F, Hayashi M, et al: The role of gamma knife surgery in the treatment of severe epilepsies. Epileptic Disord 2:113, 2000.

182. Unger F, Schrottner O, Haselsberger K, et al: Gamma knife radiosurgery for hypothalamic hamartomas in patients with medically intractable epilepsy and precocious puberty. Report of two cases. J Neurosurg 92:726, 2000.

183. Rodriguez-Arias C, Martinez R, Rey G, Bravo G: Recurrence in a different location of a cerebral arteriovenous malformation in a child after radiosurgery. Childs Nerv Syst 16:363, 2000.

184. Unger F, Schrottner O, Haselsberger K, et al: Gamma knife radiosurgery for hypothalamic hamartomas in patients with medically intractable epilepsy and precocious puberty. J Neurosurg 92:726, 2000.

185. Lunsford LD, Kondziolka D, Bissonette DJ, et al: Stereotactic radiosurgery of brain vascular malformations. Neurosurg Clin North Am 3:79, 1992.

186. Kimovec M, Monma D, Meyer R, Helenowski T: Anesthesia for gamma knife radiotherapy. Anesthesiology 77:A1179, 1992.

187. Beynen FM, Tarhan S: Anesthesia for the surgical repair of congenital heart defects in children. In Tarhan S (ed): Cardiovascular Anesthesia and Postoperative Care. 2nd ed. Chicago, Year Book Medical Publishers, 1989, p 105.

188. Hall SC: Anesthetic management. In Mavroudis C, Backer CL (eds): Pediatric Cardiac Surgery. St. Louis, Mosby, 1994, p 72.

189. Salem MR, Hall SC, Motoyama EK: Anesthesia for thoracic and cardiovascular surgery. In Motoyama EK, Davis PJ (eds): Smith's Anesthesia for Infants and Children. 5th ed. St. Louis, CV Mosby, 1990, p 518.

190. Fleischer F, Polarz H, Lang J, Bohrer H: Changes in oxygen saturation following low-dose intramuscular ketamine in paediatric cardiac surgical patients. Paediatr Anaesth 1:33, 1991.

191. Lebovic S, Reich DL, Steinberg LG, et al: Comparison of propofol versus ketamine for anesthesia in pediatric patients undergoing cardiac catheterization. Anesth Analg 74:490, 1992.

192. Crean P, Koren G, Goresky G, et al: Fentanyl-oxygen versus fentanyl-N2O/oxygen anaesthesia in children undergoing cardiac surgery. Can Anaesth Soc J 33:36, 1986.

193. Greeley WJ, Bushman GA, Davis DP, Reves JG: Comparative effects of halothane and ketamine on systemic arterial oxygen saturation in children with cyanotic heart disease. Anesthesiology 65:666, 1986.

194. Morgan P, Lynn AM, Parrot C, Morray JP: Hemodynamic and metabolic effects of two anesthetic techniques in children undergoing surgical repair of acyanotic congenital heart disease. Anesth Analg 66:1028, 1987.

195. Laishley RS, Burrows FA, Lerman J, Roy WL: Effect of anesthetic induction regimens on oxygen saturation in cyanotic congenital heart disease. Anesthesiology 65:673, 1986.

196. Rautiainen P: Alfentanil infusion for sedation in infants and small children during cardiac catheterization. Can J Anaesth 38:980, 1992.

197. Kao YJ, Norton RG: Propofol in cardiac catheterization [letter]. Anesth Analg 75:859, 1992.

198. Singh A, Girotra S, Mehta Y, et al: Total intravenous anesthesia with ketamine for pediatric interventional cardiac procedures. J Cardiothorac Vasc Anesth 14:36, 2000.

199. Hickey PR, Wessel DL, Streitz SL, et al: Transcatheter closure of atrial septal defects: hemodynamic complications and anesthetic management. Anesth Analg 74:44, 1992.

200. Hall SC: Children with congenital heart disease undergoing noncardiac surgery. Semin Anesth 12:8, 1993.

201. Rao PS: Balloon pulmonary valvuloplasty: a review. Clin Cardiol 2:55, 1989.

202. Choy M, Beekman RH, Rocchini AP, et al: Percutaneous balloon valvuloplasty for valvar aortic stenosis in infants and children. Am J Cardiol 59:1010, 1987.

203. Beekman RH, Rocchini AP, Dick M, et al: Percutaneous balloon angioplasty for native coarctation of the aorta. J Am Coll Cardiol 10:1078, 1987.

204. Rao PS, Chopra PS: Role of balloon angioplasty in the treatment of aortic coarctation. Ann Thorac Surg 52:621, 1991.

205. Hellenbrand WE, Fahey JT, McGowan FX, et al: Transesophageal echocardiographic guidance of transcatheter closure of atrial septal defect. Am J Cardiol 66:207, 1990.

206. Rome JJ, Keane JF, Perry SB, et al: Double-umbrella closure of atrial defects. Circulation 82:751, 1990.

207. Bridges ND, Perry SB, Keane JF, et al: Preoperative transcatheter closure of congenital muscular ventricular defects. N Engl J Med 324:1312, 1991.

208. Latson LA, Hofschire PJ, Kugler JD, et al: Transcatheter closure of patent ductus arteriosus in pediatric patients. J Pediatr 115:549, 1989.

209. Lavoie J, Walsh EP, Burrows FA, et al: Effects of propofol or isoflurane anesthesia on cardiac conduction in children undergoing radiofrequency catheter ablation for tachydysrhythmias. Anesthesiology 82:884, 1995.

210. Lai LP, Lin JL, Wu MH, et al: Usefulness of intravenous propofol anesthesia for radiofrequency catheter ablation in patients with tachyarrhythmias: infeasibility for pediatric patients with ectopic atrial tachycardia. Pacing Clin Electrophysiol 22:1358, 1999.

211. Wu MH, Lin JL, Lai LP, et al: Radiofrequency catheter ablation of tachycardia in children with and without congenital heart disease: indications and limitations. Int J Cardiol 72:221, 2000.

212. Besag FMC, Singh MP, Whitelaw AGL: Surgery of the ill, extremely low birthweight infant: should transfer to the operating theatre be avoided? Acta Paediatr Scand 73:594, 1984.

213. Coster DD, Gorton ME, Grooters RK, et al: Surgical closure of the patent ductus arteriosus in the neonatal intensive care unit. Ann Thorac Surg 48:386, 1989.

214. Oxnard SC, McGough EC, Jung AL, et al: Ligation of the patent ductus arteriosus in the newborn intensive care unit. Ann Thorac Surg 23:564, 1977.

215. Anand KJS, Sippell WG, Aynsley-Green A: Randomised trial of fentanyl anaesthesia in preterm babies undergoing surgery: effects of the stress syndrome. Lancet 1:243, 1987.

216. Friesen RH, Henry DB: Cardiovascular changes in preterm neonates receiving isoflurane, halothane, fentanyl, and ketamine. Anesthesiology 64:238, 1986.

217. Robinson S, Gregory GA: Fentanyl-air-oxygen anesthesia for ligation of patent ductus arteriosus in preterm infants. Anesth Analg 60:331 1981.

218. Yaster M: The dose response of fentanyl in neonatal anesthesia. Anesthesiology 66:433, 1987.

219. Hall SC: Neonatal surgical emergencies. Adv Anesth 9:27, 1992.

220. Gibson DL, Sheps SB, Uh SH, et al: Retinopathy of prematurity-induced blindness: birth weight-specific survival and the new epidemic. Pediatrics 86:405, 1990.

221. Alexander CM, Gross JB: Sedative doses of midazolam depress hypoxic ventilatory responses in humans. Anesth Analg 67:377, 1988.

222. Yaster M, Nichols DG, Deshpande JK, Wetzel RC: Midazolam-fentanyl intravenous sedation in children: case report of respiratory arrest. Pediatrics 86:463, 1990.

223. Cohen MD: Pediatric sedation. Radiology 175:611, 1990.

224. Schecter NL, Berde CB, Yaster M: Pain in Infants, Children, and Adolescents. Baltimore, Williams & Wilkins, 1993, p 145.

225. Schutzman SA, Liebelt E, Wisk M, Burg J: Comparison of oral transmucosal fentanyl citrate and intramuscular meperidine, promethazine, and chlorpromazine for conscious sedation of children undergoing laceration repair. Ann Emerg Med 28:385, 1996.

226. Kennedy RM, Porter FL, Miller JP, Jaffe DM: Comparison of fentanyl/midazolam with ketamine/midazolam for pediatric orthopedic emergencies. Pediatrics 102:337, 1998.

227. Marx CM, Stein J, Tyler MK, et al: Ketamine-midazolam versus meperidine-midazolam for painful procedures in pediatric oncology patients. J Clin Oncol 15:94, 1997.

228. Petrack EM, Marx CM, Wright MS: Intramuscular ketamine is superior to meperidine, promethazine, and chlorpromazine for pediatric emergency department sedation. Arch Pediatr Adolesc Med 150:676, 1996.

229. Auden SM, Sobczyk WL, Solinger RE, Goldsmith LJ: Oral ketamine/midazolam is superior to intramuscular meperidine, promethazine, and chlorpromazine for pediatric cardiac catheterization. Anesth Analg 90:299, 2000.

230. Snodgrass WR, Dodge WF: Lytic "DPT" cocktail: Time for rational and safe alternatives. Pediatr Clin North Am 36:1285, 1989.

231. Terndrup TE, Cantor RM, Madden CM: Intramuscular meperidine, promethazine, and chlorpromazine: analysis of use and complications in 487 pediatric emergency department patients. Ann Emerg Med 18:528, 1989.

232. Spear RM, Yaster M, Berkowitz ID, et al: Preinduction of anesthesia in children with rectally administered midazolam. Anesthesiology 74:670, 1991.

233. Gutstein HB, Johnson KL, Heard MB, Gregory GA: Oral ketamine preanesthetic medication in children. Anesthesiology 76:28, 1992.

234. Beebe DS, Belani KG, Chang P, et al: Effectiveness of preoperative sedation with rectal midazolam, ketamine, or their combination in young children. Anesth Analg 75:880, 1992.

235. Goldstein-Dresner MC, Davis PJ, Kretchman E, et al: Double-blind comparison of oral transmucosal fentanyl citrate with oral meperidine, diazepam, and atropine as preanesthetic medication in children with congenital heart disease. Anesthesiology 74:28, 1991.

236. Reeves ST, Wiedenfeld KR, Wrobleski J, et al: A randomized double-blind trial of chloral hydrate/hydroxyzine versus midazolam/acetaminophen in the sedation of pediatric dental outpatients. ASDC J Dent Child 63:95, 1996.

237. Needleman HL, Joshi A, Griffith DG: Conscious sedation of pediatric dental patients using chloral hydrate, hydroxyzine, and nitrous oxide—a retrospective study of 382 sedations. Pediatr Dent 17:424, 1995.

238. McCann W, Wilson S, Larsen P, Stehle B: The effects of nitrous oxide on behavior and physiological parameters during conscious sedation with a moderate dose of chloral hydrate and hydroxyzine. Pediatr Dent 18:35, 1996.

239. Wilson S, Matusak A, Casamassimo PS, Larsen P: The effects of nitrous oxide on pediatric dental patients sedated with chloral hydrate and hydroxyzine. Pediatr Dent 20:253, 1998.

240. Ariffin SA, Whyte JA, Malins AF, Cooper GM: Comparison of induction and recovery between sevoflurane and halothane supplementation of anaesthesia in children undergoing outpatient dental extractions. Br J Anaesth 78:157, 1997.

241. Sams DR, Thornton JB, Wright JT: The assessment of two oral sedation drug regimens in pediatric dental patients. ASDC J Dent Child 59:306, 1992.

242. Hartgraves PM, Primosch RE: An evaluation of oral and nasal midazolam for pediatric dental sedation. ASDC J Dent Child 61:175, 1994.

243. Gonzalez-Arrieta ML, Juarez Melendez J, Silva Hernandez J, et al: Total intravenous anesthesia with propofol vs. propofol/midazolam in oncology patients. Arch Med Res 26:75, 1995.

244. Litman RS: Conscious sedation with remifentanil and midazolam during brief painful procedures in children. Arch Pediatr Adolesc Med 153:1085, 1999.

245. Graff KJ, Kennedy RM, Jaffe DM: Conscious sedation for pediatric orthopaedic emergencies. Pediatr Emerg Care 12:31, 1996.

246. Rauch DA: Use of ketamine in a pain management protocol for repetitive procedures. Pediatrics 102:404, 1998.

247. Goad RN, Webster D: Sedation, analgesia, and anesthesia issues in the pediatric patient. Clin Podiatr Med Surg 14:131, 1997.

248. Sandler ES, Weyman C, Conner K, et al: Midazolam versus fentanyl as premedication for painful procedure in children with cancer. Pediatrics 89:631, 1992.

249. Schwartz S, Bevan JC, Roberts G, Dean DM: Midazolam sedation and local anaesthesia compared with general anaesthesia for paediatric outpatient dental surgery. Paediatr Anaesth 2:309, 1992.

250. Sievers TD, Yee JD, Foley ME, et al: Midazolam for conscious sedation during pediatric oncology procedures: safety and recovery parameters. Pediatrics 88:1172, 1991.

251. Tolia V, Brennan S, Aravind MK, Kauffman RE: Pharmacokinetic and pharmacodynamic study of midazolam in children during esophagogastroduodenoscopy. J Pediatr 119:467 1991.

252. Latson LA, Cheatham JP, Gumbiner CH, et al: Midazolam nose drops for outpatient echocardiography sedation in infants. Am Heart J 121:209, 1991.

253. Guidon-Attali C, Mouillac F, Quilichini D, et al: Propofol as the main anaesthetic agent in dental surgery. Acta Anaesthesiol Scand 34:397, 1990.

254. Hasty MF, Vann WF, Dilley DC, Anderson JA: Conscious sedation of pediatric dental patients: an investigation of chloral hydrate, hydroxyzine pamoate, and meperidine vs. chloral hydrate and hydroxyzine pamoate. Pediatr Dent 13:10, 1991.

255. Bauchner H, May A, Coates E: Use of analgesic agents for invasive medical procedures in pediatric and neonatal intensive care units. J Pediatr 121:647, 1992.

256. McDowall RH, Scher CS, Barst SM: Total intravenous anesthesia for children undergoing brief diagnostic or therapeutic procedures. J Clin Anesth 7:273, 1995.

257. Cote CJ, Notterman DA, Karl HW, et al: Adverse sedation events in pediatrics: a critical incident analysis of contributing factors. Pediatrics 105:805, 2000.

258. Malviya S, Voepel-Lewis T, Tait AR: Adverse events and risk factors associated with the sedation of children by nonanesthesiologists. Anesth Analg 85:1207, 1997.

259. Pena BM, Krauss B: Adverse events of procedural sedation and analgesia in a pediatric emergency department. Ann Emerg Med 34:483, 1999.

260. Chuang E, Wenner WJ Jr, Piccoli DA, et al: Intravenous sedation in pediatric upper gastrointestinal endoscopy. Gastrointest Endosc 42:156, 1995.

261. Liacouras CA, Mascarenhas M, Poon C, Wenner WJ: Placebo-controlled trial assessing the use of oral midazolam as a premedication to conscious sedation for pediatric endoscopy. Gastrointest Endosc 47:455, 1998.

262. Marx CM, Stein J, Tyler MK, et al: Ketamine-midazolam versus meperidine-midazolam for painful procedures in pediatric oncology patients. J Clin Oncol 15:94, 1997.

263. Parker RI, Mahan RA, Giugliano D, Parker MM: Efficacy and safety of intravenous midazolam and ketamine as sedation for therapeutic and diagnostic procedures in children. Pediatrics 99:427, 1997.

264. Tobias JD, Phipps S, Smith B, Mulhern RK: Oral ketamine premedication to alleviate the distress of invasive procedures in pediatric oncology patients. Pediatrics 90:537, 1992.

265. Oei-Lim VL, White M, Kalkman CJ, et al: Pharmacokinetics of propofol during conscious sedation using target-controlled infusion in anxious patients undergoing dental treatment. Br J Anaesth 80:324, 1998.

266. Zacharias M, Bridgman J, Parkinson R: Two methods of administration of propofol for dental sedation. Br J Oral Maxillofac Surg 36:19, 1998.

267. Pomeranz ES, Chudnofsky CR, Deegan TJ, et al: Rectal methohexital sedation for computed tomography imaging of stable pediatric emergency department patients. Pediatrics 105:1110, 2000.

268. Green SM, Rothrock SG, Harris T, et al: Intravenous ketamine for pediatric sedation in the emergency department: safety profile with 156 cases. Acad Emerg Med 5:971, 1998.

269. Green SM, Rothrock SG, Lynch EL, et al: Intramuscular ketamine for pediatric sedation in the emergency department: safety profile with 1,022 cases. Ann Emerg Med 31:688, 1998.

270. Dachs RJ, Innes GM: Intravenous ketamine sedation of pediatric patients in the emergency department. Ann Emerg Med 29:146, 1997.

271. Havel CJ Jr, Strait RT, Hennes H: A clinical trial of propofol vs midazolam for procedural sedation in a pediatric emergency department. Acad Emerg Med 6:989, 1999.

272. Krauss B, Zurakowski D: Sedation patterns in pediatric and general community hospital emergency departments. Pediatr Emerg Care 14:99, 1998.

273. Pruitt JW, Goldwasser MS, Sabol SR, Prstojevich SJ: Intramuscular ketamine, midazolam, and glycopyrrolate for pediatric sedation in the emergency department. J Oral Maxillofac Surg 53:13, 1995.

274. McGlone RG, Ranasinghe S, Durham S: An alternative to "brutacaine": a comparison of low dose intramuscular ketamine with intranasal midazolam in children before suturing. J Accid Emerg Med 15:231, 1998.

275. Parker RI, Mahan RA, Giugliano D, Parker MM: Efficacy and safety of intravenous midazolam and ketamine as sedation for therapeutic and diagnostic procedures in children. Pediatrics 99:427, 1997.

276. Vade A, Sukhani R: Ketamine hydrochloride for interventional radiology in children: is it sedation or anesthesia by the radiologist? AJR Am J Roentgenol 1171:265, 1998.

277. Litman RS, Kottra JA, Verga KA, et al: Chloral hydrate sedation: the additive sedative and respiratory depressant effects of nitrous oxide. Anesth Analg 86:724, 1998.

278. Shapiro BS, Cohen DE, Covelman KW, et al: Experience of an interdisciplinary pediatric pain service. Pediatrics 88:1226, 1991.

279. Donen N, King F, Reid D, Blackstock D: Canadian anesthesia physician resources: 1996 and beyond. Can J Anaesth 46:962, 1999.

280. Hoffreumon P, Lescrenier N, Baele P: Current anesthesia manpower in Belgium in relation to anesthesia work locations. Acta Anaesthesiol Belg 49:185, 1998.

281. Joint Commission on the Accreditation of Healthcare Organizations: Joint Commission Accreditation Manual Or Hospitals. Vol III. Oak Brook Terrace, IL, Joint Commission on the Accreditation of Healthcare Organizations, 1992.

282. Epstein BS, Schyve PM: Anesthesiologist's interaction with other medical departments outside the operating room [letter]. Anesth Analg 75:633, 1992.

283. Cappiello J, Wise R: Anesthesia Care: Survey Process. Oak Brook Terrace, IL, Joint Commission on the Accreditation of Healthcare Organizations, 1999.

284. Feldscot AF: The new regulations on conscious sedation. N Y State Dent J 55:8, 1989.

285. Fleischer D: Monitoring the patient receiving conscious sedation for gastrointestinal endoscopy: issues and guidelines. Gastrointest Endosc 35:262, 1989.

286. Committee on Drugs, American Academy of Pediatrics: Guidelines for monitoring and management of pediatric patients during and after sedation for diagnostic and therapeutic procedures. Pediatrics 89:1110, 1992.

287. Rosenberg MB, Campbell RL: Guidelines for intraoperative monitoring of dental patients undergoing, conscious sedation, deep sedation, and general anesthesia. Oral Surg Oral Med Oral Pathol 71:2, 1991.

288. Practice guidelines for sedation and analgesia by non-anesthesiologists. A report by the American Society of Anesthesiologists Task Force on Sedation and Analgesia by Non-Anesthesiologists. Anesthesiology 84:459, 1996.

289. Keengwe IN, Hegde S, Dearlove O, et al: Structured sedation programme for magnetic resonance imaging examination in children. Anaesthesia 54:1069, 1999.

290. Egelhoff JC, Ball WS Jr, Koch BL, Parks TD: Safety and efficacy of sedation in children using a structured sedation program. AJR Am J Roentgenol 168:1259, 1997.

291. American Society of Anesthesiologists: Standards for Basic Intraoperative Monitoring. Park Ridge, IL, American Society of Anesthesiologists, 1998.

292. Cote CJ: Sedation for the pediatric patient: a review. Pediatr Clin North Am 41:31, 1994.

293. Innes G, Murphy M, Nijssen-Jordan C, et al: Procedural sedation and analgesia in the emergency department. Canadian Consensus Guidelines. J Emerg Med 17:145, 1999.

294. Cote CJ: Sedation protocols—why so many variations? [editorial]. Pediatrics 94:281, 1994.

295. Wright SW: Conscious sedation in the emergency department: the value of capnography and pulse oximetry. Ann Emerg Med 21:551, 1992.

296. Tobias JD. End-tidal carbon dioxide monitoring during sedation with a combination of midazolam and ketamine for children undergoing painful, invasive procedures. Pediatr Emerg Care 15:173, 1999.

297. Croswell RJ, Dilley DC, Lucas WJ, et al: A comparison of conventional versus electronic monitoring of sedated pediatric dental patients. Pediatr Dent 1995; 17:332, 1995.

29

Pediatric Intensive Care

ROBERT C. PASCUCCI

◆   ◆   ◆

Care of the critically ill child is closely related to the care provided by the anesthetist in the operating room. These children present from the operating room, the emergency room, other hospital wards, or the transport service to a setting designed for optimal care of the sick child.

Most hospitals have found it best to concentrate the resources necessary to provide such care in a central location. Although it is possible to care for critically ill children and adults together in general-purpose intensive care units (ICUs), it is preferable to have a separate pediatric ICU (PICU) where the specialized equipment, environment, and personnel needed for optimal care of children can be concentrated.[1, 2]

ORGANIZATION AND ADMINISTRATION

The overall responsibility for the PICU frequently rests with an ICU committee, an advisory group with representatives from the physician and nursing staffs, administration, legal counsel, and other consultative and support services as appropriate for the institution. Broad issues of policy and the integration of the ICU into the overall mission of the hospital are rightly the function of this committee. However, the daily management of the unit and the development of policies affecting patient care must be performed by the physician and nursing director of the unit.

Nursing

Nurses trained and experienced in the care of acutely ill infants and children are key to the operation of the successful PICU.[3–5] The nursing staff must be large enough to provide safe one-on-one (or greater) coverage of the most critically ill patients, yet flexible enough to allow for occasional assignments of each individual nurse to a less stressful environment. Proper staffing allows the development of special areas of interest within the nursing staff, a primary care pattern of nursing assignments, the development of research opportunities for nursing participation, and enough diversity to minimize or postpone "burnout."

The director of nursing must be skilled not only in pediatric intensive care but also in education, leadership, and in personnel and financial management. An ongoing educational program within the unit, organized by the director or by a clinical nurse specialist, will help others develop and maintain their critical care skills and must be readily available to the staff to provide support, assistance, and encouragement where needed.

Physicians

A physician or team of physicians skilled in the resuscitation and emergency treatment of children and familiar with the patients currently in the unit must be immediately available to the ICU at all times. Optimal care is provided if a dedicated house staff team is assigned to the service, with leadership provided by an attending physician trained and skilled in pediatric intensive care. This physician should have primary responsibility for the patients in the unit and will coordinate each child's care in consultation with all services involved in the individual case. In this fashion, true multidisciplinary intensive care is provided to the patient while still allowing the focus of responsibility to fall on one individual—the ideal situation for patients, parents, and caretakers alike.

The medical director of the unit should have special expertise and training in pediatric critical care.[1] The director must represent the ICU to the rest of the hospital, integrate the mission of the ICU with that of the hospital as a whole, ensure that the ICU facility is available to all those who require it, and function as arbiter and patient advocate.

The Physical Facility

A well-designed environment for intensive care enhances the care provided and helps to reduce stress on the caretakers, patients, and families alike.[6] Adequate physical space is needed at and between each bedspace to comfortably allow use of needed equipment, minimize spread of nosocomial infection, and to provide some sense of privacy. Isolation areas are particularly needed in pediatric units because of the frequency of communicable diseases. The unit as a whole must be large enough to allow separate, defined "escape" areas for parents, visitors, and staff use. Parent and visitor space should include public and private areas. Facilities should be designed to encourage parental participation in the child's care. Charting, conference, sleeping, storage, and supply space must be part of the design, not an afterthought.

Each bedspace in the unit must be outfitted with a basic complement of patient care and monitoring equipment; additional and backup equipment must be immediately available. Central monitoring stations, commonly installed in adult ICUs, have a lesser place in pediatric units, where dysrhythmias are less often a problem and patient care is more bedside oriented. Computer workstations with Internet access, image-retrieval terminals, and hospital network interfaces are becoming more and more essential, as medical documentation becomes more "paperless" and as clinical, laboratory, and patient-monitor data become more integrated.[7–9] Gas, vacuum, lighting, and electrical outlets never seem adequate or appropriately placed; care in planning will minimize this quandary. Bedside television sets, VCRs, toys, and other facilities for entertaining children should be provided; often their use, coupled with parental reassurance, obviates the need for heavy pharmacologic sedation.

Costs and Reimbursement

Intensive care is expensive. Centralization of resources within a given hospital and regionalization of health care within a geographic area are likely to improve patient care and ensure better utilization of resources, but at the same time they place a larger burden of expense on the tertiary care center called on to provide these resources.[10–13] Adequate and appropriate reimbursement for care provided in one setting may be totally inappropriate and inadequate for care provided in another setting. Tertiary level referral centers are often essential for the critically ill child but are also the most costly setting in which to provide care. Cost consciousness must therefore be a part of one's orientation when intensive care is provided. Timely discharge or transfer of patients out of the intensive care environment

or back to the referral hospital when appropriate may reduce cost to the patient while providing suitable care in a location more convenient to the family.[14]

Excellent care must continue to be provided to those children who require it, and the cost/benefit ratio of so doing usually falls in favor of benefit.[15, 16] Appropriate use of resources, elimination of unnecessary laboratory tests, and further use of noninvasive monitoring of gas exchange contribute to small but real reductions in the cost of care for almost every patient in the ICU. The intensivist must carefully evaluate new technology as it becomes available, adopting only those devices or techniques that offer true improvement in patient care or that can provide such care more efficiently. Excellent intensive care is provided by people, not machines; the physician must continue to rely on clinical skills and an understanding of pathophysiology in caring for the seriously ill.

RESUSCITATION, STABILIZATION, AND TRANSPORT

The most acute condition with which children present is that of cardiopulmonary arrest, either in the emergency room or on the general hospital ward (see Chapter 7). Immediate, coordinated response by a trained team of physicians, nurses, and allied personnel is needed to deal with such emergencies. The pediatric anesthesiologist or intensivist is often a key member of such a team and may be asked to participate in training its members. Familiarity with the pathophysiology of cardiopulmonary arrest in children and with its management is therefore essential.

Etiology of Cardiopulmonary Arrest

It is important to stress that the etiology of cardiopulmonary arrest in most children is different from that in adults, and that the differences affect not only the conduct of resuscitation but also the long-term outlook for the patient.[17–27] The typical adult arrest victim presents after sudden collapse, often the result of an acute ventricular dysrhythmia related to coronary or other preexisting cardiac disease. This has been termed a primary cardiac arrest. The focus of resuscitation in adults is on rapid correction of the dysrhythmia.[28–34] If the rhythm disturbance is promptly corrected, recovery of spontaneous circulation is rapid, and the underlying disease is not severe, the adult patient has an excellent chance of good survival.

Children, except in unusual circumstances such as preexisting heart disease, blunt chest trauma,[35] or drug overdose,[36, 37] rarely present with ventricular dysrhythmias or primary cardiac arrest. In the previously healthy child, cardiac arrest is usually secondary to some other disease process. Most often, a primary respiratory event leads to loss of the airway or respiratory insufficiency; progressive hypoxemia and acidosis ensue and, over an extended period of time, lead to a secondary cardiac arrest. Trauma, asphyxia, central nervous system (CNS) disorders, drug overdose, sepsis, and other causes can have the same result.

Attention must therefore be directed toward evaluation and correction of the primary cause of the arrest as well as toward its result. Often, particularly if the primary cause is respiratory, simple restoration of the airway, oxygenation, and ventilation are all that is needed to restore cardiac function. Unfortunately, although return of spontaneous circulation (ROSC) is often quite easily achieved in children, the extended period of hypoxemia and ischemia before presentation may result in a poor outcome, especially in terms of neurologic function.[24, 38, 39] Emphasis is properly placed, in pediatric life support training, on the early recognition of impending cardiac or respiratory failure. Such early recognition allows appropriate intervention before the child progresses to frank cardiopulmonary arrest.[26, 27]

Physiology of Cardiopulmonary Resuscitation

The mechanism of blood flow and its distribution during cardiopulmonary resuscitation (CPR) have been extensively investigated.[28, 40, 41] An early assumption, accepted since Kouwenhoven et al.'s initial description of closed-chest CPR in 1960,[42, 43] was that forward blood flow during CPR is generated by the compression of the heart between the sternum and spine. More recent evidence suggests that in larger animals and in adult humans, thoracic rather than direct cardiac compression is the driving force for blood flow: a general increase in intrathoracic pressure, generated by chest compression, forces blood outward through the aorta. Flow is predominantly in a forward direction for three reasons: (1) valves in the jugular venous system prevent retrograde flow through that system, (2) the veins at the thoracic inlet collapse, and (3) greater pressure develops in the arterial tree compared with the venous system. The distribution of this blood flow, especially to the coronary and cerebral circulations, is both critical and complex.[44–48] Coronary perfusion is dependent on the generation of an adequate aortic diastolic (i.e., the relaxation phase of chest compression) pressure; a sufficient aortic-to-right-atrial pressure difference is necessary to create flow. Cerebral blood flow is influenced by multiple factors (transmission of intrathoracic pressure swings to the intracranial space, age, chest geometry, vascular tone, duration of resuscitation, use of medications), and is therefore more difficult to quantify. Some techniques believed to increase intrathoracic pressure and therefore improve forward blood flow may actually impede cerebral perfusion.

It is possible that circulation of blood during CPR occurs by both thoracic and cardiac pump mechanisms, the dominant mechanism being determined by the patient's size and anatomy. The thoracic pump mechanism may be operative in adults. Chest compression in children, because of their smaller and more compliant thoracic cavity, may produce direct cardiac compression.[47, 49, 50] New techniques for chest compression, based on these mechanisms, have been investigated.[51–53] The clinician should use caution here: new techniques that have theoretical appeal may not prove to be clinically better than conventional CPR, particularly in infants and small children.[49, 53]

Relevant studies are reviewed and revised guidelines for cardiopulmonary resuscitation are published approximately every 6 years by national research and consensus conferences. The following recommendations are based on the 2000 conferences and guidelines,[54] but emphasize the in-hospital situations and techniques likely to be encountered by the anesthesiologist or intensivist.

Airway, Breathing, Circulation

Loss of the airway is frequently the primary cause of a pediatric arrest, and the first priority is to establish an open airway. Assuming that there is no question of cervical spine injury, the head is placed in a "sniffing" position and the mandible is displaced anteriorly—a simple jaw-lift maneuver.[55] Hyperextension of the neck, which may compress and occlude the trachea, should be avoided. These maneuvers will relieve soft tissue airway obstruction in most children. If necessary, an oral or nasal airway can be inserted. The oral airway should just encircle the tongue; one too long or too short will worsen rather than improve the obstruction. Nasal airways must be gently placed to avoid trauma and bleeding from the child's vascular adenoid bed.

If the child does not make adequate respiratory efforts after these interventions, mouth-to-mouth or bag-and-mask ventilation is begun. Standard basic life support (BLS) protocols call for two effective breaths (1 to 1.5 seconds per breath), attempting to reexpand the lungs and restore functional residual capacity (FRC). For mouth-to-mouth ventilation in the infant, a better seal can usually be achieved by applying the mouth over both the nose and the mouth of the infant.

Bag-and-mask ventilation with 100 percent oxygen should be started as soon as possible. A self-inflating bag/valve system is useful because of its ability to function without a fresh gas source; if the device has a pop-off valve, the rescuer must be able to bypass the pop-off if higher airway pressure is needed to achieve ventilation. Most experienced rescuers prefer to use some variation on the Mapleson or Ayre's T-piece system to allow better control of FIO_2 and airway pressures. The rate, volume, and force of ventilation must be varied according to the patient's size to achieve adequate chest expansion without causing gastric distention.

If the rescuer is unable to ventilate the patient's lungs with a reasonable amount of pressure, an obstruction of the airway must be assumed. The obstructed airway should be cleared by one or more of the following maneuvers: (1) improving head and jaw position; (2) clearing of the oropharynx by suctioning and removal of foreign material, using laryngoscopy as needed; (3) if aspiration of a foreign body is suspected, a series of five abdominal thrusts (a modification of the Heimlich maneuver) or, if the victim is less than 1 year old, five back blows and five chest thrusts; (4) intubation of the trachea and, if necessary, endoscopic removal of foreign material.[25, 27] In the rare circumstance when none of these maneuvers effectively clears an obstructed airway, an emergency cricothyrotomy with transtracheal ventilation may be required.

As resuscitation progresses, ventilation should be continued with bag and mask until all is ready for tracheal intubation. A common mistake, particularly in the less controlled surroundings of the emergency room or ward, is to rush to intubate the trachea without adequate equipment, preparation, or assistance. Ventilation and oxygenation come first; tracheal intubation is a relatively elective procedure. Time is required to assemble the correct endotracheal tube, laryngoscope and blade, suction apparatus, and related materials (Table 29–1). Skilled assistance from a respiratory therapist or other trained individual is invaluable. An oral endotracheal tube (ETT) is the best choice in most emergency situations; it can be exchanged for a nasal tube when the child is more stable. If intubation is difficult, the insertion of an LMA may stabilize the situation, allow immediate ventilation, and provide a route for later fiberoptic intubation. Once the ETT is in place, adequacy of bilateral ventilation may be confirmed by auscultation, observation of chest motion and, if circulation is present, end-tidal CO_2 detection.[56] Even if correctly placed, the endotracheal tube can easily become obstructed or displaced; frequent reassessment is wise.

As soon as the patient's lungs are ventilated effectively, the patient should be assessed for signs of circulation (breathing, coughing, movement, pulse). In the infant, the pulse can best be felt in the brachial or femoral artery. If signs of circulation are lacking or doubtful, the child should be immediately placed on a firm surface and chest compressions begun. The chest is compressed by applying pressure over the lower third of the sternum, just below the level of the nipples, depressing it approximately one third to one half of the anteroposterior diameter of the chest.[27, 57] In the older child, two-hand compression is used as in the adult; in the younger child, one-hand compression usually suffices. For the small infant, better compression may be accomplished by placing both thumbs over the midsternum and encircling the chest with both hands (Fig. 29–1).[58, 59] The rate of cardiac compression should be a minimum of 100 beats/min (bpm) (faster in infants), with a compression/relaxation ratio of 1:1. The compression/ventilation ratio is 5:1, with a pause after every fifth compression to allow the breath to be delivered over approximately 1 to 1.5 seconds. With effective cardiac compression, pulses should be palpable in major arteries.

Advanced Life Support

Basic CPR must be continued during advanced life support measures. Coordination of efforts, clearly identified leadership, and communication between team members is important.[60] One physician should direct the resuscitation. This individual should not personally perform tasks but should oversee and assign duties as needed, and is able to stand back and evaluate the progress of the resuscitation as a whole.

Venous access is needed for fluid and drug administration, and should be achieved using the technique with which the clinician is most experienced. Peripheral veins can be used; if peripheral venous access is delayed, one should proceed to deep venous or intraosseous sites with minimal delay.[61–64] Suggested deep venous sites include the antecubital, saphenous, jugular, subclavian, and femoral veins. The femoral site is safe, relatively easy to cannulate, and sufficiently distant from the airway and chest that cannulation can proceed quickly without interrupting ongoing resuscitation efforts.[65] Intraosseous access, using a bone marrow needle placed through the anterior surface of the tibia, is excellent for emergency infusion of fluids, blood products, and medications.[26, 27, 64, 66–71] The intraosseous technique is especially useful in dehydrated infants. If vascular access is delayed, doses of epinephrine, atropine, lidocaine, and naloxone can be diluted in sterile water and administered through the ETT.[66, 72, 73]

The child in arrest may be hypovolemic. If so, aliquots of 10 to 20 ml/kg of an isotonic solution (normal saline, lactated Ringer's) should be administered rapidly to correct the hypovolemia. Hypotonic solutions should not be used for volume restoration because of their potential to induce hyponatremia if given rapidly or in large quantity. Should a large volume of crystalloid be found necessary, one may move to colloids or blood products as clinically indicated. Rapid or massive infusion of blood products in small infants may lead to hyperkalemia and to chelation (by the products' anticoagulant) of calcium, resulting in functional hypocalcemia.

Temperature should be measured during resuscitation with a thermometer capable of registering temperatures as low as 20°C. Children are difficult to resuscitate until their temperature is above 30°C. With severe hypothermia, it is best to continue good basic CPR, refrain from repeated drug administration, and direct attention to rewarming the child with warming lights, warmed respiratory gases and intravenous (IV) fluids, gastric or colonic irrigation with

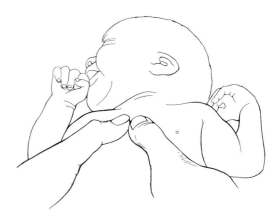

FIGURE 29–1. Method of cardiac compression in infants.

T A B L E   2 9 – 1

PEDIATRIC RESUSCITATION ENDOTRACHEAL TUBE SIZES

Age	Tube Size*	Laryngoscope Blade
Premature neonate	2.5 mm ID	Miller 0
Term neonate	3.0 mm ID	Miller 0 or 1
6 mo	3.5 mm ID	Miller 1
1 yr	4.0 mm ID	Miller 1, Wis-Hipple 1.5
18 mo	4.5 mm ID	Miller 1, Wis-Hipple 1.5
2 yr and above	$\dfrac{16 + \text{age (yr)}}{4}$	Miller 1 or 2, Wis-Hipple 1.5, Macintosh 2 or 3

* Uncuffed tube <8 years old or <6 mm ID; cuffed tube >8 years old or >6 mm ID.

warmed solutions, warmed peritoneal dialysis, or heat exchange by an extracorporeal circuit.[74]

An electrocardiogram (ECG) monitor will document the cardiac rhythm. The most common patterns seen in pediatric arrests are asystole or a very slow idioventricular rhythm.[68] These rhythms do not respond to defibrillation, and blind defibrillation is therefore not indicated in children.[27, 75] Documented ventricular fibrillation or pulseless ventricular tachycardia, unusual rhythms in children, should be managed with defibrillation, initially at 2 J/kg, increasing to 4 J/kg for a second or third shock. Automated external defibrillators,[76] becoming common for use in adults, may have application in children as well, but detailed studies have not yet been performed. Other aspects of dysrhythmia treatment are discussed below.

Medications

Restoration of oxygenation and ventilation, with a short period of effective basic CPR, may be all that is required to restore spontaneous cardiac function. Should this fail, pharmacologic therapy may be needed. Although a number of drugs are discussed below, the indications for their use vary and are rather specific. Data supporting efficacy in many cases are limited, and a given drug might be clearly indicated (an American Heart Association Class I recommendation) in one circumstance and clearly not indicated (American Heart Association Class III in another circumstance.[54]) Dosages are summarized in Table 29–2.

Epinephrine

Epinephrine is clearly the most useful of all resuscitation drugs. Although the drug has both α- and β-adrenergic stimulating effect, there is much evidence to suggest that the α (vasoconstrictive)-effect is the one of greatest importance in restoring cerebral and coronary perfusion.[45, 46, 77, 78] Epinephrine should be one of the first drugs given for cardiac arrest; specific indications include asystole, bradyarrhythmias, fine ventricular fibrillation, and (as an infusion) for pressor support after resuscitation. The goal is to restore and maintain adequate coronary perfusion pressure.[79] Although the intravenous or intraosseous route is preferable, the drug may be administered via the ETT if necessary.[80] The use of "high-dose" (from 2 to 20 times the "standard" dose) epinephrine for patients in whom the standard dose has failed to achieve return of spontaneous circulation, although based on good theoretical grounds, has met with mixed success.[81–90] Although ROSC may be achieved in a few more patients with high-dose rather than standard-dose epinephrine, ultimate survival rates are not significantly better, and there is some postresuscitation toxicity (severe tachycardia, hypertension) from the large doses administered. The current recommendation[26, 27, 68] for pediatric resuscitation is to administer epinephrine at the standard dose (10 μg/kg), and to consider 10 times that dose (100 μg/kg, 0.1 mg/kg) for subsequent doses if response to the standard dose is inadequate. If the endotracheal route is used, all doses should be "high-dose" (0.1 mg/kg) to ensure adequate drug delivery.

Atropine

Atropine should not be used for the initial resuscitation from asystole or severe bradycardia; these events indicate severe asphyxia, and epinephrine is a better choice. Once resuscitation is underway and ROSC has been obtained, atropine may be useful. Infants and small children have little ability to increase stroke volume owing to their small, relatively noncompliant ventricles, and tend to be dependent on heart rate for cardiac output. Atropine can be used to increase heart rate in bradycardic children and to provide protection against the vagal stimulation of laryngoscopy and intubation.

Bicarbonate

Administration of sodium bicarbonate to correct acidosis has been a longstanding practice, with little documentation of benefit and some evidence of possible risk. The definitive treatment of the acidosis that occurs during cardiac arrest is to provide effective CPR and to restore spontaneous circulation as quickly as possible.

Should bicarbonate be given to ameliorate the acidosis while resuscitation attempts continue? Some studies have suggested beneficial effects[91–93] and others caution of possible detrimental consequences.[94–96] Debate continues, but the balance of evidence suggests that bicarbonate is not indicated as a routine drug in resuscitation.[97] The drug may be considered for specific indications, such as renal tubular acidosis or profound diarrhea, which are associated with significant bicarbonate losses. A small initial dose of bicarbonate (1 mEq/kg or less) may be indicated in these children. Subsequent doses should be administered on the basis of results of blood gas determinations. Bicarbonate is also indicated in the management of hyperkalemia, hypermagnesemia, and tricyclic antidepressant (TCA) overdose. Overzealous administration of bicarbonate may lead to detrimental side effects of hyperosmolarity, hypernatremia, and metabolic alkalosis.

Calcium

Calcium has no role in routine resuscitation; there is little documentation of its efficacy and some concern about its potential for aggravation of postresuscitation disease.[98, 99] Calcium is indicated for hypocalcemia, hyperkalemia, hypermagnesemia, and calcium channel blocker overdose. It is also useful for short-term inotropic support. There is evidence that there may be developmental changes in calcium flux and its relation to myocardial function, perhaps making the infant more dependent on extracellular calcium concentration.[100–103] Infants less than 1 year of age seem particularly sensitive to the effect of calcium channel blocking agents, and these drugs are contraindicated in that age group.

Dextrose

Hypoglycemia is common during acute illness in small children because of their limited glycogen stores. The presence of hypoglycemia during resuscitation is easily detected with a blood-glucose test strip; if the child is

T A B L E   2 9 – 2
RESUSCITATION DRUGS AND ELECTROSHOCK*

Treatment	Dose	Route
Atropine	0.02 mg/kg	IM/IV/IT/IO
Adenosine	0.1–0.2 mg/kg	IV rapidly
Amiodarone	5 mg/kg	IV/IO slowly
Bicarbonate	1 mEq/kg	IV/IO
Calcium		
Calcium chloride	10–30 mg/kg	IV
Calcium gluconate	30–90 mg/kg	IV
Dextrose	0.5–1 g/kg	IV/IO
Epinephrine		
Low dose	10 μg/kg (0.01 mg/kg)	IV/IO
High dose	100 μg/kg (0.1 mg/kg)	IV/IO/IT
Lidocaine	1 mg/kg	IV/IT/IO
Verapamil (contraindicated in infants < 1 y of age)	0.05–0.1 mg/kg	IV/IO
Naloxone	0.1 mg/kg	IV/IO/IT (titrate to desired effect, often much less than 0.1 mg/kg)
Infusions		
Dopamine	2–20 μg/kg/min	IV/IO
Dobutamine	2–20 μg/kg/min	IV/IO
Epinephrine	0.1–1.0 μg/kg/min	IV/IO
Norepinephrine	0.1–1.0 μg/kg/min	IV/IO
Isoproterenol	0.1–1.0 μg/kg/min	IV/IO
Nitroprusside (average dose = 3 g/kg/min)	1–7 μg/kg/min	IV/IO
PGE$_1$	0.05–0.1 μg/kg/min	IV/IO
Lidocaine	15–50 μg/kg/min	IV/IO
Electroshock (Standard Waveform)		
Defibrillation	2–4 J/kg	Sync off
Cardioversion	0.5–2 J/kg	Sync on

* All doses and drug choices must be selected in light of the clinical condition of the patient; many are indicated in certain circumstances but contraindicated in others. See text for details.

hypoglycemic, glucose administration may dramatically improve the child's condition. Empiric glucose administration once during resuscitation is acceptable, but one should avoid inducing hyperglycemia because it may cause hyperosmolarity and may increase CNS damage in the postresuscitation period.[104–107]

Vasopressin

Vasopressin (40 units IV) has been included as an alternative to epinephrine in the adult algorithm for resuscitation from shock-resistant ventricular tachycardia (VT) or ventricular fibrillation (VF). It is a powerful vasoconstrictor which is thought to duplicate the positive but not the adverse effects of epinephrine. There are inadequate data to support its efficacy and safety in infants and children at present, but further study may support such use.

Antiarrhythmics

If the patient's condition is unstable and poorly perfused, electrical cardioversion should be used for emergent management of both supraventricular and ventricular tachy-dysrhythmias. Pharmacologic treatment, however, may be less injurious to the heart and is a better choice if the child's clinical condition allows.

Adenosine

Supraventricular tachycardia, with a rate typically greater than 220 bpm in infants, or greater than 180 bpm in older children, may be managed with adenosine 0.1 to 0.2 mg/kg injected rapidly intravenously, preferably through a central venous catheter.[108–110] Although there may be transient bradycardia following its administration, adenosine is generally thought to be safe and effective in terminating supraventricular tachycardia, and may help elucidate its origin.

Lidocaine

Lidocaine may be useful for management of ventricular ectopy and as an adjunct to defibrillation. Persistent dysrhythmias are uncommon during the postresuscitation period, presumably because previously healthy children lack coronary disease and myocardial damage; the need for a lidocaine infusion is uncommon. Persisting dysrhythmias suggest the presence of a metabolic or toxic etiology needing further investigation.

Amiodarone

Amiodarone (5 mg/kg over several minutes) may be considered for VT or VF resistant to multiple shocks and epinephrine, or in termination of certain supraventricular dysrhythmias. This recommendation is based on adult resuscitation data, together with limited experience with its use in pediatric cardiac critical care; data in pediatric resuscitation is limited. There is risk of hypotension if the drug is rapidly infused. Consultation with a pediatric cardiologist should be considered. Bretylium, formerly indicated for resistant VF, is no longer recommended because of the risk of hypotension and the lack of documented effectiveness in children.

Continued Cardiovascular Support

Infusions of catecholamines and other drugs to support the circulation are often required during the postresuscitation period. Their use is discussed later in the chapter. Support of ventilation, oxygenation, and intravascular volume will assist in maintaining cardiovascular stability as preparations are made for transfer of the patient to an ICU for further care.

Transport

After stabilization, arrangements must be made for transfer of the patient to an appropriate intensive care facility, either within the same hospital or at a regional referral center. The greatest risk to the patient may occur during transport from one facility to another. It is incumbent on physicians caring for the child to ensure adequate monitoring and continuing intensive care en route.

Many tertiary medical centers operate a pediatric transport service as an adjunct to their PICUs; such services provide high-level intensive care in a mobile environment.[111-115] The pediatric anesthetist in a regional center may be called on to assist in training the members of these transport teams or to provide actual care for particularly ill children during transport.

The essence of such care is the provision of trained, experienced personnel (physician, nurse, paramedic, or other specialist), equipment, and supplies for continuous travel with the patient during the transport. Team members must be trained and experienced not only in critical care but in the adaptation of critical care techniques to the moving environment.[116] Physiologic alterations, particularly the hypoxemia and gas expansion associated with decreased atmospheric pressure sometimes encountered in air transport, must be anticipated.[117] An increased F_{IO_2} may be needed, and closed gas-containing spaces, such as a pneumothorax, must be vented before transport at altitude. The transport team must also recognize the effect of hypoxemia, fatigue, motion, and spatial disorientation on their own performance. Equipment for monitoring, for infusion of medications, and for patient ventilation must be reliable and portable, with sufficient battery power or gas supply to function independent of external sources for an extended period of time. The team should be able to provide, within limitations of space and weight, a level of support similar to that provided in a good PICU, with the goal of presenting the transported patient to that ICU in a state of relative physiologic stability.

MONITORING

Anticipation and early recognition of physiologic abnormalities are major functions of an ICU. Precise, extensive, accurate, and reliable monitoring of multiple variables in the children admitted to an ICU is integral to this provision of anticipatory care.

The objectives of monitoring are to safely provide accurate and useful information to the clinician in a timely and easily interpretable fashion. This information becomes part of the database from which decisions on diagnosis, prognosis, and therapy are made. All such data must be integrated with the history, physical examination, and careful clinical judgment to achieve optimal patient care. There are multiple components to measurements of physiologic variables: (1) the actual physiologic changes in the patient; (2) the transduction, processing, and display of the physiologic variables affected by those changes; and (3) the selective interpretation of the presented information by the physician. This last component is most important. If clinical data disagree with that from monitoring equipment, it should be determined why. Data from the monitors may be wrong.

Respiratory Function

Careful observation and physical examination should always be the first line of monitoring and a constant reference against which the validity of other data must be assessed. The color of skin and mucous membranes gives an indication of blood oxygenation. Adequacy of ventilation can be estimated from respiratory frequency, chest expansion, and breath sounds. Increased work of breathing is indicated by tachypnea, nasal flaring, grunting, retractions, use of accessory muscles, or gasping. Upper airway obstruction can be detected by the presence of stridor or prolonged inspiration; lower airway obstruction is marked by the presence of wheezing or prolonged exhalation. Localized pathologic processes within the lung can be detected by regionally increased or diminished breath sounds, and by the presence of rales or rhonchi.

Radiologic examination of the chest is an essential element in respiratory evaluation and should be considered an extension of the physical examination.[118] For the patient with severe respiratory impairment, a chest film is generally indicated daily and for any unexplained deterioration.[119] The chest film gives information about the adequacy of lung expansion, the presence of abnormal lung densities, the presence of air or fluid within the pleural space, and the position of the ETT or tracheostomy tube.

Monitors of airway pressure and gas flow provide continuous, real-time calculation of inspiratory and expiratory tidal volumes. Modern technology has allowed these measurements to be made even in small infants with low flow rates, and has greatly improved our ability to monitor and care for severely ill infants and children.[120-122] Graphic displays of inspiratory and expiratory flows, volumes, and pressures are particularly useful for judging proper inspiratory and expiratory times, and allow optimal adjustment of ventilator time/cycle settings.

Oxygenation is monitored continuously by pulse oximeter, providing early warning of desaturation and allowing rapid bedside adjustments of F_{IO_2} and other variables affecting Pa_{O_2}.[123-125] The device has limitations: it requires pulsatile flow, and may be less accurate when saturations are very low or when abnormal hemoglobin is present.[120, 121, 126-128] Nevertheless, it is convenient to use, and there is good correlation with Pa_{O_2} under most conditions. Continuous fiberoptic oximetry may be used to monitor mixed-venous P_{O_2} in pulmonary artery (PA) blood or in the venous return line of an extracorporeal membrane oxygenation (ECMO) circuit.[129]

Continuous monitoring of PET_{CO_2} has become a standard in the operating room and has similar application in the ICU. The technique is well correlated with Pa_{CO_2} under most circumstances. Significant discrepancy between the Pa_{CO_2} and PET_{CO_2} is often a marker of physiologic dysfunction, such as increased alveolar dead space or decreased pulmonary perfusion; the latter is a useful marker for successful resuscitation from cardiac arrest.[130-134] Capnography (the display and interpretation of the CO_2 waveform) provides additional information on specific changes in patient condition,[130] but there is significant potential for artifact, especially with the sidestream technique of gas sampling.[135-137]

Arterial blood gas (ABG) concentrations are a valuable indicator of respiratory function. Samples can be obtained from an arterial catheter or by intermittent arterial puncture; the former is safe, much easier, more reliable, and less traumatic for the child. Intermittent ABG sampling does not allow the immediate feedback that continuous monitors provide and, although ABG remain the "gold standard," minute-to-minute patient care is best guided by pulse oximetry and capnometry.

Cardiovascular Function

Clinical indices of cardiac function, such as physical exam and urine output, are complemented by invasive and noninvasive monitoring. The bedside monitor documents ECG, heart rate, and rhythm and allows setting of alarm parameters. These devices often measure respiratory rate (detecting chest wall movement by impedance pneumography) as well. Data trending and analysis may be performed at the bedside, and data are frequently output to a centralized storage and analysis system. Arrhythmia detection modules are not commonly needed in routine pediatric critical care. Noninvasive measurement of arterial blood pressure is usually accomplished by automated oscillometric measurements, which correlate well with direct arterial pressure measurements; they may be less accurate in small premature infants.[138]

An arterial line is inserted in most patients admitted to a PICU. Direct measurement of intra-arterial systolic, diastolic, and mean pressure provides reliable data when noninvasive methods cannot. Additional information on contractility and volume status can be inferred from the shape of the waveform and from patterns of fluctuation with the respiratory cycle. The systems transducing the pressure waveform are complex, however, with many physical variables (resonance, compliance, harmonics of the system, position of the catheter within the vascular tree) contributing to the waveform pattern finally displayed.[139, 140] The relatively fast heart rates of children make artifact more likely, and some caution must be exercised to avoid overinterpretation of the information presented.[141-143] Insertion of an arterial catheter should be possible in virtually any infant or child. Cannulation can be aided by Doppler flow detection or by transillumination with a cold-light source. Collateral flow is usually excellent in children, and distal ischemic complications are rare. The most commonly used sites are the radial, posterior tibial, and dorsalis pedis arteries; some favor the axillary artery.[144] Cannulation of the temporal artery is less desirable because of reported cerebrovascular complications.[145, 146]

A central venous catheter allows measurement of the central venous pressure (CVP) and provides secure vascular access. Multilumen catheters are commonly used, even in small infants. Possible insertion sites include the jugular veins (both external and internal, the internal being more successful but also more risky), the subclavian, and the femoral vein[147-150]; of these, the femoral vein is most commonly used, easily taught, and safe.[151-153] The ideal location for the catheter tip is in the inferior or superior vena cava. Positioning of the catheter tip in the right atrium may be necessary in certain circumstances but carries the risk of perforation of the heart.[154, 155] Catheter materials are thrombogenic, and clot formation and possible venous occlusion should be anticipated.[156, 157] Heparinization of the line will help.[158] Similarly, infection is also a risk that must be accepted, and routine exchange or replacement of central catheters does not seem to reduce this.[152, 159-162]

The CVP waveform is measured and displayed by an electronic transducer/amplifier system. If high airway pressures are used, the intrapleural or esophageal pressure can be measured and subtracted from the intravascular pressure to account for transmission of airway pressure to the vascular space.[163] There is no absolute "normal" value for the CVP. It should be used as a trend monitor; the change in CVP after a volume infusion, for example, will suggest to the clinician the current volume status of the patient.

A more accurate and complete hemodynamic assessment can be obtained from a thermodilution pulmonary artery catheter, which is placed using the same technique as in adults. Although this is neither routine nor without risk,[164, 165] the correct interpretation of data obtained can assist in patient management. Measurement of the pulmonary capillary "wedge" pressure provides an approximation of left ventricular preload[166] and may be a better guide to intravascular volume status than the CVP, especially in children with pulmonary hypertension or other conditions that elevate right atrial pressure. The PA catheter also allows cardiac output to be measured by the thermodilution technique. Carefully performed, such cardiac output measurements are well correlated with those obtained by the Fick and dye-dilution techniques, even in small infants.[167-169] Knowing cardiac output, one can calculate systemic and pulmonary vascular resistances and more precisely adjust therapy to achieve effective cardiovascular function.

Neurologic Function

The clinical neurologic examination—evaluating pupillary response, global level of consciousness, and noting the presence of focal findings and stereotypic responses to pain—allows an excellent assessment of the CNS. Unfortunately, much of what we do in the ICU (sedation, paralysis, restraint) compromises our ability to complete a satisfactory neurologic exam. Specialized neurologic monitoring, designed to measure intracranial pressure (ICP) or to otherwise monitor brain function, can help in these cases.[170–172]

Indications for direct ICP monitoring include a reasonable expectation that the ICP may be elevated, that treatment for this elevation will be available, effective, and possibly improve outcome, and that the clinical examination will be unable to provide similar information. The etiology of the brain dysfunction must be considered. In general, children with head injury have a good prognosis, and ICP monitoring is often helpful in their care.[173] Other injuries, especially severe hypoxic/ischemic insults, have a less optimistic prognosis, and ICP monitoring and control do not yield a better ultimate outcome.

ICP may be measured using an intraventricular catheter, a subarachnoid bolt, or an implantable transducer.[174, 175] Each method has advantages and drawbacks. An intraventricular catheter allows both measurement of pressure and therapeutic removal of cerebrospinal fluid (CSF). It is usually the best option if the ventricles are large, but is difficult to insert if they are small or shifted. The subarachnoid bolt is a screw placed through the skull, with an opening made through the dura and arachnoid (Fig. 29–2). This device allows transmission of a pressure wave by a fluid-filled column to a standard transducer/amplifier system. It is easily inserted, and penetration of the brain is not required. It does not allow drainage of CSF, and may malfunction if its lumen becomes occluded with blood or brain tissue. Implantable transducers, of either the epidural (Ladd transducer) or intraparenchymal (Camino catheter) design, are becoming more widely used and are supplanting the use of the subarachnoid bolt.[174–177] Although these are complex designs requiring specialized electronics, they are reliable and cannot become occluded with tissue.

The exact relationship of the pressure monitored by any of these devices to the "true" ICP is not always clear. The intraventricular device is probably the most universally reliable reporter of global ICP. The bolt and implanted devices may be significantly affected by local phenomena, and may be unable to detect increases in pressure in more distant regions of the brain.[178]

Measurement of ICP provides some indication of the physical well-being of the brain by allowing approximation of the pressure differential between the intracranial space and the arterial inflow pressure. A minimal cerebral perfusion pressure (CPP), 45 to 50 mm Hg in the adult but not well-defined in infants or children, is necessary for adequate brain perfusion. The minimal CPP for infants and children has not been well defined but is probably less.

Because ICP does not necessarily reflect brain function, attention has been devoted in recent years to physiologic monitors of CNS activity. Monitoring of both spontaneous (electroencephalogram [EEG]) and stimulated (evoked potentials) neuroelectric activity is useful in evaluation of patient status. When the results are interpreted in conjunction with the clinical exam and overall patient condition, physiologic monitoring provides a more complete picture of the functional status of neural tissues and may provide some information about level of sedation.[170, 179, 180]

Typical EEG abnormalities associated with global CNS dysfunction are slow rhythms with variable changes in amplitude. Seizure activity, sometimes difficult to demonstrate clinically, can often be documented by the EEG. Continuous monitoring of the raw multichannel EEG, however, is somewhat unwieldy and produces large amounts of data. Devices to reduce, process, and present these data in a format more useful to the clinical intensivist include the cerebral function monitor (CFM) and its more complex alternate, the compressed spectral array (CSA).[170] The CFM receives raw EEG data from a single lead; it filters, analyzes, and averages the signal over time, and presents a trend recording of the average frequency and amplitude. It is a simple system but useful for an overall approximation of cerebral electrical activity. The CSA is a more complex processor, transforming raw EEG data into a display of the power present in each of several frequency bands. These power and frequency spectra are displayed graphically against time in a three-dimensional plot. The advantage of the CSA, like the CFM, is that a large amount of data is compiled into a format that is easily and quickly interpretable at the bedside.

Evoked potential monitoring summates, records, and displays the electrical signals generated in response to an external stimulus. As these signals pass from the site of stimulus to the brain, distinct waveforms are generated by each portion of the nerve tract. These waveforms are then analyzed for their pattern and, more importantly, for the conduction time (latency time between the individual wave peaks in temporal sequence). Delayed conduction

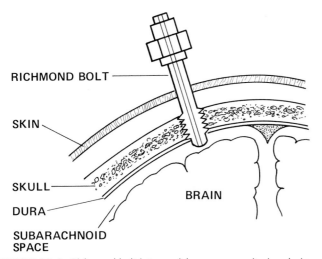

FIGURE 29–2. Richmond bolt intracranial pressure monitoring device.

in any given segment of the pattern implies physiologic dysfunction in the corresponding anatomic structure.

Evoked potentials can be generated by auditory, visual, or somatosensory stimuli; localization of dysfunction to specific brain regions is best accomplished by combining information obtained from several of these procedures. Brain stem auditory evoked potentials (BAEPs) provide information about brain stem integrity; the auditory apparatus must be intact for valid testing. Somatosensory evoked potentials (SSEPs) test more central conduction pathways and may provide more information about cortical function. Both are relatively resistant to suppression by barbiturates.

Evoked potentials may be capable of defining marginally functional neurons whose function cannot be detected by other means, and provide some information about a patient's prognosis.[181-187] Combination of the information from multimodality testing is useful: for example, a patient with intact auditory evoked potentials (preserved brain stem function) but abnormal or absent central conduction (as tested by SSEPs) might be expected to survive, but in a vegetative state. SSEPs, in particular, are becoming a useful tool to help judge prognosis.[184, 186, 187] Additional studies will be necessary before truly definitive interpretations can be given.

Near-infrared spectroscopy (NIRS) is a new technique for assessing cerebral oxygenation.[188-192] Near-infrared light, which can pass through skin, bone, and other tissues, is transmitted through the skull. Its reflectance and absorptive pattern are then analyzed to provide information on the relative quantities of oxyhemoglobin and deoxyhemoglobin present and on the redox state of cytochrome in the brain. This technique is still in early development and has been most widely applied to neonates in a variety of clinical settings, but holds promise for wider application in the future.

Finally, measurement of jugular venous bulb oxygen saturation ($Sjvo_2$) provides a global approximation of cerebral oxygen delivery and consumption.[193, 194] The procedure involves placement of a continuously-monitoring O_2 saturation catheter into the jugular venous bulb, typically from the internal jugular vein; this can be readily accomplished in the clinical setting of the ICU. Continuous monitoring of $Sjvo_2$ allows detection and possible correction of episodes of cerebral hypoxia. Although the technique is limited by inability to detect ischemia in regional areas of the brain, it has been found helpful when used in concert with other assessments of brain function.

MULTIDISCIPLINARY INTENSIVE CARE

The critically ill child often has multisystem disease. It is useful to approach pediatric intensive care in a systems-oriented fashion, affording detailed attention to the many components of the child's physiology. The ICU attending physician must ensure that care is coordinated with the many other physicians and disciplines involved, allowing focus on individual systems but maintaining an overview of the child as a whole.

Cardiovascular Support

Healthy children have a remarkable ability to compensate for circulatory dysfunction, but the stress of major trauma, surgery, or illness may exceed this ability and lead to acute circulatory failure. The clinician must recognize actual or impending circulatory failure promptly, assess it thoroughly, and provide support to restore adequate tissue perfusion.[27] Circulatory failure is manifest as the clinical syndrome of shock, with signs and symptoms of circulatory inadequacy and of the child's attempts to compensate for that inadequacy by sympathetic stimulation, catecholamine release, and vasoconstriction. A sample classification of the causes of circulatory failure is given in Table 29–3.

Although a number of measurements are made to support the impression of shock or circulatory failure, the history and physical examination remain the basis for diagnosis.[195, 196] Children in poorly compensated shock are anxious, irritable, or lethargic; they have tachycardia and tachypnea, poor peripheral pulses, peripheral cyanosis or pallor, and cool, pale extremities. Urine output is decreased, often to less than 0.5 to 1 ml/kg/h. Perfusion of central organs is maintained by distributing flow away from peripheral tissues, such as muscle and skin. This intense vasoconstriction sustains the central pressure, such that hypotension is a late sign of shock in children. Indeed, the presence of hypotension, apnea, or obtundation suggests impending cardiovascular collapse.

Once the diagnosis of circulatory failure is suspected, resources are available to confirm the diagnosis and to investigate its cause. ABGs are useful to assess the adequacy of cardiopulmonary function. In addition to documenting gas exchange, the pH of the blood may reveal metabolic acidosis, a marker of inadequate tissue perfusion. The routine chest radiograph provides information on cardiac size and pulmonary vascular markings; the 12-lead ECG documents cardiac rhythm, and may suggest ventricular strain, chamber enlargement, pericardial disease, or electrolyte disorders. These examinations, although not very specific, are readily available and may guide the initial approach to therapy.

More detailed information is available from echocardiography and Doppler blood flow analysis.[196-200] M-mode

TABLE 29–3
ETIOLOGY OF CIRCULATORY FAILURE IN CHILDREN

Hypovolemia: inadequate circulating blood volume
  True hypovolemia: loss of volume
    Blood loss (trauma, surgical)
    Plasma loss (burns, capillary leak, third-spacing)
    Water loss (vomiting, diarrhea/dehydration)
  Relative hypovolemia: no volume loss, but vasodilation
    Anaphylaxis, drug intoxication
    Sepsis
    Neurogenic: sympathetic blockade, dysautonomia

Normovolemia: volume status OK, but inadequate pump function
  Myocardial dysfunction
    Myocarditis, cardiomyopathy
    Hypoxia, acidosis, electrolyte disturbance, toxins
    Postoperative ventriculotomy
  Anatomic obstruction to inflow/outflow
  Physiologic obstruction to outflow
    Increased systemic or pulmonary resistance
  Shunt lesions (e.g., large AV malformations)
  Dysrhythmias
    Bradycardia, extreme tachycardia, ectopy

echocardiography provides a single-plane view of cardiac motion over time, allowing assessment of wall motion and changes in ventricular size during each cardiac cycle. Its high sampling frequency provides excellent time resolution, allowing precise measurements of dimension changes and temporal events.[199] The M-mode echocardiogram also detects collections of pericardial fluid, and allows the measurement of the left ventricular (LV) shortening fraction (LVSF: diastolic-to-systolic change in LV internal diameter/diastolic internal diameter). Normal LVSF is greater than 30 percent; values of less than 28 percent indicate reduced contractility. Analysis of the diastolic (relaxation) phase of the cardiac cycle is also performed echocardiographically.[201–203] Abnormalities in relaxation impair ventricular filling and are seen in children who have received cardiotoxic chemotherapy or who have other factors limiting compliance.

Two-dimensional echocardiography is used to establish a bedside diagnosis in suspected cases of anatomic congenital heart disease.[197, 199] When coupled with color Doppler blood flow measurements, the direction and velocity of flow through shunts and valvular lesions can be ascertained, yielding particularly useful data to guide the care of newborns with pulmonary hypertension. Transesophageal echocardiography may be used to measure flow velocity in the aorta and pulmonary artery. Although cardiac output can be approximated from these measurements, this requires accurate estimation of vessel diameter.[196, 198] The transesophageal approach is most useful in the intra- and postoperative management of the cardiac surgical patient.[198, 200]

Treatment of Circulatory Insufficiency

When there is insufficient cardiac output, a rapid but organized approach should be taken to improve circulation.[204–207] Cardiac output is the product of heart rate and stroke volume, and can be increased by modifying either of these components. Noninvasive and invasive diagnostic techniques, as outlined above, are helpful in establishing a diagnosis and may suggest specific therapeutic interventions and provide immediate, on-line assessment of the response to those interventions. Clarification of a diagnosis by monitoring the response to treatment is central to the practice of anesthesia and intensive care, and to some extent distinguishes those specialties from all others in clinical medicine.

Heart Rate and Rhythm

Bradycardia is poorly tolerated in infants and small children because stroke volume does not increase proportionately as heart rate decreases. This is because of their small, relatively noncompliant ventricles and to their decreased and poorly organized myocardial muscle mass.[208] Increasing the heart rate (within the physiologic range) is therefore a useful means of augmenting cardiac output. Infants and small children tolerate heart rates up to 200 bpm, with proportional increases in cardiac output.[209]

Bradycardia may be caused by an abnormally slow intrinsic cardiac pacemaker or by impaired conduction of pacemaker impulses. Slowing of the sinus node pacemaker may be caused by damage to the sinoatrial node or its blood supply by drugs, toxins, or pathophysiologic factors, the most common being severe hypoxia. Sinus bradycardia can be treated by removing the cause (e.g., hypoxia), by vagal blockade with an anticholinergic (atropine), or by a chronotropic agent (epinephrine, isoproterenol). If this is unsuccessful, or when a conduction defect is present, an artificial pacing device may be required.

Pacemaker leads can be attached directly to the myocardium at thoracotomy or can be placed in the right ventricle via a central venous approach.[210] Transvenous or external placement is used in an emergency. Ventricular pacing is usually adequate to restore cardiac output. At times, the use of a sequential atrioventricular (AV) pacer, which stimulates first the atrium and then the ventricle, may be required. This method enables atrial contraction to augment ventricular filling, providing 15 to 20 percent more cardiac output than that produced by ventricular pacing alone.

Tachydysrhythmias are less common in children than in adults but are occasionally seen, especially in those with preexisting heart disease.[211–213] Fortunately, infants and children tolerate rapid rates well and do not show evidence of diminished cardiac output or congestive heart failure unless the heart rate exceeds 250 bpm or there is an anatomic cardiac defect.

Hypoxia, hypercarbia, acidosis, or electrolyte disturbances may cause dysrhythmias. Initial management should include identification and correction of these factors. History or circumstances may suggest that a preexisting disease is the cause. Patients with prior atrial surgery (e.g., the Mustard procedure for transposition of the great arteries) commonly develop AV conduction defects and may present with complete heart block, ventricular tachydysrhythmias, or both.[212] The patient with Wolff-Parkinson-White (WPW) syndrome may present with supraventricular tachycardia.[213] Children with hereditary prolongation of the QT interval may have ventricular dysrhythmias presenting as seizure-like episodes.[214–216]

Atrial or supraventricular tachydysrhythmias (SVTs) are the most common types of tachydysrhythmia in children. When the underlying cause cannot be readily corrected and physiologic deterioration occurs or is likely to occur, immediate treatment is indicated. If cardiac output is seriously impaired, electrical cardioversion is used; the starting dose is 0.5 J/kg. If the patient is stable and time permits, maneuvers to increase vagal tone, such as carotid sinus massage, gagging, a Valsalva maneuver, stimulation of the posterior pharynx by a suction catheter, or eliciting the diving reflex by immersing the child's face in ice water may slow the rate by vagal stimulation. More likely, however, a trial of drug therapy with one or more antiarrhythmic agents will be indicated.[217]

Adenosine. Adenosine is now the drug of choice for treatment of supraventricular tachycardia.[108–110, 218–220] An IV dose of 0.1 mg/kg, administered rapidly (preferably through a central line), produces transient slowing of the sinus rate and of AV nodal conduction, and has a very high success rate in termination of SVT. High-degree AV nodal block may occur but is not a clinical problem because of adenosine's ultrashort duration of action (measured in seconds). The drug can be administered several times in succession if needed, with incremental increases of dose to 0.2 or 0.3 mg/kg.

Verapamil. Verapamil (0.1 mg/kg) is a useful treatment for SVT in older children. It is contraindicated in infants less than 1 year of age, however, because of the unique sensitivity of immature myocardium to calcium deficiency.[101-103, 221-224] Its effect is potentiated by the concomitant use of β-blockers.

Ventricular tachydysrhythmias are decidedly less common in children than those of supraventricular origin, but they usually require immediate treatment. If the patient is unstable, immediate cardioversion is indicated. If the situation is less acute, pharmacologic treatment may be administered. Lidocaine (1 mg/kg), bretylium (5 mg/kg), and procainamide (5 to 10 mg/kg, infused slowly) are the agents commonly used to treat ventricular tachycardia.[209, 225, 226]

Augmentation of Stroke Volume

Further augmentation of cardiac output is accomplished by increasing the stroke volume. Stroke volume may be increased by three mechanisms: (1) increasing preload (the end-diastolic volume of the ventricle) within certain limits; (2) increasing myocardial contractility; and (3) decreasing afterload, the resistance against which the ventricle must pump blood.

Increasing Preload. The volume of blood ejected by the ventricle during systole is proportional, within certain limits, to its filling during diastole.[227, 228] The Starling curve (Fig. 29–3) describes the relationship between ventricular end-diastolic volume and stroke volume. The limit of increasing stroke volume is reached when the ventricle becomes so distended that myocardial fibers are overstretched, impairing contractility. Overzealous fluid administration can also lead to pulmonary edema, generally seen when pulmonary capillary pressure exceeds 18 to 20 mm Hg but possible at even lower pressures if the pulmonary capillaries are abnormally permeable, if the plasma colloid osmotic pressure is low, or if lymphatic drainage of the lung is impaired.[229]

In clinical practice, the diastolic filling pressure is generally substituted for the diastolic volume, as pressure is much easier to measure than volume. Aliquots of 10 to 20 mL/kg of an isotonic solution are given and the patient's

response is observed. Clinical improvement (better perfusion, decreased heart rate, restored urine output) accompanied by modest increases in filling pressures is the desired response to volume infusion. Sudden or large increases in filling pressure suggest that intravascular volume is replete and that other measures may be needed to improve the patient's condition.

The substitution of pressure for volume measurement may be deceiving, as many factors other than volume may affect the measured pressure. Myocardial dysfunction, decreased chamber compliance, increased afterload, and pericardial constriction or tamponade are examples of factors that may increase the measured pressure independent of true changes in preload. The optimal filling pressure for an individual patient is unique and may change if the elasticity, tone, or compliance of the ventricle changes. The physician must titrate volume administration (or diuresis) against the patient's response rather than to some absolute number. By examining the pattern of response, insight is gained into that particular patient's ventricular pressure–volume–cardiac performance relationship.[230]

Respiratory and ventricular interactions must be considered in judging proper management. As an example, consider a patient with severe pulmonary disease and elevated pulmonary vascular resistance (PVR). Because of the increased PVR, right-sided pressures will be high even if intravascular volume is not. If volume is restricted or withheld, blood return to the left side of the heart will be reduced and systemic cardiac output will be compromised. Left-sided return may be even further compromised if the elevated right ventricular (RV) end-diastolic pressure (RVEDP) causes leftward shift of the interventricular septum, elevating LVEDP and impeding LV filling. It is difficult to make the "right" choice in clinical situations such as this. An attempt to reduce the PVR should be undertaken. Volume may be needed to maintain systemic output, even if high RVEDP causes peripheral edema, hepatomegaly, ascites, or pleural effusions.

Increasing Myocardial Contractility. Most children respond well to measures to optimize heart rate and volume, with improved peripheral perfusion and better urine output. In children with insufficient response, attention is next directed to improving cardiac contractility. Increased myocardial contractility may be represented on the Starling curve as an upward shift (Fig. 29–4), indicating a

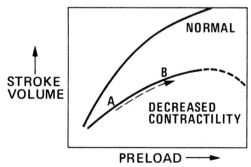

FIGURE 29–3. Frank-Starling relation. Increasing preload from point *A* and *B* results in increased stroke volume.

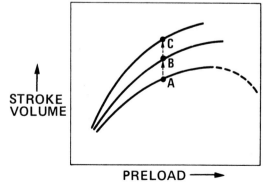

FIGURE 29–4. Effect of an inotropic agent. Stroke volume can be augmented by increasing myocardial contractility from a subnormal (*A*) to a normal (*B*) or even a supranormal level (*C*).

greater stroke volume for any given diastolic volume or pressure.

The initial step in improving contractility is to correct any negative inotropic factors such as hypoxemia, acidosis, hypocalcemia, hypoglycemia, circulating endotoxin or cardiodepressant drugs.[195, 231] Improved oxygenation and ventilation, treatment with calcium or glucose, and hemofiltration or dialysis often dramatically improve contractility and obviate the need for positive inotropic drugs. The choice of inotrope, pressor, or vasodilator and its dosage will depend on the desired effect on both contractility and vascular tone. Commonly used drugs and dosages are listed in Table 29–4.

Dopamine. Dopamine is commonly used for moderate circulatory insufficiency in pediatrics. It has a direct effect on myocardial β-receptors and also stimulates norepinephrine release from cardiac sympathetic fibers.[226, 232, 233] Although it provides only modest inotropic support, it is used because it provides support without undue tachycardia and because it improves urine output.[234, 235] The mechanism of this latter effect is complex, with contributions from selective increases in renal blood flow, from globally improved cardiac output, and from intrarenal mechanisms that enhance natriuresis.[236–241] There may be maturational changes in dosage and receptor sensitivity, but drug clearance follows first-order kinetics and seems adequate, even in ill neonates.[239, 242] Severe hepatic or renal dysfunction may prolong plasma half-life.[243]

Circulatory support from dopamine is best obtained in its middose range—typically 10 to 20 μg/kg/min. At high doses, the beneficial effects of dopamine are overcome by its vasoconstrictive effects. Therefore, if greater inotropic effect is needed than can be obtained with a moderate dose of dopamine, it may be beneficial to add another drug such as dobutamine or epinephrine, or to consider the addition of a vasodilator. By blocking undesirable vasoconstriction, the combination of an inotrope and a vasodilator may produce a more beneficial effect than either drug alone.[244]

Dobutamine. Dobutamine, at doses of 5 to 15 μg/kg/min, can provide good inotropic support without causing severe peripheral vasoconstriction or tachycardia.[245, 246] Because it does not increase afterload, it is particularly useful in supporting patients with severe myocardial dysfunction. It is effective in premature infants.[247] Dobutamine does not have any specific beneficial effect on renal perfusion but is often used in concert with low-dose dopamine to provide good inotropic support (dobutamine) and renal perfusion (dopamine).

Epinephrine. Epinephrine has potent inotropic and chronotropic effects and balanced α- and β-adrenergic effects on the vasculature.[248] It is the drug of choice for treatment of severe circulatory failure, particularly following cardiac arrest or severe hypoxemia/ischemia.[27, 68, 226] In low to moderate dosage (0.05 to 1.0 μg/kg/min), it effectively supports critically ill patients, often when other drugs have failed. The risk of extreme vasoconstriction exists, but only at higher doses; if the dose is moderate, the drug can be effectively used without undue risk. Elimination is by first-order kinetics and at a rate similar to that of dopamine and dobutamine.[249]

Isoproterenol. Isoproterenol is a pure β-agonist with potent inotropic, chronotropic, and vasodilatory effects.[248] It is especially useful in increasing heart rate, and its clinical use is generally limited to short-term use as a chronotropic agent in children with bradydysrhythmias such as complete heart block. Although it can be used as an inotrope, the associated vasodilation, potential for inducing hypotension, and increased myocardial oxygen consumption suggest extreme caution in its use. Administration to volume-depleted patients or to those with compromised myocardial perfusion or oxygenation may lead to myocardial ischemia or necrosis.

Decreasing Afterload. Alterations in heart rate, ventricular filling, and contractility may not restore tissue perfusion in seriously ill children, and further intervention may be necessary. Reduction in the tension that must be generated by the ventricle to eject blood during systole (ventricular afterload reduction) may allow the heart with limited contractility to empty more fully[250–255] (Fig. 29–5). A number of components contribute to the impedance or dynamic resistance to flow against which the ventricle must work. One that is relatively easy to modify is the systemic vascular resistance (SVR). Reducing SVR reduces afterload, increasing stroke volume without increasing the oxygen demand of the myocardium. This technique is especially useful in patients with severely limited ventricular contractility (e.g., myocarditis or cardiomyopathy) or

TABLE 29–4
DRUGS TO IMPROVE CONTRACTILITY

Drug	Dose (μg/kg/min)	Peripheral Vascular Effect			Cardiac Effect	
		α	β_2	Dopaminergic	Inotropy	Rate
Epinephrine	0.05–0.1	++	+	0	++,+++	++
	>0.10	++++	0	0	++++	+++
Dopamine	2–5	0	0	++	0,+	0
	5–20	+	++	++	+,++	+
	>20	++,+++	0	0	++	+,++
Isoproterenol	0.1–0.5	0	++++	0	++++	++++
Dobutamine	2.5–15	+	+,++	0	++	+

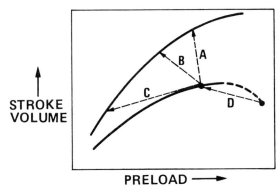

FIGURE 29–5. Effect of vasodilator drugs. (*A*) Primarily arteriolar dilator, effect similar to inotrope. (*B*) Mixed arteriolar and venous dilator; increase in stroke volume may be partially offset by decreased preload. (*C*) Primarily venous dilator; major effect may be decreased preload and decreased stroke volume. (*D*) If the heart is markedly overdistended, a venous dilator may increase stroke volume by "unloading" excessive preload.

in those with markedly increased SVR (e.g., hypertension or the later stages of septic shock).

Nitroglycerin, Sodium Nitroprusside. Nitroprusside, 0.5 to 10 µg/kg/min (typically 3 µg/kg/min), has been used extensively in children for acute short-term afterload reduction.[244, 251, 252, 254] Nitroprusside is a balanced vasodilator, with effects on both resistance and capacitance vessels.

Dilation of the systemic arterioles (resistance vessels) reduces LV afterload. Dilation of the capacitance vessels (capillaries and veins) may be helpful if the heart is over-filled, but careful attention must be paid to maintaining adequate preload. Excessive arteriolar dilation also may reduce coronary perfusion pressure, further compromising myocardial performance. Monitoring of cyanide and thiocyanate levels is recommended, although toxicity is uncommon at infusion rates less than 2 to 3 µg/kg/min. Nitroglycerin (1 to 20 µg/kg/min) is a vasodilator whose primary effect is on capacitance vessels, and which effectively reduces preload. The consequent reduction in ventricular size, wall tension, and myocardial oxygen consumption is beneficial in patients with impaired coronary perfusion. Nitroglycerin has been used in children after cardiac surgery to reduce SVR and PVR, thus improving cardiac output.

Amrinone, Milrinone. Amrinone and milrinone are phosphodiesterase inhibitors that produce both systemic vasodilation and inotropic support. These drugs act independently of the adrenergic receptors to increase intracellular cyclic adenosine monophosphate (cAMP); thus increasing intracellular calcium availability in the myocardium and enhancing relaxation of vascular smooth muscle. They are effective in improving cardiac output in infants and children, particularly where elevated afterload is a major component of the low-output state.[255-261] A loading dose of approximately 1 to 3 mg/kg (amrinone) or 50 µg/kg (milrinone) is administered over 20 to 30 minutes, followed by an infusion of 5 to 10 µg/kg/min (amrinone) or 3 µg/kg/min (milrinone); doses are adjusted to clinical effect. Unlike many other short-acting inotropic

agents, the half-life of these drugs is 4 to 6 hours. Acute vasodilation and hypotension may be noted immediately after the loading dose has been infused, but this is usually easily prevented or corrected by volume administration to maintain preload; cardiac output is often improved despite this transient hypotension. Thrombocytopenia may be seen with amrinone, and milrinone is now more commonly used.

Other agents may be useful in specific clinical settings. If abnormal vasodilation is present—in sepsis or anaphylaxis, for example—the use of norepinephrine (with its relatively greater increase in vascular tone) instead of epinephrine, or even a pure vasoconstrictor, such as phenylephrine, might be chosen. It is very common, in caring for critically ill infants and children, to administer multiple inotropic and vasoactive drugs simultaneously. The clinician should not hesitate to try different combinations and dosages of durgs in an attempt to match the type of support to the particular needs of the patient at that time. Consideration must be given to each drug's effects on contractility, myocardial oxygen supply and demand, and vascular tone in attempting to make the best selection, realizing that the situation is dynamic and that what works at one point may not continue to be effective as the patient's situation changes.

Mechanical Support. Intra-aortic balloon pumping, left ventricular assist devices, and ECMO can be used to reduce afterload, augment coronary perfusion, or fully support children with acute myocardial failure.[252, 262-264] Full discussion of these is beyond the scope of this chapter. There are technical difficulties in applying these techniques to small children (difficult access, size of catheters/balloons, anticoagulation) but these are not insurmountable. The use of these devices is best left to centers with great experience in the care of critically ill children and in the use of the device to be employed.

Hypertension

Hypertension is frequently seen in the PICU. Normative standards for blood pressure in infants and children have been developed,[265, 266] with hypertension defined as an average (over at least three determinations) systolic or diastolic pressure equal to or greater than the 95th percentile for age and sex. Moderate hypertension may simply reflect pain, anxiety, or awareness, and is then most appropriately treated with reassurance, sedation or anxiolytics, and analgesics or regional techniques for pain relief. Other causes for hypertension in the ICU are renal dysfunction, hypoxia or hypercarbia, fluid overload, and catecholamine excess secondary to physiologic stress. If sedation and diuresis are ineffective in controlling pressure, specific antihypertensive therapy to achieve vasodilation or a modest and controlled negative inotropic effect on the heart is indicated.

Fluid overload is common because of the salt- and water-avid state of the critically ill patient. Diuresis, usually with furosemide 0.5 to 1 mg/kg, is often effective. If further therapy is needed, vasodilation is a reasonable next step. Nitroprusside, as used above, or intermittent doses of hydralazine 0.1 to 0.3 mg/kg, is appropriate here. Unwanted tachycardia may ensue from the use of pure vasodilators, however. Therefore short- or medium-acting β-blockers have seen increasing use in children. Esmolol (optional load 500 μg/kg, infusion 50 to 300 μg/kg/min), a cardioselective β_1-adrenergic blocker, is effective and has the advantage of a very short half-life (β-elimination $t_{1/2}$ of 9 minutes).[267] Labetalol (0.25 to 0.5 mg/kg load, 0.25 to 1.5 mg/kg/h as an infusion; can also be given on a q6h schedule) has mixed α_1-, β_1-, and β_2-receptor blockade and a more prolonged duration of action (β-elimination $t_{1/2}$ 5.5 hours).[268] It is useful for extended control of hypertension but may present some difficulty because of the wider range of receptors blocked. Finally, chronic control of hypertension is sometimes best achieved with oral or sublingual agents such as captopril (an angiotensin converting enzyme [ACE] inhibitor) or nifedipine (a calcium channel blocker).[269, 270] Consultation with the renal or hypertension service is probably wise before such management is undertaken.

Respiratory Care

Infants and young children have less respiratory reserve than older children or young adults, and many patients admitted to the PICU have either a primary respiratory disorder or a respiratory component to their disease. The potential causes of respiratory insufficiency are many (Table 29–5).

The initial history and physical examination should identify the location, type, and severity of the lesion so that appropriate treatment can be provided. Bedside examination of vital signs, retractions, stridor, adequacy of air entry on both sides of the chest, clarity and quality of breath sounds, and the like will begin to narrow one's focus on the specific problem. This initial impression may be clarified by the diagnostic procedures and laboratory evaluations previously discussed.

The diagnosis of respiratory failure is somewhat arbitrary and must be made in the context of the individual patient. In general, inability to maintain a Pa_{O_2} of at least 60 mm Hg in an F_{IO_2} of 0.60 or less, or inability to maintain Pa_{CO_2} below 60 mm Hg may be considered respiratory failure. The patient's history and preexisting disease may suggest that some of the insufficiency is chronic in nature. Respiratory failure can occur with or without respiratory distress, if distress is defined as active struggling or increased difficulty in breathing. For example, a patient who is hypoventilating because of narcotic depression might well be in respiratory failure but would not be likely to display signs of distress.

The respiratory effort being exerted by the patient must be evaluated to determine how long it can be sustained before intervention is required or improvement occurs. If further decompensation is expected, or if there is disease of other organ systems that would be benefited by respiratory intervention, one should proceed with prompt, aggressive but careful support of airway, oxygenation, and ventilation. Fortunately, tremendous advances in nursing care, respiratory therapy, and in our understanding and management of pulmonary pathophysiology have recently been made, allowing us to support children in severe

T A B L E   2 9 – 5
CAUSES OF RESPIRATORY INSUFFICIENCY IN CHILDREN

Airway obstruction
  Upper airway
    Croup (laryngotracheobronchitis)
    Bacterial tracheitis
    Epiglottitis
    Foreign body
    Congenital anomalies
    Vocal cord paralysis, granuloma, or papilloma
    Burns
    Postintubation edema, granulation tissue, or scarring
    Vascular ring
    Tumor: intrinsic or extrinsic
  Lower airway
    Asthma
    Bronchiolitis
    Foreign body
    Lobar emphysema
    Cystic fibrosis

Alveolar or interstitial disorders
  Pneumonia
    Infectious: bacterial, viral, fungal, pneumocystis
    Chemical: aspiration, hydrocarbon, smoke inhalation
  Pulmonary edema: cardiogenic, noncardiogenic
  Massive atelectasis
  ARDS
  Oxygen toxicity, drug or radiation toxicity
  Pulmonary contusion
  Pulmonary hemorrhage

Impaired control of ventilation
  Head trauma
  Intracranial hemorrhage
  Increased intracranial pressure
  CNS infections
  "Ondine's curse"
  Drug intoxication
  Status epilepticus
  Apnea of prematurity
  RSV infection

Neuromuscular disorders
  High cervical cord injury
  Poliomyelitis
  Guillain-Barré syndrome
  Neurodegenerative diseases (e.g., Werdnig-Hoffmann syndrome)
  Muscular dystrophies and myopathies
  Myasthenia gravis
  Botulism
  Tetanus
  Phrenic nerve injury

Structural impairment
  Severe kyphoscoliosis
  Flail chest
  Pneumothorax or pneumomediastinum
  Large intrathoracic tumor
  Large pleural effusion, hemothorax, empyema
  Severe abdominal distention
  Severe obesity

respiratory failure and to achieve good survival in children who most certainly would have died just a decade ago.[271]

Respiratory Support

Airway

Patency of the upper airway may be lost because of an impaired state of consciousness or because of any of the obstructive lesions listed in Table 29–5.[272–274] Simply positioning the head and jaw as described for CPR may temporarily clear the airway but is impractical for prolonged periods and does not protect the airway from aspiration. An artificial airway is indicated for prolonged maintenance or, in the case of obstruction, to bypass a lesion that cannot be removed or otherwise corrected.[275] Other indications for an artificial airway include the need for mechanical ventilation or constant distending pressure, inability of the patient to protect the airway, and the need for access to remove secretions.

Two types of artificial airways are in common use, the endotracheal tube and the tracheostomy. In the past, an ETT was used only for temporary airway maintenance, but with improved materials and technique it is now considered safe to use an ETT for at least 2 weeks in most situations[276]; it is not uncommon for children to be safely maintained with an ETT for a month or more before tracheostomy is considered necessary. Tracheostomy is indicated only when endotracheal intubation is impossible, is contraindicated by the disease process, or where airway access is needed for an extended period of time.

Orotracheal intubation is indicated initially in most emergencies because it is easier and quicker to perform. When an ETT is required for many hours or days, it is common to change to a nasotracheal tube, which is often better tolerated by the patient, is easier to fix securely, and allows better oral hygiene during prolonged endotracheal intubation. Nasotracheal intubation is contraindicated in patients with nasopharyngeal obstruction, in those with midfacial fractures, and in patients with a coagulation disorder such that they may bleed excessively from trauma to the nasopharyngeal mucosa. There is an increased incidence of sinusitis with nasotracheal tubes.[277, 278] Nevertheless, apparent increased stability and decreased likelihood of accidental extubation with nasal placement argue for its use; unfortunately, no convincing data supporting one choice over the other exist.[279]

An ETT should be made of implant-tested, nonreactive material.[276] It is important to select the proper size tube (i.e., one that fits into the child's trachea easily and has a small air leak around it at 20 to 30 cm H_2O airway pressure). A tube that is too large is likely to produce mucosal erosion and subsequent scarring in the delicate subglottic region; one that is too small may compromise the ability to ventilate or to maintain PEEP and FRC. For children less than 8 years of age, uncuffed tubes are generally used. For older children, a cuffed ETT with a low-pressure balloon is usually preferred. Proper tube position places the distal tip of the endotracheal tube 1 to 2 cm above the carina. Positioning should be confirmed by observing bilateral chest movement, by auscultation of the lungs, and by chest radiograph. To minimize the chance of accidental extubation, the tube should be carefully affixed with waterproof tape to clean, dry, benzoin-prepared skin. Proper humidification and good nursing care should then minimize complications, such as accidental dislodgement of the tube, endobronchial intubation, and obstruction of the tube with secretions or blood.

Tracheostomy is indicated as an elective procedure when an ETT has been in place for several weeks and there is no likelihood of imminent removal, when a lesion such as a tumor, trauma, or infectious process in the pharynx or larynx precludes endotracheal intubation, or when a child known to be a difficult intubation will require multiple surgical procedures within a relatively short time. Tracheostomy tubes should be of nonreactive polyvinyl chloride or Silastic to conform to the child's tracheal anatomy. Proper humidification and suctioning have made the use of an inner cannula unnecessary in most cases. Cuffed tubes are used only in older children. Emergency tracheostomy may be necessary when acute airway obstruction occurs and endotracheal intubation is impossible. It should be remembered that oxygenation, even if the child remains apneic, can be provided through a transtracheal catheter inserted through the cricothyroid membrane.[280]

Support of Oxygenation

Adequacy of oxygenation is determined by the concentration of oxygen inspired and by the effectiveness of oxygen transfer from the inspired gas to the blood. The blood leaving well-ventilated and well-perfused alveoli is mixed with that coming from nonventilated or poorly ventilated alveoli. The resulting arterial Po_2 therefore depends on the inspired oxygen concentration and the proportion of pulmonary blood flow that is "shunted" through the lung without being oxygenated.

The most immediate method for increasing arterial oxygenation is to increase the inspired oxygen concentration. An Fio_2 of 1.0 is appropriate in the initial stabilization of the child with respiratory insufficiency. A high Fio_2 over a prolonged period of time is toxic to the lung, however, causing loss of surfactant activity, decreased compliance, alveolar collapse, pulmonary edema, and alveolar exudate.[281–284] Alveoli filled with high concentrations of oxygen may collapse as oxygen is removed by capillary blood, leading to further intrapulmonary shunting. Concern for oxygen toxicity should not be a justification for inadequate arterial and tissue oxygenation, but efforts must be made to reduce the Fio_2 as soon as possible to the lowest level that provides an adequate Pao_2.

Although supplemental oxygen compensates for impaired gas exchange, it does little to treat alveolar collapse and ventilation/perfusion ($\dot{V}/\dot{Q}$) mismatch. Recruitment of alveoli and restoration of FRC are necessary to allow adequate oxygenation at a lower Fio_2. There are a number of techniques for this; all are variations on increasing the mean airway pressure (MAP).[285–287] Continous positive airway pressure (CPAP) and positive end-expiratory pressure (PEEP), by maintaining positive airway pressure throughout the respiratory cycle, diminish atelectasis, increase the FRC above the closing volume, and prevent small airway closure during exhalation.[288, 289] Mechanical ventilation, applied in a number of ways, further assists the patient by providing the mechanical force needed to move gas into and out of the alveoli. The proper application of these techniques is discussed below.

Mechanical Ventilation

Ventilatory failure occurs when the work required for adequate ventilation exceeds that which the patient can accomplish. This may be because the patient cannot perform a normal amount of respiratory work, as in neuromuscular disease, or because the amount of work required for adequate ventilation is greater than normal because of decreased compliance or increased resistance. The respiratory bellows function of small infants has limited reserve and is particularly vulnerable to increases in the work of breathing.[290] Mechanical ventilation provides the necessary work of breathing, either by applying positive pressure to the airway or by applying negative pressure to a closed chamber surrounding the patient's chest.

Negative-pressure ventilation, developed during the mass polio epidemics, has largely been supplanted by positive-pressure ventilation in acute care settings. Negative-pressure ventilation is still useful in the chronic support of patients with neuromuscular disease.[291-293] The greatest difficulty in achieving satisfactory negative-pressure ventilation in children is adapting the devices to their size. Negative-pressure support can be provided by the classic tank or "iron lung" apparatus or by newer, more portable cuirass or "raincoat" negative-pressure generators. The latter have made it possible to conveniently and economically provide ventilatory support to children at home.

Positive-pressure ventilators employ a piston, bellows, or compressed gas source to supply the work required to inflate the lungs; exhalation is entirely passive and depends on the elastic recoil of the lung and chest wall. Conventional pediatric ventilators are either time-cycled, pressure-limited, or volume-preset machines; newer machines can be set to operate in either mode.[271, 294, 295] It is common practice to use time-cycled, pressure-limited ventilators for infants less than 10 kg and volume-preset machines for older children.

Time-cycled ventilators deliver gas at a predetermined flow rate until the preset inspiratory time has elapsed. If the machine is also pressure-limited, the peak inflating pressure (PIP) will not exceed the preset limit, but flow may continue until the end of the inspiratory time, potentially increasing tidal volume without increasing PIP. Pressure-limited ventilators have the advantage of compensating for small leaks in the system such as might occur around an uncuffed ETT. The tidal volume, however, may vary considerably with changes in compliance or airway resistance. Standard models offer a continuous flow of fresh gas, allowing the infant to breathe spontaneously between mandatory ventilator breaths (continuous-flow intermittent mandatory ventilation [IMV]). They have low internal compliance and can function reliably at fast respiratory rates.

A volume-limited ventilator delivers a preset tidal volume over a given inspiratory time, using whatever peak pressure is necessary to do so. In practice, a pressure limit or pop-off pressure is generally set to prevent excessive pressure within the system, but so long as this limit is not exceeded, the delivered tidal volume is relatively constant. Although a volume ventilator is much less affected than a pressure-limited ventilator by changes in compliance or resistance, it cannot recognize or correct for a variable leak around the ETT.

For infants and small children, the use of a volume ventilator does not guarantee delivery of a constant tidal volume to the patient.[295, 296] All ventilators lose some of the generated tidal volume by compression of gas within the ventilator, humidifier, and delivery tubing. The magnitude of loss (the "compression volume") varies considerably among ventilators and is directly related to the peak pressure; the compression volume (volume lost per unit pressure generated) can be from 2 to 10 ml/cm H_2O pressure. This may result in a marked difference between set tidal volume and that actually delivered to the patient. For example, if a 5-kg infant is ventilated with a set tidal volume of 50 ml, using a ventilator with a compliance of 2 ml/cm H_2O pressure and a peak pressure of 20 cm H_2O, the compression volume is 2×20, or 40 ml—80 percent of the set tidal volume. This amount would have to be added to the set tidal volume to deliver the intended 50 ml to the patient. Any change in compliance or resistance will alter the peak pressure generated, and therefore the compression volume and the effective tidal volume as well.

The method for providing gas flow for spontaneous breaths is a matter of particular concern in infants and children. Demand-flow IMV is now the norm in adult ventilators. With this system, gas flow enters the patient circuit only during mechanical breaths or when the machine senses that the patient is trying to breathe. This technique conserves gas and allows synchronization of the machine to the patient, increasing patient comfort and facilitating ventilation. It is difficult for infants and small children to trigger the demand valve that controls gas flow, which is conventionally activated by sensing changes in pressure within the patient circuit at the Y-piece just proximal to the ETT. A small drop in pressure (typically–2 cm H_2O), caused by the patient's attempt to breathe, signals the demand valve to open, providing flow to accommodate the desired breath. The patient must inhale sufficient volume from the circuit—often a quantity near or equal to an infant's entire tidal volume—to generate the necessary pressure drop. This requires an excessive amount of work for a sick infant. This work is magnified by the resistance to gas flow across small ETTs.[297, 298]

Conventional, pressure-triggered demand-flow systems are inappropriate for use in small children because of this workload. Continuous-flow IMV, in which gas is always flowing through the circuit and is immediately available to the patient, minimizes work of breathing but is wasteful of fresh gas and does not allow patient/machine synchronization or the ability to provide pressure support of spontaneous breaths. Several recent developments, however, have led to broader applicability of the demand-flow system, allowing its use even in small infants. It has been shown that other means of controlling the demand valve (e.g., by monitoring diaphragmatic motion, by monitoring airway flow rather than pressure, or by monitoring fluctuations in pressure distal to the ETT [i.e., just above the carina]) allow precise cycling of the valve with greatly reduced patient effort.[299-303] Of these, the practical clinical application of flow-synchronization has been most effective. With flow-synchronization, a small pneumotach, sensitive to flow rates as low as 400 to 600 ml/min, is placed in the airway at the proximal end of the ETT. The unique sensitivity of these devices allows the infant to trigger the ventilator, enabling synchronized intermittent mandatory ventilation (SIMV), pressure-support, and assist/control modes to be used freely, even in small infants.

Complications of positive-pressure ventilation may occur if excessive volumes (volutrauma) or pressures (barotrauma) are used (Table 29–6). Alveoli may be overdistended and rupture, leading to pulmonary interstitial air, pneumothorax, or pneumomediastinum.[304–312] Excessive PEEP or CPAP may overdistend the lung, reducing compliance and interfering with ventilation. Increased airway pressure may be transmitted to intrathoracic vascular structures and diminish venous return to the heart, impede pulmonary blood flow, and compromise cardiac output and oxygen delivery.[313, 314] In the child with an intracardiac right-to-left shunt, excessive intrathoracic pressure may increase pulmonary vascular resistance, increase right-to-left shunting, and decrease pulmonary blood flow.

Application of Respiratory Support Techniques

The child who requires an artificial airway to bypass an upper airway lesion, but who has normal lungs and mechanical function, usually does well if allowed to breathe spontaneously in a mist tent and oxygen. A small amount of constant distending pressure may be added if alveolar collapse occurs, but it is our practice not to do this unless necessary; the tubing and additional equipment required tether the ETT to the bed, making the chance of an accidental extubation greater.

If the patient's disease process causes a significant degree of alveolar collapse, several methods are available to restore lost alveolar volume. If the child is sufficiently strong to breathe spontaneously, CPAP is added to achieve this goal. CPAP may be increased in 2-cm H_2O increments while the patient's respiratory rate and mechanics are observed and oxygenation is monitored. The correct level of CPAP is that which optimizes lung volume and allows adequate oxygenation with an FiO_2 of 0.60 or less. With spontaneous ventilation, the correct amount of CPAP is manifested by a decreased respiratory rate, diminished intercostal retractions, and lessened respiratory distress. Excessive CPAP overdistends the lung, increases the work of breathing, and may induce apnea. It may also compromise cardiac output and reduce tissue oxygen delivery.

Controlled Ventilation

If the patient is unable to sustain the required work of breathing, mechanical support to supply part or all of the work is required. Seriously ill children may require full mechanical ventilatory support. During such controlled ventilation (CV), the ventilator performs all the inspiratory work. Mechanical breaths are delivered under volume or pressure control (see below). The patient cannot breathe spontaneously between machine breaths; attempting to do so ("fighting the ventilator") markedly interferes with effective ventilation and increases the risk of barotrauma. CV is typically used with sedative or neuromuscular block-

T A B L E   2 9 – 6
COMPLICATIONS OF RESPIRATORY SUPPORT

Source	Problem	Prevention/Treatment
Airways		
Endotracheal tube	Trauma (e.g., to larynx, pharynx, lips, teeth)	Proper intubation technique
	Occlusion of tube with secretions, blood	Proper humidification and suctioning
	Accidental extubation	Proper fixation of tube; restraint or sedation
	Endobronchial intubation	Confirmation of correct position by direct vision, auscultation, x-ray films
	Erosion of subglottic mucosa, granuloma formation, scarring, subglottic stenosis	Use of proper tube size, avoiding excessive movement, minimizing duration of intubation
Tracheostomy	Pneumothorax	Proper surgical technique, avoiding low insertion, care in changing tube
	Granuloma formation	Proper tube size, avoiding excessive movement
Oxygen	Oxygen toxicity	Minimizing concentration and duration of oxygen
Barotrauma	Pneumothorax, pneumomediastinum, pulmonary interstitial emphysema, subcutaneous emphysema	Avoiding excessive airway pressures
Atelectasis; lobar collapse	Increased intrapulmonary shunting	Use of adequate tidal volume, judicious use of CPAP or PEEP, periodic hyperinflation and suctioning, proper humidification
Infection	Pneumonia, sepsis, tracheitis	Use of sterile technique
Fluid retention	Pulmonary interstitial edema, congestive heart failure	Careful fluid balance; judicious use of diuretics
Circulatory compromise	Decreased cardiac output	Avoid airway overdistention; circulatory and volume support
Mechanical complications	Disconnection, power failure, excessive pressure, overheating, valve failure, etc.	Selection of good equipment, proper maintenance of equipment, experienced personnel, proper use of alarms and monitors

ing drugs to minimize fighting and to maximize patient comfort, and is often necessary in the acute phase of severe respiratory failure.

There is no universally applicable formula for initiating mechanical ventilation in the child. It is best to begin with reasonable settings and to immediately assess clinical adequacy of chest expansion and gas entry. Changes are then made until one is satisfied that oxygenation and ventilation are adequate. The patient without significant lung disease can usually be managed with volume control ventilation. In general, we favor tidal volumes of 6 to 8 ml/kg at relatively low rates, typically two thirds of the "normal" respiratory rate for age. If the lungs are normally compliant, this produces an inflating pressure of 15 to 20 cm H_2O. If compliance is reduced or the airway resistance markedly increased, the peak pressure must increase proportionally to deliver the same tidal volume.

Recent evidence suggests that too large a tidal volume will overdistend compliant portions of the lung, possibly lead to barotrauma or volutrauma, and not improve gas exchange.[308, 309, 315, 316] How aggressive should one be in correcting defects in oxygenation and ventilation? The goal should be to achieve acceptable—not normal—gas exchange, while minimizing potential toxicity from therapy. Pa_{O_2}s in the 60s, oxygen saturations in the low 90s, and Pa_{CO_2}s in the 60s (with corresponding pHs of 7.25 to 7.35)—parameters commonly used in "permissive hypercapnia"—are reasonable goals in children being treated for acute respiratory failure.[317, 318] In our experience, this level of gas exchange in children with sufficient cardiac output and hemoglobin concentration to ensure oxygen delivery is perfectly adequate to achieve good recovery.

Inadequate oxygenation usually responds to increased MAP, which can be applied in several ways. PEEP prevents alveolar collapse at the end of exhalation, restoring the FRC to normal and improving lung compliance. Care must be taken not to overdistend the lung, as outlined above. PEEP can be adjusted to achieve maximal compliance, which correlates well with optimal cardiopulmonary function.[319] A reasonable bedside calculation of static respiratory compliance is the following:

$$C = \frac{TV}{(P_{plat}-PEEP)}$$

where P_{plat} is the inspiratory plateau pressure, obtained by brief occlusion of the expiratory limb of the ventilator circuit just after the completion of a mechanical inspiration.

The volume-control mode is usually satisfactory for children with minimal lung disease. In patients with more severe difficulty in oxygenation or ventilation, one may switch from volume to pressure-controlled ventilation. Pressure control allows reshaping of the breath, with a rapid inflow of gas to quickly increase the airway pressure to the present level and then an extended "hold" at this level. The technique may allow significant increases in MAP, alveolar recruitment, and oxygenation without undue increases in peak pressure. Long inspiratory times or inverse I:E ratios (inspiration longer than exhalation) allow additional time for gas to diffuse into the periphery of the lung. The extreme of this technique is so-called CPAP with

release (or airway pressure release ventilation [APRV])—not commonly used in children—in which a moderately high airway pressure is sustained continuously with timed, brief interruptions to a lower pressure level to allow rapid exhalation.[320]

Adjustments to the rate and pattern of ventilation are made according to the patient's condition. Long inspiratory times, although good for oxygenation, unfortunately reduce the time allotted to exhalation. Patients with small-airway disease or diffusely increased airway resistance (see "Status Asthmaticus," below) will require a prolonged expiratory time to allow adequate exhalation and CO_2 removal. Too rapid a respiratory rate will lead to "stacking" of breaths, in which a second breath is delivered before the lungs have emptied to FRC. This, in turn, will lead to overdistention ("auto-PEEP") and will hinder rather than augment CO_2 removal.[321-323] These children are often extremely difficult to ventilate.

Some cases of acute respiratory failure cannot be reversed despite maximal conventional support. High-frequency ventilation (HFV) is the logical next step for children failing aggressive conventional support, and is now part of routine care in many pediatric intensive care units. The term "high-frequency ventilation" encompasses a number of ventilatory techniques which, although distinct, share a common feature: the delivery of low-tidal-volume breaths at rates in excess of the physiologic range. Several mechanisms of gas exchange may be operative in HFV. Dispersion of gas from proximal to distal airways and from one region of the lung to another occurs not only by conventional bulk movement of large volumes of gas but also by enhanced diffusion of gas molecules. This diffusion is augmented by turbulence, by the branching architecture of the tracheobronchial tree, and by the interaction of the advancing and recessing high-frequency wavefront with the molecules along its path.[295, 324, 325]

The three modes of high-frequency ventilation presently available can be categorized according to their method of producing a breath and the rate at which they do so. High-frequency positive-pressure ventilation (HFPPV) devices generate small tidal volumes in the manner of a conventional ventilator but at rates of 100 to 120 breaths/min. High-frequency jet ventilation (HFJV) devices inject gas directly into the trachea through a special cannula at rates of 60 to several hundred breaths/min; the Venturi effect augments the delivered tidal volume. High-frequency oscillatory ventilation (HFOV) produces an active to-and-fro cycling of respiratory gases at rates of 300 to 1,000 + breaths/min (5 to 20 Hz). HFPPV and HFJV depend on the passive recoil of the respiratory system for exhalation, whereas the HFOV produces an active exhalation.

The clinical hope for HFV has been to provide improved ventilatory support for seriously ill patients while avoiding or minimizing barotrauma caused by high peak airway pressures. It is clear that HFV has a definite place in the management of pulmonary air leaks.[326] By providing adequate gas exchange and simultaneously reducing peak airway pressure, gas leakage through bronchopleural fistulae is reduced and the leaks are allowed to seal. This application of HFV, which may be termed the "low-volume," "low-pressure," or "air-leak," protocol, is useful in certain settings, but we have found HFV, and specifically

HFOV, to be even more widely useful in achieving oxygenation and alveolar recruitment.

HFOV has received considerable evaluation in neonates and limited use in older children. The neonatal experience has been mixed, with some trials showing no benefit[327] and others notable improvement.[328, 329] The difference appears to lie in the ventilatory strategy employed; HFOV protocols that seek higher MAPs and vigorously pursue alveolar recruitment seem to be successful; those that favor reduced MAP fail.[330, 331] HFOV, using a "high-volume" or "alveolar recruitment" strategy, is generally successful in older children with diffuse alveolar disease.[332, 333] When placing a child failing conventional pressure-controlled ventilation on HFOV, MAPs are initially set at a significantly higher level than they had been on conventional ventilation. As alveolar recruitment takes place, the FIO_2 is progressively reduced to less than 0.60 and, when that goal has been achieved, the MAP is reduced slowly as tolerated. Typically, after the first 24 hours on HFOV, gas exchange is adequate, the FIO_2 has been reduced to a safe value and, although the MAP is at a level somewhat higher than it had been on conventional ventilation, the volume and pressure shifts during each cycle are minimal, presumably resulting in less barotrauma, volutrauma, and toxicity to the lung.

Failure to achieve sufficient gas exchange with HFOV or one of the conventional ventilatory techniques may prompt the use of ECMO, perfluorocarbon-assisted gas exchange, nitric oxide, or other newer or experimental modalities. These will be discussed briefly below.

Supported Spontaneous Ventilation

Controlled ventilation is used only when required by the severity of the illness. As there is benefit to spontaneous ventilation in terms of patient comfort, $\dot{V}/\dot{Q}$ matching, and reduced barotrauma, allowing the patient to breathe spontaneously while supplying sufficient support to minimize the work of breathing may be preferable in suitable patients. IMV is a commonly used mode of ventilatory support in children. IMV allows the patient to breathe at any time, receiving gas from a constant-flow or demand-valve source. At predetermined intervals, the ventilator delivers a breath at a preset tidal volume or peak pressure. Some level of PEEP is generally incorporated as well; the threshold-resistor is preferable to the flow-resistor type of PEEP valve.[295, 334] With more sophisticated ventilators, the intermittent breaths are synchronized with the patient's own respiratory efforts.

The ability to adequately support the child's own respiratory efforts is crucial when allowing spontaneous ventilation in children with lung disease. Pressure support, a hybrid of continuous distending pressure with mechanical ventilation, provides a variable degree of pressure assistance to patients during spontaneous inspiration.[335–337] The machine, sensing the child's desire for a breath (see "Mechanical Ventilation," above), provides just enough positive pressure to overcome the resistance of the endotracheal tube and to compensate for the additional work of breathing resulting from lung disease. The breath is terminated when the gas flow rate into the lungs decreases to a preset percentage of its peak. The child retains control of the size and rate of each spontaneous breath.

Pressure support can be used as the primary ventilatory support mode, allowing the child to breathe fully on his or her own with no mechanical mandatory rate. We have found this to be useful in children who are awake, calm, and cooperative and who have good bellows function and neurologic control of breathing. The mode seems to be more comfortable for the child, with less "fighting" the ventilator. Airway pressures are minimized, with the hope that this will help avoid barotrauma or other complications of mechanical ventilation. Pressure-supported spontaneous ventilation, used in conjunction with a "kinder, gentler" philosophy of permissive hypercapnia, is now a widely used technique, even in newborn infants, and will likely lead to less acute toxicity and better overall outcome.[338–341]

Pressure support can also be used in combination with a fixed mechanical rate (IMV plus pressure support), gradually weaning the IMV rate as tolerated. This is an especially effective way to maintain alveolar expansion as patients are weaned from full mechanical to full spontaneous ventilation. A gradual reduction in the number of mechanical breaths allows patients to progressively exercise respiratory muscles as they resume spontaneous breathing while ensuring adequate tidal volume and avoiding atelectasis.[342–345]

The criteria for extubation are presented in Table 29–7. A mask, hood, or other means for oxygen administration should be ready, as well as equipment and personnel for bag-and-mask ventilation or reintubation should this become necessary. If the course of intubation has been long, or if there is evidence that the fit of the endotracheal tube is particularly tight, the use of parenteral corticosteroids several hours before extubation in patients may be considered.[346, 347] Nebulized racemic epinephrine may also be administered immediately after the ETT is withdrawn. When the ETT has been removed the patient is placed in an oxygen concentration approximately 10 percent higher than that used before extubation and observed closely for signs of upper airway obstruction or inadequate ventilation. ABGs should be measured approximately 15 to 20 minutes after extubation. If the patient does well, the inspired oxygen concentration is decreased as tolerated.

T A B L E   2 9 – 7
CRITERIA FOR EXTUBATION

Acceptable ABG on FIO_2 of 0.40 or less with CPAP of 5 cm H_2O or less* and pressure support no greater than needed to overcome resistance of ETT

Comfortable breathing pattern, without tachypnea, retractions, or excessive work of breathing

Able to maintain and protect airway

Able to cough, breathe deeply, and clear secretions

No major instability of other organ systems

Able to generate an inspiratory force of −20 to −30 cm H_2O (if measurable)

* Acceptable ABG would generally include a PaO_2 of 60–80 mm Hg (except in children with cyanotic heart disease) and a $PaCO_2$ within 20 percent of the child's baseline.

Deep breathing, coughing, and chest physiotherapy are generally continued to facilitate removal of secretions and prevent atelectasis, which is common after extubation. The patient should not be allowed to eat or drink for several hours after extubation because the glottis may not be competent to prevent aspiration for a period of time.

Additional or Experimental Techniques of Respiratory Support

ECMO may be life-saving in children with severe cardiac or respiratory dysfunction who cannot be supported by conventional means. ECMO is addressed elsewhere in this text (see Chapter 13), and will not be further reviewed here.

Helium administration may be beneficial to the patient with airway obstruction. Its effect is thought to be caused by the decreased density provided by the addition of helium to the breathing mixture, resulting in a reduction in turbulent flow in the airway. Helium has been found helpful to reduce dyspnea and improve CO_2 elimination in patients with both upper and lower airway obstruction.[348-352] Although it is possible to blend pure helium and oxygen together at the time of administration, it is usual and safer to use a premixed gas source such as Heliox, a blend of 30 percent oxygen and 70 percent helium providing sufficient helium to achieve the desired effect while helping to avoid the accidental administration of a hypoxic mixture. Limitations to helium's usefulness include the necessity of administering a high inspired fraction of helium (<60 to 70 percent helium has little benefit), therefore limiting the F_{IO_2} to 0.30 to 0.40, and the short-lived nature of the effect; once helium is removed from the breathing mixture, its beneficial effect rapidly dissipates.

The administration of exogenous surfactant has become an established practice in the care of preterm neonates with respiratory distress.[353, 354] Many studies have established its efficacy in this setting.[355-359] Ongoing refinements are defining the proper mode of administration, single versus multiple dosing, prophylactic versus therapeutic administration, and type of preparation to be used. There are limited data suggesting that surfactant replacement is useful in term neonates with pneumonia or meconium aspiration.[360, 361] There is also evidence that endogenous pulmonary surfactant is deficient or ineffective in acute respiratory distress syndrome (ARDS), and replacement therapy with exogenous surfactant might be helpful.[362-369] Despite the good theoretical grounds for its use, however, clinical success has been limited and, at present, surfactant might best be considered as potentially helpful in individual cases, but not as a standard of care.

Intratracheal pulmonary ventilation (ITPV) attempts to drastically reduce pulmonary dead space, improving the efficiency of CO_2 elimination from the lungs. A blind-tipped catheter is placed within the ETT to a point just above the carina, and gas is insufflated through the catheter at high flow rates. Gas entrainment by the Venturi principle augments gas flow in and out of the lung. ITPV has shown considerable promise in correcting severe hypercapnia without unduly high airway pressures in animal models.[370-375] Preliminary data suggest that the technique may be useful in infants with severely compromised CO_2 excretion.[376]

Partial liquid ventilation is an experimental technique. Oxygen is highly soluble in fluorochemicals, and there has been interest in using these liquids to augment gas exchange in the lungs for some time.[377] Pure liquid ventilation, filling the entire tracheobronchial tree and ventilating apparatus with liquid chemical, has been shown to be effective in animals and in a very small number of otherwise terminal infants,[378] but is an impractical technique for clinical use. Partial liquid ventilation, combining use of the chemical with standard gas ventilation, is under active investigation.[379-388] Perfluorocarbons are instilled into the lung, but ventilation is achieved with a conventional ventilator. The precise quantity of fluorochemical to be administered[389] and its distribution in the lung[390, 391] are still under investigation, with particular interest in the chemical's effect on pulmonary blood flow and $\dot{V}/\dot{Q}$ matching.[392] Partial liquid ventilation seems quite effective in supporting gas exchange. There has been some evidence that perfluorochemicals can interact with or substitute for surfactant,[393, 394] with additional data that the inflammatory response in the alveoli might be tempered by the chemical as well.[395-398]

Nitric oxide (NO) is synthesized in the vasculature from L-arginine; the synthesis is catalyzed by nitric oxide synthase, which exists in two isoforms: "constitutive," or calcium-dependent, and "inducible," or calcium-independent. NO stimulates the production of cyclic guanosine monophosphate (cGMP) in vascular smooth muscle, leading to smooth muscle relaxation and, in the lung, to pulmonary vasodilation.[295] Endogenous NO synthesis can be supplemented by the administration of the drug as a gas, through the patient's breathing circuit.

NO inhalation for critically ill infants and children has generated a great deal of excitement, enthusiasm, and interest over the past several years, and with understandable reason—it may well be the selective pulmonary vasodilator that physicians caring for these patients have been seeking for years.[399-401] This enthusiasm must be tempered by the reality that much more work needs to be done to better define the patient population that might be expected to benefit,[402-409] the dosing necessary,[410-414] and the adverse effects of NO treatment.[407, 409, 415-420] In general, a beneficial effect has been more clearly demonstrated in newborns than in older children and adults. Although an acute improvement in oxygenation, sometimes modest and sometimes dramatic, is often seen after NO administration, sustained improvement or a better ultimate outcome for the patient are less clearly demonstrated.

NO is administered via the ventilator circuit, with continuous monitoring of the concentrations of NO and nitrogen dioxide (NO_2), a toxic metabolite.[295, 421] The response may be varied. In some patients—particularly newborns with persistent pulmonary hypertension and postoperative cardiac surgical patients—there is a dramatic reduction in pulmonary artery pressure. In others, there is an improvement in oxygenation without a notable change in PA pressure; in these patients, the mechanism of response is thought to be an improvement in $\dot{V}/\dot{Q}$ matching, with NO entering open, ventilated alveoli inducing an increase in blood flow to those alveoli. NO may be administered in conjunction with conventional ventilation, with high-frequency ventilation,[422, 423] or with other pulmonary vasodilators[424]; in general, ventilatory strategies that improve lung expansion improve the delivery of the drug to its alveolar site of action.

In brief, NO is a valuable adjunct in caring for patients in severe respiratory failure, particularly those in whom pulmonary hypertension is an important factor. It is not, however, a panacea for multisystem disease or even for all respiratory diseases. It has become evident that very low doses—often less than 5 ppm, and considerably less than the 80 ppm used in earlier studies—are effective in many cases. Additional experience and study will define the role of NO in the field of therapies effective in managing respiratory failure.

Respiratory Supportive Care

Meticulous supportive care is as important as the mechanical aspects of ventilation and oxygenation. Inspired gases should be warmed and fully humidified to prevent obstruction of the airway by thick, tenacious secretions and to minimize damage to the airway mucosa and ciliary function. Secretions must be removed by suctioning the airway at regular intervals. The patient should be well oxygenated and ventilated before and after suctioning. Saline 0.5 to 2 ml is instilled and careful, gentle suctioning, using sterile technique, is performed. The duration of suctioning should be limited to 10 to 15 seconds. The lungs must be reexpanded after suctioning because suctioning reduces FRC. In some circumstances, such as in patients on high-frequency oscillation, interruption of ventilatory support for suctioning is potentially detrimental and should be performed only when clinically indicated and not on a regular schedule.

Prone positioning has been shown to improve oxygenation in patients with severe acute respiratory failure (ARF).[425–429] The mechanism of its benefit seems to be in the recruitment of previously collapsed dorsal alveoli, improving $\dot{V}/\dot{Q}$ matching and decreasing shunt.[430] The technique is simple and noninvasive, though it does complicate nursing care to some extent; it may be used alone or in conjunction with other adjuncts such as nitric oxide.[425, 428]

Chest physiotherapy is helpful to aid in removal of secretions and to reverse or prevent atelectasis. Physiotherapy techniques commonly employed include postural drainage, percussion of the chest wall, vibration, and assisted coughing. Suctioning and chest physiotherapy are stressful procedures, particularly for infants.[345, 431]

Fluid retention is common during mechanical ventilation. Careful fluid balance is necessary to prevent fluid overload and maximize gas exchange. If humidification of inspired gases is adequate, the insensible water loss from the respiratory tract is eliminated, and the usual daily water requirement may be decreased by approximately 20 percent. Fluid restriction or the use of a diuretic, such as furosemide, is often necessary.[432, 433]

Agitation and discoordinated respiratory efforts interfere with effective ventilation. Sedation, analgesia, and neuromuscular blockers may be required. The variety of drugs used in the operating room for this purpose are used in similar doses in the ICU; midazolam and fentanyl for short-term sedation, and lorazepam and morphine for long-term use are common choices. Although propofol may be used for short periods of time, it is specifically not recommended for long-term sedation in children because of reported adverse effects, although the exact mechanism of this toxicity remains uncertain.[434–437] When muscle relaxants are used, the patient must be carefully attended and reliable alarm systems must be in use, since ventilator disconnection or malfunction will result in apnea.

Special Considerations

Laryngotracheobronchitis

Viral laryngotracheobronchitis, or croup, is a common cause of upper airway obstruction in children. It can be caused by a number of different viruses, most frequently parainfluenza 3. Children in the 6-month to 3-year age group are affected most frequently, although croup can be seen in older children as well. A history of recurrent severe croup suggests the possibility of an anatomic airway abnormality (e.g., mild subglottic stenosis) that may be asymptomatic between episodes.

Croup must be differentiated from other obstructive lesions, particularly epiglottitis (Table 29–8). Croup usually occurs during or after a typical upper respiratory infection with low-grade fever, rhinorrhea, and cough. Symptoms of upper airway obstruction begin 1 to 3 days after the onset of other symptoms and may persist with variable severity for 7 to 10 days. Inflammation and edema of the mucosa extend from the pharynx down into the small airways. The narrowing of the airway is most significant in the immediate subglottic trachea, and can be demonstrated on lateral neck radiographs.[438] Biphasic stridor, retractions, hoarseness, and a barking cough are present and are more severe when the child is upset or distressed.

Mild viral croup is a self-limited process that can often be treated on an outpatient basis.[439] If the patient is seen in the emergency room (ER), cool mist, with supplemental

TABLE 29–8
DIFFERENTIATION OF CROUP AND EPIGLOTTITIS

	Croup	Epiglottitis
Incidence	More common	Less common
Site of obstruction	Subglottic	Supraglottic
Etiology	Viral	Bacterial
Age	6 mo–3 yr	2–6 yr
Recurrence	More frequent	Rare
Onset	Gradual (days)	Sudden (h)
Progression	Slow, variable	Rapid
Position	Can lie down	Sitting forward
Dysphagia	Absent	Severe
Drooling	Absent	Present
Cough	Barking	Suppressed
Voice	Hoarse	Muffled
Respiratory pattern	Rapid, struggling	Slow, usually quiet

O₂ if needed, is given. If respiratory distress is significant, a topical vasoconstrictor aerosol, such as racemic epinephrine, is administered[440] (Table 29–9). Racemic epinephrine may be given as frequently as every 1 to 2 hours, monitoring for undue tachycardia. The durg has a relatively short duration of action and obstructive symptoms may "rebound" or recur after initial improvement. For this reason, the need for racemic epinephrine has been used as an indication to admit the child to hospital. More recent practice, however, has been to observe the child for 2 to 4 hours following racemic epinephrine administration and, if the child appears well and good follow-up can be ensured, the child may be sent home.[441–444]

Corticosteroids are effective in reducing the airway edema of croup,[445–447] and the risk of short-term administration of steroids is small compared with that of endotracheal intubation and mechanical ventilation. Once reserved for patients to be admitted to the hospital, steroids are now commonly used in the outpatient setting. Parenteral and oral dexamethasone are the most commonly used drugs, although there is evidence supporting the use of inhaled budesonide as well.[448, 449]

An occasional patient with severe croup does not respond adequately to initial treatment, and insertion of an artificial airway is needed.[450] Endotracheal intubation is indicated, although one must realize that the ETT will be resting in an already inflamed portion of the trachea and that the tube's presence may initially increase the mucosal edema. The patient's trachea should be intubated carefully, under controlled circumstances, preferably under general anesthesia. An ETT that will pass through the glottis without excessive pressure should be selected. A tube 0.5 to 1 mm smaller in diameter than usual is used, and may still be a snug fit; attention should also be given to the length of the tube, as the smaller tubes commonly needed may be too short for older children.

Once the obstruction is bypassed, most children are able to breathe spontaneously, with humidified oxygen in appropriate concentration provided by a mist tent. If necessitated by fatigue, atelectasis, or lower airway disease, mechanical ventilatory support is provided. Antibiotics are not indicated in the treatment of viral croup unless there is evidence of bacterial superinfection. Bacterial tracheitis, characterized by high fever and copious purulent tracheal secretions, is occasionally seen, and is most commonly of staphylococcal origin.

Supportive care is continued for at least 72 hours before extubation is attempted. The appearance of an air leak around the ETT is a good sign that airway edema is resolving and that extubation may be successfully accomplished. If signs of severe obstruction recur after extubation, the trachea is reintubated as atraumatically as possible. Extubation is then attempted again in another 2 to 3 days. If unsuccessful at this point, a tracheostomy may be considered.

Epiglottitis (Supraglottits)

Epiglottitis is an acute, life-threatening cause of upper airway obstruction. The classic case results from infection of the upper airway with *Haemophilus influenzae,* which produces marked inflammatory edema of the epiglottis and other supraglottic structures.[451] The incidence is highest in the 2- to 6-year age group, but cases have been reported from infancy to adulthood. The onset is relatively sudden, with only a few hours of symptoms before signs of severe obstruction occur. A high fever and severe sore throat are present, such that the child refuses to eat or drink. Dysphagia is often so severe that the child drools continually, unable to swallow saliva. The patient becomes acutely ill, with inspiratory stridor and a toxic, cyanotic, or ashen gray appearance. Acute airway obstruction and cardiopulmonary arrest can occur at any time; it is this unpredictability that mandates urgent tracheal intubation.

The introduction of *H. influenzae* vaccine into pediatric practice has dramatically decreased the incidence of invasive *H. influenzae* disease, including epiglottitis.[452–455] The pattern of epiglottitis is now more like that described in adults, with a broader range of organisms (*Candida,* group A β-hemolytic *Streptococcus, Staphylococcus,* and others) being causal.[456, 457] The epiglottis appears thickened, boggy, or edematous rather than exhibiting the classic "beefy red" swelling associated with *H. influenzae.* Airway management remains as in classic epiglottitis.

Epiglottitis is a clinical diagnosis and a true emergency; radiographs are not necessary to confirm it.[458] Lateral neck films may be helpful in doubtful cases (Fig. 29–6), but the patient should never be sent unattended for radiographic examinations or forced to lie down for these procedures. Oxygen is administered by mask continuously from the time the diagnosis is suspected. The child must be accompanied by a physician capable of performing either endotracheal intubation or emergency tracheostomy; equipment for these procedures, along with appropriate resuscitative equipment, should also be kept with the patient.

Because of the potential for sudden complete obstruction, an artificial airway should be inserted in all patients with epiglottitis.[459–462] Intubation is best performed under general anesthesia in the operating room. Unnecessary procedures, such as blood sampling or attempts at visualization of the epiglottis, should be deferred until the patient is adequately anesthetized in the operating room.

Postoperatively, the child should be physically restrained and sedated before coming to the ICU; airway management is as noted above for croup. Initial antibiotic treatment should be broad-spectrum in nature; a cephalosporin such as ceftriaxone or cefotaxime is reasonable, perhaps with the addition of vancomycin if resistant gram-positive organisms are a concern. When culture results are available, the choice of antibiotics is adjusted according to the observed sensitivity pattern. *H. influenzae* is an invasive

TABLE 29–9
RACEMIC EPINEPHRINE: AEROSOL DOSAGE*

0–1 yr	0.2 ml of 2.25% soln
1–3 yr	0.3 ml of 2.25% soln
3–6 yr	0.4 ml of 2.25% soln
> 6 yr	0.5 ml of 2.25% soln

* All doses are diluted in 2 ml of normal saline and are administered by nebulizer.

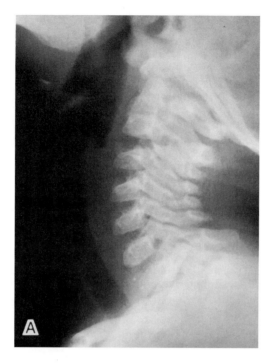

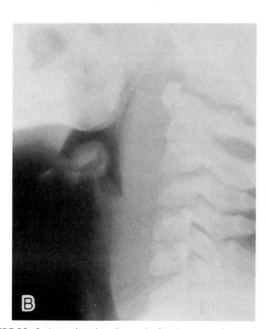

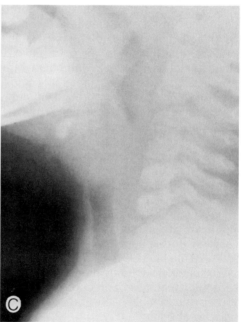

FIGURE 29–6. Lateral neck radiographs for diagnosis of epiglottitis. *A,* Child with pharyngitis but normal epiglottis. *B,* Epiglottitis of moderate severity. *C,* Severe epiglottitis with marked swelling of epiglottis and other supraglottic structures.

organism, and infection may include pneumonia, joint involvement, or meningitis. Pulmonary edema is a well-described complication of the relief of upper-airway obstruction; its treatment includes CPAP and diuresis.[463, 464] After 24 to 48 hours of antibiotic treatment, extubation is considered. The patient's fever should have decreased and some air leakage may have appeared around the ETT. Laryngoscopy can be performed if there is a question as to readiness for extubation. Extubation is usually accomplished in the ICU, although some may prefer to move the patient to the operating room.

Bronchiolitis

The management of bronchiolitis, an acute viral respiratory infection manifested by coryza, pneumonitis, wheezing, and occasional apnea (in infants <2 months old), is similar to that outlined below for asthma.[465] Oxygen and mist are standard therapy; bronchodilators are often effective; steroids are not generally used.[466] There is some evidence that aerosolized racemic epinephrine, a mixed α- and β-receptor agonist, is more beneficial than a pure β-agonist, presumably because of reduction of edema by vasoconstriction.[467] Heliox may be quite effective in relieving acute respiratory distress.[349]

Bronchiolitis is predominantly caused by respiratory syncytial virus (RSV). The virus is ubiquitous and is a pathogen in all ages, but serious lower respiratory tract disease is confined to infancy.[468] There is some evidence that RSV infection in infancy may predispose to wheezing later in life,[469–471] but the issue is complex and not clearly understood.[472–474] Ribavirin, a synthetic nucleoside, has been shown effective in enhancing clearance of RSV. The drug is not indicated in otherwise healthy children, in whom RSV infection is usually self-limited, but may be used for acute RSV infection in compromised children (e.g., those with immunodeficiencies or chronic cardiopulmonary disease). It is administered by aerosolization, either continuously or intermittently; the latter may help to reduce environmental exposure of health care workers to the drug.[475, 476] Particular caution must be taken to prevent mechanical dysfunction if the drug is to be administered through a ventilator.[477]

Status Asthmaticus

Asthma is the most common chronic respiratory disorder in children and is a leading cause of childhood disability.[465, 478] The morbidity and mortality associated with asthma are significant, and status asthmaticus is a frequent cause for admission to the ICU.

The acute asthma attack includes contraction or spasm of bronchial smooth muscle, mucosal inflammation and edema, and increased airway secretions. These changes markedly increase airway resistance and work of breathing. Occlusion of airways, segmental atelectasis, and poor matching of perfusion and ventilation cause an increase in intrapulmonary shunting, often producing marked hypoxemia.[479, 480] During an acute attack, asthmatic patients attempt to hyperventilate to compensate for hypoxemia and altered lung mechanics. Arterial blood gases demonstrate hypoxemia and a low or normal $Paco_2$; the appearance of CO_2 retention indicates severe disease and impending respiratory failure.

Chronic management of asthma has evolved to focus on inflammation as central to the pathogenesis of the disease, and anti-inflammatory treatment, in addition to bronchodilation, has become essential to the care of these children.[481–483] The administration of cromolyn or steroids (inhaled or systemic, preferably the former) is now considered first-line management of all but very mild or intermittent cases of asthma. Bronchodilation is achieved with β-adrenergic agents, either by inhalation or orally; theophylline is used with decreasing frequency because of its narrow therapeutic index.

The management of a child with status asthmaticus is fashioned along the same line of thinking, although the initial emphasis is placed on bronchodilation to relieve acute distress.[484] The administration of oxygen and an inhaled bronchodilator is begun first (Table 29–10). Terbutaline (Brethine) and albuterol (Ventolin) are β₂-selective agents with long duration (4 to 6 hours) and are good choices in this setting. Many children respond to this ther-

TABLE 29–10. INHALED BRONCHODILATORS FOR USE IN ASTHMA

Drug	β-Selectivity	Duration	Dose
Isoproterenol (Isuprel)	$\beta_1 > \beta_2$	1–2 h	0.5% solution (5 mg/ml) 0.05–0.1 mg/kg/dose (0.01–0.02 ml/kg/dose)
Isoetharine (Bronkosol)	$\beta_2 > \beta_1$	1–2 h	1% solution (10 mg/ml) 0.1–0.2 mg/kg/dose (0.01–0.02 ml/kg/dose)
Terbutaline (Brethine)	$\beta_2 \gg \beta_1$	4–6 h	0.1% solution (1 mg/ml) 0.1–0.3 mg/kg/dose (0.1–0.3 ml/kg/dose)
Albuterol (Ventolin)	$\beta_2 \gg \beta_1$	4–6 h	0.5% solution (5 mg/ml) 0.05–0.15 mg/kg/dose (0.01–0.03 ml/kg/dose) 0.3–0.5 mg/kg/h (continuous nebulization)

apy in the emergency room, and hospitalization may be avoided.

Should further treatment be needed, more aggressive use of the β₂-agonists is indicated. The dose and frequency of administration of nebulized drug can be increased to every 20 minutes for the initial few hours of emergency treatment.[485–487] It is probably more effective and cost-efficient, however, to move to continuous nebulization in the ICU setting; the continuous administration of albuterol at 0.3 to 0.5 mg/kg/h is often very effective and is not associated with any greater toxicity than intermittent dosing.[488–493] Parenteral corticosteroids (e.g., methylprednisolone 1 mg/kg q6h or hydrocortisone 5 mg/kg q4–6h) are also commonly given to the asthmatic in status.[465, 494, 495] There should be no hesitation in beginning steroids early in the hospital course, as it will take several hours for a beneficial effect to be seen. Ipratoprium bromide, an inhaled anticholinergic, may be beneficial when used with other bronchodilators.[496–498] This "package" of inhaled β-agent, ipratroprium, and steroids is typical therapy administered to the child admitted to the ICU for moderate to severe status asthmaticus.[499] Intravenous aminophylline, once the mainstay of treatment, is now considered an alternative or additional treatment. Typically, a loading dose of 5 to 6 mg/kg (less if the patient is already taking theophylline) is given over 15 to 20 minutes, followed by a continuous infusion of approximately 1 mg/kg/h to maintain a blood level of 10 to 20 mg/L; the clearance is quite variable and the therapeutic index narrow.[500] Finally, there is some evidence that magnesium (administered as 25 to 50 mg/kg of $MgSO_4$) may help attenuate a severe attack of asthma.

An alternative to the aggressive use of nebulized β-agonists is their intravenous administration, particularly if adequate delivery cannot be achieved by the inhaled route.[501–503] Terbutaline is the most commonly used agent for this purpose, but dosages in the literature vary widely. Loading doses range from 2 to 10 μg/kg, given over 20 to 30 minutes, followed by a continuous infusion at a rate ranging from 0.1 to 10 μg/kg/min; the typical infusion settles out at 2 to 4 μg/kg/min. Close monitoring to ensure adequate gas exchange, blood pressure, and perfusion are necessary. There is some risk of cardiac ischemia with aggressive use of β-agents; ECG monitoring is essential, and many centers monitor serum creatine kinase (CK), particularly the MB fraction, although data to establish the significance of the CK values are lacking. Hypokalemia is sometimes seen with the use of β-agonists; potassium supplementation may be given as needed.

In addition to drug therapy, a number of supportive measures are indicated. Because intrapulmonary shunting is markedly increased during a severe asthma episode, adequate supplemental oxygen must be given and oxygen saturation should be monitored continuously. A helium-oxygen mixture such as Heliox may acutely relieve respiratory distress, markedly improve CO_2 excretion, and forestall intubation in severe asthma.[348–352] As the necessity of administering a high concentration of helium limits the F_{IO_2}, helium therapy may be limited in its use in patients requiring more than 30 to 40 percent oxygen. Children with asthma often present in a dehydrated state; adequate parenteral hydration and humidification of inspired gases should correct this problem. Overhydration should be avoided, since it may contribute to edema of the airway mucosa and pulmonary interstitium, worsening both airway resistance and lung compliance. Although many children with status asthmaticus are markedly anxious, it should be remembered that acute anxiety and restlessness may be caused by hypoxia or retention of CO_2. Sedative drugs are relatively contraindicated until these abnormalities are excluded. Close monitoring is essential if sedation is given, and facilities for mechanical ventilation must be immediately available.

Mechanical ventilation may be required in the most severe cases. Careful intubation under adequate anesthesia (usually ketamine) is crucial, as bronchospasm may be made considerably worse by the reflex response to stimulation of the trachea. If the patient is also hypovolemic, severe hypotension may ensure. The clinician should be prepared to augment intravascular volume by rapid fluid administration and to provide inotropic support if needed. Bronchodilator drugs must be continued during mechanical ventilation; lidocaine, either intravenously or via the endotracheal tube, may reduce the bronchospastic response. A low respiratory rate and a long expiratory time are generally best for ventilating the asthmatic child. Clinical examination, aided by on-line monitors of airway flow, volume, and pressure, will aid in adjusting respiratory rate and bronchodilator support. Paralysis is usually recommended, as high inflating pressures are commonly required, although there is limited experience with supported spontaneous ventilation[504]; a permissive hypercapnic approach is taken. Asthma patients are at great risk from barotrauma during mechanical ventilation, and sudden deterioration of either respiratory or cardiac function should suggest pneumothorax or other gas leak.

An additional or alternative mode of therapy in the severely ill asthmatic is the administration of an inhala-tional anesthetic such as Forane (isoflurane). The bronchodilating qualities of these agents are well known, and they can be effective in reversing bronchospasm in patients who have failed to respond to all other forms of therapy.[505–509] They may be continued for an extended period of time, often several days, and then gradually discontinued. If use has been prolonged, a withdrawal syndrome of agitation and increased bronchospasm must be anticipated and managed with alternate forms of therapy.[507] The potential complications and adverse effects of these drugs are not different from those associated with their use in the operating room. Ketamine may also be useful in the management of status asthmaticus, dosed either intermittently (e.g., in anticipation of suctioning) or as a continuous infusion.[510]

Acute Respiratory Distress Syndrome

ARDS in children is defined in the same fashion as in adults: severe acute lung injury (ALI) with impaired oxygenation and diffuse pulmonary infiltrates not explained by left atrial hypertension.[511, 512] Childhood ARDS occurs in clinical settings similar to those in adults: sepsis, low-output states, and trauma are common examples.[511, 513, 514] The mortality rate is high despite aggressive management, and efforts are ongoing to better define prognostic variables so that newer or alternative forms of therapy can be offered to those at the greatest risk.[515, 516]

ARDS is predominantly a restrictive lung disease.[517] Oxygenation improves with increased MAP so long as overdistention is avoided[316]; as described above, PEEP, CPAP, long inspiratory times, inspiratory plateaus, pressure-controlled ventilation, and HFOV all achieve this increase in MAP and restoration of lost FRC. CO_2 removal is augmented by longer expiratory times, bronchodilators, clearance of secretions, and HFOV. Proper cardiac and systemic support will allow optimal oxygen delivery and minimize oxygen consumption and CO_2 production. The clinician treating severe respiratory failure should not attempt to maintain "normal" blood gases, as to do so will subject the child to overly aggressive management. We have found it acceptable and safe to maintain Pa_{O_2}s of 50 to 55 mm Hg (O_2 saturations 90 to 92 percent) and Pa_{CO_2}s of 60 to 80 mm Hg for extended periods of time in an effort to minimize iatrogenic damage.

The administration of steroids to patients with ARDS has been attempted; the idea is attractive, given the diffuse inflammatory nature of the lung pathology. There have been mixed results, but recent data suggest that the administration of methylprednisolone for an extended period of time (32 days) to patients with unresolving ARDS achieves improvement.[518, 519]

Surfactant replacement, NO inhalation, and ECMO may all have some place in the management of individual patients with ARDS, but their exact roles have not yet been defined.[520–522] Surfactant replacement requires further work to better define the exact preparation, dosage, and manner of administration. NO, a naturally occurring endothelium-derived vasodilator, has been shown to reduce pulmonary artery pressure and intrapulmonary shunt, acutely improving oxygenation; outcome data are lacking. ECMO can clearly provide limited-term support for children with

ARDS; its success in improving outcome depends on appropriate patient selection.

Pulmonary Hypertension

Pulmonary hypertension is seen in two settings: ARF in older children and persistent pulmonary hypertension of the newborn (PPHN). Acute pulmonary hypertension accompanies the pulmonary vasoconstriction, vascular occlusion, and intrapulmonary shunting in ARF.[522, 523] PPHN is a syndrome in which pulmonary vascular resistance remains elevated after birth, resulting in decreased pulmonary blood flow and shunting of blood from right to left across the ductus arteriosus, a patent foramen ovale, or other communication between the pulmonary and systemic circulations. It occurs either alone or in association with a number of neonatal diseases, including congenital diaphragmatic hernia, meconium aspiration, and sepsis.

The etiology of PPHN is multifactorial. Developmental anatomic abnormalities have been described in the muscularization of pulmonary arteries.[524] Abnormal elevations of prostanoids, particularly the thromboxanes, have been described in neonates with the syndrome.[525] Pulmonary hypoplasia, with poorly developed alveolar and vascular architecture, may also contribute to decreased pulmonary blood flow and right-to-left shunt.

Clinically, these infants present with marked hypoxemia. A ductal shunt, with a difference in PaO_2 of 20 mm Hg or more between arterial blood samples drawn from the right radial artery and from the descending aorta, is often present. The shunt may be episodic, with sudden changes in pulmonary vascular resistance decreasing pulmonary blood flow. These episodes are often associated with stress. We have found it beneficial to maintain the infants in as stress-free a state as possible by sedation and analgesia.

An alkalotic pH relaxes the pulmonary vasculature and increases pulmonary blood flow. One approach to infants with PPHN has been to aggressively seek a pH greater than 7.55 by use of hyperventilation and alkalinizing drugs.[526] Although sometimes successful, the extremes of ventilator pressure and rate required have resulted in much barotrauma and other adverse effects.[527] There is now renewed interest in more conservative management, with encouraging results.[528, 529] Attempts to reduce pulmonary hypertension by use of systemic vasodilators have generally been ineffective, as systemic hypotension commonly occurs. Initial experience with inhaled nitric oxide (see above) has been encouraging. NO can be delivered effectively to pulmonary vessels but does not reach the systemic circulation because of rapid inactivation by hemoglobin, thus allowing it to act as a relatively selective pulmonary vasodilator.[530, 531]

Chronic Respiratory Support, Noninvasive Ventilation

Bronchopulmonary dysplasia (BPD) is a form of chronic pulmonary disease seen in infants after a course of acute neonatal respiratory insufficiency. Many etiologic factors have been described, the most frequently noted of which are the use of high inspired oxygen concentrations and high airway pressures in the treatment of neonatal respiratory failure. Radiographically, these children have areas of hyperinflation alternating with areas of atelectasis. The pathologic appearance is one of smooth-muscle hyperplasia, fibrotic proliferation, and scarring, mixed with regions of emphysema. The clinical result is high airway resistance, increased work of breathing, and increased physiologic dead space.

These children often require prolonged ventilatory support to maintain reasonable gas exchange and to decrease the caloric cost of breathing, allowing better somatic growth.[532, 533] They are often readmitted to intensive care when an acute illness—even just a viral upper respiratory infection (URI)—interferes with their ability to maintain adequate gas exchange. Bronchospasm and fluid retention are common, and most children require bronchodilators (usually inhaled β-agonists) and diuretics.[534] The typical problems of chronic BPD include infection, nutritional support, and the need for innovative approaches to minimize developmental delays and maximize each child's potential.

Chronic ventilatory support may also be needed for children with neuromuscular diseases that impair bellows function, such as spinal muscular atrophy, myelitis, and muscular dystrophies. These children do well with levels of support varying from nighttime-only negative pressure ventilation to full-time positive-pressure support. If provided with such support, intellectually normal youngsters can lead productive and fulfilling lives.[535–538] Although occasional hospitalization is needed, most of these children are very well cared for at home.

It has become more common to employ noninvasive modes of ventilation in the acute pediatric ICU setting. Bilevel positive airway pressure ventilation (BiPAP), applied through a nasal or face mask, provides a modest level of ventilatory support.[539–541] It may be used in cases of mild upper airway obstruction to help "splint" open the airway, in cases of inadequate respiratory drive, or in children immediately following extubation and needing a short period of airway support as a "bridge" to tolerating a completely unsupported airway. BiPAP can also provide ventilatory assistance to patients in acute respiratory distress who are not candidates for tracheal intubation and ventilation. The terminally ill patient with cancer or cystic fibrosis, for example, who does not wish full mechanical ventilation but is thought to have a potentially reversible, short-term respiratory decompensation, might benefit from a period of noninvasive support.

Management of Fluids and Nutrition

The daily management of fluids and electrolytes in the ICU is much the same as in the perioperative period. Special consideration must be given, however, to providing nutrition, and to the disorders of fluid balance that occur in ICU patients.

Nutritional Support

Adequate nutrition is essential to allow growth and to ensure recovery from critical illness. Inadequate nutrition may impair wound healing and decrease resistance to infection.[542, 543] The prevalence of malnutrition in PICU populations has been estimated to be 15 to 20 percent,[544] and nutritional deficiency may predate the ICU admission in many patients.

The daily energy requirement is the sum of the requirements for basal metabolism, voluntary muscle activity, the specific dynamic action of the food being ingested, and growth.[544–546] Ideally, one would assess each child's needs by indirect calorimetry,[547] but this is often impractical and estimates are therefore made. Infants and children have a higher metabolic rate than adults. This, together with the nutritional requirements for growth, increases their need for both calories and protein. Newborn infants require 100 to 120 kcal/kg/day for normal growth, compared with 35 to 45 kcal/kg/day in the adult. Protein requirements in the newborn average 2 to 3 g/kg/day, whereas the adult may require no more than 0.5 g/kg/day.[544, 546, 548] Fat requirements for infants may be as much as 4 to 5 g/kg/day, whereas older children and adolescents may require 2 to 4 g/kg/day. Stress, such as that induced by trauma, sepsis, or major elective surgery, increases energy expenditure by 20 to 50 percent or more and induces a catabolic state in which fat stores and protein are broken down to supply the increased energy requirements.[549–552]

As a general rule, enteral nutrition is preferable to parenteral, and should be used unless contraindicated. Enteral feedings are certainly more "physiologic" and avoid the potential complications of parenteral feeding. Enteral nutrition supports the gut mucosa, maintaining a barrier against bacterial translocation from the gut into the bloodstream.[553–555] The caloric density and the protein per unit volume of administered fluid are generally higher for enteral feeding. There is some evidence that enteral feedings may speed maturation of the preterm infant's gut. If breast milk is used, there is additional protection against necrotizing enterocolitis.[556, 557]

Enteral alimentation can be provided to patients with good absorptive capacity by mouth, by nasogastric tube, by gastrostomy, or by a catheter manipulated into the jejunum.[558, 559] Use of fine, soft, Silastic feeding tubes minimizes the risk of erosion, ulceration, or perforation of the stomach or bowel; pH monitoring from the tip of the tube during manipulation is helpful in seeking placement in the small intestine. The risk of aspiration can be minimized by giving relatively small, frequent feedings, by continuously infusing the formula, and by use of the nasojejunal route.

A large variety of commercially prepared formulas are available. These include general maintenance formulas, those that are high in calories and protein, some that do not contain specific ingredients (e.g., lactose or cow's milk protein), chemically defined or elemental formulas, and modular formulas that allow separate introduction and adjustment of various components.[546, 558] Because of the variety and complexity of such products, it is best to select a few basic preparations for routine use and to seek nutritional consultation when selecting a formula for specific problems.

When enteral feeding is impossible or poorly tolerated, it is generally possible to supply nutritional requirements by the parenteral route[546, 548, 560] (Table 29–11). Limited parenteral nutrition can be administered by peripheral

TABLE 29–11
ESTIMATED DAILY REQUIREMENT FOR TOTAL PARENTERAL NUTRITION*

Age	0–1 yr	1–4 yr	5–18 yr
Calories (kcal/kg)	100–140	90–100	40–80
Water: 100 ml/kg (first 10 kg) + 50 ml/kg (next 10 kg) + 20 ml/kg (all kg over 20)			
Protein (g/kg)	2–3	1.5–3	1–2
Fat (g/kg)	0.5–3	0.5–3	0.5–2
Sodium (mEq/kg)	2–4	2–4	2–4
Potassium (mEq/kg)	2–3	2–3	2–3
Chloride (mEq/kg)	2–3	2–4	2–4
Calcium (mEq/kg)	3–4	2–3	0.5–2.5
Calcium (mg/kg)	60–80	40–60	10–50
Phosphate (mmol/kg)	1.5–2.25	1–2	1–2
Magnesium (mEq/kg)	0.25–1	0.25–1	0.25–1
Zinc (μg/kg)	400	300	100
Copper (μg/kg)	20	20	20
Manganese (μg/kg)	2–10	2–10	2–10
Chromium (ng/kg)	150–200	150–200	150–200

* Parenteral nutrition solutions are prepared by the hospital pharmacy, under the guidance of the hospital's nutrition support service. Exact compositions and formulations may vary, and the above should be treated as a general guideline. Multivitamins are routinely added. The balance between acetate and chloride salts may be varied to improve the patient's acid–base balance or chloride deficit.

vein, but the glucose concentration must be limited to 10 to 12 percent; higher glucose solutions are irritating to veins and are prone to cause phlebitis. Use of a central catheter allows higher caloric intake and long-term support. Central venous lines for parenteral nutrition can be inserted either percutaneously or by cutdown into the internal or external jugular, subclavian, saphenous, or femoral veins. Surgical insertion of a tunneled, soft silastic catheter provides prolonged function with low risk of infection.[561]

Solutions for parenteral administration may contain from 10 to 30 percent glucose and 1 to 4 percent amino acids, vitamins, and trace minerals. The concentration of glucose is increased gradually to avoid hyperglycemia and potential osmotic diuresis. Maximal benefit is attained when the infusion rate approaches the maximal rate at which glucose can be directly oxidized to provide energy. In adults, this is typically a glucose infusion rate of 3 to 4 mg/kg/min (5 to 6 g/kg/day); premature infants may tolerate up to 7 mg/kg/min.[548, 562] Lipids are added from a separate emulsion, supplied in a 10 or 20 percent concentration. Lipid emulsions have exceptional caloric density; a 10 percent solution of fat provides twice as many calories per unit volume as 10 percent glucose. Lipid suspensions are generally given by piggyback infusion, initially at 0.5 to 1 g/kg/day and gradually increased to 4 g/kg/day if required and tolerated. Excessive amounts of lipid may cause hyperlipemia, the risk for which is uncertain. Although pulmonary lipid deposition has been documented in neonates,[563] no deleterious effect on blood pH and (A–a)Do_2 was noted when lipid at 4 g/kg/day was infused into low-birth-weight infants.[564] It is recommended that lipid infusion rate not exceed 0.17 g/kg/h (4 g/kg/24 h).[565]

The "average" total parenteral nutrition solution provides energy requirements in an approximate 60:40 balance of glucose/fat. Administration of large quantities of glucose may increase CO_2 production and ventilatory requirements. If respiratory compromise makes CO_2 elimination difficult, energy requirements may be better supplied by increasing fat and decreasing glucose, thereby decreasing CO_2 production and the respiratory quotient (RQ).[566–568]

Disorders of Fluid Balance

The stressed patient responds with activation of a variety of autonomic mechanisms to maintain intravascular volume. Catecholamines increase vascular tone and may induce renal vasoconstriction, decreasing renal plasma flow and urine output. Volume depletion stimulates release of antidiuretic hormone (ADH, vasopressin), which causes the renal tubules to increase their reabsorption of water. Cortisol release and aldosterone production are increased. Stressed patients are therefore in a salt- and water-avid state that may persist even after intravascular volume is restored, and total body fluid overload is common in children after serious illness or major trauma.

Although careful attention to fluid administration and judicious use of diuretics are adequate for the management of most patients, the clinician should be alert to specific disorders of fluid homeostasis. Three of the most commonly seen are detailed below. Laboratory and clinical findings to differentiate these are presented in Table 29–12.

Syndrome of Inappropriate Antidiuretic Hormone

If extracellular fluid (ECF) volume is high and serum sodium normal to low, ADH secretion by the posterior pituitary, which is modulated by stretch receptors in the left atrium, should be low. This decrease in ADH decreases free water reabsorption in the kidney, resulting in excretion of large volumes of dilute urine. ECF volume and serum sodium concentration are thus returned toward normal.

The syndrome of inappropriate antidiuretic hormone (SIADH) is present when free water is retained despite an already dilute and overexpanded intravascular space. The diagnosis is usually a clinical one, as ADH levels are not commonly measured. SIADH develops in a variety of clinical settings: CNS infections or trauma, pulmonary disease, mechanical ventilation, and after surgery, particularly scoliosis repair.[569–572] Patients with SIADH excrete small quantities of concentrated urine in the face of a normal or increased intravascular volume.

The common (and usually appropriate) response to decreased urine output in postoperative patients is to administer a volume bolus. The clinician should keep the possibility of SIADH in mind, however. If all other evidence (heart rate, perfusion, filling pressures) indicates that volume status is adequate, SIADH might be the cause of the decreased urine output, and additional fluid will not improve matters.

Hyponatremia is often present in children with SIADH, but not if the diagnosis is suspected early and fluid restriction is begun. Anticipation of potential SIADH in susceptible children will allow early fluid restriction to 50 to 60 percent of normal "maintenance" amounts, minimizing the development of hypervolemia and hyponatremia. Fluid restriction alone is usually adequate to manage SIADH. If hyponatremia is present and its duration is uncertain, it is generally best to correct serum sodium slowly to minimize the risk of developing a CNS demyelinating syndrome, seen with rapid correction of low osmolality in patients who have chronic hypotonicity.[573] In the occasional patient with symptomatic hyponatremia (obtundation, seizures), the risk of cerebral edema outweighs the risk of osmotic demyelination, and rapid correction with 3 percent saline (513 mEq Na/L) to restore serum sodium to a reasonable value of 125 mEq/L is appropriate.[574, 575] The calculation is straightforward:

$$Na \text{ (mEq needed)} = 0.6 \times wt \text{ (kg)} \times (125 - \text{measured } [Na]).$$

Cerebral Salt Wasting

Certain patients with neurologic injury, particularly those with CNS hemorrhage, exhibit severe urinary salt wasting. The etiology of cerebral salt wasting (CSW) is uncertain, but there is evidence suggesting that it is preceded by high levels of atrial natriuretic peptide (ANP) and may involve the interaction of other neural or humoral factors as well.[576–581] The presence of marked hyponatremia may initially lead to the diagnosis of SIADH, but there are several distinct differences. Children with SIADH are often volume overloaded; those with CSW are dehydrated, with negative water balance. Assessment of central venous pressure may help in this determination.[582] The urine is concentrated in both SIADH and CSW, but urine volume is much greater in CSW than in SIADH. The treatment is volume resuscitation and administration of sufficient sodium to replace the deficit and compensate for continuing losses, which may be enormous; the use of hypertonic saline is nearly always required. Frequent monitoring of urine and serum electrolytes is critical.

Diabetes Insipidus

Diabetes insipidus (DI) is most common in the setting of CNS surgery (especially suprasellar surgery), CNS trauma,

T A B L E 2 9 – 1 2			
DISORDERS OF FLUID BALANCE			
Test/Finding	**SIADH**	**CSW**	**DI**
Urine output	Decreased	Increased	Increased
Urine osmolarity	Increased	Increased	Decreased
Urine Na⁺	Increased	Increased	Decreased
Serum osmolarity	Decreased	Decreased	Increased
Serum Na⁺	Decreased	Decreased	Increased
Intravascular volume	Increased	Decreased	Decreased

SIADH, syndrome of inappropriate ADH; CSW, cerebral salt wasting; DI, diabetes insipidus.

or global brain injury; it is often seen in brain death.[583, 584] The syndrome may result from inadequate production of ADH ("central" DI), the form most commonly seen in the ICU setting, or from inadequate renal response to adequate levels of ADH ("nephrogenic" DI), which is much less common. The diagnosis is made clinically by noting an excessive flow of dilute urine. The kidney, either lacking ADH or unable to respond to it, is unable to increase reabsorption of free water. If untreated, dehydration and hyperosmolarity result.

Children with chronic DI have learned to regulate their fluid balance nicely; they liberally drink water as needed to maintain osmolar balance, and should be allowed to self-regulate if possible. Unfortunately, their clinical condition when admitted to the ICU may preclude this, and the clinician must manage water balance for them. Initial management may involve simply volume restoration and then continued administration of free water in sufficient quantity to maintain fluid balance. This is conceptually simple but practically difficult. Urine flow may be several hundred milliliters per hour or more, necessitating rapid IV replacement. If dextrose-containing fluids are used, hyperglycemia and subsequent osmolar diuresis may occur, compounding the problem. A more effective approach for ICU management of central DI is administration of low-dose aqueous vasopressin (ADH) as a continuous infusion (0.5 to 3 mU/kg/h).[569, 585, 586] The ADH infusion is carefully adjusted to reduce but not completely stop urine flow; a goal of 1 to 2 mL/kg/h is reasonable. Continued monitoring of serum electrolytes, urine output, and specific gravity is essential. Acute DI is usually transient, and the patient can be weaned from the infusion after a day or two. If chronic treatment is needed, nasal DDAVP may be used.

Diabetic Ketoacidosis

Improved long-term management of children with diabetes has resulted in a decreased frequency of diabetic ketoacidosis (DKA), but this complication still occurs and may be life threatening. DKA may result from infection or from failure to take prescribed insulin, and may occur as the initial presentation in as many as 30 percent of new-onset diabetics.

The biochemical events that lead to ketoacidosis are caused by insulin deficiency.[569] Glucose does not enter the cells, depriving them of their primary source of energy. Fat and protein are metabolized for energy instead, and the by-products of this metabolism (e.g., ketones and organic acids) accumulate in the serum. Hyperglycemia causes glucosuria and an osmotic diuresis with loss of water, sodium, and potassium; dehydration may be worsened by vomiting and decreased oral intake. Intravascular volume depletion may become severe enough to cause impaired tissue perfusion. Severe metabolic acidosis depletes the body's bicarbonate and other buffer systems. The respiratory system attempts to compensate for the decreased pH by hyperventilation, leading to the Kussmaul respiratory pattern of DKA.

Assessment of the diabetic patient should begin with a history and physical examination, with particular reference to the details of previous diabetic management, recent fluid intake, normal weight, and any possible precipitating factors. Polydipsia, polyuria, polyphagia, and weight loss are common symptoms in the new-onset case; headache, abdominal pain, vomiting, and lethargy are also frequently seen. The severity of dehydration should be estimated from the physical findings and the difference between the normal and present weight; a dehydration of 10 to 12 percent is common.

The serum electrolytes, glucose, pH, and ketone levels should be measured immediately and every 1 to 2 hours initially. An arterial or central venous catheter makes the required frequent blood sampling easier and less traumatic. The urine volume should be measured hourly and tested for glucose and ketones. Cultures of the blood, throat, urine, and other possible sites of infection should be obtained. If a likely source of infection is found, antibiotic therapy should be started immediately.

The patient with severe DKA should be admitted to an ICU for monitoring and treatment, particularly if there are signs of volume depletion or an impaired state of consciousness. Rapid volume expansion, if needed, is achieved with saline or lactated Ringer's solution, but only to the point of ensuring adequate perfusion. Continued fluid administration should proceed slowly and should be designed to replace the estimated fluid deficit over 48 hours and to provide maintenance requirements and replacement of continuing urine losses.[587–589]

The goal of insulin therapy is to correct the energy deficit, to restore acid–base balance, and to clear the ketoacidosis. Too rapid a correction of blood glucose may induce a rapid change in osmolarity, potentially aggravating cerebral edema (see below). Continuous insulin infusion is the preferred method of treatment because of the gradual response it produces. Some clinicians administer an initial loading dose of 0.1 U/kg of regular insulin, although many do not because of concern that the blood glucose concentration might decrease too quickly.[590] Continuous infusion of insulin is begun at about 0.1 U/kg/h and then titrated to effect.[591] A decrease in serum glucose of 50 to 100 mg/dl/h is ideal, although the change in the first hour of treatment is often greater because of the effects of rehydration. Glucose is added to the IV fluids when the serum glucose reaches 250 to 300 mg/dl. The insulin infusion is continued until the acidosis is corrected and the serum is clear of ketones, after which a sliding scale for subcutaneous regular insulin is begun. Bicarbonate, given to correct acidosis, is probably not helpful.[592]

Although the initial serum potassium level may be normal or near normal, total body potassium is depleted because of the osmotic diuresis. Correction of acidosis and hyperglycemia will result in hypokalemia if potassium replacement is not begun early in the course of treatment. As soon as intravascular volume is restored and adequate urine output is ensured, potassium is added to the IV fluids in a concentration of 20 to 40 mEq/L. Because of concurrent phosphate depletion in DKA, it is useful to administer approximately half the required potassium as the phosphate salt and the remainder as the chloride.

Cerebral edema is an infrequent but serious complication of DKA, particularly in younger children, and is responsible for the bulk of the mortality and morbidity seen in this condition.[593–597] The edema may be because of rapid movement of water into brain cells as the plasma osmolality decreases during treatment, and overly rapid hydration or too rapid a decrease in plasma glucose therefore must be avoided. It is probably too simplistic, however, to cite this as the only factor in developing cerebral edema; the complication is seen in children who have been well-managed, and there are case reports suggesting its occurrence even before treatment.[598, 599] Reliable predictors to suggest the specific children at risk of developing cerebral edema are not available.[569, 589, 595, 597] Other intracranial events, particularly infarction from hyperviscosity, may also occur in the absence of edema.[600] Close monitoring of all children in DKA is essential, with rapid evaluation and intervention if signs of neurologic deterioration should occur.

Poisoning

Accidental ingestion of or other exposure to toxic chemicals represents a major cause of serious illness and death in children, particularly those in the 1- to 5-year age group; the use of child-proof containers has improved but not completely eliminated the problem.[601–605] It has been estimated that more than 500,000 incidents of potentially toxic ingestion occur in children each year, of which only approximately 100,000 are actually reported. A variety of drugs and toxic agents are involved in poisoning episodes in children.[127, 598, 599, 601–604, 606–629, 629–643] (Table 29–13).

The general approach to the patient who has had a significant exposure to a potentially toxic compound is as follows:

Identify the poison and its potential effects
Prevent absorption
Increase the rate of elimination
Prevent metabolism or binding
Administer specific antagonists
Provide general supportive care
Counseling and other measures to prevent recurrence

T A B L E   2 9 – 1 3
COMMON POISONS IN CHILDREN

Medications
  Acetaminophen[601, 603, 606]
  Salicylates[603, 607, 608, 967]
  Iron, fluoride[609, 610, 638]
  Sedatives, tranquilizers, psychotropics[611, 620, 621]
  Opiates[601, 603]
  Digitalis, other cardiac medications[612–615]
  Tricyclic antidepressants[616, 617, 618, 642, 643]
  Antihistamines[619]
  Theophylline[622]

Commercial products
  Petroleum products[623, 624]
  Cleaning agents, bleaches, corrosives[601]
  Pesticides[626]
  Alcohols, glycols[627, 628]
  Lead, heavy metals[609, 629]

Gases
  Carbon monoxide[630, 639]
  Toxic smoke[647]

Plants[631]

Because of the tremendous variety of chemical products, both man-made and natural, that can cause toxicity in children, it is necessary to have available extensive reference sources to determine the level of potential toxicity and the likely adverse effects of any compound. Such references include standard texts, the reference card system supplied by the National Clearinghouse for Poison Control Centers, and microfiche systems. The MICRO-MEDEX databases, including POISINDEX and a number of other drug- and toxin-related systems, are now available as an intranet package for installation and use within a health-care system.[644] In addition, the clinician should enlist the aid of the nearest Poison Control Center, whose staff can provide advice and follow-up.[635]

If the poison has been ingested orally, efforts should be made to decrease its absorption by removing it from the stomach, by using a cathartic agent to hasten its transit through the gastrointestinal (GI) tract, or by administering an agent such as activated charcoal, which may adsorb the toxin and diminish its availability for absorption. The use of syrup of ipecac to induce vomiting, although still indicated for use at home immediately after a drug ingestion, is no longer recommended for use in the emergency room; the efficacy of such induced vomiting is highly variable, it decreases with time since ingestion, and the risk of aspiration is real.[632] Vomiting should never be induced if a caustic or corrosive agent or a volatile petroleum product has been ingested. Gastric lavage should not be considered unless a patient has ingested a potentially life-threatening amount of a poison and the procedure can be undertaken within 60 minutes of ingestion.[633] If the patient is not fully conscious, the airway must be protected by inserting an ETT to prevent aspiration of stomach contents. Activated charcoal 1 g/kg, administered enterally as soon as possible, is effective in binding toxin and decreasing its availability for absorption.[604, 634] A cathartic, typically sorbitol, can be administered concomitantly to speed GI transit time. If the drug or toxin is known to have a significant enterohepatic circulation (absorption → excretion by the liver → reabsorption), repeated doses of charcoal should be considered.

Elimination of some poisons can be enhanced by increasing the rate of excretion in the urine. Most drugs are of small molecular size and are therefore filtered into the urine at the glomerulus. Once in the tubule, reabsorption into the blood can occur only if the drug is a nonionized, relatively lipophilic form. Elimination of some drugs can therefore be increased by ensuring good urine flow and by modifying the pH of the urine to increase the fraction of the drug existing in the ionized form.[603, 604] Excretion of weak bases can be enhanced by acidifying the urine with ascorbic acid or ammonium chloride, whereas weak acids may be eliminated more rapidly if the urine is alkalinized with bicarbonate.

Dialysis, hemoperfusion, or plasmapheresis may help to eliminate some drugs and toxins.[636, 645] The efficiency of drug removal by these techniques is influenced by the volume of distribution of the drug, the size of the molecule, the degree of protein binding, and other factors (Fig. 29–7). When a drug is widely distributed in the body, a relatively small amount is available in the plasma at any given time, making its removal by extracorporeal techniques

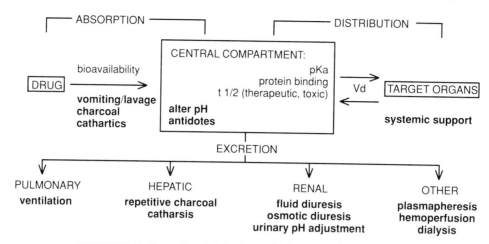

FIGURE 29–7. Absorption, distribution, and elimination of drugs or toxins.

less efficient. Drugs that are highly protein bound do not move across a dialysis membrane but may be removed by plasmapheresis.

The potential adverse effects of some drugs or toxins can be blocked or altered. Toxins that are metabolized to even more toxic by-products may have that metabolism blocked or inhibited. Ethanol can be used to decrease the rate of conversion of methanol or ethylene glycol to more toxic oxidation products,[627] although a specific inhibitor of alcohol dehydrogenase has been used more recently.[628, 640] Another method of blocking the effect of a toxic agent is to administer compounds that bind the offending toxin and render it inactive. Examples include giving a sulfhydryl donor, such as *N*-acetylcysteine, to bind acetaminophen metabolites,[625, 646] giving sodium nitrite and thiocyanate to react with cyanide,[647] using chelating agents such as ethylenediaminetetra-acetic acid (EDTA) or dimercaprol to bind heavy metals,[629] using desferoxamine to bind iron,[638] and administering specific antibodies to bind digoxin.[604, 612–614] For a few potentially toxic medications, relatively specific antagonists block some or all of the adverse effects. Examples are naloxone, which reverses opioid intoxication, and atropine, which treats intoxication with cholinesterase inhibitors.

Good supportive care, efforts to decrease the absorption and increase the elimination of drug, and specific antidotal therapy must be administered simultaneously. Details of the management of specific poisonings are available in the references in Table 29–13; particularly common ingestions include acetaminophen and the tricyclic antidepressants. Recommendations are frequently updated; the most current information and advice are available through the Poison Control Center network.

Hematology

The blood performs many functions. Oxygen transport and coagulation are among those that may be affected by disease and that are amenable to therapy in the ICU.

Oxygen Transport

Oxygen transport from the alveoli to the tissues depends on both cardiopulmonary function and the oxygen carry-

ing capacity of the blood. Although much of our focus in anesthesia and intensive care is on optimizing cardiopulmonary performance, it is equally important to ensure correct function of the gas transport medium.[648]

Under normal conditions, only a small quantity of oxygen is dissolved in the plasma during its path through the pulmonary capillaries. The bulk of the needed supply is bound to hemoglobin. Fully saturated, 1 g of normal hemoglobin (HbA) carries 1.34 mL of oxygen. The oxygen content of blood can be derived from a simple expression:

$$O_2 \text{ content (ml/dl)} = [1.34 \times Hb \text{ (g/dl)} \times \% \text{ sat}] + (0.0031 \times Pa_{O_2})$$

The first portion of the expression represents the oxygen bound to hemoglobin; the second is the oxygen dissolved in plasma. At a Pa_{O_2} of 100 mm Hg, for example, the amount of oxygen dissolved in 100 ml of blood is 0.31 ml, or approximately 1.5 percent of the usual 20 ml/dl oxygen content. Studying this relationship makes it clear that providing an adequate quantity of functional hemoglobin (e.g., transfusion to correct anemia) will improve oxygen content much more than simply raising the Pa_{O_2}.

Anemia

Anemia is characterized as an inadequate amount of circulating hemoglobin or red blood cells (RBCs) to meet the patient's oxygen transport needs. The actual hemoglobin or hematocrit level at which a child is considered "anemic" is relative to the child's age, the disease process, the cardiorespiratory status, and the expected course. Transfusion of RBCs is given more readily to children acutely ill with respiratory dysfunction than to those who are stable and have normal gas exchange. The lowest hematocrit or hemoglobin an individual patient can tolerate is difficult to define.[649, 650] Individual organs may be capable of autoregulation of blood flow or oxygen extraction to achieve stable oxygen delivery over a range of hematocrits.[651, 652]

The risks of blood transfusion (transmission of infectious disease, transfusion reaction, and sensitization to blood antigens) must be weighed against the benefit of increased oxygen-carrying capacity.[653, 654] These issues are particularly acute in sick newborns, who frequently require red cell transfusion but whose relatively immature immune function may make them more at risk for complications. Transfusion practices vary widely in this age group.[655, 656] Fortunately, the use of erythropoietin (EPO) has decreased their need for transfusion.[657–659] Elective surgical patients may benefit from predonation of autologous blood, preadministration of EPO, and the judicious use of hemodilution and autotransfusion.[660, 661]

Packed red blood cells (PRBCs) are the best product for treatment of anemia in most circumstances, although massive transfusion during rapid blood loss may be better done with fresh whole blood. Most blood centers use a citrate-phosphate-dextrose (CPD) anticoagulant for blood preservation.[662] Citrate anticoagulates the blood by binding calcium; phosphate and dextrose augment red cell adenosine triphosphate (ATP) and 2,3-diphosphoglycerate (2,3-DPG) to minimize storage loss of RBC function. Many centers add adenine in various concentrations (CPD-A1 or A2) to extend useful storage life from 21 to 35 days.[663, 664] Rapid or massive transfusion of banked blood may cause chelation of calcium, functional hypocalcemia, and myocardial dysfunction; in small children one may also encounter hyperkalemia, hypothermia, microemboli, and late-onset metabolic alkalosis.[665] Stored whole blood and PRBCs contain few functional platelets and decreased concentrations of clotting factors, and massive transfusion of these products can lead to a dilutional coagulopathy. The clinician must anticipate these complications.

Hemoglobin/RBC Dysfunction

Several alternate hemoglobins are seen in children. Fetal hemoglobin (HbF) has an increased affinity for oxygen, with 50 percent saturation (P_{50}) at a Po_2 of 19 mm Hg; fetal RBCs are also deficient in 2,3-DPG.[666] Both factors contribute to difficulty in releasing oxygen from hemoglobin at the tissue level in infants.

Oxidation of the ferrous (Fe^{2+}) ion in hemoglobin to the ferric (Fe^{3+}) form results in the formation of methemoglobin, which is unable to transport oxygen.[667] Methemoglobinemia may be congenital, which is usually asymptomatic, or may be acquired by ingestion of potent oxidizing agents such as nitrites or sulfonamides. Treatment includes oxygen, IV administration of methylene blue, and occasionally exchange transfusion.

Carbon monoxide (CO) inhalation occurs with exposure to heavy concentrations of smoke or exhaust fumes. The affinity of CO for hemoglobin is roughly 200 times that of oxygen, and CO therefore readily displaces oxygen from hemoglobin. The resulting carboxyhemoglobin is unable to transport oxygen. If carboxyhemoglobin concentrations are greater than 20 percent of total hemoglobin, oxygen transport may be compromised despite adequate Pao_2 and absence of clinical cyanosis. CO-intoxicated patients should receive 100 percent oxygen to reduce the half-life of carboxyhemoglobin from 4 hours (in room air) to 45 minutes. Hyperbaric oxygen therapy, if available, may further improve oxygen utilization at the mitochondrial level.[630]

Sickle cell anemia (SS disease) is a chronic hemolytic disease in which the abnormal hemoglobin (HbS) "gels" when deoxygenated, leading to cell sickling and occlusion of small vessels. Patients with SS disease often present with acute vaso-occlusive crises, leading to ischemia or infarction of the occluded organ[668]; the most serious of these is stroke, a complication that may be preventable, but with some risk, by chronic transfusion.[669–671] Younger patients may present with critical splenic sequestration, a massive engorgement of the spleen accompanied by intravascular volume depletion. Aplastic and hemolytic crises, with acutely decreased production or increased destruction of RBCs, occur less often.

Acute management of SS patients requires supplemental oxygen, generous hydration, and adequate pain control with systemic analgesics or regional techniques. Respiratory decompensation and desaturation in acute chest syndrome (ACS), a syndrome of fever, chest pain, leukocytosis, and a new pulmonary infiltrate in patients with sickle cell disease, is a common reason for ICU admission, and may occur in the perioperative period.[672–675] Transfusion is a potential hazard in sickle cell patients because of a high incidence of alloimunization against minor RBC antigens.[671] Nevertheless, severe crises (stroke, ACS with hypoxemia) may require simple or partial exchange transfusion to decrease the HbS concentration and to reduce sludging and vascular occlusion.[668, 676] Nitric oxide also may prove to be of benefit in ACS and other vaso-occlusive processes, although only preliminary evidence is available to support its use.[677, 678]

Coagulation

A properly functioning coagulation system allows rapid but modulated conversion of its elements between fluid and solid phases in response to injury. The process of clot formation is a phasic interaction of vessel wall, platelets, circulating coagulation factors, and anticoagulant proteins,[679, 680] and this mechanism may be immature in newborn infants.[681]

The interaction of platelets with collagen exposed by damage to the vessel wall initiates the clotting process. Platelets adhere to the damaged area and release adenosine diphosphate, serotonin, thromboxane A_2, and other mediators of vasoconstriction and adhesion, stimulating further aggregation of platelets. The platelet plug formed allows temporary hemostasis. Full clot formation occurs over the next few minutes as the activated platelet membrane stimulates the formation of thrombin by activation of the various elements of the clotting cascade. Fibrinogen is hydrolyzed by thrombin to yield fibrin monomers, which are then polymerized into fibrin and stabilized into a clot by factor XIII. Fibrinolytic control mechanisms exist to limit the extent of clot propagation and to provide for its eventual dissolution.

Under normal conditions, the ongoing processes of thrombosis and fibrinolysis are well balanced. Disorders of coagulation are commonly seen in critically ill children, either as the primary disease or as a manifestation of multisystem pathology. A complete review of the coagulation process and its potential dysfunction is beyond the scope of this chapter but is available for interested readers elsewhere.[679, 680, 682, 683] A functional approach to the support of the system with appropriate blood products is presented here.

Platelets

Platelets may be decreased in number or in function. Laboratory assessment consists of measurement of the platelet count and, if platelet dysfunction is suspected, the template (Ivy) bleeding time.

Dilutional or consumptive thrombocytopenia is not uncommon in the critically ill patient. A decision to transfuse platelets in these patients should be made on the basis of the platelet count and the presence of clinical bleeding.[684, 685] Platelet counts in excess of 50,000/mm³, assuming no other abnormality, are adequate for normal hemostasis; if bleeding is present in such a patient, it is unlikely that platelet transfusion alone will provide hemostasis. Recent or pending surgery may require maintaining the platelet count between 50,000 and 100,000/mm³. Prophylactic administration of platelets to prevent bleeding in patients with ongoing thrombocytopenia, such as children undergoing neoplastic chemotherapy, is often used, with the goal being to maintain a platelet count of 20,000/mm³ or greater. If the disorder is one of platelet function rather than number, platelet transfusion is usually beneficial. The indication for transfusion in this circumstance is abnormal bleeding and a standardized template bleeding time of at least twice the upper limit of normal.[685]

Platelets are available as a pooled product, composed of platelets separated from whole-blood donations of multiple donors, or as single-donor platelets obtained by plateletpheresis. The pooled product is more readily available and is the one usually chosen. Patient response varies, but a general rule is that 0.1 U/kg will raise the platelet count by 25,000/mm³. Alloimmunization to platelet antigens is common in patients who receive repeated platelet transfusions, and is a real risk of platelet therapy.[686–688] These patients fail to achieve the usual "bump" in platelet count after transfusion, but may respond better to HLA-matched single-donor platelets.

Coagulation Factors

Circulating coagulation factors are necessary for conversion of the temporary platelet plug to fibrin clot and for eventual dissolution of that clot. Inadequate quantities of these factors may be present for a number of reasons. Congenital deficiency of factor VIII:C (hemophilia A) or factor IX (Christmas disease; hemophilia B) may be present. Von Willebrand's factor (vWF), necessary for normal platelet function and factor VIII:C transport, may be deficient. Massive transfusion with banked blood can lead to a dilutional loss of all coagulation factors. Severe liver disease impairs production of many factors (II, V, VII, IX, XII, XIII, XXI). Finally, disseminated intravascular coagulation (DIC) is associated with increased consumption of factors.

Laboratory measurement of each of the coagulation factors is possible, but routine clinical care is based on measurement of the prothrombin time (PT), the activated partial thromboplastin time (aPTT), and the fibrinogen level (Table 29–14). The PT assesses the activity of the extrinsic pathway of coagulation (liver-dependent factors predominate), whereas the aPTT measures intrinsic pathway activity (measuring all factors except factor VII).

TABLE 29–14 TESTS OF CLOTTING FUNCTION*		
Test	**Typical Normals**	**Interpretation**
Platelet count	100,000–400,000/µl	Values <50,000 may be inadequate for surgical hemostasis; values <20,000 may lead to spontaneous bleeding
Bleeding time	2–9 min	Prolongation reflects deficiency in platelets (number or function) or abnormality in vessel wall
PT	10–12.5 sec	Tests extrinsic and common pathways; prolonged in liver disease, vitamin K deficiency, DIC
aPTT	25–36 sec	Tests intrinsic and common pathways; prolonged in DIC, liver disease, hemophilia A, von Willebrand's disease
Fibrinogen	200–400 mg/dl	Depleted in liver disease, DIC
FSPs, FDPs	Positive test: >40 µg/ml *or* titer 1:50	Elevated in DIC or other fibrinolytic process
D-dimer	positive test: <1 mg/ml	Indicates simultaneous activity of thrombin and plasmin; (+) in DIC

* Normal ranges for these tests may vary slightly from laboratory to laboratory.

Vitamin K may be deficient in newborns, malnourished patients, or those with liver disease. A prolonged PT suggests depletion of the liver-dependent factors, and administration of vitamin K 0.5 to 1 mg may be helpful. Fresh-frozen plasma (FFP) contains all plasma coagulation factors, and may be used for the nonspecific treatment of factor deficiencies such as in dilutional coagulopathy and DIC (see below). Patients with moderate to severe hemophilia A (factor VIII:C level <5 percent) are best managed with factor VIII concentrates (Table 29–15). These products are pooled from many donors, and therefore have potential for transmitting infection. Recent advances in their purification and processing, however, have dramatically reduced that risk; a recombinant product is also available.[689–693] Factor IX deficiency is managed with factor IX concentrates in similar fashion. Severe bleeding in von Willebrand's disease is managed with cryoprecipitate, which is a concentrated source of vWF, factor VIII, and fibrinogen.[684, 694–696] Less severe bleeding in von Willebrand's disease (type 1) and in milder hemophiliacs may respond to DDAVP (desmopressin), either therapeutically or as preoperative prophylaxis.[694, 696–698]

Acute, massive hemorrhage in all patients may require transfusion of all blood components; fresh whole blood, if truly fresh, is a useful source. As fresh blood is often not available, individual components are commonly used. RBC administration to maintain a hematocrit of approximately 30 percent is a reasonable approach. Loss/transfusion of greater than 1.5 to 2 blood volumes will usually

TABLE 29–15
BLOOD COMPONENT THERAPY

Product	Dose	Comments
Packed RBCs	5–10 ml/kg	Ongoing blood or volume loss makes precise calculation impossible; aim for hematocrit 35%
Platelets	0.1 U/kg will increase platelet count by 25,000/mm³	Administer slowly to avoid histamine-induced hypotension
Factor VIII concentrate	1 U/kg will increase level by 2%; half-life 12 h	Initial goal is to raise level to 100%; Not useful in von Willebrand's disease, as vWF is removed by purification process
Factor IX concentrate	1 U/kg will increase level by 1%; half-life 24 h	Same: may also be used to improve clotting in hemophilia A patients with factor VIII inhibitors
Cryoprecipitate	1–2 bags/5 kg	Specifically useful in von Willebrand's disease (contains vWF) and to replace fibrinogen; dosage is approximate, based on each bag containing 300 mg of fibrinogen; much variability exists
FFP	10–20 ml/kg	Should be used immediately after thawing; contains all factors, including antithrombin III and other necessary anticoagulants

cause a dilutional loss of platelets and clotting factors; specific replacement with platelets and FFP is indicated in these cases.[684]

Disseminated Intravascular Coagulation

A number of clinical conditions lead to the final common pathway of DIC.[679, 680, 699] Sepsis, major trauma (particularly head trauma),[700] low-output states, malignancies, vasculopathies, transfusion reactions, and other settings are ripe for the development of the syndrome. In such settings, large quantities of phospholipid are released into the circulation from disruption of endothelium, tissue, and platelets, activating the coagulation cascade in an unregulated fashion. Control of hemostasis is lost, and diffuse microvascular clotting, thrombosis, and fibrinolysis occur.

DIC should be suspected in any clinical situation in which there was a likely precipitating event and when abnormal bleeding, signs of multiple organ dysfunction, or hemolysis are present. The most common initial signs are abnormal bleeding from puncture sites or surgical incisions and the appearance of petechiae or purpura.

Confirmatory laboratory tests include elevated PT and PTT, a decreased fibrinogen and platelet count, positive tests for fibrin split products and D-dimers, and evidence of RBC fragmentation on blood smear.

The most effective method for treating DIC is reversal of the underlying cause; it is unlikely that treatment of DIC will be successful unless the primary disease can be corrected. Other aspects of treatment are controversial. The bleeding diathesis can be treated by transfusing platelets and FFP in quantities sufficient to control abnormal bleeding. This should be done aggressively, aiming for correction as rapidly as possible. DIC and abnormal bleeding may coexist with signs of fluid overload, and it may be difficult to infuse enough volume to definitively correct the coagulopathy. If so, an isovolumic partial exchange transfusion or plasmapheresis may allow correction of the clotting defects without incurring further volume overload.[701] Heparinization, once recommended for DIC alone, is now reserved for patients with severe thromboembolic manifestations (see below).

Purpura Fulminans

Most often seen in the setting of sepsis, particularly meningococcal sepsis, and generally in concert with DIC, purpura fulminans (PF) is a widespread deposition of clot in the microvasculature, particularly that of the skin and extremities. The resultant interruption of blood flow leads to patchy areas of ischemia in the skin and extremities. If flow is not restored, these may progress to necrosis and amputation may be required.[702] Although the syndrome may be seen in previously normal children, it may also be a marker for the presence of an inherited deficiency of one of three normally present anticoagulant proteins: protein C, protein S, and antithrombin III.[703–706]

The diagnosis is a clinical one, based on an examination consistent with skin/extremity ischemia in the setting of sepsis. Laboratory abnormalities consistent with DIC may be noted, and DIC management should proceed as usual. Although no longer advocated for uncomplicated DIC, heparinization, together with adequate factor replacement to ensure the presence of sufficient anticoagulant proteins (antithrombin III [AT-III], proteins C and S), is specifically indicated for purpura fulminans. The severe morbidity associated with PF has led to many novel techniques for its management, unfortunately with little solid data or large controlled trials to provide guidance. In addition to conventional means used to restore perfusion, attempts to vasodilate ischemic areas with vasodilator agents or sympathetic blockade may be considered. Topical nitroglycerin therapy has been useful in decreasing dermal ischemia in some cases.[707–709] Preliminary reports in the literature suggest that specific administration of AT-III, protein C, or low-molecular-weight fragments of heparin may be helpful.[680, 710–713] Although risky because of the possiblity of inducing uncontrolled hemorrhage, recombinant tissue plasminogen activator (rt-PA) administration may restore perfusion to areas of threatened necrosis and tissue loss.[714]

Vascular Thrombosis

Clot formation in major vessels is not uncommon in pediatric critical care, although the approach to its management is controversial.[715-717] Predisposing factors for thrombosis include low-flow states, trauma to vessel walls, and the presence of indwelling catheters. Clinical examination is the principal basis for suspecting thrombosis. Laboratory demonstration of unexplained platelet consumption or persistent septicemia with no obvious source may raise suspicion of clot. Ultrasonographic examinations may confirm the diagnosis. Dye studies can be performed but are often unnecessary.

Heparinization may prevent further clot formation but does not remove any clot already present. Fibrinolytic therapy with streptokinase 1,000 U/kg load, followed by 1,000 U/kg/h or urokinase 4,400 U/kg load followed by 4,400 U/kg/h for short periods of time (12 to 48 hours) may dissolve clot.[680, 718, 719] Such fibrinolytic therapy carries considerable risk of systemic bleeding and is relatively contraindicated in patients with recent surgery or ongoing hemorrhage.[720] Finally, surgical excision of clot is an extreme therapy but may be life saving.

Infectious Disease

Infections, particularly those of the respiratory or central nervous system, are common reasons for admission to the PICU. Nosocomial infection is similarly common in patients receiving the aggressive, invasive care provided in such a unit. A brief consideration of the common infections seen in this setting is therefore in order.

Infections Commonly Found in Children Admitted to the PICU

Children can develop severe infection from almost any viral or bacterial pathogen, and often therapy must be begun without a specific etiologic diagnosis or, in some circumstances, without a complete work-up.[721] Although some useful generalizations can be made, the clinical presentation, likely site or source of infection, and exact organisms involved vary with the age group. The infant and young child do not localize infection well, making specific clinical diagnosis more difficult. Nonspecific signs of infection (e.g., temperature instability [high or low], apnea, tachypnea, tachycardia, vasomotor instability, and metabolic abnormalities [hypoglycemia, metabolic acidosis]) are markers of sepsis in these children. The clinician must maintain a high index of suspicion to make a timely diagnosis of infection. This is especially true of young children with meningitis, who cannot give a history and often lack classic meningeal signs on physical examination.

Common Bacterial Infections

If sepsis is suspected and the physical examination fails to reveal a source, the clinician must often begin empiric antimicrobial therapy without confirmation of the diagnosis. Cultures should be obtained from blood, urine, spinal fluid, trachea, and other possible sites, and broad-spectrum antibiotic therapy instituted immediately. If the child is ill and appropriate specimens cannot be obtained (e.g., suspected meningitis in a child too ill to undergo lumbar puncture), therapy must begin without delay even though an accurate microbiologic diagnosis may be sacrificed.

Broad-spectrum antibiotic therapy once begun should continue for 2 to 3 days to allow time for culture results to become available. If a pathogen is isolated, antibiotic coverage is targeted at that organism. If cultures are negative, clinical judgment should guide the decision to stop antibiotics or to continue for a full course of therapy. Some laboratories offer rapid diagnostic testing for certain bacterial antigens in serum, urine, or spinal fluid; these may yield a specific diagnosis even if cultures remain negative.

There is a pattern to the pathogens commonly seen in children Table 29–16. In general, neonates become septic with organisms acquired from the maternal vaginal/perineal area; enteric organisms and group β-streptococci predominate.[722] Older children acquire infection by respiratory or contact spread from the community. H. influenzae type B used to be a very significant pathogen in younger children, but recent introduction of an effective vaccine has dramatically decreased the incidence of invasive H. influenzae disease.[452, 454, 455, 723] Invasive group A streptococcal disease, however, has become more prominent, with septic and toxic shock syndromes now occasionally seen.[457, 724] Finally, pneumococcal infections remain a major cause of serious bacterial illness in children, and their developing pattern of resistance to penicillin and other drugs is problematic.[725-728]

Broad-spectrum empiric therapy for children with suspected bacterial sepsis or meningitis may be prescribed based on a similar pattern of assumptions[729-732] (Table 29–17). The clinician should realize that all recommendations for antibiotic choices, such as those in this text and in the tables, should be interpreted to be guidelines. Local and institutional factors, nosocomial data, patient history and susceptibility, and continually changing patterns of sensitivity and resistance all must be considered when making a therapeutic choice for a particular child and clinical setting.

The septic infant (until age 6 to 8 weeks) is best treated with ampicillin and an aminoglycoside, usually gentamicin, to ensure coverage of Listeria (ampicillin) and enteric organisms (aminoglycoside). Although gentamicin has traditionally been administered in divided doses, new pharmacokinetic studies suggest that once-daily dosing is preferable, with a single daily dose ranging from 3 to

T A B L E   2 9 – 1 6
COMMON BACTERIAL PATHOGENS BY AGE

Neonate	Infant/Older Child
Group B streptococci	S. pneumoniae
E. coli	S. aureus
Klebsiella/Enterobacter	Group A streptococci
S. aureus	N. meningitidis
S. epidermidis	Enterobacteriaceae (e.g., Salmonella)
Listeria monocytogenes	Enterococcus
	H. influenzae, type B

T A B L E   2 9 – 1 7
EMPIRIC ANTIBIOTIC TREATMENT*

Infants <6 wk	Ampicillin + aminoglycoside
	Ampicillin + cefotaxime
6 wk to 3 mo	Ampicillin + cefotaxime *or* ampicillin +
	ceftriaxone
	Ampicillin + chloramphenicol
3 mo to 5 yr	
Non-CNS	
	Ampicillin/sulbactam
	Cefotaxime *or* ceftriaxone
	Ampicillin + chloramphenicol
CNS	
	Cefotaxime *or* ceftriaxone
	Ampicillin + chloramphenicol
5 yr to adult	
Non-CNS	
	Ampicillin/sulbactam
	Cefotaxime *or* ceftriaxone
CNS	
	Cefotaxime *or* ceftriaxone

* These are suggested antibiotic combinations for initial therapy of previously healthy, nonimmunocompromised infants and children. If the patient has a CVL, VP shunt, or other indwelling device, vancomycin might be added for *S. epidermidis* coverage.[968, 969] Extended *Pseudomonas* coverage can be obtained with ticarcillin, piperacillin/tazobactam, ceftazidime, aztreonam, or the aminoglycosides.[970, 971]

7.5 mg/kg/day depending on gestational age and renal function.[733] An alternative plan would be to use ampicillin and a third-generation cephalosporin (cefotaxime). Although the third-generation cephalosporins are excellent drugs with good cerebrospinal fluid (CSF) penetration, concern for the development of resistance may suggest their secondary rather than primary use.

Older infants and children are less likely to harbor enteric organisms. Concern in these children is for good coverage of gram-positive organisms and of *H. influenzae.* If serious, invasive, or CNS pneumococcal infection is likely, vancomycin should be added; the vancomycin should be discontinued as soon as sensitivities indicate that it is not needed, as increasing microbial resistance to drugs is a growing problem and their prudent use is essential.[734, 735] It has been standard therapy in the past, recognizing the incidence of ampicillin-resistant *H. influenzae,* to begin treatment with ampicillin and chloramphenicol. Because of concern about chloramphenicol toxicity, however, this combination is now often replaced by a third-generation cephalosporin (typically cefotaxime or ceftriaxone) or an antibiotic/β-lactamase inhibitor combination (e.g., ampicillin/sulbactam [Unasyn]).[736–739] Ceftazidime, a third-generation cephalosporin, adds coverage for *Pseudomonas* if needed. These drugs provide good coverage of all common pathogens in older infants and children; CSF penetration of ampicillin/sulbactam is uncertain. As specific culture information becomes available, coverage should be narrowed and pinpointed to the known pathogen (Table 29–18).

Antibiotic treatment of bacterial meningitis carries the caveat that adequate drug penetration into the CNS to ensure rapid sterilization of the CSF is critical.[740–742] Neurologic sequelae of meningitis, especially hearing loss, are thought to be a consequence not only of the bacterial invasion but also of the inflammatory response engendered.[743] The early administration of dexamethasone to children with *H. influenzae* meningitis has been shown to reduce the inflammatory response and to lower the incidence of hearing loss[744–748]; data are less clear, but probably supportive, of the use of steroids in pneumococcal meningitis.[749–751] There is some evidence that the concomitant use of steroids might alter the CSF penetration of vancomycin.[752]

Common Viral Infections

Although bacterial infection is often more acute or severe than viral disease, viral infection is more common, can be quite severe, and is often cause for ICU admission. Respiratory infections (RSV, parainfluenza, influenza), meningoencephalitis (often enterovirus), and multisystem disease (herpes simplex, cytomegalovirus) may all require cardiorespiratory support for successful treatment and recovery. An extensive discussion of these is beyond the scope of this chapter, but a few pertinent comments are in order.

Respiratory Viral Infections

RSV accounts for a large portion of acute lower airway disease in young children. Manifesting as bronchiolitis or pneumonia, RSV appears in winter to early spring outbreaks and infects essentially all children during their first 3 years of life.[753] Breast-feeding may be protective.[754] Severely infected infants are hospitalized with symptoms of cough, wheezing, impaired gas exchange and, in the youngest infants, apnea.[755, 756] These infants may require intensive care and mechanical ventilatory support, and there is some evidence of association with increased airway reactivity in later childhood.[757, 758]

Management of RSV infection is to a large degree symptomatic. Oxygen supplementation is provided by mist tent, and some infants improve with bronchodilators.[759, 760] Ribavirin, a synthetic nucleoside resembling guanosine, has been shown effective in ameliorating the course of RSV infection and in shortening the time span of viral shedding if administered early in the course of the disease.[753, 761] It is administered by aerosolization into the patient's mist tent several times daily.[476] The drug may be hazardous to health care personnel, and precautions to limit exposure are advised.[762] Ribavirin is generally recommended for use only in infants at particularly high risk for morbidity from the disease, such as those with preexisting cardiac or pulmonary disease or immunodeficiency. Even in these patients, use of the drug is controversial.[472, 763–766] The intensivist must exercise caution in using the drug for patients receiving mechanical ventilation, as the aerosolized particles can precipitate and lead to malfunction of the expiratory valve. Such administration can be accomplished safely, but only if meticulous attention is paid to ventilator maintenance.[475, 477]

Parainfluenza types 1 to 3 are common causes of croup, the management of which has been discussed previously in this chapter. Influenza viruses, both A and B, can cause lower airway disease. Although this disease is usually mild to moderate, diffuse primary influenza pneumonia can be extremely severe and life threatening.[767]

T A B L E   2 9 – 1 8
TYPICAL ANTIBIOTIC SPECTRA*

Antibiotic	Organism†														
	SA	SE	GAS	GBS	GDS	LM	EC	PROT	KLEB	ENT	SERR	PSD	MENG	HIB	BF
Penicillin G	0	0	+	+	+	+	0	0	0	0	0	0	+	0	+
Ampicillin	0	0	+	+	+	+	±	0	0	0	0	0	+	(+)	+
Ticarcillin	0	0	+	+	+	+	+	+	0	+	+	+	+	+	+
Mezlocillin	0	0	+	+	+	+	+	+	+	+	+	+	+	+	+
Ampicillin + sulbactam	+	0	+	+	+	+	±	+	+	+	0	0	+	+	+
Imipenem	±	+	+	+	+	+	+	+	+	+	+	+	+	+	+
Oxacillin	+	0	+	+	0	0	0	0	0	0	0	0	+	0	0
Cephalothin (1)	+	0	+		0	0	+	0	0	0	0	0	+	±	0
Cefoxitin (2)	+	0	+		0	0	+	0	±	0	0	0		0	+
Cefotaxime (3)	±	0	+	+	0	0	+	+	+	+	+	0	+	+	0
Ceftriaxone (3)	+	0	+	+	0	0	+	+	+	+	+	0	+	+	0
Ceftazidime (3)	±	0	+		0	0	+	+	+	+	+	+	+	+	0
Chloramphenicol	±	0	+	+	0		+	0	0	0	0	0	+	+	+
Gentamicin	±			+	0		+	+	+	+	+	+			0
Amikacin	±			+	0		+	+	+	+	+	+			0
Aztreonam	0	0	0	0	0	0	+	+	+	+	+	+	+	+	0
Vancomycin	+	+	+	+	+	0	0	0	0	(+)	0	0	0	0	
Clindamycin	+	0	+	+			0	0	0		0	0			±

* +, usually sensitive; 0, usually resistant; ±, intermediate or variable; (+), increasing resistance (ampicillin/HIB); (+), sensitive if used in combination with aminoglycoside (vancomycin/*Enterococcus*). Therapy for meningitis must be based on CSF penetration as well as sensitivities. (1), (2), (3), First, second, third-generation cephalosporins
† SA, *S. aureus;* SE, *S. epidermidis;* GAS, group A streptococci; GBS, group B streptococci; GDS, group D streptococci (anaerobes); LM, *Listeria monocytogenes;* EC, *E. coli;* PROT, *Proteus mirabilis;* KLEB, *Klebsiella;* ENT, *Enterobacter;* SERR, *Serratia;* PSD, *Pseudomonas;* MENG, *Neisseria meningitidis;* HIB, *Haemophilus influenzae;* BF, *Bacteroides fragilis.*

CNS and Systemic Viral Infections

Viral meningitis, often caused by enteroviral infection,[768] is particularly common in the summer months. Symptoms of fever, malaise, headache, and fever are present; meningeal signs are present on physical examination. The CSF white count is elevated, typically in the hundreds; although classically there is a predominance of lymphocytes, this is not the case early in the disease, when polymorphonucleocytes may predominate. CSF glucose and protein are usually normal. No specific therapy is available; fortunately, the disease is usually benign and self-limited.

Herpes simplex viruses (HSV-1, nongenitally transmitted, and HSV-2, transmitted venereally and during childbirth) can cause encephalitis in all age groups. HSV encephalitis is characterized by variable fever, changes in mental status, and sometimes convulsions and meningeal signs; the presentation is variable and nonspecific enough to require a high index of suspicion for diagnosis. Laboratory findings include CSF with a predominance of red cells and evidence of localized brain disease (particularly temporal) on electroencephalography (EEG) or imaging studies. Viral cultures are rarely positive, but polymerase chain reaction (PCR) testing for CSF samples is available and usually diagnostic. HSV infection in the newly born or in immunocompromised hosts can present as an overwhelming, disseminated infection with viremia, hepatic failure, coagulopathy, CNS disease, and pneumonia. The potential for significant morbidity and mortality in both encephalitis and disseminated herpes is such that treatment with acyclovir should be begun immediately, before the definitive diagnosis has been established; acyclovir may be continued or omitted subsequently based on clinical course and results from laboratory testing.

Cytomegalovirus (CMV) infection, often subclinical and asymptomatic in normal individuals, can present as serious infection in immunocompromised patients, particularly following organ transplantation. CMV pneumonia and hepatitis are the most common syndromes, although systemic infection involving many organ systems is not uncommon. Viral culture and antibody/antigen testing of urine and blood will usually confirm the diagnosis, and treatment with ganciclovir is indicated.

Nosocomial Infection

Infection can develop after admission to the ICU.[769] The transmission of infection from one patient to another, or from the ICU staff to a patient, is largely preventable by good handwashing, cohorting of infected patients, and appropriate immunization of health care workers.[770–772] Ongoing quality assurance programs to monitor and control nosocomial infection should be in place.

Indwelling venous catheter infections are a significant source of ICU morbidity and expense.[773] The most common organism isolated in line-related bloodstream infection is *S. epidermidis,* although other coagulase-negative staphylococci, *S. aureus,* gram-negative organisms, and *Candida* species are occasionally seen[773–776]; the latter is more likely in patients receiving parenteral nutrition and in those who are immunosuppressed, and is a major cause of morbidity in contemporary critical care. Care in insertion and in site protection and minimizing entrance into the catheter and its tubing should minimize the risk of infection.[774, 777] Although the likelihood of catheter-related infection does increase with time in use, there are no data to support the practice of routinely changing the catheter or site when there is no evidence of infection present.[777–782] Impregnation of the catheter with antiseptics[783] or, better still, antibiotics[784–786] has been shown to reduce the incidence of nosocomial bloodstream infections.

Nosocomial pneumonia in pediatric care is frequently viral, with RSV (spread by health care workers) a common pathogen, especially in winter months.[774] Bacterial infection is seen as well, particularly in those with instrumented airways, prolonged hospitalization, and immunosuppression. Differentiation between colonization and true infection is often difficult, with the decision to begin antibiotic therapy based on a number of factors, including clinical change, radiographic abnormalities, fever, leukocytosis, tracheal aspirate Gram's stains and cultures, and clinical judgment.[769] Bronchoscopy and BAL can be helpful in making this decision, but are costly and often impractical in infants and small children. A number of preventive strategies have been described in adults, focusing on minimizing bacterial colonization and preventing aspiration of contaminated material.[787, 788]

Septic Shock

Septic shock is a syndrome of perfusion deficits and vasomotor collapse associated with the presence of microorganisms, endotoxin, or vasoactive mediators in the bloodstream.[789, 790] It represents the host's response to infection.[791, 792] The syndrome is most often seen with bacterial infection, but it may also occur with other infectious agents. Both gram-positive and gram-negative organisms can lead to the syndrome of septic shock. The cytokine response of tumor necrosis factor (TNF), interleukins (IL-1, followed by IL-6, IL-8, and IL-10), and eicosanoids triggered by gram-negative endotoxin also may be initiated by cell wall components of gram-positive organisms, but not in precisely the same fashion.[793–796] The cytokines initiate a vasculopathy, damaging capillary endothelium throughout the body. Vascular permeability increases, and there is massive fluid loss into interstitial spaces. Vasodilation and intravascular fluid depletion, in addition to myocardial depression, are therefore a primary cause of circulatory insufficiency in sepsis.[797, 798]

Shock and mortality in gram-positive infections correlate with the quantity of organisms per milliliter of blood as well as with humoral mediators of hypotension.[790, 799] Although excessive elaboration of TNF, interleukins, and other cytokines leads to the pathologic state known as septic shock, smaller or physiologic quantities may be essential for appropriate host response to bacterial invasion.[800–803] A number of studies have been conducted to determine therapeutic approaches that might intervene in

and modulate the inflammatory response and its triggers, but none have been globally successful, although occasional benefit is seen in small subgroups of patients. Monoclonal antibodies to endotoxin, for example, have improved survival in selected subgroups of patients, but there is no experience with their use in children.[804–807] The pathophysiologic heterogenicity of patients with the same clinical presentation of sepsis, but differing abnormalities in the details of inflammatory response, may be the root cause of this lack of broader success. Continued work is needed, with an emphasis on selection of patients by enrollment criteria that are more specific and detailed.[808]

The early phase of septic shock is vasodilation, with warm, flushed skin, tachycardia, a normal or slightly decreased blood pressure, a wide pulse pressure, and an increased cardiac output.[809] The patient is febrile and is often disoriented or agitated. Urine output may be decreased despite normal or increased cardiac output. This constellation of signs and symptoms is warm shock. As sepsis progresses, massive intravascular fluid loss and myocardial depression lead to decreased cardiac output. The induced sympathetic response causes vasoconstriction and increased SVR. As compensation is lost, blood pressure can no longer be maintained, the pulse becomes weak, and the skin is pale, mottled, and cool. Urine output decreases markedly and may cease entirely. Inadequate tissue perfusion and oxygen delivery lead to metabolic acidosis. There is an apparent impairment of cell metabolism and oxygen consumption in septic shock, and oxygen consumption may sometimes appear to be directly related to oxygen delivery.[810–812] The exact mechanism of altered oxygen utilization in sepsis is not known.[809, 813, 814]

Therapy includes measures to treat the infection and to support the failing circulation.[815, 816] Vigorous intravascular volume expansion replaces fluid lost because of capillary leak; close monitoring of cardiac output and filling pressures may be assisted by placement of a PA catheter.[164, 165] If volume infusion alone does not restore tissue perfusion, an inotrope is started. In early shock with decreased SVR, the judicious use of a vasoconstrictor may increase perfusion pressure. This should not be undertaken without first adequately replacing volume, and the SVR should not be increased above low normal levels. In later shock, elevated SVR and decreased myocardial contractility are the norm, and the use of a combined inotrope/vasodilator may improve cardiac output and perfusion. The use of steroids in septic shock, although theoretically attractive, has not proven effective in improving overall outcome.[817, 818] Their use is probably best reserved for specific indications such as adrenal insufficiency.[819]

Meningococcemia

Infection with *Neisseria meningitidis,* a frequent cause of septic shock, may produce a fulminant and fatal infection.[820] The most common presentation of meningococcemia is sudden onset of fever, toxicity, and a petechial or purpuric rash. Shock may be present on initial presentation, but more commonly the patient appears alert and hemodynamically stable, only to suddenly, rapidly, and unpredictably have their condition deteriorate a few hours later. ICU admission, in anticipation of this decompensation, is indicated.

Endotoxin release, adrenal hemorrhage or insufficiency, and myocardial depression are possible factors here.[821] Children with severe meningococcal disease have a decreased cortisol response to exogenously administered adrenocorticotropic hormone (ACTH).[822] Steroids in stress doses may be specifically indicated in these children.[206] Early and severe myocardial depression is seen in children with meningococcemia because of myocarditis and direct myocardial invasion by bacteria.[823, 824] Finally, skin and organ necrosis are seen in severe cases of meningococcemia; the management is discussed above (see "Purpura Fulminans").

Immunodeficiency

Many children in the PICU are immunocompromised, either because of a primary immune deficiency (congenital or acquired) or as a consequence of chemotherapy, malnutrition, or chronic disease. These children are at risk for a number of opportunistic infections. A detailed consideration of these disorders is beyond the scope of this chapter, but several specific diagnoses have significance for the intensivist.

Human Immunodeficiency Virus/Acquired Immunodeficiency Syndrome

A number of features of human immunodeficiency virus (HIV) infection are more prominent in children than in adults. In addition to the defects in cell-mediated immunity described in adults, pediatric cases of HIV infection are notable for failure to thrive, chronic diarrhea, progressive neurologic defects, and cardiomyopathy. A chronic lymphocytic interstitial pneumonitis is present in many children with HIV. Finally, there is a unique abnormality in B-cell function as well, with large, polyclonal increases in immunoglobulins but deficient immune globulin function. There is an inability to synthesize specific antibodies in response to new antigens. The clinical correlate is a marked increase in susceptibility to common bacterial infections.

PICU management of the disease is largely treatment of its infectious complications. The prognosis for long-term survival in HIV infection has improved, particularly for those who have not progressed to the full syndrome of acquired immunodeficiency syndrome (AIDS). Prevention of opportunistic infection is ideal,[825] but infectious and noninfectious causes of acute respiratory failure (Pneumocystis, bacterial pneumonia, CMV, lymphoid interstitial pneumonitis [LIP], mycobacterial disease, Candida, and nonspecific etiologies) often occasion ICU admission.[826] Aggressive care, including tracheal intubation and ventilatory support, is usually indicated and appropriate, but the mortality rate of ARF in AIDS is high.[826, 827]

Prevention of disease transmission is also of concern in critical care. Although voluntary deferment of donation by high-risk groups, meticulous screening of blood, and new methods of processing blood products have decreased the likelihood of HIV transmission by blood products, one cannot say that it has been completely eliminated. The clinician must now weigh even more carefully for each patient the risk/benefit ratio of transfusion of blood products. The risk to health care personnel from exposure to blood products, needle sticks, and patients and their body fluids is higher in the ICU than in a less acute setting. Scrupulous attention to hygiene and technique, with careful handwashing, gown-glove-mask technique, and full eye protection are essential during contact with the HIV-infected patient. Not all HIV-infected patients are known, however, and the adoption of universal precautions is essential for true protection of personnel.[828] If accidental exposure occurs, personnel should follow institutional protocol. Immediate prophylactic administration of the reverse transcriptase inhibitors zidovudine (AZT) and lamivudine (3TC) with the protease inhibitor indinavir is currently recommended, in most cases, by the U.S. Public Health Service.[829, 830]

Opportunistic Infections

Pneumocystis carinii pneumonia (PCP) is characterized by marked hypoxemia and tachypnea in a patient who appears otherwise well and has a paucity of pulmonary findings on physical exam. The chest film demonstrates a nonspecific, diffuse interstitial pattern. The disease is common in immunosupressed patients and may be the first manifestation of AIDS.

The diagnosis can be confirmed only by observing the presence of pneumocysts in large numbers in the alveoli. An adequate sample may be obtained by endotracheal[831] or, more reliably, bronchoalveolar[832-834] lavage. Treatment, in addition to respiratory support, is trimethoprim/sulfamethoxazole. If improvement does not occur within a reasonable time, pentamidine may be substituted; IV administration of pentamidine is safe if it is slow and controlled.[835] Early administration of steroids has been shown to improve survival and decrease morbidity in AIDS patients with PCP and is considered standard therapy.[836-838]

Fungal infections are a risk to immunocompromised children, particularly when invasive devices or catheters are in use. Persistent or unexplained fever, neutropenia or leukocytosis, unusual platelet consumption, or other nonspecific signs may be the only indication of candidiasis or other fungal infection. Definitive diagnosis may be difficult, and often therapy must be begun based on a combination of culture results, identification of fungal antigens in serum, and clinical suspicion. Experience suggests that earlier institution of therapy, before definitive diagnosis, may be more successful. Quantitative fungal cultures may be helpful.[839] Treatment is typically with amphotericin B, fluconazole, or 5-fluorocytosine[840-843]; liposomal or a lipid emulsion of amphotericin may reduce nephrotoxicity.[844-846]

Viral pneumonia after organ or bone marrow transplantation may lead to respiratory failure and ICU admission. The organisms most commonly seen are CMV and parainfluenza virus.[847-849] Ganciclovir is effective in preventing serious CMV disease when given prophylactically to bone marrow transplant recipients with evidence of CMV activation.[848, 849]

Neurologic Critical Care

A patient's prognosis for recovery from neurologic injury is determined by the nature of the injury or illness that caused admission and by the speed and efficacy of resuscitation and care received thereafter. Primary injury is that which has injured the CNS before presentation. This is classically described in head trauma,[850] where physical injury has occurred at a specific time prior to medical intervention, but the concept can also apply to injury from a hypoxic/ischemic event or other brain insult. There is little we can do at present to reverse primary injury, but we can attempt to prevent secondary injury from occurring during our care by ensuring good gas exchange and CNS perfusion, minimizing metabolic abnormalities, and allowing the brain the maximum opportunity to heal.[851] Unfortunately, further cellular injury may occur during the period of reperfusion following resuscitation from hypoxic or ischemic insults, including irregularities of regional cerebral blood flow, accelerated production of lactic acidosis in ischemic areas, calcium influx into the cytosol, and liberation of arachidonic acid metabolites and free radicals.[852–854] The process is complex and poorly understood and, despite much effort to develop them, there are no proven methods to ameliorate neuronal damage after global ischemic injury.[853, 855–859]

An accurate admission history and thorough physical examination are invaluable to plan care and to estimate the patient's prognosis. If trauma is the cause of the brain injury, the possibility that the injury was not accidental and may represent child abuse should be entertained.[860, 861] The Glasgow Coma Scale (Table 29–19) is useful as a standard against which the patient's global condition can be compared. Scores less than 8 indicate severe CNS dysfunction. Focal neurologic signs must be appreciated as indicators of possible specific sites of CNS injury. Finally, evaluation of brain stem reflexes assists in defining prognosis and the need for airway protection.

Laboratory testing complements the clinical examination: the most important single test is the computed tomographic (CT) scan of the brain.[862] Although it is helpful in assessing a number of abnormalities, its most important use is to determine if there is a lesion that can be treated

surgically. If so, significant improvement may come from timely surgical intervention; if not, medical management is continued.

Increased Intracranial Volume

The intracranial vault has a defined, limited capacity. If the volume of its contents should increase beyond that capacity, increased ICP may ensue, limiting brain perfusion and further damaging neurons. Successfully managing the volume of the intracranial contents will forestall this form of secondary injury.

The relationship between intracranial volume and pressure is complex. A simple but limited diagrammatic interpretation of the relationship is presented in Figure 29–8. The figure is oversimplified, because the response in pressure to increases in volume is presented as a single curve, whereas the true relationship is modified by the time course over which the volume change occurs (more gradual volume change induces less pressure change) and by the exact location of the volume increment.[175, 863] Clinical reduction of ICP is achieved by reducing the volume of the intracranial components, shifting the patient's position on the curve downward and to the left. The total volume of the intracranial contents is the sum of the volumes of its components:

$$V_{total} = V_{brain} + V_{blood} + V_{CSF} + V_{other}$$

where V_{brain}, V_{blood}, and V_{CSF} represent the volumes of brain, blood, and CSF. V_{other}, not always present, represents an abnormal space-occupying lesion (e.g., tumor or blood clot) for which surgical removal is therapeutic. V_{CSF} can be reduced by decreasing CSF production (not a commonly used approach) or by increasing its removal (shunts, external drains).[864] A number of therapies exist to reduce the V_{blood} or V_{brain}; these will be discussed below.

Management Strategies

The decision as to the level of support and monitoring required for a specific patient is complex and is based on history, global neurologic function, expected prognosis, and need for other therapy that might cloud the clinical examination. Good general ICU care is provided to all patients. The various components of therapy directed spe-

T A B L E 2 9 – 1 9
GLASGOW COMA SCALE

Criterion	Score*
Best motor response	
Obeys verbal command	6
Localizes stimulus	5
Withdraws from noxious stimulus	4
Abnormal flexion (decorticate)	3
Abnormal extension (decerebrate)	2
No response (flaccid)	1
Best verbal response	
Oriented, appropriate	5
Confused conversation	4
Inappropriate words	3
Incomprehensible sounds	2
No response	1
Eye opening	
Spontaneous	4
To speech	3
To pain	2
None	1

* Total score correlates with overall neurologic status. Maximum score = 15; minimum score = 3.

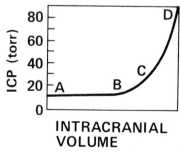

FIGURE 29–8. Intracranial pressure–volume relation. Under normal circumstances, small increases in the volume of intracranial contents (point A to B) cause only minimal increases in ICP. In pathologic conditions that increase the volume of intracranial contents, a small further increase in volume (point C and D) causes a marked increase in ICP.

cifically at reducing ICP or ensuring adequate CPP are applied more selectively and sequentially, titrated against clinical examination, ICP, CPP, and electrophysiologic monitors. A child with head trauma probably has a good prognosis, especially if there has been no intervening hypoxia or ischemia; an aggressive approach to monitoring and support are indicated. A child resuscitated after a prolonged hypoxic/ischemic event, with no mitigating circumstances such as hypothermia, generally has a poor prognosis. It is unlikely that strict control of ICP, even if successful, will improve that prognosis in any significant fashion, and invasive monitoring or extremes of therapy are probably not indicated.

Control of gas exchange is one method of cerebral blood flow (CBF) regulation. CBF must satisfy cerebral oxygen demands; if the patient is anemic or poorly oxygenated, flow must increase to compensate for the reduced arterial oxygen content (CaO_2). CaO_2, then, inversely affects CBF.[865, 866] We therefore strive to maintain a normal hemoglobin concentration and a PaO_2 of about 100 mm Hg to provide a margin of safety. Similarly, CBF is linearly and directly related to $PaCO_2$ between 20 and 80 mm Hg. We maintain a slightly lowered $PaCO_2$ (34 to 36 mm Hg) as a baseline, reserving more aggressive hypocarbia for use only as emergent therapy for acute elevations of ICP. Prolonged severe hyperventilation may be hazardous and is not recommended.[867-872]

Control of brain edema reduces V_{brain}. Although emphasis has been placed in the past on fluid restriction and on keeping patients with potential cerebral edema "dry," it is probably better to focus on maintenance of euvolemia instead, ensuring good perfusion while avoiding fluid excess. Excessive administration of free water may indeed be detrimental and should be avoided. Mannitol, an osmotic diuretic, is commonly used to control ICP.[873] It has both rheologic and diuretic effects. Mannitol induces plasma expansion, reducing blood viscosity and resulting in increased CBF; this increase in CBF may lead to cerebral vasoconstriction and consequent reduction in cerebral blood volume (CBV) and ICP.[874-876] Mannitol's diuretic effect is to generate an osmotic gradient between blood and brain, enhancing removal of water from the brain and its subsequent excretion via the kidney.[871, 877]

One approach is to initiate diuresis early in the course of therapy with mannitol and then to maintain serum osmolarity at 290 to 310 mOsm by careful fluid administration, using isotonic solutions and avoiding fluid excess. Repeated doses of mannitol should not be given on a routine basis, as such administration may lead to an accumulation of mannitol in the brain[878]; repeat doses of mannitol may be given on an as-needed basis if ICP acutely increases or if serum osmolarity has decreased below the desired range. Attention also should be directed to the possible pathologic alterations in fluid balance that are associated with brain injury. Diabetes insipidus, SIADH, and cerebral salt wasting may all occur and complicate ICP control. Evaluation and treatment are as previously discussed (Table 29–12).[569, 574, 577, 583, 879] The use of hypertonic saline maintenance fluid to improve ICP and CPP in head-injured children has had equivocal results.[880, 881]

Head position may enhance or occlude jugular venous drainage, thus affecting CBV. The ideal position is with the head midline and elevated about 30 degrees from the horizontal; this should minimize ICP while allowing good CPP.[882]

Hyperthermia increases cerebral metabolic rate and thus CBF. Fever should be evaluated and infection treated in the usual manner. Temperature control is important, and can be achieved with antipyretics or a cooling mattress, although the latter approach may require simultaneous muscle relaxation or a phenothiazine to block the shivering response. One randomized adult trial of actively induced hypothermia (32° to 33°C) following traumatic brain injury has demonstrated improved outcome at follow-up.[883] Further study is needed to provide the data necessary to clarify the role of this technique in children.

Seizure activity can dramatically increase brain O_2 consumption. Anticonvulsants, usually phenytoin or fosphenytoin, are indicated for patients with active seizure activity and are usually given prophylactically to patients after severe head trauma.[884] Appropriate monitoring of the EEG is required to ensure control of seizure activity in patients who are paralyzed.[885]

Analgesia and sedation should be provided to children in the PICU even when they appear comatose. Painful or noxious stimuli can increase cerebral electrical activity and ICP even in seemingly unresponsive patients. Such stimuli should be minimized and, if unavoidable, blocked with narcotics and hypnotics (see below). Although the use of narcotics, such as fentanyl, may be associated with a transient elevation of ICP and decrease in CPP, CBF appears to be preserved and cerebral ischemia avoided.[886-889]

Steroids have been shown to be effective for reduction of vasogenic edema around brain tumors. They are of no benefit in intracerebral hemorrhage, and may be harmful.[890] A recent meta-analysis of their use in acute traumatic brain injury, although demonstrating considerable uncertainty, provides no evidence to support their use in that setting.[891] High-dose methylprednisolone (30 mg/kg bolus, followed by 5.4 mg/kg/h for 23 hours or longer, instituted within 8 hours of injury) has been shown to improve neurologic outcome following acute traumatic spinal cord injury.[892-894]

Muscle relaxants may be required to achieve adequate ventilation, to prevent coughing or bucking on the endotracheal tube, and to improve cerebral venous drainage by decreasing thoracic and abdominal muscle tone.[895, 896] If paralysis is required, much of the clinical examination is lost, and direct ICP and EEG monitoring may be particularly helpful.

Barbiturates are indicated to reduce ICP if other methods are incompletely effective.[175, 897] Thiopental 2 to 4 mg/kg can be administered as a single dose for acute elevations in ICP. If this is effective, a pentobarbital infusion, using a 10 to 20 mg/kg loading dose administered over 1 to 2 hours, followed by an infusion of 1 to 2 mg/kg/h, may achieve sustained reduction in ICP. The infusion is titrated to achieve satisfactory reduction in ICP or to burst suppression on EEG, whichever comes first. Myocardial depression may appear if higher doses of drugs are used, and care must be taken to avoid compromising CPP by a decrease in cardiac output. Appropriate cardiovascular monitoring and support are therefore required. There is no question of the effectiveness of barbiturates in the control of ICP. Successful ICP control, in and of itself, however, is not predictive of good outcome, as the primary injury may be so severe as to mandate a poor prognosis. The treatment of increased ICP, although an essential part of preserving brain function and preventing secondary brain damage, should not become an endpoint in itself.

The prognosis of any given brain injury is difficult to predict. If secondary injury is avoided, children with head trauma have generally good prognoses. Those with severe hypoxic/ischemic injury have a poor one. There are no absolutes. Many factors affect the primary insult and the ultimate outcome, including severity of the insult, promptness and effectiveness of resuscitation, presence of hypothermia, preexisting disease, and coexisting injuries. Decisions made by the care team are often difficult because they must be made with incomplete information and uncertainty. Efforts to better define prognosis can be made using electrophysiologic monitoring to complement the clinical exam. BAEPs and SSEPs are useful in this regard, particularly in those patients with traumatic coma.[898] Bilaterally absent SSEPs imply severe cortical damage and a poor prognosis.

Special Considerations

Status Epilepticus

Seizure activity that continues for more than 30 minutes or that recurs so frequently that the patient does not regain consciousness between episodes is defined as status epilepticus.[899–901] Status epilepticus may occur in a patient with a known seizure disorder, particularly if anticonvulsant medications are stopped abruptly, or may be the first evidence of a seizure disorder. After seizures are controlled, the etiology should be investigated with careful physical examination, laboratory studies as below, CT scan, and usually a lumbar puncture. EEG studies are useful to guide anticonvulsant treatment, but the acute EEG may not be helpful in determining cause.

Status epilepticus requires emergency treatment. Respiration may be compromised, and prolonged seizure activity, even when adequate gas exchange is ensured, may cause brain damage. The amount of oxygen and energy substrate consumed by the brain during a seizure may be enormous. Such increased consumption may exceed the body's capacity to increase the delivery of oxygen and nutrients. Portions of the brain may become ischemic and sustain permanent damage. It is essential to ensure adequate oxygenation during the convulsive activity and to stop the seizure as soon as possible.

The first step is to ensure an adequate airway, oxygenation, and ventilation. Some patients may require endotracheal intubation and controlled ventilation, particularly if the seizure activity is prolonged or multiple doses of anticonvulsants are administered. Cardiovascular compromise is unusual in status epilepticus when gas exchange is adequate, although hypertension or other signs of autonomic stimulation may be present.

When IV access is established, blood samples are sent for determination of electrolyte, glucose, calcium, and magnesium concentrations; a screen for toxins also may be indicated. The blood glucose can be rapidly determined by strip test. If the patient is hypoglycemic, glucose 0.5 g/kg should be given immediately, followed by a glucose-containing IV solution. This measure should correct hypoglycemia and stop the seizure if hypoglycemia is the cause. If hypocalcemia is present, calcium (10 to 20 mg/kg of calcium chloride or 30 to 60 mg/kg of calcium gluconate) can be given.

Intravenous benzodiazepines are probably the most rapid and reliable drugs for acutely stopping seizure activity. Lorazepam 0.1 mg/kg or diazepam 0.1 to 0.2 mg/kg is typically used. To minimize potential respiratory depression or apnea, benzodiazepines should be given in small incremental doses; multiple doses may be required. Equipment and personnel should be present to manage respiratory depression or arrest. Midazolam 0.1 mg/kg is acceptable for acute use, but has a very short duration of action; a midazolam infusion, however, may be useful in subsequent management of refractory status epilepticus.[902, 903] A longer acting anticonvulsant should be started in the acute setting as well. Phenytoin or fosphenytoin (10 to 20 mg/kg phenytoin or phenytoin equivalents [PE] loading dose, given over 20 to 30 minutes) or phenobarbital (10 to 20 mg/kg) are the most common choices for initial and subsequent maintenance therapy. If seizure control is inadequate with a single drug, both can be used.

If seizures continue despite therapeutic levels of phenytoin (10 to 20 mg/L) and phenobarbital (15 to 40 mg/L), rectal paraldehyde (0.3 ml/kg) can be given. If control is still inadequate, neurologic consultation should be sought and consideration given to other drugs or to escalating therapy to "coma" levels; both pentobarbital and midazolam can be used for this purpose.[902] Continuous EEG monitoring is necessary should the latter course be chosen. Ventilatory and cardiac support are provided as needed.

Near-Drowning

Drowning accidents are the second most common cause of accidental death in children. Young infants and children may drown in home swimming pools or bathtubs; older children in lakes, ponds, rivers, canals, or irrigation ditches. Teenagers, usually boys, are injured in water sports such as swimming, diving, scuba diving, or sailing.

The pathophysiology of near-drowning has two major components, asphyxia and pulmonary aspiration, and most patients have evidence of both insults.[904] The pulmonary injury occurs as a result of aspiration of water and, often, foreign material or stomach contents. Water aspirated into the lung, whether salt or fresh, causes pulmonary edema, atelectasis, and alveolar capillary membrane injury. The tonicity of the aspirated solution affects the degree of injury: water is more injurious than saline solutions.[905] Aspirated stomach contents or other foreign material may cause chemical pneumonitis. The physiologic changes are decreased compliance and an increase in intrapulmonary shunting. Patients are typically dyspneic, with hypoxia on room air and a large alveolar–arterial gradient when breathing oxygen. Physical examination reveals retractions, cyanosis, rales, and wheezing. The chest film shows evidence of diffuse or patchy infiltrates; severe cases progress to ARDS. Aggressive respiratory care to restore FRC is as described above. Prophylactic administration of steroids or antibiotics is not indicated. The probability of secondary pulmonary infection is high, however, and appropriate cultures and antibiotic treatment should be started promptly if signs of infection appear.

Death from respiratory failure alone is possible but relatively uncommon in near-drowning patients who are appropriately managed. The severity of the anoxic insult to the brain usually determines the outcome. Although it is possible, in specific circumstances, for the degree of injury to be modified by such factors as hypothermia,[906, 907] for the most part near-drowning injuries must be viewed as hypoxic/ischemic events with their relatively poor prognosis.[908–910]

Analgesia and Sedation

An intensive care environment is filled with discomfort, painful procedures, and terrifying experiences. It is mandatory that those providing care recognize this and that adequate pain relief, pharmacologic sedation, and psychological support be provided.[911, 912] A detailed review of analgesia and sedation in children is presented elsewhere in this text and need not be repeated here. However, a few comments concerning their necessity are appropriate.

It is best to approach this issue as one does in the operating room. When confronted with an anxious, uncomfortable, agitated child, one must first be sure that pathophysiologic abnormalities causing such agitation (e.g., hypoxia, hypercarbia, airway obstruction, distended bladder) are not present or are properly treated. One should then attempt to determine which components of "anesthesia"—analgesia, amnesia, sedation, relief of anxiety—are needed for patient comfort and optimal care.

Analgesia can be provided systemically or by regional techniques. The most commonly used systemic analgesics in our unit are morphine and fentanyl. Administration is by bolus or continuous infusion, as appropriate for the clinical situation; patient-controlled analgesia is often used. The neonate and the very young infant may have difficulty clearing morphine, and occasionally will be noted to have respiratory or even cardiovascular instability when given repeated doses of the drug.[913–916] Fentanyl is well-tolerated in infants, however, even in large doses.[917] Careful tapering from narcotics is necessary; narcotic withdrawal and occasional movement disorders are seen after extended narcotic use in the PICU.[911, 918] Ketorolac, usually 0.5 mg/kg, is an excellent alternative to narcotics for short-term administration in postoperative patients.[919, 920]

Regional analgesia can be provided using techniques described elsewhere in this text. Pain relief provides comfort for the child and improves cooperation during chest physiotherapy. The child is able to cough and to breathe deeply without pain, even after a major abdominal or thoracic surgical procedure. This increased cooperation allows improved pulmonary toilet and resolution of atelectasis, which might otherwise require tracheal intubation and positive-pressure ventilation. Occasionally, sympathetic blockade is useful in improving blood flow to an extremity after microvascular anastomoses or arteriospasm.

Amnesia, sedation, and relief of anxiety are typically provided by the benzodiazepines (diazepam, midazolam, lorazepam), although chloral hydrate and barbiturates are occasionally administered instead. There is some experience with the prolonged administration of isoflurane for sedation; it appears safe and effective, although there may be issues related to withdrawal after extended use.[921–923] It is helpful to maintain a day–night cycle of activity and medication, so that the child is sedated more heavily in the evening for sleep but less so in the daytime to encourage weaning, physical therapy, and social interaction.

With advances in ventilator design allowing support of spontaneous ventilation in the majority of patients, the need for heavy sedation and muscle relaxation has markedly decreased. Nevertheless, muscle relaxants may be necessary as adjuncts to mechanical ventilation[924] or to facilitate tracheal intubation.[925] Clearly, the child who receives mechanical ventilation aided by a muscle relaxant must also receive analgesia and sedation. The extended use of relaxants has been associated with prolonged paralysis; careful monitoring, either clinically or with nerve stimulation, is recommended.[926–929]

Brain Death

Brain death is a clinical diagnosis of the irretrievable absence of brain stem and cortical functions.[930] The necessity of defining death according to CNS criteria is a consequence of our advances in the support of other organ systems. It is generally conceded by medical, legal, and ethical authorities that prolonged support of a brain-dead patient is of no benefit to anyone and is therefore not indicated (see Chapter 1).

The intensivist is often the physician who establishes the diagnosis of brain death.[931] The determination must be made according to criteria satisfactory to the physician and consistent with the guidelines of the institution. The clinical examination, demonstrating no cortical or brain stem function, is the most important component. Laboratory tests (e.g., EEG, radionuclide CBF study, evoked potentials, Doppler flow studies) may be used as adjuncts to confirm the clinical diagnosis.[932–934] Nevertheless, if the clinical examination is unequivocal and the cause and irreversibility of the clinical findings are established, laboratory tests are unnecessary.[935]

As greater experience is accumulated with brain death in children, the concept becomes more difficult. It is both bothersome and reassuring that the diagnosis is not always as clear-cut as one would like.[936, 937] An accurate diagnosis of brain death does not necessarily imply cessation of all intracranial function.[938–940] Islands of functioning neurons may remain, with consequent minimal but present registration of electrical activity on EEG or of blood flow on scan. The diagnosis of brain death is, in truth, a statement by a knowledgeable physician that an individual's brain has been so severely damaged that there is no hope of prolonged survival or even short-term independent survival. It is this irretrievable loss of the ability to survive without artificial life support, together with a loss of the capacity for consciousness, that defines death. If one is comfortable that this is the case, then the ambiguity or inconsistency of individual laboratory tests or other small pieces of data should not deter one from declaring the diagnosis with equanimity.

The determination of brain death in a child is always an emotionally difficult matter for everyone involved. Once the diagnosis is made, however, another obligation falls on the practitioner: the request for organ donation. The death of organs suitable for transplantation, together with an increasing number of suitable recipients and an improving medical ability to sustain them for a limited time, make consideration of each opportunity for organ harvest imperative.[941, 942] If medical circumstances permit donation, the physician caring for the child must discuss the possibility with the family. It is not unusual for the suggestion to be welcomed as an opportunity for some good to come from an otherwise painful and tragic loss.

PSYCHOSOCIAL AND ETHICAL CONSIDERATIONS

Confining a child in an ICU is a stressful situation for all involved. For the child, it represents a set of new and largely unpleasant experiences.[943] He or she is removed from the normal environment and placed in a strange ward filled with unfamiliar people, equipment, sounds, and routines. The child generally does not feel well and often is subjected to many painful or otherwise unpleasant procedures. Normal patterns of waking and sleeping are disturbed, and sleep deprivation may lead to disorientation. Confined to bed, restrained, or even paralyzed by drugs, the child inevitably develops a sense of powerlessness and lack of control. The parents represent the major source of security but may be kept away when support is needed most. For the child old enough to understand something of the seriousness of illness, there is always the underlying, and often realistic, fear of death.

The parents endure all these same stresses vicariously through the child.[944, 945] They experience a similar feeling of helplessness, being able to do little, if anything, to influence the outcome of the illness. An overwhelming sense of guilt may result, usually having no basis in fact. They may understand very little about the nature of the child's illness and may be afraid or unable to ask appropriate questions. Even worse, they may obtain entirely different opinions from various sources, leaving them even more confused about the seriousness of the illness and the child's prognosis. These stresses may lead to a variety of responses that the PICU staff may regard as "abnormal" or difficult[946, 947] (e.g., withdrawal, anger, hypercritical involvement in details, unrealistic optimism, or even hysteria).

PICU personnel are by no means immune to stress.[3, 948] The pediatric ICU is a very stressful environment in which to work. The work is difficult, and the hours are long. The staff must perform painful procedures and treatments on children. They must make difficult decisions, often with incomplete information, and then bear the blame for the inevitable mistakes that occur. The outcome of many illnesses is uncertain and often tragic, and a sense of powerlessness may overwhelm the physician or nurse at times, just as it does the patient or parent.[949]

Efforts can be made to reduce the stress on all. The child should, within individual ability to understand, receive an explanation of the nature of the illness and the reason for all procedures. Idle talk among staff members at the beside should be discouraged to avoid any misunderstanding by the child or a neighboring patient. Parents should spend as much time as possible at the bedside during the PICU stay.

Stress for parents can be minimized by making sure that they understand as much as possible about their child's illness and its treatment, and by giving them confidence that everything possible is being done to obtain a good outcome. They should be allowed to participate in the child's care wherever possible. When ICU care is prolonged, the parents must be encouraged to look after their own physical and psychological health and that of siblings and other family members by taking time away to eat, sleep, and deal with other everyday matters. Parental stress reactions must be handled with patience and empathy. Listening to criticisms and complaints, giving careful explanations, and allowing time for psychologic adjustment to the stressful situation is all that is required for most problems. If problems seem beyond the ability of the PICU staff to handle, professional consultation should be requested.

Siblings, like parents, experience stress, often believing themselves responsible in some way for the child's illness. The staff must anticipate this and offer guidance to the family. Siblings and close friends should generally be encouraged to visit.[950] Although one may be concerned about a child's reaction to a critically ill brother or sister, it is likely that their fears and imaginary visions have been worse than the reality. We have found such a visit to be immensely useful for relieving stress on the family. Children handle the encounter exceedingly well and, especially if the patient should not survive, the visit provides the siblings a chance to settle themselves in their relationship with the patient and a chance to say goodbye in an understanding, open, truthful, and supportive atmosphere.

Stress and conflict among personnel can be reduced by a number of means. Training and supervision of staff members must be sufficient so that each feels competent to perform the tasks required. Residents rotating through the ICU, present for only a short time and needing to perform at a high level, are particularly vulnerable to stress.[951] Communication among staff members must be encouraged. It is also helpful to establish a mechanism for staff members to express their concerns and criticisms. The goal is to maintain the concept of an intensive care team composed of individual members, each with a well-defined role, working together to provide optimal care for the child.

Care of the Terminally Ill

The outcome of pediatric intensive care is generally good.[952] There are, however, a small number of children who are imminently terminally ill. The caretakers' responsibility to these children does not lessen, but its emphasis changes from medical efforts to promote survival to those necessary to comfort the child and to allow death.[953]

The decision to limit or withdraw support from such patients is commonly made in the PICU.[954-957] The physician analyzes the pertinent data, discusses the case with all involved caretakers and, together with the care team, comes to a decision that such limitation or withdrawal is appropriate and in the child's best interest. This is then communicated to the family as the team's recommendation as to what is best for the child, based on the medical facts of the case, trying not to base it on the personal values of the physician or team members.[958] It is important that the information be presented as the caretaker's definitive plan for care: "This is what we should do." The parents, of course, may disagree and ask that another course be followed, but presenting the information as a decision made by the physician and the care team removes the parents from having to themselves actively decide to discontinue support.

Difficulties arise if there is disagreement between team and family as to what should be done, leading to much discussion about "futility" and reasonableness of care.[959-961] These are serious and arduous conflicts, and much effort must be directed at coming to an ethically defensible and mutually satisfying agreement.[962] Hospital ethics committees are a resource available to both family and care team, and should be consulted freely as necessary.

Once the decision to withdraw support has been made, it is then the physician's responsibility to ensure that it is done sensitively and that the child experiences no discomfort. This often implies administration of sedatives or analgesics before removing mechanical or pharmacologic support.[963-966] Physicians and other caretakers occasionally feel uncomfortable in so doing, but should feel strengthened in that, as in all of pediatric intensive care, they are doing what is best for the child.

RENAL CARE

Diuretics

The use of diuretics to assist in maintaining proper fluid balance and in removing excess fluid from the body is standard practice in contemporary critical care. Even in patients with normal renal function, it is often beneficial to induce additional natriuresis and fluid excretion to assist in the management of cardiorespiratory dysfunction. The loop diuretics, and particularly furosemide (Lasix), are most commonly used for this purpose.

Although there may be beneficial extrarenal vasodilatory effects of Lasix administration even before diuresis begins,[972-974] there is a threshold quantity of drug that must be delivered to the site of action in the ascending limb of the loop of Henle to effect diuresis.[975] The drug is secreted into the tubular lumen by proximal tubular cells, reaching the loop by way of the tubular fluid. The "standard" dose of Lasix is 1 mg/kg, but individual patient response varies, and one should endeavor to administer the lowest dose that elicits maximal response. In patients with established renal insufficiency, a larger dose is usually necessary to achieve an effective amount of diuretic in the tubular fluid. Continuous infusion of Lasix, maintaining an effective amount of drug at the site of action at all times, may offer a small but clinically important increase in diure-

sis.[976-982] In hypoalbuminemic patients, the delivery of the diuretic to renal secretory sites may be diminished, and the administration of 25 percent albumin (typically in a dose of 0.5 to 1.0 g/kg, either just before or simultaneously with the diuretic) may augment the diuretic effect.[975, 982-985]

Acute Renal Failure

The critically ill child with multisystem involvement may be at risk for developing ARF, the abrupt onset of renal dysfunction sufficient to prevent removal of nitrogenous wastes and to interfere with fluid and electrolyte homeostasis. Insufficient renal blood flow, certain drugs and toxins, and inflammatory or autoimmune processes may cause renal structural damage and dysfunction. Prevention of ARF by maintaining adequate intravascular volume and perfusion is the physician's first priority. Failing this, the physician must recognize when ARF is present and then manage fluids, electrolytes, and other aspects of care in a manner consistent with impaired renal function.

ARF is characterized by both decreased glomerular filtration rate (GFR) and paralysis of tubular function.[986] Histologic changes of swelling or necrosis may be seen in the renal tubules but are not always present. Abnormalities in renal blood flow may be related to systemic hypoperfusion or to local phenomena mediated by prostaglandins or the renin-angiotensin system. Peritubular edema or accumulation of intraluminal debris may continue to obstruct urine flow even after perfusion is restored. These anatomic and functional changes are usually reversible, but recovery may require several days or weeks.

Clinical Characteristics

ARF can result from parenchymal renal damage or from prerenal or postrenal factors.[987,988] *Prerenal* azotemia results from decreased renal perfusion. If renal blood flow is promptly restored, renal function is often rapidly improved. Intrinsic, *parenchymal*, or "true" renal filure can result from a prolonged period of hypoperfusion or from direct injury from drugs, toxins, autoimmune, or other causes. *Postrenal* oliguria is due to obstruction of urine flow distal to the kidney. Typical lesions include posterior urethral valves and ureteral obstruction. Obstructive lesions generally cause dilation of the proximal collecting system, which can be detected by palpation of the abdomen, ultrasound examination, or IV or retrograde pyelography. Relieving the obstruction usually restores renal function. ARF may also be characterized by the volume of urine output. *Nonoliguric* renal failure, characterized by azotemia and signs of tubular dysfunction with normal or increased urine volume, is more common and may have a better prognosis than *oliguric or anuric* ARF patients (with urine output of <0.5 ml/kg/h).[989] Further aid in making the precise diagnosis may be gained by examining the urine (Table 29–20).

In impending renal failure, restoration of circulating blood volume and renal perfusion are the first priority. After this is accomplished, some clinicians administer a diuretic to attempt to preserve renal function and increase urine flow; mannitol or a potent loop diuretic such as furosemide can be tried. The efficacy of diuretics in this

TABLE 29–20
LABORATORY DIFFERENTIATION OF OLIGURIA

Test	Prerenal Oliguria	Intrinsic Renal Failure
Urine		
Na+	Low (<20 mEq/L)	High (>40 mEq/L)
Specific gravity	High (>1.020)	Low (<1.010)
Osmolality	High (>500 mOsm/L)	Low (<350 mOsm/L)
Urine/plasma ratios		
Osmolality	>1.3:1	<1.3:1
Urea nitrogen	>20:1	<10:1
Creatinine	>40:1	<20:1
Urine sediment	Normal	Proteinuria; hematuria; granular, RBC, or tubular casts
Fractional excretion of sodium (FE$_{Na}$)		
FE$_{Na}$*	<1%	>2%

* FE$_{Na}$ (fractional excretion of sodium) = $(U_{Na}/P_{Na})/(U_{cr}/P_{cr}) \times 100$. Urine sodium values are altered (and data therefore not valid) if samples are obtained within 4 to 6 hours of Lasix administration.

situation is not proven, and their use remains controversial.[989,990] Mannitol increases renal blood flow, GFR, and urine flow by its osmolar effect. It may prevent renal failure when administered prophylactically before aortic cross-clamping, when given immediately after crush injury or rhabdomyolysis, or when large pigment or urate loads are presented to the kidney.[991] There is no benefit and some risk in administering mannitol in established renal failure; if the drug cannot be excreted it will remain in the intravascular space, where its osmolar load may excessively expand intravascular volume. Large doses of furosemide improve urine output in established renal failure in adults.[975,992] Such use does not necessarily reduce the need for dialysis or the duration of renal failure. High doses of furosemide may cause ototoxicity or potentiate toxic effects of other drugs (e.g., aminoglycoside antibiotics).

Management

When the underlying cause of acute renal failure is reversible, patients have an excellent chance of surviving and recovering renal function.[993] Treatment is directed at correcting impaired water and electrolyte balance, impaired acid–base status, hypertension, impaired excretion of protein catabolites, impaired drug excretion, and decreased resistance to infection.

When renal function is impaired, the patient is subject to fluid overload and electrolyte abnormalities, especially hyperkalemia. The patient's fluid and electrolyte intake must be controlled to prevent these abnormalities. Daily fluid intake should be limited to replacement of insensible losses (300 to 400 ml/m^2/day) plus urine output and other measured losses. Intake, output, and weight must be monitored meticulously. Potassium administration is eliminated completely, and sodium intake is limited to replacement of estimated or measured urine and GI losses.

Fluid overload may be indicated by an increase in body weight, by hyponatremia, by edema, and by hypertension; extreme overload can produce congestive failure, with a gallop rhythm, tachypnea, rales, and hepatomegaly. Excessive fluid restriction, on the other hand, is indicated by weight loss exceeding 1 percent per day, by an increase in serum osmolality, and by signs of intravascular volume depletion (e.g., tachycardia, diminished peripheral pulses, and poor perfusion). If hypoproteinemia or capillary leak is present, edema and weight gain may coexist with inadequate intravascular volume. Invasive monitoring may be necessary to accurately assess volume status.

A potentially life-threatening electrolyte abnormality seen in ARF is *hyperkalemia*. The ability to excrete potassium is markedly reduced. Acidosis potentiates hyperkalemia by shifting potassium from the intracellular to the extracellular space. The major risk of hyperkalemia is potentiation of cardiac arrhythmias. Moderate hyperkalemia causes peaked T waves, depressed ST segments, and prolonged QRS complexes. More extreme hyperkalemia causes conduction abnormalities, bradycardia, "sine wave" complexes, ventricular fibrillation, or asystole.

Immediate treatment of severe hyperkalemia may include any or all of the following agents: (1) calcium chloride 10 to 20 mg/kg IV or calcium gluconate 30 to 60 mg/kg IV; (2) sodium bicarbonate 1 to 2 mEq/kg IV; or (3) glucose 1 to 2 g/kg IV with insulin 1 unit per 4 g of glucose, IV. Calcium antagonizes some of the cardiac electrophysiologic effects of potassium, while bicarbonate and glucose/insulin cause K+ to move intracellularly. None of these maneuvers actually removes K+ from the body. An ion-exchange resin (e.g., Kayexalate) does remove potassium from the body, exchanging K+ for an equimolar quantity of Na+. Kayexalate is usually administered orally or per rectum as a suspension (1 to 2 g/kg in 10 percent sorbitol); it requires 1 to 2 hours to take effect.

Hyponatremia or hypernatremia may occur in renal failure, and commonly indicate excessive or insufficient water intake, not a deficit or excess of total body sodium. Hypernatremia is treated by giving more free water, unless the patient also has signs of fluid excess. Hyponatremia is treated by fluid restriction, with a goal of slow correction over several days. If hyponatremia is so severe that acute disorientation, seizures, coma, or cerebral edema are present, however, it may be necessary to rapidly increase the serum sodium concentration by administering hypertonic saline. These problems seldom arise unless the serum sodium is less than 120 mEq/L.

Acute renal failure reduces clearance of metabolic acids. Progressive metabolic acidosis develops, with a decrease in serum bicarbonate concentration of 1 to 2 mEq/L/day. Supplemental bicarbonate can be given, but this treatment is limited by the sodium load. The most effective method for treating progressive acidosis is dialysis.

Hypertension may occur during ARF by at least two mechanisms: volume overload and excessive plasma renin. Hypertensive encephalopathy or cardiovascular decompensation may occur. A useful approach to treating hypertension is to reduce preload, afterload, and sometimes myocardial contractility.[989] Preload reduction is most easily accomplished by avoiding volume overload. Once hypervolemia is present, fluid removal by diuresis (if possible), hemofiltration or dialysis is considered. Afterload reduction is accomplished by vasodilators (hydralazine, nitroprusside), and controlled reduction of contractility by β-blockers (propranolol, esmolol) as previously described. Calcium channel blockers may be considered; nifedipine is preferable to verapamil because the latter's myocardial depressant effect may be particularly severe in infants and children. ACE inhibitors, blocking conversion of angiotensin I to the vasoconstrictor angiotensin II, are useful; captopril or enalapril are commonly used, although they are relatively contraindicated if renal artery stenosis is present because they may induce or worsen renal failure in that setting. Diazoxide or nitroprusside are commonly administered in hypertensive emergencies. Combinations of drugs are usually more efficacious than single agents.

The accumulation of nitrogenous by-products of protein metabolism is termed *azotemia*. Severe azotemia causes a number of adverse effects, including platelet and CNS dysfunction. The rate of accumulation of nitrogenous by-products depends not only on the severity of renal dysfunction but also on the catabolic state of the patient. In a noncatabolic state, the blood urea nitrogen (BUN) usually increases by 10 to 20 mg/dl/day. In a severely catabolic state, as may occur with massive trauma or infection, the BUN may increase at two or three times this rate. Serum creatinine may rise by 1 to 2 mg/dl/day, with greater rates of rise being one of the indicators for dialysis.[994]

Clearance of many drugs from the body is dependent on renal function. Doses of renally excreted drugs must be adjusted to the decreased clearance rate by either decreasing the dose or increasing the interval between doses.[995] Blood levels of specific drugs should be monitored whenever possible to regulate the dose most accurately.

Maintenance of adequate *nutrition* is another important aspect of managing ARF and may be difficult, given the necessary restrictions on fluid and electrolytes.[996–1000] Enteral feedings, if tolerated, provide greater caloric density than parenteral nutrition. The sodium and potassium content of foods and fluids must be carefully regulated. The amount of protein must also be limited to reduce azotemia and acidosis. If parenteral nutrition is necessary, special "renal failure" solutions of glucose and essential amino acids are available.[1001] If adequate nutrition cannot be maintained because of fluid or electrolyte imbalance, ultrafiltration or dialysis may be necessary and indicated.[989]

Renal Replacement Therapy

Conservative management for ARF, as outlined above, is often adequate. Acute volume overload, hyponatremia, severe hypertension, hyperkalemia unresponsive to usual treatment, intractable acidosis, and severe or rapidly progressive azotemia are all indications for dialysis or other extracorporeal treatment. Options include peritoneal dialysis, traditional hemodialysis, or a continuous-perfusion technique, with the choice governed by the needs of the individual patient and by the experience and resources available at the particular center.[988, 1002]

In many centers, *peritoneal dialysis* is preferred to hemodialysis in small children because it is simpler, can be quickly instituted and managed in the ICU, and is usually effective.[989, 1003, 1004] Peritoneal dialysis is contraindicated in patients with intra-abdominal infections or multiple intra-abdominal adhesions.

A soft, multihole catheter is placed through the abdominal wall into the peritoneal cavity. The dialysate solution is then infused into the peritoneal cavity, where it equilibrates with the plasma and extracellular fluid across the peritoneal membrane surfaces. The period during which equilibration is allowed to take place is the "dwell time," after which the fluid is drained and replaced with fresh dialysate.

The content of the dialysate is tailored to specific patient needs. The solutions generally contain sodium 130 to 135 mEq/L, chloride 95 to 105 mEq/L, acetate or lactate 35 mEq/L, calcium 3.5 mEq/L, magnesium 1.5 mEq/L, and glucose. If the patient is hyperkalemic, no potassium is added to the dialysate initially. As the serum K^+ approaches the desired concentration, potassium in a concentration of 3.5 to 4 mEq/L is added to the dialysate to prevent systemic hypokalemia. The concentration of glucose is altered to change the osmolarity of the dialysate and the amount of ultrafiltration to be achieved. When it is desirable to remove intravascular water rapidly, a more hypertonic glucose solution (usually 4.25 percent) is used; otherwise a 1.5 percent solution is employed; even the 1.5 percent solution is hypertonic and can produce dehydration. Systemic absorption of large amounts of glucose with resultant hyperglycemia is occasionally seen.

The rapid infusion of large amounts of dialysate into the peritoneal cavity may be uncomfortable and may compromise ventilation. To minimize this discomfort, the solution should be warmed to body temperature and the volume infused for each "run" gradually increased, beginning with 10 to 20 ml/kg and increasing to about 50 ml/kg as tolerated. It is important to drain fluid adequately after each cycle so that volume does not accumulate within the abdominal cavity. Although manual peritoneal dialysis is acceptable, it is time consuming, labor intensive, and subject to error. Automated machinery to perform and control peritoneal dialysis is now readily available and is preferable.

Infection is a potential complication of peritoneal dialysis, and peritonitis or systemic sepsis is a constant risk. For this reason, frequent cultures of the dialysate must be obtained and any suspected infection treated promptly, either systemically or by inclusion of antibiotics in the dialysate itself. Peritoneal dialysis may also be complicated by hemorrhage, perforation of a viscus, or by respiratory insufficiency caused by impairment of diaphragmatic motion by large intraperitoneal volumes.

Hemodialysis is the treatment of choice when dialysis is needed, adequate vascular access is available, and the treatment center is staffed and equipped to handle small children. Its advantages include finer control, greater effectiveness and efficiency, and the ability to simultaneously transfuse blood products and remove fluid (thus avoiding volume overload). Dialysis catheters can be placed percutaneouly for short-term use or surgically for longer periods of support; rather large catheters are necessary to achieve adequate flow rates.

Several new methods of providing artificial renal support on a continuous rather than intermittent basis are available. Although there is an alphabet soup of acronyms for these techniques (e.g., CAVH, CAVHD, CVVH, CVVHD), they are all variations of *extracorporeal hemofiltration*.[988, 1002, 1005, 1006] Blood is removed from the patient, circulated through an external filter, and then returned to the patient. The acronyms, referring to catheter placement and type of filtration or dialysis, can be decoded as follows:

C, continuous
AV, arteriovenous
VV, venovenous
H, hemofiltration (isotonic fluid removal, minimal solute clearance)
HD, hemofiltration with dialysis

Venovenous circuits require an external pump to circulate and control blood flow through the filter; AV circuits do not. Filters are available in different sizes and membrane surface areas to accommodate patients from infancy to adulthood. Patients must be heparinized, with activated clotting times (ACTs) maintained at 180 to 200 seconds. All circuits allow separate control of blood flow and filtrate flow, so that filtration can be interrupted or regulated without altering blood flow through the circuit. As blood flows through the filter, an ultrafiltrate of fluid, electrolytes, and all solutes less than 50,000 daltons is passed through the membrane and removed. If desired, the outer surface of the membrane can be perfused with dialysate solution (hemodiafiltration), converting the system from simple ultrafiltration to true dialysis, with active diffusion of solutes along a concentration gradient.

Experience suggests that continuous filtration techniques can provide effective partial renal replacement therapy in critically ill infants and children, allowing fluid and electrolyte removal and permitting the fluid administration needed for aggressive nutritional support.[1007-1009] Continuous rather than intermittent therapy allows continual and substantial fluid removal without the hemodynamic instability sometimes associated with intermittent dialysis, and is an excellent choice for children who are unable to tolerate conventional hemodialysis.

Recovery from acute renal failure may require several days to weeks, and in some patients permanently impaired renal function may result. The return of normal or even excessive urine output generally precedes a decrease in BUN and serum creatinine. Tubular function, especially the ability to concentrate the urine and to excrete an acid load, may require an even longer period for recovery.

Hemolytic-Uremic Syndrome

The hemolytic-uremic syndrome (HUS) is an acute illness characterized by hemolytic anemia, thrombocytopenia, and acute renal failure.[1010-1012] There are a number of apparent etiologies, but the typical case is associated with a verotoxin-producing strain of *E. coli*, *E. coli* 0157:H7.[1012-1018] The organism is found in raw beef, and there is evidence of transmission in day-care settings.[1015, 1019, 1020] The common clinical picture is that of an infant or young child who initially has nonspecific gastroenteritis, followed by abdominal pain, bloody stools, and pallor. Laboratory testing reveals a hemolytic anemia and thrombocytopenia. Oliguria develops, indicating the onset of acute renal failure.

Severe hypertension may occur, even in the early stages of renal failure. Neurologic abnormalities are sometimes seen, including seizures, lethargy, impaired mental status, and coma.

Pathologically, there is evidence of a diffuse injury to the endothelium of small arteries and arterioles with subsequent activation of the clotting mechanism, producing intravascular thrombi and various degrees of vascular occlusion. Widespread occlusion of small vessels in the glomeruli is responsible for the renal dysfunction.[1021] In the most severe cases, bilateral renal cortical necrosis may result. The microvascular changes appear to account for the consumption of platelets and the microangiopathic-hemolytic anemia associated with the syndrome. Although the primary focus in HUS is often on the renal pathology, there is widespread involvement of small vessels in other organs as well, particularly in the gut and brain.

The diagnosis of HUS is made on the basis of the typical history. It is confirmed by laboratory findings of thrombocytopenia, anemia with microangiopathic changes, and azotemia. Stool cultures may be positive for *E. coli* 0157:H7, but only early in the course of the disease; enzyme-linked immunosorbent assay (ELISA) to detect verotoxin in fecal filtrates may confirm the etiology even after cultures cease to be positive.[1022] The urine findings are typical of acute renal failure and include decreased volume, proteinuria, hematuria, and casts.

The hematologic/angiopathic basis for HUS is under investigation. The soluble clotting factors do not appear to be dramatically affected, although fibrin split products may be present. Some investigators suspect an endothelial defect in prostacyclin production, so that prostaglandin I_2, a potent vasodilator and inhibitor of platelet aggregation, is deficient.[1011] An inhibitor of fibrinolysis (plasminogen activator inhibitor 1) has been identified in the plasma of patients with HUS.[1023] Finally, the presence of the P1 blood group antigen is thought to be protective. Verotoxin binds to the P1 antigen, and may be less available to damage the endothelial cells if there is strong expression of P1 on the patient's red cells.[1024]

Treatment of HUS includes all the basic elements of managing ARF, as described above. Dialysis is often required, and hypertension may be severe and difficult to control. Platelet transfusions should probably not be given unless there is evidence of bleeding. There is some evidence that plasmapheresis may help to reverse the underlying pathogenic process in HUS and hasten recovery. Such therapy is theoretically attractive, and has been found helpful in a similar disease, adult thrombotic thrombocytopenic purpura.[1025] Unfortunately, conclusive evidence of its effectiveness in typical diarrhea-associated HUS is still lacking.[1018, 1026] Severe neurologic involvement may lead to a poor outcome. Most patients recover renal function,[1027] though a small percentage do progress to chronic renal failure[1028] or subclinical renal dysfunction.[1027]

REFERENCES

1. Bergeson PS, Holbrook PR: Committee on hospital care and pediatric section of the Society of Critical Care Medicine: guidelines for pediatric intensive care units. Pediatrics 72:364, 1983.

2. Committee on Hospital Care, American Academy of Pediatrics: Hospital Care of Children and Youth. Elk Grove Village, IL, American Academy of Pediatrics, 1986.
3. Hazinski MF: Physician-nurse interaction in the intensive care unit. *In* Holbrook PR (ed): Textbook of Pediatric Critical Care. Philadelphia, WB Saunders Company, 1993, p 1166.
4. Lappe DG: Pediatric intensive care nursing. *In* Rogers MC, Nichols DG (eds): Textbook of Pediatric Intensive Care. 3rd ed. Baltimore, Williams & Wilkins, 1966, p 1597.
5. Curley MAQ: The essence of pediatric critical care nursing. *In* Curley MAQ, Smith JB, Moloney-Harmon PA (eds): Critical Care Nursing of Infants and Children. Philadelphia, WB Saunders Company, 1996, p 3.
6. Levin DL: The physical setting. *In* Levin DL, Morriss FC, Moore GC (eds): A Practical Guide to Pediatric Intensive Care. 2nd ed. St. Louis, CV Mosby, 1984, p 473.
7. Huang HK, Wong ST, Pietka E: Medical image informatics infrastructure design and applications. Med Inform (Lond) 22:279, 1997.
8. Labreze L, Lagouarde P, Dakin C, et al: A web interface for multimedia electronic patient record: consensual validation of the Aquitaine Health Information Network prototypes. Med Inform (Lond) 23:75, 1998.
9. Smith MS, Feied CF: The next-generation emergency department. Ann Emerg Med 32:65, 1998.
10. Lagoe RR, Milliren JW, Baader MJ: Impact of selected diagnosis-related groups on regional neonatal care. Pediatrics 77:627, 1986.
11. Broyles RS, Tyson JE, Swint JM: Have Medicaid reimbursements been a credible measure of the cost of pediatric care? Pediatrics 99:E8, 1997.
12. Anonymous: Issues in the application of the resource-based relative value scale system to pediatrics: a subject review. American Academy of Pediatrics. Resource-Based Relative Value Scale Project Advisory Committee. Pediatrics 102(4 pt 1):996, 1998.
13. Harris BH, Bass KD, O'Brien MD: Hospital reimbursement for pediatric trauma care. J Pediatr Surg 31:78, 1996.
14. Phibbs CS, Mortensen L: Back transporting infants from neonatal intensive care units to community hospitals for recovery care: effect on total hospital charges. Pediatrics 90:22, 1992.
15. Walker DJ, Vohr BR, Oh W: Economic analysis of regionalized neonatal care for very low-birth-weight infants in the state of Rhode Island. Pediatrics 76:69, 1985.
16. Meert K, Lieh-Lai M, Sarnaik I, et al: The role of intensive care in managing childhood cancer. Am J Clin Oncol 14:379, 1991.
17. Eisenberg M, Bergner L, Hallstrom A: Epidemiology of cardiac arrest and resuscitation in children. Ann Emerg Med 12:672, 1983.
18. Torphy DE, Minter MG, Thompson BM: Cardiorespiratory arrest and resuscitation of children. Am J Dis Child 138:1099, 1984.
19. Orlowski JP: The effectiveness of pediatric cardiopulmonary resuscitation. Am J Dis Child 138:1097, 1984.
20. O'Rourke PP: Outcome of children who are apneic and pulseless in the emergency room. Crit Care Med 14:466, 1986.
21. Lewis JK, Minter, Eshelman SJ, et al: Outcome of pediatric resuscitation. Ann Emerg Med 12:297, 1983.
22. Zaritsky A, Nadkami V, Getson P, et al: CPR in children. Ann Emerg Med 16:1107, 1987.
23. Fiser DH, Wrape V: Outcome of cardiopulmonary resuscitation in children. Pediatr Emerg Care 3:235, 1987.
24. Schindler MB, Bohn D, Cox PN, et al: Outcome of out-of-hospital cardiac or respiratory arrest in children. N Engl J Med 335:1473, 1996.
25. Nadkarni V, Hazinski MF, Zideman D, et al: Pediatric resuscitation: an advisory statement from the pediatric working group of the international liason committee on resuscitation. Circulation 95:2185, 1997.
26. Anonymous: Instructor's Manual, Pediatric Advanced Life Support. Dallas, TX, American Heart Association, 1997.
27. Anonymous: Textbook of Pediatric Advanced Life Support. Dallas, TX, American Heart Association, 1997.
28. Niemann JT: Cardiopulmonary resuscitation. N Engl J Med 327:1075, 1992.
29. White RD, Hankins DG, Bugliosi TF: Seven years experience with early defibrillation by police and paramedics in an emergency medical services system. Resuscitation 39:145, 1998.
30. de Vreede-Swagemakers JJ, Gorgels AP, Dubois-Arbouw WI, et al: Circumstances and causes of out-of-hospital cardiac arrest in sudden death survivors. Heart 79:356, 1998.
31. Valenzuela TD, Roe DJ, Cretin S, et al: Estimating effectiveness of cardiac arrest interventions: a logistic regression survival model. Circulation 96:3308, 1997.
32. Herlitz J, Bang A, Holmberg M, et al: Rhythm changes during resuscitation from ventricular fibrillation in relation to delay until defibrillation, number of shocks delivered and survival. Resuscitation 34:17, 1997.
33. Kloeck W, Cummins RO, Chamberlain D, et al: Early defibrillation: an advisory statement from the Advanced Life Support Working Group of the International Liaison Committee on Resuscitation. Circulation 95:2183, 1997.
34. Barton CW, Manning JE: Cardiopulmonary resuscitation [review]. Emerg Med Clin North Am 13:811, 1995.
35. Maron BJ, Poliac LC, Kaplan JA, et al: Blunt impact to the chest leading to sudden death from cardiac arrest during sports activities. N Engl J Med 333:337, 1995.
36. Frommer DA, Kulig KW, Marx JA, et al: Tricyclic antidepressant overdose. A review. JAMA 257:521, 1987.
37. Shannon M, Liebelt EL: Toxicology reviews: targeted management strategies for cardiovascular toxicity from tricyclic antidepressant overdose: the pivotal role for alkalinization and sodium loading. Pediatr Emerg Care 14:293, 1998.
38. Torres AJ, Pickert CB, Firestone J, et al: Long-term functional outcome of inpatient pediatric cardiopulmonary resuscitation. Pediatr Emerg Care 13:369, 1997.
39. Slonim AD, Patel KM, Ruttimann UE, et al: Cardiopulmonary resuscitation in pediatric intensive care units. Crit Care Med 25:1951, 1997.
40. Sanders AB, Meislin HW, Ewy GA: The physiology of cardiopulmonary resuscitation; an update. JAMA 252:3283, 1984.
41. Rogers MC: New developments in cardiopulmonary resuscitation. Pediatrics 71:655, 1983.
42. Kouwenhoven WB, Jude JR, Knickerbocker GG: Closed-chest cardiac massage. JAMA 173:1064, 1960.
43. Sladen A: Closed-chest massage after twenty-five years. JAMA 251:3137, 1984.
44. Sanders AB, Ewy GA, Taft TV: Prognostic and therapeutic importance of the aortic diastolic pressure in resuscitation from cardiac arrest. Crit Care Med 12:871, 1984.
45. Koehler RC, Michael JR, Guerci AD, et al: Beneficial effect of epinephrine infusion on cerebral and myocardial blood flows during CPR. Ann Emerg Med 14:744, 1985.
46. Schleien CL, Dean JM, Koehler RC, et al: Effect of epinephrine on cerebral and myocardial perfusion in an infant animal preparation of cardiopulmonary resuscitation. Circulation 73:809, 1986.
47. Schleien CL, Kuluz JW, Shaffner DH, et al: Cardiopulmonary resuscitation. *In* Rogers MC, Nichols DG (eds): Textbook of Pediatric Intensive Care. 3rd ed. Baltimore, Williams & Wilkins, 1996, p 3.
48. Schleien CL, Rogers MC: CPR in infants and children. *In* Kaye W, Bircher NG (eds): Clinics in Critical Care Medicine. New York, Churchill Livingstone, 1989, p 135.
49. Berkowitz ID, Chantarojanasiri T, Koehler RC: Blood flow during cardiopulmonary resuscitation with simultaneous compression and ventilation in infant pigs. Pediatr Res 26:558, 1989.
50. Dean JM, Koehler RC, Schleien CL: Age-related changes in chest geometry during cardiopulmonary resuscitation. J Appl Physiol 62:2212, 1987.
51. Halperin HR, Weisfeldt ML: New approaches to CPR: four hands, a plunger, or a vest. JAMA 267:2940, 1992.
52. Cohen TJ, Tucker KJ, Lurie KG: Active compression-decompression a new method of cardiopulmonary resuscitation. JAMA 267:2916, 1992.
53. Krischer JP, Fine EG, Weisfeldt ML: Comparison of prehospital conventional and simultaneous compression-ventilation cardiopulmonary resuscitation. Crit Care Med 17:1263, 1989.
54. Emergency Cardiac Care Committee and Subcommittees AHA: Guidelines for cardiopulmonary resuscitation and emergency cardiac care. JAMA 268:2171, 1992.
55. Roth B, Magnusson J, Johansson I, et al: Jaw lift—a simple and effective method to open the airway in children. Resuscitation 39:171, 1998.
56. Bhende MS, Thompson AE: Evaluation of an end-tidal CO2 detector during pediatric cardiopulmonary resuscitation. Pediatrics 95:395, 1995.
57. Finholt DA, Kettrick RG, Wagner HR, et al: The heart is under the lower third of the sternum. Am J Dis Child 140:646, 1986.

58. David R: Closed chest cardiac massage in the newborn infant. Pediatrics 81:552, 1988.
59. Houri PK, Frank LR, Menegazzi JJ, et al: A randomized, controlled trial of two-thumb vs two-finger chest compression in a swine infant model of cardiac arrest. Prehosp Emerg Care 1:65, 1997.
60. Hoff WS, Reilly PM, Rotondo MF, et al: The importance of the command physician in trauma resuscitation. J Trauma 43:772, 1997.
61. Fleisher G, Caputo G, Baskin M: Comparison of external jugular and peripheral venous administration of sodium bicarbonate in puppies. Crit Care Med 17:251, 1989.
62. Kanter RK, Zimmerman JJ, Strauss RH, et al: Pediatric emergency intravenous access: evaluation of a protocol. Am J Dis Child 140: 132, 1986.
63. Rosen KR, Rosen DA: Comparative flow rates for small bore peripheral intravenous catheters. Pediatr Emerg Care 2:153, 1986.
64. Brunette DD, Fischer R: Intravascular access in pediatric cardiac arrest. Ann Emerg Med 6:577, 1988.
65. Abdulla F, Dietrich KA, Pramanik AK: Percutaneous femoral venous catheterization in preterm neonates. J Pediatr 117:788, 1990.
66. Orlowski JP: My kingdom for an intravenous line. Am J Dis Child 138:803, 1984.
67. Berg RA: Emergency infusion of catecholamines into bone marrow. Am J Dis Child 138:810, 1984.
68. Anonymous: Guidelines 2000 for cardiopulmonary resuscitation and emergency cardiovascular care: International consensus on science. Circulation 102 (suppl I):I-1 through I-384, 2000.
69. Neish SR, Macon MG, Moore JWM, et al: Intraosseous infusion of hypertonic glucose and dopamine. Am J Dis Child 142:878, 1988.
70. Orlowski JP, Julius CJ, Petras RE, et al: The safety of intraosseous infusions: risks of fat and bone marrow emboli to the lungs. Ann Emerg Med 18:1062, 1989.
71. Glaeser PW, Losek JD, Nelson DB: Pediatric intrasseous infusions: impact on vascular access time. Am J Emerg Med 6:330, 1988.
72. Greenberg MI, Roberts JR, Baskin SI: Endotracheal naloxone reversal of morphine-induced respiratory depression in rabbits. Ann Emerg Med 9:289, 1980.
73. Roberts JR, Greenberg MI, Knaub MA: Blood levels following intravenous and endotracheal epinephrine administration. J Am Coll Emerg Phys 8:53, 1979.
74. Harnett RM, Sias FR, Pruitt JR: Resuscitation from hypothermia: a literature review. Report CG-D-26-79. Springfield VA, US Department of Transportation, United States Coast Guard, National Technical Information Center, 1979.
75. Losek JD, Hennes H, Glaeser PW: Prehospital countershock treatment of pediatric asystole. Am J Emerg Med 7:571, 1989.
76. Mancini ME, Kaye W: In-hospital first-responder automated external defibrillation: what critical care practitioners need to know. Am J Crit Care 7:314, 1998.
77. Holmes HR, Babbs CF, Voorhees WD: Influence of adrenergic drugs upon vital organ perfusion during CPR. Crit Care Med 8:137, 1980.
78. Otto CW, Yakaitis RW, Blitt CD: Mechanism of action of epinephrine in resuscitation from asphyxial arrest. Crit Care Med 9:321, 1981.
79. Paradis NA, Martin GB, Rivers EP: Coronary perfusion pressure and the return of spontaneous circulation in human cardiopulmonary resuscitation. JAMA 263:1106, 1990.
80. Mielke LL, Frank C, Lanzinger MJ, et al: Plasma catecholamine levels following tracheal and intravenous epinephrine administration in swine. Resuscitation 36:187, 1998.
81. Ornato JP: High-dose epinephrine during resuscitation. JAMA 265:1160, 1996.
82. Paradis NA, Martin GB, Rosenberg J: The effect of standard and high-dose epinephrine on coronary perfusion pressure during prolonged cardiopulmonary resuscitation. JAMA 265:1139, 1991.
83. Callaham ML, Barton CW, Kayser S: Potential complications of high-dose epinephrine therapy in patients resuscitated from cardiac arrest. JAMA 265:1117, 1991.
84. Callaham ML, Madsen CD, Barton CW: A randomized clinical trial of high-dose epinephrine and norepinephrine vs standard-dose epinephrine in prehospital cardiac arrest. JAMA 268:2667, 1992.
85. Goetting MG, Paradis NA: High-dose epinephrine in refractory pediatric cardiac arrest. Crit Care Med 17:1258, 1989.
86. Stiell IG, Hebert PC, Weitzman BN: High-dose epinephrine in adult cardiac arrest. N Engl J Med 327:1045, 1992.
87. Brown CG, Martin DR, Pepe PE: A comparison of standard-dose and high-dose epinephrine in cardiac arrest outside the hospital. N Engl J Med 327:1051, 1992.
88. Berg RA, Otto CW, Kern KB, et al: A randomized, blinded trial of high-dose epinephrine versus standard-dose epinephrine in a swine model of pediatric asphyxial cardiac arrest. Crit Care Med 24:1695, 1996.
89. Cairns CB, Niemann JT: Hemodynamic effects of repeated doses of epinephrine after prolonged cardiac arrest and CPR: preliminary observations in an animal model. Resuscitation 36:181, 1998.
90. Gueugniaud PY, Mols P, Goldstein P, et al: A comparison of repeated high doses and repeated standard doses of epinephrine for cardiac arrest outside the hospital. European Epinephrine Study Group. N Engl J Med 339:1595, 1998.
91. Sessler D, Mills P, Gregory G: Effects of bicarbonate on arterial and brain intracellular pH in neonatal rabbits recovering from hypoxic lactic acidosis. J Pediatr 111:817, 1981.
92. Vukmir RB, Bircher N, Safar P: Sodium bicarbonate in cardiac arrest: a reappraisal [review]. Am J Emerg Med 14:192, 1996.
93. Vukmir RB, Bircher NG, Radovsky A, et al: Sodium bicarbonate may improve outcome in dogs with brief or prolonged cardiac arrest. Crit Care Med 23:515, 1995.
94. Graf H, Leach W, Arieff AI: Evidence for a detrimental effect of bicarbonate therapy in hypoxic lactic acidosis. Science 227:754, 1985.
95. von Planta M, Weil MH, Gazmuri RJ: Myocardial acidosis associated with CO_2 production during cardiac arrest and resuscitation. Circulation 80:684, 1989.
96. Hein HA: The use of sodium bicarbonate in neonatal resuscitation: help or harm? Pediatrics 91:496, 1993.
97. Levy MM: An evidence-based evaluation of the use of sodium bicarbonate during cardiopulmonary resuscitation. Crit Care Clin 14: 457, 1998.
98. Stueven H, Thompson BM, Aprahamian C, et al: Use of calcium in prehospital cardiac arrest. Ann Emerg Med 12:136, 1983.
99. Stempien A, Katz AM, Messineo FC: Calcium and cardiac arrest. Ann Intern Med 105:603, 1986.
100. Nakanishi T, Jarmakani JM: Developmental changes in myocardial mechanical function and subcellular organelles. Am J Physiol 246:H615, 1984.
101. Artman M, Graham TPJ, Boucek RJ Jr: Effects of postnatal maturation on myocardial contractile responses to calcium antagonists and changes in contraction frequency. J Cardiovasc Pharmacol 7:850, 1985.
102. Rebeyka IM, Yeh TJ, Hanan SA, et al: Altered contractile response in neonatal myocardium to citrate-phosphate-dextrose infusion. Circulation 82(Suppl):IV-367, 1990.
103. Uemura S, Young H, Matsuoka S, et al: Calcium paradox in the neonatal heart. Can J Cardiol 1:114, 1985.
104. Pulsinelli WA, Waldman S, Rawlinson D, et al: Moderate hyperglycemia augments ischemic brain damage: a neuropathologic study in the rat. Neurology 32:1239, 1982.
105. Farias LA, Willis M, Gregory GA: Effects of fructose-1,6-diphosphate, glucose, and saline on cardiac resuscitation. Anesthesiology 65:595, 1986.
106. Nakakimura K, Fleischer JE, Drummond JC: Glucose administration before cardiac arrest worsens neurologic outcome in cats. Anesthesiology 72:1005, 1990.
107. Hoffman WE, Braucher E, Pelligrino DA: Brain lactate and neurologic outcome following incomplete ischemia in fasted, nonfasted, and glucose-loaded rats. Anesthesiology 72:1045, 1990.
108. Crosson JE, Etheridge SP, Milstein S, et al: Therapeutic and diagnostic utility of adenosine during tachycardia evaluation in children. Am J Cardiol 74:155, 1994.
109. Ralston MA, Knilans TK, Hannon DW, et al: Use of adenosine for diagnosis and treatment of tachyarrhythmias in pediatric patients. J Pediatr 124:139, 1994.
110. Reyes G, Stanton R, Galvis AG: Adenosine in the treatment of paroxysmal supraventricular tachycardia in children. Ann Emerg Med 21:1499, 1992.
111. Dobrin RS, Block B, Gilman JI, et al: The development of a pediatric emergency transport system. Pediatr Clin North Am 27:633, 1980.
112. Day SE: Intra-transport stabilization and management of the pediatric patient. Pediatr Clin North Am 40:263, 1993.
113. Anonymous: Handbook of Pediatric and Neonatal Transport Medicine. Philadelphia, PA, Hanley & Belfus (a division of Mosby, St. Louis), 1996.

114. McCloskey KAL, Orr RA: Pediatric Transport Medicine. St. Louis, Mosby-Year Book, 1995.
115. Aoki BY, McCloskey KAL: Evaluation, Stabilization, and Transport of the Critically Ill Child. St. Louis, Mosby-Year Book, 1992.
116. Hageman JR, Fetcho S: Transport of the Critically Ill. Crit Care Clin 8:465, 1992.
117. McNeil EL: Airborne Care of the Ill and Injured. New York, Springer-Verlag, 1982.
118. Goldman HS: Pediatric pulmonary radiology. In Scarpelli EM, Auld PA, Goldman HS (eds): Pulmonary Disease of the Fetus, Newborn and Child. Philadelphia, Lea & Febiger, 1978.
119. Hauser GJ, Pollack MM, Sivit CJ: Routine chest radiographs in pediatric intensive care: a prospective study. Pediatrics 83:465, 1989.
120. Meliones JN, Wilson BG, Cheifetz IM, et al: Respiratory monitoring. In Rogers MC, Nichols DG (eds): Textbook of Pediatric Intensive Care. Baltimore, Williams & Wilkins, 1996, p 331.
121. Tobin MJ: Respiratory monitoring. JAMA 264:244, 1990.
122. Baboolal R, Kirpalani H: Measuring on-line compliance in ventilated infants using hot-wire anemometry. Crit Care Med 18:1070, 1990.
123. Jennis MS, Peabody JL: Pulse oximetry: an alternative method for the assessment of oxygenation in newborn infants. Pediatrics 79:524, 1987.
124. Hay WW, Brockway JM, Eyzaguirre M: Neonatal pulse oximetry: accuracy and reliability. Pediatrics 83:717, 1989.
125. Harris AP, Sendak MJ, Donham RT: Absorption characteristics of human fetal hemoglobin at waveforms used in pulse oximetry. J Clin Monit 4:175, 1988.
126. Watcha MF, Connor MT, Hing AV: Pulse oximetry in methemoglobinemia. Am J Dis Child 143:845, 1989.
127. Barker SJ, Tremper KK, Hyatt J: Effects of methemoglobinemia on pulse oximetry and mixed venous oximetry. Anesthesiology 70:112, 1989.
128. Brown M, Vender JS: Noninvasive oxygen monitoring. Crit Care Clin 4:493, 1988.
129. Mault JR, Santoro-Nease A, Leonard RA: Continuous fiberoptic venous oximetry during neonatal ECMO: analysis of accuracy and longevity [abstract]. Crit Care Med 20:S11, 1992.
130. Swedlow DB: Capnometry and capnography: the anesthesia disaster early warning system. Semin Anesth 5:194, 1986.
131. Barton C, Callaham ML: Lack of correlation between end-tidal carbon dioxide concentrations and PaCO2 in cardiac arrest. Crit Care Med 19:108, 1991.
132. Gazmuri RJ, von Planta M, Weil MH, et al: Arterial PCO2 as an indicator of systemic perfusion during cardiopulmonary resuscitation. Crit Care Med 17:237, 1989.
133. Burrows FA: Physiologic dead space, venous admixture, and the arterial to end-tidal carbon dioxide difference in infants and children undergoing cardiac surgery. Anesthesiology 70:219, 1989.
134. Fletcher R: The relationship between the arterial to end-tidal PCO2 difference and hemoglobin saturation in patients with congenital heart disease. Anesthesiology 75:210, 1991.
135. Badgewell JM, Heavner JE, May WS: End-tidal PCO2 monitoring in infants and children ventilated with either a partial rebreathing or a non-rebreathing circuit. Anesthesiology 66:405, 1987.
136. From RP, Scamman FL: Ventilatory frequency influences accuracy of end-tidal CO2 measurements. Anesth Analg 67:884, 1988.
137. Pascucci RC, Schena JA, Thompson JE: Comparison of a sidestream and mainstream capnometer in infants. Crit Care Med 17:560, 1989.
138. Briassoulis G: Arterial measurement in preterm infants [abstract]. Crit Care Med 14:S735, 1986.
139. Fry DL: Physiologic recording by modern instruments with particular reference to pressure recording [abstract]. Physiol Rev 40:753, 1960.
140. Geddes LA: Handbook of Blood Pressure Measurement. Clifton, NJ, Humana Press, 1991.
141. Fiser DH, Graves SA, van der Aa J: Catheters for arterial pressure monitoring in pediatrics. Crit Care Med 13:580, 1985.
142. Swedlow DB, Cohen DE: Invasive assessment of the failing circulation. In Swedlow DB, Raphaely RC (eds): Cardiovascular Problems in Pediatric Critical Care. New York, Churchill Livingstone, 1986, p 129.
143. Gerber MJ, Hines RL, Barash PG: Arterial waveforms and systemic vascular resistance: is there a correlation? Anesthesiology 66:823, 1987.
144. Greenwald BM, Notterman DA, DeBruin WJ, et al: Percutaneous axillary artery catheterization in critically ill infants and children. J Pediatr 117:442, 1990.
145. Simmons MA, Levine RL, Lubchenco LO: Warning: serious sequelae of temporal artery catheterization. J Pediatr 92:284, 1978.
146. Prian GW: Complications and sequelae of temporal artery catheterization in the high-risk newborn. J Pediatr Surg 12:829, 1977.
147. Nicolson SC, Sweeney MF, Moore RA, et al: Comparison of internal and external jugular cannulation of the central circulation in the pediatric patient. Crit Care Med 13:747, 1985.
148. Lloyd TR, Donnerstein RL, Berg RA: Accuracy of central venous pressure measurement from the abdominal inferior vena cava. Pediatrics 89:506, 1992.
149. Chathas MK, Paton JB, Fisher DE: Percutaneous central venous catheterization. Am J Dis Child 144:1246, 1990.
150. Agee KR, Balk RA: Central venous catheterization in the critically ill patient. Crit Care Clin 8:677, 1992.
151. Goldstein AM, Weber JM, Sheridan RL: Femoral venous access is safe in burned children: an analysis of 224 catheters. J Pediatr 130:442, 1997.
152. Stenzel JP, Green TP, Fuhrman BP, et al: Percutaneous central venous catheterization in a pediatric intensive care unit: a survival analysis of complications. Crit Care Med 17:984, 1989.
153. Kanter RK, Zimmerman JJ, Strauss RH, et al: Central venous catheter insertion by femoral vein: safety and effectiveness for the pediatric patient. Pediatrics 77:842, 1986.
154. Bar-Joseph G, Galvis AG: Perforation of the heart by central venous catheters in infants: guidelines to diagnosis and management. J Pediatr Surg 18:284, 1983.
155. Duntley P, Siever J, Korwes ML: Vascular erosion by central venous catheters. Chest 101:1633, 1992.
156. Jackson JC, Truog WE, Watchko JF: Efficacy of thromboresistant umbilical artery catheters in reducing aortic thrombosis and related complications. J Pediatr 110:102, 1987.
157. Beck C, Dubois J, Grignon A, et al: Incidence and risk factors of catheter-related deep vein thrombosis in a pediatric intensive care unit: a prospective study. J Pediatr 133:237, 1998.
158. Randolph AG, Cook DJ, Gonzales CA, et al: Benefit of heparin in central venous and pulmonary artery catheters: a meta-analysis of randomized controlled trials. Chest 113:165, 1998.
159. Furfaro S, Gauthier M, Lacroix J: Arterial catheter-related infections in children. Am J Dis Child 145:1037, 1991.
160. Albrecht R, Hudson-Civetta J, Baker M, et al: Catheter related infection with multiple guidewire exchanges in critically ill patients [abstract]. Crit Care Med 20:S37, 1992.
161. Eyer S, Brummitt C, Crossley K: Catheter-related sepsis: prospective, randomized study of three methods of long-term catheter maintenance. Crit Care Med 18:1073, 1990.
162. Lee RB, Buckner M, Sharp KW: Do multi-lumen catheters increase central venous catheter sepsis compared to single-lumen catheters? J Trauma 28:1472, 1988.
163. Downs JB, Douglas ME: Assessment of cardiac filling pressure during continuous positive pressure ventilation. Crit Care Med 8:285, 1980.
164. Vender JS: Resolved: a pulmonary artery catheter should be used in the management of the critically ill patient. Pro. [review]. J Cardiothorac Vasc Anesth 12(Suppl 1):9, 1998.
165. Becker K Jr: Resolved: a pulmonary artery catheter should be used in the management of the critically ill patient. Con. [review]. J Cardiothorac Vasc Anesth 12(Suppl 1):13, 1998.
166. Teboul JL, Zapol WM, Brun-Buisson C: A comparison of pulmonary artery occlusion pressure and left ventricular end-diastolic pressure during mechanical ventilation with PEEP in patients with severe ARDS. Anesthesiology 70:261, 1989.
167. Freed MD, Keane JF: Cardiac output measured by thermodilution in infants and children. J Pediatr 92:39, 1978.
168. Jensen JR, Schreuder JJ, Bogaard JM: Thermodilution technique for measurement of cardiac output during artificial ventilation. J Appl Physiol 51:584, 1981.
169. Stevens JH, Raffin TA, Mihm FG: Thermodilution cardiac output measurement: effects of the respiratory cycle on its reproducibility. JAMA 253:2240, 1985.
170. Filloux F, Dean JM, Kirsch JR: Monitoring the central nervous system. In Rogers MC, Nichols DG (eds): Textbook of Pediatric Intensive Care. 3rd ed. Baltimore, Williams & Wilkins, 1996, p 667.
171. Greenberg RP, Ward JD, Lutz H: Advanced monitoring of the brain: In Grenvik A, Safar P (eds): Clinics in Critical Care Medicine: Brain Failure and Resuscitation. New York, Churchill Livingstone, 1981, p 67.

172. Sloan TB: Neurologic monitoring. Crit Care Clin 4:543, 1988.
173. Saul TG, Ducker TB: Effect of intracranial pressure monitoring and aggressive treatment on mortality in severe head injury. J Neurosurg 56:498, 1982.
174. Rogers AT, Stump DA: Cerebral physiologic monitoring. Crit Care Clin 5:845, 1989.
175. Poss WB, Brockmeyer DL, Clay B, et al: Pathophysiology and management of the intracranial vault. *In* Rogers MC, Nichols DG (eds): Textbook of Pediatric Intensive Care. Baltimore, Williams & Wilkins, 1996, p 645.
176. Tasker RC, Matthew DJ: Cerebral intraparenchymal pressure monitoring in non-traumatic coma: clinical evaluation of a new fibreoptic device. Neuropediatrics 22:47, 1991.
177. Gambardella G, Zaccone C, Cardia E, et al: Intracranial pressure monitoring in children: comparison of external ventricular device with the fiberoptic system. Childs Nerv Syst 9:470, 1993.
178. Mindermann T, Reinhardt H, Gratzl O: Significant lateralization of supratentorial ICP after blunt head trauma. Acta Neurochir 116:60, 1992.
179. Cascino GD: Neurophysiological monitoring in the intensive care unit. J Intensive Care Med 3:215, 1988.
180. Veselis RA, Reinsel R, Alagesan R: The EEG as a monitor of midazolam amnesia: changes in power and topography as a function of amnesic state. Anesthesiology 74:866, 1991.
181. Fisher B, Peterson B, Hicks G: Use of brainstem auditory-evoked response testing to assess neurologic outcome following near drowning in children. Crit Care Med 20:578, 1992.
182. Goodwin SR, Friedman WA, Bellefleur M: Is it time to use evoked potentials to predict outcome in comatose children and adults? Crit Care Med 19:518, 1991.
183. Reid KH, Mullins ER, Iyer VG: Changes in brainstem auditory evoked response latency predict survival after CPR in a rat model of cardiac arrest and resuscitation. Resuscitation 36:65, 1998.
184. Ruiz-Lopez MJ, deAzagra AM, Serrano A, et al: Brain death and evoked potentials in pediatric patients. Crit Care Med 27:412, 1999.
185. Flannery AM: Brain death and evoked potentials in pediatric patients. Crit Care Med 27:264, 1999.
186. Moulton RJ, Brown JI, Konasiewicz SJ: Monitoring severe head injury: a comparison of EEG and somatosensory evoked potentials. Can J Neurol Sci 25:S7, 1998.
187. Konasiewicz SJ, Moulton RJ, Shedden PM: Somatosensory evoked potentials and intracranial pressure in severe head injury. Can J Neurol Sci 21:219, 1994.
188. Brazy JE: Cerebral oxygen monitoring with near infrared spectroscopy: clinical application to neonates. J Clin Monit 7:325, 1991.
189. Edwards AD, Brown GC, Cope M: Quantification of concentration changes in neonatal human cerebral oxidized cytochrome oxidase. J Appl Physiol 71:1907, 1991.
190. von Siebenthal K, Bernert G, Casaer P: Near-infrared spectroscopy in newborn infants. Brain Dev 14:135, 1992.
191. Faris F, Rolfe P, Thorniley M: Non-invasive optical monitoring of cerebral blood oxygenation in the foetus and newborn: preliminary investigation. J Biomed Eng 14:303, 1992.
192. Hirtz DG: Report of the national institute of neurologic disorders and stroke workshop on near infrared spectroscopy. Pediatrics 91:414, 1993.
193. Robertson CS, Gopinath SP, Goodman JC, et al: SjvO2 monitoring in head-injured patients. J Neurotrauma 12:891, 1995.
194. Feldman Z, Robertson CS: Monitoring of cerebral hemodynamics with jugular bulb catheters [review]. Crit Care Clin 13:51, 1997.
195. Crone RK: Acute circulatory failure in children. Pediatr Clin North Am 27:525, 1980.
196. Schieber RA: Noninvasive recognition and assessment of the failing circulation. *In* Swedlow DB, Raphaely RC (eds): Clinics in Critical Care Medicine: Cardiovascular Problems in Pediatric Critical Care. New York, Churchill Livingstone, 1986, p 87.
197. Sherman FS, Sahn DJ: Pediatric Doppler echocardiography 1987: major advances in technology. J Pediatr 110:333, 1987.
198. Heitmiller ES, Wetzel RC: Hemodynamic monitoring considerations in pediatric critical care. *In* Rogers MC, Nichols DG (eds): Textbook of Pediatric Intensive Care. Baltimore, Williams & Wilkins, 1996, p 607.
199. Colan SD: Echocardiography. *In* Chang AC, Hanley FL, Wernovsky G, et al (eds): Pediatric Cardiac Intensive Care. Baltimore, Williams & Wilkins, 1998, p 425.
200. Frommelt MA, Frommelt PC: Advances in echocardiographic diagnostic modalities for the pediatrician. Pediatr Clin North Am 46:427, 1999.
201. Goldberg SJ, Hutter JJ Jr, Feldman L, et al: Two sensitive echocardiographic techniques for detecting doxorubicin toxicity. Med Pediatr Oncol 11:172, 1983.
202. Nishimura RA, Housmans PR, Hatle LK, et al: Assessment of diastolic function of the heart: background and current applications of Doppler echocardiography. Part I: Physiologic and pathophysiologic features. Mayo Clin Proc 64:71, 1989.
203. Nishimura RA, Abel MD, Hatle LK, et al: Assessment of diastolic function of the heart: background and current applications of Doppler echocardiography. Part II: Clinical studies. Mayo Clin Proc 64:181, 1989.
204. Perkin RM, Levin DL: Shock in the pediatric patient. Part I. J Pediatr 101:163, 1982.
205. Perkin RM, Levin DL: Shock in the pediatric patient. Part II: Therapy. J Pediatr 101:319, 1982.
206. Perkin RM: Shock states. *In* Fuhrman BP, Zimmerman JJ (eds): Pediatric Critical Care. St. Louis, Mosby Year Book, 1992, p 287.
207. Tobin JR, Wetzel RC: Shock and multi-organ system failure. *In* Rogers MC, Nichols DG (eds): Textbook of Pediatric Intensive Care. 3rd ed. Baltimore, Williams & Wilkins, 1996, p 555.
208. Friedman W: The intrinsic physiologic properties of the developing heart. Prog Cardiovasc Dis 15:87, 1972.
209. Wetzel RC, Stiff JC, Rogers MC: Heart rate and rhythm as determinants of cardiac output. *In* Swedlow DB, Raphaely RC (eds): Clinics in Critical Care Medicine: Cardiovascular Problems in Pediatric Critical Care. New York, Churchill Livingstone, 1986, p 257.
210. Jafri SM, Kruse JA: Temporary transvenous cardiac pacing. Crit Care Clin 8:713, 1992.
211. Rocchini AP, Chun PO, Dick M: Ventricular tachycardia in children. Am J Cardiol 47:1091, 1981.
212. Duster MC, Bink-Boelkens MT, Wampler D: Long-term follow-up of dysrhythmias following the Mustard procedure. Am Heart J 109:1323, 1985.
213. Perry JC, Giuffre RM, Garson A: Clues to the electrocardiographic diagnosis of subtle Wolff-Parkinson-White syndrome in children. J Pediatr 117:871, 1990.
214. Bricker JT, Garson A Jr, Gillette PC: A family history of seizures associated with sudden cardiac deaths. Am J Dis Child 138:866, 1984.
215. Davis AM, Wilkinson JL: The long QT syndrome and seizures in childhood [review]. J Paediatr Child Health 34:410, 1998.
216. Ackerman MJ: The long QT syndrome [review]. Pediatr Rev 19:232, 1998.
217. Perry JC, Walsh EP: Diagnosis and management of cardiac arrythmias. *In* Chang AC, Hanley FL, Wernovsky G, et al (eds): Pediatric Cardiac Intensive Care. Baltimore, Williams & Wilkins, 1998, p 461.
218. Pinski SL, Maloney JD: Adenosine: a new drug for acute termination of supraventricular tachycardia. Cleve Clin J Med 57:383, 1990.
219. Overholt ED, Rheuban KS, Gutgesell HP: Usefulness of adenosine for arrhythmias in infants and children. Am J Cardiol 61:336, 1988.
220. Rossi AF, Steinberg LG, Kipel G: Use of adenosine in the management of perioperative arrhythmias in the pediatric cardiac intensive care unit. Crit Care Med 20:1107, 1992.
221. Porter CJ, Garson A Jr, Gillette PC: Verapamil: an effective calcium blocking agent for pediatric patients. Pediatrics 71:748, 1983.
222. Leitner RP, Hawker RE, Celermajer JM: Intravenous verapamil in the treatment of paroxysmal supraventricular tachycardia in children. Aust Paediatr J 19:40, 1983.
223. Garland JS, Berens RJ, Losek JD, et al: An infant fatality following verapamil therapy for supraventricular tachycardia: cardiovascular collapse following intravenous verapamil. Pediatr Emerg Care 1:198, 1985.
224. Epstein ML, Kiel EA, Victorica BE: Cardiac decompensation following verapamil therapy in infants with supraventricular tachycardia. Pediatrics 75:737, 1985.
225. Wetzel RC, Rogers MC: Dysrhythmias and their management. *In* Rogers MC (ed): Textbook of Pediatric Intensive Care. 2nd ed. Baltimore, Williams & Wilkins, 1992, p 532.
226. Ushay HM, Notterman DA: Pharmacology of pediatric resuscitation. Pediatr Clin North Am 44:207, 1997.
227. Braunwald E: Regulation of the circulation. Parts I and II. N Engl J Med 290:1124, 1974.

228. Sarnoff SJ, Berglund E: Ventricular function. Circulation 9:706, 1954.
229. Gabel JC, Drake RE: Pulmonary capillary pressure and permeability. Crit Care Med 7:92, 1979.
230. Raphaely RC, Browning RA: The role of preload in the manipulation of the failing circulation. *In* Swedlow DB, Raphaely RC (eds): Clinics in Critical Care Medicine: Cardiovascular Problems in Pediatric Critical Care. New York, Churchill Livingstone, 1986, p 205.
231. Perkin RM, Anas NG: Nonsurgical contractility manipulation of the failing circulation. *In* Swedlow DB, Raphaely RC (eds): Clinics in Critical Care Medicine: Cardiovascular Problems in Pediatric Critical Care. New York, Churchill Livingstone, 1986, p 229.
232. Zaritsky A, Chernow B: Use of catecholamines in pediatrics. J Pediatr 105:341, 1984.
233. Scholz H: Inotropic drugs and their mechanisms of action. J Am Coll Cardiol 4:389, 1984.
234. Padbury JF, Agata Y, Baylen BG: Dopamine pharmacokinetics in critically ill newborn infants. J Pediatr 110:293, 1986.
235. Tulassay T, Seri I: Acute oliguria in preterm infants with hyaline membrane disease: interactions of dopamine and furosemide. Acta Paediatr Scand 75:420, 1986.
236. Hughes A, Thom S, Martin G: The action of a dopamine (DA-1) receptor agonist, fenoldopam, in human vasculature in vivo and in vitro. Br J Clin Pharmacol 22:535, 1986.
237. Hilberman M, Maseda J, Stinson EB: The diuretic properties of dopamine in patients after open-heart operation. Anesthesiology 61:489, 1984.
238. Miller ED: Renal effects of dopamine. Anesthesiology 61:487, 1984.
239. Pelayo JC, Fildes RD, Jose PA: Age-dependent renal effects of intrarenal dopamine infusion. Am J Physiol 247:R212, 1984.
240. Seri I: Dopamine and natriuresis. Am J Hypertens 3:82S, 1990.
241. Cuevas L, Yeh TF, John EG: The effect of low-dose dopamine infusion on cardiopulmonary and renal status in premature newborns with respiratory distress syndrome. Am J Dis Child 145:799, 1991.
242. Padbury JF, Agata Y, Baylen BG: Pharmacokinetics of dopamine in critically ill newborn infants. J Pediatr 117:472, 1990.
243. Zaritsky A, Lotze A, Stull R, et al: Steady-state dopamine clearance in critically ill infants and children. Crit Care Med 16:217, 1988.
244. Benzing G III, Helmsworth JA, Schreiber JT, et al: Nitroprusside and epinephrine for treatment of low output in children after open-heart surgery. Ann Thorac Surg 27:523, 1979.
245. Perkin RM, Levin DL, Webb R: Dobutamine: a hemodynamic evaluation in children with shock. J Pediatr 100:977, 1982.
246. Habib DM, Padbury JF, Anas NG: Dobutamine pharmacokinetics and pharmacodynamics in pediatric intensive care patients. Crit Care Med 20:601, 1992.
247. Stopfkuchen H, Queisser-Luft A, Vogel K: Cardiovascular responses to dobutamine determined by systolic time intervals in preterm infants. Crit Care Med 18:722, 1990.
248. Luchessi BR: Inotropic agents and drugs used to support the failing heart. *In* Antonaccio M (ed): Cardiovascular Pharmacology. New York, Raven Press, 1977, p 337.
249. Fisher DG, Schwartz PH, Davus AL: Pharmacokinetics of exogenous epinephrine in critically ill children. Crit Care Med 21:111, 1993.
250. Mason DT: Afterload reduction and cardiac performance. Physiologic basis of systemic vasodilators as a new approach in treatment of congestive heart failure. Am J Med 65:106, 1978.
251. Appelbaum A, Blackstone EH, Kouchoukos NT, et al: Afterload reduction and cardiac output in infants early after intracardiac surgery. Am J Cardiol 39:445, 1977.
252. Steward DJ: Afterload: nonsurgical manipulation of the failing circulation. *In* Swedlow DB, Raphaely RC (eds): Clinics in Critical Care Medicine: Cardiovascular Problems in Pediatric Critical Care. New York, Churchill Livingstone, 1986, p 221.
253. LeJemtel TH, Katz SD, Sonneblick EH: Peripheral circulatory response in cardiac failure. Hosp Pract 26:75, 1991.
254. Lewis AB: The failing myocardium. *In* Chang AC, Hanley FL, Wernovsky G, et al (eds): Pediatric Cardiac Intensive Care. Baltimore, Williams & Wilkins, 1998, p 483.
255. Shekerdemian LS, Redington A: Cardiovascular pharmacology. *In* Chang AC, Hanley FL, Wernovsky G, et al (eds): Pediatric Cardiac Intensive Care. Baltimore, Williams & Wilkins, 1998, p 45.
256. Lawless S, Burckart G, Diven W: Amrinone in neonates and infants after cardiac surgery. Crit Care Med 17:751, 1989.
257. Berner M, Jaccard C, Oberhansli I, et al: Hemodynamic effects of amrinone in children after cardiac surgery. Intensive Care Med 16:85, 1990.
258. Lawless ST, Zaritsky A, Miles M: The acute pharmacokenetics and pharmacodynamics of amrinone in pediatric patients. J Clin Pharmacol 31:800, 1991.
259. Shipley JB, Tolman D, Hastillo A, et al: Milrinone: basic and clinical pharmacology and acute and chronic management [review]. Am J Med Sci 311:286, 1996.
260. Bailey JM, Miller BE, Lu W, et al: The pharmacokinetics of milrinone in pediatric patients after cardiac surgery. Anesthesiology 90:1012, 1999.
261. Leier CV, Binkley PF: Parenteral inotropic support for advanced congestive heart failure [review]. Prog Cardiovasc Dis 41:207, 1998.
262. Pollock JC, Charlton MC, Williams WG: Intraaortic balloon pumping in children. Ann Thorac Surg 29:522, 1980.
263. del Nido PJ, Duncan BW, Mayer JEJ, et al: Left ventricular assist device improves survival in children with left ventricular dysfunction after repair of anomalous origin of the left coronary artery from the pulmonary artery. Ann Thorac Surg 67:169, 1999.
264. Hetzer R, Loebe M, Potapov EV, et al: Circulatory support with pneumatic paracorporeal ventricular assist device in infants and children. Ann Thorac Surg 66:1498, 1998.
265. AAP Task Force on Blood Pressure Control in Children: Report of the second task force on blood pressure control in children—1987. Pediatrics 79:1, 1987.
266. Park MK, Lee DH: Normative arm and calf blood pressure values in the newborn. Pediatrics 83:240, 1989.
267. Kaplan JA: Dupont Critical Care Lecture: role of the ultrashort-acting b-blockers in the perioperative period. J Cardiothorac Anesth 2:683, 1988.
268. Bunchman TE, Lynch RE, Wood EG: Intravenously administered labetalol for treatment of hypertension in children. J Pediatr 140:1203, 1992.
269. Siegler RL, Brewer ED: Effect of sublingual or oral nifedipine in the treatment of hypertension. J Pediatr 112:811, 1988.
270. Hanna JD, Chan JCM, Gill JR: Hypertension and the kidney. J Pediatr 118:327, 1991.
271. Curley MAQ, Thompson JE, Molengraft J, et al: Oxygenation/ventilation. *In* Curley MAQ, Smith JB, Moloney-Harmon PA (eds): Critical Care Nursing of Infants and Children. Philadelphia, WB Saunders Company, 1996, p 249.
272. Backofen JE, Rogers MC: Upper airway disease. *In* Rogers MC (ed): Textbook of Pediatric Intensive Care. 2nd ed. Baltimore, Williams & Wilkins, 1992, p 231.
273. Killham H, Gillis J, Benjamin B: Severe upper airway obstruction. Pediatr Clin North Am 34:1, 1987.
274. Denison C: My first intubation of the larynx; recovery. (Reprinted in JAMA 257:1564, 1987). JAMA 7:342, 1887.
275. Houck CS: Access to the airway. *In* Holbrook PR (ed): Textbook of Pediatric Critical Care. Philadelphia, WB Saunders Company, 1993, p 430.
276. Berlauk JF: Prolonged endotracheal intubation vs. tracheostomy. Crit Care Med 14:742, 1986.
277. Seiden AM: Sinusitis in the critical care patient [review]. New Horiz 1:261, 1993.
278. Pedersen J, Schurizek BA, Melsen NC, et al: The effect of nasotracheal intubation on the paranasal sinuses. A prospective study of 434 intensive care patients. Acta Anaesthesiol Scand 35:11, 1991.
279. Spence K, Barr P: Nasal vs oral intubation for mechanical ventilation of newborn infants. The Cochrane Database of Systemic Reviews, 1999. URL:http://grover.tch.harvard.edu/ovidweb/ovidweb.cgi.
280. Cote CJ, Eavey RD, Todres ID, et al: Cricothyroid membrane puncture: oxygenation and ventilation in a dog model using an intravenous catheter. Crit Care Med 16:615, 1988.
281. Raffin TA: Oxygen toxicity: etiology. Int Anesth Clin 19:169, 1981.
282. Miller JN, Winter PM: Clinical manifestations of pulmonary oxygen toxicity. Int Anesth Clin 19:179, 1981.
283. Jackson RM: Pulmonary oxygen toxicity. Chest 88:900, 1985.
284. Tsan MF: Superoxide dismutase and pulmonary oxygen toxicity [review]. Proc Soc Exp Biol Med 214:107, 1997.
285. Marini JJ, Ravenscraft SA: Mean airway pressure: physiologic determinants and clinical importance—part I: physiologic determinants and measurements. Crit Care Med 20:1461, 1992.
286. Marini JJ, Ravenscraft SA: Mean airway pressure: physiologic determinants and clinical importance—part 2: clinical implications. Crit Care Med 20:1604, 1992.

287. Ciszek TA, Modanlou HD, Owings D, et al: Mean airway pressure—significance during mechanical ventilation in neonates. J Pediatr 99:121, 1981.

288. Kumar A, Falke KJ, Geffin B: Continuous positive-pressure ventilation in acute respiratory failure. N Engl J Med 283:1430, 1970.

289. Gregory GA, Kitterman JA, Phibbs RH: Treatment of the idiopathic respiratory-distress syndrome with continuous positive airway pressure. N Engl J Med 284:1333, 1971.

290. Nichols DG: Respiratory muscle performance in infants and children. J Pediatr 118:493, 1991.

291. Garay SM, Turino GM, Goldring RM: Sustained reversal of chronic hypercapnia in patients with alveolar hypoventilation syndromes. Long-term maintenance with noninvasive nocturnal mechanical ventilation. Am J Med 70:269, 1981.

292. Frates RC Jr, Splaingard ML, Smith EO, et al: Outcome of home mechanical ventilation in children. J Pediatr 106:850, 1985.

293. Splaingard ML, Frates RC Jr, Jefferson LS: Home negative pressure ventilation: report of 20 years of experience in patients with neuromuscular disease. Arch Phys Med Rehab 66:239, 1985.

294. Miyasaka K: Mechanical ventilation. In Holbrook PR (ed): Textbook of Pediatric Critical Care. Philadelphia, WB Saunders Company, 1993, p 442.

295. Martin LD, Bratton SL, Walker L: Principles and practice of respiratory support and mechanical ventilation. In Rogers MC, Nichols DG (eds): Textbook of Pediatric Intensive Care. 3rd ed. Baltimore, Williams & Wilkins, 1996, p 265.

296. Haddad C, Richards CC: Mechanical ventilation of infants: significance and elimination of ventilator compression volume. Anesthesiology 29:365, 1968.

297. Farstad T, Bratlid D: Effects of endotracheal tube size and ventilator settings on the mechanics of a test system during intermittent flow ventilation. Pediatr Pulmonol 11:15, 1991.

298. Weissman C: Flow-volume relationships during spontaneous breathing through endotracheal tubes. Crit Care Med 20:615, 1992.

299. Banner MJ, Kirby RR, Blanch PB: Site of pressure measurement during spontaneous breathing with continuous positive airway pressure: effect on calculating imposed work of breathing. Crit Care Med 20:528, 1992.

300. Banner MJ, Blanch PB, Kirby RR: Imposed work of breathing and methods of triggering a demand-flow, continuous positive airway pressure system. Crit Care Med 21:183, 1993.

301. Nishimura M, Hess D, Kacmarek RM: The response of flow-triggered infant ventilators. Am J Respir Crit Care Med 152(6 pt 1):1901, 1995.

302. Nishimura M, Imanaka H, Yoshiya I, et al: Comparison of inspiratory work of breathing between flow-triggered and pressure-triggered demand flow systems in rabbits. Crit Care Med 22:1002, 1994.

303. Sassoon CS, Del Rosario N, Fei R, et al: Influence of pressure- and flow-triggered synchronous intermittent mandatory ventilation on inspiratory muscle work. Crit Care Med 22:1933, 1994.

304. Connolly JP: Hemodynamic measurements during a tension pneumothorax. Crit Care Med 21:294, 1993.

305. Baumann MH, Sahn SA: Tension pneumothorax: diagnostic and therapeutic pitfalls. Crit Care Med 21:177, 1993.

306. Taylor J, Dibbins A, Sobel DB: Neonatal pneumomediastinum: indications for, and complication of, treatment. Crit Care Med 21:296, 1993.

307. Powner DJ: Pulmonary barotrauma in the intensive care unit. J Intensive Care Med 3:224, 1988.

308. Parker JC, Hernandez LA, Peevy KJ: Mechanism of ventilator-induced lung injury. Crit Care Med 21:131, 1993.

309. Lee KH, Lim TK: Ventilatory strategies for acute respiratory distress syndrome [review]. Ann Acad Med Singapore 27:409, 1998.

310. Fukunaga T, Davies P, Zhang L, et al: Prolonged high intermittent positive-pressure ventilation induces airway remodeling and reactivity in young rats. Am J Physiol 275(3 pt 1):L567, 1998.

311. Gannon CM, Wiswell TE, Spitzer AR: Volutrauma, PaCO2 levels, and neurodevelopmental sequelae following assisted ventilation [review]. Clin Perinatol 25:159, 1998.

312. Finfer S, Rocker G: Alveolar overdistension is an important mechanism of persistent lung damage following severe protracted ARDS. Anaesth Intensive Care 24:569, 1996.

313. Dorinsky PM, Hamlin RL, Gadek JE: Alterations in regional blood flow during positive end-expiratory pressure ventilation. Crit Care Med 15:106, 1987.

314. Lamm WJE, Kirk KR, Hanson WL: Flow through zone 1 lungs utilizes alveolar corner vessels. J Appl Physiol 70:1518, 1991.

315. Kiiski R, Takala J, Kari A, et al: Effect of tidal volume on gas exchange and oxygen transport in the adult respiratory distress syndrome. Am Rev Respir Dis 146:1131, 1992.

316. Carlton DP, Cummings JJ, Scheerer RG: Lung overexpansion increases pulmonary microvascular protein permeability in young lambs. J Appl Physiol 69:577, 1990.

317. Ring JC, Stidham GL: Novel therapies for acute respiratory failure [review]. Pediatr Clin North Am 41:1325, 1994.

318. Tuxen DV: Permissive hypercapnic ventilation [review]. Am J Respir Crit Care Med 150:870, 1994.

319. Suter PM, Fairley B, Isenberg MD: Optimum end-expiratory airway pressure in patients with acute pulmonary failure. N Engl J Med 292:284, 1975.

320. Martin LD, Wetzel RC, Bilenki AL: Airway pressure release ventilation in a neonatal lamb model of acute lung injury. Crit Care Med 19:373, 1991.

321. Simbruner G: Inadvertent positive end-expiratory pressure in mechanically ventilated newborn infants: detection and effect on lung mechanics and gas exchange. J Pediatr 108:589, 1986.

322. Bancalari E: Inadvertent positive end-expiratory pressure during mechanical ventilation. J Pediatr 108:567, 1986.

323. Hess DR, Medoff BD: Mechanical ventilation of the patient with chronic obstructive pulmonary disease [review]. Respir Care Clin North Am 4:439, 1998.

324. Rossing TH, Slutsky AS, Lehr JL: Tidal volume and frequency dependence of carbon dioxide elimination by high-frequency ventilation. N Engl J Med 305:1375, 1981.

325. Sjostrand UH, Smith RB: Overview of high frequency ventilation. Int Anesth Clin 21:1, 1983.

326. Carlon GC, Ray C Jr, Klain M, et al: High-frequency positive-pressure ventilation in management of patient with bronchopleural fistula. Anesthesiology 52:160, 1980.

327. Anonymous: High-frequency oscillatory ventilation compared with conventional mechanical ventilation in the treatment of respiratory failure in preterm infants. The HIFI study group. N Engl J Med 320:88, 1989.

328. Froese AB, Butler PO, Fletcher WA, et al: High-frequency oscillatory ventilation in premature infants with respiratory failure: a preliminary report. Anesth Analg 66:814, 1987.

329. Plavka R, Kopecky P, Sebron V, et al: A prospective randomized comparison of conventional mechanical ventilation and very early high frequency oscillatory ventilation in extremely premature newborns with respiratory distress syndrome. Intensive Care Med 25:68, 1999.

330. Bryan AC, Froese AB: Reflections on the HIFI trial. Pediatrics 87:565, 1991.

331. Cools F, Offringa M: Meta-analysis of elective high frequency ventilation in preterm infants with respiratory distress syndrome. Arch Dis Child Fetal Neonatal Ed 80:F15, 1999.

332. Kinsela JP, Clark RH: High-frequency oscillatory ventilation in pediatric critical care. Crit Care Med 21:174, 1993.

333. Arnold JH, Hanson JH, Toro-Figuero LO, et al: Prospective, randomized comparison of high-frequency oscillatory ventilation and conventional mechanical ventilation in pediatric respiratory failure. Crit Care Med 22:1530, 1994.

334. Rasanen J, Leijala M: Breathing circuit respiratory work in infants recovering from respiratory failure. Crit Care Med 19:31, 1991.

335. MacIntyre NR: Respiratory function during pressure support ventilation. Chest 89:677, 1986.

336. Kanak R, Fahey PJ, Vanderwarf C: Oxygen cost of breathing. Changes dependent upon mode of mechanical ventilation. Chest 87:126, 1985.

337. Tokioka H, Nagano O, Ohta Y, et al: Pressure support ventilation augments spontaneous breathing with improved thoracoabdominal synchrony in neonates with congenital heart disease. Anesth Analg 85:789, 1997.

338. Ng SP, Tan TH, Gomez JM: A retrospective study of infants with severe persistent pulmonary hypertension (PPHN) managed without extracorporeal membrane oxygenation (ECMO). Ann Acad Med Singapore 27:366, 1998.

339. Wilson JM, Lund DP, Lillehei CW, et al: Congenital diaphragmatic hernia—a tale of two cities: the Boston experience. J Pediatr Surg 32:401, 1997.

340. Azarow K, Messineo A, Pearl R, et al: Congenital diaphragmatic hernia—a tale of two cities: the Toronto experience. J Pediatr Surg 32:395, 1997.
341. Schindler MB: Strategies to prevent chronic neonatal lung disease [review]. J Paediatr Child Health 32:477, 1996.
342. MacIntyre NM: Respiratory function during pressure support ventilation. Chest 89:677, 1986.
343. MacIntyre NM: Pressure support ventilation: effects on ventilatory reflexes and ventilatory-muscle workloads. Respir Care 32:447, 1987.
344. Viale JP, Annat GJ, Bouffard YM: Oxygen cost of breathing in postoperative patients. Chest 93:506, 1988.
345. Akashi M, Sakanaka K, Noguchi H, et al: Flow-regulated continuous positive airway pressure to minimize imposed work of breathing. Crit Care Med 18:999, 1990.
346. Anene O, Meert KL, Uy H, et al: Dexamethasone for the prevention of postextubation airway obstruction: a prospective, randomized, double-blind, placebo-controlled trial. Crit Care Med 24:1666, 1996.
347. Shemie S: Steroids for anything that swells: dexamethasone and postextubation airway obstruction. Crit Care Med 24:1613, 1996.
348. Habib DM, Garner SS, Brandeburg S: Effect of helium-oxygen on delivery of albuterol in a pediatric, volume-cycled, ventilated lung model. Pharmacotherapy 19:143, 1999.
349. Hollman G, Shen G, Zeng L, et al: Helium-oxygen improves Clinical Asthma Scores in children with acute bronchiolitis. Crit Care Med 26:1731, 1998.
350. Tobias JD: Heliox in children with airway obstruction [review]. Pediatr Emerg Care 13:29, 1997.
351. Kudukis TM, Manthous CA, Schmidt GA, et al: Inhaled helium-oxygen revisited: effect of inhaled helium-oxygen during the treatment of status asthmaticus in children. J Pediatr 130:217, 1997.
352. Carter ER, Webb CR, Moffitt DR: Evaluation of heliox in children hospitalized with acute severe asthma. A randomized crossover trial. Chest 109:1256, 1996.
353. AAP Committee on Fetus and Newborn: Surfactant replacement therapy for respiratory distress syndrome. Pediatrics 87:946, 1991.
354. Avery ME, Merritt TA: Surfactant-replacement therapy. N Engl J Med 324:910, 1991.
355. Couser RJ, Ferrara B, Ebert J: Effects of exogenous surfactant therapy on dynamic compliance during mechanical breathing in preterm infants with hyaline membrane disease. J Pediatr 116:119, 1990.
356. Bose C, Corber A, Bose G: Improved outcome at 28 days of age for very low birth weight infants treated with a single dose of a synthetic surfactant. J Pediatr 117:947, 1990.
357. Kendig JW, Notter RH, Cox C: A comparison of surfactant as immediate prophylaxis and as rescue therapy in newborns of less than 30 weeks' gestation. N Engl J Med 324:865, 1991.
358. Dunn MS, Shennan AT, Zayack D, et al: Bovine surfactant replacement therapy in neonates of less than 30 weeks' gestation: a randomized controlled trial of prophylaxis versus treatment. Pediatrics 87:377, 1991.
359. Merritt TA, Hallman M, Berry C: Randomized, placebo-controlled trial of human surfactant given at birth versus rescue administration in very low birth weight infants with lung immaturity. J Pediatr 118:581, 1991.
360. Auten RL, Notter RH, Kendig JW: Surfactant treatment of full-term newborns with respiratory failure. Pediatrics 87:101, 1991.
361. Lotze A, Knight GR, Martin GR: Improved pulmonary outcome after exogenous surfactant therapy for respiratory failure in term infants requiring extracorporeal membrane oxygenation. J Pediatr 122:261, 1993.
362. Lachmann B: Animal models and clinical pilot studies of surfactant replacement in adult respiratory distress syndrome [abstract]. Eur Respir J 2:98s, 1989.
363. Baker CS, Evans TW, Randle BJ, et al: Damage to surfactant-specific protein in acute respiratory distress syndrome. Lancet 353:1232, 1999.
364. Lutz C, Carney D, Finck C, et al: Aerosolized surfactant improves pulmonary function in endotoxin-induced lung injury. Am J Respir Crit Care Med 158:840, 1998.
365. Robertson B: Surfactant inactivation and surfactant therapy in acute respiratory distress syndrome (ARDS) [review]. Monaldi Arch Chest Dis 53:64, 1998.
366. Gregory TJ, Steinberg KP, Spragg R, et al: Bovine surfactant therapy for patients with acute respiratory distress syndrome. Am J Respir Crit Care Med 155:1309, 1997.
367. Evans DA, Wilmott RW, Whitsett JA: Surfactant replacement therapy for adult respiratory distress syndrome in children [review]. Pediatr Pulmonol 21:328, 1996.
368. Walmrath D, Gunther A, Ghofrani HA, et al: Bronchoscopic surfactant administration in patients with severe adult respiratory distress syndrome and sepsis. Am J Respir Crit Care Med 154:57, 1996.
369. Anzueto A, Baughman RP, Guntupalli KK, et al: Aerosolized surfactant in adults with sepsis-induced acute respiratory distress syndrome. Exosurf Acute Respiratory Distress Syndrome Sepsis Study Group. N Engl J Med 334:1417, 1996.
370. Bancalari E: Intratracheal pulmonary ventilation in neonatal respiratory failure. Crit Care Med 27:18, 1999.
371. Schnitzer JJ, Thompson JE, Hedrick HL: A new ventilator improves CO2 removal in newborn lambs with congenital diaphragmatic hernia. Crit Care Med 27:109, 1999.
372. Rossi N, Kolobow T, Aprigliano M, et al: Intratracheal pulmonary ventilation at low airway pressures in a ventilator-induced model of acute respiratory failure improves lung function and survival. Chest 114:1147, 1998.
373. Handman H, Rais-Bahrami K, Rivera O, et al: Use of intratracheal pulmonary ventilation versus conventional ventilation in meconium aspiration syndrome in a newborn pig model. Crit Care Med 25:2025, 1997.
374. Barnes SD: Intratracheal pulmonary ventilation versus conventional ventilation in a model of meconium aspiration: searching for a safer and more efficient ventilation modality. Crit Care 25:1947, 1997.
375. Giacomini M, Kolobow T, Reali-Forster C, et al: Intratracheal pulmonary ventilation and continuous positive airway pressure in a sheep model of severe acute respiratory failure. Chest 112:1060, 1997.
376. Makhoul IR, Bar-Joseph G, Blazer S, et al: Intratracheal pulmonary ventilation in premature infants and children with intractable hypercapnia. ASAIO J 44:82, 1998.
377. Clark LC: Survival of mammals breathing organic liquids equilibrated with oxygen at atmospheric pressure. Science 152:1755, 1966.
378. Greenspan JS, Wolfson MR, Rubenstein SD, et al: Liquid ventilation of human preterm neonates. J Pediatr 117:106, 1990.
379. Fuhrman BP, Paczan PR, DeFrancisis M: Perfluorocarbon-associated gas exchange. Crit Care Med 19:712, 1991.
380. Bartlett RH: Liquid ventilation: background and clinical trials [review]. Pediatr Pulmonol Suppl 18:182, 1999.
381. Day SE, Gedeit RG: Liquid ventilation [review]. Clin Perinatol 25:711, 1998.
382. Greenspan JS, Cleary GM, Wolfson MR: Is liquid ventilation a reasonable alternative? [review]. Clin Perinatol 25:137, 1998.
383. Greenspan JS, Fox WW, Rubenstein SD, et al: Partial liquid ventilation in critically ill infants receiving extracorporeal life support. Philadelphia Liquid Ventilation Consortium. Pediatrics 99:E2, 1997.
384. Weis CM, Wolfson MR, Shaffer TH: Liquid-assisted ventilation: physiology and clinical application [review]. Ann Med 29:509, 1997.
385. Pranikoff T, Gauger PG, Hirschl RB: Partial liquid ventilation in newborn patients with congenital diaphragmatic hernia. J Pediatr Surg 31:613, 1996.
386. Leach CL, Greenspan JS, Rubenstein SD, et al: Partial liquid ventilation with perflubron in premature infants with severe respiratory distress syndrome. The LiquiVent Study Group. N Engl J Med 335:761, 1996.
387. Arnold JH: Liquid breathing: stretching the technological envelope. Crit Care Med 24:4, 1996.
388. Gauger PG, Pranikoff T, Schreiner RJ, et al: Initial experience with partial liquid ventilation in pediatric patients with the acute respiratory distress syndrome. Crit Care Med 24:16, 1996.
389. Cannon ML, Cheifetz IM, Craig DM, et al: Optimizing liquid ventilation as a lung protection strategy for neonatal cardiopulmonary bypass: full functional residual capacity dosing is more effective than half functional residual capacity dosing. Crit Care Med 27:1140, 1999.
390. Meaney JF, Kazerooni EA, Garver KA, et al: Acute respiratory distress syndrome: CT findings during partial liquid ventilation. Radiology 202:507, 1997.
391. Garver KA, Kazerooni EA, Hirschl RB, et al: Neonates with congenital diaphragmatic hernia: radiographic findings during partial liquid ventilation. Radiology 200:219, 1996.
392. Doctor A, Ibla JC, Grenier BM, et al: Pulmonary blood flow distribution during partial liquid ventilation. J Appl Physiol 84:1540, 1998.

393. Moya FR, Lanos AJ, Rios AM, et al: Repeated doses of the perfluoro-carbon FC-100 improve lung function of preterm lambs. Pediatr Res 42:893, 1997.

394. Steinhorn DM, Leach CL, Fuhrman BP, et al: Partial liquid ventilation enhances surfactant phospholipid production. Crit Care Med 24:1252, 1996.

395. Bruch LA, Flint A, Hirschl RB: Pulmonary pathology of patients treated with partial liquid ventilation. Mod Pathol 10:463, 1997.

396. Colton DM, Till GO, Johnson KJ, et al: Neutrophil accumulation is reduced during partial liquid ventilation. Crit Care Med 26:1716, 1998.

397. Rotta AT, Steinhorn DM: Partial liquid ventilation reduces pulmonary neutrophil accumulation in an experimental model of systemic endotoxemia and acute lung injury. Crit Care Med 26:1707, 1998.

398. Quintel M, Heine M, Hirschl RB, et al: Effects of partial liquid ventilation on lung injury in a model of acute respiratory failure: a histologic and morphometric analysis. Crit Care Med 26:833, 1998.

399. Roberts JD, Polaner DM, Lang P, et al: Inhaled nitric oxide in persistent pulmonary hypertension of the newborn. Lancet 340:818, 1992.

400. Atz AM, Adatia I, Lock JE, et al: Combined effects of nitric oxide and oxygen during acute pulmonary vasodilator testing. J Am Coll Cardiol 33:813, 1999.

401. Russell IA, Zwass MS, Fineman JR, et al: The effects of inhaled nitric oxide on postoperative pulmonary hypertension in infants and children undergoing surgical repair of congenital heart disease. Anesth Analg 87:46, 1998.

402. Dobyns EL, Cornfield DN, Anas NG, et al: Multicenter randomized controlled trial of the effects of inhaled nitric oxide therapy on gas exchange in children with acute hypoxemic respiratory failure. J Pediatr 134:406, 1999.

403. Bohn D: Nitric oxide in acute hypoxic respiratory failure: from the bench to the bedside and back again [review]. J Pediatr 134:387, 1999.

404. Bland RD: Inhaled nitric oxide: a premature remedy for chronic lung disease? Pediatrics 103:667, 1999.

405. Banks BA, Seri I, Ischiropoulos H, et al: Changes in oxygenation with inhaled nitric oxide in severe bronchopulmonary dysplasia. Pediatrics 103:610, 1999.

406. Cheung PY, Peliowski A, Robertson CM: The outcome of very low birth weight neonates (< /=1500 g) rescued by inhaled nitric oxide: neurodevelopment in early childhood. J Pediatr 133:735, 1998.

407. Greene JH, Klinger JR: The efficacy of inhaled nitric oxide in the treatment of acute respiratory distress syndrome. An evidence-based medicine approach. Crit Care Clin 14:387, 1998.

408. Nelin LD, Hoffman GM: The use of inhaled nitric oxide in a wide variety of clinical problems [review]. Pediatr Clin North Am 45:531, 1998.

409. Kinsella JP, Abman SH: Controversies in the use of inhaled nitric oxide therapy in the newborn [review]. Clin Perinatol 25:203, 1998.

410. Ream RS, Hauver JF, Lynch RE, et al: Low-dose inhaled nitric oxide improves the oxygenation and ventilation of infants and children with acute, hypoxemic respiratory failure. Crit Care Med 27:989, 1999.

411. Tibby S, Shemie S: Low-dose inhaled nitric oxide and oxygenation in pediatric hypoxic respiratory failure. Wrong bullet, wrong target. Crit Care Med 27:871, 1999.

412. Tang SF, Sherwood MC, Miller OI: Randomised trial of three doses of inhaled nitric oxide in acute respiratory distress syndrome. Arch Dis Child 79:415, 1998.

413. Lum LC, Tan PS, Saville A, et al: Occult nitric oxide inhalation improves oxygenation in mechanically ventilated children. J Pediatr 133:613, 1998.

414. Okamoto K, Hamaguchi M, Kukita I, et al: Efficacy of inhaled nitric oxide in children with ARDS. Chest 114:827, 1998.

415. Rosenberg AA: Inhaled nitric oxide in the premature infant with severe hypoxemic respiratory failure: a time for caution. J Pediatr 133:720, 1998.

416. Christou H, Magnani B, Morse DS, et al: Inhaled nitric oxide does not affect adenosine 5'-diphosphate-dependent platelet activation in infants with persistent pulmonary hypertension of the newborn. Pediatrics 102:1390, 1998.

417. Moenkhoff M, Schmitt B, Wohlrab G, et al: Electroencephalogram changes during inhalation with nitric oxide in the pediatric intensive care patient—a preliminary report. Crit Care Med 26:1887, 1998.

418. Kochanek PM, Venkataraman S, Whalen MJ, et al: Is the administration of inhaled nitric oxide (NO) associated with electroencephalogram abnormalities? There is NO harm in looking [review]. Crit Care Med 26:1788, 1998.

419. Hallman M, Bry K, Turbow R, et al: Pulmonary toxicity associated with nitric oxide in term infants with severe respiratory failure. J Pediatr 132:827, 1998.

420. George TN, Johnson KJ, Bates JN, et al: The effect of inhaled nitric oxide therapy on bleeding time and platelet aggregation in neonates. J Pediatr 132:731, 1998.

421. Sokol GM, Van Meurs KP, Wright LL, et al: Nitrogen dioxide formation during inhaled nitric oxide therapy. Clin Chem 45:382, 1999.

422. Kinsella JP, Abman SH: High-frequency oscillatory ventilation augments the response to inhaled nitric oxide in persistent pulmonary hypertension of the newborn: Nitric Oxide Study Group. Chest 114(Suppl):100S, 1998.

423. Hoehn T, Krause M, Hentschel R: High-frequency ventilation augments the effect of inhaled nitric oxide in persistent pulmonary hypertension of the newborn. Eur Respir J 11:234, 1998.

424. Ziegler JW, Ivy DD, Wiggins JW, et al: Effects of dipyridamole and inhaled nitric oxide in pediatric patients with pulmonary hypertension. Am J Respir Crit Care Med 158(1 pt 1):1388, 1998.

425. Martinez M, Diaz E, Joseph D, et al: Improvement in oxygenation by prone position and nitric oxide in patients with acute respiratory distress syndrome. Intensive Care Med 25:29, 1999.

426. Jolliet P, Bulpa P, Chevrolet JC: Effects of the prone position on gas exchange and hemodynamics in severe acute respiratory distress syndrome. Crit Care Med 26:1977, 1998.

427. Trottier SJ: Prone position in acute respiratory distress syndrome: turning over an old idea [review]. Crit Care Med 26:1934, 1998.

428. German P, Poschl G, Leitner C, et al: Additive effect of nitric oxide inhalation on the oxygenation benefit of the prone position in the adult respiratory distress syndrome. Anesthesiology 89:1401, 1998.

429. Dries DJ: Prone positioning in acute lung injury [review]. J Trauma 45:849, 1998.

430. Pappert D, Rossaint R, Slama K, et al: Influence of positioning on ventilation-perfusion relationships in severe adult respiratory distress syndrome. Chest 106:1511, 1994.

431. Yeh TF, Lilien LD, Leu ST, et al: Increased O2 consumption and energy loss in premature infants following medical care procedures. Biol Neonate 46:157, 1984.

432. McCann EM, Lewis K, Deming DD: Controlled trial of furosemide therapy in infants with chronic lung disease. J Pediatr 106:957, 1985.

433. Kao LC, Warburton D, Sargent CW: Furosemide acutely decreases airways resistance in chronic bronchopulmonary dysplasia. J Pediatr 103:624, 1983.

434. Trotter C, Serpell MG: Neurologic sequelae in children after prolonged propofol infusion. Anaesthesia 47:340, 1992.

435. Bray RJ: Propofol infusion syndrome in children [review]. Paediatr Anaesth 8:491, 1998.

436. Cray SH, Robinson BH, Cox PN: lactic acidemia and bradyarrhythmia in a child sedated with propofol [review]. Crit Care Med 26:2087, 1998.

437. Susla GM: Propofol toxicity in critically ill pediatric patients: show us the proof [review]. Crit Care Med 26:1959, 1998.

438. Mills JL, Spackman TJ, Borns P: The usefulness of lateral neck roentgenograms in laryngotracheitis. Am J Dis Child 133:1140, 1979.

439. Skolnik NS: Treatment of croup—a critical review. Am J Dis Child 143:1045, 1989.

440. Gardner HG, Powell KR, Roden VJ: The evaluation of racemic epinephrine in the treatment of croup. Pediatrics 52:52, 1973.

441. Schweich PJ, Smith KM, Dowd MD, et al: Pediatric emergency medicine practice patterns: a comparison of pediatric and general emergency physicians. Pediatr Emerg Care 14:89, 1998.

442. Rizos JD, DiGravio BE, Sehl MJ, et al: The disposition of children with croup treated with racemic epinephrine and dexamethasone in the emergency department. J Emerg Med 16:535, 1998.

443. Thomas LP, Friedland LR: The cost-effective use of nebulized racemic epinephrine in the treatment of croup. Am J Emerg Med 16:87, 1998.

444. Kunkel NC, Baker MD: Use of racemic epinephrine, dexamethasone, and mist in the outpatient management of croup. Pediatr Emerg Care 12:156, 1996.

445. Kairys SW, Olmstead EM, O'Connor GT: Steroid treatment of laryngotracheitis: a meta-analysis of the evidence from randomized trials. Pediatrics 83:683, 1989.

446. Smith DS: Corticosteroids in croup: a chink in the ivory tower? J Pediatr 115:256, 1989.
447. Super DM, Cartelli NA, Brooks LJ: A prospective randomized double-blind study to evaluate the effect of dexamethasone in acute laryngotracheitis. J Pediatr 115:323, 1989.
448. Geelhoed GC: Croup [review]. Pediatr Pulmonol 23:370, 1997.
449. Fitzgerald D, Mellis C, Johnson M, et al: Nebulized budesonide is as effective as nebulized adrenaline in moderately severe croup. Pediatrics 97:722, 1996.
450. McEniery J, Gillis J, Kilham H, et al: Review of intubation in severe laryngotrachetis. Pediatrics 87:847, 1991.
451. Margolis CZ, Coletti RB, Grundy G: Haemophilus influenza, type B: the etiologic agent in epiglottitis. J Pediatr 87:322, 1975.
452. AAP Committee on Infectious Diseases: Haemophilus influenzae type b conjugate vaccines: recommendations for immunization with recently and previously licensed vaccines. Pediatrics 92:480, 1993.
453. Murphy TV, White KE, Pastor P: Declining incidence of Haemophilus influenzae type B disease since introduction of vaccination. JAMA 269:246, 1993.
454. Adams WG, Deaver KA, Cochi SL: Decline of childhood haemophilus influenzae type B (Hib) disease in the Hib vaccine era. JAMA 269:221, 1993.
455. Broadhurst LE, Erickson RL, Kelley PW: Decreases in invasive haemophilus influenzae diseases in US Army children, 1984 through 1991. JAMA 269:227, 1993.
456. Shapiro J, Eavey RD, Baker AS: Adult supraglottitis: a prospective analysis. JAMA 259:563, 1988.
457. Givner LB, Abramson JS, Wasilauskas B: Apparent increase in the incidence of invasive group A b-hemolytic streptococcal disease in children. J Pediatr 118:341, 1991.
458. Rapkin RH: The diagnosis of epiglottitis: simplicity and reliability of radiographs of the neck in the differential diagnosis of the croup syndrome. J Pediatr 80:96, 1972.
459. Kilham H, Gillis J, Benjamin B: Severe upper airway obstruction. Pediatr Clin North Am 34:1, 1987.
460. Duncan PG: Management of upper airway disease in children. In Gregory GA (ed): Clinics in Critical Care Medicine: Respiratory Failure in the Child. New York, Churchill Livingstone, 1981, p 66.
461. Rapkin RH: Tracheostomy in epiglottitis. Pediatrics 52:426, 1973.
462. Rapkin RH: Nasotracheal intubation in epiglottitis. Pediatrics 56:110, 1975.
463. Warner LO, Beach TP, Martino JD: Negative pressure pulmonary oedema secondary to airway obstruction in an intubated infant. Can J Anaesth 35:507, 1988.
464. Galvis AG: Pulmonary edema complicating relief of upper airway obstruction. Am J Emerg Med 5:294, 1987.
465. Helfaer MA, Nichols DG, Rogers MC: Lower airway disease: bronchiolitis and asthma. In Rogers MC, Nichols DG (eds): Textbook of Pediatric Intensive Care. 3rd ed. Baltimore, Williams & Wilkins, 1996, p 127.
466. Berger I, Argaman Z, Schwartz SB, et al: Efficacy of corticosteroids in acute bronchiolitis: short-term and long-term follow-up. Pediatr Pulmonol 26:162, 1998.
467. Sanchez I, DeKoster J, Powell RE: Effect of racemic epinephrine and salbutamol on clinical score and pulmonary mechanics in infants with bronchiolitis. J Pediatr 122:145, 1993.
468. LaVia WV, Marks MI, Stutman HR: Respiratory syncytial virus puzzle: clinical features, pathophysiology, treatment, and prevention. J Pediatr 121:503, 1992.
469. Pullan CR, Hey EN: Wheezing, asthma, and pulmonary dysfunction 10 years after infection with respiratory syncytial virus in infancy. BMJ 284:1665, 1982.
470. Garofalo R, Kimpen JLL, Welliver RC, et al: Eosinophil degranulation in the respiratory tract during naturally acquired respiratory syncytial virus infection. J Pediatr 120:28, 1992.
471. Sorkness R, Lemanske RF Jr, Castleman WL: Persistent airway hyper-responsiveness after neonatal viral bronchiolitis in rats. J Appl Physiol 70:375, 1991.
472. Rodriguez WJ, Arrobio J, Fink R, et al: Prospective follow-up and pulmonary functions from a placebo-controlled randomized trial of ribavirin therapy in respiratory syncytial virus bronchiolitis. Ribavirin Study Group. Arch Pediatr Adolesc Med 153:469, 1999.
473. Martinez FD, Stern DA, Wright AL, et al: Differential immune responses to acute lower respiratory illness in early life and subsequent development of persistent wheezing and asthma. J Allergy Clin Immunol 102(6 pt 1):915, 1998.
474. Oymar K, Bjerknes R: Differential patterns of circulating adhesion molecules in children with bronchial asthma and acute bronchiolitis. Pediatr Allergy Immunol 9:73, 1998.
475. Smith DS, Frankel LR, Mathers LH: A controlled trial of aerosolized ribavirin in infants receiving mechanical ventilation for severe respiratory syncytial virus infection. N Engl J Med 325:24, 1991.
476. Englund JA, Piedra PA, Jefferson LS: High-dose, short-duration ribavirin aerosol therapy in children with suspected respiratory syncytial virus infection. J Pediatr 117:313, 1990.
477. Outwater KM, Meissner HC, Peterson MB: Ribavirin administration to infants receiving mechanical ventilation. Am J Dis Child 142:512, 1988.
478. Nelson DR, Sachs MI, O'Connell EJ: Approaches to acute asthma and status asthmaticus in children. Mayo Clin Proc 64:1392, 1989.
479. Downes JJ, Heiser MS: Status asthmaticus in children. In Gregory GA (ed): Clinics in Critical Care Medicine: Respiratory Failure in the Child. New York, Churchill Livingstone, 1981, p 107.
480. Cohen NH, Eigen H, Shaughnessy TE: Status asthmaticus [review]. Crit Care Clin 13:459, 1997.
481. Barnes PJ: A new approach to the treatment of asthma. N Engl J Med 321:1517, 1989.
482. Larsen GL: Asthma in children. N Engl J Med 326:1540, 1992.
483. McFadden ER, Gilbert IA: Asthma. N Engl J Med 327:1928, 1992.
484. Nichols DG: Emergency management of status asthmaticus in children. Pediatr Ann 25:394, 1996.
485. Schuh S, Parkin P, Rajan A: High- versus low-dose, frequently administered, nebulized albuterol in children with severe, acute asthma. Pediatrics 83:513, 1989.
486. Schuh S, Reider MJ, Canny G: Nebulized albuterol in acute childhood asthma: comparison of two doses. Pediatrics 86:509, 1990.
487. Kelly HW, McWilliams BC, Katz R, et al: Safety of frequent high dose nebulized terbutaline in children with acute severe asthma. Ann Allergy 64:229, 1990.
488. Portnoy J, Aggarwal J: Continuous terbutaline nebulization for the treatment of severe exacerbations of asthma in children. Ann Allergy 60:368, 1988.
489. Craig VL, Bigos D, Brilli RJ: Efficacy and safety of continuous albuterol nebulization in children with severe status asthmaticus. Pediatr Emerg Care 12:1, 1996.
490. Khine H, Fuchs SM, Saville AL: Continuous vs intermittent nebulized albuterol for emergency management of asthma. Acad Emerg Med 3:1019, 1996.
491. Moler FW, Johnson CE, Van Laanen C, et al: Continuous versus intermittent nebulized terbutaline: plasma levels and effects. Am J Respir Crit Care Med 153(3 pt 1):602, 1995.
492. Katz RW, Kelly HW, Crowley MR, et al: Safety of continuous nebulized albuterol for bronchospasm in infants and children [published erratum appears in Pediatrics 93(2):A28, 1994]. Pediatrics 92:666, 1993.
493. Papo MC, Frank J, Thompson AE: A prospective, randomized study of continuous versus intermittent nebulized albuterol for severe status asthmaticus in children. Crit Care Med 21:1479, 1993.
494. Tal A, Levy N, Bearman JE: Methylprednisolone therapy for acute asthma in infants and toddlers: a controlled clinical trial. Pediatrics 86:350, 1990.
495. Ratto D, Alfaro C, Sipsey J: Are intravenous corticosteroids required in status asthmaticus? JAMA 260:527, 1988.
496. Gross NJ: Ipratropium bromide. N Engl J Med 319:486, 1988.
497. Freeman J, Landau LI: The effects of ipratropium bromide and fenoterol nebulizer solutions in children with asthma. Clin Pediatr 28:556, 1989.
498. Beakes DE: The use of anticholinergics in asthma [review]. J Asthma 34:357, 1997.
499. McDowel KM, Chatburn RL, Myers TR, et al: A cost-saving algorithm for children hospitalized for status asthmaticus. Arch Pediatr Adolesc Med 152:977, 1998.
500. Levy J, Kolski GB: The use of theophylline clearance in pediatric status asthmaticus. II: The choice of appropriate dose for the intravenous theophylline infusion. Am J Dis Child 141:288, 1987.
501. Fuglsang G, Pedersen S, Borgstrom L: Dose-response relationships of intravenously administered terbutaline in children with asthma. J Pediatr 114:315, 1989.

502. Stephanopoulos DE, Monge R, Schell KH, et al: Continuous intravenous terbutaline for pediatric status asthmaticus. Crit Care Med 26:1744, 1998.
503. DeNicola LK, Monem GF, Gayle MO, et al: Treatment of critical status asthmaticus in children. Pediatr Clin North Am 41:1293, 1994.
504. Wetzel RC: Pressure-support ventilation in children with severe asthma. Crit Care Med 24:1603, 1996.
505. O'Rourke PP, Crone RK: Halothane in status asthmaticus. Crit Care Med 10:341, 1982.
506. Schwartz SH: Treatment of status asthmaticus with halothane. JAMA 251:2688, 1984.
507. Arnold JH, Truog RD, Rice SA: Prolonged administration of isoflurane to pediatric patients during mechanical ventilation. Anesth Analg 76:502, 1993.
508. Rice M, Hatherill M, Murdoch IA: Rapid response to isoflurane in refractory status asthmaticus [letter]. Arch Dis Child 78:395, 1998.
509. Tobias JD, Garrett JS: Therapeutic options for severe, refractory status asthmaticus: inhalational anaesthetic agents, extracorporeal membrane oxygenation and helium/oxygen ventilation. Paediatr Anaesth 7:47, 1997.
510. Nehama J, Pass R, Bechtler-Karsch A, et al: Continuous ketamine infusion for the treatment of refractory asthma in a mechanically ventilated infant: case report and review of the pediatric literature [review]. Pediatr Emerg Care 12:294, 1996.
511. Sachdeva RC, Guntupalli KK: Acute respiratory distress syndrome [review]. Crit Care Clin 13:503, 1997.
512. Bernard GR, Artigas A, Brigham KL, et al: The American-European Consensus Conference on ARDS. Definitions, mechanisms, relevant outcomes, and clinical trial coordination [review]. Am J Respir Crit Care Med 149(3 pt 1):818, 1994.
513. Fraisse A, Paut O, Viard L, et al: Recent developments in the treatment of pediatric acute respiratory distress syndrome [review] [in French]. Arch Pediatr 5:1107, 1998.
514. Beaufils F, Mercier JC, Farnoux C, et al: Acute respiratory distress syndrome in children [review]. Curr Opin Pediatr 9:207, 1997.
515. Timmons OD, Dean JM, Vernon DD: Mortality rates and prognostic variables in children with adult respiratory distress syndrome. J Pediatr 119:896, 1991.
516. Tamburro RF, Bugnitz MC, Stidham GL: Alveolar-arterial oxygen gradient as a predictor of outcome in patients with nonneonatal pediatric respiratory failure. J Pediatr 119:935, 1991.
517. Newth CJ, Stretton M, Deakers TW, et al: Assessment of pulmonary function in the early phase of ARDS in pediatric patients. Pediatr Pulmonol 23:169, 1997.
518. Meduri GU, Headley AS, Golden E, et al: Effect of prolonged methylprednisolone therapy in unresolving acute respiratory distress syndrome: a randomized controlled trial. JAMA 280:159, 1998.
519. Meduri GU, Tolley EA, Chinn A, et al: Procollagen types I and III aminoterminal propeptide levels during acute respiratory distress syndrome and in response to methylprednisolone treatment. Am J Respir Crit Care Med 158(5 pt 1):1432, 1998.
520. Richman PS, Spragg RG, Robertson B: The adult respiratory distress syndrome: first trials with surfactant replacement [abstract]. Eur Respir J 2:109s, 1989.
521. Morton NS: Exogenous surfactant treatment for the adult respiratory distress syndrome? A historical perspective. Thorax 45:825, 1990.
522. Rossaint R, Falke KJ, Loez F: Inhaled nitric oxide for the adult respiratory distress syndrome. N Engl J Med 328:399, 1993.
523. Zapol WM, Snider MT: Pulmonary hypertension in severe acute respiratory failure. N Engl J Med 296:476, 1977.
524. Gegel RL, Murphy JD, Langleben D: Congenital diaphragmatic hernia: arterial structural changes and persistent pulmonary hypertension after surgical repair. J Pediatr 107:457, 1985.
525. Hammerman C, Lass N, Strates E: prostanoids in neonates with persistent pulmonary hypertension. J Pediatr 110:470, 1987.
526. Weigel TJ, Hageman JR: National survey of diagnosis and management of persistent pulmonary hypertension of the newborn. J Perinatol 10:369, 1990.
527. Bifano EM, Pfannenstiel A: Duration of hyperventilation and outcome in infants with persistent pulmonary hypertension. Pediatrics 81:657, 1988.
528. Dworetz AR, Moya FR, Sabo B: Survival of infants with persistent pulmonary hypertension without extracorporeal membrane oxygenation. Pediatrics 84:380, 1989.
529. Marron MJ, Crisafari MA, Driscoll JM Jr: Hearing and neurodevelopmental outcome in survivors of persistent pulmonary hypertension of the newborn. Pediatrics 90:392, 1992.
530. Vane JR, Anggard EE, Botting RM: Regulatory functions of the vascular endothelium. N Engl J Med 323:27, 1990.
531. Dinh-Xuan AT, Higenbottam TW, Clelland CA: Impairment of endothelium-dependent pulmonary artery relaxation in chronic obstructive lung disease. N Engl J Med 324:1539, 1991.
532. Schreiner MS, Donar ME, Kettrick RG: Pediatric home mechanical ventilation. Pediatr Clin North Am 34:47, 1987.
533. Morray JP, Fox WW, Kettrick RG, et al: Clinical correlates of successful weaning from mechanical ventilation in severe bronchopulmonary dysplasia. Crit Care Med 9:815, 1981.
534. Gomez-Del Rio M, Gerhardt T, Hehre D: Effect of a b-agonist nebulization on lung function in neonates with increased pulmonary resistance. Pediatr Pulmonol 2:287, 1986.
535. Gilgoff IS, Kahlstrom E, MacLaughlin E, et al: Long-term ventilatory support in spinal muscular atrophy. J Pediatr 115:904, 1989.
536. Heckmatt JZ, Loh L, Dubowitz V: Nocturnal hypoventilation in children with nonprogressive neuromuscular disease. Pediatrics 83:250, 1989.
537. Fields AI, Rosenblatt A, Pollack MM, et al: Home care cost-effectiveness for respiratory technology-dependent children. Am J Dis Child 145:729, 1991.
538. Quint RD, Chesterman E, Crain LS: Home care for ventilator-dependent children. Am J Dis Child 144:1238, 1990.
539. O'Neill N: Improving ventilation in children using bilevel positive airway pressure [review]. Pediatr Nurs 24:377, 1998.
540. Villa MP, Dotta A, Castello D, et al: Bi-level positive airway pressure (BiPAP) ventilation in an infant with central hypoventilation syndrome. Pediatr Pulmonol 24:66, 1997.
541. Elixson EM, Myrer ML, Horn MH: Current trends in ventilation of the pediatric patient [review]. Crit Care Nurs Q 20:1, 1997.
542. Puri S, Chandra RK: Nutritional regulation of host resistance and predictive value of immunologic tests in assessment of outcome. Pediatr Clin North Am 32:499, 1985.
543. Sheridan R, Remensnyder J, Prelack K, et al: Treatment of the seriously burned infant. J Burn Care Rehabil 19:115, 1998.
544. Pollack MM: Nutritional failure and support in pediatric intensive care. In Shoemaker WC, Thompson WL, Holbrook PR (eds): Textbook of Critical Care. Philadelphia, WB Saunders Company, 1984, p 694.
545. Kinney JM: Nutrition in the intensive care patient. Crit Care Clin 3:1, 1987.
546. Haber BA, Deutschman CS: Nutrition and metabolism in the critically ill child. In Rogers MC, Nichols DG (eds): Textbook of Pediatric Intensive Care. 3rd ed. Baltimore, Williams & Wilkins, 1996, p 1141.
547. Witte MK: Metabolic measurements during mechanical ventilation in the pediatric intensive care unit [review]. Respir Care Clin North Am 2:573, 1996.
548. Zlotkin SH, Stallings VA, Pencharz PB: Total parenteral nutrition in children. Pediatr Clin North Am 32:381, 1985.
549. Tilden SJ, Watkins S, Tong TK, et al: Measured energy expenditure in pediatric intensive care patients. Am J Dis Child 143:490, 1989.
550. Curley MA, Castillo L: Nutrition and shock in pediatric patients [review]. New Horiz 6:212, 1998.
551. Teitelbaum DH, Coran AG: Perioperative nutritional support in pediatrics [review]. Nutrition 14:130, 1998.
552. Schears GJ, Deutschman CS: Common nutritional issues in pediatric and adult critical care medicine [review]. Crit Care Clin 13:669, 1997.
553. Deitch EA, Berg R: Bacterial translocation from the gut: a mechanism of infection. J Burn Care Rehabil 8:475, 1987.
554. Deitch EA, Winterton J, Li MA, et al: The gut as a portal of entry for bacteremia. Role of protein malnutrition. Ann Surg 205:681, 1987.
555. Alverdy JC, Aoys E, Moss GS: Total parenteral nutrition promotes bacterial translocation from the gut. Surgery 104:185, 1988.
556. Berseth CL: Effect of early feeding on maturation of the preterm infant's small intestine. J Pediatr 120:947, 1992.
557. Eibl MM, Wolf HM, Furnkranz H, et al: Prevention of necrotizing enterocolitis in low-birth-weight infants by IgA-IgG feeding. N Engl J Med 319:1, 1988.
558. Moore MC, Greene HL: Tube feeding of infants and children. Pediatr Clin North Am 32:401, 1985.

559. Verger J: Nutrition. *In* Curley MA, Smith JB, Moloney-Harmon PA (eds): Critical Care Nursing of Infants and Children. Philadelphia, WB Saunders Company, 1996, p 410.

560. Canete A, Duggan C: Nutritional support of the pediatric intensive care unit patient [review]. Curr Opin Pediatr 8:248, 1996.

561. Sadiq HF, Devaskar S, Keenan WJ, et al: Broviac catheterization in low birth weight infants: incidence and treatment of associated complications. Crit Care Med 15:47, 1987.

562. Lafeber HN, Sulkers EJ, Chapman TE, et al: Glucose production and oxidation in preterm infants during total parenteral nutrition. Pediatr Res 28:153, 1990.

563. Schulman RJ, Langston C, Schanler RJ: Pulmonary vascular lipid deposition after administration of intravenous fat to infants. Pediatrics 79:99, 1987.

564. Brans YW, Dutton EB, Andrew DS: Fat emulsion tolerance in very low birth weight neonates: effect on diffusion of oxygen in the lungs and on blood pH. Pediatrics 78:79, 1986.

565. Pierro A, Carnielli V, Filler RM: Metabolism of intravenous fat emulsion in the surgical newborn. J Pediatr Surg 24:95, 1989.

566. Hagerdal M, Caldwell CB, Gross JB: Intraoperative fluid management influences carbon dioxide production respiratory quotient. Anesthesiology 59:48, 1983.

567. Delafosse B, Bouffard Y, Viale JP, et al: Respiratory changes induced by parenteral nutrition in postoperative patients undergoing inspiratory pressure support. Anesthesiology 66:393, 1987.

568. Piedboeuf B, Chessex P, Hazan J: Total parenteral nutrition in the newborn infant: energy substrates and respiratory gas exchange. J Pediatr 118:97, 1991.

569. Kohane DS, Tobin JR, Kohane IS: Endocrine, mineral, and metabolic disease in pediatric intensive care. *In* Rogers MC, Nichols DG (eds): Textbook of Pediatric Intensive Care. 3rd ed. Baltimore, Williams & Wilkins, 1996, p 1247.

570. Burrows FA, Shutack JG, Crone RK: Inappropriate secretion of antidiuretic hormone in a postsurgical pediatric population. Crit Care Med 11:527, 1983.

571. Bell GR, Gurd AR, Orlowski JP, et al: The syndrome of inappropriate antidiuretic hormone secretion following spinal fusion. J Bone Joint Surg 68:720, 1986.

572. Brazel PW, McPhee IB: Inappropriate secretion of antidiuretic hormone in postoperative scoliosis patients: the role of fluid management. Spine 21:724, 1996.

573. Lauriat SM, Berl T: The hyponatremic patient: practical focus on therapy. J Am Soc Nephrol 8:1599, 1997.

574. Arieff AI: Treatment of symptomatic hyponatremia: neither haste nor waste. Crit Care Med 19:748, 1991.

575. Sarnaik AP, Meert K, Hackbarth R, et al: Management of hyponatremic seizures in children with hypertonic saline: a safe and effective strategy. Crit Care Med 19:758, 1991.

576. Wijdicks EF, Ropper AH, Hunnicutt EJ: Atrial naturietic factor and salt wasting after aneurysmal subarachnoid hemorrhage. Stroke 22:1519, 1991.

577. Diringer M, Ladenson PW, Borel C: Sodium and water regulation in a patient with cerebral salt wasting. Arch Neurol 46:928, 1989.

578. Zafonte RD, Mann NR: Cerebral salt wasting syndrome in brain injury patients: a potential cause of hyponatremia. Arch Phys Med Rehabil 78:540, 1997.

579. Uygun MA, Ozkal E, Acar O, et al: Cerebral salt wasting syndrome [review]. Neurosurg Rev 19:193, 1996.

580. Kappy MS, Ganong CA: Cerebral salt wasting in children: the role of atrial natriuretic hormone [review]. Adv Pediatr 43:271, 1996.

581. Levin ER, Gardner DG, Samson WK: Natriuretic peptides. N Engl J Med 339:321, 1998.

582. Damaraju SC, Rajshekhar V, Chandy MJ: Validation study of a central venous pressure-based protocol for the management of neurosurgical patients with hyponatremia and natriuresis. Neurosurgery 40:312, 1997.

583. Weise K, Zaritsky A: Endocrine manifestations of critical illness in the child. Pediatr Clin North Am 34:119, 1987.

584. Outwater KM, Rockoff MA: Diabetes insipidus accompanying brain death in children. Neurology 34:1243, 1984.

585. Baylis PH, Cheetham T: Diabetes insipidus [review]. Arch Dis Child 79:84, 1998.

586. Lugo N, Silver P, Nimkoff L, et al: Diagnosis and management algorithm of acute onset of central diabetes insipidus in critically ill children. J Pediatr Endocrinol Metab 10:633, 1997.

587. Brink SJ: Diabetic ketoacidosis [review]. Acta Paediatr Suppl 88:14, 1999.

588. Klekamp J, Churchwell KB: Diabetic ketoacidosis in children: initial clinical assessment and treatment. Pediatr Ann 25:387, 1996.

589. Rosenbloom AL, Hanas R: Diabetic ketoacidosis (DKA): treatment guidelines [review]. Clin Pediatr 35:261, 1996.

590. Glaser NS, Kuppermann N, Yee CK, et al: Variation in the management of pediatric diabetic ketoacidosis by specialty training. Arch Pediatr Adolesc Med 151:1125, 1997.

591. Menon RK, Sperling MA: Diabetic ketoacidosis. *In* Fuhrman BP, Zimmerman JJ (eds): Pediatric Critical Care. St. Louis, Mosby Year Book, 1992, p 797.

592. Green SM, Rothrock SG, Ho JD, et al: Failure of adjunctive bicarbonate to improve outcome in severe pediatric diabetic ketoacidosis [review]. Ann Emerg Med 31:41, 1998.

593. Rosenbloom AL, Rilery WJ, Weber FT: Cerebral edema complicating diabetic ketoacidosis in childhood. J Pediatr 96:357, 1980.

594. Krane EJ, Rockoff MA, Wallman KK, et al: Subclinical brain swelling in children during treatment of diabetic ketoacidosis. N Engl J Med 312:1147, 1985.

595. Rosenbloom AL: Intracerebral crises during treatment of diabetic ketoacidosis. Diabet Care 13:22, 1990.

596. Smedman L, Escobar R, Hesser U, et al: Sub-clinical cerebral oedema does not occur regularly during treatment for diabetic ketoacidosis. Acta Paediatr 86:1172, 1997.

597. Hale PM, Rezvani I, Braunstein AW, et al: Factors predicting cerebral edema in young children with diabetic ketoacidosis and new onset type I diabetes. Acta Paediatr 86:626, 1997.

598. Glasgow AM: Devastating cerebral edema in diabetic ketoacidosis before therapy [letter]. Diabetes Care 14:77, 1991.

599. Couch RM, Acott PD, Wong GW: Early onset fatal cerebral edema in diabetic ketoacidosis [letter]. Diabetes Care 14:78, 1991.

600. Roe TF, Crawford TO, Huff KR, et al: Brain infarction in children with diabetic ketoacidosis. J Diabetes Complications 10:100, 1996.

601. Thompson WL: Recognition, treatment, and prevention of poisoning. *In* Shoemaker WC, Thompson WL, Holbrook PR (eds): Textbook of Critical Care. Philadelphia, WB Saunders Company, 1984, p 801.

602. US Centers for Disease Control: Unintentional ingestions of prescription drugs in children under five years old. MMWR Morb Mortal Wkly Rep 36:124, 1987.

603. Woolf AD, Berkowitz ID, Liebelt EL, et al: Poisoning and the critically ill child. *In* Rogers MC, Nichols DG (eds): Textbook of Pediatric Intensive Care. 3rd ed. Baltimore, Williams & Wilkins, 1996, p 1315.

604. Vernon DD, Gleich MC: Poisoning and drug overdose [review]. Crit Care Clin 13:647, 1997.

605. Lembersky RB, Nichols MH, King WD: Effectiveness of child-resistant packaging on toxin procurement in young poisoning victims [review]. Vet Hum Toxicol 38:380, 1996.

606. Rumack BH: Acetaminophen overdose in children and adolescents. Pediatr Clin North Am 33:691, 1986.

607. Snodgrass WR: Salicylate toxicity. Pediatr Clin North Am 33:381, 1986.

608. Pinsky PF, Hurwitz ES, Schonberger LB, et al: Reye's syndrome and aspirin: evidence for a dose-response effect. JAMA 260:657, 1988.

609. Banner W, Tong TG: Iron poisoning. Pediatr Clin North Am 33:393, 1986.

610. Augenstein WL, Spoerke DG, Kulig KW: Fluoride ingestion in children: a review of 87 cases. Pediatrics 88:907, 1991.

611. Bertino JS, Reed MD: Barbiturate and non-barbiturate sedative hypnotic intoxication in children. Pediatr Clin North Am 33:703, 1986.

612. Smith TW, Burler VP, Haber E: Treatment of life-threatening digitalis intoxication with digoxin specific FAB antibody fragments. N Engl J Med 307:1357, 1982.

613. Zucker AR, Lacina SJ, DasGupta DS: FAB fragments of digoxin-specific antibodies used to reverse ventricular fibrillation induced by digoxin ingestion in a child. Pediatrics 70:468, 1982.

614. Woolf AD, Wenger T, Smith TW, et al: The use of digoxin-specific FAB fragments for severe digitalis intoxication in children. N Engl J Med 326:1739, 1992.

615. Fiser DH, Moss M, Walker W: Critical care for clonidine poisoning in toddlers. Crit Care Med 18:1124, 1990.

616. Frommer DA, Kulig KW, Rumack B: Tricyclic antidepressant overdose. JAMA 257:521, 1987.

617. Braden NJ, Jackson JE, Walson PD: Tricyclic antidepressant overdose. Pediatr Clin North Am 33:287, 1986.

618. Boehnert MT, Lovejoy FH: Value of the QRS duration versus the serum drug level in predicting seizures and ventricular arrhythmias after an acute overdose of tricyclic antidepressants. N Engl J Med 313:474, 1985.

619. Hestand HE, Teske DW: Diphenhydramine hydrochloride intoxication. J Pediatr 90:1017, 1977.

620. Knight ME, Roberts RJ: Phenothiazine and butyrophenone intoxication in children. Pediatr Clin North Am 33:299, 1986.

621. Kulberg A: Substance abuse: clinical identification and management. Pediatr Clin North Am 33:325, 1986.

622. Shannon M, Lovejoy FH: Effect of acute versus chronic intoxication on clinical features of theophylline poisoning in children. J Pediatr 121:125, 1992.

623. Klein BL, Simon JE: Hydrocarbon poisonings. Pediatr Clin North Am 33:411, 1986.

624. Mack RB: Hydrocarbon ingestion—to Eyre is human. Contemp Pediatr 12:47, 1991.

625. Rumack BH: Acetaminophen overdose in children and adolescents. Pediatr Clin North Am 33:691, 1986.

626. Mortensen ML: Management of acute childhood poisonings caused by selected insecticides and herbicides. Pediatr Clin North Am 33:421, 1986.

627. Litovitz T: The alcohols: ethanol, methanol, isopropanol, ethylene glycol. Pediatr Clin North Am 33:311, 1986.

628. Galliot M, Astier A, Vu B: Treatment of ethylene glycol poisoning with intravenous 4-methylpyrazole. N Engl J Med 319:97, 1988.

629. Chisolm JJ: Poisoning due to heavy metals. Pediatr Clin North Am 17:591, 1970.

630. Myers RAM, Snyder SK, Emhoff TA: Subacute sequelae of carbon monoxide poisoning. Ann Emerg Med 14:1163, 1985.

631. Lampe KF: Systemic plant poisoning in children. Pediatrics 54:347, 1974.

632. Krenzelok EP, McGuigan M, Lheur P: Position statement: ipecac syrup. American Academy of Clinical Toxicology; European Association of Poisons Centres and Clinical Toxicologists [review]. J Toxicol Clin Toxicol 35:699, 1997.

633. Vale JA: Position statement: gastric lavage. American Academy of Clinical Toxicology; European Association of Poisons Centres and Clinical Toxicologists [review]. J Toxicol Clin Toxicol 35:711, 1997.

634. Chyka PA, Seger D: Position statement: single-dose activated charcoal. American Academy of Clinical Toxicology; European Association of Poisons Centres and Clinical Toxicologists [review]. J Toxicol Clin Toxicol 35:721, 1997.

635. Burda AM, Burda NM: The nation's first poison control center: taking a stand against accidental childhood poisoning in Chicago [review]. Vet Hum Toxicol 39:115, 1997.

636. Parekh RS, Bunchman TE: Dialysis support in the pediatric intensive care unit [review]. Adv Renal Replace Ther 3:326, 1996.

637. Radovsky A, Safar P, Angelos M, et al: Histopathologic confirmation that standard external cardiopulmonary resuscitation (SECPR) can maintain brain viability in prolonged ventricular fibrillation (VF) cardiac arrest (CA) in dogs [abstract]. Crit Care Med 20:S25, 1992.

638. McGuigan MA: Acute iron poisoning [review]. Pediatr Ann 25:33, 1996.

639. Ernst A, Zibrak JD: Carbon monoxide poisoning. N Engl J Med 339:1603, 1998.

640. Brent J, McMartin K, Phillips S, et al: Fomepizole for the treatment of ethylene glycol poisoning. Methylpyrazole for Toxic Alcohols Study Group. N Engl J Med 340:832, 1999.

641. Hollander JE: The management of cocaine-associated myocardial ischemia [review]. N Engl J Med 333:1267, 1995.

642. Liebelt EL, Ulrich A, Francis PD, et al: Serial electrocardiogram changes in acute tricyclic antidepressant overdoses. Crit Care Med 25:1721, 1997.

643. Boehnert MT, Lovejoy FH Jr: Value of the QRS duration versus the serum drug level in predicting seizures and ventricular arrhythmias after an acute overdose of tricyclic antidepressants. N Engl J Med 313:474, 1985.

644. MICROMEDEX Healthcare Series. 1999. www.MICROMEDEX.com.

645. Pearson-Shaver AL, Steinhart CM: Evaluation of the poisoned child. In Holbrook PR (ed): Textbook of Pediatric Critical Care. Philadelphia, WB Saunders Company, 1993, p 982.

646. Jones AL: Mechanism of action and value of N-acetylcysteine in the treatment of early and late acetaminophen poisoning: a critical review [review]. J Toxicol Clin Toxicol 36:277, 1998.

647. Baud FJ, Barriot P, Toffis V: Elevated blood cyanide concentrations in victims of smoke inhalation. N Engl J Med 325:1761, 1991.

648. Yu CW, Sung RY, Fok TF, et al: Effects of blood transfusion on left ventricular output in premature babies. J Paediatr Child Health 34:444, 1998.

649. Welch HG, Meehan KR, Goodnough LT: Prudent strategies for elective red blood cell transfusion. Ann Intern Med 116:393, 1992.

650. Hebert PC, Wells G, Blajchman MA, et al: A multicenter, randomized, controlled clinical trial of transfusion requirements in critical care. N Engl J Med 340:409, 1999.

651. Holzman IR, Tabata B, Edelstone DI: Blood flow and oxygen delivery to the organs of the neonatal lamb as a function of hematocrit. Pediatr Res 20:1274, 1986.

652. Holzman IR, Tabata B, Edelstone DI: Effects of varying hematocrits on intestinal oxygen uptake in neonatal lambs. Am J Physiol 248:G432, 1985.

653. Simon TL, Alverson DC, AuBuchon J, et al: Practice parameter for the use of red blood cell transfusions: developed by the Red Blood Cell Administration Practice Guideline Development Task Force of the College of American Pathologists. Arch Pathol Lab Med 122:130, 1998.

654. Goodnough LT, Brecher ME, Kanter MH, et al: Transfusion medicine—part I. N Engl J Med 340:438, 1999.

655. Bednarek FJ, Weisberger S, Richardson DK, et al: Variations in blood transfusions among newborn intensive care units. SNAP II Study Group. J Pediatr 133:601, 1998.

656. Widness JA, Seward VJ, Kromer IJ, et al: Changing patterns of red blood cell transfusion in very low birth weight infants. J Pediatr 129:680, 1996.

657. Maier RF, Obladen M, Kattner E, et al: High-versus low-dose erythropoietin in extremely low birth weight infants. The European Multicenter rhEPO Study Group. J Pediatr 132:866, 1998.

658. Ohls RK, Harcum J, Li Y, et al: Serum erythropoietin concentrations fail to increase after significant phlebotomy losses in ill preterm infants. J Perinatol 17:465, 1997.

659. Ohls RK, Harcum J, Schibler KR, et al: The effect of erythropoietin on the transfusion requirements of preterm infants weighing 750 grams or less: a randomized, double-blind, placebo-controlled study. J Pediatr 131:661, 1997.

660. Helfaer MA, Carson BS, James CS, et al: Increased hematocrit and decreased transfusion requirements in children given erythropoietin before undergoing craniofacial surgery. J Neurosurg 88:704, 1998.

661. Goodnough LT, Brecher ME, Kanter MH, et al: Transfusion medicine—part II. N Engl J Med 340:525, 1999.

662. Perkins HA: Preserving blood. JAMA 250:1902, 1983.

663. Sladen RN: The oxyhemoglobin dissociation curve. In Brodsky JB (ed): International Anesthesiology Clinics: Clinical Aspects of Oxygen. Boston, Little, Brown, 1981, p 39.

664. Heaton A, Keegan T, Holme S: In vivo regeneration of red cell 2,3-diphosphoglycerate following transfusion of DPG-depleted AS-1, AS-3, and CPDA-1 red cells. Br J Haematol 71:131, 1989.

665. Patterson A: Massive transfusion. Int Anesth Clin 25:61, 1983.

666. Dallman PR: Developmental changes in red blood cell production and function. In Rudolph AM (ed): Rudolph's Pediatrics. 19th ed. Norwalk, CT, Appleton & Lange, 1991, p 1091.

667. Mentzer WC: Methemoglobinemia. In Rudolph AM (ed): Rudolph's Pediatrics. 19th ed. Norwalk, CT, Appleton & Lange, 1991, p 1140.

668. Steinberg MH: Management of sickle cell disease. N Engl J Med 340:1021, 1999.

669. Adams RJ, McKie VC, Hsu L, et al: Prevention of a first stroke by transfusions in children with sickle cell anemia and abnormal results on transcranial Doppler ultrasonography. N Engl J Med 339:5, 1998.

670. Cohen AR: Sickle cell disease—new treatments, new questions. N Engl J Med 339:42, 1998.

671. Vichinsky E, Earles A, Johnson RA, et al: Alloimmunization in sickle cell anemia and transfusion of racially unmatched blood. N Engl J Med 322:1617, 1990.

672. Delatte SJ, Hebra A, Tagge EP, et al: Acute chest syndrome in the postoperative sickle cell patient. J Pediatr Surg 34:188, 1999.

673. Golden C, Styles L, Vichinsky E: Acute chest syndrome and sickle cell disease [review]. Curr Opin Hematol 5:89, 1998.

674. Martin L, Buonomo C: Acute chest syndrome of sickle cell disease: radiographic and clinical analysis of 70 cases. Pediatr Radiol 27:637, 1997.
675. Vichinsky EP, Styles LA, Colangelo LH, et al: Acute chest syndrome in sickle cell disease: clinical presentation and course. Cooperative Study of Sickle Cell Disease. Blood 89:1787, 1997.
676. Mallouh AA, Asha M: Beneficial effect of blood transfusion in children with sickle cell chest syndrome. Am J Dis Child 142:178, 1988.
677. Atz AM, Wessel DL: Inhaled nitric oxide in sickle cell disease with acute chest syndrome. Anesthesiology 87:988, 1997.
678. Gladwin MT, Schechter AN, Shelhamer JH, et al: The acute chest syndrome in sickle cell disease. Possible role of nitric oxide in its pathophysiology and treatment [review]. Am J Respir Crit Care Med 159(5 pt 1):1368, 1999.
679. Petrovitch C: Evaluation and management of coagulation abnormalities. In Anonymous. 48th Annual Refresher Course Lectures. Chicago, American Society of Anesthesiologists, 1997.
680. Eskenazi AE, Bernstein ML, Gordon JB: Hematologic disorders in the pediatric intensive care unit. In Rogers MC, Nichols DG (eds): Textbook of Pediatric Intensive Care. 3rd ed. Baltimore, Williams & Wilkins, 1996, p 1395.
681. Bleyer WA, Hakami N, Shepard TH: The development of hemostasis in the human fetus and newborn infant. J Pediatr 79:838, 1971.
682. Dallman PR: Disorders of coagulation. In Rudolph AM, Hoffman JE, Rudolph CD (eds): Pediatrics. 19th ed. Norwalk, CT, Appleton & Lange, 1991, p 1162.
683. Parker RI: Etiology and treatment of acquired coagulopathies in the critically ill adult and child. Crit Care Clin 13:591, 1997.
684. Nacht A: The use of blood products in shock. Crit Care Clin 8:255, 1992.
685. Aster RH: NIH consensus conference: platelet transfusion therapy. JAMA 257:1777, 1987.
686. Webb IJ, Anderson KC: Risks, costs, and alternatives to platelet transfusions [review]. Leuk Lymphoma 34:71, 1999.
687. Cahill MR, Lilleyman JS: The rational use of platelet transfusions in children [review]. Semin Thromb Hemost 24:567, 1998.
688. Novotny VM: Prevention and management of platelet transfusion refractoriness [review]. Vox Sang 76:1, 1999.
689. Morfini M, Manucci PM, Longo G: Comparative evaluation of the pharmacokinetics of three monoclonal factor VIII concentrates. Thromb Res 61:285, 1991.
690. Schwartz RS, Abildgaard CF, Aledort L: Human recombinant DNA-derived antihemophilic factor (factor VIII) in the treatment of hemophilia A. Recombinant Factor VIII Study Group. N Engl J Med 323:1800, 1990.
691. Lusher JM, Salzman PM: Viral safety and inhibitor development associated with factor VIIIC ultra-purified from plasma in hemophiliacs previously unexposed to factor VIIIC concentrates. The Monoclate Study Group. Semin Hematol 27(Suppl 2):1, 1990.
692. Aygoren-Pursun E, Scharrer I: A multicenter pharmacosurveillance study for the evaluation of the efficacy and safety of recombinant factor VIII in the treatment of patients with hemophilia A. German Kogenate Study Group. Thromb Haemost 78:1352, 1997.
693. Kelly KM, Butler RB, Farace L, et al: Superior in vivo response of recombinant factor VIII concentrate in children with hemophilia A. J Pediatr 130:537, 1997.
694. Aledort LM: Treatment of von Willebrand's disease. Mayo Clin Proc 66:841, 1991.
695. Smith MP, Rice KM, Bromidge ES, et al: Continuous infusion therapy with very high purity von Willebrand factor concentrate in patients with severe von Willebrand disease. Blood Coagul Fibrinolysis 8:6, 1997.
696. Mannucci PM: Treatment of von Willebrand disease [review]. Haemophilia 4:661, 1998.
697. Manucci PM: Desmopressin (DDAVP) for treatment of disorders of hemostasis. Prog Hemost Thromb 8:19, 1986.
698. Rose EH, Aledort LM: Nasal spray desmopressin (DDAVP) for mild hemophilia and von Willebrand disease. Ann Intern Med 114:563, 1991.
699. Buchanan GR, Lucey JF: The bleeding child. In Dickerman JD (ed): The Critically Ill Child: Diagnosis and Medical Management. 3rd ed. Philadelphia, WB Saunders Company, 1985, p 212.
700. Miner ME, Kaufman HH, Graham SH: Disseminated intravascular coagulation fibrinolytic syndrome following head injury in children: frequency and prognostic implications. J Pediatr 100:687, 1982.
701. Kevy S, Fosburg M, Wayne A: Intensive plasma exchange (IPE) and manual whole blood exchange (WBE) support for patients in acute hepatic failure, abstracted. Transfusion 31(Suppl):22S, 1991.
702. Cohen JR, Lackner R, Keller A, et al: The surgical implications of purpura fulminans. Ann Vasc Surg 4:276, 1990.
703. Madden RM, Gill JC, Marlar RA: Protein C and protein S levels in two patients with acquired purpura fulminans. Br J Haematol 75:112, 1990.
704. Marlar RA, Montgomery RR, Broekmans AW: Diagnosis and treatment of homozygous protein C deficiency. Report of the Working Party on Homozygous Protein C Deficiency of the Subcommittee on Protein C and Protein S, International Committee on Thrombosis and Haemostasis. J Pediatr 114:528, 1989.
705. Marlar RA, Mastovich S: Hereditary protein C deficiency: a review of the genetics, clinical presentation, diagnosis and treatment. Blood Coagul Fibrinolysis 1:319, 1990.
706. Darmstadt GL: Acute infectious purpura fulminans: pathogenesis and medical management [review]. Pediatr Dermatol 15:169, 1998.
707. Irazuzta J, McManus ML: Use of topically applied nitroglycerin in the treatment of purpura fulminans. J Pediatr 117:993, 1990.
708. Meyer MT, Irazuzta JE, Tozibikian H: Topical nitroglycerin and pain in purpura fulminans. J Pediatr 134:639, 1999.
709. Irazuzta J, Jarrell J, Portillo A, et al: Compared contralateral application of topical nitroglycerin on purpura fulminans. W V Med J 94:29, 1998.
710. Nowak-Gottl U, Groll A, Kreuz WD: Treatment of disseminated intravascular coagulation with antithrombin III concentrate in children with verified infection. Klin Padiatr 204:134, 1992.
711. Gerson WT, Dickerman JD, Bovill EG, et al: Severe acquired protein C deficiency in purpura fulminans associated with disseminated intravascular coagulation: treatment with protein C concentrate. Pediatrics 91:418, 1993.
712. Rintala E, Seppala OP, Kotilainen P, et al: Protein C in the treatment of coagulopathy in meningococcal disease. Crit Care Med 26:965, 1998.
713. Smith OP, White B, Vaughan D, et al: Use of protein-C concentrate, heparin, and haemodiafiltration in meningococcus-induced purpura fulminans. Lancet 350:1590, 1997.
714. Aiuto LT, Barone SR, Cohen PS, et al: Recombinant tissue plasminogen activator restores perfusion in meningococcal purpura fulminans. Crit Care Med 25:1079, 1997.
715. Various: Practical treatment guidelines: publications of the thrombosis interest group of Canada. Thrombosis Interest Group of Canada, 1999. URL:http://is.dal.ca/~mscully/ptg.html.
716. Streif W, Mitchell LG, Andrew M: Antithrombotic therapy in children [review]. Curr Opin Pediatr 11:56, 1999.
717. Leaker M, Massicotte MP, Brooker LA, et al: Thrombolytic therapy in pediatric patients: a comprehensive review of the literature [review]. Thromb Haemost 76:132, 1996.
718. Gal P, Ransom JL: Neonatal thrombosis: treatment with heparin and thrombolytics. Drug Intell Clin Pharm 25:853, 1991.
719. Kirk CR, Qureshi SA: Streptokinase in the management of arterial thrombosis in infancy. Int J Cardiol 25:15, 1989.
720. Guidry JR, Raschke RA, Morkunas AR: Anticoagulants and thrombolytics: risks and benefits. Crit Care Clin 7:533, 1991.
721. Needleman JP, Ackerman AD: Overwhelming sepsis. In Rogers MC, Nichols DG (eds): Textbook of Pediatric Intensive Care. 3rd ed. Baltimore, Williams & Wilkins, 1996, p 1011.
722. McKenna DS, Iams JD: Group B streptococcal infections [review]. Semin Perinatol 22:267, 1998.
723. Gonzalez VH, Wald ER, Rose E, et al: Epiglottitis and Haemophilus influenzae immunization: the Pittsburgh experience—a five-year review. Pediatrics 96(3 pt 1):424, 1995.
724. Montgomery VL, Bratcher D: Complications associated with severe invasive streptococcal syndrome. J Pediatr 129:602, 1996.
725. Orenstein JB: Invasive pneumococcal infection in a community hospital, 1993 to 1995. Characteristics of resistant strains. Arch Pediatr Adolesc Med 150:809, 1996.
726. Silverstein M, Bachur R, Harper MB: Clinical implications of penicillin and ceftriaxone resistance among children with pneumococcal bacteremia. Pediatr Infect Dis J 18:35, 1999.
727. Deeks SL, Palacio R, Ruvinsky R, et al: Risk factors and course of illness among children with invasive penicillin-resistant Streptococcus pneumoniae. The Streptococcus pneumoniae Working Group. Pediatrics 103:409, 1999.

728. Bradley JS, Kaplan SL, Tan TQ, et al: Pediatric pneumococcal bone and joint infections. The Pediatric Multicenter Pneumococcal Surveillance Study Group (PMPSSG). Pediatrics 102:1376, 1998.

729. Rhodes KH, Henry NK: Antibiotic therapy for severe infections in infants and children. Mayo Clin Proc 67:59, 1992.

730. McCracken GH, Saez-Llorens X: Initial management of bacterial meningitis: steroids and antibiotics. Resid Staff Phys 39:25, 1993.

731. Stutman HR: Therapy for bacterial meningtis: which drugs, and for how long? J Pediatr 110:812, 1987.

732. Dagbjartsson A, Ludvigsson P: Bacterial meningitis: diagnosis and initial antibiotic therapy. Pediatr Clin North Am 34:219, 1987.

733. Hayani KC, Hatzopoulos FK, Frank AL, et al: Pharmacokinetics of once-daily dosing of gentamicin in neonates. J Pediatr 131(1 pt 1):76, 1997.

734. Anonymous: Therapy for children with invasive pneumococcal infections. American Academy of Pediatrics Committee on Infectious Diseases. Pediatrics 99:289, 1997.

735. Smith TL, Pearson ML, Wilcox KR, et al: Emergence of vancomycin resistance in Staphylococcus aureus. Glycopeptide-Intermediate Staphylococcus aureus Working Group. N Engl J Med 340:493, 1999.

736. Marks WA, Stutman HR, Marks MI: Cefuroxime versus ampicillin plus chloramphenicol in childhood bacterial meningitis: a multicenter randomized controlled trial. J Pediatr 109:123, 1986.

737. Rubin LG: b-Lactamase inhibitors: how they work, when to use them. Contemp Pediatr 6:44, 1989.

738. Yogev R: A strategy for evaluating which of the new cephalosporins to use. Pediatr Ann 15:470, 1986.

739. Masur H: Principles of antimicrobial therapy. In Holbrook PR (ed): Textbook of Pediatric Critical Care. Philadelphia, WB Saunders Company, 1993, p 883.

740. Lebel MH, McCracken GH: Delayed cerebrospinal fluid sterilization and adverse outcome of bacterial meningitis in infants and children. Pediatrics 83:161, 1989.

741. Schaad UB, Suter S, Gianella-Borradori A: A comparison of ceftriaxone and cefuroxime for the treatment of bacterial meningitis in children. N Engl J Med 322:141, 1990.

742. Quagliarello V, Scheld WM: Bacterial meningitis: pathogenesis, pathophysiology, and progress. N Engl J Med 327:864, 1992.

743. Saez-Llorens X, McCracken GH: Mediators of meningitis: therapeutic implications. Hosp Pract 1:68, 1991.

744. Lebel MH, Freij BJ, Syrogiannopoulos GA, et al: Dexamethasone therapy for bacterial meningitis: results of two double-blind, placebo-controlled trials. N Engl J Med 319:964, 1988.

745. Havens PL, Wendelberger KJ, Hoffman GM: Corticosteroids as adjunctive therapy in bacterial meningitis. Am J Dis Child 143:1051, 1989.

746. Kennedy WA, Hoyt MJ, McCracken GH: The role of corticosteroid therapy in children with pneumococcal meningitis. Am J Dis Child 145:1374, 1991.

747. Odio CM, Faingezicht I, Paris M: The beneficial effects of early dexamethasone administration in infants and children with bacterial meningitis. N Engl J Med 324:1525, 1991.

748. Schaad UB, Kaplan SL, McCracken GH Jr: Steroid therapy for bacterial meningitis [review]. Clin Infect Dis 20:685, 1995.

749. Rappaport JM, Bhatt SM, Burkard RF, et al: Prevention of hearing loss in experimental pneumococcal meningitis by administraction of dexamethasone and ketorolac [published erratum appears in J Infect Dis 179:735, 1999]. J Infect Dis 179:264, 1999.

750. Arditi M, Mason EOJ, Bradley JS, et al: Three-year multicenter surveillance of pneumococcal meningitis in children: clinical characteristics, and outcome related to penicillin susceptibility and dexamethasone use. Pediatrics 102:1087, 1998.

751. McIntyre PB, Berkey CS, King SM, et al: Dexamethasone as adjunctive therapy in bacterial meningitis. A meta-analysis of randomized clinical trials since 1988. JAMA 278:925, 1997.

752. Ahmed A, Jafri H, Lustar L, et al: Pharmacodynamics of vancomycin for the treatment of experimental penicillin- and cephalosporin-resistant pneumococcal meningitis. Antimicrob Agents Chemother 43:876, 1999.

753. AAP Committee on Infectious Diseases: Ribavirin therapy of respiratory syncytial virus. Pediatrics 79:475, 1987.

754. Holberg CJ, Wright AL, Martinez FD: Risk factors for respiratory syncytial virus associated lower respiratory illnesses in the first year of life. Am J Epidemiol 133:1135, 1991.

755. Church NR, Anas NG, Hall CB, et al: Respiratory syncytial virus related apnea in infants. Am J Dis Child 138:247, 1984.

756. Kneyber MC, Brandenburg AH, de Groot R, et al: Risk factors for respiratory syncytial virus associated apnoea. Eur J Pediatr 157:331 1998.

757. McBride JT: Pulmonary function changes in children after respiratory syncytial virus infection in infancy. J Pediatr 135:S28, 1999.

758. Kattan M: Epidemiologic evidence of increased airway reactivity in children with a history of bronchiolitis. J Pediatr 135:S8, 1999.

759. Soto ME, Sly PD, Uren E: Bronchodilator response during acute viral bronchiolitis in infancy. Pediatr Pulmonol 1:85, 1985.

760. Rodriguez WJ: Management strategies for respiratory syncytial virus infections in infants. J Pediatr 135:S45, 1999.

761. Hall CB, McBride JT, Gala CL: Ribavirin treatment of respiratory syncytial viral infection in infants with underlying cardiopulmonary disease. Am J Dis Child 254:3047, 1985.

762. Kacmarek RM: Care-giver protection from exposure to aerosolized pharmacologic agents. Is it necessary? Chest 100:1104, 1991.

763. Pollack MM: An RSVP to RSV (respiratory syncytial virus): declining mortality rates. Crit Care Med 20:1375, 1992.

764. Moler FW, Khan AS, Meliones JN: Respiratory syncytial virus morbidity and mortality estimates in congenital heart disease patients: a recent experience. Crit Care Med 20:1406, 1992.

765. Law BJ, Wang EE, MacDonald N, et al: Does ribavirin impact on the hospital course of children with respiratory syncytial virus (RSV) infection? An analysis using the pediatric investigators collaborative network on infections in Canada (PICNIC) RSV database. Pediatrics 99:E7, 1997.

766. Ottolini MG, Hemming VG: Prevention and treatment recommendations for respiratory syncytial virus infection. Background and clinical experience 40 years after discovery [review]. Drugs 54:867, 1997.

767. Henderson FW: Viral respiratory infections. In Rudolph AM, Hoffman JIE, Rudolph CD (eds): Rudolph's Pediatrics. 20th ed. Stamford, CT, Appleton & Lange, 1996, p 671.

768. Rotbart HA: Enteroviruses. In Rudolph AM, Hoffman JIE, Rudolph CD (eds): Rudolph's Pediatrics 20th ed. Stamford, CT, Appleton & Lange, 1996, p 633.

769. Merritt WT, Green M: Nosocomial infections in the pediatric intensive care unit. In Rogers MC, Nichols DG (eds): Textbook of Pediatric Intensive Care. 3rd ed. Baltimore, Williams & Wilkins, 1996, p 975.

770. Gaynes RP, Solomon S: Improving hospital-acquired infection rates: the CDC experience. J Comm J Qual Improv 22:457, 1996.

771. Gaynes RP, Edwards JR, Jarvis WR, et al: Nosocomial infections among neonates in high-risk nurseries in the United States. National Nosocomial Infections Surveillance System. Pediatrics 98(3 pt 1):357, 1996.

772. Adal KA, Flowers RH, Anglim AM, et al: Prevention of nosocomial influenza. Infect Control Hosp Epidemiol 17:641, 1996.

773. Cunha BA: Intravenous line infections. Crit Care Clin 14:339, 1998.

774. Stein F, Trevino R: Nosocomial infections in the pediatric intensive care unit. Pediatr Clin North Am 41:1245, 1994.

775. Levy I, Rubin LG, Vasishtha S, et al: Emergence of Candida parapsilosis as the predominant species causing candidemia in children. Clin Infect Dis 26:1086, 1998.

776. Girmenia C, Martino P, De Bernardis F, et al: Rising incidence of Candida parapsilosis fungemia in patients with hematologic malignancies: clinical aspects, predisposing factors, and differential pathogenicity of the causative strains. Clin Infect Dis 23:506, 1996.

777. Civetta JM, Hudson-Civetta J, Ball S: Decreasing catheter-related infection and hospital costs by continuous quality improvement. Crit Care Med 24:1660, 1996.

778. O'Leary M, Bihari D: Central venous catheters—time for a change? If you put them in properly you don't need to change them routinely. BMJ 316:1918, 1998.

779. Badley AD, Steckelberg JM, Wollan PC, et al: Infections rates of central venous pressure catheters: comparison between newly placed catheters and those that have been changed. Mayo Clin Proc 71:838, 1996.

780. Anonymous: Guidelines for prevention of intravascular device-related infections. Part II. Recommendations for the prevention of nosocomial intravascular device-related infections. Hospital Infection Control Practices Advisory Committee [review]. Am J Infect Control 24:277, 1996.

781. Cobb DK, High KP, Sawyer RG, et al: A controlled trial of scheduled replacement of central venous and pulmonary-artery catheters. N Engl J Med 327:1062, 1992.

782. Eyer S, Brummitt C, Crossley K, et al: Catheter-related sepsis: prospective, randomized study of three methods of long-term catheter maintenance. Crit Care Med 18:1073, 1990.

783. Maki DG, Stolz SM, Wheeler S, et al: Prevention of central venous catheter-related bloodstream infection by use of an antiseptic-impregnated catheter. A randomized, controlled trial. Ann Intern Med 127:257, 1997.

784. Wenzel RP, Edmond MB: The evolving technology of venous access. N Engl J Med 340:48, 1999.

785. Darouiche RO, Raad II, Heard SO, et al: A comparison of two antimicrobial-impregnated central venous catheters. Catheter Study Group. N Engl J Med 340:1, 1999.

786. Raad I, Darouiche R, Dupuis J, et al: Central venous catheters coated with minocycline and rifampin for the prevention of catheter-related colonization and bloodstream infections. A randomized, double-blind trial. The Texas Medical Center Catheter Study Group. Ann Intern Med 127:267, 1997.

787. Kollef MH: The prevention of ventilator-associated pneumonia. N Engl J Med 340:627, 1999.

788. Craven DE, Steger KA: Ventilator-associated bacterial pneumonia: challenges in diagnosis, treatment, and prevention. New Horiz 6(Suppl):S30, 1998.

789. Mariscalco MM: Infection and the host response. In Fuhrman BP, Zimmerman JJ (eds): Pediatric Critical Care. St. Louis, Mosby Year Book, 1992, p 917.

790. Karakusis PH: Considerations in the therapy of septic shock. Med Clin North Am 70:933, 1986.

791. Anderson MR, Blumer JL: Advances in the therapy for sepsis in children. Pediatr Clin North Am 44:179, 1997.

792. Carcillo JA, Cunnion RE: Septic shock. Crit Care Clin 13:553, 1997.

793. Sullivan JS, Kilpatrick L, Costarino AT Jr: Correlation of plasma cytokine elevations with mortality rate in children sepsis. J Pediatr 120:510, 1992.

794. Riesenfeld-Orn I, Wolpe S, Garcia-Bustos JF: Production of interleukin-1 but not tumor necrosis factor by human monocytes stimulated with pneumococcal cell surface components. Infec Immun 57:1890, 1989.

795. Sriskandan S, Cohen J: Gram-positive sepsis. Mechanisms and differences from gram-negative sepsis [review]. Infect Dis Clin North Am 13:397, 1999.

796. Blanco A, Solis G, Arranz E, et al: Serum levels of CD14 in neonatal sepsis by Gram-positive and Gram-negative bacteria. Acta Paediatr 85:728, 1996.

797. Zimmerman JJ, Dietrich KA: Current perspectives on septic shock. Pediatr Clin North Am 34:131, 1987.

798. Jacobs ER, Bone RC: Clinical indicators in sepsis and septic adult respiratory distress syndrome. Med Clin North Am 70:921, 1986.

799. McCabe WR, Treadwell TL, DeMaria A Jr: Pathophysiology of bacteremia. Am J Med 78:7, 1983.

800. Herdegen JJ, Casey LC: The role of tumor necrosis factor in infections: pathophysiology and clinical implications. Infect Med 10: 27, 1993.

801. Michie HR, Manogue KR, Spriggs DR: Detection of circulating tumor necrosis factor after endotoxin administration. N Engl J Med 318:1481, 1988.

802. Dinarello CA, Wolff SM: The role of interleukin-1 in disease. N Engl J Med 328:106, 1993.

803. Girardin E, Roux-Lombard P, Grau GE: Imbalance between tumour necrosis factor-α and soluble TNF receptor concentrations in severe meningococcaemia. The J5 study group. Immunology 76:20, 1992.

804. Greenman RL, Schein RM, Martin MA: A controlled clinical trial of E5 murine monoclonal IgM antibody to endotoxin in the treatment of gram-negative sepsis. JAMA 266:1097, 1991.

805. Bone RC: Monoclonal antibodies to endotoxin: new allies against sepsis? JAMA 266:1125, 1991.

806. Warren HS, Danner RL, Munford RS: Anti-endotoxin monoclonal antibodies. N Engl J Med 326:1153, 1992.

807. Wenzel RP: Anti-endotoxin monoclonal antibodies—a second look. N Engl J Med 326:1151, 1992.

808. Nasraway SA: Sepsis research: we must change course. Crit Care Med 27:427, 1999.

809. Parker MM: Pathophysiology of cardiovascular dysfunction in septic shock [review]. New Horiz 6:130, 1998.

810. Pollack MM, Fields AI, Ruttimann UE: Sequential cardiopulmonary variables of infants and children in septic shock. Crit Care Med 12:554, 1984.

811. Astiz ME, Rackow EC, Falk JL, et al: Oxygen delivery and consumption in patients with hyperdynamic septic shock. Crit Care Med 15:26, 1987.

812. Rackow EC, Astiz ME: Pathophysiology and treatment of septic shock. JAMA 266:548, 1991.

813. Dobb GJ, Faragher EB: The relationship between oxygen uptake and delivery. Int Care World 7:131, 1990.

814. Hotchkiss RS, Karl E: Reevaluation of the role of cellular hypoxia and bioenergetic failure in sepsis. JAMA 267:1503, 1992.

815. Parker MM: Current management of septic shock. Infect Med 6:47, 1989.

816. Wheeler AP, Bernard GR: Treating patients with severe sepsis. N Engl J Med 340:207, 1999.

817. Sprung CL, Caralis PV, Marcial EH: The effects of high-dose corticosteroids in patients with septic shock: a prospective, controlled study. N Engl J Med 311:1137, 1984.

818. Lefering R, Neugebauer EA: Steroid controversy in sepsis and septic shock: a meta-analysis. Crit Care Med 23:1294, 1995.

819. Duggan M, Browne I, Flynn C: Adrenal failure in the critically ill. Br J Anaesth 81:468, 1998.

820. Bausehr JC, Baker RC: Early prognostic indicators in acute meningococcemia: implications for management. Pediatr Emerge Care 2: 176, 1986.

821. Neveling U, Kaschula RO: Fatal meningococcal disease in childhood: an autopsy study of 86 cases. Ann Trop Paediatr 13:147, 1993.

822. Wajchenberg B, Leme CE, Tambascia M: The adrenal response to exogenous adrenocorticotropin in patients with infections due to Neisseria meningitidis. J Infect Dis 138:387, 1978.

823. Boucek MM, Boerth RC, Arthman M: Myocardial dysfunction in children with acute meningococcemia. J Pediatr 105:538, 1984.

824. Monsalve F, Rucabado L, Salvador A: Myocardial depression in septic shock caused by meaningococcal infection. Crit Care Med 12:1021, 1984.

825. Kaplan JE, Masur H, Holmes KK: 1999 USPHS/IDSA Guidelines for the Prevention of Opportunistic Infections in Persons infected with Human Immunodeficiency Virus. MMWR Recommendations and Reports 48(RR-10):1, 1999.

826. Cowan MJ, Shelhamer JH, Levine SJ: Acute respiratory failure in the HIV-seropositive patient [review]. Crit Care Clin 13:523, 1997.

827. Wachter RM, Luce JM, Hopewell PC: Critical care of patients with AIDS. JAMA 267:541, 1992.

828. Lewandowski C, Ognjan A, Rivers E: Health care worker exposure to HIV-1 and HTLV I-II in critically ill, resuscitated emergency department patients. Ann Emerg Med 21:1353, 1992.

829. de la Tribonniere X, Dufresne MD, Alfandari S, et al: Tolerance, compliance and psychological consequences of post-exposure prophylaxis in health-care workers. Int J STD AIDS 9:591, 1998.

830. Anonymous: Public Health Service guidelines for the management of health-care worker exposures to HIV and recommendations for postexposure prophylaxis. Centers for Disease Control and Prevention. MMWR Morb Mortal Wkly Rep 47(RR-7):1, 1998.

831. Karpel JP, Prezant D, Appel D, et al: Endotracheal lavage for the diagnosis of Pneumocystis carinii pneumonia in intubated patients with acquired immune deficiency syndrome. Crit Care Med 14:741, 1986.

832. Levine SJ, Shelhamer JH: Fiberoptic bronchoscopy in patients with HIV infection. AIDS Reader 1:51, 1991.

833. Frankel LR, Smith DW, Lewiston NJ: Bronchoalveolar lavage for diagnosis of pneumonia in the immunocompromised child. Pediatrics 81:785, 1988.

834. Guerra LF, Baughman RP: Use of bronchoalveolar lavage to diagnose bacterial pneumonia in mechanically ventilated patients. Crit Care Med 18:169, 1990.

835. Mallory DL, Parrillo JE, Bailey KR: Cardiovascular effects and safety of intravenous and intramuscular pentamidine isethionate. Crit Care Med 15:503, 1987.

836. NIH-University oCEP: Consensus statement on the use of corticosteroids as adjunctive therapy for pneumocytsis pneumonia in the acquired immunodeficiency syndrome. N Engl J Med 323:1500, 1990.

837. Bozzette AA, Sattler FR, Chiu J: A controlled trial of early adjunctive treatment with corticosteroids for Pneumocystis carinii pneumonia in the acquired immunodeficiency syndrome. N Engl J Med 323:1451, 1990.

838. Gagnon S, Boota AM, Fischl MA: Corticosteroids as adjunctive therapy for severe Pneumocystis carinii pneumonia in the acquired immunodeficiency syndrome. N Engl J Med 323:1444, 1990.

839. Telenti A, Steckelberg JM, Stockman L: Quantitative blood cultures in candidemia. Mayo Clin Proc 66:1120, 1991.

840. Baley JE, Meyers C, Kliegman RM: Pharmacokinetics, outcome of treatment, and toxic effects of amphotericin B and 5-fluorocytosine in neonates. J Pediatr 116:791, 1990.

841. Terrell CL, Hughes CE: Antifungal agents used for deep-seated mycotic infections. Mayo Clin Proc 67:69, 1992.

842. Schwarze R, Penk A, Pittrow L: Administration of fluconazole in children below 1 year of age [review]. Mycoses 42:3, 1999.

843. Aspesberro F, Beghetti M, Oberhansli I, et al: Fungal endocarditis in critically ill children. Eur J Pediatr 158:275, 1999.

844. Noskin G, Pietrelli L, Gurwith M, et al: Treatment of invasive fungal infections with amphotericin B colloidal dispersio in bone marrow transplant recipients [review]. Bone Marrow Transplant 23:697, 1999.

845. Ringden O, Andstrom EE, Remberger M, et al: Prophylaxis and therapy using liposomal amphotericin B (AmBisome) for invasive fungal infections in children undergoing organ or allogeneic bone-marrow-transplantation. Pediatr Transplant 1:124, 1997.

846. Walsh TJ, Finberg RW, Arndt C, et al: Liposomal amphotericin B for empirical therapy in patients with persistent fever and neutropenia. National Institute of Allergy and Infectious Diseases Mycoses Study Group. N Engl J Med 340:764, 1999.

847. Wendt CH, Weisdorf DJ, Jordan MC: Parainfluenza virus respiratory infection after bone marrow transplantation. N Engl J Med 326:921, 1992.

848. Schmidt GM, Horak DA, Niland JC: A randomized, controlled trial of prophylactic ganciclovir for cytomegalovirus pulmonary infection in recipients of allogeneic bone marrow transplants. N Engl J Med 324:1005, 1991.

849. Goodrich JM, Mori M, Gleave CA: Early treatment with ganciclovir to prevent cytomegalovirus disease after allogeneic bone marrow transplantation. N Engl J Med 325:1601, 1991.

850. Allen EM, Boyer R, Cherny WB, et al: Head and spinal cord injury. In Rogers MC, Nichols DG (eds): Textbook of Pediatric Intensive Care. 3rd ed. Baltimore, Williams & Wilkins, 1996, p 809.

851. Chesnut RM: Secondary brain insults after head injury: clinical perspectives. New Horiz 3:366, 1995.

852. Milde LN: Pathophysiology of ischemic brain injury. Crit Care Clin 5:729, 1989.

853. Haun SE, Kirsch JR, Dean JM: Theories of brain resuscitation. In Rogers MC, Nichols DG (eds): Textbook of Pediatric Intensive Care. 3rd ed. Baltimore, Williams & Wilkins, 1996, p 699.

854. Rolfsen ML, Davis WR: Cerebral function and preservation during cardiac arrest. Crit Care Med 17:283, 1989.

855. Shin'oka T, Nagashima M, Nollert G, et al: A novel sialyl Lewis X analog attenuates cerebral injury after deep hypothermic circulatory arrest. J Thorac Cardiovasc Surg 117:1204, 1999.

856. Sirin BH, Yilik L, Coskun E, et al: Pentoxifylline reduces injury of the brain in transient ischamemia. Acta Cardiol 53:89, 1998.

857. du Plessis AJ: Cerebral hemodynamics and metabolism during infant cardiac surgery. Mechanisms of injury and strategies for protection [review]. J Child Neurol 12:285, 1997.

858. Matsumoto M, Iida Y, Sakabe T, et al: Mild and moderate hypothermia provide better protection than a burst-suppression dose of thiopental against ishemic spinal cord injury in rabbits. Anesthestiology 86:1120, 1997.

859. White BC, Grossman LI, O'Neil BJ, et al: Global brain ischemia and reperfusion [review]. Ann Emerg Med 27:588, 1996.

860. Jenny C, Hymel KP, Ritzen A, et al: Analysis of missed cases of abusive head trauma. JAMA 281:621, 1999.

861. Nimkin K, Kleinman PK: Imaging of child abuse [review]. Pediatr Clin North Am 44:615, 1997.

862. Hershey BL, Zimmerman RA: Pediatric brain computed tomography. Pediatr Clin North Am 32:1477, 1985.

863. Rogers MC, Traystman RJ: An overview of the intracranial vault. Crit Care Clin 1:195, 1985.

864. Guertin SR: Cerebrospinal fluid shunts: evaluation, complications, and crisis management. Pediatr Clin North Am 34:203, 1987.

865. Jones MD Jr, Traystman RJ, Simmons MA, et al: Effects of changes in arterial O2 content on cerebral blood flow in the lamb. Am J Physiol 240:H209, 1981.

866. Brown MM, Wade JP, Marshall J: Fundamental importance of arterial oxygen content in the regulation of cerebral blood flow in man. Brain 108:81, 1985.

867. Muizelaar JP, Marmarou A, Ward JD: Adverse effects of prolonged hyperventilation in patients with severe head injury: a randomized clinical trial. J Neurosurg 75:731, 1991.

868. Manley GT, Pitts LH, Morabito D, et al: Brain tissue oxygenation during hemorrhagic shock, resuscitation, and alterations in ventilation. J Trauma 46:261, 1999.

869. Schneider GH, Sarrafzadeh AS, Kiening KL, et al: Influence of hyperventilation on brain tissue-PO2, PCO2, and pH in patients with intracranial hypertension. Acta Neurochir Suppl 71:62, 1998.

870. Thiagarajan A, Goverdhan PD, Chari P, et al: The effect of hyperventilation and hyperoxia on cerebral venous oxygen saturation in patients with traumatic brain injury. Anesth 87:850, 1998.

871. Allen CH, Ward JD: An evidence-based approach to management of increased intracranial pressure [review]. Crit Care Clin 14:485, 1998.

872. Marion DW, Firlik A, McLaughlin MR: Hyperventilation therapy for severe traumatic brain injury [review]. New Horiz 3:439, 1995.

873. Paczynski RP: Osmotherapy. Basic concepts and controversies [review]. Crit Care Clin 13:105, 1997.

874. Muizelaar JP, Wei EP, Kontos HA, et al: Mannitol causes compensatory cerebral vasconstriction and vasodilation in response to blood viscosity changes. J Neurosurg 59:822, 1983.

875. Rosner MJ, Coley I: Cerebral perfusion pressure: a hemodynamic mechanism of mannitol and the postmannitol hemogram. Neurosurgery 21:147, 1987.

876. Takayasu M, Dacey RG: Effects of mannitol on intracerebral arteriolar diameter in vitro: extraluminal and intraluminal application. Neurosurgery 25:747, 1989.

877. Bullock R: Mannitol and other diuretics in severe neurotrauma [review]. New Horiz 3:448, 1995.

878. Kaufmann AM, Cardoso ER: Aggravation of vasogenic cerebral edema by multiple-dose mannitol. J Neurosurg 77:584, 1992.

879. Ganong CA, Kappy MS: Cerebral salt wasting in children. Am J Dis Child 147:167, 1993.

880. Simma B, Burger R, Falk M, et al: A prospective, randomized, and controlled study of fluid management in children with severe head injury: lactated Ringer's solution versus hypertonic saline. Crit Care Med 26:1265, 1998.

881. Clark RSB, Kochanek PM: Pass the salt? Crit Care Med 26:1161, 1998.

882. Feldman Z, Kanter MJ, Robertson CS, et al: Effect of head elevation on intracranial pressure, cerebral perfusion pressure, and cerebral blood flow in head-injured patients. J Neurosurg 76:207, 1992.

883. Marion DW, Penrod LE, Kelsey SF, et al: Treatment of traumatic brain injury with moderate hypothermia. N Engl J Med 336:540, 1997.

884. Temkin NR, Haglund MM, Winn HR: Causes, prevention, and treatment of post-traumatic epilepsy [review]. New Horiz 3:518, 1995.

885. Sloan TB: Electrophysiologic monitoring in head injury [review]. New Horiz 3:431, 1996.

886. Albanese J, Viviand X, Potie F, et al: Sufentanil, fentanyl, and alfentanil in head trauma patients: a study on cerebral hemodynamics. Crit Care Med 27:407, 1999.

887. Bedell EA, DeWitt DS, Prough DS: Fentanyl infusion preserves cerebral blood flow during decreased arterial blood pressure after traumatic brain injury in cats. J Neurotrauma 15:985, 1998.

888. de Nadal M, Ausina A, Sahuquillo J, et al: Effects on intracranial pressure of fentanyl in severe head injured patients. Acta Neurochir Suppl 71:10, 1998.

889. Lauer KK, Connolly LA, Schmeling WT: Opioid sedation does not alter intracranial pressure in head injured patients. Can J Anaesth 44:929, 1997.

890. Poungvarin N, Bhoopat W, Viriyavejakul A: Effects of dexamethasone in primary supratentorial intracerebral hemorrhage. N Engl J Med 316:1229, 1987.

891. Alderson P, Roberts I: Corticosteroids in acute traumatic brain injury: systematic review of randomised controlled trials. BMJ 314:1855, 1997.

892. Bracken MB: Pharmacological interventions for acute spinal cord injury (Cochrane Database of Systematic Reviews). The Cochrane Library, 1999. URL.

893. Bracken MB, Shepard MJ, Collins WF, et al: A randomized, controlled trial of methylprednisolone or naloxone in the treatment of acute spinal-cord injury. Results of the Second National Acute Spinal Cord Injury Study. N Engl J Med 322:1405, 1990.

894. Bracken MB, Shepard MJ, Holford TR, et al: Administration of methylprednisolone for 24 or 48 hours or tirilazad mesylate for 48 hours in the treatment of acute spinal cord injury. Results of the Third National Acute Spinal Cord Injury Randomized Controlled Trial. National Acute Spinal Cord Injury Study. JAMA 277:1597, 1997.

895. Fanconi S, Duc G: Intratracheal suctioning in sick preterm infants: prevention of intracranial hypertension and cerebral hypoperfusion by muscle paralysis. Pediatrics 79:538, 1987.

896. Prielipp RC, Coursin DB: Sedative and neuromuscular blocking drug use in critically ill patients with head injuries [review]. New Horiz 3:456, 1995.

897. Wilberger JE, Cantella D: High-dose barbiturates for intracranial pressure control [review]. New Horiz 3:469, 1995.

898. Attia J, Cook DJ: Prognosis in anoxic and traumatic coma. Crit Care Clin 14:497, 1998.

899. Rawal K, D'Souza BJ: Status epilepticus. Crit Care Clin 1:339, 1985.

900. Tasker RC, Dean JM: Status epilepticus. In Rogers MC, Nichols DG (eds): Textbook of Pediatric Intensive Care. 3rd ed. Baltimore, Williams & Wilkins, 1996, p 747.

901. Weise KL, Bleck TP: Status epilepticus in children and adults [review]. Crit Care Clin 13:629, 1997.

902. Holmes GL, Riviello JJ Jr: Midazolam and pentobarbital for refractory status epilepticus [review]. Pediatr Neurol 24:259, 1999.

903. Pellock JM: Use of midazolam for refractory status epilepticus in pediatric patients [review]. J Child Neurol 13:581, 1998.

904. Orlowski JP: Drowning, near-drowning, and ice-water submersion. Pediatr Clin North Am 34:75, 1987.

905. Orlowski JP, Abulleil MM, Phillips JM: Effect of tonicities of saline solutions on pulmonary injury in drowning. Crit Care Med 15:126, 1987.

906. Suominen PK, Korpela RE, Silvast TG, et al: Does water temperature affect outcome of nearly drowned children? Resuscitation 35:111, 1997.

907. Biggart MJ, Bohn DJ: Effect of hypothermia and cardiac arrest on outcome of near-drowning accidents in children. J Pediatr 117(2 pt 1):179, 1990.

908. DeNicola LK, Falk JL, Swanson ME, et al: Submersion injuries in children and adults [review]. Crit Care Clin 13:477, 1997.

909. Spack L, Gedeit R, Splaingard M, et al: Failure of aggressive therapy to alter outcome in pediatric near-drowning. Peddiatr Emerg Care 13:98, 1997.

910. Christensen DW, Jansen P, Perkin RM: Outcome and acute care hospital costs after warm water near drowning in children. Pediatrics 99:715, 1997.

911. Marx CM, Rosenberg DI, Ambuel B: Pediatric intensive care sedation: survey of fellowship training programs. Pediatrics 91:369, 1993.

912. Movius AJ, Martin LD: Sedation, analgesia, and neuromuscular blockade during pediatric mechanical ventilation [review]. Respir Care Clin North Am 2:509, 1996.

913. Lynn AM, Slattery JT: Morphine pharmacokinetics in early infancy. Anesthesiology 66:136, 1987.

914. Bhat R, Chari G, Gulati A: Pharmacokinetics of a single dose of morphine in preterm infants during the first week of life. J Pediatr 117:477, 1990.

915. Bhat R, Abu-Harb M, Chari G, et al: Morphine metabolism in acutely ill preterm newborn infants. J Pediatr 120:795, 1992.

916. McRorie TI, Lynn AM, Nespeca MK: The maturation of morphine clearance and metabolism. Am J Dis Child 146:972, 1992.

917. Arnold JA, Truog RD, Scavone JM, et al: Changes in the pharmacodynamic response to fentanyl in neonates during continuous infusion. J Pediatr 119:639, 1991.

918. Lane JC, Tennison MB, Lawless ST: Movement disorder after withdrawal of fentanyl infusion. J Pediatr 119:649, 1991.

919. Olkkola KT, Maunuksela EL: The pharmacokinetics of postoperative intravenous ketorolac tromethamine in children. Br J Clin Pharmacol 31:182, 1991.

920. Watcha MF, Jones MB, Laguerela RG: Comparison of ketorolac and morphine as adjuvants during pediatric surgery. Anesthesiology 76:368, 1992.

921. Breheny FX, Kendall PA: Use of isoflurane for sedation in intensive care. Crit Care Med 20:1062, 1992.

922. Tanigami H, Yahagi N, Kumon K, et al: Long-term sedation with isoflurane in postoperative intensive care in cardiac surgery. Artif Organs 21:21, 1997.

923. McBeth C, Watkins TG: Isoflurane for sedation in a case of congenital myasthenia gravis. Br J Anaesth 77:672, 1996.

924. Klessig HT, Geiger HJ, Murray MJ, et al: A national survey on the practice patterns of anesthesiologist intensivists in the use of muscle relaxants. Crit Care Med 20:1341, 1992.

925. Barrington KJ, Finer NN, Etches PC: Succinylcholine and atropine for premedication of the newborn infant before nasotracheal intubation: a randomized, controlled trial. Crit Care Med 17:1293, 1989.

926. Fiamengo SA, Savarese JJ: Use of muscle relaxants in intensive care units. Crit Care Med 19:1457, 1991.

927. Rossiter A, Souney PF, McGowan S, et al: Pancuronium-induced prolonged neuromuscular blockade. Crit Care Med 19:1583, 1991.

928. Agoston S: Paralysis after long-term administration of vecuronium [letter, with reply]. Anesthesiology 74:792, 1991.

929. Pascucci RC: Prolonged weakness after extended mechanical ventilation in a child. Crit Care Med 18:1181, 1990.

930. Vernon DD, Grant MJ, Setzer NA: Brain death, organ donation, and withdrawal of life support. In Rogers MC, Nichols DG (eds): Textbook of Pediatric Intensive Care. 3rd ed. Baltimore, Williams & Wilkins, 1996, p 893.

931. Harrison AM, Botkin JR: Can pediatricians define and apply the concept of brain death? Pediatrics 103:e82, 1999.

932. Ahmann PA, Carrigan TA, Carlton D: Brain death in children: characteristic common carotid arterial velocity patterns measured with pulsed Doppler ultrasound. J Pediatr 110:723, 1987.

933. Ruiz-Lopez MJ, Martinez DA, Serrano A, et al: Brain death and evoked potentials in pediatric patients. Crit Care Med 27:412, 1999.

934. Qian SY, Fan XM, Yin HH: Transcranial Doppler assessment of brain death in children. Singapore Med J 39:247, 1998.

935. Ad Hoc Committee on Brain Death TCHB: Determination of brain death. J Pediatr 15:1103, 1987.

936. Shewmon DA: Chronic "brain death": meta-analysis and conceptual consequences. Neurology 51:1538, 1998.

937. Truog RD: Is it time to abandon brain death? [review]. Hastings Cent Rep 27:29, 1997.

938. Drake B, Ashwal S, Schneider S: Determination of cerebral death in the pediatric intensive care unit. Pediatrics 78:107, 1986.

939. Fackler JC, Rogers MC: Is brain death really cessation of all intracranial function? J Pediatr 110:84, 1987.

940. Truog RD, Fackler JC: Rethinking brain death. Crit Care Med 20:1705, 1992.

941. Spital A: The shortage of organs for transplantation. Where do we go from here? N Engl J Med 325:1243, 1991.

942. Veatch RM: Routine inquiry about organ donation—an alternative to presumed consent. N Engl J Med 325:1246, 1991.

943. Smith JB, Browne AM: Critical illness and intensive care during infancy and childhood. In Curley MA, Smith JB, Moloney-Harmon PA (eds): Critical Care Nursing of Infants and Children. Philadelphia, WB Saunders Company, 1996, p 15.

944. Rothstein P: Psychological stress in families of children in a pediatric intensive care unit. Pediatr Clin North Am 27:613, 1980.

945. Curley MA, Meyer EC: The impact of the critical care experience on the family. In Curley MA, Smith JB, Moloney-Harmon PA (eds): Critical Care Nursing of Infants and Children. Philadelphia, WB Saunders Company, 1996, p 47.

946. Rothstein P: Family reaction to acute overwhelming illness in children. Crit Care Med 7:130, 1979.

947. Groves JE, Beresin EV: Difficult patients, difficult families. New Horiz 6:331, 1998.

948. Frader JE: Difficulties in providing intensive care. Pediatrics 64:10, 1979.

949. Waller DA, Todres ID, Cassem NH: Coping with poor prognosis in the pediatric intensive care unit. Am J Dis Child 133:1121, 1979.

950. Meyer EC, Kennally KF, Zika-Beres E, et al: Attitudes about sibling visitation in the neonatal intensive care unit. Arch Pediatr Adolesc Med 150:1021, 1996.

951. Stern TA, Jellinek MS: Training issues in the intensive care unit. New Horiz 6:398, 1998.

952. Butt W, Shann F, Tibballs J: Long-term outcome of children after intensive care. Crit Care Med 18:961, 1990.

953. Wanzer SH, Federman DD, Adelstein SJ: The physician's responsibility toward hopelessly ill patients. N Engl J Med 320:844, 1989.

954. Mink RB, Pollack MM: Resuscitation and withdrawal of therapy in pediatric intensive care. Pediatrics 89:961, 1992.

955. Lantos JD, Berger AC, Zucker AR: Do-not-resuscitate orders in a children's hospital. Crit Care Med 21:52, 1993.

956. Todres ID: Ethical dilemmas in pediatric critical care. Crit Care Clin 8:219, 1992.

957. Todres ID, Armstrong A, Lally P, et al: Negotiating end-of-life issues. New Horiz 6:374, 1998.

958. Truog RD: "Doctor, if this were your child, what would you do"? Pediatrics 103:153, 1999.

959. Nelson LJ, Nelson RM: Ethics and the provision of futile, harmful, or burdensome treatment to children. Crit Care Med 20:427, 1992.

960. Tomlinson T, Brody H: Futility and the ethics of resuscitation. JAMA 264:1276, 1990.

961. Truog RD, Brett AS, Frader JE: The problem with futility. N Engl J Med 326:1560, 1992.

962. Nelson RM: Ethics in the intensive care unit. Creating an ethical environment [review]. Crit Care Clin 13:691, 1997.

963. Truog RD: Allowing to die. Crit Care Med 18:790, 1990.

964. Safar P, Winter P: Helping to die. Crit Care Med 18:788, 1990.

965. Truog RD, Berde CB: Pain, euthanasia, and anesthesiologists. Anesthesiology 78:353, 1993.

966. Jonsen AR: To help the dying die—a new duty for anesthesiologists? Anesthesiology 78:225, 1993.

967. Belay ED, Bresee JS, Holman RC, et al: Reye's syndrome in the United States from 1981 through 1997. N Engl J Med 340:1377, 1999.

968. Patrick CC: Coagulase-negative staphylococci: pathogens with increasing clinical significance. J Pediatr 116:497, 1990.

969. Wilhelm MP: Vancomycin. Mayo Clin Proc 66:1165, 1991.

970. Brewer NS, Hellinger WC: The monobactams. Mayo Clin Proc 66:1152, 1991.

971. Edson RS, Terrell CL: The aminoglycosides. Mayo Clin Proc 66:1158, 1991.

972. Haugan K, Petersen JS, Spannow J, et al: Antihypertensive action of nonnatriuretic doses of furosemide in Dahl salt-sensitive rats. J Hypertens 15:775, 1997.

973. Abrahams Z, Pang MY, Lam EK, et al: What is the plasma cofactor required by diuretics for direct vascular relaxant effect in vitro? J Hypertens 16:801, 1998.

974. Pickkers P, Dormans TP, Russel FG, et al: Direct vascular effects of furosemide in humans. Circulation 96:1847, 1997.

975. Brater DC: Diuretic therapy. N Engl J Med 339:387, 1998.

976. Pivac N, Rumboldt Z, Sardelic S, et al: Diuretic effects of furosemide infusion versus bolus injection in congestive heart failure. Int J Clin Pharmacol Res 18:121, 1998.

977. Eades SK, Christensen ML: The clinical pharmacology of loop diuretics in the pediatric patient [review]. Pediatr Nephrol 12:603, 1998.

978. Schuller D, Lynch JP, Fine D: Protocol-guided diuretic management: comparison of furosemide by continuous infusion and intermittent bolus. Crit Care Med 25:1969, 1997.

979. Luciani GB, Nichani S, Chang AC, et al: Continuous versus intermittent furosemide infusion in critically ill infants after open heart operations. Ann Thorac Surg 64:1133, 1997.

980. Klinge JM, Scharf J, Hofbeck M, et al: Intermittent administration of furosemide versus continuous infusion in the postoperative management of children following open heart surgery. Intensive Care Med 23:693, 1997.

981. Aaser E, Gullestad L, Tollofsrud S, et al: Effect of bolus injection versus continuous infusion of furosemide on diuresis and neurohormonal activation in patients with severe congestive heart failure. Scand J Clin Lab Invest 57:361, 1997.

982. Kellum JA: Use of diuretics in the acute care setting [review]. Kidney Int Suppl 66:S67, 1998.

983. Fliser D, Zurbruggen I, Mutschler E, et al: Coadministration of albumin and furosemide in patients with the nephrotic syndrome. Kidney Int 55:629, 1999.

984. Pichette V, Geadah D, Du SP: Role of plasma protein binding on renal metabolism and dynamics of furosemide in the rabbit. Drug Metab Dispos 27:81, 1999.

985. Pichette V, Geadah D, Du SP: The influence of moderate hypoalbuminaemia on the renal metabolism and dynamics of furosemide in the rabbit. Br J Pharmacol 119:885, 1996.

986. Gaudio KM, Siegel NJ: Pathogenesis and treatment of acute renal failure. Pediatr Clin North Am 34:771, 1987.

987. Osofsky SG, Lewy JE, Lucey JF: Acute renal failure. In Dickerman JD (ed): Smith's the Critically Ill Child: Diagnosis and Medical Management. 3rd ed. Philadelphia, WB Saunders Company, 1985, p 287.

988. Stewart CL, Barnett R: Acute renal failure in infants, children, and adults. Crit Care Clin 13:575, 1997.

989. Hand MM, McManus ML, Harmon WE: Renal disorders in pediatric intensive care. In Rogers MC, Nichols DG (eds): Textbook of Pediatric Intensive Care. 3rd ed. Baltimore, Williams & Wilkins, 1996, p 1217.

990. Badr KF, Ichikawa I: Prerenal failure: a deleterious shift from renal compensation to decompensation. N Engl J Med 319:623, 1988.

991. Better OS, Stein JH: Early management of shock and prophylaxis of acute renal failure in traumatic rhabdomyolysis. N Engl J Med 322:825, 1990.

992. Brown CB, Ogg CS, Cameron JS: High dose furosemide in acute renal failure: a controlled trial. Clin Nephrol 15:90, 1981.

993. Counahan R, Cameron JS, Ogg CS: Presentation, management, complications, and outcome of acute renal failure in childhood. BMJ 1:599, 1977.

994. Safi HJ, Harlin SA, Miller CC, et al: Predictive factors for acute renal failure in thoracic and thoracoabdominal aortic aneurysm surgery [published erratum appears in J Vasc Surg 25:93, 1997]. J Vasc Surg 24:338, 1996.

995. Bennett WM, Singer I, Golper T: Guidelines for drug therapy in renal failure. Ann Intern Med 86:754, 1977.

996. Takala J: Nutrition in acute renal failure. Crit Care Clin 3:155, 1987.

997. Mouser JF, Hak EB, Kuhl DA, et al: Recovery from ischemic acute renal failure is improved with enteral compared with parenteral nutrition. Crit Care Med 25:1748, 1997.

998. Riella MC: Nutrition in acute renal failure [review]. Ren Fail 19:237, 1997.

999. Ikizler TA, Himmelfarb J: Nutrition in acute renal failure patients [review]. Adv Ren Replace Ther 4(Suppl 1):54, 1997.

1000. Alvestrand A: Nutritional aspects in patients with acute renal failure/multiorgan failure [review]. Blood Purif 14:109, 1996.

1001. Abitol CL, Holliday MA: Total parenteral nutrition in anuric children. Clin Nephrol 5:153, 1976.

1002. Parekh RS, Bunchman TE: Dialysis support in the pediatric intensive care unit [review]. Adv Ren Replace Ther 3:326, 1996.

1003. Gerber DR, Bekes CE: Peritoneal catheterization. Crit Care Clin 8:727, 1992.

1004. Anonymous: Proceedings of workshop: status of peritoneal dialysis in the United States. National Institute of Diabetes and Digestive and Kidney Diseases, National Institutes of Health [review]. Adv Ren Replace Ther 4:297, 1997.

1005. Mendley SR, Langman CB: Acute renal failure in the pediatric patient [review]. Adv Ren Replace Ther 4(Suppl 1):93, 1997.

1006. Zobel G, Rodl S, Urlesberger B, et al: Continuous renal replacement therapy in critically ill patients [review]. Kidney Int Suppl 66:S169, 1998.

1007. Paganini EP: Continuous renal prosthetic therapy in acute renal failure: an overview. Pediatr Clin North Am 34:165, 1987.

1008. Pascual JF, Lopez JD, Molina M: Hemofiltration in children with renal failure. Pediatr Clin North Am 34:803, 1987.

1009. Alexander SR, Leone MR, Jenkins RD, et al: Early experience with continuous arteriovenous hemofiltration (CAVH) in critically ill pediatric patients. Crit Care Med 14:1058, 1986.

1010. Fong JS, deChadarevian JP, Kaplan BS: Hemolytic-uremic syndrome: current concepts and management. Pediatr Clin North Am 29:835, 1982.

1011. Friedman AL: Acute renal disease. In Fuhrman BP, Zimmerman JJ (eds): Pediatric Critical Care. St. Louis, Mosby Year Book, 1992, p 723.

1012. Trachtman H, Christen E: Pathogenesis, treatment, and therapeutic trials in hemolytic uremic syndrome [review]. Curr Opin Pediatr 11:162, 1999.

1013. Whittam TS, Wachsmuth IK, Wilson RA: Genetic evidence of clonal descent of Escherichia coli 0157:H7 associated with hemorrhagic colitis and hemolytic uremic syndrome. J Infect Dis 157:1124, 1988.

1014. Coad NA, Marshall T, Rowe B, et al: Changes in the postenteropathic form of the hemolytic uremic syndrome in children. Clin Nephrol 35:10, 1991.

1015. Doyle MP: Escherichia coli 0157:H7 and its significance in foods. Int J Food Microbiol 12:289, 1991.

1016. Bitzan M, Moebius E, Ludwig K: High incidence of serum antibodies to Escherichia coli 0157 lipopolysaccharide in children with hemolytic-uremic syndrome. J Pediatr 119:380, 1991.

1017. Rowe PC, Orrbine E, Wells GA, et al: Epidemiology of hemolytic-uremic syndrome in Canadian children from 1986 to 1988. J Pediatr 119:218, 1991.

1018. Gordjani N, Sutor AH, Zimmerhackl LB, et al: Hemolytic uremic syndromes in childhood [review]. Semin Thromb Hemost 23:281, 1997.

1019. Martin DL, MacDonald KL, White KE: The epidemiology and clinical aspects of the hemolytic uremic syndrome in Minnesota. N Engl J Med 323:1161, 1992.

1020. Spika JS, Parsons JE, Nordenberg D: Hemolytic uremic syndrome and diarrhea associated with Escherichia coli 0157:H7 in a day care center. J Pediatr 109:287, 1986.

1021. Inward CD, Howie AJ, Fitzpatrick MM, et al: Renal histopathology in fatal cases of diarrhoea-associated haemolytic uraemic syndrome. British Association for Paediatric Nephrology. Pediatr Nephrol 11:556, 1997.

1022. Rosenweig JN, Gourley GR: Verotoxic Escherichia coli in human disease. J Pediatr Gastroenterol Nutr 12:295, 1991.

1023. Bergstein JM, Riley M, Bang NU: Role of plasminogen-activator inhibitor type 1 in the pathogenesis and outcome of the hemolytic uremic syndrome. N Engl J Med 327:755, 1992.

1024. Taylor CM, Milford DV, Rose PE: The expression of blood group P1 in post-enteropathic haemolytic uraemic syndrome. Pediatr Nephrol 4:59, 1990.

1025. Rock G, Shumak K, Kelton J: Thrombotic thrombocytopenic purpura: outcome in 24 patients with renal impairment treated with plasma exchange. Transfusion 32:710, 1992.

1026. Ruggenenti P, Remuzzi G: Pathophysiology and management of thrombotic microangiopathies [review]. J Nephrol 11:300, 1998.

1027. Trompeter RS, Schwartz R, Chantler C, et al: Haemolytic-uraemic syndrome: an analysis of prognostic features. Arch Dis Child 58:101, 1983.

1028. Gagnadoux MF, Habib R, Gubler MC, et al: Long-term (15–25 years) outcome of childhood hemolytic-uremic syndrome. Clin Nephrol 46:39, 1996.

APPENDIX

LYNNE M. REYNOLDS

Medication	Indications	Dose and Route of Administration	Side Effects (partial list)
Adenosine	Acute paroxysmal supraventricular tachycardia	0.05 mg/kg IV—may double dose q 1–2 min until effective (maximum single dose: 0.3 mg/kg) Doses greater than 12 mg are not recommended	Bradycardia, hypotension
Acetaminophen	Pain	10–15 mg/kg PO or 45 mg/kg PR q 4–6 h (maximum dose: 2.6 gm/24 h)	Hepatic necrosis with overdose; blood dyscrasias
Albuterol	Bronchospasm	Inhaled nebulization: 2.5 mg diluted with NSS for 0.83 mg/ml q 4–6 h	Arrhythmias, hypertension, tachycardia
Amrinone	Heart failure	Load: 1–2 mg/kg IV; Maintenance: 5–10 μg/kg/min IV	Arrhythmias, hypotension
Aminophylline	Severe bronchospasm	Load: If no current theophylline (theo) therapy: 7.5 mg/kg IV Load: If current theophylline therapy: weight (in kg) × 1.6 (target theophylline level–current theo level) = mg aminophylline IV Maintenance: <9 yr: 1–2 mg/kg/h IV 9–12 yr: 0.9–1 mg/kg/h IV 12–16 yr: 0.6–0.7 mg/kg/h IV	Tachyarrhythmias, seizures, tremors
Atracurium	Induction of neuromuscular blockade to facilitate intubation	0.5 mg/kg IV	Apnea, paralysis
Atropine	Bradycardia	0.02–0.04 mg/kg IV or intratracheal (recommended minimum dose: 0.1 mg & maximum dose: 1 mg)	Mydriasis, tachyarrhythmias
	To blunt muscarinic effects during antagonism of neuromuscular blockade	0.02 mg/kg IV	
Bicarbonate (NaHCO$_3$)	Metabolic acidosis	0.5–1 mEq/kg IV or mEq HCO$_3$ IV = (base deficit in mEq/L) × (1/3 weight in kg)	Acute (transient) PaCO$_2$ elevation
Bretylium	Refractory ventricular fibrillation; refractory ventricular tachycardia	5 mg/kg IV over 5 min; then 10 mg/kg IV q 15 min prn (recommended maximum: 30 mg/kg)	Arrhythmias

Table continued on following page

USEFUL DRUGS IN THE PERIOPERATIVE PERIOD *Continued*

Medication	Indications	Dose and Route of Administration	Side Effects (partial list)
Caffeine	Neonatal apnea; postoperative apnea of the newborn	Load: 10 mg/kg PO, IM, IV; Maintenance: 2.5 mg/kg PO q day	Seizures, tachyarrhythmias
Calcium	Hypotension, hypocalcemia, hyperkalemia, hypermagnesemia, and rapid administration of citrate-containing blood products	Calcium gluconate 60 mg/kg IV or calcium chloride 20 mg/kg IV	Arrhythmias, especially bradycardia
Chloral hydrate	Sedation	20–50 mg/kg PO (recommended maximum dose: 1 g)	Respiratory depression, excitement
Codeine	Pain	0.5–1.0 mg/kg PO or IM (recommended maximum dose: 30 mg/dose)	Apnea
Dantrolene	Malignant hyperthermia	Load: 1–4 mg/kg IV then 2 mg/kg IV q 6 h	Apnea, seizures, tachycardia
Diphenhydramine	Allergic reactions (treatment & prophylaxis)	1–2 mg/kg IV (recommended maximum: 300 mg/24 h)	Bronchospasm, hypertension, mydriasis, tachycardia
Dobutamine	Hypotension, heart failure	2.5–15 μg/kg/min IV	Arrhythmias, hypotension, tachycardia
Dopamine	Hypotension, heart failure	2.5–15 μg/kg/min IV	Arrhythmias, hypertension
Digoxin	Heart failure, supraventricular tachycardia	Digitalization: Preterm infant: 25 μg/kg IV Term infant to 2 yr: 50 μg/kg IV 2–10 yr: 25 μg/kg IV 10 yr to adult: 0.5–1 mg/kg IV	Arrhythmias, worsening CHF Note: Digoxin toxicity is worsened by hypokalemia.
Droperidol	Postoperative nausea and vomiting	15 μg/kg IV (recommended maximum dose: 0.625 mg)	Hypotension, extrapyramidal symptoms, sedation, tachycardia
Edrophonium	Antagonism of neuromuscular blockade	0.5–1.0 mg/kg IV—must be given with atropine	Cholinergic crisis including severe bradycardia
Ephedrine	Hypotension	0.2–0.3 mg/kg IV (recommended maximum dose: 0.5 mg)	Arrhythmias, hypertension, tachycardia
Epinephrine	Asystole or profound bradycardia, anaphylaxis Heart failure, hypotension Airway edema	10 μg/kg IV or intratracheal q 3–5 min prn 0.1–1 μg/kg/min IV Inhaled nebulization: 0.5 ml of 2.25% soln in 3 ml NSS q 4 h	Arrhythmias, hypertension, tachycardia
Esmolol	Tachycardia, hypertension	300 μg/kg IV and increase by 50–100 μg/kg/min IV q 10 min	Bradycardia
Etomidate	Induction of general anesthesia	0.3–0.4 mg/kg IV	Apnea, hypotension, painful injection, muscle movement compensatory tachycardia
Fentanyl	Pain Adjuvant to general anesthesia	1–2 μg/kg IV 5–10 μg/kg IV; up to 75–150 μg/kg for cardiac surgery or ECMO	Apnea, bradycardia, chest wall rigidity, tolerance
Furosemide	Pulmonary edema, hypervolemia	Preterm infants: 1–2 mg/kg IV; Other children: 1 mg/kg IV	Hypokalemia, hypovolemia
Glucose (10% dextrose)	Asymptomatic hypoglycemia Symptomatic hypoglycemia	4 mg/kg/min IV 200 mg/kg IV followed by 4 mg/kg/min IV	Hyperglycemia
Glycopyrrolate	To blunt muscarinic effects during antagonism of neuromuscular blockade	0.01 mg/kg IV	Tachyarrhythmias
Ibuprofen	Pain	10–15 mg/kg PO q 8 h	Hepatotoxicity, inhibition of platelet aggregation, renal failure
Isoproterenol	Bradycardia	0.1–1.5 μg/kg/min IV	Tachyarrhythmias
Ketamine	Premedication/preinduction Induction of general anesthesia	0.5–1 mg/kg IV or 3–5 mg/kg IM 1–2 mg/kg IV or 5–10 mg/kg IM	Arrhythmias, hemodynamic instability, hallucinations, apnea
Ketorolac	Pain	0.5–1 mg/kg IM or IV	Inhibition of platelet aggregation, renal failure
Labetalol	Hypertension	0.5 mg/kg IV	Bradycardia

Table continued on opposite page

USEFUL DRUGS IN THE PERIOPERATIVE PERIOD *Continued*

Medication	Indications	Dose and Route of Administration	Side Effects (partial list)
Lidocaine	Ventricular ectopy, ventricular arrhythmias	1 mg/kg IV or intratracheal q 5 min (recommended maximum dose: 5 mg/kg) Maintenance: 20–50 μg/kg/min	Heart block, seizures
Meperidine	Pain	1–1.5 mg/kg IV or IM	Apnea
Metaproterenol	Bronchospasm	Inhaled nebulization: Infants: 6 mg/dose over 5 min Children: 0.5 mg/kg/dose q 4–6 h (recommended maximum: 15 mg/dose)	Arrhythmias, hypertension, tachycardia
Methohexital	Premedication/preinduction	25–30 mg/kg PR	Apnea, hypotension
Midazolam	Premedication/preinduction Anxiety	0.5 mg/kg PO 0.1–0.2 mg/kg IV	Apnea, hypotension
Mivacurium	Induction of neuromuscular blockade to facilitate intubation	0.3 mg/kg IV	Apnea, paralysis, hypotension
Morphine	Pain	0.1–0.2 mg/kg IV or IM	Apnea, histamine release
Naloxone	Narcosis	1–10 μg/kg IV or SC q 2–3 min prn	Arrhythmias, hypertension, pulmonary edema
Neostigmine	Antagonism of neuromuscular blockade	0.07 mg/kg IV—Must be given with atropine or glycopyrrolate	Cholinergic crisis including severe bradycardia and cardiac arrest
Nifedipine	Hypertension	0.25–0.5 mg/kg PO or SL	Hypotension
Nitroglycerin	Pulmonary hypertension, inadequate coronary artery perfusion	1–5 μg/kg/min IV	Hypotension
Nitroprusside	Hypertension	0.5–10 μg/kg/min IV (recommended maximum for neonates: 6 μg/kg/min; others 10 μg/kg/min)	Cyanide toxicity, hypotension
Norepinephrine	Hypotension associated with low systemic vascular resistance	0.1–1 μg/kg/min IV	Hypertension, severe peripheral vasoconstriction
Ondansetron	Postoperative nausea and vomiting	0.1 mg/kg IV (recommended maximum dose: 4 mg)	Hypotension, tachycardia
Pancuronium	Induction of neuromuscular blockade to facilitate intubation	0.1 mg/kg IV	Apnea, paralysis, tachycardia
Pentobarbital	Premedication Sedation	3–4 mg/kg PO 4 mg/kg IV; additional 2 mg/kg IV q 2 min prn (recommended maximum dose of 10 mg/kg)	Apnea, hypotension
Phenylephrine	Hypotension associated with low systemic vascular resistance	Bolus: 5–20 μg/kg IV or 0.1 mg/kg IM; Infusion: 0.1–0.5 μg/kg/min IV	Bradycardia, hypertension
	TET spell (hypercyanotic episodes of tetralogy of Fallot)	Bolus: 10–100 μg/kg IV	
Procainamide	Refractory symptomatic ventricular tachycardia	Load: 3–5 mg/kg IV over 5–10 min; Maintenance: 20–60 μg/kg/min IV (recommended maximum dose: 100 mg/dose or 2g/24h)	Arrhythmias, blood dyscrasias hypotension
Propofol	Induction of anesthesia	Load: 1–5 mg/kg IV; Maintenance: 100–250 μg/kg/min IV	Apnea, hypotension, painful injection, muscle movement
Propranolol	Tachyarrhythmias, hypertension	0.01–0.1 mg/kg IV (recommended maximum of 1 mg/dose)	Bronchospasm, heart block, heart failure, hypotension
Prostaglandin E_1	To maintain pulmonary vasodilation	0.05–0.1 μg/kg/min IV	Apnea, bradycardia, hypotension, seizures
Rocuronium	Induction of neuromuscular blockade to facilitate intubation	0.5–1 mg/kg IV	Apnea, paralysis, tachycardia
Succinylcholine	Laryngospasm	4 mg/kg IM or 1–2 mg/kg IV Recommended simultaneous administration of atropine 0.2 mg/kg IM or IV	Acute rhabdomyolysis, apnea, bradycardia, cardiac arrest, histamine release, hyperkalemia, paralysis
	Rapid sequence induction of neuromuscular blockade	2 mg/kg IV	

Table continued on following page

USEFUL DRUGS IN THE PERIOPERATIVE PERIOD *Continued*

Medication	Indications	Dose and Route of Administration	Side Effects (partial list)
Terbutaline	Bronchospasm	<12 years of age: (1) 0.05–0.15 mg/kg PO q 8 h (recommended maximum: 5 mg/24 h) (2) 0.3 mg/kg inhaled as nebulization q 4 h (recommended maximum: 10 mg q 4 h) (3) 5–10 μg/kg SC q 15 min × 3 doses (recommended maximum: 0.4 mg/dose) >12 years of age: (1) 2.5–5 mg PO q 8 h (2) 2 inhalations from metered dose inhaler q 4 h (3) 0.25 mg SC q 15 min × 1 dose (recommended maximum: 0.5 mg q 4 h)	Arrhythmias, tachycardia, tremors
Thiopental	Induction of anesthesia	2–5 mg/kg IV	Apnea, hypotension
Tromethamine (THAM)	Refractory metabolic acidosis especially when $NaHCO_3$ is contraindicated	ml tromethamine = (weight in kg) × (base deficit in mEq/L) [Note: Supplied as 0.3 mEq tromethamine/ml]	Alkalosis, respiratory depression, thrombosis, venospasm
Vecuronium	Induction of neuromuscular blockade to facilitate intubation	0.1 mg/kg IV	Apnea, paralysis
Verapamil	Hypertension, tachycardia	0.05–0.2 mg/kg IV q 15–30 min (recommended maximum: 5 mg/dose)	Bradycardia, heart block, heart failure, hypotension
Other	Bacterial Endocarditis (SBE) Prophylaxis 1. Procedure: dental, oral, upper respiratory tract, or esophageal procedures Standard (oral) prophylaxis:	 First Choice: Amoxicillin 50 mg/kg PO (max 2 g) 1 h preop Alternative 1: Clindamycin 20 mg/kg PO (max 600 mg) 1 h preop Alternative 2: Cephalexin or cefadroxil 50 mg/kg PO (max 2 g) 1 h preop Alternative 3: Azithromycin or clarithromycin 15 mg/kg PO (max 500 mg) 1 h preop	
	Unable to take oral medications:	First Choice: Ampicillin 50 mg/kg IM or IV (max 2 g) within 30 min preop Alternative 1: Clindamycin 20 mg/kg IV (max 600 mg) within 30 min preop Alternative 2: Cefazolin 25 mg IM or IV (max 1 g) within 30 min preop	

Table continued on opposite page

USEFUL DRUGS IN THE PERIOPERATIVE PERIOD *Continued*

Medication	Indications	Dose and Route of Administration	Side Effects (partial list)
	2. Procedure: genitourinary or non-esophageal gastrointestinal procedures		
	High-risk patients:	First Choice: Ampicillin 50 mg/kg IM or IV (max 2 g) plus gentamicin 1.5 mg/kg IV or IM (max 120 mg) within 30 min of incision (6 h following initial dose: ampicillin 25 mg/kg IM/IV or amoxicillin 25 mg/kg PO) Alternative 1: Vancomycin 20 mg/kg (max 1 g) IV over 1 h plus gentamicin 1.5 mg/kg IV or IM (max 120 mg)—complete within 30 min of incision	
	Moderate-risk patients:	First Choice: Amoxicillin 50 mg/kg PO (max 2 g) 1 h preop or ampicillin 50 mg/kg IM or IV (max 2 g) within 30 min of incision Alternative 1: Vancomycin 20 mg/kg (max 1 g) IV over 1 h— complete within 30 min of incision	

IM, intramuscular; IV, intravenous; PO, oral; PR, per rectum; SC, subcutaneous; SL, sublingual.

References:
Medication package inserts.
Benitz WE, Tatro DS (eds): The Pediatric Drug Handbook. Chicago, Year Book Medical Publishers, 1988.
Bunchman TE, Lynch RE, Wood EG: Intravenously administrated labetalol for treatment of hypertension in children. J Pediatric 120:140, 1992.
Dajani AS, Taubert KA, Wilson W, et al: Prevention of bacterial endocarditis—recommendations by the American Heart Association. JAMA 277:1794, 1997.
Deal JE, Barratt TM, Dillon MJ: Management of hypertensive emergencies. Arch Dis Child 67:1089, 1992.
Feld LH, Negus JB, White PF: Oral midazolam preanesthetic medication in pediatric outpatients. Anesthesiology 73:831, 1990.
Forbes RB, Murray DJ, Dillman JB, Dull DL: Pharmacokinetics of two per cent rectal methohexitone in children. Can J Anaesth 36:160, 1989.
Lillen LD, Pildes RS, Srinivasan G, et al: Treatment of neonatal hypoglycemia with minibolus and intravenous glucose infusion. J Pediatr 97:295, 1980.
Liu LMP, Goudsouzian HG, Liu PL: Rectal methohexital premedication in children, a dose-comparison study. Anesthesiology 55:343, 1980.
Liu LMP, Gaudreault P, Friedman PA, et al: Methohexital plasma concentrations in children following rectal administration. Anesthesiology 62:567, 1985.
McMillan CO, Spahr-Schopfer IA, Sikich N, et al: Premedication of children with oral midazolam. Can J Anaesth 39:545, 1992.
Nicolson SC, Betts EK, Jobes DR, et al: Comparison of oral and intramuscular preanesthetic medication for pediatric inpatient surgery. Anesthesiology 71:3, 1989.
Trippel DL, Wiest DB, Gilletter PC: Cardiovascular and antiarrhytmic effects of esmolol in children. J Pediatr 119:142, 1991.
Watcha MF, Jones MB, Lagueruela RG, et al: Comparison of ketorolac and morphine as adjuvants during pediatric surgery. Anesthesiology 76:368, 1992.
Weldon BC, Watcha MF, White PF: Oral midazolam in children: effect of time and adjunctive therapy. Anesth Analg 75:51, 1992.
Wiest DB, Trippel DL, Gillette PC, Garner SS: Pharmacokinetics of esmolol in children. Pharmacol Ther 49:618, 1991.

APPENDIX

LYNNE M. REYNOLDS

Test–Serum Unless Stated	Reference Range*	SI Units
Alanine aminotransferase (ALT, SGPT)		
Newborn	25–65 U/L	25–65 U/L
Thereafter	10–40 U/L	10–40 U/L
Albumin—plasma		
Premature, birth	1.8–3.0 g/dl	18–30 g/L
Term <1 week old	2.5–3.4 g/dl	25–34 g/L
<5 years old	3.9–5.0 g/dl	40–50 g/L
Thereafter	4.0–5.3 g/dl	40–53 g/L
Alkaline phosphatase (ALT)		
≤12 years old	25–350 U/L	25–350 U/L
Thereafter:		
Male	25–100 U/L	25–100 U/L
Female	25–90 U/L	25–90 U/L
Ammonia nitrogen		
Newborn	90–150 μg N/dl	64–107 μmol N/L
0–2 weeks old	79–129 μg N/dl	56–92 μmol N/L
>4 weeks old	29–70 μg N/dl	21–50 μmol N/L
Adult	15–45 μg N/dl	11–32 μmol N/L
Aspartate aminotransferase (AST, SGOT)		
Newborn	25–65 U/L	25–65 U/L
Thereafter	10–40 U/L	10–40 U/L
Bicarbonate		
Arterial	21–28 mEq/L	21–28 mEq/L
Venous	22–29 mEq/L	22–29 mEq/L
Bilirubin, total		
Preterm:		
≤24 hours old	<8 mg/dl	<137 μmol/L
1–2 days old	<12 mg/dl	<205 μmol/L
2–5 days old	<16 mg/dl	<274 μmol/L
Term:		
≤24 hours old	<6 mg/dl	<103 μmol/L
1–2 days old	<8 mg/dl	<137 μmol/L
2–5 days old	<12 mg/dl	<205 μmol/L
Thereafter	≤1.2 mg/dl	20.5 μmol/L
Bilirubin, conjugated	≤0.2 mg/dl	≤3.4 μmol/L
Calcium, ionized		
<24 hours old	4.3–5.1 mg/dl	1.07–1.27 mmol/L
<48 hours old	4.0–4.7 mg/dl	1.00–1.17 mmol/L
Thereafter	4.8–4.92 mg/dl	1.12–1.23 mmol/L
Calcium, total		
Premature: <1 week old	6–10 mg/dl	1.5–2.5 mmol/L
Term: <48 hours old	7–12 mg/dl	1.75–3.0 mmol/L
Child	8.8–10.8 mg/dl	2.2–2.7 mmol/L
Thereafter	8.4–10.2 mg/dl	2.1–2.55 mmol/L

Table continued on following page

NORMAL LABORATORY VALUES *Continued*

Test—Serum Unless Stated	Reference Range*	SI Units
Chloride		
Newborn	97–110 mEq/L	97–110 mEq/L
Thereafter	98–106 mEq/L	98–106 mEq/L
Creatinine		
Newborn	0.3–1.0 mg/dl	27–88 μmol/L
Infant	0.2–0.4 mg/dl	18–35 μmol/L
Child	0.3–0.7 mg/dl	27–62 μmol/L
Adolescent	0.5–1.0 mg/dl	44–88 μmol/L
Adult:		
Male	0.6–1.2 mg/dl	53–106 μmol/L
Female	0.5–1.1 mg/dl	44–97 μmol/L
Fibrin degradation products—whole blood	<10 μg/ml	<10 mg/L
Fibrinogin		
Newborn	125–300 mg/dl	1.25–3 g/L
Thereafter	200–400 mg/dl	2–4 g/L
Gamma-glutamyl transferase (GGT, GGTP)		
<1 month old	13–147 U/L	13–147 U/L
1–2 months old	12–123 U/L	12–123 U/L
2–4 months old	8–90 U/L	8–90 U/L
4 months–10 years old	5–32 U/L	5–32 U/L
10–15 years old	5–24 U/L	5–24 U/L
Thereafter:		
Male	≤40 U/L	≤40 U/L
Female	≤25 U/L	≤25 U/L
Glucose		
Newborn:		
24 hours old	40–60 mg/dl	2.2–2.3 mmol/L
>24 hours old	50–90 mg/dl	2.8–5.0 mmol/L
Child	60–100 mg/dl	3.3–5.5 mmol/L
Thereafter	70–105 mg/dl	3.9–5.8 mmol/L
Hemoglobin—whole blood		
1–3 days old	14.5–22.5 g/dl	2.25–3.49 mmol/L
2 months old	9.0–14.0 g/dl	1.40–2.17 mmol/L
6–12 years old	11.5–15.5 g/dl	1.78–2.40 mmol/L
12–18 years old:		
Male	13.0–16.0 g/dl	2.02–2.48 mmol/L
Female	12.0–16.0 g/dl	1.86–2.48 mmol/L
18–49 years old:		
Male	13.5–17.5 g/dl	2.09–2.27 mmol/L
Female	12.0–16.0 g/dl	1.86–2.48 mmol/L
Lactate dehydrogenase (LD)		
Neonate	160–1500 U/L	160–1500 U/L
<1 year	170–580 U/L	170–580 U/L
1–9 years	150–500 U/L	150–500 U/L
10–19 years	120–330 U/L	120–330 U/L
Magnesium		
<1 week old	1.2–2.6 mg/dl	0.48–1.05 mmol/L
<2 years old	1.6–2.6 mg/dl	0.65–1.05 mmol/L
2–14 years old	1.5–2.3 mg/dl	0.60–0.95 mmol/L
Osmolality	275–295 mOsm/kg H_2O	
Potassium		
<2 years old	3.0–6.0 mEq/L	3.0–6.0 mmol/L
2–12 years old	3.5–7.0 mEq/L	3.5–7.0 mmol/L
Thereafter	3.5–5.0 mEq/L	3.5–5.0 mmol/L
Sodium		
Newborn:		
Premature	128–148 mEq/L	128–148 mmol/L
Term	134–144 mEq/L	134–144 mmol/L
Thereafter	136–146 mEq/L	136–146 mmol/L
Urea nitrogen		
Newborn:		
Premature	3–25 mg/dl	1.1–9 mmol/L
Term	3–12 mg/dl	1.1–4.3 mmol/L
Thereafter	5–18 mg/dl	1.8–6.4 mmol/L

* The reader is reminded that reference ranges are a function of the testing method. Individual laboratory values must be interpreted according to the reference range provided by the laboratory performing the test.

References:
Behrman RE, Kleiegman RM, Nelson WE, Vaughan III VC (eds): Nelson Textbook of Pediatrics. Philadelphia, WB Saunders Company, 1992.
Howanitz JH, Howanitz PJ (eds): Laboratory Medicine—Test Selection and Intrepretation. New York, Churchill Livingstone, 1991.

Index

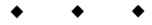

Note: Page numbers followed by f refer to figures; page numbers followed by t refer to tables.

907

Pain (*Continued*)
assessment of, 750
chronic, 758–766
after amputation, 762
"benign" recurrent, 758–760
transcutaneous electrical nerve
stimulation in, 765
definition of, 749
from pneumatic tourniquets, 643
hemodynamic response to, 474–476
in neonates, 749–750
neuropathic, 749, 758, 760–761
postoperative, 241–242
Pain management, 749–766
cognitive-behavioral therapy in, 765
complementary/alternative, 765–766
developmental issues in, 750
for painful procedures, 758
in burns, 740–741
in cancer, 762–764
in cystic fibrosis, 764
in intensive care unit, 874
in poorly understood conditions,
764–765
in reflex sympathetic dystrophy,
761–762
in sickle cell disease, 764
nonopioid analgesics in, 750–752, 751t
opioid analgesics in, 752–755, 754t–755t.
See also Opioid(s).
patient-controlled analgesia in, 755, 755t
postoperative, in outpatient anesthesia,
781–783
psychological treatment in, 765
Palate
cleft, 715, 717f
reconstruction of, 724–726, 726f
anesthesia for, 731f, 731–732
embryology of, 708–709, 710f
Pancreatic transplantation, 562–563
Pancuronium
for intravenous anesthesia, 234
in congenital heart disease, 495
neuropharmacology of, 392–393
perioperative use of, 901t
properties of, 30–31
Pao₂ (arterial oxygen pressure),
transcutaneous oxygen pressure and,
257f, 257–258
Papilloma, laryngeal, laser surgery for,
687–688
Parallel circulation, single ventricle and, 510t,
510–512, 511f, 512t
Fontan procedure for, 512–517, 514f,
515t–516t. *See also* Fontan procedure.
Paralysis, familial periodic, 654
Paramyotonia congenita, 653
Parasitic disease(s), transfusion-transmitted,
119
Paravascular block, inguinal, 295–296
Paravertebral thoracic block, 289–291, 290f
anatomic considerations in, 290
anesthetic dosage and solution for,
290–291
complications of, 291
indications for, 290
technique of, 290, 290f
Parent(s)
as blood donors, 121–122
conflicts with, ethical issues concerning,
10–11
consent by, 3–4
involvement of, during preinduction, 219,
778
outpatient anesthesia and, 774, 785

Parent(s) (*Continued*)
presence of
during induction of anesthesia, 219,
613–614, 778
in postanesthesia care unit, 239
psychological adjustment of, to child's
surgery, 176–177
relationship with, 177–178
requests for cessation of treatment by, 10
stress in, in intensive care unit, 875
Parenteral fluid(s). *See also* Fluid(s); Fluid
therapy.
maintenance, 90–91, 90t–91t
Parkland formula, for fluid resuscitation,
734
Partial liquid ventilation, 851
Parvovirus B19 infection, transfusion-
transmitted, 119
Patent ductus arteriosus
anesthesia in, 526–527
heart rate in, 356, 357t
in premature infants, 349f, 349–350
occlusion devices for, insertion of, 505
pathophysiology of, 526
Patient-controlled analgesia (PCA), 755, 755t
for cancer pain, 763
PCACD (phased chest abdominal
compression-decompression)
cardiopulmonary resuscitation, 154
PCP (Pneumocystis carinii) pneumonia, 870
Pectus carinatum, 449
Pectus excavatum, 447–448, 448f
Pediatric anesthesiologist(s), competency of,
14–15
Pediatric anesthesiology
definition of, 14
history of, 13–14
practice of, settings for, 14–16
quality assurance in, 14
recent changes in, 16–18, 17t
regional care centers providing, 17
standards of care for, 16, 17t
training facilities for, 14
training programs in, 15–16
Pediatric intensive care unit. *See* Intensive
care unit (ICU).
PEEP. *See* Positive end-expiratory pressure
(PEEP).
Penile block, 301–302, 302t, 303f
dorsal, 301–302, 302t
for outpatient surgery, 782
subcutaneous ring, 302
subpubic, 302, 303f
Penis, topical analgesia for, 302–303
Pentastarch, 109
during supratentorial craniotomy, 404
Pentobarbital
during computed tomography, 811
perioperative use of, 901t
Pentolinium, for controlled hypotension,
328
Percutaneous administration route, 20–21
Perfection, parental expectations of, 10
Periodic breathing, in expremature infants,
378
Peripheral airway(s), abnormalities of, 670
Peripheral nerve block(s), 289–291, 290f
Peripheral nerve stimulator(s), for placement
of nerve block, 273–274, 274f
Peritoneal dialysis, 605, 878
Peritonsillar abscess, 676
Peroneal nerve(s), blockade of, 306–307
Persistent fetal circulation, 425
Persistent pulmonary hypertension of
newborn (PPHN), 425, 857

Perspiration
during general anesthesia, 70, 70f
in premature infants, 347
physiology of, 67–68
P_ETCO₂. *See* End-tidal Co₂ (P_ETCO₂).
pH
and drug ionization, 19
and serum potassium, 99, 99t
gastric, 20
homeostasis of, 598
of blood, monitoring of, 257f, 257–258
sodium bicarbonate and, 157–158
Phantom limb pain, 762
Pharmacokinetics, 24t, 24–25, 25f
gastrointestinal effects of, 571t
Pharyngeal flap, for velopharyngeal
incompetence, 726, 726f
Phased chest abdominal compression-
decompression (PCACD)
cardiopulmonary resuscitation, 154
Phenobarbital, metabolism of, 36
Phenylephrine
and coronary blood flow, during
cardiopulmonary resuscitation, 155
for myocardial dysfunction, 469, 470t
for strabismus surgery, 690
perioperative use of, 901t
Phosphate, homeostasis of, in neonates, 100
Phospholipase A₂, and muscle contractions, in
malignant hyperthermia, 54, 55f
Physical therapy, for reflex sympathetic
dystrophy, 762
Pierre-Robin syndrome, 643t
Plasma
fresh frozen, transfusion of, 134–135
during liver transplantation, 550
viscosity of, 318
volume of, 91–93
Plasma half-life, 24, 24t
Plasma protein(s), binding of drugs to, 22t,
22–23
Plasmin, and inhibition of coagulation, 129
Plastic surgery, 707–741. *See also* Burn(s);
Craniofacial reconstruction.
Platelet(s)
in hemostasis, 127
transfusion of, 132–134, 134f, 864. *See also*
Transfusion, of platelets.
Platelet-activating clotting test (PACT), 131
Platelet function
aspirin and, 129
evaluation of, 131
hypothermia and, 74
in fresh whole blood, 124
Platelet-related sepsis, 119
Pleuroperitoneal membrane, embryology of,
and congenital diaphragmatic hernia, 434
Pneumatic tourniquet(s)
for intravenous regional anesthesia,
305–306
in orthopaedic surgery, 642–644
Pneumocystis carinii (PCP) pneumonia, 870
Pneumonia
nosocomial, 869
Pneumocystis carinii, 870
Pneumonitis, from amiodarone, 163
Pneumothorax, from intercostal nerve block,
305
Poisoning, 861t, 861–863, 862f
activated charcoal for, 861
agents causing, 861t
drug distribution in, 861–862, 862f
drug inactivation in, 862
incidence of, 861
induced vomiting in, 861